GENERAL

AND

APPLIED TOXICOLOGY

GENERAL AND APPLIED TOXICOLOGY

SECOND EDITION

EDITORS

Bryan Ballantyne
MD, DSc, PhD, FFOM, FACOM, FAACT, FATS, FRCPath, FIBiol, MRCS
Director of Applied Toxicology
Union Carbide Corporation, Danbury, Connecticut, USA
Adjunct Professor of Pharmacology and Toxicology
West Virginia University, USA

Timothy C. Marrs
MD, DSc, MRCP, FRCPath, FIBiol
Senior Medical Officer
Joint Food Safety and Standards Group
London, UK

Tore Syversen
MSc, DrPhil
Professor of Toxicology
Norwegian University of Science and Technology
Trondheim, Norway

VOLUME 3

Published in the United Kingdom by
MACMILLAN REFERENCE LTD., 1999
25 Eccleston Place, London, SW1W 9NF
Basingstoke and Oxford

Companies and representatives throughout the world.

http://www.macmillan-reference.co.uk

Distributed in the UK and Europe by
Macmillan Distribution Ltd.,
Brunel Road, Houndmills,
Basingstoke, Hampshire, RG21 2XS, England

General and Applied Toxicology - 2nd ed.
1. Toxicology
I. Ballantyne, Bryan.   II. Marrs, Timothy C.   III. Syversen, Tore L. M.
615.9
ISBN 0-333-698681

Published in the United States and Canada by
GROVE'S DICTIONARIES INC., 1999
345 Park Avenue South, 10th Floor
New York, NY 10010-1707, USA

ISBN 1-56159-242-0

A catalog record for this book is available from the Library of Congress

Typeset by Kolam Information Services Ltd, India
Printed and bound in the UK by Bath Press, Bath

Contents

VOLUME 1

PART ONE: BASIC SCIENCE

VOLUME 2

PART FOUR: TARGET ORGAN AND TISSUE TOXICITY

PART FIVE: GENETIC TOXICOLOGY, CARCINOGENICITY, REPRODUCTIVE AND DEVELOPMENTAL TOXICOLOGY

PART SIX: ENVIRONMENTAL TOXICOLOGY

VOLUME 3

LIST OF CONTRIBUTORS

Lisbeth Aasmoe, *MSc, PhD*
Department of Clinical Pharmacology, University
Hospital of Tromso, N-9038 Tromso, Norway

Gerald E. Adams, *PhD, DSc, FACR*
Medical Research Council Radiobiology Unit,
Chilton, Didcot, Oxfordshire OX11 ORD, UK
Professor Adams died in 1998

Catrine Ahlen,
Senior Scientist, SINTEF UNIMED, Department
of Extreme Work Environment, N-7489
Trondheim, Norway

Antero Aitio, *MD, PhD*
Programme for Chemical Safety, World Health
Organization, Avenue Appia 20, Geneva 27
CH-1211, Switzerland

Diana Anderson, *BSc, MSc, PhD, Dip Ed,
FRCPath, FIBiol, FIFST, FATS*
Senior Associate, Coordinator External Affairs,
BIBRA International, Woodmansterne Road,
Carshalton, Wallington, Surrey SM5 4DS, UK

Charles M. Auer, *BSc*
Director, Chemical Control Division, Office
of Pollution Prevention and Toxics, US
Environmental Protection Agency (7405), 401 M
Street SW, Washington DC 20460, USA

Ronald C. Backer, *PhD, DABFT*
Universal Toxicology Laboratories, 10210 West
Highway 80, Midland, Texas 79706, USA

Bryan Ballantyne, *MD, DSc, PhD, FFOM,
FACOM, FAACT, FATS, FRCPath, FIBiol, MRCS*
Director of Applied Toxicology, Union Carbide
Corporation, 39 Old Ridgebury Road, Danbury,
Connecticut 06817-0001, USA

Steven I. Baskin, *PharmD, PhD, FCP, FACC,
DABT, FATS*
Team Leader and Principal Investigator, Division
of Pharmacology, U.S. Army Medical Research
Institute of Chemical Defense, 3100 Ricketts
Point Road, Aberdeen Proving Ground, Edgewood
Area, Maryland 21010-5400, USA

D. Nicholas Bateman, *BSc, MD, FRCP*
Director, Scottish Poisons Information Bureau,
Royal Infirmary, 1 Lauriston Place, Edinburgh
EH3 9YW, UK

George S. Behonick, *BS, MS, PhD*
NRC/NAS Research Associate, U.S. Army Medical
Research Institute of Chemical Defense, 3100
Ricketts Point Road, Aberdeen Proving Ground,
Edgewood Area, Maryland 21010-5400, USA

Sir Colin Berry, *DSc, MD, PhD, FRCP, FRCPath,
FFPM, FFOM*
Professor of Morbid Anatomy and Histopathology,
Department of Morbid Anatomy, Institute of
Pathology, Royal London Hospital, Whitechapel,
London E1 1BB, UK

Chantal Bismuth, *MD*
Professor of Medicine, Medical and Toxicological
Intensive Care Unit, Hôpital Lariboisière,
Université Paris VII, 2 rue Ambroise Paré, 75010
Paris, France

Olav Bjørseth, *MSc, PhD*
Associate Professor, Department of Industrial
Economics and Technology Management,
Norwegian University of Science and Technology,
A Getz vl, N-7491 Trondheim, Norway

Stephen W. Borron, *MD, MS*
Associate Clinical Professor of Emergency
Medicine, School of Medicine, George Washington
University, 1215 Seventeenth Street NW,
Washington DC 20036-3008; Visiting Researcher,
Hôpital Lariboisière, Université Paris VII, 2 rue
Ambroise Paré, 75475 Paris, France

Joan M. Braganza, *DSc, MSc, FRCP, FRCPath*
Pancreato-Biliary Service, Manchester Royal
Infirmary, Oxford Road, Manchester M13 9WL,
UK

John Caldwell, *PhD, DSc, FIBiol, HonMRCP*
Section of Molecular Toxicology, Division of
Biomedical Sciences, Imperial College School of
Medicine, South Kensington, London SW7 2AZ,
UK

Flemming R. Cassee, *PhD*
Laboratory for Health Effects Research, National
Institute for Public Health and the Environment,
P.O. Box 1, NL-3720 BA Bilthoven, The
Netherlands

Cheryl E.A. Chaffey, *BSc*
Head, Health Re-evaluation Section, Pest
Management Regulatory Agency, Health Canada,
2250 Riverside Drive, 6606E1 Ottawa, Ontario
K1A 0K9, Canada

John J. Clary, *PhD, FATS*
BioRisk, P.O. Box 2326, 2407 Oakfield Drive,
Midland, Michigan 48641, USA

Mary E. Clinton, *MD*
Clinical Professor, Department of Neurology,
School of Medicine, Vanderbilt University, 2100
Pierce Avenue, Medical Center South, Nashville,
Tennessee 37232, USA

David M. Conning, *OBE, MB, BS, FRCPath,
FIBiol, FIFST*
Blacksmith's Cottage, Totnor, Brockhampton,
Hereford HR1 4TJ, UK

Philip T. Copestake, *BSc, MSc*
Information and Advisory Service, BIBRA
International, Woodmansterne Road, Carshalton,
Surrey SM5 4DS, UK

Ian A. Cotgreave, *PhD*
Associate Professor, Division of Biochemical
Toxicology, Institute of Environmental Medicine,
Karolinska Institute, Box 210, S-17177 Stockholm,
Sweden

P.F. D'Arcy, *OBE, BPharm, PhD, DSc, DSc(Hon),
FRPharmS, CChem, FRSC, FPSNI*
Emeritus Professor, School of Pharmacy, The
Queen's University of Belfast, Medical Biology
Centre, 97 Lisburn Road, Belfast BT9 7BL,
Northern Ireland, UK

Susan Davies, *BPharm, MRPS, MBIRA*
Head of Regulatory Affairs, Schering Health Care
Ltd., The Brow, Burgess Hill, West Sussex RH15
9NE, UK

Rebecca J. Dearman, *BSc, PhD*
Research Toxicology Section, AstraZeneca Central
Toxicology Laboratory, Alderley Park,
Macclesfield, Cheshire SK10 4TJ, UK

Anthony P. DeCaprio, *BS, PhD, DABT*
Associate Professor, School of Public Health,
University at Albany, State University of New
York, One University Place, Rensselaer, New York
12144, USA

Wolf-D. Dettbarn, *MD*
Professor, Departments of Pharmacology and
Neurology, School of Medicine, Vanderbilt
University, 2100 Pierce Avenue, Medical Center
South, Nashville, Tennessee 37232, USA

Ian C. Dewhurst, *BSc, PhD*
Mallard House, Kings Pool, 3 Peasholme Green,
York YO1 7PX, UK

Geoff E. Diggle, *MB, BS, DipPharmMed, FFPM*
97 Bennetts Way, Croydon, Surrey CR0 8AG, UK

Virginia A. Dobozy, *VMD, MPH*
Office of Pesticide Programs, Health Effects
Division (7509C), US Environmental Protection
Agency, 401 M Street SW, Washington DC 20460,
USA

Lennart Dock, *PhD*
National Institute of Environmental Medicine,
Karolinska Institute, Box 210, S-17177 Stockholm,
Sweden

Gareth O. Evans, *BSc, MSc*
Principal Clinical Pathologist, Clinical Pathology,
Astra Safety Assessment, Astra Charnwood,
Bakewell Road, Loughborough LE11 5RH, UK

Steven Fairhurst, *BSc, PhD*
Head of Toxicology, Toxicology Unit, Health and
Safety Executive, Room 156, Magdalen House,
Trinity Road, Bootle, Merseyside L20 3QZ, UK

Victor J. Feron, *PhD*
Emeritus Professor of Biological Toxicology, Toxicology Division, TNO Nutrition and Food Research Institute, P.O. Box 360, NL-3700 AJ Zeist, The Netherlands

Robin J. Fielder, *BSc, PhD, DipToxRCPath*
Department of Health, Skipton House, 80 London Road, London SE1 6LW, UK

Brent L. Finley, *PhD, DABT*
Exponent, 149 Commonwealth Drive, Menlo Park, California 74025, USA

Trond Peder Flaten, *PhD*
Department of Chemistry, Norwegian University of Science and Technology, N-7491 Trondheim, Norway

Frode Fonnum, *BSc, PhD*
VISTA Professor, Forsvarets forskninsinstitutt, Postboks 25, N-2007 Kjeller, Norway

Andrew Forge, *BSc, MSc, PhD*
Institute of Laryngology and Otology, University College London, 330-332 Gray's Inn Road, London WC1X 8EE, UK

John R. Foster, *BSc, PhD, DipRCPath, FRCPath*
Senior Pathologist, AstraZeneca Central Toxicology Laboratory, Alderley Park, Macclesfield, Cheshire SK10 4TJ, UK

Etienne Fournier, *MD*
Professor Emeritus of Clinical Toxicology, Clinique Toxicologique, Hôpital Fernand Widal, 200 rue du Faubourg-St-Denis, 75475 Paris, Cedex 10, France

Arthur Furst, *PhD, ScD*
Institute of Chemical Biology, Harney Science Center, University of San Francisco, San Francisco, California 94117-1080, USA

Shayne C. Gad, *PhD, DABT*
Gad Consulting Services, 1818 White Oak Road, Raleigh, North Carolina 27608, USA

Sharat D. Gangolli, *BSc PhD, MChemA, CChem, FRSC, FRCPath*
157 Old Lodge Lane, Purley, Surrey CR8 4AU, UK

Michael L. Gargas, *PhD*
ChemRisk, The Courtland East Building, 29225 Chagrin Boulevard, Cleveland, Ohio 44122, USA

David G. Gatehouse, *CBiol, BSc, PhD, FIBiol, FRCPath*
Department of Genetic Toxicology, Preclinical Safety Sciences, Glaxo Wellcome Research and Development Ltd., Park Road, Ware, Hertfordshire SG12 ODP, UK

Paul Grasso, *BSc, MD FRCPath, DCP, DTM&H*
Robens Institute, University of Surrey, Guildford, Surrey GU2 5XH, UK

Peter Greaves, *MB, ChB, FRCPath*
Head of Safety of Medicines, Safety of medicines, AstraZeneca, Mereside, Alderley Park, Macclesfield, Cheshire SK10 4TG, UK

John P. Groten
Department of Explanatory Toxicology, TNO Nutrition and Food Research Institute, PO Box 360, 3700 AJ Zeist, The Netherlands

Ramesh C. Gupta, *DVM, PhD, DABT*
Professor and Head of Toxicology, Toxicology Department, Breathitt Veterinary Center, Murray State University, P.O. Box 2000, 715 North Drive, Hopkinsville, Kentucky 42241-2000, USA

Güneyt Güzey, *MD*
Institute of Cancer Research and Molecular Biology, Medical Technical Research Centre, Norwegian University of Science and Technology, N-7005 Trondheim, Norway

Hakam Hadidi, *MD, PhD*
Associate Professor, Department of Pharmacology, Faculty of Medicine, Jordan University of Science and Technology, P.O. Box 3030, Irbid, Jordan

Roy Hamlet, *BSc, PhD, CBiol, MIBiol*
Department of Health, Skipton House, 80 London Road, London SE1 6LW, UK

Ernest S. Harpur, *BSc, PhD, MRPharmS*
Department of Toxicology, Sanofi Research, Alnwick Research Centre, Willowburn Avenue, Alnwick, Northumberland NE66 2JH, UK

Jan G. Hengstler, *MD*
Institute of Toxicology, University of Mainz, Obere Zahlbacher Strasse 67, D-55131 Mainz, Germany

Steven J. Hermansky, *MS, PharmD, PhD, DABT*
Principal Toxicologist, Schering-Plough HealthCare Products, 3030 Jackson Avenue, Memphis, Tennessee 38151, USA

Paul M. Hext, *BSc, PhD*
AstraZeneca Central Toxicology Laboratory, Alderley Park, Macclesfield, Cheshire SK10 4TJ, UK

Elwood F. Hill, *BA, PhD*
Wildlife Toxicologist, Adjunct Professor, University Center for Environmental Sciences and Engineering, University of Nevada, Reno, Nevada USA; P.O. Box 1615, Gardnerville, Nevada 89410, USA

Richard H. Hinton, *BA, PhD, FRCPath*
School of Biological Science, University of Surrey, Guildford, Surrey GU2 5XH, UK

Bo Holmberg, *PhD*
Professor Emeritus, Department of Toxicology and Chemistry, National Institute for Working Life, S-17184 Solna, Sweden

William J.M. Hrushesky, *MD*
Professor of Medicine, Department of Medicine, Stratton Veterans Affairs Medical Centre and Albany Medical College, Albany, New York 12208, USA

Deborah J. Hussey, *BSc*
Mallard House, Kings Pool, 3 Peasholme Green, York YO1 7PX, UK

Jeffrey R. Idle, *PhD, CChem, FRSC*
Professor in Medicine and Molecular Biology, Institute for Cancer Research and Molecular Biology, Norwegian University of Science and Technology, Medisinsk Teknisk Senter, 7005 Trondheim, Norway

H. Paul A. Illing, *PhD, FIBiol, FRSC, FRIPHH, FIOSH*
Centre for Occupational and Environmental Health, Medical School, University of Manchester, Stopford Building, Oxford Road, Manchester M13 9PT, UK

Imran Imam
Research Service, Stratton Veterans Affairs Medical Centre, Albany, New York 12208, USA

Bengt Jernström, *PhD*
Associate Professor, Division of Biochemical Toxicology, Institute of Environmental Medicine, Karolinska Institute, Box 210, S-17177 Stockholm, Sweden

Sam Kacew, *PhD, FATS*
Department of Pharmacology, University of Ottawa, 451 Smyth Road, Ottawa, Ontario K1H 8M5, Canada

James P. Kehrer, *PhD*
Professor and Head, Division of Pharmacology and Toxicology, College of Pharmacy, The University of Texas at Austin, Austin, Texas 78712-1074, USA

Ian Kimber, *BSc, MSc, PhD*
Research Manager, AstraZeneca Central Toxicology Laboratory, Alderley Park, Macclesfield, Cheshire SK10 4TJ, UK

Alan B.G. Lansdown, *BSc, PhD, FRCPath, FIBiol, MIMgt*
Hon.Senior Lecturer and Research Fellow, Skin Research and Wound Healing Laboratory, Clinical Chemistry, Division of Investigative Sciences, Imperial College School of Medicine, London W6 8RP, UK

Peter N. Lee, *MA, FSS, CStat*
P. N. Lee Statistics and Computing Ltd., Hamilton House, 17 Cedar Road, Sutton, Surrey SM2 5DA, UK

Hon-Wing Leung, *PhD, DABT, CIH*
Union Carbide Corporation, 39 Old Ridgebury Road, Danbury, Connecticut 06817-0001, USA

David W. Lincoln II, *PhD*
Research Service, Stratton Veterans Affairs Medical Centre, Albany, New York 12208, USA

Edward A. Lock, *MIBiol, PhD, FRCPath*
AstraZeneca Central Toxicology Laboratory,
Alderley Park, Macclesfield, Cheshire SK10 4TJ,
UK

Thomas F. Long, *MS*
Senior Health Scientist, ChemRisk, McLaren Hart
Inc., 5900 Landerbrook Drive, Suite 100,
Cleveland, Ohio 44124, USA

David P. Lovell, *BSc, PhD, FSS, CStat, MBiol,
CBiol*
BIBRA International, Woodmansterne Road,
Carshalton, Surrey SM5 4DS, UK

Timothy C. Marrs, *MD, DSc, MRCP, FRCPath,
FIBiol*
Joint Food Safety and Standards Group, Skipton
House, 80 London Road, London SE1 6LH, UK

Robert L. Maynard, *BSc, MB, BCh, MRCP,
FRCPath, FFOM, FIBiol*
Department of Health, Skipton House, 80 London
Road, London SE1 6LH, UK

Patricia R. McElhatton, *MSc, PhD, CBiol, FIBiol*
National Teratology Information Service, Regional
Drug and Therapeutics Centre, Wolfson Unit,
Claremont Place, Newcastle-upon-Tyne NE2 4HH,
UK

Douglas McGregor, *PhD, FIBiol, FRCPath*
International Agency for Research on Cancer, 150
Cours Albert Thomas, 69372 Lyon, Cedex 08,
France

Clive Meredith, *MA, MSc, PhD*
Immunotoxicology Department, British Industrial
Biological Research Association International,
Woodmansterne Road, Carshalton, Surrey SM5
4DS, UK

Klara Miller, *ChemEng, MSc, PhD, FRCPath*
Consultant, Immunotoxicology, Food Science and
Biotechnology, 35D Arteberry Road, Wimbledon,
London SW20 8AG, UK

Jeremy J. Mills, *BSc, PhD*
Section of Molecular Toxicology, Division of
Biomedical Sciences, Imperial College School of
Medicine, South Kensington, London SW7 2AZ,
UK

Neil A. Minton, *BSc, MD, MRCP, MFPM*
Medical Toxicology Unit, Guy's Hospital, London
SE1 9RT, UK

Karl E. Misulis, *PhD, MD*
Clinical Professor, Department of Neurology,
School of Medicine, Vanderbilt University, 2100
Pierce Avenue, Medical Center South, Nashville,
Tennessee 37232, USA

Ralf Morgenstern, *PhD*
Associate Professor, Institute of Environmental
Medicine, Karolinska Institute, Box 210, S-17177
Stockholm, Sweden

Roy C. Myers, *BS, DABT*
Manager, Risk Assessment Information Group,
Union Carbide Corporation, 39 Old Ridgebury
Road, Danbury, Connecticut 06817-0001, USA

B.K. Nelson, *PhD, MSc, BSc*
Research Toxicologist, Division of Biomedical and
behavioral Science (C-24), National Institute for
Occupational Safety and Health, Centers for
Disease Control and Prevention, 4676 Columbia
Parkway, Cincinnati, Ohio 45226, USA

James C. Norris Jr., *PhD, DABT, MS, BS*
Head, Inhalation Toxicology, Covance Laboratories
Ltd., Otley Road, Harrogate, North Yorkshire HG3
1PY, UK

Frederick W. Oehme, *DVM, PhD*
Professor of Toxicology, Pathobiology, Medicine
and Physiology, Comparative Toxicology
Laboratories, Kansas State University, 1800
Denison Avenue, Manhattan, Kansas 66506-5606,
USA

Franz Oesch, *PhD*
Professor, Director, Institute of Toxicology,
University of Mainz, Obere Zahlbacher Strasse 67,
D-55131 Mainz, Germany

Eugene J. Olajos, *BA, MS, PhD*
US Army SBCCOM, Edgewood Chemical
Biological Center, Office of Director, Research and
Technology Directorate, Aberdeen Proving
Ground, Maryland 21010-5424, USA

Sten G. Orrenius, *MD, PhD*
Professor, Institute of Environmental Medicine, Karolinska Institute, Box 210, S-17177 Stockholm, Sweden

Alan J. Paine, *DSc, PhD, FRCPath, FIBiol*
Department of Toxicology, School of Medicine and Dentistry, Queen Mary and Westfield College, University of London, Charterhouse Square, London EC1M 6BQ, UK

Dennis J. Paustenbach, *PhD, DABT*
Group Vice President and Principal, Environmental Group, Exponent, 149 Commonwealth Drive, Menlo Park, California 94025, USA; Adjunct Professor of Toxicology, University of Massachusetts, Amherst, USA

Ellen K. Pedersen, *MSc*
Research Fellow, Department of Pharmacology and Toxicology, School of Medicine, Norwegian University of Science and Technology, N-7489 Trondheim, Norway

Alphonse Poklis, *PhD, DABFT, DABCC-TC*
Professor, Departments of Pathology and Pharmacology/Toxicology, Medical College of Virginia Campus at Virginia Commonwealth University, Richmond, Virginia 23298-0165, USA

Frances D. Pollitt, *MA, DipRCPath*
Department of Health, Skipton House, 80 London Road, London SE1 6LH, UK

Christopher J. Powell, *PhD, DipRCPath(Tox), MSc, BSc, FRCPath*
Vanguard Medica, Chancellor Court, Surrey Research Park, Guildford, Surrey GU2 5SF, UK

B.V. Rama Sastry, *DSc, PhD*
Professor of Pharmacology Emeritus, Adjunct Professor of Anesthesiology, Vanderbilt University Medical Center, 209 Oxford House, Nashville, Tennessee 37232-4245, USA

Jennifer M. Ratcliffe, *PhD, MSc, BSc*
Senior Epidemiologist, Statistics and Public Health Research Division, Analytical Sciences Inc., 2605 Meridian Parkway, Durham, North Carolina 27713, USA

Sidhartha D. Ray, *PhD, FACN*
Associate Professor, Division of Pharmacology, Toxicology and Medicinal Chemistry, Arnold and Marie Schwartz College of Pharmacy and Health Sciences, Long Island University, University Plaza, Brooklyn, New York 11201, USA

Daniel F. Reidy, *PhD, JD*
Attorney at Law, Suite 825, 545 Sansome Street, San Francisco, California 94111, USA

Andrew G. Renwick, *BSc, PhD, DSc*
Professor of Biochemical Pharmacology, Clinical Pharmacology Group, School of Medicine, Biomedical Sciences Building, University of Southampton, Bassett Crescent East, Southampton S016 7PX, UK

Christopher Rhodes, *BSc, PhD, DABT*
Safety of Medicines Department, AstraZeneca, Mereside, Alderley Park, Macclesfield, Cheshire SK10 4TG, UK

Ian R. Rowland, *BSc, PhD*
Professor of Human Nutrition, Northern Ireland Centre for Diet and Health, School of Biomedical Sciences, University of Ulster, Coleraine BT52 1SA, Northern Ireland, UK

Wilson K. Rumbeiha, *BVM, PhD, DABVT, DABT*
Assistant Professor of Clinical Toxicology, Animal Health Diagnostic Laboratory, Michigan State University, G303 VMC, East Lansing, Michigan 48824-1314, USA

Harry Salem, *BA, BSc, MA, PhD, FNYAS, FCP, FATS, FACT*
Chief Scientist, Research and Technology Directorate, US Army SBCCOM, Edgewood Chemical and Biological Center, 5183 Blackhawk Road, Aberdeen Proving Ground, Maryland 21010-5424, USA

Jeffrey D. Simon, *PhD*
Political Risk Assessment Company, P.O. Box 82, Santa Monica, California 90406-0082, USA

Robert Snyder, *PhD*
Environmental and Occupational Health Sciences Institute, Rutgers University, 170 Frelinghuysen Road, Piscataway, New Jersey 08854-8020, USA

Patricia J. Sparks, *MD, MPH*
Private Consultant, 7683 SE 27th Street, Suite 291, Mercer Island, Washington 98040, USA

Maria A. Stander, *MSc*
SASOL Center for Chemistry, Potchefstroom University, Private Bag X60001, Potchefstroom 2520, Republic of South Africa

Eiliv Steinnes, *DrPhil*
Department of Chemistry, Norwegian University of Science and Technology, N-7491 Trondheim, Norway

Pieter S. Steyn, *MSc, PhD*
Director of Research, Division of Research Technology, University of Stellenbosch, Stellenbosch 7600, Republic of South Africa

Tim R. Stiles, *MBA*
Stiles Quality Associates, 1 Old Farm Close, Needingworth, Huntingdon, Cambridgeshire PE17 3SG, UK.

Michael D. Stonard, *BSc, PhD*
Independent Toxicology Consultant, 4A Somerset Close, Congleton, Cheshire CW12 1SG, UK

Jürgen Sühnel
Biocomputing, Institute of Molecular Biotechnology, Beutenbergstr. 11, D-07745 Jena, Germany

Frank M. Sullivan, *BSc Hons*
National Teratology Information Service, Regional Drug and Therapeutic Centre, Wolfson Unit, Claremont Place, Newcastle-upon-Tyne NE2 4HH, UK

F. William Sunderman, Jr., *MD*
Department of Chemistry and Biochemistry, Bicentennial Hall, Middlebury College, Middlebury, Vermont 05753, USA

Tore Syversen, *MSc, DrPhilos*
Professor of Toxicology, Department of Pharmacology and Toxicology, School of Medicine, Norwegian University of Science and Technology, N-7489 Trondheim, Norway

Hanna S. E. Tahti, *PhD*
Research Director, Medical School, University of Tampere, P.O. Box 607, FIN-33101 Tampere, Finland

John A. Thomas, *PhD, FATS*
Professor Emeritus, Department of Pharmacology, Health Science Center, University of Texas, 219 Wood Shadow, San Antonio, Texas 78216, USA

Michael J. Thomas, *MD, PhD*
Department of Internal Medicine, Division of Endocrinology, School of Medicine, University of North Carolina, Chapel Hill, North Carolina 27599-7170, USA

John A. Timbrell, *BSc, PhD, DSc, MRCPath, FIBiol, FRSC*
Biochemical Toxicology, Pharmacy Department, King's College London, Franklin Wilkins Building, Stamford Street, London SE1 8WA, UK

John A. Tomenson, *BSc, DipStat (Cantab), PhD*
ICI Epidemiology Unit, Brunner House, P.O. Box 7, Winnington, Northwich, Cheshire CW8 4DJ, UK

David J. Tweats, *CBiol, BSc, PhD, FIBiol, FRCPath*
Director, Preclinical Safety Sciences UK, Glaxo Wellcome Research and Development Ltd., Park Road, Ware, Hertfordshire SG12 ODP, UK

Rochelle W. Tyl, *PhD, DABT*
Director, Center for Life Sciences and Toxicology, Chemistry and Life Sciences Division, Research Triangle Institute, 3040 Cornwallis Road, P.O. Box 12194, Research Triangle Park, North Carolina 27709-2194,USA

Tipton R. Tyler, *PhD, DABT*
Associate Director, Corporate Applied Toxicology, Union Carbide Corporation, 39 Old Ridgebury Road, Danbury, Connecticut 06817-0001, USA

Marie Vahter, *PhD*
Professor, National Institute of Environmental Medicine, Karolinska Institute, Box 210, S-17177 Stockholm, Sweden

John P. Van Miller, *PhD, DABT*
Associate Director of Applied Toxicology, Union Carbide Corporation, 39 Old Ridgebury Road, Danbury, Connecticut 06817-0001, USA

Duncan W. Vere, *MD, FRCP, FFPM*
14 Broadfield Way, Buckhurst Hill, Essex IG9 5AG, UK

David Walker, *BVSc, CBiol, FIBiol, FRCVS*
APT Consultancy, Old Hawthorn Farm, Hawthorn Lane, Four Marks, Alton, Hampshire GU34 5AU, UK

Robert E. Waller, *BSc*
72 King William Drive, Charlton Park, Cheltenham, Gloucester GL53 7RP, UK

Simon P.F. Warren, *CBiol, MIBiol, BSc, MSc, DIBT, DABT, DipRCPath*
Mallard House, Kings Pool, 1-3 Peasholme Green, York Y01 2PX, UK

Catherine J. Waterfield, *BSc, PhD*
Senior Principal Toxicologist, General and Reproductive Toxicology, Glaxo Wellcome Research and Development Ltd., Park Road, Ware, Hertfordshire SG12 0DP, UK (for all correspondence); Department of Pharmacy, King's College London, Manresa Road, London SW3 6LX, UK

Mike Watson, *BSc*
Ricerca Inc., 7528 Auburn Road, PO Box 1000, Painesville, Ohio 44077-1000, USA

Gregory P. Wedin, *PharmD, DABAT*
Hennepin Regional Poison Center, Hennepin County Medical Center, 701 Park Avenue, Minneapolis, Minnesota 55415, USA

Bernard Weiss, *PhD*
Professor of Environmental Medicine and Pediatrics, Department of Environmental Medicine, School of Medicine and Dentistry, University of Rochester, Rochester, New York 14642, USA

Peter G. Wells, *BSc, MSc, PhD*
Research Scientist, Coastal Ecosystems, Environment Canada, Environmental Conservation Branch, 45 Alderney Drive, Dartmouth, Nova Scotia B2Y 2N6, Canada; Associate Professor, School for Resource and Environmental Studies, Dalhousie University, Halifax, Nova Scotia B3H 3E2, Canada

Randy D. White, *PhD*
Director, Toxicology, Corporate Research and Technical Services, Baxter HealthCare Corporation, Round Lake, Illinois 60073, USA

Martin F. Wilks, *MD, PhD*
Zeneca Agrochemicals, Fernhurst, Haslemere, Surrey GU27 3JE, UK

Angela Wilson, *BSc, PhD*
Medical Research Council Radiobiology Unit, Chilton, Didcot, Oxfordshire OX11 ORD, UK

Patricia A. Wood, *MD, PhD*
Associate Professor of Medicine, Department of Medicine and Experimental Pathology, Stratton Veterans Affairs Medical Centre and Albany Medical College, Albany, New York 12208, USA

Kevin N. Woodward, *BA, BSc, MSc, PhD, DipRCPath, EurChem, CChem, FRSC, EurBiol, CBiol, FIBiol, MBIRA*
Schering-Plough Animal Health, Breakspear Road South, Harefield, Uxbridge, Middlesex UB9 6LS, UK

FREQUENTLY USED ABBREVIATIONS

Most abbreviations, either standard or infrequently used, are defined by authors in individual chapters. For ease of reference, the most frequently used abbreviations are listed below.

ACGIH	American Conference of Governmental Industrial Hygienists
ACh	acetylcholine
AChE	acetylcholinesterase (specific cholinesterase)
ACTH	adenocorticotrophic hormone
ADH	antidiuretic hormone
ADI	acceptable daily intake
ADME	absorption, distribution, metabolism and excretion
ADR	adverse drug reaction
ALAD	δ-aminolevulinic acid dehydratase
ALT	alanine aminotransferase
ANOVA	analysis of variance
ANSI	American National Standards Institute
APase	alkaline phosphatase
APTT	activated partial thromboplastin time
ASR	acoustic startle response
AST	aspartate aminotransferase
ATP	adenosine triphosphate
ATPase	adenosine triphosphatase
ATSDR	Agency for Toxic Substances and Disease Registry (US)
AUC	area under the curve
BAC	blood alcohol concentration
BAL	biological action level
BBB	blood-brain barrier
BCF	bioconcentration factor
BChE	butyryl cholinesterase (non-specific cholinesterase; pseudocholinesterase)
BEI	biological exposure index
BMD	bench mark dose
BOD	biological oxygen demand
BP	blood pressure; boiling point
BrDU	bromodeoxyuridine
BUN	blood urea nitrogen
CA	chromosomal aberration
CalEPA	California Environmental Protection Agency
CAM	chorioallantoic membrane
CAS	Chemical Abstracts Service
cAMP	cyclic adenosine monophosphate
ChE	cholinesterase
CHO	Chinese hamster ovary
CK	creatine kinase
CL	confidence limit(s)
CNS	central nervous system
CO	carbon monoxide
COHb	carboxyhaemoglobin
CPSC	Consumer Product Safety Commission (US)
CSF	cerebrospinal fluid
Ct (or CT)	inhalation exposure dosage (atmospheric concentration x time)
CVS	cardiovascular system
CW	chemical warfare
DHHS	Department of Health and Human Services (US)
DNA	deoxyribonucleic acid
DNase	deoxyribonuclease
DOT	Department of Transportation (US)
EAC	endocrine-active compound
EC	effective concentration [with respect to a particular (specific) end-point]
EC_{50}	effective concentration producing (or calculated to produce) a 50% response for the specific end-point
ECG	electrocardiogram
EDSTAC	Endocrine Disrupter Screening and Testing Advisory Committee (US)
EEG	electroencephalogram
EGF	epidermal growth factor
ELISA	enzyme-linked immunosorbent assay
EM	electron microscopy
EMEA	European Medicines Evaluation Agency
EMG	electromyogram
ER	endoplasmic reticulum
ERG	electroretinogram
ESR	erythrocyte sedimentation rate
ETS	environmental tobacco smoke
EU	European Union
FAD	flavine adenine dinucleotide
FAO	Food and Agricultural Organisation of the United Nations
FAS	foetal alcohol syndrome
FDA	Food and Drug Administration (US)
FEV	forced expiratory volume
FEV_1	forced expiratory volume in one second
FGF	fibroblast growth factor
FID	flame ionization detector
FIFRA	Federal Insecticide, Fungicide and Rodenticide Act (US)
FMO	flavin-containing monooxygenase
FOB	functional observation battery

FRC	functional residual capacity	IOP	intraocular pressure
FSH	follicle stimulating hormone	ip	intraperitoneal
FVC	forced vital capacity	IPCS	International Programme on Chemical Safety (WHO)
GABA	γ-aminobutyric acid		
GATT	General Agreement on Tariffs and Trade	IRIS	Integrated Risk Information System
GC	gas chromatography	ISO	International Standards Organization
GC-MS	gas chromatography - mass spectrometry	iv	intravenous
GD (gd)	gestational day	JECFA	Joint Expert Committee on Food Additives
GFR	glomerular filtration rate		
GGT	γ-glutamyl transferase	JMPR	Joint Meeting on Pesticide Residues
GH	growth hormone	K_D	dissociation constant
GI	gastrointestinal	K_M	Michaelis constant
GLC	gas-liquid chromatography	K_{ow}	octanol-water partition coefficient
GLP	good laboratory practice	LAA	laboratory animal allergy
GOT	glutamate-oxaloacetate transaminase (now referred to as AST, qv)	LAP	leucine aminopeptidase
		LC	lethal concentration (atmosphere or liquid)
GPT	glutamate-pyruvate transaminase (now referred to as AST, qv)		
		LC_{50}	concentration causing (or calculated to cause) 50% mortality in population studied
GRAS	generally recognised as safe		
GSH	glutathione		
GST	glutathione-*S*-transferase	$L(Ct)_{50}$	inhalation dosage causing (or calculated to cause) 50% mortality in population studied
G6P	glucose-6-phosphate		
G6Pase	glucose-6-phosphatase		
G6PD	glucose-6-phosphate dehydrogenase		
6TG	6-thiogaunine	LD	lethal dose
Hb	haemoglobin	LD_{50}	dose causing (or calculated to cause) 50% mortality in the population studied
HDLP	high density lipoprotein		
HDN	hyaline droplet nephropathy		
HGH	human growth hormone	LDH	lactate dehydrogenase
HGPRT	hypoxanthine-guanine-phosphoribosyl transferase	LDLP	low-density lipoprotein
		LH	luetinizing hormone
HIV	human immunodeficiency virus	LLNA	local lymph node assay
HPLC	high performance liquid chromatography	LOAEL	lowest observed adverse effect level
HPV	high production volume	LVET	low volume eye test
HSE	Health and Safety Executive (UK)	MAO	monoamine oxidase
HVAC	heating, ventilation and air control	MAT	mean absorption time
5-HT	5-hydroxytryptamine (serotonin)	MCA	Medicines Control Agency (UK)
ia	intra-arterial	MCH	mean (red blood cell) corpuscular haemoglobin
IARC	International Agency for Research on Cancer		
		MCHC	mean (red blood cell) corpuscular haemoglobin concentration
ic	intracerebral		
IC	incapacitating concentration	MCS	multiple chemical sensitivity
ICH	International Conference on Harmonization	MCV	mean (red blood cell) corpuscular volume
		MEST	mouse ear swelling test
ICRP	International Commission on Radiological Protection	metHb	methaemoglobin
		MFO	mixed function oxidase
ICSH	interstitial cell stimulating hormone	MMAD	mass median aerodynamic diameter
IC_{50}	concentration causing (or calculated to cause) 50% incapacitation in the population studied	MN	micronucleus
		MP	melting point
		MRC	Medical Research Council (UK)
ID	inhibitory dose	MRL	maximum residue level
ID_{50}	dose causing (or calculated to cause) 50% inhibition in the population studied	mRNA	messenger ribonucleic acid
		MRT	mean residue time
		MS	mass spectometry
Ig	immunoglobulin	MSDS	material safety data sheet
IL	interleukin	MTD	maximum tolerated dose
im	intramuscular	MW	molecular weight
		NAD	nicotine adenine dinucleotide

NADH	reduced nicotine adenine dinucleotide	REM	rapid eye movement
NAG	*N*-acetyl-β-D-glucosaminidase	RER	rough endoplasmic reticulum
NDA	new drug application	RfC	reference concentration
NIEHS	National Institute of Environmental Health and Safety (US)	RfD	reference dose
		RIA	radioimmunoassay
NIOSH	National Institute of Occupational Safety and Health (US)	RR	relative risk
		rRNA	ribosomal ribonucleic acid
NKC	natural killer cell	RTECS	Registry of Toxic Effects of Chemical Substances
NLM	National Library of Medicine (US)		
NMR	nuclear magnetic resonance	RV	residual volume
NOAEL	no observed adverse effect level	SAR	structure-activity relationship
NOEL	no observed effect level	SBS	sick building syndrome
NRC	National Research Council (US)	sc	subcutaneous
NSAID	nonsteroidal anti-inflammatory drug	SCE	sister chromatid exchange
5NT	5-nucleotidase	SD	standard deviation
NTE	neurotoxic esterase	SDH	sorbitol dehydrogenase
NTP	National Toxicology Program (US)	SE	standard error
OC	organochlorine	SEM	standard error of the mean
OECD	Organization for Economic Cooperation and Development	SER	smooth endoplasmic reticulum
		SG	specific gravity
OEL	occupational exposure limit	SIDS	screening information dab set
OP	organophosphate	SMR	standardized mortality ratio
OSHA	Occupation Safety and Health Administration (US)	SOP	standard operating procedure
		STEL	short-term exposure limit
OTC	over-the-counter	T_3	3,5,3′-tridothyronine
PAH	polycyclic aromatic hydrocarbons	T_4	3,5,3′,5′-tetraiodothyronine (thyroxine)
PAS	periodic acid-Schiff reaction	TCA	tricarboxylic acid
PBPK	physiologically based pharmacokinetics	TGF	transforming growth factor
pc	percutaneous	TK	thymidine kinase
PCB	polychlorinated biphenyls	TLC	thin layer chromatography
PCD	programmed cell death	TLV	threshold limit value
PCV	packed (red blood) cell volume	TOS	toxic oil syndrome
PEL	permitted exposure level	TNF	tumour necrosis factor
PMN	premanufacturing (premarketing) notification	tRNA	transfer ribonucleic acid
		TSCA	Toxic Substances Control Act (US)
PMR	proportionate mortality ratio	TSH	thyroid stimulating hormone
PMS	postmarketing surveillance	UDP	uridine diphosphate
PND (pnd)	postnatal day	UDPG	uridine diphosphate glucuronide
PNS	peripheral nervous system	UDS	unscheduled DNA synthesis
po	peroral	USDA	United States Department of Agriculture
PSD	Pesticides Safety Directorate (UK)	US EPA	United States Environmental Protection
PSI	peripheral sensory irritation	(EPA)	Agency
PTH	parathyroid hormone	USP	United States Pharmacopiea
QA	quality assurance	VMD	Veterinary Medicines Directorate (UK)
QSAR	quantitative structure-activity relationship	VOC	volatile organic compound
RAST	radioallergosorbent test	VP	vapour pressure
RBC	red blood cell	WBC	white blood cell
RD	depression of respiration	WHO	World Health Organization
RD_{50}	inspired concentration of material producing (or calculated to produce) a 50% decrease in respiratory rate	WTO	World Trade Organization

PART SEVEN

SPECIALIZATION

Chapter 64

Pharmaceutical Toxicity

P.F. D'Arcy

C O N T E N T S

INTRODUCTION

The development of potent and effective drugs continues to be associated with a concern regarding their safety. The administration of biologically active compounds to man must always be accompanied by some element of risk that cannot be avoided even by the most careful and exhaustive scientific and clinical tests of the new drug before it is introduced on to the therapeutic market. Safety, quality and efficacy are the three statutory requirements in the UK guiding the evaluation and approval for subsequent use of any pharmaceutical product, and these requirements are universal to drug regulatory bodies in other countries.

Regulations in the pharmaceutical industry arose out of the concept of protecting the population—indeed, safeguarding the public health is the first objective stated in the Directive 65/65 of the European Community—but predating this Directive is the accepted medical concept of 'first do no harm'.

It is salutary to look back into recent times and recall that the Committee on Safety of Drugs (the Dunlop Committee), which was established on a voluntary basis in the UK in 1963, was not directly concerned with drug efficacy. The voluntary arrangements with the pharmaceutical industry were dominated by safety; the Committee's remit did not impose upon it any responsibility to consider the efficacy of drugs except in so far as their safety was concerned. Even today, the successors of this group, the Medicines Control Agency and its attendant Medicines Commission and the

Committee on Safety of Medicines, are precluded from judgements of relative efficacy between candidate medicines and their established competitors in the evaluation processes.

It is only since 1971 that an integrated regulatory system concerned with the three requirements—safety, efficacy and quality of medicinal products—was established in the UK through the implementation of the Medicines Act of 1968. This enactment placed special emphasis on considerations of safety in relation to the issue of both Clinical Trials Certificates (Section 36.2) and Product Licences (Section 19.1). In contrast with its provisions in respect of efficacy, the Medicines Act allowed the Licensing Authority to take account of comparative safety (Section 19.2) in judging applications. Moreover, the Act took a broad view of safety by including not only potential dangers to patients themselves, but also hazards to the community and to those administering the drugs; it also covered interference with diagnosis, treatment or prevention of disease (Section 13.2). Comparable requirements within the European Community are contained in the relevant EEC Directives (Commission of the European Communities, 1984); matters which have potential financial implications such as clinical need and comparative efficacy are specifically excluded from both the Medicines Act and the EEC Directives.

In attempting to ensure the safety of medicines, the Licensing Authority and the Committee on Safety of Medicines in the UK rely on three strategies—the control of quality, rigorous pre-marketing safety studies and post-marketing surveillance. Quality is controlled in relation to both manufacture and wholesale selling and, as a consequence, toxicity due to product defects is now exceptional (Rawlings, 1989).

There are no priorities within safety, quality and efficacy, for all three requirements are equally weighted. Default in any one will jeopardize marketing approval or continuation of clinical use. Stephens (1988) summed up the situation thus: 'in future it will be no longer sufficient for pharmaceutical companies to plan their clinical trial programme for a new drug on the basis of showing that it is efficacious and that secondarily no adverse drug reactions (ADRs) were noted. The cost half of the cost/benefit ratio now demands that equal effort must be put into active research for adverse reactions as in the proof for efficacy'. Thus the evaluation of the toxic potential of a new medicine must be an active search, not merely a passive observation of what toxicity emerges during preliminary studies and subsequent clinical use.

The original chapter on Pharmaceutical Toxicology was written over 5 years ago for the First Edition of this book and during that time there have been a number of developments in the international scene regarding the safety testing of medicines. Foremost among these are the guidelines of the International Conference on Harmonization of Technical Requirements for Registration of Pharmaceuticals for Human Use (D'Arcy and Harron, 1992, 1994, 1996, 1998) and the guidelines issued by the European Committee for Proprietary Medicinal Products (CPMP), which has recently issued its Note for Guidance on The Investigation of Drug Interactions (Committee for Proprietary Medicinal Products, 1997).

Broadly similar guidance has been given by the US Food and Drug Administration (FDA) on approaches to *in vitro* studies of drug metabolism and interaction (Center for Drug Evaluation and Research, 1997). Discussions on the influence of these guidelines on current practices of safety assessment are given later in this chapter.

RESPONSIBILITY

The discovery of the ADR profile of a new drug prior to marketing lies entirely within the sphere of the pharmaceutical company and, therefore, the company has the responsibility for obtaining and then providing adequate information. After a new medicine is marketed, the responsibility for extending the knowledge base of its adverse reactions spreads also to all prescribers of the medicine, and also to specific organizations set up for that purpose.

Drug–drug interactions are an unfortunate facet of potent therapy with modern drugs and in the not so distant past the recognition and subsequent avoidance of drug–drug interactions were largely the concern of the clinician treating patients in the clinic. The manufacturer had a minor role. This field has developed so greatly in

extent and complexity that it is now predominantly a matter for the drug manufacturer to investigate prior to marketing. The influence of the European and American guidelines on the investigation of drug interactions has changed the focus of drug interaction studies from post-marketing largely *ad hoc* observational studies to pre-marketing rationally and scientifically designed programmes of investigation. Further discussion will be given to this later.

The predominant objective of all national and international drug regulations is to ensure the safety of marketed medicinal products during normal conditions of use. It could be defined as protecting the public health and safeguarding the public purse, for such procedures also ensure that the patient gets value for money spent on medication.

DRUG DISASTERS (PRE- AND POST-THALIDOMIDE)

Modern drug regulation in the UK was conceived in the aftermath of the thalidomide disaster. There is evidence that earlier disasters were equally troublesome, although perhaps not so well publicized as thalidomide (see **Table 1**). For example, jaundice and hepatic necrosis ('yellow atrophy of the liver') reached epidemic levels following the use of organo-arsenicals such as salvarsan to treat syphilis in soldiers returning from World War 1.

Amidopyrine was commonly used as an antipyretic and analgesic and it took almost half a century of common use to recognize that it caused agranulocytosis.

The ill-fated 'elixir of sulfanilamide' produced by the old-established Massengil Company in the USA not only heralded the new era of the sulphonamide drugs, but also during September and October 1937 directly caused at least 76 deaths owing to the renal toxicity of its 72% content of the solvent diethylene glycol; many of the victims were children. The sulphanilamide disaster shocked the country and was instrumental in Congress reacting by passing the Food, Drug and Cosmetic Act in 1938, which required all new drugs to be demonstrated to be safe (Wax, 1995).

One would have thought that the attendant publicity of this poisoning with diethylene glycol would have made an indelible impression on pharmaceutical manufacturers. However, from January 1990 until December 1992, 429 children were admitted to the renal unit of Dhaka Shishu Childrens' Hospital in Bangladesh. The cause of renal failure was identified in 90 of these patients (21%). Because ingestion of a toxic substance was suspected, special attention was directed towards identifying medicines taken before renal failure developed. Paracetamol elixir was identified as the medicine most commonly taken and samples tested showed that 19 out of the 69 elixirs examined contained diethylene glycol as

Table 1 Notable drug disasters or discovery of important adverse effects

1920s	Organo-arsenicals (jaundice and hepatic necrosis)
1933	Amidopyrine (agranulocytosis)
1937	'Elixir of Sulfanilamide'—Massengil (fatal diethylene glycol toxicity)
1957	Stalinon (raised intracranial pressure)
1960s	Phenacetin (renal damage)
1960s	Thalidomide (teratogenicity)
1960s	Clioquinol (subacute myelo-opticoneuropathy)
1967	Phenytoin (rickets, osteomalacia)
1970s	Practolol (oculomucocutaneous syndrome)
1970s	Metamizol (novaminsulfon) (blood dyscrasias)
1979–91	Triazolam (Halcion) (excitation reactions and acute psychic derangement)
1982	Benoxaprofen (Opren) (photosensitivity, oncholysis, fatal hepatic reactions in the elderly)
1983	Indoprofen (Flosint) (GI tract disorders and carcinogenicity)
1983	Osmosin (indomethacin dumping, ulceration and intestinal perforation, some cases fatal)
1983	Zimeldine (Zelmid) (neurotoxicity)
1983	Zomepirac (Zomax) (serious allergic and anaphylactic reactions)
1984	Alphaxalone (anaphylaxis)
1984	Fenclofenac (Flenac) (skin rashes, gastrointestinal disorders and suspected carcinogenicity)
1984	Feprazone (Methrazone) (skin rashes, gastrointestinal disorders, thrombocytopenia and haemolytic anaemia)
1984	Oxyphenbutazone (haematology, GI tract disorders)
1986	Domperidone injection (benzamide) (cardiotoxicity)
1986	Guanethidine eye drops (ophthalmological)
1986	Nomifensine (Merital) (immune haemolytic anaemia)
1986	Suprofen (Suprol) (reversible renal insufficiency)
1990	Propess (controlled-release PGE2, dinoprostone) (uterine hypotonus and foetal distress syndrome)
1990–92	Paracetamol elixir (fatal diethylene glycol toxicity in children in Bangladesh)
1991	Terolidine (Micturin) (cardiac arrhythmias)
1992	Elixirs (fatal diethylene glycol toxicity in children in Nigeria)
1992	Propofol (Diprivan) (fatal neurological, cardiac and renal toxicity and hyperlipidaemia in children)
1992	Medicinal products containing extracts from the plant germander (*Teucrium* spp.) (hepatitis)
1992	MMR vaccines (Pluserix-MMR, Immravax) (meningitis caused by mumps vaccine component in children)
1992–96	Terfenadine (Triludan, Seldane) (ventricular arrhythmias particularly *torsade de pointes*, potentiation by liver enzyme inhibitors (e.g. ketoconazole, and related antifungals, erythromycin and related macrolide antibiotics and grapefruit juice); changed to POM status in UK, withdrawn in USA)
1995	Desogestrel and gestodene-containing oral contraceptives (twofold risk of thromboembolism compared with older (second generation) OCs
1996	Amidarone (Cordarone X) (eye, lung, liver, thyroid and peripheral nervous system toxicity, skin reactions associated with photosensitivity)
1997	Paracetamol (concern about association with accidental or deliberate overdosage with liver toxicity, often fatal)
1997	Combination therapy with anorectic agents (e.g. fenfluramine or dexfenfluramine and phentermine (valvular heart disease)
1997	Protease inhibitors [e.g. indinavir (Crixivan), ritonavir (Norvir) and saquinavir (Invirase) (caused hyperglycaemia and caused new-onset diabetes mellitus, or exacerbated existing cases)]
1997	Pemoline (Volital) (hepatotoxicity, withdrawn in UK and USA)
1997	Phenolphthalein (FDA stated that when used as a laxative it poses a relevant carcinogenic risk for humans, alleged mechanism thought to be genetic mutations in the *p53* gene).

the sole diluent. The remaining 50 had propylene glycol or glycerin as the diluent. Three of the elixirs containing diethylene glycol were from the stock of the hospital's pharmacy, four were purchased from three different pharmacies and 12 were obtained from patients. The government of Bangladesh, with the assistance of WHO, subsequently analysed 104 different brands of paracetamol elixir available in the country and found five brands containing diethylene glycol. A total of 51 children died in this outbreak (Hanif *et al.*, 1995).

There is absolutely no excuse for formulating any elixir with diethylene glycol, which is a higly toxic organic solvent. It has a notorious history, as the early 'elixir of sulfanilamide' so clearly demonstrated. Even if this early disaster is forgotten, a 1992 report of mass diethylene glycol poisoning among 40 Nigerian children should serve as a very pertinent reminder of the criminal, if not murderous, practice of formulating any elixir with diethylene glycol (Okuonghae *et al.*, 1992).

The government of Bangladesh banned the sales of paracetamol elixirs in December 1992 and then cases of renal failure declined. However, there was obviously something wrong with the governmental drug administration and drug control laboratories that an outbreak of diethylene glycol poisoning could have occurred in children and continued for at least 35 months before it was recognized. In Nigeria, the outbreak of diethylene glycol toxicity was attributed to wholesale distributors fraudently substituting diethylene glycol for the more expensive propylene glycol. Obviously something was wanting in the quality control and drug regulations in that country to allow such criminal activity to be perpetrated.

Returning to **Table 1**, Stalinon, a preparation designed to treat boils, led to a 2 year prison sentence for its French inventor; it contained diiodoethyl tin and isolinoleic esters and was associated with raised intracranial pressure. The product was alleged to have killed 102 people and permanently affected 100 more, some survivors having residual paraplegia.

Phenacetin was first used in 1887 and is an effective analgesic and antipyretic. Unfortunately, however, it also has a long and somewhat controversial association with chronic renal disease, especially in the Swedish town of Huskvarna, where local custom amongst the munition workers involved the frank abuse of Hjorton's Powders, which contained caffeine, phenacetin and phenazone.

The subacute myelo-opticoneuropathy (SMON) epidemic in Japan, due to the use of clioquinol for enteric disorders, has received much publicity and was directly responsible for a greater awareness among the public of adverse drug reactions and led demand through their legislators for stricter controls over medicines.

Practolol, a very useful member and forerunner of the beta-blockers, gave rise to an oculomucocutaneous syndrome and was withdrawn from general use some 5 years after its introduction into the therapeutic market place.

Metamizol (novaminsulfon), a non-steroidal anti-inflammatory agent, was associated with blood dyscrasias.

The hypnotic agent triazolam, a benzodiazepine derivative, was associated with excitation reactions and acute psychic derangement, reactions that were complicated in 1979 by media-induced suggestion and excitement in the Netherlands—the so-called 'Halcion story'. This led to the suspension of triazolam in the Netherlands, although it was subsequently reapproved in 1990. The drug, however, remained somewhat controversial and the Licensing Authority withdrew this medicine from the UK market in October 1991 and some other countries followed at about the same time. Opinions still remain divided over its adverse effects.

Osmosin is worthy of particular mention because it was the formulation and not its indomethacin content that was the problem. This sustained-action (release) formulation 'dumped' its contents into the gut, causing ulceration and fatal intestinal perforation.

The non-steroidal anti-inflammatory agents (NSAIDs) have been singularly unfortunate in terms of their marketing history. Benoxaprofen caused fatal hepatic reactions in elderly patients and photosensitivity and oncholysis on a massive scale. It had a very short market life and well illustrated the suddenness with which a true epidemic of adverse events can occur. Zomepirac, another NSAID, was withdrawn because of the large number of incidents of serious anaphylaxis and allergic reactions that were associated with its use, and fenclofenac was withdrawn from the UK market in 1984 owing to a cluster of ADRs, including skin rashes, gastrointestinal disorders, thrombocytopenia and haemolytic anaemia.

Other problems with marketed drug products have followed in succeeding years. For example, in recent times amiodarone, a proven drug to treat supraventricular and ventricular arrhythmias, has been available since 1980 for oral and intravenous use and serious adverse reactions of various types have been recognized. Between 1980 and 1995, the Committee on Safety of Medicines in the UK received 1383 reports describing 2084 reactions, of which 65 were fatal, for oral amiodarone, and 77 reports of 117 reactions, of which four were fatal, for intravenous injection of the drug. The main organs affected by serious ADRs were lung (125 reports, 27 fatal), liver (78 reports, 17 fatal), peripheral nervous system (84 reports), eye (101 reports), thyroid gland (185 reports, four fatal) and skin (35 reports) with associated photosensitivity. This drug should be initiated only under hospital or specialist supervision for severe rhythm disorders unresponsive to other therapy or when other treatments cannot be used (Committee on Safety of Medicines/Medicines Control Agency, 1996).

On 15 October 1995, the Chairman of the UK Committee on Safety of Medicines (CSM) (Professor M. D. Rawlins) sent a letter to all doctors and pharmacists in the UK stating that the Committee had recently become aware of the results of three (then unpublished) epidemiological studies on the safety of oral contraceptives in relation to venous thromboembolism (deep venous thrombosis and pulmonary embolism). All three studies were reported to indicate that combined oral contraceptives containing desogestrel and gestodene were associated with a twofold increase in the risk of thromboembolism compared with those containing other progestogens. There was insufficient information to know whether or not norgestimate was also associated with an increased risk of thromboembolism. In the light of this new evidence, the Committee advised that combined oral contraceptives containing desogestrel or gestodene should not be used by women with risk factors for venous thrombosis and that they should only be used by women who were intolerant to other contraceptives and were prepared to accept an increased risk of thromboembolism.

There was some controversy over this advice and warning from doctors, patients and of course the media, not the least being that the three incriminating reports had not yet been published. However, when publications did appear a short while later they fully confirmed the action that had been taken by the CSM and its Chairman (Blomenkamp *et al.*, 1995; Jick *et al.*, 1995; World Health Organization, 1995a, b; Lewis *et al.*, 1996; McPherson, 1996; Spitzer *et al.*, 1996). All the studies indicated a statistically significant doubling of the adjusted ratios for venous thromboembolism in women taking third – rather than second – generation oral contraceptives.

Also in recent times, problems have emerged with terfenadine, a non-sedating antihistamine. It is a prodrug which is converted to fexofenadine as it passes through the liver after absorption from the gut. Generally it is fully metabolized in its first pass and is not present in the systemic circulation. However, if metabolism is inhibited or overloaded, for example by inhibitors of hepatic metabolism, then the parent drug reaches the circulation and prolongs the electrocardiograph QT interval. This predisposes to ventricular arrhythmias, particularly *torsade de pointes*, which may progress to ventricular fibrillation and death. Terfenadine should not be taken by patients with cardiac or hepatic disease and it should not be taken at the same time as a number of drugs which inhibit its hepatic metabolism, namely ketoconazole, itraconazole and related imidazole antifungals, erythromycin, clarithromycin and related macrolide antibiotics, or with grapefruit juice (Bailey *et al.*, 1991, 1993, 1994; Soons *et al.*, 1991; Ahmad, 1992; Committee on Safety of Medicines, 1992; Ducharme *et al.*, 1993; Benton *et al.*, 1994; Merkel *et al.*, 1994; Proppe *et al.*, 1995; Kupferschmidt *et al.*, 1995; Honig *et al.*, 1996). Grapefruit juice inhibits the cytochrome P450 enzyme systems (CYP3A4) via the active principles of its bitter flavonoids naringin, naringenin, quercetin and kaempferol, an effect that is not apparently caused by other citrus fruits or their juices.

The CSM has recently reviewed the safety of terfenadine in relation to cardiac arrhythmias and was concerned that serious adverse reactions to terfenadine continued to be reported. From 1982, when the drug was first marketed in the UK, up to April 1997, the CSM had received 33 reports of serious cardiac arrhythmias, 14 of which were fatal. Until recent times in the UK this antihistamine was classified as a pharmacy medicine (P), but it has now been reclassified as a prescription-only medicine (POM). Other countries have also taken legislatory action, e.g. the US FDA has removed products containing terfenadine from the US market, a decision which was influenced by the successful introduction of fexofenadine, a metabolite of terfenadine, which it is claimed provides the benefits of terfenadine without the cardiotoxic risks. The French authorities have likewise withdrawn terfenadine and the Committee on Proprietary Medicinal Products (CPMP), which advises the European Licensing Authority, has the drug under consideration (Anon., 1997a–e).

The FDA has associated the laxative phenolphthalein with a risk of cancer in humans. The alleged risk is thought to be caused by mutation of the *p53* gene (Vogel, 1997). This is surprising in view of the long and widespread use (ingredient of the chocolate-based X-Lax) of this laxative, which has not hitherto been associated with cancer during almost 100 years of use. It is, however, well known for causing fixed drug eruptions of the skin.

The thalidomide tragedy looms so ponderously over this catalogue of adverse drug reactions that it causes other events that have occurred since to pale into insignificance and even suggests that since 1961 the worst of the problems have been solved. This is just not so! The number of patients gravely injured or killed in epidemics of drug-induced disease since then is a vast multiple of the number of thalidomide victims. Although much information has been gained about the circumstances leading to these individual disasters, there is little in this collection of data that will serve to prevent other drug disasters occurring that are qualitatively different from those that have gone before. The range of injuries produced is so wide that no single solution to the detection of future drug-induced disasters before they occur seems likely to emerge. At best, this catalogue of disasters has fine tuned the mechanisms by which drug regulatory bodies respond to early warnings of serious ADRs so that they can limit damage by quickly withdrawing the offending drug.

REGULATIONS CONCERNED WITH SAFETY

Pharmaceutical toxicology is a different field from industrial or pesticide toxicity evaluations. The techniques employed and the methodology used are similar but the orientation is different. Since there is no way of providing the absolute safety of a new medicine before it comes into widespread use, it becomes a question of the stage of development at which the risks should be defined. The easy answer is, as soon as possible, so that as few patients as possible are exposed to unnecessary risks. The regulatory authority must therefore weigh the advantages of the efficacy of a new drug, compared with the normal prognosis of the disease with known therapy, against the risks involved in marketing the new drug without full knowledge of its adverse reaction burden. At the same time, the regulatory authority has to decide whether to leave the detection of the rarer side-effects to be discovered by the present testing systems or whether they should institute a major surveillance programme so that these risks may become known earlier.

The regulation of medicines by society has been expressed by Lasagna (1989) as being time-bound, country-bound and person-bound. It is time-bound both because of what are thought to be socially necessary changes over the years and because the sciences of medicine and pharmacology are constantly evolving. It is country-bound because each nation, in setting up its own regulatory system, will be guided by the particular needs of its citizens for medicines, its economy, its political philosophy and the quality and extent of its scientific establishment and its health care delivery system. It is person-bound because no matter what the letter of the law may be for regulating medicines, or the nature of the published regulations, there is always the opportunity for value judgements to be made by those implementing the laws and regulations. These comments have been somewhat modified in recent time by the success of the ICH guidelines (D'Arcy and Harron, 1992, 1994, 1996, 1998) in bringing about harmonization of drug regulations between the three major drug research and manufacturing regions, Europe, America and Japan. These guidelines have had a significant impact on the time-bound and country-bound facets of regulation.

In considering the role of regulations, it is useful to be realistic about what can and what cannot be achieved by regulations, even when based on scientific rules of evidence and on accepted approaches to decision making. Traditionally, the most ancient and in a sense the least controversial function of regulations has been to ensure that a medicine is accurately labelled as to its contents and the nature of the ingredients and their amounts (Lasagna, 1989). It is more difficult, however, to delineate the safety and efficacy of the medicine proposed for registration. Since the ability to explore the full dose–response curve for a drug's toxicity is not ethically possible in humans, it is necessary to rely to a great extent on animal studies to achieve insight into this relationship.

THE USE OF ANIMALS IN SAFETY TESTING

There are powerful scientific, ethical and regulatory reasons for exploring the effect of potential therapeutic candidates in animals before they are administered to man. There are also strong and public emotive reasons why animals should not be used. However, the low proportion of significant toxic reactions in humans with new medicines, compared with the number tested and introduced, supports the contention that toxicity studies in laboratory animals are, in the main, predictive for man.

There are also many positive occurrences between the findings in animals toxicity tests and adverse reactions in human, particularly for dose-and time-related toxic effects (**Table 2**). In contrast, there have been well publicized accounts of failure of experimental toxicology and

Table 2 Some toxic reactions that occur in both animals and man. Source: Morton (1990)

Acrylamide	Peripheral neuropathy
Aniline	Methaemoglobinaemia
Atropine	Anticholinergic effects
Benzene	Leukaemia
Bleomycin	Pulmonary fibrosis
Carbon disulphide	Nervous system toxicity
Carbon tetrachloride	Hepatic necrosis
Cis-platinum	Nephrotoxicity
Cobalt sulphate	Cardiomyopathy
Cyclophosphamide	Haemorrhagic cystitis
Cyclosporin A	Nephropathy
D&C Yellow	Eczema
Diethylene glycol	Nephropathy
Diethylaminoethoxy hexoestrol	Phospholipidosis of liver
Doxorubicin	Cardiomyopathy
Emetine	ECG abnormalities
Ethylene glycol	Obstructive nephropathy
Frusemide (furosemide)	Hypokalaemia
Gentamicin	Nephropathy and ototoxicity
Hexacarbon	Peripheral neuropathy
Hexachlorophene	Spongiform encephalopathy
Isoniazid	Peripheral neuropathy
Isoprenaline (isoproterenol)	Peripheral neuropathy
Isothiocyanates	Goitre
Isotretinoin	Multiple malformations
Kanamycin	Cochlear toxicity
Methanol	Blindness (monkey)
Methoxyflurane	Nephropathy (Fischer rat)
8-Methoxypsoralen	Photosensitivity
Methylmercury	Encephalopathy
Morphine	Physical and psychological dependence
MPTP (1-methyl-4-phenyl-1,2,5,6-tetrahydropyridine)	Parkinsonism
Musk ambrette	Photosensitivity
2-Naphthylamine	Bladder cancer (dog)
Neuroleptic drugs	Galactorrhoea
Nitrofurantoin	Testicular damage
Paracetamol (acetaminophen)	Hepatic necrosis
Paraquat	Lung damage and fibrosis
Phenformin	Lactic acidosis
Phenothiazine NP207	Retinopathy (pigmented animals)
Penicillamine	Loss of taste
Potassium (slow-release)	Intestinal ulceration
Pyridoxine	Sensory neuropathy
Scopolamine	Behavioural disturbances
Thalidomide (prenatal)	Phocomelia (monkey, rabbit)
Triparanol	Cataract
Vinyl chloride	Angiosarcoma of liver
Vitamin A	Osteopathy
Vitamin D	Nephrocalcinosis

false alarms resulting from apparently irrelevant toxicological observations in animals, a good example of this being the animal studies carried out in the USA in the late 1960s on the risks of cancer from ingesting sugar-free sweeteners. The overall success of the current pre-clinical safety evaluation process is difficult to assess. Although useful information could be obtained by retrospective analysis of data obtained for compounds that have been used extensively in the clinic, to date this has received only limited systematic study (Lumley and Walker, 1990).

In 1989, the Sixth Centre for Medicines Research (CMR), held at the Ciba Foundation, London, provided the opportunity for an international group of experts from the pharmaceutical industry, academia and the regulatory authorities to review critically and discuss past methodologies which have been employed to assess the efficacy of animal toxicity testing procedures in predicting qualitative toxicity in man. Conventional animal toxicological studies have three purposes: they attempt to define a candidate compound's general toxicological profile, they are expected to reveal those target organs/ systems demanding special study during clinical trials and, it is hoped, they will provide a basis for predicting human safety (Rawlings, 1989). A most important aspect of the correlation of toxic effects between man and animals is the selection of animal species in which the drug is absorbed, distributed, metabolized and excreted in a similar manner to man.

The value of multi-species toxicity studies and parallel metabolic studies has been well established (Morton, 1990). However, despite wide experience with animal studies, their validity remains uncertain (Zbinden, 1981). Only a few investigators (Fletcher 1978; Griffin, 1983; Laurence *et al.*, 1984) have attempted to correlate findings during human use with those observed during pre-clinical toxicity studies, and even these have been limited in scale and scope (Rawlings, 1989). Routine animal toxicity tests are most useful when there are no important qualitative differences between species and where one can make up for the difficulty in demonstrating certain adverse effects with clinically relevant doses in animals by administering the drug at very high doses, on the assumption that more sensitive individuals will respond in a similar fashion when given smaller doses of the drug (Lasagna, 1989).

INTERNATIONAL CONFERENCE ON HARMONIZATION (ICH): ITS ROLE IN DRUG SAFETY

The International Conference on Harmonization of Technical Requirements for the Registration of Pharmaceuticals for Human Use (ICH) was established in 1990 as a joint regulatory/industry project to improve,

through harmonization, the efficiency of the process for developing and registering new medicinal products in Europe, Japan and the USA. Through harmonization, it was believed, the products would become available to patients with a minimum of delay. The six parties forming ICH represented the regulatory bodies and research-based industry in the three regions, which are responsible for the major output of new medicines in the world. The Geneva-based International Federation of Pharmaceutical Manufacturers Associations (IFPMA), which represents the research-based pharmaceutical industry, world-wide, has been closely involved with ICH from the outset, and acts as coordinator for global industry and organizer for the ICH Conferences

The ICH process achieved success because it was based on scientific consensus developed between industry and regulatory experts and because of the commitment of the regulatory parties to implementing the ICH tripartite harmonized guidelines and recommendations. ICH held four Conferences, the first in Brussels in 1991, the second in Orlando in 1993, the third in Yokohama in 1995 and the fourth in Brussels in 1997; the full proceedings of these conferences have been published (D'Arcy and Harron, 1992, 1994, 1996, 1998). The prime objective of ICH was to reduce or obviate the need for duplication or even triplication of the extensive and highly expensive testing which prior to ICH was carried out separately in each of the three regions during the research, development and clinical and toxicological evaluation of the new medicines. Harmonization of animal studies formed a large part of the work of ICH, which was initially divided into considerations of Safety, Quality and Efficacy, to which latterly was added Regulatory Communications. A summary of the progress of development of ICH guidelines is shown in **Figure 1**, which shows the five steps in the ICH process for harmonization of technical issues, and **Table 3**, which shows, amongst other progress, the steps to consensus in safety topics and in reproductive toxicology. Of particular relevance also are the progress of carcinogenicity and genotoxicity studies and the single and repeat-dose studies in

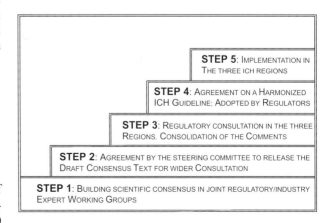

Figure 1 Five steps in the ICH process for harmonization.

Table 3 ICH progress in steps to concensus

Topic	Code	Apr-90	Apr-91	Nov-91	Mar-92	Sep-92	Mar-93	Jun-93	Oct-93	Mar-94	Oct-94	Mar-95	Jul-95	Nov-95	May-96	Jul-96	Nov-96	Mar-97	Jul-97
				ICH 1					ICH 2					ICH 3					ICH 4
Quality Topics																			
STABILITY	T1																		
Stability: drug substance and product	Q1A				STEP 2				STEP 4										STEP 5
Photostability	Q1B													STEP 2			STEP 4		STEP 5
Stability: new dosage forms	Q1C													STEP 2			STEP 4		STEP 5
SPECIFICATIONS	T2																		
Analytical validation: terminology	Q2A								STEP 2	STEP 4									STEP 5
Analytical validation: methodology	Q2B													STEP 2			STEP 4		STEP 5
Impurities: new drug substances	Q3A									STEP 2	STEP 4								STEP 5
Impurities: new drug products	Q3B													STEP 2			STEP 4		STEP 5
Residual solvent impurities	Q3C													STEP 2			STEP 2	STEP 4	STEP 5
Biotechnology: viral safety	Q5A													STEP 2					STEP 5
Biotechnology: genetic stability	Q5B											STEP 2		STEP 4					STEP 5
Biotechnology: product stability	Q5C											STEP 2		STEP 4					STEP 5
Biotechnology: cell substrates	Q5D																	STEP 2	
Specifications: chemical drug	Q6A																		
Specifications: biotech drug	Q6B																		
PHARMACOPOEIAS	Q4			T3															
Safety Topics																			
TOXICITY TESTING PROGRAMME	T1																		
Carcinogenicity: need for studies	S1A											STEP 2		STEP 4					STEP 5
Carcinogenicity: testing methodology	S1B														STEP 2				STEP 5
Carcinogenicity: dose selection	S1C								STEP 2										STEP 5
Revision of S1C	S1C/R																		
Genotoxicity: specific aspects	S2A									STEP 2			STEP 4				STEP 2		STEP 5
Genotoxicity: standard battery of tests	S2B																STEP 2		STEP 5
Toxicokinetics	S3A								STEP 2		STEP 4								STEP 5
Pharmacokinetics	S3B								STEP 2		STEP 4								STEP 5
Single and repeat-dose toxicity in rodents	S4		STEP 4																
Repeat-dose toxicity in non-rodents	S4A																		STEP 5

(Continued)

Table 3 *(Contd)*

Topic	Code	ICH/Date	Steps
REPRODUCTIVE TOXICOLOGY		T2 (Nov-91, ICH 1)	
Toxicity to reproduction	S5A		STEP 2 (Sep-92), STEP 4 (Jun-93), STEP 5 (Jul-97)
Male fertility studies	S5B		STEP 2 (Mar-95), STEP 4 (Nov-95), STEP 5 (Jul-97)
BIOTECHNOLOGY		T3 (Nov-91)	
Pre-clinical safety: biotech products	S6		STEP 2 (Nov-96), STEP 5 (Jul-97)
TIMING OF TOXICITY STUDIES		T4 (Nov-91)	
Timing of non-clinical safety studies	M3		STEP 2 (Nov-96)
Efficacy Topics			
ASSESSMENT OF CLINICAL SAFETY		T1 (Nov-91)	
Extent of population exposure	E1		STEP 2 (Oct-93), STEP 4 (Oct-94), STEP 5 (Jul-97)
Safety data: definitions and standards	E2A		STEP 2 (Jun-93), STEP 4 (Oct-94), STEP 5 (Jul-97)
Safety data: data elements	E2B		STEP 2 (May-96)
Safety data: periodic safety updates	E2C		STEP 2 (Mar-95), STEP 4 (Jul-96), STEP 5 (Jul-97)
Clinical study reports	E3		STEP 2 (Mar-95), STEP 4 (Nov-95), STEP 5 (Jul-97)
DESIGN OF DOSE–RESPONSE STUDIES		T2 (Nov-91)	
Dose-response information	E4		STEP 2 (Mar-93), STEP 4 (Oct-93), STEP 5 (Jul-97)
Ethnic factors	E5		STEP 2 (Mar-96)
GOOD CLINICAL PRACTICE		T3 (Nov-91)	
Consolidated guideline	E6		STEP 2 (Jul-95), STEP 4 (May-96), STEP 5 (Jul-97)
Addendum on investigator's brochure	E6A		STEP 2 (Oct-93), STEP 4 (Mar-95), STEP 5 (Jul-97)
Addendum on essential documents	E6B		STEP 2 (Oct-93), STEP 4 (Oct-94), STEP 5 (Jul-97)
TRIALS IN SPECIAL POPULATIONS		T4 (Nov-91)	
Special populations: geriatrics	E7		STEP 2 (Sep-92), STEP 4 (Jun-93), STEP 5 (Jul-97)
General considerations for clinical trials	E8		STEP 2 (Nov-96)
Statistical principles for clinical trials	E9		STEP 2 (Nov-96)
Choice of control group	E10		

KEY: Preliminary discussion · Step 1 · Step 3 · Next Step expected · Step-wise process does not apply rodents and non-rodents. In ICH Guideline S4, for example, it states that the LD_{50} determination should be abandoned for pharmaceuticals, as this would greatly reduce the number of small animals required for toxicity testing, as also do the further provisions of this guideline, which reduces the duration of repeat dose toxicity studies in the rat from 12 to 6 months. Space does not allow anything more than a passing reference here to these studies; the reader may, however, obtain detailed information in the published proceedings of the conferences.

CARCINOGENICITY AND MUTAGENICITY TESTING

Unfortunately, there is current reliance on carcinogenicity and mutagenicity tests whose power and reliability are in question. Morton (1990) has summarized problems with the evaluation of animal mutagenicity and carcinogenicity tests and their prediction of potential carcinogenicity in humans.

For many years, potential new medicines have been tested at high doses in long-term carcinogenicity studies in rodents prior to regulatory approval and broad clinical use. These studies have been costly in testing, chemicals, animals, laboratory facilities and staff and research time. Although the overall database on animal bioassays has been greatly expanded by the US National Cancer Institute and the National Toxicology Program, the prediction of human carcinogenicity is still problematic. In many studies, the results have varied between species, strains and sexes of the animals tested. The incidence of tumours observed has not always been dose-related and the relevance of these studies to human carcinogenesis is still not clear.

Over the last 6 years, the deliberations of ICH has led to intimate investigation of the battery of tests previously employed by the European, US and Japanese industries to predict carcinogenicity, mutagenicity and genotoxicity. As a result of this there has been considerable improvement and harmonization of testing procedures and the production of agreed guidelines which have led to a reduction in numbers of animals used, a reduction in the number of species of animals involved, a reduction in the time-scales of testing and a significant reduction in the costs of testing. The safety testing of biotechnology products, the timing of toxicity studies in relation to clinical trials and testing for carcinogenicity in pharmaceuticals are examples of other topics that have also undergone considerable discussion by the appropriate Expert Working Groups and guidelines are in the process of gaining concensus. The latter example, the testing for carcinogenicity in pharmaceuticals, has been of particular importance. It has been intensively reviewed, especially in respect to the need to carry out carcinogenicity studies in *both* mice and rats, or whether reduced testing

procedures can be accepted without jeopardizing safety.

Short-term mutagenicity tests are expected to detect genotoxic carcinogens, and a strong rationale has been developed for the use of these tests early in the process of drug development. Although neither a positive nor a negative result in short-term tests can be considered fully definitive, the International Agency for Research on Cancer has noted that the majority of chemicals that have given sufficient evidence of inducing human tumours are genotoxic (International Agency for Research on Cancer, 1987).

It has become evident within the last decade or so that the early estimates of the predictability of mutagenicity tests for the carcinogenic properties of most chemicals were to optimistic (Shelby and Stasiewicz, 1984; Tennant et al., 1987). A careful validation of in vitro tests against the results of long-term rodent carcinogenicity by Tennant et al. (1987) found that none of the short-term tests were necessarily predictive. In fact, it was suggested that no combination of the available in vitro mutgenicity tests (e.g. Ames bacterial mutation; L5178Y mammalian mutation; rat hepatocyte DNA repair; CHO cell cytogenetics) was significantly better than a single test. Furthermore, Clayson (1987) has suggested that short-term tests cannot be expected to detect all types of carcinogens, since mutations may only be related to the initiation phase of the complex process of carcinogenesis. Further evidence has been given by Morton (1990), who described and quoted mutagenicity testing in the laboratories of Eli Lilly and Company; in the validation studies most of the known human or animal carcinogens were detected in the broadly used and well accepted battery of in vitro and in vivo mutagenicity tests. However, when research compounds were tested in this tier, the number of positive findings was relatively small and in no case did a compound produce a positive response in more than one test.

The deliberations of the ICH have been especially concerned with the harmonization of carcinogenicity and genotoxicity testing and over the last 6 years several issues have been addressed which have simplified testing and its evaluation, reduced the number of animals required and eliminated the need to carry out unnecessary testing. For example, the S1 Guideline on the Need for Carcinogenicity Studies of Pharmaceuticals has been finalized. Its objective is to provide consistency in defining the circumstances under which it is necessary to undertake carcinogenicity studies on new drugs, taking account of known risk factors and the intended indications and duration of exposure. This guideline should eliminate the need to carry out unnecessary studies. The companion Guideline S1B, Testing for Carcinogenicity in Pharmaceuticals, has reviewed the scientific approach to testing pharmaceuticals for carcinogenicity especially with respect to the need to carry out such studies in *both* mice and rats, or whether reduced testing procedures could be accepted without jeopardizing safety. Guideline S1C, Dose Selection for Carcinogenicity Studies of Pharmaceuticals, was released for consultation in November 1996 and gives criteria for the selection of the high dose which is to be used in carcinogenicity studies on new therapeutic agents, in order to harmonize current practices and improve the design of studies.

In genotoxicity studies, the ICH Guideline S2A, Genotoxicity: Specific Aspects of Regulatory Tests, gives guidance and recommendations for *in vitro* and *in vivo* tests and on the evaluation of test results. It also includes a glossary of terms related to genotoxicity tests, to improve consistency in applications. The companion Guideline S2B, Genotoxicity: Standard Battery Tests, addresses two fundamental areas of genotoxicity testing: the identification of a standard set of assays to be conducted for registration and the extent of confirmatory experimentation in any particular genotoxicity assay in the standard battery.

Certainly, this harmonization of tests and testing will do much to resolve the earlier confusion and uncertainty and ensure that candidate pharmaceuticals are now tested in meaningful and necessary tests that can be easily evaluated. It must not be forgotten that the ICH guidelines are mandatory only in Europe, the USA and Japan. However, they are the major pharmaceutical-producing areas in the world and with the planned expansion of ICH activities (D'Arcy and Harron, 1998) it is likely that other countries and regions will also adopt these criteria, for example, Canada, the European Free Trade Area (EFTA) and WHO have been observers and have attended the Steering Committee Meetings and participated in the Expert Working Groups since the start of the ICH. The WHO, in particular, has the means of bringing the ICH guidances, which are applicable to 19 countries, to more than 170 member states that currently remain outside the ICH exercise.

TRANSLATION OF RESULTS FROM ANIMALS TO MAN

When one moves from animals to humans, a conservative approach is usually taken, starting with doses in healthy volunteers at only a fraction of those which produce significant toxicity in the most sensitive animal species. It is generally agreed that in these earliest human studies, and in the subsequent clinical trials in Phases 1 and II, one can gain considerable insight into those adverse reactions that occur with some frequency. However, it is usually not possible to detect in the studies the truly rare serious side-effect, to say nothing of the side-effect that is long delayed in its onset, or occurs as a result of an interaction with basic disease processes, or with other drugs. All that eventually will be known about the drug's effects, both good and bad, will never be known at

the time of initial marketing of a new medicine. The lesson is obvious: efficient and skilful post-registration observations must be relied upon to identify and prove cause–effect relationships between the taking of the medicine and the occurrence of an untoward effect.

In the UK, for example, the Committee on Safety of Medicines designates all newer medicines, of which there is limited experience of use, by an inverted arrow sign (▼). Doctors are asked to report all suspected reactions (i.e. any adverse or unexpected event, however minor, which could conceivably be attributed to the drug). Reports should be made despite uncertainty about a causal relationship, irrespective of whether the reaction is well recognized, and even if other drugs have been given concurrently.

Prospective studies designed to assess the relevance and predictive value of animal toxicity studies for man are rarely possible for ethical reasons (Brimblecombe, 1990). Substances showing marked toxicity in animals can only rarely, for ethical reasons, be administered to man. Prospective studies are, therefore, only possible with substances showing an acceptable toxicological profile in animals. In general, there is a paucity of data in this area. However, although retrospective collection and analysis of data are less satisfactory, they are none the less important alternatives. Such data are available, for example, within pharmaceutical companies, but analysis of larger databases, such as those in the files of regulatory authorities or those collected from a number of companies (e.g. by the Centre for Medicines Research), has the potential for yielding more valuable information. Brimblecome (1990) has suggested that retrospective studies can take a number of forms:

(1) Re-evaluation of data from animal studies when unwanted effects occur subsequently and unexpectedly in man.
(2) Design of specific animal studies to elucidate mechanisms of untoward effects which have been observed in man.
(3) Pooling of data from a number of sources to increase the size of the database and to enable more meaningful 'epidemiological-type' analyses to be performed.
(4) Review of the history of individual compounds which have been, or are in, development.

Bass (1990), in summarizing the toxicologist's viewpoint on what could be learned by examining the data in the files of regulatory authorities, stated that data in those files highlighted the problem areas that exist in extrapolating the results of animal studies to man. Since animal toxicity studies should be performed for the sake of man, this implied differences for each developmental product; hence it is no longer appropriate to work to generalized and rigid guidelines. Flexibility in itself seems insufficient if the pharmaceutical manufacturer does not know how the regulatory authorities will react to the test programmes envisaged, and if revision through interaction with the clinical level is not included. Bass concluded that the question to be answered is not whether studies available retrospectively have been of relevance to man and to what extent or percentage, but how to make such studies useful and relevant in the future. Thus early interactions between the pharmaceutical manufacturer and the regulatory authority may be needed case by case. This, he believes, should reduce the overall number of toxicological studies, rendering those remaining as requirements more relevant. Through the agency of ICH, these concepts have been largely achieved and there is good and early rapport between industrialists and regulators.

Fletcher (1990), expressing the clinician's viewpoint, commented on the number of guidelines that have been introduced since 1977 which were similar but not identical: the toxicological guidelines of the Committee for Proprietary Medicinal Products (CPMP); the OECD toxicity testing guidelines; the Annexes of the Sixth Amendment Directive of the EEC, which were also toxicological guidelines; and the Guidelines for Good Laboratory Practice. The problem with these is that they have codified and ritualized toxicity testing, so that there is very little flexibility. In Fletcher's view this was not ideal, for what was needed was a possibility of matching toxicological requirements to particular compounds.

Over the last 6 years, the ICH process has added new guidelines for toxicity testing which have been or will be adopted by the regulatory authorities in Europe, the USA and Japan. Certainly, they have enfolded many of the guidelines that were produced earlier and they have addressed toxicity topics such as Guidance on the Assessment of Systemic Exposure in Toxicity Studies (S3A), Guidance for Repeated Dose Tissue Distribution Studies (S3B), Single Dose and Repeat Dose Toxicity Tests (S4), Repeat-Dose Toxicity in Non-Rodents (S4A), Detection of Toxicity to Reproduction for Medicinal Products (S5A), Reproductive Toxicology; Male Fertility Studies (S5B), Safety Studies for Biotechnological Products (S6) and The Extent of Population Exposure to Assess Clinical Safety (E1). Clinical safety topics that have been addressed include Clinical Data Safety Management: Definitions and Standards for Expedited Reporting (E2A) and Data Elements for Transmission of ADR Reports (E2B), Periodic Safety Update Reports (E2C), Clinical Study Reports: Structure and Content (E3), Dose–Response Information to Support Drug Registration (E4) and Ethnic Factors in the Acceptibility of Foreign Clinical Data (E5).

The ICH did not, however, advance the case of throwing open the files of regulatory authorities. There is a great deal of potential in examining the files of regulatory authorities, as these have a unique value in that they cover a whole range of compounds and therapeutic classes, providing the full range of toxicological and clinical testing. However, access to data held by regulatory authorities is strictly limited, since any one company has access only to information on its own compounds and the only place in which the totality exists is with the regulatory authorities. Fletcher (1990) has suggested how this situation could be improved. First, the inclusion of toxicokinetics in safety evaluation studies would provide the opportunity to compare pharmacokinetics and metabolism in animals with man and could prevent inappropriate conclusions being drawn with regard to animals and human conditions. Second, there is an urgent need for closer cooperation between toxicologists and clinicians in the industry. Finally, detailed analyses of toxicological and clinical data available from regulatory authorities should be carried out.

Fletcher (1990) suggested that this could be approached by tabulating and analysing all the anatomical, physiological and toxicological findings for particular groups of chemically or therapeutically similar compounds. This would give an insight into whether they were consistent or inconsistent and what could and could not be relied upon. He also suggested an analysis of time relationships to identify situations that have proved to be consistently unreliable, inappropriate or irrelevant. This should provide evidence as to whether long-term tests, for example in dogs, were irrelevant.

From 8 September 1997, the Secretary of State for Health in England launched the remote access to marketing authorizations (RAMA) service by which pharmaceutical companies can now buy direct computer access to the Medicines Control Agency's full database on their products. They will also have access to non-confidential information on all other medicines authorized for sale in the UK. They will not have access to confidential information on other companies' products. The new service is to be provided free of charge to other European Community regulatory authorities. This is certainly a step in the right direction, but it does not go far enough. It does not give access to information on products that have failed to gain marketing authorization, and this is likely to be a fruitful source of toxicological information, and it does not give access to companies on confidential information on products other than their own.

Lumley (1990) has provided interesting information on the termination of development by companies as a result of clinical toxicity. Eighteen pharmaceutical companies in the UK, Switzerland and the USA gave information on 29 compounds for which they terminated development between 1975 and 1986. These data are summarized in **Table 4**. Almost half of the clinical effects causing termination (14) were effects that are difficult to measure in animal tests, including CNS disturbances, blood dyscrasias, skin reactions and allergies, and only two of these (both blood dyscrasias) were detected in

Table 4 Compounds: development terminated owing to clinical toxicity. Source: Lumley (1990)

Therapeutic class	Phase of testing	Approx. No./vol. of patients tested	Clinical toxicity	Predicted (Y/N) or confirmed (C) in animal tests
1 GI	Clinical trial	2000	Raised liver enzymes	C
2 CVS	n/a	n/a	Abnormal liver function tests	n/a
3 CVS	Post-marketing	–	Hepatic necrosis	N
4 CVS	Phase I/II	–	Increased transaminases	Y
5 Respiratory	n/a	n/a	Abnormal liver function tests	n/a
6 NSAID	Phase III	2000	Raised liver enzymes	N
7 –	Clinical trial	n/a	Raised liver enzymes	N
8 Antiallergy	Clinical trial	100s	Hepatotoxicity	C
9 Anti-secretory	Volunteers	–	Liver abnormalities	Y
10 CVS	Volunteers	3	Rashes	N
11 Skin	Phase II	150	Skin reactions	N
12 Prostaglandin inhibitor	n/a	n/a	Topical reaction	n/a
13 Spermicide	Volunteers	< 10	Local irritability	N
14 Antiinfective	Volunteers	–	Pain on injection	N
15 Endocrine	Phase II	35	Allergy	N[a]
16 CNS	Phase II	14	Allergy	N
17 n/a	Volunteers	–	Anaphylactic reaction	N
18 GI	Volunteers	10s	Tachycardia	N
19 –	Phase II	60	Postural hypotension	Y[b]
20 Anti-allergy	Volunteers	10s	Flushing	N
21 GI	Clinical trial	100s	Granulocytopenia	C
22 Thrombolytic	Volunteers	10s	Haemorrhage	Y
23 n/a	Phase II	200–300	Blood dyscrasias	N
24 CNS	Volunteers	40	White blood cell count decreased	N
25 GI	Volunteers	–	CNS disturbances	N
26 CNS	Phase II	40	CNS effects	N
27 Steroid	Volunteers	10	Adrenal suppression	C
28 Leukotriene-D4 antagonist	n/a	n/a	GI effects (high dose)	n/a
29 Anti-infective	n/a	n/a	n/a	n/a

n/a = Not available.
[a] Partially expected from chemical structure.
[b] Nausea/vomiting which would have limited clinical use was also observed.

animal tests. Lumley concluded from these data, that it was not possible to draw any conclusions as to why some adverse reactions were predicted and others were not. More information would be needed, for example, on numbers of animals, species used and duration of exposure to drugs in animals and man. Without these data, the predictive value of animal studies for man was doubtful.

Heywood (1990) has commented that many adverse reactions in man, in particular immunotoxicity, allergy, hypersensitivity and effects on bone marrow, are unpredictable in animal models. The correlation between target system toxicity in the rat and a non-rodent species is around 30% and the best guess for the correlation of adverse reactions in man and animal toxicity data is somewhere between 5 and 25%. **Table 5** shows major adverse reactions reported since 1975 and whether they can be predicted in animal studies; only 14% showed adverse reactions that could have been predicted.

DRUG INTERACTION PREDICTION: WHOSE RESPONSIBILITY?

Apart from the pioneering work of Conney et al. (1956, 1957) and Levy (1970), animal experimentation has not contributed much of substance to knowledge about drug–drug or drug–food interactions. Indeed, most reports of drug interactions have been from experiences in the clinical setting, but few of these have been able to indicate the precise mechanism(s) of the interaction and many are often anecdotal and uncorroborated. Current studies into drug interactions tend to concentrate on elucidating mechanisms of interaction, especially those involving the cytochrome P450 hepatic enzyme systems (D'Arcy et al., 1996). If mechanisms of interaction are fully understood then it may be possible to develop meaningful in vitro or in vivo models of interactions to which new medicines could be exposed during their development stage.

Table 5 Major adverse reactions (ADR) in man since 1960: predictability in animal tests. Source: Heywood (1990)

Drug	ADR	Predictable in animals
Anti-inflammatory drugs	Gastrointestinal	Yes
	Haematological	Yes
	Skin rashes	No
Alphaxalone	Anaphylaxis	No
Benoxaprofen	Fatal liver toxicity, skin rashes, oncholysis, photosensitivity	No
Chloramphenicol	Aplastic anaemia	No
Clioquinol	Neurotoxicity	Yes
Domperidone	Cardiotoxicity	No
Halothane	Jaundice	Yes
Lincomycin, clindamycin	Pseudomembranous colitis	No
Methysergide	Retroperitoneal fibrosis	No
Nomifensine	Immune haemolytic anaemia	No
Oral contraceptives	Thromboembolism	No
Phenacetin	Nephropathy	No
Phenformin	Lactic acidosis	No
Phenothiazines	Dyskinesia	Questionable
Phenylbutazone	Aplastic anaemia	No
Practolol	Oculomucocutaneous syndrome	No
Propandid	Allergy	No
Stilboestrol	Vaginal cancer in female offspring	No (mice)
Sulphamethoxypyridazine	Haematological, dermatology	Questionable
Sympathomimetic aerosols	Asthmatic death	No
Triazolam	Amnesia	No
Zimeldine	Neurotoxicity	No

Drug interactions are now not just the concern of clinicians treating patients in the clinic—the field has developed so greatly in extent and importance that it is now predominantly a matter for the drug manufacturer to investigate prior to marketing and the regulatory authority to assess the information presented.

This is well illustrated by the issue of a recently issued guideline by the European Committee for Proprietary Medicinal Products (CPMP), Note for Guidance on the Investigation of Drug Interactions (Committee for Proprietary Medicinal Products, 1997). In its Introduction, the guideline states, 'As a consequence of the scientific development within the areas of pharmacokinetics (particularly drug metabolism) and pharmacodynamics, the focus of interaction studies has changed from *ad hoc* observational studies to rationally designed studies. Depending on the chemical characteristics and *in vitro* data, selective *in vivo* studies are performed. Based on the results from such studies, the risk of clinically relevant interactions may be predicted. As a consequence, the information provided to the prescriber has also become more detailed and scientific'.

Within its provisions, the guideline states that, '*in vitro* data should mainly be used qualitatively due to the uncertainty of *in vitro /in vivo* correlation. Thus based on *in vitro* data, applicants (manufacturers) should design and perform relevant *in vivo* studies'. It goes on

further to state, 'Generally *in vivo* studies will be required to support a claim of "No clinically relevant interactions" in the Summary of Product Characteristics (SPC)'. Hence it is no longer sufficient for the manufacturer to seek market approval for a new product without carrying out an investigation into the extent of clinically relevant interactions and those which may be regarded as potential interactions. This is vastly different from the situation not so long ago, when manufacturers rarely carried out systematic investigations into possible drug–drug interactions during the development stage of their new drug and largely relied on the unplanned senario of the clinician discovering such interactions during the post-marketing clinical use of the drug.

The FDA guidance to industry on drug interactions (Center for Drug Evaluation and Research, 1997) would seem to be more orientated towards *in vitro* testing than the CPMP guidance; it provided suggestions on current approaches to studies *in vitro* of drug metabolism and interaction. This guidance is intended to encourage routine, through evaluation of metabolism and interactions *in vitro* whenever feasible and appropriate. As is the case for all FDA guidance documents, suggestions are not requirements, but are offered for consideration by drug development scientists as a means to address potentially important safety concerns. The FDA recognizes that the importance of any approach will vary depending on the drug in development and its intended clinical use. The FDA also recognizes that clinical observations can address some of the same issues identified in the guideline as being susceptible to *in vitro* study (Collins, 1997).

THE NUMBERS GAME

With all the reports on ADRs that appear in the literature each year from official drug regulatory bodies and from investigating clinicians, it may be difficult to understand why toxic reactions to drugs are so often undetected initially during the development stage of the drug. Some individual reasons for this can be pinpointed: for example, in most clinical trials on new drugs, patients are usually selected by criteria which may differ from those of patients treated in later clinical practice. Medicines which are to be used mainly in very old patients (e.g. benoxaprofen and other antirheumatic agents, cardiovascular agents, CNS-acting drugs) are commonly tested on much younger populations and drugs considered safe or effective in younger adults may be neither in the very old.

The 'numbers game' probably also exerts influence. If an ADR is likely to occur in $x\%$ of patients, then there is no guarantee that this probability will be uniformly distributed among the finite and relatively small population that is involved in the typical clinical trial. It is only when a large population of patients are involved that the true extent of the x percentage is revealed. It may take a period of relatively extensive clinical use before the true extent of the ADR is revealed; this was so for benoxaprofen, chloramphenicol, ticrynafen (tienilic acid), halothane, practolol and the sulphonamides and, in a different context, the same is true of the hazards of cigarette smoking. The statistics speak for themselves: in order to have a 95% chance of detecting an adverse event with an incidence of 1 per 1000, 3000 patients at risk are required. With no more than 3000–4000 individuals usually exposed to a medicinal product prior to marketing, only those adverse events with an approximately 1/1000 or greater incidence can be expected to be found (Lewis, 1981).

Furthermore, individual patients in clinical trials are generally exposed to the product for less than 1 year. Even long-duration pre-marketing clinical trials which can last several years do not provide the degree of patient exposure that will occur post-marketing with a chronically used medicine. In addition, the relatively short duration of clinical trials mitigates against the detection of adverse events with long latency. It may be an oversimplification, but it does seem that clinical trials, although satisfactory for demonstrating therapeutic efficacy, are less than efficient in demonstrating adverse events of moderate to low incidence (MedWatch, 1996).

DO MEDICINE REGULATIONS PROTECT THE PUBLIC BUT HINDER RESEARCH?

Griffin (1989) holds that medicines regulations have safeguarded the public. There is no doubt that the pharmaceutical industry has much improved its standards of toxicology screening, clinical pharmacology, pharmacokinetic studies and clinical trial evaluations as a result of the guidelines that have been laid down by the UK regulatory authorities, by the CPMP and more recently by the ICH process. It is Griffin's personal view that the safety and efficacy of medicinal products have been improved more by the pharmaceutical industry striving to adhere to the standards laid down by the test procedures than as a result of any regulatory scrutiny of the data derived therefrom. He qualifies his view, however, by adding that the fact that data are scrutinized must encourage the adherence to the standards set. He also holds that the collection of adverse reaction data is of no value if they are not analysed and interpreted adequately and are then communicated in such a form that they can modify the behaviour of the prescribing doctor.

There has been a price to pay, however, and it is evident, for example, from a review of licensing applications in the UK during the 1970s, that regulation did hinder research. Deregulation, in the form of the Clinical Trial Exemption Scheme, has provided the stimulus for innovation without presenting a hazard to the medicated population. Not only is regulation a deterrent to innovation, but also regulatory delay erodes effective patent term and reduces financial returns. Research initiatives are also reduced by high licensing fees. Furthermore, the existence in Europe of 12 regulatory authorities consumes scarce technical and scientific resources that could be better employed (Griffin, 1991).

Since Griffin expressed these views, the deliberations and guidelines of the ICH have much reduced the duplication of safety testing and regulatory requirements, not only in Europe but also between Europe, the USA and Japan.

HOW SAFE HAVE NEW MEDICINES BEEN?

Perhaps the final question to be asked in this chapter is, How safe have medicines been? In this respect, it is worth remembering the words of Inman (1980): 'No worthwhile drug is entirely without risk, but few have been responsible for large-scale disasters'. Of the more than 320 new chemical entities introduced in the USA between 1960 and 1982, only eight were removed from the market for safety reasons. That 22 year record argues that the balance between relative risk and providing new therapies is an excellent one (Spiker and Cuatrecasas, 1990).

The predominant objective of all national and international drug regulations is to ensure freedom from undue toxicity (i.e. to ensure the safety) of marketed medicinal products during normal conditions of use. Total safety is probably an untenable goal since the use of any therapeutic agent is inevitably attended by a small risk that the patient may react adversely to it. So, although absolute safety in drug treatment is probably not achievable, much can be done, and is being done, to reduce hazard.

REFERENCES

Ahmad, S. R. (1992). USA Antihistamine alert. *Lancet*, **340**, 542.

Anon. (1997a). FDA proposes withdrawal of terfenadine—no action in UK. *Pharm. J.*, **258**, 90.

Anon. (1997b). Terfenadine metabolite marketed as new antihistamine for hay fever. *Pharm. J.*, **258**, 260.

Anon. (1997c). MCA on antihistamines. *Pharm. J.*, **258**, 296.

Anon. (1997d). Pharmacists should intervene in all terfenadine sales, Society says. *Pharm. J.*, **258**, 534.

Anon. (1997e). Leading article: selling terfenadine. *Pharm. J.*, **258**, 575.

Bailey, D. G., Spence, J. D., Munoz, C. and Arnold, J. M. O. (1991). Interaction of citrus juice with felodipine and nifedipine. *Lancet*, **i**, 268–269.

Bailey, D. G., Arnold, J. M. O., Strong, H. A., Munoz, C. and Spence, J. D. (1993). Effect of grapefruit juice and naringin on nisoldipine pharmacokinetics. *Clin. Pharmacol. Ther.*, **54**, 589–594.

Bailey, D. G., Arnold, J. M. O. and Spence, J. D. (1994). Grapefruit juice and drugs: how significant is the interaction. *Clin. Pharmacokinet.*, **26**, 91–96.

Bass, R. (1990). What can be learnt by examining the data in the files of regulatory authorities?—The toxicologists viewpoint. In Lumley, C. E. and Walker, S. R. (Eds), *Animal Toxicity Studies: Their Relevance for Man*. CMR Workshop Series. Quay Publishing, Lancaster, pp. 33–39.

Benton, R., Honig, P., Zamani, K., Hewett, R. N., Cantilena, L. R. and Woosley, R. L. (1994). Grapefruit juice alters terfenadine pharmacokinetics resulting in prolongation of AT (Abstract). *Clin. Pharmacol. Ther.* **55**, 146.

Bloemenkamp, K. W. M., Rosendall, F. R., Heimerhorst, F., Buller, H. R. and Vandenbrocke, F. P. (1995). Enhancement by factor V Leiden mutation of risk of deep-vein thrombosis associated with oral contraceptives containing a third-generation progestogen. *Lancet*, **346**, 1593–1596.

Brimblecombe, R. (1990). The importance of retrospective comparisons. In Lumley, C. E. and Walker, S. R. (Eds), *Animal Toxicity Studies: Their Relevance for Man*. CMR Workshop Series. Quay Publishing, Lancaster, pp. 15–19.

Center for Drug Evaluation and Research (1997). *Drug Metabolism/Drug Interactions—In Vitro Studies*. Working Group of the Clinical Pharmacology Section of the Medical Policy Coordinating Committee in the Center for Drug Evaluation and Research, Rockville MD.

Clayson, D. B. (1987). The need for biological risk assessment in reaching decisions about carcinogens. *Mutat. Res.*, **185**, 243–269.

Collins, J. (1997). Guidance for industry: drug metabolism/drug interaction studies in the drug development process: studies *in vitro*. In *Drug–Drug Interaction*. IBC UK Conferences, Royal College of Pathologists, London.

Commission of the European Communities (1984). *The Rules Governing Medicaments in the European Communities*. Office for Official Publications of the European Communities, Luxembourg.

Committee for Proprietary Medicinal Products (1997). *Note for Guidance on the Investigation of Drug Interactions*. CPMP/EWP560/95. European Agency for the Evaluation of Medicinal Products, London.

Committee on Safety of Medicines/Medicines Control Agency (1966). Amiodarone (Cordarone X). *Curr. Probl.*, No. 22, 3.

Committee on Safety of Medicines (1992). Ventricular arrhythmias due to terfenadine and astemizole. *Curr. Probl.*, No. 35, 1–2.

Conney, A. H., Miller, E. C. and Miller, S. A. J. (1956). The metabolism of methylated aminoazo dyes. V. Evidence for the induction of enzyme synthesis in the rat by 3-methylcholanthrene. *Cancer Res.*, **16**, 450–459.

Conney, A. H., Miller, E. C. and Miller, J. A. (1957). Substrate-induced synthesis and other properties of benzpyrenehydroxylase in rat liver. *J. Biol. Chem.*, **228**, 753–766.

D'Arcy, P. F. (1996). Drug-interactions and drug-metabolising enzymes. In D'Arcy, P. F., McElnay, J. C. and Welling, P. G. (Eds), *Mechanisms of Drug Interactions*. Springer, Berlin, pp. 151–171.

D'Arcy, P. F. and Harron, D. W. G. (Eds) (1992). *Proceedings of the First International Conference on Harmonisation, Brussels, 1991*. Queen's University of Belfast and Greystone Books, Antrim, Northern Ireland.

D'Arcy, P. F. and Harron, D. W. G. (Eds) (1994). *Proceedings of the Second International Conference on Harmonisation, Orlando, Florida 1993*. Queen's University of Belfast and Greystone Books, Antrim, Northern Ireland.

D'Arcy, P. F. and Harron, D. W. G. (Eds) (1996). *Proceedings of the Third International Conference on Harmonisation, Yokohama, Japan, 1995*. Queen's University of Belfast and Greystone Books, Antrim, Northern Ireland.

D'Arcy, P. F. and Harron, D. W. G. (Eds) (1998). *Proceedings of the Fourth International Conference on Harmonisation, Brussels, 1997*. Queen's University of Belfast and Greystone Books, Antrim, Northern Ireland.

D'Arcy, P. F., McElnay, J. C. and Welling, P. G. (Eds) (1996). *Mechanisms of Drug Interactions*. Springer, Berlin.

Ducharme, M. P., Provenzano, R., Dehoorne-Smith, M. and Edwards, D. J. (1993). Trough concentrations of cyclosporin in blood following administration with grapefruit juice. *Br. J. Clin. Pharmacol.*, **36**, 457–459.

Fletcher, A. P. (1978). Drug safety testing and subsequent clinical experience. *J. R. Soc. Med.*, **71**, 693–696.

Fletcher, P. (1990). What can be learnt by examining the data in the files of regulatory authorities? The clinician's viewpoint. In Lumley, C. E. and Walker, S. R. (Eds), *Animal Toxicity Studies: Their Relevance for Man*. CMR Workshop Series. Quay Publishing, Lancaster, pp. 41–46.

Griffin, J. P. (1983). Repeat-dose long-term toxicity studies. In Balls, M., Riddell, R. J., and Worden, A. N. (Eds), *Animals and Alternatives in Toxicity Testing*. Academic Press, London, pp. 98–103.

Griffin, J. P. (Ed.) (1989). Medicines control within the United Kingdom. In D'Arcy, P. F. and Harron, D. W. G. (Exec. Eds), *Medicines, Regulation, Research and Risk*. Queen's University of Belfast, Belfast, pp. 1–25.

Griffin, J. P. (1991). Are regulations a stimulus to innovation? In Walker, S. R. (Ed.), *Creating the Right Environment for Drug Discivery*. CMR Workshop Series. Quay Publishing, Lancaster, p. 93.

Hanif, M., Mobarak, M. R., Ronan, A., Rahman, D., Donovan, J. J., Jr, and Bennish, M. L. (1995). Fatal renal failure caused by diethylene glycol in paracetamol elixir: the Bangladesh epidemic. *Br. Med. J.*, **311**, 88–91.

Heywood, R. (1990). Clinical toxicity—could it have been predicted? Post-marketing experience. In Lumley, C. E. and Walker, S. R. (Eds), *Animal Toxicity Studies: Their Relevance for Man*. CMR Workshop Series. Quay Publishing, Lancaster, pp. 57–67.

Honig, P. K., Wortham, D. C., Lazarev, A. and Cantilena, L. R. (1996). Grapefruit juice alters the systemic bioavailability and cardiac repolarization of terfenadine in poor metabolizers of terfenadine. *J. Clin. Pharmacol.*, **36**, 345–351.

Inman, W. H. W. (Ed.) (1980). The United Kingdom. In *Monitoring for Drug Safety*. MTP, Lancaster, p. 9.

International Agency for Research on Cancer (1987). *IARC Monograph on Evaluation of Carcinogenic Risks to Humans. Suppl. 7. Overall Evaluations of Carcinogenicity: an Updating of IARC Monographs*, Vols 1–42. IARC, Lyon.

Jick, H., Jick, S. S., Gurewich, V., Myers, M. W. and Vasilakis, C. (1995). Risk of idiopathic cardiovascular death and non-fatal venous thromboembolism in women using oral contraceptives with differing progestagen components. *Lancet*, **346**, 1589–1593.

Kupferschmidt, H. H. I., Ha, H. R., Ziegler, W. H., Meier, P. J. and Krähenbühl, S. (1995). Interaction between grapefruit juice and midazolam in humans. *Clin. Pharmacol. Ther.*, **58**, 20–28.

Lasagna, L. (1989). Setting the scene—the role of regulation. In Walker, S. R. and Griffin, J. P. (Eds), *International Medicines Regulations: a Forward Look to 1992*. Kluwer, Dordrecht, pp. 19–26.

Laurence, D. R., Maclean, A. and Weatherall, M. (1984). *Safety Testing of New Drugs*. Academic Press, London.

Levy, G. (1970). Biopharmaceutical considerations in dosage form and design. In Sprouls, J. B. (Ed.), *Prescription Pharmacy*, 2nd edn. Lippincott, Philadelphia, pp. 70, 75, 80.

Lewis, J. A. (1981). Post-marketing surveillance: how many patients? *Trends Pharmacol. Sci.*, **2**, 93–94.

Lewis, M. A., Spitzer, W. O., Heinemann, L. A. J., MacRae, K. D., Bruppacher, R. and Thorogood, M. (1996). Third generation oral contraceptives and risk of myocardial infarction: an international case-control study. *Br. Med. J.*, **312**, 88–90.

Lumley, C. E. (1990). Clinical toxicity: could it have been predicted? Pre-marketing experience. In Lumley, C. E. and Walker, S. R. (Eds), *Animal Toxicity Studies: Their Relevance for Man*. CMR Workshop Series. Quay Publishing, Lancaster, pp. 49–56.

Lumley, C. E. and Walker, S. R. (Eds) (1990). *Animal Toxicity Studies: Their Relevance for Man*. CMR Workshop Series. Quay Publishing, Lancaster, p. vii.

McPherson, K. (1996). Third generation oral contraceptives and venous thromboembolism. *Br. Med. J.*, **312**, 68–69.

MedWatch (1996). Premarketing human clinical studies. In *The Clinical Impact of Adverse Event Reporting*. MedWatch, October 1996. FDA, Washington, DC, pp. 1–11.

Merkel, U., Sigusch, H. and Hoffman, A. (1994). Grapefruit juice inhibits 7-hydroxylation in healthy volunteers. *Eur. J. Clin. Pharmacol.*, **46**, 75–177.

Morton, D. (1990). Expectations from animal studies. In Lumley, C. E. and Walker, S. R. (Eds), *Animal Toxicity Studies: Their Relevance for Man*. CMR Workshop Series. Quay Publishing, Lancaster, pp. 3–13.

Okuonghae, H. O., Ighogboja, I. S., Laweson, J. O. and Nwana, E. J. (1992). Diethylene glycol poisoning in Nigerian children. *Ann. Trop. Paediatr.*, **12**, 235–238.

Proppe, D. G., Hoch, O. D., McLean, A. J. and Visser, K. E. (1995). Influence of chronic ingestion of grapefruit juice on steady-state blood concentrations of cyclosporin A in renal transplant patients with stable graft function. *Br. J. Clin. Pharmacol.*, **39**, 337–338.

Rawlings, M. D. (1989). Objectives and achievements of medicines regulations in the UK. In Walker S. R. and Griffin, J. P. (Eds), *International Medicines Regulations: a Forward Look to 1992*. Kluwer, Dordrecht, pp. 93–100.

Shelby, M. D. and Stasiewicz, S. (1984). Chemicals showing no evidence of carcinogenicity in long-term two species rodent studies; the need for short-term test data. *Environ. Mutagen.*, **6**, 871–876.

Soons, P. A., Vogels, B. A. P. M., Roosmalen, M. C. M., *et al.* (1991). Grapefruit juice and cimetidine inhibit stereoselective metabolism of nitrendipine in humans. *Clin. Pharmacol. Ther.*, **50**, 394–403.

Spiker, B. and Cuatrecasas, P. (1990). *Inside the Drug Industry*. Prous Science, Barcelona, p. 53.

Spitzer, W. O., Lewis, M. A., Heinemann, L. A. J., Thorogood, M. and MacRae, K. D. (1996). Third generation oral contraceptives and risk of venous thromboembolic disorders: an international case-control study. *Br. Med. J.*, **312**, 83–88.

Stephens, M. D. B. (1988). *The Detection of New Adverse Drug Reactions*, 2nd edn. Stockton Press, New York, p.1.

Tennant, R. W., Margolin, B. H., Shelby, M. D., Zeiger, E., Haseman, J., Spalding, J., Caspary, W., Resnick, M., Stasiewicz, S. W., Anderson, B. and Minor, R. (1987). Prediction of chemical carcinogenicity in rodents from *in vitro* genetic toxicity assays. *Science*, **236**, 933–941.

Vogel, M. R. (1997). Common OTC laxative ingredient linked to cancer. *Pharm. Today*, **3**, 9.

Wax, P. M. (1995). Elixirs, diluents and the passage of the 1938 Federal Food, Drug and Cosmetic Act. *Ann. Intern. Med.*, **122**, 456–461.

World Health Organization (1995a). Collaborative study of cardiovascular disease and steroid hormone contraception: venus thromboembolic disease and combined oral contraceptives: results of international multicentre case-controlled study. *Lancet*, **346**, 1575–1582.

World Health Organization (1995b). Collaborative study of cardiovascular disease and steroid hormone contraception: effect of different progestogens in low oestrogen oral contraceptives on venous thromboembolic disease. *Lancet*, **346**, 1582–1588.

Zbinden, G, (1981). Scope and limitation of animal models for the prediction of human toxicity. In Brown, S. S. and Davies, D. S. (Eds), *Organ Directed Toxicity*. Pergamon Press, Oxford, pp. 3–7.

Chapter 65

Medical Toxicology

Chantal Bismuth, Stephen W. Borron and Etienne Fournier

C O N T E N T S

INTRODUCTION

Toxicology is the science that deals with chemical substances as causes of disease in man, defines the internal and external factors which determine and modify the harmful actions of chemical substances, investigates the biological effects of chemicals in experimental systems and assesses the risk for man.

G. Zbinden

This definition introduces medical toxicology as a science which encompasses:

1. Knowledge of those chemical substances harmful to man.
2. Knowledge of diseases (injuries, lesions) induced by chemical substances.
3. Knowledge of methods for the identification and quantitative analysis of harmful chemicals and diagnosis of chemically-induced diseases.
4. Appraisal of prognostic factors in poisoning, thus permitting an evaluation of symptomatic (toxicodynamic) or antidotal (toxicokinetic) approaches to treatment.
5. Assessment of the tangible risks imposed by chemicals in therapy, in industry and in the environment and communication of risks to other scientists, governmental authorities and the public, so that appropriate decisions regarding conditions of chemical use may be established or re-evaluated.

Toxicology was first studied by physiologists, such as Claude Bernard, who declared that an intoxicant is to the physiologist what a scalpel is to the surgeon, and by specialists in forensic medicine, such as Orfila, who in the early nineteenth century in France first proposed the use of the toxicological analysis of human tissues. During the following century, chemists, pharmacologists and biologists developed their own conceptions of toxicology.

In the last 30 years, there has been an extraordinary development of pesticides and other industrial compounds necessary to a worldwide demographic expansion, introduction into the household of products with the potential for danger, an accretion of active therapeutic drugs, including an ever-increasing number of psychotropic agents, which are utilized in attempted and completed suicides, and massive abuse of addictive substances, such as alcohol, tobacco, amphetamines, tranquillizers, heroin and cocaine. These events have fostered the development of new areas, such as environmental and occupational medicine, molecular toxicology, the isolation of toxicokinetics from pharmacokinetics (definitively separating toxicology from pharmacology) and behavioural toxicology, which has contributed to our understanding of the exciting and promising field of neurotransmitters.

The public media have become more acutely aware of human toxicological problems through a number of dramatic and highly publicized events such as the collective suicides with cyanide in Jonestown and the Temple of the Sun, the release of dioxins at Seveso in Italy and methyl isocyanate at Bhopal in India and the nuclear catastrophe at Chernobyl in Russia. These incidents have deeply impressed public opinion regarding the serious potential of toxic effects, leading to an ever-growing need by the public not only to be informed and protected, but also to have access to effective tests for detecting exposures to toxins in both their preclinical and clinical stages. This is of considerable importance since we know that some substances may be carcinogenic or mutagenic in humans.

In fact, not all of the great 'toxicological catastrophes' are industrial in origin. They may also be related to alimentary (toxic oil syndrome), therapeutic (thalidomide, sulphanilimide elixir) or environmental (automobile pollution) sources. Chemical weapons (mustard gas and anticholinesterases) must also be considered, as they pose a potential menace either through military use or by terrorists. The production and utilization of nuclear weapons extend to the most politically unstable regimes. Finally, natural disasters, such as forest fires, volcanic eruptions and sandstorms, have toxic effects, the extent of which is likely underestimated.

Toxic exposures have become the second most common cause of acute admission to hospitals in many developed countries. Trauma itself is closely linked to alcohol and drug use. Poisonings, together with accidents, are the second most common cause of death (after infectious diseases) in many developing countries in individuals between 2 and 30 years of age (Goulding, 1977). In intensive care units or emergency departments, physicians on duty often devote over 20% of their time to the evaluation and care of poisonings (Bismuth *et al.*, 1999). Every physician, therefore, whatever his or her discipline, will at some time need to cope with acute or chronic toxic diseases. It should be noted that the present frequency of these acute events presents not only a strain on health services and public health, but also both a significant social and an economic problem, (Ellenhorn and Barceloux, 1988).

MISSION OF THE MEDICAL TOXICOLOGIST

The medical toxicologist has a four-point mission:

1. To detect the secondary effects of xenobiotics and to link them to the responsible agent, which is easily accomplished only if the disposition of the chemical in man is well known (absorption, metabolism, elimination, target organs). This linkage becomes more difficult if studies surrounding the compound have been purely experimental, these difficulties being multifactorial: interspecies differences, human-specific metabolites, false-positive results in animals. The interpretation of human studies is equally complex, as non-invasive tests are limited, responses in the population are heterogeneous and exposure levels are often low in comparison with experimental studies.
2. To treat correctly the effects of xenobiotics on humans. This concerns not only supportive therapy

(symptomatic treatment) but also the employment of a toxicokinetic and toxicodynamic approach to the patient (for example, by the rational utilization of antidotes) (Baud *et al.*, 1995). In the evaluation of these therapies, the establishment of prognostic factors related to the toxin is imperative, in order to avoid incorrectly attributing therapeutic benefit to a treatment when, in fact, the outcome represents the normal evolution of the intoxication.
3. To prevent future intoxications through the proper use of 'risk assessment'. The medical impact here is unlimited. The management of chemically-induced suicides, toxic occupational exposures, criminal poisonings, atmospheric pollution, immuno-allergic reactions, addictive behaviours, application of pesticides, household and industrial products, aggressions by plant and animal toxins, etc.—all medical observation and interventions in such cases lead to information of interest to the public and, at times, help to structure restrictive regulation.
4. Finally, careful contextual analysis of observed incidents by the medical toxicologist will lead to a more balanced view of their impact and to better risk communication. Three brief examples, given below, will suffice to illustrate this point.

The term 'chemical warfare' is emotionally charged, with public fear of these weapons being fomented by recent terrorist activities, such as the use of sarin in the Tokyo subway, and continuing propaganda surrounding the production of 'weapons of mass destruction'. It should be recalled, however, that chemical weapons, with a mortality of 2%, were responsible for 1% of deaths in the First World War (Fouyn *et al.*, 1991). Clearly, this represents unnecessary deaths, but one should not lose sight of the fact that firearms, land mines and conventional weapons (with equal charges) remain the most deadly tools of war. Conventional explosive devices, not classically viewed as chemical weapons, were indeed the 'weapons of mass destruction' in the Gulf War.

In 1976, in Seveso, Italy a chemical release of between 159 g and 2 kg of tetrachlorodibenzo-*p*-dioxin occurred. Many animals died, leaves fell off the trees and people soon noticed skin lesions. The public was rightly alarmed. Dioxin has since been hailed 'the most toxic substance known to man' (Müller, 1997). In the 10 year follow-up of victims of this exposure, however, the only recognized human health effect has been the occurrence of chloracne in a small segment of the population. If one looks further back, to 1949, 13 industrial releases of dioxins have been recorded, involving over 9000 human exposures. Among these, only one death clearly related to dioxins and four deaths possibly related to dioxins have been noted (Müller, 1997). While five deaths from an industrial chemical over a 27 year period are lamentable, dioxins clearly do not pose the threat often portrayed by the media.

Asbestos-related disease and asbestos abatement are currently matters of great debate. Clearly, these mineral fibres have resulted in disease and death among poorly protected and unprotected workers having inhaled significant concentrations. However, in this 'man-made mineral fibres disease', are unprotected workers the only ones in danger? Is it scientifically plausible that those passively exposed are equally (or at all) at risk?

We hope here to remind readers of some basic concepts of nomenclature, to underline the importance of the expression of analytical results, to discuss the correlation between human and experimental toxicology and, under the rubric of 'human risk assessment', to discuss the impact of the expansion of ecotoxicology and to introduce the possible importance of the effects of small doses or 'chemical hormesis'.

NOMENCLATURE

Clear definitions are imperative: confusion between terms and their abusive extension (for example, labelling as 'chronic' an intoxication of only 2 weeks duration) render many observations useless. Misperceptions and miscommunication regarding chemical exposures and their risk may find their way into the medical literature, the lay media or organizational or official reports and lead to unwarranted fear on the part of the public and sensational regulation or sanction of products which benefit society and which may, in fact, have an acceptable safety profile.

Intoxication

An intoxication is a measurable alteration in health which results from the exposure to, and action of, an identifiable chemical product or its metabolites.

We must first insist on the fact that intoxications result in measurable alterations in health. While this appears evident, it would be inappropriate to refer even to a massive acute chemical *exposure* which has resulted in no demonstrable negative health effect as an 'acute intoxication'.

Second, it must be demonstrated that an exposure has indeed occurred—the presence of symptoms alone is insufficient to demonstrate toxicity. Apparent 'mass intoxications' have occurred where the only link between the illness and the chemical 'at fault' is the *belief* by the patients that they have been exposed (Selden, 1989). In the same vein, ascribing toxicity to an agent or agents based on the occurrence of very common syndrome complexes (headache, fatigue, nausea), in the absence of reliable physical or laboratory evidence of poisoning, is perilous. Toxicological diseases conform to the scientific postulates of proof of association. If a 'toxicological syndrome' cannot be reproduced in an animal model by

similar exposures, or a dose–effect relationship demonstrated in man, the validity of the syndrome should be questioned. This is not to say that non-reproducible associations should be summarily discarded, but that extreme caution should be exercised in their interpretation.

Clearly, the chemical product or metabolite in question should be identifiable, either in the source material or in biological media, if a causal relationship is to be firmly established. In current toxicology, the habitual causal reference is to the product absorbed. For example, one may correctly write 'intoxication by 2,4-dinitrophenol'. However, one often finds, through abusive simplification, the use of elemental nomenclature, such as 'arsenic intoxication', to refer to any of a number of arsenic-containing compounds, which differ significantly in their toxicity. The transfer of regulatory decisions to non-physician toxicologists has recently brought about the appearance of the term 'speciation', a neologism aiming at the atomic or molecular form from which the product is viewed. This term takes into account, for example, that the toxicity of hexavalent chromium ion is not the same as that of the trivalent ion. The term speciation leads to the conclusion that each product, simple or compound, should be studied specifically. The application of the grand principles of chemistry to toxicology poses problems which remain unsolved; thus, in the halogen series, the toxicities of fluorides, of bromides, of chlorides and of iodides are not comparable. Medical authors often refer casually to the dangers of 'pesticides', a term which envelopes dozens of chemical families and mechanisms of actions, and thousands of products of varying concentration, potency and indicated use. Is the cyanogen bromide used to fumigate buildings truly comparable to the pyrethroids we use to kill garden insects? Furthermore, there is an unfortunate tendency to lump intoxications involving a common compound under a familiar brand name, for example, referring to all intoxications involving paracetamol as 'Tylenol poisonings'. Such a habit not only renders a disservice to the manufacturer of the brand name product but also, of greater concern, such simplification may result in overlooking a poisoning which is due not to the principal active ingredient but to an excipient, a colourant, another ingredient or to packaging which may not even be present in the brand name product.

It is hazardous to attempt to extract conclusions regarding the toxicity of a highly purified compound on the basis of observations of toxic effects from technical products sold under a commercial name. A case in point is that of a product labelled 'trichloroethylene', which was believed to have caused hepatitis. In fact, the product involved contained not more than 60% of pure trichloroethylene and contained more than 30% of hepato- and nephrotoxic carbon tetrachloride (Conso *et al.*, 1982). Similarly, toluene was once believed to be responsible for haematological disorders. It is now appreciated that these disorders were caused by benzene, as a contaminant.

Human intoxications are, in fact, often complex: air pollution, for example, involves complex mixtures of chemical pollutants; fire smoke may contain several hundred different gases implicating, for example, not only carbon monoxide but also cyanide, among many others (Anderson, 1986; Baud *et al.*, 1991). Finally, chemical mixtures in industrial toxicology modify not only the clinical expression of the effects of the individual constituents but also their evolution over time.

The bias of impurity is common in medical toxicology when good clinical and experimental practices in studies are not respected. Conversely, the purification of certain biological products may be complex or impossible and, in such cases, experimental studies should mention a reference for purification procedures employed, or the lot and date of fabrication of commercial products, so that the experimental conditions might be reproduced and the experiment appropriately interpreted after the fact.

In the twenty-first century, toxicologists should refer only to the *absorbed* product by its exact formula, in case of a defined chemical structure, or by its exact composition (including impurities, as many products may contain 5–10% of impurities, often of undetermined toxicity, which may vary according to the synthetic and purification processes). Where the exact composition of a product is unknown, this should be stated.

Acute Intoxication

It is almost without exception the physician who provides the first description of an acute intoxication. An acute intoxication meets the criteria of the above definition of intoxication, with expression of signs and symptoms occurring within minutes to 7 days after the exposure.

Subacute (Subchronic)[1] Intoxications

The twentieth century has brought greater light to the notions of subacute (7 days to 3 months) or chronic (greater than 6 months) toxicity, of drug effects labelled 'adverse' or 'toxic/unexpected', of occupational illness (a moving term which links suffering and death with the mere human condition of work) and of drug-induced maladies termed 'iatrogenic'.

It is appropriate to underline as a primordial truth, in industrial or environmental toxicology, the differences in biological actions of pure products that are apparently very similar. Analogous groupings of compounds (the 'dioxin' of Seveso being composed of more than 200

[1] Dr. Wallace Hayes has pointed out that the term "subacute" is actually a misnomer, and that "subchronic" is more appropriate. The authors have retained the term most commonly employed, but recognise that the latter is more precise

isomers and analogues (Müller, 1997)) are unacceptable, except for those end-points which are purely socially defined, or for regulatory convenience. Such groupings are illusory in practice because they are of extremely debatable validity. While they may serve as a reassuring convenience, they are reprehensible in that they propagate a state of ignorance.

Chronic Exposure and Long-term Effects

These two terms are not equivalent. The prolonged absorption of lead oxide may provoke an acute syndrome, 'lead colic'. This is a chronic exposure which manifests itself by acute painful crises. The complete termination of exposure makes the crises disappear, so that lead colic is not a long-term effect. The inhalation of asbestos (a collective and imprecise term) may provoke pulmonary fibrosis after a delay of many years since the last exposure. This is a long-term effect generally due to a chronic exposure. Finally, crocidolite, a more precise term for one type of asbestos, may result in a long-term effect (mesothelioma) after even a relatively brief, intense exposure.

Effects at extreme long term (life-long) on the immune system, on the process of reproduction, the maintenance of the genome and cancerous degeneration of cell growth came to light essentially during the twentieth century and will predominate thinking for decades to come.

This ensemble constitutes the toxicological part of classical pharmacology. Many of the medications available in the nineteenth century were extremely toxic (the most disquieting ones being labeled 'heroic' without a clear distinction as to who the hero was in the affair), as were other forms of chemical products employed during the explosion of modern technology. Our retrospective view of the twentieth century is not sufficiently long to appreciate how much real progress we have made in preventing this type of slow pathology.

Formulation of Analytical Results (Their Expression and Units)

Common approaches to the expression of analytical results are critical to the comprehension and reproducibility of observed and measured phenomena in human toxicokinetics and toxicodynamics. The utility of this notion is perhaps best appreciated through the example of molecular therapy of human intoxication.

The molarity of a solution, defined by the number of molecules in 1 litre of solvent, is obtained by dividing the mass of the dissolved substance by its molecular weight. A molar solution contains (in mass) the molecular weight of its constituents, e.g. the molecular weight of NaCl is 58.5, hence a molar solution contains 58.5 g of the salt per litre.

Anti-digoxin Fab antibody fragments are believed to neutralize the toxin *molecule by molecule*. Accordingly, the standard approach to digoxin Fab therapy calls for equimolar neutralization. When one compares the molecular weight of therapeutic antibody fragments (approximately 50 000 Da) with that of digoxin (approximately 782 Da), it would appear that enormous quantities of foreign proteins are required to achieve equimolar action and a therapeutic effect.

There are reasons to believe that such a 'maximalist' approach to therapy may not be optimal. The administration of antidotes in doses equal to or exceeding the molar concentration of the toxin is often associated with undesirable effects. While digoxin Fab fragments have a high toxic-to-therapeutic ratio, serious side-effects, such as tachyarrhyhmias and uncovering of congestive heart failure, may occur when digoxin is rapidly removed by antibody complex formation. It is probably possible to administer smaller, less costly and perhaps less potentially dangerous quantities (for example, 0.5 molar), converting a potentially lethal intoxication (based on previously established prognostic factors) to a less serious intoxication compatible with life (Taboulet *et al.*, 1993; Borron *et al.*, 1997). Smaller doses of Fab, administered over a longer period of time, may improve the kinetics of therapy (matching circulating antibodies to digoxin redistribution) and prove to decrease the already small incidence of complications (Schaumann *et al.*, 1986).

The molar expression of toxic doses or toxic body fluid concentrations, as extensively imposed by publishers in the 1970s and 1980s, may be impractical and confusing, however. It seems that most toxicologists are more comfortable with the notion of toxic doses in the form of weight of toxin (expressed as μg or mg kg^{-1} of human body weight (or per litre of body fluid), rather than micromoles or millimoles kg^{-1}. In the interest of avoiding therapeutic errors, molar relationships may have to remain in the purely scientific background.

CORRELATIONS AND COMPARISONS BETWEEN HUMAN AND EXPERIMENTAL TOXICOLOGY

Human toxicology, just like experimental toxicology, is multidisciplinary, and composed of at least three areas of competence:

Medical. The analysis of chemical exposure data in humans and their correlation with observable effects on human health are clearly the domain of the medical toxicologist. The treatment of complex intoxications is probably best accomplished by physicians specialized in the domain, with some training in epidemiology, exposure assessment, toxicokinetics and the use of specific antidotes. Where the treatment is primarily toxicody-

namic, specialists in other domains, such as intensivists and emergency physicians, are generally well versed in poisoning management.

Chemical/analytical. The characterization of chemical products and their quantification in human tissues, along with similar analytical measures in the occupational or general environment, allow the establishment of biological exposure indices. These may be then compared with data from experimental studies in order to allow the establishment of indices of toxicity or safety. These indices can assist in the establishment of a 'dossier of toxicity' and in risk assessment, which is discussed later.

Social and regulatory. Administrators and jurists intervene in the goal of sanctioning misdeeds, reparation of damages, prevention of accidents by producers, transporters and users of chemicals and, above all, the establishment of norms for studies which must be carried out before a product may be placed on the market. The medical toxicologist is frequently called upon for advice regarding the frequency of illness related to specific toxins and preventive measures.

Viewpoints of the Biologist and the Physician

The natural tendency of the biologist is to search for understanding by undertaking measurements. The first goal of the physician is to participate in the healing process by providing appropriate care. These two procedures do not superpose themselves in a rigorous manner. Biologists search experimentally for correlations between doses and their effects, carefully controlling experimental conditions. Medical knowledge, on the other hand, must be accumulated case by case, as a collection of individual results which must subsequently be evaluated in terms of their specificity and sensitivity. This evaluation is complicated in man by multiple confounders (occupational and environmental exposures, multiple medications, use of alcohol and tobacco).

Experimental toxicology is a discipline of observation, similar to that of medical toxicology, which is likewise equipped with means of observation (poison centres, centres of toxicovigilance) and with the technical capacity of chemical analysis in biological milieu. Extrapolation to man, from data obtained in animal or *in vitro* models, however, remains problematic: there are interspecies differences, but also elementary constraints in human studies: time, dose and the absolute requirement for preservation of the integrity of the human organism. While studies on healthy human volunteers are a useful source of information in human toxicology, their application to pathological conditions is strictly limited.

In experimental toxicology, concordance is easily established between acute toxicity studies in small animals and acute effects in man. A regular, predictive correlation is constituted with much greater difficulty in subacute and chronic toxicology, the life span of laboratory animals being much abbreviated, thus often requiring exaggerated dosing schedules to induce chronic effects.

Subacute intoxications are perfectly reproducible and demonstrate, above all, cumulative effects. The dosage of the product found in the tissues and histological and biological studies confirm the toxicity. The transposition to man may be discussed after comparison of the kinetics and metabolism of the product in man and in the animal. In terms of chronic toxicity studies, it is difficult to link human epidemiological studies with experimental observations carried out on laboratory animals (e.g. over 2 years in the rat), the latter being strictly observed with application of good laboratory practice. The transposition is habitually carried out through determination of a 'no observed effect level (NOEL)' from which general regulations are derived.

This may likewise be said of tests of teratogenicity and of effects on successive generations. A large number of tests based on cellular models are proposed, in particular tests of genotoxicity and of immunotoxic effects. These models bring forth important information regarding the capacity of a chemical product to react with DNA (the Ames test) or with specific genes (p53). The multiplicity of reactive sites and the frequency with which certain results of tests are classified 'slightly positive' renders the transposition to man a delicate affair, given that those making the decisions are neither physicians nor specialized biologists. The tendency to take an attitude deemed 'precautionary' imposes a vast distance between 'political toxicology' and that of rational human toxicology.

The best available test of validity of an effect is the establishment of a quantitative relation between an effect and the dose administered, according to an empirical approach—the dose–effect relation—where the dose is expressed in weight for an ingested toxin, in concentration/surface area for dermal exposures and in concentration/litre of air (or m^3) in the case of inhalation.

Profile of Toxicity—New Chemical Product

Based on the information obtained from the experimental toxicologist, and from medical observations, a toxicological profile, which should include all raw data obtained about the product, may be formulated.

The advice of the expert is a result of the validation of the facts in the dossier and the analysis of those facts once validated.

Validation is composed of a criticism of techniques, putting those results judged abnormal into context with 'norms' in the studied species (or race, if it is pure), while keeping in mind the fluctuations of the observations of the laboratory.

In the practice of such validations, toxicologists utilize essentially animal models, believed to be homologous with humans, and complete bioclinical studies (specialized veterinarians) as detailed as possible by quantification (specialized analytical chemistry) of the chemical structure in the different milieu where it may be detected.

The practical result of such experimental observations may be very divergent owing to ideological, political, or simply historical biases. For example, strict health and safety regulations relating to drinking water and to the composition of artificial food products have been based on such experimental studies. However, it would be absurd to believe that a minor modification of these figures (allowance of 200 rather than 150 μg of manganese per 100 g of food or 7 rather than 5 μg of cadmium per litre of drinking water) would pose a toxic risk to the population. Toxic chronic doses are often unknown, except with a large margin of uncertainty. Coefficients (factors) of safety of 10, 100 or even 1000 are often used by legislators for arriving at norms.

Although applying a safety factor is prudent, the levels frequently proposed in modern chemical regulation (e.g. less than 1 ppb or 1 μg kg^{-1}) are arrived at by linear extrapolation, and are completely nonsensical in a biological sense, because toxic effects cannot be demonstrated *in vivo* at such concentrations. Such an approach represents sociological appeasement. Applied to the speed of automobiles, extremely dangerous at 200 km h^{-1}, this would correspond to proposing a speed limit of 200 m h^{-1}.

TOXICOLOGICAL FACTSHEETS AND DATABASES

Unlike the toxicological profile, toxicological factsheets (material safety data sheets, for example) present summary data, which are practical for conveying toxicological information to non-toxicologists but which may be subject to misinterpretation (not only of the information that they do contain but also of that which they do not). Such accessible sources of information are growing at a rapid pace. Many sources of toxicological summary data are found on the Internet or in public libraries.

Factsheets are often employed as tools by individuals not well informed in the interpretation of toxic effects, in the same way that a 'breathalyser' is utilized by a police officer (who may have little understanding of the kinetics of alcohol metabolism) in deciding whether or not to arrest a driver. While it is important that regulatory bodies, politicians, media and the public have free access to chemical information, this information should not be interpreted in a vacuum, but should be accompanied by appropriate education and consultation.

One of the great difficulties encountered in the organization of meetings between consultants and experts for the purpose of arriving at a 'consensus' is related to the fact that there now exist, in regular function and daily practice, few experts independent of industrial, commercial, governmental or political structures. Clinical toxicology is an applied discipline which can only be taught in organizations which directly observe intoxications. Chronic toxicology deals with rare diseases that are only observed in practice at poorly protected worksites or in polluted sites (geographic 'hotspots' of pollution), with frequent illnesses due to auto-exposure to pollution, such as the lung cancers in a smoking populations, or with frequent common illnesses, such as lymphomas (of which the majority are not of toxic origin). In each case, the epidemiologist should take into account all possible causes in the establishment of questionnaires (for example, in childhood leukaemia: benzene, X-rays, gamma-rays, radon other radioactive products), which is rarely the case. Most of these studies are content to target a single physical or chemical parameter and to draw conclusions therefrom.

With the progression of information technology, we shall probably see the development of 'networks' in toxicology involving input from experts in the medical, analytical and socio-political arenas, where progression in understanding leads to intersections more and more numerous and finally to a body of information the use of which depends only on the pertinence of the data and the degree of competence of the manipulator of these data. This is the ideal domain of expert systems. In other words, almost anyone, particularly someone with an introduction to the process of scientific thought, might be able to read and process these toxicological data sources after a brief apprenticeship. However, the continued development and utility of such an expert system is inextricably dependent on a permanent acquisition of new medical, scientific and regulatory data, and thus on input by experts.

HUMAN RISK ASSESSMENT: HOW DO WE EVALUATE THE POTENTIAL AND ACTUAL HAZARDS FOR MAN?

'Hazard' touches on the notion of 'real danger', rather than a phenomenon of probability. A hazardous substance is one which, under conditions of routine use, poses a danger to the user and must be manipulated with caution.

'Risk' is the calculable probability or estimate of danger. The term hazard applies more to the prevention of danger, whereas risk applies to the evaluation of potential danger.

Evaluation of the Probability of Danger (Risk)

It is in these terms that one speaks of 'risk assessment'. The situation of the expert in this evaluation varies greatly, depending on whether or not validated human observations of intoxication induced by the product in question are available.

Almost every reference text of modern medical toxicology is based on collections of medical observations alone. Their validation, through procedures of toxicovigilance and pharmacovigilance, introduces them into the human risk assessment dossier, which must be complemented by evaluations based on doses absorbed by man and by experimental doses at the limit of danger (NOEL). From these figures, one can define a threshold dose that is probably without danger for man, for example 1% of the NOEL.

The reasoning remains valid, regardless of the illness under observation. Whether we may apply this methodology practically to immunotoxicology and to carcinogenesis remains a matter of debate among medical toxicologists.

Where there are no human observations, risk assessment rests on validated experimental toxicology performed using good laboratory practice. Even in the case where the animal is biologically substantially different from man (absence of a reactive enzyme in one of the two species, very different kinetics, different target organs), the transcription may be possible if one adds an inter-species factor of security.

In the absence of human or animal data, risk assessment is impossible and, if published, is simply a calculated guess.

Cellular and subcellular *in vitro* toxicological studies and mathematical analysis of chemical structures (quantitative structure–activity relationships or QSAR) are increasingly common and at times are more numerous, or supplant entirely, experimental studies on the whole animal. One must keep in mind, however, that the mammal is the sole conceivable model for the study of subacute or chronic effects, the aforementioned tests being limited to the identification of reactive sites for the chemical products and totally incapable of accounting for protective and reparative mechanisms found in the intact animal.

Evaluation of Danger in a Given Situation (Hazard)

The situation of the observer in this case is very different from that of a risk assessment expert, in the sense that the situation must take into account the product, its use and its material and human 'environment'.

Driving a truck filled with nitroglycerine does not invoke the same concerns regarding a 'hazard' as the absorption of a nitroglycerine tablet by a patient with angina. The product in question is, nonetheless, the same.

In the matter of manipulation of dangerous products, it would be useful to research incidents, unexpected events which could have provoked damage, but which took place without consequence, not in order to compare them with true accidents but rather to utilize them in the name of prevention, in particular against the adverse effects of medications and of household products used in everyday life. The decrease of incidents by reasonable regulatory actions reduces considerably the number of accidents which occur, in general, as a result of multiple forms of negligence. The suppression of a single possible act of negligence reduces the global risk. It is in this domain that one finds preoccupations with storage, transport, labelling and protection of consumers and of the environment.

In evaluating a hazard, it is important to distinguish the hazard under conditions of everyday use from accident conditions. If one puts aside those hazards which occur by 'accident' (explosion, fire, sudden releases or spills of large quantities), one can find again the orientations toward the systematic epidemiology of toxic phenomena already known and validated or suspected on the basis of validated experimental observations.

Prognostic Criteria and Factors

Epidemiological Criteria

Prognostic criteria are not applicable to the individual but to the study of groups, essentially in order to appreciate the validity of certain parameters. These parameters are generally 'hard data': the initial blood pressure and heart rate, the plasma concentration of the drug, the serum potassium, etc. Establishment of prognostic factors is critical if medical toxicologists are to assess appropriately the efficacy of their treatments. It is not uncommon to read reports of invasive therapeutic manoeuvres, such as haemofiltration or dialysis, resulting in 'lifesaving' improvement, without any consideration or discussion of the normal temporal evolution of similar intoxications. While the tincture of time cures many initially serious intoxications, one prefers to credit medical technology, and sometimes without good evidence.

Semi-quantitative Criteria

These 'soft data' tend to group the ill according to positive criteria and the healthy according to negative criteria. They are employed with increasing frequency, asking the subject to represent him-or herself along a scale of the type:

| Do you feel fatigued? | Not at all | A little | A lot |
| Do your eyes burn at work? | Not at all | A little | A lot |

In principle, statistical manipulation of semi-quantitative criteria is fairly simple. In practice, immediate difficulty is encountered in understanding where these results lie in comparison with ranges considered to be normal:

- Among analytical laboratories;
- In the population;
- In an identifiable group (e.g. a group of healthy voluntary male Caucasians 20–25 years of age).

The quantification quickly degenerates when one attempts to look at standard medical nomenclature and diagnosis of the illnesses, their gravity and their evolution. Such scales are also plagued by recall bias and biases introduced by the investigator in wording the questions, question order, etc. Except in the case of a few classical situations, where the incidence of toxicity is high (lung cancer and tobacco use, bladder cancer and aromatic amines in non-smoking workers) or the manifestation is rare in the general population (pleural mesotheliomas among asbestos workers), much information obtained by this type of data-gathering tool is biased by coincidences or non-causal associations.

There has been a recent focus in human toxicology on 'multiple chemical sensitivity (MCS)', essentially a sensory and, above all, olfactory phenomenon, which is based largely on such subjective semi-quantitative criteria. While this syndrome defies classical toxicological methods of reproducibility, dose–response and physical expression of signs of toxicity, it has generated intense public interest and the support of a portion of the medical community known as 'clinical ecologists' and has become a compensated occupational illness in some locales (Gots, 1995). MCS and similar 'toxic syndromes' will no doubt pose a great challenge to toxicologists, physicians and public policy makers in the twenty-first century.

ECOTOXICOLOGY

Regardless of their competence, or lack thereof, in the domain of ecotoxicology, physicians are increasingly implicated in the discussions raised by this applied science, which reunites two fundamental disciplines (biology and chemistry) with the following goals:

1. The understanding of negative effects (noxious or adverse) of all chemical products, natural or not, on every living being.
2. The evaluation of practical consequences of this understanding on the actual state and probable evolution of the health of living beings (regulatory protection), on the equilibria existing between living

beings and their planetary niche (ecology and ecotoxicology).

A global mastery of negative effects based on short-term tests, interpreted as predictive of long-term effects, is elusive, given the absence of models with which to test the predictions and also the high degree of inability on the part of man to prevent in an effective way dramatic modifications due to climatic changes, natural catastrophes, or even man-made perturbations (demographic or occupational). The so-called 'mathematical modelling' of variable complexity utilizes formulae extending from the simplest calculations to integration of very diverse parameters. These models tend to be substituted for first-hand medical studies and may employ mediocre second-hand documents to arrive at recommendations which are often as ineffectual for the public health as they are costly to taxpayers. Take, for example, the 'greenhouse effect'. There remains great debate about the consequences of this issue. We cannot, at present, be certain that greenhouse gases will be detrimental to the biosphere and to man over the long term. Will the slow rise of the oceans prove to be beneficial rather than harmful to ocean flora and fauna?

EFFECTS OF SMALL DOSES

The study of effects associated with small doses (chemical hormesis) (Fournier, 1993) will be one of the challenges of toxicology in the decades to come, as are the treatments called 'homeopathic' in modern medicine.

Let us remember that Hahnemann, father of the utilization of extremely dilute solutions, had involuntarily poisoned his wife by the prescription of arsenic derivatives for their tonic effects. Physicians and apothecaries of the age were little embarrassed by such 'therapeutic accidents' but Hahnemann felt real chagrin and, in applying himself to the subject, made the remark that in lowering the doses, catastrophes disappeared. What remained was an apparently beneficial effect of a preparation which had become toxicologically tolerable.

A similar effect has been the subject of recent observations which are enveloped under the term 'hormesis' or 'stimulation' for low doses, the term stimulation indicating, in general, an effect in the opposite sense of what one observes with classical toxic doses, considered as causes of deficits. In the case of medications, we generally accept that at low doses effects are beneficial, and that at high doses effects are negative, and that there exists some threshold dose for toxic effects. We also recognize that the absence of a substance to which the organism has become accustomed (barbiturates) or which constitutes a normal physiological requirement (vitamin A) can also lead to negative effects (withdrawal or deficiency syndromes). This concept is demonstrated by the so-called U-curve, which represents a significant departure from the dose–effect theory of linear extrapolation to zero **(Figure 1)**.

The discussion of benefit becomes more delicate when we speak of xenobiotics without any known therapeutic benefit, where we are only familiar with their adverse effects. However, we should also recognize a double ignorance in this regard, one being that we have voluntarily forgotten past therapeutic effects of some substances. The salts of lead and antimony and dinitrocresol were medications in the nineteenth and twentieth centuries, and we should temper the reputation of comic idiocy of those physicians who preceded us, because nothing has proved that current representatives of the species have become superior, any more so in medicine than in biology; the other is the volition with which we denigrate chemical products, a rich fraction of the politico-social themes of ecologists of a 'purified world'.

What is certain is that the low portion (the favourable portion) of the U-curve is fairly close to the average band of normality, whereas the zone of classical toxicity is radically separated from it.

The theoretical importance of these studies is linked to the observation of a dose 'at least without adverse effects', which comes back to the recognition of the existence of a threshold of action, regardless of the chosen end-point, which is in concordance with the fundamental physiological notion of the regulation of all living organisms.

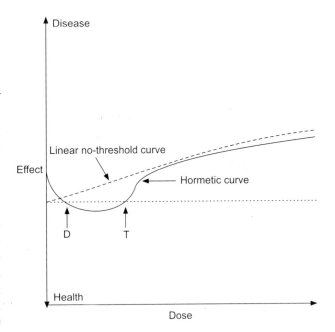

Figure 1 Dose–effect relationships. Hormesis versus linear extrapolation to zero. Generalized biological response to chemical and physical agents. Deficiency symptoms are caused by a deficit of an agent (dose less than D). Small doses (between D and T) are vital for good health. Doses higher than T cause toxic or other harmful effects. Adapted from Jaworowski (1997), with permission.

U models have been well demonstrated for certain neurophysiological parameters, such as latency of evoked potentials compared with the blood lead level, and observations of the same type seem to have been noted in the prevalence of leukaemia in the course of exposure to small doses of ionizing radiation (Jaworowski, 1997).

More evident, perhaps, are the observations of effects judged favourable from very small doses of alcohol and nicotine on certain biological parameters. The reduction of serious cardiovascular complications by the moderate absorption of alcohol is one of the classics of modern paramedical literature.

CONCLUSION AND CURRENT TRENDS

The veritable explosion of human toxicology is palpable in the demand for more physician-experts in toxicology in all domains — not only in health care, but also in the defence, food, chemical, pharmaceutical and cosmetics industries, which in developed societies or those becoming so are caught between greater demands for their products and shrinking tolerance of their presence.

Goldfrank (1994) proposed a history of chemical catastrophes that is instructive. One by one he evokes a long series: gas disasters, food disasters, alcohol and elicit drug disasters, therapeutic drug disasters, chemical group suicides and homicides, occupational toxic epidemics and environmental disasters, each of them being the subject of multiple examples, with diagnostic misadventures sometimes prolonged, their weight in human lives and sequellae and the difficulties of toxicologists and their social partners to deal with these problems.

Medical skills for the diagnosis and management of poisoned patients will always be an essential quality for human toxicologists, but simultaneously they will have to devote more time and competence to epidemiological studies, post-market surveillance of chemicals (toxicovigilance), risk assessment and communication, in order to meet the needs of the twenty-first century.

The World Health Organization has instituted a major focus on medical toxicology with the formation of the International Programme for Chemical Safety (IPCS). Among their many activities, the IPCS is taking a more critical look at the many substances which have been historically termed 'antidotes' (Pronczuk de Garbino *et al.*, 1997) and is promoting the international collection of toxicological data (Meredith and Haines, 1996). Accreditation processes are coming about in medical toxicology, both in terms of physicians and specialized treatment centres (Anony, 1993). These data collection activities, in concert with the processes of certification of medical toxicologists developing in various countries, should result in a veritable expertise which is currently still sparse and will hopefully help to ensure that chemical safety for man in the twenty-first century is more advanced than it was in the twentieth.

REFERENCES

Anderson, R. C. (1986). Fire gases. In Curry, A. S. (Ed.), *Analytical Methods in Human Toxicology*. Macmillan, London, pp. 289–317.

Anon. (1993). American Academy of Clinical Toxicology: facility assessment guidelines for regional toxicology treatment centers. *Clin. Toxicol.*, **31**, 211–217.

Baud, F. J., *et al.* (1991). Elevated blood cyanide concentrations in victims of smoke inhalation. *N. Engl. J. Med.*, **325**, 1761–1766.

Baud, F. J., *et al.* (1995). Modifying toxicokinetics with antidotes. *Toxicol. Lett.*, **82/83**, 785–793.

Bismuth, C., *et al.* (1999). *Toxicologie Clinique*, 5th edn. Flammarion, Paris. In press.

Borron, S. W., *et al.* (1997). Advances in the management of digoxin toxicity in the older patient. *Drugs Aging*, **10**, 18–33.

Conso, F., *et al.* (1982). Hépatonéphrite et hépatite toxiques par inhalation de trichlorethylène frauduleux. *Gastroenterol. Clin. Biol.*, **6**, 539.

Ellenhorn, M. J. and Barceloux, D. G. (1988). *Medical Toxicology: Diagnosis and Treatment of Human Poisoning*. Elsevier, New York.

Fournier, E. (1993). *Toxicologie*. Ellipses, Paris.

Fouyn, T. *et al.* (1991). Management of chemical warfare injuries. *Lancet*, **337**, 121–122.

Goldfrank, L. R. (Ed.) (1994). *Goldfrank's Toxicological Emergencies*. Appleton and Lang, Norwalk, CT.

Gots, R. E. (1995). Multiple chemical sensitivies — public policy. *Clin. Toxicol.*, **33**, 111–113.

Goulding, R. (1997). Lecture at the Royal Society of Medicine, London.

Jaworowski, Z. (1997). Beneficial ionizing radiation. In Bate, R. (Ed.), *What Risk? Science, Politics, and Public Health*. Butterworth–Heinemann, Oxford, pp. 151–172.

Meredith, T. and Haines, J. (1996). International data collection and evidence-based clinical toxicology. *Clin. Toxicol.*, **34**, 647–649.

Müller, H. E. (1997). The risks of dioxin to human health. In: Bate, R. (Ed.), *What Risk? Science, Politics, and Public Health*. Butterworth–Heinemann, Oxford, pp. 201–217.

Pronczuk de Garbino, J., *et al.* (1997). Evaluation of antidotes: activities of the International Programme on Chemical Safety. *Clin. Toxicol.*, **35**, 333–343.

Schaumann, W., *et al.* (1986). Kinetics of the Fab fragments of digoxin antibodies and of bound digoxin in patients with severe digoxin intoxication. *Eur. J. Clin. Pharmacol.*, **30**, 527–533.

Selden, B. S. (1989). Adolescent epidemic hysteria presenting as a mass casualty, toxic exposure incident. *Ann. Emerg. Med.*, **18**, 892–895.

Taboulet, P., *et al.* (1993). Clinical features and management of digitalis poisoning: rationale for immunotherapy. *Clin. Toxicol.*, **31**, 247–260.

Chapter 66

Occupational Toxicology *

Eugene J. Olajos and Harry Salem

C O N T E N T S

INTRODUCTION

Occupational toxicology is defined as that branch of toxicology concerned with the hazards from potential occupational exposure to biological, chemical and physical agents in the workplace. These hazards may be determined toxicologically and epidemiologically. The toxicological framework used in risk assessment and characterization is utilized, occupational exposure limits are established, preventive and control measures are implemented as well as training/educational programmes in the risk management and risk communication process.

In 1971, the US Congress created the Occupational Safety and Health Administration (OSHA) in response to the passage of the Occupational Safety and Health Act of 1970 (PL 91-596). OSHA was to assure, as far as possible, every working man and woman in the United States safe and healthful working conditions. As a result, OSHA issues and enforces regulations in many diverse industrial settings, both large and small. Each state is also encouraged to develop its own approved safety and

health plans, which must be at least as stringent as the federal requirements.

This chapter discusses occupational toxicology in its widest sense, which includes diverse areas such as industrial exposures, exposures of individuals in the service industries (e.g. health care industry, clinical/diagnostic laboratories, automotive repair, dry cleaning, painting, cosmetic/hairdressing, florists, printing/duplication services), chemical industry, agriculture-related occupations, mining and smelting, metal fabrication and biotechnology. Additionally, the interface with epidemiology and occupational medicine is reviewed as well as the implications of findings in various occupational settings. Occupational health and safety issues, concerns, pollution control/abatement and regulatory requirements as related to service industries, particularly small business enterprises and emerging biotechnology industry, are discussed. Reproductive hazards in the workplace are discussed as representative of challenging issues/concerns requiring the integrative efforts of the toxicology, epidemiology, industrial hygiene, medical, and regulatory communities in order to assure a safe work environment for both female and male employees. The roles of hazard evaluation, risk assessment and relevant regulations are also presented.

* The views of the authors do not purport to reflect the position of the Department of Defense. The use of trade names does not constitute an official endorsement or approval of the use of such commercial hardware or software.

SMALL INDUSTRY

Occupational exposure to chemical and physical agents is not confined to chemical industries but encompasses numerous occupational settings ranging from agriculture to mining. No occupational setting or workplace is too small to utilize one or more chemical agents and small industries (manufacturing or service) are bound to OSHA regulations, standards and compliance. Of considerable importance and implication to the occupational health and regulatory communities is the ever-increasing number of service industries, which, aside from the health care industry, are considered small enterprises. In the USA, Japan and Western European countries, a substantial number of the working population is no longer employed in agriculture or industry but in occupations generally defined as 'services' or in emerging industries such as biotechnology. Chemicals of all kinds are widely distributed to small industry concerns whether involved in manufacturing of consumer goods or in providing a service to the consumer (e.g. automotive repair, dry cleaning, hair/beauty establishments). The potential health risks from chemical and physical agents in such occupational settings may be greater than that encountered in much larger industrial establishments. The infrastructure to monitor and assure worker safety and health may be limited and in most instances absent altogether. A number of resources (consultative assistance, technical and management assistance, training, seminars and conferences and information resources) at the federal and state level are available to small industries in striving to provide safe working conditions.

BIOTECHNOLOGY

Biotechnology is a rapidly developing enterprise with a vast potential for application towards various manufacturing and industrial processes yet with the benefits come the challenges in providing a safe work environment where biotechnology processes and/or their products are utilized. Biotechnology, as defined by Liberman *et al.* (1991), is 'The application of natural or engineered biological organisms to technical and industrial processes'. The biotechnology industry had its origin in the early 1970s and comprises the following areas: (1) recombinant DNA technology, (2) hybridoma technology, (3) enzyme engineering and (4) protein engineering. Biotechnology has major implications not only in terms of technical and manufacturing processes but also in terms of health and safety issues for a diverse array of industries (e.g. clinical/diagnostics, health care, agriculture, chemical and petroleum, food processing, mining). Biotechnology presents new challenges to the toxicology, epidemiology and risk assessment/risk management communities. One of the critical challenges is to keep pace with an industry that is rapidly evolving and emerging and/or integrated into existing companies. Demain (1991) estimated that by the late 1980s, there were 400 biotechnology companies and about 70 pharmaceutical/chemical companies in the USA alone dedicating resources to biotechnology. The emergence of many small biotechnology enterprises presents an extraordinary challenge to occupational toxicologists, health professionals and regulatory officials in developing and implementing safety strategies that assure the health of the worker because such establishments usually lack the infrastructure or are ill-prepared to respond adequately to health-related disease or injuries. A brief overview will be presented highlighting the various areas within biotechnology and the potential health hazards and ways to mitigate/control hazards associated with biotechnology processes and products.

The following areas of biotechnology may be categorized as follows: (1) recombinant DNA technology, (2) vaccine development and production and (3) diagnostic tests/monoclonal antibodies/DNA probe technologies. Recombinant DNA technology, which is utilized in the production of mammalian peptides (e.g. somatostatin, insulin, growth hormone, interferons, interleukins) and growth factors [e.g. epidermal growth factor (EGF), fibroblast growth factor (FGF), transforming growth factors (TGF-α, TGF-β)] is a significant component of the biotechnology industry. Vaccine production also represents a major component of biotechnology. Monoclonal antibodies/DNA probes which have major applications in the diagnostic arena (e.g. genetic and infectious diseases), therapy (e.g. transplant rejection, autoimmune diseases) and in protein purification are likewise major components of the biotechnology industry (see Kingsbury, 1987). The application of biotechnology in the agricultural domain is a major thrust and effort of biotechnology. The use of recombinant DNA technology has led to the development of modified plants resistant to disease, insects, frost, etc. Within the food processing industry, biotechnology has contributed significantly—primarily in the utilization of microbial enzymes, as partial or full replacement of plant and animal enzymes in various foods processing steps.

The modern biotechnology industry employs thousands of workers and the number of toxicants (chemical and biological) encountered is substantial. The occupational toxicologists and allied personnel are faced with formidable tasks in the identification, monitoring and abatement/control related to occupational hazards in the biotechnology industry. Potential chemical exposures/hazards may arise from the following: (1) cell culture additions, (2) chemicals used in the extraction of nucleic acids, (3) in the identification of nucleic acids, (4) chemicals used in the sequencing procedures, (5) sterilization procedures and (6) products of biotechnology. Related to cell culture preparation, the major potential health hazard stems from the use of methotrexate, which is a common addition in all cultures. Methotrexate, which is highly cytotoxic, is a hepatotoxin and nephrotoxin, and exposure has been associated with immunosuppression. Furthermore, it is a known teratogen, even at therapeutic doses (Shepard, 1986). **Table 1** presents a synopsis of various chemicals used in biotechnology and their potential health risks. Chemical extraction of nucleic acids can be performed with a wide array of solvents and precipitating agents (extractants), some of which are highly toxic (e.g. cyanogen bromide, hydrazine, dimethyl sulphate). The identification of nucleic acids is based primarily on the utilization of high-performance liquid chromatography (HPLC), and potential chemical exposures are associated with the use of HPLC reagents and column materials. Chemicals utilized in the sequencing operations may be significant sources of exposure to and include such chemicals as acrylamide, dimethyl sulphate, ethidium bromide, hydrazine, hydrofluoric acid, piperidine and tetramethylenediamine. Most notable is the potential for peripheral neuropathy from acrylamide exposure (LeQuesne, 1980). Sterilization processes used in biotechnology can be achieved with heat, radiation and a number of chemicals, which can pose an occupational hazard. The products of biotechnology, not necessarily perceived as potential sources of hazard, are

potentially sources for health effects. Products of biotechnology include a wide variety of materials which include insulin, interferons, growth hormones, cell stimulating factors, anti-clotting agents, enzyme inhibitors, synthetic hormones, etc. Even minute quantities of a final product may cause adverse effects; notable examples are adrenocortical suppression in the manufacture of synthetic glucocorticosteroids (Newton *et al.*, 1978) and gynaecomastia in males associated with the manufacturing of oestrogen-containing oral contraceptives (Harrington *et al.*, 1978).

INTERFACE WITH EPIDEMIOLOGY

The critical goals of an occupational health programme are the prevention of illnesses/injuries among workers and the creation of a safe work environment. Success in attaining the above goals is dependent on the interaction between the toxicologist, epidemiologist, industrial hygienist, physician, safety engineer and regulatory specialist. The interface with the epidemiologist is increasingly crucial in assuring a safe work environment.

Table 1 Biotechnology processes/procedures as potential sources of xenobiotic exposure[a]

Biotechnology processes[b]

Cell culture procedures		Extraction procedures		Identification procedures		Sequencing procedures	
Chemicals	Primary risks	Chemicals	Primary risks	Chemicals	Primary risks	Chemicals	Primary risks
Antimetabolites cytotoxins		**Solvents**		**HPLC reagents**		Acrylamide Ethidium bromide	Carcinogen Mutagen
		Benzene	Carcinogen	Acetonitrile	Severe irritant	Hydrazine Hydrofluoric acid	Carcinogen Corrosive
Actinomycin	Teratogen	Chloroform	Carcinogen	Chloroform	Carcinogen	Piperidine	Carcinogen
Adriamycin	Tumorigen	Ethanol	CNS effects	Dimethyl formamide	Irritant	Urea	Carcinogen
Bleomycin	Respiratory	Naphthalene	CNS effects	Ethanolamine	Severe irritant		
Methotrexate	Carcinogen	Toluene	CNS effects	Hexane	CNS effects		
Vincristine	Neurotoxin			Pyridine	Severe irritant		
		Extractants/ precipitating agents		**Column materials**			
Antibiotics				Silica	Irritant		
				Fluorocarbons	Irritant		
Neomycin	Hepatotoxin	Dimethyl sulphate	Irritant	Octadecysilane	Irritant		
Rifampin	Reproductive	Hydrazine	Carcinogen				
Strepotomycin	Reproductive	Perchloric acid	Corrosive				
		Cyanogen bromide	Severe irritant				
Hormones		Formic acid	Severe irritant				
Growth homones							
Prednisone	Reproductive						

a Partial listing of chemicals provided for each of the biotechnology procedures indicated.
b Chemical sterilants are also used in biotechnology (e.g. formaldehyde, ethylene oxide, hydrogen peroxide, phenol). Toxic effects: formaldehyde (carcinogenic); ethylene oxide (carcinogenic and neurotoxic); hydrogen peroxide (corrosive); and phenol (severe irritant, carcinogenic).

Whether from an occupational or environmental perspective, methods used for assessing human risks should be supported by human data. In an occupational setting, the exposure assessment, including the determination of significant exposure levels, to a given chemical and associated effects is dependent on both toxicological and epidemiological data. High reliability in the health risk assessment and the development of a meaningful safety standard for a chemical are inseparable from robust databases comprising both epidemiological and toxicological information. Unfortunately, epidemiological data for many industrial chemicals is non-existent. However, when such data are available, its incorporation into the risk assessment/risk characterization paradigm has often resulted in a much improved risk assessment process. Occupational toxicology and occupational epidemiology are inter-linked, multifaceted disciplines that draw upon the knowledge, developments, and techniques of allied/adjunct disciplines such as industrial hygiene, biology, biochemistry, biotechnology, chemistry, pharmacology and mathematics/statistics. Collective efforts, with the integration of the various approaches, are essential to the accurate and successful identification, assessment, and characterization of occupationally related physiological effects, diseases and injuries.

Occupational epidemiology is the study of the distribution and determinants of a physiological condition or disease among a working population. Occupational toxicology and epidemiology have become important and integral components of occupational health, and seek to identify the relationships between occupational exposures and diseases as well as the identification of high-risk subgroups (susceptible populations). Generally, epidemiological approaches toward the identification of chemically induced altered physiological functions/states and diseases have been highly useful. Early epidemiological studies demonstrated the health risks associated with coal dusts, asbestos and other occupational exposures. Epidemiological studies, for example, were instrumental in establishing the relationship between vinyl chloride and hepatic cancer (angiosarcoma) among plastic manufacturing workers (Waxweiler et al., 1976) and the association between cancer and formaldehyde in the resin manufacturing industry (Bertazzi et al., 1986). Epidemiological studies have also provided data in establishing the linkage between occupational exposure and non-cancer effects, for example, the development of heart disease and carbon disulphide exposure (Balcarova and Halik, 1991), genotoxicity and toluene exposure (Maki-Paakkanen et al., 1986) and hepatoxicity and toluene exposure (Boewer et al., 1988).

As in toxicity studies, exposure and manifestations (outcomes), appropriate controls and appropriate statistical measures are critical to epidemiological studies. Sacks and Schenker (1990) have identified three types of epidemiological studies, namely descriptive, analytical and experimental. Bang (1996), in an overview of the applications of occupational epidemiology, focused on observational epidemiological studies, the most common, and for the purposes of our discussions highly suitable in illustrating the role and relationships of epidemiology in the occupational setting and in occupational toxicology. Observational epidemiological studies include the following: cohort, case-control, cross-sectional, occupational surveillance, meta-analysis, molecular epidemiology and ecological. In general, the most common epidemiological studies are of the cohort or case-control types. Only a very brief description of the various occupational epidemiological approaches are presented and the reader is referred to one or more of the texts on epidemiology for details. Morbidity and mortality cohort studies (prospective or retrospective) are useful and effective. In the prospective cohort (follow-up) study, rates of diseases can be derived in both exposed and unexposed groups. Excess risk can be expressed in either absolute or relative terms (Breslow et al., 1983). An example of prospective cohort mortality studies is the study of lung cancer among formaldehyde workers (Blair et al., 1990). Illustrative of prospective cohort morbidity studies is the morbidity study on the respiratory effects associated with toluene diisocyanate exposure (Wegman, 1982) and a study of pulmonary function in wood workers exposed to formaldehyde (Alexanderson and Hedenstierna, 1989). In case-control studies (effect to cause), individuals with disease are selected for comparisons with individuals without the disease (Schlesselman, 1982). Cases and controls are compared with regard to exposures associated with the disease under study. Case-control studies are relevant in circumstances when several occupations or substances are associated with the disease of interest. Illustrative of case-control studies is the study on the relationship between laryngeal cancer and exposure to machining fluids among autoworkers (Eisen et al., 1994). Cross-sectional (survey or prevalence) studies are those that examine the association between disease and other variables as they exist in a defined population at one specific point in time (Last, 1995). Cross-sectional study designs are most appropriate in situations where subtle, subclinical health effects are under consideration. The prevalence of the health effect is compared among subgroups with various occupational exposures, age differences, medical conditions/histories, etc. Illustrative of a cross-sectional study was a respiratory survey of agricultural workers—the findings implicated exposure to agriculture chemicals and respiratory distress (Senthilselvan et al., 1992). The meta-analysis approach relies on a variety of statistical techniques in the analyses of data derived from separate studies (Hedges and Olkin, 1985; Labbe et al., 1987; and Chalmers, 1991) and has been applied to occupational studies with divergent findings. Illustrative of the application of the meta-analysis approach to an occupational setting is the meta-analysis of studies on lung cancer among silicotics (Smith *et al.*, 1995). The case-crossover approach and its potential application to occupational settings, particularly in regard to occupational injuries, were discussed by Mittleman *et al.* (1997).

TRENDS IN OCCUPATIONAL EPIDEMIOLOGY: MOLECULAR EPIDEMIOLOGY

The term 'molecular epidemiology' was coined by Higginson (1967) and has been used in the literature since the late 1970s. For example, Lower *et al.* (1979) used the term in describing a study on *N*-acetyltransferase phenotype and urinary bladder cancer risk. Molecular epidemiology came about because epidemiology has evolved more and more as a science of methods due in part to the need to address adequately the concerns and outcomes regarding exposures that elicit less obvious health effects and produce smaller increases in risk than those in the past. Many advances in molecular biology/biochemistry have been integrated into the fields of epidemiology, medicine and toxicology (Ahmed, 1995a, b). In the field of epidemiology, the application of such advances has resulted in the evolution of molecular epidemiology as an integral part of occupational epidemiology. Molecular epidemiology, an integral part of occupational epidemiology, has expanded the capabilities as well as providing a means for overcoming limitations of classical epidemiology through the use of biological and biochemical measurements collected from individuals/sub-populations exposed to toxicants (Marx, 1991; Schulte and Perera, 1993). Advances in molecular epidemiology have helped to identify metabolic pathways, enzymes and genes, that play an important role in diseases (Hemminki, 1992). Molecular epidemiology has provided useful insights related to occupational exposures and effects and will have an increasing role in occupational epidemiology, occupational medicine, occupational toxicology and risk assessment/characterization/management. Critical to the success and utility of molecular epidemiology was the development and integration of biomarker technology into the practice of occupational empidemiology, and this is highlighted below.

Molecular/biochemical biomarkers are of great interest because perturbations at the molecular/biochemical level are sensitive measures of exposure and effect. In many instances, biochemical markers are usually the most immediate and quantifiable responses to toxicant exposure and as indicators of early adverse health effects. Thus, biochemical measures have become reliable and useful tools for the detection and documentation of exposure and the effects of chemical exposure in the workplace. Biological markers, in particular molecular/biochemical, have been developed to augment various epidemiological strategies; for example, the use of exposure biomarkers in case-control and cohort studies, the utilization of markers in disease classification, and the use of biomarkers to ascertain genetic susceptibility enabling the identification of sensitive individuals/subpopulation(s). In occupational epidemiology, exposure biomarkers have contributed in the following ways: (1) have enhanced the exposure assessment in cases where there were insufficient details of exposure, (2) have provided a basis for validation of other sources of information, (3) have allowed the documentation of target tissue exposure and (4) have helped in the quantification of biological load from an exposure (dosimetry) (Stein and Hatch, 1987).

Biomarkers of exposure and effect have provided useful information in the specification of disease entities and in the identification of susceptible individuals (Axelson and Soderkvist, 1991). Tissue levels of toxicant have been used as biological dosimeters in establishing the association between organohalide body burden and cancer of the lung (Austin *et al.*, 1989). Aflatoxin exposure, common in the agricultural industry, has been associated with a mutation specific to the *p53* tumour suppressor gene (Greenblatt *et al.*, 1994). Oncogene (*ras*) activation has been linked with solvent exposure in cases of acute myeloid leukaemia (Taylor *et al.*, 1992). Considerable interest and effort have been directed to the development and use of macromolecular adducts (DNA, RNA, and protein), particularly the identification of chemical adducts to DNA in various occupational groups. Macromolecular adducts, the products of the interactions between reactive xenobiotics and/or their metabolites with DNA, RNA or proteins, have emerged as highly useful biomarkers of exposure. Research on macromolecular adducts dates to the 1970s—the development and application to risk assessment have been amply reviewed (Farmer and Bailey, 1989; Skipper and Tannenbaum 1990; Chang *et al.*, 1994). The use of protein adducts as surrogates for DNA adducts as indicators of exposure to chemical carcinogens has been espoused by Calleman *et al.* (1978). Haemoglobin adducts have been shown to be highly useful exposure biomarkers (Pereira and Chang, 1981). The adducts of DNA can be thought of as markers of exposure, of effects including early adverse effects, or as susceptibility markers (Axelson, 1994).

CASE STUDY: TRANSFORMING INDUSTRIAL HYGIENE DATABASE ON CHROMIUM AND INTEGRATION INTO EPIDEMIOLOGICAL STUDIES

Health effects related to chromium and chromium-containing compounds have been the subject of numerous animal and epidemiological studies. Concern has centred on hexavalent chromium (Cr^{6+}), a demonstrated animal carcinogen, suspect human carcinogen, and mutagen. The toxicology of chromium with respect to speciation has been reviewed (Katz and Salem, 1993). The hazards of occupational exposure to chromium and/or chromium-containing compounds has been extensively studied in particular as related to Cr^{6+}. With increasing frequency, epidemiological studies are being utilized to characterize worker exposures, in risk assessment/risk management paradigms, and in the development of occupational exposure standards. Thus, epidemiologists have placed much emphasis on the quantitative characterization of exposures and quantifiable end-points on occupational epidemiology studies. However, for a considerable number of chemicals, substantial industrial hygiene and epidemiological data exist that are flawed to a lesser or greater degree and/or lack robust exposure data. Interest exists in the transformation of such data with potential utilization in other study designs and/or evaluation of the workplace environment. Approaches such as that described by Pastides *et al.* (1994) attempt to utilize such data for exposure reconstruction by careful evaluation and data transformation. Pastides *et al.* examined the available industrial hygiene records and past exposure data on Cr^{6+}. Cumulative exposure estimates were derived by summing time-weighted values related to each job in a worker's employment history. Such approaches enhance the range of options related to workplace evaluation and occupational study designs.

RELATIONSHIP BETWEEN OCCUPATIONAL TOXICOLOGY AND OCCUPATIONAL MEDICINE

Occupational health is dependent on the integrative efforts of the occupational physician, the industrial hygienist, the toxicologist and ancillary safety and health professionals. Occupational medicine is a subspecialty of preventive medicine and is concerned with the appraisal, maintenance, restoration and improvement of worker health. It is also engaged in the promotion of a productive and fulfilling work environment for the employee. The occupational physician is responsible for providing an occupational health programme to protect the employee from health and safety hazards in the workplace that may stem from a chemical, physical or biological hazard, or a combination thereof. This is accomplished via utilization of the knowledge and insights of the industrial hygienist concerning manufacturing processes and health background of an employee's job. Information provided by the industrial hygienist also enables the physician to correlate employee concerns with potential job health hazards. The toxicologist augments the physician's knowledge on cause–effect relationships of chemicals and signs and symptoms of

toxicant exposure. The toxicologist also functions in the following capacities: (1) involved in data collection and interpretation concerning chemical exposures and effects, (2) provides information on the most recent developments related to the assessment/evaluation of toxicant-induced effects, (3) provides information pertaining to experimental studies in animals, (4) contributes to epidemiological study designs, (5) contributes to biological monitoring programmes and (6) contributes to the design and development of medical control measures.

OCCUPATIONAL LEGISLATION: OSHA, TSCA

The US Congress enacted protective federal legislation related to the workplace, namely the Occupational Safety and Health Act (OSHAct) of 1970. This legislation established the occupational safety and health law with the following key agencies being involved: the National Institutes of Occupational Safety and Health (NIOSH) and the Occupational Safety and Health Administration (OSHA). It should also be noted that under the Occupational Safety and Health Act, individual states might establish and administer their own occupational safety and health programmes and agencies. NIOSH, a component of the Department of Health and Human Services, functions in a research capacity. OSHA is a component of the Department of Labor and its function is the setting and enforcement of safety and health standards in the workplace. OSHA is responsible for establishing and enforcing laws and standards for the regulation of health and safety in the workplace. OSHA standards can be mandatory or advisory and are categorized as follows: (1) general industry, (2) agriculture, (3) maritime and (4) construction.

A number of organizations are involved in the development of standards, namely the American Conference of Governmental Industrial Hygienists (ACGIH), the American National Standards Institute (ANSI) and the National Fire Protection Association (NFPA). Standards may be categorized as horizontal, vertical, health, permanent, emergency/temporary or voluntary standards. Horizontal standards apply to all workplaces found in Title 29 (Labor) of the Code of Federal Regulations (CFR) Parts 1900–1910 (general industry). Vertical standards apply to a particular vocation or industry. Health standards which make up approximately 85% of general industry standards regulate chemical exposure. Federal standards governing exposure levels in the workplace are Permissible Exposure Levels (PELs) and Threshold Limit Values (TLVs), which are complemented by short-term exposure limits. PELs are exposure limits for chemicals published by OSHA as legal standards. TLVs are exposure limits established by a non-governmental group (ACGIH). There are three categories of TLVs: TLV-TWA (time-weighted average concentration for an 8 h work day); TLV-STEL (maximum concentration to which a worker can be exposed for a period of up to 15 min without effect); and TLV-C (the concentration that should not be exceeded even instantaneously). Since the passage of OSHAct, both OSHA and NIOSH have been committed to establishing PELs that are more complete than the TLVs issued by the ACGIH. Workplace standards are based on the best available information from industrial experience, chemical analogy data, animal experimentation and human epidemiological data. In addition to PELs and TLVs there is the Occupational Exposure Limit (OEL). OELs are developed by manufacturers for substances that are not subject to governmental regulation. OELs may serve as a benchmarks for a healthy work environment and represent the link between risk assessment and risk management.

The employee's right-to-know as to which chemicals and materials are used is governed under the OSHA Communication Standard (1983). This standard came into effect in 1985 and was amended in 1987. Under this regulation, chemical manufacturers must evaluate or assess the hazards of chemicals which they produce or import and along with distribution provide information to other manufacturing and non-manufacturing employees. Employees must be informed about chemical hazards by way of hazard communication programme, labels, material safety data sheets (MSDSs) and training. OSHA considers the MSDS as the primary vehicle for transmitting hazard information to downstream employers and workers. The Toxic Substances Control Act (TSCA) of 1976 has considerable potential for providing protection from chemical hazards. Under TSCA, the US Environmental Protection Agency (US EPA) is empowered to require the development of adequate toxicity and environmental data on new and existing chemicals. The development of data on is the responsibility of the chemical manufacturers and processors. Furthermore, under TSCA the US EPA may prohibit or place conditions on the manufacture, distribution and use of a chemical if it possesses unreasonable risks to human health and the environment. Manufacturers are required to notify the US EPA prior to the production of any new chemical via the 'premanufacture notice' (PMN).

Biological hazards also represent significant workplace and public health issues. Numerous occupational settings (e.g. biotechnology industries, the health care industry, clinical and research laboratories, veterinary, fermentation and food processing plants, forestry products industry) are potential sources of biological hazards. The diversity of sources requires the efforts of local, state and federal governments to assure a safe work environment. OSHA has issued one standard addressing biological hazards in the work environment, namely the Bloodborne Pathogen Standard issued in December 1991. Concerns regarding recombinant DNA technology have led to the development of numerous controls and practices designed to prevent or minimize hazards. The National Institutes of Health (NIH), for example, have developed guidelines that address recombinant DNA research (US Public Health Service, National Institutes of Health, 1974, 1976, 1983, 1994). In addition, the Centers for Disease Control (CDC) have issued guidelines for various microbial agents as related to health-care facilities. States have also formulated statutes and regulations governing the handling and use of bio-hazardous agents and materials. States have also enacted public health laws that go beyond the requirements established by OSHA. Furthermore, all states have developed mandatory reporting requirements for various conditions, which facilitates the investigation and surveillance of communicable diseases.

OCCUPATIONAL HEALTH AND REGULATORY ISSUES: AGRICULTURAL BIOTECHNOLOGY

The biotechnology industry, in particular those aspects involving agricultural biotechnology, present a number of unique and challenging issues related to human health and the environment including the interface between various regulatory agencies. The concerns and issues related to field testing of biotechnologically derived agricultural products have led to a government regulatory framework involving several federal agencies (Department of Agriculture, Environmental Protection Agency, and the Food and Drug Administration). The responsibility for the regulation of agricultural biotechnology products and field testing by the above agencies is based on pre-existing statutory authority. The 'Coordinated Framework' for biotechnology regulation outlines the jurisdiction of each federal agency responsible for regulating biotechnology products and research (*Federal Register*, 51, 23302–23393, 1986). It covers the entire spectrum of biotechnology activity. The US Department of Agriculture (USDA) and the US EPA have authority over agricultural biotechnology products. The USDA's authority stems from several statutes and the major law covering biotechnology is the Plant Pest Act specifically through new legislation adopted in 1987. The US EPA's authority derives from two specific laws, namely, the Federal Insecticide, Fungicide and Rodenticide Act (FIFRA) and the Toxic Substances Control Act (TSCA). FIFRA, under which US EPA regulates all pesticides, has used this legislation to register a number of naturally occurring microbes and viruses as biological pest control agents. The US EPA is using existing regulations to review and register genetically engineered microbial pesticides and extend authority to small-scale field testing of genetically altered microorganisms.

MEDICAL SURVEILLANCE AND ENVIRONMENTAL MONITORING IN THE WORKPLACE

Controlling safety and hazards in the workplace begins with a strong medical surveillance and monitoring (biological and environmental) programme. Monitoring and surveillance are critical in the development of effective strategies to minimize and/or prevent health hazards and/or diseases in the occupational setting. After potential hazards and risks have been identified in an occupational setting, the goals and scope of a medical surveillance programme are determined. Furthermore, the surveillance programme must be in compliance with local, state and federal regulations. Medical surveillance programmes (agent specific or symptom specific) are designed to detect subtle changes indicative of exposure and are also useful to ensure that controls are effective. Medical surveillance is a complex and multifaceted process and consists of the following components: (1) pre-placement examination, (2) job requirements review, (3) occupational history review, (4) medical history, (5) screening tests, (6) biological monitoring and (7) preventive measures. Medical screening is critical from two aspects. First, it identifies pre-existing health condition(s) (e.g. underlying medical condition, medication, deficiencies in host defences and reproductive system concerns) in the worker that would increase the risk of adverse health outcome. A compromized health status would exclude a worker from a particular operation or limit the extent that a worker can engage in a particular process. Second, screening identifies early signs and symptoms of disease related to workplace exposure.

Monitoring consists of both biological monitoring (body fluids, urinalysis, hair analysis, etc.) and environmental monitoring for ambient levels of pollutants. Environmental monitoring of suspected exposure includes primarily air sampling using direct reading measurements, other sampling methods and sampling and analysis by analytical laboratory methods. Monitoring the workplace of chemical pollutant is not only an indicator of exposure but is equally important as an indicator that engineering controls and other measures are effective in maintaining the concentration of pollutant at safe levels.

MEDICAL SURVEILLANCE AND ENVIRONMENTAL MONITORING IN THE BIOTECHNOLOGY INDUSTRY

Medical surveillance and environmental monitoring in occupations utilizing biotechnology must consider not only the various chemicals used in the biotechnology industry and related fields but also biological agents, biotechnology products and radioisotopes. Biological monitoring approaches that have been developed to detect exposure to chemicals, in particular carcinogenic agents, associated with biotechnology include urinalysis for carcinogens and/or their metabolites, macromolecular adduct formation, detection of altered oncogene proteins and pre-clinical response using an array of genotoxicity bioassays [e.g. chromosomal aberrations (CA), sister chromatid exchange (SCE) and micronuclei test (McDiarmid and Emmett, 1987; Brandt-Rauf, 1988)].

RISK ASSESSMENT/RISK MANAGEMENT: HANDLING AND PRODUCTION OF INDUSTRIAL CHEMICALS

Risk assessment and risk management, critical to the assurance of a safe work environment, are the two distinct elements in the regulatory process (National Academy of Sciences, 1983). Risk assessment and risk management are multifaceted processes that are dependent on the input of scientific, social, political and economic disciplines. Risk assessment is viewed as a scientific process which characterizes risk and assesses the likelihood of its occurrence. The risk assessment paradigm consists of hazard identification, exposure assessment, dose–response assessment and risk characterization (discussed subsequently). It has been practised in the USA and other industrialized countries for about 20 years and is the framework for most occupational and environmental health regulations in the USA and elsewhere. The ultimate goal is the attainment of a comprehensive risk assessment which is dependent on the integrative efforts of the toxicology community, allied health sciences, safety and regulatory communities. Toxicology and other databases on chemicals are assessed in determining the potential adverse (unwanted) health effects to the human population in either an occupational or environmental setting. Additionally, the assessment provides a basis for implementing or modifying existing control measures associated with the handling and/or manufacturing of chemicals. The assessment of toxicological data, as a basis for predicting health risks stemming from chemical exposures, parallels federal agency (e.g. OSHA, US EPA and FDA) developments in risk assessment. Risk assessments have improved over the years owing to the integration of new/improved risk assessment techniques: (1) low-dose extrapolation modelling, (2) modelling techniques [e.g. physiologically based pharmacokinetic (PBPK) modelling] (3) absorption uptake models related to route (e.g. inhalation, dermal) or to specific chemicals (e.g. arsenic), (4) biomarkers (e.g. exposure, effect, susceptibility), (5) improved dosimetry (e.g. macromolecular adducts, dosimetry modelling), (6) mechanistic approaches, (7) improved analytical measures of exposure and (8) improved exposure assessment techniques (e.g. incorporating biomarkers). Improved exposure assessments and low-dose extrapolation models, for example, have contributed greatly to the risk assessment process. Thus, by the 1980s, occupational health standards and occupational/environmental health regulations have been based on the results of low-dose extrapolation models and improved exposure assessments (Munro and Krewski, 1981; Rodricks *et al.*, 1987). Risk assessment methodologies have been utilized to establish standards for workplace exposures, ambient air standards, pesticide residues, pharmaceuticals, food additives, contaminants in consumer products, etc.

As indicated, risk assessment is a multi-step process consisting of hazard identification, exposure assessment, dose–response evaluation and risk characterization. Hazard identification is the evaluation of data to determine if there is or is not a causal relationship between exposure to a chemical and adverse (unwanted) health effects. Exposure assessment is that part of the risk assessment process that links chemical exposure to adverse health effects and disease. It is the process that not only addresses the likelihood of xenobiotic uptake but also involves estimating the route, frequency, duration and magnitude of exposure with a chemical or physical agent. Many factors require consideration when developing an exposure assessment, namely route, duration, intermittent versus continuous exposure, target populations, sensitive sub-populations, etc. The complexities associated with this process increase when one considers multichemical/multipathway situations/scenarios (Preuss and Ehrlich, 1987). Direct (e.g. biological monitoring) and indirect (e.g. models for source release, exposure and uptake) approaches are available in estimating exposure to a chemical. The exposure estimate is linked to available epidemiological data and extrapolations from animal data to characterize the risk or hazard to obtain a meaningful perspective concerning the significance of an exposure. The dose–response component of the risk assessment process is the quantitative relationship between exposure and the occurrence of health effects. It necessitates an extrapolation from high-dose animal exposures to exposures expected from human

exposure to a chemical in an occupational or environmental setting. The key approaches in dose–response assessment include the safety (uncertainty factor) approach and the mathematical modelling approach. Improvements in these areas have provided a more scientific basis for risk assessment and consequently a risk assessment with greater predictability and less uncertainty. Risk characterization is the summary and interpretation of the information collected, which essentially identifies the limitations in databases/data sets, and uncertainties involved. It is the final step in the risk assessment process and compares the estimated level of risk to the acceptable level.

BIOMARKERS AND HEALTH RISK ASSESSMENT

Numerous biomarkers have been developed and utilized successfully to quantify toxicant-induced changes in biochemical processes/pathways, physiological functions and structure/morphology. For purposes of classification, biomarkers have been categorized as organ-specific or toxicant-specific. They have also been classified as either biochemical, physiological or histopathological. Biomarkers have augmented strategies (e.g. conventional epidemiological paradigms, conventional toxicity testing, structure–activity relationships). Furthermore, biomarkers are powerful tools for detecting and documenting exposure to, and the effects from, chemical exposure in the occupational setting. Biomarker technology has been applied to all of the various components of the risk assessment process. The greatest utility of biomarkers is the quantification of effects and providing a means for an integrated view of health status. Biomarkers are used extensively in medicine and in the evaluation of occupational health risks. Measurements in body fluids and tissue samples provide information that can be used as biomarkers of exposure and effect. A synopsis of some commonly used biomarkers and their assay potential in blood and other tissues is presented in **Table 2**. Broadly defined, biomarkers are indicators signalling events in biological systems over the entire range of biological organization from molecular to community levels.

Table 2 Assay utility of some common biomarkers in blood and other tissues

Biomarker	Preferred tissue	Assay potential (blood)	Comment
AChE[a] inhibition	Neural	Yes	RBC can be used, effect in blood is transient
ALAD[b]	Blood	Yes	Tissue of choice
Porphyrins	Liver	Unproven	Techniques under development for use in plasma
Adducts	Wide range	Yes	Haemoglobin good surrogate for DNA
Metallothioneins	Liver, kidney	None	Associated with storage in tissue
Stress proteins	Wide range	Unproven	Some database using RBC

[a] AChE = acetylcholinesterase.
[b] ALAD = δ-aminolaevulinic acid dehydratase.

Biomarkers are used to document exposure and effects and may be categorized into the broad categories of non-specific and specific biomarkers. Specific indicators may be further classified as either organ-specific or toxicant-specific. Organ-specific biomarkers (exposure and effect) exist for all of the major organ systems. The array of useful biomarkers, sensitivity, diagnostic effectiveness, utility across species and their predictive value vary considerably. Generally, the various approaches/techniques that constitute organ-specific biomarkers include organ-specific enzymes, organ function tests and histopathological end-points. Organ-specific biomarkers have been extensively used in the occupational field and a brief synopsis on biomarkers indicative of hepatic and renal dysfunction/injury will be presented.

As an organ system, the liver exhibits marked vulnerability to xenobiotic-induced dysfunction and damage. Detection and evaluation of liver dysfunction and disease have been approached from an integrative perspective to include biochemical, physiological and morphological outcomes. Despite some difficulty in the selection of appropriate assays to ascertain outcomes of chemical exposure on the hepatic system, several useful tests are available for the detection and evaluation of liver dysfunction and injury (Kachmar and Moss, 1976; Plaa and Charbonneau, 1994; Stonard and Evans, 1994). Assays used in the detection and evaluation of hepatic dysfunction and injury include serum enzyme assays, hepatic clearance/excretion assays, changes in endogenous constituents and morphological assessment of liver injury. The determination of hepatic enzyme activity in blood is a very useful tool in the detection and assessment of hepatic damage made possible by the release of tissue enzyme into the blood by the damaged liver. A number of enzyme-based assays are available and are grouped as follows: (1) assays that are somewhat non-specific (e.g. lactate dehydrogenases, transaminases), (2) assays based on enzymes localized mainly in hepatic tissue [e.g. alanine aminotransferase (ALT, ALAT, GPT)] and (3) assays based on an enzyme exclusively associated with the liver [e.g. sorbitol dehydrogenase (SDH)].

The renal system, multifunctional and critical in the control and regulation of homeostasis, is vulnerable to chemically induced dysfunction/damage. Assessment of nephrotoxicity can be accomplished via serum chemistry, urinalysis, clearance procedures and histopathological analyses (for details, see Foulkes, 1993; Davis and Berndt, 1994; Tarloff and Goldstein, 1994). Various biochemical measures in blood or urine have been successfully used as indicators of chemically induced renal dysfunction/pathology: lactate dehydrogenase, N-acetyl-β-glucosaminidase (NAG) and alkaline phosphatase. Urinary excretion of proteins has long been utilized as an indicator of renal damage. Clearance procedures to evaluate glomerular filtration rate (GFR) are conducted via monitoring the renal handling of inulin, creatinine or p-aminohippurate (PAH). Glomerular function may be assessed by monitoring blood urea nitrogen (BUN).

Toxicants manifest their effects at varying levels of biological organization and perturbations at the molecular/biochemical level represent sensitive indices of exposure and effect. Biochemical markers, extremely diverse, have been used in the assessment of occupational hazards, most notably the measurement of acetylcholinesterase (AChE) activity in the pesticides manufacturing and agriculture industries. The reader is directed to a comprehensive review on biochemical indices of chemical exposure and effect (Stegeman et al., 1992). Another excellent source of information on biochemical and cellular indices, as useful tools for monitoring toxicity, is that of Foa et al. (1987).

RISK MANAGEMENT

Risk management is that process involving the evaluation of a wide range of factors (e.g. extrascientific factors, socioeconomic issues, political aspects, economic factors and risk assessment outcome) ultimately to protect human health.

Risk Assessment and Risk Management: Biotechnology Industry

Occupational hazards associated with biotechnology include not only potential exposure to the hazards from the chemical used in biotechnology but also the use of microorganisms (genetically intact or altered) and biotechnology products (e.g. synthetic hormones, vaccines, blood products). Thus, assessing and characterizing the risks associated with biotechnology processes and products require highly integrative approaches and input from a broad spectrum of health and physical scientists. Relatively early in the emergence of the biotechnology industry, the key question was, and still is, how we could assess the risks associated with biotechnology. Prominent issues and concerns were type and degree of hazard, probability of occurrence of a hazardous event, characterization of the biology of microorganisms and outcomes including impact on foreign ecosystems. An extensive review on the use of microorganisms as related to biotechnology was conducted by the Office of Technology Assessment (US Congress) (1984). Of paramount concern are the potential hazards associated with the products of biotechnology, particularly those products that are highly physiologically active. Approaches towards dealing with these hazards varied considerably; however, a consensus among regulatory agencies was achieved, namely that these products be assessed like any other physiologically active product (Miller, 1983a). The hazards associated with biotechnology products were also addressed by the Cell Products Safety Commission of the World Health Organization (WHO) (1987). Thus, biotechnology products (e.g. human growth hormone) produced via genetic engineering should be tested for purity, chemical identity and biological activity in the same manner as those hormones derived from human tissues. The need for comprehensive product characterization and testing of biotechnology products has been emphasized by the eosinophilia myalgia epidemic that was related to an impurity in an engineered amino acid product (Roberts, 1990).

IMPLICATIONS OF FINDINGS IN THE WORKPLACE

Findings in the workplace include both negative and positive indicators as to the effectiveness of an occupational health programme within an occupational setting. The absence of negative findings is indicative that engineering controls are properly operating, that effective medical screening and surveillance programmes are in place, that appropriate protective equipment is utilized and that effective training and education programmes are in place. On the other hand, outcomes from accidental exposures, employee complaints and illnesses, positive findings from workplace monitoring (biological and/or environmental) and indicators of exposure from medical surveillance have many implications, not only for the worker but also for management and technical personnel responsible for assuring a safe work environment. Generally, implications may be of great significance to the employer in terms of resource and time or may have minimal impact. Specific implications relate to the effectiveness of monitoring programmes, effectiveness of health surveillance, effectiveness of engineering controls, the need for more stringent standards, the appropriate and effective use of protective equipment and training needs for the employee. Based on the nature of the findings, a number strategies may be implemented to ensure worker safety and health. These may include one or more of the following: more stringent exposure standards, substitution in a manufacturing process, isolation or enclosure of a process, engineering controls (initial or improved), personal protective equipment, better medical surveillance, precautionary measures, pragmatic considerations and worker training and education. It is of interest to note that in the past health and safety have utilized engineering and enforcement as the principal solutions towards correcting workplace-related exposures and violations. Recently, however, the regulatory perspective has shifted towards the incorporation of education/training of the employee as an adjunct to engineering controls and enforcement as a combined strategy to worker safety.

CHALLENGING ISSUES/PROBLEMS IN OCCUPATIONAL TOXICOLOGY: REPRODUCTIVE HAZARDS IN THE WORKPLACE

A substantial number of chemicals are known (established) reproductive toxicants and a significant number are suspected of causing adverse reproductive outcomes. Epidemiological studies (incidence surveys or linking health records with work records) have been conducted to discern the possible relationships between occupational exposures and adverse reproductive outcomes (Figa-Talamanca, 1984; McDonald et al., 1987; Savitz et al., 1989; Lindbohm et al., 1991; Peoples-Sheps et al., 1991; Sanjose et al., 1991). Reproductive risks from occupational exposures in a wide array of settings (e.g. chemical manufacturing, pesticide production, metal working, printing, agriculture, health care and biotechnology) are of great concern to the occupational health and regulatory communities, as evidenced by the many review articles, book chapters and government reports on the subject (Schrag and Dixon, 1985; Baird and Wilcox, 1986; Welch, 1986; Whorton, 1986; Paul and Himmelstein, 1988; Keleher, 1991; Giacoia, 1992; Figa-Talamanca and Hatch, 1994; Gold et al., 1994; Olshan and Mattison, 1994; Shepard, 1986). Occupational exposures to various solvents, pesticides, metals, feedstock chemicals, anaesthetic gases, cytotoxic chemicals and radiation have been associated with adverse reproductive outcomes [e.g. menstrual disorders, reduced fertility (male and female), poor semen quality] among workers. An overview is presented focusing on the effects of exposure on reproductive function, epidemiological findings, methods for the quantitative assessment of reproductive risks (methods for evaluating reproductive health), role of biomarkers in developmental and reproductive toxicology, and policy and regulatory issues related to reproductive hazards in the workplace.

The human reproductive system is highly complex, dynamic and interdependent on other organ systems such as the endocrine and, neural systems. In the male, germ cell production is continuous and, dependent on the stage of development, manifests varying degrees of susceptibility to toxicant-induced damage (e.g. stem cells less susceptible than maturing cells). In addition, one must consider the presence of a 'blood–testis' barrier, which blocks the passage of certain toxicants; however, some occupational and environmental pollutants are known to pass this barrier (e.g. some solvents, aromatic hydrocarbons and certain metals). The male reproductive system appears to be more vulnerable to xenobiotic-induced effects/damage than the female reproductive system (Figa-Talamanca and Hatch, 1994). However, Figa-Talamanca and Hatch also stressed that the prevailing view regarding reproductive function is that the ability to conceive is an attribute of the couple and that neither male nor female reproductive function is fully determinant. It should be stressed that the paternal role in abnormal reproductive outcomes is not simply related to insufficient numbers of viable sperm but in the following ways also: (1) genetic quality of male gametes is a critical determinant of the susceptibility and viability of the offspring *in utero* and after birth, (2) epigenetic changes in male gametes may be important to normal development, (3) the existence of prelesions in sperm and their repairability and (4) the father may be a source of exposure of toxicant (Wyrobek, 1994). Furthermore, the prevailing view that male-mediated developmental effects are less likely (Brown, 1985) is under challenge based on recent laboratory and epidemiological studies that reinforce previous animal data suggesting the importance of paternal exposure. Paternal occupational exposures have been associated with spontaneous abortion [e.g. anaesthetic gases, chloroprene, dibromochloropropane (DBCP), ethylene oxide and vinyl chloride and its structural analogue] (Lindbohm *et al.*, 1991; Figa-Talamanca and Hatch, 1994). Paternal exposures in the workplace have also been associated with childhood cancers [e.g. exposure to ionizing radiation and leukaemia (Sorahan and Roberts, 1993), exposure to certain hydrocarbons and leukaemia (Figa-Talmanca and Hatch, 1994), exposure to lead and Wilm's tumour (Kantor *et al.*, 1979) and exposure to aromatic hydrocarbons and Wilm's tumour (Roos *et al.*, 1992)]. Buckley (1994) has reviewed the reported linkages between paternal exposures to petroleum products and solvents and childhood cancer risk and discussed issues concerning the relative contributions of genetic and environmental factors in the aetiology of childhood cancers. In the female reproductive system, production of germ cells begins and ends prior to birth and the maturation process resumes only years later. In the female, chemicals may also interfere with reproductive processes (implantation and subsequent embryonic development). Pregnancy may enhance the woman's susceptibility to toxicants via a higher body burden of lipophilic compounds and also manifest effects in the developing conceptus and foetus. Animal and human studies have confirmed the presence and transfer through the placenta of occupational and environmental pollutants such as lead, mercury, polychlorinated biphenyls and disinfectants (Miller, 1983b). Furthermore, the altered physiology (e.g. increased ventilation) associated with pregnancy also contributes to an enhanced body burden of a chemical. Hence a pregnant woman may absorb more inhaled chemicals in the workplace.

Mechanisms of Reproductive Toxicity

Processes related to reproduction are complex and interdependent on other organ systems, particularly the neuroendocrine system for the regulation of gametogenesis, fertilization, implantation, embryogenesis, foetal growth and development. Perturbations can occur in any phase of the reproductive process, producing any number of deleterious outcomes (e.g. sperm reduction, altered sperm motility and morphology, disturbances in menstrual cycle, miscarriage, pre-term birth, low birth weight). Chemical-induced effects on reproduction can be direct or indirect (e.g. endocrine function disruption, hormonal feedback controls, glandular secretions, altered enzyme function and DNA repair mechanisms). Metals are considered direct-acting reproductive toxicants, whereas certain solvents and pesticides are categorized as indirect acting. Mechanisms of reproductive toxicity may be non-genetic, genetic or epigenetic. Generally, biochemical/molecular mechanisms of reproductive toxicity are not well understood and have been investigated for very few chemicals (Zenick, 1984).

Biomarkers in Developmental and Reproductive Toxicology

Biological markers are highly useful tools to toxicologists and epidemiologists. Numerous biomarkers have been developed and utilized successfully to quantify toxicant-induced changes in all organ systems across species from invertebrates to humans. Biomarkers are critical to the evaluation and understanding of chemically induced alterations/outcomes in developmental and reproductive processes. A number of years ago, the National Research Council (NRC) had identified biomarkers for the evaluation of reproductive toxicity (National Research Council, 1989). Specific methods for evaluating reproductive toxicity in the human male have been reviewed by Comhaire (1993) and the status of biological markers as related to assessment of male reproductive toxicity was reviewed by Wyrobek *et al.*, (1994). Biomarkers for evaluating reproductive toxicity in males include such end-points as sperm number, motility and structure, sperm penetration and interaction assays, physical characteristics of semen, chemical composition of semen, functional measures of Sertoli cells, Leydig cells, hormone levels, fertility ratio and histopathological analysis (testis). Wyrobek (1994) placed emphasis on various biomarkers that he referred to as 'bridging' biomarkers—biomarkers that enable one to make valid comparisons between human and animal responses and between *in vivo* and *in vitro* data.

Biological markers are highly useful in the evaluation of female reproductive function (e.g. ovarian function, pregnancy and foetal development) and in ascertaining outcomes resulting from physical and/or chemical exposures. Biological markers in relation to the identification and interpretation of female reproductive disorders have been reviewed by Stein and Hatch (1987). Of particular interest is the refinement and re-refinement of biomarker technology in order to enhance the specificity and sensitivity of the end-point measured. An example of this is the development and refinement of specific hormone assays such as the human chorionic gonadotropin (hCG) assay (Canfield et al., 1987). The objective was the development of an assay that would serve as a biomarker of pregnancy as well as of early foetal loss. Thus, an hCG assay has evolved from a bioassay to a sensitive enzyme immunoassay that would detect pregnancy before clinical signs (e.g. absent menstrual period) and also detect early foetal loss not detected by other procedures (e.g. radioimmunoassay). Longo (1987) reviewed technological developments in the evaluation of the foetus in utero and the development and application of biomarkers to assess physiologically foetal health and diagnosis of abnormalities and also issues such as foetal blood and tissue sampling. Promising biomarkers to assess foetal development and health include molecular probes (e.g. DNA probes) and techniques designed to measure foetal physiology (e.g. foetal breathing activity).

Occupational Hazards: Female Reproductive Processes

Many chemical and physical agents have been demonstrated to cause reproductive disorders in women exposed to pollutants in the workplace or environment. Reproductive disorders in women have resulted from occupational exposure to a wide array of chemical and physical agents [e.g. anaesthetic gases, antibiotics, solvents, industrial chemicals (see **Table 3**)]. Effects include perturbations in reproductive function, fecundity, fertility, foetal development/morphology and deleterious outcomes in offspring. Exposures in the post-conception period can result in deleterious effects on the offspring from early foetal death, prematurity, maldevelopment, congenital defects and tumours in childhood. (It should again be emphasized that developmental effects may have their aetiology as a result of occupational exposure to the father.) Generally, reproductive end-points in women include (1) menstrual function (e.g. cycle characteristics, ovulation, luteal adequacy), (2) fecundity (capacity for fertilization and implantation) and (3) fertility (development of viable offspring).

Menstrual disorders have been associated with occupational exposures to alkylating agents, chlorinated hydrocarbons, heavy metals, pesticides, radiation, synthetic hormones and other compounds (Mattison, 1985; Gold and Tomich, 1994). The association between workplace exposures and spontaneous abortion has been critically reviewed (Gold and Tomich, 1994). Occupational settings have been studied for potential risk for spontaneous abortion and linkage between exposure and spontaneous abortion was demonstrated for metals (lead and mercury) and ionizing radiation (McDonald et al., 1987; Taskinen, 1990; Figa-Talamanca and Hatch, 1994). Low

birth weights and prematurity (preterm births) as negative reproductive outcomes in relation to the work environment have also been examined. Stressors, in particular physical tasks/ergonomic factors, have been studied in relation to occupationally related causes of such outcomes and ways to identify such outcomes (Mamelle and Munoz, 1987; Axelsson et al., 1989; Hatch and Stein, 1990; Marbury, 1992; Gold and Tomich, 1994). Malformations have been shown to be related, although not consistently so, to occupational exposures. Positive associations were found for overall birth defect rates. Exposure to chemicals in industrial settings suggest an increased risk of malformations (e.g. cleft lip, cleft palate, defects involving the central nervous system, cardiac anomalies and gut atresia). The development of childhood tumours as the result of occupational exposure of one or both parents to a pollutant is of great concern to occupational health and regulatory communities. Childhood tumours may in some cases be due to workplace exposure of the mother to carcinogens. Leukaemia, the most common of childhood cancers, has been linked to the occupational exposure of parents. Carcinogens have been demonstrated to cross the placental barrier and produce cancer in the offspring of experimental animals (Miller, 1983b). A proven human transplacental carcinogen is diethylstilboestrol. Cancer-causing agents have been found in umbilical cord and in foetal tissues—DNA adducts are found in spontaneously aborted embryos (Hatch et al., 1990). Although epidemiological data for the potential association between occupational exposure and childhood tumours is at present inconclusive, the occupational setting cannot be excluded as an aetiological factor in certain childhood tumours. Epidemiological investigations of childhood cancers affords the prospect of a greater understanding of the carcinogenic process as applied to both adults and children.

Methods for Evaluation of Reproductive Health in Women

Strategies for the evaluation of the reproductive well being of the female and assessment of the consequences from exposure to chemical and physical stressors originate from either a clinical or non-clinical perspective. Many of the events related to female productive health occur without the awareness of women or the health care practitioner. Some type of biological sampling is necessary in order to evaluate the reproductive function and/or perturbations of in an accurate manner. Various end-points (e.g. ovulation, implantation, luteal function) can only be evaluated via the examination of tissue or hormone assays of blood or urine. Procedures in the clinic are not practical and/or ethical in large field studies, yet there is a need to develop strategies to evaluate the reproductive health status of women outside the clinic. Lasley and Shideler (1994), in their overview of approaches towards the assessment of female reproductive health, focused on the utilization of urine assays in the assessment of female reproductive health. The following methodologies were addressed by Lasley and Shideler as to practicality, utility and advantages over other bioassays: (1) urinary assays to detect early foetal loss, (2) urinary assays to assay ovarian function, (3) urinalysis for hormone metabolites and (4) urinary assays to assess pituitary function

Occupational Hazards: Male Reproductive Processes

Male reproductive toxicants can be identified using the following approaches: (1) clinical observations, (2) population studies, (3) epidemiological studies, (4) hormonal studies and (5) semen studies. Reproductive endpoints in the male include disturbances in sexual behaviour (e.g. potency and libido), which are generally difficult to assess, and measures of fecundity (e.g. spermatogenesis and semen quality). Research on the effects of chemicals on the male reproductive system in an occupational setting was established in the mid-1970s when Lancranjan *et al.* (1975) studied lead-exposed workers. One of the early documented workplace exposures affecting the male reproductive system was that of Whorton *et al.* (1977) that related exposure to the pesticide dibromochloropropane (DBCP) and reproductive toxicity. The initial findings by Whorton *et al.* (1977) were confirmed in other manufacturing plants (Whorton and Foliart, 1983). Follow-up of DBCP-exposed workers indicated that DBCP may permanently impair spermatogenesis (Eaton *et al.*, 1986; Potashnik and Yanai-Inbar, 1987). The study by Whorton *et al* focused attention on the effects of pesticides and other agriculture chemicals on the male reproductive system [ethylene dibromide (Wong *et al.*, 1979); carbaryl (Whorton *et al.*, 1979; Wyrobek *et al.*, 1981)]. A partial listing of chemical and physical agents encountered in an occupational setting that are associated with reproductive effects in the male is presented in **Table 3**.

To a very large extent, if animal studies have indicated that a compound is a reproductive toxicant, such studies form the basis for epidemiological and occupational research studies. As indicated previously, concluding that an association exists between male reproducive toxicants in the workplace may be identified by a number of approaches. A brief overview of how these various approaches contribute to the identification of toxicants with potential to elicit adverse reproductive effects is presented. Clinical (case) studies involve the reports by an occupational physician of worker(s) exposed to potentially toxic compounds. Although such studies may provide unique information not provided by other methodologies, such results usually serve as sentinel

Table 3 Partial listing of chemical and physical agents in the workplace that are associated with reproductive effects

Males	Females
Chemical agents	**Chemical agents**
Anaesthetic gases	Acetone
Cadmium	Anaesthetic gases
Carbaryl	Antibiotics
Dibromochloropropane	Antineoplastic agents
Ethylene dibromate	Benzene
Glycol ethers	Carbon monoxide
Lead	Ethylene oxide
Manganese	Formaldehyde
Mercury	Hydrocarbons
Perchloroethylene	Glycol ethers
Vinyl chloride	Lead
	Mercury
	Nitrous oxide
	Perchloroethylene
	Trichloroethylene
	Toluene
	Vinyl chloride
Physical agents	**Physical agents**
Electromagnetic field (EMF)	Electromagnetic field (EMF)
Elevated temperatures	Ionizing radiation
Ionizing radiation	Strenuous work

reports that initiate further studies. Epidemiological approaches to identifying reproductive hazards in the workplace include the following study designs: (1) population-based studies, (2) case-control studies and (3) cohort studies. Population-based studies link job category with reproductive outcome(s); this type of study is widely conducted in European countries where work history is a component of medical records. Such studies, however, are problematic since they preclude control for confounding factors. Case-control studies involve the comparison of workers with toxic exposure manifesting reproductive effects with those without such history. However, studies of this design may result in misleading results because of bias. Cohort studies evaluate the frequency of adverse reproductive outcome(s) between exposed and unexposed groups. Cohort studies are highly useful and involve questionnaires, semen analyses, neuroendocrine measurements, or a combination of these. Olshan and Schnitzer (1994) have extensively reviewed the epidemiological literature pertaining to paternal occupations and developmental effects, concluding that an association exists between developmental effects and workplace exposures to pesticides, solvents, metals and wood/wood products. Occupations and related exposures that warrant additional studies include textile workers, painters, forestry and logging workers, welders and electrical/electronics workers.

Male infertility—progressive decrease in the density of human sperm—is an emerging health problem (Carlsen *et al.*, 1992). Semen analysis is the primary source of information utilized in assessing male reproductive ability. Semen analysis provides information on spermatogenesis, sperm cell motility, sperm capability in penetrating and fertilizing the ovum and integrity of accessory sex glands. The effects of numerous chemical agents singly or in combination have been evaluated by analysis of human semen (Wyrobek *et al.*, 1983). A large number of sperm evaluation studies on workers exposed to various industrial chemicals (e.g. boric acid, cadmium, carbon disulphide, ethylene dibromide, glycol ethers, lead, manganese, mercury, thallium, vinyl chloride) have been conducted. Exposure to lead has been studied most frequently and damage to male reproduction has been demonstrated repeatedly. Welch *et al.* (1988) examined the effects of vinyl chloride and glycol ethers on sperm viability. Perturbations in semen quality in workers exposed to ethylene dibromide have also been reported (Ratcliffe *et al.*, 1987, 1989). Other avenues (e.g. endocrine status/hormone levels) are available to detect perturbations in male reproductive function related to occupational exposures (Schrader, 1992). Assay of endocrine status is highly useful, but unfortunately this approach is very much underutilized.

Regulatory and Policy Issues Related to Reproductive Hazards in the Workplace

Federal legislation protecting reproductive health in the workplace include the Occupational Safety and Health Act (OSHAct), the Toxic Substances Control Act (TSCA) and the Federal Insecticide, Fungicide and Rodenticide Act (FIFRA). Specialized policies, programmes, and animal tests protocols are in various stages of development to address concerns related to the assessment of reproductive toxicity. The US EPA has recently published guidelines for reproductive risk assessment (US Environmental Protection Agency, 1994). Developmental neurotoxicity guidelines have been developed for evaluating neural system damage in offspring (US Environmental Protection Agency, 1991). Within the regulatory framework, occupational health programmes related to ensuring the reproductive health of the worker requires an interdisciplinary approach with input from epidemiologists, toxicologists, occupational health physicians and industrial hygiene specialists. The issues concerning reproductive health in the workplace are very complex not only in terms of technical aspects but also in terms of economic demands, political concerns, and legal and social issues (e.g. compliance with the federal Pregnancy Discrimination Act of 1978; corporate/company policies in the workplace). Paul *et al.* (1989) examined workplace policies (corporate response) to reproductive hazards in occupational settings. As described by Saiki *et al.* (1994), elements of workplace policy as related to reproductive hazards include hazard definition, exposure assessment, hazard minimization, notification and training and

worksite modification, transfer or reassignment. Implementation of company policies may give rise to conflicts and complications. Giacoia (1992) indicated that social and corporate policies concerning reproductive hazards need to focus on eliminating hazards as contrasted to removing workers. Considerable efforts are needed to enhance our knowledge concerning reproductive hazards, in communicating information pertaining to reproductive hazards in the workplace, compliance with regulatory policies, compliance with legislation and effective and reasonable workplace policies. The processes will continue to evolve as many issues related to reproductive health in the workplace have yet to be resolved.

REFERENCES

Ahmed, F. E. (1995a). Applications of molecular biology to biomedicine and toxicology. *Environ. Carcinog. Ecotoxicol. Rev.*, **C13**, 1–51.

Ahmed, F. E. (1995b). Molecular biology as a mechanistic tool in occupational, diagnostic, and forensic medicine. *Int. J. Occup. Med. Toxicol.*, **4**, 433–452.

Alexanderson, R. and Hedenstierna, G. (1989). Pulmonary function in wood workers exposed to formaldehyde—a prospective study. *Arch. Environ. Health*, **44**, 571–575.

Austin, H., Keil, J. E. and Cole, P. (1989). A prospective follow-up study of cancer mortality in relation to serum DDT. *Am. J. Publ. Health*, **79**, 43–46.

Axelson, O. (1994). Some recent developments in occupational epidemiology. *Scand. J. Work. Environ. Health*, **20**, 9–18.

Axelson, O. and Soderkvist, P. (1991). Characteristics of disease and some exposure considerations. *Appl. Occup. Environ. Hyg.*, **6**, 428–435.

Axelsson, G., Rylander, R. and Molin, I. (1989). Outcome of pregnancy in relation to irregular and inconvenient work schedules. *Br. J. Ind. Med.*, **46**, 393–398.

Baird, D. D. and Wilcox, A. J. (1986). Effects of occupational exposures on fertility of couples. *Occup. Med. State Art Rev.*, **1**, 361–374.

Balcarova, O. and Halik, J. (1991). Ten-year epidemiological study of ischaemic heart disease (IHD) in workers exposed to carbon disulphide. *Sci. Total Environ.*, **101**, 97–99.

Bang, K. M. (1996). Applications of occupational epidemiology. *Occup. Med. State Art Rev.*, **11**, 381–392.

Bertazzi, P., Pesatori, A. C. Radice, L., *et al.* (1986). Exposure to formaldehyde and cancer mortality in a cohort of workers producing resins. *Scand. J. Work Environ. Health*, **12**, 461–468.

Blair, A., Stewart, P. A., and Hoover, R. N. (1990). Mortality from lung cancer among workers employed in formaldehyde industries. *Am. J. Ind. Med.*, **17**, 683–699.

Boewer, C. Enderlein, G. and Wollgase, U., *et al.* (1988). Epidemiological study on the hepatoxicity of occupational toluene exposure. *Int. Arch. Occup. Environ. Health*, **60**, 181–186.

Brandt-Rauf, P. W. (1988). New markers for monitoring occupational cancer. The example of oncogene proteins. *J. Occup. Med.*, **5**, 399–404.

Breslow, N. E., Lubin, J. H., Marek, P. and Langhotz, B. (1983). Multiplicative models and cohort analysis. *J. Am. Stat. Assoc.*, **78**, 1–12

Brown, N. A. (1985). Are offspring at risk from their father's exposure to toxins? *Nature*, **316**, 110.

Buckley, J. (1994). Male-mediated developmental toxicity: paternal exposures and childhood cancer. In Olshan, A. F. and Mattison, D. R. (Eds), *Male-Mediated Developmental Toxicity*. Plenum Press, New York, pp. 169–176.

Calleman, C. J., Ehrenberg, L., Jansson, B., Osterman-Golkar, S., Segerback, D., Svensson, K. and Wachtmeister, C. A. (1978). Monitoring and risk assessment by means of alkyl groups in hemoglobin in persons occupationally exposed to ethylene oxide. *J. Environ. Pathol. Toxicol.*, **2**, 427–442.

Canfield, R. E., O'Connor, J. F., Birken, S., Krichevsky, A. and Wilcox, A. J. (1987). Development of an assay for a biomarker of pregnancy and early fetal loss. *Environ. Health Perspect.*, **74**, 57–66.

Carlsen, E., Giwercman, A., Keiding, N. and Skakkebaek, N. E. (1992). Evidence for decreasing quality of semen during the past 50 years. *Br. Med. J.*, **305**, 609–613.

Chalmers, T. C. (1991). Problems induced by meta-analysis. *Stat. Methods*, **10**, 971–980.

Chang, L. W., Hsia, S. M., Chan, P., and Hsieh, L. L. (1994). Macromolecular adducts: biomarkers for toxicity and carcinogenesis. *Annu. Rev. Pharmacol. Toxicol.*, **34**, 41–67.

Comhaire, F. H. (1993). Methods to evaluate reproductive health in the human male. *Reproductive Toxicol.*, **Vol. 7**. Suppl. 1, S39–S46.

Davis, M. E. and Berndt, W. O. (1994). Renal methods for toxicology. In Hayes, A. W. (Ed.), *Principles and Methods of Toxicology*, 3rd edn. Raven Press, New York, pp. 871–894.

Demain, A. L. (1991). An overview of biotechnology. *Occup. Med. State Art Rev.*, **6**, 157–168.

Eaton, M., Schenker, M. G., Whorton, M., *et al.* (1986). Seven-year follow-up of workers exposed to 1,2-dibromo-3-chloropropane. *J. Occup. Med.*, **28**, 1145–1150.

Eisen, E. A., Tolbert, P. E., Hallock, M. F., *et al.* (1994). Mortality studies of machining fluid exposure in the automobile industry III. A case-control study of larynx cancer. *Am. J. Ind. Med.*, **26**, 185–202.

Farmer, P. B. and Bailey, E. (1989). Protein-carcinogen adducts in human dosimetry. *Arch. Toxicol.*, **13**, Suppl., 83–90.

Figa-Talamanca, I. (1984). Spontaneous abortion among female industrial workers. *Intl. Arch. Occup. Environ. Hlth.*, **54**, 163–171.

Figa-Talamanca, I. and Hatch, M. C. (1994). Reproduction and the workplace: what we know and where we go from here. *Int. J. Occup. Med. Toxicol.*, **3**, 279–303.

Foa, V., Emmett, E. A., Maroni, M. and Colomi, A. (1987). *Occupational and Environmental Chemical Hazards. Cellular and Biochemical Indices for Monitoring Toxicity*. Wiley, New York.

Foulkes, E. C. (1993). Functional assessment of the kidney. In Hook, J. B. and Goldstein, R. S. (Eds), *Toxicology of the Kidney*, 2nd edn. Raven Press, New York, pp. 37–60.

Giacoia, G. P. (1992). Reproductive hazards in the workplace. *Obstet. Gynecol. Surv.*, **47**, 679–687.

Gold, E. B. and Tomich, E. (1994). Occupational hazards to fertility and pregnancy outcome. *Occup. Med. State Art Rev.*, **9**, 435–470.

Gold, E. B., Lasley, B. L. and Schenker, M. B. (Eds) (1994). *Reproductive Hazards, Occupational Medicine. State of the Art Reviews*, Vol. 9, No. 3. Hanley and Belfus, Philadelphia, PA.

Greenblatt, M. S., Bennett, W. P., Hollstein, M. *et al.* (1994). Mutations in the p53 tumor suppresser gene: clues to cancer etiology and pathogenesis. *Cancer Res.*, **54**, 4855–4878.

Harrington, J. M., Stein, G. F., Rivers, R. V. and DeMorales, A. V. (1978). The occupational hazards of formulating oral contraceptives: a survey of plant employees. *Arch. Environ. Health*, **33**, 12–14.

Hatch, M. C. and Stein, Z. A. (1990). Work and exercise during pregnancy: epidemiologic studies. In Artal, R., Wisewell, R. and Drinkwater, B. (Eds), *Exercise and Pregnancy*, 2nd edn. Williams and Wilkins, Barltimore, pp. 279–288.

Hatch, M. C., Warburton, D. and Santella, R. M. (1990). Polycyclic aromatic hydrocarbon–DNA adducts in spontaneously aborted fetal tissue. *Carcinogenesis*, **11**, 1673–1675.

Hedges, L. V. and Olkin, I. (1985). *Statistical Methods for Meta-Analysis*. Academic Press, San Diego.

Hemminki, K. (1992). Use of molecular biology techniques in cancer epidemiology. *Scand. J. Work Environ. Health*, **18**, Suppl. 1, 38–45.

Higginson, J. (1967). The role of the pathologist in environmental medicine and public health. *Am. J. Pathol.*, **86**, 460.

Kachmar, J. F. and Moss, D. W. (1976). Enzymes. In Tietz, N. W. (Ed.), *Fundamentals in Clinical Chemistry*. W. B. Saunders, Philadelphia, PA, pp. 652–660.

Kantor, A. F., McCrea-Curnen, M. G., Meigs, J. W. and Flannery, J. T. (1979). Occupations of fathers of patients with Wilm's tumor. *J. Epidemiol. Commun. Health.*, **33**, 253–256.

Katz, S. and Salem, H. (1993). The toxicology of chromium with respect to its chemical speciation: a review. *J. Appl. Toxicol.*, **13**, 217–224.

Keleher, K. C. (1991). Occupational health: how work environments can affect reproductive capacity and outcome. *Nurse Pract.*, **16**, 23–37.

Kingsbury, D. T. (1987). DNA probes in the diagnosis of genetic and infectious diseases. *Trends Biotechnol.*, **5**, 107–111.

Labbe, K. A., Detsky, A. S. and Orourke, K. (1987). Meta-analysis in clinical research. *Ann. Intern. Med.*, **107**, 224–233.

Lancranjan, I., Popescu, H. I., Gavanescu, O., *et al.* (1975). Reproductive ability of workmen occupationally exposed to lead. *Arch. Environ. Health.*, **30**, 396–401.

Lasley, B. L. and Shideler, S. E. (1994) Methods for evaluating reproductive health of women. *Occup. Med. State Art Rev.*, **9**, 423–433.

Last, J. M. (1995). *A Dictionary of Epidemiology*, 3rd edn. Oxford University Press, Oxford.

LeQuesne, P. M. (1980). Acrylamide. In Spencer, P. H. and Schaumburg, H. A. (Eds), *Experimental and Clinical Neurotoxicology*. Williams and Wilkins, Baltimore, pp. 309–325.

Liberman, D. F., Israeli, E. and Fink, R. (1991). Risk assessment of biological hazards in the biotechnology industry. *Occup. Med. State Art Rev.*, **6**, 285.

Lindbohm, M. L., Hemminki, K., Bonhomme, M. G., Anttila, A., Rantala, K., Heikkila, P., and Rosenberg, M. J. (1991). Effects of paternal occupational exposure on spontaneous abortion. *Am. J., Publ. Health.*, **81**, 1029–1033.

Longo, L. D. (1987). Physiologic assessment of fetal compromise: biomarkers of toxic exposure. *Environ. Health Perspect.*, **74**, 93–101.

Lower, G. M., Jr, Nilsson, T., Nelson, C. E., *et al.* (1979). N-Acetyltransferase phenotype and risk in urinary bladder cancer: approaches in molecular epidemiology. *Environ. Health Perspect.*, **29**, 71–79.

Maki-Paakkanen, J., Husgafud-Pursiainen, K., Kalliomaki, P. L., *et al.* (1980). Toluene-exposed workers and chromosome aberrations. *J. Toxicol Environ. Health*, **6**, 775–781.

Mamelle, N. and Munoz, F. (1987). Occupational working conditions and preterm birth: a reliable scoring system. *Am. J. Epidemiol.*, **126**, 150–152.

Marbury, M. C. (1992). Relationship of ergonomic stressors to birthweight and gestational age. *Scand. J. Work Environ. Health.*, **18**, 73–83.

Marx, J. (1991) Zeroing in on individual cancer risk. *Science*, **253**, 612–616.

Mattison, D. R. (1985). Clinical manifestations of ovarian toxicity. In Dixon, R. L. (Ed.), *Reproductive Toxicology*. Raven Press, New York, pp. 109–130.

McDiarmid, M. D. and Emmett, E. A. (1987). Biological monitoring and medical surveillance of workers exposed to antineoplastic agents. *Semin. Occup. Med.*, **2**, 109–117.

McDonald, A. D., McDonald, J. C., Armstrong, B., Cherry, N., Delorme, C., Nolin, A. D. and Robert, D. (1987). Occupation and pregnancy outcome. *Br. J. Ind. Med.*, **44**, 521–526.

Miller, H. (1983a). *Report on the World Health Organization Working Group on Health Implications of Biotechnology*. Rec. DNA Tech. Bull. 6, World Health Organization, Geneva, pp. 65–66.

Miller, R. K. (1983b). Perinatal toxicology: its recognition and fundamentals. *Am. J. Ind. Med.*, **4**, 205–244.

Mittleman, M. A., Maldonado, G., Gerberich, S. G., Smith, G. S., and Sorock, G. S. (1997). Alternative approaches to analytical designs in occupational injury epidemiology. *Am. J. Ind. Med.*, **32**, 129–141.

Munro. I. C. and Krewski, D. R. (1981). Risk assessment and regulatory decision making. *Food Cosmet. Toxicol.*, **19**, 549–560.

National Academy of Sciences (1983). *Risk Assessment in the Federal Government: Managing the Process*. National Academy Press, Washington, DC.

National Research Council/National Academy of Sciences (1989). *Biologic Markers of Reproductive Toxicology*. National Academy Press, Washington, DC.

Newton, R. W., Browning, M. K., Ingal, J., *et al.* (1978). Adrenal cortical suppression in workers manufacturing synthetic gluococorticoids. *Br. Med. J.*, **1**, 73–75.

Office of Technology Assessment (US Congress) (1984). *Commercial Biotechnology—an International Analysis*. Government Printing Office, Washington, DC.

Olshan, A. F. and Mattison, D. R. (Eds) (1994). *Male-Mediated Developmental Toxicity*. Plenum Press, New York.

Olshan, A. F. and Schnitzer, P. G. (1994). Paternal occupation and birth defects. In Olshan, A. F. and Mattison, D. R. (Eds), *Male-Mediated Developmental Toxicity*. Plenum Press, New York, pp. 153–167.

Pastides, H., Austin, R., Mundt, K. A., Ramsey, F. and Feger, N. (1994). Transforming industrial hygiene data for use in epidemiologic studies: a case study of hexavalent chromium. *J. Occup. Med. Toxicol.*, **3**, 57–71.

Paul, M. and Himmelstein, J. (1988). What the practitioner needs to know about chemical exposures. *Obstet. Gynecol.*, **71**, 921–938.

Paul, M., Daniels, C. and Rosofsky, R. (1989). Corporate response to reproductive hazards in the workplace: results of the family, work, and health survey. *Am. J. Ind. Med.*, **16**, 267–280.

Peoples-Sheps, M. D., Siegel, E., Suckindran, C. M., Origasa, H., Ware, A. and Barakat, A. (1991). Characteristics of maternal employment during pregnancy. Effects on low birthweight. *Am. J. Publ. Health.*, **81**, 1007–1012.

Pereira, M. A. and Chang, L. W. (1981). Binding of chemical carcinogens and mutagens to rat hemoglobin. *Chem.–Biol. Interact.*, **33**, 301–306.

Plaa, G. L. and Charbonneau, M. (1994). Detection and evaluation of chemically induced liver injury. In Hayes, A. W. (Ed.), *Principles and Methods of Toxicology*, 3rd edn. Raven Press, New York, pp. 839–870.

Potashnik, G. and Yanai-Inbar, I. (1987). Dibromochloropropane (DBCP): an 8-year reevaluation of testicular function and reproductive performance. *Fertil. Steril.*, **47**, 317–323.

Preuss, P. W. and Ehrlich, A. M. (1987). The environmental protection agency's risk assessment guidelines. *J. Air Pollut. Control Assoc.*, **37**, 784–791.

Ratcliffe, J. M., Schrader, S. M., Steenland, K., *et al.* (1987). Semen quality in papaya workers with long-term exposure to ethylene dibromide. *Br. J. Ind. Med.*, **44**, 317–326.

Ratcliffe, J. M., Schrader, S. M., Clapp, D. E., *et al.*, (1989). Semen quality in workers exposed to 2-ethoxyethanol. *Br. J. Ind. Med.*, **46**, 399–406.

Roberts, L. (1990). L-Tryptophan puzzle takes a new twist. *Science*, **249**, 988.

Rodricks, J. V., Brett, S. M. and Wrenn, G. C. (1987). Significant risk decisions in federal regulatory agencies. *Regul. Toxicol. Pharmacol.*, **7**, 307–320.

Roos, S. D., Buckley, J. D., Ruccione, K., Sather, H. N., Waskerwitz, M. J., Woods, W. G. and Bunin, G. R. (1992). Paternal occupational risk factors for Wilm's tumor. Presented at the International Conference of Male-mediated Developmental Toxicity, University of Pittsburgh Medical Center, Graduate School of Public Health, September 16–19, 1992.

Sacks, S. T. and Schenker, M. B. (1990) Biostatistics and epidemiology. In LaDou, J. (Ed.), *Occupational Medicine*. Appleton and Lange, Norwalk, CT, pp. 534–554.

Saiki, C. L., Gold, E. B. and Schenker, M. B. (1994) Workplace policy on hazards to reproductive health. *Occup. Med. State Art Rev.*, **9**, 541–550.

Sanjose, S., Roman, E. and Beral, V. (1991). Low birth weight and preterm delivery, Scotland, 1981–1984: effect of parents' occupation., *Lancet*, **338**, 428–431.

Savitz, D. A., Whelan, E. A. and Klecker, R. C. (1989). Effect of parents' occupational exposures on risk of stillbirth, preterm delivery, and small-for-gestational-age infants. *Am. J. Epidemiol.*, **129**, 1201–1218.

Schlesselman, J. J. (1982). *Case-Control Studies: Design, Conduct, Analysis*. Oxford University Press, New York.

Schrader, S. M. (1992). Data gaps and new methodologies in the assessment of male fecundity in occupational field studies. *Scand. J. Work Environ. Health.*, **18**, Suppl. 2, 30–32.

Schreg, S.D. and Dixon, L. (1985). Occupational exposures associated with male reproductive dysfunction. *Am. Rev. Pharmacol. and Toxicol.*, **25**, 567–592.

Schulte, P. A. and Perera, F. P. (1993). *Molecular Epidemiology*. Academic Press, New York.

Senthilselvan, A., McDufie, H. H. and Dosman, J. A. (1992). Association of asthma with use of pesticides: results of a cross-sectional survey of farmers. *Am. Rev. Respir. Dis.*, **146**, 884–887

Shepard, T. H. (1986). *Catalog of Teratogenic Agents*, 5th edn. Johns Hopkins, Baltimore, MD.

Skipper, P. L. and Tannenbaum, S. R. (1990). Protein adducts in the molecular dosimetry of chemical carcinogens. *Carcinogenesis*, **11**, 507–518.

Smith, A. H., Lopipero, P. A. and Barroga, V. R. (1995). Meta-analysis for studies of lung cancer among silicotics. *Epidemiology*, **6**, 617–624.

Sorahan, T. and Roberts, P. J. (1993). Childhood cancer and paternal exposure to ionizing radiation: preliminary findings from the Oxford survey of childhood cancers. *Am. J. Ind. Med.*, **23**, 343–353.

Stegeman, J. J., Brouwer, M., Digiulio, R. T., Forlin, L., Fowler, B. A., Sanders, B. M. and Van Veld, P. A. (1992). In Huggett, R. J., Kimerele, R. A., Mehrle, P. M. and Bergman, H. L. (Eds), *Biomarkers: Biochemical, Physiological, and Histological Markers of Anthropogenic Stress*. Lewis, Boca Raton, FL, pp. 235–335.

Stein, Z. and Hatch, M. (1987). Biological markers in reproductive epidemiology: prospects and precautions. *Environ. Health. Perspect.*, **74**, 67–75.

Stonard, M. D. and Evans, G. O. (1994). Clinical chemistry. In Ballantyne, B., Marrs, T. and Turner, P. (Eds), *General and Applied Toxicology, 1st edn*. Macmillan, Basingstoke and Stockton Press, New York, pp. 303–332.

Tarloff, J. B. and Goldstein, R. S. (1994). *In vitro* assessment of nephrotoxicity. In Gad, S. C. (Ed.), *In Vitro Toxicology*. Raven Press, New York, pp. 149–193.

Taskinen, H. (1990). Occupational risks of spontaneous abortion and congenital malformation. *Acta Univ. Tamper., Ser. A*, **289**. Unversity of Tampere.

Taylor, J. A., Sandler, D. P., Bloomfield, C. D., *et al.*, (1992). Ras oncogene activation and occupational exposure in acute myeloid leukemia. *J. Natl. Cancer Inst.*, **84**, 1626–1632

US Environmental Protection Agency (1991). Pesticide Assessment Guidelines—Subdivision F—Hazard Evaluation: Human and Domestic Animals. Addendum 10: Neurotoxicity. Series 83-A, Developmental Neurotoxicity Study. *EPA Document 540/090910123*. Department of Commerce, National Toxicology Information Service, Springfield, VA.

US Environmental Protection Agency (1994). Draft Guidelines for Reproductive Toxicity Risk Assessment. *EPA/600/AP-94/001*. Washington, DC.

US Public Health Service, National Institutes of Health (1974). *Biohazards Safety Guidelines*. NIH, Bethesda, MD.

US Public Health Service, National Institutes of Health (1976). Guidelines for Research Involving Recombinant DNA Activity. *Fed. Regist.*, **41**, 27902.

US Public Health Service, National Institutes of Health (1983). Guidelines for Research Involving Recombinant DNA Activity. *Fed. Regist.*, **48**, 24555–24581.

US Public Health Service, National Institutes of Health (1994). Guidelines for Research Involving Recombinant DNA Activity, *Federal Register*, July 5, **Vol 59** (127), 34343–34552.

Waxweiler, K. J., Stringer, W., Wagoner, J. K., and Jane, J. (1976). Neoplastic risk among workers exposed to vinyl chloride. *Ann. NY Acad. Sci.*, **271**, 40–46.

Wegman, D. H. (1982). Accelerated loss of Fev_1 in polyurethane production workers: a four year prospective study. *Am. J. Ind. Med.*, **3**, 209–215.

Welch, L. S. (1986). Decision making about reproductive hazards. *Semin. Occup. Med.*, **1**, 97–106.

Welch, L. S., Schrader, S. M., Turner, T. W. and Cullen, M. R. (1988). Effects of exposure to ethylene glycol ethers on shipyard painters: II male reproduction. *Am. J. Ind. Med.*, **14**, 509–526.

Whorton, M. D. (1986). Male reproductive hazards. *Occup. Med. State Art Rev.*, **1**, 375–379.

Whorton, M. D. and Foliart, D. E. (1983). Mutagenicity, carcinogenicity, and reproductive effects of DBCP. *Mutat. Res.*, **123**, 13–30.

Whorton, M. D., Krauss, R. M., Marshall, S. and Milby, T. H. (1977). Infertility in male pesticide workers. *Lancet*, **ii**, 1259–1261.

Whorton, M. D., Milby, T. H., Stubbs, H. A., *et al.* (1979). Testicular function among carbaryl-exposed employees. *J. Toxicol. Environ. Health.*, **5**, 929–941

Wong, O., Utidijian, H. M. D., and Kaaraten, V. S. (1979). Retrospective evaluation of reproductive performance of workers exposed to ethylene dibromide (EDB). *J. Occup. Med.*, **21**, 98–102.

World Health Organization (WHO) (1987). *Cell Products Safety, Commission on the Development of Biological Standards, (Bulletin 68)*. Karger, Basle, p. 81.

Wyrobek, A. J. (1994). Methods and concepts in detecting abnormal reproductive outcomes of paternal origin. In Olshan, A. F. and Mattison, D. R. (Eds), *Male-Mediated Developmental Toxicity*. Plenum Press, New York, pp. 1–21.

Wyrobek, A. J., Watchmaker, G., Gordon, L., *et al.* (1981). Sperm shape abnormalities in carbaryl-exposed employees. *Environ. Health. Perspect.*, **40**, 225–265.

Wyrobek, A. J., Gordon, L. A., Burkhart, J. G., Francis, M. C., Kapp, R. W., *et al.* (1983). An evaluation of human sperm as indicators of chemically-induced alterations of spermatogenic function. A report for the U.S. Environmental Protection Agency Gene-Tox Program. *Mutat. Res.*, **115**, 73–148.

Wyrobek, A. J., Anderson, D., Lewis, S., Nagao, T., Perreault, B. and Schrader, S. (1994). Biomarkers and health end points of developmental toxicology of paternal origin: summary of working group discussions. In Olshan, A. F. and Mattison, D. R. (Eds), *Male-Mediated Developmental Toxicity*. Plenum Press, New York, pp. 359–370.

Zenick, H. (1984). Mechanisms of environmental agents by class associated with adverse male reproductive outcomes.

In Lockey, J. E., LeMasters, G. K. and Keye, W. R., Jr (Eds), *Reproduction: the New Frontier in Occupational and Environmental Health Research*. Alan R. Liss, New York, pp. 335–361.

FURTHER READING

Ashford, N. A., Spadafor, C. J., Hattis, D. B. and Caldart, C.C. (1990). *Monitoring the Worker for Exposure and Disease*. Johns Hopkins University Press, Baltimore and London.

Greenberg, M. I., Hamilton, R. J. and Phillips, S. D. (Eds.) (1997). *Occupational, Industrial, and Environmental Toxicology*. Mosby Year Book Inc., St. Louis, Missouri.

Hathway, G. J., Proctor, N. H. and Hughes, J. P. (1996). *Proctor & Hughes' Chemical Hazards of the Workplace, 4th edn*. Van Nostrand Reinhold, New York.

Howard, J. K. and Tyrer, F. H. (Eds.) (1987). *Textbook of Occupational Medicine*. Churchill Livingstone, Edinburgh.

Lauwerys, R. R. and Hoet, P. (1993). *Industrial Chemical Exposure, Guidelines for Biological Monitoring. 2nd edn*. Lewis Publishers, Boca Raton, FL.

McCunney, R. J. (1994). *A Practical Approach to Occupational and Environmental Medicine. 2nd edn*. Little, Brown and Company, Boston.

Mendelsohn, M. L., Peeters, J. P. and Normandy, M. J. (Eds.) (1995). *Biomarkers and Occupational Health. Progress and Perspectives*. Joseph Henry Press, Washington, D.C.

Raffle, P. A. B., Adams, P. H., Baxter, P. J. and Lee, W. R, (Eds.) (1994). *Hunter's Diseases of Occupations. 8th edn*. Edward Arnold, London.

Rom, W. N. (Ed.) (1992). *Environmental and Occupational Medicine*. Little, Brown and Company, Boston.

Zenz, C., Dickerson, O. B. and Horvath, E. P, Jr. (Eds.) (1994). *Occupational Medicine*. Mosby, St. Louis, Baltimore.

Chapter 67
Industrial Toxicology and Hygiene

Steven Fairhurst

CONTENTS

BASIC FEATURES

Toxicology that focuses on the hazardous properties of chemicals encountered at work and the risks of these properties being manifested under working conditions is known as occupational (in Europe) or industrial (in USA) toxicology. The discipline has important interactions with occupational or industrial hygiene which, in relation to chemicals, addresses the exposure conditions created during the manufacture and use of chemicals and the potential means of controlling and protecting against exposure. The manner in which the two disciplines interact is brought out by considering the familiar 'risk assessment paradigm' (**Figure 1**). Toxicology deals with the assessment of toxicological hazards and the risks of expression of such hazards under defined exposure conditions. Occupational or industrial hygiene deals with exposure assessment, defining what exposure conditions could or will be encountered at work and with many of the technical and practical issues arising in considering appropriate risk management measures. In this context, the shared aim of both specialisms is to develop a sound scientific and technical basis for good standards of health and effective and appropriate control measures in the workplace. Other disciplines, particularly occupational medicine but also epidemiology, chemistry and engineering, also have made and will continue to make substantial contributions to achieving this goal.

Almost every chemical substance involved in modern society has an occupational exposure context and hence potentially falls under the scrutiny of industrial toxicology and hygiene. Beyond the vast array of chemicals, such as reactants in synthetic processes, solvents, metals, oils, coatings, colourants and polymers, and the manufacturing and use situations in which they arise, conventionally thought of as 'industrial', there are other occupational exposure situations that should not be forgotten. Pharmaceuticals are made, formulated and even used by people in their work. Foods are processed, additives are added and cooking is done in an occupational context. Pesticides are made, formulated and applied by workers. Overall, there are tens of thousands of substances present in the occupational environment of most industrialized countries.

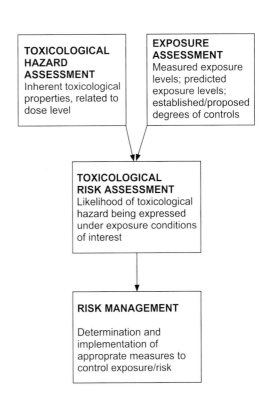

Figure 1 The risk assessment paradigm.

For most chemical substances the workplace is the situation where there is the potential for heavier exposure than in other sectors of human life. The two modes of exposure of primary interest in the workplace are inhalation of the airborne substance and surface (skin, eyes) contact with the substance. Ingestion can also be an issue, arising from contamination of material entering the mouth (food, drink, cigarettes), poor personal hygiene (hand-to-mouth transfer of chemicals) or swallowing of mucous containing inhaled substance being cleared from the respiratory tract by the mucociliary escalator.

The occupational environment holds several exposure possibilities—single short-term exposure under controlled (i.e. intended) conditions, single short-term exposure under uncontrolled (i.e. spillage, accident) conditions, occasional but repeated exposure, regular daily exposure under controlled conditions and combinations of these. Exposure concentrations and time periods will fluctuate and exposure can also occur via more than one route. The industrial hygienist needs to give consideration to all of these aspects in making exposure assessments and contemplating control measures. The industrial toxicologist needs to consider all exposure scenarios and their potential impact on health in order to gain a full appreciation of the risks of ill-health arising from encountering a substance at work.

A particular feature of occupational toxicology is the consideration of site-of-contact effects. This can be a problem, in that much conventional toxicology has been and continues to be performed using the oral (and sometimes parenteral) route(s). Alongside the possibilities arising from the absorption, distribution around the body and metabolism (to more or less toxic derivatives) of a substance, significant occupational toxicology concern surrounds the local consequences of inhalation or skin/eye contact at and around the initial point of impact. Sensory irritation (nerve stimulation), tissue inflammation and damage, sensitization, mutation and cancer can arise in the lung or skin as a result of direct exposure to some reactive industrial chemicals or their locally produced metabolites. Additionally, pH effects and particle effects in the lungs (some related more to the physical than the chemical properties of a substance) are important considerations for local toxicity.

HISTORICAL DEVELOPMENT

Observation of the adverse effects on health of occupational exposure to chemicals has a long history; brief allusions can be found in texts from ancient Greece and Rome. The classical early founders of toxicology from the sixteenth century, Paracelsus (Philippus Aureolus Theophrastus Bombastus von Hohenheim) and Georgius Agricola (Georg Bauer) documented severe occupationally induced toxicity among workers in mining and metallurgy. The contributions of other prominent historical figures followed: Bernardino Ramazzini, whose published works appeared at the beginning of the eighteenth century, Percival Pott with his observation in 1775 of soot-induced scrotal cancer in chimney sweeps and Charles Thackrah's observations of occupational lead toxicity and lung disease in the early nineteenth century.

Industrialization and the development of chemistry and the chemical industry brought about many benefits to society, but also problems, including occupational ill-health arising from exposure to industrial chemicals. One can almost go through the alphabet listing examples of adverse effects known to have arisen from the toxicity of substances to which the sufferers were exposed at work (Table 1). The number of substances known with confidence to have produced occupational ill-health runs into three figures (Hamilton and Hardy, 1983; Clayton and Clayton 1993). It should also be acknowledged that there have been and continue to be many other, less well substantiated, claims made for evidence of manifestations of toxicity arising in the working environment.

Until well into the twentieth century there was a general acceptance or tolerance by society that where such chemical-induced ill-health at work was apparent, it was unfortunate but largely inescapable. Observations of affected workers were made, but there was little or no toxicological testing of industrial chemicals, exposure assessment or pre-emptive action based on prediction of potential risks to health and aimed at prevention of toxicity arising from workplace exposures. The following quotation is illustrative of the culture prevailing in the USA in the 1930s (Patty, 1978):

During the early 1930s there were probably fewer than 50 people who were industrial hygienists working to protect the health of workers. The public was little interested in industrial hygiene, and some managers thought it was a source of trouble and a waste of money. A few physicians viewed it as an intolerable invasion of the doctor's domain and insisted that only medical doctors could express opinions regarding the effects of any material or any stress on the human body. Unions were more interested in getting hazardous pay than in controlling the environment, and the workers were kept in the dark, uninformed about the actual hazards. Gradually and gratifyingly, a light began to shine in the darkness. It has been a slow but positive evolution.

The first rudimentary toxicity testing of chemicals for the purposes of better understanding and controlling the risks to health involved in their industrial use was carried out by Lehmann in Germany in the late nineteenth century. These studies, principally on gases, involved only short-term exposure of animals and humans and were primitive in their design and conduct, but they did establish a baseline which was important to later investigators. Similar studies were performed by others in the early

Table 1 Confirmed examples of toxicity that have been seen as a result of occupational exposure

Substance	Effects seen
Asbestos (amphiboles and chrysotile)	Lung fibrosis, lung cancer, mesothelioma
Benzene	Aplastic anaemia, leukaemia
Cadmium metal and compounds	Acute lung inflammation, chronic lung and kidney damage
Dichloromethane	Acute CNS depression
Ethylenediamine	Respiratory sensitization
Formaldehyde	Irritation, skin sensitization
Grain dust	Respiratory sensitization
n-Hexane	Peripheral neuropathy
(Di)isocyanates	Skin and respiratory sensitization
Kaolin	Lung inflammation
Lead metal and compounds	Colic, anaemia, nervous system damage, kidney toxicity, testicular toxicity
Mercury metal and compounds	Nervous system damage
Nitroglycerin	Vasodilation producing severe headache
Organophosphorus pesticides	Acute anticholinesterase poisoning
Phosphorus (white elemental)	Jawbone necrosis
Quartz	Acute and chronic silicosis
Rosin-based solder flux fume	Respiratory sensitization
Sulphuric acid	Irritation/corrosion
Trichloroethylene	Acute (fatal) CNS depression
Uranium metal and compounds	Kidney damage
Vinyl chloride	Liver cancer
Wood dusts	Nasal cancer, respiratory sensitization
Xylenes	Skin defatting (liquid); sensory irritation, CNS depression (vapour)
Zinc chloride	Irritation/corrosion

part of the twentieth century, although the range of substances covered remained small. The findings were laid out in standard textbooks of the time (Henderson and Haggard, 1927; Flury and Zernik, 1931).

Toxicological investigations on industrial chemicals became more regular and refined from the 1940s. Nevertheless, it is generally true that the enormous and rapid expansion in the last 50 years in the number of chemical substances potentially in the occupational environment has occurred largely in the absence of programmes specifically requiring the gathering and critical assessment of detailed and comprehensive toxicological data. Hence even in the early 1970s, the American Conference of Governmental Industrial Hygienists (ACGIH) (see Emergence of Early OEL Lists) recommended a Threshold Limit Value for vinyl chloride as high as 500 ppm (8 h time-weighted average), commensurate with a substance being viewed as of low toxicity. Soon afterwards, vinyl chloride was clearly shown to be genotoxic and unfortunately to have already produced cancer in humans (Purchase *et al.*, 1987). In the mid-1970s, workers were grossly exposed and consequently severely poisoned by Kepone (chlordecone) in Hopewell, VA, USA, although this was perhaps more a failure to implement sensible industrial hygiene measures than an absence of toxicological knowledge (Reich and Spong, 1983). And then there is asbestos; in the 1990s, in the UK alone over

1000 deaths per year are occurring due to earlier occupational exposure to at least one of the several forms of this natural mineral fibre.

Accepting the history, replete with accounts of industrial chemical toxicity that are both fascinating but also somewhat gloomy or even tragic from a worker health standpoint, much has been done in the last two to three decades to improve the understanding and control of the risks to health posed by occupational exposures. Nevertheless, it is still true to say that the toxicology of industrial chemicals has been examined in a patchy fashion. A minority of substances have been well investigated. However, most substances of interest in relation to occupational exposure do not have extensive, detailed toxicological data on them, and many have still not been investigated at all (National Academy of Sciences, 1984).

Having made this point, it should be acknowledged that in some circumstances it could be deemed to be unnecessary or uneconomical to generate toxicological data on an industrial chemical. Where only small quantities of a substance are being manufactured and used, it is often more realistic to approach risk management by applying very stringent controls to achieve negligible exposure, rather than investing the time, effort and money necessary to acquire a clear understanding of the toxicology.

One feature of the industrial toxicology and hygiene professions is that there has in the past been a heavy reliance on what might be called 'classical' textbook sources of industrial toxicology information. Publications such as Sax and Lewis's *Dangerous Properties of Industrial Materials* (Sax and Lewis, 1996) and *Patty's Industrial Hygiene and Toxicology* (Clayton and Clayton, 1993) have often been the first and only port of call for those seeking toxicological information on industrial chemicals. Such sources have been and will continue to be extremely helpful as brief, general synopses of the known properties of some substances. They are readily at hand and the convenience and attraction of their use is obvious. However, they do not cover all substances. Also, where a substance is covered, there can on occasion be problems concerning the identification of the original source and underpinning evidence for some of the statements made. Furthermore, there is a tendency in such abbreviated presentations not to make clear what is not known (i.e. where there are no data) for the substance in question. One should always keep firmly in mind the degree to which the information source being used meets requirements, in terms of being up-to-date and thorough, and whether or not it incorporates the important feature of critical appraisal of the data being presented.

Almost anecdotal but seemingly definitive statements of the type, 'Exposure to 20–50 ppm of substance A produces no adverse effects in workers' or 'Workers exposed to 10 ppm of substance Z experienced headache, nausea and fatigue' abound in the industrial toxicology and hygiene literature. Even brief reflection on these statements should raise many questions, to which answers should be available if the information is to be used in decision making—The original source of the data? The reliability of the atmospheric concentrations in terms of the actual conditions experienced by the workers? The duration of exposure? The nature and extent of the health investigations made? The number of subjects involved? The presence of potential confounding factors? It is still too often the case that statements such as those above are propagated through industrial toxicology and hygiene networks without proper scrutiny.

FRAMEWORK FOR MANAGING THE POTENTIAL THREAT TO HEALTH POSED BY OCCUPATIONAL EXPOSURE TO CHEMICALS: WHO SHOULD DO WHAT?

The general philosophy applied to the risk management of chemicals in the workplace can be described in the following terms (**Figure 1** is again relevant). Suppliers are held responsible for determining the hazardous prop-

erties of the chemical(s) being supplied. This toxicological information should be conveyed, in a suitably interpretable manner, to recipients/users of the chemical(s). Regulators have developed classification systems that provide criteria by which to allocate substances to particular hazard categories denoted by symbols and phrases appearing on labels. Users are held responsible for understanding the intended local conditions of use of the chemical and setting this knowledge, with its implications for levels, routes and frequencies of exposure, alongside the hazard information. In doing so, the user is required to make a situation-specific risk assessment and draw conclusions regarding the appropriate risk management measures to apply. In attempting to help the user, regulatory authorities have established some general risk management measures, chiefly by extolling adherence to specified occupational exposure limits for the airborne substance.

TOXICOLOGICAL HAZARD IDENTIFICATION: CLASSIFICATION AND LABELLING

One of the central principles of the regulation of industrial chemicals is that their hazardous properties are categorized in accordance with a classification system. The act of 'classification' can determine what information about the toxicological characteristics of a substance appears on the label placed on the substance during its transport and supply to users. Classification systems can also represent a gateway to other elements of the regulatory framework that selectively pick up substances with particular hazardous properties such as carcinogenicity, reproductive toxicity or high acute toxicity. For example, in the European Union (EU), substances classified as 'category 1' or 'category 2' carcinogens fall under the Carcinogens Directive (EEC, 1990).

The European Union (EU) Classification and Labelling Scheme

For the supply of chemicals to be used in workplaces (and elsewhere) in the EU, there is a regulatory requirement to classify and label substances, and formulations thereof, in accordance with the EU-wide system described in EC Directives (and their Amendments) on the Classification and Labelling of Dangerous Substances and Preparations, together with their accompanying Annexes (EEC, 1967, 1988). In the UK, this system is implemented through the Chemicals (Hazard Identification and Packaging) (CHIP) Regulations (CHIP, 1993); other EU Member States have their own national legislation implementing these Directives.

Importantly, the primary purpose of the scheme, as originally conceived, is harmonization of trade across the EU; the intention is that a substance is similarly (and appropriately) labelled wherever it is supplied within the EU, irrespective of the particular country or company involved.

The EU Classification and Labelling system requires that identified hazardous toxicological properties, from whatever test situation used or observations made, are considered in terms of their relevance to human health and the classification and labelling ultimately derived should reflect this relevance. All the data available on the chemical, including both experimental animal and human findings, needs to be taken into account. The system encompasses all toxicological end-points: acute toxicity arising from single exposure; skin, eye and upper respiratory tract irritancy; skin and respiratory sensitization; long-term toxicity arising from repeated exposure; mutagenicity; carcinogenicity; and reproductive toxicity, covering both effects on adult reproductive function and effects on the developing foetus and newborn offspring. For some issues, such as acute toxicity or skin irritation, the criteria are relatively straightforward and easy to apply. In other areas, such as carcinogenicity or reproductive toxicity, things can become more difficult and/or controversial, with much greater scope and need for careful consideration and interpretation.

The detailed criteria against which the toxicological (and physicochemical and ecotoxicological) properties of a substance are compared in order to determine its classification are given in Annex VI to the Directive dealing with substances. Preparations containing one or more hazardous substances are classified either by comparing the toxicological properties of the preparation against the same criteria or by a series of rules based on the concentrations of individual substances present in the preparation. There are three components to the classification and label ultimately derived—danger symbols, R-phrases and S-phrases. A typical label is shown in **Figure 2**. The danger symbol is intended to give an easily recognizable warning via a pictogram. Brief statements about the toxicological (or physicochemical or ecotoxicological) properties of the substances are also given. An unfortunate and potentially confusing aspect of the scheme is that these are termed 'R' or 'Risk' phrases. The phrases describe hazard, not risk—the reasons for this misnaming stem from the lack of clear discrimination between these terms, both historically when the scheme was first developed in the 1960s and in different European languages. The third element is 'S' or 'Safety' phrases, which give some basic, precautionary instructions to encourage safe use.

The EU Classification and Labelling scheme applies to all substances supplied into the EU workplace, other than those classes of substance covered by their own specific regulatory programmes, such as pharmaceuticals.

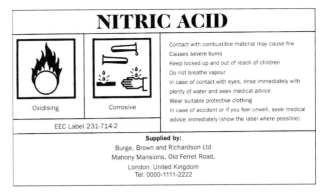

Figure 2 Example of a typical label for supply of a dangerous substance under the EU Classification and Labelling system.

However, the scheme in itself does not specify an information requirement. Rather, it is a set of criteria against which should be compared the observed or predicted toxicological properties of a substance, however extensive or sparse the available data.

Other Hazard Classification Systems

There are other classification and labelling systems in use in different parts of the world, which categorize industrial chemicals according to one or more of their toxicological hazards. In the USA, the Hazard Communication Standard administered by the Occupational Safety and Health Administration (OSHA) requires that all industrial chemicals meeting established criteria for various toxicological end-points are labelled to indicate these properties and have appropriate material safety data sheets (Department of Labour, Occupational Safety and Health Administration, 1987). Canada has a classification system via the Controlled Products Regulations Under the Hazardous Products Act, which implement the regulatory requirements placed on industrial chemical suppliers by the Canadian Workplace Hazardous Material Information System (WHMIS) (Canadian Controlled Products Regulations Under the Hazardous Products Act, 1987). Other systems exist, for example, in Japan, Switzerland and Australia.

Furthermore, two major non-regulatory institutions primarily associated with the development and exposition of occupational exposure limits, the US ACGIH and the German MAK Commission (see User-side Risk Assessment/Risk Management for Industrial Exposure to Chemicals) have developed their own classification systems denoting the carcinogenic hazard of industrial chemicals (ACGIH, 1997; DFG, 1997). Also in the carcinogenicity area, the International Agency for Research on Cancer (IARC) has its system for categorizing substances in accordance with the strength of evidence for their carcinogenicity.

Global Harmonization of Classification Systems

Recognizing the existence of different hazard classification systems around the world, not only for industrial chemicals but also for other groupings of substances, and the difficulties thereby created, in terms of confusion, dispute, inadequate communication of information and problems for trade, the 1992 United Nations Conference on Environment and Development (UNCED; also known as the Rio 'Earth Summit') agreed, amongst many other things, to pursue the following aim:

> *A globally harmonized hazard classification and compatible labelling system, including material safety data sheets and easily understandable symbols, should be available, if feasible, by the year 2000.*

Regulatory toxicologists, particularly those in the occupational field, are currently working together under the direction of the Organization for Economic Cooperation and Development (OECD) in pursuit of this objective.

Material Safety Data Sheets (MSDSs)

Along with labelling, the provision of Material Safety Data Sheets (MSDSs) is a universally recognized, important means by which toxicological information on and advice for safe handling of substances and formulation at work should be conveyed from suppliers to users. In many countries the issuing of an MSDS by suppliers of chemical products is legally required where the properties are deemed to meet various categories of toxicological hazard. For example, in the EU, the supplier of any substance or preparation deemed to be 'dangerous for supply' (i.e. its toxicological properties satisfy one or more of the classification categories in the EU Classification and Labelling system) must provide the industrial recipient with an MSDS containing information under a list of headings (EC, 1993):

1. Identification of the substance/preparation and company.
2. Composition/information on ingredients.
3. Hazards identification.
4. First-aid measures.
5. Fire-fighting measures.
6. Accidental release measures.
7. Handling and storage.
8. Exposure controls/personal protection.
9. Physical and chemical properties.
10. Stability and reactivity.
11. Toxicological information.
12. Ecological information.
13. Disposal considerations.
14. Transport information.
15. Regulatory information.
16. Other information.

There is clearly a need for industrial toxicologists and hygienists to work together in contributing to the MSDS, particularly in relation to several of these points.

The concept of an MSDS is a good one. However, in reality there are a number of contentious issues surrounding it, for both industrial toxicology and industrial hygiene, relating to the quantity and quality of the information provided. A central problem is the question of who is being addressed and what it is that they are expected to assimilate. Most chemical-receiving companies do not employ toxicologists and most will not have hygienists; hence overly scientific/technical language might well be a problem. There is something of a conflict for the MSDS between effective communication with the recipient (pressures for clarity, brevity and simplicity of messages) and insuring against the possibility, should things go wrong, of legal challenge at some later date for 'not telling all' (pressures for extensive, detailed, technically precise and hence often complex information). These issues are worthy of further attention, as research has shown that for many industrial recipients of chemicals the MSDS is probably the most important influence in shaping their assessment of risks to health at their place of work (Research International, 1998).

SUPPLY-SIDE PROGRAMMES REQUIRING INFORMATION, ASSESSMENT AND POSSIBLE FURTHER TESTING OF INDUSTRIAL CHEMICALS

EU New Substances Programme

In recognition of the fact that the toxicology of many long-standing industrial chemicals is poorly understood, substances first introduced on to the EU market after September 1981 are subject to the notification requirements of the '7th Amendment' to the original 1967 Directive on Classification and Labelling (EEC, 1992). In the UK this programme is implemented via the Notification of New Substances (NONS) Regulations (NONS, 1993); again, other EU Member States have their own national legislation implementing this EU requirement. Among other things, this scheme requires the generation, by the manufacturer or importer, of a package of toxicity tests on the 'new substance' in question and the submission of full reports of such tests to the appropriate regulatory authority in one of the Member States. The package is assessed for conformity with requirements specifying the extent and quality of the toxicological information, and for interpretation of the findings of the tests conducted. One of the principal regulatory outcomes is the determination of the appropriate classification and labelling for the substance.

The toxicity testing of new substances must be performed in accordance with internationally recognized standard OECD guidelines. The EU Classification and Labelling scheme, as it relates to the use of experimental animal findings, is geared to accommodate most easily the results of tests conducted to these methods. Hence the results generated from the testing of new substances should readily slot into the classification and labelling criteria. Notification of the substance and an accompanying package of information to, and acceptance of it by, the regulatory authority are an essential pre-marketing requirement for new substances.

In terms of toxicological testing, for substances placed on the EU market in quantities of less than 100 kg per year, only an acute toxicity test is required. Above 100 kg per year, more toxicological work is specified and when the substance reaches the 'full notification' stage of 1 tonne per annum the toxicological requirement (the so-called 'base-set') is:

- Acute toxicity via one (for gases; inhalation) or two (for others) of the three potential exposure routes: inhalation, oral, dermal.
- Skin irritation.
- Eye irritation
- Skin sensitization
- Repeated exposure (up to at least 28 days) toxicity, via the oral route unless there are clear indications that the inhalation or dermal route would be more appropriate.
- Mutagenicity: Ames test and *in vitro* chromosome aberration test.
- Assessment of the toxicokinetics of the substance, to the extent that can be deduced from other information and test results in the package.

Therefore, although the extent of toxicity testing is limited at the initial stage, nevertheless the principle is that new substances and preparations containing them, being supplied to workplaces, arrive for the first time with some of their toxicological end-points having already been explored and, where indicated by the findings, the relevant hazardous properties shown in the MSDS and on the label.

As the quantity of a new substance on the market increases beyond this (significant thresholds being 10, 100 and 1000 tonnes per annum or 50, 500 and 5000 tonnes in total), then consideration is given to more extensive testing, embracing a wider range of potential end-points and greater depth of detail. The results of earlier tests are an influential factor in the approach

taken to further toxicity testing. Again, the EU classification and labelling criteria are applied to the results of such testing to update the position regarding hazard identification.

A further requirement of the 'New Substances' legislation is the need for a risk assessment. At each trigger tonnage level, the notifier company and the regulatory authority interact in producing an assessment of the risks to health that could arise during the life cycle of the substance, including its use in industry. The specifications for such a risk assessment are given in the accompanying Risk Assessment Directive (EEC, 1993b) and an associated package of detailed technical guidance documents has also been produced.

The occupational risk assessment should combine the skills of the toxicologist and the industrial hygienist. In order to form a view on the risk to health in a particular situation, some idea of the level(s) of exposure involved is needed. For new substances, when they are first notified at the pre-marketing stage, there is the obvious problem that there is no experience in use, either of the levels of exposure arising or the impact on the exposed human population(s). Hence it is almost inevitable that for new substances, at least when they are first notified, exposure will have to be predicted/modelled based on experienced professional judgement and generic approaches.

The need to predict workplace exposure has been addressed in the UK by the development of a knowledge-based system, EASE (Estimation and Assessment of Substance Exposure) (HSE, 1995). EASE contains numerous possible exposure fields or scenarios built up of combinations of the different physical properties a substance could possess during the conditions of its manufacture and use (e.g. gas, respirable solid), the different possible patterns of use of the substance (e.g. within a matrix, wide dispersive use) and the different types of control that can be applied to industrial processes (e.g. local exhaust ventilation, full containment). Historical measurements taken under conditions characteristic of each type of scenario have been used to allocate numerical exposure ranges to each of these combinations of fields. In order then to predict occupational exposures arising from the planned introduction of a new substance on to the market, the characteristics of the substance and the envisaged conditions surrounding its manufacture and use are fed into EASE. The system then fits the data relevant to each set of conditions to the most closely fitting exposure field, with its associated numerical exposure range; this exposure range becomes the prediction for the new substance in the situation in which it is destined to occur. Predictions can be made for both inhalation and dermal exposure. However, the predicted numerical ranges are very much rough approximations and it is essential that they are considered and interpreted in context by an experienced occupational hygienist.

EU and OECD Existing Substances Risk Assessment Programmes

For existing substances, the OECD has been running a High Production Volume (HPV) chemicals programme since the late 1980s. The toxicology element of this programme is based on the principles of identifying the hazardous toxicological properties and assessing the risks to human health arising from exposure, for industrial substances in the world market at high tonnage and for which it was believed, at the time of drawing up priority lists, that few data were available. A central element in this programme is the concept of a Screening Information Data Set (SIDS), a requirement that each substance examined by the programme should have as a minimum a basic package of information, the toxicology element of which is similar to that of the EU New Substances 'base-set' (see the previous section). SIDS imposes an additional requirement, which is for some investigation of reproductive toxicity in the minimum data-set package. The programme is voluntary and thus far most of the attention has been focused on the toxicity testing required to complete the SIDS packages for individual substances; there has been little consideration of industrial exposure and risk issues.

Recently, the EU has introduced the Existing Substances Regulation (ESR) (EEC, 1993a). Similarly to the OECD HPV SIDS programme, the scope of ESR embraces the potential impact of substances on all sectors of the human population and also on the environment; industrial health and hygiene considerations form one important element. As with the OECD programmes, ESR contains the concept of a minimum data set, very similar to the SIDS package. At present, the ESR programme is also focused mainly on relatively high production industrial chemicals, on the EU market in quantities greater than 1000 tonnes per annum. ESR has an accompanying Risk Assessment Regulation (EC, 1994). The process by which substances are dealt with under ESR consists of the following stages:

(i) Collation by industry of all relevant data already available, including toxicological and exposure data, in the HEDSET (Harmonized Electronic Dataset) computerized proforma; this is then sent in to the European Commission.

(ii) Use of these data by the European Commission and EU Member States to select priority substances for regulatory assessment.

(iii) For these priority substances, identification by the regulatory authorities of essential further information required in order to complete the minimum data requirements.

(iv) Gathering this further information by industry, possibly entailing the commissioning of additional toxicity testing.

(v) Detailing by a *rapporteur* EU Member State of the hazardous properties of the substance, its dose–response characteristics, exposure data and the degree of risk judged to be involved for various sectors of the human population (and the environment) encountering the substance.

(vi) Consideration by the EU regulatory authorities of the need for still further information to clarify the picture of the potential impact of the substance on health and the environment, or the need for measures to be taken to reduce the risk of such effects.

In relation to the workplace, the regulatory outcome of the programme is determined by the picture emerging from an assessment of the risks of ill-health to all groups and types of workers believed to be exposed to the substance in industry across the EU. Again, this requires the fusion of the expertise and knowledge of industrial toxicologists and hygienists. Occupational exposure measurements for many of the circumstances that need to be considered are often lacking; the predictive and modelling skills of experienced hygienists become crucial in filling these gaps.

The EU supply-side programmes are focused on manufacturers and suppliers of substances and reflect the philosophies of product stewardship and cradle-to-grave, holistic management of chemicals. Each programme offers the regulators, as one potential outcome, the option of developing control measures to reduce the risk envisaged in any of the human exposure scenarios, including the workplace. However, from an occupational health standpoint, there is a major difficulty in identifying and characterizing from the supply point all the potential workplaces, working practices and associated exposure situations that could arise with a particular substance. The ESR programme is still in its formative stages, with very few substances having been processed through all stages.

Supply-side Testing and Risk Assessment for Industrial Chemicals in the USA

In the USA, the Toxic Substances Control Act (TSCA) is a wide-ranging piece of legislation embracing all chemical substances imported into, or manufactured or processed in the USA, with the exception of those classes of substances covered by other, more specific regulatory programmes (TSCA, 1976). TSCA confers on the US Environmental Protection Agency (US EPA) three main powers:

(i) To require toxicity testing of any industrial chemical where the scale of exposure, degree of uncertainty in the toxicological picture or indications of a concern for health are deemed sufficient to merit such further investigations.

(ii) For new substances, to require the intended manufacturer or distributor to notify the USEPA of the intention to produce or distribute the substance, and supply any pre-existing relevant data, 90 days prior to commencement of the operation. However, in contrast to the EU scheme for new substances, in the USA scheme there is no routine testing requirement imposed on all new substances.

(iii) To restrict, and in extreme cases to ban, the manufacture, processing, distribution, use or disposal of a substance where there is deemed to be an 'unreasonable risk of injury to health or environment'.

In practice, the last element of the legislation has proved to be very difficult to bring into regular use. This exemplifies a persistent feature of the regulation of industrial chemicals, not just in the USA but across the world, which sets it apart from some other areas of human exposure to chemicals, such as the intentional presence of chemicals in food or the use of pharmaceuticals. In these other areas, the onus is placed mainly on those wishing to market the product to demonstrate safety. In contrast, for industrial chemicals and the regulation of occupational exposure, the onus is often placed on those wishing to regulate to demonstrate that regulatory action is required.

Toxicity testing requirements under TSCA are determined by an Interagency Testing Committee, comprising representatives of several US agencies, which derives a recommended list of chemicals requiring testing, with the types of studies desired, and an order of priority. These are then progressed to legal requirements of industry (with the potential for legal challenge by industry), via TSCA test rules and enforceable testing consent agreements.

USER-SIDE RISK ASSESSMENT/RISK MANAGEMENT FOR INDUSTRIAL EXPOSURE TO CHEMICALS

Most industrially developed countries have general legislation requiring employers to protect their workforces from the potential adverse effects of chemicals to which they are occupationally exposed. Often this legislation is linked to the notion of regulatory authorities establishing standards for occupational exposure and employers being required to take the necessary measures to adhere to such standards. Thus, for example, the 1970 Occupational Safety and Health Act in the USA requires employers to provide employees with safe working conditions and empowers the Occupational Safety and Health Administration (OSHA) to prescribe mandatory occupational safety and health standards (OSHA, 1970).

In the UK, the 1974 Health and Safety at Work etc. Act states that 'it shall be the duty of every employer to ensure, so far as is reasonably practicable, the health, safety and welfare at work of all his employees' (HSWA, 1974). The Control of Substances Hazardous to Health (COSHH) Regulations, made under HSWA, requires employers to control the exposure of their workers to substances in accordance with standards established by the UK Health and Safety Commission (COSHH, 1994).

Such legislation embodies the following concepts. First, an employer is envisaged to have information on the toxicological hazards and associated dose–response characteristics of the substance(s) in question, either from the supplier (via the label and MSDS) or, if the substance(s) is (are) being generated on-site, from knowledge of his own product(s). It is also envisaged that the employer should know the features of the exposure situation, in terms of the numbers and characteristics of those exposed and the route(s), frequencies, durations and levels of exposure. The employer is then viewed as being in a position to use all of this information to assess the nature and extent of any risks to the health of employees and implement whatever measures are judged to be necessary to minimize the risks (see **Figure 1**). Regulatory authorities seek to enforce such obligations but also seek to assist employers in fulfilling their responsibilities by issuing information, advice, guidance and standards, adherence to which is taken to be securing appropriate control of exposure. In the EU, the emerging Chemical Agents Directive, still under negotiation at the time of writing this chapter, also embodies these principles and will apply across all EU Member States.

Within the typical 'user-side' regulatory framework, airborne occupational exposure limits (and associated notations) hold a highly significant, central position in the minds of many professionals and policymakers in the occupational health and hygiene fields. Recent research in the UK has revealed that the awareness and understanding of occupational exposure limits for many employers and employees and the significant of limits in controlling occupational exposure to chemicals, particularly in the ever-increasing small company sector is perhaps much lower than those establishing occupational exposure limits would like to believe (Research International, 1998). Nevertheless, in the context of this chapter, occupational exposure limits are worthy of detailed consideration.

Occupational Exposure Limits

What is an Occupational Exposure Limit?

Occupational Exposure Limits (OELs), their origin and basis, and differences in the numerical values of limits for the same substance in various listings have been the subject of much controversy in recent years (Castleman and Zeim, 1988, 1994; Roach and Rappaport, 1990). At the outset, it is important to consider what an OEL is, and perhaps what it is not. It is a standard intended *to play a part* in controlling the exposure of workers to an airborne substance. However, there are crucial differences between different types of OEL within the same limit-setting system and in the meaning of OELs between different limit-setting systems. Some types of OEL carry some kind of assurance of health protection; others do not. Some types of OEL are intended to be legally enforceable; others are not, being more in the way of guidance. Some types of OEL are influenced by what levels of control are deemed to be achievable with current technology and not exorbitant cost; others are more idealistic targets which, it is hoped, can be achieved at some point in the future. Hence a simple comparison of the numerical values of limits for the same substance in different OEL lists should not be taken as a reflection of the relative standards of occupational health protection in those parts of the world covered by the lists.

It is also worth remembering that the listing of an OEL in itself will achieve little, if anything. Assuming that the OEL is well founded, it will be an effective measure only if used by the occupational hygiene discipline to set in place an appropriate control regime aimed at adherence to the OEL, supported by means of establishing that such adherence has been achieved.

Emergence of Early OEL Lists

The first published OEL is held to be the value of 500 ppm carbon monoxide, put forward by Max Gruber in the late nineteenth century and derived from studies involving 12 rabbits, 2 hens and himself! (Paull, 1984). The focus was on avoidance of acute effects, as it was in the first lists of harmful concentrations of substances in air which began to appear in the first quarter of the twentieth century, mainly from toxicology work performed in Germany (see Historical Development). Almost no toxicological information beyond acute toxicity and irritancy was available for substances at this time. From the 1920s, some information became available on dose–effect relationships for long-term exposure to a few familiar toxicants—lead, mercury, crystalline silica, benzene—and the stated purpose of listing 'maximum allowable concentrations' gradually changed to one of protecting the workforce against ill-health when exposure was occurring daily over a working lifetime.

Perhaps the single most significant development in this area was the establishment, during the 1940s, of the Threshold Limits Committee of what was first the National, and then became the American Conference of Governmental Industrial Hygienists (ACGIH), in the USA. This committee used pre-existing information and its own experience to construct and adopt its first published list of Maximum Allowable Concentrations (MACs), comprising limit values for 160 substances, in 1946. The list of what soon became known as Threshold Limit Values (TLVs) was first published in 1950 (ACGIH, 1950).

In terms of health protection, the intended meaning of the TLV was:

> *That amount of gas, vapour, fumes or dust which can be tolerated by man with no bodily discomfort nor impairment of bodily function either immediately or after years of exposure.*

Subsequently, to the present day, the ACGIH TLV list has been amended and extended on an annual basis to cover now more than 600 substances (ACGIH, 1997). From 1962 onwards the list was supplemented with brief supporting documentation and references (ACGIH, 1962).

Interestingly Russia (or, formerly, the whole of the USSR) has also had a long-standing system of establishing OELs. As early as the 1930s, a list of Russian MACs was published. This system is discussed further in the section Toxicological and Industrial Hygiene Concepts Surrounding Occupational Exposure Limits.

Proliferation of OEL Lists

The ACGIH TLV Committee has remained active to the present day and its TLV list has been extremely influential in the USA and across the world, with many countries using the values listed either as guidance or as the basis for national legal standards. In USA, the Occupational Safety and Health Act of 1970 incorporated the 1968 ACGIH TLV list, along with a small number of other occupational air standards for substances, into US law. Many of these still persist in the US Occupational Safety and Health Administration's current list of Permissible Exposure Limits (PELs). In more recent times, OSHA in the USA and institutions in several other countries around the world have established their own systems for producing in-depth critical assessments of the toxicological data (and, in some cases, also occupational hygiene and analytical data), which are then considered for the purposes of establishing occupational exposure limits and other associated risk management measures. The first such system was that developed in Germany. In 1968, Germany ceased to adhere to the ACGIH TLV list and began a programme of generating its own OELs under the Maximale Arbeitskonzentrationen (MAK) Commission [the Commission for the Investigation of Health Hazards of Chemical Compounds in the Work Area, a body within the German Research Institute (Deutsche Forschungsgemeinschaft)]. The MAK Commission also produces an annual listing of its limit values (DFG, 1997).

Other systems have developed more recently, including those in The Netherlands, the UK, Nordic countries, Australia and Japan (AIHA/CMA, 1996). Furthermore, since the beginning of the 1990s, the European Union (EU), via its Directorate General V, has been developing a structure for producing EU-wide occupational exposure limits based on similar review documentation (Zielhuis *et al*, 1991; EEC, 1991; EC, 1996).

Toxicological and Industrial Hygiene Concepts Surrounding Occupational Exposure Limits

The purpose of establishing an occupational exposure limit is to signify the level of exposure to which it is suggested, hoped or legally required that exposure should be controlled. The intention is health protection, or at least management of the risk of ill-health effects to an acceptable level.

Most toxicological end-points are associated with the general concept of a threshold dose, that is, for any particular substance, the dose below which the effect will not be produced. However, this concept is often portrayed in an overly simplistic manner. Further consideration of the issues involved raises the question of just what is meant by the term 'threshold'. Taking the fictitious substance putrid obnoxide and its recognized hazardous property of producing kidney damage on repeated exposure, there are difficult questions regarding a 'threshold'. Does this mean the highest dose of putrid obnoxide at which there will be no kidney toxicity in a 'normal' (whatever that means) member of the exposed population or in any conceivable member of the exposed population? And what do we mean by 'kidney toxicity'? Does this mean any detectable perturbation in kidney appearance, biochemistry or physiology, or a change of a nature and scale deemed to represent a significant adverse effect on health? These two issues, superimposed, render the concept of a threshold difficult. Even if we can clarify what we conceive the threshold to be, the identification of where this threshold might lie is even more problematic, given that we are aiming to specify a level of exposure to putrid obnoxide which will not adversely effect the health of a relatively large number of genetically and physiologically variable humans from data often available only from a small number of relatively genetically homogeneous rodents. The usual final 'missing piece' is that we are unclear about the toxicokinetic and toxicodynamic pathways along which putrid obnoxide passes and which results in the ultimate manifestation of the kidney toxicity that has been observed.

The general manner in which the establishment of an occupational exposure limit is approached for situations where, despite the difficulties outlined above, the toxicological effects of a substance are conceived to be threshold phenomena is often as follows. From the toxicological information available, an overall No Observed Adverse Effect Level (NOAEL), the highest dose level at which no toxicological significant effects of relevance to human health have been observed, is sought;

sometimes the identification of an NOAEL from the available data is not possible, and the Lowest Observed Adverse Effect Level (LOAEL) has to suffice. Across a range of substances, the quality of data from which the respective NOAELs (or LOAELs) can be identified will be extremely variable. The conventional approach is then to derive an occupational exposure limit which is at or below the NOAEL (or below the LOAEL) and to associate with the occupational exposure limit the degree of health protection which, it is judged, adherence to this level of exposure will confer. Such occupational exposure limits are often termed 'health-based'.

The judgement as to how far below the NOAEL (or LOAEL) it is appropriate to pitch a 'health-based' OEL is influenced not only by toxicological considerations but also by the context in which the occupational exposure limit is intended to sit. Returning to the above example, with kidney toxicity being the principal effect of concern with exposure to putrid obnoxide, and with a NOAEL of 100 ppm for kidney toxicity in a 90 day inhalation study in rats, an ever-increasing degree of reassurance that the exposed human population would be protected from ill-health would be achieved by establishing the occupational exposure limit at 50, 10, 1, 0.1 or 0.01 ppm. However, in moving further and further down the exposure scale one is also increasing the technical, practical and economic difficulties of controlling such levels. One might also reach a point where there is no reliable and practical analytical technique available to measure such a low exposure.

Most 'health-based' OELs profess to offer health protection to 'nearly all' members of an exposed working population, based on 'current knowledge'; forms of words are used that concede the difficulties often caused by poor toxicological databases and a lack of understanding of the position surrounding inter-species and inter-individual variability in response to the substance in question. Examples of health-based OELs are the ACGIH TLVs, the Occupational Exposure Standard (OES) in the UK system and the MAK values from Germany (see **Table 2**).

However, differences between listings around the world in the numerical values established for health-based OELs for particular substances arise not only because of timing and interpretational differences in the most recent toxicological evaluation made, but also because of differences in the intended practicality, real-life achievability and legal enforceability of limits established within different systems. Several publications have discussed the issue of deriving health-based OELs from toxicological data and particularly the application of uncertainty factors to NOAELs (Zielhuis and van der Kreek, 1979; ECETOC, 1995; Fairhurst, 1995).

The nature of the principal toxicological effect(s) produced by a substance may necessitate specified controls for either the longer term aggregated dose (e.g. daily exposure to a concentration averaged over the workshift)

Table 2 Expressions of the degree of health protection offered by health-based OELs and the degree of confidence that such protection is assured

'Health-based OEL'	Explanatory text
ACGIH TLV	'Conditions under which it is believed that nearly all workers may be repeatedly exposed day after day without adverse health effects. Because of wide variation in individual susceptibility, however, a small percentage of workers may experience discomfort from some substances at concentrations at or below the threshold limit; a smaller percentage may be affected more seriously by aggravation of a pre-existing condition or by development of an occupational illness'
German MAK value	'The maximum concentration of a chemical substance (as gas, vapour or particulate matter) in the workplace air which generally does not have known adverse effects on the health of the employee nor cause unreasonable annoyance even when the person is repeatedly exposed during long periods'
UK OES	'The available scientific evidence allows for the identification, with reasonable certainty, of a concentration averaged over a reference period, at which there is no indication that the substance is likely to be injurious to employees if they are exposed day after day to that concentration'

or short-term exposure of only a few minutes duration, or both. An attritional effect such as liver necrosis or lung fibrosis may be adequately controlled by the former, whereas an immediate effect such as sensory irritation, more dependent on airborne concentration than on duration of exposure, requires tight control of short-term exposure. Hence occupational exposure limits are often expressed in terms of atmospheric concentrations averaged over reference periods constituting a full workshift [8 h time-weighted average (TWA)] or a short, 15 min period (short-term exposure limit, STEL). The German MAK list is accompanied by a five-category system for limiting excursions in atmospheric concentration above the 8 h TWA MAK value of 2–10-fold, for maximum periods of 5–60 min, 1–8 times during a workshift (DFG, 1997). The ACGIH TLV system has, in addition to 8 h TWA and 15 min short-term exposure limit TLVs, the additional concept of a Ceiling Value, a concentration which should not be exceeded during any period of the working day (ACGIH, 1997).

In some cases the toxicological picture, including the knowledge gaps, defeats the aim of identifying with confidence a level of exposure which is both sufficiently 'safe' and achievable in practice. This is often the situation in dealing with DNA-damaging (genotoxic) chemicals with known or suspected consequential mutagenic and/or carcinogenic potential, such as bis(chloromethyl) ether, ethylene oxide or o-toluidine. Respiratory sensitizers are another class of substances where such problems arise. The difficulty here is that there is currently no acceptable and widely used experimental test system for exploring the end-point and therefore one is reliant almost exclusively on human clinical/medical information. In most cases, this type of information does not permit the determination of dose–response characteristics for induction of a sensitized state and for triggering a response in hypersensitive individuals.

In situations such as this, several occupational exposure limit systems around the world have an alternative type of limit which is not deemed to be 'health-based', but where the numerical value is governed by what is deemed to be the most stringent level of control achievable with reasonable expenditure on currently available and practical technology and using best practice. Examples of such occupational exposure limits are the TRK (Technische Richtkonzentrationen) values in Germany or the Maximum Exposure Limit (MEL) values in the UK system (DFG, 1997; HSE, 1997).

The Russian system for developing MACs referred to above was developed independently of the ACGIH TLVs and continues to run separately from this and the later systems of other organizations/countries. Furthermore, the MACs are based on principles that are unique to that system. MACs are based exclusively on toxicological information, with no reference to industrial hygiene or other disciplines or considerations. Each MAC is set at the level which, it is judged, would correspond to a tissue burden in exposed individuals representing 'the minimum dose which triggers changes beyond the limits of physiological adaptation reactions' (Sanotsky et al., 1986). Most of the toxicological literature used in developing the MAC values is Russian in origin and the MAC values tend to be much lower than the 'health-based' OELs established elsewhere in the world. The MAC values tend to follow logically from the reported toxicological information; it is the Russian toxicological literature that tends to report biological changes arising in experimental animals at appreciably lower doses than is reported in studies elsewhere in the world. The reasons for this discrepancy are unclear. Also unclear is the degree to which such stringent MAC values can be and are enforced in Russia.

The lists of occupational exposure limits from several sources are also supplemented with additional notations. The notation 'sk' or, in German, 'H' (Haut being German for skin) denotes a substance which, under occupational exposure conditions, could be absorbed through the skin to such an extent as to contribute significantly to the total body burden of a substance achieved from exposure at work. The purpose of the notation is to indicate to industrial hygienists that attention to inhalation exposure alone might not be sufficient to guard against health effects from systemic uptake of the substance, if skin (and eye) contact with the substance in solid, liquid or vapour form is not also controlled. It is important to recognize that the notation relates to absorption through the skin, not to effects on the skin (or eyes) such as irritation, corrosion or skin sensitization.

The notation 'Sen' or, in the German system, 'Sa' or 'Sh' is to denote that the substance has sensitizing properties towards the respiratory tract or skin or both—the criteria differ in different listings. Its use is to indicate to industrial hygienists that risk management approaches considered to be adequate to protect health in non-sensitized individuals may not prevent allergic reactions from arising in those already sensitized to the agent in question.

Biological Monitoring, Biological Effect Monitoring and Health Surveillance

Biological monitoring involves the measurement of a substance and/or its metabolite(s) in body fluids (usually urine or blood) or exhaled air. Biological effect monitoring is the measurement of a biochemical change in the body caused by exposure to a substance, the degree of change being below that associated with frank ill-health. Health surveillance refers to the examination of workers for emerging signs of ill-health; in a toxicological context, adverse health effects arising from exposure to industrial chemicals.

Each of these approaches can complement risk management based on workplace air standards for industrial substances. In general, biological monitoring gives a more accurate assessment of individual intake of a substance, compared with atmospheric measurements, and it is particularly useful in the following respects:

- To assess the extent of substance intake via routes other than inhalation (skin, ingestion);
- To track the potential accumulation of substances in the body, resulting from long-term repeated exposure;
- To examine the effectiveness of personal protective equipment in guarding against exposure to, and intake of substances.

Table 3 gives some examples of the entities that are amenable to analysis in various biological media as a means of assessing the degree of exposure to, or consequential biochemical changes arising from, industrial chemicals.

The particular technique employed has to take into account the sensitivity and specificity of the measurement as a means of tracking exposure to a substance. The toxicokinetics of the substance influence the choice of biological medium and sampling regime. In addition to advantages over atmospheric measurement, there are some disadvantages with biological (effect) monitoring, not least the potential invasiveness of the sampling techniques employed and the medical confidentiality of the results obtained. Although biological (effect) monitoring forms a cornerstone of risk management for a small number of industrial exposure situations, particularly working with lead and lead compounds, there are relatively few industrial substances that have well established biological (effect) monitoring approaches.

The two best recognized systems of biological monitoring and biological effect monitoring standards are those of the ACGIH in USA and the MAK Commission in Germany. As with airborne standards, it is essential to focus not just on the numerical value of the standard but also on the associated definition of what the number represents. There are different types of biological standard.

The ACGIH proposes Biological Exposure Indices (BEIs). In most cases a BEI represents the level of a substance or its metabolite(s) which is most likely to be observed in specimens collected from a healthy worker who has been exposed to the substance to the same extent as a worker with inhalation exposure at the ACGIH TLV (ACGIH, 1997). The concept is that the BEI reflects an equivalent body burden to that received from inhalation exposure at the TLV.

The MAK Commission establishes BAT values, translated as Biological Tolerance Values for Working Materials (DFG, 1997). A BAT value is set at what is judged to be the maximum level of a substance or its metabolite in a biological medium, or the maximum extent of deviation from the norm of a biochemical parameter, which will not impair the health of a worker. Therefore, in health protection terms, measurements up to the BAT are deemed to reflect 'healthy' situations.

Table 3 Some examples of biological monitoring and biological effect monitoring measurements in use

Biological monitoring	
In blood	Lead, cadmium
In urine	Mercury, mandelic acid (from styrene), trichloroacetic acid (from trichloroethylene)
In exhaled breath	Carbon monoxide (from CO itself or from dichloromethane)
Biological effect monitoring	
For lead	Evidence for increased zinc protoporphyrin in blood
For organophosphorus pesticides	Evidence for reduction in plasma and erythrocyte cholinesterase activities

The UK has recently introduced two types of biological monitoring standards (HSE, 1997). A Health Guidance Value is the concentration of an analyte in a biological medium which is judged to reflect either the highest level deemed not to affect health, or the level that would be produced by inhalation exposure at the OES (see Toxicological and Industrial Hygiene Concepts Surrounding Occupational Exposure Limits). Alternatively, a Benchmark Value is set at approximately the 90th percentile of the available data from UK workplaces deemed to be implementing good practice and is used, for example, for substances for which health-based biological monitoring standards cannot be established (e.g. the suspect human carcinogen methylenebis-2-chloroaniline, MbOCA).

'In-house' Occupational Exposure Limits and Risk Management Banding

Lists of occupational exposure limits from around the world each cover a few hundred substances. As most of these lists were originally based on the ACGIH TLVs and still bear many of the features of this parent list, many of the substances covered by different lists are the same. This situation is set against a background of tens of thousands of chemicals being present in the occupational environment in many of the more industrially developed parts of the world. Hence, in numerical terms (although not necessarily in tonnage or industrial importance terms), most chemicals encountered in industry do not have 'official' occupational exposure limits.

Some industry sectors and/or individual companies have responded to this situation by developing their own 'in-house' occupational exposure limits. Such limits are usually derived by fusing the available toxicological information on the substance in question with practical industrial hygiene considerations. The limits are produced for application within the premises of the company(ies) generating them, and/or for onward transmission to recipients of the substances that these companies supply. Several publications have discussed the practice of establishing 'in-house' limits (McHattie *et al.*, 1988; ABPI, 1995).

However, the setting of in-house OELs, particularly via a process similar to that used by more formal limit-setting bodies, is still a resource-intensive and relatively sophisticated activity. An alternative approach has been explored in recent years by a number of groups, each seeking to embrace all substances potentially in the workplace air in a general scheme for controlling airborne exposure. Although a variety of terms have been used, the various schemes can all be regarded as forms of 'risk management banding'. The schemes recognize that industrial hygienists tend to deal in a relatively small number of different approaches to substance containment and exposure control. Consequently, the schemes allocate substances (and, for some schemes, the type of situation in which the substance occurs) into one of a limited number of bands, each of which is in turn associated with a specified hygiene approach to controlling airborne exposure.

The essence of these schemes is to take the kind of information surrounding a substance and its conditions of use that is expected to be readily available, and to link this in a straightforward manner with guidance on the appropriate industrial hygiene approach to employ. One such scheme allocates the active ingredients used in pharmaceutical manufacture to one of five categories, based on toxicological hazard data, and attaches to each hazard band a containment strategy deemed to correspond to appropriate control for the type and the degree of hazard expressed (Naumann *et al.*, 1996). Another scheme, developed by the UK Chemical Industries Association, allocates substances to one of five numerical occupational exposure bands (ranges), based on their classification for toxicological hazard under the EU Classification and Labelling scheme (CIA, 1997). The decision on how to achieve control to these ranges in any particular industrial setting is then left to the experience and expertise of the industrial hygienist.

A further scheme has been developed to secure appropriate control of exposure to chemicals in laboratory work (RSC, 1996). This combines information on toxicological hazard classification (EU criteria), the tendency of the substance to become airborne and the quantity being used to develop appropriate strategies to control the concentration of the substance present in the workplace air or coming into contact with the skin. The UK Health and Safety Executive, together with external toxicology and industrial hygiene experts, is currently attempting to develop a scheme along similar principles, which could be applied for any substance and situation across all industry (Brooke, 1998).

CURRENT PERSPECTIVES AND FUTURE PROSPECTS

Industrial toxicology has an interesting combination of features. In one sense, in terms of sophistication of regulatory structure and the typical data sets that are available for many of the substances of interest, it has been a poor relation of other areas of applied toxicology such as the approval for use of pharmaceuticals, foodstuffs or pesticides. On the other hand the occurrence of toxicity due to workplace exposure to chemicals is a genuine, real-life issue with many unfortunate examples from the past and numerous contemporary issues that still need to be addressed. Although some of the more horrendous consequences of occupational exposure to chemicals are hopefully yesterday's problem, there remain many and sometimes new issues, questions, concerns and challenges. It has to be acknowledged that even today, there is a paucity of knowledge of the scale and range of ill-health produced by occupational exposure to chemicals.

There are many examples of the ways in which the skills, knowledge and experience of industrial toxicologists and industrial hygienists have been brought together to good effect. The two disciplines are separate but, in the area of controlling occupational exposure to chemicals, they should be closely interlinked. Industrial toxicologists are endeavouring to establish a clear understanding of the potential for harm to arise from occupational exposure to chemicals. Industrial hygienists need to ensure that such information is translated into appropriate and effective control of occupational exposures.

Significant issues still remain surrounding some of the more familiar industrial chemicals and their effects. Has the threat to health from occupational exposure to asbestos now been brought under satisfactory control? What threat to the health of the developing foetus is posed by occupational exposure to lead during pregnancy? What exactly is meant by the many reports of sensory 'irritation' arising from occupational exposure to airborne industrial chemicals, as chemically disparate as chlorine and acetone, and what health significance should be accorded such phenomena? Some of the observations of such irritation that are still highly influential in industrial toxicology and hygiene were made in the 1940s and only recently are the sensations being properly characterized.

There are also newer and as yet unresolved issues to address. A major one is whether or not long-term occupational exposure to organic solvents or organophosphorus pesticides can produce chronic neurological disease. Another surrounds the regular but controversial claims made in the literature for reproductive effects arising from occupational exposure to a variety of individual organic solvents or in occupations involving organic solvent exposure. For these and a variety of other alleged associations between occupational exposure to chemicals and ill-health consequences, there is much work to be done by specialists in the relevant fields, in seeking a clearer understanding of the toxicological situation and the appropriate industrial hygiene approaches to adopt.

Important questions are also being raised about the expectations that the regulatory framework places on those using, and thereby exposed to, chemicals in industry. Is it reasonable to expect that many employers, particularly small companies, will have the awareness, understanding and ability to perform toxicological risk assessment? Are the traditional regulatory approaches, such as lists of numerical OELs or phrases such as 'possible risk of irreversible effects' on a label, effectively communicating the toxicological properties of industrial chemicals and the industrial hygiene requirements surrounding their use? There is an ever-increasing propor-tion of industry comprising small companies employing relatively few workers. Very many businesses, now and in the future, will have no individuals with knowledge of the technical aspects of toxicology and industrial hygiene. If we are to achieve more in the future in relation to the avoidance of adverse health effects from occupational exposure to chemicals, there is the enormous challenge of translating the detailed, complex, technical concepts and language of the specialisms and specialists involved into simple, accurate and pragmatic information and advice for the workforces encountering substances at work.

REFERENCES

ABPI (1995). *Guidance on Setting Occupational Exposure Limits for Airborne Therapeutic Substances and Their Intermediates*. Association of the British Pharmaceutical Industry, London.

ACGIH (1950). Threshold Limit Values for 1950. *AMA Arch. Ind. Hyg. Occup. Med.*, **2**, 98–100.

ACGIH (1962). *Documentation of the Threshold Limit Values for Substances in Workroom Air*. 1st edn. American Conference of Governmental Industrial Hygienists, Cincinnati, OH.

ACGIH (1997). *1997 TLVs and BEIs: Threshold Limit Values for Chemical Substances and Physical Agents, and Biological Exposure Indices*. ACGIH Worldwide, Cincinnati, OH.

AIHA/CMA (1996). *An International Review of Procedures for Establishing Occupational Exposure Limits*. American Industrial Hygiene Association and Chemical Manufacturers Association, AIHA, Fairfax, VA.

Brooke, I. M. (1998). A UK scheme to help small firms control health risk from chemicals. *Ann. Occup. Hyg.*, **42**, 377–390.

Canadian Controlled Products Regulations Under the Hazardous Products Act (1987). *Canadian Gazette Part II*, **122**, No. 2, adopted 31 December 1987.

Castleman, B. I. and Zeim, G. E. (1988). Corporate influence on threshold limit values. *Am. J. Ind. Med.*, **13**, 531–559.

Castleman, B. I. and Zeim, G. E. (1994). American Conference of Governmental Industrial Hygienists: low threshold of credibility. *Am. J. Ind. Med.*, **26**, 133–143.

CHIP (1993). *The Chemicals (Hazard Information and Packaging) Regulations 1993*. Statutory Instrument 1993 No. 1746. HMSO, London.

CIA (1997). *The Control of Substances Hazardous to Health (COSHH): Guidance on Allocating Occupational Exposure Bands (Regulation 7)*. Chemical Industries Association, London.

Clayton, G. D. and Clayton, F. E. (eds) (1993). *Patty's Industrial Hygiene and Toxicology*, 4th edn. Wiley, New York.

COSHH (1994). *Control of Substances Hazardous to Health Regulations 1994*. Statutory Instrument 1994 No. 3246. HMSO, London.

Department of Labor, Occupational Safety and Health Administration (1987). Hazard Communication, Final Rule, 29 CFR 1910. *Fed. Regist.*, **52**, No. 153, 24 August 1987. US Government Printing Office, Washington, DC.

DFG (1997). *Maximum Concentrations at the Workplace and Biological Tolerance Values for Working Materials*. Report

No. 33, Deutsche Forschungsgemeinschaft, Commission for the Investigation of Health Hazards of Chemical Compounds in the Work Area. VCH, Weinheim.

EC (1993). *Commission Directive 93/112/EC, amendment to the Safety Data Sheet Directive (Commission Directive 91/155/EEC)*. European Commission, Brussels.

EC (1994). *Commission Regulation (EC) No. 1488/94, Laying Down the Principles for the Assessment of Risks to Man and the Environment of Existing Substances in Accordance with Council Regulation (EEC) No. 793/93*. European Commission, Brussels.

EC (1996). *Commission Directive 96/34/EC of 18 December 1996 Establishing a Second List of Indicative Limit Values in Implementation of Council Directive 80/1107/EEC on the Protection of Workers from the Risks Related to Exposure to Chemical, Physical and Biological Agents at Work*. European Commission, Brussels.

ECETOC (1995). *Assessment Factors in Human Health Risk Assessment*. Technical Report No. 68. European Centre for Ecotoxicology and Toxicology of Chemicals, Brussels.

EEC (1967). *Council Directive 67/548/EEC on the Approximation of the Laws, Regulations and Administrative Provisions Relating to the Classification, Packaging and Labelling of Dangerous Substances*. European Commission, Brussels.

EEC (1988). *Council Directive 88/379/EEC on the Approximation of the Laws, Regulations and Administrative Provisions of the Member States Relating to the Classification, Packaging and Labelling of Dangerous Preparations*. European Commission, Brussels.

EEC (1990). *Council Directive 90/394/EEC of 28 June 1990 on the Protection of Workers from the Risks Related to Exposure to Carcinogens at Work*. European Commission, Brussels.

EEC (1991). *Commission Directive 91/322/EEC on Establishing Indicative Limit Values by Implementing Council Directive 80/1107 EEC on the Protection of Workers from the Risks Related to Exposure to Chemical, Physical and Biological Agents at Work*. European Commission, Brussels.

EEC (1992). *Council Directive 92/32/EEC, Amending for the Seventh Time Directive 67/548/EEC on the Approximation of the Laws, Regulations and Administrative Provisions Relating to the Classification, Packaging and Labelling of Dangerous Substances*. European Commission, Brussels.

EEC (1993a). *Council Regulation (EEC) No. 793/93 of 23 March 1993 on the Evaluation and Control of the Risks of Existing Substances*. European Commission, Brussels.

EEC (1993b). *Commission Directive 93/67/EEC, Laying Down the Principles for Assessment of Risks to Man and the Environment of Substances Notified in Accordance with Council Directive 67/548/EEC*. European Commission, Brussels.

Fairhurst, S. (1995). The uncertainty factor in the setting of occupational exposure standards. *Ann. Occup. Hyg.*, **39**, 375–385.

Flury, F. and Zernik, F. (1931). *Schadliche Gase*. Springer, Berlin.

Henderson, Y. and Haggard, H. W. (1927). *Noxious Gases*. Reinhold, New York.

Hamilton, A. and Hardy, H. L. (1983). *Hamilton and Hardy's Industrial Toxicology*, 4th edn. Revised by Finkel, A. J. John Wright PSG, Boston.

HSE (1995). *Risk Assessment of Notified New Substances: Technical Guidance Document*, Health and Safety Executive. HSE Books, Sudbury, Suffolk, Chapt. 3.

HSE (1997). *Occupational Exposure Limits. EH40*. Health and Safety Executive, HMSO, London.

HSWA (1974). *Health and Safety at Work etc. Act 1974*. HMSO, London, Chapt. 37.

McHattie, G. V., Rackham, M. and Teasdale, E. L. (1988). The derivation of occupational exposure limits in the pharmaceutical industry. *J. Soc. Occup. Med.*, **38**, 105–108.

National Academy of Sciences (1984). *Toxicity Testing: Strategies to Determine Needs and Priorities*. National Academy of Sciences, Washington, DC.

Naumann, B. D., Sargent, E. V., Sharkman, B. S., Fraser, W. J., Becker, G. T. and Kirk, G. D. (1996). Performance-based exposure control for pharmaceutical active ingredients. *Am. Ind. Hyg. Assoc. J.*, **57**, 33–42.

NONS (1993). *The Notification of New Substances Regulations 1993*. Statutory Instrument 1993 No. 3050. HMSO, London.

OSHA (1970). *Occupational Safety and Health Act*. 29 U.S.C. 651 *et seq.*

Patty, F. A. (1978). Industrial hygiene: retrospect and prospect. In Clayton, G. D. and Clayton, F. E. (Eds), *Patty's Industrial Hygiene and Toxicology*, 3rd edn, Vol. 1. *General Principles*. J Wiley, New York, pp. 1–21.

Paull, J. M. (1984). The origin and basis of threshold limit values. *Am. J. Ind. Med.*, **5**, 227–238.

Purchase, I. F. H., Stafford, J. and Paddle, G. M. (1987). Vinyl chloride: an assessment of the risk of occupational exposure. *Food Chem. Toxicol.*, **25**, 187–202.

Reich, M. R. and Spong, J. K. (1983). Kepone: a chemical disaster in Hopewell, Virginia. *Int. J. Health Serv.*, **13**, 227–246.

Research International (1998). *Evaluation of Industry's Perception and Use of OELs and Their Role in Risk Reduction*. Research International (UK), London.

Roach, S. A. and Rappaport, S. M. (1990). But they are not thresholds: a critical analysis of the documentation of threshold limit values. *Am. J. Ind. Med.*, **17**, 727–753.

RSC (1996). *COSHH in Laboratories*, 2nd edn. Royal Society of Chemistry, Cambridge.

Sax, N. I. and Lewis, R. J., Sr (Eds) (1996). *Dangerous Properties of Industrial Materials*, 9th edn. Van Nostrand Rheinhold, New York.

Sanotsky, I. V., Kagan, Y. S., Krasovsky, G. N., Mazaev, V. T. and Ivanov, N. G. (1986). Thresholds of harmful health effects of chemicals on animals and man; prediction of safe exposure levels. In Kasparov, A. A. and Sanotsky, I. V. (Eds), *Toxicometry of Environmental Chemical Pollutants*. United Nations Environment Programme, New York, Chapt. 9, pp. 301–336.

TSCA (1976). *Toxic Substances Control Act*. 15 U.S.C. 2601.

Zielhuis, R. L., Noordan, P. C., Maas, C. L., Kolk, J. J. and Illing, H. P. A. (1991). Harmonisation of criteria documents for standard setting in occupational health: report of a meeting. *Regul. Appl. Toxicol.*, **13**, 241–262.

Zielhuis, R. L. and van der Kreek, F. W. (1979). The use of a safety factor in setting health based permissible levels for occupational exposure. *Int. Arch. Occup. Environ. Health*, **42**, 191–201.

Chapter 68

Forensic Toxicology: A Broad Overview of General Principles

Ronald C. Backer and Alphonse Poklis

C O N T E N T S

INTRODUCTION

Toxicology is the study of poisons and how they impact on biological systems. As a science, toxicology is concerned with physical and chemical properties of toxic substances, their physiological and clinical effects and qualitative and quantitative methods for their analysis in biological and non-biological materials (Poklis, 1997). Methods of treatment for poisoning, including the development of specific antidotes, are also an important aspect of toxicology. The American Board of Forensic Toxicology defines forensic toxicology as the application of toxicology for the purposes of the law. When forensic is used as an adjective it means 'pertaining to the courts of justice' or 'to the administration of justice'. Therefore, forensic toxicology literally means the study of the effects of poisons for the administration of justice.

THE TOXICOLOGY PROCESS

Toxicology plays an important part in the medicolegal investigation of death. It answers the question of whether alcohol, other drugs and or chemical poisons were the cause or a contributory cause of the death. The laboratory can analyse biological specimens including blood, urine, vitreous, bile, tissues (liver, brain, kidney, spleen) and non-biological material such as pills, air samples and clothing for many toxicants.

Once the laboratory has determined the absence or presence of a drug or chemical toxicant, the toxicologist will render an opinion as to whether the findings are significant and how they may have been related to the death. Since drug effects may differ from individual to individual and depend on many factors (health status of an individual, age, sex, combinations of drugs detected, quantity of drug taken, manner of dosing [oral, inhalation, injection] and rate of consumption), interpretation is a difficult and complex task based on knowledge and experience.

FOUNDATIONS OF TOXICOLOGY

Knowledge about poisons existed as long ago as the ancient writings of the Egyptians which made reference to poisons from plants. A passage from an ancient papyrus has been translated as 'Speak not of the name of Yao under penalty of the peach', indicating knowledge of a poison (hydrocyanic acid) in parts of the peach tree or fruit (Gettler, 1956). The papyrus Ebers from 1500 BC also mentions antimony, copper, hyoscyamus, lead and opium as poisons. Writings from India during the period 600–100 BC mention poisons including gold, copper, iron, lead, silver and tin. Socrates was executed in 339 BC with an extract of hemlock. A book entitled *The History of Plants*, published in 300 BC by Theophrastus, refers to medicinal and poisonous plants.

Numerous poisonings have been recorded in the history of the first 1800 years after Christ. Nine of the successors of Charlemagne (Holy Roman Empire) died of poisonings before the 1400s. Famous poisonings included five popes, many cardinals, and several kings. It became common place for kings to have 'tasters' of their food. In 1552, nux vomica (strychnine) was described.

Many poisonings occurred in England, France and Italy during the sixteenth and seventeenth centuries. Spara in the 1650s was the leader of a secret poisoning society in Rome. In the 1700s, Madam Toffana of Naples poisoned over 600 victims with white arsenic. The poisons most frequently used in this period were hemlock, aconite, opium, arsenic and corrosive sublimate (mercury).

Up until the late 1700s, convictions of perpetrators of homicidal poisonings were based on circumstantial evidence. In 1781, Joseph Plenic stated that the detection and identification of the poison in the organs of the decreased was the only true sign of poisoning. Mathiew J. B. Orfila (1787–1853), a Spanish chemist who became a professor of legal medicine at the University of Paris, published the first complete work of international importance on the subject of poisons and legal medicine in 1813, entitled Traité des Poisons Tirés des Règnes Minéral Végétal et Animal ou Toxicologie Générale. Orfila is considered the 'Father of Toxicology'. He identified several different disciplines of toxicology, including pharmaceutical, clinical, industrial and environmental. He established many of the guiding principles of toxicology including the need for adequate proof of identity and quality assurances. The principles still hold true today. They are:

1. Experience is paramount for credibility and reliability.
2. All facts surrounding the case must be given to the analysts.
3. All the evidence must be submitted properly identified and labelled and sealed.
4. All tests should be run and properly recorded.
5. Reagents must be pure and control samples free of the analyte of interest must be tested.
6. All tests should be repeated and compared with specimens to which known amounts of the analytes of interest have been added.

Devising analytical methods for the determination of poisons in human organs was one of Orfila's most important accomplishments. In 1839, Orfila extracted arsenic from human tissues using a procedure for identification developed several years earlier by James Marsh. Evidence of poisoning developed by this procedure was presented in court in 1840 to convict Marie Lafarge of homicide. This was the first time that toxicological data had been used as evidence in a trial. He was also the

instructor of Robert Christison (1779–1882), an British physician who returned to Britain after his education. Christison became a professor of legal medicine at the University of Edinburgh and is considered the first British toxicologist. In 1829, he wrote the text Treatise on Poisons, which was introduced into the USA in 1845.

Some of the major events that led to the development of chemical toxicology (Gettler, 1956) were:

1. In 1836, the development of a test for arsenic by James M. Marsh.
2. In 1839, Orfila successfully applied the Marsh test to identify arsenic extracted from liver, kidneys, spleen, muscle and heart.
3. In 1844, Freenius and von Babo developed a procedure for the systematic search for all mineral poisons. The procedure used wet ashing with chlorine to destroy the sample matrix.
4. In 1850, Stas developed a procedure for the extraction of nicotine from human tissues. The method was modified in 1856 by Otto to yield purer extracts of alkaloids. This modified procedure is commonly called the Stas–Otto method.
5. In 1874, Salami proved that decomposition can create artifacts and that extreme caution must be used in identification of poisons after death.

During the period from the 1830s to the early 1900s, analysis of tissue from human organs for toxicants still remained extremely rare. Most analyses were performed on gastric contents. Likewise, most tests were only performed in a qualitative manner. However, as more procedures were developed using 'wet ashing' and the Stas–Otto technique, some quantitative procedures also began to appear. Quantitative methods for alcohol were introduced in 1852 by Cotte based on the reduction of chromic acid. Electrolytic deposition techniques for metals were first used in 1862. In 1879, a method for the quantitative determination of arsenic was devised by Gutzeit. A quantitative procedure for carbon monoxide using palladium chloride reduction was introduced in 1880 by Fodor. Quantitative methods for alkaloids were introduced in 1890.

In 1918, New York replaced its coroners' system with the Medical Examiner's Office after members of the New York Academy of Medicine demonstrated that the medico-legal investigations carried out by politically appointed coroners were not adequate to protect the public's interest. A toxicology laboratory was established immediately. The chief forensic toxicologist of this laboratory was Alexander O. Gettler, the 'Father of American Toxicology'. During the first 30 years of the laboratory, the only analytical instruments were a Duboscq colorimeter, an analytical balance, a pH meter, a filter photometer and a Van Slyke manometric gas analysis apparatus. Despite the lack of more sophisticated analytical equipment, the laboratory was able to analyse biological materials for alcohol, cyanide, fluoride, carbon monoxide and thallium and perform the micro-isolation of volatile toxic substances from tissue.

In 1935, Gettler instituted a graduate course in toxicology at New York University (NYU) Graduate School. He trained many renowned toxicologists over the years, including H. C. Freimuth, C. J. Umberger, I. Ellerbrook, A. Stolman, F. Rieders, J. O. Baine, S. Kaye, I. Sunshine, L. Goldbaum, A. Freireich, M. Feldstein and H. Schwartz.

PROFESSIONAL ORGANIZATIONS, CERTIFICATION AND INSTRUMENTATION

In 1949, the American Academy of Forensic Sciences was formed to promote the practice of the forensic sciences, including forensic toxicology. Since that time several other organizations have been formed which have only forensic toxicologists as members. Two such organizations are the International Association of Forensic Toxicologists (1963) and the Society of Forensic Toxicologists (1970).

The four decades from 1960 to the present have seen an astronomical growth in technology applied to the science of forensic toxicology. Sophisticated instrumentation including thin-layer chromatography, spectrophotometry, gas chromatography, immunoassays, mass spectrometry and high-performance liquid chromatography have all been applied successfully to analyses in the area of forensic toxicology. These analytical techniques will be discussed in the section 'Types of Testing'.

Until the early 1980s, forensic toxicology was primarily concerned with medical examiners' cases and blood alcohol concentrations (BACs) in driving under the influence (DUI) cases. However, with the advent of testing for drugs in the armed services and the workplace, the birth of a new area of forensic toxicology occurred, Forensic Urine Drug Testing (FUDT). The demand for 'certified' forensic toxicologists to direct 'accredidated forensic urine drug testing laboratories' has caused a shortage of 'Board Certified Forensic Toxicologists' in the USA. Toxicology certification is available from several sources, including the American Board of Forensic Toxicology (ABFT) and the American Association of Clinical Chemists. One of the stated objectives of the ABFT is 'to make available to the judicial system, and other publics, a practical and equitable system for readily identifying those persons professing to be specialists in forensic toxicology who possess the requisite qualifications and competence'. Those certified as Diplomats of the Board must have an earned Doctor of Philosophy or Doctor of Science degree, have at least 3 years full-time professional experience and pass a written examination. At present, there are approximately 250 Diplomats and 15 specialists certified by the Board. Additionally, ABFT

has developed an accreditation programme for laboratories performing forensic toxicology. The first post-mortem toxicology laboratories were accredited in 1997. It is anticipated that such accreditation will be a standard in the profession within a few years. Another new frontier in the 1980s for forensic toxicologists has been the testing for driving under the influence of drugs other than alcohol (DUID). This chapter will focus on traditional post-mortem forensic toxicology.

The Forensic Laboratory is responsible for demonstrating the absence or presence of chemical substances in biological and non-biological specimens in connection with medico-legal investigations. The laboratory must be capable of analysing a wide variety of toxic substances. Alcohols (methanol, ethanol, propan-2-ol), antidepressants, barbiturates and other sedative hypnotics, benzodiazepines (minor tranquillzers), carbon monoxide, chlorinated hydrocarbons, drugs of abuse (amphetamines, cocaine, phencyclidine, marijuana constituents) including so-called 'designer drugs' [methylenedioxymethamphetamine (MDMA), methylfentenyl], heavy metals (arsenic, antimony, lead, mercury), insecticides, opium alkaloids (morphine, codeine) and synthetic opiates (hydromorphone, oxycodone, pethidine), phenothiazines and other major tranquillizers are among the most frequently encountered substances in the forensic laboratory.

The toxicology laboratory is responsible for the handling of evidence and must maintain a proper chain of evidence with receipts or records for the transfer and storage of materials to be analysed. The specimens should be properly refrigerated until transported to the laboratory. Specimens must be delivered to the laboratory with proper identification of the specimen affixed to each container. The information on the container label should include the name of the deceased, the case number, date of sampling and the type of sample **(Figure 1)**. When the specimens are delivered to the laboratory, they must be accompanied by a proper transmittal form that shows the name, case number, date and types of specimens being transmitted **(Figure 2)**. This transmittal form is referred to as the 'external chain of custody'. A separate form must be created for each case. Any

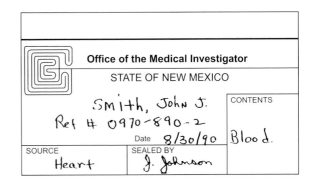

Figure 1 Specimen container label.

TOXICOLOGY SPECIMEN TRANSMITTAL FORM

NAME: SMITH, JOHN J. DOD 8/29/90
REF #: 0970–890–2
PATH: DR. VEASEY

1 FEMORAL BLOOD
1 HEART BLOOD
1 VITREOUS
1 URINE
1 WHITE POWDER

LAST PAGE OF 1 PAGE
ABOVE SPECIMENS TRANSMITTED BY J. Johnson ON 30–AUG–90
ABOVE SPECIMENS RECEIVED BY R. Backer ON 30–AUG–90

Figure 2 Toxicology specimen transmittal form.

TOXICOLOGY WORK SHEET

NAME - SMITH, JOHN J. DATE OF DEATH - 8/29/90

MEDICAL EXAMINER - S. PEASEY, M.D. DATE OF REQUEST-8/30/90

REF# - 0970–890–2 DECOMPOSED -NO

BRIEF HISTORY - FOUND WITH WHITE POWDER, RAZOR BLADE, AND STRAW AT SCENE; SUSPECT COCAINE OVERDOSE

SPECIMENS		TEST
BLOOD (HEART)	– 1	ALCOHOL -_X_
BLOOD (FEMORAL)	– 1	UR DRUG -_X_
BLOOD ( )	–	BL DRUG -_X_
URINE	– 1	OTHER (specify)
BILE	–	ANALYZE UNKNOWN WHITE POWDER
VITREOUS	– 1	
KIDNEY	–	
BRAIN	–	
OTHER ( )		

RESULTS:

ANALYSTS	DATE	TEST
J Robb	8/3/90	Ht Bld Alc 43.42 mmol/L
R Backer	9-1-90	fem bld alc 41.25 mmol/L
R Backer	9-1-90	white Powder Coc-Pos GC/MS
R Backer	9-2-90	Ht Bld Coc 19.90 uMol/L GC/MS
R Backer	9-2-90	fem Bld Coc 14.85 uMol/L GC/MS
R Backer	9-2-90	DAS urine coc present - all others -
		None detected

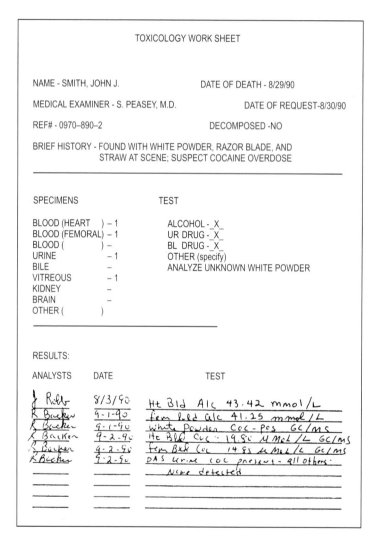

Figure 3 Toxicology laboratory work sheet.

discrepancies in the form and the samples should be noted on the transmittal form signed and dated by the receiving person in the laboratory and person making the delivery. Additional documentation includes a laboratory work sheet **(Figure 3)** and a report form **(Figure 4)**.

SPECIMEN STORAGE

Specimens are usually kept refrigerated (4 °C) during the time until they are analysed (short-term storage) and then in a freezer (−10 °C) until disposed of (long-term storage). It has been calculated that approximately

0970–890–2

Smith, John J.
2224 Saxton Court
Albuquerque, New Mexico

TOXICOLOGY REPORT
OFFICE OF THE MEDICAL INVESTIGATOR
STATE OF NEW MEXICO
University of New Mexico, School of Medicine
Albuquerque, New Mexico 87131

Age   49   Sex M   Race Anglo

Toxicology Bureau   8/30/90
Received by _____ **Date** _____

SPECIMEN:

1   Femoral Blood   1   Heart Blood
1   Vitreous   1   Urine
1   White Powder

EXAMINATION REQUESTED:

x   Alcohol   x Drugs of Abuse   x Identify White Powder

RESULTS:

Alcohol, Heart Blood, GLC
Ethanol 43.42 mmol/L

Alcohol, Femoral Blood, GLC
Ethanol 41.25 mmol/L

Drugs of Abuse, Urine, EIA
Cocaine: Present (parent and metabolites)
No other drugs detected

Basic Drug Screen, Heart Blood, GC/MS
Cocaine 19.8 mol/L; Benzoylecgonine - present
No other drugs detected

Basic Drug Screen, Femoral Blood, GC/MS
Cocaine 14.85 mol/L; Benzoylecgonine - present
No other drugs detected

X Final Report	____ Amended Report	Laboratory No. 0970–890–2	
REQUESTED BY S. Peasey, M.D.	REVIEWED 9/9/90 RCB	SIGNATURE OF TOXICOLOGIST *Ronald C. Backer, Ph.D.*	DATE 9/11/90

UNM. OMI. 010   Distribution: White - Case File: Canary - District Medical Investigator

Figure 4 Toxicology report form.

0.85 m^3 of freezer space is required to store the specimens from 500 cases (Backer, 1981). Obviously the need of freezer space will vary with the number of cases in which multiple specimens are collected.

Ideally, storage capacity should be adequate to store all specimens indefinitely. This idea is impractical since storage space is usually limited. A written policy must be established concerning disposal of samples. The policy should include the effective date of the policy, the length of time specimens will be held and a mechanism by which a request can be made for an extension of storage. **Figure 5** is an example of a form to request extended specimen

Office of the Medical Investigator
STATE OF NEW MEXICO

Universty of New Mexico
School of Medicine
Albuquerque, New Mexico 87131
(505) 277-3053

REQUEST FOR EXTENDED SPECIMEN STORAGE

DATE _____

NAME OF REQUESTOR _____

AGENCY AND MAILING ADDRESS _____

_____

NAME OF DECEASED _____ COUNTY OF DEATH _____

DATE OF DEATH _____ OMI CASE # _____

REASON FOR REQUEST _____

_____

I am aware that if a written confirmation of this request is not received within two weeks that it is my responsibility to call the Office of the Chief Forensic Toxicologist and confirm that the request has been received.

_____
Name of Requestor

Mail to: Chief Forensic Toxicologist
Office of the Medical Investigator
University of New Mexico
School of Medicine
Albuquerque, NM 87120.

Figure 5 Request form for extended storage of toxicology specimens.

storage. A reasonable length of storage is 2 years, which will allow for adjudication of most court procedings, both criminal and civil.

THE FORENSIC TOXICOLOGIST

The role of the forensic toxicologist in the forensic investigation is to determine whether various toxicants were present or absent in the specimens submitted to the laboratory. He must be a first-rate analytical chemist and be knowledgeable about the effects of poisons. He must know the 'older' techniques in addition to the newly evolving ones.

The major responsibilities of the forensic toxicologist include on-the-scene investigation, preservation of chains of evidence (external and internal), oral and written reports, consultation (pathologist, police, attorneys), expert testimony, research and development, education (self and others) and above all the ability to interpret the meaning of the concentration of the toxicant. The absence of a particular toxicant may be as important to a particular case as the detection of the substance in lethal concentrations. For example, finding sub-

therapeutic concentrations of antiepileptic drugs is important in seizure-related deaths. The presence of low concentrations of carboxyhaemoglobin in a suspected fire death always raises questions about the actual cause of death.

The forensic toxicologist is responsible for all the results that are reported by the laboratory. He must be familiar with all the procedures used by the laboratory and capable of developing new methods when they are needed. He must recognize that all laboratories have analytical limitations and be knowledgeable when and where outside sources should be utilized.

The forensic toxicologist must have the proper educational background and professional experience necessary to interpret the laboratory's results. He must be knowledgeable of the specificity and sensitivity of the equipment and procedures utilized in the analyses. The forensic toxicologist must be capable of defending the results in judicial proceedings to a reasonable degree of medical and scientific certainty. His reputation will be reinforced by his work record, evidence of professional growth through peer-reviewed publications, presentations at professional meetings, membership of professional societies, and 'Board Certifications'.

One must always remember that the most important criterion in the interpretation of results is the circumstances surrounding the death. In the case of a low carboxyhaemoglobin level in the above-mentioned example, it would be important to know if the fire victim had been given oxygen or had been doused with gasoline. In either of these two case circumstances the carboxyhaemoglobin level might be less than 10% of saturation. Another example in which the toxicology results help to complete the circumstances is as follows: a person was last seen alive 6 h prior to his body being found with a gunshot wound to the back of his head. When last seen he was sharing a marijuana joint with his friend. Analysis of the blood of the deceased revealed a concentration of 60 ng ml^{-1} of Δ^9 THC and 100 ng ml^{-1} of THC acid. This result indicates that the person had died less than 1–2 h after smoking the marijuana cigarette. This type of information aids the investigation and helps to narrow the time of death estimation.

Even in cases where circumstances make the cause of death obvious, the laboratory may be able to resolve some questions, such as: was the homicide drug related?; was the deceased sexually molested (acid phosphatase)?; was the deceased incapacitated by drugs (hypnotics, anaesthetic agents)?; or was bizarre or life-threatening behaviour prior to death due to self-intoxication with a drug of abuse such as phencyclidine or LSD?

CONSIDERATIONS IN SPECIMEN COLLECTION

Since the autopsy usually occurs before the investigation of the circumstances surrounding the death is completed, it is important to obtain adequate types and volumes of specimens at the time of the autopsy (**Table 1**). The specimens collected in a specific medical examiner's case may differ from case to case depending on the circumstances. However, in all medico-legal investigation cases a blood specimen should be obtained when blood is available. The analysis of a post-mortem specimen is only as reliable as the conditions surrounding its collection (Plueckhahn, 1968). Proper collection of specimens often requires the addition of preservatives and/or enzyme poisons to protect the specimen from postmortem changes such as bacterial production of ethanol or other alcohols or their loss. A commonly employed agent for this purpose is sodium fluoride at a concentration of at least 10 mg ml^{-1} of specimen.

Traditionally, heart blood has been collected at autopsy. However, recent studies have shown that with drugs such as propoxyphene, tricyclic antidepressants (amitriptyline, imipramine, doxepin, etc.) and many others, heart blood concentrations can increase postmortem (Bandt, 1981; Prouty and Anderson, 1984, 1990; Jones and Pounder, 1987; Andrenyak and Backer,

Table 1 Typical autopsy samples collected for toxicological analysis

Type	Quantity	Analytes
Blood (heart and femoral)[a]	20 ml	Volatile, carbon monoxide, drugs
Urine	20 ml	Drugs, heavy metals
Bile	20 ml	Opiates, other drugs
Kidney	Entire	In absence of urine
Liver	20 g	All drugs
Gastric	Total	Drugs taken orally
Vitreous humor	Both eyes	Alcohol, glucose, electrolytes

Challenging cases: exhumed, decomposed, skeletal remains:

Bone, rib and long bone	Whole	Most drugs
Hair	500 μg	Most drugs
Maggots	5–10 g	Most drugs
Nails	One whole toe	Heavy metals
Skeletal muscle	20 g	Most drugs

[a] Should contain preservative: sodium fluoride, 10 mg ml^{-1}.

1988). These reports show a relationship between postmortem interval (time from death to autopsy) and concentration increase. The concentration differences in heart blood and other peripheral sites are referred to as 'anatomical site concentration differences' or 'postmortem redistribution'. A list of some of the drugs in which anatomical site concentrations differences have been shown is given in **Table 2**. Peripheral blood concentrations have been shown to be more reliable with these drugs when compared with peri-mortem concentrations (Andrenyak and Backer, 1988; Prouty and Anderson, 1990). Therefore, in all suspected drug overdoses or in cases of unknown causes of death a femoral blood specimen should be collected and analysed

It is interesting that some drugs even within the same specimen do not show an increase whereas others do. **Table 3** shows the analytical data from an actual postmortem case study with multiple drugs, carisoprodol and propoxyphene. The carisoprodol heart/femoral concentration ratio (H/F) was 1.02 and the propoxyphene H/F

Table 2 Drugs shown to have significant anatomical site-dependent blood concentrations

Alprazolam	Diphenhydramine	Normeperidine
Amantidine	Doxepin	Norpropoxyphene
Amitriptyline	Doxylamine	Nortriptyline
Amoxapine	Fluoxetine	Phencyclidine
Amphetamine	Imipramine	Propoxyphene
Brompheniramine	Maprotoline	Propranolol
Caffeine	Meperidine	Thioridazine
Chlordiazepoxide	Methamphetamine	Trimipramine
Chlorpheniramine	Metoprodol	Verapamil
Cocaine	Nordoxepin	
Desipramine	Norfluoxetine	

Table 3 Case data showing heart and femoral concentrations (μmol l^{-1}) in a multiple drug overdose

Specimen	Carisoprodol	Propoxyphene
Heart blood	31.1	11.22
Femoral blood	30.3	5.54

was 2.03. Other authors have proposed that drug concentrations in liver specimens are a better indicator of toxicity (Apple and Bandt, 1988; Prouty and Anderson, 1990).

Some studies have reported that heart blood alcohol concentrations also change during the post-mortem interval (Bowden and McCallum, 1949; Turkel and Gifford, 1957; Briglia *et al.*, 1986). The authors of these studies recommended that femoral blood specimens be used for alcohol determinations in post-mortem cases. In several other studies it has been shown that heart blood concentrations of alcohol did not change post-mortem in intact bodies and that ethanol concentration differences in heart and femoral blood are minor and more likely represent the expected difference seen in the absorptive phase of alcohol consumption (Plueckhahn, 1968; Backer *et al.*, 1980). However, in cases where bacterial infiltration of the body is likely, a femoral specimen is recommended. Endogenous alcohol production will be proportional to glucose concentration which can be several times higher in post-mortem heart blood than femoral blood (O'Neal and Poklis, 1996).

A particular challenge to forensic toxicologists are those cases involving embalmed, exhumed, decomposed and incinerated bodies (Poklis *et al.*, 1998a). Hair analysis is a rapidly growing technique in forensic toxicology (Inoue and Seta, 1992). Hairs should be plucked from the scalp, capturing the entire shaft from root to tip. About 20–30 hairs are plucked from the back of the scalp and rolled into a clean plastic or foil sheet with an indication of the scalp ends on the attached label. The properly labelled packet is submitted to the laboratory. In the absence of scalp hair, hair from other body sites may be collected. If heavy metals such as arsenic are a consideration, nails may also be collected and analysed (Poklis and Saady, 1990).

In decomposing bodies, the absence of blood and/or the scarcity of solid tissue suitable for toxicological analysis have led to the collection and analysis of maggots (fly larvae) feeding upon the body. The fundamental premise underlying maggot analysis is that if drugs or intoxicants are detected they could only have originated from tissues upon which the larvae were feeding, i.e. the decedent (Pounder, 1991). Surprisingly, analysis of maggots has proved fairly straightforward, requiring no special methodology beyond that routinely applied in toxicology laboratories. Controlled studies that allowed maggots to feed on tissues to which drugs had been added have demonstrated the accumulation of the drugs in the larvae (Goff *et al.*, 1993). At present there is no correlation between drug concentrations in maggots and those of the human solid tissues from the corpse on which the larvae were feeding. Therefore, maggot results provide only qualitative information about drug use.

Owing to the advances in analytical sensitivity and specificity over the last decade, drug identification even in skeletal remains is not a hopeless undertaking. Any muscle tissue available and both rib and long bone specimens should be collected for analysis. Numerous drugs have been successfully identified in bone marrow and bond washings from skeletal remains, even after decomposition and burial (Noguchi *et al.*, 1978; Benko, 1985). Hair should also be collected for analysis of drugs. If the remains are suspected to be those of a particular person, hair may also be tested for any medications known to have been taken by the decedent. Soil immediately adjacent to the area of the visceral organs and maggots, if present, should also be submitted for analysis.

PROCEDURAL APPROACH

The particular approach that a laboratory takes to testing biological specimens is dictated by the type of services it provides. Therefore, a laboratory serving a hospital emergency room will be interested in rapid turnaround times for the common drugs of abuse. Laboratories testing for chemical substances in relationship to determining the cause of death typically utilize a large variety of different types of tests, including immunoassay, colorimetric, spectrophotometric and thin-layer, gas and high-performance liquid chromatographic methods. The post-mortem forensic laboratory must be prepared to analyse for a number of commonly encountered analytes. **Table 4** lists frequently encountered substances for which a post-mortem toxicology laboratory should be capable of performing qualitative and quantitative

Table 4 Commonly encountered substances in acute overdoses

A. Gases and volatiles
   Alcohols, chlorinated hydrocarbons, aromatic hydrocarbons, carbon monoxide and cyanide
B. Extractable organic acids
   Barbiturates, salicylates, acetaminophen (paracetamol)
C. Extractable organic neutrals
   Glutethimide, ethchlorvynol, meprobamate, carisoprodol
D. Extractable organic bases
   Cocaine, propoxyphene, opium alkaloids, antidepressants, benzodiazepines
E. Ionic Poisons
   Borate, bromide, cyanide, fluoride
F. Toxic Metals
   Antimony, arsenic, mercury, thallium

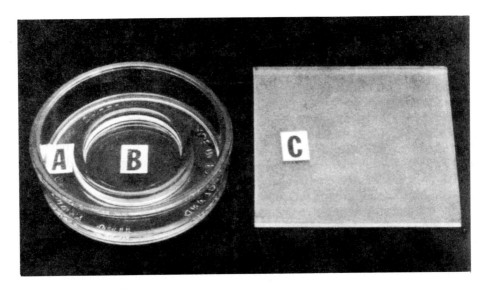

Figure 6 Conway microdiffusion dish.

analysis. The following section describes some of the commonly employed types of tests and their general applications.

TYPES OF TESTING

Colorimetric—Screening Tests

Screening tests are usually performed directly on biological specimens with little or no sample preparation (Widdop *et al.*, 1986). Some of the most common substances tested for include phenothiazines, imipramine, desipramine, trimipramine, halogenated compounds, salicylates, acetaminophen (paracetamol), ethchlorvynol (Finkle and Bath, 1971) and heavy metals (Gettler and Kaye, 1950). These tests are rapid and informative but only presumptive. Since many of them only identify a class of compounds, they usually require further identification of the specific toxicant and confirmation.

Steam Distillation

Volatile substances can be separated from blood, urine, or tissue homogenates by steam distillation. The specimen is made either acidic with hydrochloric acid or basic with solid magnesium oxide. Steam is passed into the solution and the aqueous distillate is collected by condensation. Analytes steam distilled from acidic solutions include ethanol, methanol, phenols, halogenated hydrocarbons, cyanide and ethchlorvynol. Distillates from basic solutions will contain volatile basic drugs such as amphetamines, pethidine, methadone and nicotine. The distillates can then be analysed by various techniques including colorimetric tests, immunoassays,

spectroscopy and various chromatographic methods including thin-layer, gas and liquid chromatography.

Microdiffusion

Microdiffusion is a convenient, rapid separation technique that allows for the analyte to be either detected as it is isolated (alcohols, carbon monoxide) or to be captured in an appropriate medium and tested by various techniques (cyanide, methanol, phenols, chlorinated hydrocarbons, sulphides). The technique of isolation utilizes a Conway microdiffusion dish **(Figure 6)**. A comprehensive review of microdiffusion applications has been presented by Feldstein and Klendshoj (1957). A microdiffusion method for ethchlorvynol has also been described (Peel and Freimuth, 1972).

Spectroscopy

Spectroscopy is based on the principle that substances either gain or lose energy when subjected to electromagnetic radiation. Identification of the substance may be possible by noting the wavelengths at which the energy changes take place. The energy changes are proportional to the quantity of the analyte present. The common types of spectroscopy utilized in the forensic laboratory include visible, ultraviolet, fluorimetric, atomic absorption and infrared.

Chromatography

Chromatography is a separation technique utilizing a partitioning process. Mixtures of drugs and their metabolites are commonly separated by chromatography. Chromatography requires a stationary or fixed phase which may be a liquid or solid absorbed on an inert support having a large surface area and a moving or mobile phase of a liquid or gas. In a chromatographic method, analytes within a mixture are moved by the mobile phase while the different interactions of the individual analytes with the stationary phase cause separation from other components. After separation, the components are identified by various methods including colorimetry, spectrophotometry and/or electrolytic analysis.

Most chromatographic techniques require extraction of the specimen before analysis. The extent of the 'clean-up' prior to chromatography depends on many variables, including the nature of the matrix, the concentration of the analyte of interest, and the type of chromatography. Liquid–liquid extraction is one of the most common separation techniques. Other types of extraction techniques commonly employed include liquid–solid methods such as charcoal and solid-phase extractions.

Thin-layer chromatography (TLC) is a simple separation technique which does not require expensive equipment. An extract of a biological specimen is applied as a concentrated spot at the origin of a TLC plate. The plate is placed in a developing tank with just enough solvent to submerge the bottom 1–1.5 cm. As the solvent (mobile phase) moves up the plate by capillary action, drugs and their metabolites are separated depending on the polarity of the solvent system and the solubility characteristics of the compounds in the extract. Visualization is accomplished with chromogenic reagents and long- or short-wave ultraviolet light. The distance the compound travels from the origin divided by the distance the solvent travelled from the origin is called the R_f or migration value. The R_f value along with the colour reactions are used for qualitative and semi-quantitative results.

In general, TLC is a fairly sensitive technique. The specificity of TLC can be increased by using multiple chromogenic visualization reagents. Most reagents are non-destructive and the analytes can be removed and tested by other analytical techniques. The major disadvantages of TLC include the need for extraction prior to analysis and that the experience of the chromatographer will effect the quality of the results. Some excellent reviews of different TLC separation and visualization techniques can be found in the literature (Davidow *et al.*, 1968; Bussey and Backer, 1974; Moffat, 1986).

With some drugs, confirmation tests can be performed directly on the TLC plate or the spot after removal without further extraction. A procedure for pethidine confirmation by fluorimetry directly on TLC spots without extraction is described below. The spot corresponding to pethidine is removed with a spatula and placed in a 10 ml beaker and then processed as follows: to the TLC scrap-

ings add 5 drops of Marquis reagent (8–10 drops of 40% formaldehyde in 10 ml of concentrated sulphuric acid) and heat in an oven at 110 °C for 10 min. Then add 1 ml of distilled water and observe under long-wave ultraviolet light. A blue fluorescence indicates that pethidine may be present. To confirm its presence (Dal Cortivo, 1970), add 2 ml of water and scan in a spectrofluorimeter with excitation at 270 nm and emission at 420 and 440 nm **(Figure 7)**.

TLC drug identification systems can be purchased from commercial sources. One system, Toxi-LAB, available from ANSYS Diagnostics, Lake Forest, CA, utilizes silica gel-impregnated paper and dip solutions for visualization. Its chromatogram is subjected to four visualization steps (stages) and the colours and R_f values are noted for each stage. A compendium of photographs depicting chromatograms with the R_fs and colours in

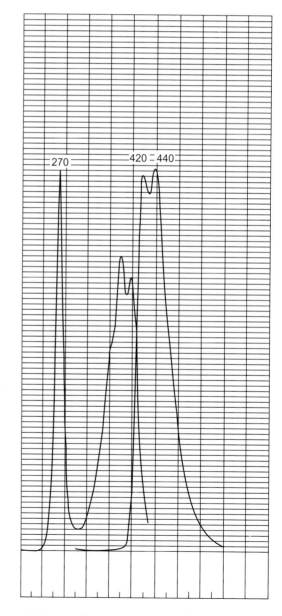

Figure 7 Spectrofluorimetric spectrum of pethidine.

each stage of development for hundreds of drugs is supplied by the manufacturer. The advantage of this type of system is that it makes everything available, including extraction tubes, visualization reagents, the photograph compendium, confirmation systems, drug standards, continual updates on new drugs and technical assistance. The disadvantage is the cost, but much of that is offset by technician time savings in not having to prepare visualization reagents and extraction tubes and that less technical training is necessary to be proficient at identification. Another similar system has been developed using a single mobile phase and multiple visualization and detection reagents (Siek *et al.*, 1997). A computer program (Spot Chek) assists in matching the data from a particular chromatogram with those obtained from known drugs from serum, urine and other specimens. The system is based on nine different colour reactions and the R_f zone for 243 drugs and metabolites.

Gas–liquid chromatography (GLC), like TLC, is a separation technique. It is one of the most widely used techniques in drug analysis. It is used for both screening and confirmation procedures. In GLC, an inert gas, such as nitrogen or helium, serves as the mobile phase. An extract of the biological specimen is dissolved in a small amount of organic solvent (usually 25–100 μl) and then injected into a heated injector. The sample is vaporized and swept on to the column by the carrier gas (mobile phase). The identification of compounds in GLC is by retention time.

The column is in an oven with a temperature controller. The vaporized sample is carried through the column by a controlled flow-rate of the mobile phase. The stationary phase interacts with the sample, causing the analytes within the mixture to separate. The retention time is a measure of the time elapsed from the injection of the extract into the gas chromatograph until the apex of the detector response.

A column's capability to separate analytes can be modified by using different types and amounts of liquid phases (stationary phases) absorbed on an inert solid phase. Types of columns used include packed and capillary columns. Packed columns are usually glass, 1–2 m in length and 3–6 mm in diameter. **Figure 8** shows a typical separation of a mixture of volatile intoxicants (alcohols and acetone) using a 2 m packed column (0.2% Carbowax 1500 on Carbopack C; Supelco, Bellefonte, PA). Capillary columns usually offer better separation than packed columns. They are commonly made of fused silica, 10–100 m in length and have a diameter between 0.25 and 0.60 mm. The stationary phase is a thin film (usually 0.25–1.0 μm). With most drugs, non-polar stationary phases such as polydimethylsiloxane or polydiphenyldimethylsiloxane are commonly employed. **Figure 9** shows a chromatogram of the separation of 'basic drugs' with a 30 m capillary column (polydiphenyldimethylsiloxane).

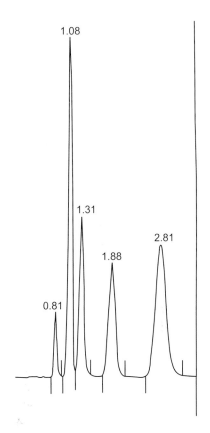

Figure 8 Separation of a volatile mixture on a packed column: methanol (0.81); acetone (1.08); ethanol (1.31); propan-2-ol (1.88); *n*-propanol (2.81 min).

There are several common types of detectors used in the toxicology laboratory. **Table 5** lists commonly utilized detectors and their relative sensitivity to commonly encountered drugs in toxicology.

Gas chromatography–mass spectrometry (GC–MS) combines the separating powers of the gas chromatography with the discriminating abilities of a mass spectrometer. Recently, the combination of a liquid chromatograph or chromatograph with two mass analysers, referred to as tandem mass spectrometry (MS–MS), has found many applications in forensic toxicology. The advantages of MS are that extracts require less purification prior to analysis and the high sensitivity of the technique. The major disadvantage is the cost of the instruments.

The basic operation of a mass spectrometer can be separated into three steps: ionization, mass filtration and detection.

In the most common mode of operation, the mass spectrometer utilizes electron impact (EI) for ionization. Neutral molecules in a gas phase are bombarded with high-energy electrons, which causes the molecules to lose an electron, so that they carry a positive charge and sufficient energy to undergo fragmentation. The fragmentation pattern always occurs in the same manner, thereby creating an identifiable spectrum. The spectrum

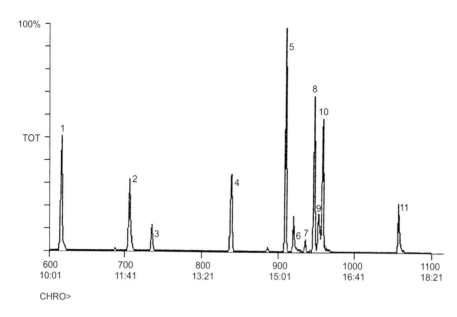

Figure 9 Separation of a 'basic drug' mixture: 1, pethidine; 2, ketamine; 3, phencyclidine; 4, methadone metabolite; 5, methadone; 6, methaqualone; 7, propoxyphene; 8, cocaine; 9, nortriptyline; 10, imipramine; 11, codeine.

Table 5 Gas chromatography detector sensitivity related to relative blood concentrations of various drugs

Detector	Drug	Blood concentration (mg l^{-1})	Relative sensitivity
Flame ionization (FID)	Ethanol	1000	g
	Valproic acid	100	mg
Nitrogen–phosphorus (NPD)	Phenobarbital	10	μg
	Pentobarbital	1	μg
	Amitriptyline	0.1	μg
Electron capture (ECD)	Flurazepam	0.01	ng
Mass spectrometer (MS)	Fentanyl	0.001	ng
MS–MS	LSD	0.0001	pg

fragmentation pattern for a given compound is its fingerprint **(Figure 10A)**.

Another mode of mass spectrometer operation is selective ion monitoring (SIM). In this mode the MS monitors the ion current of only those ions of a few masses that are characteristic for a specific drug. SIM affords a higher sensitivity for most mass spectrometers, but provides a less specific pattern for identification. Other modes of operation include positive and negative chemical ionization (CI). The spectra produced from CI are typically less complex than EI spectra and more sensitive **(Figure 10B)**.

Liquid chromatography (LC) is one of the oldest analytical separation techniques. The technique was a slow separation process when first developed because the mobile phase flowed through a column by gravity only. In the modern technique of high-performance liquid chromatography (HPLC), pumps are utilized to pass the mobile phase through columns at pressure exceeding 1000 psi. The major components of a basic high-performance liquid chromatograph are a solvent reservoir (mobile phase), a pump, a packed column (stationary phase) and a detector. There are various types of detectors, including spectrophotometric, electrochemical, fluorescence and mass spectrometric. The characteristic measurement used in HPLC is the time from injection to detection at a given flow-rate. Additionally, specificity can be added by the type of detector, on-line ultraviolet analysis or by using different wavelengths for detection.

This technique has become widespread in clinical toxicology is becoming more popular in forensic work. Reports on the use of HPLC include forensic cases involving benzodiazepines (Hoskins *et al.*, 1977; Edinboro and Backer, 1985), propoxyphene (Rio *et al.*, 1987) and marijuana (Peat *et al.*, 1983; Isenschmid and Caplan, 1986).

Immunoassays

Immunoassays are based on a competition between the drug of interest in the specimen and a 'labelled' drug added to the specimen for sites on an antibody for the drug of interest. Immunoassays are widely used for the

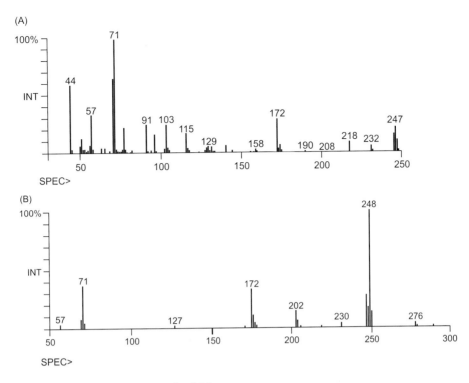

Figure 10 (A) EI and (B) positive CI mass spectra of pethidine.

direct testing of urine specimens, but in post-mortem toxicology may be used for analysis of whole blood, other body fluids and tissue homogenates. Immunoassays are commercially available for the detection of popular abused drugs and therapeutic agents which require routine plasma concentration monitoring.

Numerous immunoassays of varying selectivity and sensitivity are available to toxicologists; therefore, depending upon the purpose for testing, a positive result may be appropriate or a 'false-positive' result. For example, at present three different EMIT-d.a.u. enzyme immunoassays are available for the detection of amphetamine and/or methamphetamine in urine (Poklis and Moore, 1995). These assays have different antibody compositions and hence different stereoselectivities, analyte sensitivities and cross-reactivities with amphetamine-like compounds. The EMIT-d.a.u. Amphetamine Class Assay (EC) contains polyclonal antibodies and has a cut-off calibrator of 300 ng ml^{-1} d-amphetamine. The assay readily cross-reacts with phenylpropanolamine, ephedrine, pseudoephedrine, phentermine and other phenylisopropylamine derivatives. The EC assay is indicated when low detection limits for amphetamines and/or high cross-reactivity to other structurally related stimulants are desired, such as in post-mortem or athletic drug testing. The EMIT-d.a.u. Monoclonal Amphetamine/ Methamphetamine Assay (EM) contains monoclonal antibodies with a cut-off calibrator of 1000 ng ml^{-1} d-methamphetamine. The assay will also yield a positive result with approximately 400 ng ml^{-1} amphetamine. The EM assay displays much less cross-reactivity with

phenylisopropylamine derivatives than the EC assay except for the drug of abuse 3,4-methylenedioxy-methamphetamine (MDMA, Ecstasy) (Poklis et al., 1993a, b). EM may be appropriate when a 1000 ng ml^{-1} cut-off calibrator is required and high selectivity for not only amphetamine and methamphetamine, but also MDMA is desired. The EMIT II Amphetamine/ Methamphetamine Assay (EII) contains monoclonal antibodies with a cut-off calibrator of 1000 ng ml^{-1} d-methamphetamine, but unlike the EM assay requires 1000 ng ml^{-1} d-amphetamine to produce a positive response (Dasgupta et al., 1993). EII has low cross-reactivity to phenylisopropylamine derivatives and is configured for high-volume, high-speed analysers when high selectivity for amphetamine or methamphetamine is desired. The analyst should understand the performance characteristics of the immunoassay, particularly the cross-reactivity with 'over the counter' and prescription medications and illicit drugs of abuse.

Enzyme Immunoassay (EIA) is a homogeneous enzyme technique in which the antigen (drug) and antibody complex does not need to be separated from the matrix before assaying. The EIA system most often described is the EMIT system (Syva Corporation, Palo Alto, CA). In the EMIT assay, the label on the antigen (drug) is an enzyme. The specimen to be tested, usually urine, is mixed with a reagent containing glucose-6-phosphate (G-6-P) and antibodies to the drug of interest. A second reagent containing a drug derivative labelled with G-6-P dehydrogenase is added to the specimen. The enzyme is inactive when bound to an antibody site. If the drug of interest or its metabolite was present in the specimen then it will also react with the limited number of antibodies. This will have the effect of increasing the activity of the enzyme and allows for a semi-quantitative measurement of the concentration of the drug and/or its metabolite. A study has shown that by using a five-point calibration curve and a logit data transform, reasonable quantitative measurements of some drugs by EIA are possible (Standefer *et al.*, 1989).

Advantages of EIA include a short analysis time and minimal sample preparation. The sensitivity is adequate for most drugs of abuse. Disadvantages of the system include a lack of assay selectivity and the need to prepare supernates of blood or tissues prior to analysis (Asselin *et al.*, 1988).

A newer immunoassay similar to EIA is the 'cloned enzyme donor immunoassay' (CEDA). In this assay, the labelled drug is attached to a fragment of the enzyme β-D-galactosidase. If prevented from binding the antibody, this results in a 'freed enzyme' catalysing the cleavage of galactose from the substrate chlorophenylred-β-galactose. The substrate is a deep orange dye which turns purple after the lost of β-galactose. The resultant increase in absorbance of the sample at 550 nm is proportional to the quantity of drug in the sample. The difference between this assay and EIA is that the freed enzyme does not become active until two fragments of enzyme combine, hence the term 'donor' assay.

Another immunoassay which uses a different form of labelled drug is the 'kinetic interaction microparticles in solution' (KIMS) assay. In this assay, the labelled drug is covalently bonded to microparticles which, if no drug is present in the sample, form conjugates with the antibody. These aggregates of microparticles and antibody are of sufficient size to scatter light, thus reducing light transmission through the sample. If drug is present in the sample, aggregate formation is blocked and light transmission increased. Thus the optical density of the sample is inversely proportional to the concentration of drug present.

A variant of EIA which is gaining popularity among forensic toxicologist is the 'enzyme-linked immunosorbent assay' (ELISA). Unlike the immunoassays mentioned above, ELISAs do not require the preparation of supernates or extractions prior to the analysis of blood or tissues (Perrigo and Joynt, 1995). In this assay, the antibodies are bound to the surface of sample wells arranged on a plate. The sample and enzyme-labelled drug are added to the antibody well and incubated. The well is then washed and substrate added. After a second incubation, a stopping reagent is added and the absorbance of the well measured. If no drug is present, the antibody-bound enzyme-labelled drug will produce a coloured product. This enzyme-mediated colour reaction is blocked if drug is present. Thus, the absorbance of the reagent in the reaction wells is inversely proportional to the concentration of drug present.

Radioimmunoassay (RIA) is also a competitive reaction for antibody sites between a drug and or its metabolites and a radioactively labelled drug. Like ELISA, RIA does not require the preparation of supernates or extractions prior to the analysis of blood or tissues. After separation of the antigen–antibody complex, the radioactivity is determined on either the supernatant or the precipitated antibody. The presence or absence of the drug is indicated by the radioactivity of the sample. If the supernatant is counted, a positive specimen is one in which the radioactivity counts are equal to or greater than those of a standard. When the precipitate is counted, a positive specimen is indicated when the radioactive counts are equal to or less than those of a standard. The advantages of RIA are its sensitivity and small sample size. The disadvantages are incubation time, the need for radioactive material and the cost of reagents.

Fluorescent polarization immunoassay (FPIA) utilizes a drug labelled with a fluorescent substance. The labelled drug competes with unlabelled drug or metabolite in the specimen for an antibody site. When a fluorophore is excited by polarized light, it will emit polarized light. A larger molecule will emit a greater proportion of polarized light. The antibody–fluorescent-labelled drug complex results in a macromolecule and therefore an increase in fluorescence. The amount of drug and/or metabolite in the specimen is inversely related to the amount of fluorescent polarization. The advantages of the technique are its sensitivity and that it may be used directly to analyse body fluids and tissue homogenates (Poklis *et al.*, 1998b). The major disadvantage is the cost of the reagents.

ANALYTICAL SCHEMES FOR THE DETECTION OF POISONS

The major types of medico-legal cases include apparent natural causes of death, accidents (motor vehicle related), accidents (non-motor vehicle related), homicides, suicides and drug abuse. The circumstances surrounding the case will usually determine the types of toxicology tests that are required. In almost all cases a volatile screen (VS) will be required. Other types of protocols include a drug of abuse screen (DAS), a general drug screen (GDS), an acid neutral screen (ANS) and a basic drug screen (BDS). **Figure 11** outlines the flow of specimens through the laboratory using the protocols described below.

The most frequently requested test in a forensic toxicology laboratory is a volatile screen (VS) for ethanol. There are many different types of techniques available for ethanol determination such as oxidative, enzymatic and gas chromatographic. The most popular method in forensic applications for determining ethanol is GLC. GLC has the ability to separate commonly encountered

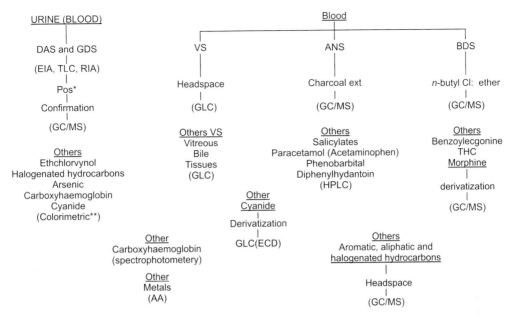

* If a drug is detected then the appropriate blood screen is initiated.
** If a colorimetric test is positive an appropriate confirmation is performed.

Figure 11 Flow diagram of laboratory protocols.

volatiles including ethanol, methanol, acetone and propan-2-ol, providing the required specificity and sensitivity to measure ethanol levels as low as 2.2 mmol l^{-1} (10mg dl^{-1}). A typical GLC procedure [with flame ionization detection (FID)] for ethanol would employ an internal standard such as n-propanol or *tert*-butyl alcohol (O'Neal et al., 1996). For quantitative determinations the peak height or area responses of ethanol to the internal standard would be compared with those for a series of aqueous standards with the same amount of internal standard. Direct injection analysis procedures for alcohols have been described (Jain, 1971; Winek and Carfagna, 1987), and also headspace procedures using both packed columns (Dubowski, 1977) and capillary columns (Penton, 1987; O'Neal et al., 1996). **Figure 8** shows a GLC trace for the analysis of a volatile mixture of alcohols and acetone from a headspace injection using n-propanol as an internal standard.

There are instances when a suitable blood specimen is not available for analysis (such as in traumatic injuries) or when the body is decomposing. Endogenous postmortem production of alcohol is a well known occurrence (O'Neal and Poklis, 1996). In cases where a suitable blood specimen is not available it may be possible to analyse various other biological specimens and estimate the blood concentration (Backer et al., 1980). Vitreous humor has been shown to be a fluid useful in the determination of alcohol in the absence of blood and in decomposing bodies (Zumwalt et al., 1982). The finding of ethanol in the vitreous humor and/or urine of a cadaver is consistent with an exogenous (ingested before death) source of alcohol. In Zumwalt's et al. study of 130 decomposing bodies, the highest concentra-

tion of endogenous ethanol was 47.8 mmol l^{-1} (220 mg dl^{-1}).

Another problem in ethanol determinations arises in embalmed cases. Embalming fluid can contain ethanol (Winek, 1984) and the embalming process has been reported to reduce the ethanol concentration by 52% when it is free of ethanol (Backer, 1989). Vitreous humor ethanol concentrations have been shown to be useful in embalmed cases. In a series of cases where pre- and post-embalmed vitreous alcohol concentrations were determined (Scott, et al., 1974. Coe, 1976), it was found that in 78% of the cases the post-embalmed concentration was within 6.5 mmol l^{-1} (30 mg dl^{-1}) of the usually higher pre-embalmed specimen's ethanol concentration. A drugs of abuse screen (DAS), which commonly tests for amphetamines, barbiturates, benzodiazepines, cocaine, marijuana, methadone, propoxyphene, phencyclidine and opiate alkaloids, is requested in most homicides and accidental deaths. The most common test is an enzyme immunoassay (EIA), usually performed on urine but also applicable to other specimens.

A general drug screen (GDS) is a broad-spectrum analysis for many drugs required when the cause of death is not clear. The GDS usually involves a TLC and/or a GLC method and is applicable to many different specimens, including urine, blood and gastric and tissue homogenates.

The acidic and neutral drug screen (ANS) usually involves a GLC and/or a GC/MS method for acidic and neutral drugs including barbiturates and non-barbiturate sedative hypnotics such as glutethimide and muscle relaxants including meprobamate and carisoprodol. The

ANS method is applicable to many types of specimens, including blood, urine and tissue homogenates.

The basic drug screen (BDS) usually involves a GC (GC–MS) method for the analysis of many basic drugs such as propoxyphene, cocaine, antidepressants, opiates (codeine, oxycodone, hydromorphone, pethidine), calcium channel blockers and many others.

Miscellaneous protocols that are also needed for other commonly encountered analytes include cyanide, carboxyhaemoglobin, arsenic and other metals, pesticides, aromatic, aliphatic and chlorinated hydrocarbons and vitreous chemistries such as sodium, chloride and glucose. There are many publications that can be referred to for protocols for these and other analytes (Sunshine, 1971; Moffat et al., 1986, Baselt and Cravey, 1989).

INTERPRETATION OF RESULTS

After the analysis of specimens is complete, the forensic toxicologist must interpret the findings as to the physiological effects of the analytes in retrospect to their concentrations. The specific questions that must be answered are whether the concentrations of any analyte or combinations of analytes were:

■ Sufficient to cause the death?
■ Sufficient to have affected the actions of the decedent so as to cause the death?
■ Insufficient to have any involvement in the cause of death?
■ Insufficient to protect the individual from an underlying mechanism of death such as an epileptic seizure?

Many factors must be taken into account, including the route of administration. The most common methods of administration of toxicants are oral, intravenous and inhalation. Since concentrations of drugs administered intravenously that result in fatalities are often much lower than those found in oral overdoses, it can be very important to know the route. In forensic cases, the route may not always be known unless evidence is found at the scene, such as a syringe and the decedent has very recent injection sites. The toxicology finding may answer some questions about the route, for example, finding a large amount of drug or even intact medication in the stomach contents is a good indication of an oral route of administration. However, some drugs are absorbed very rapidly, such as tricyclic antidepressants and even when massive overdoses are ingested only traces may be found in the gastric contents. It is important to point out that with most analytes the presence of the drug in the gastric contents is not sufficient proof that it was the agent or one of a combination of toxicants that caused the death. It must be documented that sufficient absorption of the substance occurred to result in a toxic concentration of the analyte in blood and/or liver. Other findings, such as extremely high lung concentrations of a drug or chemical, are very suggestive of an inhalation route.

It had always been assumed that the concentration of most analytes in heart blood paralleled the physiological consequences, but this premise has been shown to be untrue (Jones and Pounder, 1987; Andrenyak and Backer, 1988; Prouty and Anderson, 1990). It is now known that the concentrations of many analytes increase in both heart and peripheral blood specimens during the post-mortem interval. These anatomical site concentration differences have shown that in most cases that femoral blood is more likely to be a better indicator of the peri-mortem (at death) concentration of the analyte (Table 2). Reference to common tabulations of toxic concentrations of analytes (Baselt et al., 1975; Winek, 1976; Baselt and Cravey, 1977; Stead and Moffat, 1983) must be used with extreme caution since most are based on heart blood findings. A compilation of fatal drug concentrations in post-mortem femoral blood has been tabulated (Druid and Holmgren, 1997).

The liver concentration and/or brain concentration of an analyte may be extremely important in the determination of the involvement of an analyte in the cause of death. The toxic concentrations of many analytes in liver can be found in tabular form (Baselt and Cravey, 1977). The concentration ratio of the analyte in blood and liver is often very helpful in the interpretation of the involvement of the analyte (Apple and Bandt, 1988). With some drugs such as methadone, the therapeutic (or maintenance concentration) overlaps the concentrations found in overdoses. However, it has been postulated that the concentration ratio of 1,5-dimethyl-3,3-diphenyl-2-ethylidenepyrrolidine, a major metabolite of methadone, in the liver and kidney is always $\leqslant 1$ in case of overdose of methadone (Thompson, 1976). The ratio of blood propoxyphene concentration to its major metabolite, norpropoxyphene, has also been investigated in predicting toxicity (Caplan et al., 1977; Hartman et al., 1988).

Drugs taken in combination can be more toxic than if considered separately. Knowledge of the interaction of toxicants will be paramount to proper interpretation of the toxicity of any analyte. Most analytes are more toxic in the presence of alcohol. The toxicity of barbiturates and alcohol has been studied (Cimbura et al., 1972). Unfortunately, information about most combinations of analytes is scarce and the toxicologist must often deal with them on an individual basis. Experience with similar cases or published reports will be the only information upon which the forensic toxicologist can rely in predicting the toxicity of many analyte combinations.

Other factors that must be considered in the interpretative process by the forensic toxicologist are the age, sex, body weight, genetic factors, tolerance, environmental exposures and general health status of the individual. All of these factors can influence the response of a given concentration of an analyte or combinations of analytes. Liver disease may prevent the metabolism of an analyte, allowing multiple dosing to result in accumulation of the drug to toxic concentrations, or an underlying condition such as atherlosclotic cardiovascular disease will make the presence of analyte at a given concentration more toxic. Environmental exposure and abusive use of halogenated hydrocarbons can result in the sensitization of myocardial tissues, making an individual more susceptible to a cardiac arrthymia (Reinhardt *et al.*, 1971).

CONCLUSION

Post-mortem forensic toxicology has changed dramatically in the past 30 years. Some of the major changes have been related to analytical techniques such as immunoassays, high-performance liquid chromatography and the role of gas chromatography–mass spectrometry and tandem mass spectrometry in positive identifications of toxicants. The knowledge that the concentrations of many drugs are not stable in post-mortem specimens has caused considerable debate and change in the toxicologist's ability to interpret the analytical findings.

The increase in the requirement of laboratories to be certified will remain one of the major challenges in the new millennium, along with the need to control costs, which will result in more and more centralization of laboratories and the growth of private forensic toxicology laboratories as many governmental agencies refer toxicology services in an attempt to control expenditure.

REFERENCES

Andrenyak, D. M. and Backer, R. C. (1988). Postmortem concentrations of propoxyphene and norpropoxyphene in blood obtained from different anatomical locations. Presented at the 40th Annual Meeting of the American Academy of Forensic Sciences, Philadelphia, PA.

Apple, F. S. and Bandt, C. M. (1988). Liver and blood postmortem tricyclic antidepressant concentrations. *Am. J. Clin. Pathol.*, **89**, 794–796.

Asselin, W. M., Leslie, J. M. and McKinley, B. (1988). Direct detection of drugs of abuse in whole hemolyzed blood using Emit d.a.u. urine assays. *J. Anal. Toxicol.*, **12**, 207–215.

Backer, R. C. (1981). In Cravey, R. H. and Baselt, R. C. (Eds), *Introduction to Forensic Toxicology*. Biomedical Publications, Davis, CA, pp. 142–150.

Backer, R. C. (1989). Determination of alcohol—postmortem consideration in embalmed and decomposed cases. Presented at the 41st Annual Meeting of the American Academy of Forensic Sciences, Las Vegas, NV.

Backer, R. C., Pisano, R. V. and Sopher, I. M. (1980). The comparison of alcohol concentrations in postmortem fluids and tissues. *J. Forensic Sci.*, **25**, 327–331.

Bandt, C. M. (1981). Postmortem changes in serum levels of tricyclic antidepressants. Presented at the 33rd Annual Meeting of the American Academy of Forensic Sciences, Los Angeles, CA.

Baselt, R. C. and Cravey, R. H. (1977). A compendium of therapeutic and toxic concentrations of toxicologically significant drugs in human biofluids. *J. Anal. Toxicol.*, **1**, 81–101.

Baselt, R. C. and Cravey, R. H. (Eds) (1989). *Disposition of Toxic Drugs and Chemicals in Man*, 3rd edn. Year Book Medical Publishers, Chicago.

Baselt, R. C., Wright, J. A. and Cravey, R. H. (1975). Therapeutic and toxic concentrations of more than 100 toxicologically significant drugs in blood, plasma, or serum: a tabulation. *Clin. Chem.*, **21**, 44–62.

Benko, A. (1985). Toxicological analysis of amobarbital and glutethimide from bone tissue. *J. Forensic Sci.*, **30**, 708–714.

Bowden, K. M. and McCallum, N. E. W. (1949). Blood alcohol content: some aspects of its post-mortem uses. *Med. J. Aust.*, **2**, 76–81.

Briglia, E. J., Hauser, C., Giaquinta, P. and Dal Cortivo, L. A. (1986). Distribution of ethanol in post-mortem specimens. Presented at the International Symposium on Driving Under the Influence of Alcohol and/or Drugs, Quantico, VA.

Bussy, R. and Backer, R. C. (1974). Thin-layer chromatographic differentiation of amphetamine from other primary-amine drugs in urine. *Clin. Chem.*, **20**, 302–304.

Caplan, Y. H., Thompson, B. C. and Fisher, R. S. (1977). Propoxyphene fatalities: blood and tissue concentrations of propoxyphene and norpropoxyphene and a study of 115 medical examiner cases. *J. Anal. Toxicol.*, **1**, 27–35.

Cimbura, G., McGarry, E. and Daigle, J. (1972). Toxicological data for fatalities due to carbon monoxide and barbiturates in Ontario. *J. Forensic Sci.*, **17**, 640–644.

Coe, J. I. (1976). Comparative postmortem chemistries of vitreous humor before and after embalming. *J. Forensic Sci.*, **21**, 583–586.

Dal Cortivo, L. (1970). Fluorometric determination of microgram amounts of meperidine. *Anal. Chem.*, **42**, 941–942.

Dasgupta, A., Saldana, S., Kinnaman, G., Smith, M. and Johansen, K. (1993). Analytical performance evaluations of Emit® d.a.u. Monoclonal Amphetamine/Methamphetamine Assay. *Clin. Chem.*, **39**, 104–108.

Davidow, B., Li-Petri, N. and Quane, B. (1968). A thin-layer chromatographic screening procedure for detecting drug abuse. *Am. J. Clin. Pathol.*, **38**, 714–719.

Druid, H. and Holmgren, P. (1997). A compilation of fatal and control concentrations of drugs in postmortem femoral blood. *J. Forensic Sci.*, **42**, 79–87.

Dubowski, K. M. (1977). *Manual for the Analysis of Ethanol in Biological Liquids*, DOT-TSC-NHTS-76-4. US Department of Transportation, Washington, DC.

Edinboro, L. E. and Backer, R. C. (1985). Preliminary report on the application of a high pressure liquid chromatographic method for alprazolam in postmortem blood specimens. *J. Anal. Toxicol.*, **9**, 207–208.

Feldstein, M. and Klendshoj, N. C. (1957). The determination of volatile substances by microffusion analysis. *J. Forensic Sci.*, **2**, 39–58.

Finkle, B. S. and Bath, R. J. (1971). In Sunshine, I. (Ed.), *Manual of Analytical Toxicology*. Chemical Rubber Co., Cleveland, OH, pp. 150–151.

Gettler, A. O. (1956). History of forensic toxicology. *J. Forensic Sci.*, **1**, 3–25.

Gettler, A. O. and Kaye, S. (1950). A simple and rapid analytical method for Hg, Bi, Sb and As in biological materials. *J. Lab. Clin. Med.*, **35**, 146–151.

Goff, M. L., Brown, W. A., Omori, A. I. and LaPointe D. A. (1993). Preliminary observations of the effects of amitriptyline in decomposing tissue on the development of *Parasarcophaga ruficornis* (Diptera: Sarcophagidae) and implications of this effect to estimation of postmortem interval. *J. Forensic Sci.*, **38**, 316–322.

Hartman, B., Miyada, D., Pirkle, H., Sedgwick, P., Cravey, R., Tennant, F. and Wolen, R. (1988). Serum propoxyphene concentrations in a cohort of opiate addicts on long-term propoxyphene maintenance therapy. *J. Anal. Toxicol.*, **12**, 25–29.

Hoskins, W. M., Richardson, A. and Sanger, D. G. (1977). The use of high pressure liquid chromatography in forensic toxicology. *J. Forensic Sci. Soc.*, **17**, 185–188.

Inoue, T. and Seta S. (1992). Analysis of drugs in unconventional samples. *Forensic Sci. Rev.*, **4**, 89–107.

Isenschmid, D. S. and Caplan, Y. H. (1986). A method for the determination of 11-nor-delta-9-tetrahydrocannabinol-9-carboxylic acid in urine using high performance liquid chromatography with electrochemical detection. *J. Anal. Toxicol.*, **10**, 170–174.

Jain, N. C. (1971). Direct blood-injection method for gas chromatographic determination of alcohols and other volatile compounds. *Clin. Chem.*, **17**, 82–85.

Jones, G. R. and Pounder, D. J. (1987). Site dependence of drug concentrations in postmortem blood—a case study. *J. Anal. Toxicol.*, **11**, 184–190.

Mofatt, A. C. (1986). Thin-layer chromatography. In Moffat, A. C., Jackson, J. V., Moss, M. S. and Widdop, B. (Eds), *Clarke's Isolation and Identification of Drugs*, 2nd edn. Pharmaceutical Press, London, pp. 160–177.

Moffat, A. C., Jackson, J. V., Moss, M. S. and Widdop, B. (Eds) (1986). *Clarke's Isolation and Identification of Drugs*, 2nd edn. Pharmaceutical Press, London.

Noguchi, T. T., Nakamura, G. R. and Griesemer, E. C. (1978). Drug analyses of skeletonizing remains. *J. Forensic Sci.*, **23**, 490–492.

O'Neal, C. L. and Poklis, A. (1996). Postmortem production of ethanol and factors which influence interpretation: a critical review. *Am. J. Forensic Med. Pathol.*, **17**, 8–20.

O'Neal, C. L., Wolf, C., II, Levine, B., Kunsman, G. and Poklis, A. (1996). Gas chromatographic procedures for determination of ethanol in postmortem blood using *t*-butanol and methyl ethyl ketone as internal standards. *Forensic Sci. Int.*, **83**, 31–38.

Peat, M., Deyman, M. E. and Johnson, J. R. (1984). High performance liquid chromatography–immunoassay of delta-9-tetrahydrocannnabinol and its metabolites in urine. *J. Forensic Sci.*, **31**, 110–119.

Peel, H. W. and Freimuth, H. C. (1972). Methods for the determination of ethchlorvynol in biological tissue. *J. Forensic Sci.*, **17**, 688–692.

Penton, Z. (1987). Gas-chromatographic determination of ethanol in blood with 0.53 mm fused silica open tubular columns. *Clin. Chem.*, **33**, 2094–2095.

Perrigo, B. J. and Joynt, B. P. (1995). Use of ELISA for the detection of common drugs of abuse in forensic whole blood samples. *Can. Soc. Forensic Sci. J.*, **28**, 261–269.

Plueckhahn, V. D. (1968). The evaluation of autopsy blood alcohol levels. *Med. Sci. Law*, **8**, 168–176.

Poklis, A. (1997). Forensic toxicology. In Eckert, W. (Ed.), *An Introduction to Forensic Sciences*. CRC Press, Boca Raton, FL, pp. 107–132.

Poklis, A. and Moore, K. A. (1995). Response of Emit amphetamine immunoassay to urinary desoxyephedrine following Vicks inhaler use. *Ther. Drug Monit.*, **17**, 89–94.

Poklis, A. and Saady, J. J. (1990). Arsenic poisoning: acute or chronic, suicide or murder? *Am. J. Forensic Med. Pathol.*, **11**, 226–232.

Poklis, A., Hall, K. V., Eddleton, R. A., Fitzgerald, R. L., Saady, J. J. and Bogema, S. C. (1993a). Emit-d.a.u. Monoclonal Amphetamine/Methamphetamine Assay. I. Stereoselectivity and clinical evaluation. *Forensic Sci. Int.*, **59**, 49–62.

Poklis, A., Saady, J. J., Hall, K. V. and Fitzgerald, R. L. (1993b). EMIT-d.a.u. Monoclonal Amphetamine/Methamphetamine Assay: II. Detection of methylenedioxyamphetamine (MDA) and methlenedioxymethamphetamine/ (MDMA). *Forensic Sci. Int.*, **59**, 63–70.

Poklis, A., Sunshine, I. and Jentzen, J. (1998a). Toxicology. In Fierro, M. (Ed.), *Handbook for Postmortem Examination of Unidentified Remains*. College American Pathologist, Northfield, IL, pp. 241–247.

Poklis, A., Poklis, J. L., Trautman, D., Treece, C., Backer, R. and Harvey, C. M. (1998b). Disposition of valproic acid in a case of fatal intoxication. *J. Anal. Toxicol.*, **22**, 537–540.

Pounder, J. D. (1991). Forensic entomo-toxicology. *J. Forensic Sci. Soc.*, **31**, 469–472.

Prouty, R. W. and Anderson, W. H. (1984). Documented hazards in the interpretation of postmortem blood concentration of tricyclic antidepressants. Presented at the 36th Annual Meeting of the American Academy of Forensic Sciences, Anaheim, CA.

Prouty, R. W. and Anderson, W. H. (1990). The forensic implications of site and temporal influences on postmortem blood-drug concentrations. *J. Forensic Sci.*, **35**, 243–270.

Reinhardt, C. F., Azar, A., Maxifield, M. E., Smith, P. E. and Mullins, L. S. (1971). Cardiac arrhythmias and aerosol 'sniffing'. *Arch. Environ. Health*, **22**, 265–279.

Rio, J., Hodnett, N. and Bidanset, J. H. (1987). The determination of propoxyphene, norpropoxyphene, and methadone in post-mortem blood and tissue by high-pressure liquid chromatography. *J. Anal. Toxicol.*, **11**, 222–224.

Scott, W., Root, I. and Sanborn, B. (1974). The use of vitreous humour for determination of ethyl alcohol in previously embalmed bodies. *J. Forensic Sci.*, **19**, 913–916.

Siek, T. J., Stradling, C. W., McCain, M. W. and Mehary, T. C. (1997). Computer-aided identification of thin-layer chromatographic patterns in broad-spectrum drug screening. *Clin. Chem.*, **43**, 619–626.

Standefer, J., Backer, R. C. and Archuletta, M. S. (1989). Comparison of quantitative results: EMIT assay vs TDX for drugs of abuse. Presented at the 41st Annual Meeting of the American Academy of Forensic Sciences, Las Vegas, NV.

Stead, A. H. and Moffat, A. C. (1983). A collection of therapeutic toxic and fatal blood drug concentrations in man. *Hum. Toxicol.*, **3**, 437–464.

Sunshine, I. (Ed.) (1971). *Manual of Analytical Toxicology*. Chemical Rubber Co., Cleveland, OH.

Thompson, B. C. (1976). Chemical diagnosis of methadone related death. Doctoral Thesis. University of Maryland, Baltimore, MD.

Turkel, H. W. and Gifford, H. (1957). Erroneous blood alcohol findings at autopsy; avoidance by proper sampling technique. *J. Am. Med. Assoc.*, **164**, 1077–1079.

Widdop, B., Moffat, A. C., Jackson, J. V., Moss, M. S. and Widdop, B. (Eds) (1986). *Clarke's Isolation and Identification of Drugs*, 2nd edn. Pharmaceutical Press, London, pp. 3–34.

Winek, C. L. (1976). Tabulation of therapeutic and lethal drugs and chemicals in blood. *Clin. Chem.*, **22**, 832–836.

Winek, C. L. (1984). Reply to research query. *Soc. Forensic. Toxicol. Newsl., Toxtalk*, No. 4, 4.

Winek, C. L. and Carfagna, M. (1987). Comparison of plasma, serum, and whole blood ethanol concentration. *J. Anal. Toxicol.*, **11**, 267–268.

Zumwalt, R. E., Bost, R. O. and Sunshine, I. (1982). Evaluation of ethanol concentrations in decomposed bodies. *J. Forensic Sci.*, **27**, 547–554.

Chapter 69
Veterinary Toxicology

Frederick W. Oehme and Wilson K. Rumbeiha

CONTENTS

INTRODUCTION

Veterinary toxicology is a diverse discipline with many subspecialities dealing with the health and care of animals, the relevance of animals in studying human disease and the concern for domestic and wild animals in the environment. As these themes cannot all be addressed adequately in the space of one chapter, the focus will be on the classic role of veterinary medicine in understanding and managing chemically induced disorders of domestic animals. Domestic animals have basic anatomical, physiological and biochemical differences and it is, therefore, not surprising that each animal species may often react differently to the same toxicant. Those interspecies differences will be emphasized.

Approximately 10% of veterinary clinical practice is devoted to the diagnosis and treatment of poisonings in animals. The range of animals varies from small domestic animals, i.e. cats and dogs, to food-producing animals, i.e. dairy and beef cattle and swine, to horses, pet birds, zoo animals and occasionally wild game, such as rabbits and fish. The small animals react to chemicals more or less in the same way as humans because the species are all monogastrics. The ruminants (i.e. cattle and sheep), however, react differently from the monogastrics. The ruminants have evolved a unique digestive tract structure and microbial flora which play a major role in the fermentation of the forage ingested. The ruminant's microflora are usually capable of metabolizing toxic chemicals. As an example, cattle are more susceptible to nitrate poisoning than the horse, while dogs and cats are very resistant. Cattle are very susceptible to nitrate poisoning because the microbes in their digestive tract will convert nitrates to the proximate toxic metabolite, nitrite. Dogs, because of their relatively small gastro-intestinal microbial population, are resistant to nitrate poisoning. The horse may succumb to

nitrate poisoning because of the microorganisms in the caecum in its posterior digestive tract. However, by the time nitrate reaches the caecum, more than 70% will have been absorbed; little will be available for biotransformation into the toxic nitrite ion. The horse will therefore require threefold higher nitrate concentrations to be poisoned than will cattle.

Physiological differences among species can markedly alter the susceptibility of animals to toxicants. Birds, including pet birds, are more sensitive to toxic vapours and gases than mammals. Canaries have been used in mines to test for the presence of poisonous gases because their elaborate respiratory system will make them succumb to lower concentrations of toxic gases than humans. Biochemical differences also contribute to differential susceptibility between and within species. Cats are more susceptible to paracetamol (acetaminophen) poisoning than other domestic animals (Welch et al., 1966). The cat's glucuronyl transferase activity for conjugating paracetamol (acetaminophen) is much lower than in other domestic species and feline haemoglobin is more susceptible to oxidation than that of other animals (Rumbeiha and Oehme, 1992a). Therefore, cats given what would be considered a therapeutic dose for humans will die of methaemoglobinaemia. Biochemical differences are also found within the same species; for example, the Bedlington terrier is much more susceptible to copper poisoning than other species of dogs. Most biochemical differences are of genetic origin.

Adequate comprehension of the variability in toxicity from chemicals in the domesticated species requires understanding the anatomy, physiology and biochemistry of the affected animals. The other general factors that affect the toxicity of chemicals must also be considered when dealing with clinical toxicities in domestic animals. These factors include the animal's age, sex, health and nutritional status, concurrent exposure to other chemicals and the environment in which it lives (Osweiler *et al.*, 1985). The effects of these and other factors in modifying the outcome of poisoning can be of vital significance in determining its outcome and also indicates the appropriate management options. There is a vast literature in this area which interested readers can consult for detailed discussions (Osweiler *et al.*, 1985; Hayes, 1991).

COMMON TOXICOSES OF DOGS AND CATS

Dogs and cats are commonly poisoned by pesticides, herbicides, household products such as antifreeze, and drugs often used by humans such as paracetamol (acetaminophen). By far the most commonly reported toxicities in these small animals involve insecticides because of overzealous use of these products by owners in controlling fleas and ticks on their pets (Trammel *et al.*, 1989).

The insecticides most commonly involved in poisoning dogs and cats are organophosphates and carbamates, pyrethrins and pyrethroids, and chlorinated hydrocarbons. The organophosphate and carbamate insecticides have a common mode of action which is the inhibition of acetylcholinesterase (Fikes, 1990). Acetylcholinesterase is an enzyme which breaks down acetylcholine, a neurotransmitter in autonomic ganglia and at cholinergic nerve endings. The inhibition of acetylcholinesterase by organophosphate and carbamate compounds causes acetylcholine to accumulate and results in persistent firing of cholinergic nerve fibres. Affected animals are overexcited and show increased respiratory rates, muscle tremors and excessive salivation. Treatment of animals poisoned by organophosphate compounds involves administration of atropine and pralidoxime. Cases involving carbamates can only be treated with atropine. The organophosphate and carbamate compounds have a relatively high acute toxicity compared with chlorinated hydrocarbons but have a lower residual activity. As such, organophosphate compounds have largely replaced the organochlorines for insecticide use because of environmental concerns.

The chlorinated hydrocarbons (CH) were among the first insecticide compounds to be used, but have fallen into disfavour because of their persistence in the environment (Smith, 1991). Typical examples include DDT and lindane. The toxicity of these compounds in small animals is characterized by central nervous system (CNS) signs including ataxia and convulsions. Small animals are usually poisoned accidentally by being sprayed or by drinking concentrates of CH intended for spraying on crops. Although most of the organochlorines are burned or their use is highly restricted in Western countries, they are still widely used in developing countries. Therefore, cases of chlorinated hydrocarbon insecticide poisoning are still present mainly in developing countries.

Another class of insecticides which is increasingly commonly involved in small animal poisoning involves plant products: pyrethrins and their synthetic congeners the pyrethroids. These products are currently enjoying a resurgence because of their selective insecticidal properties and absence of environmental persistence (Valentine, 1990). These compounds are metabolized in the body mainly in the liver by glucuronidation. The cat is the most sensitive domesticated animal to pyrethrin toxicity because of the low activity of the glucuronide conjugating system in this species. Young cats, less then 6 weeks of age, are the most sensitive. We are seeing frequent toxicosis in cats from the pyrethroid products when they are used enthusiastically on cats for flea control or when products formulated for dogs are applied to cats or cats sleeping with treated dogs lick the pyrethroid product from their companion dog's haircoat. Pyrethroid compounds formulated with the insect repellant diethyltoluamide (DEET) were responsible for numerous deaths in cats and dogs in the early 1980s. Pyrethroids interfere with sodium channels in nerves causing them to fire repetitively (Casida *et al.*, 1983). Clinical signs of pyrethroid poisoning in small animals include muscle fasciculations and tremors, ataxia and excitement. There is no antidote for pyrethrin poisoning but treatment consists of symptomatic treatment such as decontamination procedures and sedation (Valentine, 1990).

Rodenticides

Rodenticide poisoning is commonly encountered in small animals. Rodenticides are widely used around farm houses to control rodents such as rats and mice which destroy property and farm produce. Several classes of rodenticides are currently in use. These include the anticoagulant rodenticides (warfarin and the second generation rodenticides such as brodifacoum), zinc phosphide, strychnine, compound 1080, and arsenic compounds. Small animals are poisoned either by consuming baits directly or through consumption of carrion of animals which have died of rodenticide poisoning. The clinical signs will vary with the compound involved and in the majority of cases occur in dogs because of their indiscriminate eating habits. Strychnine and anticoagulant rodenticides are the most frequently reported offenders. Strychnine poisoning in dogs is a rapidly developing syndrome characterized by tonic–clonic seizures. These signs are a result of strychnine competitively blocking the inhibitory neurones in the brain (Heisser *et al.*, 1992). The animals start showing signs within 20 min to 1 h of ingesting strychnine and if the animal has ingested a sufficient amount, death from anoxia occurs fairly acutely. Anoxia results from paralysis of respiratory muscles. Treatment of strychnine poisoning is symptomatic and involves general decontamination procedures, use of sedatives such as phenobarbitone (phenobarbital) and diazepam, maintenance of adequate urine output and respiratory support. The sedatives control the seizures and cause muscles to relax (Maron *et al.*, 1971; Boyd and Spyker, 1983).

The anticoagulant rodenticides have been in use for a fairly long time. Because of the long time required to take effect, some strains of rats became genetically resistant to the so-called first-generation anticoagulant rodenticides, such as warfarin. This led to the introduction of second-generation rodenticides, such as brodifacoum. Unlike the first-generation rodenticides which took at least 24–48 h to take effect, the second-generation rodenticides act fairly acutely; clinical signs can be evident within a few hours and have a long residual action. These anticoagulant rodenticides act by inhibiting vitamin K-dependent factors (VII, IX and X), decreasing prothrombin synthesis and by directly damaging blood capillaries (Coon and Wallis, 1972). Clinically, animals poisoned by anticoagulant rodenticides are weak, have swollen joints because of bleeding into the joint cavities, may show bleeding from the nostrils and may pass blood-stained faeces. Treatment of anticoagulant rodenticide poisoning involves blood transfusions if the bleeding is severe or heparin and vitamin K_1 injections. Early intervention involves general decontamination procedures to limit further absorption of toxicants, especially in the case of exposure to second-generation rodenticides, followed by vitamin K_1 therapy (Pelfrene, 1991).

The toxicity of zinc phosphide is due to phosphine gas which is produced by acid hydrolysis in the stomach. Animals with partially filled stomachs are more sensitive to zinc phosphide poisoning than those on empty stomachs because of higher acid secretion precipitated by the presence of food. Phosphine gas is then absorbed systemically and exerts its effects in the lungs. Poisoned animals exhibit respiratory difficulties because of the build-up of fluid in the lungs. The cause of death is respiratory failure (Stephenson, 1967). Supportive therapy, including respiratory support, is recommended in cases of zinc phosphide poisoning but the prognosis is poor as no effective antidote is available.

Compound 1080 (sodium fluoroacetate) is a very lethal toxicant which acts by blocking the Embden–Meyerhof pathway, thereby depriving cells of energy. *In vivo*, fluoroacetate is metabolized to fluorocitrate, which inhibits mitochondrial aconitase. This blocks ATP production (Buffa and Peters, 1950). Affected animals are initially uneasy, become excitable and will run in one direction and finally fall down in seizures and die of anoxia. There is no antidote to Compound 1080 and, invariably, poisoned animals die.

Cholecalciferol (Quintox) is a rodenticide which has been reported to be widely involved in the poisoning of dogs. The compound alters calcium homeostasis by promoting calcium absorption from the gut and also by mobilizing calcium from bones. Consequently, poisoned animals have increased blood calcium levels. The calcium is subsequently deposited in soft tissues, such as muscle, liver, heart and kidneys. Mineralization of soft tissue interferes with normal function of these organs. Clinically the animals do not show signs until 24–48 h after ingestion of the bait. The affected animals are depressed, have reduced urine production and the urine is of low specific gravity. Severely poisoned animals have haematemesis, azotaemia and cardiac arrhythmias (Dorman, 1990). Animals with renal impairment are more susceptible to cholecalciferol poisoning than those with normal renal function. Cholecalciferol poisoning requires protracted treatment which may last as long as 3 weeks in severe intoxications (Livezey *et al.*, 1991). The treatment consists of fluid therapy to assist the kidneys excrete calcium, corticosteroids to depress inflammation, and calcitonin to enhance calcium resorption into bones.

Several other rodenticides can cause poisoning in small animals but less frequently because these rodenticides are used less often. Red squill and thallium have been used as rodenticides for a very long time. Red squill acts as a cardiotoxicant and causes death by cardiac arrest. Red squill also causes convulsions and paralysis. Thallium is a general systemic toxicant. It has a high affinity for sulphydryl groups throughout the body. Thallium causes cracking at the corners of the lips and also hair loss. α-Naphthylthiourea (ANTU) causes death by inducing lung oedema, subsequently leading to anoxia. White phosphorus is a hepatorenal toxicant. Animals poisoned by white phosphorus have severe abdominal pain, hepatomegaly and signs of hepatic insufficiency such as prolonged bleeding and hypoglycaemia. In general, cases of rodenticide poisoning in small animals should be regarded as emergencies. General decontamination procedures such as vomiting induced with either hydrogen peroxide or apomorphine, use of activated charcoal to bind the unabsorbed toxicants, or enterogastric lavage should be employed to minimize absorption of the toxicant.

Herbicides

Herbicides are not widely involved in small animal toxicity despite their frequent use around farms. However, toxicity in dogs arising from consumption of concentrates of herbicides during mixing is occasionally reported. The triazine herbicides act by inhibiting photosynthesis and are generally safe products. The LD_{50} of these compounds in the rat is at least 1900 mg (kg body weight)$^{-1}$. Therefore, toxicity in dogs can only occur following ingestion of large doses of concentrates. In experimental situations, triazine herbicide-poisoned dogs become either excited or depressed, have motor incoordination and may show clonic–tonic spasms. Some inorganic arsenic compounds are used as herbicides. Inorganic arsenicals are general protoplasmic poisons and are therefore hazardous to both plant and animal life. Affected dogs have severe abdominal pain, bloody diarrhoea and vomiting and the vomitus may contain mucous shreds from erosion of the intestinal epthelium.

Paraquat, although restricted in use in Western countries, is a very toxic herbicide which is readily available in developing tropical countries. Following intake, paraquat is rapidly metabolized in the liver and lungs with secondary oxygen radical production. It is these secondary radicals which cause injury to tissues, especially the lungs. Poisoned animals die of acute respiratory failure (see Chapter 94).

Unlike other animals, the dog appears to be sensitive to chlorphenoxy herbicides such as 2,4-D. In the dog the oral LD_{50} is 100 mg (kg body weight)$^{-1}$. Ventricular fibrillation is the cause of death in severely poisoned dogs. Ingestion of sublethal doses induces myotonia, stiff extremities, ataxia, paralysis, coma and subnormal temperatures (Stevens and Sumner, 1991).

Chlorates are herbicides which have been used on roadsides. Chlorates are rapidly metabolized in the liver to the chlorate ion, which induces methaemoglobinaemia in both cats and dogs. Cats, however, because of the greater susceptibility of their haemoglobin molecule to oxidation, are more susceptible to chlorate poisoning than dogs. Organophosphate herbicides, e.g. glyphosate and merphos, are weak cholinesterase inhibitors and are of moderate toxicity in dogs and cats. Carbamate herbicides are not inhibitors of acetylcholinesterase and are moderately toxic in dogs. The LD_{50} of most of the carbamate herbicides is at least 5000 mg (kg body weight)$^{-1}$.

Household Chemicals

Antifreeze is one of the household products most commonly involved in small animal poisoning. The active ingredient in antifreeze is ethylene glycol. The characteristic sweet taste of this compound makes it very attractive to small animals. Ethylene glycol is metabolized in the liver by the alcohol dehydrogenase pathway into glycollic acid and oxalate and the former contributes to acidosis which is characteristic of ethylene glycol poisoning. The oxalic acid binds calcium in the blood to produce calcium oxalate crystals, which are filtered in the glomerulus into renal tubules where they cause blockage of the tubules (Grauer and Thrall, 1982). Consequently, affected animals have renal failure characterized by anuria and uraemia. The binding of blood calcium to oxalate causes hypocalcaemia which, if severe, can lead to death. Ethylene glycol poisoning is traditionally treated by giving ethanol if the animal is presented within 4–8 h of suspected ingestion and by giving fluids containing

sodium bicarbonate to facilitate flushing out the calcium oxalate crystals from the kidney and also to correct the acid–base imbalance. Alcohol dehydrogenase, an enzyme which breaks down ethanol to acetic acid and water, prefers ethanol to ethylene glycol and in the presence of both substrates will metabolize ethanol, leaving ethylene glycol to be excreted unchanged in the urine. 4-Methylpyrazole has recently been confirmed to have excellent antidotal properties against ethylene glycol toxicosis in dogs (Connally et al., 1996). It has fewer side-effects than ethanol and works by reversibly blocking the conversion of ethylene glycol to glycollic acid and oxalate by alcohol dehydrogenase. It is effective if administered up to 12 h after the consumption of the antifreeze, but because of species differences in enzyme specificity it is of no benefit to cats poisoned with ethylene glycol. Ethanol is still the preferred treatment for ethylene glycol intoxication in cats (Dial et al., 1994).

Household products such as sink cleaners, dish washing detergents and toilet cleaners are common causes of poisoning in small animals. The majority of the cleaning detergents are corrosive compounds which contain either strong alkali, acids or phenolic compounds (Coppock et al., 1988). These compounds therefore act as contact poisons, causing coagulative necrosis of the tissues which they contact. Following ingestion of these products the dog or cat will vomit, have severe abdominal pain and may have diarrhoea. The vomitus and faeces may be bloody. Animals may also show other signs depending on the specific ingredients of the offending products. For example, products containing phenolic derivatives will cause acidosis and hepatotoxicty. In general, treatment following ingestion of household products is symptomatic and involves the administration of adsorbents such as activated charcoal, gastro-intestinal protectants such as peptobismol and correction of systemic disturbances such as the acidosis which may accompany the poisoning. Animals should also be administered plenty of glucose and fed a high-protein diet.

Garbage Poisoning

Garbage poisoning is a frequently encountered problem in small animals. This condition is also referred to as enterotoxicosis or endotoxaemia, depending on whether poisoning is from bacterial infection or ingestion of bacterial endotoxins. Dogs that are not well fed and/or not closely supervised may eat garbage. Cats may also be affected but only rarely because they are discriminate eaters. The bacteria most commonly involved are coliforms, staphylococci, *Salmonella* and occasionally *Clostridium botulinum*. In enterotoxaemia affected animals develop a bacteraemia after eating infected carrion, clinical signs normally appearing at least 24–48 h after ingestion of the infected carrion. The condition is characterized by severe abdominal pain, anorexia, fever, vomiting and a bloody diarrhoea. In endotoxaemia the poisoning results from the bacterial endotoxins which are normally present in bacterial cell walls. The clinical signs are generally indistinguishable from those of enterotoxaemia, except that in the later there is no bacteraemia (which can be ruled out by culturing the blood). Although rare in occurrence, botulism is a rapidly developing fatal disease which can result from ingesting bones contaminated with *Clostridium botulinum*. In small animals the disease is characterized by an ascending paralysis. At first there is weakness and incoordination in the muscles of the hind limbs and as the paralysis progresses anteriorly there are dyspnoea and convulsions.

Garbage poisoning is rarely a severe condition in small animals because the animals invariably vomit and reduce the amount of toxicant ingested. However, in severe cases medical attention will be required. If the cat or dog is presented early after ingestion then general decontamination procedures should be instituted. Anti-inflammatory corticosteroids and antibiotics should be given, further treatment involving tender supportive therapy.

Heavy Metals

Lead and arsenic are the heavy metals most frequently involved in small animal poisoning, although zinc intoxication is unique and seen in dogs with increasing frequency. Lead poisoning is more commonly reported in the dog than the cat, but both are susceptible. The sources of lead poisoning in the dog include ingested leaded objects such as lead weights and paint chips in old houses that are being renovated. The clinical signs of lead poisoning in the dog primarily involve the CNS. The dogs often present with abdominal pains, diarrhoea and CNS involvement. Lead poisoning is a chronic disease in dogs but the overt central nervous signs may appear suddenly. Lead poisoning causes blood dyscrasia characterized by reticulocytosis and occasionally anaemia. Similar clinical signs are elicited in the cat. Treatment consists of giving chelating agents such as calcium disodium EDTA, dimercaprol (BAL), succimer (DMSA) or D-penicillamine.

Arsenic is the active ingredient in some insecticides, rodenticides and herbicides. Inorganic arsenic and the aliphatic organic arsenicals are rapidly absorbed from the gut, skin and lungs and are more toxic than cyclic organic arsenicals which are used as feed additives (Furr and Buck, 1986). Trivalent arsenic is the proximate toxicant of the pesticide arsenicals and it reacts with the sulphydryl groups of proteins throughout the body. It is therefore a general poison, inhibiting all sulphydryl-containing enzymes. The clinical signs of inorganic arsenic poisoning in dogs include severe abdominal pain, bloody diarrhoea, anorexia and hair loss etc., as discussed earlier under herbicides. Treatment involves decontamination, chelation therapy with BAL and supportive therapy.

The playful mouthing and swallowing behaviour of dogs results in their swallowing coins that in the acidity of the stomach release zinc. The absorbed zinc causes chronic liver damage and red blood cell destruction, presenting as a haemolytic anaemia. The often puzzling clinical illness responds quickly to removal of the dissolving coins from the stomach and appropriate supportive care for several days.

Plant and Mushroom Poisonings

Although one would not expect dogs and cats to eat plants (toxic or non-toxic), plant poisoning is surprisingly often reported in these species (Fowler, 1981). Because of their exploratory nature, puppies and kittens are most often involved. Boredom and change of environment are some of the predisposing factors to plant ingestion in dogs and cats. Poisonous ornamental plants, e.g. *Rhododendron*, and plants used around fences such as cassia and oak are mostly involved. The subject of poisonous plants is a vast one and because the clinical signs are similar in food-producing and small animals, this subject will be dealt with extensively under food-producing animals. In addition, interested readers may consult a good review of plant poisonings in small companion animals (Fowler, 1981).

Occasionally dogs or cats will eat or be fed poisonous mushrooms by uninformed owners. *Amanita muscaria* and *A. pantherima* are acutely toxic and induce signs within 15–30 min of ingestion. These two mushroom species cause nervous signs which include salivation, pupillary constriction, muscular spasms, drowsiness or excitement and eventually coma and death, in severe intoxications. Ibotenic acid and muscimol are the active ingredients. However, *A. phaloides*, *A. virosa* and *A. verna* induce gastro-intestinal signs which are evident 6–12 h after ingestion. The signs include violent vomiting, diarrhoea, dehydration and muscle cramps, and these mushrooms also cause hepatic insufficiency. Phalloidin and alpha- and beta-amanitine are the principal poisons in this group (Fowler, 1981).

COMMON TOXICOSES IN FOOD-PRODUCING ANIMALS

This section will address toxicoses commonly encountered in cattle, swine and small ruminants. Swine differ from all other animals in this category in that they have a simple stomach (monogastrics) whereas the rest have a compound stomach. Most of the toxicants discussed under small animals also affect food-producing animals but there are some toxicants which are peculiar or predominantly seen only in food-producing animals. Toxicoses which are frequently encountered in ruminants include non-protein nitrogen toxicoses, copper, lead, arsenic, mycotoxicoses, nitrite poisoning, plant poisoning and algae poisoning. In swine, salt poisoning, mycotoxicoses, organic arsenicals, plant poisoning and gases generated in swine-confinement operations are often involved.

Poisoning by Non-Protein Nitrogen Compounds

Non-protein nitrogenous sources in food-producing animals include urea, biuret, and ammoniated feeds. These compounds are cheap sources of nitrogen, which is required by the animals for protein synthesis. Non-protein nitrogen poisoning is a common problem and is often seen in animals that are not gradually introduced to diets containing these compounds. It is an acute fatal condition which is characterized by bloating, intense abdominal pain, ammonia on the breath, frequent urination and frenzy. Often several animals will be affected. In ruminant animals the rumen microflora normally convert urea to ammonia, and the ammonia is rapidly utilized by the liver for protein synthesis. However, in cases of excess ammonia production, the blood ammonia concentration builds up to toxic levels very quickly and induces CNS derangement (Lloyd, 1986). Therefore, in addition to gastro-intestinal signs, the animals will show fulminating central nervous signs. Treatment of the condition involves giving a weak acid such as vinegar and plenty of cold water orally. The rationale behind giving cold water and acetic acid is to slow the action of urease, the enzyme responsible for breaking down urea to ammonia, which requires high temperature and pH for optimal function. The cold water lowers the temperature and the acetic acid lowers the pH. Infusions of calcium and magnesium solutions should be given to alleviate tetany (Osweiler et al., 1985; Lloyd, 1986).

Other sources of non-protein nitrogen (urea) poisoning in ruminants involve accidental ingestion of nitrogen-based fertilizers, such as ammonium phosphate (Gosselin et al., 1976). Occasionally cattle break into drums or bags of fertilizers containing these nitrogen-based compounds. Prognosis is grave in most cases if several animals are affected. In cases where only a few valuable animals are affected, a rumenotomy can be performed. Although small ruminants have the same anatomical predisposition to suffer from non-protein nitrogen poisoning, they are rarely involved probably because they are not often fed rations containing these compounds.

Nitrate–Nitrite Poisoning

Excessive exposure of ruminants to nitrates causes nitrite toxicity, an acute, rapidly fatal disease. The commonest source of nitrates in ruminants is through consumption of forage grown on heavily fertilized fields that have accumulated a lot of nitrates (Ridder and Oehme, 1974). All common animal feeds such as sorghum, alfalfa and milo etc. can accumulate excessive amounts of nitrates (Clay et al., 1976). Another common source of nitrates is contaminated drinking water. Nitrates are highly water soluble and underground water contamination can occur from heavily fertilized fields (Menzer, 1991). Run-off from fertilized fields is another source of contamination to surface pools and ponds. Nitrates are broken down to nitrites by rumen microflora, and under normal circumstances the nitrite ion is rapidly utilized for ammonia synthesis, but in cases of excessive acute intake of nitrate, the nitrite ion is absorbed into the blood stream. In blood the nitrite ion reacts with haemoglobin to form methaemoglobin. Methaemoglobin is incapable of oxygen transport and the animal compensates for the anoxia by increasing the respiratory rate. Therefore, affected animals will be hyperventilating, have brownish mucous membranes, and will be weak. Chronic intake of nitrates has been reported to cause reproductive problems, such as abortion, but experimental results are inconclusive (Osweiler et al., 1985). Besides reacting with haemoglobin, the nitrite ion also replaces iodine in the thyroid gland, thereby interfering with the function of the thyroid hormone. Treatment of nitrate/nitrite poisoning involves intravenous infusion of 1% methylene blue at a dose of 1.5 mg (kg body weight)$^{-1}$ and withdrawal of the offending feed.

Copper-Molybdenum Poisoning

Sheep are more susceptible to copper poisoning than cattle but cattle are more sensitive to molybdenum poisoning than sheep. The in vivo relationship between copper and molybdenum is well understood, copper excess inducing molybdenum deficiency and vice versa. The most frequent cause of copper poisoning in sheep is feeding them, by uninformed farmers, feed meant for cattle. Copper is an essential element for cattle and is usually added to their feeds, but molybdenum is not considered essential and is therefore not added. Cattle feeds therefore have high copper and no molybdenum and feeding this ration to sheep upsets the normal copper/molybdenum ratio in vivo. Copper toxicity in sheep is an acute condition which develops after a chronic copper intake. During the chronic phase copper is stored in the liver until a certain critical concentration is reached and, following stressful conditions such as transportation or insufficient feed or water intake, a massive hepatic release of copper may be triggered, producing a haemolytic crisis (Osweiler et al., 1985). Affected sheep have haemoglobinuria, are weak and death occurs acutely. The massive release of haemoglobin can block the renal tubules inducing renal failure and the prognosis is poor for animals already showing clinical signs. Chelation therapy using D-penicillamine is recommended for exposed animals not showing clinical signs.

In cattle molybdenosis is characterized by a foamy diarrhoea which may be bloody; affected cattle also have depigmented hair. Molybdenosis is a subacute to chronic condition and occurs when the copper/molybdenum ratio is 2:1 or less. The condition has a geographical distribution and occurs in areas deficient in copper or where there is an excess of molybdenum, in parts of the USA (California, Oregon, Nevada and Florida) (Buck, 1986). Treatment of this condition involves copper supplementation in the feed.

Lead Poisoning

Despite an awareness of the dangers of lead poisoning in humans and domestic species, it is surprisingly the most frequently encountered heavy metal toxicity in food-producing animals. Lead poisoning is more commonly seen in cattle than in other food-producing animals. Young animals are mostly affected because of their curiosity and indiscriminate feeding habits. There are several sources of lead for cattle and discarded batteries and leaded water pipes are the commonest sources. Often uninformed owners will discard or store old batteries in farm environments and cattle will lick them. Discarded leaded pipes, especially those used around oil wells, are a common source of lead poisoning (Blood and Rodostits, 1989). Lead interferes with haem synthesis and causes renal and CNS lesions as in small animals. Affected animals are initially anorectic. They may become belligerent and blind at the terminal stages of the disease. Once the CNS signs have appeared the prognosis is poor but treatment with chelating agents, e.g. calcium disodium EDTA and DMPS, may be of value.

Arsenic

Arsenic poisoning is second to lead as the most frequently reported heavy metal toxicant in food-producing animals. Arsenic is present in the environment in two forms: inorganic and organic. Inorganic arsenic is often incorporated into pesticides, which are the most common sources of arsenic poisoning in cattle. Inorganic arsenicals are also used as herbicides and cattle are sometimes exposed by eating grass clippings from recently sprayed forage. Inorganic arsenic poisoning is a rapidly developing and fatal disease (Radeleff, 1970). Affected animals show severe gastro-intestinal abnormalities with minor CNS involvement, and have severe abdominal pain, haemorrhagic diarrhoea, and are depressed. Usually these signs appear 24–36 h after exposure.

Phenylarsonic arsenicals are less toxic to mammals than the inorganic arsenicals. Phenylarsonic compounds are usually incorporated into swine and poultry feed for disease-control purposes and also to improve weight gain. Examples of these compounds include arsenilic acid, 3-nitroarsenilic acid and 4-nitroarsenilic acid. Organic arsenicals are also available as trivalent and pentavalent compounds, the trivalent forms being more toxic than the pentavalent compounds. These phenylarsonic compounds are peripheral nervous system (PNS) toxicants. They cause demyelination of the peripheral nerve fibres leading to ataxia and paralysis of the hind quarters. The condition occurs frequently in swine kept on feed containing 10 000 ppm arsenic for at least 10 days or 200 ppm arsenic for 30 days. Therefore, unlike inorganic arsenic poisoning, which is an acute form of the disease, poisoning by phenylarsonic compounds has an insidious onset. In addition, organic arsenic is commonly involved in toxicities in swine because of its incorporation into swine feeds, whereas inorganic arsenic poisoning is commonly seen in cattle.

Treatment of inorganic poisoning is by decontamination procedures and the use of BAL antidote. Use of demulcent to coat the gastro-intestinal tract and antibiotics is also recommended. Treatment of organic arsenic poisoning involves withdrawal of the feed involved. Severely affected pigs should be culled.

Selenium Poisoning

Selenium poisoning is a regional problem occurring in areas where the selenium content in soil is high. Selenium is absorbed and concentrated by selenium-accumulating plants such as *Astragalus*. Cattle, sheep, goats and swine are exposed by consuming these indicator plants and acute selenium poisoning occurs when animals consume plants containing more than 10 000 ppm. This is characterized by sudden death or the animal may have laboured breathing, abnormal movement and posture, frequent urination, diarrhoea and death. Because plants containing high selenium concentration are unpalatable they are rarely consumed by animals so that acute selenium poisoning is rare. However, chronic selenium poisoning is common. Chronic consumption of plants containing as low as 50 ppm of selenium can cause chronic poisoning. Affected animals are anorexic, have impaired vision, wander, salivate excessively, are emaciated, lame and lose hair. Removal of animals from pastures that have high selenium concentrations is the recommended cure (Muth and Binns, 1964).

Mycotoxins

Some of the mycotoxins of veterinary interest include aflatoxins, deoxynivalenol (DON), diacetoxyscirpenol (DAS), T-2, zearalenone, ochratoxins and fumonism B_1

(Cheeke and Shull, 1985; Keller *et al.*, 1990). Mycotoxins are especially a common problem in warm climates where high temperatures and relative humidity support fungal growth and favour mycotoxin production. All food-producing animals are susceptible and clinical signs will depend on the mycotoxins involved. Rarely is only one mycotoxin involved because several species of fungi, e.g. *Fusarium*, *Penicillium* and *Aspergillus*, coexist and often produce more than one type of mycotoxin. The common sources of aflatoxins to food-producing animals include corn and oats. When aflatoxins are ingested in parts per million quantities acute death can occur with the affected animals showing severe gastrointestinal pain and haemorrhage. Aflatoxins are severe hepatotoxicants; therefore hepatomegaly and jaundice may be observed in severe subacute cases. Quite often, however, aflatoxin poisoning is insidious following a chronic intake of parts per billion concentrations of aflatoxin over a prolonged period of time. Clinical signs include poor weight gain, decreased milk production and poor reproductive performance, including abortions. Virtually every organ function is affected by aflatoxins. The immune system of affected animals is impaired and they succumb to infectious diseases (Pier, 1981).

Toxicity due to T-2 mycotoxins has been reported in North America and some other parts of the world, including Germany, Hungary, France and South Africa. It is less common than aflatoxin toxicity. T-2 acts by interfering with the blood clotting mechanism. Affected animals have gastro-intestinal bleeding and will pass blood-stained faeces. The animals will perform poorly, i.e. have low weight gain, decreased milk production and decreased food intake. T-2 is also an immunosuppressant. All food-producing animals are susceptible to T-2 mycotoxicosis. Treatment consists of withdrawal of the contaminated feed and supportive care.

Zearalenone is an oestrogenic mycotoxin which often causes toxicity in swine, prepubertal swine being mostly affected. Swine are affected by consuming contaminated corn. Affected females show swelling of the vulva and excessive straining which may cause vaginal prolapse. In male animals zearalenone will cause decreased libido. There is no effective treatment apart from withdrawing the contaminated feed.

Other mycotoxins, including DON, DAS and ochratoxin, are not of major economic importance although they can be toxic to food-producing animals. DAS causes necrosis and erosion of the oral mucous membranes. Consequently, affected animals may refuse to feed and have impaired growth. DON also induces vomiting and feed refusal in swine. Ochratoxins cause renal problems including hydronephrosis, especially in swine. Ergot poisoning is occasionally encountered in livestock fed grain screenings contaminated with *Claviceps purpurea*. The active ingredients are ergotoxin and ergotamine, which are vasoactive compounds. These compounds cause vasoconstriction of the peripheral vessels, especially those of the extremities, causing necrosis and gangrene of hooves and tail. Abortions and agalactia have been reported in cattle fed contamined feed. Therapy consists of discontinuation of the source of the toxicant and antibiotics to prevent secondary bacterial infection in necrotic tissues (Cheeke and Shull, 1985). Fumonisin B_1 is produced by *Fusarium moniliforme*, a worldwide fungus which predominantly grows on corn. Fumonisin B_1 causes pulmonary oedema and respiratory distress in swine. Deaths have been reported in swine fed contamined corn screenings (Colvin and Harrison, 1992). This mycotoxin is also responsible for numerous sporadic outbreaks of CNS disease in horses characterized by an encephalomalacia and is epidemiologically associated with high incidences of human oesophageal cancer in cultures that have corn as a dietary staple.

Blue–Green Algae

Blue–green algae poisoning occurs late in summer and early autumn when algae form a scum on pond water. Because of husbandry practices cattle are most frequently involved. Algae of the genus *Anabaena* are the ones most frequently involved. There are two distinct syndromes in blue–green algae poisoning: hepatotoxic and neurotoxic. The neurotoxic type is peracute, and cattle that drink water containing the neurotoxic principle anatoxin A can die within a few minutes and are found close to the pond. On the other hand, the hepatotoxic type causes an acute poisoning characterized by lethargy and jaundice (Beasley *et al.*, 1989) and death may occur within 2–3 days after drinking contaminated water. Blue–green algae poisoning has been reported in North America and the UK. Treatment involves supportive therapy in animals affected with the liver syndrome. Because of the peracute nature of the blue–green algae-induced neurological syndrome there is hardly time for treatment and the prognosis is poor.

Toxic Gases

Toxic gases are of primary concern in closed animal housing, especially swine operations. In intensive swine confinement operations, with buildings designed to save on energy, toxic gases can accumulate in swine houses, causing serious health consequences in cases of ventilation failure. These toxic gases are generated from the decomposition of urine and faeces, respiratory excretion, and operation of fuel-burning heaters. The most important gases are ammonia, carbon monoxide, methane and hydrogen sulphide. A number of vapours which cause odours of manure decomposition, such as organic acids, amines, amides, alcohols, carbonyls and sulphides, are also produced. Respirable particles may be loaded with endotoxins and are also a major health problem in swine and animal caretakers in confinement operations (Osweiler *et al.*, 1985).

Ammonia is highly lipid soluble and will react with the mucous membranes of the eyes and respiratory passages. At 100 ppm or greater, ammonia toxicosis will show as excessive tearing, shallow breathing and clear or purulent nasal discharge. The irritation of the respiratory tract epithelium leads to bronchoconstriction and shallow breathing. Hydrogen sulphide poisoning is responsible for more animal deaths than any other gas and, at 250 ppm and above, hydrogen sulphide causes irritation of the eyes and respiratory tract and pulmonary oedema. Concentrations of hydrogen sulphide above 500 ppm cause marked nervous system stimulation and acute death (O'Donogue, 1961). To prevent hydrogen sulphide poisoning, manure pits should be agitated when pigs are not in the premises and proper ventilation should always be in place.

Carbon monoxide is produced by incomplete combustion of hydrocarbon fuels. Poisoning by carbon monoxide is caused by operating improperly vented space heaters or furnaces in poorly ventilated buildings. Carbon monoxide binds to haemoglobin forming carboxyhaemoglobin, thereby reducing the oxygen-carrying capacity of the blood and subsequently causing hypoxia. Concentrations of carbon monoxide greater than 250 ppm cause hyperventilation and respiratory distress; stillbirths have been reported (Carson and Dominick, 1982).

Nitrogen dioxide is a very poisonous gas which is responsible for causing silo fillers' disease in humans and the gas is also very toxic to animals. Nitrogen dioxide is produced during the first 2 weeks after the silage has been cut and put in the silo. Highest concentrations of the gas are reached during the first 48 h after filling the silo. Nitrogen dioxide dissolves in water to form nitric acid, which is very corrosive to the respiratory tract and the lungs. As low as 4–5 ppm nitrogen dioxide can cause respiratory system disturbances (Osweiler *et al.*, 1985).

Exposure to sulphur dioxide at 5 ppm or higher causes irritation and salivation in swine. The gas is soluble in water forming the more toxic sulphuric acid, which causes eye and nasal irritation, and in severe cases haemorrhage and emphysema of the lungs (Osweiler *et al.*, 1985).

The effects of these toxicants singly and in combination is a hypofunctional respiratory system, and affected animals are predisposed to respiratory tract infections. The end result is retarded performance of the affected animals. It is therefore important to ensure that animal housing is adequately ventilated to provide animals with a healthy environment.

Toxic Plants

Plant poisoning is very common in areas where open grazing is practised, such as in South America and Africa. Interestingly, though, plant poisoning is also widely reported in North America during the spring and autumn. The subject of poisonous plants is a wide one which cannot be adequately summarized here. However, the toxicity of some selected poisonous plants is summarized in **Tables 1–8**. In these tables the plants are discussed on the basis of the organs most prominently affected. It is important to realize, however, that these plants rarely affect only one organ. This presentation is an attempt to summarize the vast amount of literature on the subject.

Interested readers should consult the relevant literature for detailed discussions (Kingsburry, 1964; Cheeke and Shull, 1985). It is important to remember that the toxicity of a given plant can vary widely depending on the prevailing natural conditions. It is therefore not surprising that a given toxic plant may be toxic under certain conditions, e.g. during stressful drought conditions, but safe during other times.

Salt Poisoning

Salt poisoning is frequently encountered in swine operations but can also occur in feedlot cattle. The causes of this condition are twofold. Most commonly, the pigs will be on a ration containing the recommended concentration of sodium chloride but management failure can favour conditions that can cause salt poisoning to occur. These poor management conditions include the sudden absence of water, e.g. by freezing in winter or breakdown of the water supply, and the possibility of the accidental addition of excessive amounts of salt to the ration. Salt poisoning has also been reported in swine operations even when the management situation is satisfactory, the only change being that the animals were moved into a new housing facility, as occurs after weaning. Apparently, the animals were not used to the new watering facilities in the new buildings and they did not know how to obtain the water and went without water while feeding on a normal ration. Clinically, salt poisoning is a neurological disorder and the syndrome is acute. Affected pigs will spin on their hind quarters and fall down in convulsions. The pigs will also show a characteristic rhythmic pattern of convulsions which occur every 3–5 min. Several pigs will be affected at the same time. The condition is corrected by provision of adequate but restricted amounts of water (Dunn and Leman, 1975).

COMMON TOXICOSES OF HORSES

In comparison with cats and dogs and food-producing animals, horses are less frequently poisoned. The most commonly encountered equine toxicoses involve pesticides, snake bites, arsenic, selenium, monensin,

Table 1 Toxic plants affecting the gastro-intestinal tract of food-producing animals

Scientific name	Common name	Species commonly affected	Toxic parts and principle(s)	Clinical signs
Ricinus communis	Castor oil plant	Cattle, pigs	Seeds, leaves Ricin	Abdominal pain, vomiting, convulsions, dullness
Robinia pseudocacia	Black locust	Cattle, sheep	Bark, foliage, seed Robin, robitin, phasin	Anorexia, lassitude, posterior paralysis, cold extremities, dilated pupils
Phoradendron spp.	Mistletoe	Cattle, sheep	Berries. β-Phenylethylamine, choline, tyramine	Vomiting, diarrhoea, bradycardia, sudden death
Ranunculus spp.	Buttercup	Cattle, goats, swine	Fresh foliage Protoanemonin	Blisters on lips, salivation, diarrhoea, tucked abdomen
Phytolacca dodecandra	Pokeweed	Cattle, sheep, swine	Foliage, unripe berries. Oxalic acid, phytolaccotoxin, phytolaccin	Diarrhoea, dyspnoea, spasms, reduced milk, convulsions, ataxia
Sesbania spp.	Rattlebox	All	Seeds, foliage Sesbanine	Haemorrhagic diarrhoea, severe abdominal pain, coma, death
Agrostemma githago	Corn cockle	Cattle, swine	Seeds. Githagenin	Diarrhoea, arched back
Quercus spp.	Oak	Cattle, sheep, swine	Acorns, buds, young leaves, flowers, seeds, stem Tannic acid, gallic acid	Abdominal pain, constipation or bloody diarrhoea
Euphorbia spp.	Spurge	Cattle, sheep	Whole plant Euphoron, euphorbin, cyanide	Diarrhoea (haemorrhagic or not), blisters of skin and oral mucous membranes, salivation, abdominal pain
Xanthium spp.	Cocklebur	Pigs, cattle, sheep	Seeds, cotyledons Carboxyatractlyloside	Anorexia, vomiting, tucked abdomen, depression, severe hypoglycaemia, weakness, convulsions

cantharidin and mycotoxins (Oehme, 1987a). Most plants discussed earlier with regard to food-producing animals are also toxic to horses, but less frequently. Horses are very sensitive to monensin and cantharidin poisoning.

The pesticides most frequently encountered in equine poisoning are the organophosphate, carbamate, and chlorinated hydrocarbon insecticides. Both the organophosphates and the carbamates are acetylcholinesterase inhibitors and the clinical presentation is similar to that of food-producing animals. Affected animals salivate profusely, and show muscle incoordination and ataxia. The chlorinated hydrocarbons are central nervous system stimulants and affected horses become excited, alert, and in extreme cases go into convulsions. In the majority of cases the mode of exposure to pesticides is topical (Oehme, 1987b).

Horses are highly susceptible to monensin poisoning in comparison with other domesticated animals. Monensin and other ionophores are commonly incorporated into cattle and poultry feeds to provide improved growth efficiency by enhancing the absorption of calcium and sodium from the gut. Horses are easily poisoned by accidentally consuming cattle or poultry feed containing recommended amounts of monensin. Affected animals can die suddenly without any premonitory signs. Monensin affects the cardiac and skeletal muscles and heart failure is the cause of death (Amend *et al.*, 1980).

Cantharidin is the toxic agent found in blister beetles. Several species of blister beetles are known and only a few contain cantharidin. Blister beetles are abundant in July–September at the time that hay is harvested in North America. Horses may be poisoned by eating hay containing swarms of blister beetles. Affected horses show severe colic and will kick at their belly and roll; they may die of shock. There is no effective therapy for affected horses but treatment involves the use of pain killers such as banamine hydro-chloride (Schmitz and Reagor, 1987) and intensive electrolyte therapy.

Lead poisoning in horses is characterized by neurological abnormalities. Affected horses may be either depressed or excited. Colic and diarrhoea are also observed. Horses poisoned by lead also have difficult respiration with roaring because of laryngeal nerve paralysis. Abortions are also common.

Arsenic poisoning in horses is caused by consumption of foliage which has recently been sprayed with arsenic herbicides and the condition is normally acute and characterized by intense colic and haemorrhagic diarrhoea. As in food-producing animals, inorganic arsenic poisoning does not involve the nervous system which helps differentiate this condition from organophosphate or carbamate poisoning.

Toxic Plants

Selenium is an essential element but is toxic when excessive quantities are ingested. Exposure is usually through

Table 2 Toxic plants primarily affecting the liver of food-producing animals

Scientific name	Common name	Species commonly affected	Toxic parts and principle(s)	Clinical signs
Senecio spp.	Groundsel	Cattle, sheep, goats	Foliage Several alkaloids, e.g. jacobine, jacodine	Dullness, aimless walking, weakness, increased pulse, rapid respiration
Crotolaria sagitallis and *C. spectabilis*	Rattlebox	Cattle and swine mainly, but all species affected	Foliage and seeds Monocrotaline	Loss of appetite, weakness, emaciation incoordination, excitability, nervousness
Amsinkia intermedia	Fiddleneck	Pigs mainly but also sheep and cattle	Seeds Intermidine, lycopsamine, sincamidine	Unthrifty, icteric, haemorrhages of the gastro-intestinal tract and subcutaneous tissues
Echium plantagineum	Viper's bugloss	Sheep mainly but also cattle and pigs	All parts are toxic Echiumine, echimidine	As for *Amsinkia*; contact dermatitis
Heliotropium	Heliotrope	Sheep	All parts Heliotrine, lasiocarpine, heleurine	As for *Amsinkia*; secondary photosensitization
Trichodesma europeum	–	All	Foliage Unidentified pyrolizidine alkaloids	As for *Amsinkia*
Lantana camara	–	Cattle, sheep, goats	All parts but especially foliage and berries Lantadine A and B	Severe gastroenteritis, bloody watery faeces, jaundice, secondary photosensitization
Helenium spp.	Sneezeweeds	Sheep and goats mainly but also cattle	All parts but especially leaves and flowers Helenaline, helanine, dugaldine	Severe abdominal pain, bloating, CNS involvement, e.g. head pressing
Hymenoxys	Bitterweed	Sheep, cattle, goats	All parts. Hymenoxon	Unthriftiness, inappetence, salivation
Kochia scoporia	Kochia	Cattle	Foliage Unidentified alkaloids + oxalates, nitrates and a thiamine antagonist	Unthriftiness, CNS signs, bleeding disorders, photosensitization
Agave lechaguilla	Agave	Sheep, goats, but also cattle	Foliage Unidentified saponins	Listlessness, primary photosensitization
Trifolium hybridum	Alsike clover	Pigs, sheep, cattle	Foliage. Unidentified saponins	Listlessness
Lotus corniculatus	Birdsfoot trefoil	Cattle	Foliage. Unidentified principles	Listlessness, bloat

consumption of seleniferous (indicator) plants, e.g. *Astragalus*. Exposure to high quantities of selenium over a short period of time causes diarrhoea, which may be foul smelling and contain air bubbles, and neurological, cardiovascular and respiratory signs. Death in these animals is from respiratory failure. Chronic exposure to excessive selenium is characterized by hoof abnormalities at the coronary bands and discoloration and loss of hair. The hoof deformities and pain cause lameness (Hultine *et al.*, 1979).

The other plant poisonings commonly encountered in horses are those that cause gastro-intestinal problems, liver damage, primary or secondary nervous system involvement, and sudden death. Plants such as castor bean, oleander and bracken fern cause colic and diarrhoea, Oleander also causing heart failure. Prolonged ingestion of some plants for several weeks can lead to liver damage and hepatic cirrhosis. Examples of commonly involved hepatotoxic plants include *Amsinckia*, *Senecio* and *Crotolaria* (Rumbeiha and Oehme, 1992b). Liver damage may compromise the ability of the horse to detoxify ammonia which accumulates *in vivo*, leading to

CNS involvement. Plants that commonly cause CNS stimulation include larkspur, locoweed, lupin, water hemlock and fitweed. Common plants that cause CNS depression include black locust, bracken fern, horsetail, milkweed and white snake root. Like ruminants, horses will avoid eating toxic plants because they are not palatable. Therefore, consumption of poisonous plants will occur during drought conditions when the animals lack suitable pasture. Sudden death in horses can be caused by the consumption of cyanide-containing plants such as sorghum. The cyanide ion forms a complex with cytochrome oxidase, which prevents transportation of electrons and utilization of oxygen by tissues throughout the body. As a consequence, blood is well oxygenated and cherry red. Treatment for this condition is an emergency and in the USA involves giving both sodium thiosulphate and sodium nitrite (other antidotes are used in other countries).

Horses, like other monogastrics, are more resistant to nitrate/nitrite poisoning than ruminants. However, horses can reduce nitrates to nitrites in the caecum but it takes three times more nitrate to produce a similar effect in the horse as in the ruminants.

Table 3 Toxic plants primarily causing CNS effects in food-producing animals

Scientific name	Common name	Species commonly affected	Toxic parts and principle(s)	Clinical signs
Dicentra cucullaria	Dutchman's breeches	Cattle	All parts but especially leaves and bulbs. Isoquinaline-type alkaloids, e.g. apomorphine	Initially abdominal pain and diarrhoea; ataxia, trembling, respiratory distress, convulsions
Cicuta spp.	Water hemlock	Cattle, sheep, goats, pigs less often	Roots, stem base Cicutoxin, cicutol	Muscular spasms and spasmodic convulsions
Corydalis spp.	Fitweed	Sheep mostly but also cattle	Foliage Unidentified alkaloids	Clonic seizures, twitching of facial muscles
Asclepsia spp.	Milk weed	All	Foliage Cardenolides	Severe depression, ataxia, dilated pupils, laboured respiration
Gelsemium spp.	Carolina jessamine	Cattle, sheep, goats	Foliage, flowers Gelsemine and other strychnine-related alkaloids	Depression, muscle weakness, respiratory failure, convulsive movements preceding death
Calycanthus spp.	Sweet shrub	Cattle	Seeds Calycanthine	Seizures, severe tetanic spasms, muscular fasciculations
Eupatropium rugosum	White snakeroot	Young cattle, sheep	Foliage, passes in milk Tremetol	Depression, listlessness, trembling, laboured breathing
Haplopappus heterophylus	Rayless goldenrod	Cattle, sheep, goats	Foliage Tremetol	Depression, trembling, rare limb weakness
Sophora spp.	Mescal beans	Sheep mostly but also cattle and goats	All parts but seeds especially Cytisine, sophorine and nicotinic alkaloids	Nervousness, exercise-induced violent tremors, stiff gait
Xanthium spp.	Cocklebur	Pigs mostly but also cattle and sheep	Seeds, cotyledons Carboxyatractyloside	Depression, prostration, hunched posture, severe hypoglycaemia, extreme hypersensitivity, convulsions when recumbent
Ranunculus spp.	Buttercup	Cattle mostly but also sheep, goats, pigs	Fresh foliage Protoanemonin	Irritation of oral tissues, salivation, nervousness, paralysis, depression or excitement and convulsions

Mycotoxins

Contaminated grains are sources of mycotoxin exposure in horses. The effects of mycotoxins are similar in the horse as for food-producing animals, the most commonly involved mycotoxins being aflatoxins, T-2 and fumonisin B_1. Aflatoxins will cause non-specific signs such as poor thriving, haemorrhages and abortions. T-2 is a trichothecene mycotoxin which causes prolonged bleeding time in affected animals. A specific mycotoxin affecting horses is fumonisin B_1 which is produced by *Fusarium moniliforme* and has been responsible for the condition called equine leucoencephalomalacia. Horses are affected by the consumption of mouldy corn and become anorectic and initially depressed, but as the condition progresses animals become blind, walk aimlessly and may show head pressing, have difficulties with swallowing and eventually die (Wilson *et al.*, 1990).

COMMON TOXICOSES OF POULTRY

This section will mainly address toxicoses in chicken, ducks and turkeys. However, there is much interest in the toxicology of wild birds, especially those kept in zoos, as well as pet birds. This discussion will emphasize toxicoses encountered in poultry. Readers interested in the general subject of avian toxicology are referred to LaBonde (1991).

Chemotherapeutic Drugs

Sulphonamides have been used as coccidiostats in poultry for four decades. Although sulphonamides have inhibitory action against coccidia and other pathogenic agents, they can be toxic to the host. In poultry, sulphonamide toxicity is characterized by blood dyscrasia, and renal and liver dysfunctions, and feeding chicken a mash containing as low as 0.2% sulphonamides for 2 weeks is toxic. Clinically affected birds have ruffled feathers, are depressed, pale, icteric, have poor weight gain and prolonged bleeding time. In laying birds, sulphonamides cause a marked decrease in egg production, thin rough shells and depigmentation in brown eggs. The temperature of affected birds is often elevated. At post mortem, haemorrhages are found in the skin, muscles (especially those of thighs and breast) and in internal organs. Once

Table 4 Toxic plants affecting the autonomic nervous system of food-producing animals

Scientific name	Common name	Species commonly affected	Toxic parts and principle(s)	Clinical signs
Datura stramonium	Jimsonweed, thorn apple	Pigs mostly; sheep goats, cattle	All parts but especially seeds Atropine, scopolamine, hyoscyamine	Anticholinergic signs, e.g. dilated pupils, dry mouth, muscle twitching, incoordination, paralysis
Hyoscyamus niger	Henbane	All	Seed. Hyoscyamine	As for *D. stramonium*
Solanum spp.	Nightshades	Pigs mostly; sheep, goats	Foliage, berries Solanine, dihydrosolanine, chaconine	Apathy, depression, dilated pupils, trembling, incoordination, muscular weakness, paralysis, convulsions
Physalis spp.	Groundcherry	Sheep	Tops and unripe berries. Solanine and atropine-like alkaloids	Diarrhoea, trembling, hyperthermia, weakness, paralysis
Gelsemium spp.	Carolina jessamine	Cattle, sheep, goats	(see 'plants causing CNS effects')	
Lycium spp.	Matrimony vine	Calves and sheep	Foliage Unidentified solanaceous alkaloids	Excitement, convulsion
Lobelia spp.	Wild tobacco	Sheep, cattle, goats	Foliage and green fruits Lobeline and lobelidine	Profuse salivation, dilated pupils, narcosis
Conium maculatum	Poison hemlock	Cattle, pigs	Seeds most toxic; fresh Nicotinic alkaloids, e.g. coniine	Muscle tremors, ataxia, muscle weakness, frequent urination and defecation, respiratory failure
Lupinus spp.	Lupine	Sheep	Pods (seeds). Nicotinic alkaloids, lupinine, lupanine	Laboured breathing, depression, salivation, ataxia, seizures
Sophora spp.	Mescal beans	(see 'plants causing CNS effects')		

Table 5 Toxic plants affecting the reproductive system of food-producing animals[a]

Scientific name	Common name	Species commonly affected	Toxic parts and principle(s)	Clinical signs
Veratrum californicum	False hellebore	Sheep	Roots and rhizomes mainly, but all parts are toxic. Jervin, veratrosin, cyclopamine	Cyclopian-type congenital malformation, anophthalmia, cleft palate
Festuca arundinacea	Tall fescue	Sheep, cattle	Foliage. Endophyte alkaloids, e.g. perlolidine, perloline	Abortion, still births, agalactia
Pinus ponderosa	Ponderosa	Cattle, sheep	Pine needles Unidentified	Last trimester abortions, stillbirths, premature deliveries, retained placenta
Gutierrezia microcephala	Broomweed	All	Foliage Unidentified saponins	Abortions, premature delivery, swelling of vulva
Cupressus macrocarpa	Monterey cypress	Cattle	Foliage Unidentified	Last trimester abortions, weakness, ataxia, death
Iva augatifolia	Sumpweed	Cattle	Foliage Unidentified	Abortion in last half of gestation

[a] Other plants that cause abortion include those containing nicotinic alkaloids (such as poison hemlock and tobacco), nitrate-accumulating plants (such as locoweed), cyanogenic plants (such as sorghum) and oestrogenic plants (such as clovers and wheat germ).

these signs are noticed, the concentration of sulphonamides in the ration should be checked and the feed involved withdrawn (Peckham, 1978).

Other chemotherapeutic agents sometimes involved in poisoning poultry include coccidiostats such as nicarbazine, zoalene (3, 5-dinitro-*o*-toluamide) and nitrophenide and the ionophore monensin. As little as 0.006% nicarbazine causes mottled yolks and at 0.02% there is a depressed rate of growth and depressed feeding efficiency. Feeding 0.025% nicarbazine to day-old chicks for 1 week results in dullness, listlessness, weakness and ataxia. Feeding zoalene at twice the recommended level of 0.025% will cause nervous signs and depressed growth and feeding efficiency. The nervous signs include stiff neck, staggering and tumbling over when the birds are excited. Nitrophenide possesses marked electrostatic properties and therefore sticks to the walls of the feed mixer. The last part of feed in the feed mixer will normally contain a high concentration of nitrophenide and has caused disturbances in posture and locomotion, retarded growth and mortality in chickens. Postural disturbances include a tilted position of the head, tremor of the neck and difficulty in the righting reflex (Peckham, 1978).

Table 6 Toxic plants affecting the cardiovascular system of food-producing animals[a]

Scientific name	Common name	Species commonly affected	Toxic parts and principle(s)	Clinical signs
Digitalis purpurea	Foxglove	All (see 'plants causing CNS effects')		
Nerium oleander	Common pink oleander	All	Foliage and flowers Several digitoxin-like glycosides	Cardiac arrhythmias, unconsciousness, hypotension, dyspnoea
Convalaria spp.	Lily-of-the-valley	All	All parts. Convallarine, convallatoxin, convallamarin	Tachycardia, diarrhoea, anorexia
Apocynum spp.	Dogbane	Cattle, sheep	All parts. Cardiac glycosides, e.g. apocynamarin	Cardiac arrhythmias, fever, gastro-intestinal pain, fever, gastric upset
Taxus spp.	Yew	All, but swine most sensitive	Foliage, bark, seeds Taxine	Acute heart failure (bradycardia)
Zygadenus spp.	Death camas	Sheep, cattle	All parts. Zygacine	Lowered blood pressure, salivation
Brassica spp.	Kale, rape	Cattle, sheep, goats	Foliage S-Methylcysteine sulphoxide	Haemolytic anaemia, weakness, fast respiration, haemoglobinuria, staggering, collapse
Onion	Onion	All	All parts. *n*-Propyl disulphide	As for *Brassica* spp.

[a] Several nitrate-accumulating plants, e.g. *Astragalus*, sudan grass, sorghum, corn and pigweed, cause methaemoglobinaemia. Some other plants, including sudan grass and sorghum, affect the cardiovascular system by virtue of their cyanogenic properties (see text).

Table 7 Toxic plants affecting renal function of food-producing animals

Scientific name	Common name	Species commonly affected	Toxic parts and principle(s)	Clinical signs
Beta vulgaris	Beet	Sheep and cattle	Sugar beet tops. Oxalates	Muscle tetany, renal failure
Rheum rhaponticum	Rhubarb	All	Foliage Oxalic acid, oxalates	Irritation of oral cavity and digestive tract, renal failure, death in convulsions
Halogeton spp.	Halogeton	All	Foliage and seeds Oxalates	Renal failure, dullness, weakness, slobbering
Sarobatus vermiculatus	Black grease-wood	Sheep, cattle	Foliage. Oxalates	As for *Halogeton*
Rumex spp.	Curlydock	Sheep, cattle	Foliage. Oxalic acid	As for *Halogeton*
Chenopodium spp.	Lambsquarters	All	All parts. Oxalic acid	As for *Halogeton*
Amaranthus spp.	Rough pigweed	Pigs, cattle, sheep	Foliage. Unidentified	Non-specific but related to perirenal oedema and nephrosis
Quercus spp.	Oak	Cattle, sheep	Young leaves, acorn, flowers, stem. Tannic acid, gallic acid	Abdominal pain, constipation, frequent urination, renal failure

In general, poultry are more resistant to monensin toxicity than mammals. There have been reports of monensin toxicity in turkeys accidentally fed rations containing 250 ppm monensin. There is a big difference in species susceptibility among poultry to monensin poisoning. Chickens and turkeys less than 2 weeks old are more resistant than older birds but keets (young guinea fowl) seem to be more susceptible than adult guinea fowl and the young of other species. For example, monensin at 200 ppm was not toxic for poults whereas 100 ppm was toxic for keets.

Cresol

Cresol was a commonly used disinfectant in poultry houses but has been gradually withdrawn and replaced by safer disinfectants. Nevertheless, cresol is still used in some countries. In chickens cresol poisoning usually occurs at 3–6 weeks of age. Affected chicks are depressed and have a tendency to huddle. There are signs of respiratory problems such as rales, gasping and wheezing, and in the event of prolonged exposure some chicks will have oedema of the abdomen.

Sodium Chloride

All poultry and pigeons are susceptible to salt poisoning, young birds being more susceptible than adults. Although both acute and chronic forms of salt poisoning can occur, the chronic form is more commonly encountered and results from prolonged ingestion of feed containing a high salt content. Levels of 0.5% and above in drinking water or 5–10% in feed cause death in baby

Table 8 Toxic plants causing primary photosensitization of food-producing animals

Scientific name	Common name	Species commonly affected	Toxic parts and principle(s)	Clinical signs
Hypericum perforatum	St. John's wort	Cattle, sheep, goats	Foliage Hypericin	Acute: increased respiration and heart rate, mild dermatitis Chronic: photosensitization of unpigmented areas of the skin, photophobia
Agave lecheguilla	Agave	Sheep, goats, cattle	Foliage. Unidentified	As for *H. perforatum*
Fagopyrum esculantum	Buckwheat	All	All parts and seeds. Fagopyrin	As for *H. perforatum*
Cymopterus watsonii	Spring parsley	Sheep, cattle	Foliage. Psolalens	As for *H. perforatum*
Trifolium hybrium[a]	Alsike clover	Pigs, sheep, cattle	Foliage and seeds. Unidentified	As for *H. perforatum*

[a] May be a secondary photosensitizer.

chicks. Signs of salt poisoning in poultry include anorexia, thirst, dyspnoea, opisthotonos, convulsions and ataxia. Increased water consumption may be the most significant early indicator of salt poisoning in poultry (Peckham, 1978).

Insecticides

Chlorinated hydrocarbon insecticides and organophosphate compounds are sometimes used inappropriately around poultry houses to control external parasites (LaBonde, 1991). Commonly involved organochlorine insecticides include chlordane, dieldrin, DDT, heptachlor and lindane. Occasionally birds are exposed by gaining access to sprayed grounds, such as golf courses. Chlordane causes chicks to chirp nervously, rest on their hocks and lie on their sides. The birds then become hyperexcitable as the condition progresses. In adult birds there is reduced food consumption, decreased body weight and a fall in production. Consumption of seeds dressed with dieldrin has been a source of exposure in wild birds. Affected birds are listless, have coordination problems while alighting, and severely poisoned birds show nervous signs characterized by lateral movements of the head and tremors of the head and neck. Birds die of violent convulsions. DDT toxicity in chickens is characterized by hyperexcitability and fine tremors in severe cases. Moderate cases are characterized by loss of weight, moulting and reduced egg production. Lindane dust is frequently used in chicken houses. Adult chickens poisoned by lindane become anorectic, manifest opisthotonos, flapping of the wings and clonic muscle spasms, and they die in coma (Peckham, 1978).

The organophosphate compounds commonly involved include diazinon, malathion and parathion. Diazinon is used for chicken premises but is very toxic to ducklings; when used at rates recommended for chicken, 100% mortality occurred in 1–2-week-old ducklings. Experimental studies suggest that goslings are three times more sensitive than ducks, chickens and turkeys. Poisoned birds are unable to stand, salivate profusely, and manifest tremors of the head and neck. Brain cholinesterase levels in birds that die of organophosphate poisoning are on average 69% less than controls. Other organophosphate compounds commonly used in chicken premises include dichlorvos, malathion and parathion. Birds poisoned by these compounds manifest similar signs to diazinon. Other signs that may be encountered include birds being depressed, ataxic and reluctant to move, paralysis, lachrymation, gasping, diarrhoea, crop stasis and dyspnoea (Mohan, 1990). In general, ducks are more sensitive to organophosphate poisoning than chickens and care should be exercised when using this product in premises holding ducks (Mohan, 1990).

The carbamate insecticide carbaryl is widely used as a poultry insecticide. This compound is relatively safe to use but deaths have been reported in turkey poults kept in premises where the product had been applied at 10 times the recommended rate. The clinical signs are similar to those caused by organophosphate poisoning.

Heavy Metals

Lead poisoning is not as common in poultry as in wild birds. Lead poisoning is the most common toxicity reported in avian species (LaBonde, 1991). Lead shot has caused losses in waterfowl populations in North America. All birds are susceptible to lead poisoning but most losses are reported in waterfowl because their feeding habits predispose them to lead ingestion. Characteristic signs of lead poisoning are those related to CNS derangement, such as ataxia, depression, paralysis of wings or convulsions. In some cases the birds present anaemic, emaciated, regurgitating and weak. Green diarrhoea has also been reported in some affected birds (LaBonde, 1991).

Yellow phosphorus is a highly toxic element used as a rodenticide. Poultry and wild birds can be intoxicated by consumption of bait intended for rodents. Fragments of fireworks also are a common source of poisoning in free range birds. Affected birds are depressed, anorectic, have increased water consumption and manifest diarrhoea, ataxia, paralysis, coma and death (Peckham, 1978).

Rodenticides

The effects of yellow phosphorus have been discussed in the preceding section. All rodenticides are potentially toxic to poultry and other birds. The clinical signs caused by rodenticides are similar to those in small animals. Birds occasionally consume baits containing anticoagulant rodenticides. The more potent second generation rodenticide-containing baits such as brodifacoum are especially dangerous to birds. These coumarin anticoagulants act by interfering with vitamin K recycling causing bleeding because of depletion of vitamin K-dependent clotting factors. Poisoned birds bleed from nares and subcutaneously, and have oral petechiae; often they are also weak and depressed.

Of special interest, however, is secondary intoxication from consumption by free range birds of carrion of animals that died of rodenticide poisoning. Strychnine and sodium mono-fluoroacetate are compounds commonly involved because they cause acute death in primary victims and are present in high concentrations in carrion. Strychnine-poisoned birds manifest clinical signs within 2 h of ingesting the product. The birds become apprehensive, nervous and show violent tetanic convulsions which cause the birds to become exhausted and die of hypoxia. Sodium monofluoroacetate causes overstimulation of the CNS and also myocardial depression. Cardiac failure is the cause of death and this occurs within 1 h of consuming the product or contaminated carcasses (Peckham, 1978).

Mycotoxins

Mycotoxicoses are a common problem in the poultry industry in developing countries in the tropics. Aflatoxins are the most commonly involved mycotoxins and poultry are normally exposed by consumption of contaminated feed, especially corn. Some developing countries lack the resources to screen contaminated corn adequately. In some cases poultry feed is made from poor quality corn which has been rejected for human consumption, and often this poor quality feed is contaminated. Aflatoxicosis in poultry can be either acute or chronic depending on the exposure dose. Ducklings are more susceptible to aflatoxin than turkeys, pheasants or chickens (Butler, 1974). In acute cases affected birds become lethargic, their wings droop and they manifest nervous signs, such as opisthotonos, and die with legs rigidly extended backward. Chronic consumption of at least 2.5 ppm aflatoxin in the diet causes a significant

drop in performance, such as weight gain and egg production. Perhaps more important is the increased susceptibility of the affected flock to infection because chronic consumption of aflatoxins lowers the immunity of the birds. Aflatoxicosis is therefore a disease of serious economic consequences to the poultry industry in developing countries such as Uganda, both through lowered productivity and the death of affected birds.

Ergot poisoning has been reported in Europe where rye is commonly used as a feed. In acute ergot poisoning the comb is cold, wilted and cyanotic. The birds are weak, thirsty and have diarrhoea. In severe cases the birds go into convulsions, paralysis and death. Ochratoxins have been reported to cause renal toxicity in poultry.

SUMMARY

In this chapter we have summarized the broad discipline of veterinary toxicology. We have given brief accounts of some selected common toxicities among different animal species so as to draw the attention of the reader to similarities and differences in their reaction to toxicants. Because some animals are more sensitive than others given the same toxicant, the diagnosis of some toxicoses may require the help of specialists within the veterinary profession. This chapter was not intended to be a detailed source of reference for diagnosis and treatment of animal poisonings, nor was it meant to be all inclusive. Rather it is a summary of the commonly encountered toxicoses in the veterinary profession. We suggest that interested readers consult the relevant references given in order to gain in-depth knowledge on subjects of interest. From the general overview of the subject it should be clear that all animals are susceptible to some type of toxicants and that some toxicants are toxic to all animals (including humans). It is therefore important to be cautious when handling chemicals around animals and we also need to provide a clean environment to all animals. Animals should be fed well balanced, quality food from reputable sources and suspect feed should be either avoided or checked for suspected toxicants before feeding. It is also vitally important to remember that all chemicals are poisons if the exposure is high enough. Therefore, even some of the useful compounds we use around animals, e.g. growth promoters, can be fatal if used excessively or if given to species for which they are not intended. The susceptibility of sheep to feed containing copper that was intended for cattle, or of monensin in horses fed poultry feeds, are cases in point.

REFERENCES

Amend, J. F., Mellon, F. M. and Wren, W. B. (1980). Equine monensin toxicosis: some experimental clinicopathologic observations. *Comp. Contin. Ed. Pract. Vet.*, **2**, S175–S183.

Beasley, V. R., Dahlem, A. M., Cook, W. O., Valentine, W. M., Lovell, R. A., Hooser, S. B., Harada, K., Suzuki, M. and Carmichael, W. W. (1989). Diagnositic and clinically important aspects of cyanobacterial (blue-green) algae toxicoses. *J. Vet. Diagn. Invest.*, **1**, 359–365.

Blood, D. C. and Rodostits, O. M. (1989). *Veterinary Medicine.* Baillière Tindall, London, pp. 1241–1249.

Boyd, R. E., and Spyker, D. A. (1983). Strichnine poisoning: recovery from profound lactic acidosis, hyperthermia and rhabdomyolysis. *Am. J. Med.*, **74**, 507–512.

Buck, W. B., (1986). Copper–molybdenum. In Howard, J. L. (Ed.), *Current Veterinary Therapy: Food Animal Practice 2.* W. B. Saunders, Philadelphia, pp. 437–439.

Buffa, P. and Peters, R. A. (1950). The *in vivo* formation of citrate induced by fluoroacetate poisoning and its significance. *J. Physiol. (Lond.)*, **110**, 488–500.

Butler, W. H. (1974). Aflatoxin. In Purchase I. F. H. (Ed.), *Mycotoxins.* Elsevier, Amsterdam, pp. 1–28.

Carson, T. L. and Dominick, M. A. (1982). Diagnosis and experimental reproduction of carbon monoxide induced fetal death in swine. *Am. Assoc. Vet. Lab. Diagn.*, **25**, 403–410.

Casida, J. E., Gammon, D. W., Glickman, A. H. and Lawrence, L. J. (1983). Mechanisms of selective action of pyrethroid insecticides. *Annu. Rev. Pharmacol. Toxicol.*, **23**, 413–438.

Cheeke, P. R. and Shull, L. R. (1985). Mycotoxins. In Cheeke, P. R. and Shull, L. R. (Eds), *Natural Toxicants in Feeds and Poisonous Plants.* AVI Publishing, Storrs, CT, pp. 393–476.

Clay, B. R., Edwards, W. C. and Peterson, D. R. (1976). Toxic nitrate accumulation on sorghums. *Bovine Pract.*, **11**, 28–32.

Colvin, B. M. and Harrison, L. R. (1992). Fumonisin-induced pulmonary edema and hydrothorax in swine. *Mycopathologia*, **117**, 79–82.

Connally, H. E., Thrall, M. A., Forney, S. D., Grauer, G. F. and Hamar, D. W. (1996). Safety and efficacy of 4-methylpyrazole for treatment of suspected or confirmed ethylene glycol intoxication in dogs: 107 cases (1983–1995). *J. Am. Vet. Med. Assoc.*, **209**, 1880–1883.

Coon, W. W. and Wallis, P. W. (1972). Some aspects of pharmacology of oral anticoagulants. *Clin. Pharmacol. Ther.*, **11**, 312–336.

Coppock, R. W., Monstrom, M. S. and Lillie, L. E. (1988). The toxicology of detergents, bleaches, antiseptics and disinfectants in small animals. *Vet. Hum. Toxicol.*, **30**, 463–473.

Dial, S. M., Thrall, M. A. and Hamar, D. W. (1994). Comparison of ethanol and 4-methylpyrazole as treatments for ethylene glycol intoxication in cats. *Am. J. Vet. Res.*, **55**, 1771–1782.

Dorman, D. C. (1990). Anticoagulant, cholecalciferol, and bromethalin-based rodenticides. In Beasley, V. R. (Ed.), *The Veterinary Clinics of North America. Small Animal Practitioner. Toxicology of Selected Pesticides, Drugs and Chemicals*, Vol. 20, pp. 339–352.

Dunn, H. W. and Leman, A. D. (Eds) (1975). *Diseases of Swine*, 4th edn. Iowa State University Press, Ames, IA, pp. 854–860.

Fikes, J. D. (1990). Organophosphorus and carbamate insecticides. In Beasley, V. R. (Ed.), *The Veterinary Clinics of North America. Toxicology of Selected Pesticides, Drugs and Chemicals*, Vol. 20, pp. 353–367.

Fowler, M. E. (1981). *Plant Poisoning in Small Companion Animals.* Ralston Purina, St Louis, MO, pp. 1–4.

Furr, A. and Buck, B. W. (1986). Arsenic. In Haward, J. L. (Ed.), *Current Veterinary Therapy: Food Animal Practice 2.* W. B. Saunders, Philadelphia, pp. 435–437.

Gosselin, R. E., Hodge, H. C., Smith, R. P. and Gleason, M. N. (Eds) (1976). Ammonia. In *Clinical Toxicology of Commercial Products*, 4th edn. Williams and Wilkins, Baltimore, pp. 20–24.

Grauer, G. F. and Thrall, M. A. (1982). Ethylene glycol (antifreeze) poisoning in the dog and cat. *J. Am. Anim. Hosp. Assoc.*, **18**, 492–497.

Hayes, W. J. Jr. (1991). Dosage and other factors influencing toxicity. In Hayes, W. J., Jr, and Laws, E. R., Jr (Eds), *Handbook of Pesticide Toxicology.* Academic Press, San Diego, pp. 39–105.

Heisser, J. M., Doya, M. R., Magnussen, A. R., Norton, R. L., Spyker, D. A., Allen, D. W. and Krasselt, W. (1992). Massive strichnine intoxication: serial blood levels in a fatal case. *Clin. Toxicol.*, **30**, 269–283.

Hultine, J. D., Mount, M. E., Easiley, K. J. and Oehme, F. W. (1979). Selenium toxicosis in the horse. *Equine Pract.*, **1**, 57.

Keller, W. C., Beasley, V. R. and Robens, J. F. (1990). In *Proceedings of the Symposium on Public Health Significance of Natural Toxicants in Animal Feeds*, Alexandria, Virginia, February 1989, pp. 1–111.

Kingsburry, J. M. (1964). *Poisonous Plants of the United States and Canada.* Prentice-Hall, Englewood Cliffs, NJ.

LaBonde, J. (1991). Avian toxicology. *Vet. Clin. N. Am. Small Anim. Pract.*, **21**, 1329–1342.

Lloyd, W. E. (1986). Urea and other non-protein nitrogen sources. In Howard, J. L. (Ed.), *Current Veterinary Therapy: Food Animal Practice 2.* W. B. Saunders, Philadelphia, pp. 354–356.

Livezey, K. L., Dorman, D. C., Hooser, S. B. and Buck, W. B. (1991). Hypercalcemia induced by vitamin D_3 toxicosis in two dogs. *Canine Pract.*, **16**, 126–132.

Maron, B. J., Krupp, J. R. and Tune, B. (1971). Strychnine poisoning successfully treated with diazepam. *J. Pediatr.*, **78**, 697–699.

Menzer, R. E. (1991). Water and soil pollutants. In Amdur M. O., Doull, J. and Klaassen C. D. (Eds), *Casarett and Doull's Toxicology, the Basic Science of Poisons*, 4th edn. Pergamon Press, New York, pp. 872–902.

Mohan, R. (1990). Dursban toxicosis in a pet bird breeding operation. In *Proceedings of Association of Avian Veterinary Conference*, Phoenix, AZ, pp. 112–114.

Muth, O. H. and Binns, W. (1964). Selenium toxicity in domestic animals. *Ann. N. Y. Acad. Sci.*, **3**, 583–590.

O'Donohue, J. G. (1961). Hydrogen sulfide poisoning in swine. *Can. J. Comp. Med. Vet. Sci.*, **25**, 217–219.

Oehme, F. W. (1987a). Toxicosis commonly observed in horses. In Robinson, N. E. (Ed.), *Current Therapy in Equine Medicine 2.* W. B. Saunders, Philadelphia, pp. 649–653.

Oehme, F. W. (1987b). Insecticides. In Robinson, N. E. (Ed.), *Current Therapy in Equine Medicine 2.* W. B. Saunders, Philadelphia, pp. 656–660.

Osweiler, G. D., Carson, T. L., Buck, W. B. and Van Gelder, G. A. (Eds) (1985). *Clinical and Diagnostic Veterinary Toxicology*, 3rd edn. Kendal/Hunt, Dubuque, IA, pp. 27–39, 160–166.

Peckham, M. C. (1978). Poisons and toxins. In Hofstad, M. S., Calnek, B. W., Hemboldt, C. F., Reid, W. M. and Yonder,

H. W., Jr (Eds), *Diseases of Poultry*. Iowa State University Press, Ames, IA, pp. 895–933.

Pelfrene, A. F. (1991). Synthetic organic rodenticides. In Hayes, W. J., Jr, and Laws, E. R., Jr (Eds), *Handbook of Pesticide Toxicology*. Academic Press, San Diego, pp. 1271–1316.

Pier, A. C. (1981). Mycotoxins and animal health. *Adv. Vet. Sci. Comp. Med.*, **25**, 185–243.

Radeleff, R. D. (1970). *Veterinary Toxicology*. Lea and Febiger, Philadelphia, pp. 158–161.

Ridder, W. E. and Oehme, F. W. (1974). Nitrate as an environmental animal and human hazard. *Clin. Toxicol.*, **7**, 145.

Rumbeiha, K. W. and Oehme, F. W. (1992a). Methylene blue can be used to treat methemoglobinemia in cats without inducing Heinz body hemolytic anemia. *Vet. Hum. Toxicol.*, **34**, 120–122.

Rumbeiha, K. W. and Oehme, F. W. (1992b). Emergency procedures for equine toxicoses. *Equine Pract.*, **14**, 26–30.

Rumbeiha, W. K., and Oehme, F. W. (1997). Fumonisin exposure to Kansans through consumption of corn-based market foods. *Vet. Hum. Toxicol.*, **39**, 220–225.

Schmitz, D. G. and Reagor, J. C. (1987). Cantharidine (blister beetle) toxicity. In Robinson, N. E. (Ed.), *Current Therapy in Equine Medicine 2*. W. B. Saunders, Philadelphia, pp. 120–122.

Smith, A. G. (1991). Chlorinated hydrocarbon insecticides. In Hayes, W. J., Jr, and Laws, E. R., Jr (Eds), *Handbook of Pesticide Toxicology*. Academic Press, San Diego, pp. 731–916.

Stephenson, J. P. B. (1967). Zinc phosphide poisoning. *Arch. Environ. Health*, **15**, 83–88.

Stevens, J. T. and Sumner, D. D. (1991). Herbicides. In Hayes, W. J., Jr, and Laws, E. R., Jr (Eds), *Handbook of Pesticide Toxicology*. Academic Press, San Diego, pp. 1317–1408.

Trammell, H. L., Dorman, D. C., and Beasley, V. R. (1989). *Ninth Annual Report of the Illinois Animal Poison Information Center*, Kendal/Hunt, Dubuque, IA.

Valentine, W. M. (1990). Pyrethrin and pyrethroid insecticides. In Beasley, V. R. (Ed.), *The Veterinary Clinics of North America: Toxicology of Selected Pesticides, Drugs and Chemicals*, vol. 20, pp. 375–385.

Welch, R. M., Conney, A. H. and Burns, J. J. (1966). The metabolism of acetophenetidin and *N*-acetyl-*p*-aminophenol in the cat. *Biochem. Pharmacol.*, **15**, 521–531.

Wilson, T. M., Ross, P. F., Rice, L. G., Osweiler, G. D., Nelson, H. A., Owens, D. L., Platner, R. D., Reggiardo, C., Noon, T. H. and Pickrell, J. W. (1990). Fumonisin B_1 levels associated with an epizootic of equine leucoencephalomalacia. *J. Vet. Diagn. Invest.*, **2**, 231–216.

Chapter 70
Epidemiology in Relation to Toxicology

John A. Tomenson

CONTENTS

INTRODUCTION

Epidemiology is sometimes simply defined as the study of patterns of health in groups of people (Paddle, 1988). Behind this deceptively simple definition lies a surprisingly diverse science, rich in concepts and methodology. For instance, the group of people might consist of only two people. Goudie *et al.* (1985) described a father suffering from rheumatoid arthritis and his daughter with vertigo. In both father and daughter the pattern of affected areas was remarkably similar, which might suggest that the distribution of joint lesions in rheumatoid arthritis is genetically determined.

At the opposite extreme, studies of the geographic distribution of diseases using national mortality and cancer incidence rates have provided clues about the aetiology of several diseases such as cardiovascular disease and stomach cancer. The patterns of health studied are also wide-ranging, and may include the distribution, course and spread of disease. The term 'disease' also has a loose definition in the context of epidemiology, and might include ill-defined conditions such as organic solvent and sick building syndromes or consist of an indirect measure of impairment such as biochemical and haematological parameters or lung function measurements.

McMahon and Pugh (1970) observed that epidemiology has evolved from the study of striking outbreaks of disease or epidemics, and noted that modern epidemiology can still be regarded as the study of epidemics if a broad view is taken as to what constitutes an epidemic. Clearly epidemiology has a very wide scope, but the aim of this chapter is to describe the relationship between epidemiology and toxicology. For this reason, discussion will be mainly limited to the role epidemiology plays alongside toxicology in the assessment of the hazards of chemical and physical agents and the recommendation of safe conditions under which we may come into contact with them.

Both toxicology and epidemiology are considered by many to be relatively new scientific disciplines. Toxicology, however, has a longer tradition and in the twentieth century it has come to be regarded as a science in its own right and not simply a branch of pharmacology. In order to survive, our prehistoric ancestors had to be aware of which foods were harmful, and they were naturally led to experiment in order to cure natural ailments or develop antidotes to poisons. There is evidence that poisons were used for hunting and fishing and that prehistoric man was aware of the therapeutic benefits of certain natural substances. There are many early examples of toxicological writings such as the Papyrus Ebers of the ancient Egyptians, written about 1500 BC, and the Sanskrit medical writings in the Ayur Veda, which date back to around 900 BC. Decker (1987) provides a good description of the early history of the science of poisons and the rapid development of analytical toxicology during the nineteenth and twentieth centuries. In contrast, epidemiologists can quote Hippocrates to demonstrate that the ancient Greeks were aware that health may be connected with a person's environment.

However, there the similarity with toxicology ends, for it was not until the seventeenth century that the beginnings of quantitative epidemiology started to appear. John Graunt, who in 1662 published his *Natural and Political Observations . . . on the Bills of Mortality*, is often credited as being the pioneer of quantitative epidemiology, although McMahon and Pugh (1970) noted that, since the techniques of Graunt saw no further epidemiological application for almost 200 years, it is more appropriate to regard Graunt as a forerunner than a founder of epidemiology. Although the nineteenth century saw important work by people such as William Farr and John Snow, most of the theory and quantitative methods of epidemiology have really only come into being during the past four decades.

Epidemiology and toxicology differ in many other ways but principally in that epidemiology is essentially an observational science, in contrast to the experimental nature of toxicology. The opportunistic approach of epidemiology has been commented upon by several authors (e.g. Utidjian, 1987; Paddle, 1988). The epidemiologist often has to make do with historical data which have been collected for reasons which have nothing to do with epidemiology. Nevertheless, the availability of personnel records such as lists of new starters and leavers, payrolls and work rosters and exposure monitoring data collected for compliance purposes has enabled many epidemiological studies to be conducted in the occupational setting. Thus, the epidemiologist has no control over who is exposed to an agent, the levels at which they are exposed to the agent of interest or the other agents to which they may be exposed. The epidemiologist has great difficulty in ascertaining what exposure has taken place and certainly has no control over lifestyle variables such as diet and smoking.

Despite the lack of precise data, the epidemiologist has one major advantage over the toxicologist: an epidemiology study documents the actual health experiences of human beings subjected to real-life exposures in an occupational or environmental setting. Indeed, Smith (1988) has expressed the view that uncertainty in epidemiology studies resulting from exposure estimation may be equal to or less than the uncertainty associated with extrapolation from animals to man. Regulatory bodies such as the US Environmental Protection Agency (US EPA) are starting to change their attitudes towards epidemiology and recognize that it has a role to play in the process of risk assessment. However, there is also a complementary need for epidemiologists to introduce more rigour into the conduct of their studies and to introduce standards akin to the Good Laboratory Practice standards under which animal experiments are performed.

HISTORY OF EPIDEMIOLOGY

As noted in the Introduction, awareness of certain epidemiological principles can be traced back to the days of Hippocrates, but it was a further 2000 years before epidemiology truly began to emerge. The analysis by John Graunt of the weekly Bills of Mortality and christenings recorded in the parish registers of London is generally regarded to be the first example of an epidemiological study. He reported higher death rates and birth rates for males than for females, and examined the influence of various factors on the spread of the plague. However, the greatest achievement of Graunt was to recognize the importance of studying biological phenomena in groups of people. Edmund Halley, the English Astronomer

Royal, was another seventeenth century scientist who was interested in population mortality rates. Halley made a study of the records of births and deaths kept in the Silesian city of Breslau (now Wrocław in Poland) since 1584 and drew up a life-table which was published in 1693. Casina Stabe, a seventeenth century Italian physician, has received comparatively little recognition. However, the following extract from *Demorbis artificum* (*Diseases of Workers*) written by Ramazzini in 1713 (Ramazzini, 1964), demonstrates clearly that Stabe understood the basic principles of epidemiology:

> *A few years ago a violent dispute arose between a citizen of Finale, a town in the dominion of Modena, and a certain businessman, a Modenese, who owned a huge laboratory at Finale where he manufactured sublimate. The citizen of Finale brought a lawsuit against this manufacturer and demanded that he should move his workshop outside the town or to some other place, on the ground that he poisoned the whole neighbourhood whenever his workmen roasted vitriol in the furnace to make sublimate. To prove the truth of his accusation he produced the sworn testimony of the doctor of Finale and also the parish register of deaths, from which it appeared that many more persons died annually in that quarter and in the immediate neighbourhood of the laboratory than in other localities. Moreover, the doctor gave evidence that the residents of that neighbourhood usually died of wasting disease and disease of the chest; this he ascribed to the fumes given off by the vitriol, which so tainted the air near by that it was rendered unhealthy and dangerous for the lungs. Dr Bernardino Corradi, the commissioner of ordnance in the Duchy of Este, defended the manufacturer, while Dr Casina Stabe, then the town physician, spoke for the plaintiff. Various cleverly worded documents were published by both sides, and this dispute which was literally 'about the shadow of smoke', as the saying is, was hotly argued. In the end the jury sustained the manufacturer, and vitriol was found not guilty. Whether in this case the legal expert gave a correct verdict, I leave to the decision of those who are experts in natural science.*

During the nineteenth century, modern epidemiological theory began to take shape. In 1836 the registration of births, marriages and deaths became compulsory in England, and William Farr, appointed Registrar General for England and Wales in 1839, established a pattern for the reporting of mortality data which has continued to this day. Farr looked at mortality in a variety of occupational settings and established a procedure for linking mortality data to occupational groupings derived from census data. Another Victorian pioneer in epidemiology was John Snow, who is famous for demonstrating the relationship between the incidence of cholera in certain London boroughs and faecal contamination of the water supply. The work of Farr and Snow is extremely well known but there were also many other excellent epidemiological studies conducted during the nineteenth century. Florence Nightingale, well known as the Lady of the Lamp, was also a reformer who knew how medical statistics could benefit her causes. She was a firm friend of William Farr, and one example of her work was a mortality table for hospital nurses and attendants showing a greatly increased prevalence of communicable diseases (Newell, 1984).

Having given due recognition to the nineteenth century fathers of epidemiology such as Farr and Snow, it is still fair to say that epidemiology has only begun to develop as a science in the last 40 years. The post-World War II period has seen a tremendous upsurge in epidemiological activity and a parallel rise in concern over environmental and occupational health matters. The work of Doll and Hill (1950, 1954) was of great importance in demonstrating that cigarette smoking causes lung cancer, but it also established the methodology of case-control and cohort studies. The bladder cancer study by Case et al. (1954) was extremely influential in establishing the credibility of the historical cohort study. Not only does the work of Case et al. stand up to scrutiny more than 40 years later, but also this study and the work of Cornfield (1951) on case-control studies have legitimized the use of retrospectively collected data and led to the historical cohort and case-control studies becoming the major techniques in modern cancer and mortality epidemiology.

The Framingham Heart Study initiated in 1949 to study risk factors for cardiovascular diseases was another major landmark in the development of epidemiology as a science. In addition to making a significant contribution to our understanding of the aetiology of cardiovascular disease, the Framingham study spurred the development of a large body of epidemiological methodology (e.g. Cornfield, 1962). However, despite the undoubted progress during the last 40 years, the science of epidemiology is still in its infancy. Rothman and Greenland (1998) note that 'Clear concepts of causation and related ideas such as induction period are as fundamental to an understanding of epidemiologic research as the definition of basic measures. Nevertheless, even these underpinnings have not yet been fully integrated into the conceptual bedrock of the discipline'. They also discuss disagreements about basic concepts and methodology which lead to profound differences in the interpretation of data. Feinstein (1988) notes that, despite peer review approval, current epidemiological methods need substantial improvement to produce trustworthy scientific evidence.

EPIDEMIOLOGICAL END-POINTS

The end-points studied by epidemiologists and toxicologists serve to illustrate some of the major differences between the two sciences. An excellent review of epidemiological end-points and their measurement is provided in a WHO publication on guidelines on studies in environmental epidemiology (WHO, 1983). The end-points studied by epidemiologists and toxicologists are broadly similar, e.g. organ malfunction, death, carcinogenesis, birth defects and mutagenesis. However, only in the case of cancer is the epidemiologist likely to obtain the same quality of information about the end-point as is the toxicologist. An epidemiologist conducting a study of workers exposed to a hepatotoxin will be reliant on haematology and clinical chemistry laboratory test results. The toxicologist will of course also make use of the same indicators of liver malfunction but will also have access to other measures of subacute or chronic toxicity such as the organ weight at necropsy and histopathology. Even in the case of a discrete end-point such as death, the epidemiologist is reliant on death certificates for information. Many studies of the accuracy of death certificates have shown that the individual causes listed on the certificate are often identified incorrectly. The quality and limitations of death registration data are discussed in the decennial occupational mortality supplement of the Office of Population Censuses and Surveys (OPCS), in England and Wales, (1986). It is noted there that the errors are generally greater for deaths of the elderly and for deaths from certain conditions, notably cerebro-vascular disease. As an illustration, Doll and Peto (1981) argued that in recent years the old have received increasingly careful medical attention, which must affect artefactually the trends in cancer death certification rates. Consequently, they restricted a study of trends in cancer incidence to people under the age of 65.

The epidemiologist is not at a total disadvantage, for there are certain health responses that the toxicologist would find difficult to measure in experimental studies of animals. The neurobehavioural tests for studies of organic solvent syndrome are one such example (WHO, 1985). Results in human studies cannot usually be replicated or explored in animal models, because we do not know how animals 'think' or 'feel'. However, the study of reproductive disorders typifies the difficulties that epidemiologists sometimes face in obtaining health, response data. The toxicological approach to the study of reproductive effects is described in Chapter 52 and is a well established feature of regulatory submissions for agrochemicals and pharmaceutical products. The epidemiologist has considerable difficulty in measuring the reproductive efficiency of couples. Male functional performance has been measured in some industry studies using semen collected from workforce volunteers (e.g. Lahdetie, 1995; Bonde et al., 1996), but such an approach would be unacceptable in occupational and environmental studies in many countries. However, such studies have become of great interest in recent years because of the regulatory focus on environmental oestrogens (Colborn et al., 1996). Decreased libido and functional disorders may be revealed by questionnaires, but the value of such an approach has yet to be proven. Questionnaires have also been used to measure the reproductive efficiency of couples (Joffe, 1997). Kallen (1988) comprehensively reviews the end-points studied in reproductive epidemiology and the methods for collecting and interpreting data on spontaneous abortion and malformations. However, foetal loss rates are extremely difficult to quantify and the event may not even be noticed by the woman herself in the first trimester.

Questionnaires have been described in the discussion of reproductive epidemiology and represent another major difference between toxicology and epidemiology. The use of symptom questionnaires is widespread in epidemiology and makes it possible to compare symptom prevalence in groups of individuals exposed to different agents. In the case of respiratory and cardiovascular epidemiology, standardized questionnaires are an extremely important research tool and considerable efforts have been made to ensure their validity and reproducibility (e.g. MRC, 1976; Rose et al., 1982). Questionnaires are also used to quantify a number of ill-defined conditions such as stress (Goldberg, 1972), sick building syndrome (Finnegan et al., 1984) and allergy to laboratory animals (Botham et al., 1987). They also form an important component of the range of neurological examination methods and the techniques used in epidemiological studies for assessing neurotoxic effects.

MEASUREMENT OF EXPOSURE

Wegman and Eisen (1988) made the valid point that epidemiologists have placed much greater emphasis on the measure of response than on the measure of exposure. They claimed that this is because most epidemiologists have been trained as physicians and are consequently more oriented towards measuring health outcomes. It is certainly true that a modern textbook of epidemiology such as that by Rothman and Greenland (1998) says very little about how exposure is assessed in epidemiology studies. However, this is probably as much a reflection of the historical paucity of quantitative exposure information as a reflection on the background of epidemiologists. Nevertheless, it is surprising how many epidemiological studies do not contain even a basic qualitative assessment of exposure. **Table 1** shows the quality of exposure data in 52 mortality studies of pesticide applicators reviewed by Brown (1990). Almost half (24) do not even specify the pesticides to which applicators were potentially exposed.

The contrast between epidemiology and toxicology is never more marked than in the area of dose response. In a toxicology study the conditions of the exposure to the agent of interest can be carefully controlled. In addition, the toxicologist can usually be sure that the animals have

Table 1 Quality of exposure data in 52 mortality studies of pesticide applicators (Brown, 1990)

Information on exposure	Number
Do not specify compounds or give exposure assessments	24
Compounds named (no exposure assessment)	10
Exposure assessment by questionnaire (personal or next of kin)	14
Exposure assessment by hygiene measurements	3
Biological monitoring data	1

not come into contact with any other toxic agents. However, this is not always the case (Sharpe et al., 1998). The industrial epidemiologist conducting the study of workers exposed to a hepatotoxin described in the previous section will certainly have to control for alcohol intake and possibly for exposure to other hepatotoxins in the work and home environment. Nevertheless, it can be argued that epidemiology studies more accurately measure the effect on human health of 'real-life' exposures.

In occupational studies, it is often necessary to assess exposure retrospectively. Few companies have either recorded or kept quantitative exposure data over even the working lifetimes of their current employees. Most manufacturing processes change considerably over time, as do the exposures experienced by the workforce. In addition, the ingredients and chemical reactions may not be well documented and can greatly complicate the characterization of exposure. Often the epidemiologist has to rely on anecdotal evidence and careful detective work by an industrial hygienist to construct a matrix of exposures by job title and time period. Occasionally attempts are made to estimate past exposures by reconstructing redundant industrial processes. Ayer et al. (1973) described the reconstruction of an old granite shed to estimate dust levels. The principles of exposure assessment in epidemiology studies were well described by Armstrong et al. (1992).

Even if quantitative exposure data are available, obtained by either static monitor or personal sampler, it will almost certainly have been collected to determine compliance with internal or external regulations. More emphasis is placed on recording the higher levels which occur after spillages and plant malfunction, and this may render the exposure data inappropriate for use to define normal exposures encountered in the jobs. It is to be hoped that, in future, epidemiologists and hygienists can develop sampling strategies that generate exposure data suitable for both compliance and epidemiological purposes.

In recent years, considerable interest has focused upon the investigation of the human health effects of pollutants in the environment. In the past it has been extremely difficult to obtain detailed exposure information. However, the characteristic biological changes associated with exposure to pollutants, or biomarkers, present major opportunities to measure long-term exposure to carcinogens, neuro- and developmental toxins and hormonally active substances (WHO Regional Office for Europe, 1995; IEH, 1996). Biomarkers will be discussed in more detail later in this chapter.

EPIDEMIOLOGICAL STUDY DESIGNS

This section provides a brief introduction to the most important types of studies conducted by epidemiologists. It is an attempt to describe briefly the principles of the major types of epidemiological studies in order to assist the toxicologist to understand the reporting of epidemiological studies and the assumptions made by epidemiologists. The next section discusses the similarities and differences between the methodologies of toxicology and epidemiology.

Cohort Studies

Historical Cohort Study

When the need arises to study the health status of a group of workers, there is often a large body of historical data which can be utilized. If sufficient information exists on individuals exposed in the past to a potential workplace hazard, then it may be possible to undertake a retrospective cohort study. The historical data will have been collected for reasons which have nothing to do with epidemiology. Nevertheless, the availability of personnel records such as starters' and leavers' registers, payrolls, work rosters and individuals' career records has enabled many epidemiological studies to be conducted, in particular mortality studies.

The principles of a historical cohort study can also be applied to follow a cohort of workers prospectively. This approach will be discussed further in the next subsection, although it should be emphasized that many historical data studies have a prospective element in so far as they are updated after a further period of follow-up. The discussion of historical cohort studies in this section will concentrate on mortality and cancer incidence studies. However, there is no reason why hearing loss, lung function, or almost any measure of the health status of an individual should not be studied retrospectively if sufficient information is available.

Mortality and cancer incidence studies are unique among retrospective cohort studies in that they can be conducted using national cancer and mortality registers even if there has been no medical surveillance of the workforce. A historical cohort study also has the advantages of being cheaper and providing estimates of the potential hazard much earlier than a prospective study. However, historical cohort studies are beset by a variety of problems. Principal among these is the problem of determining which workers have been exposed and, if so, to what degree. In addition, it may be difficult to decide what is an appropriate comparison group. It should also be borne in mind that in epidemiology, unlike animal experimentation, random allocation is not possible and there is no control over the factors which may distort the effects of the exposure of interest, such as smoking and standard of living.

The principles of historical cohort studies as they apply within a large chemical company in the UK are described in the following subsections.

Cohort Definition and Follow-up Period

A variety of sources of information are used to identify workers exposed to a particular workplace hazard, to construct an occupational history and complete the collection of information necessary for tracing (see below). It is essential that the cohort be well defined and that criteria for eligibility be strictly followed. This requires that a clear statement be made about membership of the cohort so that it is easy to decide whether an employee is a member or not. It is also important that the follow-up period be carefully defined. For instance, it is readily apparent that the follow-up period should not start before exposure has occurred. Furthermore, it is uncommon for the health effect of interest to manifest itself immediately after exposure, and allowance for an appropriate biological induction (or latency) period may need to be made when interpreting the data.

Tracing

In the UK the vital status (alive, dead, emigrated or untraced) and the causes of death of members of a cohort study are ascertained by use of the National Health Service Central Register (NHSCR) of the UK. In the authors' company it is also possible to ascertain the vital status of a large proportion of cohort members by use of company mortality registers and personnel records. NHSCR provides assistance to a wide variety of medical research projects in the UK. In addition to ascertaining the status of an individual on a given date, NHSCR will also flag live individuals and notify the study manager when they die. Consequently, it is a relatively simple matter to update a mortality study after a further period of follow-up.

Comparison Subjects

The usual comparison group for many studies is the national population. However, it is known that there are marked regional differences in the mortality rates for many causes of death. Regional mortality rates are often available but have to be used with caution because they are often based on small numbers of deaths and estimated population sizes. In some situations the local rates for certain causes may be highly influenced by the mortality of the workforce being studied. Furthermore, it is not always easy to decide what the most appropriate regional rate for comparison purposes is, as many employees may reside in a different region from that in which the plant is situated. An alternative or additional approach is to establish a cohort of unexposed workers for comparison purposes. However, workers with very low exposures to the workplace hazard will often provide similar information.

Analysis and Interpretation

In a cohort study, the first stage in the analysis consists of calculating the number of deaths expected during the follow-up period. In order to calculate the expected deaths for the cohort, the survival experience of the cohort is broken down into individual years of survival known as 'person-years'. Each person-year is characterized by the age of the cohort member and the time-period when survival occurred and the sex of the cohort member. The person-years are then multiplied by age, sex and time-period specific mortality rates to obtain the expected number of deaths. The ratio between observed and expected deaths is expressed as a standardized mortality ratio (SMR) as follows:

$$SMR = 100 \times \frac{\text{observed deaths}}{\text{expected deaths}}$$

Thus, an SMR of 125 represents an excess mortality of 25%. An SMR can be calculated for different causes of death and for subdivisions of the person-years by factors such as level of exposure and time since first exposure.

Interpretation of cohort studies is not always straightforward, and there are a number of selection effects and biases that must be considered (Rothman and Greenland, 1998). Cohort studies routinely report that the mortality of active workers is less than that of the population as a whole. This is not an unexpected finding, since workers usually have to undergo some sort of selection process to become or remain workers. Nevertheless, this selection effect, known as the 'healthy worker' effect, can lead to considerable arguments over the interpretation of study results, particularly if the cancer mortality is as expected, but the all-cause mortality is much lower than expected. However, even an experimental science such as toxicology is not without a similar problem of interpretation, viz. the problem of distinguishing between the effects of age and treatment on tumour incidence (Peto et al., 1980).

Proportional Mortality Study

There are situations where one has no accurate data on the composition of a cohort but does possess a set of death records (or cancer registrations). Under these circumstances a proportional mortality study may sometimes be substituted for a cohort study. In such a mortality study the proportions of deaths from a specific cause among the study deaths is compared with the proportion of deaths from that cause in a comparison population. The results of a proportional mortality study are expressed in an analogous way to those of the cohort study with follow-up. Corresponding to the observed deaths from a particular cause, it is possible to calculate an expected number of deaths based on mortality rates for that cause and all causes of death in a comparison group and the total number of deaths in the study. The ratio between observed and expected deaths from a certain cause is expressed as a proportional mortality ratio (PMR) as follows:

$$PMR = 100 \times \frac{\text{observed deaths}}{\text{expected deaths}}$$

Thus, a PMR of 125 for a particular cause of death represents a 25% increase in the proportion of deaths due to that cause. A proportional mortality study has the advantage of avoiding the expensive and time-consuming establishment and tracing of a cohort, but the disadvantage of little or no exposure information.

Prospective Cohort Study

Prospective cohort studies are no different in principle from historical cohort studies in terms of scientific logic, the major differences being timing and methodology. The study starts with a group of apparently healthy individuals whose health and exposure are studied over a period of time. As it is possible to define in advance the information that is to be collected, prospective studies are theoretically more reliable than retrospective studies. However, long periods of observation may be required to obtain results and the results may be difficult to interpret.

Case-Control Study

In a case-control study (also known as a case-referent study), two groups of individuals are selected for study. One group has the disease whose causation is to be studied (the cases) and the other does not (the controls). In the context of the chemical industry, the aim of a case-control study is to evaluate the relevance of past exposure to the development of a disease. This is done by obtaining an indirect estimate of the rate of occurrence of the disease in an exposed and unexposed group by comparing the frequency of exposure among cases and controls.

Principal Features

Case-control and cohort studies complement each other as types of epidemiological study. In a case-control study the groups are defined on the basis of the presence or absence of a given disease and, hence, only one disease can be studied at a time. The case-control study compensates for this by providing information on a wide range of exposures which may play a role in the development of the disease. In contrast, a cohort study generally focuses on a single exposure but can be analysed for multiple disease outcomes. A case-control study is a better way of studying rare diseases because a very large cohort would be required to demonstrate an excess of a rare disease. In contrast, a case-control study is an inefficient way of assessing the effect of an uncommon exposure, when it might be possible to conduct a cohort study of all those exposed.

The complementary strengths and weaknesses of case-control and cohort studies can be used to advantage. Increasingly, mortality studies are being reported which utilize 'nested' case-control studies to investigate the association between the exposures of interest and a cause of death for which an excess has been discovered. However, case-control studies have traditionally been held in low regard, largely because they are often badly conducted and interpreted. There is also a tendency to over interpret the data and misuse statistical procedures. In addition, there is still considerable debate among leading epidemiologists themselves as to how controls should be selected (e.g. Poole, 1986; Schlesselman and Stadel, 1987).

Analysis and Interpretation

In a case-control study, it is possible to compare the frequencies of exposures in the cases and controls. However, what one is really interested in is a comparison of the frequencies of disease in the exposed and the unexposed. The latter comparison is usually expressed as a relative risk (RR), which is defined as

$$RR = \frac{\text{rate of disease in exposed group}}{\text{rate of disease in unexposed group}}$$

It is clearly not possible to calculate the RR directly in a case-control study, since exposed and unexposed groups have not been followed in order to determine the rates of occurrence of the disease in the two groups. Nevertheless, it is possible to calculate another statistic, the odds ratio (OR), which, if certain assumptions hold, is a good estimate of the RR. For cases and controls the exposure odds are simply the odds of being exposed, and the OR is defined as

$$OR = \frac{\text{cases with exposure/cases without exposure}}{\text{controls with exposure/controls without exposure}}$$

An OR of 1 indicates that the rate of disease is unaffected by exposure. An OR greater than 1 indicates an increase in the rate of disease in exposed workers.

Matching

Matching is the selection of a comparison group that is, within stated limits, identical with the study group with respect to one or more factors such as age, years of service and smoking history, which may distort the effect of the exposure of interest. The matching may be done on an individual or group basis. Although matching may be used in all types of study, including follow-up and cross-sectional studies, it is more widely used in case-control studies. It is common to see case-control studies in which each case is matched to as many as three or four controls.

Nested Case-Control Study

In a cohort study the assessment of exposure for all cohort members may be extremely time-consuming and demanding of resources. If excess mortality or incidence has been discovered for a small number of conditions, it may be much more efficient to conduct a case-control study to investigate the effect of exposure. Thus, instead of all members being studied, only the cases and a sample of non-cases would be compared with regard to exposure history. Hence there is no need to investigate the exposure histories of all those who are neither cases nor controls. However, the nesting is only effective if there are a reasonable number of cases and sufficient variation in the exposure of the cohort members.

Other Study Designs

Descriptive Studies

There are large numbers of records in existence which document the health of various groups of people. Mortality statistics are available for many countries and even for certain companies (e.g. Pell et al., 1978; Paddle, 1981). Similarly, there is a wide range of routine morbidity statistics, in particular, those based on cancer registrations (Waterhouse et al., 1982). These health statistics can be used to study differences between geographic regions [e.g. maps of cancer mortality and incidence (Boyle et al., 1989)], occupational groups and time periods. Investigations based on existing records of the distribution of disease and of possible causes are known as descriptive studies. It is sometimes possible to identify hazards associated with the development of rare conditions from observation of clustering in occupational or geographical areas. The report by Creech and Johnson (1974) on three cases of haemangiosarcoma in vinyl chloride workers at the B. F. Goodrich Chemical Company is a good example. At that time only 25 cases a year of haemangiosarcoma were reported for the whole of the USA. However, much more detailed information on the population at risk (age, sex, size, etc.) and valid comparison rates are usually required to allow sensible interpretation of mortality and morbidity statistics.

Cross-sectional Study

Cross-sectional studies measure the cause (exposure) and the effect (disease) at one point in time. They compare the rates of diseases or symptoms of an exposed group with an unexposed group. Strictly, the exposure information is ascertained simultaneously with the disease information. In practice, such studies are usually more meaningful from an aetiological or causal point of view if the exposure assessment reflects past exposures. Current information is often all that is available but may still be meaningful, because of the correlation between current exposure and relevant past exposure.

Cross-sectional studies are widely used to study the health of groups of workers who are exposed to possible hazards but do not undergo regular surveillance. They are particularly suited to the study of subclinical parameters such as blood biochemistry and haematological values. Cross-sectional studies are also relatively straightforward to conduct in comparison with prospective cohort studies and are generally simpler to interpret.

Intervention Study

Not all epidemiology is observational, and experimental studies have a role to play in evaluating the efficiency of an intervention programme to prevent disease, e.g. fluoridation of water. An intervention study at one extreme may closely resemble a clinical trial with individuals randomly selected to receive some form of intervention, e.g. advice on reducing cholesterol levels. However, in some instances it may be a whole community that is selected to form the intervention group. The selection may or may not be random. The toxicologist might argue that even if selection was random, such a study of two communities, each consisting of many individuals, was in a sense a study of only two subjects. However, it can also be argued that the 'three rats to a cage' design of many subacute toxicity studies does not really generate three independent responses per cage.

THE EPIDEMIOLOGY–TOXICOLOGY INTERFACE

The protection of human health from chemicals in the workplace, market place and environment has become a universally recognized goal. The approach towards this goal has developed over time and can be roughly characterized by three processes (Friess, 1987): (1) the development of some form of human dose–response relationship for an adverse health effect; (2) the assessment of risk for that effect under specific exposure conditions; and (3) the setting of permissible exposure limits for the chemical in various exposure scenarios. At the beginning of the twentieth century the US government passed the first Food and Drug Act, aimed at regulating the widespread adulteration of food with chemical additives. To identify some chemicals and to emphasize the problems, Dr Harvey Wiley conducted the first toxicology studies for regulatory purposes on behalf of the Bureau of Chemistry (which subsequently became the Food and Drug Administration) by setting up feeding experiments with 12 healthy male volunteers (Glocklin, 1987). It soon became apparent that there were insidious, even life-threatening, toxicities lurking in foodstuffs and patent medicines which went far beyond the transient gastro-intestinal upsets or general malaise that Dr Wiley's so-called 'poison squad' would have been willing to accept. The ethical concerns with human studies quickly led to the use of animals in safety testing. By developing strains of laboratory animals and maintaining them in good health and in a controlled environment, it was possible to carry out reproducible experiments, and the science of experimental toxicology came into existence (Zapp, 1981). However, ever since toxicologists came to rely on surrogate models for man, arguments about trans-species prediction in assessing human health hazards have been a major issue (Brown and Paddle, 1988).

Although the epidemiology–toxicology interface in the area of risk assessment has often been confrontational in the past, there are encouraging signs that toxicologists and epidemiologists are now moving towards much more productive collaborations. In recent years, there has been an upsurge in mechanistic work to explain species differences (e.g. Green, 1997; Green et al., 1997). However, the most important development is the explosion of interest in the application of biomarkers in epidemiology or molecular epidemiology as it is sometimes described (e.g. Grandjean, 1995; IARC, 1997). Biomarkers offer considerable opportunities to characterize exposure better, to understand the relationship between exposure and disease, and to identify susceptible individuals.

A good example of the realization that epidemiologists and toxicologists need to work together to resolve public health issues is provided by Wilks et al. (1996). They make a strong argument for an infrastructure to encourage and fund cooperative studies between toxicology and epidemiology, in particular, to resolve health issues related to the so-called 'environmental oestrogens'. Wilks et al. (1996) note that toxicologists know that there are many chemicals, synthetic as well as naturally occurring, which can modulate endocrine function. A number of reproductive function and cancer end-points have been linked to 'environmental oestrogens' (e.g. Sharpe and Skakkebaek, 1993; Crisp et al., 1998). Toxicologists also know a lot about the mechanisms by which they may modulate endocrine function and their potency relative to 'natural' endocrine modulators. However, relative potency may have little value in assessing the biological effect of chemicals which may be affected by the extent of protein binding, chemical interactions, pharmacokinetics and other factors. Hence it may be simple for the toxicologist to design *in vitro* assays which demonstrate whether a chemical does or does not have an endocrine effect, but it is much more difficult to assess the relevance of this information to human risk assessment. In contrast, epidemiologists have a lot of human data relating to the end-points linked with 'environmental oestrogens' but much of this is descriptive (e.g. Carlsen *et al.*, 1992) and is difficult to interpret. Furthermore, it sheds little light on causality. The danger with endocrine modulators is that 'toxicologists will continue to do experiments, and epidemiologists will continue to collect data, but they will fail to constructively interact with each other'.

Methodological Differences

The interface between epidemiology and toxicology has sometimes been fraught in the past. The toxicologist argues that the tighter specification of animal studies, and the absence of the social and environmental factors which confuse the issue in human studies, should lead one to regard the animal studies as more informative. However, the epidemiologist would counter that the greater relevance of the species, and the greater relevance of the dose in that species, make the epidemiological data more informative.

The toxicologist will have noticed certain similarities between the prospective cohort study and the carcinogenesis bioassay and other approaches to chronic toxicity testing. The use of national mortality statistics for comparison purposes may seem odd to the toxicologist, but is analogous to the use of historical information in toxicology studies. The most obvious difference, however, is the inability of the epidemiologist randomly to assign workers to the different exposure groups. Randomization does play a part in epidemiology, as can be seen in the description of intervention studies. The cross-sectional study will also be recognized by the toxicologist as being the analogue of a subacute toxicity study. Although many of the study end-points are similar (e.g. haematology and clinical chemistry test results), the epidemiologist will also study a much larger range of health effects such as respiratory function (lung function testing and X-ray changes) and blood pressure. However, unlike the toxicologist, the epidemiologist is unable to look for histopathological changes in the tissues of subjects. The studies that will seem most alien to the toxicologist are the retrospective studies. They clearly have no counterpart in toxicology or any other experimental science, although it is interesting to note that Schlesselman (1982) claims that the case-control approach was formalized within the field of sociology during the 1920s.

The major differences between the methodologies of laboratory and epidemiological studies are summarized in **Table 2**. The differences become most apparent when one considers carcinogens. It is both unethical and impractical to expose humans to compounds and wait and see (typically 15–30 years) whether cancers result. Animal studies are not so constrained by either ethics or time. A rodent bioassay can be completed within 3 years (animal life-span = 2 years; pathological and quantitative analyses up to 1 year) and therefore toxicology may be described as a prospective study, while epidemiology is largely retrospective. Chapters 33–47 of this book will also testify to the more sophisticated techniques that are afforded to animal toxicology for individual organ analyses, be they ongoing, interim or final evaluations. The poorer quality of some epidemiological end-points, particularly those based on death certification, has already been discussed. The epidemiologist has little control over the health of subjects on entry but, as noted previously, the health of an employee at recruitment is likely to be better than average. However, the health of a subject at recruitment will be one factor that influences the response of the subject to exposure to the agent under study. In addition, there may be many other confounding factors such as age, smoking habits, alcohol consumption, diet and exposure to other hazards at work and at home. By comparison, the toxicologist can be confident of minimal confounding effects and pure compound exposure, and has the reassurance provided by his trial control data of detecting genuine compound-related effects.

A further difference between the two types of study is in the pattern and level of exposure. Both animal and human studies may be investigating the same chemical but the means to the end is quite different. Suppose that the compound of interest is a pesticide used in spraying corn (maize). Then two potential human groups to study would be (1) applicators, having exposure seasonally to significant amounts, then periods of no exposure at all (i.e. pulse doses), and possibly concurrent exposure to other chemicals, and (2) the general population, who may consume the product on average twice a week in only very small amounts as a food contaminant. Not only is the pattern and level of exposure different for the two groups of humans potentially at risk, but also the routes of exposure are dissimilar. The applicators are exposed by skin absorption, inhalation and oral routes to more than one pesticide, while the general population is exposed by the oral route. The toxicology study, however, would be conducted as a 7 days a week, lifetime feeding study with the only control variable being the single pesticide of interest. Dose levels would be defined around the maximum tolerance dose (MTD) and some subfraction thereof.

Three different exposure scenarios, (1) human, 'pulse dose' to more than one chemical, (2) human, intermittent very low doses, and (3) animal, constant high levels, exemplify how exposure patterns, levels and routes can vary not only within a species, but also between species. Epidemiologists of necessity study populations of great

Table 2 Differences between animal and human studies

Parameter	Animal study	Human study
Ethics	Provided that governmental animal cruelty/rights acts are not contravened, then it is perfectly acceptable knowingly to expose the animal to carcinogens, mutagens, teratogens, etc.	It is unethical to knowingly and deliberately expose humans to carcinogens, mutagens, teratogens, etc
Conduct	Good laboratory practice (strict adherence to GLP)	Protocol for study (protocol may change during study)
Subject observation	Monitored case histories (record of animal health throughout study)	Exhaustive follow-up (sometimes subjects are untraceable/disappear)
Dose	Regulated exposure (defined dose at defined intervals)	Defined exposed group (it may only be known whether there was a potential for exposure but not at what level)
Length of exposure	Depending on the suspected effect of the chemical (generally lifetime for carcinogens, throughout organogenesis for teratogens, generations for reprotoxins)	Various (depending on whether chemical is an occupational, market place or environmental hazard)
Pattern of exposure	Single chemicals at around the maximum tolerated dose, dose levels constant	Mixed exposure at varied levels (usually 'pulse' exposure)
Comparison groups	Randomized uniformity (control group known to have no exposure, otherwise identical with exposed group)	Valid unexposed group (it can only be assumed that the only different variable is exposure)
Genetic homogeneity	Generally 'inbred' strain used; hence, high degree of genetic homogeneity	High level of inaccuracy; High degree of heterogeneity
Death	Standardized necropsy (every animal subject to pathological examination)	Not applicable
Relevance	Extremely relevant to the species in which data were generated (trans-species relevance unknown)	Extremely relevant to man

genetic heterogeneity and of wide age distribution (at least within 16–65 years for industrial working age range and lifetime years for environmental agents). They are populations exposed intermittently to largely unknown concentrations of the toxicant of interest, by an ill-defined combination of routes, almost never in isolation, for outcomes or effects which are rarely determinable or even definable in the precise terms which are demanded of animal studies (Utidjian, 1987).

Hazard Identification and Risk Assessment

A major challenge for toxicologists and epidemiologists, is to give appropriate weight to information produced by both disciplines in the hazard identification and risk assessment processes. Toxicologists have devoted much energy to demonstrating the effectiveness of experimental animal studies in identifying carcinogens. However, as long ago as 1984, the eminent epidemiologist Sir Richard Doll noted that most recognized occupational cancers could have been avoided if modern toxicological techniques had been employed to test the substances used

before humans were exposed to them in the industrial environment (Doll, 1984). Nevertheless, he noted that most had been discovered as a result of clinical intuition or epidemiological observation. Virtually all of the chemicals that have been demonstrated to be causative agents of cancer in humans also produce cancer in a variety of animal models (Huff, 1993). Furthermore, Huff (1993) noted that evidence of carcinogenicity in experimental animals preceded that observed in humans for nearly 30 agents; examples of this are vinyl chloride (Maltoni, 1977) and bis(chloromethyl) ether (Van Duuren et al., 1972). On the basis of this substantial background of evidence that human carcinogens can be revealed in animal models, it has been widely assumed that chemicals that are carcinogenic in animal models are likely to be potential cancer hazards to man.

Some evidence of the predictability of carcinogenicity from species to species is provided by comparisons between rats and mice. Gold et al. (1991) reviewed 533 chemicals that are carcinogenic in at least one species. They reported that 76% of rat carcinogens are positive in mice and 71% of mouse carcinogens are positive in rats. Since about 50% of test chemicals are positive in each species, by chance alone one would expect a predictive value of about 50%. Gold *et al.* (1991) also reported a high degree of agreement on target site; 52% of rat carcinogens are positive in the same site in mice and 48% of mouse carcinogens are positive in the same site in rats. However, Gold *et al.* (1991) did not calculate a comparison figure for the level of agreement expected by chance.

The International Agency for Research on Cancer (IARC, 1987) classified 50 chemicals and industrial processes as human carcinogens, and of these there was sufficient evidence to classify 21 as carcinogenic to both humans and experimental animals. **Table 3** shows that at least 16 of these 21 agents could be considered to exhibit site concordance of tumours in test animals and humans. However, many of these agents produce tumours at several sites and there is agreement in respect of only one site. Nevertheless, compounds for which tumours are induced in the animals but at sites not in accordance with the human data can generally be reasoned by virtue of differential metabolism, e.g. benzidine and 2-naphthylamine. It is apparent that human carcinogens are generally characterized by overt genetic toxicity (Shelby, 1988) and that tumour induction for genotoxins is ubiquitously trans-species.

Although it may be possible to examine the sensitivity of experimental testing in animals as an indicator of carcinogenicity in humans, it is extremely difficult to examine its specificity. The IARC (1987) classifies only

Table 3 Site concordance between man and rat and/or mice for 21 compounds with sufficient evidence of carcinogenicity in humans and experimental animals (IARC, 1987)

Agree	Disagree	Debatable
Aflatoxins	Benzene	2-Naphthylamine[b]
4-Aminobiphenyl	Benzidine	Nickel and nickel
	Melphalan[a]	compounds[c]
Asbestos		
Bis(chloromethyl)ether and chloromethyl methyl ether (technical grade)		
Chlorambucil		
Chromium compounds, hexavalent		
Coal-tar pitches		
Coal tars		
Cyclophosphamide		
Diethylstilboestrol		
Erionite		
Methoxsalen + UV-A		
Mineral oil, untreated and mildly treated		
Shale oils		
Tobacco smoke		
Vinyl chloride		

a Acute non-lymphocytic leukaemia in man and lymphosarcomas in rats and mice.
b Bladder cancer reported in one rat study.
c Nickel carbonyl and nickel acetate produced lung tumours in rats and mice, respectively.

one chemical, caprolactam, as probably not carcinogenic. Other agents are classified as having evidence suggesting lack of carcinogenicity in experimental animals, but no agent (including caprolactam) is classified as such in terms of human carcinogenicity. Hence we cannot estimate how many times animal testing wrongly predicts carcinogenicity in humans.

Quantitative risk assessment based on animal data has caused considerable debate over the scientific merits and shortcomings of the methodology among toxicologists (e.g. Olin *et al.*, 1997). Epidemiologists often feel that insufficient weight is given to epidemiology data where it is available and which is often dismissed because of lack of power or poor exposure data. The situation has not been helped by attempts to demonstrate that epidemiology findings are compatible with predictions from animal-based risk assessment models which demonstrably overestimate human risks. A good illustration in the case of methylene chloride is provided by Tollefson *et al.* (1990) and Stayner and Bailer (1993), who attempt to justify OSHA's multistage models of risk based on liver and lung cancer in mice in the face of negative epidemiology. However, in the case of saccharin, epidemiologists have argued that the epidemiology is compatible with a small but undetectable risk of bladder cancer even though toxicologists have shown that the mechanism for the production of bladder tumours in rats is not relevant to man (Hertz-Picciotto and Neutra, 1994; Wilson, 1995).

The literature is scattered with examples that reveal either marked under or overestimation of the risks for man. Formaldehyde is an example where risk assessments based on animal data have overestimated the risks for man. The dose levels at which animal tumours were observed (Kerns *et al.*, 1983) resulted in overestimation of the risks for man (US EPA, 1987), which directly conflict with several epidemiology studies (Acheson *et al.*, 1984; Blair *et al.*, 1986). On the other hand, there are examples where epidemiology has revealed toxic effects in man at far lower levels than the animal models would predict, e.g. vinyl chloride (Purchase, 1985) and benzene (Wong, 1987).

Prediction of human cancer risk from the results of rodent bioassays requires two types of extrapolation: a qualitative extrapolation from short-lived rodent species to long-lived humans, and a quantitative extrapolation from near-toxic doses in the bioassay to low-level human exposures (Gold *et al.*, 1992). Fortunately, in recent years more constructive efforts have been made to address these deficiencies and incorporate epidemiological data in the risk assessment. Metabolic and biochemically orientated investigations of species differences are resulting in greater understanding of anomalies between toxicology and epidemiology studies. In the case of methylene chloride, Green (1997) has shown that the liver tumours in mice result from interactions between metabolites of the glutathione *S*-transferase pathway and DNA. The tumours were not increased in rats or hamsters and the species specificity is thought to be a direct consequence of the very high activity and specific cellular and nuclear localization of a theta class glutathione S-transferase enzyme which is unique to the mouse. The mouse lung tumours are believed to have resulted from damage to the mouse lung Clara cells and increased cell division. Green concluded that the mouse is unique is its response to methylene chloride and that it is an inappropriate model for human health assessment. However, as Kaiser (1996) noted, the story does not end there, as a very small proportion of humans carry two copies of a gene, *GSTTI*, that makes them produce more glutathione pathway enzymes (see also Casanova *et al.*, 1997).

Biomarkers in Epidemiology

A report on a workshop held at the IARC, (1997) defines a biological marker (commonly abbreviated, for convenience, to biomarker) as any substance, structure or process that can be measured in the human body or its products and may influence or predict the outcome of disease. Although biomarkers have been used in epidemiological studies for many years, interest has exploded in the last 10 years (e.g. Hulka *et al.*, 1990; Schulte and Perera, 1993; IEH, 1996). Biomarkers are often separated into three categories of exposure, effect and susceptibility and represent real opportunities for effective collaboration between epidemiologists and toxicologists. The assumption underlying biomarker research is that environmentally induced diseases start with measurable subclinical changes that may eventually induce persistent organ dysfunction. Thus, the value of a biomarker to the epidemiologist is its ability to predict backwards towards exposure and forwards to clinical outcome (Silbergeld and Davis, 1994). Rothman (1993) described biomarkers as a biological footprint that intermediates the causal action. Research in mechanistic toxicology is providing a range of useful biomarkers which should lead to an improved understanding of pathogenesis. Biomarkers offer the epidemiologist an opportunity to move away from 'black box' risk factor epidemiology (Skrabenek, 1994).

Biomarker research is starting to answer a huge range of questions. For example, a number of epidemiology studies have shown that underground miners are at increased risk of lung cancer (Lubin *et al.*, 1995). However, the relative contributions of radon, cigarette smoking and other pollutants such as diesel exhausts have not been clear. However, biomarkers can answer the question of whether the lung cancer of a miner is due to radon or cigarette smoking (Semenza and Weasel, 1997). Mutations in p53 have also established links between dietary aflatoxin exposure and liver cancer, exposure to ultraviolet light and skin cancer, smoking and cancer of the lung and bladder and vinyl chloride and liver cancer (Semenza and Weasel, 1997). Benefits in assessing the susceptibility of individuals to exposure are also becoming clear (Warren and Sheilds, 1997), although it is important to recognize the distinction between rare inherited somatic mutations that initiate cancer and much more common metabolic polymorphisms that predispose only if the right exposure occurs (Venitt, 1994). Hayes (1995) lists a number of examples of genetic susceptibility factors that influence metabolism of some common occupational exposures.

Biomarkers have started to have a considerable impact on improving the quality of exposure assessment and identifying population subgroups at increased susceptibility to exposure-related disease. However, there have been far fewer successes in the use of biomarkers as early outcome measures to predict the occurrence of clinical disease and to elucidate the biological mechanism of pathogenesis. McMichael and Hall (1997) have split the 'effect' role of biomarkers in epidemiology research into two components. The first use is as a basis for differentiating disease subtypes with potentially different aetiologies, e.g. the differentiation of radon and smoking-related lung cancers described above. The second use is as a measure of early outcome with known (or presumed) predictive significance. They argued that this latter role is far less well developed although of great potential value.

There can be little doubt that the potential benefits of constructive collaboration between toxicologists and epidemiologists are huge. However, transitional studies provide a good illustration of where integration may not be easy. Transitional studies require both laboratory and epidemiological expertise as they are studies that bridge the gap between laboratory experiments and population-based epidemiology (Schulte and Perera, 1997). They involve the first field testing of the markers and Schulte and Perera (1997) discussed the problems that arise in such collaborations, many of which result from the different assumptions, paradigms and language of the two disciplines as described earlier in this chapter. Wilcox (1995) also discussed these culture problems and identified other areas of possible misunderstanding between the two disciplines in molecular epidemiology. Smith and Suk (1994) noted that epidemiologists want well characterized and reproducible assays that can be applied in large studies (hundreds or thousands of subjects). In contrast, laboratory scientists have little interest in running large numbers of assays but wish to refine methods to stay at the cutting edge. However, the recommendations produced by an IARC workshop on the application of biomarkers in cancer epidemiology (IARC, 1997) clearly show that epidemiologists and toxicologists have recognized the value of effective collaboration.

CONCLUSION

Utidjian (1987) provided, for several compounds, a comprehensive review of the ways in which epidemiology has historically interacted with animal toxicity studies. Utidjian concluded that epidemiology has started to lose its historic role as the initiating or hypothesis-generating discipline and has become a secondary tool to confirm, refute or quantify human carcinogenic effects, the animal carcinogenesis bioassay being responsible for this change in role. This is undoubtedly true to some degree, and Utidjian cited acrylonitrile, formaldehyde, ethylene oxide and acrylamide as examples where the results of animal carcinogenesis bioassays have triggered a flurry of epidemiology studies. However, cancer is not the only health effect of interest to medical investigators and regulators. For instance, Axelson *et al.* (1976) first described the syndrome now known as organic solvent syndrome or 'Danish painters' disease' and a tentative association between the syndrome and chronic exposure to solvents. The report not only led to much epidemiological work, but also stimulated toxicologists to take a greater interest in neurobehavioural effects. Even in the case of carcinogenesis, the increasing interest taken by IARC in occupations and mixtures is likely to strengthen the hand of epidemiology. It is clear in the case of nickel and chromium that epidemiological evidence first indicated that certain nickel and chromium compounds must be carcinogens. However, the early studies led to much speculation as to what the specific carcinogenic agent or agents might be. Animal studies were conducted in an attempt to clarify the situation, and the combination of evidence from the two disciplines has led to the identification of certain chromium compounds as human carcinogens, although the nickel debate continues. Epidemiology will undoubtedly continue to point the first finger of suspicion at occupations or processes that involve a mixture of compounds. The case-control study has an important role to play as a hypothesis generator and is a particularly potent research tool in the Scandinavian countries, where there exist computerized record systems linking census information and health data.

There can be little doubt that the relationship between epidemiology and toxicology should be an interaction. Although the two disciplines are methodologically very different and sometimes generate conflicting results, they should be seen as complementary. In this chapter we have tried to describe the strengths and weaknesses of each discipline and to indicate the need for cooperation between epidemiologists and toxicologists. Both share a common goal—human health protection. Toxicology in essence is animal epidemiology, and epidemiology can be viewed as an opportunistic analysis of the inadvertent exposure of humans to toxicants. Kamrin (1988) goes further when describing the different types of toxicity testing, and includes epidemiology as the fourth major study design alongside acute toxicity testing, subacute toxicity testing and chronic toxicity testing in animal experiments. Fortunately, in recent years advances in mechanistic research and biomarker development have resulted in epidemiologists and toxicologists working more closely together to (i) obtain a better understanding of causal mechanisms, (ii) produce improved risk assessments and (iii) obtain greater sensitivity of detection and quantification of adverse effects (Hattis, 1991).

In conclusion, Sir Richard Doll (1981), in an article on the relevance of epidemiology to policies for the prevention of cancer, concluded that '. . . no rational person would want to learn by counting dead bodies if he could possibly learn by other means how their particular causes of death could have been avoided' and 'Epidemiology may not be the method of choice for the discovery of preventative measures, as it requires some people to have been affected before it can be employed; but at present its use is essential . . .'. These remarks clearly indicate the need for both toxicologists and epidemiologists to be aware of the contributions their respective disciplines can make in assessing human health hazards.

REFERENCES

Acheson, E. D., Barnes, H. R., Gardner, M. J., Osmond, C., Panett, B. and Taylor, C. D. (1984). Formaldehyde in the British chemical industry. *Lancet*, **i**, 611–616.

Armstrong, B. K., White, E. and Saracci, R. (1992). Principles of exposure measurement in epidemiology. *Monographs in Epidemiology and Biostatistics*, Vol. 21. Oxford University Press, New York.

Axelson, O., Haue, M. and Hogstedt, C. (1976). A case-referent study on neuropsychiatric disorders among workers exposed to solvents. *Scand. J. Work Environ. Health*, **2**, 14–20.

Ayer, H. E., Dement, J. M., Busch, K. A., Ashe, H. B., Levadie, B. T. H., Burgess, W. A. and Diberardins, L. (1973). A monumental study: reconstruction of a 1920 granite shed. *Am. Ind. Hyg. Assoc. J.*, **34**, 206–216.

Blair, A., Stewart, P., O'Berg, M., Gaffey, W., Walrath, J., Ward, J., Bales, R., Kaplan, S. and Cubitt, D. (1986). Formaldehyde. *J. Natl. Cancer Inst.*, **76**, 1071–1084.

Bonde, J. P., Giwercman, A. and Ernst, A. (1996). Identifying environmental risk to male reproductive function by occupational sperm studies: Logistics and design options. *Occup. Environ. Med.*, **53**, 511–519.

Botham, P. A., Davies, G. E. and Teasdale, E. L. (1987). Allergy to laboratory animals: a prospective study of its incidence and of the influence of atopy on its development. *Br. J. Ind. Med.*, **44**, 627–632.

Boyle, P., Muir, C. S. and Grundmann, E. (1989). *Cancer Mapping*. Springer, Berlin.

Brown, L. P. (1990). *A Review of the Mortality and Morbidity of Pesticide Manufacturers and Applicators*. Internal Report, British Agrochemicals Association, Peterborough.

Brown, L. P. and Paddle, G. M. (1988). Risk assessment: animal or human model? *Pharm. Med.*, **3**, 361–374.

Carlsen, E., Giwercman, A., Keiding, N. and Skakkebaek, N. E. (1992). Evidence for decreasing quality of semen during past 50 years. *Br. Med. J.*, **305**, 609–613.

Casanova, M., Bell, D. A. and Heck, H. D. (1997). Dichloromethane metabolism to formaldehyde and reaction of formaldehyde with nucleic acids in hepatocytes of rodents and humans with and without glutathione S-transferase T1 and M1 genes. *Fundam. Appl. Toxicol.*, **37**, 168–180.

Case, R. A. M., Hosker, M. E., McDonald, D. B. and Pearson, J. T. (1954). Tumours of the urinary bladder in workmen engaged in the manufacture and use of certain dyestuff intermediates in the British chemical industry. Part 1. The role of aniline, benzidine, alpha-naphthylamine and beta-naphthylamine. *Br. J. Ind. Med.*, **11**, 75–104.

Colborn, T., Dumanoski, D. and Myers, J. P. (1996). *Our Stolen Future. Are We Threatening Our Fertility, Intelligence and Survival?—A Scientific Detective Story*. Little, Brown, Boston.

Cornfield, J. (1951). A method of estimating comparative rates from clinical data. Applications to cancer of the lung, breast and cervix. *J. Natl. Cancer Inst.*, **11**, 1269–1275.

Cornfield, J. (1962). Joint dependence of risk of coronary heart disease on serum cholesterol and systolic pressure: a discriminant function analysis. *Fed. Proc.*, **2**, 58–61.

Creech, J. L. and Johnson, M. N. (1974). Angiosarcoma of the liver in the manufacture of vinyl chloride. *J. Occup. Med.*, **16**, 150–151.

Crisp, T. M., Glagg, E. D., Cooper, R. L., Wood, W. P., Anderson, D. G., Baetche, K. P., Hoffmann, J. L., Morrow, M. S., Rodier, D. J., Schaeffer, J. E., Touart, L. W., Zeeman, M. G. and Patel, Y. M. (1998). Environmental endocrine disruption: an effects assessment and analysis. *Environ. Health Perspect.*, **106**, 11–56.

Decker, W. J. (1987). Introduction and history. In Haley, T. J. and Berndt, W. O. (Eds), *Toxicology*. Hemisphere, Washington, DC, pp. 1–19.

Doll, R. (1981). Relevance of epidemiology to policies for the prevention of cancer. *J. Occup. Med.*, **23**, 601–609.

Doll, R. (1984). Epidemiological discovery of occupational cancers. *Scand. J. Work Environ. Health*, **10**, 121–138.

Doll, R. and Hill, A. B. (1950). Smoking and carcinoma of the lung. Preliminary report. *Br. Med. J.*, **iii**, 739–748.

Doll, R. and Hill, A. B. (1954). The mortality of doctors in relation to their smoking habits. A preliminary report. *Br. Med. J.*, **ii**, 1451–1455.

Doll, R. and Peto, R. (1981). The causes of cancer: quantitative estimates of avoidable risks of cancer in the United States today. *J. Natl. Cancer Inst.*, **66**, 1191–1308.

Feinstein, A. R. (1988). Scientific standards in epidemiologic studies of the menace of daily life. *Science*, **242**, 1257–1263.

Finnegan, M. J., Pickering, C. A. C. and Burge, P. S. (1984). The sick building syndrome: prevalence studies. *Br. Med. J.*, **289**, 1573–1575.

Friess, S. L. (1987). History of risk assessment. In Rohlich, G. (Ed.), *Pharmokinetics in Risk Assessment. Drinking Water and Health*, Vol. 8. National Academy of Science, Washington, DC, pp. 3–7.

Glocklin, V. C. (1987). Current FDA perspective on animal selection and extrapolation. In Roloff, M. V. (Ed.), *Human Risk Assessment: the Role of Animal Selection and Extrapolation*. Taylor and Francis, London, pp. 15–22.

Gold, L. S., Slone, T. H., Manley, N. B. and Bernstein, L. (1991). Target organs in chronic bioassays of 533 chemical carcinogens. *Environ. Health Perspect.*, **93**, 233–246.

Gold, L. S., Manley, N. B. and Ames, B. N. (1992). Extrapolation of carcinogenicity between species: qualitative and quantitative factors. *Risk. Anal.*, **12**, 579–588.

Goldberg, D. (1972). *The Detection of Psychiatric Illness by Questionnaire*. Maudsley, London.

Goudie, R. B., Jack, A. S. and Goudie, B. M. (1985). Genetic and developmental aspects of pathological pigmentation patterns. *Curr. Top. Pathol.*, **74**, 132–138.

Grandjean, P. (1995). Biomarkers in epidemiology. *Clin. Chem.*, **41**, 1800–1803.

Green, T. (1997). Methylene chloride induced mouse liver and lung tumours: an overview of the role of mechanistic studies in human safety assessment. *Hum. Exp. Toxicol.*, **16**, 3–13.

Green, T., Mainwaring, G. W. and Foster, J. R. (1997). Trichloroethylene-induced mouse lung tumors: studies of the mode of action and comparisons between species. *Fundam. Appl. Toxicol.*, **37**, 125–130.

Hattis, D. (1991). Use of biological markers and pharmacokinetics in human health risk assessment. *Environ. Health Perspect.*, **90**, 229–238.

Hayes, R. B. (1995). Genetic susceptibility and occupational cancer. *Med. Lav.*, **86**, 206–213.

Hertz-Picciotto, I. and Neutra, R. R., (1994). Resolving discrepancies among studies: the influence of dose on effect size. *Epidemiology*, **5**, 156–163.

Huff, J., (1993). Chemicals and cancer in humans: first evidence in experimental animals. *Environ. Health Perspect.*, **100**, 201–210.

Hulka, B. S., Wilcosky, T. C. and Griffith, J. D. (Eds) (1990). *Biological Markers in Epidemiology*. Oxford University Press, New York.

IARC (1987). *Evaluation of Carcinogenic Risks to Humans. Overall Evaluations of Carcinogenicity: an Updating of IARC Monographs Vols 1–42*. IARC Monographs, Suppl. 7. International Agency for Research on Cancer, Lyon.

IARC (1997). Workshop Report. In *Applications of Biomarkers in Cancer Epidemiology*. IARC Scientific Publications, No. 142. International Agency for Research on Cancer, Lyon, pp. 1–18.

IEH (1996). *IEH Report on the Use of Biomarkers in Environmental Exposure Assessment*. Report R5. Institute for Environment and Health, Leicester.

Joffe, M. (1997). Time to pregnancy: a measure of reproductive function in either sex. Asclepios Project. *Occup. Environ. Med.*, **54**, 289–295.

Kaiser, J. (1996). New data help toxicologists home in on assessing risks. *Science*, **272**, 200.

Kallen, B. (1988). *Epidemiology of Human Reproduction*. CRC Press, Boca Raton, FL.

Kamrin, M. A. (1988). *Toxicology*. Lewis, Chelsea, MI.

Kerns, W. D., Pavkov, K. L., Donofrio, D. J., Gralla, E. J. and Swenberg, J. A. (1983). Carcinogenicity of formaldehyde in rats and mice after long term inhalation exposure. *Cancer Res.*, **43**, 4382–4392.

Lahdetie, J. (1995). Occupation and exposure-related studies on human sperm. *J. Occup. Environ. Med.*, **37**, 922–930.

Lubin, J. H., Boice, J. D., Jr, Edling, C., Hornung, R. W., Howe, G. R., Kunz, E., Kusiak, R. A., Morrison, H. I., Radford, E. P. and Samet, J. M. (1995). Lung cancer in radon-exposed miners and estimation of risk from indoor exposure. *J. Natl. Cancer Inst.*, **87**, 817–827.

Maltoni, C. (1977). Vinyl chloride carcinogenicity: an experimental model for carcinogenesis studies. In Hiatt, H. H., Watson, J. D. and Winsten, J. A. (Eds), *Origins of Human*

Cancer. Cold Spring Harbor Laboratory Press, Cold Spring Harbor, NY, pp. 119–146.

McMahon, B. and Pugh, T. F. (1970). *Epidemiology, Principles and Methods*. Little, Brown, Boston.

McMichael, A. J. and Hall, A. J. (1997). The use of biological markers as predictive early-outcome measures in epidemiological research. In *Applications of Biomarkers in Cancer Epidemiology*. IARC Scientific Publications, No. 142. International Agency for Research on Cancer, Lyon, pp. 281–290.

MRC (1976). *Questionnaire on Respiratory Symptoms and Instructions for Its Use*. Medical Research Council, London.

Newell, D. J. (1984). Present position and potential developments: some personal views. Medical statistics. *J. R. Statist. Soc. A*, **147**, 186–197.

Olin, S. S., Neumann, D. A., Foran, J. A. and Scarano, G. J. (1997). Topics in cancer risk assessment. *Environ. Health Perspect.*, **105**, 117–126.

OPCS (1986). *Occupational Mortality. The Registrar General's Decennial Supplement for Great Britain, 1979–80, 1982–83*. Series DS No. 6. HMSO, London.

Paddle, G. M. (1981). A strategy for the identification of carcinogens in a large, complex chemical company. In Peto, R. and Schneiderman, M. (Eds), *Quantification of Occupational Cancer: Banbury Report 9*. Cold Spring Harbor Laboratory Press, Cold Spring Harbor, NY, pp. 177–186.

Paddle, G. M. (1988). Epidemiology. In Anderson, D. and Conning, D. M. (Eds), *Experimental Toxicology: the Basic Principles*. Royal Society of Chemistry, London, pp. 436–456.

Pell, S., O'Berg, M. and Karrh, B. (1978). Cancer epidemiologic surveillance in the Du Pont Company. *J. Occup. Med.*, **20**, 725–740.

Peto, R., Pike, M. C., Day, N. E., Gray, R. G., Lee, P. N., Parish, S., Peto, J., Richards, S. and Wahrendorf, J. (1980). Guidelines for simple, sensitive significance tests for carcinogenic effects in long-term animal experiments. *IARC Monographs on the Evaluation of Carcinogenic Risks of Chemicals to Man*, Suppl. 2, International Association for Research on Cancer, Lyon, pp. 311–426.

Poole, C. (1986). Exposure opportunity in case-control studies. *Am. J. Epidemiol.*, **123**, 352–358.

Purchase, I. F. H. (1985). Carcinogenic risk assessment: a toxicologist's view. In Hoel, D. G. (Ed.), *Risk Quantitation and Regulatory Policy: Banbury Report 19*. Cold Spring Harbor Laboratory Press, Cold Spring Harbor, NY, pp. 175–186.

Ramazzini, B. (1964). *Demorbis artificum diatriba (Diseases of Workers)*. Translated from the Latin text of 1713 by Wright, W. C., Hafner, New York.

Rothman, K. J. (1993). Methodologic frontiers in environmental epidemiology. *Environ. Health Perspect.*, **101**, 19–21.

Rothman, K. J. and Greenland, S. (1998). *Modern Epidemiology*, 2nd edn. Lipincott-Raven, Philadelphia.

Rose, G. A., Blackbum, H., Gillum, R. A. and Pricas, R. J. (1982). *Cardiovascular Survey Methods*, 2nd edn. Monograph Series No. 56. WHO, Geneva.

Schlesselman, J. J. (1982). *Case-Control Studies: Design, Conduct, Analysis*. Oxford University Press, New York.

Schlesselman, J. J. and Stadel, B. V. (1987). Exposure opportunity in epidemiologic studies. *Am. J. Epidemiol.*, **125**, 174–178.

Schulte, P. A., Perera, E. P. (Eds) (1993). *Molecular Epidemiology: Principles and Practices*. Academic Press, San Diego.

Schulte, P. A. and Perera F. P. (1997). Transitional Studies. In *Applications of Biomarkers in Cancer Epidemiology*. IARC Scientific Publications, No. 142. International Agency for Research on Cancer, Lyon, pp. 19–29.

Semenza, J. C. and Weasel, L. H. (1997). Molecular epidemiology in environmental health: The potential of tumor suppressor gene p53 as a biomarker. *Environ. Health Perspect.*, **105**, 155–163.

Sharpe, R. M. and Skakkebaek, N. E. (1993). Are oestrogens involved in falling sperm counts and disorders of the male reproductive tract? *Lancet*, **341**, 1392–1395.

Sharpe, R. M., Turner, K. J. and Sumpter, J. P. (1998). Endocrine disruptors and testis development. *Environ. Health Perspect.*, **106**, A220–A221.

Shelby, M. D. (1988). The genetic toxicity of human carcinogens and its implications. *Mutat. Res.*, **204**, 3–15.

Silbergeld, E. K. and Davis, D. L. (1994). Role of biomarkers in identifying and understanding environmentally induced disease. *Clin. Chem.*, **40**, 1363–1367.

Skrabenek, P. (1994). The emptiness of the black box. *Epidemiology*, **5**, 553–555.

Smith, A. H. (1988). Epidemiologic input to environmental risk assessment. *Arch. Environ. Health*, **43**, 124–127.

Smith, M. T. and Suk, W. A. (1994). Application of molecular biomarkers in epidemiology. *Environ. Health Perspect.*, **102**, 229–235.

Stayner, L. T. and Bailer, A. J. (1993). Comparing toxicologic and epidemiologic studies. Methylene chloride—a case study. *Risk Anal.*, **13**, 667–673.

Tollefson, L., Lorentzen, R. J., Brown, R. N. and Springer, J. A. (1990). Comparison of the cancer risk of methylene chloride predicted from animal bioassay data with the epidemiologic evidence. *Risk. Anal.*, **10**, 429–435.

US EPA (1987). *Environmental Protection Agency Assessment of Health Risks to Garment Workers and Certain Home Residents from Exposure to Formaldehyde*. Office of Pesticides and Toxic Substances, Washington, DC.

Utidjian, H. M. D. (1987). The interaction between epidemiology and animal studies in industrial toxicology. In Ballantyne, B. (Ed.), *Perspectives in Basic and Applied Toxicology*. Wright, Bristol, pp. 309–329.

Van Duuren, B. L., Katz, C., Goldschmidt, B. M., Frenkel, K. and Sivak, A. (1972). Carcinogenicity of halo-ethers. II. Structure–activity relationships of analogs of bis(chloromethyl) ether. *J. Natl. Cancer Inst.*, **48**, 1431–1439.

Venitt, S. (1994). Mechanisms of carcinogenesis and individual susceptibility to cancer. *Clin. Chem.*, **40**, 1421–1425.

Warren, A. J. and Sheilds, P. G. (1997). Molecular epidemiology: carcinogen–DNA adducts and genetic susceptibility. *Proc. Soc. Exp. Biol. Med.*, **216**, 172–180.

Waterhouse, J. A. H., Muir, C. J., Shanmugaratnam, K. and Powell, J. (Eds.) (1982). *Cancer Incidence in Five Continents*, Vol. IV. IARC Scientific Publication, No. 42. International Agency for Research on Cancer, Lyon.

Wegman, D. H. and Eisen, E. A. (1988). Epidemiology. In Levy, B. S. and Wegman, D. H. (Eds), *Occupational Health. Recognizing and Preventing Work-Related Disease*. Little, Brown, Boston, pp. 55–73.

WHO (1983). *Guidelines on Studies in Environmental Epidemiology*. Environmental Health Criteria Series, No. 27. World Health Organization, Geneva.

WHO (1985). *Neurobehavioural Methods in Occupational and Environmental Health*. World Health Organization, Copenhagen.

WHO Regional Office for Europe (1995). Guiding principles for the use of biological markers in the assessment of human exposure to environmental factors: An integrative approach of epidemiology and toxicology. Report on a WHO consultation. *Toxicology*, **101**, 1–10.

Wilcox, A. J. (1995). Molecular epidemiology: collision of two cultures. *Epidemiology*, **6**, 561–562.

Wilson, J. D. (1995). Predicting responses in humans using animal study results. *Epidemiology*, **6**, 92–93.

Wilks, M. F., Volans, G. N. and Smith, L. L. (1996). Environmental endocrine modulators—where toxicology meets epidemiology. *Hum. Exp. Toxicol.*, **15**, 692–693.

Wong, O. (1987). An industry-wide study of chemical workers occupationally exposed to benzene. II. Dose–response analyses. *Br. J. Ind. Med.*, **44**, 348–395.

Zapp, J. A. (1981). Industrial toxicology, retrospective and prospect. In Clayton, G. D. and Clayton, F. E. (Eds), *Patty's Industrial Hygiene and Toxicology*, 3rd edn, Vol. 2A. Wiley, Chichester, pp. 1197–1219.

PART EIGHT
REGULATORY TOXICOLOGY

Chapter 71
Overview of Regulatory Affairs*

G. Diggle

CONTENTS

PATTERNS OF REGULATION

Most regulatory systems for chemical products fall into one of a small number of standard patterns. The principal patterns are pre-marketing authorization schemes, schemes based on lists of permitted (or proscribed) ingredients, notification schemes and voluntary schemes. A given category of products is usually controlled by means of the same type of regulatory system from country to country. Individual pharmaceutical products, for example, are subject to pre-marketing authorization in the EU, the USA, Japan and other trading regions. In contrast, most countries control cosmetics by means of ingredient lists. The principal regulatory patterns are as follows:

Pre-marketing authorization. Individual authorization must be obtained before any product can be marketed. Widely applied to pesticides and pharmaceuticals.

Permitted/proscribed lists. Products can be marketed without individual authorization, provided that the ingredients conform to official lists. Widely applied to relatively safe products for which limited ranges of ingredients are used, such as cosmetics and food additives.

Notification schemes. Substances and their basic properties must be notified, the aim being to ensure that safe conditions for use are established, rather than to control marketing authorization. Industrial chemicals constitute the major category regulated in this way.

Voluntary schemes. These non-statutory arrangements are sometimes used before decisions about the need for more formal systems are taken, or as temporary measures while statutory systems are being prepared. Novel foods have been subject to voluntary controls in various countries, although formal systems are now being introduced.

Although regulatory systems conform to a limited number of basic patterns, there is great variation of detail and terminology. For example, the terminology associated with pre-marketing authorization schemes varies considerably from country to country, even for a given class of products: pharmaceuticals, for example, require *licences* in the UK, but need *approvals* in the USA (although *approvals* are granted for pesticides in the UK). Within a given country, variations in terminology are seen; in the UK, for example, trials of experimental new pesticides require *permits*, while trials of new pharmaceuticals require *certificates*. With the subtlety so favoured in the UK (Shah, 1988), an alternative scheme for clinical trials has been provided, which allows for applications to be made for *exemption* from the need to hold a certificate; in practice, this exemption scheme has proved to be so popular that most applications are now for exemptions rather than certificates.

The many terms in use include licence, clearance, approval, authorization, certification, notification, permission and registration. It seems reasonable to expect that terms such as *licence* will be used consistently. After all, driving licences, dog licences and product licences can be seen to possess some common features. These seem to reflect a general principle of English law which avers that a licence is something which allows someone to do something which, without the licence, would be unlawful. But a permit, clearance or authorization may function in a very similar way, and indeed these expressions are often defined in terms of one another (James, 1986; Saunders, 1988). The meanings of these terms in ordinary English are not always applicable in the regulatory context, usually because of derivation from legal usage in other, earlier statutory contexts. Special meanings have developed, sometimes over centuries, in areas quite different

---

* The views expressed in this chapter are the author's and are not necessarily those of any government department or regulatory agency.

to the markets for chemical products. *Clearance*, for instance, is derived from customs law (James, 1986). While knowledge of these derivations is helpful in understanding the origins of regulatory systems and their apparent differences, it must be emphasized that the only safe definitions are those provided by the relevant legislation itself, in each case. The need for this cautious approach is illustrated by misunderstandings about the meaning of *registration*, as discussed elsewhere in this chapter.

Pre-marketing Authorization

Regulatory systems such as those which authorize the marketing of individual pesticides and pharmaceuticals make use of well established procedures: application, registration, assessment, representations (if required) and decision. The pre-marketing application is usually required to be in a prescribed format, giving details of the proposed product and its intended uses. In general the formal application must be accompanied by scientific data, the detailed requirements being indicated by the agency's guidelines. When an application is submitted, the agency first decides whether it is adequate for assessment (whether, for example, the documentation is clear, in an approved language, etc). If the application is adequate for further consideration, it is registered for formal evaluation. This is carried out by the agency's expert assessors and, in most systems, there is also provision for independent expert advice. If the results of assessment are favourable, marketing authorization is granted. If it is not, it is usually possible for the applicant to make representations, involving the submission of arguments, with or without new scientific data. In general, it is only when all rights to make representations have been exhausted, without success, that an application is formally refused. Once granted, a marketing authorization may be revoked or suspended, for example when a previously unrecognized safety problem comes to light.

Pre-marketing authorization systems are illustrated by the existing regulatory arrangements for pharmaceutical products in the EU, the USA and Japan. In the EU, Council Directive 65/65 provides the basis for the control of medicines in the Member States. Subsequent development in the Community eventually produced a 'decentralized' procedure, incorporating an agreed method of binding arbitration, for the authorization of conventional medicines in more than one Member State. There is also a centralized procedure for innovative medicines. In the USA the controls provided by the Food and Drugs Act 1906 were greatly strengthened 32 years later (following the 'Elixir of Sulfanilamide' tragedy) when the Food, Drug and Cosmetic Act 1938 was enacted; this statute has been amended subsequently on a number of occasions. In Japan, medicinal products are regulated by means of the Pharmaceutical Affairs Law. Further details of these important systems are provided elsewhere in this chapter and in other specialized chapters.

Methods and standards of assessment vary considerably throughout the world. In some developing countries, criteria are less stringent; sometimes the fact that a product is authorized for the market in one or more developed countries is sufficient, and there is little independent assessment of data. In Norway, by contrast, conditions for the authorization of pharmaceuticals are particularly demanding, and include criteria for safety, effectiveness, quality, cost and need. Differences in standards are reflected in different rates of toxicological injury and mortality. For pesticides, these rates are much higher in countries where legislation concerning marketing and occupational safety is less stringent and/or is enforced less rigorously.

A particular chemical may be used as the active ingredient in different products, belonging to different regulatory classes. A given anti-fungal compound may, for example, be used in medicines, pesticides and veterinary drugs. Requirements for pre-marketing authorization are unlikely to be identical in the different regulatory environments concerned, one reason for this being the different risk–benefit ratios which will apply.

Written authorizations to place chemical products on the market are given different names according to the countries and classes of products concerned. In the case of pharmaceuticals, the term New Drug Approval (NDA) is used in the USA, while the British equivalent is the Product Licence (PL). PLs in the UK are valid for only 5 years, whereas in the USA, NDAs do not have this limitation. The general term used at Community level in the EU is Marketing Authorization.

Permitted and Proscribed Lists

Permitted and proscribed lists, sometimes known as positive and negative lists, are used very widely. Such lists are particularly useful where a relatively small number of ingredients, which may be used in a large number of marketed products, is to be controlled. For example, certain pesticide ingredients are prohibited in the EU by means of a negative list, under Directive 79/117/EEC. Cosmetic ingredients are regulated in many countries by means of this approach: ingredients which are not permitted (or are no longer permitted) to be used in cosmetics are placed on a negative list, while those which are permitted are included in a positive list. Lists may be further sub-divided into various categories of ingredients. Other important categories controlled with the help of lists include food colouring agents, other food additives and food processing agents.

Ingredient lists are not, however, the only forms in which permitted and proscribed lists are used for regulatory purposes. In many countries negative lists are used which contain those medicinal products for which national health insurance systems will not pay. Products are listed according to such criteria as relative cost and relative efficacy. If a listed product is prescribed, reimbursement is not available through the national insurance system, and the patient must pay the full cost. The products on these negative lists may include some which possess marketing authorizations and some which lie in the borderline area between medicines and foods, for which pharmaceutical marketing authorizations are not required. In the EU, the Transparency Directive (Council Directive 89/105/EEC) requires that a statement of the reasons, which must be based on objective and verifiable criteria, must be provided when a product is placed on a negative list. Regulatory agencies must also publish a statement of the criteria which they use when deciding whether products are to be listed.

Other special forms of negative lists appear in legislation designed to prevent drug misuse. In the UK, for example, the relevant regulations (made under the Misuse of Drugs Act 1971) make use of no less than nine negative lists of 'controlled' drugs. In five of these lists, 'scheduled' drugs are placed according to the applicable levels of control over manufacture, prescribing, custody, record-keeping, etc., which apply. Schedule 1 is a list of substances which are not used medicinally (cannabis, lysergide, etc.). Schedule 2 is a list of drugs to which the greatest restrictions apply (diamorphine and other opiates, cocaine, amphetamine, glutethimide, certain barbiturates, etc.). A further three negative lists contain drugs according to their harmfulness. The most harmful are placed in class A, which is a list including diamorphine, lysergide, methylenedioxymethamphetamine (MDMA, '*ecstasy*') and phencyclidine (PCP, '*angel dust*'). Class B is a list which includes cannabis, cannabis resin and oral amphetamines. Finally, doctors in the UK are required to provide the regulatory agency (in this case the Home Office) with details of patients they attend whom they believe to be addicted to a drug on a list of 14 'notifiable' substances (including diamorphine and cocaine).

Notification Schemes

There is a fundamental distinction between *notification* and *pre-marketing authorization*. Pre-marketing authorization systems allow products (such as a pesticides and medicines) to be placed on the market once evidence of safety and other criteria have been assessed and found to be acceptable. Notification schemes, on the other hand, may require no more than that basic data about a compound (such as an industrial chemical), be supplied to the regulatory agency before marketing commences. The purpose of a notification scheme is not to enable an agency to decide whether or not products such as industrial chemicals should be allowed on to the market, but to enable them to be registered with the agency, which then ensures that they are used safely.

In the case of industrial chemicals, this is generally achieved by means of basic toxicological testing, classification and labelling, by setting exposure limits in the workplace and by ensuring adequate methods for storage, handling, disposal and the treatment of accidental spillages and of injuries caused by the chemical.

In the USA, the Environmental Protection Agency regulates chemicals (particularly new industrial chemicals) which are not controlled by other laws, by means of a notification scheme under the powers of the Toxic Substances Control Act 1976. Two laws involving notification schemes regulate industrial chemicals in Japan, and separate compliance with both of them is mandatory.

There are numerous minor differences between the notification schemes which have been developed in different countries. In the USA, notification must take place before *manufacture* of an industrial chemical commences, whereas the European approach specifies notification before *marketing*. In the European and Japanese approaches, the submission of standardized sets of basic data is required, whereas the US Environmental Protection Agency (US EPA) does not possess this power, although it can request specific data on an individual-case basis (if it is considered that there is need to evaluate a potential hazard) before granting manufacturing approval. In the European schemes, notification that production has reached specified annual tonnages is required, and this may trigger further data requirements.

In the Member States of the EU, notification schemes for industrial chemicals have been introduced into domestic law in accordance with Council Directive 79/831. This is known universally as 'the sixth amendment' because it amends for the sixth time Council Directive 67/548 (otherwise known as 'the dangerous substances directive') which deals with the classification, packaging and labelling of industrial chemicals. In the UK, for example, the legal basis for the notification scheme has been provided by means of regulations made under the Health and Safety at Work Etc. Act 1974, which is implemented by the Health and Safety Executive.

Voluntary Schemes

An important distinction is to be made between *statutory* and *voluntary* pre-marketing schemes. In the former, details of a product must be assessed and deemed satisfactory before marketing can take place. In the latter, there are no specific legal requirements and the submission of safety data by organizations is not enforceable. Once it becomes clear that some sort of supervision is needed, it is not unusual for regulatory procedures to be introduced after consideration by a committee of inquiry. The inquiry stage may be followed by an interim period of voluntary self-regulation, before formal legislative provisions and statutory bodies are introduced.

In many instances, regulatory agencies have adopted an initial voluntary approach and, when this has been seen to be inadequate, have moved to a statutory one. Sometimes voluntary schemes are introduced as temporary measures while statutory systems are being prepared. The development of the new market for so-called '*functional foods*' will afford an opportunity to observe the evolution of controls. At present, as the need for the regulation of these products is being recognized, some manufacturers argue that voluntary systems will suffice, whereas other interest groups consider that pre-marketing approval systems should be established in the first instance.

Controls for novel foods and food ingredients are making the transition away from voluntary systems. Although a legislative approach has for some time been used in The Netherlands, other countries have relied on voluntary systems. In the EU, a new Regulation is being incorporated into the domestic law of Member States, providing statutory control at Community level for novel foods and food ingredients. The European Parliament considered the draft Regulation in October 1993 and suggested some revisions, including the adoption of a single common (centralized) assessment procedure. The Regulation has provided, in its final form, for a Europe-wide pre-marketing authorization system.

In many countries, voluntary approaches were applied to both pharmaceuticals and to pesticides before statutory arrangements were introduced. In the UK in 1957 a voluntary approach, the Pesticide Safety Precautions Scheme (PSPS), for ensuring the safe use of pesticides was set up following the deaths of workers exposed to dinitro compounds. The PSPS was later superseded by statutory controls under the Control of Pesticides Regulations enacted under the Food and Environmental Protection Act 1985. Under the voluntary scheme, trade associations had agreed that their member companies would submit data to, and obtain *clearances* from, the regulatory agency before marketing new products. Following the thalidomide tragedy, a voluntary scheme for medicines operated in the UK from 1963. Pharmaceutical companies were invited to seek the advice of the Committee on Safety of Drugs (the so-called 'Dunlop Committee') before launching new products. The voluntary scheme for medicines was superseded when a statutory system of pre-marketing authorization was eventually introduced in September 1971, when *licensing* under the Medicines Act 1968 was implemented.

Certification

A certificate is a document which attests to a particular fact (James, 1986; Saunders, 1988), for example, the fact that the clinical trial of a pharmaceutical has been authorized. In some countries the procedures involved in applications for clinical trial authorization resemble those used to obtain marketing authorization, with provisions for making representations when applications are not immediately successful. In other countries, notification schemes operate.

The control of pharmaceutical testing in *healthy human volunteers* (as opposed to patients) varies considerably from country to country. In the USA, statutory controls relating to volunteers are included in the regulations for Investigational New Drugs (INDs), which provides a form of certification, whereas in the UK there is no statutory system.

Registration

In the UK, *registration* has a specific meaning in company law (James, 1986), although it is used more widely in ordinary British English (Saunders, 1988) to mean the placement of something on some sort of register. In regulatory affairs, registration is sometimes used as a synonym for *notification*, in relation to the control of industrial chemicals, for example. In this case the register concerned is the resister of notified chemicals. The word is also used in relation to pre-marketing approval systems, where it may refer either to a register of authorized products or to a register of products which have been submitted for consideration. Thus, a registered product may mean one which has been allowed on to the market, or it may mean a product which is awaiting assessment. It all depends on which register is implied: the register of authorized products, or the register of products awaiting assessment. This ambiguity has caused problems in international regulatory affairs on several occasions. One such case concerned a medicinal product which, for safety reasons, had been withdrawn from use in developed countries. Marketing authorization was then sought in a less developed country, where the regulatory agency was assured that the product was 'registered' in one of the developed countries, and the application was based on that claim. Fortunately, the agency in the less developed country made appropriate checks before proceeding. It found that, in the developed country, all medicinal products submitted for assessment are immediately and routinely 'registered', that is, placed on a register of products awaiting assessment. It emerged that this was the true status of the product concerned, for which a renewed application for authorization had been submitted following withdrawal.

The word registration is enshrined in the title of the International Conferences for the Harmonization of Technical Requirements for the Registration of Pharmaceuticals for Human Use. Many companies possess registration departments, which deal with regulatory systems of all kinds. In practice, therefore, this flexible word is firmly entrenched. It is useful to recall that any statement that a product is registered merely means that it has been placed on a register; this causes no difficulty when it is clear to all concerned which register is implied.

National Approaches

The value of internationally consistent standards and data requirements is now well appreciated and is receiving much attention. Before the current era of international harmonization, however, regulatory arrangements were for the most part established at national level and the approaches adopted often owed much to national circumstances and history. Sometimes the emphasis reflected earlier toxicological incidents in the countries concerned. In Japan, for example, particular legislative attention was paid to the problem of environmental pollution by industrial chemicals, following incidents in which pollutants reached foodstuffs and produced serious illness.

The legislative background of a country inevitably influences the development of its regulatory approach. In France, for example, studies of drug pharmacokinetics in healthy human volunteers were not permitted because, under the Code Napoléon, a citizen's body is the property of the state, and may not be endangered. Changes in the law removed this restriction in the late 1980s. In relation to *in vitro* fertilization (IVF), French law prohibits the creation of human embryos specifically for research purposes; however, a couple may now agree to studies in some circumstances, provided that they have a therapeutic purpose and do not harm the embryo.

Major tragedies which are not in themselves related to toxicity may influence the development of higher standards across broad areas, chemical safety among them. On 21 October 1966, in the Welsh village of Aberfan, 116 children were killed when their school was buried under spoil from a coalmine which had been dumped over a mountain spring above the school, and had subsequently slipped. This event provided a major spur for the development of the Health and Safety at Work Etc. Act 1974, which put the obligation of employers to take reasonable and practicable steps to ensure the safety of the public and employees on a statutory basis.

PRODUCT CATEGORIES

Today, substances which are known to be toxic to humans are used in individual restraint, riot control and judicial execution. In some countries drugs, such as suxamethonium and apomorphine, have been (and perhaps are) used for torture. Substances with much greater human toxicity have been used in warfare. It has been appreciated for millenia that medicinal and toxic substances have much in common, although it was left to the great Paracelsus (1493–1541) to remind Western science

of this. By the Hellenic period the Greek word *pharmakon* (φαρμακon) had already come to mean both drug and poison. The Greek *toxon* means the archer's bow and, because arrows were sometimes tipped with poison, the Greek *toxicon pharmakon* was used to denote arrow poison. The English word *toxicology* is in turn derived from this.

In this chapter, of course, the focus is upon product categories which pose *unintended* toxicological hazards to humans. Yet there are several boundary areas in which the proper regulatory category may not be immediately clear. Problems of classification apply particularly to some of the interfaces between medicines and food products. Sometimes the same active ingredient forms the basis of products belonging to different regulatory types, leading to further problems of categorisation. Finally, all chemical products start life as industrial chemicals, but are later regulated as pesticides, drugs etc, so that the stage at which re-classification occurs must be considered. In addition to products, agencies are also concerned with chemical contaminants.

Pesticides

Pesticides are chemical products which are designed to possess toxic properties, and which are used to control unwanted living organisms. Ideally, pesticides would possess highly selective toxicity, and affect only the target species (i.e. the animals or plants deemed in the circumstances to be pests). In practice, this ideal is rarely achieved, and many pesticides are toxic to wide ranges of animal and plant species. For insecticides, the mammalian selectivity ratio (MSR) provides a crude measure of relative (acute) toxicity. The MSR is the ratio of the topical LD_{50} in the female housefly to the oral LD_{50} in the mouse. It has been known for several decades that the MSR varies widely (from less that 1.0 to more than 1000) from one well known insecticide to another (Metcalf, 1972). Inter-species differences in mechanisms, xenobiotic biotransformation, target enzymes, etc., have been shown in some cases to account for toxicological differences, but much research is needed in this area. Pesticides are ubiquitous and, as many different types are in use and large numbers of non-target species are affected, much more knowledge of their differential toxicology is needed. This is also necessary for the development of new generations of selective pesticides. Categories of pesticides are named according to the groups of animals or plants which they are used to control: rodenticides, insecticides, acaricides, molluscicides, nematocides, herbicides, fungicides, algicides and so forth. By convention, products used for the control of micro-organisms are not classed as pesticides: bactericides, disinfectants, antibacterials and antibiotics are regarded as distinct groups and are not included in the category.

Pesticides are used for several reasons, one of the major ones being the need to protect food-producing plants. These agricultural pesticides or plant-protection products may be designed to control unwanted plants (weeds, fungi, etc.) or animals (e.g. insects, rodents). Other reasons for the use of pesticides include the need to protect timber, to prevent the fouling of ships by marine growths and to prevent algal and other growths on masonry. Some pesticide ingredients are also used in other categories: malathion and carbaryl, for example, are used in both human medicines and pesticides. The organochlorine lindane is used both in agricultural pesticides for plant protection and in veterinary medicines, and some organophosphates are used as pesticides and as veterinary medicines for the treatment of farm animals infested with ectoparasites. Pesticides constitute a category within a very broad group of products, agrochemicals. Other categories which are regarded as agrochemicals include fertilizers and plant growth regulators. Related products include those marketed for use in aquaculture, fish farming, etc., and are categorized and regulated according to their precise functions.

Many pesticides are able to produce toxicological effects in a wide range of species, including humans, and human exposure can occur through several routes. Occupational exposure affects agricultural workers, who are often required to work with more concentrated formulations. Residues of pesticides occur in foodstuffs, including but not limited to those to which pesticides have been applied intentionally. Finally, residues of pesticides are able to enter the environmental media (water, soil and air) in sufficient amounts to harm wide ranges of non-target plant and animal life. As some pesticidal compounds are stable and non-biodegradable, they are able, having entered the environment, to remain unchanged for long periods and to produce ecological changes. Problems of this kind have been posed by various organochlorine insecticides, one of the best known being DDT, which was introduced in the early 1940s and which is no longer used. DDT is very persistent, exerts weak oestrogenic actions and is said to produce eggshell thinning in predatory birds, although good evidence of causality for the latter effect is not available.

The regulatory control of agricultural pesticides therefore presents particular challenges. The safety of agricultural workers using pesticides is addressed by measures similar in principle to those required in other working environments where industrial chemicals are used but, in this case, the workplace is not a factory; both measures and their enforcement have to be adapted realistically to field conditions if safe agricultural practice is to be ensured. Occupational exposure accounts for practically all the mortality and serious morbidity attributable to pesticides, and practically all cases occur in less developed countries. The safety of food consumers is protected by regulations which aim to limit pesticide residues in foodstuffs to levels which are well below those at which any toxicological effect can occur, and incidents involving consumers are rare. In one unusual incident in 1985, there were more than 250 reports of illness in Oregon associated with contamination of watermelons by the carbamate aldicarb, which has a high level of acute oral toxicity. Similar outbreaks in which aldicarb has been implicated have occurred in Canada and Ireland in recent years. Regulations must, of course, be underpinned by effective systems for sampling and residue measurement. The escape of pesticides into environmental water is limited by measures such as special requirements for drainage and disposal. Dispersal by air in the form of spray drift and the accumulation of soil residues are limited by the enforcement of good agricultural practice.

Pharmaceuticals

Many pharmaceuticals for human use are marketed for the treatment or prevention of disease, although some are approved for other purposes. These include contraceptives, anaesthetics and radiological contrast media. Pharmaceutical products designed for specialized diagnostic uses include pentagastrin preparations for studying gastric secretion and radioactive vitamin B_{12} products for use in the diagnosis of pernicious anaemia by means of the Schilling test. Other products are used to modify normal physiological functions, as when bromocriptine is used to suppress puerperal lactation, or when mydriatics are used to facilitate ophthalmological examinations.

Medicines comprise a very wide variety of product types. These include preparations of fine chemicals and substances of biological origin, ranging from blood products (such as factor VIII for the treatment of haemophilia-A) to antibiotics. Pharmaceutical products of biotechnology are emerging slowly. Although genes responsible for many disorders have been identified and sequenced, the application of this knowledge in ways which are useful in clinical practice is proceeding more gradually; the popular idea that the required gene can be delivered to the appropriate cells in the body, made to function and thereby cure the disease, is misleadingly optimistic. Nevertheless, emerging products of biotechnology range from hormones to new vaccines containing genetically modified microorganisms. Special considerations apply to the testing and regulation of biotechnological products, as has been reflected, for example, in the establishment of centralized arrangements for their control in the EU.

Medical devices may also be regulated by agencies responsible for the control of medicines. A wide range of devices may be dealt with in this way or, in other countries, the scope of medicinal controls may only be extended to a limited range of devices such as intra-uterine contraceptives and some absorbable surgical products. As with other categories of products, the raw materials from which medicines and medical devices are manufactured start life as industrial chemicals. The same bulk chemicals may in some cases also be supplied for the manufacture of other, unrelated products. During the production of the bulk material, it is subjected to the controls which apply to industrial chemicals. When the bulk material is supplied to the manufacturer of a medicinal product or medical device, it continues to be controlled as an industrial chemical in the workplace, but also becomes subject to the requirements for safety testing, good manufacturing practice, etc., which apply to the category to which the finished product will belong.

Although many of the uses of pharmaceuticals in veterinary practice are analogous to those in human medicine (treatment, prevention and diagnosis of disease, etc.), some animal medicines are used for special commercial purposes in food-producing animals. Although these products are relatively few in number, the market for them is very large. These include products designed to increase lactation, promote growth, modify the timing of oestrous, etc. The use of some of these special animal products is controversial. For some of these non-therepeutic products, different positions have been taken by major regulatory agencies and this has led to difficulties in international trade. The use of hormonal growth promoters in food-producing animal species is, for example, prohibited in the EU, whereas it is permitted in the USA. The same scientific data are available to all the agencies concerned, but fundamental differences in political factors influencing risk perception ultimately underlie the different positions taken.

The safety of a medicinal product must be considered in the light of its effectiveness or efficacy. Safety is therefore relative and wise prescribing is indispensable. Some medicines produce toxic effects (which may be substantial for some drugs, such as cytotoxic agents used in the treatment of cancer), but these effects are considered to be an acceptable price to pay for the therapeutic benefits obtainable. In such cases the risk of the anticipated adverse effects (i.e. their likelihood) is high. Here, high risk means that an unwanted effect will probably occur, and not necessarily that the effect is a life-threatening one. Toxic or other unwanted effects are much less tolerable in medicines used only for minor conditions, and those possessing little efficacy. In all cases, what is required is a sensible balance between safety and efficacy. In addition to the two principal criteria of safety and efficacy, quality constitutes a third criterion. Questions of quality (e.g. impurities, stability and chemical specifications) are of importance mainly because of their implications for the safety and efficacy of the product.

The unwanted effects associated with medicines may be of a relatively predictable nature associated with the pharmacodynamic or physiological actions of the drug; examples include sinus bradycardia in a patient receiving digoxin, tachycardia following treatment with liothyronine and hypoglycaemia induced by an insulin preparation. Such effects are relatively common and can be minimized by good clinical management. They tend to be dose-related and are more likely to occur when the therapeutic index is small, as with the cardiac glycosides. Some unwanted effects only emerge after prolonged use, such as skin atrophy following the long-term use of a topical corticosteroid. Others appear when the drug is discontinued, as may occur following the withdrawal of a benzodiazepine.

Effects which are unpredictable in the individual patient include those due to genetic polymorphisms such as acetylator status and to hypersensitivity reactions and other idiosyncrasies. These effects may be very difficult to attribute to the drug, unless the clinician is aware of the phenomenon. Examples of these phenomena include the oculomucocutaneous syndrome caused by practolol and the neutropenia which may be induced by carbimazole. An idiosyncratic effect is much more likely to be attributed correctly to its cause when it is of a kind known to be associated with drugs (e.g. bone marrow depression) or known to be linked either with the drug in question or its close relatives. If the effect is a reversible one, it may be helpful to observe the effects of withdrawal and re-challenge. Sometimes the timing of the unwanted effect will provide a useful clue to causality, if the delay is a characteristic one. Examples include anaphylaxis immediately following an antibiotic injection and serum sickness a few days after the administration of an anti-toxin. Some of the most serious unwanted drug effects are only apparent after a long delay. These include teratogenesis (e.g. resulting from the use of a retinoid in a woman of child-bearing potential) and carcinogenesis (e.g. liver cancer following the use of anabolic steroids).

As all practising clinicians are aware, people have an irresistible tendency to take medicines of one kind or another. If the doctor is not inclined to prescribe a medicine, perhaps explaining that it is not appropriate in the circumstances, some patients may not be able to resist a little self-medication, perhaps some garlic capsules, or 50 mg tablets of vitamin B_6, or a ginseng elixir. One of the great physicians of the last century wrote:

> '... man has an inborn craving for medicine ... the desire to take medicine is one feature which distinguishes man the animal from his fellow creatures. It is really one of the most serious difficulties with which we have to contend ... the doctor's visit is not thought to be complete without a prescription ...' (Osler, 1894).

As a result of this irrepressible tendency, there is an enormous market for preparations which, although they might not sail through placebo-controlled, randomized, double-blind trials with flying colours, are generally (but not always) quite safe. They include various kinds of 'alternative' remedies including homoeopathics, herbals, anthroposophics and health supplements. Some of these preparations have been approved for marketing as medicines with relatively few formalities, especially when there is a history of safe use. Others escape medicinal controls by avoiding any overt claims of a medicinal nature, and are often marketed through health food stores and by mail order. These products are discussed elsewhere in this chapter.

In recent years, regulators and heavily loaded clinicians in various countries have recognized that it would be sensible to extend the range of genuinely effective medicines available to the public without prescription. The preparations affected include anti-histamines, topical corticosteroid preparations and the non-steroidal anti-inflammatory agent ibuprofen. These changes have been of considerable benefit to both patients and their doctors.

Drugs in a well recognized group tend to be obtained illegally and misused. Some misused drugs have been in clinical use in the past (e.g. lysergide, methylenedioxy-methamphetamine [MDMA] and phencyclidine). Some are authorized for medicinal use in some administrations, but not in others (e.g. diamorphine). Some have no history of medicinal use (e.g. 'freebase' cocaine). Others are currently authorized for use in clinical medicine in many administrations (e.g. amyl nitrate, amphetamine sulphate).

Cosmetics

Cosmetics are preparations for application to the surface of the body, for specified non-medicinal purposes. They are usually classified as part of a larger category, consumer products, which in many jurisdictions also includes household detergents, cleaning and washing aids, disinfectants, toiletries, etc. The recognized purposes for which cosmetics are used generally include improving appearance, cleaning, maintaining condition, protecting, perfuming, deodorizing and inhibiting perspiration. The range of cosmetic products is wide, and different agencies have not always adopted identical criteria for categorization. In some interesting cases it may not be immediately obvious whether a particular product should be treated as a cosmetic. One group of such products for example, consists of eye drops which exert vasoconstrictor effects and so increase the whiteness of the conjunctiva. Another group consists of tablets which, when taken orally, change the skin colour to simulate a suntan. It has been necessary to develop precise legal definitions, taking account both of function and anatomical site of application, to ensure that products are consistently categorized.

The definitions developed in the EU, the USA and Japan are now similar. They contain descriptions of anatomical sites and the purposes for which products may be marketed, if they are to be recognized as cosmetics. In European law, cosmetics are as defined in Directive 76/768. In the UK, the definition provided in the Cosmetic Products (Safety) Regulations 1989 (made under the Consumer Protection Act) is consistent with the Directive, and states:

'Cosmetic product' means any substance or preparation intended to be applied to any part of the external surfaces of the human body (that is to say, the epidermis, hair system, nails, lips and external genital organs) or to the teeth or buccal mucosa wholly or mainly for the purpose of cleaning, perfuming or protecting them or keeping them in good condition or changing their appearance or combating body odour or perspiration, except where such cleaning, perfuming, protecting, keeping, changing or combating is wholly for the purpose of treating or preventing disease. 'Cosmetic product intended to come into contact with the mucous membranes' means a cosmetic product intended to be applied in the vicinity of the eyes, on the lips, in the oral cavity or to the external genital organs, and does not include any cosmetic product which is intended to come into only brief contact with the skin.

In general, cosmetic ingredients are relatively safe substances from the toxicological point of view. Substances with appreciable toxicity have been used in the past, e.g. certain hair dyes. Innovatory substances appear from time to time. Examples include mitogens, which increase proliferation in the stratum germinativum and so change the appearance of the skin, and careful safety assessments are needed in such cases. Many cosmetics are able to cause local hypersensitivity reactions in susceptible individuals and, as a result, there is a market for 'non-allergenic' products.

Industrial Chemicals

Industrial chemicals constitute the raw materials used in the manufacture of chemical products, ranging from pharmaceuticals and pesticides to plastics. It is therefore in the workplace (rather than the marketplace) that their safety aspects are especially important, although escapes to the environment (e.g. in wastewater) are also taken very seriously. Industrial chemicals are not the only category which poses problems of occupational safety. Finished chemical products, such as pesticides and pharmaceuticals, can of course harm those who work with them. This applies to the nurse who handles cytotoxic medicines and to the agricultural operator who applies pesticides.

The toxicity of industrial chemicals spans the widest possible range; some (such as deionized water) can hardly be regarded as toxic at all, while others (such as vinyl chloride) are very hazardous. In itself, toxicity does not determine whether a chemical can be used in industry; rather, it determines the kind and degree of safeguards required. There are many recognized industrial chemicals and the total continues to increase as new substances are added, and there are many ways in which exposures can occur in the working environment throughout industry. Some of these chemicals are, of course, used in extremely large quantities.

Once the basic toxicological properties of a new industrial chemical are known, appropriate classification and labelling are applied. In the interests of occupational safety, exposure limits in the workplace are set and adequate methods for handling, storage and disposal laid down. Appropriate protective clothing and other special means of protection may be required and must be specified, as must methods for dealing with accidental spillages. Facilities for the treatment of injuries caused by the chemical must be provided.

Although many industrial chemicals pose very little toxicological hazard, for example those used as ingredients for cosmetics and in the manufacture of processed foods, others, such as ingredients for pesticides, may be more toxic. Some useful industrial chemicals are extremely toxic and necessitate the most stringent precautions. Toxicity may not, of course, be immediately apparent, as with some carcinogens. This point may be illustrated by reviewing briefly the properties of vinyl chloride, the monomer from which the widely used plastic polyvinyl chloride (PVC) is manufactured. Vinyl chloride is a flammable gas at room temperature, and it is usually handled in liquid form in factories. The acute toxicity is not particularly great and vinyl chloride was at one time considered as a possible inhalational anaesthetic. In the early 1970s it became clear that occupational exposure was responsible for angiosarcomas developed in workers engaged in the manufacture of PVC. Vinyl chloride was formerly used as an aerosol propellant in household consumer products, and residues have been found in drinking water. In the manufacture of a plastic, the toxicological hazards posed by the product of the polymerization reaction are generally very different from those of the monomer, and quite different safety requirements will be applicable when, for example, polymer resin pellets are used in the manufacture of specific plastic goods.

Food Products

In most countries, there are basic legal provisions which apply to all foods, while specific regulations exist to control additives, processing aids, etc. Some food products which fall into more or less distinct categories, such

as slimming aids, dietary and 'health' supplements, are not yet controlled by specific regulations in most countries and are subject only to basic food law. New legislation is being created to take account of technical progress and market developments, for example in the area of novel foods and food ingredients. Some products, used in the management of specific disorders, fall into the borderline area between foods and medicines. Future developments may require new legislative approaches, for example, in relation to so-called *functional foods.* Specific regulations frequently exist to control the maximum permitted levels of contaminants in foodstuffs, although controls are generally undeveloped in relation to natural toxins. Basic food law imposes minimum obligations on those who market food. Typically, offences include selling food which is not what the purchaser asked for, or which does not comply with relevant safety requirements, or which has been made injurious to health. If it is to be enforced effectively, basic food law must be backed by positive political will, as well as adequate resources. In many instances of injury to health, the cause is microbiological contamination. In this chapter, the focus is on toxicological hazards which pose threats to consumers. Chemical contamination is sometimes found to be responsible for serious outbreaks of food poisoning associated with a major food product.

A very serious incident of this kind came to light in May 1981, in Spain. More than 20 000 people were affected by a condition which came to be called the toxic oil syndrome (TOS). There was injury to many tissues and organs, a consistent feature being damage to the endothelium of arteries. Several hundred died within 12 months. Ultimately, thousands were incapacitated and more than 800 died. The victims of the tragedy had ingested colza (rapeseed) oil, which had earlier been denatured with 2% aniline to ensure that it would be fit only for industrial use. However, the oil had later undergone some form of clandestine re-processing in an attempt to remove the adulteration and to enable it to be marketed illicitly as cooking oil. It emerged that the oil had been sold by itinerant salesmen or at local markets in unlabelled plastic containers. Neither the identity of the toxic agent nor the pathological mechanism have been elucidated (Diggle, 1995). Toxicologically, a non-necrotizing arteritis (mainly affecting the intima) is a consistent feature in the many organs affected, but toxicological studies in animals have been unrevealing.

Food supplements, such as vitamins and minerals, are necessary in certain circumstances, for example to prevent or treat deficiency diseases which occur mainly in certain less developed countries. Iron deficiency is the most prevalent problem of micronutrient malnutrition worldwide, and deficiencies of vitamin A and iodine are also common. There is a high mortality associated with iron deficiency anaemia, while low intakes of vitamin A and iodine are responsible for high prevalences of blindness and cretinism, respectively, in some countries. In developed countries, the situation is different. Throughout the post-war years economic growth, advances in knowledge and the development of cheap methods for mass production have ensured that supplies of nutritious foodstuffs are now readily available. There has been continuous improvement in the safety, nutritional value, economy and variety of foodstuffs available to whole populations. Poor nutritional habits and failure to eat healthy mixed diets often result from reasons other than economic ones, such as lack of nutritional understanding and unwillingness to apply available knowledge. There is less need for dietary supplements (with the possible exception of slimming aids) than for sensible, informed dietary practices. Many governments are therefore pursuing active programmes of public education, and are encouraging manufacturers to improve the nutritional quality of confectionery and other food products. At the same time, a food supplement market has developed, which attracts disposable income from consumers for whom there are few economic barriers to adequate diets. Toxicological hazards arise from excessive intakes of some micronutrients. Human teratogenic effects have been associated with excessive vitamin A intakes during pregnancy, and women who are (or who may become) pregnant are advised not to take vitamin A supplements, except on medical advice. There is a dangerous fallacy along the lines that if a little is good, then a lot must be better. This is well illustrated by the problem of vitamin B_6 (pyridoxine). About 1.5 mg day^{-1} is required to maintain good health, and this is provided by a balanced diet. Intakes of 50 mg day^{-1} and above have been associated with neurotoxic effects (peripheral neuropathy). Yet vitamin B_6 supplements consisting of tablets containing up to 100 mg per tablet are on sale in various countries, with no controls other than those provided by general food law.

Fortified foods enable dietary supplements to be provided in the form of additives. This has been shown to be of real value in overcoming iodine deficiency in areas where populations have been dependent on locally produced food and there is little iodine in the soil, as in some inland regions. One approach has been to add iodide to table salt, in order to reduce the incidence of hypothyroidism and cretinism which can result from iodine deficiency. Fortification is of real value today in areas where micronutrient deficiencies are common. Recent examples include the fortification of sugar with vitamin A, iron and zinc in Brazil, the fortification of condensed milk with vitamin A in Thailand and the fortification of noodle seasoning powder with iron, iodine and vitamin A in various countries. In the more affluent conditions of developed countries, the fortification of breakfast cereals with iron and vitamins has been found to be important for marketing reasons.

'Health' supplements consist of a very varied and ill-defined assortment of products. They include substances of animal, plant and mineral origins, with some having known health associations, such as fish liver oils, kelp and various vitamin and mineral preparations. In other cases, knowledge of the toxicology and pharmacology of health products (such as ginseng) is limited. For some, there is no confirmed evidence of benefit and some herbal products, including broom, mistletoe, comfrey and sassafras, are known to contain toxic ingredients. Serious toxicological effects in consumers have been produced by bizarre health supplements, which have been marketed with no regulatory control other than that provided by general food law. Recent examples include the amino acid L-tryptophan and germanium compounds, as discussed elsewhere in this chapter.

Functional foods is an American term meaning a particular category of food products. The term is a poor one, since all foods exert physiological functions. The Japanese term is better: Foods for Specific Health Uses (FOSHUs). As to a formal definition, it is worth stating that functional foods fall into two categories:

- Those from which a deleterious component has been eliminated or replaced with a beneficial one.
- Those to which a beneficial component not normally present is added or, if normally present, is increased in its normal inherent concentration.

Direct medicinal claims are of course avoided. As with health supplements, however, claims are *implied* or intimated by indirect means. While a tablet containing, for example pyridoxine might be presented as a health supplement, a live yoghurt might be marketed as a functional food, the implied claim being that the bacteria present confer health-giving effects. Other examples include margarines claimed to reduce serum cholesterol (and, by implication, atherogenesis) and foods with added cellulose providing all the health benefits of fibre. In most countries, there are no specific controls for functional foods. Japan is an exception.

Food additives include specified colouring agents, sweeteners, flavourings, preservatives, antioxidants, emulsifiers, stabilizers, flour treatment agents, solvents, enzymes, modified starches and bulking agents. These useful substances are generally regulated by means of permitted list systems. Additives have received particular regulatory attention for many years in the USA, where stringent controls have been enforced. Carcinogenic potential has been a particular concern and this led to an important change in US food law in 1960 when the Food, Drug and Cosmetic Act was amended to incorporate a provision which has become known as the Delaney clause. This prevented the regulatory approval of any food additive which had been shown to be carcinogenic in animals. However the amendment made no allowance for any species-specificity shown by the carcinogenic effect, whether or not it was genotoxic, its mechanism, the dosage level required to produce tumours, the type of tumours produced or the tissue sites at which they occurred. Some 200 colouring agents were placed on a provisional list pending assessment of carcinogenicity. The intense sweetener saccharin, which has been used widely and safely since the turn of the century, was affected by the Delaney clause, because sodium saccharin administered in feed is able to produce tumours in the rat. However this only occurs in male animals and only at one site, the bladder. Moreover, the effect only appears when the concentration in the diet exceeds the very high level of 1%, and when this dosage is started immediately after birth and maintained for the lifespan of the animal. Saccharin was banned in the USA, but was later returned to the market when the US Congress agreed to allow a moratorium on the ban. There are ongoing uncertainties in the USA about several additives which are now permitted in other countries. One of these is the red colouring agent erythrosine (FD&C Red 3), which produces thyroid tumours in laboratory rodents. Erythrosine (E127 in the EU) is permitted in the Community, where it is used to enhance the colour of glacé cherries.

Novel foods comprise a broad category for which there is as yet no comprehensive international definition. As generally understood, it includes foods and ingredients which have not been consumed to a significant degree in the country concerned, or have been produced by new or significantly modified processes. A system of pre-marketing authorization is being introduced for novel foods and food ingredients in the EU. Novel foods range from fruits unfamiliar in the country concerned (although widely and safely consumed for long periods elsewhere) to completely new organisms produced by extensive genetic modification.

Products of biotechnology have been the cause of much public anxiety in some countries, although it is worth recalling that plant breeding and other traditional methods of genetic modification have been used with great benefit since time immemorial. Breeding techniques have been used to select and perpetuate desirable characteristics, for example, the changing of breeding seasons in order to increasing the number of crops which can be harvested. New strains have been developed by means of these techniques of artificial selection, increasing the variety of available foodstuffs. Improvements in resistance to plant diseases and to insect pests have been achieved by means of breeding techniques, as has the elimination of inherent toxicants (such as solanine in potatoes, gossypol in cotton seed and cyanide in cassava). Methods, such as mutagenesis, for increasing artificially the variability of species have been used to provide wider ranges upon which artificial selection could operate. However, inability to induce directed genetic changes by such means and difficulties of selection have limited these methods. Recombinant DNA (rDNA) methods now enable specific and precise modifications to be made rapidly to plants and microorganisms for food purposes. A range of approaches is being developed; for example, simple ingredients such as amino acids can be produced by microorganisms, while the genomes of higher plants can be modified to confer advantages for food purposes. One of the best known examples is the slow-softening tomato. Delayed ripening of the tomato allows it to be harvested later, thus providing more time for the development of natural flavour and colour. Crop plants, modified by rDNA techniques, can produce greater yields. It is also possible to achieve increased insect resistance, although it remains to be seen whether such approaches will achieve permanent reductions in pesticide usage, or whether they will be negated by ecological adaptations such as the acquisition of resistance by insect pests themselves. Until more experience and knowledge are gained, the safety evaluation of foods and ingredients produced by means of biotechnology must err on the side of caution and allow for the unexpected. It might be supposed that the ingestion of a common amino acid produced by well characterized, genetically modified bacteria would be unlikely to lead to a serious safety problem, yet the association of eosinophilia–myalgia syndrome with the consumption of L-tryptophan (used in the manufacture of approved medicines and of food supplements) provided a timely lesson, as discussed elsewhere in this chapter.

Borderline products occupy territory between food products and medicines. These preparations provide nutrition in specific diseases or conditions in which the consumer is unable to tolerate or to metabolize certain normal food constituents. Many food products are available for special diets, and several illustrative examples are included here. Gluten-free carbohydrate products are used in coeliac disease, in which enteropathy results from sensitivity to gluten. Soya-based milks are produced for children having intolerance to cow's milk or to lactose. Phenylalanine-free amino acid mixtures are available for use in phenylketonuria, a condition in which an inborn error of metabolism prevents the normal metabolism of phenylalanine. Products are available for use in renal disease, which provide non-protein calories in the form of fat emulsions or glucose solutions, together with amino acids, which both prevent tissue breakdown and obviate the need for ingested protein. Products containing medium-length triglycerides can be helpful in the management of biliary and pancreatic disorders, as these mixtures provide a source of energy and are absorbed in the absence of bile salts.

Food contaminants include chemicals leaching from packaging and other food-contact materials, residues of agrochemicals including pesticides, fertilizers and veterinary drugs and unwanted industrial and other chemicals entering food from environmental media. In many countries, levels of contaminants in foodstuffs are monitored to ensure that they do not exceed statutory levels, as described elsewhere in this chapter.

Some toxic contaminants are ubiquitous and may be very difficult to eliminate completely from the diet. These include several groups of chlorinated, fat-soluble, environmentally persistent compounds, which accumulate in fatty foods such as milk. Examples include dioxins, polychlorinated biphenyls (PCBs) and organochlorine pesticides. Dioxins (more correctly, compounds based on substituted dioxane) are produced by industrial processes, particularly incomplete incineration, and by natural combustion. The most toxic is 2,3,7,8-tetrachlorodibenzo-p-dioxin (TCDD), which has an oral LD_{50} of 0.001 mg kg^{-1} in the guinea pig and is a potent, but atypical, carcinogen. PCBs are non-flammable, non-conducting liquids which were much used as coolants in heavy electrical equipment, as heat exchangers and as hydraulic fluids. The acute toxicity of the PCBs is generally low, although longer term effects are appreciable in various species and include hepatotoxicity and chloracne in man. Most applications of PCBs have been abandoned because of their environmental persistence and chronic toxicity.

Natural toxins include substances which arise as inherent constituents of food-producing plants themselves (such as solanine in potatoes), and also those from external sources, such as mycotoxins produced by moulds. Natural toxins inherently present in novel foods pose particular problems.

Chemical contamination is sometimes responsible for episodes of food poisoning, although the commonest causes are microbiological. The presenting clinical features may provide valuable clues as to whether the aetiological agent is a chemical and, if it appears that it is, to the class of toxic substance concerned. Clinical signs may be pathognomonic in some cases, as when outbreaks of atropinization have resulted from the use of comfrey tea contaminated with *Atropa belladonna* L. Careful questioning of affected subjects and the preparation of detailed diet diaries may be needed before a particular foodstuff can be implicated. In many cases, the nature of a chemical contaminant can be elucidated. However, this is not always possible (Diggle, 1995), as in the case of the Spanish toxic oil tragedy. In the absence of diagnostic pointers in the symptomatology, chemical screening procedures for known contaminants may be particularly useful. The standard methods for heavy metals are available in many laboratories. Assays are available for estimating agents such as saxitonin, which is responsible for the well recognized picture of paralytic shellfish poisoning. Tests for beta-agonists and anabolic steroids can be used when the illegal use of growth promoters in beef cattle is suspected; such studies are not necessarily restricted to individual compounds and group tests may be used, but the analyst must of course decide, if only in broad terms, what to look for.

In order to test hypotheses, special investigations may be carried out on affected subjects. If, for example, organophosphate pesticide residues are suspected, cholinesterase levels can be measured, although this is only likely to be useful if moderately severe poisoning has occurred and when samples are taken and assayed promptly (as problems of *in vivo* and *ex vivo* reactivation are likely to occur). Also, organophosphates such as tri-o-cresyl phosphate lack the anticholinesterase potency to depress the enzyme significantly. Many food toxins produce short-lived effects and testing may produce negative results if it is not carried out promptly; for example, elevated histamine levels following the consumption of scombrotoxic tuna and mackerel often return rapidly to normal. Contamination incidents may be unpredictable and may draw on a surprisingly wide variety of legal powers for their resolution. One such incident occurred in October 1989, when a large quantity of cattle feed became contaminated with lead-bearing ore in the hold of a ship. Although the feed was condemned, it found its way on to the UK market and, before illegal sale could be prevented, caused large-scale lead contamination of milk and beef. Regulatory action included prohibition of the movement of livestock, milk, other dairy products and beef until concentrations of lead had fallen to safe levels in these foodstuffs. The measures required drew upon an extraordinary range of legal provisions.

THE DEVELOPMENT OF REGULATORY SYSTEMS

In this section, selected regulatory developments in the three main trading regions (the EU, the USA and Japan) and the Nordic countries are discussed, and examples are provided to illustrate the distinctive characters which regulatory systems have acquired in these regions. One of the influences which affects the development of a regulatory style is the background of toxicological incidents in the country or region concerned; because of such incidents, certain aspects of regulatory toxicology often acquire particular emphasis.

In the EU, a long-standing aim of community-minded Europeans has been the achievement of mutual recognition for the marketing authorizations of individual Member States. In the following section on the European Union, particular attention is paid to the progress which has been made in the development of Europe-wide systems for the regulation of chemical-based products. The section on the US FDA provides a brief outline of the historical milestones which mark the development of this unique agency. It focuses also on the special balance needed by FDA, with its unique reputation for guarding the safety of consumers and patients, but which must also ensure that unnecessary regulatory burdens are not imposed on industry. In Japan, incidents in which the environment and the human food chain were contaminated by toxic elements (e.g. the heavy metals cadmium and lead) carried in industrial effluents led to serious concerns in the post-war years, and to the creation of particularly thorough legislation in this area. Some unusual toxicological incidents involving chemical-based products (e.g. clioquinol, germanium, tryptophan) have also influenced the development of controls in these areas. Unusual if not unique incidents took place in 1994 at Matsumoto and in 1995 at Tokyo, in which terrorists using the nerve agent sarin attacked civilian populations; seven died in the first incident and eight in the second. More recently, considerations of international trade have influenced the pace of change for the regulation of chemical products in Japan. This applies in particular to the influence of the International Conferences for Harmonization on controls in the pharmaceutical sector. The section on the Nordic countries provides a brief outline of the exceptionally close cooperation which exists in this unique region, and notes the special arrangements which apply in Norway to pharmaceuticals.

The European Union (EU)

In many regulatory contexts, especially where European legislation is involved, it is more appropriate to refer to the European Community (EC) than to the EU. This is because legislation is a matter for the EC, rather than the EU.

The *Treaty on European Union* was signed by the Member States at Maastricht on 7 February 1992. Before it could come into force, however, ratification was required by the individual countries, and this was far from uneventful in some cases. In Germany, there was a legal challenge on the grounds that ratification would alter the country's constitution, but this argument was not upheld by the constitutional court. In France, public opinion was finely balanced and a referendum was held, which narrowly favoured ratification. In Denmark, public opinion was clearly divided and a referendum rejected ratification, after which new concessions were agreed and a second referendum secured approval. In Britain, political opinion was sharply divided but no referendum was held and, after lengthy exchanges of views within the governing party, it was not until 2 August 1993 that ratification was agreed. The Treaty on European Union came into force on 1 November 1993. This established the European Union (EU), and made it clear that the EU is 'founded on the European Communities', which had their origin in 1952.

Background to the EU

In 1952, the European Communities (referred to in the 1992 Treaty of Maastricht, and on which the EU is founded) had their inception with the creation of the European Coal and Steel Community (ECSC). The ECSC was established by the six founding member states (see 'The Six' below) with the overriding aim of putting the major materials required for warfare under a common system of supra-national control, open to any country in Europe, using the economic approach devised by Robert Schuman and Jean Monnet. It was clear to the western allies that the post-war arrangements concerning Germany must be very different from those specified by the Treaty of Versailles of 1919. An important extension of this approach occurred in 1957 with the establishment of the European Atomic Energy Community (EURATOM). The *Treaty of Rome* established the European Economic Community (EEC) in 1957. The UK applied for membership of the Community first in 1961 and, again, in 1967; both applications were vetoed by France on the grounds that the current and future commitment of the UK to the Community could not be assured, because of the existing strong links between the UK and other English-speaking countries. Ten years later the EEC, the ECSC and EURATOM, were merged in 1967 to form the European Community (EC). The progress of the Community towards the goals set by the founding fathers, Schuman and Monnet, has been slow and many difficulties have had to be overcome. The 1970s saw tangible progress in the form of a voluntary agreement on foreign policy, which was subsequently improved and extended. The European monetary system (EMS) was set up in 1979, as a preparation for eventual monetary union. The EMS aims to prevent as far as possible wild currency fluctuations and to create a zone of financial stability. The EMS therefore is an important step on the path towards the long-term goals of economic and monetary union. In 1987, the Single European Act came into force. It confirmed the creation of a European Union as the broad objective and set out a framework for a single market by 1992. Provisions were introduced for closer cooperation on foreign policy, and on policies affecting technology, the environment and research. The 1957 Treaty of Rome contained no specific provisions concerning chemical safety, but it became apparent at an early stage that a good deal of 'harmonization' would be required to ensure that national differences in the regulatory control of chemical products would not restrict the free movement of these goods. The on-going programme of EC legislation which originated from this requirement has resulted in the present large body of European law concerning chemical safety. This is of great importance in regulatory toxicology, as European law takes precedence over domestic statutes in the Member States.

By the end of 1995, the Member States comprising the Union were as shown in the table below, which also gives their accession dates. Dependent territories belonging to member states were generally included in the membership arrangements. The Union includes a large piece of territory in South America, French Guiana, which is a Département of France and has the status of an EU region. Greenland, a Danish possession, entered the Community with Denmark.

The 'Six' (the Founder Members)

1	France	1951
2	Germany (FRG)	1951
3	Italy	1951

The Benelux countries

4	Belgium	1951
5	The Netherlands	1951
6	Luxembourg	1951

Later members

7	United Kingdom	1973
8	Ireland	1973
9	Denmark	1973
10	Greece	1981
11	Spain	1986
12	Portugal	1986
13	Austria	1995
14	Sweden	1995
15	Finland	1995

THE EU AND THE EC

It is important to note that the EC has not been replaced by the EU. The EC is one of three 'pillars' which comprise the EU. The three pillars are:

- The EC. The EC is an international legal entity which can, for example, unlike the EU, legislate, enter into legal obligations and despatch and receive legations.
- The Common Foreign and Security Policy (CFSP). Statements of policy (e.g. at the United Nations) are now made in the name of the EU. However, legal instruments (e.g. treaties, memoranda of understanding) must continue to be signed by member states, alone or alongside the EC.
- Justice and Home Affairs.

As a result of the Treaty on European Union signed at Maastricht on 7 February 1992, the Council of Ministers has become 'the Council of the EU'. The Commission of the European Communities has become the European Commission; whether the Commission is an institution of the Communities or of the EU has not been specified. Heads of government continue to meet as the European Council. Arrangements and understandings concerning future membership exist with many countries. Eventual admission has been promised to Turkey, Cyprus and Malta, subject to certain conditions. Hungary, Poland and the Czech and Slovak Republics have applied for membership, and their applications are under consideration. Cooperation agreements exist with Bulgaria, Romania and various countries of the former Soviet Union. More limited cooperation agreements with Russia and the Ukraine were made in 1994. Norway declined an offer of membership in 1994, following a referendum. Although no arrangements for withdrawal from the Communities were included in the treaties, this does not of course mean that withdrawal is impossible, and it did not prevent the departure of Greenland. Greenland, as a possession of Denmark, had joined in 1973, but conducted a referendum in 1982 which resulted in a majority against continued membership. It was then agreed that Greenland would secede from the EC on 1 January 1995, although it retains the status of an associated overseas territory.

The aims of the EU are pursued through the introduction by the EC of laws and other instruments. These instruments are Regulations, Directives, Recommendations and Opinions. Member states must obey Regulations as they stand, while Directives set out general principles which are incorporated by Member States into new 'domestic' legislation. Recommendations and Opinions are, as their names imply, not binding on Member States. Council Directives must be agreed by the Council of Ministers, while Commission Directives are issued by the officials of the EC, the European Commission. The essential powers for the regulation of chemicals are provided by Council Directives. For example, the framework for the regulation of pharmaceuticals is set out in Council Directive 65/65, while a daughter instrument (Council Directive 75/319) provides for advisory machinery and multi-state applications. Commission Directives do not require Council approval, and deal with more detailed matters such as methods of analysis and technical advances; for example, Commission Directives are used to promulgate revisions of the lists of substances annexed to the Council Directive on cosmetics, 76/768.

Industrial Chemicals

Industrial chemicals are subject to a number of important Council Directives, which ensure a considerable degree of harmonization throughout the EU. The Dangerous Substances Directive 67/548 is fundamental to the system. The sixth amendment to this directive (79/831) sets out a notification scheme which covers all new chemicals (i.e. those not already included in the EU inventory), other than those which are dealt with under separate provisions for product categories such as pharmaceuticals, pesticides, cosmetics and food additives. The purpose of the scheme is to ensure that member states are aware of new chemicals entering the market at a rate greater than 1 tonne per year. The scheme does not provide for the grant of any form of marketing authorization. New chemicals are understood to be those not included in an official inventory of existing substances, the European Inventory of Existing Commercial Chemical Substances (EINECS). EINECS contains the names of some 100 000 substances which were marketed for commercial uses between 1 January 1971 and 18 September 1981 (when the sixth amendment was adopted). Notifications are made to the 'competent' authority of the Member State in which the chemical is first marketed. The notification must be submitted at least 45 days before marketing. Basic toxicity and ecotoxicity data must accompany the notification; requirements include information on acute toxicity, eye and skin irritancy, skin sensitization, 28 day repeated dose toxicity and mutagenicity studies. The competent authority must be informed when the marketing rate reaches 10, 100 and 1000 tonnes per year, when further data requirements are invoked. It may be mentioned in passing that the EU approach differs from that adopted in the USA, where the Environmental Protection Agency (US EPA) regulates industrial chemicals under the provisions of the Toxic Substances Control Act (TOSCA). In the USA, manufacturers must submit to the US EPA a pre-manufacturing notice at least 90 days before commencing production of chemicals whereas, in the EU, manufacture (but not marketing) can take place before notification. Under TOSCA, the US EPA cannot demand a basic set of data on each chemical, although it can specify studies which must be performed on a case-by-case basis before granting marketing authorization.

Returning now to industrial chemicals in the EU, classification and labelling are controlled with by two Directives, one dealing with 'substances' (defined as 'chemical elements and their compounds, as they occur in the natural state or produced by industry') and the other with 'preparations' ('mixtures or solutions composed of two or more substances'). For substances and preparations the labelling requirements, and the classification system upon which they are based, are fully harmonized throughout the EU. The system provides criteria for nine categories of hazard: harmful, toxic, very toxic, irritant, corrosive, flammable, very flammable, oxidizing and explosive. Labelling phrases and symbols are specified for each category. Although the classification of substances and preparations has the same basis, allowance is made for the dilution of hazardous substances in preparations by means of concentration cut-off limits. Preparations covered by other provisions (such as pharmaceuticals) are, of course, excluded from the scheme.

Pesticides

Attempts to achieve harmonized regulatory arrangements for the marketing of pesticides in the Community have encountered some difficulties. Existing pre-marketing authorization systems used in individual Member States differ considerably. Reluctance to surrender domestic powers and resistance to change led to the rejection of a system for the mutual recognition of national pre-marketing authorizations proposed by the Commission in 1976. This outcome contrasts with the early harmonization achieved for other classes of

products such as cosmetics. For cosmetics, national approaches favour lists of permitted and prohibited ingredients, and the present European approach to pesticide control utilizes a system of this kind. It was decided to adopt such a system for agricultural pesticides (or 'plant protection products'), as a compromise, when it became clear that mutual recognition of national pre-marketing authorizations would not be easy to achieve. Council Directive 79/117, the so-called 'prohibition' Directive for pesticides, came into effect in 1981 and provided for negative lists of chemicals which could not be used as ingredients in plant protection products. The prohibited substances include persistent organochlorines, mercury compounds, nitrofen (a herbicide) and the fumigants ethylene oxide, ethylene dichloride and ethylene dibromide. It was not until 1991 that arrangements for positive lists were agreed: Council Directive 91/414, known as the 'authorization' Directive for pesticides, provides for lists of those chemicals which are to be permitted in plant protection products. Member States will continue to grant marketing authorizations on an individual product basis for products containing active ingredients on the accepted list (EC, 1991), but will be required to observe agreed principles when doing so. There will be an expectation that a product which receives authorization in one Member State will also receive it in another, unless there are local differences in safety and efficacy considerations. Fuller details of these developments, and of progress towards harmonized arrangements for non-agricultural pesticides, are given in another chapter.

Pharmaceuticals

In 1965, Directive 65/65/EEC, known as the 'first pharmaceutical Directive', provided definitions and set out an initial framework and basis for the marketing authorization of pharmaceutical products within member states. General requirements, notably the requirement that the safety, efficacy and quality of a product must be established before it could be authorized, were set out in this Directive.

In 1975, Directive 75/318/EEC provided detailed norms and protocols and standards for testing; this is sometimes referred to as the 'norms and protocols' Directive. In the same year, Directive 75/319/EEC (the 'second' Directive) established the Committee on Proprietary Medicinal Products (CPMP) to provide expert advice at Community level. This Directive further defined the general framework provided by 65/65/EEC: the CPMP would be notified of suspensions, revocations and refusals; the Committee would be consulted about products of new technology. CPMP could advise on multi-state applications and could require expert reports, but its opinions would not be binding. Hence this Directive prepared the ground for the forthcoming 'multi-state authorization procedure'.

For veterinary medicines, parallel developments were taking place at the same time. Council Directive 81/851 laid down the regulatory requirements and 81/852 set out toxicological, pharmacological and analytical guidelines. In some Member States systems of pre-marketing authorization were introduced for the first time, in order to meet the requirements of European law, with adequate time being allowed in such cases for the introduction of new measures. This is illustrated by developments in Ireland. Although limited controls on the sale of veterinary drugs in Ireland were available under the Animal Remedies Act 1956, this statute did not empower Ministers to establish a modern system of pre-marketing authorization in Ireland. In 1987, temporary measures were introduced under new powers provided by European law, until the enactment of the Animal Remedies Act 1993. This Act was passed by the Dail in June 1993 and by the Senate in July 1993. It provides a comprehensive range of controls on manufacture, import, distribution, supply and use of veterinary medicines. It also provides controls on foodstuffs of animal origin. The Act makes comprehensive powers available to authorized officers of the Garda Siochana and customs service to enforce its provisions, and provides substantial penalties with a maximum fine of £250 000 and up to 10 years imprisonment for the most serious offences.

Returning now to medicines for human use, Directive 83/570/EEC provided a basis for a multi-state authorization procedure in 1983, which would allow a company already holding an authorization in one Member State to seek authorization in at least five (later reduced to at least two) additional Member States. The multi-state procedure required that the agency in the Member State which first authorized the product would act as a 'rapporteur' in dealing with the other Member States in which marketing authorization was sought. The other Member States would receive copies of the essential documents, in particular the applicant's dossier, a summary of product characteristics, an independent expert report commissioned by the applicant and the CPMP assessment report. The other Member States, acting separately and independently, would assess the application and be able to raise any 'reasoned objections', which would then be passed to the CPMP. The Committee would provide its opinion, which would not, however, be a binding one. Member States, acting separately, would then decide on the application, taking any CPMP opinion into account.

When the multi-state procedure was implemented, it was found, in practice, that a CPMP opinion was needed in more than two thirds of cases. It was found, even after the minimum number of additional Member States in which authorization could be sought had been reduced from five to two, that very few applications escaped objections from those States. There were particular difficulties in obtaining agreement across the Community about the product particulars to be included in data-sheets. There were many complaints about undue delays, poor arrangements for representations, etc. Nevertheless, the multi-state procedure provided valuable lessons. It was clear that better communications between assessment processes conducted in different countries would be needed if differences in *medical culture* (however minor in objective terms) were not to impair progress. Also, it was clear that, if some form of mutual recognition was to be feasible, binding arbitration would be unavoidable.

In 1987, Directive 87/22/EEC was introduced to provide special arrangements for products of biotechnology and those in other innovatory and high-technology categories. These arrangements were known as the 'concertation procedure'. The procedure would be obligatory for biotechnological products (known as list A products) but would be optional for other innovatory and high technology products, which comprise list B. The procedure required that a non-binding CPMP opinion be obtained before any Member State could authorize marketing, even if marketing was only sought in a single Member State. The applicant would apply to a chosen national agency, which would then act as *rapporteur*. A copy of the application would go to the CPMP, and summaries to the other Member States. The *rapporteur* agency would make a detailed assessment of the application and send its assessment report and recommendations to the other Member States. Any concerns of the other Member States would then be passed by the *rapporteur* agency to the applicant. The *rapporteur* agency would then assesses the applicant's responses. The CPMP would issue a Community-wide opinion before the *rapporteur* agency determined the application. Although the CPMP opinion would be non-binding, it was intended that it would routinely take account, at an early stage, of the questions and concerns of Member States, and so facilitate the approach to a common view before there was any hardening of positions. It was intended that, when the *rapporteur* agency determined favourably, authorization would be granted in that Member State, and would be expected to follow without undue difficulty in the others. The performance of the concertation procedure was encouraging; this is due in part to the implementation of lessons learned from experience with the multi-state procedure initiated in 1983.

In October 1993, following a meeting between heads of government, agreement was announced about the development of future systems. There was to be:

- A 'centralised' authorization procedure, which would enable single, Europe-wide authorizations to be sought, for products of biotechnology. For such products, this procedure would be mandatory. Other innovatory products could also be dealt with by this procedure, although this would not be mandatory.
- A 'decentralized' authorization procedure, which would enable marketing authorization in more

than one Member State to be sought, for pharmaceutical products in general, other than those for which the centralized procedure was mandatory. This procedure would incorporate a system of binding arbitration.

- A 4 year transition period to allow for the introduction of the new arrangements
- A European Medicines Evaluation Agency (EMEA), based in London

The UK Licensing Authority and its independent advisory groups, including the Committee on Safety of Medicines **(Figure 1)**, with their reputation for fairness and sound science, have provided important role models for various components of the new European arrangements.

The forerunner of the centralized procedure was the relatively successful concertation procedure introduced in 1987. The concertation procedure worked better than the multi-state procedure initiated in 1983. Although the concertation procedure was concerned with complex, innovatory pharmaceuticals, numerous products were processed successfully through the system. Much attention has therefore been paid to the differences between the concertation and multi-state systems, and the lessons learned have been applied in the development of the new centralized and decentralized systems. The decentralized procedure makes use of binding arbitration by the CPMP when Member States are unable to reach agreement. This binding arbitration is the essential difference between the decentralized procedure and the 1983 multi-state procedure; it is this which has allowed a form of mutual recognition to be created. The decentralized procedure was implemented in January 1995 and was voluntary until January 1998, when it became compulsory. In broad outline, the major steps involved in the procedure are:

- An applicant first obtains marketing authorization in one Member State, which then acts as *rapporteur*.
- The *rapporteur* sends an assessment to other Member States.
- The other Member States may at this stage express concerns having health implications.
- If there are such concerns, the *rapporteur* will discuss them with the Member States concerned.
- If agreement cannot be reached, CPMP will provide an opinion for binding arbitration.
- When the CPMP's opinion is unfavourable to the application, the applicant may appeal to the Committee, which must then provide a second opinion.
- Any Member State is free to raise any new safety issue if it is considered to be of important public health significance. This may then result in further consideration by the CPMP.

Cosmetics

Cosmetics are regulated at Community level by means of a system of positive and negative lists for ingredients. Individual cosmetics themselves are not subject to individual product authorizations in any Member State, and

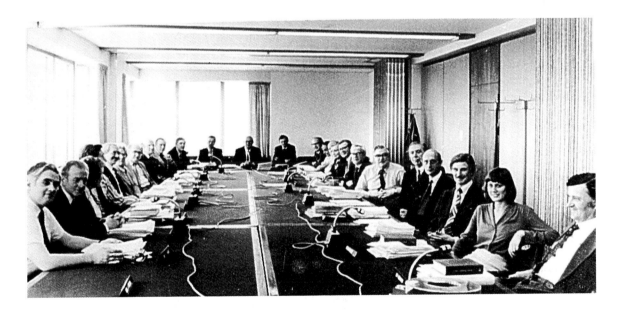

Figure 1 Committee on Safety of Medicines Meeting on 26 June 1980. Members and Secretariat, from left to right: Dr G. Diggle (DHSS), Dr R. Corcoran (DHSS), Dr L. Hill (DHSS), Professor M. Rawlins, Dr F. Fish, Dr M. Richards, Professor A. Read, Professor A. Goldberg, Professor D. G. Grahame-Smith, Dr J. Griffin (DHSS), Dr Gerald Jones (DHSS—Medical Assessor), Professor Sir Eric Scowen (Chairman), Mr P. Allen (DHSS—Secretary), Mr N. Williams (DHSS), Professor W. J. Cranston, Professor F. A. Jenner, Professor B. M. Hibbard, Dr J. M. Holt, Professor J. H. Girdwood, Professor J. W. Dundee, Mr R. Butcher (DHSS), Mr M. Parke (DHSS), Dr J. Calderwood (DHSS), Dr N. Taylor (DHSS) and Dr G. Venning (DHSS). © Crown Copyright.

it was possible to achieve complete harmonization for the regulation of this class at an early stage. The Cosmetics Directive, 76/768/EEC, provides positive lists of preservatives, colouring agents, ultraviolet filters, etc., which are permitted for use in cosmetic products. In some cases permitted substances may only be used as ingredients on a provisional basis, until further toxicological data are provided; in such cases, the additional data must be submitted within a specified timespan. There is also a negative list of prohibited substances which may not be used as ingredients. The lists, which appear as annexes to the Directive, are brought up to date by means of new Commission Directives which adapt the Cosmetics Directive to technical progress. An expert committee, the Scientific Committee on Cosmetology (SCC), provides advice on the chemicals in the lists, although individual products are not considered by the Committee.

Food Chemicals

The foundations of the single market in foodstuffs are now in place. The Community's food law harmonization programme has helped to set higher standards of food safety and improved food labelling. The main framework Directives on labelling, additives, flavourings, contact materials, special dietary foods and food inspection have already been adopted, as have other important Directives, for example on nutrient labelling, lot marking and extraction solvents.

Expert advice is provided by the Scientific Committee for Food (SCF), which consists of experts from the Member States and advises on food safety, including the safety of additives. The role of the SCF is illustrated by the part played by the Committee in the addition of a new additive to a permitted list. When the Committee considers that an additive is acceptable, an acceptable daily intake (ADI) is recommended. If the anticipated exposure is likely to approach the ADI, a list of foods to which it must be restricted is also provided. The recommendations of the SCF are then submitted to a working group of national representatives which decides (by a system of voting) whether the additive will be added to the appropriate positive list. Member States may suspend authorizations temporarily if information becomes available suggesting that the substance may endanger human health, but other Member States must be informed and reasons provided.

A Regulation (258/97) for the control of novel foods and food ingredients was introduced in 1997. Its aim is to provide a single safety assessment for food materials which are novel, including those whose production involves the use of genetically modified organisms (GMOs). The Regulation is concerned with the marketing within the Community of foods and food ingredients which are in the following categories and which have not been used for human consumption to a significant degree in the Community:

(a) Foods and food ingredients containing, or consisting of, GMOs.
(b) Foods and food ingredients produced from, but not containing, GMOs.
(c) Foods and food ingredients having a new or intentionally modified primary molecular structure.
(d) Foods and food ingredients consisting of, or isolated from, microorganisms, fungi or algae.
(e) Foods and food ingredients consisting of (or isolated from) plants, except for those obtained by traditional propagation or breeding practices, and having a safe history of use. Food ingredients isolated from animals, except for those obtained by traditional breeding practices, and having a safe history of use.
(f) Foods and food ingredients to which has been applied a production process which is not in current use, and which gives rise to significant changes in composition or structure, which affect levels of undesirable substances, nutritional value or metabolism.

The Regulation requires that the regulated products must not present any danger to, or mislead, the consumer. These products must not differ from those which they are intended to replace to such an extent that their normal consumption would be nutritionally disadvantageous. The SCF will advise on all questions having public health implications. Detailed procedures for marketing authorization under the Regulation are available. It is envisaged that applications will be made to a single Member State, and will include information necessary to demonstrate that the products are safe and do not mislead the consumer and that consumers would not be disadvantaged by their consumption. If the novel food or food ingredient is a GMO, data to establish environmental safety must be included. Evaluations of applications will be performed within a Member State by a competent assessment body, which will have 3 months prepare its assessment. This is then circulated to other Member States, which have 2 months to submit comments and objections. Cases in which there are objections are referred to the SCF for advice. The authorization decision can establish, among other things, conditions of use and labelling requirements. The Regulation specifies labelling requirements additional to those imposed by other requirements of Community law. If, for example, the novel product is not equivalent to an existing one, then this must be made clear to the consumer. A simplified procedure is provided for foods and food ingredients having only a minor degree of novelty and being substantially equivalent to existing products. The Regulation does not cover additives, flavourings and extraction solvents, as these are dealt with by other Community legislation.

The US Food and Drugs Administration (FDA)

If there is a single organization which is seen, worldwide, as the quintessential regulatory agency, it is the long-established Food and Drugs Administration (FDA) in the USA. Yet the FDA is, in some respects, unique. When, for example, an applicant seeks approval for a new drug, on-going discussions between the agency and the company are a normal part of the process. The discussions deal with, among other things, the way in which guidelines (which are binding on FDA but not on applicants) are to be interpreted in the circumstances. If the company elects to use a test method set out in a guideline, then FDA must accept the study for assessment. However, an alternative approach may be agreed. In addition to meetings with FDA officials on the interpretation of guidelines, an applicant's on-going development programme may be discussed with FDA's advisory committees. Because of the FDA approach, the development of the work programme on a new drug, and the contents of the application, may be influenced substantially. This contrasts with approaches used in other countries. In the EU system, for example, this interactive process between an agency and a company is not seen, and development programmes are not influenced through any such continuous dialogue. Although the guidelines issued by EU Member States are not legally binding, agencies do expect them to be observed, unless departures from them are justified and explained in the application. In Japan, guidelines on the studies needed in the development of new pharmaceuticals are seen rather as lists of minimum requirements; applicants who do not wish to be seen to be lacking or unwilling, can carry out work in excess of that specified. Other important differences between the FDA and corresponding agencies in other countries stem from the US Freedom of Information Act, which has no counterpart elsewhere.

The FDA is, deservedly, renowned for the efficiency with which it pursues the safety of the products which it regulates, and ensures protection of the public. It is supported by effective legislation and has excellent resources to enable it to carry out its protective role. The FDA has a cautious approach and maintains the highest precautionary standards for all the product categories with which it is concerned. This cautious stance is conditioned by extensive experience over most of the present century. The agency points to a long history of unsafe products and fraudulent claims, and considers that such a stance is no more than prudent. The interesting question here is whether conditions in other countries are so different that arrangements of this kind are not necessary. This is a controversial question, but it cannot be denied that many FDA initiatives are, sooner or later, adopted worldwide. The example most relevant in the present context is Good Laboratory Practice (GLP). GLP was introduced by the FDA when it came to light that much falsified toxicological data had been submitted for regulatory purposes.

In addition to its responsibility for public protection, the FDA must also ensure that inappropriate regulatory burdens are not imposed on industry. To achieve a balance which can be accepted as fair and reasonable by all parties may be easier said than done, for example, in relation to the risks associated with trace quantities of carcinogens in foodstuffs. The FDA has responded to considerable public concern about this problem (as the Environment Protection Agency has responded to similar concerns about environmental media), and several unique approaches have emerged as a result. One approach was the introduction of special legislative measures (such as the Delaney clause in the Food, Drugs and Cosmetics Act). Another has been the attempt to develop methods for quantitative carcinogenic risk estimation, for regulatory purposes.

The FDA enjoys an unusual degree of independence from interest groups (representing both consumer and commercial interests), and also relative independence from government departments. This arrangement may be compared with the pattern in many EU Member States where, in the area of food safety, for example, responsibility is borne directly by government departments (and often with major degrees of responsibility resting with agriculture departments). Nevertheless, regulatory principles which have been adopted in numerous countries have followed many of the approaches pioneered by the FDA. The following review outlines some of the agency's developmental milestones and current tasks.

The Food and Drugs Act 1906 was the first US statute to regulate these products, although the powers provided by the Act were very limited. Fraud was particularly prevalent, and there was a great need for measures to protect the public from products containing harmful adulterants and those which did not contain the claimed ingredients, as well as devices such as the 'orgone box' of Wilhelm Reich which was claimed to be an effective treatment for cancer. No pre-marketing approval was required under the 1906 Act, and the onus of proof rested firmly on the government departments. Moreover, there were no requirements for safety testing by manufacturers. There was little to protect the public from products such as Radiothor Certified Radioactive Water: this 'tonic', which contained a significant amount of radium, was the cause of an unknown number of fatal cancers (Macklis, 1990). The enactment of the 1906 statute was the direct result of intense pressure of the US Department of Agriculture (USDA) which had submitted more than 100 Bills to Congress proposing regulatory controls. The efforts of the USDA were further rewarded in 1927 by the creation of the Food, Drug and Insecticide Administration, the precursor of the present FDA. The long-standing concerns of the USDA, arising from the large numbers of dangerous and quack products on the market, were seen to be fully justified in 1937, when more than 100 people died as a result of taking a medicine labelled 'Elixir of Sulfanilamide'. The account of the investigation, and of the behaviour of those involved, is compelling reading (Secretary of Agriculture, 1937). It emerged that diethylene glycol (now used as an antifreeze) had been used as the solvent in the formulation, sulphanilamide being insoluble in aqueous solvents. The product had not undergone safety testing, but had merely been examined for colour, flavour and smell. The only legal basis for action available to the FDA under the 1906 Act was that the product did not contain a claimed ingredient (traditionally, 'elixirs' are expected to contain ethanol, but diethylene glycol was used instead in this case). In a press statement, the manufacturer, the S. E. Massengill Company of Tennessee, denied responsibility (Secretary of Agriculture, 1937), claiming that the deaths must have been caused by sulphanilamide, and could not have been foreseen. The statement by Dr Massengill included the following:

'My chemists and I deeply regret the fatal results, but there was no error in the manufacture of the product. We have been supplying legitimate professional demand and not once could have foreseen the unlooked for results. I do not feel that there was any responsibility on our part. The chemical sulphanilamide had been approved for use and had been used in large quantities in other forms, and now its many bad effects are developing'.

A most important result of this tragedy was the enactment of the Food, Drug and Cosmetic Act 1938. This law contained major new provisions, including the requirement for safety testing, although there was still no requirement for the submission of the test data to the FDA before marketing could be authorized. Other improvements included requirements for manufacturer registration and factory inspection. There were also new provisions to permit the seizure of products which did not meet the new requirements, by means of court injunctions. The 1938 Act was amended in 1951, to include controls for prescription drugs (the Durham–Humphrey amendment).

It was not until 1962 that the Act was further modified (the Kefauver–Harris amendment) to include requirements for the submission of data on safety and efficacy, before marketing authorization could be granted. This major advance was an immediate result of the thalidomide tragedy, in which thousands of neonates throughout Western Europe were found to be affected by the normally rare limb-reduction deformity phocomelia ('seal-limb'), as a result of the use of this tranquillizer in the early weeks of pregnancy. It is to the great credit of the FDA's medical staff that the incidence of thalidomide-induced phocomelia in the USA was relatively very small. Marketing authorization had never been granted,

and women of child-bearing potential were excluded from the clinical trials which had been permitted in the USA. The only cases of phocomelia which did occur involved patients whose doctors had not supervised this criterion adequately. The FDA commenced a large-scale review of 'over-the-counter' pharmaceuticals in 1966. In 1976 the Medical Device amendments were introduced; this improvement was made as a result of continuing concerns about the availability of fraudulent and unsafe products of this kind. The present procedure for the marketing authorization of pharmaceuticals in the US implements the Kefauver–Harris amendment. A new drug application (NDA) is approved only when the FDA is satisfied that the criteria of safety, effectiveness and quality have been met adequately. Neither relative effectiveness (in comparison with other drugs) nor price can be taken into account by the review team, which generally consists of doctor, pharmacologist, toxicologist, chemist, statistician and pharmacist. Although independent views may be obtained from expert advisory committees, their advice is not binding on the FDA. If the FDA is satisfied with the application, an 'approval letter' is issued and the product may then be marketed. Alternatively, the FDA may issue an 'approvable' letter indicating that marketing authorization would be granted if specified additional data were submitted or conditions met. However, if the FDA does not consider that the NDA can be granted, a 'not approvable' letter is issued. Information submitted to the FDA is confidential, with the exception of data which can be released under the Freedom of Information Act; FDA staff prepare and publish a 'summary basis for approval' for each new chemical entity. FDA procedures for regulating pharmaceuticals differ in some respects from those used by other countries. For example, the FDA has long required that original patient documentation, duly signed by the investigating physicians, be submitted in support of NDAs. This is now becoming a requirement in other countries, with the development of Good Clinical Practice.

The history of the FDA's role in ensuring the safety of the American food supply has been similar in many ways to that relating to medicines. This is illustrated by the FDA's activities in the area of food additives. The legal basis is the 1958 Food Additive Amendment of the 1938 Act. Statutory responsibility is vested in regulatory agencies within some individual states, in addition to the FDA itself (most States have adopted the provisions of the 1958 amendment into their own legislation). New food additives are subject to a system of pre-marketing approval, under which the substance must be shown to be 'safe'. In this context 'safe' means not injurious to the health of humans or animals and, in particular, not carcinogenic. Approximately 3000 substances have been approved for use in food under this procedure. Some substances added to food do not fall within the legal definition of 'food additives'. These exceptions include substances which are 'generally recognized as safe' (GRAS), substances which were in use before 6 September 1958, and pesticides on or in raw foods.

The 'Delaney clause', added to the Food Drugs and Cosmetics Act in 1958, prohibits the addition to food products of any chemical shown to be carcinogenic in animals or man. The clause makes no reference to the carcinogenic mechanism involved, to the dosage level required to produce tumours, to the type or tissue site of tumours produced in animals, to the species specificity of the phenomenon or to whether the substance is genotoxic. In the years since the introduction of the Delaney clause, laboratory methods for detecting contaminants have become much more sensitive. Today, limits of detection of one part per billion or lower are not unusual. Also, there are many pesticides, food additives and other man-made substances which appear in foodstuffs that do produce tumours in animals at high doses. Since the Delaney clause was introduced, therefore, it has been appreciated that various widely used chemicals do, under a literalist interpretation of the clause, require prohibition. Once it has been shown, by modern chemical methods, that these substances are present in foodstuffs or the wider environment, it only requires the assumption of low-dose linearity in mathematical modelling (discussed elsewhere in this chapter) to establish the existence of apparently finite risks to consumers. Nevertheless, for many of these substances, prohibition has not taken place. However, although the pragmatic position adopted by agencies is underpinned by sound scientific arguments (reviewed elsewhere in this chapter), this does not change the law. Revision of statutory provisions is not a matter for regulatory agencies; if scientific advance indicates a need for changes in the law, then it is for the legislature to make those changes. Yet no-one has been eager to seize the initiative, because of the political courage required to depart from what appears to be the uncompromising wholesomeness and apparent commonsense of the Delaney clause.

Chemical contaminants in food, as distinct from additives, demand a good deal of FDA attention. The major health concerns associated with contaminants in fresh fruits and vegetables arise from pesticide residues. The FDA is responsible for ensuring compliance with maximum residue limits (MRLs), which are discussed elsewhere in this chapter, under the 1938 Act (Pesticide Chemical Amendment 1954). It is the EPA, however, and not the FDA, which sets pesticide MRLs under the provisions of the Insecticide, Fungicide and Rodenticide Act. The FDA carries out random testing of many thousands of shipments of raw food commodities, including fruit and vegetables, each year. When illegal pesticide residue levels are detected, the FDA is able to seize the commodity, impose an injunction and prosecute the seller. Commodities can also be turned away at ports of entry. There are two special circumstances in which pesticides are regarded, for the FDA's purposes, as food

additives: first, when the concentration of the residue becomes greater in the final food product itself, as during the formation of raisins; and second, when the pesticide is applied to the final food product (rather than the crop) after harvesting. For veterinary drug residues, on the other hand, tolerance levels in meat and poultry are set by the FDA and not by the US EPA. However, monitoring and testing for chemical and microbiological contamination are carried out in accordance with the animal drug residues programme of the Food Safety Inspection Service (US Department of Agriculture), under powers provided by the Meat Inspection Act and the Poultry Products Inspection Act. Nevertheless, when veterinary drug residues in excess of tolerance levels are detected, it is the FDA which takes enforcement action.

Good Laboratory Practice

Good Laboratory Practice (GLP) was devised by the FDA and was proposed formally in 1976, when Congressional hearings and investigations by officials established that fraudulent data relating to a number of toxicological studies on pharmaceuticals had been submitted to the FDA. Since then, this approach for ensuring the integrity of toxicological data produced for regulatory purposes has been introduced throughout the world.

The specific instances which, when publicly exposed in the USA, caused such concern resulted in criminal charges of fraud against a number of contract laboratory officials. Some of these were convicted and received prison sentences. Several laboratories were compelled to abandon their pre-clinical work programmes, including one of the largest establishments of this kind in the world. Large numbers of studies which had been submitted in support of the safety of drugs, food additives, pesticides, etc., had to be reviewed again by the FDA (or by the US EPA, as appropriate) and many were found to be invalid. It was because the problem was considered to be so widespread and serious that the introduction of far-reaching general measures was considered to be needed. The GLP approach was devised to meet this need. Although the dramatic public disclosures which took place in the USA were not duplicated in other countries, it was clear that the problem was not a uniquely American one. One commentary on quality assurance in toxicology which was published in the UK at that time was ominously entitled *The Seven Deadly Sins* (Griffin, 1977). Although, in the first instance, GLP was applied only to pharmaceuticals in the USA, it was later extended to the *other products* about which toxicological data are generated for regulatory purposes.

GLP consists essentially of a set of principles, first embodied in regulations brought into force by the FDA in 1979. Many of these principles merely reflect the requirements which must be met by *any* scientific study if it is to be of unquestionable quality, and to be reported with such integrity that similar results would be expected if the work were repeated in another laboratory. The requirements of GLP, which are largely based on scientific common sense, were first enforced in the USA by the FDA and, later, by means of a separate inspectorate, by the US EPA. Since then, programmes for GLP monitoring, in which compliance with appropriate criteria is ensured by well informed inspectorates, have been introduced by many countries.

GLP criteria cover record-keeping and reporting, identification and control of test substances, equipment and facilities, written operating procedures and protocols. In addition to such criteria, which any well organized university laboratory, for example, would be expected to meet, further security is ensured by several requirements which go beyond the basics of scientific methodology. These include the need for an independent quality assurance unit which enjoys the unequivocal backing of senior management. Another criterion is that there should be a fully empowered, named Study Director for every study.

As in so many areas, the lead established by FDA was followed in many other countries. The European Community signalled its official recognition of the advent of GLP in 1979, when Council Directive 79/831 (widely known as 'the sixth amendment') required that toxicology data on industrial chemicals should 'comply with the principles of good current laboratory practice' (although no definition of this new term was offered). The OECD (discussed elsewhere in this Chapter) did much to coordinate the international harmonization of GLP, as it did to encourage the standardization of toxicological test methods. It was the OECD, in particular, which fostered the concept of mutual acceptance of data (MAD). In 1981, the OECD council recommended to member countries that '... the data generated in the testing of chemicals in an OECD member country, in accordance with OECD Test Guidelines and OECD principles of Good Laboratory Practice, shall be accepted in other member countries for purposes of assessment and other uses relating to the protection of Man and the environment...' (OECD, 1981). In 1987–88, changes in European law required that all Member States establish their own GLP monitoring authorities (87/18/EEC) and programmes of compliance (88/320/EEC) covering all categories of chemical products. After years of patient international negotiation, the OECD achieved agreement on MAD between those participating countries which possessed GLP monitoring authorities and programmes of compliance, in 1989. In 1990, the EC endorsed the OECD position and incorporated it into Directive 90/18/EEC. Compliance with GLP, then, ensures the integrity, reproducibility and proper documentation of data generated to establish the toxicological properties of chemicals used in all chemical products for which regulatory approval is required. Today, GLP monitoring authorities and programmes of compliance ensure, throughout the developed world,

that toxicological studies performed for regulatory purposes, whether conducted 'in-house' or elsewhere under contract, comply in full with GLP requirements.

Background to Regulatory Developments in Japan

Industrial Chemicals

In Japan, particular attention has for many years been paid to the environmental effects of industrial chemicals, which must satisfy the requirements of two separate statutes, one of which emphasizes testing for bioaccumulation and biodegradability. This legislative approach can be understood historically in the light of several serious episodes in which heavy metal contamination of the environment resulted from industrial effluents, leading in turn to serious effects in human populations.

Cadmium toxicity appeared shortly after the end of World War II, in the form of a mysterious illness which became known as the *itai-itai* (or 'pain-pain') disease, which was seen in the region of Fuchu and the Jintsu river. Itai-itai disease primarily affected middle-aged to elderly multiparous women. The condition was characterized by signs of nephrotoxicity (proteinuria and glycosuria), osteomalacia and associated fractures and joint pains. The cause was eventually traced to the contamination of dietary rice by cadmium. Cadmium-containing effluents from smelter waste had entered rice paddy fields and thus passed into the diet. The source of the smelter waste was found to be a mine producing cadmium, lead and zinc, upstream of the paddies. This incident triggered valuable research into the effects of long-term, low-level cadmium ingestion. This work showed, among other things, that proximal tubular damage results from such exposure and that signs of nephrotoxicity appear when a critical no-effect level of a protein–cadmium complex is exceeded (hepatic synthesis of the binding protein metallothionein is induced by cadmium, zinc and mercury).

Mercury toxicity is associated in the minds of toxicologists with Minamata, a small coastal village on the west coast of Kyushu, where a serious episode of mercury poisoning appeared in 1953 and continued for some 10 years. This became the best known example of mercury release into the environment from industrial sources. The source of contamination was traced to industrial effluents from plant at which mercury was used as a catalyst. These effluents produced high levels of methylmercury in the coastal waters; bioconcentration of mercury, up to 1 mg kg^{-1}, then occurred in fish and molluscs. These were consumed in considerable quantities, sometimes every day, by the local fishermen and their families, resulting in deaths and serious disablement. The clinical features were those of mercury neurotoxicity. The widely known episode at Minamata was followed soon afterwards by another in the vicinity of Niigata, a coastal town on the west coast of Honshu. Altogether these two episodes led to a total of 1200 case reports. They stimulated much research into the toxicokinetics of methylmercury. Today in Japan, as in other highly developed countries, industrial wastewater is subjected to specific treatment processes before discharge into the environment. Treatments are designed according to the particular toxic wastes present, which may include carcinogens, radioactive substances and heavy metals.

Following these episodes, there developed a regulatory approach based on two separate statutes. First, there is the Chemical Substances Control Law 1986, sometimes called Law 44. This is implemented jointly by the Ministry of International Trade and Industry (MITI) and the Ministry of Health and Welfare (MHW). The second is the Industry Safety and Health Law 1972, which is administered by the Ministry of Labour (MOL). Separate compliance with both laws is required before a new industrial chemical can be marketed. The emphasis of Law 44 is on the prevention of adverse human effects occurring indirectly, via the environment. Under Law 44, new compounds must be tested for biodegradation. No further testing is required for substances which are found to biodegrade readily to produce safe degradation products. Compounds which do not, however, must be tested for bioaccumulation potential and must undergo basic toxicological testing. A preliminary estimate of potential for bioaccumulation is provided by the octanol–water partition coefficient, which depends on the hydrophilic–lipophilic balance of the chemical. As in the USA (but not the EU), pre-manufacturing notification is required in Japan for industrial chemicals. The requirements of the Industrial Safety and Health Law also include pre-marketing notification and basic toxicological testing. More recently there have been particular concerns in Japan about possible effects on male fertility, not only by heavy metals, but also environmental contaminants which contain a phenolic ring which is able to some extent to mimic the A ring of the steroid nucleus and which possess some weak oestrogenic actions. The sources of such compounds include pesticide residues (e.g. DDT), domestic sewage (e.g. contraceptive steroids) and industrial effluents (e.g. PCBs, bisphenol-A and other plasticizers). There is recent evidence that such compounds, which may possess both hormonal and anti-hormonal actions, are able to affect reproductive physiology in fish (Lye et al., 1997) and other aquatic animals (Vonier et al., 1996). Although these 'environmental oestrogens' possess only low hormonal (or anti-hormonal) potency, there is cause for concern because there are large numbers of them, many of them are able to accumulate in fatty tissues and many are persistent in the environment.

Pharmaceuticals

In Japan, as in other highly developed countries, the evolution of controls for pharmaceuticals is influenced by adverse effects that occur unexpectedly from time to time. A recent example involved a new anti-viral agent, sorivudine, a synthetic derivative of thymidine, which is active against Herpes varicella-zoster. The drug was withdrawn from the Japanese market following the deaths of patients as a result of an unpredicted interaction between sorivudine and 5-fluorouracil in patients receiving both drugs concomitantly (Yawata, 1993). Particular emphasis is being placed on interaction studies following this incident.

When serious adverse reactions affecting many people emerge, they can be expected to occur in all the countries in which the drug is marketed; it is not to be expected that this would occur in only one such country. Nevertheless, this is what appears to have happened in the case of the drug clioquinol. Before reviewing the present arrangements for the control of pharmaceuticals in Japan, an outline of the tragic episode of neurotoxicity associated with the use of this drug in Japan will be given. Clioquinol, an iodine-containing 8-hydroxyquinoline, was synthesized in Germany at the beginning of the present century. Clioquinol preparations were restricted to topical uses at first, but oral preparations were for many years used to treat travellers' diarrhoea and other abdominal complaints, despite the high frequency of abdominal symptoms caused by the drug. It was eventually recognized that these preparations also produced serious neurotoxic effects, especially at doses exceeding 2 g per day. The neuropathology consists of a central distal axonopathy, together with degenerative changes affecting the visual pathways (Rose and Gawel, 1984). Affected subjects complained of bladder disturbances and bilateral ascending paraesthesia and weakness of the legs, with increased reflexes. Visual impairment was frequent. This was usually bilateral, and was mild in some cases, while total blindness due to atrophy of the optic nerve occurred in others.

Historically, Vioform and Entero-Vioform were the best known proprietaries containing clioquinol. Vioform was marketed widely by a Swiss company as a topical antibacterial. Around 1930, Entero-Vioform was first marketed for internal use to treat diarrhoea and amoebic dysentery. When the patents expired, many other brands appeared. Commercially, clioquinol products were so successful that the annual production of the compound at one stage far exceeded 1000 tons (Gholz and Arons, 1964). There were sporadic reports of adverse neurological effects in the medical and veterinary literature during the 1960s (Gholz and Arons, 1964; Schantz and Wikstrom, 1965; Hangartner, 1980). In 1966, Berggren and Hanssen, discussing the treatment of childhood zinc deficiency syndrome (acrodermatitis enteropathica), reported a case in which clioquinol, used in an attempt to relieve the chronic diarrhoea associated with this condition, appeared to have induced optic atrophy.

In Japan, an unfamiliar neurological syndrome began to occur with increasing frequency from the mid-1950s.

From 1957, there were several epidemics of this myelitis-like condition. It was soon realized that optic nerve damage was a frequent component of the syndrome, which was appropriately termed subacute myelo-optico-neuropathy (SMON) at a meeting of Japanese physicians in 1964 (Kono, 1975). It was found that a very steep rise in the Japanese sales of clioquinol products throughout the 1960s was closely matched by the soaring incidence of SMON. It is clear that there was a period of immense enthusiasm for clioquinol in Japan, although it is difficult to pinpoint a reason for this, especially as the drug was long known to cause abdominal symptoms—for which the drug was promoted. The Japanese Ministry of Health and Welfare (MHW) acted promptly to prohibit further marketing of clioquinol-containing medicines (in September 1970) and the appearance of new cases soon ceased. The initial recognition of the causal link between clioquinol and SMON (Tsubaki *et al.*, 1971) was underpinned by numerous surveys, and it was established that the severity of the response was dose-related. The neurotoxicity of clioquinol was subsequently confirmed in animal studies (Tateshi, 1980). A detailed review has been provided by Mann (1986). At least 10 000 cases of SMON occurred in Japan, where 20 companies had been involved in the manufacture and sale of clioquinol-containing preparations (KICADIS, 1979). The evolution of the Pharmaceutical Affairs Law in Japan was greatly influenced by the SMON tragedy. Only sporadic cases were reported in other countries.

Another iodinated 8-hydroxyquinoline, iodoquinol, has also been associated with optic nerve atrophy and blindness, although it is considered to be safer than clioquinol. Iodoquinol is available in the USA as the proprietary medicines Yodoxin and Moebiquin.

The present system for the regulatory control of pharmaceuticals in Japan possesses major features in common with systems in the EU and US. Japanese controls are based on pre-marketing authorization under the Pharmaceutical Affairs Law (PAL). The Pharmaceutical Affairs Bureau (PAB) of the Ministry of Health and Welfare (MHW) acts as the regulatory agency for medicines. A marketing authorization, usually translated as 'approval', is issued in the name of the Minister. A normal application by a Japanese pharmaceutical company for the approval of a new drug is submitted to the government of the prefecture in which the applicant's head office or relevant manufacturing plant is located (Japan is a geographically elongated country, being some 2000 km in length, and many administrative functions, which in other countries are concentrated in the capital, are carried out at prefectural level). The application is passed by the prefectural government to the PAB, where an examiner carries out a preliminary review. The review establishes whether all required data have been included, whether the data meet the relevant requirements and whether a suitable outline (*gaiyo*) has been provided. The review therefore ascertains the completeness of the

application and identifies any deficiencies in it. The applicant then has an opportunity to attend a meeting with the examiner, who provides a list of the deficiencies identified to enable the applicant to make the necessary improvements. Further meetings of this kind may take place until the application is suitable for consideration by the Central Pharmaceutical Affairs Council (CPAC). Committees and specialized sub-committees (*chsakai*) comprise the CPAC, and the application is first considered by one or more of the latter, with the help of the PAB examiner. Direct contact between the applicants and sub-committees does not normally occur. The sub-committee may recommend approval or it may issue a further list of deficiencies which is then passed back to the applicant, who has the opportunity to make the necessary improvements. This process, like the preliminary review, is an iterative one. This feature of the Japanese system gives an applicant continuing opportunities to improve the application, although each cycle is time consuming as the sub-committees are extremely busy. When the application is considered by the sub-committee to be suitable for approval, it is passed to two senior committees, the Special Committee and the Executive Committee. It is usual for these senior committees to endorse sub-committees' recommendations for approval. It then only remains for MHW to respond to the advice of CPAC by transmitting a notice of approval to the prefectural government, which then informs the applicant.

In Japan applications concerning new active substances are, as elsewhere, the most demanding. It has been possible for many years to apply for approval to import a foreign pharmaceutical, i.e. a medicine manufactured in another country. In 1983, the PAL was amended so that facilities could be provided to allow foreign companies to apply for approval to manufacture in Japan. A foreign manufacturing approval requires the appointment of an 'in-country caretaker' for the product concerned, that is, a responsible person qualified in an appropriate sphere, such as pharmaceutical medicine or pharmacy. This person is responsible for ensuring that all requirements of the PAL are satisfied for the product concerned throughout its development and subsequent marketing.

In summary, three types of approvals are available in the Japanese system:-

- Manufacturing Approvals, for normal Japanese pharmaceutical products.
- Importation Approvals, for products manufactured in foreign countries and imported into Japan.
- Foreign Manufacturing Approvals, for products manufactured in Japan by foreign companies, which must appoint in-country caretakers.

In broad terms, data requirements are similar to those of other developed countries, but they are not identical. During the independent evolution of the Japanese requirements for toxicological testing following the thalidomide tragedy, there was some divergence between developments in Japan and in other countries. In the case of genotoxicity studies, the Japanese battery does not include the test for gene mutation in eukaryotic cells which is required in the EU. Also, although testing for gene mutation in bacteria is specified in Japan, it must be carried out in both *Salmonella typhimurium* and *Escherichia coli*, whereas only one species is required in the EU. Furthermore, whereas the *in vivo* test included in the EU requirements is not specified in detail (the requirement being worded merely as 'an *in vivo* test for genetic damage'), the Japanese guidelines ask specifically for a micronucleus test in the mouse. The scientific justification for the Japanese battery is considered to be superior by some Western experts (Scales and Mahoney, 1991).

It is in the area of reproductive toxicological testing where divergence between the requirements of Japan and of other countries has become best known. One of the differences relates to the period of dosing in the Segment I study, widely known as the fertility study. The Japanese guidelines specify that dosing is to cover the period of gametogenesis (excluding the first part of meiosis I in females) and to cease around implantation. In the EU, however, dosing is continued throughout pregnancy and lactation, reflecting the complete European title of this study: the fertility and general reproductive performance test. A major divergence developed between Japanese and non-Japanese requirements for Segment II, often termed the teratology study. The EU guidelines specify that all foetuses are to be necropsied at the end of pregnancy. However, half the foetuses are allowed to reproduce and rear offspring in Japan, where Segment II is seen as a test for a wide range of possible embryotoxic effects, including those which manifest late.

As these examples show, there are no substantial scientific reasons why common positions cannot be achieved in the course of the ICH process. As differences in preclinical requirements are resolved, agreed amendments will be incorporated into official guidelines in the three regions, in accordance with the stepwise procedure adopted to achieve harmonized guidelines. Studies in humans, however, both volunteers and patients, present special problems. There may be differences in clinical response to drugs by Japanese, as compared with Western subjects, because of inter-ethnic genetic differences and differences in environmental influences, such as diet. The Japanese guidelines therefore require that certain work be carried out in Japanese subjects. There has been little systematic scientific study in the areas of comparative kinetics, pharmacogenetics, etc. However, several studies have been published in which data, provided by companies on drugs which have been studied in accordance with both Western and Japanese guidelines, have been compared (Walker *et al.*, 1994). Few differences have been observed and those which were seen may have been attributable to cultural factors, including aspects of medical practice. As yet, therefore, no firm conclusions can be drawn and it is clear that systematic research will be needed, if a definitive answer to the question of inter-ethnic clinical responsiveness is to be obtained.

Food Products

A number of unusual food products have emerged in Japan, including various health and dietary supplements, and a new category which became known in the USA as '*functional foods*'. A market for these products was created in Japan in the late 1980s, and the Japanese government established the Committee on Foshu to provide expert advice. '*Foshu*' reveals an interesting use of the acronym (Shah, 1988) when foshu is interpreted to mean *Foods for Specified Health Uses*. This title better reflects the claims made for these products than the American term. Functional foods are discussed in more detail elsewhere in this chapter.

An unusual health supplement, tablets containing germanium compounds, was marketed in Japan and then more widely in other countries in the 1980s. These products, in common with many health supplements, had the appearance of medicines: they were in tablet form, they were supplied in bottles of the kind used for medicinal tablets and they bore directions about dosage régimes. However they were not authorized for marketing as medicines, and were classified variously as health or food supplements and (in the UK) as novel foods. Germanium supplements were developed for the health market when the use of the element in the solid-state electronics industry declined steeply after silicon-based devices had been found to be superior for many types of transistors and, later, for integrated circuits. In November 1980, a book was published advocating germanium sesquioxide as a 'miracle cure' (Asai, 1980). At a conference on germanium compounds in 1984 (Lekim and Samochowiec 1985), various toxicological effects, including teratogenicity (Dluzniewski, 1985), were described. There had also been a clinical report in 1985 about a long-term user of germanium who died of acute renal failure (Nagata *et al.*, 1985). Nevertheless, tablets containing germanium compounds, including the sesquioxide and the dioxide, were marketed worldwide. No overt medicinal claims were attached directly to these products, ensuring their immunity from pharmaceutical controls. Popular literature was circulated about what was termed the new miracle cure, and a book was published in the UK on the new 'health and life enhancer' (Goodman, 1988). Although relatively costly, germanium tablets with their medicine-like appearance were particularly sought for self-medication by sufferers from serious conditions such as AIDS and cancer. The germanium episode appeared in its most serious form in Japan, where a wave of enthusiasm was stimulated by imaginative claims in popular publications. Further case reports of renal damage in patients began to appear in the literature (Matsusaka *et al.*, 1988; Obara *et al.*, 1988; Sanai *et al.*, 1990a). Animal studies confirmed and progressively elucidated the nephrotoxicity of germanium compounds (Cremer and Aldridge, 1964; Schroeder and Balassa, 1967; Sanai *et al.*, 1990b). From the regulatory standpoint there were difficulties in dealing with germanium tablets. While it was clear that purchasers' enthusiasm arose from belief in the amazing medicinal powers of germanium, manufacturers took care to ensure that the product literature itself contained no such claims. Instead, promotion was indirect: optimistic articles in popular health magazines, leaflets distributed in health food shops, etc. The germanium episode highlighted the need for more effective controls for supplements in many countries, and not only in Japan.

This need was re-emphasized with the appearance in 1989 of the serious and previously unknown condition eosinophilia–myalgia syndrome (EMS), which was associated with the ingestion of the amino acid L-tryptophan allegedly produced by a Japanese source using recombinant DNA technology. EMS shares major features with the Spanish toxic oil syndrome of 1981 (Diggle, 1995), which is discussed elsewhere in this chapter, including intense eosinophilia, severe myalgia and multi-system involvement with long-term complications. The mortality and morbidity figures have fortunately been much smaller than those for the toxic oil syndrome. As a normal constituent of food proteins, tryptophan could not be expected to produce toxicological effects, even when large amounts were ingested. The EMS-associated tryptophan had been included as an ingredient in a variety of food and medicinal products and, through a variety of routes, reached those who developed the syndrome throughout the world. EMS first appeared in the USA in November 1989 and most cases occurred there. Affected products included dietary supplements used by body-builders who believed that an amino acid supplement would help their efforts, and pharmaceuticals authorized for use as sedatives. No satisfactory animal model has been developed for EMS; a particular strain of rat can be used to distinguish between EMS-associated and control L-tryptophan, but only when high doses are employed, and it does not constitute a model for the condition.

The Nordic Council

The Nordic Council is a vehicle for cooperation between the governments of the Nordic countries. It was created in 1952 by Denmark, Iceland, Norway and Sweden. Finland joined in 1955 and Greenland has been represented since 1984. Recommendations are made to the Nordic Council of Ministers (founded in 1971), which ensures that appropriate action is taken by the national governments (each government appoints a minister for Nordic cooperation). Some 60 joint institutions and committees deal with specific subjects, including food safety and the testing of drugs.

Denmark, Sweden and Finland are members of the EU and the other Nordic countries have entered into various agreements with the Community. These links are helping to maintain common approaches to shared areas of concern, such as food safety. There is extensive trade in food between the EU and the Nordic countries, and the EU's work in the field of food safety regulation has been allowed to exert an influence on the inter-Nordic programme of food safety cooperation (Nordisk Ministerrad, 1988). The Nordic Working Group on Food Toxicology (NMT) is responsible for coordinating methods for assessing the health problems arising from contaminants, including residues of pesticides, veterinary and radioactive materials.

Despite the considerable degree of cooperation which exists between Nordic regulatory agencies, their approaches are by no means identical in every respect, and some of the existing systems possess a great deal of individuality. Norway, which has not joined the EU, is noteworthy for its approach to the regulation of medicines. In Norway, the authorization system for pharmaceuticals pre-dates the major tragedies ('*Elixir of Sulfanilamide, thalidomide* etc.) which triggered such profound legislative changes elsewhere. Moreover, the criteria laid down by the Norwegian statute enacted in 1928 were unprecedented. These were safety, efficacy, quality, medical need and cost. In 1958, the wholesale supply of medicines in Norway was nationalized, with the establishment of Norsk Medisinaldepot, the state-owned supplier. The legislation was revised and consolidated by means of the Poison and Drug Act 1964 and a reorganization of the regulatory agency, the Norwegian Medicines Control Authority, was undertaken in 1974. Although the cost of a product is a criterion for final marketing authorization, it is only considered after the other criteria have been assessed and found to be satisfactory. The Authority is assisted in its work by a number of expert advisory committees, including the Specialities Committee, which approves new products. The members are specialists in medicine and pharmacy and are appointed by the Minister of Social Affairs; the committee is chaired by the Director General of Public Health. The Norwegian legislation is unusual in that it contains a 'need' clause. This states that marketing authorization will '... only be granted for preparations which are medically justified and which are considered to be needed ...'. The need clause allows the relative effectiveness of different products to be taken into account when they are assessed for marketing authorization. This is generally not possible under the legislation of other countries. Another practical effect of the need clause is to limit the number of products on the market containing any particular active ingredient, the number of products in each case depending on the size of the patient population requiring the drug. The marketing of 'me-too' and combination products is particularly limited. The stated intentions of this approach are to reduce costs, to promote rational therapy and to reduce confusion among prescribers, patients and distributors. Physicians can obtain special licences which enable them to prescribe unauthorized products for particular uses in named patients.

Unlike Norway, no Member State of the EU has gone so far as to introduce a 'need' criterion for marketing authorizations, to accompany the three widely established criteria of safety, efficacy and quality. Moreover, compliance with a cost criterion does not constitute a condition for marketing approval in the EU. However, some government health insurance systems within the Community regulate the pricing of medicines once they have entered the market and determine which of those products used by patients will be paid for by the national insurance system. The National Health Service in the UK, for example, issues a list of products for which reimbursement is not available. Although it employs a *negative* list, this is referred to as the *Selected* List Scheme. Denmark, Sweden and Finland, as members of the EU, are subject to the provisions of Council Directive 89/105/EEC, which ensures the openness of procedures for adding products to such negative lists (the 'Transparency' Directive).

Despite the individuality of the Norwegian regulatory system for pharmaceuticals, the Nordic guidelines on the evaluation of drugs (Nordic Council on Medicines, 1986) ensure uniformity of the data requirements for marketing authorization throughout the region. Moreover, a medical prescription issued in one Nordic country is recognized in all others.

International Organizations

Various organizations within the framework of the United Nations and its associated bodies are of particular relevance in the context of this chapter. These are the World Trade Organization (WTO), the Codex Alimentarius Commission (CAC), the Organization for Economic Cooperation and Development (OECD), the International Programme on Chemical Safety (IPCS), the International Agency for Research on Cancer (IARC), the International Register of Potentially Toxic Chemicals (IRPTC) and the International Environmental Information System (INFOTERRA). Other relevant bodies include the International Courts and the Council of Europe.

The World Trade Organization (WTO)

The General Agreement on Tariffs and Trade (GATT) was created by the United Nations in 1948 to liberalize trade in the post-war era. Since then, a series of on-going international negotiations known as 'rounds' have taken place. The last of these, the Uruguay round, was finalized on 15 April 1994 in Marrakesh, Morocco, after negotiations lasting 7 years. The agreements reached have been incorporated into the Final Act of the Uruguay round. To replace GATT, the Act established a World Trade Organization (WTO) whose 139 member countries are putting into practice the agreed provisions and principles. It is intended that the work of WTO will result in substantial cuts in world tariffs and the wider opening of markets to imported goods including human foodstuffs.

WTO has recently concluded an Agreement on Technical Barriers to Trade. This, together with the recent Agreement on Sanitary and Phytosanitary Measures, necessitates the global adoption of agreed standards for food safety. It is clear that an international system of standards, such as that provided by the Codex Alimentarius (discussed below), is needed. Recently, the WTO has called upon member countries to play a full part in Codex activities. Member nations are required to apply the same standards to imported and domestically produced foodstuffs. If a country imposes stricter standards than others, the WTO will require proper scientific justification. National measures are expected to be arrived at by open and transparent procedures, and the WTO expects member nations to ensure that technical barriers are based on sound scientific principles and risk assessment.

One of the components of the Final Act of the Uruguay round is an agreement which will affect trade in chemical-based products. This is the Agreement on Trade-related Aspects of Intellectual Property Rights (TRIPS). Patent arrangements for chemical-based products will be affected by TRIPS, although the impact will vary considerably from country to country. This can be seen in the pharmaceutical field, for example, in the elimination of the long-standing international division between countries which grant patents for new active substances and those which do not. The TRIPS agreement requires that all WTO member countries establish at least 20 years' patent protection. However, the Agreement also grants WTO member countries the right to so-called 'compulsory' marketing licences when a patent holder refuses to make a product available under 'reasonable' voluntary licence arrangements (Correa, 1996). Other grounds on which the Agreement grants WTO members the right to compulsory marketing licences are:

- To adopt measures to protect public health and nutrition, and to promote the public interest . . .' (Article 8);
- To prevent anti-competitive practices and abuses of dominant market positions;
- For public, non-commercial use;
- In national emergencies and circumstances of extreme urgency (Article 31b).

WTO members had a 1 year transition period within which to meet their obligations under the TRIPS

Agreement, which became effective on 1 January 1996. Developing countries which join the WTO have an additional 4 years (5 years altogether), and least-developed countries have an additional 10 years (11 years altogether) to meet the provisions of the Agreement.

The Codex Alimentarius Commission (CAC)

The term *Codex Alimentarius* translates roughly from the Latin as 'food code'. Although the Codex Alimentarius Commission (CAC) is not in itself a regulatory agency, it is responsible for a system of standards, guidelines and codes of practice which many agencies throughout the world use, to different degrees, in formulating their regulations.

The Codex Alimentarius Commission was established in 1962 and is based in Rome. It is a subsidiary body of both the Food and Agriculture Organization of the United Nations (FAO) and the World Health Organization (WHO). Membership is available to all nations having full or associate membership of either FAO or WHO. At present there are 156 members of Codex Alimentarius.

The Codex system is well suited to the emerging needs of the WTO. The CAC is charged especially with quality controls for food, in particular controls related to consumer safety, health and trade. Codex provisions exist for inspection, labelling, certification systems, food additives, pesticide residues, sampling and analysis. The Codex approach is a flexible one; for example, methods of analysis are required only to be equivalent, and not necessarily identical (although results must, of course, be verifiable).

In carrying out its work, the Commission is assisted by a network of committees. One group of committees deals with specific commodities, such as the Codex Committee on Fats and Oils, which is hosted by the UK and first met in 1964. A second group of Codex committees deals with general subjects, such as food labelling. Three of the committees in this second group are of especial importance in the present context. These are the Codex Committee on Food Additives and Contaminants (CCFAC), the Codex Committee on Pesticide Residues (CCPR) and the Codex Committee on Residues of Veterinary Drugs in Foods (CCRVDF). The CCFAC is hosted by the government of The Netherlands and the first session took place in 1964. The CCPR is also hosted by the government of The Netherlands and the initial meeting occurred in 1966. The terms of reference of CCPR also include 'environmental and industrial contaminants showing chemical or other similarity to pesticides'. The CCRVDF first met in 1986 in the USA and it is hosted by the government of that country. Expert advice on scientific aspects, including toxicology, is required in conjunction with the work of these three committees, which are made up of government representatives and trade delegations. In the case of CCFAC and CCRVDF, independent specialist advice is provided by the Joint (FAO/WHO) Expert Committee on Food Additives (JECFA). The Joint Meeting on Pesticide Residues (JMPR) plays a similar part in relation to the work of CCPR. The advice of these expert committees is addressed to the Directors General of FAO and WHO.

New Codex standards are 'elaborated' by the appropriate committee (together with the relevant expert group) and, following a series of consultative steps, are sent by the Codex Commission to governments for acceptance. The work of elaborating a new standard may follow a decision either of the Commission or of the committee concerned. Such standards include, for example, maximum residue levels (MRLs) for pesticide residues in specific food commodities and tolerances for veterinary drug residues in the carcasses of food-producing animals. Individual governments may or may not choose to accept Codex standards. Countries which decide upon full acceptance may implement Codex standards by incorporating them into their own national legislation. Joint decisions on acceptance may, of course, be taken by inter-governmental groups, such as the EU.

The Organization for Economic Cooperation and Development (OECD)

More than 20 countries, including the USA, Japan and the EC Member States, take part in the work of the OECD. The organization is based in Paris and was established in 1960. The OECD plays a particularly valuable role as a facilitator for agreements between member countries. Most recently, in 1997, the organization made important contributions to the negotiations between the USA and the EU for a mutual recognition agreement for pharmaceutical authorizations.

For many years the OECD chemicals programme has formed an important part of the OECD's work and, in 1984, a cooperative agreement with the three United Nations agencies which sponsor the IPCS was signed. An important aspect of the OECD chemicals programme relates to the harmonization of test methods for assessing health effects, environmental effects (ecotoxicity and accumulation/degradation) and physicochemical properties. To this end, the OECD has published guidelines on the testing of chemicals for toxicity, and these are updated as necessary. Guidance on the principles and monitoring of good laboratory practice (which is discussed elsewhere in this chapter) have also been published by OECD. The Mutual Acceptance of Data Agreement has done much to reduce the duplication of studies and unnecessary testing. This agreement requires OECD member countries to accept data provided that they conform with the relevant OECD test guidelines, and are generated in compliance with the OECD principles of GLP (OECD, 1981).

Industrial chemicals are the subject of several OECD initiatives. The exchange of information on banned and severely restricted substances is encouraged by OECD. Member countries receive assistance in examining and refining their risk management policies. This work includes case studies of risk management approaches to specific chemicals and chemical groups. The Organization's EXICHEM database is used to assist member countries to identify opportunities for cooperation in the investigation of specific existing chemicals and to facilitate negotiations about the conduct of such work. EXICHEM is available on media for personal computers. The secretariat examines the database twice yearly and makes suggestions on potential candidate chemicals for cooperative work. Such work is undertaken as part of the OECD 'clearing house' function. In 1989, the OECD compiled a list of chemicals which are produced in large quantities and which have been examined for data availability. Additional data required for hazard assessment is being identified and accorded priorities.

The Council of Europe (COE)

The COE was founded in 1949, is based in Strasbourg and has a membership more than 20 European governments. It cooperates closely with other international organizations, including the UN, the EC and the OECD. One of the Council's objectives is the introduction of uniform health regulations and 12 of the member countries cooperate particularly closely to encourage protection against food contamination and to support harmonization of legislation in this field. Aspects of this work include flavourings, packaging materials and pesticide and veterinary drug residues. The COE has also been involved in safety-related work on toxic substances in cosmetics and adverse effects of medicines and detergents. Seventeen of COE's member countries cooperate in producing the *European Pharmacopoeia*.

The International Programme on Chemical Safety (IPCS)

The IPCS is based in Geneva and was sponsored jointly by three specialized agencies of the United Nations, the World Health Organization, the International Labour Organization and the UN Environment Programme. Its major aim is to assess the effects of chemicals on health and on the environment and to publish these assessments. In support of this aim, the IPCS is also developing risk assessment, laboratory and epidemiological methods which are intended to give internationally comparable results. Other activities include the development of toxicological expertise in these areas, in the follow-up of chemical accidents and in mechanistic aspects of toxicology. IPCS produces numerous publications in its 'Environmental Health Criteria' and 'Health and Safety Guide' series, and it has recently started to publish a companion series of International Chemical Safety Cards (ICSC). The IPCS also collaborates with the European Commission in the evaluation of antidotes used in the treatment of poisoning and the results of these evaluations are published jointly.

The International Agency for Research on Cancer (IARC)

The IARC is an international research organization based in Lyon, France, concerned with the identification of environmental causes of human cancer. It carries out both laboratory work and epidemiological studies in various parts of the world where different environmental conditions apply. The research programme is particularly concerned with aetiological factors in carcinoma of the stomach, the oesophagus and other important sites, and with exploring the possible role of pesticides and viruses in human cancer.

The IARC was the first international biomedical body and was the outcome of a French proposal. The founding countries were France, the UK, the USA, the former West Germany and Italy. The IARC was established in 1965 (during the 18th World Health Assembly) as an autonomous body within the World Health Organization. In addition to the founding members, many other countries participate today. The IARC Monographs provide authoritative, up-to-date assessments of the carcinogenic potential for humans associated with a wide range of compounds.

International Register of Potentially Toxic Chemicals (IRPTC)

The IRPTC was founded in 1976 and is based in Geneva. Its objective is to reduce the risks associated with chemical contamination of the environment and it constitutes a valuable source of information about regulations and standards. The IRPTC exists within the framework of the United Nations Environment Programme and it is particularly concerned with the needs of developing countries. It provides a query–response service and general information on many chemicals. The IRPTC Bulletin is published twice a year and there is a unique series of monographs on the hazards of pesticides and other chemicals. The IRPTC has also developed a computerized registry of chemicals which have been tested for topical effects, in conjunction with the IPCS.

International Environmental Information System (INFOTERRA)

INFOTERRA is an environmental information network, involving more than 100 countries, founded in 1977 as part of the United Nations Environment Programme. Major centres are located in Geneva and Nairobi. It possesses a register of information sources and its major function is to refer enquiries to the appropriate sources (Ekstrom and Kidd, 1989), rather than providing detailed technical information. INFOTERRA's international directory contains descriptions of some 6000 sources and there is a network of national focal points in the participating countries.

The International Courts

Although there are major differences between international courts, they all become involved with regulatory affairs from time to time.

The European Court of Justice, based in Luxembourg, was set up under the terms of the Treaty of Rome and is the judicial body of the EU. Its judgements overrule those of the national courts and it ensures that Member States incorporate into national laws the intentions of the Directives, including those concerned with chemical safety. The court also ensures that new domestic legislation of this kind, and also the Regulations of the EU itself, are enforced.

The International Court of Justice, or 'World Court', based in The Hague, is the principal judicial body of the UN. Its work includes the provision of legal advice to UN bodies including the World Health Organization and its agencies.

The European Court of Human Rights, based in Strasbourg, has been the guardian of the European Convention on Human Rights since its creation in 1953. It became involved in a prominent toxicological issue when it upheld the right of a British newspaper to publish information about the thalidomide tragedy. Following the 1997 election in the UK, the new government announced that the Convention would be incorporated into UK domestic law.

DATA REQUIREMENTS

The toxicological information required by regulatory agencies in support of applications and notifications varies between countries. The degree of difference varies from one category of products to another, being relatively small in the case of industrial chemicals and larger in the case of pharmaceuticals. Differences in data requirements give rise to repetition of studies, leading to the unnecessary use of animals and other toxicological resources. This in turn increases costs unnecessarily and has implications for trade. Although the desirability of consistency without loss of flexibility is not in dispute, it is difficult to achieve in practice. That it is possible, given clear political will and a suitable administrative–legal framework, is shown by the harmonization achieved within the EU. The consistency of the guidelines issued by the Member States of the EU has improved considerably for all the categories of regulated chemicals as a result of the ongoing programme of European legisla-

tion, and complete harmonization has been achieved for some categories of chemical-based products. The benefits of consistency have also been realised to a very considerable degree between the nations which comprise the Nordic Community, three of which (Denmark, Sweden and Finland) are now members of the EU. On a wider scale, many regulatory agencies throughout the world have recognized the advantages of allowing their guidelines and toxicological requirements to be influenced by those which have been published by the OECD (OECD, 1981). For the categories of pesticides and industrial chemicals, an important comparison was made between the requirements published by the OECD and by the relevant agencies in the EU, the USA and Japan (ECETOC, 1985). The authors considered that the OECD guidelines were the most widely recognized internationally, and made various recommendations for ensuring common approaches without loss of flexibility.

The International Conference on Harmonization (ICH)

During the 1990s, an important dialogue known as the International Conference on Harmonization of Technical Requirements for the Registration of Pharmaceuticals for Human Use (ICH) has been sponsored by the EU, the USA and Japan. Representatives of both regulatory and commercial interests are provided by each of the three regions. The first meeting (known as ICH-1) took place in 1991, and has been followed by others at two-yearly intervals:

ICH-1	Brussels	November 1991
ICH-2	Orlando	October 1993
ICH-3	Yokohama	November 1995
ICH-4	Brussels	July 1997

ICH provides a forum for dialogue between regulatory agencies and the pharmaceutical industry on the differences in the data requirements for marketing authorization in the three regions. It is therefore concerned with the requirements for testing in human volunteers and patients, as well as those relating to animal testing. The conference considers how mutual acceptance of different research approaches and agreed modifications of data requirements might lead to more economical use of human, animal and material resources, without compromising safety. ICH is an informal process in that it produces recommendations. These propose specific improvements in harmonization for data requirements and for the interpretation and application of guidelines. A promising start has been made on the requirements for pre-clinical testing, where differences in medical culture exert relatively little influence. The work of ICH has already done much to prepare the ground for removing the inconsistencies and international anomalies in guidelines noted by Alder and Zbinden in 1988. Once the current exercise has been completed, and harmonized pre-clinical guidelines have been adopted by the agencies, a continuation of the ICH process by means of some form of on-going review process would be beneficial, to take account of technical progress and prevent the unnecessary expansion of requirements.

The working procedure adopted by ICH commences with Step 1, the identification of a topic or concept to be dealt with. A paper is prepared by any party and, after approval by the Steering Committee, serves to initiate discussion on the topic. The procedure concludes with Step 5, the adoption of a harmonized tripartite guideline on the topic by the regulatory agencies, following official publication and consultation on the proposal in the countries concerned.

After a topic has been identified, it is considered in conference until a draft consensus paper can be agreed by the six parties (Step 2). The draft is then circulated for consultation in the countries concerned and is re-drafted as necessary by the three regulatory participants (Step 3). After further consideration in conference, the draft harmonized tripartite guideline can be agreed by the three industry participants. This stepwise procedure was developed from that employed by UN agencies, for example, in the processes of the Codex Alimentarius Commission, as described elsewhere in this chapter.

For the topic of general toxicity, it has been agreed that the LD_{50} test should be abandoned and that the durations of repeated-dose studies in rodents should be reduced. Consideration of the duration of general toxicity studies in dogs continues. In the area of mutagenicity (genotoxicity) testing, it was recognized that terminological difficulties still occur in this area. An ICH glossary has therefore been produced. Agreement has been reached on the evaluation of *in vitro* and *in vivo* test results, which should facilitate the assessment of applications. The question of which tests should comprise the standard battery is under discussion, and consideration is being given to the value of the gene mutation test in mammalian cells. The guidelines on the *in vivo* test are receiving attention, and the need to make the requirement relate more specifically to methods using cytogenetic changes in rodent bone-marrow cells is being considered. The objectives of reproductive toxicity testing in mammals have been clarified. It has been accepted that by applying a scientific approach to these objectives, the repetition of studies (which has been necessitated by differences in the existing guidelines) should no longer be required. Consideration is being given to the harmonization of protocols for three-segment toxicity studies, based on understandable scientific principles, but without excessive rigidity.

For carcinogenicity testing, it has been agreed that the use of the maximum tolerated dose of a non-toxic compound in the highest dose group is not necessary. Several alternative criteria for the selection of the highest dose have been agreed. Circumstances in which carcinogenicity studies are (and are not) considered to be necessary have been defined. Consideration of the need for two rodent species continues (for some years a consensus has been developing that a mouse study can rarely add greatly to the information provided by a rat study, and that the development of liver and lung tumours in the mouse, in response to non-genotoxic compounds, can be misleading). Consideration is being given to the value of short-term studies (e.g. specific transgenic mouse models). This approach would enable specific mechanisms to be studied, and a number of transgenic models are under investigation.

ICH is also addressing the need to harmonize guidelines on testing for efficacy, which has been emphasised by pharmaceutical physicians for many years. Some controversy is anticipated in this area, which involves questions of good clinical practice and of ethnic factors in the acceptability of foreign clinical data. Considerations in the design and conduct of clinical trials on which there is much need for agreement include the size and composition of trial populations (in terms of gender, age, racial origin, general and specific medical history, etc.), the duration of testing, the choice of active comparators, the circumstances in which the use of placebos are appropriate and the use of historical comparators. Although therapeutic efficacy, as such, is outside the scope of this book, it is the benefit with which the toxicological hazard inherent in a medicine must always be compared. Much of the cost of developing a new medicine is expended on clinical testing, and international harmonization would bring considerable benefits.

TOXICOLOGICAL RISK

Risk Assessment

In the context of this chapter, the risk associated with a chemical means the likelihood that it will be toxicologically harmful in some specified way within a human population. However, the likelihood (i.e. the *probability*) that toxic harm will occur is often very difficult to determine in quantitative terms. It is fortunate, therefore, that much of the work of regulatory agencies can be carried out without numerical risk estimates. The term *risk assessment* is used widely in regulatory toxicology, but often not to signify a procedure for estimating risk quantitatively; the term must therefore be interpreted with caution. A general procedure developed in the USA (National Research Council, 1983) has been adapted with various modifications for use in many other countries. This is outlined here; special considerations which apply to carcinogens are discussed later. When the toxicological hazards posed by a chemical have been identified, it may be clear that one or more of these has relevance for humans. If sufficient data are available, dose–response relationships are developed for these end-points in man. Unfortunately, however, the available epidemiological and other human data are usually inadequate and an indirect approach, using the results of testing in laboratory animals, is frequently used. When sufficient information from animal studies is available, dose–response relationships in those species may be constructed. Then, using available comparative information about the test species and man, attempts are made to predict a dose–response relationship for man. This approach can be applied to toxicological end-points of various kinds (e.g. liver damage, teratogenesis, skin effects). The predicted dose–response relationship for man can then be used, in conjunction with exposure information, to forecast effects in people. This general procedure can be applied to chemicals encountered in products, in occupational exposure and in the wider environment. It enables Acceptable Daily Intakes (ADIs) for potentially toxic chemicals to be agreed, but it does not provide a numerical indication of risk when intake exceeds ADI.

Risk Management

Once the dose–response relationships for the toxicological effects of a chemical have been estimated for humans, it is often possible to set a regulatory standard by applying an appropriate safety factor. The area of food chemical toxicology provides many examples of regulatory standards for use in the work of *risk management*. These include MRLs for pesticides and for veterinary drugs in foodstuffs and the ADIs of these residues and of substances intentionally present in food, such as additives. The ADI is the upper limit of lifetime exposure to the chemical which is acceptable on public health grounds. In the case of residues and other food contaminants, this figure may be referred to as the *tolerable daily intake* (TDI). When it is known that the toxicological phenomena associated with a compound only appear above a certain daily dosage level, the procedure followed is straightforward and makes use of the concept of the 'no observed adverse effect level' (NOAEL), which is determined in the most sensitive species by means of the most discriminating test. In such cases, the regulatory standard is generally derived from the NOAEL, after a safety factor has been applied to it.

These principles are well illustrated by the standard approach to risk management applied to food chemicals possessing NOAELs, such as additives. Here, the ADI is obtained by dividing the NOAEL by the chosen safety factor. There are several ways in which this approach can be used. In the case of a *new* additive, the regulatory agency decides the safety factor; the NOAEL is then divided by this factor to give the ADI. Food consumption data are taken into account, and are used to estimate the maximum likely daily intake which would occur if the chemical was present in the types of food and at the concentrations proposed. A comparison between the maximum total intake expected and the ADI provides the measure of safety which constitutes the basis for regulatory decisions about the foods and the concentrations in which the additive may be used. In the case of an *existing* additive, the procedure is necessarily different. Here, a comparison is made between the known dietary intake and the ADI. If the difference is not judged to be adequate, then regulatory action may be taken.

For residues of veterinary drugs in human food, the regulatory standard is the MRL. The MRL is based on the NOAEL divided by a safety factor (i.e. on the ADI), together with data on food consumption. The MRL might, for example, refer to the maximum limit for the residue of an antibacterial in pig carcass muscle. The time–concentration (depletion) curve in the living pig is then used to determine the minimum period between the last administration of the drug and slaughter (i.e. the 'withdrawal' period for the drug) which must be enforced in order to ensure that the MRL is not exceeded. For pesticides the MRL is also the regulatory standard, although it is determined by field trials in which the pesticide is used in accordance with good agricultural practice (GAP). It is also essential that the pesticide MRL satisfies the criterion of consumer safety as well as GAP. Consumer exposure is calculated (on the basis of MRL and food intake data) and compared with the ADI, which is again derived by applying a safety factor to the NOAEL. Regulatory agencies are responsible for establishing and enforcing conditions of pesticide use which ensure that exposures do not exceed ADIs. The ADI approach can be applied to any unwanted effect, provided that a NOAEL can be established, but it must be stressed that this approach does not provide any means for the calculation of risk (i.e. *probability* of toxicological harm) when the ADI is exceeded by any particular amount. In other words, the probability that the relevant toxicological effect will occur cannot be calculated from the amount by which actual intake exceeds the ADI. There should, of course, be no excess risk at all if the ADI is not exceeded. Moreover, the safety factors used in setting ADIs should be sufficiently large to ensure that there is unlikely to be any appreciable added risk if ADIs are exceeded by only small amounts, or for only short periods.

Carcinogens in Trace Quantities

The approach described above can be reasonably applied to many substances, traces of which occur in foodstuffs and in the wider environment. However, for chemicals which produce cancer in laboratory animals, there are problems with this approach. Although a NOAEL may appear in a bioassay, the possibility that this dose (or even a lower one) would produce a carcinogenic effect detectable in a larger group of animals can rarely be excluded. Even when the human exposure level would be well below the bioassay NOAEL, the numbers of individuals exposed are likely to be large. In view of these uncertainties, there are obvious difficulties with an approach in which an arbitrary safety factor is used in conjunction with the results of an animal study. In order to circumvent this problem, attempts have been made to estimate quantitatively the risks to man posed by traces of carcinogens by means of mathematical methods which model the probability of carcinogenesis as a function of dose. A mathematical model of this kind utilizes as 'input' the data from an animal bioassay. The results of such modelling depend on a range of assumptions, some of which are often fragile, so that levels of uncertainty may be very high indeed. Assumptions about the shape of the dose–response curve in the low-dose region are crucial, but neither animal nor human data are usually available to validate the model's prediction in this region, yet it is this portion of the curve that corresponds to the doses in food and the environment to which human populations are actually exposed, and for which reliable answers are needed. Another difficulty is that the available mathematical models provide risk estimates which vary widely. It is often very difficult to decide which model, if any, can be used for a particular chemical with some hope of validity. The problem is illustrated in simplified form in **Figure 2**.

Figure 2 shows coordinates against which probability of carcinogenesis is plotted against dose. The results of a rodent carcinogenicity bioassay, using three dose levels, are represented by three asterisks. Two graphs are shown, representing two alternative models. One is linear, the other sub-linear. The enlarged portion of the figure shows the region relevant to human exposures, the low-dose region. To produce a given probability of carcinogenesis, p_1, very different doses, either d_1 or d_2, are required depending on which model is chosen. A valid choice of model requires a knowledge of the mechanisms of carcinogenesis operating at low exposure levels, which is often unavailable. Agencies which routinely use models are therefore often compelled, in ignorance, to adopt default assumptions (such as low-dose linearity) to ensure that risks are not underestimated. The results are sometimes claimed to overestimate risk to a degree which decreases confidence in the regulatory process. Similar comments apply to inappropriate selection of models (e.g. models providing non-zero estimates in the low-dose region for non-genotoxic or secondary carcinogens having clear thresholds).

In addition to the major problem of interpolating from high to low doses, there are great difficulties in extrapolating from laboratory animal species to man. Models can only make use of the data provided by an animal carcinogenicity study. Although additional data may be highly relevant (e.g. information about mechanisms,

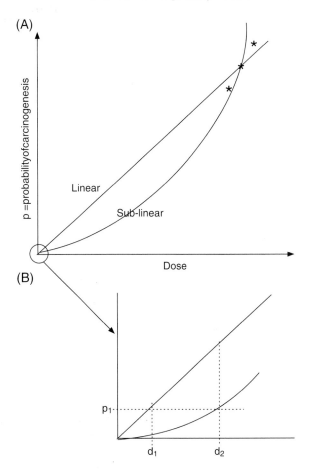

Figure 2 (A) The asterisks represent the results of an animal carcinogenicity study. **(B)** The 'acceptable' risk, p_t, is attained at a dose of either d_1 or d_2, according to which model is used.

mutagenicity, toxicokinetics and toxicity), they cannot be included in the modelling process. In some cases additional data would suggest that risks are lower than those predicted by modelling: perhaps the chemical can be absorbed from the animal but not the human gastrointestinal tract; perhaps it is broken down completely and rapidly by a metabolizing enzyme present in man but not in the test species. Data of this kind might provide a degree of reassurance. When adequate information about the carcinogenic mechanism is available, this too may provide assurance that low levels of exposure would pose no excess risk to man.

Because of these difficulties, results derived from mathematical models must be accompanied by carefully worded cautions about the uncertainties involved. Unfortunately, these cautions are often lost in transmission and do not appear in versions carried by popular media, in political controversies and in the arguments of interest groups. In recent years, the serious limitations of mathematical models for human carcinogenesis based on animal testing have been better appreciated (Department of Health, 1991; Krewski *et al.*, 1993a, b; Park and Hawkins, 1995; Lovell and Thomas, 1996; McDonald *et al.*, 1996). This has led to a better appreciation of the need to base assessments on *all* available data and to a greater reluctance to issue quantitative carcinogenicity estimates. Pragmatic approaches to the prioritization of food carcinogens have been developed which do not rely on modelling, but make use of all existing toxicological data and all available information about exposure (McDonald *et al.*, 1996).

Statements About Risk

Regulatory agencies must often issue statements about risks. Sometimes the circulation of information is limited, for example, to interest groups representing consumers and manufacturers. Sometimes it is very wide, with the intention of bringing the information to the widest possible public audience; here it may be desirable to inform health professionals before releasing information to the public, in order to ensure that they are in a position to answer questions, although efficient communication networks are needed for this. In other cases there is no proactive announcement, but briefing is provided so that questions can be dealt with as they arise. The preparation of statements about risks is a special skill. Many agencies employ experienced press officers with backgrounds in journalism and broadcasting. Often a balance must be struck between the prevention of unnecessary alarm and the clear transmission of necessary information. Professional press officers, who are also keenly aware of political climates, are able to make valuable contributions in this area. Particular skill and experience are needed in dealing with the media, as anyone can confirm who has experience of interviewers seeking 'scare' stories. The press officer is an essential participant on such occasions; it is the press officer, for example, who knows which people can be trusted to respect confidential background briefing and the rules of attribution.

When a public statement about a new risk is issued, it will immediately provoke questions about the scale of the problem. Words such as 'serious' are sometimes used ambiguously in relation to risks. If a risk is said to be serious, does this mean that it is likely to occur? Or does it mean that the adverse event concerned is a serious one, albeit very unlikely? In some cases it may be possible to give answers about probability. For questions about the relative risks of fatal lung cancer in smokers and non-smokers, for example, it is possible to draw upon reliable numerical data and to formulate answers in clear, quantitative terms. In many cases however, the threat cannot be quantified and, however much 'risk assessment' has been carried out, the probability of the adverse event cannot be expressed in figures. The only alternative is words. Here there is a serious problem of consistency. Different sources tend to use different forms of words when referring to risk in a particular scenario. This leaves the way open for complaints that one source has tried to underplay the danger, or that another has sought to exaggerate it. In the development of the British BSE problem, the following comments were made by different political sources: the risk is very small; the risk is negligible; there is no risk; there is no significant risk; the risk is minimal; the risk is remote; it is perfectly safe; it is acceptably safe; the risk is unknown; the risk is unknown but is probably very small; the risk is less than that of crossing the road. This example suggests several ways in which progress can be made. First, avoidance of sweeping statements of the form 'so-and-so presents no risk or is perfectly safe' unless, of course, they can be substantiated. Second, willingness to use the word 'unknown', where it accurately describes the situation. This may be more difficult than it sounds, because of the temptation to apply numbers even without evidence to justify them. An instance of this phenomenon was documented recently: when pressed for a quantitative estimate for the risk of BSE at a meeting of the Royal Statistical Society in the UK on 26 November 1996, Professor Adrian Smith, the President of the Society, was quoted as saying that the risk might be between zero and millions (Anon., 1996). However, the report of the meeting in the *Independent* newspaper led with a headline claiming that 'hundreds' would die. Third, agreement on how certain words might correspond consistently with numerical statements; proposals for clarifying the language of risk have been put forward for discussion (Calman, 1996). Fourth, the use of the simple concept of relative risk to indicate how an unknown risk compares with an everyday known risk. In some cases, although the size of a risk is not known, there may nevertheless be sufficient knowledge to *rank* it in relation to other, known, risks. Known risks can be arrayed on a scale from high to low. If it is possible to place a risk of death of unknown size between two of the known ones, this can be very helpful to those who find it difficult to judge the seriousness of the problem in broad, familiar terms. Suppose, for example, that the unknown risk can be positioned between the known annual risks of death from a traffic accident and from smoking 10 cigarettes per day. The available information is then presented with clarity and simplicity. When the size of a risk is known, then it can of course be positioned with precision on the scale. Various risk scales have been developed (British Medical Association, 1990; Paulos, 1990), but they tend to be too complicated to meet the needs of the ordinary person. The levels of sophistication required to satisfy the expert statistician, on the one hand, and to be useful as an aid to public communication, on the other, are very different. For the latter, a simple 10-point scale on which known, common risks can be set out in order would be helpful **(Figure 3)**. Risks on the 10-point scale are represented by a risk factor, a number between 1 and 10: the greater the risk, the closer the risk factor is to 10. The mathematical derivation of the risk factor should be as simple as possible, and accessible to non-mathematicians. It starts from the

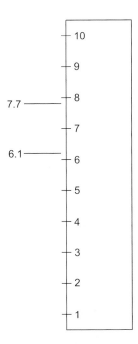

Figure 3 Scale 1–10 for risk factor *R*.

Two examples illustrate the use of the risk factor. Suppose that one in 8000 people dies in a traffic accident each year, so that the annual risk for an individual is 1 in 8000. Substituting 8000 for *N* in Equation 1 gives 6.1 as the risk factor *R*. A greater annual risk of death is undertaken by the individual smoking 10 cigarettes per day: if this risk is 1 in 200, Equation 1 gives 7.7 as the value of *R* (see **Figure 3**).

Risk perception is sometimes dismissed as subjective, but it is worth remembering that what subjects perceive is their reality. People take into account a wide range of factors which are of importance to them personally, and which influence their perception of risk. People arrive at their own judgements when balancing risk against benefit, and this too influences risk perception. It is arrogant to dismiss the psychological aspects of risk perception as irrationality. People (rightly) make their own assessments, using a broader basis than experts, and take account of a wide variety of related questions, often unconsciously, which might include: Do I have confidence in the agency? Is an 'unfair' risk being imposed? Can I avoid the risk if I choose? Can the agency control the risk? Do the experts agree? Are children at risk? Is there a risk of cancer, AIDS, etc.? Judgements about what constitutes 'benefit' vary considerably between individuals. Sometimes considerable danger is confronted without hesitation (e.g. in sports) when the benefit or objective is all-important. Lack of control often makes a risk less tolerable and even risks which are (in objective terms) very small may give rise to greater distress for this reason. If the problem concerns an individual food product, for example, consumers can exercise control in choosing alternatives, but if the water supply is contaminated, self-determination is more difficult. The belief (albeit often a flawed one) that they are in control is one of the reasons why smokers continue with a habit known to carry high risk. Risks affecting practically any aspect of *human reproduction* cause particular concern. A risk is perceived as greater when it involves something unexpected, unfair, exotic or alien, unnatural or synthetic, or something particularly dreaded, such as congenital deformity.

It is essential that those responsible for communicating risk-related information should understand something of the factors which determine how the information will be perceived, as risks are generally perceived to be greater when, in addition to the reasons mentioned above, the individual lacks trust, or believes that there is lack of openness, undue secrecy or authoritarianism. Confidence in an official source of information reduces perceived risk. When a regulatory agency enjoys wide public trust, perceived risk will not be amplified by fears that the problem is being underplayed or covered up. Trust is fostered by a policy of openness. If an agency statement is straightforward but non-patronizing, and does not shrink from admissions of ignorance where information is simply not available, it is more likely to

assumption that the form 'a chance of 1 in *N*' is straightforward and widely understood. It should be applicable to a sufficiently wide range of possible risks to meet the needs of everyday discussion and comparison. Such an approach would make it much easier for many people to develop their own ranking of the different risks which concern them. Equation 1 enables *R*, a risk factor which meets these criteria, to be calculated. Where the risk is 1 in *N*, the equation enables the risk factor *R* to be calculated for any value of *N* within a wide range. Any value of *N* from a billion (10^9) (i.e. 'extremely' unlikely) to 1 (i.e. complete certainty) can be substituted in Equation 1 to give a value between 1 and 10 for the risk factor *R*.

$$R = 10 - \log_{10} N \qquad (1)$$

Values of *R* corresponding to a wide range of values for *N* are given in **Table 1**.

Table 1 Values of risk factor *R* corresponding to different values of *N*

N	R
1	10
10	9
100	8
1000	7
10 000	6
100 000	5
1 000 000	4
10 000 000	3
100 000 000	2
1 000 000 000	1

be respected. Authoritarianism is to be avoided. In developed countries today, the public is well informed and is unlikely to accept unsubstantiated assertions without question. Official attitudes suggesting that the authorities know best, have an automatic right to public respect and cannot be expected to explain things openly are most inadvisable. Whatever may have been tolerated in the past, such attitudes are not acceptable today. They increase the perception of risks and create suspicions that authorities are either covering something up or do not understand the problem as well as they imply. Unwillingness to provide information, without a reasonable explanation, results in distrust and such reticence may engender suspicions that secrecy is being used to protect some interest at the expense of public safety. Seen from the inside, it is often perfectly clear that there are no sinister connotations, but this does not resolve the problem of public perception. A declared policy of openness is belied if unnecessary secrecy occurs in practice. There are, of course, categories of information which an agency cannot properly divulge. In addition to material classified for reasons of national security, this includes certain kinds of commercially sensitive material. However, the variation in the restrictions which apply between different countries is very wide, and has become more so with the enactment of the Freedom of Information Act in the USA. Unnecessary secrecy, like authoritarianism, has an adverse effect on risk perception.

FOUNDATIONS OF EFFECTIVE REGULATION

The term *regulatory agency* is more a product of American English than British usage. The great American regulatory agencies are known throughout the world, and the term is a convenient single expression encompassing the many types of organisation included in this chapter. In the UK it has been more usual to use expressions such as *the authorities* and, in the formal terminology of the EU, the generic term is the *competent authorities*. An agency is an organization which carries out specified functions on behalf of someone else, sometimes at a distance. A regulatory agency, strictly, carries out particular, limited, regulatory functions on behalf of government. It usually does this by acting as an agent for one or more government departments. In many countries functions traditionally carried out directly by government departments are increasingly being delegated to newly created agencies, set up to provide services on commercial lines. One example in the UK is the Medicines Control Agency (MCA), established in 1989 to deal with the regulatory control of pharmaceuticals on behalf of the Secretary of State for Health, a function previously carried out directly by a division of the Department of Health. Following the 1997 election in the UK, the new government announced that an independent agency concerned with food standards and safety would be established. When regulators are asked what qualities an agency should possess, several factors are mentioned regularly. Although expressed in different forms, these factors can be resolved into three essentials: scientific competence, public credibility and a firm but impartial approach *to regulatory affairs*.

Scientific competence is ensured by providing the resources and selection procedures needed to provide the agency with professional staff of adequate calibre in the relevant fields: medicine and other biosciences, risk assessment, etc. First-class recruits are more likely to be attracted to agencies with reputations for providing good career opportunities for those wishing to remain in regulatory affairs. Equally, an agency is more likely to recruit first-class people who are not committed to long-term regulatory affairs when its reputation suggests that the experience gained will confer career advantages.

Agencies also need independent advisers of outstanding expertise and impeccable objectivity. The use of advisory committees, consisting of well balanced combinations of experts, including academics, is a well tried approach for the provision of independent advice. An advantage of this collective approach is the tendency for peer interactions to make idiosyncratic outcomes less likely. Several core specialities are likely to be needed on most committees concerned with chemical products: toxicologists are usually included and the importance of expertise in risk assessment is being increasingly recognized. Other specialities represented depend on the product categories on which advice is given. Factory inspectors and engineers, as well as toxicologists, are likely to be needed on committees dealing with industrial chemicals. Practising clinicians are needed on committees which consider pharmaceuticals. Committees concerned with pesticides must include experts on occupational and environmental aspects. It is sometimes difficult in very specialized fields to recruit first-class advisers who are not also acting for other interested parties, such as manufacturers and consumer protection groups; there must, therefore, be a clear policy on potential conflicts of interests (and on procedures to be followed when interests are declared). The extent to which regulatory affairs are influenced by the contributions of advisory committees varies considerably from country to country. In some cases, specialist advice from a committee will simply be one of the several contributions taken into account by an agency when formulating its decision. In other cases the conclusions of committees amount almost to *de facto* regulatory decisions. It is hardly necessary to add that, if the expertise of an advisory committee does not extend to regulatory affairs and legal aspects (being limited, for example, to biomedical and other scientific matters), then care is needed to ensure that proper attention is paid to these aspects before final decisions are taken.

Public credibility is elusive. Trust is lost rapidly when it appears that an agency has not responded adequately to some threat to public safety, and especially when it appears that earlier knowledge of the threat was concealed: whether that was what *really* happened is another matter; once lost, credibility is difficult to restore and the distrust becomes generalized. On the other hand, a few instances which are seen as panicky over-reactions, leading to unnecessary scares and fears, may be sufficient to damage the credibility of an agency in the opposite sense: it is seen as over-protective, fussy and not to be taken seriously. Regulatory responses should be visibly in proportion to the seriousness of the issues concerned, yet both types of mis-perception (that the agency underplays real threats; that the agency is responsible for unnecessary scares) may result from poor risk communication. It is important to recognize that risk assessment is an immature science and that risk communication is an undeveloped art. However, there is no doubt that several improvements can be introduced to improve clarity and reduce misunderstanding. One is attention to the language of risk (Calman, 1996). The other is a simple risk scale, as discussed earlier in this chapter.

As regulatory agencies do not operate in isolation, they are influenced by the cultures within which they exist, including the political forces affecting the governments for which they act as agents. Many different interests exert political pressures, all of which are reflected by the media. There are lobbies which urge that levels of protection for consumers, the environment, patients, etc., should be more thorough. There are lobbies which demand that regulatory burdens on industry should be lighter. All these, of course, have legitimate expectations and agencies must endeavour to conduct regulatory affairs with impartiality and firmness. Moreover, agencies must steer this steadfast course in the face of arguments which are are often emotive and, while appearing to be scientific, are sometimes little more than assertions with limited objective or verifiable foundation.

The effectiveness of an agency is influenced by the political climate. Two primary needs depend upon the political environment: first, appropriate legislation to provide the powers needed by the agency; second, the political will and resources needed for the effective implementation and enforcement of the legislation. Given these primary requirements, it is for the agency to win its reputation for scientific competence, regulatory fairness and public credibility in regulatory affairs.

REFERENCES

Alder, S. and Zbinden, G. (1988). *National and International Drug Safety Guidelines*. MTC Verlag Zollikon, Zollikon.

Anon. (1996). Editorial. *Lancet*, **348**, 1529.

Asai, K. (1980). *Miracle Cure: Organic Germanium*, 1st edn. Japan Publications, ISBN 0 87040 474 1. Distributed by International Book Distributors Hemel Hempstead.

Berggren, L. and Hanssen O. (1966). Treating acrodermatitis enteropathica. *Lancet*, **i**, 52.

British Medical Association (1990). *The BMA Guide to Living with Risk*. Penguin, London.

Calman, K. C. (1996). Cancer: science and society and the communication of risk. *Br. Med. J.*, **313**, 799–802.

Correa, C. M. (1996). *The Uruguay Round and Drugs*. WHO Task Force on Health Economics: Action Programme on Essential Drugs. WHO, Geneva.

Cremer, J. E. and Aldridge, N. (1964) Toxicological and biochemical studies on some tri-alkyl-germanium compounds. *Br. J. Ind. Med.*, **21**, 214–217.

Department of Health (1991). *Committee on Carcinogenicity of Chemicals in Food, Consumer Products and the Environment: Guidelines for the Evaluation of Chemicals for Carcinogenicity*. Department of Health Report on Health and Social Subjects, No. 42. HMSO, London.

Diggle, G. E. (1995). The toxic oil syndrome: a continuing challenge. *Adverse Drug React. Toxicol. Rev.*, **14**, 11–35.

Dluzniewski, A. (1985). Die teratogenen Eigenschaften von Sanugerman in Ratten. In Lekim, D. and Samochowiec, L. (Eds), *Germanium in Biologischen Systemen: Benicht der Ersten Internationalen Tagung über Germanium, Gehalten in Hannover am 12 und 13 Oktober, 1984*. Semmelweis-Verlag, Hannover, pp. 115–128.

EC (1991). Council Directive of 15th July 1991 Concerning the Placing of Plant Protection Products on the Market. *Off. J. Eur. Commun.*, **230**, 1–31.

ECETOC (1985). *Recommendations for the Harmonisation of International Guidelines for Toxicity Studies*. Monograph No. 7. European Chemical Industry Ecology and Toxicology Centre, Brussels.

Ekstrom, G. and Kidd, H. (Eds) (1989). *World Directory of Pesticide Control Organisations*, 1st edn. Royal Society of Chemistry, Cambridge.

Gholz, L. M. and Arons, W. L. (1964). Prophylaxis and therapy of amoebiasis and shigellosis: iodochlorhydroxyquine. *Am. J. Trop. Med. Hyg.*, **13**, 396–401.

Goodman, S. (1988). *Germanium: the Health and Life Enhancer*. Thorsons, Wellingborough, England.

Griffin, J. P. (1977). The seven deadly sins: a UK view. In *Quality Control in Toxicology*. MTP Press, Lancaster.

Hangartner, P. (1980). Clinical study of clioquinol intoxication in dogs and cats. In Soda, T. (Ed.), *Drug-induced Sufferings*. Excerpta Medica, Amsterdam, pp. 459–463.

James, J. S. (Ed.) (1986). *Stroud's Judicial Dictionary*, 5th edn. Sweet and Maxwell, London.

KICADIS (1979). *Decision of the Tokyo District Court on 3 August 1978 Regarding SMON Patients vs. the State, Ciba-Geigy (Japan) Ltd, Takeda Chemical Industries Ltd, Tanabe Seiyaku Co. Ltd, et al*. Organizing Committee of the Kyoto International Conference Against Drug-induced Sufferings (KICADIS), Tokyo.

Kono, R. (1975). Introductory review of SMON and its studies done by the SMON Research Commission. *Jpn. J. Med. Sci. Biol.*, **28**, Suppl. 1–21.

Krewski, D., Gaylor, D. W., Soms, A. P. and Szyszkowicz, M. (1993a). Correlation between carcinogenic potency and maximum tolerated dose: implications for risk assessment. In

Issues in Risk Assessment. National Academy Press, Washington, DC.

Krewski, D., Gaylor D. W., Soms, A. P. and Szyszkowicz, M. (1993b). An overview of the report: Correlation Between Carcinogenic Potency and Maximum Tolerated Dose: Implications for Risk Assessment. *Risk Anal.*, **13**, 383–397.

Lekim, D. and Samochowiec, L. (Eds) (1985). *Germanium in Biologischen Systemen: Bericht der Ersten Internationalen Tagung über Germanium, Gehalten in Hannover am 12 und 13 Oktober, 1984.* Semmelweis-Verlag, Hannover.

Lovell, D. P. and Thomas, G. (1996). Quantitative risk assessment and the limitations of the linearised multistage model. *Hum. Exp. Toxicol.*, **15**, 87–104.

Lye, C. M., Frid, C. L. J., Gill M. E. and McCormick, D. (1997). Abnormalities in the reproductive health of the flounder *Platichthys flesus* exposed to effluent from sewerage treatment works. *Mar. Pollut. Bull.*, **34**, 34–41.

Macklis, R. M. (1990). Radiothor and the era of mild radium therapy. *J. Am. Med. Assoc.*, **264**, 614–618.

Mann, R. D. (1986). Drug-induced disorders of CNS function In Griffin, J. P. and D'Arcy, P. F. (Eds), *Iatrogenic Diseases*, 3rd edn. Oxford University Press, Oxford, pp. 604–612.

Matsusaka, T., Fujii, M., Nakano, T., Terai, T., Kurata, A., Imaizumi, M. and Abe, H. (1988). Germanium-induced nephropathy: report of two cases and review of the literature. *Clin. Nephrol.*, **30**, 341–345.

McDonald, A. L., Fielder, R. J., Diggle, G. E., Tennant, D. R. and Fisher, C. E. (1996). Carcinogens in food: priorities for regulatory action. *Hum. Exp. Toxicol.*, **15**, 739–746.

Metcalf, R. L. (1972). Development of selective and biodegradable pesticides. In *Pest Control Strategies for the Future.* National Research Council, Washington, DC.

Nagata, N., Yoneyama, T., Yanagida, K., Ushio, K., Yanagihara, S., Matsubara, O. and Eishi, Y. (1985). Accumulation of germanium in the tissues of a long-term user of germanium preparation who died of acute renal failure. *J. Toxicol. Sci.*, **10**, 333–341.

National Research Council (1983). Committee on the Institutional Means for Assessment of Risks to Public Health. *Risk assessment in the Federal Government: Managing the Process.* National Academy Press, Washington, DC.

Nordic Council on Medicines (1986). *Evaluation Reports on Propriety Medicinal Products.* NLL Publication 17, 1st edn., Nordic Council on Medicines, Uppsala.

Nordisk Ministerrad (1988). *The Nordic Programme of Cooperation in the Field of Foodstuffs.* Nordisk Ministerrad, Copenhagen.

Obara, K., Akiyu, N., Sato, H., Saito, T., Miura, Y., Yoshinaga, M., Tada, K., Tsukamoto, T. and Hongo, M. (1988). Two cases with various symptoms and renal dysfunction induced by long-term germanium intake. *J. Jpn. Soc. Intern. Med.*, **77** (11), 68–73.

OECD (1981). *Decision of the OECD Council Concerning the Mutual Acceptance of Data in the Assessment of Chemicals.* C-81-30-final OECD, Paris.

Osler, W. (1894). Quoted in: Laurence, D. R. and Bennett, P. N. (1987). *Clinical Pharmacology*, 6th edn. Churchill Livingstone, London, p. 11.

Park, C. N. and Hawkins, N. C. (1995). Cancer risk assessment. In Cralley, L. J., Cralley, L. V. and Bus, J. S. (Eds), *Patty's Industrial Hygiene and Toxicology*, 3rd edn, Vol. 3, Part B. Wiley, New York, pp. 275–318.

Paulos, J. A. (1990). *Innumeracy.* Penguin, London.

Rose, E. C. and Gawel, M. (1984). *Clioquinol neurotoxicity: an overview. Acta Neurol. Scand.*, **70**, Suppl. 100, 137–145.

Sanai, T., Okuda, S., Onoyama, K., Oochi, N., Oh, Y., Kobayashi, K., Shimamatsu, K., Fujimi, S. and Fujishima, M. (1990a) Germanium dioxide-induced nephropathy: a new type of renal disease. *Nephron*, **54**, 53–60.

Sanai, T., Oochi, N., Okuda, S., Osato, S., Kiyama, S., Komota, T., Onoyama, K. and Fujishima, M. (1990b) Subacute nephrotoxicity of germanium dioxide in the experimental animal. *Toxicol. Appl. Pharmacol.*, **103**, 345–353.

Saunders, J. B. (Ed.) (1988). *Words and Phrases Legally Defined*, 3rd edn. Butterworths, London.

Scales, M. D. C. and Mahoney, K. (1991). Animal toxicology studies on new medicines and their relationship to clinical exposure: a review of international recommendations. *Adverse Drug React. Toxicol. Rev.*, **10**, 155–168.

Schantz, B. and Wikstrom, B. (1965). Suspected poisoning with oxychinoline preparation in dogs. *Svensk. Vet. Tidn.*, **17**, 106.

Schroeder, H. A. and Balassa, J. J. (1967) Abnormal trace metals in man; germanium. *J. Chron. Dis.*, **20**, 211–224.

Secretary of Agriculture (1937). Report of the Secretary of Agriculture submitted in response to resolutions in the House of Representatives and Senate. *J. Am. Med. Assoc.*, **109**, 1985*ff*.

Shah, I. (1988). *The natives are Restless.* Octagon Press, London.

Tateshi, J. (1980). Reproduction of experimental SMON in animals by oral administration of clioquinol. In Soda, T. (Ed.), *Drug-induced Sufferings.* Excerpta Medica, Amsterdam, pp. 464–469.

Tsubaki, T., Honma, Y. and Hoshi, M. (1971). Neurological syndrome associated with clioquinol. *Lancet*, **i**, 696–697.

Vonier, P. M., Crain, D. A., McLeachlan, J. A., Guilette, L. J. and Arnold, S. F. (1996). Interaction of environmental chemicals with the estrogen and progesterone receptors from the oviduct of the American alligator. *Environ. Health Perspect.*, **104**, 1318–1322.

Walker, S. R., Lumley, C. E. and McAuslane, J. A. N. (Eds) (1994). *The Relevance of Ethnic Factors in the Clinical Evaluation of Medicines.* Kluwer, Dordrecht.

Yawata, M. (1993). Deaths due to drug interaction. *Lancet*, **342**, 1166.

Chapter 72

Regulation of Industrial Chemicals in the USA and the European Union*

C. M. Auer and R. J. Fielder

CONTENTS

INTRODUCTION

This chapter focuses on the regulation of industrial chemicals, first by the US Environmental Protection Agency (US EPA) and second in the European Union (EU). The harmonization of the laws and regulations of industrial chemicals of the numerous states and legal jurisdictions of the EU has been necessarily a complicated process, for which reason this chapter cites a great number of European Directives. On the other hand, the legal framework for chemicals regulation in the USA involves national (federal) regulation, with only limited instances of state legislation and is therefore simpler. However, the objective in both the USA and the EU has been basically the same, namely to ensure the protection of the general public, workers and the environment from toxic chemicals.

CHEMICAL REGULATION IN THE USA

The fundamental piece of legislation governing the regulation of industrial chemical in the USA is the Toxic Substances Control Act (TSCA) (USA, 1976). However, certain major non-TSCA industrial chemical federal regulatory programs and voluntary initiatives are also relevant and are discussed below.

By enacting TSCA, the US Congress established a number of new requirements and authorities for identifying and controlling existing and potential

* The views expressed in this chapter are those of the authors and do not commit any government department or agency

toxic chemical risks to human health and the environment. Programmes now exist within the US EPA under TSCA to gather information about the toxicity of chemicals and the extent to which people and the environment are exposed to them, to assess whether they cause unreasonable risks to humans and the environment and to institute appropriate control actions after weighing their potential risks against their benefits to the economic and social well being of the USA. The TSCA programmes are implemented by the US EPA's Office of Pollution Prevention and Toxics.

Generally, TSCA gives the US EPA authority to gather certain kinds of basic data relevant to determining chemical risks from those who manufacture and process chemicals. The law also enables the US EPA to require companies to test chemicals for toxic effects and requires the agency to review most new chemicals before they are manufactured commercially. To prevent unreasonable risks, the US EPA may select from a broad range of control actions under TSCA, from requiring hazard-warning labels to outright bans on manufacture and/or use. The US EPA may regulate a chemical's risks at any stage of its life cycle: at manufacture, processing, distribution in commerce, use or disposal.

TSCA coverage does not extend to the following product categories, which are excluded from TSCA authority: tobacco, nuclear materials, munitions, food additives, drugs, cosmetics and substances used solely as pesticides. These substances fall under the jurisdiction of other federal laws and are reviewed by other federal programmes.

NEW CHEMICALS REGULATORY PROGRAM

Section 5 of TSCA provides the US EPA with the authority to regulate new chemical substances prior to their commercial manufacture. Anyone who plans to manufacture or import a new chemical substance for a commercial purpose is required to provide the US EPA with a pre-manufacture notice (PMN) at least 90 days prior to the activity.

Section 5 of TSCA gives the US EPA the role of gatekeeper between the laboratory and the commercial marketplace. The New Chemicals Program reviews the PMN to determine whether the manufacture, processing, distribution in commerce, use or disposal of the substance 'may present an unreasonable risk' to human health or the environment, or cause exposures of concern. The Program's assessment includes exposures and risks to workers, consumers and the general population (for example, from drinking water or fish consumption), as well as risks to wildlife, including endangered species. From its inception in 1979, the Program has reviewed over 30 000 new chemical notices and taken action to control or require testing on approximately 10% of those chemicals.

Information Required in a PMN

PMN submissions require all available data on chemical identify, production volume, byproducts, use, environmental release, disposal practices and human exposure. The submitter is also required to provide all existing health and environmental data in the possession of the submitter.

Exemptions from PMN Reporting

Some new chemical substances are not subject to PMN reporting. These substances are either exempt from TSCA, or the US EPA has determined that they do not warrant review or require only a short review. The following are excluded from PMN reporting under certain conditions: products of incidental reactions, products of end-use reactions, mixtures, by-products, substances manufactured solely for export, non-isolated intermediates and substances formed during the manufacture of an article.

The US EPA has more limited PMN reporting requirements for new chemical substances in the following cases:

- The substance is manufactured in small quantities for research and development;
- 10 000 kg or less of the substance will be manufactured or imported each year;
- The substance is expected to have low releases and low exposures;
- The substance is being manufactured or imported for test marketing; or
- The substance is a polymer that meets certain specified criteria where the substance is not considered chemically active or bioavailable.

Evaluation of the New Chemical Substance

EPA toxicologists, chemists, biochemists, engineers and experts in other disciplines work together to assess the potential risks to humans or the environment from each new substance. In doing so, they draw on data submitted with the PMN form, other information available to the Agency and exposure and release modelling. TSCA does not require prior testing of new chemicals. A limited amount of toxicity data is typically submitted with PMNs, although approximately 50% of submissions contain no test data. Thus, the US EPA bases its health and environmental toxicity review of new substances primarily on structure–activity relationships (SARs) (Auer et al., 1994; Zeeman et al., 1995). The review of each chemical substance in a PMN submission can be characterized as a review of the life cycle of the chemical, including manufacture, processing, use, worker exposure, environmental release and disposal.

Potential Regulatory Outcomes of the PMN Review

Almost 90% of the PMNs submitted to the Program complete the review process without being restricted or regulated in any way; 10% of the PMNs, however, are regulated by the US EPA, (under a Section 5(e) consent order or by a Significant New Use Rule (SNUR)), or are voluntarily withdrawn by the submitter often in the face of pending regulation.

During PMN review, the US EPA may determine that 'the information available . . . is insufficient to permit a reasoned evaluation' of the new chemical substance that is the subject of the PMN. At the same time, the US EPA may determine, based on SAR analysis (or data submitted with the PMN), that activities involving the new substance 'may present an unreasonable risk of injury to health or the environment' (referred to as a risk-based finding). When the US EPA makes these two findings, it acts under Section 5(e) of TSCA to regulate the new substance. In the most such circumstances, the US EPA believes that it is appropriate to negotiate an order (known as a 'consent order') under Section 5(e) with the PMN submitter to control human exposure and/or environmental releases until test data or other information sufficient to assess the potential risks adequately become available. Section 5(e) consent orders have specified a variety of control measures, including protective equipment, use limitations, process restrictions, labelling requirements and limits on environmental release. Some consent orders include testing requirements that are triggered and must be met when specified levels of production volume or other indices of increased exposure are reached.

In other instances, the US EPA may determine that a new substance will be produced in substantial quantities (currently set at 100 000 kg year^{-1}) and there is or may be significant or substantial human or environmental exposure to the substance (referred to as an exposure-based finding) and that the available information is insufficient to determine the effects of the substance. Consent orders issued to address exposure-based concerns include testing requirements, record keeping provisions and production volume limits. The testing is similar to the Minimum Pre-market Dataset (MPD) used in the EU, although in many cases certain of the tests will not be required by the US EPA.

Section 5(e) orders apply only to the submitter of the PMN. When a PMN submitter commences commercial manufacture of the substance and submits a Notice of Commencement of Manufacture to the US EPA, the US EPA adds the substance to the TSCA Chemical Substance Inventory maintained pursuant to Section 8(b) of TSCA. When a substance is listed in the Inventory, it is no longer a 'new chemical substance' for which a PMN would be required under Section 5(a)(1)(A). Thus, other persons are able to manufacture, import or process the substance without the US EPA review and without the restrictions imposed on the PMN submitter by the Section 5(e) order.

Under TSCA Section 5(a)(2), the US EPA may determine that a use of a chemical substance is a 'significant new use'. The US EPA must make this determination by issuing a Significant New Use Rule (SNUR), after which TSCA requires persons to submit a significant new use notice (SNUN) to the US EPA at least 90 days before they manufacture, import or process the chemical substance for that use. The US EPA may take regulatory action under TSCA to control the activities for which it has received a SNUN before they begin, if appropriate. The US EPA can use its SNUR authority to extend limitations in Section 5(e) orders to other manufacturers, importers and processors of the PMN chemical. These SNURs are framed so that non-compliance with the control measures or other restrictions in the Section 5(e) consent orders is defined as a 'significant new use'. Thus, other manufacturers, importers and processors of the substances must either observe the SNUR restrictions or submit a SNUN to the US EPA at least 90 days before initiating activities that deviate from the restrictions.

Accomplishments

Since 1979, the US EPA has reviewed over 30 000 new chemical substances. This figure includes over 25 000 PMNs that have undergone full review and approximately 7000 low-volume, test-market and polymer exemptions (**Table 1**). In that time, the agency has taken

Table 1 Chemical substances renewed by the US EPA since 1979

Type of submission	No. submitted
Pre-manufacture notices	25547
Low-volume exemptions	3999
Test-market exemptions	636
Polymer exemptions	2334
Total	32516

action to prevent potential risks to people and the environment on nearly 3000 new substances.

Pollution Prevention in the New Chemicals Program

By assessing new chemical substances before they are manufactured or imported, the New Chemicals Program is actively carrying out the US EPA's strategy to prevent pollution before it can occur. In addition to its role as a 'gatekeeper', the US EPA also acts as a guide or advocate for safer or less polluting new chemicals. This aspect of the New Chemicals Program supports the development of safer chemical substances by minimizing or eliminating regulatory burdens on new chemicals if they represent an improvement compared with riskier substances already in the marketplace.

The New Chemicals Program strongly encourages industry efforts to prevent pollution and reduce risk through innovation. One of the ways this is accomplished is through the PMN form, which requests industry to provide voluntarily information about steps taken to reduce exposures to or releases of chemical substances. During the PMN review, the US EPA carefully considers this information in evaluating potential risks. A guidance document on how to report pollution prevention activities is included as an attachment to the PMN Instruction Manual. The US EPA also has programmes to recognize publicly new chemicals that demonstrate significant pollution prevention improvements; this is known as the 'Pollution Prevention Recognition Program'.

EU/US Structure–Activity Relationship/ Minimum Pre-marketing Data Set Study (SAR/MPD Study)

As noted above, the US EPA does not receive any test data with most PMNs. When data are submitted, they often do not go beyond acute toxicity end-points. (Quantitative) structure–activity relationships or (Q)SARs are the technique, that the US EPA uses to carry out preliminary hazard/risk assessments of new chemicals in the absence of test data. These (Q)SARs are predictive methods which estimate the properties of a chemical, e.g. melting point, vapour pressure, toxicity and ecotoxicity, on the basis of its structure and test data on analogous chemicals. Based on the recommendation of a 1989 OECD workshop on new chemical notification systems, a joint USA/EU study was initiated to evaluate the predictive power of (Q) SARs by applying (Q) SAR methods to chemicals for which minimum pre-marketing data sets (MPD) were already available in the EU and then comparing the properties predicted by (Q) SAR with the properties observed from MPD testing (OECD, 1994). Analysis of the results of this study showed that while this SAR approach has largely been successful in identifying chemicals of concern, the process could be improved by selectively incorporating specific testing schemes into the process. Results from such schemes would serve two purposes: to gain insight into chemical toxicities and to improve predictive capabilities. Improving predictive capabilities would result in better hazard assessment for new chemicals by providing a richer data base upon which to base predictions as to their fate and effects. These enhanced capabilities would also serve to avoid questionable testing requirements and thus spare manufacturers the cost of such testing while not compromising worker, consumer or environmental safety. Such a focused effort would provide valuable data while not presenting large overall cost implications.

Biotechnology—New Microorganisms

TSCA defines 'chemical substance' broadly and in terms which cover microorganisms in addition to traditional chemicals. Examples of microorganisms that are subject to TSCA are those that are used in the industrial production of enzymes and other specialty chemicals, as biofertilizers and in bioremediation. Microorganisms are regulated under specific regulations (USA, 1997b) under the Toxic Substances Control Act. The rule established notification procedures for review of certain new microorganisms before they are introduced into commerce. 'New' microorganisms are those formed by deliberate combinations of genetic material from organisms classified in different taxonomic genera; these microorganisms are termed 'intergeneric'. The rule implements the application of TSCA Section 5 to microorganisms.

New microorganisms that are manufactured for commercial purposes are subject to TSCA Section 5 reporting requirements. A commercial activity is one that is undertaken with the purpose of obtaining an immediate or eventual commercial advantage. This definition extends to some research and development activities. Similar to the filing of a PMN, any manufacturer, processor or importer of a new viable microorganism must file a Microbial Commercial Activity Notice (MCAN) with the US EPA 90 days before commencing the activity. The US EPA can take control action where warranted using the authorities described above.

There are a number of exemptions to the requirements to submit a MCAN:

(1) Non-commercial R&D uses of microorganisms.
(2) Contained R&D activities subject to the jurisdiction of other federal programmes or agencies.
(3) R&D activities conducted under contained conditions when certain conditions are met.
(4) TSCA Experimental Release Application (TERA). Rather than submitting a MCAN for research and development activities that are not exempted, manufacturers may submit a TERA.
(5) Test marketing of new microorganisms.
(6) Tier I exemption. Intergeneric constructs of certain microorganisms are not subject to MCAN reporting if exemption criteria (including limitations on introduced genetic material and containment and control technologies) are met.
(7) Tier II exemption. Persons who intend to manufacture new microorganisms that meet the Tier I exemption criteria except for the specific containment and control technologies may submit a Tier II exemption request. The request must include information on production volume and process and containment procedures.

Chemical Testing Program

Section 2 of TSCA states that 'It is the policy of the United States that adequate data be developed with respect to the effect of chemical substances and mixtures on health and the environment and that development of such data be the responsibility of those who manufacture [and import] and those who process such chemicals and mixtures'. Section 4 of TSCA provides to the US EPA the authority to issue rules to require chemical producers, importers and processors to conduct specified testing for health and environmental effects as well as chemical fate and exposure.

Approach

The statutory 'findings' that the US EPA must make in order to require chemical testing under a TSCA Section 4 Test Rule are:

■ A chemical may present an unreasonable risk (known as a risk finding) [TSCA Section 4(a) (1) (A) (I)]; *and/or*
■ A chemical is or will be produced in substantial quantities, and it enters or may be expected to enter the environment in substantial quantities, *or* there is or may be substantial or significant human exposure to such substance (known as the exposure finding) [TSCA Section 4 (a) (1) (B) (I)]; *and*

■ Existing data are inadequate [TSCA Section 4 (a) (1) (A) (ii) or (B) (ii)]; *and*

■ Testing is necessary [TSCA Section 4 (a) (1) (A) (iii) or (B) (iii)].

As a result of litigation in the 1980s, the US EPA, industry and environmental NGOs developed an alternative to the TSCA Section 4 rule-making process. This alternative involves the negotiation of formal TSCA Section 4 'Enforceable Consent Agreements' (ECAs). The ECA process provides for and encourages public participation in the development of ECAs.

The US EPA also looks to voluntary industry testing initiatives to supplement its TSCA Chemical Testing Program. A primary example of such a voluntary initiative is the 'Screening Information Data Set' (SIDS) Program, an important programme focused on the testing of international high production volume (HPV) chemicals. The programme is operated under the auspices of the Organization for Economic Cooperation and Development (OECD).

Product Stewardship Agreements between the US EPA and industry incorporating testing and other risk management provisions are additional mechanisms used by the Agency. A noteworthy example of this approach is a 'Memorandum of Understanding' (MOU) between the US EPA and the Dow Corning Corporation. Under this MOU, Dow Corning agreed to develop and implement a comprehensive product stewardship and toxicity/exposure testing programme for six siloxanes, all of which are key materials in the silicone industry. It is estimated that the voluntary toxicity testing programme alone will cost in excess of US$30 000 000 and will take more than 6 years to complete.

Master Testing List

In the early 1990s, the US EPA also developed a Master Testing List (MTL) to establish clearly the agenda and priorities for the TSCA Chemical Testing Program. The MTL serves as the corner-stone of the US EPA's TSCA Chemical Testing Program policy by presenting the 'universe' of chemicals that deserve the highest consideration and have the greatest need for testing. Since its initial release in 1992, all of the US EPA's TSCA testing actions have come from the MTL.

The MTL is used to establish the US EPA's TSCA Chemical Testing Program agenda and priorities by:

■ Identifying the chemical testing *needs* of the Federal Government and international programmes of interest to the USA (e.g., the OECD's 'Screening Information Data Set' (SIDS) programme);

■ Focusing the US EPA's resources on the highest priority chemical testing needs, especially those for US HPV chemicals (i.e. those produced and/or imported in amounts greater than 500 tons per year);

■ Publicizing the US EPA's chemical testing priorities;

■ Obtaining broad public input; and

■ Encouraging voluntary industry initiatives to conduct needed testing.

Results

Thus, the US EPA relies on a mix of TSCA Section 4 test rules, enforceable consent agreements/orders and voluntary testing agreements. Together, these tools add flexibility to the US EPA's TSCA Chemical Testing Program; one mechanism may be used if the Agency encounters impediments to testing under another. Since 1979, approximately 550 chemicals have been the subject of final testing actions. Virtually all of the actions taken to date have involved US HPV chemicals and more than 50% of the testing actions taken to date have been developed since 1990.

Today's TSCA Chemical Testing Program is best characterized by the following:

■ The US EPA has established and maintains a clear testing agenda via use of the Master Testing List which presents a consolidated list of priority high production volume industrial chemica testing needs of the US EPA and other federal agencies.

■ More chemical testing is being conducted—if one projects out to the year 2000, the second decade pace of testing activity is expected to be two and possibly three times that of the first decade.

■ The US EPA will continue to use a mix of testing actions (TSCA Section 4 Test Rules, TSCA Section 4 Enforceable Consent Agreements/Orders and Voluntary Testing Agreements).

■ The US EPA's continued use of TSCA Section 4 Enforceable Consent Agreements and Voluntary Testing Agreements offers an increased role for voluntary pollution prevention and risk reduction measures as an offset to some testing.

■ International efforts such as the voluntary OECD/SIDS testing programme will continue to play an integral role in the US EPA's TSCA Chemical Testing Program. The US EPA will continue to encourage US industry participation in this very important international cooperative effort.

■ There appears to be a continuing willingness on the part of many US chemical companies to conduct needed toxicological testing on the substances that they produce, import and process and to establish voluntary product stewardship programmes for those chemicals.

■ The US EPA is working hard to improve public access to testing data and other information submitted under TSCA [e.g. TSCA Section 8(d) health and safety data submissions and TSCA Section 8 (e) substantial risk information notices].

Other recent developments related to the Chemical Testing Program are discussed in the section on Existing Chemicals.

TSCA Information Gathering Authorities

TSCA Section 8 record keeping and data gathering authorities provide access to data that the US EPA and others need to identify, assess, manage and reduce actual or potential risks posed by exposure to chemical substances.

- Section 8(a) allows the US EPA to require chemical manufacturers, importers and processors of chemical substances to maintain records and/or report data on a wide range of subjects, including chemical identity, trade names, molecular structure, categories of use, quantity manufactured or processed, individuals exposed and methods of disposal.
- Section 8 (c) regulations require chemical manufacturers, importers and certain processors of chemical substances and mixtures to keep records concerning 'allegations of significant adverse reactions' and report them to the US EPA if needed.
- Section 8 (d) allows the US EPA to require chemical manufacturers, importers and processors to submit lists and/or copies of ongoing and completed health and safety studies.
- Section 8 (e) requires persons who manufacture, process or distribute in commerce a chemical substance or mixture and who obtain information which reasonably supports the conclusion that such substance or mixture presents a substantial risk of injury to health or the environment to inform the US EPA immediately of such information unless such persons have actual knowledge that the US EPA has been adequately informed of such information.

EXISTING CHEMICALS PROGRAM

The Existing Chemicals Program develops and evaluates strategies for preventing pollution and reducing the risks associated with chemicals currently in production or use.

Approach

A chemical generally enters the US EPA Existing Chemicals Program when it is selected for a screening level assessment known as Risk Management One (RM1). The primary purpose of RM1 is to determine which chemicals are likely to present unreasonable risks to

human health or the environment, to spend a minimal amount of resources doing so and to make the results of the assessment available to the public. An RM1 assessment:

- Contains basic information on uses, hazards, and exposures;
- Relies on readily available data;
- Generally is completed in about 1 month.

At the end of RM1, a management decision is made either to drop the chemical from further review, recommend testing or proceed to RM2.

RM2 is also a screening level assessment, but is more in-depth than RM1 and is generally focused on specific concerns. The purpose of the RM2 assessment is to improve the understanding of chemical hazards and exposures and to identify feasible risk management paths. An RM2 assessment:

- Contains information on uses, substitutes, and a more detailed analysis of hazards and exposures;
- Uses readily available data and information, but considers the information in greater depth;
- Involves the stakeholders having an interest in the case in locating additional sources of existing information;
- Includes stakeholder briefings;
- Identifies risk management strategies and possible options including pollution prevention opportunities;
- Identifies key data gaps;
- Generally is completed in about 6 months.

At the end of RM2, a management decision is made either to drop the chemical from further review, gather more information to fill in the data gaps or pursue one or more of the risk management strategies identified in the assessment.

In post-RM2, a specific risk management strategy is considered in-depth. Risk management options are developed, selected and implemented. The nature of post-RM2 activities varies greatly, depending on the strategy selected. If a decision is made to seek voluntary action by industry, initiate a public awareness campaign or implement other non-regulatory strategies, the US EPA will continue to involve stakeholders and will publically report on the outcomes.

If a regulatory path is followed, an in-depth analysis is performed to supplement the findings from RM2. Data gaps may be addressed through collecting data from primary sources or requiring testing under Section 4. Stakeholder involvement is much greater and procedural rules for regulation development must be followed.

Actions to control chemical risk can be taken under TSCA Section 6 where the US EPA makes a finding of 'unreasonable risk' to health or the environment. Section

6 requires that the US EPA weighs various factors in making this determination, including health and environmental effects, exposures, benefits, availability of substitutes and economic impacts. The US EPA is also required to chose the least burdensome approach to address risks adequately. This process, in practice, has proven to be difficult and resource intensive. Owing in part to the limitations in Section 6, the Existing Chemicals Program has increasingly used voluntary measures to promote pollution prevention and reduce risk.

Examples of Existing Chemical Programme Activities

Acrylamide

Acrylamide is a known human neurotoxicant and has been classified by the US EPA as a probable human carcinogen. The people at risk, approximately 1000 grouting workers, face very high individual neurotoxic and cancer risks. Acrylamide grouts are used primarily to seal leaks in sewers and manholes.

Neurotoxic margins of exposure for these workers are less than 10, and the estimated individual risk of cancer is somewhat greater than 1 in every 100 workers engaged in sewer grouting and 4 in every 100 engaged in manhole grouting. Based upon the US EPA's investigation, which concluded that the unavoidable exposures associated with grouting work precluded any solution short of a ban, the Agency proposed a rule under TSCA Section 6 that would ban all uses of acrylamide grout. The proposed rule would also ban N-methylolacrylamide (NMA) grouts 3 years following promulgation. NMA, a derivative of acrylamide, produces the same health effects, but with an order of magnitude less potency. The US EPA expected to finalize the rule in late-1999.

Benzidine-based Dyes

Benzidine is classified by the US EPA as a known human carcinogen. Further, studies have demonstrated that benzidine-based dyes are highly potent carcinogens. The US EPA believes that benzidine and benzidine-based dyes may present a risk of bladder cancer to humans in occupational and other settings.

The US EPA completed an RM1 analysis which confirmed its initial cancer and other health concerns. In RM2, the US EPA successfully took steps to persuade the few remaining distributors or importers to stop selling benzidine-based dyes in the USA. Additionally, the US EPA has been negotiating with industry to reduce or eliminate the risks associated with certain benzidine congener dyes (o-tolidine and non-metallized o-dianisidine). Product stewardship programmes developed by two companies making several of these dyes were accepted. The agreements include exposure controls, medical monitoring, customer product stewardship programmes and product phase-outs.

As a regulatory measure to ensure that the US EPA has an opportunity to review and take action before any new use of benzidine-based dyes occurs again, the US EPA issued a Significant New Use Rule (SNUR) under TSCA Section 5. This rule requires notification to the US EPA prior to commercial manufacture, import or processing of benzidine-based dyes. After reviewing any SNUR notice, the US EPA may take additional regulatory action to regulate the substance, if appropriate.

Chemical Hazard Data Availability Study

In an Earth Day 1998 announcement, US Vice President Gore and US EPA Administrator Browner committed the US EPA to testing initiatives aimed at strengthening the public's right and ability to know about the potential health and environmental risks from existing HPV chemicals. The US EPA will be increasing critical testing for 3000 HPV chemicals and pursuing new rules to guarantee that the chemicals children are exposed to are fully tested for their health effects. These initiatives build on OPPT's existing right-to-know and TSCA programmes.

The announcement on the testing of HPV chemicals is a direct result of the US EPA's recent analysis of the public availability of basic testing and screening information on chemicals produced or imported at more than 500 tons/year. In the US EPA's Chemical Hazard Data Availability Study, the US EPA researched public information sources for data contained in the internationally agreed-upon Screening and Information Data Set (SIDS), considered the minimum set of tests that can allow an informed screening-level evaluation of a chemical's hazards.

The study found that of the 3000 US HPV chemicals, a full set of SIDS testing was publicly available for only 7% of them and that no SIDS data were available for 43%. The report also considers specific subsets of chemicals including the US EPA's Toxic Release Inventory-listed Chemicals, those with occupational exposure standards and consumer chemicals, and examines the proportion of SIDS data end-points available for US HPV chemicals for each manufacturer/importer of the chemicals.

The US EPA is taking action to secure these data so that individuals and communities can evaluate better the chemical hazards and risks they face. Because of Vice President Gore's initiative, the USA will expect to complete SIDS testing and assessment on all US HPV chemicals by early in the next century. It is also hoped that the US action will spur other countries to step up their rate of testing. Implementation plans include both a voluntary programme and the promulgation of test rules to accomplish the goal.

The children's testing initiative will focus on consumer chemicals and chemicals with large environmental releases. Testing will be required by a forthcoming TSCA Section 4 test rule. Testing requirements have not been defined but will probably involve confirmatory testing, including a two-generation reproductive effects study, two-species developmental toxicity testing and subchronic toxicity testing.

Common Sense Initiative

The Common Sense Initiative (CSI) is a government reinvention activity begun by the Agency in 1995. An innovative approach to environmental protection and pollution prevention, CSI addresses environmental management by industrial sector rather than by environmental medium (air, water, land). The CSI goal is to find 'cleaner, cheaper, smarter' ways for both industry and government to operate. The US EPA selected six industries to serve as CSI pilots:

Automobile manufacturing
Computer and electronics
Iron and steel
Metal finishing
Petroleum refining
Printing

These six sectors were chosen because they comprise over 11% of the US gross national product, employ over 4 million people and account for over 12% of the toxic releases reported by American industry. As such, these sectors present excellent opportunities to test and refine CSI concepts, to create environmental solutions that can operate across industries and to expand CSI to other industrial sectors. Since beginning their work in January 1995, the sector subcommittees have initiated nearly 40 projects involving over 150 stakeholders who actively participate in sector subcommittees and subcommittee work groups. Using a consensus approach to decision making, the sector subcommittees address diverse topics such as pollution prevention, environmental reporting requirements and public access to environmental information.

Benefits of the CSI approach are apparent. In addition to producing specific products and tools in each of the sectors, CSI has established a forum for a cooperative dialogue among parties whose previous interactions were predominantly adversarial. By involving all of the interested groups in a consensus-based process, CSI allows for the development of balanced solutions to environmental problems. Change can happen faster and along a wider front with a greater degree of buy-in from very disparate viewpoints.

Polychlorinated Biphenyls (PCBs) Risk Management

In TSCA, PCBs were specifically singled out for both immediate regulation and phased withdrawal from the market. The US EPA may authorize certain uses of PCBs and may exempt, pursuant to certain TSCA Section 6 (e) criteria, specific activities involving manufacture, processing and distribution in commerce of the substances. PCBs are of concern because exposure may cause cancer, developmental, reproductive and other effects and they are known to persist in the environment and bioaccumulate. The US EPA has implemented a broadly based regulatory programme to prohibit or otherwise manage PCB manufacture, import, processing, use, distribution in commerce and disposal.

Exports and Imports

Under TSCA Section 12(b), if a person intends to export a chemical substance which is the subject of certain actions under TSCA (e.g. a test rule, SNUR or Section 6 control action), the person must notify the US EPA. The US EPA is then responsible for notifying the importing country's government of the export, the regulatory action triggering the notification and, in certain cases, the availability of information.

Regarding imports, TSCA Section 13 prohibits the import of chemical substances, mixtures and articles containing substances or mixtures into the USA if the shipment fails to comply with TSCA requirements. Importers are required to certify compliance with TSCA upon a shipment's import. More can be found about TSCA and other US EPA activities on the US EPA's Internet home page on the World Wide Web at http://www.epa.gov.

Occupational and Consumer Protection

Worker Protection

In the USA, federal and state governments work in partnership with 6.5 million employers and over 100 million working men and women to protect their health and safety. The Occupational Safety and Health Act of 1970 is the primary worker protection statute in the USA (USA, 1970). The Occupational Safety and Health Administration (OSHA) is the leading federal agency on worker protection issues. The OSHA is in the Department of Labor and is responsible for creating and enforcing workplace safety and health regulations. The OSHA and its state partners have approximately 2100 inspectors, plus complaint discrimination investigators, engineers, physicians, educators, standards writers and other technical and support personnel spread over more than 200 offices throughout the country. Workplace inspections are one of the OSHA's principal activities. The OSHA's most significant work to protect workers from chemical risks is to set permissible exposure limits (PELs) to protect workers against the health effects of exposure to hazardous substances. PELs are regulatory limits on the amount or concentration of a substance in air. They may also may limit skin exposure. PELs are enforceable and are usually based on an 8 h time-weighted average (TWA) exposure.

The OSHA has many other federal government partners in its efforts to protect workers. These partners include the US Environmental Protection Agency (US EPA), the National Institute for Occupational Safety and Health (NIOSH), the Mine Safety and Health Administration (MSHA) and the Department of Transportation (DOT). These partners often have specific and narrowly defined roles in protecting workers and assisting OSHA.

The National Institute for Occupational Safety and Health (NIOSH) is part of the Centers for Disease Control and Prevention (CDC), which is in the Department of Health and Human Services and is responsible for conducting research and making recommendations for the prevention of work-related illnesses and injuries. NIOSH identifies the causes of work-related diseases and injuries and the potential hazards of new work technologies and practices. With this information, NIOSH determines new and effective ways to protect workers from chemicals, machinery and hazardous working conditions. Creating new ways to prevent workplace hazards is the job of NIOSH.

The Mine Safety and Health Administration (MSHA) administers the provisions of the Federal Mine Safety and Health Act of 1977 (Mine Act) and enforces compliance with mandatory safety and health standards as a means to eliminate fatal accidents, to reduce the frequency and severity of non-fatal accidents, to minimize health hazards and to promote improved safety and health conditions in the nation's mines.

The Department of Transportation (DOT) operates many programmes that protect the health and safety of US workers. Most notably, the Office of Hazardous Materials Safety, which is within DOT's Research and Special Programs Administration, is responsible for coordinating a national safety programme for the transportation of hazardous materials by air, rail, highway and water.

Consumer Protection

The US Consumer Product Safety Commission (CPSC) is the leading Federal Agency on consumer protection issues, including risks posed by chemicals. The CPSC is an independent, federal, regulatory agency that was created in 1972 by Congress in the Consumer Product Safety Act. In that law, Congress directed the Commission to 'protect the public against unreasonable risks of injuries and deaths associated with consumer products'.

The CPSC has jurisdiction over about 15 000 types of consumer products, from automatic-drip coffee makers,

through toys to lawn mowers. CPSC has many other federal government partners in its efforts to protect the health and safety of consumers. Some types of products, however, are covered by other federal agencies. For example, cars, trucks and motorcycles are covered by the DOT; drugs and cosmetics are covered by the FDA; and alcohol, tobacco and firearms are within the jurisdiction of the Department of the Treasury. The US Environmental Protection Agency has special responsibilities in protecting consumers from potential chemical risks. It plays an especially significant role in the control of chemical and pesticide risks.

The CPSC works to reduce the risk of injuries and deaths from consumer products by:

- Developing voluntary standards with industry;
- Issuing and enforcing mandatory standards;
- Banning consumer products if no feasible standard would adequately protect the public;
- Obtaining the recall of products or arranging for their repair;
- Conducting research on potential product hazards;
- Informing and educating consumers through the media, state and local governments, private organizations, and by responding to consumer inquiries.

Consumer Labeling Initiative (CLI)

The CLI is a voluntary partnership between the US EPA, other government agencies, companies that make and distribute household hard surface cleaners and pesticides and other stakeholders, including consumer groups. The CLI focuses on consumer needs, helping them find, read and understand labelling information, so they can compare products and use them safely and effectively. The CLI started in 1996. In Phase I, the CLI partners researched ways to improve consumer package labels, solicited consumers' ideas for better labels, reviewed the existing labelling research literature and published a research report and other information about the progress of CLI. In Phase II, the CLI will engage in additional research to assess consumers comprehension, attitudes, behaviour and satisfaction with labelling and evaluate alternatives, research the potential standardization of language and format on labels to facilitate comparisons and location of important information, work to develop new storage and disposal language to facilitate appropriate disposal, identify more understandable first aid statements, identify what types of ingredient information are useful and continue to expand outreach efforts.

Toxic Release Inventory

The US EPA requires annual reports of toxic chemical releases and transfers under Section 313 of the

Emergency Planning and Community Right-to-Know Act (EPCRA). These reports are submitted on the US EPA Form R, the Toxic Release Inventory (TRI) Reporting Form. The reports provide the public with information on the releases of 600 listed toxic chemicals and chemical categories in their communities. Additionally, the information is used by the US EPA in supporting the development of TSCA and other regulations/programmes. Generally, facilities must report the quantities of both routine and accidental releases of listed toxic chemicals, and also the maximum amount of the listed toxic chemical on-site during the calendar year and the amount in wastes transferred off-site.

The TRI database has been used by government, industry and communities to help identify and assess chemical releases better. With this information, communities know what toxic chemicals are present in their neighbourhoods, emergency planners understand what potential threats they must be prepared to handle and facility managers can identify opportunities for source reduction. Based on the principle that people have the 'right to know' this information, the TRI programme has become a model worldwide.

REGULATION OF INDUSTRIAL CHEMICALS IN THE EUROPEAN UNION

There is a strong European dimension to regulatory activity on industrial chemicals in Member States of the EU. The majority of national legislation on chemical safety now relates to the implementation of EU Directives. This is particularly well illustrated with new chemicals, where there is a requirement to notify competent authorities within Member States when such chemicals are placed on the market and to provide adequate data for a risk assessment to be carried out; the latter covers occupational and also, if appropriate, consumer exposure. Another example of a harmonized approach across the EU is the classification and labelling of dangerous substances and preparations (i.e. mixtures of substances). More recently, EU activity has extended to 'old' chemicals already on the market before the notification scheme was established. This is by the Existing Substances Regulation, which required producers or importers of chemicals in the EU to provide data directly to the Commission of the European Communities on compounds produced at levels of 10 tonnes p.a. or more. Detailed risk assessments are being carried out on priority chemicals. In addition, there is increasing activity at the EU level in the field of occupational exposure limits.

This review will concentrate on those areas covered by EU activities, rather than on national legislation in individual Member States, much of which is specifically to implement these Directives. A key Directive in this regard is Directive 67/548/EEC on the approximation of laws, regulations and administrative provisions relating to the classification, packaging and labelling of dangerous substances, commonly referred to as the Dangerous Substances Directive (EEC Council, 1967), and its subsequent amendments.

NEW SUBSTANCES NOTIFICATION

A Notification Scheme for new substances placed on the market in any Member State of the EU has been in operation for many years. This scheme was first introduced by the Sixth Amendment to the Dangerous Substances Directive which was agreed by Member States as Directive 79/831/EEC in 1979 (EEC Council, 1979). This was implemented in the UK by the Notification of New Substances Regulations 1982 made by the Health and Safety Executive (HSE), the agency responsible for all matters relating to occupational health and safety. The competent authority in the UK is the HSE and what was then the Department of the Environment (now the Department of Environment, Transport and Regions). Under this scheme, a new substance is defined as any substance placed on the market which is not on the EU's list of existing substances, called the European Inventory of Existing Commercial Chemical Substances or EINECS (CEC, 1990). This lists all those substances placed on the market for commercial purposes between 1 January 1971 and 18 September 1981; substances on this list are known as 'existing' substances. This notification scheme was modified by the Seventh Amendment to the Dangerous Substances Directive adopted in 1992 (EEC Council, 1992). This was implemented in the UK by the Notification of New Substances Regulations 1993. The most important change was the requirement that Competent Authorities carry out a risk assessment on notified new substances. It was stated that this should follow the principles set out in the risk assessment Directive (EEC Council, 1993).

The Notification Scheme requires manufacturers/importers of new chemicals to notify the competent authority in the Member State in which the chemical is first manufactured or imported. There are exceptions for substances used solely in areas covered by other Directives requiring safety clearance (e.g. human and veterinary medicines, pesticides, food additives). The objective of the Notification Scheme is to ensure that the potential of any new substance to cause harm to humans or the environment is assessed before being placed on the market.

The full notification requirements apply to substances placed on the market in amounts greater than 1 tonne p.a. Some more limited data, primarily relating to identity and quantity, are required on new substances placed on the market in smaller amounts; these are referred to as 'Limited Announcements'. In the case of substances placed on the market in amounts in the range 100–1000 kg year^{-1}, the following toxicity data are required: acute toxicity using two routes, skin and eye irritancy, skin sensitization and a bacterial assay for mutagenicity. There are also special provisions relating to chemicals supplied solely for commercial development, but these only apply for 1 year, and an undertaking has to be given by each recipient company that the substance will only be handled by their employees and that it will not be made available to the general public.

Initial or 'Base-set' Data Requirements

Suppliers of substances that are subject to full notification procedure are required to provide a technical dossier of physico-chemical, toxicity and ecotoxicity data (the 'base-set' data) to the Competent Authority of the EEC Member State in which the substance is first marketed. This dossier must be submitted at least 45 days prior to marketing; the 45 day time-period starts from the time the Competent Authority receives a notification that complies with the requirements of the Directive. This allows a summary of the data to be circulated to the Competent Authorities of other Member States, via the CEC, so that all Member States are aware of the data and can raise any queries if necessary. The supplier will then not have to renotify when the substance is marketed in other Member States.

The 'base-set' toxicity data comprise the following studies. First, acute toxicity investigations are required in a single species (preferably the rat) by at least two routes, one being the oral route and the second being dependent on the intended use and the physico-chemical properties of the substance. However, gases and highly volatile liquids need to be investigated by the inhalation route. Skin and eye irritancy data are required, preferably using the rabbit, and skin sensitization in the guinea pig. Regarding the latter study, the Magnusson–Kligman maximization test is the preferred method for detecting skin sensitization potential, although it is accepted that other methods may be appropriate in certain cases. Assessment of repeated-dose effects is by a 28 day study, preferably in the rat and using the oral or inhalation route, depending on the likely exposure and the physico-chemical properties of the substance. Screening tests for genotoxicity and potential carcinogenicity with information on two end-point—namely gene mutation and chromosome aberrations—are also required. This should be obtained from *in vitro* tests (unless scientific justification can be given to indicate that an *in vivo* assay is essential). This requirement was a change from the earlier Sixth Amendment Notification Scheme when an *in vivo* assay for clastogenicity was allowed. This reflected the fact that it was now felt by Member States possible to screen for mutagenic potential using *in vitro* methods and thus the use of an *in vivo* animal model could not be justified for routine screening.

Indeed, there is an EU Directive covering animal welfare issues that specifically prohibits the use of animal tests if an adequately validated and practical alternative is available (EEC Council, 1986). Information on exposure estimates (both in the work environment and the general population) is also required to enable the risk assessment to be carried out.

Although the 'base-set' toxicity data given above list those studies that would normally be expected, there is flexibility: where a supplier considers that it would not be technically possible to carry out a specific test, or it does not appear that the results of a test are necessary for the evaluation of the potential hazards of the substance, omission of the study would be considered by the Competent Authority, provided that scientific justification was given. Furthermore, the Competent Authority may require further tests, depending on the results of the 'base-set' tests, and having regard to all current knowledge of the substance, quantity to be supplied, known and planned uses and the costs involved.

Requirement for Further Data

Notifiers are required to inform the Competent Authority when tonnage levels increase to 10, 100 or 1000 tonnes p.a. when further testing may be required. The Competent Authority will take into account the results of the initial base-set studies, the known and planned uses and all current knowledge of the substance, when considering what data are necessary.

The Sixth Amendment Directive outlines what studies may be needed at Level 1 (i.e. 10–100 tonnes p.a.)—namely teratogenicity and fertility studies, 90 day repeated-dose studies and further mutagenicity data—and at Level 2 (i.e. 1000 tonnes p.a.)—namely further reproductive toxicity studies, chronic studies, studies in a second species and toxicokinetic data. However, it is anticipated that any further information considered appropriate will be identified on a case-by-case basis, after consultation and dialogue with the relevant Competent Authority.

It is important to note that there is continual consideration of any notified substance as the tonnage increases and, in general, the total number of exposed persons increases. The substance is always considered 'new'. This should ensure that an appropriate toxicity profile will be built up to permit an adequate hazard assessment, thus ensuring that the exposed population is not subject to any unacceptable risk.

Toxicity Test Methods

In order to support the data requirements of the Sixth Amendment Directive, the CEC published guidance on test methods to use in 'Annex V' to the Dangerous

Substances Directive. Methods for the 'base-set' tests were outlined in Part A of Directive 84/449/EEC (EEC Commission, 1984) and methods for the Level 1 and 2 tests in Part B in Directive 87/307/EEC (EEC Commission, 1987). The 'base-set' methods were updated in 1992 (EEC Commission, 1992). However, the importance of harmonization of test methods in the wider international context is recognized, to avoid the needless duplication of tests with minor variations for different countries. In this regard, the OECD test guidelines play a key role. Member countries of the OECD have agreed to accept data if done to an OECD test method and in compliance with the OECD principles of Good Laboratory Practice (GLP); this is spelt out in their Council Decision on the Mutual Acceptance of Data (OECD, 1981). Since all Member States of the EU are also members of the OECD, it is reasonable that they look to the well established updating mechanism of the OECD for the technical updating of the Annex V test methods. The EU intends to publish further updates of its Annex V guidelines, but these will be based technically on the OECD methods, with conversion into the Annex V format and publication in the *Official Journal* in all the Community languages. This is a slow process and no updates have been published since 1992.

EXISTING CHEMICALS

Prior to 1993, there were no requirements for the notification of data on existing chemicals (i.e. those on EINECS). However, this changed with the adoption of the Council Regulation on the evaluation and control of the risks of existing substances in March 1993 (EC Council, 1993). This required manufacturers or importers of chemicals in quantities of 10 tonnes p.a. or more to send a package of data directly to the EC (since this was a Regulation and not a Directive to Member States). Priority was given to HPV chemicals, i.e. those produced or imported in quantities of 1000 tonnes p.a. or more. Annex 1 to the Directive listed about 2000 chemicals for which data needed to be sent within 1 year of publication of the Regulation. Other chemicals produced in these amounts needed to be notified by March 1995. Data on the chemicals produced or imported in quantities in the range 10–1000 tonnes p.a. needed to be provided during the period March 1995–February 1998.

The information to be sent to the Commission on the HPV chemicals included the chemical name and EINECS number, quantity produced or imported, classification, information on reasonable foreseeable uses, physico-chemical data, data on environmental pathways and ecotoxicity and on acute, sub-acute and reproductive toxicity, as well as mutagenicity and carcinogenicity. It was stated in the Regulation that manufacturers and importers must make all reasonable efforts to obtain existing data regarding the toxicity and ecotoxicity but

that they were not bound to carry out further testing to complete any specific data sets. A reduced data package (only the first four items listed above) was required on the 10–1000 tonne p.a. chemicals.

This measure was somewhat unusual in that it was a Regulation rather than a Directive and also because industry was required to provide the data on diskette using a specially designed EC computer program. In practice, this produced a great deal of difficulty due to problems with the program.

Priority lists of chemicals have been drawn up on an annual basis for substances to be examined in detail and risk assessments carried out. To date, three lists have been published, each of about 40 chemicals. These have been divided between the Competent Authorities of the Member States who designate a *rapporteur* for each substance. If necessary, the EU will draw up proposals to control the risks. The scheme is complex and introduced a number of relatively novel approaches (e.g. provision of data in electronic format) and progress on agreeing risk assessments at Community level has been slow. It was hoped that summaries of the first few completed risk assessments would be published in the *Official Journal* in 1999.

In addition to providing a formal procedure whereby the EU can assess priority existing chemicals and identify those for which further controls may be justified, the scheme also has a wider international component. The products of the EU scheme, prior to finalization, are considered as the EU's contribution to the OECD's HPV chemical programme. These risk assessments form a key contribution to the ambitious targets set by the Intergovernmental Forum on Chemical Safety (IFCS, 1994) for expanding and accelerating the international assessment of chemical risks. The IFCS is the intergovernmental body which oversees the implementation of the programme of the safe management of chemical risks agreed at the United Nations Conference on Environment and Health (UNCED) and spelt out in Chapter 19 of Agenda 21, a programme for sustainable development. The other two types of document that are recognized by the IFCS for this purpose are the Environmental Health Criteria documents produced by IPCS (the International Programme on Chemical Safety, a joint venture of WHO, ILO and UNEP) and the IPCS/OECD Concise International Chemical Assessment Documents (CICADs).

Classification and Labelling of Dangerous Substances Directive

The labelling of substances (and preparations) supplied within the European Union (either for use at work or to the general public) provides a primary route for giving essential information about any potential hazard. This is an important area of harmonization under Directive 67/548/EEC, 'The Dangerous Substances Directive' (EEC Council, 1967). Substances are considered dangerous within the meaning of this Directive if classified in one of the following categories: explosive, oxidizing, extremely flammable, highly flammable, flammable, very toxic, toxic, harmful, corrosive, irritant and dangerous to the environment. It is pertinent to note that classification is on the basis of hazard, an inherent property of the substance, rather than risk in use. The criteria to be used for classification in each category are given in the European Commission's Labelling Guide, i.e. Annex VI of Directive 67/548/EEC as last adapted to technical progress by Directive 93/21/EEC; classification in any category results in the substance being considered as dangerous and covered by the Dangerous Substances Directive. In the UK this is implemented by the Health and Safety Commission's (HSC) Chemicals (Hazard Information and Packaging for Supply) Regulations 1994. Detailed guidance on the general principles of classification and labelling for supply is given in an approved guide, based on the EU's Labelling Guide (HSC, 1994).

Regarding the classifications covering the toxic properties of the substance, the criteria for very toxic, toxic and harmful are based on acute toxicity data, repeated-dose effects, or carcinogenic, mutagenic or reproductive toxicity. Although there are only three classification classes covering 'systemic' toxicity (namely very toxic, toxic and harmful, requiring the symbols skull and crossbones plus, skull and crossbones and St Andrew's Cross, respectively), there are numerous different risk phrases, agreed in all of the nine Community languages, appropriate for each type of toxic effect.

The criteria for classification based on acute toxic properties are based on the LD_{50} values, as given in **Table 2**.

Regarding effects other than lethality, substances are regarded as very toxic, toxic or harmful if there is strong evidence that irreversible damage (other than that due to carcinogenic, mutagenic and reproductive effects, which are considered separately) is likely to be caused by a single exposure by an appropriate route, usually in the dose ranges given in **Table 2**. Substances are also considered harmful if serious damage ('clear functional disturbance or morphological changes which have

toxicological significance') is likely to be caused by repeated exposure by an appropriate route at levels of the order of 50 mg kg^{-1} day^{-1} or less for the oral route, 100 mg kg^{-1} day^{-1} for the percutaneous route and 0.5 mg l^{-1} per 4h day^{-1} for exposure by inhalation. If such effects are likely to occur at 'significantly lower' dose levels, the substance should be regarded as toxic.

Classification on the basis of carcinogenic, mutagenic or effects on the reproductive system are considered separately. Regarding carcinogenicity, there are three categories, depending on whether the substance is known to be carcinogenic in man, or whether there is sufficient evidence for a strong presumption that the substance will be carcinogenic to man or, finally, where substances give concern owing to possible carcinogenic effects in man. For labelling purposes the first two categories are treated in an identical fashion, requiring classification as toxic and the use of the risk phrase R45 (namely 'may cause cancer'). The third category is classified as harmful, with the risk phrase R40 (namely 'possible risk of irreversible effects'). Similarly, there are three categories for mutagenic properties: first, chemical substances that are known human mutagens (there are no substances that meet this criterion); second, substances for which the evidence provides a strong presumption from animal studies, and other relevant data, that the substance may result in the development of heritable genetic damage; and third, substances that give rise to concern (in this case category 2 mutagens are considered harmful, but require the risk phrase R46, i.e. 'may cause heritable genetic damage'); category 3 mutagens require the risk phrase R40, similar to category 3 carcinogens. There are two categories of reproductive toxin—effects on the reproductive system (fertility) and on developmental toxicity. Each is subdivided into known human and suspect human reproductive toxins.

Dangerous Preparations (The Preparations Directive)

The EEC Directive considered above applies to dangerous substances as opposed to preparations (i.e. products containing mixtures of substances). Prior to 1988 there were a number of EC Directives covering specific areas of 'industrial'-type products, for example, solvents (EEC Council, 1973) and paints, varnishes, printing inks, adhesives and similar products (EEC Council, 1977). However, in 1988 agreement was reached on a general Preparations Directive (EEC Council, 1988a) which replaces these more limited Directives and covers essentially all general preparations containing 'dangerous' substances, as defined by the Dangerous Substances Directive. It applies to all preparations supplied within

Table 2 Classification of categories of exposure

Category of exposure	Oral LD_{50} in rat (mg kg^{-1})	Percutaneous LD_{50} in rat (mg kg^{-1})	Inhalation LD_{50}, 4 h exposure (mg l^{-1})
Very toxic	25	50	0.5
Toxic	25–200	50–400	0.5–2
Harmful	200–2000	400–2000	2–20

the Community apart from those covered by specific Directives involving some form of authorization or clearance, e.g. human and veterinary medicines, cosmetics, pesticides and foodstuffs.

The basis of the Preparations Directive is to use the same basic criteria as in the Dangerous Substances Directive but with a calculation method being recommended for assessing the classification of preparations containing dangerous substance(s) based on concentration limits or cut-off values. With regard to acute toxicity, if the substance itself is classified as very toxic, then preparations containing concentrations of 7% or more are classified as very toxic, 1–7% as toxic and 0.1–1% as harmful. If the preparation contains more than one substance that is classified on the basis of acute lethality, a calculation method based on simple additivity is proposed, using the percentage present and consideration of the appropriate concentration limits. Similar calculations apply to all the other parameters used for classification on the basis of the toxicity profile, with specific concentration limits being given for very toxic, toxic and harmful in the Preparations Directive. The calculation assuming additivity is only used for the acute lethality and the corrosive and irritant properties.

The Preparations Directive thus adopts a pragmatic approach to the classification of preparations, based on a calculation method aimed at reducing the animal testing needed on the vast number of preparations involved. However, the relatively rigid system has two important provisos. First, where the toxicological properties of a preparation have been established by both the calculation method and testing in animals using the Annex V test method, the latter may be used for classification of the preparation, except when carcinogenic, mutagenic or effects on the reproductive system are involved. In the latter cases the calculation approach, with cut-off limits, must be used. Second, human experience takes precedence, provided that it is based on good-quality data, including full details of exposure conditions—i.e. the human data must be sound. It is accepted that the calculation method being recommended assumes that there is no potentiation of effect in mixtures. However, if this is known to occur, account should be taken of this when classifying the preparation.

In summary, the objective of the Preparations Directive is to harmonize labelling of products as far as possible throughout the Community. The recommended approach is based on consideration of classification of each dangerous substance present, and the use of a calculation method for classification of the preparation. However, if results from testing the preparation itself are available these may be used, except for carcinogenicity, mutagenicity and effects on the reproductive system. Furthermore, sound data in humans takes precedence.

Occupational Exposure Levels

Individual Member States of the EU have their own procedures for establishing occupational exposure limits. When a specific compound has not been assessed in a given country, it is common to use the extensive list of Threshold Limit Values (TLVs) recommended by the American Conference of Government Industry Hygienists (ACGIH). A brief outline of some of the most established systems in various countries of the EU is given below.

Germany publishes its own list of MAK (Maximale Arbeitsplatz Konzentrationen) values (Deutsche Forschungsgemeinschaft, 1996). There is a two-step procedure. In the first stage, a non-government scientific committee (the DFG Commission) evaluates all the available data on a given compound and produces a scientific document with a proposal for an occupational exposure limit. In the second stage, a government committee (Ausschuss für Gefahrstoffe, AGS), with representatives of all interested society groups, gives an opinion on the economic, technical and analytical feasibility. The Ministry of Labour publishes the annually revised list of MAK values and may, on rare occasions, change a proposed limit on the basis of socioeconomic factors. For carcinogens and agents with reproductive effects, no MAK values are set, but TRK (Technische Richtkonzentrationen) are established by the AGS Committee. MAK values are considered as indicative of 'commonly accepted medical and hygiene rules', and as such have legal force for application by the Industrial Inspection Board.

In The Netherlands, ACGIH values were used up to 1978, but since then an expert committee produces an evaluation report and a recommended value based exclusively on health aspects. The government agency, in parallel with this work, reports on technical and economic aspects. Based on the two reports, a suggested value is considered by a tripartite body, before it is definitively adopted by the Director General of Labour. In most other cases the ACGIH values are used.

In the UK, the Health and Safety Executive publish lists of occupational exposure limits annually (HSE, 1997). Initially these consisted of Control Limits and Recommended Limits. However, since the Control of Substances Hazards to Health (COSHH) Regulations came into force (UK, 1994) two different types of exposure limit are specified, namely Maximum Exposure Limits (MELs) and Occupational Exposure Standards (OESs). Advice on both exposure limits is provided by a tripartite committee, the Advisory Committee on Toxic Substances (ACTS), which considers comprehensive reviews of the toxicity data and also information on technical and analytical feasibility together with economic facts. If an MEL is agreed, this is specified in a Schedule to the COSHH regulations, and the limit, so far as inhalation of the substance is concerned, must not be exceeded. Furthermore, exposure should be reduced, so far as is reasonably practical, below the limit. Regarding the OES, control to that level is regarded as adequate, so far as inhalation of the substance is concerned. This level should be achieved, so far as is reasonably practical, by means other than personal protective equipment.

Hence, the system adopted for setting occupational exposure limits varies between Member States. However, this is an area of increasing EU-wide activity in an attempt to provide greater harmonization of systems.

EU Activity on Occupational Exposure Limits

The framework for EU activity in this area was laid by Directive 80/117/EEC, which set out measures for the control of risks relating to chemical, physical and biological agents (EEC Council, 1980). This was amended in 1988 by the adoption of Directive 88/642/EEC, which outlined the mechanism for recommending indicative exposure limits (EEC Council 1988b). It is also pertinent to note here Council Directive 90/394/EEC on carcinogens at work, which includes provision for setting binding limit values. At EU level there are thus two types of exposure limit, binding limit values which reflect both scientific data and socioeconomic considerations and which must be transposed into national legislation as a minimum requirement and indicative limits. At present there are binding values for vinyl chloride monomer (7 ppm), lead and its ionic compound (0.15 mg m^{-3}) and asbestos (chrysotile 0.6 fibres ml^{-1}; other forms 0.3 fibres ml^{-1}. Indicative limit values are adopted by the Commission after obtaining an opinion from the European Commission's relevant expert advisory committee, the Scientific Committee for Occupational Exposure Limits to Chemical Agents (SCOEL). Member States are required to take these indicative limits into account when they adopt national measures for the protection of workers. The procedures by which the European Commission arrives at these occupational exposure limits have recently been outlined (Hunter *et al.*, 1997). At present there are indicative values for about 30 substances.

Other EU Activities Relating to Chemicals

This review does not attempt to cover all the areas being considered by the EEC relating to occupational safety, but has aimed at giving an indication of the extent to which harmonized procedures have already been adopted, particularly with regard to classification and labelling and notification of new substances. The schemes described do not control the marketing of substances within the Community, but this can be done, on a case-by-case basis, by use of another Directive. This is EEC Council Directive 76/769/EEC, on the approximation of the laws, regulations and administrative provisions of Member States relating to restrictions on the marketing and use of certain dangerous substances and preparations. Amendments to this Directive have introduced controls on the marketing of a number of substances at the Community level, e.g. polychlorinated and polybrominated biphenyls, certain lead compounds, mercury, arsenic and benzene.

In addition, this Directive has introduced a general prohibition of the use in consumer products of chemicals classified as category 1 and 2 carcinogens, mutagens, or on the basis of toxicity to the reproductive system. In the future, it is anticipated that this Directive will be the vehicle by which controls are introduced following the risk assessments carried out on priority chemicals under the Existing Substances Regulations, if the outcome indicates that further controls are appropriate.

Regulations in the UK

Finally, although this review is concerned primarily with the harmonization of requirements throughout the EU, it is pertinent to outline the framework that exists for controlling industrial chemicals in the UK.

The Health and Safety Executive is the UK Government Agency that has the responsibility for all aspects of occupational safety in England, Wales and Scotland, while a division of the Department of Economic Development performs similar functions in Northern Ireland. The work of the Executive is 'overseen' by the Health and Safety Commission (HSC), a body with representatives from government, trade unions and industry. The HSE is funded by the Department of the Environment, Transport and the Regions (DETR), and the Director General of the HSE is responsible to the Secretary of State of that Department. On matters relating to the toxicity of chemicals, the HSC is advised by the Advisory Committee on Toxic Substances, which has representatives from industry, trade unions and local authorities, together with government and independent experts. The two principal pieces of legislation governing the work of the HSE are outlined below.

Health and Safety at Work Act 1974

The Health and Safety at Work Act (1974) established the HSC and the HSE. It is a very wide-ranging piece of 'enabling' legislation covering all aspects of safety at work.

The general provisions of Section 2 of this Act require employers to protect workers' health, so far as is reasonably practical—in particular, by the use of proper plant, systems of work, safe handling, storage and transport, provision of information, instruction and training.

The Act also covers responsibilities of workers (Section 4) and of persons not employed at the site, but who may be affected by work activities. Thus, Section 3 of the Act requires employers and the self-employed to conduct their undertakings in such a way as to ensure, so far as is reasonably practical, that persons not in their employment who may be affected by these work activities are not thereby exposed to risks to their health and safety.

Section 5 of the Act places a general duty on persons in control of certain premises in relation to harmful emissions to the atmosphere, which relates to best practical means for preventing emissions into the atmosphere of noxious or offensive substances, and for rendering such substances harmless and inoffensive.

Regarding chemical safety at work, Section 6(4) of the Act is the most relevant, as this relates to the duties regarding substances. Thus, Section 6 (4) states: 'It shall be the duty of any person who manufactures, imports or supplies any substance for use at work to ensure, as far as is reasonably practical, that the substance is safe and without risk to health when properly used'. Section 6 then goes on to explain that this duty may be fulfilled by providing adequate information on the results of relevant tests. No detailed guidance is given on the extent of toxicity testing necessary in order to provide adequate information to enable the substance to be used safely. This is the responsibility of the manufacturer, importer or supplier.

Control of Substances Hazardous to Health (COSHH) Regulations 1994

The Control of Substances Hazardous to Health (COSHH) Regulations and subsequent amendments require employers, in any situation where hazardous substances are used at work, to carry out an assessment of the health risks involved (UK, 1994). A substance is regarded as hazardous to health if it would be classified as very toxic, toxic, harmful, corrosive or irritant, using the criteria used for the EEC Dangerous Substances Directive (67/548/EEC). Following the assessment of the risks, the employer is required to determine what action is necessary to prevent the risks or, where this is not reasonably practical, to ensure that there are adequate controls, using, where possible, means other than personal protective equipment. The major duties that are placed on an employer are thus as follows: the need to gather data on the substances used and to evaluate their risks to health; to decide on what precautions are necessary, including the need to conform with any maximum exposure limit or occupational exposure limit; to monitor exposure levels; to provide information, instructions and training to persons who may be exposed; to record the assessment; and to decide when the assessment would need to be updated.

To summarize, the Health and Safety at Work Act, together with the COSHH Regulations, provides a comprehensive framework of legislation to ensure that, so far as is reasonably practical, substances used at work do not pose any undue risks to the health of employees.

CONCLUSION

This chapter has described major components of the US programmes to assess and manage the risk of industrial chemicals. The contrasting situation in the EU, where the regulations of the various Member States are being harmonized, seems likely to be repeated as the North Atlantic Free Trade Area (NAFTA) and the EU and other organizations, as well as countries outside trading blocks, such as Japan, in turn, attempt to reconcile their different approaches in this area of regulatory toxicology.

REFERENCES

Auer, C. M., Zeeman, M., Nabholz, J. V. and Clements, R. G. (1994). SAR—the US regulatory perspective. *SAR QSAR Environ. Res.*, **2**, 29–38.

CEC (1990). European Inventory of Existing Commercial Substances (EINECS). *Off. J. Eur. Commun.*, No. C146, 15 June 1990.

Deutsche Forschungsgemeinschaft (1996). *List of MAK and BAT values*. VCH, Weinheim.

EEC Commission (1984). Directive 84/449/EEC Adapting to Technical Progress for the Sixth Time Council Directive 67/548/EEC on the Approximation of the Laws, Regulations and Administrative Provisions Relating to the Classification, Packaging and Labelling of Dangerous substances. Annex V test methods. Part B. Methods for the determination of toxicity. *Off. J. Eur. Commun.*, No. L251, 19 September 1984.

EEC Commission (1987). Directive 87/302/EEC adapting to technical progress for the ninth time Council Directive 67/548/EEC on the approximation of the laws, regulations and administrative provisions relating to the classification packaging and labelling of dangerous substances. Annex V test methods. Part B. Methods for the determination of toxicity. *Off. J. Eur. Commun.*, No. L133/11, 30 May 1988.

EEC Commission (1991). Directive 91/325/EEC of 1 March 1991 adapting to technical progress for the 12th time Council Directive 67/548/EEC on the approximation of the laws, regulations and administrative provision relating to the classification packaging and labelling of dangerous substances. *Off. J. Eur. Commun.*, No. L80, 8 July 1991.

EEC Commission (1992). Directive 92/69/EEC adapting to technical progress for the 17th time Council Directive 67/548/EEC on the approximation of the laws, regulations and administrative provisions relating to the classification, packaging and labelling of dangerous substances. *Off. J. Eur. Commun.*, No. L383A, 29 December 1992.

EEC Council (1967). Directive 67/548/EEC on the approximation of the laws, regulations and administrative provisions relating to the classification packaging and labelling of dangerous substances. *Off. J. Eur. Commun.*, No. 196/1, 16 August 1967.

EEC Council (1973). Directive 73/173/EEC of 4th June 1973 on the approximation of the laws, regulations and administrative provisions relating to the classification packaging and labelling of dangerous preparations (solvents). *Off. J. Eur. Commun.*, No. L189, 11 June 1973.

EEC Council (1977). Directive 77/728/EEC of 7th November 1977 on the approximation of the laws, regulations and administrative provisions relating to the classification, packaging and labelling of paints, varnishes, printing inks adhesives and similar products. *Off. J. Eur. Commun.*, No. L303, 28 November 1977.

EEC Council (1979). Directive 79/831/EEC adopting for the sixth time Council Directive 67/584/EEC on the approximation of the laws, regulations and administrative provisions relating to the packaging and labelling of dangerous substances. *Off. J. Eur. Commun.*, No. L259, 15 October 1979.

EEC Council (1980). Directive 80/117/EEC of 27th November 1980 on the protection of workers from the risks related to exposure to chemical, physical and biological agents at work. *Off. J. Eur. Commun.*, No. L327, 3 December 1980.

EEC Council (1986). Directive 86/609/EEC of 24th November 1986 on the approximation of the laws, regulations and administrative provisions of the Member States regarding the protection of animals used for experimental and other scientific purposes. *Off. J. Eur. Commun.*, No. L358, 18 December 1986.

EEC Council (1988a). Directive 88/379/EEC of 7th June 1988 on the approximation of the laws, regulations and administrative provisions of the member states relating to the classification, packaging and labelling of dangerous preparations. *Off. J. Eur. Commun.*, No. L187/14, 16 July 1988.

EEC Council (1988b). Directive 88/642/EEC of 16th December 1988 amending Directive 80/1107/EEC of 27th November 1989 on the protection of workers from the risks relating to exposure to chemical, physical and biological agents at work. *Off. J. Eur. Commun.*, No. L356, 24 December 1988.

EEC Council (1990). Directive 90/394/EEC of 28th June 1990 of the protection of workers from the risks related to exposure to carcinogens at work. *Off. J. Eur. Commun.*, No. L196, 26 July 1990.

EEC Council (1992). Directive 92/32/EEC of 30th April 1992 amending for the seventh time Directive 67/548/EEC on the approximation of the laws, regulations and administrative provisions relating to the classification packaging and label-

ling of dangerous substances. *Off. J. Eur. Commun.*, No. L154/1, 5 June 1992, 65–80.

EEC Council (1993). Regulation (EEC) No. 793/93 of 23rd March 1993 on the evaluation and control of the risks of existing substances. *Off. J. Eur. Commun.*, No. L84, 5 April 1993.

EPA (1998). Chemical Hazard Data Availability Study, April 1998. Available on the internet at http://www.epa.gov/opptintr/chemtest/hazchem.htm.

HSC (1994). *Approved Guide to the Classification and Labelling of Substances and Preparations Dangerous for Supply*, 2nd edn. Chemical (Hazard Information and Packaging for Supply) Regulations 1994. CHIP2. Guidance on Regulations L63. HSE Books, Sudbury.

HSE (1997) EG40/97. *Occupational Exposure Limits 1997*. HSE Books, Sudbury.

Hunter, W. J., Aresini, F., Haigh, R., Papadopoulos, P. and Van der Hund, W. (1997). Occupational Exposure Limits for Chemicals in the European Union. *Occup. Environ. Med.*, **54**, 217–222.

IFCS (1994). *Intergovernmental Forum on Chemical Safety: Background, Purpose, Function*. WHO, Geneva.

OECD (1981). *Decision of the OECD Council Concerning the Mutual Acceptance of Data in the Assessment of Chemicals*. C-81–30. Organization for Economic Cooperation and Development, Paris.

OECD (1994). *US EPA/EC Joint Project on the Evaluation of (Quantitative) Structure–Activity Relationships*. OECD Environment Monographs, No. 88. Organization for Economic Cooperation and Development, Paris.

UK (1994). *Control of Substances Hazardous to Health Regulations 1994 (SI 1994 3246) as Amended by the Control of Substances Hazardous to Health Regulations (Amendment) Regulations (SI 1996/3/38) and the Control of Substances Hazardous to Health Amendment Regulations 1997 (SI 1997/11)*. HMSO, London.

USA (1970). *Occupational Safety and Health Act*. USC 29 Section 651 *et seq.*

USA (1976). *Toxic Substances Control Act*. USC 15 Section 2601–2629.

USA (1997). *Microbial Products of Biotechnology; Final Regulation Under the Toxic Substances Control Act*. 62 FR 17932, 11 April 1997.

Zeeman, M., Auer, C. M., Clements, R. G., Nabholz, J. V. and Boethling, R. S. (1995). U. S. EPA regulatory perspectives on the use of QSAR for new and existing chemical evaluations. *SAR QSAR Environ. Res.*, **3**, 179–201.

Chapter 73
Pesticide Regulation

Cheryl E. A. Chaffey, Virginia A. Dobozy and Deborah J. Hussey

CONTENTS

NORTH AMERICA

History and Legislation

USA

Pesticide regulation in the USA has evolved from an original focus on protecting pesticide users from fraudulent claims about efficacy to its current focus on protecting human health and the environment. The authority for pesticide regulation is intertwined in several statutes which have been administered by multiple government agencies. The first federal food legislation was the Pure Food and Drug Act of 1906 which guaranteed the wholesomeness and truthfulness of labelling of foods, drugs and cosmetics (USA, 1906). The first federal pesticide legislation was the Insecticide Act of 1910, which was administered by the US Department of Agriculture (USDA) (USA, 1910). It was intended to prevent the manufacture, sale or transportation of impure or improperly labelled insecticides and fungicides. In 1938, the Federal Food, Drug and Cosmetic Act (FFDCA), which included regulation of pesticides on food, was passed (USA 1938). The present statute under which pesticides are regulated, the Federal Insecticide, Fungicide and Rodenticide Act (FIFRA) was passed in 1947 (USA, 1947). It extended coverage to include herbicides and rodenticides. USDA was required to register all pesticides sold interstate; however, registrations could not be denied. The 1954 Miller amendment to FFDCA stipulated the establishment of tolerances (maximum legal residue concentrations) for pesticide residues on food and animal feed. Public interest in environmental issues was ignited by the 1962 publication of *Silent Spring* by Rachel Carson (Carson, 1962), which warned about the persistence and magnification of organochlorines in the food chain. With the 1964 amendment to FIFRA, USDA was given the authority to deny, cancel or suspend pesticide registrations to protect public health. In 1970,

FIFRA administration was transferred to the newly formed US Environmental Protection Agency (US EPA). Authority to establish tolerances on food was transferred from the Food and Drug Administration (FDA) to the US EPA, but tolerance enforcement remained with FDA.

A complete overhaul of FIFRA followed in 1972. Included in the legislation was the designation of two classes of pesticides, general and restricted use. Only certified applicators were permitted to apply restricted-use pesticides. Companies proposing to register pesticides were required to supply scientific evidence that the pesticide would present 'no unreasonable adverse effect' to crops, livestock, non-target organisms and the environment. The next major amendment to FIFRA, passed in 1988, required the acceleration of pesticide reregistration for active ingredients registered prior to 1984. The US EPA was directed to perform a comprehensive re-evaluation of these pesticides, which were registered when registration standards were less stringent. Previously registered pesticides are reviewed to ensure they measure up to current scientific and regulatory standards. The 1996 Food Quality Protection Act amended both FFDCA and FIFRA with sweeping changes in how pesticides safety should be assessed by the US EPA (USA, 1996). The safety standard for pesticides in food was changed from 'no unreasonable adverse effect' to 'reasonable certainty of no harm'. In establishing tolerances, the US EPA was directed to provide for the protection of potentially sensitive populations, such as infants and children. The statute specified that risk from pesticide exposure should be assessed from total exposure from all non-occupational sources, i.e. through the diet, drinking water and as a result of household pesticide use. In addition, the US EPA was instructed to assess the effects of exposure to multiple pesticides with a common mechanism of toxicity, the effects of *in utero* exposure to pesticides and the potential effects of pesticides on the endocrine system.

Canada

Pesticides first became subject to regulation in Canada in 1927 under the Agricultural Pests' Control Act, administered by the Department of Agriculture. That Act was revised in 1939 and became the Pest Control Products Act (PCPA). It was recognized in the mid-1960s that a more sophisticated law was needed to manage the more complex and emerging class of synthetic organic pesticides. In 1969, a revised PCPA was passed by Parliament and brought into force by the adoption of Regulations in 1972 (Canada, 1985a). Departments of Health, Environment and Natural Resources (Forestry, Fisheries) served in an advisory capacity to the Department of Agriculture. The Department of Health maintained authority for establishing maximum residue limits for pesticides on food under the Food and Drugs Act, last revised in 1964 (Canada, 1985b). The Food and Drugs Act, originally promulgated in 1920, was the first Canadian legislation dealing with food adulteration and the authority under this Act was the Department of Health.

After the Canadian government committed itself to implement the recommendations of a 1990 Pesticide Registration Review, conducted by 12 multi-stakeholder representatives, the Pest Management Regulatory Agency (PMRA) was established within Health Canada in 1995. Authority for the administration of the PCPA was transferred from the Department of Agriculture to that of Health and the expertise and functions from all of the participating departments were convened within the PMRA. The Agency's mandate is twofold: to protect human health and the environment by minimizing risks associated with pest control products; and to ensure that users have access to pest management tools, that is, pest control products and pest management strategies. The main purpose of the PCPA is to ensure the safety, merit and value of pesticide products, through pre-market assessment. Additional legislation impacting on the use and regulation of pesticides can be found at the federal, provincial and municipal level.

Definition of Pesticide

In both the USA and Canada, the term pesticide applies to a similar range of products including, but not limited to, herbicides, fungicides, insecticides and biocides. In the USA, the definition of pesticide under FIFRA is (1) any substance or mixture of substances intended for preventing, destroying, repelling or mitigating any pest and (2) any substance or mixture of substances intended for use as a plant regulator, defoliant or desiccant. In Canada, the PCPA defines a control product as any product, device, organism, substance or thing that is manufactured, represented, sold or used as a means for directly or indirectly controlling, preventing, destroying, mitigating, attracting or repelling any pest.

Types of registrations

USA

In the USA, the type of pesticide registration is usually denoted by the applicable section of FIFRA. Section 3 of FIFRA describes the information and data required for a full registration of a new active ingredient. With an unconditional Section 3 registration, the application for registration is complete and the US EPA has determined the product will perform its intended purpose without unreasonable effects on the environment. A conditional Section 3 registration may be granted for a limited time period in certain circumstances, usually to allow the generation of additional data, but only if the use of the pesticide is in the public interest and will not cause any unreasonable effects on the environment. Experimental Use Permits (EUPs), issued under Section 5 of FIFRA, allow prospective registrants of pesticides to generate the data necessary for a Section 3 registration. Pesticides under EUPs may not be sold or distributed, except by participants to be used only at an application site and in accordance with the terms and conditions of the EUP. Section 18 of FIFRA authorizes the US EPA to exempt a state or federal agency from the provisions of the law if an emergency pest condition exists. The exemption is limited to a 1 year period. Under Section 24(c) of FIFRA, a state may provide registration for additional needs provided that a tolerance exists if the additional use is for food or feed.

Canada

Currently in Canada, several registration types are accommodated under the PCPA. Once the safety, value and merit of a pesticide have been satisfactorily addressed, it is eligible for a full registration, whereby a registration number is assigned prior to the introduction to the marketplace. Registration numbers are assigned to both a technical product (usually containing only the active ingredient and related impurities) and to all end-use products which must then contain a registered technical product in addition to any non-pesticidal components (also known as formulants). Full registrations are valid for a period of 5 years, after which renewal of registration is necessary. Temporary registrations, that are limited to a period not exceeding 1 year, can be granted in situations where additional scientific or technical information is forthcoming from the applicant; this information is usually non-pivotal in so far as safety is concerned. A temporary registration can also be issued for the emergency control of infestations that are seriously deterimental to public health, domestic animals or natural resources. Products used for research purposes are exempt from registration but must still undergo an approval process if the research is conducted on premises not owned or operated by the researcher. The PCPA also has a provision that allows products to be exempt from registration provided that they meet the conditions set forth in a specified schedule that accompanies the Regulations. If the safety of the pesticide or its merit or value for its intended purposes is deemed to be no longer acceptable, the PCPA allows for the cancellation or suspension of a registration, subject to appeal from the registrant and reconsideration.

Data requirements

In both the USA and Canada, applications for new pesticide products are submitted with a dossier of information. Basic elements of this dossier include labelling and product chemistry information, human and environmental safety data, relevant application fees and, in Canada, data pertaining to value (specifically efficacy data). Efficacy data are required in the USA for products intended for use against public health pests, including bacteria, viruses, mosquitoes, ticks, cockroaches, fleas, rats and mice. Product chemistry information is required on technical active ingredients and formulated products with respect to the identity, manufacturing processes, specifications, presence of toxic impurities, analytical methodologies and chemical properties. Wherever it is possible that a product can enter the environment, it is necessary to determine the risk to the environment as assessed through environmental fate and toxicity data.

Of particular interest here are the requirements for toxicological testing that allow a determination of human risk and safety. In general, both countries accept studies that follow guidelines established by the US EPA or Organization for Economic Cooperation and Development (OECD). Slight differences between the guidelines are due primarily to when the guidelines were established or revised; however, quality data are required that should comply with principles of Good Laboratory Practice (GLP). Studies that are submitted in support of applications are performed either by the applicant's own laboratories or contract laboratories. The regulatory toxicologist performs a detailed evaluation of the studies in order to gain a thorough understanding of the risks associated with any given pesticide.

For traditional agricultural chemical pesticides, the basic requirements for toxicology testing are similar in both the USA and Canada. For both technical active ingredients and formulations, acute studies by the oral, dermal and inhalation routes and also skin and eye irritation and dermal sensitization studies are required. These studies are used primarily to identify relative hazards of products for classification and labelling. More comprehensive study is undertaken of the technical active ingredient in order to identify end-points of toxicological concern. Toxicokinetic data (absorption, distribution, metabolism and excretion) are required to provide a basic knowledge of how a pesticide is handled in animal systems, including detoxification mechanisms. Short-term repeated-dose studies are useful in elucidating cumulative action, variation in species sensitivity and identification of organ effects, in addition to providing guidance for selection of doses for chronic studies. Short-term studies are performed via oral, dermal and/or inhalation routes, often for periods of varying duration and sometimes with a withdrawal period to assess reversibility of observed effects. Long-term studies are required to address the potential for chronic toxicity and oncogenicity when the product is administered over the normal life span of the animal. In order to delineate the inherent hazard of the product, dosages for the long-term studies are selected that sufficiently challenge the animals while not compromising their longevity. A battery of genotoxicity studies that address the potential of a product to affect either the gene or the chromosome are required to supplement assessments of oncogenicity. Multi-generation reproduction studies are required to provide information on the potential effects on reproductive capacities of treated animals and also any effects on resulting offspring. These studies are useful in determining any particular sensitivity of the young. Additionally, required teratology studies provide data on the potential of a product to cause or alter the incidence of congenital malformations or affect other developmental parameters. Neurotoxicity testing is particularly important for pesticides such as organophosphates and carbamates which are known to have neurotoxic potential. More refined testing methods are now available that allow for neurobehavioural observation following acute or short-term exposure or exposure during reproductive testing. Current areas of interest with respect to the development of study guidelines and regulatory requirements include immunotoxicity and endocrine modulation.

Although the studies outlined above are typically required for a new chemical pesticide, both countries are flexible in the information that is requested. Where an applicant considers that it is not technically feasible to carry out a specific study or that the results of the study are not necessary for the hazard or risk evaluation, both the US EPA and the PMRA in Canada consider waiving studies, provided that adequate scientific justification exists to support the waiver. Given this flexibility, the US EPA has embraced a tiered approach to data generation for certain product types, most notably antimicrobial products. The Canadian government is currently considering this approach for antimicrobial products demonstrating a low potential for exposure. Canada has tiered data requirements for products used for research purposes. Data requirements for other groups of products, such as microbial products and pheromones, are generally harmonized between the countries and are tailored to address the unique features of these products. In general, the toxicology data requirements are not as extensive as those for agricultural chemicals.

Occupational and Bystander Risk Assessment

The evaluation of the toxicity data is one of two critical elements for the determination of occupational and/or bystander (residential) risk. The second critical element is the assessment of occupational and/or bystander exposure. Both the US EPA and the PMRA in Canada impose regulatory requirements for applicants to address occupational and bystander exposure and accept quantification of exposure based on actual studies conducted with the product under typical use conditions. Exposure can be quantified through biological or ambient monitoring. Biological monitoring, which provides a direct measurement of chemical in the body fluids or tissues (e.g. blood, urine) of exposed individuals, is useful where the pharmacokinetics of the product are uncomplicated and well understood. Ambient monitoring, conducted through dermal and inhalation dosimeters, is used more frequently and measures the amount of substance available for uptake. Surrogate data from a different pesticide can also be used to quantify exposure provided that the pesticides have similar attributes (e.g. formulation type, vapour pressure) and similar uses (e.g. rates of application, application equipment).

Occupational exposure can also be quantified through modelling techniques. The Agencies, in collaboration with the American Crop Protection Association (ACPA), have produced a generic database, namely the Pesticide Handlers Exposure Database (PHED). This database is a compilation of numerous exposure studies utilizing ambient monitoring that enables users to sort by criteria such as formulation type, application method and clothing and protective equipment in order to generate exposure estimates for relevant scenarios.

Applicants are also required by both Agencies to quantify post-application or reentry exposure to workers (e.g. harvesters) and to individuals exposed at home. The USA and Canada cooperate in the development of post-application exposure study guidelines outlining methodologies and sampling strategies in Task Forces generating generic databases.

Once an exposure estimate has been obtained, the toxicity database is evaluated for the most relevant end-points for risk assessment. Critical factors that are considered in the toxicology end-point selection process include the duration of exposure, route of exposure and relevance of end-point. The most relevant No Observed Effect Level (NOEL) from a toxicity study is divided by the exposure estimate to yield a Margin of Exposure (MOE). The acceptability of an MOE is influenced by the severity of the toxicity end-point selected, the sensitivity of the population that will be exposed and deficiencies in the database. Under the requirements of the Food Quality Protection Act in the USA, aggregate exposures to a chemical must be included in the risk

assessment. The dietary exposure (food and water) must be combined with possible non-occupational non-dietary exposure (residential, lawn and garden, turf).

Dietary Risk Assessment

In both countries, dietary exposure is estimated by multiplying the maximum residue limit or the tolerance of a pesticide on a food by the consumption of the food divided by body weight. In the USA, food consumption data are obtained from the USDA National Food Consumption Survey conducted in 1977–78 (USDA, 1983). In this survey, both 3-day mean consumption and single-day consumption information were recorded for the US population and 22 demographic and socio-economic subpopulations. In Canada, disappearance values are normally used in lieu of food consumption data, although actual food consumption data are available from the 1972 Nutrition Canada Survey (Canada, 1975). Disappearance figures reflect the disappearance of food products from the market and are taken from food balance sheet data supplied by Statistics Canada. The maximum residue limit or the tolerance of a pesticide is derived from representative field trial data reflecting the maximum application rate, the maximum number of applications and the minimum pre-harvest interval. With an additional assumption of 100% of a crop treated with the pesticide, a 'worst case scenario' or the first estimate of exposure is derived. In the USA, this estimate is referred to as the Theoretical Maximum Residue Contribution of the residue. In Canada, the exposure estimate is referred to as the Potential Daily Intake (PDI). Although producing a more conservative exposure estimate due to the use of disappearance values, this estimate is roughly equivalent to the Theoretical Maximum Residue Contribution used in the USA. Internationally, both estimates are equivalent to the National Theoretical Maximum Daily Intake or NTMDI.

Further refinement of these estimates can be accomplished by using additional field trial data, monitoring data or consumer survey data to provide a more realistic estimate of the actual pesticide residues as they relate to actual human consumption. In the USA, this refined dietary exposure estimate is referred to as the Anticipated Residue Contribution and may also include consideration of the percentage of crop treated and average processing factors. In Canada, this refined dietary exposure estimate or 'best estimate' may also incorporate processing factors and any other data available to refine the dietary exposure assessment. Internationally, both estimates are roughly equivalent to the National Estimated Daily Intake or NEDI.

The risk of both acute and chronic (i.e. non-acute) dietary exposure to pesticides is estimated in both countries. A computer program used in the US EPA, the Dietary Risk Evaluation System, links consumption and residue data with toxicological endpoints to provide a dietary exposure and risk estimate. For acute dietary risk assessments, Canada and the USA take similar approaches. The NOEL from an acute or subacute toxicity study is divided by an appropriate uncertainty factor to derive an Acute Reference Dose (acute RfD). Although uncertainty factors of 100 (10 × for inter-species extrapolation and 10 × for intra-species extrapolation) are typically used, the factors may be modified in the light of considerations such as the availability of human data, the quality of the database and the type and significance of the toxic response. In Canada, the PDI for acute effects must not exceed the values established for the acute RfD and thus influences the allowable Maximum Residue Limit established for a given commodity. If no appropriate acute end-point is identified, an acute dietary risk assessment is not necessary in either country.

For chronic dietary exposure, the NOEL from the most appropriate toxicity study divided by the appropriate safety factor determines the Reference Dose (RfD) in the USA or the Acceptable Daily Intake (ADI) in Canada. For the chronic dietary risk assessment in the USA, the sum of the exposure from each crop is divided by the RfD to obtain a percentage of the RfD for the overall US population and for each of the 22 subgroups. In Canada, as with the acute dietary exposure, the PDI for chronic effects must not exceed the values established for the ADI.

With the passage of the Food Quality Protection Act in the USA, the US EPA is required to factor all sources of pesticide exposure into decisions on establishing and reassessing tolerances, including drinking water exposure. Likewise, where it has been determined that pesticides from this source could contribute to overall exposure potential, a risk assessment is required in Canada. Two methods of determining exposure are employed. The first is to measure or monitor directly actual drinking water for pesticide contamination. At present, there are no national, comprehensive, appropriate databases of pesticide concentrations in drinking water. Most of the monitoring data are for a small number of pesticides with a history of intensive use on major agricultural crops. Therefore, most drinking water concentration estimates rely on simulation or modelling. In the USA, the primary use of these models at present is to provide a coarse screen for identifying those pesticides for which there is a human health drinking water level of concern (DWLOCs). A human health DWLOC is the concentration of a pesticide in drinking water which would result in unacceptable aggregate risk, after having factored in all food exposures and other non-occupational exposures.

In Canada, generally 10% of the ADI is allocated to exposure from drinking water sources. Based on this value and water consumption patterns for various Canadian subpopulations, federal guideline values may be set for pesticides in drinking water.

Classification, Labelling and Packaging Requirements

USA

In the USA, a pesticide product may be classified for general or restricted use based on its potential as a hazard to humans and/or non-target species. When classified for restricted use, a pesticide product must be applied by or under the supervision of a certified applicator. Training and certification of applicators are usually carried out under a state plan authorized by the US EPA. A pesticide may be classified for both general and restricted uses, depending on the product formulation and its toxic potential.

Human hazard signal words (Danger, Warning, Caution) are required based on a pesticide product's oral, inhalation or dermal acute toxicity, in the USA. The word 'Poison' with a skull and crossbones must also appear on products labelled with the 'Danger' signal word. In addition, precautionary statements are required, indicating the particular hazard, route(s) of exposure and precautions to be taken to avoid injury, based on the acute toxicity profile. Criteria for requiring precautionary labelling for environmental and physical or chemical hazards also exist.

Labelling specifications are also included in the US EPA's Worker Protection Standard, regulations designed to reduce risks of illnesses or injury to workers and handlers of pesticides involved in agricultural production (USA, 1997). Required labelling information includes restricted-entry intervals, use of personal protective equipment and notification of pesticide application.

The US EPA, in conjunction with industry, trade associations and other federal agencies, recently undertook a project to improve labelling of household products. The Consumer Labelling Initiative focuses on indoor and outdoor pesticides and household hard surface cleaners. The goal of the project is to design labels so that consumers have the type of information that will enable them to make informed choices among products and to use chosen products safely as directed.

Child-resistant packaging is required in the USA if a pesticide product meets certain toxicity criteria and is expected to have residential use. The packaging must be designed and constructed to be significantly difficult for children under 5 years of age to open or obtain a toxic or harmful amount of the substance contained therein within a reasonable time, and is not difficult for normal adults to use properly.

Canada

In Canada, the primary consideration in classifying pesticides is the use for which they are intended. In addition, classification is characterized by product-specific toxicological, environmental and packaging criteria. There are three classes for end-use products: Domestic, Commercial and Restricted classes. These typically reflect an ascending degree of hazard. Domestic products are marketed to consumers for use in and around a dwelling. Generally, their toxicity is low, no special precautions or protective equipment are required, disposal can be via household garbage and packaging can be limited to single season use. Commercial products, which include those with an Agricultural, Industrial or Institutional designation, are indicated for farming, commercial pest control or industrial activities. Owing to toxicity considerations and volumes of use, some limitations are often indicated for commercial products with respect to use and disposal practices. Restricted products are considered the most hazardous because of inherent toxicity or intended use in environmentally sensitive areas. Additional limitations respecting the display, distribution, use or operator qualifications may be required to ensure human and environmental safety. Training and certification of pesticide applicators is a provincial responsibility and their programmes conform to national standards. A fourth class of product, Manufacturing, allows for the manufacturing, formulating or repackaging into end-use products in Canada.

Canadian labelling regulations require similar information to that required in the USA and stipulate that pesticide labels must contain the following type of information: identification and guarantee (name, contents of active ingredient, net quantity), class designation, registration number, name and address of registrant, directions for use, nature and degree of hazard (including signal words and symbols), hazard mitigation and decontamination/disposal measures and first aid instructions. Specific criteria determines the level, type and placement of information.

To date, no generic requirements for child-resistant containers exist for Canadian pesticides; however, this area will warrant consideration in the future. Currently, child-resistant packaging is undertaken voluntarily by the manufacturer or is required on a product specific basis. More focus has been placed in the area of worker protection with specialized packaging requirements such as water-soluble bags designed to minimize exposure through handling.

Future Directions

Changes to pesticide regulatory regimes are occurring at a rapid rate with the increasing globalization of pesticide markets and constraints on regulatory resources. The most notable change is the current focus on harmonization.

USA Food Quality Protection Act

With the passage of the Food Quality Protection Act in the USA, complex scientific issues have been raised that will ultimately influence the regulatory process in both Canada and the USA. Issues such as the sensitivity of the young, aggregate exposure, exposure to multiple pesticides with common mechanisms of action, *in utero* exposure to pesticides and endocrine disruption will require the development of new policies and evaluation methods.

NAFTA

The USA, Canada and Mexico have made commitments under the North American Free Trade Agreement (NAFTA) to (1) share the work of regulation, (2) harmonize scientific and policy considerations and (3) reduce trade barriers. Biannual meetings are held to monitor the progress and guide efforts on these commitments. The countries also liase regularly on a more informal level, on matters that include joint reviews of pesticide products, guideline development, guideline requirements and a variety of other issues.

Wider Harmonization

Harmonization within the international community also represents a challenge for North America. Participation in various OECD activities including guideline development and harmonization of hazard classification is essential for ensuring that all countries benefit from uniform procedures and practices in assessing and communicating pesticide risk. The USA and Canada are contributing to the identification and implementation of risk reduction initiatives under the OECD framework. Collaborative efforts with the European Union are focusing on issues such as standardization of dossier preparation and electronic submission and review formats. Work sharing has expanded beyond the North American borders and has been initiated with other OECD countries (see Chapter 71).

Conclusion

In conclusion, the North American regulatory processes are committed to ensuring the safety of pesticide products entering the marketplace. The ongoing challenge is continually to refine the methods for assessing potential risk in light of new scientific knowledge or awareness and to do so recognizing the principles of efficiency and harmonization.

THE EUROPEAN UNION

The authorization of pesticides in the European Community is governed by two main Directives, namely

Directive 91/414/EEC concerning the placing of plant protection products on the market (EEC Council, 1991) and a new Directive covering similar provisions for biocidal products (European Parliament and EC Council 1998). Where appropriate, these Directives call on existing Community legislation in related areas such as classification, packaging and labelling and maximum residue levels (MRLs).

Plant Protection Products Directive (91/414/EEC)

Prior to the introduction of Directive 91/414/EEC, the various Member States of the European Community had their own national registration schemes which, owing to their differing requirements, represented a barrier to trade both of plant protection products and of plant products within the Community. A proposal for a Directive intended to achieve the harmonization of pesticide regulation was actively examined between 1977 and 1983, but reservations on the part of a number of Member States prevented adoption. As part of the provisions for the creation of the internal market, detailed negotiations resumed in 1989 and led to the adoption of an amended proposal (Directive 91/414/EEC) which came into force in July 1993 (EEC Council, 1991).

Plant protection products are defined as chemical or biological products intended to: protect plants or plant products against harmful organisms; influence the life processes of plants, other than as a nutrient (e.g. growth regulators); preserve plant products; destroy undesired plants or parts of plants; and check or prevent undesired growth of plants.

Directive 91/414/EEC lays down harmonized procedures for the authorization of plant protection products that must be followed by all Member States. It provides for the establishment of a positive list of active substances (Annex I to the Directive) which may then be incorporated into products intended for use within the Community. Only substances which can be shown to the satisfaction of the Standing Committee on Plant Health (SCPH) to be without danger to human and animal health or to the environment, on the basis of a comprehensive data package, will be entered in Annex I.

Annexes II and III to Directive 91/414/EEC give details of the data requirements for active substances and plant protection products respectively, for both chemicals and micro-organisms, under the general headings given in **Table 1**. The introductions to Annexes II and III allow applicants to submit a justification in place of data where they believe certain pieces of information would not be necessary owing to the nature of the substance or its proposed uses. To date, further guidance on these requirements and details of test guidelines to be followed have been provided for chemical substances and preparations in a series of amending Directives

(EEC Commission, 1993a; EC Commission, 1994a, b, 1995a, b, 1996a–c). The third of these Directives (94/79/EC) gives the expanded details for toxicological and metabolism studies and the headings from this are reproduced in **Table 2**. The majority of test guidelines referred to in this Directive are for methods given in Annex V of the Dangerous Substances Directive (67/548/EEC). Details of the toxicity test guidelines are given in the 9th, 17th, 18th and 22nd adaptations to Directive 67/548/EEC (EEC Commission, 1987, 1992a, 1993b; EC Commission, 1996d). Many of these methods have been adapted from those of other international organizations, such as the OECD. The toxicological information provided must be sufficient to permit an evaluation to be made as to the risks for man associated with the handling and use of plant protection products containing the active substance and the risk for man arising from residual traces remaining in food and water. In addition, the information provided must be sufficient to establish a relevant acceptable daily intake level (ADI) for man, and establish acceptable operator exposure levels (AOELs).

Further guidance covering the requirements for microorganisms and viruses is currently being developed; the details for toxicity, pathogenicity and infectivity studies taken from the current proposal are given in **Table 3**. It is proposed that a tiered testing system will apply to studies on microorganisms and plant protection products containing them and that the appropriate test programmes for specific applications will need to be decided on a case-by-case basis.

Individual Member States retain powers in respect of the national authorization of plant protection products. As such they will be responsible for making judgements regarding the safety and efficacy of preparations containing those active substances in Annex I of Directive 91/414/EEC. To ensure a consistent approach, Member States have agreed the uniform principles (Annex VI to the Directive), or rules which must be observed in authorizing plant protection products. Annex VI was published as Directive 97/57/EC (EC Council, 1997a) and came into force immediately.

New Active Substances

An applicant wishing to market a plant protection product containing an active substance new to the Community must submit a 'dossier' in line with the requirements of Annexes II and III (data requirements for active substances and plant protection products). The Commission has produced guidelines for industry on the preparation and presentation of dossiers (EC Commission, 1997a). Once a dossier has been submitted, it has to be confirmed as complete to the satisfaction of the SCPH. By early 1998, there had been positive votes at the SCPH on the completeness of over 30 dossiers for new active substances. These details are published as Commission Decisions. When a dossier has been confirmed as complete, the appointed

Table 1

Annex II—Requirements for the dossier to be submitted for the inclusion of an active substance in Annex I

Introduction
1. Identity of the active substance/organism
2. Physical and chemical properties/biological properties
3. Further information on the active substance
4. Analytical methods
5. Toxicological studies
6. Residues in or on treated products, food and feed
7. Fate and behaviour in the environment
8. Ecotoxicological studies
9. Classification and labelling proposals

Annex III—Requirements for the dossier to be submitted for the authorization of a plant protection product

Introduction
1. Identity of the plant protection product
2. Physical, chemical or technical properties
3. Data on application
4. Further information on the plant protection product
5. Analytical methods
6. Efficacy data
7. Toxicological studies
8. Residues in or on treated products, food and feed
9. Fate and behaviour in the environment
10. Ecotoxicological studies
11. Further information, e.g. authorizations in other countries, classification and labelling proposals

Table 2

Annex II, Part A—Chemical Substances

Section 5—Toxicological studies on the active substance

5.1   Studies on absorption, distribution, excretion and metabolism in mammals
5.2   Acute toxicity: oral; percutaneous; inhalation; skin irritation; eye irritation; skin sensitization
5.3   Short-term toxicity: oral 28-day study; oral 90-day study; other routes
5.4   Genotoxicity testing: *in vitro* studies; *in vivo* studies in somatic cells; *in vivo* studies in germ cells
5.5   Long-term toxicity and carcinogenicity
5.6   Reproductive toxicity: multi-generation studies; developmental toxicity studies
5.7   Delayed neurotoxicity studies
5.8   Other toxicological studies: toxicity studies of metabolites; supplementary studies on the active substance
5.9   Medical data: medical surveillance on manufacturing plant personnel; direct observation, e.g. clinical cases and poisoning incidents; observations on exposure of the general population and epidemiological studies if appropriate; diagnosis of poisoning (determination of active substance, metabolites), specific signs of poisoning, clinical tests; proposed treatment (first aid measures, antidotes, medical treatment); expected effects of poisoning
5.10   Summary of mammalian toxicity and overall evaluation

Annex III, Part A—Chemical Preparations

Section 7—Toxicological studies on the plant protection product

7.1   Acute toxicity: oral; percutaneous; inhalation; skin irritation; eye irritation; skin sensitization; supplementary studies for combinations of plant protection products
7.2   Data on exposure: operator exposure (estimation of operator exposure, measurement of operator exposure); bystander exposure; worker exposure (estimation of worker exposure, measurement of worker exposure)
7.3   Dermal absorption
7.4   Available toxicological data relating to non-active substances

Table 3

Annex II, Part B—Microorganisms and viruses

Section 5—Toxicological, pathogenicity and infectivity studies

5.1   Step I—Basic studies
5.1.1   Acute toxicity, pathogenicity and infectivity: acute oral toxicity, pathogenicity and infectivity; acute inhalation toxicity, pathogenicity and infectivity; intraperitoneal/subcutaneous single dose; skin irritation; eye irritation; skin sensitization
5.1.2   Genotoxicity testing: *in vitro* studies; *in vivo* studies in somatic cells
5.1.3   Cell culture study
5.1.4   Short-term toxicity, pathogenicity and infectivity
5.1.5   Pathogenicity and infectivity under immunosuppression
5.2   Step II—Additional studies
5.2.1   Acute percutaneous toxicity, pathogenicity and infectivity
5.2.2   Genotoxicity—*in vivo* studies in germ cells
5.3   Step III—Specific toxicity, pathogenicity and infectivity studies
5.4   Medical data
5.4.1   Medical surveillance on manufacturing plant personnel
5.4.2   Sensitization/allergenicity observations, if appropriate
5.4.3   Direct observations, e.g. clinical cases
5.4.4   Observations on exposure of the general population and epidemiological studies if appropriate
5.4.5   Proposed treatment: first aid measures, medical treatment
5.5   Summary of mammalian toxicity, pathogenicity and infectivity and overall evaluation

Annex III, Part B—Preparations of microorganisms or viruses

Section 7—Toxicological and/or pathogenicity and infectivity studies

7.1   Step I—Basic acute toxicity studies
7.1.1   Acute oral toxicity
7.1.2   Acute inhalation toxicity
7.1.3   Acute percutaneous toxicity
7.2   Step II—Additional acute toxicity studies
7.2.1   Skin irritation
7.2.2   Eye irritation
7.2.3   Skin sensitization
7.3   Data on exposure
7.4   Available toxicological data relating to non-active substances
7.5   Supplementary studies for combinations of plant protection products
7.6   Summary and evaluation of health effects

rapporteur Member State has 12 months in which to evaluate it. The result of the *rapporteur* work is a draft evaluation or 'monograph' prepared in accordance with the Commission's guidelines (EC Commission, 1997b). By April 1998, monographs for more than 10 new active substances had been delivered to the Commission.

The final decision on the inclusion of an active substance in Annex I of Directive 91/414/EEC will normally be taken by the Commission after obtaining a favourable opinion from the SCPH. This opinion is delivered by Member States in the SCPH following consideration in full working group meetings (attended by representatives from all 15 Member States) and is reached by qualified majority voting.

In order to help the decision-making process, the Commission has established procedures for the review of monographs before their submission to the SCPH. Since September 1996, the UK Pesticides Safety Directorate (PSD) and the German Biologische Bundesanstalt für Land-und Forstwirtschaft (BBA) have been con-

tracted to organize a series of European Community Coordination (ECCO) peer review meetings to undertake this work. To date, each ECCO meeting has considered a section of the monograph (physical and chemical properties; environmental fate and behaviour; ecotoxicology; mammalian toxicology; and residues) followed by an overview meeting. Up to seven experts from different Member States have been invited to attend each meeting, which lasts approximately 4 days and examines five or six monographs.

Once a round of ECCO meetings is complete, a report of the discussions and conclusions for each active substance is circulated to all Member States and to the applicant, together with an invitation to submit their comments to the Commission. A proposal for the decision on the active substance is then prepared, accompanied by a comprehensive report which gives the basis for the decision. By April 1998, reports and proposed decisions for five new active substances had been prepared and discussed at full working group meetings and a decision had been taken by the SCPH on inclusion of one new active substance, azoxystrobin, in Annex I.

If so requested by an applicant, once the Commission has confirmed the completeness of a new active substance dossier, Member States may proceed to issue provisional authorizations for use of plant protection products containing the substance. Provisional authorization can be granted for up to 3 years (renewable once) to allow these new products to be made available in individual member states while consultations for Annex I listing progress.

Reviews

Directive 91/414/EEC provides for the establishment of a review programme of 'old' active substances, that is, substances on the Community market in plant protection products when Directive 91/414/EEC came into force (approximately 800 chemical substances and 20 microorganisms and viruses). Following the compilation of a list of these substances, the Commission selected 90 which were to be reviewed first. These substances were then allocated to *rapporteur* member states. The number of reviews given to each Member State varies; for example, France, Germany, Italy and the UK are each carrying out 11 reviews from the first list of 90 compounds. Details of the substances on this first review list, and of the *rapporteurs* and procedures for the review programme, are given in Regulations 3600/92 and 933/94 (EEC Commission, 1992b; EC Commission, 1994c). *Rapporteur* responsibilities for the active substances under review were reallocated following the accession to the Community of three new Member States (Austria, Finland and Sweden) on 1 January 1995; details are set out in Regulation 491/95 (EC Commission, 1995c). It was originally intended that further lists of about 90 substances would be published annually until the review programme was completed. However, the next phases of the review programme have yet to be finalized.

Industry has supported 86 of the substances from the first priority list. Notifiers were originally required to have submitted their review dossiers by 30 April 1995. However, extensions to this deadline were requested for several active substances by notifiers. These requests were forwarded to the Commission for consideration, and the substances for which an extension was granted (until 31 October 1995) were listed in Regulation 2230/95 (EC Commission, 1995d).

Community procedures have been established for Member States to check the review dossiers for completeness, to ensure that they meet the requirements laid down in Regulation 3600/92 and that sufficient information has been received to allow evaluation to start. Assuming that a satisfactory dossier has been received, Member States have 12 months in which to undertake the detailed evaluation and submit their draft monograph to the Commission. By early 1998, a total of 45 review monographs had been submitted to the Commission.

Monographs for reviews follow the same route as those for new substances, via the ECCO peer review meetings. Once a round of ECCO meetings is complete, and following consultation with all Member States and the notifiers, a proposal for the Annex I listing of the active substance is prepared (or, where necessary, a decision on suspension, withdrawal or postponement). This proposal is accompanied by a comprehensive 'review report' which gives the basis for the decision. As with the reports for new substances, the finalized review report will include the monograph and ECCO report as background documents. The reports for both new and reviewed active substances will be made available by Member States for consultation by any interested parties. By April 1998, review reports and proposed decisions for several active substances had been prepared and discussed at full working group meetings and a decision had been taken on the inclusion of one active substance, imazalil, in Annex I. Conditions attached to the Annex I inclusion of substances are published as Commission Directives.

Plant Protection Products

Plant protection products which were on the Community market when Directive 91/414/EEC came into force may continue to be marketed and used under national rules until their active substances are reviewed. Once an active substance has been entered in Annex I, products containing it must be assessed by Member States to ensure that they comply with the conditions attached to the Annex I listing and with the uniform principles, and that all data requirements and any data protection provisions are satisfied. Once a product is re-registered satisfactorily, it can continue to be marketed and used, subject to a 10-yearly review.

The uniform principles encompass evaluation and decision-making for the authorization of plant protection products in the following areas: efficacy; absence of unacceptable effects on plants or plant products; impact on vertebrates to be controlled; impact on human or animal health; influence on the environment; analytical methods; and physical and chemical properties. Operator exposure likely to occur under the proposed conditions of use (including in particular dose, application method and climatic conditions) is evaluated preferably by using realistic exposure data or, if such data are not available, a suitable, validated calculation model. Similarly, the possibility of exposure of bystanders or workers exposed after the application of the plant protection product (such as realistic re-entry periods) is also evaluated. Authorization is not granted if the extent of exposure under the proposed conditions of use exceeds the acceptable operator exposure level (AOEL). The uniform principles require the estimation of the potential exposure of consumers through diet and, if applicable, other routes, using a suitable calculation model. Taking into account all the registered uses (including residues arising from other plant protection products containing the same active substance or giving the same residue), the proposed use cannot be authorized if the most realistic estimate of dietary exposure exceeds the acceptable daily intake (ADI). It is hoped that discussions will lead to a harmonized EC approach to consumer risk assessment by 1998–99. At present calculations on dietary exposure are done in a stepwise fashion leading to an increasingly realistic prediction of intake, based on the following endpoints: ADI; acute reference dose (ARfD); maximum residue level (MRL); supervised trials median residue (STMR); theoretical maximum daily intake (TMDI); international estimated daily intake for the European diet (IEDI); and acute exposure. The principles behind these estimates are described in a report published by the Food and Agriculture Organization and the World Health Organization (WHO, 1995). The uniform principles also require the assessment of the concentrations of active substances or of relevant metabolites, degradation or reaction products in groundwater and surface water. Reference is made to Council Directive 80/778/EEC relating to the quality of water intended for human consumption (EEC Council, 1980). This Directive sets a maximum admissible concentration of 0.1 μg l^{-1} for individual pesticides and 0.5 μg l^{-1} for total pesticides and related substances.

Once an active substance has been entered in Annex I, Directive 91/414/EEC allows for the mutual recognition of products containing that active ingredient. A Member State would not be permitted to refuse the authorization of a plant protection product already authorized in another Member State if all agricultural, plant health and environmental considerations relevant to the use of the product were comparable. Several Member States have been involved in drafting Commission guidance for both applicants and registration authorities on assessing the comparability of these conditions. General concern over the reduction in availability of minor use recommendations as the Community review programme progresses has led to the Commission, Member States and industry working to develop proposals for an equivalent to 'voluntary mutual recognition' of such uses.

Directive 91/414/EEC also makes provision for the use of unauthorized plant protection products in research and development and in emergency situations. Any experiment or test involving the release into the environment requires authorization and may only be carried out under controlled conditions and for limited quantities and areas. Member States may also authorize a plant protection product for a period of up to 120 days for a limited and controlled use if such a measure appears necessary because of an unforeseeable danger which cannot be contained by other means.

Other Provisions

Formal information exchange between Member States and the Commission is an important aspect of Directive 91/414/EEC. Since the Directive came into force, Member States have circulated hardcopy sources of information such as annual lists of product authorization details and results of residues surveillance schemes. There has been some progress within the Commission to develop IT systems to support this information exchange.

The Commission has initiated guidance in other areas to assist with the implementation of Directive 91/414/EEC. For example, a guideline detailing the GLP requirements for all studies listed in Annexes II and III has been issued (EC Commission, 1995e), while a document giving guidance on establishing acceptable operator exposure levels (AOELs) is currently under consideration by Member States and industry. The Commission is also funding the development and maintenance of models for use in the risk assessment of pesticides, such as the European predictive operator exposure model (EUROPOEM).

On an international scale, the guidelines for industry and Member States on the preparation and presentation of dossiers and monographs have also been taken up by the OECD's Pesticide Forum to develop guidelines for wider use. In addition, the CADDY project (computer-aided dossier and data supply) to develop a CD-ROM based electronic format for dossier submission is nearing completion. This has been a joint venture between industry, the Commission, Member States and representatives from the North American regulatory authorities. The Commission does not propose to make submission of data on CD-ROM obligatory, but the CADDY system became available for all applicants who may wish to use this medium from the end of 1997 onwards.

Classification, Packaging and Labelling

The Dangerous Substances Directive (67/548/EEC) covers the hazard classification, packaging and labelling of substances dangerous to humans and the environment which are placed on the market in the Community. The Directive defines substances as 'dangerous' if they are explosive, oxidizing, extremely flammable, highly flammable, flammable, very toxic, toxic, harmful, corrosive, irritant, sensitizing, carcinogenic, mutagenic, toxic for reproduction or dangerous to the environment. Annexes to Directive 67/548/EEC describe the test methods to be used for assessing these properties (Annex V) together with the relevant classification criteria and the associated labelling requirements (Annex VI), including both symbols (Annex II) and risk and safety phrases (Annexes III and IV). Details of these Annexes are given in the 9th, 17th, 18th and 22nd adaptations to the Directive (EEC

Commission, 1987, 1992a, 1993b; EC Commission, 1996d).

At present, plant protection products are subject to some of the hazard classification and labelling requirements of Directive 67/548/EEC, as modified in part by specific provisions of a 'daughter' Directive (78/631/EEC) covering pesticide preparations (EEC Council, 1978). For example, under the former Directive the cut-off points specified as the basis for toxicity classification are the same for both solids and liquids, whereas Directive 78/631/EEC specifies different values for the toxicity of solid and liquid preparations.

In 1991, another classification, packaging and labelling Directive (88/379/EEC) came into force: this covers most dangerous preparations, with some exceptions such as medicinal, veterinary or plant protection products (EEC Council, 1988). Directive 88/379/EEC provides calculation methods for assessing the hazard classification of a product where test data are not available, for example for carcinogenic, mutagenic or reprotoxic effects. A Commission proposal for a new directive to amend Directive 88/379/EEC has been published recently (EC Commission, 1996e). Amongst other changes, this proposal annuls Directive 78/631/EEC and includes pesticide products in the general requirements for classification, packaging, labelling and safety data sheets. It is likely that this new Directive will be adopted by the end of 1998, following which a period of up to 5 years has been proposed for implementation. Member States and industry are currently involved in negotiations to ensure that this implementation is achieved in such a way as to be compatible with the provisions of Directive 91/414/EEC.

Labelling requirements for plant protection products under Directive 91/414/EEC include the following: trade name; name and address of the authorization holder; authorization number of the product; active substance content; hazard classification details and information on first aid; other risk and safety phrases; directions for use (including any special agricultural, plant health and environmental conditions under which the product should not be used); safety intervals (such as harvesting and re-entry intervals); and directions for safe disposal of the product and its packaging.

Maximum Residue Levels (MRLs)

To date, MRLs have been set through the mechanisms provided for in specific Directives, primarily for trade purposes but occasionally as a measure to protect human health. MRLs are designed to ensure that users of pesticides comply with good agricultural practice (GAP). The MRL Directives place obligations on Member States to monitor treated produce for residues of pesticides as a key mechanism to ensure compliance. The establishment of MRLs is also an integral

part of the authorizations process under Directive 91/414/EEC.

Community activity to harmonize national MRLs in Member States started in 1975 with negotiations on a Directive (76/895/EEC) which fixed harmonized maximum levels for residues in and on fruit and vegetables (EEC Council, 1976). Implementation of the MRLs set in this Directive was optional on Member States, who were constrained only by the fact that they could not establish national MRLs which were lower than the levels in the Directive, since these might act as trade barriers. In the mid-1980s, the Commission and Member States advanced the work by agreeing two framework Directives (86/362/EEC and 86/363/EEC) which fixed obligatory MRLs for cereals and foodstuffs of animal origin, respectively (EEC Council, 1986a, b). In 1990, a further Directive (90/642/EEC) was adopted which provided an obligatory framework for the setting of MRLs in a much wider range of products of plant origin, which included fruit and vegetables (EEC Council, 1990).

Since the establishment of these framework Directives there has been an ambitious programme in the Community to establish harmonized MRLs for approximately 100 active substances in four separate priority lists. This intensive scientific and legislative exercise has resulted in two Directives per year between 1993 and 1996 which establish obligatory MRLs in the three framework Directives (EEC Council 1993a, b; EC Council, 1994a, b, 1995a, b, 1996a, b). The MRL Directives also set residue data requirements (i.e. 'open positions') which are reviewed after 4 years when trials data become available. At least two further proposals for MRL Directives are anticipated before the separate MRL setting programme is completed.

A further landmark MRL Directive (97/41/EC) has recently been adopted (EC Council, 1997b). This Directive must be brought into force by Member States by the end of 1998 and will achieve the following: speed up the agreement of straightforward MRL proposals, by transferring power from the Council to the SCPH; introduce a conciliation agreement for trade disputes; extend the scope of the MRLs Directives to include selected processed and composite foods; formalize arrangements whereby the Commission may recommend annual programmes for monitoring treated foods for residues; and provide for transitional arrangements for implementing MRLs to allow the marketing of previously treated produce.

It has been recognized that the continuation of two separate Community initiatives on pesticides, namely the MRL setting programme and reviews under Directive 91/414/EEC, is potentially inefficient in the use of Member State, Commission and industry resources. The Commission has already started integrating these programmes by transferring the responsibility for reviewing data in support of 'open positions' in the priority lists of

MRLs to the review *rapporteurs* where practical. It is likely that, once the next list of active substances to be reviewed under Directive 91/414/EEC is published, the two programmes will run in parallel. Thus the Member State appointed to act as *rapporteur* for the review under Directive 91/414/EEC would maintain 'cradle to grave' responsibility for all aspects of the substance, including MRLs.

Biocidal Products Directive (98/8/EC)

A proposal for a Directive concerning the placing of biocidal products on the market was first published in 1993 and detailed negotiations led to its adoption (Directive 98/8/EC) by the European Parliament and Council in April 1998). Member states have 2 years from this date in which to implement Directive 98/8/EC. The Directive covers a wide range of product types, including (target organisms in parentheses): disinfectants (bacteria and viruses), e.g. used in hospitals or in the home; preservatives (mould, fungi and insects), e.g. for use in paints, carpets, clothes or wood; public hygiene insecticides (e.g. flies, mosquitoes and ants); rodenticides (rats and mice); and antifouling preparations, which are used against barnacles and other marine organisms on the hulls of ships.

The Biocidal Products Directive complements Directive 91/414/EEC and indeed has very similar requirements in many respects. Active substances will be evaluated at the Community level by the Standing Committee on Biocides for inclusion in a positive list (Annex I to the Directive). The review of existing active substances, which are already on the market in products when the Directive comes into force, will last for 10 years and will be controlled by an EC Regulation (yet to be written). During the transition period, existing national rules in Member States with regard to the marketing of biocidal products containing existing active substances, will continue to apply until such time as the active substances are added to, or refused entry to, Annex I. Risk assessment and authorization of individual biocidal products will be carried out at Member State level based on common principles (Annex VI) to ensure a consistent approach. There is also a requirement for mutual recognition of authorized products throughout the Community.

However, the Biocidal Products Directive also contains some additional facilities and requirements which are not found in Directive 91/414/EEC. It provides simplified procedures for 'low-risk' substances and also contains provisions on comparative assessment. The application of comparative assessment means that the inclusion of an active substance in Annex I may be refused or reviewed if another substance presents significantly less risk to health or the environment.

REGULATION OUTSIDE NORTH AMERICA AND THE EUROPEAN UNION

Formerly, most countries regulated pesticides independently of their neighbours. The major trading blocks, NAFTA, EU, etc., increasingly regulate pesticides trans-nationally. Moreover, smaller groups of countries also do so. For example, since the Australian National Registration Authority (NRA) was established in 1992, there has been significant progress in joint initiatives between this Authority and the Agricultural Compound Unit (ACU) in New Zealand. In the central and eastern European states with aspirations for future EU membership, there are now moves to bring pesticide registration requirements into line with Directive 91/414/EEC and Directive 98/8/EC. Harmonization is also being addressed within regional groupings in southern and central America and Africa, although progress has been slow in some of these areas.

INTERNATIONAL HARMONIZATION IN PESTICIDE REGULATION

At an international level, the Food and Agriculture Organization (FAO), World Health Organization (WHO) and Organization for Economic Cooperation and Development (OECD) are actively involved in initiatives of relevance to pesticide regulation.

Joint FAO/WHO Meeting on Pesticide Residues (JMPR) and Other WHO Programmes

Since the 1960s, the FAO and WHO has convened meetings of panels of experts who serve in their personal capacities and evaluate selected pesticide residues on the basis of available data. A major role of the JMPR is the determination of acceptable daily intakes (ADIs) and maximum residue levels (MRLs) for pesticides. The JMPR decisions are then used as the basis of MRLs produced by the FAO/WHO Codex Alimentarius Commission on Pesticide Residues (CCPR). Since the Uruguay round of GATT (General Agreement on Tariffs and Trade) negotiations on free trade and the agreement on preventing the use of sanitary and phytosanitary measures as barriers to trade, the decisions made by the JMPR and CCPR have taken on added importance.

The WHO panel which sets ADIs works by a form of peer review. A monograph is prepared by an independent 'temporary adviser' from study reports submitted by the pesticide manufacturer and from data in the public domain, often papers in peer-reviewed journals. The reports should cover: absorption and metabolism; single-and repeat-dose toxicity, including genotoxicity, carcinogenicity, reproduction; and any human data. The adviser summarizes the studies and proposes No Observed Adverse Effect Levels (NOAELs). The adviser's draft monograph is then reviewed by an 'invited expert' before being discussed at the JMPR meeting. If the database is deemed to be acceptable by the JMPR, an ADI can be proposed and allocated. The outcomes of the Meetings are published in the form of reports (e.g. FAO/WHO, 1998a, 1999) and more detailed evaluations (e.g. FAO/WHO, 1998b).

The acceptability or otherwise of pesticide treatments used on produce going into international trade is determined by comparing ADIs with estimated intakes derived by the FAO panel, using residues data and information on food consumption in different areas of the world. The guidelines currently used for estimating dietary pesticide residues have been reviewed at two Joint FAO/WHO Consultations with the objective of obtaining more realistic estimates of human exposure (WHO, 1995, 1997). The Consultations focused mainly on the issues of residue levels in foods, exposure assessment related to both acute and chronic toxicity and food consumption. However, it was recognized that other potential contributions to pesticide dietary intake from sources such as drinking water may need to be considered.

The work of the JMPR is supported by WHO's International Programme on Chemical Safety (IPCS). The IPCS produces a useful range of publications entitled Environmental Health Criteria. The series comprises comprehensive reviews of chemicals, including pesticides, as well as guidelines and principles on assessment. One of the latter publications outlines the principles used by JMPR (IPCS, 1990). It has been recognized that there is considerable duplication of effort on an international scale in multiple assessments of the same data for a pesticide submitted to different regulatory authorities. In a move to reduce this, the IPCS has introduced a programme for the production of 'concise international core assessment documents' (CICADS). These will be produced by one regulatory authority or consultant for review by a core assessment panel and, if acceptable, could then be used by other regulatory authorities for the purposes of human and environmental risk assessment in place of their own extensive review of individual study reports.

Organization for Economic Cooperation and Development (OECD)

The OECD plays an important role in harmonizing the safety assessment of pesticides on a global scale. Since their development in 1981, the OECD's Test Guidelines have become the internationally recognized reference tool for those working on the testing of chemicals and the assessment of their potential hazards. Following an agreement on mutual acceptance of data, any studies performed to the minimum requirements of the OECD Test Guidelines should be accepted by regulatory authorities in all signatory countries (OECD, 1981). This agreement has benefits particularly with respect to animal welfare as there should be no need to repeat studies for submission to different authorities.

In 1992, the OECD set up the 'Pesticide Forum', a meeting of regulatory authorities from member countries, industry, the EC Commission and organizations such as WHO and FAO. The Forum aims to find common approaches to a range of topics relevant to the assessment of pesticides (both plant protection and biocidal products). Its work programme includes: data requirements (including the development of data requirements for new types of pesticides such as pheromones); risk assessment and reduction (such as the development of pesticide risk indicators); and registration matters (including guidance documents for industry data submissions and country review reports and the procedures for the exchange of data and reports to reduce duplication). One important link with other OECD work is for the Forum to identify specific test procedures relevant to pesticides (e.g. delayed neuropathy tests) and to determine whether these are a high priority for the OECD to devise an internationally accepted Test Guideline.

REFERENCES

Canada (1975). *Food Consumption Patterns Report: a Report from Nutrition Canada*. Bureau of Nutritional Sciences. Department of National Health and Welfare, Canada, Ottawa.

Canada (1985a). *Pest Control Products Act. Revised Statutes of Canada, 1985. c. P-9. Pest Control Product Regulations 1988*. The Queen's Printer, Ottawa.

Canada (1985b). *Food and Drugs Act. Revised Statutes of Canada, 1985. c. F-27. Food and Drug Regulations. 1979*. The Queen's Printer, Ottawa.

Carson, R. (1962). *Silent Spring*. Hamish Hamilton, London.

EC Commission (1994a). Directive 94/37/EC of 22 July 1994 amending Council Directive 91/414/EEC concerning the placing of plant protection products on the market. *Off. J. Eur. Commun.*, No. L194, 29.7.94, 65–81.

EC Commission (1994b). Directive 94/79/EC of 21 December 1994 amending Council Directive 91/414/EEC concerning the placing of plant protection products on the market. *Off. J. Eur. Commun.*, No. L354, 31.12.94, 16–31 (corrigenda: *Off. J. Eur. Commun.*, No. L280, 23.11.95, 58).

EC Commission (1994c). Regulation (EC) No. 933/94 of 27 April 1994 laying down the active substances of plant protection products and designating the rapporteur member states for the implementation of Commission Regulation (EEC) No. 3600/92. *Off. J. Eur. Commun.*, No. L107, 28.4.94, 8–18.

EC Commission (1995a). Directive 95/35/EC of 14 July 1995 amending Council Directive 91/414/EEC concerning the placing of plant protection products on the market. *Off. J. Eur. Commun.*, No. L172, 27.7.95, 6–7.

EC Commission (1995b). Directive 95/36/EC of 14 July 1995 amending Council Directive 91/414/EEC concerning the placing of plant protection products on the market. *Off. J. Eur. Commun.*, No. L172, 27.7.95, 8–20.

EC Commission (1995c). Regulation (EC) No. 491/95 of 3 March 1995 amending Regulation (EEC) No. 3600/92 and Regulation (EC) No. 933/94, in particular with regard to the integration of the designated public authorities and the producers in Austria, Finland and Sweden in the implementation of the first stage of the programme of work referred to in Article 8 (2) of Council Directive 91/414/EEC concerning the placing of plant protection products on the market. *Off. J. Eur. Commun.*, No. L49, 4.3.95, 50–52.

EC Commission (1995d). Regulation (EC) No. 2230/95 of 21 September 1995 amending Regulation (EC) No. 933/94 laying down the active substances of plant protection products and designating the rapporteur member states for the implementation of Commission Regulation (EEC) No. 3600/92. *Off. J. Eur. Commun.*, No. L225, 22.9.95, 1–3.

EC Commission (1995e). Guideline developed within the SCPH with regard to the applicability of GLP to data requirements according to Annexes II, Part A, and III, Part A, of Council Directive 91/414/EEC. Commission Document 7109/VI/94 rev. 6 cl, 14.7.95.

EC Commission (1996a). Directive 96/12/EC of 8 March 1996 amending Council Directive 91/414/EEC concerning the placing of plant protection products on the market. *Off. J. Eur. Commun.*, No. L65, 15.3.96, 20–37.

EC Commission (1996b). Directive 96/46/EC of 16 July 1996 amending Council Directive 91/414/EEC concerning the placing of plant protection products on the market. *Off. J. Eur. Commun.*, No. L214, 23.8.96, 18–24.

EC Commission (1996c). Directive 96/68/EC of 21 October 1996 amending Council Directive 91/414/EEC concerning the placing of plant protection products on the market. *Off. J. Eur. Commun.*, No. L277, 30.10.96, 25–34.

EC Commission (1996d). Directive 96/54/EC of 30 July 1996 adapting to technical progress for the twenty-second time Council Directive 67/548/EEC on the approximation of the laws, regulations and administrative provisions relating to the classification, packaging and labelling of dangerous substances. *Off. J. Eur. Commun.*, No. L248, 30.9.96, 1–230.

EC Commission (1996e). Commission proposal for a European Parliament and Council Directive concerning the approximation of the laws, regulations and administrative provisions of the member states relating to the classification, packaging and labelling of dangerous preparations. *Off. J. Eur. Commun.*, No. C283, 26.9.96, pp. 1–54.

EC Commission (1997a). Guidelines and criteria for the preparation and presentation of complete dossiers and of summary dossiers for the inclusion of active substances in Annex I of Directive 91/414/EEC (Article 5.3 and 8.2). Commission Document 1663/VI/94 rev. 7.6, 31.10.97.

EC Commission (1997b). Guidelines and criteria for the evaluation of dossiers and for the preparation of reports to the European Commission by rapporteur member states relating to the proposed inclusion of active substances in Annex I of Directive 91/414/EEC. Commission Document 1654/VI/94 rev. 6.4, 31.10.97.

EC Council (1994a). Council Directive 94/29/EC of 23 June 1994 amending the Annexes to Directives 86/362/EEC and 86/363/EEC on the fixing of maximum levels for pesticide residues in and on cereals and foodstuffs of animal origin respectively. *Off. J. Eur. Commun.*, No. L189, 23.7.94, 67–69.

EC Council (1994b). Council Directive 94/30/EEC of 23 June 1994 amending Annex II to Directive 90/642/EEC relating to the fixing of maximum levels for pesticide residues in and on certain products of plant origin, including fruit and vegetables, and providing for the establishment of a first list of maximum levels. *Off. J. Eur. Commun.*, No. L189, 23.7.94, 70–83.

EC Council (1995a). Council Directive 95/38/EC of 17 July 1995 amending Annexes I and II to Directive 90/642/EEC on the fixing of maximum levels for pesticide residues in and on certain products of plant origin, including fruit and vegetables, and providing for the establishment of a list of maximum levels. *Off. J. Eur. Commun.*, No. L197, 22.8.95, 14–28.

EC Council (1995b). Council Directive 95/39/EC of 17 July 1995 amending the Annexes to Directives 86/362/EEC and 86/363/EEC on the fixing of maximum levels for pesticide residues in and on cereals and foodstuffs of animal origin. *Off. J. Eur. Commun.*, No. L197, 22.8.95, 29–31.

EC Council (1996a). Council Directive 96/32/EC of 21 May 1996 amending Annex II to Directive 76/895/EEC relating to the fixing of maximum levels for pesticide residues in and on fruit and vegetables and Annex III to Directive 90/642/EEC relating to the fixing of maximum levels for pesticide residues in and on certain products of plant origin, including fruit and vegetables. *Off. J. Eur. Commun.*, No. L144, 18.6.96, 12–34.

EC Council (1996b). Council Directive 96/33/EC of 21 May 1996 amending the Annexes to Directives 86/362/EEC and 86/363/EEC on the fixing of maximum levels for pesticide residues in and on cereals and foodstuffs of animal origin. *Off. J. Eur. Commun.*, No. L144, 18.6.96, 35–38.

EC Council (1997a). Directive 97/57/EC of 22 September 1997 establishing Annex VI to Council Directive 91/414/EEC concerning the placing of plant protection products on the market. *Off. J. Eur. Commun.*, No. L265, 27.9.97, 87–109.

EC Council (1997b). Council Directive 97/41/EC of 25 June 1997 amending Directives 76/895/EEC, 86/362/EEC, 86/363/EEC and 90/642/EEC relating to the fixing of maximum levels for pesticide residues in and on, respectively, fruit and vegetables, cereals, foodstuffs of animal origin, and certain products of plant origin, including fruit and vegetables. *Off. J. Eur. Commun.*, No. L184, 12.7.97, 33–49.

EEC Commission (1987). Directive 88/302/EEC of 18 November 1987 adapting to technical progress for the ninth time Council Directive 67/548/EEC on the approximation of the laws, regulations and administrative provisions relating to the classification, packaging and labelling of dangerous substances. *Off. J. Eur. Commun.*, No. L133, 30.5.88, 1–127 (corrigendum: *Off. J. Eur. Commun.*, No. L136, 2.6.88, 20).

EEC Commission (1992a). Directive 92/69/EEC of 31 July 1992 adapting to technical progress for the seventeenth time Council Directive 67/548/EEC on the approximation of the laws, regulations and administrative provisions relating to the classification, packaging and labelling of dangerous substances. *Off. J. Eur. Commun.*, No. L383, 29.12.92, 113–114; No. L383A, 29.12.92, 1–235.

EEC Commission (1992b). Regulation (EEC) No 3600/92 of 11 December 1992 laying down the detailed rules for the implementation of the first stage of the programme of work referred to in Article 8(2) of Council Directive 91/414/EEC concerning the placing of plant protection products on the market. *Off. J. Eur. Commun.*, No. L366, 15.12.92, 10–16.

EEC Commission (1993a). Directive 93/71/EEC of 27 July 1993 amending Council Directive 91/414/EEC concerning the placing of plant protection products on the market. *Off. J. Eur. Commun.*, No. L221, 31.8.93, 27–36 (corrigenda: *Off. J. Eur. Commun.*, No. L4, 6.1.96, 16).

EEC Commission (1993b). Directive 93/21/EEC of 27 April 1993 adapting to technical progress for the eighteenth time Council Directive 67/548/EEC on the approximation of the laws, regulations and administrative provisions relating to the classification, packaging and labelling of dangerous substances. *Off. J. Eur. Commun.*, No. L110, 4.5.93, 20–21; No. L110A, 4.5.93, 1–86.

EEC Council (1976). Directive 76/895/EEC of 23 November 1976 relating to the fixing of maximum levels for pesticide residues in and on fruit and vegetables. *Off. J. Eur. Commun.*, No. L340, 9.12.76, 26–31.

EEC Council (1978). Directive of 26 June 1978 on the approximation of the laws of the Member States relating to the classification, packaging and labelling of dangerous preparations (pesticides), *Off. J. Eur. Commun.*, No. L206, 29.7.78, 13–25.

EEC Council (1980). Directive 80/778/EEC of 15 July 1980 relating to the quality of water intended for human consumption, *Off. J. Eur. Commun.*, No. L229, 30.8.80, 11–29.

EEC Council (1986a). Directive 86/362/EEC of 24 July 1986 on the fixing of maximum levels for pesticide residues in and on cereals. *Off. J. Eur. Commun.*, No. L221, 7.8.86, 37–42.

EEC Council (1986b). Directive 86/363/EEC of 24 July 1986 on the fixing of maximum levels for pesticide residues in and on foodstuffs of animal origin. *Off. J. Eur. Commun.*, No. L221, 7.8.86, 43–47.

EEC Council (1988). Directive of 7 June 1988 on the approximation of the laws, regulations and administrative provisions of the member states relating to the classification, packaging and labelling of dangerous preparations. *Off. J. Eur. Commun.*, No. L187, 16.7.88, 14–30.

EEC Council (1990). Directive 90/642/EEC of 27 November 1990 on the fixing of maximum levels for pesticide residues in and on certain products of plant origin, including fruit and vegetables. *Off. J. Eur. Commun.*, No. L350, 14.12.90, 71–79.

EEC Council (1991). Directive 91/414 of 15 July 1991 concerning the placing of plant protection products on the market. *Off. J. Eur. Commun.*, No. L230, 19.8.91, 1–32 (corrigenda: *Off. J. Eur. Commun.*, No. L170, 25.6.92, 40).

EEC Council (1993a). Council Directive 93/57/EEC of 29 June 1993 amending the Annexes to Directives 86/362/EEC and 86/363/EEC on the fixing of maximum levels for pesticide residues in and on cereals and foodstuffs of animal origin respectively. *Off. J. Eur. Commun.*, No. L211, 23.8.93, 1–5.

EEC Council (1993b). Council Directive 93/58/EEC of 29 June 1993 amending Annex II to Directive 76/895/EEC relating to the fixing of maximum levels for pesticide residues in and on fruit and vegetables and the Annex to Directive 90/642/EEC relating to the fixing of maximum levels for pesticide residues in and on certain products of plant origin, including fruit and vegetables, and providing for the establishment of a first list of maximum levels. *Off. J. Eur. Commun.*, No. L211, 23.8.93, 6–39.

European Parliament and EC Council (1998). Directive 98/8/EC of 16 February 1998 concerning the placing of biocidal products on the market. *Off. J. Eur. Commun.*, No. L123, 24.4.98, 1–63.

FAO/WHO (1998a). *Pesticide Residues in Food—1997. Report 1997*. Joint Meeting of the FAO Panel of Experts and the WHO Core Assessment Group: Lyon, 22 September–1 October 1997. World Health Organization, Geneva.

FAO/WHO (1998b). *Pesticide Residues in Food—1997. Evaluations 1997, Part II Toxicological*. Joint Meeting of the FAO Panel of Experts and the WHO Core Assessment Group: Lyon, 22 September–1 October 1997. World Health Organization, Geneva.

FAO/WHO (1999). *Pesticide Residues in Food—1998. Report 1998*. Joint Meeting of the FAO Panel of Experts and the WHO Core Assessment Group: Rome, 21–30 September 1998. World Health Organization, Geneva.

IPCS (1990). *Principles for the Toxicological Assessment of Pesticide Residues in Food*. Environmental Health Criteria 104. World Health Organization, Geneva.

OECD (1981). *Decision of the OECD Council Concerning the Mutual Acceptance of Data on the Assessment of Chemicals, C-81-30 Final*. OECD, Paris.

USA (1906). Pub. L. 59–384, 34 Stat. 768. Pure Food and Drug Act of 1906.

USA (1910). Pub. L. 6–152, 36 Stat. 331. Insecticide Act of 1910.

USA (1938). Federal Food, Drug and Cosmetic Act, 21, U.S.C. 321 *et seq*.

USA (1947). Federal Insecticide, Fungicide and Rodenticide Act, 7 U.S.C 136 *et seq*.

USA (1996). Pub. L. 104–70. Food Quality Protection Act of 1996.

USA (1997). *Code of Federal Regulations 40, Part 170—Worker Protection Standard, July 1, 1997*. US Government Printing Office, Washington, DC.

USDA (1983). *US Department of Agriculture. National Food Consumption Survey. Nutrient Intakes: Individuals in 48 States, Year 1977–78. Report No. I–1*. Consumer Nutrition Division, Human Nutrition Information Service, Hyattsville, MD.

WHO (1995). *Recommendations for the Revision of the Guidelines for Predicting Intake of Pesticide Residues. Report of an FAO/WHO Consultation*. World Health Organization, Geneva.

WHO (1997). *Food Consumption and Exposure Assessment of Chemicals. Report of an FAO/WHO Consultation*, World Health Organization, Geneva.

Chapter 74

Regulation of Pharmaceuticals

Susan Davies and Mike Watson

CONTENTS

INTRODUCTION

The aim of this chapter is to give a broad overview of drug licensing procedures in the USA and EU, in order to put the role of toxicology into context. The emphasis is on the toxicological aspects of drug licensing.

Most developed nations regulate pharmaceuticals by premarketing authorization, i.e. the regulatory authority has to be satisfied on a number of accounts that the product is safe and efficacious and sometimes also that it is necessary. In the USA there is a system of regulatory control, more or less uniform throughout the country, whereas the EU has had the difficult task of bringing together the disparate regulatory systems of the Member States. At the present time, the EU system is in a process of transition and therefore somewhat complex for which reason the European section of this chapter focuses on the evolving regulatory system, whereas the USA section concentrates on regulatory toxicology requirements.

Trading blocks such as the EU and countries such as the USA and Japan are increasingly harmonizing their requirements for registration at the International Conference on Harmonization (ICH). The process is discussed at the end of this chapter.

REGULATION IN THE USA

Regulatory control of pharmaceuticals in the USA is the responsibility of the Food and Drug Administration (FDA). It is the mission of the FDA's Center for Drug Evaluation and Research (CDER) to ensure that safe and effective drugs are available to the American population.

During the early, preclinical, development of a new drug, the primary goal is to determine if the potential drug product is reasonably safe for initial use in humans, and that the compound exhibits pharmacological activity that justifies commercial development. When a product is identified as a viable candidate for further development, attention must be focused on gathering data to ensure that the product will not expose humans to undue risk in limited, early-stage clinical studies. The Investigational New Drug Application (IND) is the first result of a successful drug development programme. The IND is not an application for marketing approval—technically it is a request for an exemption from the Federal law that prohibits an unapproved drug being shipped in interstate commerce. In effect, the IND is the vehicle through which the drug developer advances to the next stage of the development process.

The complete commercial approval of new drugs in the USA is based on the New Drug Application (NDA). Since 1938 (when the Food Drug and Cosmetic Act was passed into law), every new drug has been the subject of an approved NDA before commercial sale in the USA. The NDA has evolved considerably during its history. Initially NDAs were only required to contain evidence of safety of the new drug. In 1962 the law was amended to require NDAs also to contain evidence that the new drug was effective for its intended use and that the established benefits of the drug outweighed its known risks. Further amendment in 1985 (the 'NDA rewrite') modified content requirement, but was primarily intended to restructure information organization in order to expedite review of NDAs at the FDA.

The type of information to be submitted to the FDA will be dependent upon the stage of development of the drug, for example, clinical data will not be available at the IND stage. However, the format and content of FDA submissions (FDA, 1998a) is generally constant and would include:

- Index and summary;
- Chemistry, manufacturing and control information;
- Samples, method validation and labelling;
- Non-clinical pharmacology and toxicology;
- Human pharmacokinetics and bioavailability;
- Clinical data.

Non-clinical Safety Studies Required to Support the Conduct of Clinical Trials

General Principles

The development of a pharmaceutical product is a step-wise process, involving the evaluation of all available data at every stage. The goals of the non-clinical safety evaluation include characterization of toxic effects with respect to target organs, the dose dependence, the relationship to exposure time and potential reversibility. This information is important for the estimation of an initial safe starting dose for the human trials and the identification of parameters for clinical monitoring for potential adverse effects. Human clinical trials are conducted to demonstrate the efficacy and safety of a pharmaceutical, starting with a relatively low exposure in a small number of subjects. This is followed by clinical trials in which exposure usually increases by dose, duration and/or size of the exposed patient population. Clinical trials are extended based on the demonstration of adequate safety in the previous clinical trial(s) as well as additional non-clinical safety information that is available as the clinical trials proceed. Clinical trials are conducted in phases for which different terminology has been utilized in various geographical regions. The purpose and objectives may be used to group clinical trials. The first human exposure studies are generally single-dose studies, followed by dose escalation and short-term repeated-dose studies to evaluate pharmacokinetic parameters and tolerance. These are referred to as Phase I studies or Human Pharmacology studies. These studies are often conducted in healthy volunteers but may also include patients. The next phase of trials consists of exploratory efficacy and safety studies in patients. These are referred to as Phase II studies or Therapeutic Exploratory studies. These are followed by confirmatory clinical trials for efficacy and safety in patient populations referred to as Phase III studies or Therapeutic Confirmatory studies.

The extent of data required will generally increase as progress is made through the different phases. Information will generally be needed in each of the areas specified below (FDA, 1997a).

Safety Pharmacology

Safety pharmacology refers to the assessment of effects on vital functions, such as cardiovascular, central nervous and respiratory systems. These screening tests for possible effects should be evaluated in animals prior to human exposure. These evaluations may be conducted as additions to toxicity studies or as separate studies.

Toxicokinetic and Pharmacokinetic Studies

Exposure data in animals should be evaluated prior to human clinical trials. Further information on absorption, distribution, metabolism and excretion in animals should be made available to compare human and animal metabolic pathways. Appropriate information should usually be available by the time the Phase I (Human Pharmacology) studies have been completed.

Single-dose Toxicity Studies

The single-dose (acute) toxicity for a pharmaceutical should be evaluated in two mammalian species prior to the first human exposure (FDA, 1996a). Acute toxicity studies should usually be conducted using two routes of drug administration—the intended human administration route and also intravenous administration if feasible. A dose escalation study is considered an acceptable alternative to the single-dose design. Studies should usually be conducted in two mammalian species, including a non-rodent when reasonable. The design of these studies follows conventional acute toxicity testing procedures, although the use of large numbers of animals to determine LD_{50} values is not required.

Repeated-dose Toxicity Studies

All repeated-dose toxicity studies are generally conducted in animals using the proposed route of human administration. The recommended duration of the repeated-dose toxicity studies is usually related to the duration, therapeutic indication and scale of the proposed clinical trial. In principle, the duration of the animal toxicity studies conducted in two mammalian species (one non-rodent) should be equal to or exceed the duration of the human clinical trials up to the maximum recommended duration of the repeated-dose toxicity studies. In certain circumstances, where significant therapeutic gain has been shown, trials may be extended beyond the duration of supportive repeated-dose toxicity studies on a case-by-case basis.

A repeated-dose toxicity study in two species (one non-rodent) for a minimum duration of 2–4 weeks would support Phase I (Human Pharmacology) and Phase II (Therapeutic Exploratory) studies up to 2 weeks in duration. Beyond this, and into Phase III clinical studies, 1-, 3- or 6-month toxicity studies would support these types of human clinical trials for up to 1, 3 or 6 months, respectively. Six-month rodent and chronic non-rodent studies would support clinical trials of longer duration than 6 months. The duration of studies required is summarized in **Table 1** (FDA, 1997b).

Local Tolerance Studies

Local tolerance should be studied in animals using routes relevant to the proposed clinical administration. The

Table 1 Duration of repeated-dose toxicity study required to support clinical trials

Duration of clinical trials	Minimum duration of repeat dose toxicity studies	
	Rodents	Non-rodents
Single dose/up to 2 weeks	2–4 weeks[a]	2 weeks[a]
Up to 1 month	1 month	1 month
Up to 3 months	3 months	3 months
Up to 6 months	6 months	6 months
> 6 months	6 months	Chronic (9 months)

[a] In the USA, as an alternative to 2 week repeat-dose studies, single-dose toxicity studies with extended examinations can support single-dose human trials. Extended examinations would include clinical pathology, at the time of peak effect and following recovery from drug effect, and histopathology on animals killed at termination.

evaluation of local tolerance should be performed prior to human exposure. The assessment of local tolerance may be part of other toxicity studies.

Genotoxicity Studies

Prior to first human exposure, *in vitro* tests for the evaluation of mutations and chromosomal damage are generally needed. If an equivocal or positive finding occurs, additional testing should be performed. The complete standard battery of tests for genotoxicity should be completed prior to the initiation of Phase II studies. FDA guidelines state that the following standard test battery is recommended (FDA, 1997c):

- A test for gene mutation in bacteria;
- An *in vitro* test with cytogenetic evaluation of chromosomal damage with mammalian cells or an *in vitro* mouse lymphoma tk assay;
- An *in vivo* test for chromosomal damage using rodent haematopoietic cells.

For compounds giving negative results, the completion of this three-test battery usually is considered to provide a sufficient level of safety to demonstrate the absence of genotoxic activity. Compounds giving positive results in the standard test battery may, depending on their therapeutic use, need to be tested more extensively. Assessment of the genotoxic potential of a compound should take into account the totality of the findings and acknowledge the value and limitations of both *in vitro* and *in vivo* tests (FDA, 1996b). The test battery approach is designed to reduce the risk of false-negative results for compounds with genotoxic potential. A single positive result in any assay for genotoxicity does not necessarily mean that the test compound is considered to pose a genotoxic hazard to humans.

Carcinogenicity Studies

Completed carcinogenicity studies are not usually needed in advance of the conduct of clinical trials unless there is cause for concern.

Reproduction Toxicity Studies

Reproduction toxicity studies should be conducted as is appropriate for the population that is to be exposed.

Men
Men may be included in Phase I and II trials, prior to the conduct of the male fertility study, since an evaluation of the male reproductive organs is performed in the early repeated-dose toxicity studies. A male fertility study should be completed prior to the initiation of Phase III trials.

Women Not of Childbearing Potential
Women not of childbearing potential (i.e. permanently sterilized, postmenopausal) may be included in clinical trials without reproduction toxicity studies provided that the relevant repeated-dose toxicity studies (which include an evaluation of the female reproductive organs) have been conducted.

Women of Childbearing Potential
For women of childbearing potential there is a high level of concern for the unintentional exposure of an embryo/foetus before information is available concerning the potential benefits versus potential risks. There are currently regional differences in the timing of reproduction toxicity studies to support the inclusion of women of childbearing potential in clinical trials. In the USA, women of childbearing potential may be included in early, carefully monitored studies without reproduction toxicity studies provided that appropriate precautions are taken to minimize risk. These precautions include pregnancy testing, use of a highly effective method of birth control and entry after a confirmed menstrual period. Continued testing and monitoring during the trial should be sufficient to ensure compliance with the measures not to become pregnant during the period of drug exposure (which may exceed the length of study). To support this approach, informed consent should include any known pertinent information related to reproductive toxicity, such as a general assessment of potential toxicity of pharmaceuticals with related structures or

pharmacological effects. If no relevant information is available, the informed consent should clearly note the potential for risk. In the USA, assessment of female fertility and embryo–foetal development should be completed before women of childbearing potential using birth control are enrolled in Phase III trials. The pre- and postnatal development study should be submitted for marketing approval or earlier if there is cause for concern. All female reproduction toxicity studies and the standard battery of genotoxicity tests should be completed prior to the inclusion, in any clinical trial, of women of childbearing potential not using highly effective birth control or whose pregnancy status is unknown.

Pregnant Women

Prior to the inclusion of pregnant women in clinical trials, all the reproduction toxicity studies and the standard battery of genotoxicity tests should be conducted. In addition, safety data from previous human exposure are generally needed.

Supplementary Studies

Additional non-clinical studies may be needed if previous non-clinical or clinical findings with the product or related products have indicated special safety concerns.

Clinical Trials in Children

When paediatric patients are included in clinical trials, safety data from previous adult human exposure would usually represent the most relevant information and should generally be available before paediatric clinical trials. The necessity for adult human data would be determined on a case-by-case basis. In addition to appropriate repeated-dose toxicity studies, all reproduction toxicity studies and the standard battery of genotoxicity tests should be available prior to the initiation of trials in paediatric populations. Juvenile animal studies should be considered on an individual basis when previous animal data and human safety data are insufficient. The need for carcinogenicity testing should be addressed prior to long term exposure in paediatric clinical trials considering the length of treatment or cause for concern.

Additional Non-clinical Safety Studies Required to Support Marketing Approval

In a conventional drug development programme, most of the non-clinical safety studies required to support marketing approval would have been conducted in order to support the longer, more extensive clinical trials. The only possible area requiring special attention is that of carcinogenicity testing. Since this is a contentious area, special attention will be devoted to the need for carcinogenicity testing and the regulatory guidance available for design and conduct of these experiments.

Need for Long-term Rodent Carcinogenicity Testing of Pharmaceuticals

There are certain fundamental considerations in assessing the need for performing carcinogenicity studies on pharmaceuticals, as detailed below (FDA, 1996c).

Duration of Treatment

Carcinogenicity studies should be performed for any pharmaceutical whose expected clinical use is continuous for at least 6 months. Certain classes of compounds may not be used continuously over a minimum of 6 months but may be used repeatedly in an intermittent manner. It is difficult to determine and to justify scientifically what time represents a clinically relevant treatment period for frequent use with regard to carcinogenic potential, especially for discontinuous treatment periods. For pharmaceuticals used frequently in an intermittent manner in the treatment of chronic or recurrent conditions, carcinogenicity studies are generally needed. Examples of such conditions include allergic rhinitis, depression and anxiety. Carcinogenicity studies may also need to be considered for certain delivery systems that may result in prolonged exposures. Pharmaceuticals administered infrequently or for short duration of exposure (e.g. anaesthetics and imaging agents) do not need carcinogenicity studies unless there is cause for concern.

Cause for Concern

Criteria for defining these cases need to be very carefully considered because this is the most important reason to conduct carcinogenicity studies for most categories of pharmaceuticals. A number of factors which could be considered may include:

- Previous demonstration of carcinogenic potential in the product class that is considered relevant to humans;
- Structure–activity relationship suggesting carcinogenic risk;
- Evidence of preneoplastic lesions in repeated-dose toxicity studies;
- Long-term tissue retention of parent compound or metabolite(s) resulting in local tissue reactions or other pathophysiological responses.

Genotoxicity

Unequivocally genotoxic compounds, in the absence of other data, are presumed to be trans-species carcinogens, implying a hazard to humans. Such compounds need not be subjected to long-term carcinogenicity studies. However, if such a drug is intended to be administered chronically to humans, an extended chronic toxicity study (up to 1 year) may be necessary to detect early tumourigenic effects.

Indication and Patient Population

For pharmaceuticals developed to treat certain serious diseases, carcinogenicity testing need not be conducted before market approval although these studies should be conducted post- approval. This speeds the availability of pharmaceuticals for life-threatening or severely debilitating diseases, especially where no satisfactory alternative therapy exists. In instances where the life expectancy in the indicated population is short (i.e. less than 2–3 years), long-term carcinogenicity studies may not be required. For example, anti-cancer agents intended for treatment of advanced systemic disease do not generally need carcinogenicity studies. In cases where the therapeutic agent for cancer is generally successful and life is significantly prolonged, there may be later concerns regarding secondary cancers. When such pharmaceuticals are intended for adjuvant therapy in tumour-free patients or for prolonged use in non-cancer indications, carcinogenicity studies are usually needed.

Guidelines for Conduct of Long-term Rodent Carcinogenicity Testing of Pharmaceuticals

Long-term rodent carcinogenicity studies for assessing the carcinogenic potential of chemicals (including pharmaceuticals) to humans are currently receiving critical examination. Since the early 1970s, many investigations have shown that it is possible to provoke a carcinogenic response in rodents by a diversity of experimental procedures, some of which are now considered to have little or no relevance for human risk assessment. Positive results in long-term carcinogenicity studies that are not relevant to the therapeutic use of a pharmaceutical present a dilemma to all parties involved in drug development and regulatory control. Recent FDA draft guidelines offer a new, flexible approach to the design of carcinogenicity studies for the testing of pharmaceuticals (FDA, 1998b). The basic scheme comprises one long-term rodent carcinogenicity study plus one other study to provide additional information not generally available from the standard long-term assay. This additional study should be selected so as to provide insight into carcinogenic end-points. Examples include models of initiation–promotion in rodents or models of carcinogenesis using transgenic or neonatal rodents. FDA guidelines call for flexibility and judgement in selecting a test method which can contribute information valuable to the overall 'weight of evidence' for the assessment of carcinogenic

potential. The guidance also stresses the use of mechanistic information in providing a perspective on the relevance of all test results to human risk assessment. FDA guidelines also present information useful in the design of conventional carcinogenicity studies.

Route of Exposure

The route of exposure in animals should be the same as the intended clinical route when feasible. If similar metabolism and systemic exposure can be demonstrated by differing routes of administration, carcinogenicity studies should only be conducted by a single route, recognizing that it is important that relevant organs for the clinical route (e.g. lung for inhalational agents) be adequately exposed to the test material. Evidence of adequate exposure may be derived from pharmacokinetic data.

Selection of Dose Levels

Traditionally, carcinogenicity studies for chemical agents have relied upon the maximally tolerated dose (MTD) as the standard method for high dose selection The MTD is generally chosen based on data derived from toxicity studies of 3 months' duration. For pharmaceuticals with low rodent toxicity, use of the MTD may result in the administration of very large doses in carcinogenicity studies, often representing high multiples of the clinical dose. For nongenotoxic substances where thresholds may exist and carcinogenicity may result from alterations in normal physiology, linear extrapolations from high dose effects have been questioned. This has led to the concern that exposures in rodents greatly in excess of the intended human exposures may not be relevant to human risk, because they so greatly alter the physiology of the test species that the findings may not reflect what would occur following human exposure. There are guidelines for dose selection (FDA, 1995).

Ideally, the doses selected for rodent bioassays for non-genotoxic pharmaceuticals should provide an exposure to the agent that:

- Allows an adequate margin of safety over the human therapeutic exposure;
- Is tolerated without significant chronic physiological dysfunction and is compatible with good survival;
- Is guided by a comprehensive set of animal and human data that focus broadly on the properties of the agent and the suitability of the animal;
- Permits data interpretation in the context of clinical use.

Recent FDA guidance proposes that any one of several approaches may be appropriate and acceptable for dose selection, and should provide for a more rational approach to dose selection for carcinogenicity studies for pharmaceuticals. These include:

- Toxicity-based end-points;
- Pharmacokinetic end-points;
- Saturation of absorption;
- Pharmacodynamic end-points;
- Maximum feasible dose;
- Additional end-points.

Toxicity End-points

The FDA has agreed to continue use of the MTD as an acceptable toxicity-based end-point for high dose selection for carcinogenicity studies. The following definition of the MTD is considered consistent with those published previously by international regulatory authorities: the top dose or maximum tolerated dose is that which is predicted to produce a minimum toxic effect over the course of the carcinogenicity study. Such an effect may be predicted from a 90-day dose range-finding study in which minimal toxicity is observed. Factors to consider are alterations in physiological function that would be predicted to alter the animal's normal life span or interfere with interpretation of the study. Such factors include: no more than 10% decrease in body weight gain relative to controls; target organ toxicity; and significant alterations in clinical pathological parameters.

Pharmacokinetic End-points

A systemic exposure representing a large multiple of the human AUC (at the maximum recommended daily dose) may be considered an appropriate end-point for dose selection for carcinogenicity studies for non-genotoxic pharmaceuticals which have similar metabolic profiles in humans and rodents where high doses are well tolerated in rodents. The level of animal systemic exposure, should be sufficiently great, compared with human exposure, to provide reassurance of an adequate test of carcinogenicity. The selection of a high dose for carcinogenicity studies which represents a 25-fold ratio of rodent to human plasma AUC of parent compound and/or metabolites is considered pragmatic.

Saturation of Absorption

High dose selection based on saturation of absorption measured by systemic availability of drug-related substances is acceptable. The middle and low doses selected for the carcinogenicity study should take into account saturation of metabolic and elimination pathways.

Pharmacodynamic End-points

The utility and safety of many pharmaceuticals depend on their pharmacodynamic receptor selectivity. Pharmacodynamic end-points for high dose selection will be highly compound specific and are considered for individual study designs based on scientific merits. The high dose selected should produce a pharmacodynamic response in dosed animals of such magnitude as would preclude further dose escalation. However, the dose should not produce disturbances of physiology or homeostasis which would compromise the validity of the study. Examples include hypotension and inhibition of blood clotting (because of the risk of spontaneous bleeding).

Maximum Feasible Dose

Currently, the maximum feasible dose by dietary administration is considered 5% of diet. International regulatory authorities are re-evaluating this standard. It is believed that the use of pharmacokinetic end-points (AUC ratio) for dose selection of low-toxicity pharmaceuticals should significantly decrease the need to select high doses based on feasibility criteria. When routes other than dietary administration are appropriate, the high dose will be limited based on considerations including practicality and local tolerance.

Selection of Middle and Low Doses in Carcinogenicity Studies

Regardless of the method used for the selection of the high dose, the selection of the middle and low doses for the carcinogenicity study should provide information to aid in assessing the relevance of study findings to humans.

Conclusion

There are four basic regulatory questions for a drug product that the FDA must answer in an NDA assessment:

- Is it safe?
- Is it effective?
- What is the dose?
- Does it have good quality?

Studies must always be designed and conducted, using good science as the guiding principle, with the intention of providing answers to these questions. Applicants to the FDA can be aided by knowledge of the basic working rules of any regulator in performing a risk assessment:

- What do we want to know?
- What assumptions are we prepared to make?
- How sure do we want to be?

REGULATION IN THE EUROPEAN UNION

European Legislation

The European Economic Community (EEC) was established in 1957 by the signing of the Treaty of Rome by the six original Member States (France, The Netherlands, Luxembourg, Belgium, Germany and Italy). Subsequently, four basic types of legislation implemented the Treaty. *Regulations* are binding on all Member States and are effective without the need for national legislation. *Directives* lay down the objectives of the legislation, which are binding in all Member States but allow their implementation to be transposed nationally. *Decisions* are binding on those individuals or bodies to whom they are addressed. *Recommendations* provide advice, which is not binding.

The law-making institutions established by the Treaty of Rome include the Council of Ministers and the Commission. The *Council* is composed of Ministers from the government of each Member State with a rotating presidency on a 6-monthly basis. It is the decision-making body of the EU. The *Commission* is the policy-making body in the EU which also ensures that treaty legislation is implemented. It acts like a civil service for the EU and is composed of 17 Commissioners, each with responsibility for a particular policy area.

The texts of the legislation relating to medicinal products have been compiled in the publication *Rules Governing Medicinal Products in the European Union*, Vol. I (EU, 1998a). This publication is recommended reading because it shows how the basic legislation, Directives laid down in 1965 and 1975, has been subsequently amended. The original text of each piece of legislation can be found in the *Official Journal of the European Communities* as referenced. The primary purpose of the legislation is to safeguard public health without hindering the development of the pharmaceutical industry or trade in medicinal products within the Community. Directive 65/65/EEC (EU, 1998b) sets out the general framework of the European system for marketing authorization of medicinal products. It defines a medicinal product as follows:

> Any substance or combination of substances presented for treating or preventing disease in human beings or animals. Any substance or combination of substances which may be administered to human beings or animals with a view to making a medical diagnosis or to restoring, correcting or modifying physiological functions in human beings or animals.

This Directive established that before a medicinal product could be marketed, it must have a marketing authorization, which has been approved on the basis of safety, quality and efficacy.

Subsequent Directives built on this general framework. Directive 75/318/EEC (EU, 1998c) established the analytical, pharmaco-toxicological and clinical standards for testing medicinal products. Directive 75/319/EEC (EU, 1998d) established the Committee for Proprietary Medicinal Products (CPMP), which is responsible for giving opinions on whether a medicinal product fulfils the requirements relating to safety, quality and efficacy. The CPMP is composed of representatives from each of the Member State authorities. Regulation 2309/93 (EU, 1998e) and Directive 93/39/EEC (European Council, 1993) amend Directives 65/65/EEC, 75/318/EEC and 75/319/EEC. Council Regulation 2309/93/EEC laid down the Community procedures for authorization and supervision of medicinal products and established the European Agency for the Evaluation of Medicinal Products (EMEA), which is situated in London.

Notice to Applicants

The Notice to Applicants (NTA) is an official guide for the pharmaceutical industry and other interested parties on how the requirements should be met. It has been prepared by the European Commission to represent the harmonized views of the Member States and the EMEA. The NTA is Volume 2 in the series *The Rules Governing Medicinal Products in the European Union*. There are two parts: part 2A describes the procedures for marketing authorization and part 2B gives guidance on the format and content of marketing authorization applications. This series was published initially in 1989 and has been updated since, with the most recent edition in 1998. The format and content of marketing authorization applications are standard throughout Europe and are described later in this chapter. Prior to the application for a marketing authorization, certain aspects of the drug development process are regulated by legislation.

Good Laboratory Practice

Legislation (Directive 91/507/EEC) (European Commission, 1991) has been put in place with the aim of ensuring that safety tests are conducted in conformity with good laboratory practice (GLP) as laid down by Directives 87/18/EEC (European Council, 1987) and 88/320/EEC (European Council, 1988) (see also Chapter 21). In the context of this requirement, the following are considered as safety tests, which must conform to GLP: single- and repeated-dose toxicity; reproductive (including embryo/foetal and perinatal) toxicity; tests for mutagenic and carcinogenic potential; local tolerance studies; toxicokinetic studies which provide systemic exposure data for the aforementioned studies and pharmacodynamic studies designed to investigate potential adverse side-effects. Furthermore, studies which provide general or specific data for safety assessment, e.g. validation of virus removal or inactivation for biological/biotechnological products, should also be carried out in accordance with GLP.

The principles of GLP should ensure that the results produced by these tests are comparable and of high quality. Tests do not have to be repeated within the EC because there are no differences in laboratory practice. This reduces animal experimentation in accordance with Directive 86/609/EC (European Council, 1986), regarding the protection of animals used for experimental and other scientific purposes. Directive 88/320/EC established the necessity for a harmonized system for study audit and laboratory inspection to ensure that GLP is being applied. Member States are required to designate authorities responsible for monitoring GLP compliance. Guidance for compliance monitoring procedures and the conduct of laboratory inspections and study audits is given in the Annex to this Directive.

Clinical Trials

During the development of a medicinal product, the first regulatory hurdle is met when the drug is first tested in man. Statutory requirements for clinical trials currently vary throughout Europe and the sponsor is required to observe the national requirements within the country concerned before proceeding with clinical trials in humans.

Clinical pharmacology studies in human volunteers do not require regulatory authority authorization, in the UK for example, but must comply with the Declaration of Helsinki and its subsequent amendments (World Medical Association, 1996), and GMP (Good Manufacturing Practice), GLP and GCP (Good Clinical Practice) requirements.

Within Europe, although the data requirements are generally harmonized (CPMP, 1995a), the format of the application for permission to undertake clinical trials varies. In most Member States, there is a requirement either to notify or to receive approval from the competent authority before a clinical trial can start in that Member State. In the UK, for example, before clinical trials can start, approval must be obtained from the licensing authority in the form of a Clinical Trial Certificate (CTC) or, more commonly, a Clinical Trials Exemption (CTX) (UK, 1995a, b). Application for a CTX requires the submission of all chemical, pharmaceutical, pharmacotoxicological and any clinical data, in a summarized format.

The aim of the toxicological development of a drug is to investigate the safety in the clinical population to be treated as it is to be used when the drug is marketed. Animal toxicological studies provide information prior to testing in man and this testing is continued during human trials of the drug to cover the full duration of use in the population to be treated and to investigate further any safety issues which arise during human trials. The toxicological data requirements will depend therefore on a number of factors, including the chemical nature and biological activities of the drug substance,

the proposed dosage and duration of treatment in man, the severity of the disease and the population to be treated (male, female, paediatric, etc.). *Medicines Act Leaflet, MAL 4*, (MCA, 1996) gives basic guidance on the toxicological data requirements for clinical trials in the UK. Deviation from these guidelines should be justified. As a general guidance, the toxicological data should include single-dose acute toxicity studies in two mammalian species by the route of administration in the proposed clinical trial and by a route which ensures systemic exposure. Normally, repeat-dose studies with duration at least as long as the proposed duration of treatment with the drug in the clinical trial are required (minimum 14-day toxicity studies) for early phase clinical studies. For larger, less closely monitored trials (some Phase II and Phase III) and/or where there is evidence of prolonged retention in the body, the duration of toxicity studies should be the same as is required for Marketing Authorization (MA) in the EC. The number of species and the mode of conduct of the studies should be the same for clinical trials as for Marketing Authorization applications (EU, 1998i).

As regards genotoxicity tests, the basic requirement is that the results of a bacterial mutation test (or *in vitro* mammalian cell mutation test) and a chromosomal damage test should be available prior to human exposure. Before starting Phase II trials, the standard battery of genotoxicity tests, (CPMP, 1995c) is required.

Results of completed carcinogenicity studies are not required during clinical development except where there are suspicions about the drug, for example based on mutagenicity results or histopathological findings in repeat toxicity studies.

For women of childbearing potential, embryo-foetal development studies should be completed prior to Phase I clinical trials and female fertility studies prior to Phase III trials. Prior to the inclusion, in any clinical trial, of women of childbearing potential, not using highly effective birth control or whose pregnancy status is unknown, all female reproduction toxicity studies (EU, 1998k) and the standard battery of genotoxicity tests (CPMP, 1995c) should be completed.

The biological safety testing of biopharmaceuticals was one of the topics for harmonization in the International Conference on Harmonization (ICH) process. However, it has proved difficult to reach a consensus on the test packages required. This is reflected in the CPMP guideline on biological safety testing on medicinal products derived from biotechnology products (EU, 1998f).

It is often necessary to carry out clinical testing in 2000–3000 human subjects to prove safety and efficacy in MA applications for a new active substance. This means that multicentre, multinational trials are common. As stated previously, statutory requirements and therefore the format of the application and the time taken for approval are different in each of the different

Member States. Setting up the necessary multicentre, multinational trials is therefore complex and lengthy.

It is proposed to standardize clinical trial regulations within Europe by means of a new Directive (EU, 1997). A proposal for the Directive has been published which specifies the requirements for the implementation of Good Clinical Practice (GCP). The Directive also seeks to lay down the procedures to be followed before a clinical trial may be initiated, whereby the sponsor submits an application to the Member State competent authority and authorization should be given unless the Member State raises objections within a specified period of time. Detailed guidance on the format and contents of the application including the documentation to be supplied on toxicological and pharmacological tests are to be drawn up by the Commission.

Commission Directive 91/507/EEC (European Commission, 1991) requires that all phases of clinical trials should be carried out and reported in accordance with GCP. GCP includes the provision of an investigator brochure (IB) using a standard format (CPMP, 1995b). The IB is a compilation of the clinical and non-clinical (pharmacology, pharmacokinetics and toxicology) data. Its purpose is to provide the trial investigators with sufficient information to aid understanding of the protocol rationale and to enable them to make their own risk–benefit assessment of the appropriateness of the clinical trial. The IB includes the results of the non-clinical studies and any clinical data available, giving information on the methodology used and a discussion of the relevance of the findings with regard to the proposed therapeutic use in man.

Marketing Authorization Applications— Procedures

In most circumstances, toxicity studies are continued while the clinical phases of human trials proceed to produce sufficient clinical data at the time of the MA. As stated previously, Directive 65/65/EC (EU, 1998b) established the requirement for a Marketing Authorization (MA) before a medicinal product can be sold or supplied in any Member State. The MA once granted includes an approved Summary of Product Characteristics (SmPC). The SmPC is the basic source of information to the prescriber and provides the platform for promotion of the product. In fact, the product cannot be promoted outside the remit of the approved SmPC. The following details of the product are included on the SmPC in a specified format: name, composition, pharmaceutical form, clinical particulars (indications, dose, contraindications, precautions and warnings, interactions, use in pregnancy and lactation, effects on ability to drive and use machines, undesirable effects, information on overdose), pharmacological properties (pharmacodynamic, pharmacokinetic and preclinical safety data) and information on shelf-life and storage instructions. Applications for marketing authorisation can be made in Europe using one of three procedures: the centralized procedure, the mutual recognition procedure (a decentralized procedure) and national procedures.

The Centralized Procedure

Council Regulation (EEC) No. 2309/93 (EU, 1998e) established a centralized Community procedure for marketing authorization of medicinal products whereby a single application is made. There is a single evaluation which, if favourable, results in a single authorization. This allows direct access to the single European market. The Regulation also established the EMEA (see above) which receives the application and coordinates the assessment through the CPMP using the scientific resources made available by the Member State competent authorities. The centralized procedure can only be used for certain categories of products. These are listed in Parts A and B of the Annex to Regulation 2309/93.

Part A. the centralized procedure must be used for products developed by the following biotechnological processes:

- Recombinant DNA technology;
- Controlled expression of genes coding for biologically active proteins in prokaryotes and eukaryotes including transformed mammalian cells;
- Hybridoma and monoclonal antibody methods.

Part B. Applications for medicinal products containing a new active substance may use the centralized procedure. Additionally, applications for innovatory medicinal products may, at the request of the applicant, be accepted for consideration under the centralized procedure. An innovatory product is defined in Part B of Annex to Regulation 2309/93 and includes: novel delivery systems; new indications of significant therapeutic interest; medicinal products based on radio-isotopes which are of significant therapeutic interest; medicinal products derived from human blood or plasma; medicinal products manufactured by an innovative process or one of significant technical advance.

Prior to submission of the application, the applicant liases with the EMEA so that a *Rapporteur* can be appointed. The *Rapporteur* is a CPMP member and is appointed by the CPMP. A second member, to act as a *Co-Rapporteur*, may also be appointed. The role of the *Rapporteur* is to lead and coordinate the scientific evaluation of the application. Before the application is submitted the *Rapporteur* will nominate certain European experts to evaluate the application. These European experts are selected from a list provided by the Member States. Following submission and validation of the application, a timetable for evaluation is prepared by the

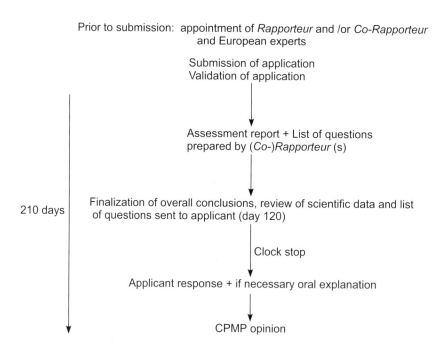

Figure 1 Flow diagram of the centralized procedure for marketing authorizations.

EMEA secretariat in consultation with the *Rapporteur* and *Co-Rapporteur*. This ensures that the CPMP will deliver a scientific opinion on the application within 210 days. During this time the *(Co-)Rapporteur*(s) prepare an assessment report and list of questions for review by the other members of the CPMP. These are finalized by the CPMP and sent to the applicant. Time is then allowed for the applicant to respond (clock stop). The clock is restarted on receipt of the response. If necessary, the applicant may provide an oral explanation to the CPMP. Following consideration of the applicant response, the CPMP should then be in a position to provide an opinion by the end of the 210-day period. The centralized procedure can be briefly summarized as shown in **Figure 1**.

In the event of a favourable opinion, the CPMP may require the applicant to undertake certain follow-up measures or specific obligations as a condition of the marketing approval. These will be annexed to the opinion and a timetable for completion and review will be agreed. Non-fulfilment of specific obligations or follow-up measures may result in a variation/suspension /withdrawal of the marketing authorization. A further step is necessary to convert a favourable opinion into a binding decision for marketing authorization. The power to make these decisions, which are legally binding on all Member States, lies with the Commission and, if necessary, the Council. The procedure for the decision-making process can be described briefly as follows.

Decision-making Process

The process is initiated when the opinion of the EMEA's scientific committee, the CPMP, is transmitted to the Commission together with various annexes in all languages of the Community (Summary of Product Characteristics, manufacturing authorization, labelling, user leaflet). Within 30 days of receipt of the valid opinion, the Commission prepares a draft decision. The next step is a written procedure in which the draft decision is forwarded to the Standing Committee which is the Regulatory Committee of the pharmaceutical sector and is composed of representatives from the Member States. The Committee makes its decision by a qualified majority. Member States have 30 days to respond. If the opinion is favourable, the Commission will proceed to the next stage of taking its decision. This written procedure may not be possible if the Commission's decision differs from the CPMP's opinion, in which case the Commission must immediately call a meeting of the Standing Committee. A meeting may also be called at the written request of a Member State. If a Member State makes written comments which, in the Commission's opinion, raise new scientific issues, a request for a further opinion is sent to the CPMP.

If the Standing Committee's opinion is favourable, the Commission will proceed with the decision-making process. Following internal procedures, the Commissioner signs the decision. If the Standing Committee's is not favourable, the Commission must submit the matter to the Council. Within 3 months of submission, the Council either makes a decision on the Commission's proposal with a qualified majority or against the proposal by a simple majority. If the Council does not make a decision, the Commission adopts the proposed decision. The decision-making process is represented very briefly in **Figure 2**.

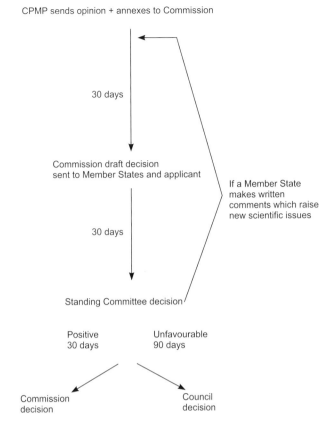

CPMP sends opinion + annexes to Commission

30 days

Commission draft decision
sent to Member States and applicant

If a Member State
makes written
comments which raise
new scientific issues

30 days

Standing Committee decision

Positive
30 days

Unfavourable
90 days

Commission
decision

Council
decision

Figure 2 Flow diagram of the decision-making process following the centralized procedure for marketing authorizations.

European Public Assessment Report (EPAR)

Article 12 of Council Regulation (EEC) No. 2309/93 requires that the EMEA should make available the assessment report of the medicinal product by the Committee giving the reasons for advising the approval of the marketing authorization (after deletion of any information of a commercially confidential nature). This document is called the European Public Assessment Report (EPAR). The EPAR is prepared by the EMEA in parallel to the decision-making phase so that it can be made available to the public as soon as the Commission decision has been made.

The Mutual Recognition Procedure

This procedure (sometimes called the decentralized procedure) has been available since 1 January 1995 and the legal basis for it is set out in Directives 65/65/EEC and 75/319/EEC as amended. A pharmaceutical company with a marketing authorization in one Member State (the Reference Member State) can request one or more other Member States mutually to recognize, within 90 days, the marketing authorization granted by the Reference Member State. A Member State can also request mutual recognition and after 1 January 1998, initiation of mutual recognition should be automatic. This applies when one Member State has already authorized the

medicinal product and therefore becomes the Reference Member State. When more than one Member State has authorized the product (independently of the mutual recognition procedure) the Concerned (i.e. subsequent) Member State(s) will each select the Reference Member State upon which to base its mutual recognition. In the case where no Member State has authorized the product, the first Member State, which approves the marketing authorization automatically, becomes the Reference Member State.

To allow mutual recognition to proceed, the Marketing Authorization Holder must give an assurance that the SmPC and the supporting dossier in the concerned Member State(s) are the same as the one in the Reference Member State. The Reference Member State has 90 days to update and issue the assessment report to the concerned Member States. Within 90 days of receipt of the assessment report, the concerned Member State can either recognize the decision of the first Member State and grant a marketing authorization with an identical SmPC or, on grounds relating to a risk to public health, ask for arbitration. During the 90-day period, the concerned Member States are required to raise their objections by day 60. This gives the applicant time to resolve the issues by day 90. To aid the process, the Mutual Recognition Facilitation Group (MRFG) meets at around day 75 to discuss the resolution of any outstanding issues. The MRFG is an informal liaison group, which meets during the week of the CPMP meeting. If serious objections remain by day 90, the application will be referred for arbitration. For ease of reference, a brief summary of the mutual recognition procedure is given in **Figure 3**.

Arbitration

In the event of a disagreement between Member States about the safety, quality or efficacy of a medicinal product, a scientific evaluation of the issue is undertaken by the CPMP, resulting in an opinion. This opinion is then converted into a Commission Decision which is legally binding on all Member States. There are a number of circumstances where such a disagreement can arise and these include community referral in accordance with Directive 75/319/EC under Articles 10 (risk to public health), 11 (divergent decisions), 12 (Community interest) or 15a (protection of public health). The arbitration procedure is laid down in Directive 75/319/EEC, as amended Articles 13 and 14.

A *Rapporteur* is chosen for the procedure by the CPMP and a timetable is drawn up whereby the CPMP reach an opinion within 90 days. During the 90 days, the clock may be stopped to allow the applicant to prepare a response to the questions raised by the CPMP and to prepare for an oral explanation if necessary. The applicant has the opportunity to appeal against the CPMP opinion. In this case, the applicant should notify the EMEA of grounds for appeal. The CPMP then has 60

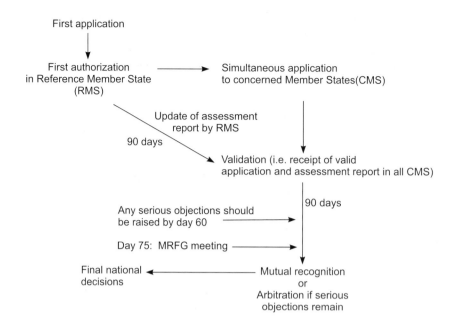

Figure 3 Flow diagram of the mutual recognition procedure for marketing authorizations

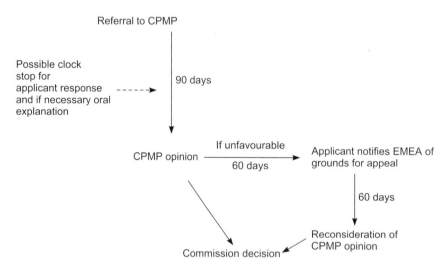

Figure 4 Flow diagram for the arbitration system following the mutual recognition procedure for marketing authorizations.

days in which to reconsider its opinion. The final opinion is then forwarded to the Commission for a legally binding Commission Decision. This decision making process has been described previously in the section above on the Centralized Procedure. The decision is binding on all Member States including the Reference Member State in cases of arbitration arising from a mutual recognition application. An overview of the process of arbitration is presented diagrammatically in **Figure 4**.

National Procedures

The centralized and mutual recognition procedures were initiated in January 1995 with a 3-year transition period. From 1 January 1998, all applications should be processed through either the centralized or the mutual recognition procedures. National applications for marketing authorization are in principle limited to the initial phase of the mutual recognition procedure (i.e. obtaining authorization in the reference Member State) and medicinal products intended to be marketed in one Member State only. For mutual recognition of an existing national marketing authorization to be possible, the dossier and Summary of Product Characteristics (SmPC), submitted in the concerned Member States (CMS) must be identical to that approved in the reference Member State (RMS). The complexities of this and how it can be applied in different situations, for example for generic applications or line extensions, is described in a Commission Communication dated July 1998 (European Commission, 1998a).

It is important to note that the European procedures have evolved from the separate national procedures. The European system evolved to date is essentially a coordination by the EMEA of the existing national agencies. In the UK, for example, the Marketing Authorization, which is usually referred to as the Product Licence (PL), is granted by the Licensing Authority, defined in the 1968 Medicines Act (UK, 1968) as UK Health and Agriculture Ministers. A Department of Health Agency, The Medicines Control Agency (MCA), is responsible for administering the system. The MCA contains a professional secretariat, which fully evaluates each valid application. If the Licensing Authority wishes to reject the application on grounds of safety, quality or efficacy or submit it for further assessment, it will refer the application to a Committee, established under Section 4 of the Medicines Act (UK, 1968), usually the Committee on Safety of Medicines (CSM). Under the centralized procedure, the CSM can be consulted by the Licensing Authority whether or not the UK is *Rapporteur* or *Co-Rapporteur*. The CSM also advises the Licensing Authority on matters of pharmacovigilance, legal classification of medicines and various policy issues such as guidelines.

Format and Content of Marketing Authorization Applications

There are two types of application: new active substance (chemical or biological/biotechnology) and abridged.

New Active Substance Application

The format of the application is standard throughout Europe and comprises four parts:

Part I: Summary of the application
Part II: Chemical/pharmaceutical documentation
Part III: Preclinical documentation
Part IV: Clinical documentation

The CPMP has prepared guidelines on the quality, safety and efficacy of medicinal products. These guidelines are intended to harmonize the data requirements to promote mutual recognition amongst the Member States. Where guidelines are available, these should be followed, unless justified in the expert report. Many guidelines are already published in *The Rules Governing Medicinal Products in the European Community*, Vol. III (1998) (EU, 1998g). Other guidelines approved by the CPMP are available from the EMEA (7 Westferry Circus, Canary Wharf, London E14 4HB, UK). Many of these originate from ICH (International Conference on Harmonization) (see below).

Part I: Summary of the Application

This includes the application form, the proposed Summary of Product Characteristics (SmPC) proposed package labelling, Patient Information Leaflet and three expert reports. The expert reports are as follows:

- Expert Report on the chemical, pharmaceutical and biological documentation.
- Expert Report on the toxico-pharmacological (pre-clinical) documentation.
- Expert Report on the clinical documentation.

Directive 75/319/EC, as amended, established the requirement for expert reports. The expert reports play an important role within the application. They provide an expert overview of the data presented in Parts II, III and IV and in particular are an unbiased critique of the data. They should discuss and justify any deviation from relevant community guidelines or omission of particular studies, e.g. oncogenicity/carcinogenicity studies. Furthermore, the experts should give a justification for the SmPC texts based on the submitted data. The expert must be suitably qualified and should provide a curriculum vitae with the signed and dated expert report.

The expert reports are designed to give a critical overview of the whole application to the assessors, which highlights any important issues and cross-refers (via tabulated summaries) to the full reports in Parts II, III and IV of the application. A good, critical expert report is likely to form the basis of the assessor's own report and will be beneficial to the application. Conversely, a poor expert report, for example one which ignores significant issues, will delay and may adversely affect assessment.

The preclinical expert report should comment on the GLP status of the safety studies submitted with the application. There should be relevant links between the preclinical expert report and the pharmaceutical and clinical expert reports. For example, if signs of potential toxicity were seen in animal studies, it is important that such potential toxicity is investigated in clinical trials. This should be discussed in both the preclinical and clinical expert reports. Similarly, a critical assessment of the impurities in the active substance should be included in the preclinical expert report together with a justification for the standardized impurity profile described in the pharmaceutical expert report. An evaluation of the possible risks to the environment (during use/disposal) and recommendations for labelling to reduce the risk should be included.

Hence it is important that the expert reports should not be written in isolation and the correlation between them should reflect the development of the product by showing how any toxicity issues are further investigated in the clinical studies and if necessary reflected in the proposed SmPC.

Part II: Chemical, Pharmaceutical and Biological Documentation

Part II contains detailed data on the composition, development and manufacture of the formulation. The chemistry of the active substance is described including the synthesis, physicochemical characteristics and impurities. The quality specifications and analytical methods used to control all ingredients are specified. Details of the package (primary and secondary containers) and quality control of the finished product (specifications and analytical methods) must also be given. Stability data are provided to support the shelf-life and storage precautions in the SmPC. The manufacturing process and all analytical methods used are validated. Data on the environmental risk assessment for products containing or consisting of genetically modified organisms (GMOs) are contained in this part of the dossier (EU, 1998t). For biological medicinal products, data on viral safety should also be included.

Part III: Toxico-pharmacological Documentation

Part III should contain information in a specific format and this is presented below. Where guidelines on data requirements are available, these should be followed. The currently-available guidelines are as described, while general guidance is available on the preclinical evaluation of anticancer products (CPMP, 1998).

(A)   Toxicity (single and repeat dose)

Single-dose toxicity guidelines (EU, 1998h) require that these tests should reveal signs of acute toxicity and determine the mode of death. A quantitative evaluation of the approximate lethal dose and the dose–effect relationship should be made, although a high level of precision is not required. The studies should be designed so that the maximal amount of necessary information is obtained from the smallest number of animals. Single-dose toxicity tests may give some indication of the likely effects of acute overdose in humans. Repeat-dose toxicity guideline (EU, 1998i) states that the duration of dosing should be related to the intended duration of human exposure as indicated in **Table 2**.

Repeat-dose toxicity testing should be carried out in at least two species, one being a non-rodent. The species should be selected on the basis of their similarity to man

Table 2 Recommended duration of toxicity studies in relation to duration of treatment in humans

Proposed duration of human treatment	Recommended duration of repeated dose toxicity studies
One or several doses within one day	2 weeks
Repeated doses up to 7 days	4 weeks
Repeated doses for up to 30 days	3 months
Repeated doses beyond 30 days	6 months

Source: EU (1998i)

with regard to pharmacokinetics. The pharmacodynamic effects of the drug should, if possible, demonstrated in at least one of the species. Guidelines on repeated dose distribution studies (EU, 1998j) should also be taken into account.

(B)   Reproductive function (fertility and general reproductive performance), and

(C)   Embryo-foetal and perinatal toxicity.

Guidelines on reproduction studies (EU, 1998k). These should be taken into account and in general these state that effects on reproduction should be studied for all new drugs so that any effect on fertility (including male fertility), mating behaviour, foetal loss, foetal abnormality and damage to offspring in later life is detected. Guidance is given for a flexible scheme for testing mammalian reproduction, from conception in one generation to conception in the following generation.

(D)   Mutagenic potential (in vitro and in vivo)

The first CPMP guideline (EU, 1998l) has been largely superseded by a more recent guideline (EU, 1998m). A further guideline (CPMP, 1995c) gives recommendations for a standard battery of genotoxicity testing based on current knowledge.

(E)   Carcinogenic potential

The first guideline (EU, 1998n) can largely be replaced by two more recent guidelines (EU, 1998o, p). These give guidance on the need for carrying out carcinogenicity studies, approaches for evaluating carcinogenic potential and dose selection. The guideline on dose selection is supplemented by a further addendum (CPMP, 1996). There is a further guideline, which originated from ICH and has been finalized more recently (CPMP, 1995d).

(F)   Pharmacodynamics (pharmacodynamic effects relating to the proposed indications/general pharmacodynamics/drug interactions)

No specific guidelines on pharmacodynamics are available but some information is included in the guidelines for certain therapeutic classes of drugs.

(G)   Pharmacokinetics (after single and repeat doses, distribution in normal and pregnant animals, biotransformation)

General guidance on absorption, distribution, excretion and metabolism studies is available (EU, 1998q). A guideline (EU, 1998r) has been developed to provide guidance on toxicokinetics.

(H)   Local tolerance (where appropriate)

Guidance is available (EU, 1998s) which states that the purpose of such studies is to ascertain whether medicinal products (i.e. the proposed formulation for marketing) are tolerated at sites of the body which it is envisaged will come into contact with the product during clinical use.

(Q)   Other information (e.g. biological safety testing of biotechnology products)

The difficulties in standardizing a test package is recognized in the guideline on preclinical biological safety testing on medicinal products derived from biotechnology products (EU, 1998f). It is recommended that this guideline be taken into consideration when deciding which preclinical safety testing is appropriate. The guideline categorizes biotechnology-derived products into groups (e.g. hormones, cytokines and other regulatory factors, blood products, monoclonal antibodies and vaccines) and provides a summary of strategies for safety testing requirements.

(R)   Environmental risk assessment/ecotoxicity
Data on the environmental risk assessment of products containing genetically modified organisms (GMOs) is included in Part II of the application. An environmental risk assessment of non-GMO products should be included in Part III. This particularly applies to new active substances and live vaccines

Part IV: Clinical Documentation

Clinical testing should take into account any significant findings noted during toxicity testing. The first section covers clinical pharmacology (pharmacodynamics and pharmacokinetics). The second section contains details of all clinical trials carried out. Any information on post-marketing experience, published and unpublished studies, ongoing and incomplete trials is presented subsequently.

Abridged Applications

The above information refers to an application for a new drug substance for which the maximum documentation is required. Abridged applications vary considerably in the content and amount of documentation required. An application for a generic product, whose use in clinical practice is well established for 6–10 years within the European Community, will not need any preclinical or clinical documentation apart from brief preclinical and clinical expert reports, which verify that the product is well established. In certain circumstances, preclinical data may be needed to support an abridged application. Examples of such circumstances include an application for a well established product to be administered via a new route, whereby data from toxicology studies carried out using the new route would need to be presented. Another example would be if the drug substance has been manufactured using a new synthesis, which has resulted in a different impurity profile.

Post-Marketing Authorisation Procedures

Pharmacovigilance

Following grant of a Marketing Authorisation (MA), the holder of the MA has responsibilities to gather, evaluate and act upon any information which relates to the risk: benefit assessment of the medicine. This includes spontaneous suspected adverse reaction reports, peri-odic safety updates, published literature, clinical and epidemiological studies and any other relevant information. Such procedures must be carried out on a global level.

Periodic Safety Updates

Following Marketing Authorization (MA), the responsibilities of the holder of the MA involve the submission of periodic safety update reports (PSURs). In Europe, these updates must be provided every 6 months for the first 2 years of marketing, annually for the three following years and then once every 5 years. This is in accordance with Council Directive 93/39/EC and Council Regulation 2309/93. Essentially, these updates review all new clinical and preclinical data, including spontaneously reported adverse reactions to the marketed product, and re-evaluate the risk–benefit in the conclusion of the report. Guidance notes for PSURs are available (CPMP, 1995e), which is an ICH Harmonised Tripartate Guideline, effective from 18 June 1997 in Europe. Within this report, all completed studies yielding safety information (with potential impact on product information) should be discussed. Furthermore, any new studies specifically planned or conducted to examine a safety issue should be described. Published literature should be documented and discussed.

Renewals

According to Directive 65/65/EEC, Article 10 (EU, 1998b) and Council Regulation (EEC) No. 2309/93 (EU, 1998e) a marketing authorization is valid for 5 years, at which time it is renewable. A renewal application must be made at least 3 months before expiry.

Variations

Any changes (variations) to the Marketing Authorization require approval in accordance with Commission Regulation (EC) No. 541/95 (European Commission, 1995a) as amended by (EC) No. 1146/98 (European Commission, 1998b) for marketing authorizations granted under the mutual recognition procedure and Commission Regulation (EC) No. 542/95 (European Commission, 1995b) as amended by (EC) No. 1069/98 (European Commission 1998c) for marketing authorizations granted under the centralized procedure. Variations will need to go through the same procedure (mutual recognition or centralized) as the original marketing authorization. Variations are classified into two types: Type I (listed in Annex 1 of the Regulations) and Type II (all other changes which do not require a new application). Approval is required before the change can be implemented. Type I variations are simpler and can be approved within 30 days. Type II variations can be approved within 90 days. Provision has been made for an urgent safety restriction to be made to the SmPC, where this is deemed necessary for safe use of the product.

A variation (or suspension or withdrawal) to a Marketing Authorisation which has been authorised by Mutual Recognition can be Member State initiated (Community referral) in accordance with Article 12 (Community interest) and Article 15 (protection of Public health) of Directive 75/319/EC.

INTERNATIONAL CONFERENCE ON HARMONIZATION

ICH is the International Conference on Harmonization of Technical Requirements for Registration of Pharmaceuticals for human use. It brings together the regulatory authorities of Europe, Japan and the USA together with pharmaceutical industry experts with the aim of harmonizing product registration requirements in the three regions. The process has primarily focused on the development of harmonized tripartite guidelines in five steps. Step 1 is when a consensus has been reached by a selected group of experts and at Step 2 the consensus is released for consultation. This is followed (Step 3) by consultation outside ICH with the aim of finalizing the guideline (Step 4). Step 5 is the incorporation of the finalized guideline into the national/regional regulations.

To date, the Fourth International Conference held in July 1997 concluded the first phase of the harmonization process with respect to developing detailed technical guidelines. At the end of Phase 1, there were 27 harmonized tripartite guidelines and nine further finalized guidelines (i.e. at Step 4) which require implementation in the three regions. Currently, a number of ICH safety guidelines have been adopted in Europe. One further guideline on the duration of chronic toxicity testing in animals has been recently finalised (Step 4). This guideline states that a duration of 9 months for chronic testing in non-rodent species is acceptable in the three regions.

The second phase of ICH aims to harmonize a common technical document to enable pharmaceutical companies to submit data of a common format and content for new medicinal products in a Marketing Authorization Application in the three regions. It is hoped that a final consensus could be achieved by the year 2000.

REFERENCES

CPMP (1995a). Note for guidance on non-clinical safety studies for the conduct of human clinical trials for pharmaceu-

ticals (CPMP/ICH/286/95). European Medicines Evaluation Agency, London.

CPMP (1995b). Note for guidance on Good Clinical Practice (CPMP/ICH/135/95). European Medicines Evaluation Agency, London.

CPMP (1995c). Note for guidance on genotoxicity: a standard battery for genotoxicity testing of pharmaceuticals (CPMP/ICH/174/95). European Medicines Evaluation Agency, London.

CPMP (1995d). Note for guidance on carcinogenicity: testing for carcinogenicity of pharmaceuticals (CPMP/ICH/299/95). European Medicines Evaluation Agency, London.

CPMP (1995e) Note for guidance on clinical safety data management: periodic safety update reports for marketed drugs (CPMP/ICH/288/95). European Medicines Evaluation Agency, London.

CPMP (1996). Addendum to Note for guidance on dose selection for carcinogenicity studies of pharmaceuticals (addition of a limit dose and related notes) (CPMP/ICH/366/96). European Medicines Evaluation Agency, London.

CPMP (1998). Note for guidance on the preclinical evaluation of anticancer medicinal products EMEA 23 July 1998 CPMP/SWP/997/96. European Medicines Evaluation Agency, London.

EU (1997). Proposal for a European Parliament and Council Directive on approximation of provisions laid down by regulation or administrative action relating to the implementation of Good Clinical Practice in the conduct of clinical trials on medicinal products for human use (COM (97) 369). *Off. J. Eur. Commun.*, C306.

EU (1998a). Rules Governing Medicinal Products in the European Union, Vol. 1. Office for Official Publications of the European Union, Luxembourg.

EU (1998b). Council Directive 65/65/EC of 26 January 1965, Rules Governing Medicinal Products in the European Union, Vol. 1. Office for Official Publications of the European Union, Luxembourg, pp. 3–12; *Off. J. Eur. Commun.*, 1965, L22.

EU (1998c). Council Directive 75/318/EEC of 20 May 1975, Rules Governing Medicinal Products in the European Union, Vol. 1, Office for Official Publications of the European Union, Luxembourg, pp. 13–40; *Off. J. Eur. Commun.*, 1975, L147.

EU (1998d). Council Directive 75/319/EEC of 20 May 1975, Rules Governing Medicinal Products in the European Union, Vol. 1, Office for Official Publications of the European Union, Luxembourg, pp. 41–64; *Off. J. Eur. Commun.*, 1975, L147.

EU (1998e). Council Regulation 2309/93/EEC of 22 July 1993, Rules Governing Medicinal Products in the European Union, Vol. 1, Office for Official Publications of the European Union, Luxembourg, pp. 133–168; *Off. J. Eur. Commun.*, 1993, L214.

EU (1998f). Pre-clinical biological safety testing on medicinal products derived from biotechnology products, (3B315a), Rules Governing Medicinal Products in the European Union, Vol. III B, Office for Official Publications of the European Union, Luxembourg, pp. 117–129.

EU (1998g). Rules Governing Medicinal Products in the European Union, Vol. III, Guidelines on the quality, safety and efficacy of medicinal products for human use. Office for Official Publications of the European Union, Luxembourg.

EU (1998h). Single Dose Toxicity (3B301A), Rules Governing Medicinal Products in the European Union, Vol. IIIB, Office for Official Publications of the European Union, Luxembourg, pp. 3–7.

EU (1998i). Repeated Dose Toxicity (3B302A), Rules Governing Medicinal Products in the European Union, Vol. IIIB, Office for Official Publications of the European Union, Luxembourg, pp. 9–20.

EU (1998j). Repeated Dose Tissue Distribution Studies (3B303A) (CPMP/ICH/385/95), Rules Governing Medicinal Products in the European Union, Vol. IIIB, Office for Official Publications of the European Union, Luxembourg, pp. 21–24.

EU (1998k). Detection of Toxicity to Reproduction for Medicinal Products (3B305A) (CPMP/ICH/386/95) including Toxicity to Male Fertility (3B306A) (CPMP/ICH/136/95), Rules Governing Medicinal Products in the European Union, Vol. IIIB, Office for Official Publications of the European Union, Luxembourg, pp. 25–44.

EU (1998l). Testing of Medicinal Products for their Mutagenic Potential (3B307A), Rules Governing Medicinal Products in the European Union, Vol. IIIB, Office for Official Publications of the European Union, Luxembourg, pp. 45–50.

EU (1998m). Genotoxicity: Guidance on Specific aspects of Regulatory Genotoxicity Tests for Pharmaceuticals (3B308A) (CPMP/141/95), Rules Governing Medicinal Products in the European Union, Vol. IIIB, Office for Official Publications of the European Union, Luxembourg, pp. 51–62.

EU (1998n). Carcinogenic Potential (3B309A), Rules Governing Medicinal Products in the European Union, Vol. IIIB, Office for Official Publications of the European Union, Luxembourg, pp. 63–71.

EU (1998o). The Need for Carcinogenicity Studies of Pharmaceuticals (3B310A) (CPMP/ICH/140/95), Rules Governing Medicinal Products in the European Union, Vol. IIIB, Office for Official Publications of the European Union, Luxembourg, pp. 73–78.

EU (1998p). Dose Selection for Carcinogenicity Studies of Pharmaceuticals (3B311A) (CPMP/ICH/383/94), Rules Governing Medicinal Products in the European Union, Vol. IIIB, Office for Official Publications of the European Union, Luxembourg, pp. 79–88.

EU (1998q). Pharmacokinetics and Metabolic Studies in the Safety Evaluation of new drugs in animals, (3B313A), Rules Governing Medicinal Products in the European Union, Vol. IIIB, Office for Official Publications of the European Union, Luxembourg, pp. 103–106.

EU (1998r). The assessment of Systemic Exposure in Toxicity Studies (3B312A) (CPMP/ICH/384/95), Rules Governing Medicinal Products in the European Union, Vol. IIIB, Office for Official Publications of the European Union, Luxembourg, pp. 89–101.

EU (1998s). Non-Clinical Local Tolerance Testing of Medicinal Products (3B314A), Rules Governing Medicinal Products in the European Union, Vol. IIIB, Office for Official Publications of the European Union, Luxembourg, pp. 107–116.

EU (1998t). Environmental Risk Assessment of Human Medicinal Products Containing or Consisting of GMOs, Rules Governing Medicinal Products in the European Union, Vol. IIIB, Office for Official Publications of the European Union, Luxembourg, pp. 133–146.

European Commission (1991) Commission Directive 91/507/EEC of 19 July 1991. *Off. J. Eur. Commun.*, L270.

European Commission (1995a) Commission Regulation 541/95/EC. *Off. J. Eur. Commun.*, L55.

European Commission (1995b) Commission Regulation 542/95/EC. *Off. J. Eur. Commun.*, L55.

European Commission (1998a) Commission Communication of 22 July 1998. *Off. J. Eur. Commun.*, L229.

European Commission (1998b) Commission Regulation 1146/98EC. *Off. J. Eur. Commun.*, L159.

European Commission (1998c) Commission Regulation 1069/98EC. *Off. J. Eur. Commun.*, L153.

European Council (1986). Council Directive 86/609/EEC of 24 November 1986. *Off. J. Eur. Commun.*, L358.

European Council (1987) Council Directive 87/18/EEC of 18 December 1986. *Off. J. Eur. Commun.*, L15.

European Council (1988) Council Directive 88/320/EEC of 9 June 1988. *Off. J. Eur. Commun.*, L145.

European Council (1993). Council Directive 93/39/EEC of 14 June 1993. *Off. J. Eur. Commun.*, L214.

FDA (1995). Department of Health and Human Services, Food and Drug Administration: International Conference on Harmonization, Guidance on Dose Selection for Carcinogenicity Studies of Pharmaceuticals. *Fed. Regist.*, **60**, 40.

FDA (1996a). Department of Health and Human Services, Food and Drug Administration: Single Dose Acute Toxicity Testing for Pharmaceuticals. *Fed. Regist.*, **61**, 166.

FDA (1996b). Department of Health and Human Services, Food and Drug Administration: International Conference on Harmonization, Guidance on Specific Aspects of Regulatory Genotoxicity Testing for Pharmaceuticals. *Fed. Regist.*, **60**, 80.

FDA (1996c). Department of Health and Human Services, Food and Drug Administration: International Conference on Harmonization, Final Guidance on the Need for Long Term Rodent Carcinogenicity Studies for Pharmaceuticals. *Fed. Regist.*, **61**, 42.

FDA (1997a). Department of Health and Human Services, Food and Drug Administration: International Conference on Harmonization, Guidance on Nonclinical Safety Studies for the Conduct of Human Clinical Trials for Pharmaceuticals. *Fed. Regist.*, **62**, 227.

FDA (1997b). Department of Health and Human Services, Food and Drug Administration: International Conference on Harmonization, Draft Guidance on the Duration of Chronic Toxicity testing in Animals (Rodent and Nonrodent Toxicity Testing). *Fed. Regist.*, **62**, 222.

FDA (1997c). Department of Health and Human Services, Food and Drug Administration: International Conference on Harmonization, Guidance on Genotoxicity—A Standard Battery for Genotoxicity Testing for Pharmaceuticals. *Fed. Regist.*, **62**, 225.

FDA (1998a). *The CDER Handbook*. Department of Health and Human Services, Food and Drug Administration, Center for Drug Evaluation and Research, Washington, DC.

FDA (1998b). Department of Health and Human Services, Food and Drug Administration: International Conference on Harmonization, Guidance on Testing for Carcinogenicity of Pharmaceuticals. *Fed. Regist.*, **63**, 34.

MCA (1996). *Medicines Act Leaflet, MAL 4, Guidance Notes on Applications for Clinical Trial Exemptions and Clinical Trial Certificates*. Medicines Control Agency, London.

UK (1968). *The Medicines Act 1968*. HMSO, London.

UK (1995a). *The Medicines (Exemption from Licences) (Clinical Trials) Order 1995 (SI 1995/2808)*. HMSO, London.

UK (1995b). *The Medicines (Exemption from Licences and Certificates) (Clinical Trials) Order 1995 (SI 1995/2809)*. HMSO, London.

World Medical Association (1996). Declaration of Helsinki. Recommendations guiding physicians in Biomedical Research in human subjects. *J. of Am. Med. Assoc.*, **277**, 925–926.

Chapter 75
Regulation of Veterinary Drugs

K.N. Woodward

CONTENTS

- Introduction
- Regulation in the United States
- Regulation in Europe
- International Aspects
- Conclusions
- References

INTRODUCTION

The evolution of legislation governing veterinary medicines, human medicines and indeed other classes of chemical has taken a similar route in almost all countries. An event, usually an adverse event, has led to the establishment of a national registration scheme under national law that has then gradually been modified over time to reflect developments in science, or indeed further accidents or tragedies. This has led to formation of regulatory schemes on a worldwide basis. Some countries still maintain only a rudimentary regulatory authority whereas others, including the USA and most European countries, have more complex and refined systems in place. This chapter will examine two of these for veterinary medicines, the US model and the European systems.

For both human and veterinary medicines, the three major criteria are safety, quality and efficacy (see **Table 2**). It is worth pointing out that safety of human medicines is concerned primarily with the safety of the product to the patient. This is also true to some extent for veterinary drugs, particularly for those medicines intended for use in companion animals such as cats and dogs. However, farm animals are usually destined to be eaten by human beings and so safety here is focused on the safety of residues of the drug in food of animal origin, such as meat, offal, eggs, milk and honey, to the consumer.

REGULATION IN THE UNITED STATES

As we shall see later, the situation in the USA is simpler than that which pertains in the European Union (EU), in that many of its systems are at least seemingly less bureaucratic. On the other hand, complications are introduced by the fact that medicines in the USA are divided into three distinct groups and are handled under separate legislation and by separate agencies.

The standard pharmaceuticals intended for use in animals, such as antibiotics, anti-inflammatory drugs, anthelmintics and anaesthetics, are dealt with through the Food and Drug Administration (FDA) and its Center for Veterinary Medicine (CVM). However, ectoparasiticides intended for use on animals are regarded as pesticides and are authorized through the US Environmental Protection Agency (US EPA). Finally, the US Department of Agriculture (USDA) deals with vaccines. All three classes are dealt with under separate legislation covered in separate areas of the Code of Federal Regulations (CFR), as shown in **Table 1**.

The pharmaceutical group is by far the largest group in terms of diversity of products and complexity of types, whereas the ectoparasiticides, although they may form one of the largest groups in terms of quantities used, are

Table 1 Regulation of veterinary products in the USA

Type	Examples	Agency	Legislative base
Pharmaceuticals	Antimicrobials Anthelmintics Anti-inflammatory drugs Analgesics Anaesthetics Anti-fungal drugs	FDA (CVM)	21 CFR[a]
Ectoparasiticides	Sheep and cattle dips Pour-on formulations Ear tags for cattle Formulations to treat fleas on cats and dogs	EPA	40 CFR
Biologicals[b]	Vaccines, sera, toxins	USDA	9 CFR

[a] The Code of Federal Regulations is published by the Office of the Federal Register, National Archives and Records Administration, as a Special Edition of the Federal Register (Washington, DC).
[b] For more information on this topic in the USA, see Espeseth (1997).

more restricted in type, largely to organophosphorus compounds, carbamates and synthetic pyrethroids. From the point of toxicology and human safety, the vaccines in general are often outside of the scope of such considerations. As a consequence of these considerations, this section will focus largely on the pharmaceuticals and the part played and taken by the CVM.

Historical Perspective

Although there were numerous reasons behind the passing of legislation on drugs, as in many other countries, including the UK (see later), it took a series of disasters for the USA to focus on the need for specific laws on drug regulation. For example, over 100 people died of renal failure following the consumption of sulphanilamide-containing medicines made up in ethylene glycol. There then followed an investigation that led in turn to the Food, Drug and Cosmetic Act of 1938. This in itself did not prevent medical disaster, but wider powers were applied following further events, largely caused by the concealment of adverse reaction in humans by drug manufacturers in the USA. These included aplastic anaemia induced by chloramphenicol, ocular toxicity due to triparanol and blood dycrasias due to amphenidone. Finally, the events surrounding thalidomide (see later) provided the impetus for the passing of legislation which required that new drugs must be both safe and effective. In 1972, further amendments to the legislation were made and these required that for new veterinary drugs, the following must be provided (Davis, 1988):

- Data to demonstrate target species safety;
- Therapeutic efficacy data;
- Satisfactory analytical method for detecting residues in animal tissues and products;
- Data to determine a withdrawal period.

The current scientific requirements for veterinary drug registration in the USA are very similar to those which now pertain in the EU and which will be described later.

In the USA now, veterinary medicines are subject to registration under the FDA, through the CVM, which is based near Washington, DC. The assessment system differs slightly from that in the EU. In the EU and its Member States, there is a wide dependence on extensive committee procedures, particularly those composed of external experts, often from organizations independent of government. On the other hand, the US system is more dependent on assessments by government-employed staff (Guest, 1990).

There are two basic types of authorization within the US FDA system. The New Animal Drugs Application (NADA) is the major route for placing new products on the US market, while the Investigational New Animal Drugs (INAD) application allows for the generation of data to support NADAs.

New Animal Drugs Application (NADA)

The NADA must consist of all the proposed product literature and labelling information, residues, safety, efficacy and quality data and, in addition, a Freedom of Information Summary. Efficacy studies make use of dose titration experiments using three drug levels, and, in addition, clinical field trials are required. The quality data requirements are similar to those demanded in the EU, with emphasis on production and manufacture, purity, stability and proof of identity. To ensure safety to the target animal, toxicity studies in the proposed indicated species are required at 0, 1, 3 and 5 times the intended therapeutic dose for 3 times the recommended treatment period. As with the EU procedures, the toxicological and residues evaluations for food safety assessment are of paramount importance, and the FDA produces a number of Guidelines ranging from toxicological testing to establishing a withdrawal period, for use by prospective drug sponsors (Bloomfield, 1989).

Investigational New Drugs Application (INAD)

The INAD is a specific exemption aimed at allowing the generation of data for a New Animal Drug Application. Protocols of studies to demonstrate efficacy or target animal safety are examined by CVM staff, who also keep records of those conducting the studies. All animals which are treated in the investigations must be accounted for and the trials are conducted under the supervision of the FDA, the US Department of Agriculture (USDA) and the drug sponsor. If the safety data from laboratory animal studies are satisfactory, food derived from treated animals may be allowed to enter the food chain, but if there are elements missing from the package of safety data, extended withdrawal periods may be required before this is allowed to occur (Farber, 1985).

Food Safety Assessment

The FDA employs a six-step evaluation procedure when examining food safety data for a NADA. These are outlined below (Bloomfield, 1989; Guest, 1990).

(1) Metabolism study: so that residues of toxicological concern may be identified.
(2) Comparative metabolism studies: to determine the appropriate species for toxicological testing.

(3) Toxicity tests: to determine the toxicological profile of the drug, to establish safe levels and to identify no-effect levels.

(4) Metabolism study: to identify the target tissue for residues, the marker residue and the tolerance (or maximum residue limit).

(5) Development of a regulatory assay: to allow for monitoring of the marker residue in produce.

(6) Establishment of a withdrawal period.

By use of this procedure, the identity and nature of residues likely to be found in animal products can be established and the conditions for safe use identified. Moreover, decisions can be taken on whether or not residues require regulatory surveillance and, if so, what method of monitoring should be used.

Toxicological Testing

The primary package of toxicological tests for a NADA may be summarized as follows: a battery of genetic toxicity tests; a 90 day feeding study in a rodent (usually the rat) and a non-rodent mammalian species (usually the dog); and other specialized toxicity testing, as necessary.

The studies need to be in compliance with Good Laboratory Practice, and should be conducted according to protocols contained in the 'Redbook' published by the FDA (Farber, 1985). The 'other specialized toxicity testing' category is intended to allow for the conduct of further studies which might be necessary as indicated by the results of those listed above. These include such examples as immunotoxicity, hormonal effects, chronic bioassays, 1 year feeding studies in a rodent species (rat) and 1 year feeding studies in a non-rodent (dog), a teratology study in a second species, studies of neurotoxicity and *in utero* studies and teratology in other species (Farber, 1995). Moreover, the FDA has established cut-off levels for maximum residues in animal products above which further testing is required. These are currently 3 mg kg^{-1} in muscle and 1 mg kg^{-1} in milk and eggs, and the further testing requirements include lifetime studies in two different rodent species, a 6 month study in a non-rodent mammal and a three-generation reproduction study with a teratology investigation. A threshold assessment of carcinogenicity activity is essential, as part of the initial NADA to determine whether carcinogenicity studies in two rodent species is required. The residues cut-off assessment described above is but a part of the threshold assessment, and structure–activity relationships, general biology and the results of genetic toxicity testing contribute to the final decision on carcinogenicity testing, as do the identity and biological properties of the main metabolite(s) present as residues (Food and Drug Administration, 1987).

The FDA has produced extensive guidelines for toxicity and residues assessment. The major ones are as follows:

Guideline	
	General Principles for Evaluating the Safety of Compounds used in Food-producing Animals
I	Guideline for metabolism studies and for selection of residues for toxicological testing.
II	Guideline for toxicological testing
III	Guideline for threshold assessment
IV	Guideline for establishing a tolerance (now, Guideline for establishing a safe concentration)
V	Guideline for approval of a method of analysis for residues
VI	Guideline for establishing a withdrawal period
VII	Guideline for new animal drugs and food additives derived form fermentation
VIII	Guideline for the human food safety evaluation of bound residues derived form carcinogenic drugs
26	Guidelines for the preparation of data to satisfy the requirements of Section 512 of the Act regarding minor species
	Microbiological testing of antimicrobial residues in food

Acceptable Daily Intake, Safe Concentration and Tolerance

The acceptable daily intake (ADI), as with ADIs determined by other regulatory bodies, is calculated by dividing the no-effect level (no-observed effect level; NOEL) from the most sensitive and appropriate toxicity test by a suitable safety factor. The FDA specifies safety factors that it will normally employ, and these depend on the type of test. NOELs determined in chronic toxicity studies or in reproductive and/or teratology studies, where there is clear evidence of maternal toxicity, are normally divided by a factor of 100 to give the ADI. However, if the no-effect level is derived from a 90 day study and there is no reassuring evidence from chronic studies, a 1000-fold safety factor may be used. Similarly, if there is no evidence of maternal toxicity in the reproductive/teratology studies where an effect is seen, again a 1000-fold safety factor will probably be used in the calculation of the ADI.

A safe concentration of the drug or its metabolite(s) is calculated (Teske, 1992; Weber 1992). This is a function of the NOEL and a safety factor, i.e. the ADI, and the standard adult weight (60 kg) divided by the product of a food factor and meat intake factor. The daily intake of meat is taken as being one third of the total solid diet intake of 1500 g (i.e. 500 g). The food factor is normally 1 for bovine, ovine and porcine muscle, 3 for milk, $\frac{1}{3}$ for eggs, 2–5 for liver and 3–5 for kidney, depending on the species. Hence,

$$\text{safe concentration} = \frac{\text{ADI } (\mu\text{g kg}^{-1}\text{day}^{-1}) \times 60}{\text{food factor} \times 500\text{g day}^{-1}}$$

A tolerance or maximum residue limit for the marker residue can be derived for each edible tissue from each species, by establishing a safe concentration for each. The safe concentration or tolerance must not result in intakes of drug residues that would lead to an intake in excess of the ADI (Teske, 1992).

Interestingly, the CVM has adopted a different approach to microbiologically active residues compared with that used in the EU (see later). In the guideline published in 1993, it opted for a 'maximum safe concentration' of 0.1 ppm in the total adult diet. For anti-microbial compounds, this would equate to $1.5 \, \mathrm{mg \, day^{-1}}$ or $0.025 \, \mathrm{mg \, (kg \, body \, weight)^{-1} \, day^{-1}}$ (Kidd, 1994; Food and Drug Administration, 1996). In this guideline, the FDA recognized the shortcomings of the test systems for microbiologically active substances. However, it went on to indicate that the cut-off of 1 ppm might be reconsidered on the basis of experimental data provided.

As part of the NADA, drug sponsors must submit a method for regulatory surveillance of residues to ensure that violations of the tolerance are not occurring in use. There are three steps in the adoption of the residues monitoring method. First, the sponsor must develop a method in accordance with the FDA's Guidelines. Second, the FDA determines its suitability for an inter-laboratory study. Finally, an interlaboratory study is initiated to ensure that the method performs as claimed by the sponsor, and that it is suitable as a regulatory surveillance instrument. In this way, the procedure differs from the situation in the EU. As described later, although Council Regulation 2377/90 (Council of the European Communities, 1990) includes a requirement for companies to submit a proposed regulatory method as part of application for Community-wide maximum residue limits (MRLs), there is currently no demand for the actual testing of these methods.

Withdrawal Periods

Metabolism studies and, more specifically, residues depletion studies are used to determine the withdrawal period for a new drug. Simplistically, the study is conducted in a group of target animals using four or five points for serial slaughter, in such a way that the residues depletion passes through the tolerance. The 99% statistical tolerance, with 95% confidence limits, can be determined and from the intercept with the tolerance, the withdrawal period can be determined from the time axis (Weber, 1990a, 1992).

Bound Residues

To a large extent, the proposals put forward by the FDA in its draft guideline on bound residues are similar to those proposed by the Joint FAO/WHO Expert Committee on Food Additives (JECFA) (Joint FAO/WHO Expert Committee on Food Additives, 1990). The essentials are that the drug sponsor determines the bioavailability and toxicological potential of the bound residues, then estimates the reversibility of adduct formation and proposes a mechanism of bound residue formation (Weber, 1990b).

The draft guideline to some extent assumes that if residues are not absorbed following ingestion, their relevance is lessened, but it does take note of possible direct effects on the gastrointestinal tract. As such, it does not merely take into account the absorption of bound residues if the concern is due to carcinogenic potential, because of possible local carcinogenic effects on the gastrointestinal system. Genotoxicity studies may prove useful as one example of investigating the toxicological properties of residues, albeit in a very specific area, in these circumstances. Studies with enzymatic and chemical methodologies can provide some information on the possibility of the regeneration of toxic reactive species from bound residues. Hence, the reversibility—or otherwise—of adduct formation is important in the overall assessment of hazards posed by bound residues.

Ectoparasiticides

As mentioned earlier, ectoparasiticides are regulated by the US EPA, under the Federal Insecticide, Fungicide and Rodenticide Act (FIFRA). This requires that pesticides, including ectoparasiticides, be given prior approval before they can be legally used in the USA (US Environmental Protection Agency, 1996).

Toxicity data (and related information such as metabolism and physicochemical data) are required, in the same way that similar information is demanded for veterinary drug registration through the FDA. Moreover, on a global basis, the toxicological requirements for pesticide registration have many similarities (Schmidt-Bleek and Marchal, 1993). For residues issues, the ADI concept is generally used along with the establishment of tolerances, in a manner, once again, similar to that adopted by the FDA (National Research Council, 1987).

As with the FDA, guidelines are available on toxicity testing and requirements and, in many cases, 'public draft' guidelines are also available. This is because there is currently an exercise within the US EPA to harmonize guidelines, particularly with those of the OECD (Environmental Protection Agency, 1996). Some current public drafts include the following:

Guideline	Date
Acute dermal irritation	June 1996
Acute inhalation toxicity	June 1996
Skin sensitization	June 1996
Preliminary developmental toxicity screen	June 1996
Subchronic inhalation toxicity	June 1996
Reproduction and fertility effects	February 1996
Chronic toxicity	June 1996
Carcinogenicity	June 1996
Delayed neurotoxicity (organophosphorus compounds)	June 1996
Neurotoxicity screening battery	June 1996
Neurophysiology	June 1996
Immunotoxicity	June 1996
Various genotoxicity studies	June 1996

Residues Monitoring

The National Residue Program carried out by the Food Safety and Inspection Service of the USDA offers a comprehensive system of residues monitoring in the USA. This programme examines not only veterinary drugs, but also pesticides (including ectoparasiticides) and other chemical contaminants, in meat and other animal products (Cordle, 1988; United States Department of Agriculture, 1989). Compounds are chosen by a ranking system which takes into account the amount used, the conditions of use, the potential for misuse, metabolism in animals and the toxicity of the residues (United States Department of Agriculture, 1989). The residues monitoring system is extremely comprehensive. Raw meat containing residue levels above the permitted tolerance is designated adulterated and thus it violates Federal inspection laws (Pullen 1990). Past experience suggests that in the USA, as with several other countries, residues violations are low for veterinary drugs in general, but sulphonamides in pigs prove to be notable exceptions (Cordle, 1988; United States Department of Agriculture, 1989).

Other Aspects of Drug Control in the USA

Unlike the UK, where there is a close relationship between the Licensing Authority for veterinary medicines and the government agency responsible for worker safety, the Health and Safety Executive, there appears to be a much more distant collaboration in the USA between the respective agencies. However, as in the European systems, medicines are evaluated on the basis of toxicity data and potential for worker exposure. Drugs that are thought to offer an unacceptable operator risk are assigned prescription drug category. As is the case in many other countries, there are specific controls on drugs

with abuse potential (Davis, 1988). The CVM receives and analyses reports of suspected adverse reactions as a contribution to post-marketing surveillance.

REGULATION IN EUROPE

The UK system serves as a good model of what can be achieved and, some would say, of what should be achieved. It is among the more sophisticated regulatory regimes currently operating within the EU and it will be used here to illustrate the role of the regulatory authority in an EU Member State, and how it fits in turn with the EU functions and requirements.

The thalidomide episode and the events surrounding it led directly to the regulation of human and veterinary medicines in the UK, although there had previously been attempts to control 'drugs' as early as the reign of Henry VIII, while the Food and Drugs Act of 1925 placed a degree of control over the quality of medicinal products (Cuthbert et al., 1978; Harrison, 1986a).

However, following on from the disaster surrounding thalidomide, the Committee on Safety of Drugs, usually referred to as the Dunlop Committee after its Chairman, Sir Derrick Dunlop, was established. This Committee had no regulatory powers, but it worked with the pharmaceutical industry in a voluntary manner with an equally voluntary system of registration, product assessment and post-marketing surveillance for medicinal products used in humans. Following further consideration by the Joint Subcommittee of the English and Scottish Standing Medical Advisory Committees, which had initially recommended the establishment of the Dunlop Committee, further, and this time legislative, measures were examined, and this ultimately resulted in the passing by Parliament of the Medicines Act 1968. Until relatively recently, this formed the basis of the regulation of both veterinary and human medicinal products in the UK (Cuthbert et al., 1978).

Until the Medicines Act 1968, veterinary drugs had also been controlled in the UK by a voluntary scheme, largely aimed at adequate safety labelling, under the auspices of the Ministry of Agriculture, Fisheries and Food (MAFF). The basic goal then, as now, was to protect human beings, livestock, domestic animals and wildlife against any harmful effects. MAFF was advised on these aspects by the Veterinary Products Committee (VPC) and by the Advisory Committee on Pesticides and Other Toxic Chemicals, because many veterinary drugs were similar to related pesticidal products.

After the introduction of the Medicines Act, the advisory structure became more formal. Expert advice on veterinary medicines is now provided largely by the VPC, the veterinary counterpart of the better known Committee on Safety of Medicines (CSM) for human medicinal products. Both committees were established under Section 4 of the Medicines Act (1968). The members of these advisory committees, and their chairmen, are drawn from academia, research institutes and other independent centres. They therefore provide a source of independent and unbiased advice for government ministers (Harrison, 1986b; Woodward, 1993a).

Applications for marketing authorizations are dealt with by two executive agencies in the UK. The Medicines Control Agency (MCA) handles applications for human pharmaceuticals and biological products, while the Veterinary Medicines Directorate (VMD) deals with those for veterinary medicines including pharmaceuticals, including ectoparasiticides, and biological products, with advice on authorization of these being provided by the VPC. Although under the jurisdiction of the Department of Health (DH) for human medicines and MAFF and DH for veterinary medicinal products, the two organizations come together with the Medicines Commission under Section 2 of the Medicines Act 1968 and indeed, the Licensing Authority in the Act is defined as the UK Health and Agriculture Ministers acting jointly (Woodward, 1991a, 1993a).

The European Dimension: Pre-1995

As noted earlier, European regulatory systems tend to be more complex and bureaucratic than the US counterparts. This may be because US legislation has been established in what is already a federal system, whereas in Europe, there has been a need to harmonize requirements across 15 separate and independent Member States. Some of those systems were very different from each other.

Regardless, there is now a comprehensive system of regulation for veterinary drugs in the EU. Directive 65/65/EEC of 1965 was the first of the pharmaceutical directives and it formed the basis of subsequent directives and regulations which now govern the authorization of both veterinary and human medicinal products in the EU (Cartwright, 1991). The two major Directives that formed the backbone of the European legislation on veterinary medicines are Directives 81/851/EEC and 81/852/EEC, both of which have been amended several times. The former established the basic regulatory framework for veterinary medicines in the EU while the latter set out the testing requirements to ensure safety, quality and efficacy—the three criteria on which human and veterinary medicines are assessed. Examples of aspects of each of these are given in **Table 2**.

Importantly, Directive 81/851/EEC also created provision for the major European advisory committee on veterinary medicines, the Committee for Veterinary Medicinal Products (CVMP), which was established in 1983. The legislative provisions of Directives 81/851/EEC and 81/852/EEC were subsumed into the legal frameworks of the Member States. In the UK, this meant legislation in the form of Statutory Instruments under

Table 2 Examples of the major elements of quality, efficacy, safety and residue data

Quality	Manufacturing methods and dosage form
	Analysis
	Composition
	Control of starting materials
	Control of finished product
	Stability/shelf-life
	Containers/cartons and packaging
	Labelling/literature
	Quality relating to safety (toxic degradation products or contaminants)
Efficacy	Pharmacodynamics
	Pharmacokinetics
	Laboratory studies e.g. *in vitro* effects on pathogens
	Laboratory trials of efficacy
	Clinical field trials
Safety	Consumer safety[a]
	Operator safety[b]
	Environmental safety[c]
	Target animal (patient) safety
Residues	Pharmacokinetics
	Residues depletion studies
	Methods for residues surveillance

[a] Largely toxicological data.
[b] Largely toxicological and operator exposure data.
[c] Environmental toxicological, exposure and persistence/degradation data.

the Medicines Act (1968). Hence the legislative framework and the testing requirements for safety, quality and efficacy in European Member States stemmed from these two key directives.

For the most part, applications were considered and authorizations granted in Member States, for example, as product licences in the UK. However, two European Community procedures were available. Once of these, known as the concertation procedure, was introduced by Directive 87/22/EEC. This procedure was compulsory for so-called high-technology products such as those derived from recombinant DNA technology or from methods involving hybridoma or monoclonal antibody techniques. The procedure was optional for other products including products containing substances new to veterinary medicine in Europe. Concertation procedure applications were considered by the CVMP meeting in Brussels, under the auspices of Directorate General (DG) III of the European Commission (Commission of the European Communities, 1993). What emerged was an opinion of the CVMP that could include a recommendation that the product should be authorized. However, this opinion was not legally binding on Member States and they could, if they so wished, ignore it.

The other procedure was the so-called multi-state procedure that was based on a provision in Directive 81/851/EEC as amended by Directive 90/676/EEC. Here a marketing authorization was first obtained from one of the Member States in accordance with national procedures.

The holder of the authorization could then apply to at least two other Member States using the dossier approved by the first as the basis for the subsequent applications. It was then up to those subsequent Member States to grant the authorizations or to give reasoned objections as to why they would not. Under the latter circumstances, the matter was referred to the CVMP for an opinion. Again, this opinion was not legally binding (Commission of the European Communities, 1993).

It was probably the lack of binding opinions which resulted in a relatively poor uptake of both procedures by the veterinary pharmaceutical industry. For example, it meant that if the CVMP issued an opinion that a product should be authorized, but a Member State took the opposite view, then that Member State could not be compelled to authorize the product. Fewer difficulties appeared to be encountered by the human pharmaceutical industry, which made far greater use of these procedures under the corresponding provisions governing human pharmaceutical products (Jefferys, 1995).

A third procedure, which for obvious reasons has no counterpart on the human side, was the introduction of a Council Regulation for establishing MRLs. Council Regulation (EEC) No 2377/90 was introduced on 26 June 1990 and it brought with it European Community requirements for the establishment of MRLs, based on toxicology and residue data, for drugs used in food-producing animals. This will be discussed in more depth later.

The New Procedures

Council Regulation (EEC) No 2309/93 introduced some of the most fundamental changes affecting veterinary (and human) medicines in the EU since the introduction of Directives 81/851/EEC and 81/852/EEC more than a decade before. This regulation introduced radically new procedures for medicinal products and established the European Medicines Evaluation Agency (EMEA) (Jefferys, 1995).

As is now widely known, the EMEA started to operate in January 1995, as an agency of the European Commission. In doing so, the EMEA took over the responsibility for the assessment of medicinal products, both veterinary and human, from the Commission. As a consequence, the CVMP and its counterpart for human drugs, the Committee for Proprietary Medicinal Products (CPMP), and all of their working parties, including the one that deals with residues and MRLs, now meet at the EMEA. This is based in Canary Wharf in London's Docklands area, rather than in Brussels. The only committee which continues to meet in Brussels is the so-called Regulatory Committee (or Standing Committee), as this is a legal instrument of the European Commission, which adopts CVMP (and CPMP) opinions on MRLs and authorizations into EU law.

The role and composition of the CVMP (and CPMP) have also changed. Previously, the committee consisted of two representatives from each Member State who represented their national authorities. Now, the members are appointed experts from each country who, although they may still be chosen from national authorities, nevertheless serve as individual experts in their own right. As a result, the role of the committee has changed in a subtle manner. Whereas previously the Committee advised on scientific, policy and legislative matters, it now concerns itself almost exclusively with scientific advisory issues. Policy inputs and advice on legislative matters now come from the Veterinary Pharmaceutical Committee. This is an *ad hoc* advisory committee which meets under the auspices of the Commission (DG III) in Brussels, and it should not be confused with the Regulatory Committee mentioned in the previous paragraph (Woodward, 1997).

The Centralized System

This evolved from the old concertation procedure. Its legal basis is set out in Regulation No. 2309/93. Unlike the concertation procedure, the outcome is binding in Member States (Council of the European Communities, 1998; Jefferys, 1995). In fact, it goes beyond the scope of the old concertation procedure. The outcome of the centralized procedure is, in fact, an EU-wide marketing authorization issued by the European Commission through the EMEA, and on the basis of a scientific assessment by the CVMP, and the adoption of the CVMP's subsequent scientific opinion by the Regulatory Committee.

The assessment of centralized applications for veterinary medicinal products is dealt with using the rapporteur and co-rapporteur system. The rapporteur and the co-rapporteur, chosen from the CVMP's membership, can appoint assessment teams of up to three members each from a list of 'European Experts' held by the EMEA. These experts may tackle the general areas of safety, quality and efficacy or they may examine more detailed aspects of these issues such as residues depletion, analytical methods or ecotoxicity. The applications must be in accordance with the general requirements of Articles 5, 5a and 7 of Directive 81/851/EEC and be accompanied by supporting data on safety, quality and efficacy as set out in Directive 81/852/EEC as amended by Directive 92/18/EEC. As with the MRL procedure, scientific advice is given by the CVMP and the decision is adopted into EU law through the Regulatory Committee procedure.

Products which go through the centralized procedure must have MRLs (see later) if they are intended for use in food-producing animals. Applicants can choose to obtain the MRL (or Annex II entry—see later) first, or they can submit a simultaneous application for the MRL or Annex II entry with the centralized procedure application. However, in the latter case, the applications are dealt with separately, as each has its own separate legal basis.

The scope of the centralized procedure is detailed in Regulation (EEC) No. 2309/93 in its Annex. Products that fall into Part A of the Annex must follow this route; there is no choice. These include products derived from recombinant DNA technology, for the controlled expression of genes in prokaryotes and eukaryotes and from hybridoma and monoclonal antibody methods. In addition, for veterinary medicines, products intended to promote growth, or to enhance yield (for example, of milk), must follow the centralized route.

The centralized route is optional for products covered by Part B of the Annex. For veterinary medicinal products these options include:

- Products developed from biotechnology which, in the opinion of the EMEA, constitute a significant innovation;
- Products administered by means of a new delivery system which, in the opinion of the EMEA, constitute a significant innovation;
- Products presented for an entirely new indication which, in the opinion of the EMEA, is of significant therapeutic interest;
- Products, the manufacture of which employs processes which, in the opinion of the EMEA, demonstrate a significant advance such as two-dimensional electrophoresis under microgravity;
- Products intended for use in animals, containing a new active substance which, on the date of entry into force of the regulation, was not authorized in any Member State.

It is also possible to make minor amendments to marketing authorizations under another regulation, Commission Regulation (EEC) No. 542/95 (Commission of the European Communities, 1995). This views variations as minor (Type I) and major (Type II). Minor variations are listed in Annex I to the Commission Regulation and include, for example, change of name of the product, change of name and/or address of the authorization holder, deletion of an indication, deletion of a route of administration, change in batch size, extension of shelf-life (as foreseen at initial authorization) and change in container shape. Type II variations are more substantial and include any not covered in Annex I as Type I or in Annex II of the Regulation as requiring a new application. Examples of this latter category include changes to the active substance, changes to the therapeutic indications, changes to strength, pharmaceutical form and route of administration and, for veterinary drugs, an addition or changes in target species.

Article 41 of Regulation (EEC) No. 2309/93 introduces a requirement for pharmacovigilance or the monitoring of suspected adverse reactions under the centralized procedure. Responsibility for this also lies with the EMEA but, obviously, the Agency will need to rely on Member States for information from national pharmacovigilance systems. However, it is the duty of the authorization holder to appoint a person responsible for pharmacovigilance matters within the company and to provide necessary reports on adverse reactions to both the national authorities and to the EMEA.

The benefits of the centralized procedure are obvious. Applicants can pay a single fee to a single agency and obtain an authorization for a product in all 15 Member States. Indeed, as already mentioned, the result of the procedure is a European-wide marketing authorization issued by the European Commission. The disadvantage is the not inconsiderable fee that currently applies, but this can be offset against the sum of the national fees. In addition, there is the advantage of discussions with only one set of officials rather than 15, and the pleasure of having to deal with just one set of queries and questions, again rather than 15. At the time of writing in early 1999, only twelve veterinary products had been dealt with through this procedure, although several more were under evaluation. However, the experience so far suggests that this will be a useful and successful method for obtaining EU-wide marketing authorizations.

The Mutual Recognition (Decentralized) Procedure

The mutual recognition procedure, or decentralized procedure as it is often (and incorrectly) known, is allowed for under Article 17 of Directive 81/851/EEC (as amended). Under this procedure, the applicant obtains initial authorization in one EU Member State, the so-called Reference Member State (RMS) through the national procedure in that State (including any national fee payable), and then requests mutual recognition of this authorization in the other Member States of interest, which are known as the Concerned Member States (CMS).

The mutual recognition procedure replaces the old multi-state procedure and, unlike the latter, the decision is binding on Member States. It enables an applicant to obtain a marketing authorization in more than one Member State without (in theory at least) the complexities of multiple applications at the national level. The procedure can be initiated by a Member State where parallel multiple applications are made by the applicant to several Member States. If the applicant of such multiple applications informs a Member State, that Member State may choose to suspend its own procedures and recognize the authorisation granted by another Member State. Alternatively, and more likely, the applicant may initiate the procedure and ask one or more Member

States (the CMS) to recognize an authorization granted in the RMS. Under these circumstances, the assessment report produced by the RMS must be updated (on the basis of data supplied by the applicant) and this must be supplied to each CMS. On receipt of the assessment report, the CMS should then mutually recognize the application granted in the RMS.

It is important to recognize that the EMEA is not usually concerned with this procedure. With one major exception, it is the sole province of the EU Member States. The exception arises when Member States cannot agree on aspects of safety, quality and efficacy and mutual recognition cannot be achieved. In this case, the application will go to arbitration through the EMEA and the opinion of the CVMP will be sought. The outcome of this arbitration is binding on Member States and it can affect the application even in the RMS or other Member States where the authorization has already been granted. At its worst, if the arbitration decision was that the product should not be authorized, then not only would the CMS not grant the application, but the RMS would need to revoke the existing authorization. It is also important to recognize that for products intended for use in food-producing animals, EU MRLs must be in force before mutual recognition can begin, or the applicant be able to verify that the pharmacologically active substance concerned was in use in each CMS, in the species of interest, before 1 January 1992, when Regulation (EEC) No. 2377/90 came into effect.

Until the end of 1997, the mutual recognition procedure was optional for all applications for which the centralized procedure was not compulsory. However, from 1 January 1998, the procedure became mandatory for all applications made in more than one Member State.

Obviously, the system requires an unprecedented degree of cooperation between the RMS, the CMS and the applicant. An absolute degree of trust and willingness is also needed if the procedure is to work at the Member State level.

Its is important to realize at this stage that no regulatory differences are recognized under EU legislation between pharmaceuticals, ectoparasiticides and vaccines (often referred to as immunological products). All are covered by the EU legislation on medicines and the EMEA, CVMP and the new procedures apply to all three categories of product. This also applies generally in all EU Member States, although some countries still retain a division of responsibility. For example, in Ireland, the Irish Medicines Board deals with pharmaceuticals (including ectoparasiticides) whereas vaccines are handled by the Department of Agriculture and Food, although this situation is set to change. In general, vaccines have little or no toxicological significance for human food safety assessment (see below) and they are not mentioned in any depth in this chapter. The reader interested in the EU regulatory aspects of vaccines is referred elsewhere (Brunko, 1997).

Maximum Residue Limits

The situation with respect to MRLs is more complex in the EU than it is in the US regulatory system. Council Regulation No. (EEC) 2377/90 is an item of European Legislation the effects of which have been profound and long lasting for both veterinary pharmaceutical manufacturers and for regulatory authorities within the EU (Council of the European Communities, 1990). For the former, it has introduced a wide-ranging review of the toxicology and residue depletion profiles of pharmacologically active ingredients used in food-producing animals and, for the latter, it has imposed a heavy burden of scientific assessments in order that MRLs can be established. It is important to recognize that in addition to active ingredients, the MRL legislation affects all pharmacologically active substances, including solvents and other excipients, including those found in vaccines and other immunological products.

The scope and implications of Council Regulation No. (EEC) 2377/90 are indeed more comprehensive than at first it might appear. There are four annexes to the Regulation, as follows:

Annex I	Full MRLs
Annex II	No MRLs required
Annex III	Provisional MRLs
Annex IV	No MRLs possible on consumer safety grounds

Annex I is self-explanatory. These are full MRLs for which no further action is imminent **(Table 3)**. Annex III, on the other hand, is for provisional MRLs where further scientific information is considered necessary by the CVMP. They can be established for periods of up to 5 years and extended for a further 2 year period. In general, the expiry date is established on the basis of the time period thought likely by the CVMP to be needed for the industry to complete the required work. Substances in Annex II are those for which it is considered that there is no undue risk to human health, either because the substance is of low toxicity, or it is used in small numbers of animals, or it is rapidly detoxified and excreted, or a combination of these factors. Annex IV is the destiny of those substances which are considered to pose a risk to consumer safety or where there is insufficient data to assuage concerns over specific issues (Woodward, 1992a).

The Annex entries are significant because of the legislative implications involved. As from the data of entry into force of the Regulation, veterinary medicines intended for use in food-producing animals and containing a new active ingredient may not be authorized in the EU until MRLs have been established for drug in that species. Furthermore, MRLs must be established for 'old' molecules prior to 2000, or their use in food-producing species will be lost in the EU.

Table 3 Examples of veterinary drugs in Annexes I–IV of Council Regulation (EEC) No. 2377/90

Annex I—full MRLs

Pharmacologically active substance	Marker residue	Animal species	MRL (μg kg^{-1})	Target tissue
Difloxacin	Difloxacin	Chicken, turkey	1900	Liver
			600	Kidney
			300	Muscle
			400	Skin/fat
Vedaprofen	Vedaprofen	Horse	1000	Kidney
			100	Liver
			50	Muscle
			20	Fat
Eprinomectin	Eprinomectin B1$_a$	Cattle	30	Muscle
			30	Fat
			600	Liver
			100	Kidney
			30	Milk

Annex II—no MRLs required

Pharmacologically active substance	Animal species	Other provisions
Tau fluvalinate	Bees	
Corticotropin	All food producing	
Chlorhexidine	All food producing	Topical use only
Thiomersal	All food producing	For use only as a preservative in multi-dose vaccines at a concentration not exceeding 0.02%
Praziquantel	Sheep	Non-lactating sheep only
Natamycin	Bovine, equidae	Topical use only
Echinaceae purpurea	All food producing	Topical use only
Pyrethrum extract	All food producing	Topical use only

Annex III—provisional MRLs

Pharmacologically active substance	Marker residue	Animal species	MRL (μg kg^{-1})	Target tissue	Expiry
Moxidectin	Moxidectin	*Equidae*	50	Muscle	Jan. 2000
			500	Fat	
			100	Liver	
			50	Kidney	
Carprofen	Carprofen	Bovine	1000	Liver	Jan. 2000
				Kidney	
			500	Muscle	
				Fat	
Teflubenzuron	Teflubenzuron	*Salmonidae*	500	Muscle/skin	Jul. 1999
Penethamate	Benzylpenicillin	Ovine	50	Muscle	Jan. 2000
				Fat	
				Liver	
				Kidney	
			4	Milk	

Annex IV—no MRLs can be established (prohibited in food-producing animals)

Furazolidone	Chloramphenicol	Colchicine
Other nitrofurans	Dimetridazole	Chlorpromazine
Dapsone	Metronidazole	Chloroform
Ronidazole	*Aristolochia* spp.	

The Annex entries are published in the *Official Journal of the European Communities* (*OJ*) as amending Commission Regulations to the original Council Regulation and at the time of writing there have been over 50 such amendments. Examples of how the entries appear in the *OJ* are given in **Table 3** (the headings, where necessary, will be explained later in the text).

The EMEA has also taken over the work on MRLs. MRLs for new substances under Article 6 of Regulation 2377/90 are now dealt with directly by the CVMP. However, MRLs for existing substances, under Article 7 of the Regulation, continue to be dealt with by the Working Group on the Safety of Residues, which then passes its recommendations to the CVMP for ratification.

Elaboration of MRLs

A requirement of the Regulation is to supply a safety file and residue file. The former is primarily a package of toxicology studies, whereas the latter details the residues depletion, that is, the time-dependent disappearance of residues from the animal by metabolism and excretion. It also includes the analytical data, including a method for routine surveillance of residues of the drug involved. These requirements are set out in some detail in Annex V to the regulation and are set out more fully in Directive 81/852/EEC as amended by Directive 92/18/EEC. The requirements are given in detail in **Table 4** (Commission of the European Communities, 1991). It is worth commenting on some of these aspects.

There is a formal requirement for acute toxicity studies, but little emphasis is placed on this from the point of view of MRLs, as residues are unlikely to reach concentrations at which an acute effect could be elicited through the ingestion of food. However, the same data package, or at least major parts of it, is used to assess user/worker safety aspects of applications and acute toxicity often has more relevance here. Like many other regulatory systems, less emphasis is now placed on LD_{50} values and other, more modern, approaches are acceptable.

Similarly, although there is a formal requirement for two species repeated dose studies of at least 90 days duration, again some flexibility is given so that other, equally valid, subchronic studies may be used in the evaluation. This might be to accept a 90 day study in one species plus a 28 day in another *in lieu*, or to accept a 90 day study in one species and a carcinogenicity (or a combined carcinogenicity–chronic toxicity) study in other species. Similarly, there is a requirement for teratology studies in two species, a rodent and non-rodent, usually the rabbit. However, this too may be waived provided that good justification is given. For example, antibiotics are often highly toxic to rabbits because of effects on the gut flora and under these circumstances a second rodent species might be considered. Alternat-

ively, for veterinary drugs, which have also been used as human drugs and where there is a long history of safe use in pregnancy, good human epidemiological data are accepted in place of a second animal species.

There is also a specific requirement for carcinogenicity studies but these are only expected or demanded if the drug has a close structural analogy with a known carcinogen, if data from genotoxicity studies suggest there is a concern and if 'suspect' signs have been seen during toxicity testing. The last aspect might include peroxisome proliferation or renal damage suggestive of the potential for non-genotoxic carcinogenesis but, apart from this, little emphasis is placed on this category of carcinogen in terms of testing. However, where substances are confirmed to be non-genotoxic carcinogens, emphasis is placed on evaluating the mechanisms of carcinogenicity so that suitable thresholds and NOELs can be identified. Indeed, the NOEL is the basis for the MRL elaboration as this in turn forms the basis for the calculation of the ADI. In this respect, the EU approach has much in common with that in the USA and, indeed, the scientific requirements are very similar.

It is worth noting at this point that the ADI concept was developed in 1957 by the JECFA (World Health Organization, 1987) and is calculated in the same way that it is by other regulatory regimes, i.e. the NOEL is divided by a suitable safety factor, usually 100, to give the ADI. As the NOEL is usually identified in terms of mg drug per kg body weight per day mg (kg body weight)$^{-1}$ day^{-1}, the ADI takes similar units:

$$ADI = \frac{NOEL}{100} \, mg \, (kg \, body \, weight)^{-1}$$

It is often considered useful to factor in the average human adult body weight, for this purpose taken to be 60 kg, to give the ADI in terms of mg person^{-1}:

$$ADI = \frac{NOEL \times 60}{100} \, mg \, person^{-1}$$

The concept of the 100-fold safety factor, which is empirical, arose from the contention that there is a 10-fold intra-species variability in toxicity and a 10-fold animal–human variability, giving an overall factor of 100. However, in practice, this factor of 100 is often increased by a further factor to take account of flaws in the data package or because of some concern over the nature of the toxic event seen (e.g. irreversible effects, such as teratogenicity). Thus, higher safety factors, usually 200, 500 or 1000, are sometimes used. Conversely, if the data are derived from observations in humans, and if these data are robust, a lower safety factor, usually 10, may be used to calculate the ADI (Woodward, 1991b).

On occasions, a pharmacological effect (or effects) may be the most relevant 'adverse' effect, for example

Table 4 Data requirement for Safety and Residues File under Regulation No. (EEC) 2377/90

A		**Safety File**
A.0		**Expert Report**
A.1		**Precise identification**
	1.1	International non-proprietary name (INN)
	1.2	IUPAC name
	1.3	Chemical Abstract Service name
	1.4	Classification
		—therapeutic
		—pharmacological
	1.5	Synonyms and abbreviations
	1.6	Structural formula
	1.7	Molecular formula
	1.8	Molecular weight
	1.9	Degree of impurity
	1.10	Qualitative and quantitative composition of impurities
	1.11	Description of physical properties
		—melting-point
		—boiling-point
		—vapour pressure
		—solubility in water and organic solvents
		—density
		—refractive index, rotation, etc.
A.2		**Pharmacology**
A.2.1		**Pharmacodynamics in laboratory species**
A.2.2		**Pharmacokinetics in laboratory species**
A.3		**Toxicological studies**
	3.1	Single dose (at least two mammalian species)
	3.2	Repeated dose (at least two mammalian species, at least 90 day duration)
	3.3	Tolerance in target species
	3.4	Reproductive toxicity, including teratogenicity
	3.4.1	Study of the effects on reproduction
	3.4.2	Embryotoxicity/foetoxicity, including teratogenicity, at least two species, preferably one rodent and the rabbit
	3.5	Genotoxicity
	3.6	Carcinogenicity
A.4		**Studies of other effects**
	4.1	Immunotoxicity
	4.2	Microbiological properties of residues
	4.2.1	Potential effects on the human gut flora
	4.2.2	Potential effects on food processing
	4.3	Observations in humans
B		**Residue File**
B.0		**Expert Report**
B.1		**Precise identification**
		– as for residues file at A.1
B.2		**Residue studies**
	2.1	Pharmacokinetics in target species
	2.2	Depletion of residues
	2.3	Elaboration of MRLs
B.3		**Routine analytical Methods**
	3.1	Description of the method
	3.2	Validation of the method
		—specificity
		—accuracy
		—precision
		—limit of detection
		—limit of quantitation (determination/qualification)
		—practicability and applicability
		—susceptibility to interference

with some anaesthetics, analgesics, hormones and β-agonist drugs. Here, it is the convention to determine a no-pharmacological effect level and to use this as the basis of the ADI, if it is lower than the toxicological ADI, or if it is considered to be more relevant than the toxicological response for human hazard and risk assessment. For many hormonal substances, and particularly for the synthetic anabolic steroid hormones such as the congeners of testosterone, progesterone and 17β-oestradiol, ADIs have been established on the basis of no-hormonal effect levels in suitable animal models. Although the ADI concept and the magnitude of the safety factor have been addressed and refined by Renwick and others in recent years, the considerations have yet to be extended to ADIs calculated for veterinary drugs (Rubery *et al.*, 1990; Renwick, 1991).

In recent years, the problem of microbiological endpoints has arisen for residues of drugs with antimicrobial properties. The concerns here for the consumer are four-fold (Woodward, 1992b, 1998; Boisseau, 1993). Such residues may:

- Perturb the bacterial ecology of the colon;
- Weaken the barrier effect of the gastrointestinal flora allowing the influx and growth of potential pathogens;
- As a result, increase the vulnerability of the consumer to pathogenic bacteria;
- Provide conditions that could lead to the development of bacterial resistance to antibiotics.

Although it is accepted that therapeutic doses of anti-microbial drugs in humans can perturb the human gut flora, sometimes dramatically, there is no firm evidence that residues present in food of animal origin can have such an effect. Nevertheless, it is considered prudent to consider the potential of drug residues to exert adverse effects through antimicrobial mechanisms (Woodward, 1998).

There are no validated experimental models for this approach, but several options are available (Rumney and Rowland, 1995):

- Studies in humans;
- Studies in gnotobiotic animals;
- Studies in conventional animals;
- *In vitro* studies.

The first three involve the treatment of groups of animals (or humans) with the antimicrobial substance of interest, followed by the analysis of faecal specimens and comparisons with pretreatment situations. The *in vitro* systems involve the determination of the so-called MIC_{50} (minimal inhibitory concentration), either through serial dilution methods or using continuous culture methods that aim to model microflora interactions and ecology in the human colon.

All the methods have drawbacks. For example, studies in humans are difficult to conduct and are often considered to be unethical for the purposes of establishing the safety of veterinary drugs. Studies in gnotobiotic animals (germ-free animals carrying gut flora other than their own) inoculated with human gut flora [human flora-associated (HFA) animals] are very difficult to interpret, not least because host–bacterial reactions may be greater than the effects of any drug. However, a recent study has demonstrated the utility of such an approach with HFA rats. Low concentrations of tilmicosin or spiramycin were found to have transient effects on tilmicosin or spiramycin-resistant organisms in such a model (Rumney *et al.*, 1998). Studies in conventional animals are no better as the gut flora in dogs and rodents, as examples, are extremely different and the relevance to human risk assessment is difficult to identify. This leaves *in vitro* studies. These are often difficult to relate to safety as MIC_{50} values, or indeed any measure of inhibition in *in vitro* systems, are almost impossible to relate to the *in vivo* situation.

Nevertheless, an equation has been developed by the CVMP to calculate the ADI for these *in vitro* studies:

$$A = \frac{\dfrac{B \times CF_2(\mu g\, ml^{-1})}{CF_1} \times C}{D \times E}$$

where A = weight of microbiological ADI μg (kg body weight)$^{-1}$, B = geometric mean MIC_{50}, C = daily faecal bolus, D = fraction of oral dose available to microorganisms, E = human body weight (60 kg) and CF_1 and CF_2 are correction factors.

The correction factors CF_1 and CF_2 are used to account for the range of MIC_{50} values (i.e. the numbers of bacterial species representative of the human gut flora, actually tested), the risk of selection of multi-resistant bacteria and the induction of colonization resistance. In addition, factors that may affect bacterial growth, such as pH, anaerobiosis and the effects of population density, can also be taken into account. The weight of the daily faecal bolus, a somewhat arbitrary factor, has been established at 150 g, which some biologists consider to be rather low. The above equation is subject to constant review and modification and other factors are added or substituted from time to time.

Finally, MRLs must be set so that the potential effects of antimicrobial substances on processes used in food production are not disrupted. For this reason, the CVMP has recently focused on the effects of antimicrobial drugs on microorganisms used in yoghurt and cheese starter cultures. The effect of NOELs derived from these types of study has often been to lower dramatically the MRL value.

Most drugs examined so far in the EU's programme tend to have toxicological and microbiological effects or toxicological and pharmacological effects. Nevertheless, it cannot be ruled out that some might have all three activities. Whatever, in general, the lowest ADI from the three possible end-points, toxicological, pharmacological or microbiological, is usually chosen as the definitive ADI, unless there are valid reasons not to do so, e.g. if a pharmacological or toxicological effect seen in animals is shown not to occur in humans.

Once an ADI, whatever its background, has been established, it can be used to elaborate the MRLs. However, it is important to recognize that there is no simple equation, such as that used to determine the ADI, which can be employed to calculate MRLs. It is a much more iterative approach. This is because the magnitudes of the MRLs in the various tissues and other products of animal origin are not only based on the ADI, and the requirement that this is not exceeded, but must also take into account the pharmacokinetics, and particularly the distribution of the drug. It is of little practical use to set an MRL for muscle if residues of the drug do not occur in muscle. Similarly, it is contrary to logic and practicality to establish an MRL for the drug in liver with twice the magnitude of that for kidney if tissue distribution dictates that the situation should be the other way around.

Some indication of distribution and metabolism is provided by the pharmacokinetic studies in the target species. However, the main information comes from the so-called residue depletion studies. Here, groups of target animals (i.e. cattle, sheep, pigs, etc.) are given doses of the drug, preferably the intended in-use dose, and preferably by the in-use route of administration, and these groups are then sequentially slaughtered at various times after cessation of drug treatment (usually at 6, 12 and 24 h and 1, 2, 3, etc., days afterwards), so that a comprehensive picture of the residues depletion profile is built up.

Two important concepts are involved in this. The first is that of the target tissue. This is the edible tissue chosen to monitor residues. Usually, but not always, it is the tissue with the slowest residue depletion rate. In practice, it is usual to set MRLs for the four major edible tissues, namely fat, kidney, liver and muscle. For pigs and poultry, where skin is also eaten, fat and skin taken together in natural proportions are considered, whereas for fish, where skin is also often eaten, skin and muscle in natural proportions are specified. For other food of animal ori-

gin the target 'tissue' is more readily identified, e.g. for milk of lactating animals, eggs of laying birds and honey.

To estimate whether or not the ADI is likely to be exceeded, and therefore to establish appropriate MRLs, some idea about typical food (meat) consumption must also be available and must be taken into account. It is difficult to estimate factors for the whole of Europe, and indeed this is made difficult by ethnic variations and 'extreme' consumers such as those who eat only liver each day, and do so in large quantities. As a result, rather arbitrary 'food factors' or daily consumption factors have been derived as part of the so-called 'market basket' approach. They are set out in **Table 5**.

The other major concept is the marker residue. This is the residue whose concentration is known in relation to the concentration of the total residue in the various target tissues and which, therefore, could serve as the analytical marker for residue monitoring. Its depletion is usually typical and characteristic of that for residues of the drug as a whole. Examples of the target tissue and the marker residue concepts are included in **Table 2**.

As MRLs are subject to surveillance and monitoring, there is a requirement for companies to supply a suitable analytical method which can be used or adapted for this purpose. Under the terms of the Regulation, MRLs must be 'practicable', and this is interpreted to mean that there is such a method and that suitable analytical standards are available, if necessary, from the applicant (Woodward and Shearer, 1995).

As in other areas of chemical analysis, the method must meet criteria of accuracy, precision and susceptibility, but it must also be specific. Hence a method developed for the determination of a β-lactam antibiotic would not be considered acceptable if it was not specific for that drug and if other β-lactam antibiotics were found to interfere with quantification or detection. Similarly, the limits of quantification of the assay in each target tissue must be such that they are below the MRL in each tissue. For example, if the MRL is $10\ \mu g\ (\text{kg tissue})^{-1}$, the limit of quantification should be below this, and preferably the limit of quantification should be half the MRL, i.e. in this case $5\ \mu g\ \text{kg}^{-1}$. MRLs may need to be adjusted to take into account the limits of quantification of the assay, bearing in mind the constraints of the ADI and tissue distribution. If the MRLs cannot be adjusted, a

Table 5 Daily food factors (g) used in the EU

Large animals		Poultry		Fish/bees	
Muscle	300	Muscle	300	Muscle/skin[b]	300
Liver	100	Liver	100	Honey	20
Kidney	50	Kidney	10		
Fat	50[a]	Fat/skin[b]	90		
Milk	1500	Egg	100		

[a] For pigs, skin and fat in natural proportions.
[b] In natural proportions.

better analytical method may be required as the method demanded by the Regulation is intended for routine monitoring of residues in food—it is destined to become the so-called regulatory method.

Progress In Establishing MRLs and Their Roles in Legislation

There has been considerable progress in the development of MRLs (or Annex II entries) over the last few years. When Annex entries are made, so-called summary documents are produced by the CVMP setting out briefly the results of the toxicology and residues studies and outlining the reasons for the decisions taken. Where no annex entry can be made, a status report is produced instead, again summarizing the data but also outlining the reasons why an annex entry cannot be made. With these, and indeed with summary documents supporting provisional MRLs in Annex III, lists of questions are sent to the applicant which, if answered satisfactorily, would lead to Annex I or Annex II entries. Summary documents (and other CVMP/EMEA information) are available on the Internet.

Towards the beginning of the exercise, applicants were required to submit 'intentions to apply' for existing drugs that would later be followed by the MRL application itself. Of these, 171 did not materialize as applications and should MRLs still be required for these, new applications would now be required.

It is important to recognize that MRLs have several useful purposes. The main reason, of course, is to protect the consumer by ensuring that residues of veterinary drugs consumed by way of food of animal origin do not exceed the ADI for that drug.

To achieve this, the withdrawal period (withhold period) concept is employed. Here, studies are performed in which groups of target animals are treated with a drug using the commercial formulation and then slaughtered at intervals for residue analysis. The withdrawal period, the period between the last treatment and when the animal may be slaughtered for human consumption, is derived from the point when residues deplete to below the MRL in all target tissues in all the animals in a group. Similar concepts apply for milk and eggs, although here, of course, residues do not deplete and the food has to be discarded until residues fall below the milk or egg MRLs. Honey often presents a particular problem, as bees, which are treated on a hive basis, often need medication during the period of maximum honey flow. If this results in residues above the MRL, it will mean that the affected honey is unusable, as residues will not deplete. Consequently, medicines for the treatment of diseases in bees need to be designed and formulated so that the MRLs for honey are not exceeded in the first place. Fish are poikilothermic (cold-blooded) animals and

their rates of metabolism and indeed the nature of their metabolism can vary with the temperature, depending on the species of fish (Kleinhow et al., 1992). Hence, whereas withdrawal periods for mammals and avian species are quoted in days, those for fish are quoted in degree days (Woodward, 1996) to take account of the dual effects of time and temperature.

Withdrawal periods are legal requirements and, in the EU, the withdrawal period, even if it is zero, must appear in the product literature and on the label for veterinary medicines intended for use in food-producing animals. However, it is futile to impose withdrawal periods if these are not observed on the farm. As with traffic speed limits, withdrawal periods, and the MRL, must be monitored and enforced!

Directive 86/469/EEC introduced requirements on EU Member States to conduct surveillance on their territories for residues in red meat. This is not only to find and quantify residues that violate the MRL, but also to detect prohibited drugs. During 1995, some 47 000 samples of red meat (i.e. meat and offal from mammals) were taken in the UK and examined for MRL violations and the detection of prohibited drugs under UK legislation implementing Directive 86/469/EEC (Veterinary Medicines Directorate, 1996). Samples are taken from slaughterhouses and later examined in the laboratory.

Less than 0.15% of the total number of these samples were found to contain residues above the MRL. Of this 0.15%, a major contributory element arose from residues of antimicrobials and sulphonamides in pig kidney. Several factors account for this, apart from failure to observe withdrawal periods. These include:

■ Deficiencies in handling medicated feed on farms;
■ Low-level cross-contamination of feed during manufacture;
■ Cross-contamination between medicated and non-medicated pigs during transport and at abattoirs, e.g. through urine or faeces from pigs medicated with antimicrobials.

However, the numbers of violations have been much higher in previous years and it is clear that tight regulation combined with publicity campaigns continue to contribute to annual reductions.

Directive 86/469/EEC currently applies only to red meat. However, Directive 96/23/EEC repeals Directive 86/469/EEC and extends surveillance to poultry and farmed fish from 1 January 1998 (Council of the European Communities, 1996a). The Directive also covers surveillance in milk, eggs and honey. Furthermore, Directive 96/22/EEC confirms the existing ban on hormones used for growth promotion and on thyrostatic compounds and extends it to cover β-agonist drugs except when used in companion animals and in cattle during calving. Member States are currently introducing measures to enshrine these two Directives into their national laws (Veterinary Medicines Directorate, 1998).

The UK has also, for several years, conducted a non-statutory surveillance scheme independent of EU legislation and in 1995 a total of 3600 samples of home-produced and imported food of animal origin were examined and especially those not covered by Directive 86/469/EEC. The most significant findings here were of residues of an unauthorized drug, malachite green, in farmed trout and of ivermectin, a drug only authorized in mammalian species, in farmed salmon. Both aspects are currently being investigated (Woodward, 1996). Indeed, follow-up actions are often pursued (depending on individual findings and circumstances) either by visits to farms where these can be traced or, in extreme cases with persistent offenders, through prosecution.

Residue monitoring exists not only to assess if violations of MRL values are occurring, but also to determine if illegal drugs are being used in food production. Previously, there have been a number of legislative measures introduced into the EU to ban specific types of drug for use in food animals, but recently a consolidating Directive, Directive 96/22/EEC, which prohibits the use of certain substances having hormonal or thyrostatic activity and the use of certain β-agonist drugs, has been introduced (Council of the European Communities, 1996b).

Other Uses of Toxicity Data

In addition to being used to derive MRLs which are compound specific, toxicity data are required as part of the safety package in the safety, quality and efficacy requirements. Here, more emphasis is usually given to the safety of the formulation rather than to that of the active ingredient alone. The toxicity data are also used to assess hazards for workers through exposure to potentially toxic materials, so that recommendations for operator safety, e.g. for protective clothing or face masks, can be made.

Feed Additives

The feed additives are an important group of substances (or organisms) which are added to animal feed, generally for the purpose of better growth performance, although many are used to improve the physical characteristics of the feed. This improved performance may stem from higher nutritional value imparted by the additive, for example, by a vitamin. Alternatively, it may arise because the additive has growth-promoting properties. In this latter category are included the growth-promoting antibiotics such as virginiamycin. Substances of this type are regulated in the EU under Directive 70/524/EEC and not under Directive 81/851/EEC. Rather incongru-

ously, the anticoccidial drugs, if given in feed, are also controlled under Directive 70/524/EEC rather than under the veterinary medicines legislation.

The feed additives are largely evaluated in the same way as conventional drugs with safety, efficacy and quality being important aspects. However, the legislation operates under the auspices of Directorate General VI (Agriculture) rather than DGIII within the European Commission, and currently there is no equivalent of the MRL process that applies to drugs regulated under Directive 81/851/EEC. Scientific advice is provided by the Scientific Committee on Animal Nutrition and not by the CVMP, and the process does not operate through the EMEA. Instead, it works through the traditional Brussels EU systems but, like the CVMP routes, the results of its deliberations are published in the OJ (Woodward, 1993a).

There are intentions to update the system and the first moves have come through Directive 96/51/EC that extensively amends Directive 70/524/EEC. Most notably, it will review those substances authorized some time ago (prior to January 1988) and update their safety evaluations (Council of the European Communities, 1996c). Further amending Directives may introduce requirements for MRLs for this group of substances.

Four of the antibiotic growth promoters, spiramycin, tylosin, bacitracin and virginiamycin used as feed additives have recently been banned by the European Commission because of fears over the induction of resistance and the possible threat to human health. This is despite a lack of any evidence to this effect. Another two antimicrobial growth promoters, carbadox and olaquindox were also banned because of concerns over carcinogenicity and genotoxicity (Editorial Reports, 1998a, 1999).

INTERNATIONAL ASPECTS

Whatever else MRLs and tolerances may achieve, they can act as barriers to international trade. Countries may prohibit the import of meat if the exporting country has an MRL value for a certain drug which differs from their own and it is even worse if a drug has an MRL in one country but is banned in another. Hence it is to everyone's benefit if MRLs (and even prohibitions) are harmonized at the international level.

To this end, JEFCA, referred to earlier, began its evaluation of the toxicity and residues depletion of veterinary drugs in the mid-1980s, meeting either in Rome (at the Food and Agriculture Organization) or in Geneva (at the World Health Organization). The MRLs developed are taken into the United Nations' Codex Alimentarius system through the Codex Committee on Residues of Veterinary Drugs in Food. These are then adopted through the Codex step procedure and finally published as Codex food standards for international adoption. Such steps should help to protect the health of consumers internationally, while preventing barriers to trade and international trade disputes (Woodward, 1991c, 1993b). Similar initiatives exist for the harmonization of pesticide MRLs through the Joint FAO/WHO Meeting on Pesticide Residues (JMPR) and the Codex Committee on Pesticide Residues (Herrman, 1993). This, along with the JECFA efforts, should eventually lead to international harmonization for MRLs for ectoparasiticides, as several trading blocks, including the EU and the USA, are committed to the adoption of Codex Standards, including MRLs.

Recent suggestions have been made that there should be comparisons of MRLs between countries. This would ensure that ADI values are not exceeded, and it might offer another route to resolve trade disputes raised by the existence of differing MRL values across different countries (Fitzpatrick *et al.*, 1995).

These moves towards harmonization of MRLs are mirrored by developments in related areas. For example, the USA and the EU have recently arrived at a mutual recognition agreement for Pharmaceutical Good Manufacturing Practices (European Society of Regulatory Affairs, 1998). However, the main mechanism for change is likely to be the Veterinary International Cooperation on Harmonization (VICH). This is, as the title suggests, an international effort involving the regulatory agencies in Japan, the USA and the EU and the veterinary pharmaceutical industries, to achieve harmonization on the regulatory and testing requirements for applications for veterinary drugs at the world-wide level (Editorial Report, 1998b). It parallels developments in the better known International Conference on Harmonization (ICH) for human pharmaceuticals (D'Arcy and Harron, 1994). Significant progress has already been made on guidelines for stability and photostability, and those on pharmacovigilance, ecotoxicity testing and aspects of toxicity testing are in development. Furthermore, some trading blocks have already made significant contributions to local harmonization initiatives, for example, those accepted between the North American Free Trade Area (NAFTA) countries.

Together, these initiatives should contribute to the wider acceptance of data generated in one country in another territory which will reduce costs and bureaucracy and have the added benefit of reducing the numbers of animals used in experimental studies.

CONCLUSIONS

There is a sophisticated system governing the approval of veterinary drugs in the USA. The basic philosophies of drug assessment here are also similar to those used in many countries, including the EU Member States. These are based around the toxicological assessment of veterinary drugs and their metabolites, the assessment of their depletion in food-producing animals and their products

and the establishment of withdrawal periods. In both the EU and the USA, there is a complex system of residues monitoring to ensure that consumers are not exposed to undue violative or unsafe levels of veterinary drug residues.

A complex and comprehensive system for the granting of marketing authorizations for veterinary medicinal products also exists in the EU and this is reflected in the legislation of Member States, including that of the UK. This system endeavours to ensure the quality, efficacy and safety of veterinary drugs. Currently there is no examination of 'socio-economic' factors such as whether or not a particular product is needed. Safety to consumers and occupational health considerations are of extreme importance, and these require careful assessment of pharmacological, toxicological, microbiological and residue data.

Progress within the Codex Alimentarius system should also ensure advancement of the issues involved and, moreover, will assist developing countries, some of which may lack the necessary expertise, in establishing MRLs of veterinary drugs. At the same time it should assist in removing barriers to international trade, as various trading blocks adopt Codex Standards. The role of the Codex is likely to grow. Until 1995, the standards that it promulgated were not binding. However, since then the General Agreement on Tariffs and Trade (GATT), the evolution through the Uruguay Round and the influence of the World Trade Organization (WTO) have led to Codex standards gaining much more weight. Since the Agreement on the Application of Sanitary and Phytosanitary Measures through the WTO, objections to various issues and standards, including MRLs, can only be raised by countries if these are science based. Hence, refusal to adopt each other's MRLs on 'socio-economic' grounds or for other political or domestic reasons is groundless under WTO rules. If countries persist, financial sanctions can be brought to bear against them.

Such difficulties have been highlighted by the dispute between the European Commission (EC) and the USA over growth-promoting hormones and bovine somatotropin (BST), a milk production enhancer. This has led in turn to a trade dispute between the EU and the USA.

The EU banned both the hormones and BST for what were widely regarded as politically motivated reasons masquerading as consumer safety issues. However, these substances were authorized in the USA for growth promotion or milk yield enhancement. Hence a trade dispute arose, largely involving the hormone growth promoters, as the export of US meat from treated animals into the EU was adversely affected. Unfortunately for the EC and the EU, JECFA evaluated the toxicology and residues data for these drugs and concluded that they did not pose a risk to consumers, and the Codex ratified this view. As a result of this, the WTO ruled against the

EU and threatened it with financial sanctions if the ban on the import of US beef was not lifted.

Hence, in the future, the WTO–JECFA–Codex alliance can be expected to develop increased powers and will be used more often in the resolution of trade issues in the veterinary drug and in other sectors. Toxicology will play an increasingly important part in the resolution of such issues.

REFERENCES

Bloomfield, G. (1989). *Veterinary Drug Residues*. Animal Pharm; PJB Publications, Richmond, Surrey, pp. 40–49.

Boisseau, J. (1993). Basis for the evaluation of the microbiological risks due to veterinary drug residues in food. *Vet. Microbiol.*, **35**, 187–192.

Brunko, P. (1997). Procedures and technical requirements in the European Union. In Pastoret, P. -P., Blancou, J., Vannier, P. and Verscheuren, C. (Eds), *Veterinary Vaccinology*. Elsevier, Oxford, pp. 674–679.

Cartwright, A. C. (1991). Introduction and history of pharmaceutical regulation. In Cartwright, A. C. and Matthews, B. R. (Eds), *Pharmaceutical Product Licensing. Requirements for Europe*. Ellis Horwood, New York, pp. 29–45.

Commission of the European Communities (1991). *The Rules Governing Medicinal Products in the European Community. Volume VI. Establishment by the European Community of Maximum Residue Limits (MRLs) for Residues of Veterinary Medicinal Products in Foodstuffs of Animal Origin*. Commission of the European Communities, Luxembourg.

Commission of the European Communities (1993). *The Rules Governing Medicinal Products in the European Community. Volume VB. Notice to Applicants for Marketing Authorization for Veterinary Medicinal Products in the European Community*. Commission of the European Community, Luxembourg.

Commission of the European Communities (1995). Commission Regulation (EC) No. 541/95 of 10 March 1995 concerning the examination of variations to the terms of a marketing authorisation granted by a competent authority of a Member State. *Off. J. Eur. Commun.*, No. L55, 7–14.

Commission of the European Communities (1998). *The Rules Governing Medicinal Products in the European Union. Volume VIA. Notice to Applicants. Veterinary Medicinal Products Procedures for Marketing Authorisation*. European Commission, Luxembourg.

Cordle, M. K. (1988). USDA regulation of residues in meat and poultry products. *J. Anim. Sci.*, **66**, 413–433.

Council of the European Communities (1990). Council Regulation (EEC) No. 2377/90 of 26 June 1990 laying down a Community procedure for the establishment of maximum residue limits of veterinary medicinal products in foodstuffs of animal origin. *Off. J. Eur. Commun.*, No. L224, 1–8.

Council of the European Communities (1993). Council Regulation (EEC) No. 2309/93 of 22 July 1993 laying down Community procedures for the authorization and supervision of medicinal products for human and veterinary use and establishing a European Agency for the Evaluation of Medicinal Products. *Off. J. Eur. Commun.*, No. L214, 1–30.

Council of the European Communities (1996a). Council Directive 96/23/EC of 29 April 1996 on measures to monitor certain substances and residues thereof in live animals and animal products and repealing Directives 85/358/EEC and 86/469/EEC and Decisions 89/187/EEC and 91/664/EEC. *Off. J. Eur. Commun.*, No. L125, 10–31.

Council of the European Communities (1996b). Council Directive 96/22/EC of 29 April 1996 concerning the prohibition of the use in stock farming of certain substances having a hormonal or thyrostatic action and of beta-agonists, and repealing Directives 81/602/EEC, 88/146/EEC and 88/299/EEC. *Off. J. Eur. Commun.*, No. L125, 3–9.

Council of the European Communities (1996c). Council Directive 95/51/EC of 23 July 1996 amending Directive 70/524/EEC concerning additives in feedingstuffs. *Off. J. Eur. Commun.*, No. L235, 39–58.

Cuthbert, M. F., Griffin, J. P. and Inman, W. H. W. (1978). The United Kingdom. In Wardell, W. M. (Ed.), *Controlling the Use of Therapeutic Drugs. An International Comparison*. American Institute for Public Policy Research, Washington, DC, pp. 99–134.

D'Arcy, P. F. and Harron, D. W. G. (Eds) (1994). *Proceedings of the Second International Conference on Harmonisation*, Queen's University of Belfast, Belfast.

Davis, L. E. (1988). Legal control of drugs in the USA. In Booth, N. H. and McDonald, L. E. (Eds), *Veterinary Pharmacology and Therapeutics*, 6th edn. Iowa State University, Ames, IA, pp. 9–13.

Editorial Report (1998a). EU acts in haste, may repent at leisure. *Animal Pharm.*, No.. 411, 1–2.

Editorial Report (1998b). VICH expects major progress in 98. *Animal Pharm.*, No. 392, 14.

Editorial Report (1999). Short-term view means long-term rue, says NOAH. *Animal Pharm.*, No. 413, 5–6.

Environmental Protection Agency (1996). *Guidelines and Guideline Harmonization*. Environmental Protection Agency, Washington, DC.

Espeseth, D. (1997). Procedures and norms in the United States. In Pastoret P.-P., Blancou, J., Vannier, P. and Verscheuren, C. (Eds), *Veterinary Vaccinology*. Elsevier, Oxford, pp. 680–686.

European Society of Regulatory Affairs (1998). *Rapporteur*, **5**, 29.

Farber, T. M. (1985). Regulatory requirements for the approval of drugs used in food producing animals. In Homburger, F. and Marquis, J. K. (Eds), *Chemical Safety and Compliance*. Karger, London, pp. 11–23.

Farber, T. M. (1995). Current testing procedures for residues and contaminants. *Drug Metab. Rev.*, **27**, 543–548.

Fitzpatrick, S. C., Brynes, S. D. and Guest, G. B. (1995). Dietary intake estimates as a means to the harmonisation of maximum residue levels for veterinary drugs. I. Concept. *J. Vet. Pharmacol. Ther.*, **18**, 325–327.

Food and Drug Administration (1987). Sponsored compounds in food-producing animals; criteria and procedures for evaluating the safety of carcinogenic residues; animal drug safety policy. *Fed. Regist.*, **52**, 49572–49588.

Food and Drug Administration (1996). *Guidance: Microbiological Testing of Antimicrobial Drug Residues in Food*. Center for Veterinary Medicine, Rockville, MD.

Guest, G. B. (1990). Veterinary drug registration in the United States. In Simon F., Lees, P. and Semjen, G. (Eds), *Veter-*

inary Pharmacology, Toxicology and Therapy in Food Producing Animals. Unipharma, Budapest, pp. 269–272.

Harrison, I. H. (1986a). Historical background and introduction. In *The Law on Medicines. A Comprehensive Guide*, Vol. 1. MTP Press, Lancaster, pp. 1–16.

Harrison, I. H. (1986b). The administration of the Act. In *The Law on Medicines. A Comprehensive Guide*, Vol. 1. MTP Press, Lancaster, pp. 17–32.

Herrman, J. (1993). The role of the World Health Organization in the evaluation of pesticides. *Regul. Toxicol. Pharmacol.*, **17**, 282–286.

Jefferys, D. B. (1995). The new pharmaceutical regulatory procedures for Europe. *Trends Pharm. Sci.*, **16**, 226–231.

Joint FAO/WHO Expert Committee on Food Additives. (1990). *Evaluation of Certain Veterinary Drug Residues.* Thirty-sixth Report of the Joint FAO/WHO Expert Committee on Food Additives. Technical Report Series 799, World Health Organization, Geneva.

Kidd, A. R. M. (1994). *The Potential Risk of Effects on Antimicrobial Residues on Human Gastro-intestinal Microflora.* Report prepared at the invitation of Fédération Européene de la Santé Animale (FEDESA), FEDESA, Brussels, Belgium.

Kleinhow, K. M., James, M. O. and Lech, J. J. (1992). Drugs pharmacokinetics and metabolism in food-producing fish and crustaceans: methods and examples. In Hutson, D. H., Hawkins, D. R., Paulson, G. D. and Struble, C. B. (Eds), *Xenobiotics in Food Producing Animals. Metabolism and Residues.* ACS Symposium Series, Vol. 503, American Chemical Society, Washington, DC, pp. 98–130.

National Research Council (1987). *Regulating Pesticides in Food. The Delaney Paradox.* Committee on Scientific and Regulatory Issues Underlying Pesticide Use Patterns and Agricultural Innovation. Board on Agriculture. National Research Council, National Academy Press, Washington, DC.

Pullen, M. M. (1990). Residues. In Pearson, A. M. and Dutson, Y. R. (Eds), *Meat and Health. Advances in Meat Research*, Vol. 6, Elsevier Applied Science, London, pp. 135–156.

Renwick, A. G. (1991). Safety factors and establishment of acceptable daily intakes. *Food Addit. Contam.*, **7**, 135–150.

Rubery, E. D., Barlow, S. M. and Steadman, J. H. (1990). Criteria for setting quantitative estimates of intakes of chemicals in food in the U.K. *Food Addit. Contam.*, **7**, 287–302.

Rumney, C. J. and Rowland, I. R. (1995). Microbiological endpoint testing for veterinary antimicrobials—setting MRLs. *Food Addit. Contam.*, **33**, 331–333.

Rumney, C. J., Coutts, J. T., Smith, J. S. and Rowland, I. R. (1998). Microbiological end-point determination of antibiotics. *Microbiol. Ecol. Health Dis.*, **10**, 3–11.

Schmidt-Bleek, F. and Marchal, M. M. (1993). Comparing regulatory regimes for pesticide control in 22 countries: Towards a new generation of pesticide regulation. *Regul. Toxicol. Pharmacol.*, **17**, 282–286.

Teske, R. H. (1992). Chemical residues in food. *J. Am. Vet. Med. Assoc.*, **201**, 253–256.

United States Department of Agriculture (1989). *Compound Evaluation and Analytical Capability. National Residue Program Plan, 1989.* United States Department of Agriculture, Washington, DC.

Veterinary Medicines Directorate (1996). *Annual Report on Surveillance for Veterinary Residues in 1995.* Veterinary Medicines Directorate, Addlestone.

Veterinary Medicines Directorate (1998). *Annual Report on Surveillance for Veterinary Residues in 1997.* Veterinary Medicines Directorate, Addlestone.

Weber, N. E. (1990a). Pharmacokinetics, use in approval of new and generic animal drugs in the United States. In Haagsma, N., Ruiter, A. and Czedik-Eyesenberg, P. B. (Eds), *Residues of Veterinary Drugs in Food*, Proceedings of the EuroResidue Conference, Noordwijkerhout, The Netherlands, 1990, pp. 399–403.

Weber, N. E. (1990b). Safety assessment of bound residues, the draft FDA Guidelines. In Haagsma, N., Ruiter, A. and Czedik-Eyesenberg, P. B. (Eds), *Residues of Veterinary Drugs in Food*, Proceedings of the EuroResidue Conference, Noordwijkerhout, The Netherlands, 1990, pp. 405–410.

Weber, N. E. (1992). Use of xenobiotics in food-producing animals in the United States. Regulatory Aspects. In Hutson, D. H., Hawkins, D. R., Paulson, G. D. and Struble, C. B. (Eds), *Xenobiotics and Food-Producing Animals. Metabolism and Residues.* ACS Symposium Series, Vol. 503, American Chemical Society, Washington, DC, pp. 17–25.

Woodward, K. N. (1991a). The licensing of veterinary medicinal products in the United Kingdom—the work of the Veterinary Medicines Directorate. *Biologist*, **38**, 105–108.

Woodward, K. N. (1991b). Choice of safety factors in setting acceptable daily intakes for veterinary drugs. *Regul. Affairs J.*, **2**, 787–790.

Woodward, K. N. (1991c). The use and regulatory control of veterinary products in food production. In Creaser, C. and Purchase, R. (Eds), *Food Contaminants. Sources and Surveillance.* Royal Society of Chemistry, Cambridge, pp. 99–108.

Woodward, K. N. (1992a). Veterinary medicines—regulation in Europe and the importance of pharmacokinetic studies. In Hutson, D. H., Hawkins, D. R., Paulson, G. D. and Struble, C. B. (Eds), *Xenobiotics in Food Producing Animals. Metabolism and Residues.* ACS Symposium Series, Vol. 503, American Chemical Society, Washington, DC, pp. 26–36.

Woodward, K. N. (1992b). The uses of veterinary drugs. In Hutson, D. H., Hawkins, D. R., Paulson, G. D. and Struble, C. B. (Eds), *Xenobiotics in Food Producing Animals. Metabolism and Residues.* ACS Symposium Series, Vol. 503, American Chemical Society, Washington, DC, pp. 2–16.

Woodward, K. N. (1993a). Regulation of Veterinary Drugs in Europe, including the UK. In Ballantyne, B., Marrs, T. C. and Turner, P. (Eds), *General and Applied Toxicology*, 1st edn. Macmillan, Basingstoke, pp. 1105–1128.

Woodward, K. N. (1993b). Maximum residue limits—the impact of UK and EC legislation. In Garnsworthy, P. C. and Cole, D. J. A. (Eds), *Recent Advances in Animal Nutrition.* Nottingham University Press, Nottingham, pp. 165–172.

Woodward, K. N. (1996). The regulation of fish medicines—UK and European Union aspects. *Aquacult. Res.*, **27**, 725–734.

Woodward, K. N. (1997). Regulation of veterinary drugs in the European Union—the new procedures. *Br. Inst. Regul. Affairs J.*, **14**, 13–20.

Woodward, K. N. (1998). The use of microbiological endpoints in the safety evaluation and elaboration of maximum residue limits for veterinary drugs intended for use in food-producing animals. *J. Vet. Pharmacol. Ther.*, **21**, 47–53.

Woodward, K. N. and Shearer, G. (1995). Antibiotic use in animal production in the European Union—regulation and current methods of detection. In Oka, H., Nakazawa, H., Harada, K. and MacNeil, J. D. (Eds), *Chemical Analysis for Antibiotics Used in Agriculture*. AOAC International, Arlington, VA, pp. 45–76.

World Health Organization. (1987). *Principles for the Safety Assessment of Food Additives and Contaminants in Food, Environmental Health Criteria 70*. World Health Organization, Geneva.

Chapter 76

Regulation of Food Additives and Food Contact Materials

Frances D. Pollitt

CONTENTS

INTRODUCTION

The manufacture of attractive, processed foods would not be possible without the use of a group of chemicals known as food additives to add flavour, colour and stability or to act as preservatives. Similarly, many foods could not be transported and stored effectively without the use of packaging materials to keep the foods fresh and free from microbiological contamination. Clearly, regulatory controls are needed to ensure that the additives and packaging materials used do not pose a risk to human health. The purpose of this chapter is to give an overview of the regulation of food additives and of materials used for packaging food. The chapter will define and describe these groups of substances and describe the legislation and the approval and advisory systems to which they are subject in Europe and North America.

EUROPE

Definitions

Food Additive

A definition of a food additive can be found in European Community (EC) Directive 89/107/EEC. This is the 'Framework Directive' under which other EC directives controlling the use of food additives are made (Commission of the European Communities, 1989a). It defines a food additive as follows:

'any substance not normally consumed as a food in itself and not normally used as a characteristic ingredient of food, whether or not it has nutritive value, the inten-

tional addition of which to food for a technological purpose in the manufacture, processing, preparation, treatment, packaging, transport or storage of such food results, or may reasonably be expected to result, in it or its by-products becoming directly or indirectly a component of such foods'.

There are several different functional classes of food additives, the major classes of which are as follows:

Artificial sweeteners—Used to impart a sweet taste to food or to provide the sweetness in table-top sweeteners. There are two types of artificial sweeteners: the intense sweeteners, such as saccharin or aspartame, which need to be used in only tiny amounts, and the bulk sweeteners, such as sorbitol or xylitol.

Colours—Used for the primary purpose of adding or restoring colouring in a food. Among the better known examples are tartrazine, cochineal and β-carotene.

Preservatives—Used to prolong the shelf-life of food by protecting it against deterioration caused by micro-organisms. Examples are sulphur dioxide, sulphites and sodium and potassium benzoate.

Emulsifiers and stabilizers—These are substances which are used to aid the formation of, or to maintain, the uniform dispersion of two or more immiscible substances, such as oil and water, in a food.

There are also a number of lesser classes of food additives such as bulking agents, antioxidants, flavour enhancers, modified starches and glazing agents. These tend to be referred to commonly as miscellaneous additives (although it should be noted that, in UK law, this term applies to all regulated food additives other than colours and sweeteners).

Approximately 350 substances falling within the EC definition of a food additive are permitted for use within the EC.

In addition, there is a far larger class of chemical substances which are added to food and which could be considered to come under the definition of food additives, were they not specifically excluded by Directive 89/107/EEC. These are the food flavourings, which are used in food to impart odour, taste or both. Flavourings fall into four main categories, as follows:

Chemically defined flavouring substances, which can be subdivided further into (i) natural flavours, which are found in nature and extracted from natural sources for use in food; (ii) artificial flavours, which are chemically synthesized flavouring substances which are not found in nature; and (iii) nature-identical flavours, which are chemically synthesised but identical with flavouring substances occurring naturally in plant and animal products or in natural flavouring preparations.

Flavouring preparations, which are complex mixtures of aromatic products obtained from material of animal or vegetable origin.

Process flavourings, such as thermal process flavourings, enzymatically or microbiologically derived flavourings and flavourings obtained as products of biotechnology which are not covered by the two categories above.

Smoke flavourings, derived from smoke extracts and condensates which are used to mimic the effects of traditional food smoking.

Food Contact Materials

The definition in EC law of what constitutes a food contact material is vague. The relevant EC Framework Directive, EC Directive 89/109/EEC (Commission of the European Communities, 1989b, c), refers to 'food contact materials and articles', and these are generally considered to include all types of food packaging, cookware, cutlery, tableware, work surfaces and food processing machinery and equipment. It specifically excludes covering or coating substances, such as the substances covering cheese rinds, prepared meat products or fruit, which form part of foods and may be consumed together with those foods. The term 'food contact materials' generally refers to packaging materials used to wrap or cover food. The main classes of food contact materials, as listed in Annex 1 of EC Directive 89/109/EEC, are given in **Table 1**.

The use of food contact materials is a potential hazard to human health because some chemicals in the materials can migrate from packaging into foods. While many chemicals migrate in only negligible amounts, others can migrate in larger quantities, in some cases matching, or even exceeding, the amounts of other chemicals present in foods from their deliberate use as food additives. The task of evaluating the safety-in-use of food contact materials is large and complex. For example, within the EC, only one class of food contact materials—plastics—has been subject to a detailed evaluation so far. However,

Table 1 Major classes of food contact materials

Plastics, including varnishes and coatings
Regenerated cellulose
Elastomers and rubber
Paper and board
Ceramics
Glass
Metals and alloys
Wood, including cork
Textile products
Paraffin waxes and microcrystalline waxes

the substances evaluated include over 1200 monomers and other starting materials used in the manufacture of the plastics, and over 1000 additives which are added to plastics to modify the properties of the material. This indicates the size of the task involved in regulating these materials.

Control of Food Additives and Food Contact Materials in Europe

Legislative Framework

Additives Other than Flavourings

Within the EC, the Framework Directive 89/107/EEC is the enabling legislation under which more specific regulations on the marketing and use of food additives within the EC are drawn up. This directive lists the categories to which food additives may belong and lays down general criteria for the use of food additives. Among the general criteria is the stipulation that food additives can only be approved provided that:

—it can be demonstrated that there is a reasonable technological need and the purpose cannot be achieved by other means which are economically and technologically practicable;
—they present no hazard to the health of the consumer at the level of use proposed, so far as can be judged on the scientific evidence available; and
—they do not mislead the consumer.

In the mid-1990s, the control of the use of food additives within the Member States of the EC was further harmonized with the adoption of three more EC Directives (Commission of the European Communities, 1994a, b, 1995a, b). The purpose of harmonization was to facilitate trade among EC Member States—it is easier for food manufacturers to manufacture and sell their products within the EC if there is common agreement about which food additives may be permitted in food within Member States. The three directives specify which additives may be used in food, the foods in which they may be used and the maximum levels allowed in the foods as sold. They also assign to each additive a unique EEC number (or E number) by which it can be identified on food labels (in many cases, it is more convenient for a food manufacturer to put the E number on a label than the name of the additive, as it takes up less space). Further directives lay down specific criteria of purity for those substances permitted for use in food and, where necessary, the methods of analysis needed to verify that the criteria of purity are satisfied (Commission of the European Communities, 1995c, d).

Flavourings

The total number of individual flavouring substances available for use in food manufacture vastly outnumbers the other classes of food additives and has been estimated at around 3500 (Ministry of Agriculture, Fisheries and Food, 1995). Also, flavouring preparations, thermal process flavourings and smoke flavourings are complex mixtures which are difficult to characterize chemically. For these reasons, most European countries have been slow to regulate flavourings by means of a permitted list. Some EC countries have regulated artificial flavourings by means of a permitted (positive) list, and other chemically defined flavourings by a negative list, i.e. one which prohibits certain flavouring substances from use in foodstuffs or which permits their use in only a limited, defined way.

EC legislation on flavourings is also currently limited. As in the case of food additives, there is a Framework Directive (Commission of the European Communities, 1988) which defines flavourings and lays down general principles which should be observed in the marketing and use of flavourings in the EC. The Framework Directive also prohibits the use of certain 'biologically active principles' (BAPs) as flavouring substances. BAPs are inherent toxicants, such as coumarin or pulegone, found in some natural flavouring preparations derived from plant source materials. Where these BAPs are present as part of a natural flavouring preparation, they may be added to a foodstuff, but the Directive places a limit on the levels in the foodstuff to which the flavouring is added.

Article five of Directive 88/388/EEC states that it is the intention of the European Council to 'adopt appropriate provisions' on the various categories of flavourings defined in it. The first such provision, which covers chemically defined flavouring substances, is laid out in EC Regulation No. 2232/96 (Commission of the European Communities, 1996). Under the provisions of this regulation, the Commission intends to establish a register of substances which are currently used in EC Member States, and then to draw up and carry out a safety evaluation programme with the aim of adopting a positive list in the year 2004.

Food Contact Materials

The Framework Directive for food contact materials, EC Directive 89/109/EEC, sets out a number of general requirements which must be met by all food contact materials. In essence, it requires that all materials should be manufactured in accordance with good manufacturing practice so that they do not transfer their constituents into food in such a way that they endanger human health or bring about organoleptic or other unacceptable changes in the nature, substance or quality of the food. It provides for further, specific directives to be drawn up to cover the individual classes of food contact materials given in **Table 1** and for these directives to establish a positive list of substances which are authorized for use in that class of food contact material.

The only class of food contact materials for which there is substantive, specific EC legislation at present is plastics. EC Directive 90/128/EEC (Commission of the European Communities, 1990a), as amended, defines the meaning of plastic for the purpose of the directive and lists what substances are included or excluded from this area. It sets general migration limits for constituents migrating from materials and provides a positive list of monomers and other starting substances to be used in the manufacture of plastics. It also provides an incomplete list of additives to be used in the manufacture of plastics. This is not a positive list to be used to the exclusion of all others, but is simply a list approved by the Scientific Committee for Food (see below). Other 'safe' additives can continue to be used and are regulated by national law until the EC Commission is able to propose a positive list.

Approval and Advisory Systems

Food Additives Other than Flavourings

There are two routes by which the manufacturer of a novel food additive can seek authorization to market a new food additive in the EC. The first is to seek to obtain Community-wide approval by applying to the European Commission to have the novel food additive included on the list of permitted EC additives. In order to achieve this, the Commission and Member States will need to be reassured as to the safety of the additive. The Commission seeks advice on such matters from the Scientific Committee for Food (SCF).

The SCF was set up in 1974 to provide expert advice to the Commission on matters of food safety. It was originally appointed by the Industry Directorate General, DG III, but was transferred in 1997 to the Directorate General for Consumer Policy and Health Protection, DG XXIV. The SCF comprises about 20 members, who are individuals working in Member States either in academia, Government service or as independent consultants. In the past, this one committee has advised the Commission on a wide range of food safety issues, chemical, microbiological and nutritional, and has comprised individuals with expertise in all these areas. In recent years, a number of working groups has been formed to provide a mechanism to co-opt additional expertise in each of these areas and in new fields such as genetic modification. The important working group in respect of food additives is the SCF Working Group on Food Additives. The working groups report through the main plenary SCF committee, which delivers its advice in the form of 'Opinions'. These are published in the Commission series *Reports of the Scientific Committee for Food*, published by the Office for Official Publications of the European Community, Luxembourg.

If the SCF delivers a favourable opinion on a new food additive for which an application for approval has been made, the Commission will seek to amend the relevant directive, through a procedure laid down in EC Directive 89/107/EEC, so that the novel additive may be included in the permitted list.

EC Directive 89/107/EEC also allows an individual Member State to permit the marketing and use of a new food additive within its own territory on a temporary basis for a maximum period of 2 years. During the 2 year period the Member State can ask the Commission to include the additive in the permitted EC list. The Commission would then put the additive through the usual approval system, seeking the advice of the SCF on safety issues. If approval is not gained within the 2 year period, the Member State must cancel the temporary approval of the additive on its territory. In practice, it is probably more cost effective for any manufacturer seeking to gain approval of a novel additive to apply to the Commission for EC-wide approval in the first place.

If a Member State decides at any stage to suspend approval of a food additive because it considers that continued use presents an unacceptable risk to human health, it can do so provided that it informs the Commission and other Member States immediately, giving the reasons for the decision. The Commission will then examine the evidence on which the decision was made, seeking advice as necessary from the SCF, and decide whether or not to amend the relevant directive or to take other measures, as appropriate. In practice, this situation is unlikely to arise, given the innocuous nature of most permitted food additives.

The type of technological information required in a food additive submission is summarized in **Table 2** and the type of toxicological studies which are generally required on an additive with the potential for extensive use are outlined in **Table 3**. The actual data required on any new additive will vary and any manufacturer wishing to apply for approval would be well advised to discuss with the relevant regulatory authority at an early stage what the data requirements are likely to be. In particular, it should not be assumed that a submission which has been designed to satisfy one regulatory authority will automatically satisfy all others. The manufacturer should design an appropriate programme of toxicological testing which is likely to provide reassurance as to the

Table 2 Technological data required on a new food additive

Chemical name and structure
Specification
Method of manufacture
Technological function(s) and proposed level(s) of use
Method of analysis
Stability data
Estimated intakes
Toxicological data

Table 3 Toxicological data required on a new food additive

Absorption, distribution, metabolism, excretion
Genotoxicity studies
90 day studies in two species
1 year study in two species
Carcinogenicity studies in two rodent species
Teratology studies
Multigeneration studies in rodents
Short-term human studies

safety of the additive, depending on features such as its chemical structure, its likely absorption through the gastro-intestinal tract, its metabolism and the predicted intake levels.

In most cases in which an additive is considered acceptable for use in food, the SCF will assign to the additive an acceptable daily intake (ADI), which is defined as the amount of a food additive, expressed on a body weight basis, that can be ingested daily over a lifetime without appreciable health risk (World Health Organization, 1987). The conditions of use in the relevant directive, i.e. the foods in which the additive may be used and the levels at which it may be used, will then be set such that the ADI is not exceeded by an individual consuming those foods.

Flavourings

At present, with the exception of the general provisions in EC Directive 88/388/EEC, there are no specific, EC-wide controls on the use of flavourings in food or a list of permitted flavourings. Therefore, there is no EC-wide requirement at present to seek specific approval for a novel flavouring substance or preparation. However, within the EC, some individual Member States either have statutory controls on specific groups of flavourings or operate an advisory system to guide manufacturers, for example, in the case of flavourings about which there are some safety concerns.

As described above, the European Commission intends to introduce specific controls on the use of flavouring substances, beginning with a positive list of chemically defined flavouring substances in 2004. Given the large number of substances in use, and the limited exposure and toxicological data on most of them, this will be a considerable undertaking. It is only likely to succeed if a pragmatic approach is taken which recognizes that the intake of most chemically defined flavouring substances is so low that they are unlikely to constitute a significant risk to health. The evaluation procedure is likely to make full use of existing safety evaluations, such as those of the Council of Europe Committee of Experts on Flavouring Substances (CEFS) and the Joint Expert Advisory Committee on Food Additives (see below; World Health Organisation, 1996, 1998). The CEFS, whose membership includes both EC and non-EC countries, is the only European body which has carried out, as far as possible, a systematic evaluation of flavourings in use in food manufacture in Europe. The CEFS evaluations are published in a document commonly referred to as the 'Blue Book'. The most recent evaluation of chemically defined flavouring substances was published in 1992 in the Fourth Edition of Volume 1 of the Blue Book (Council of Europe, 1992a). The CEFS has also produced sets of guidelines on smoke flavour on thermal process flavourings, and on certain flavouring preparations (Council of Europe, 1992b, 1994, 1995, 1998).

Food Contact Materials

Within the EC, evaluation of food contact materials is carried out by the SCF Working Group on Food Contact Materials. To date, as stated above, only monomers and other starting materials and additives used in plastics have been subject to detailed evaluation. SCF opinions on individual substances in plastics are set out in the form of classifications into one of ten different lists, numbered 0–9 (Barlow, 1993). Substances on which there are adequate toxicity data to make a proper safety assessment are classified into one of the first six lists, i.e. 0–4 and occasionally 5. Substances on which there are inadequate data to make a proper safety assessment are classified into Lists 6–9. A summary of the classification scheme is given in **Tables 4** and **5**.

Within EC legislation, substances classified in Lists 0–4 are authorized for use, provided that they comply with any specific restrictions. No further toxicity data are required on them unless they are classified as only temporarily acceptable or tolerable for use in food. List 5 substances are excluded from the positive lists in the EC

Table 4 SCF classification scheme for substances used in food packaging materials: data sufficient for evaluation

List	ADI	TDI	Explanation
0	–	–	Food ingredients or normal body metabolites
1	+	+	Or temporary ADI, MTDI, PMTDI, PTWI set by SCF or JECFA
2	–	+	Or temporary TDI set by SCF
3	–	–	Use self-limiting or very low migration
4	–	–	Migration not detectable
5	–	–	Bioaccumulate or too toxic for use

Table 5 SCF classification scheme for substances used in food packaging materials: data insufficient for evaluation

List	Explanation
6	Insufficient/no data
	Suspect toxicity:
	A carcinogenicity
	B other toxicity
7	Some useful toxicity data but insufficient to set an ADI. SCF specifies required data
8	Insufficient/no data
	Data needed according to guidelines
9	Inadequate chemical specification

directives. For substances classified in Lists 6–9 there are insufficient data for the SCF to give an opinion as to their safety-in-use. In fact, approximately 80% of monomers and 60% of additives are classified in these lists. These substances are included in a sub-section of the positive list in the relevant EC directives, as substances which may continue to be used pending a decision on whether they can considered fully authorized for use. However, in order to retain these substances in the relevant directives, the data required by the SCF must be submitted according to deadlines laid down by the European Commission.

The SCF published guidance on the toxicological tests required for the evaluation of food contact materials in 1990, with minor revisions in 1991 (Commission of the European Communities, 1990b, 1991). The guidelines employ a graded approach, whereby the amount of toxicity testing required depends on the likely migration of the substance from the packaging material into foods. For example, for substances with very low migration, less than 0.05 mg kg^{-1} of food, the only tests required are three mutagenicity tests to establish that the substance is free of genotoxic potential. For substances migrating in higher amounts more toxicity data are required, possibly including reproduction, teratogenicity and long-term toxicity tests. The SCF has also set an overall limit for all substances migrating out of any food packaging of 60 mg kg^{-1} food or food simulant (a simulant is a product which is used to represent a range of food products for migration testing, e.g. olive oil is the simulant for fatty foods).

The Council of Europe is also active in this area. Its Committee of Experts on Materials and Articles Coming into Contact with Food prepares resolutions and guidelines on food contact materials. Although these resolutions are recommendations which have no legal basis, they are often quoted as specification requirements, which are often adopted as legislation by non-EC countries and may form the basis of EC directives. A number of activities are currently under way in the Council of Europe Committee, including drafting of resolutions on paper and board, printing inks and rubbers.

NORTH AMERICA

United States

Legislation

In the USA, the relevant legislation for food additives and food contact materials is the Federal Food, Drug and Cosmetic (FD&C) Act 1938, as amended. Formal control of food additives as a class began with the 1958 Food Additives Amendment of this Act. The categorization of food additives in the USA is different to that in Europe. In general, substances added to food in the USA fall into one of three categories:

1. *Generally recognized as safe (GRAS)*. This concept is described in more detail below.
2. *Food additives*. Under 201(s) of the FD&C Act, a food additive is defined as 'any substance the intended use of which results or may reasonably be expected to result, directly or indirectly, in its becoming a component or otherwise affecting the characteristics of any food'. Food additives are further divided into:
    Direct food additives, which are deliberately added to food and include all the classes of substances considered as food additives in Europe, with the exception of colours, and also include flavourings, or
    Indirect food additives, which include food contact materials, or
3. *Colour additives*. Additives other than GRAS additives are tightly regulated and require rigorous evidence of safety based on toxicological testing and premarketing approval by the Food and Drug Administration (FDA). Amendments to the permitted list of additives, or extension of the foods in which an additive may be used, require specific regulations to be issued by the FDA. A regulation may specify the amount of the substance which may be present in or on the foods, the foods in which it is permitted, the manner of use and any special labelling requirements. Detailed instructions on preparing a food additive petition and on the general principles used in evaluating the safety of food additives are laid down in FDA regulations. These are published in the *Code of Federal Regulations* (CFR) with regulations on food additives in Title 21, CFR, Volume 3, Parts 170–199.

The concept of 'generally recognized as safe' or GRAS additives was introduced at the time of the 1958 amendment to deal with those chemicals which were used extensively in food prior to 1958 and whose use was generally recognized as safe under the conditions of intended use by a panel of experts appropriately 'qualified by training and experience'. It has been most widely used in the case of flavourings and flavouring ingredients. The original GRAS listing by FDA for flavourings contained only 265 natural and 27 artificial flavouring substances, far less than are actually in use. This prompted the US flavouring industry's trade association, the Flavor and Extract Manufacturers' Association (FEMA), to set up its own panel of independent experts to review and evaluate all flavouring substances for GRAS status. The Panel meets regularly and has published its own GRAS lists of almost 2000 flavourings in total. This initiative was possible because the 1958 Amendment did not specifically state that GRAS status should be determined solely by the FDA. Although the FDA has not adopted this list into regulation, it has officially recognized it. A manufacturer's independent determination of GRAS status exempts them from the need to carry out extensive toxicological testing on an additive and to seek formal FDA approval, which may take many years to obtain.

If a manufacturer wishes to obtain affirmation of the GRAS status of a substance from the FDA, there are two ways in which it may be obtained. The first is to establish that the product was used commonly in the food supply prior to 1958. The second is to submit a GRAS affirmation petition to the FDA for approval, but in this case the quality and quantity of toxicological studies required are likely to be similar to those required for a new food additive. The FDA is currently considering a GRAS reform proposal which would introduce a new procedure for obtaining GRAS affirmation. Under this new procedure, the manufacturer would be required to submit summaries of toxicological and other studies on a substance. The FDA would then have a fixed time period—90 days—in which to notify the manufacturer of any problems with their GRAS determination. If no notification is made, the product would obtain GRAS affirmation by default.

One further important legislative instrument relating to food additives in the US is the 'Delaney Clause' in the 1960 Color Additive Amendments to the FD&C Act. This provides that no food additive may be found safe if it produces cancer when ingested by man or animals, or if it is shown by other appropriate tests to be a cancer-producing agent. Although this might have been a reasonable requirement at the time it was introduced in view of the state of toxicological knowledge at that time, it could be regarded as unnecessarily restrictive today. It is generally accepted nowadays that not all chemicals which are carcinogenic in animal bioassays are necessarily a carcinogenic risk to man. In some cases, for non-genotoxic carcinogens, the mechanism of action may not be relevant to man or a threshold may exist for the toxicological effect which leads to cancer. For example, in the case of the artificial sweetener saccharin, it is accepted in Europe that the bladder tumours produced in male rats at high doses are not relevant to man and that saccharin is not a carcinogenic risk to man. However, in the USA, because of the Delaney Clause, saccharin is still legally regarded as a carcinogenic risk to man and is only permitted by means of a specific Act of Congress.

Toxicological Requirements for Direct Food Additives and Colour Additives

The FDA has published detailed guidance on its toxicological testing requirements for direct food additives and for colour additives in what is generally known as the 'Redbook' (Food and Drug Administration, 1982). These guidelines provide guidance on toxicological testing and set out a tiered system of information requirements for additives in food. This priority ranking system is based on chemical structure and likely human exposure. Based on these two parameters, substances are assigned to one of three different 'concern levels'. For Concern Level 1, i.e. substances with a simple chemical structure and very low potential exposure, toxicity testing requirements are few. However, as structure becomes more complex and/or potential exposure increases, the amount of toxicity testing required increases.

The guidelines are currently undergoing revision by the FDA to take account of developments in toxicological knowledge in the last 20 years or so.

Threshold of Regulation

'Threshold of regulation' is a concept introduced by the FDA to aid its consideration of petitions for the use of chemicals as components of food contact materials (Food and Drug Administration, 1993, 1995). The intention is to avoid the unnecessary use of limited resources by carrying out toxicological studies and evaluating food additive petitions in cases where the risk to the public is likely to be minimal. The concept embodies the principle that a dietary concentration of a chemical of unknown toxicity can be specified, which can be considered for practical purposes as toxicologically insignificant and thus pose no unacceptable risk to the consumer. Under this procedure, information about the proposed use of a substance undergoes an abbreviated review by the FDA, as opposed to the extensive review and formal issue of a regulation normally required for food additives.

The threshold of regulation was chosen after review of existing acute and chronic toxicity data on a large number of representative chemicals. It is set at 0.5 ppb, i.e. it applies to substances for which the petition shows that migration data obtained under worst case conditions give a dietary concentration below 0.5 ppb and where there is no reason, on the basis of chemical structure, to suspect the substance is a carcinogen. The dietary concentration of 0.5 ppb is equivalent to a maximum intake of 1.5 μg person^{-1} day^{-1}, assuming that a person eats 1.5 kg of solid food and 1.5 kg of liquid food per day. If a untested substance should, in fact, be a carcinogen and is inadvertently accepted, the FDA has estimated that, at the 0.5 ppb level of exposure, there would be an 85% upper bound probability that the lifetime cancer risk to man would not exceed one in a million.

Canada

In Canada, the relevant legislation for food additives are the Food and Drug Regulations made persuant to the Food and Drugs Act 1920, last revised 1964 (Canada, 1985). The Regulations define the term 'food additive' in Canadian law and contain tables of permitted food additives. The original Food Additive Tables in Division 16 of the Regulations were established in 1964 and contained 317 additives. Any petitioner seeking to have the tables amended to include a new additive or to extend the list of foods in which the additive may be used must supply supporting information to the Health Protection Branch (HPB) of Health Canada in the form of a food additive submission. The Food and Drug Regulations set out the basis for the petitioning process (Section B.16.002) and provide guidance on what is required in the submission.

In Canada (unlike the USA), food packaging materials are, by definition, excluded from food additive status and therefore are not subject to preclearance procedures. Regulation of food contact materials is limited. The relevant regulation states: 'No person shall sell any food in a package that may yield to its contents any substance that may be injurious to the health of a consumer of the food'. The main approval process is non-statutory and involves the issuing of a 'letter of opinion' from the Health Protection Branch, on request, for a new food packaging additive after a review of the proposed use, results of solvent extractions of the packaging material and toxicity data.

JOINT WHO/FAO EXPERT COMMITTEE ON FOOD ADDITIVES (JECFA)

No discussion of international regulatory and advisory systems for food additives would be complete without mention of the Joint Expert Committee on Food Additives (JECFA). JECFA serves as a scientific advisory body to the Food and Agriculture Organization and the World Health Organization (WHO), their Member States and the Codex Alimentarius Commission on the safety of food additives, residues of veterinary drugs, naturally occurring toxicants and contaminants in food. JECFA publishes specifications for food additives and prepares toxicological monographs on substances which it has considered. The conclusions of JECFA meetings are published in the WHO Technical Report Series and toxicological monographs in the WHO Food Additives Series under the auspices of the International Programme on Chemical Safety. JECFA is commonly used as the source of toxicological and technological advice on food additives and contaminants in those countries which do not have sophisticated regulatory systems for these classes of chemicals.

ACKNOWLEDGEMENTS

I am grateful to Dr David Hattan, Dr Bruce Lauer and Ms Elizabeth Vavasour for their help during the preparation of the manuscript.

REFERENCES

Barlow, S. M. (1993). The role of the Scientific Committee for Food in evaluating plastics for packaging. *Food Addit. Contamin.*, **11**, 249–259.

Canada (1985). *Food and Drugs Act Revised Statutes of Canada, 1985*. CF–27. Food and Drug Regulations. The Queen's Printer, Ottawa.

Commission of the European Communities (1988). Council Directive of 22 June 1988 on the approximation of the laws of Member States relating to flavourings for use in foodstuffs and to source materials for their production (88/388/EEC). *Off. J. Eur. Commun.*, No. L184, 61–66.

Commission of the European Communities (1989a). Council Directive of 21 December 1988 on the approximation of the laws of the Member States concerning food additives authorized for use in foodstuffs intended for human consumption (89/107/EEC). *Off. J. Eur. Commun.*, L40, 27–33.

Commission of the European Communities (1989b). Council Directive of 21 December 1988 on the approximation of the laws of the Member States relating to materials and articles intended to come into contact with foodstuffs (89/109/EEC). *Off. J. Eur. Commun.*, L40, 38–44.

Commission of the European Communities (1989c). Corrigendum to Council Directive 89/109/EEC of 21 December 1988 on the approximation of the laws of the Member States relating to materials and articles intended to come into contact with foodstuffs. *Off. J. Eur. Commun.*, L347, 37.

Commission of the European Communities (1990a). Commission Directive of 23 February 1990 relating to plastics materials and articles intended to come into contact with foodstuffs (90/128/EEC). *Off. J. Eur. Commun.*, L75, 19–40.

Commission of the European Communities (1990b). Guidelines for presentation of data for toxicological evaluation of a substance to be used in materials and articles intended to come into contact with foodstuffs. Note for guidance of applicants for presentation of a request for assessment of a substance to be used in plastics materials and articles intended to come into contact with foodstuffs. III/3568/89-Final, 25–35. DGIII/C/1, Brussels.

Commission of the European Communities (1991). Guidelines for presentation of data for toxicological evaluation of a substance to be used in materials and articles intended to come into contact with foodstuffs. Note for guidance of applicants for presentation of a request for assessment of a substances to be used in plastics materials and articles intended to come into contact with foodstuffs. CS/PM/1025, 28–41. DGIII/C/1, Brussels.

Commission of the European Communities (1994a). European Parliament and Council Directive 94/35/EC of 30 June 1994 on sweeteners for use in foodstuffs. *Off. J. Eur. Commun.*, L237, 3–12.

Commission of the European Communities (1994b). European Parliament and Council Directive 94/36/EC of 30 June 1994 on colours for use in foodstuffs. *Off. J. Eur. Commun.*, L237, 13–29.

Commission of the European Communities (1995a). European Parliament and Council Directive No. 95/2/EC of 20 February 1995 on food additives other than colours and sweeteners. *Off. J. Eur. Commun.*, L61, 1–40.

Commission of the European Communities (1995b). Corrigendum to European Parliament and Council Directive No. 95/2 EC on food additives other than colours and sweeteners. *Off. J. Eur. Commun.*, L248, 60.

Commission of the European Communities (1995c). Commission Directive 95/31/EC of 5 July 1995 laying down specific criteria of purity concerning sweeteners for use in foodstuffs. *Off. J. Eur. Commun.*, L178, 1–19.

Commission of the European Communities (1995d). Commission Directive 95/45/EC of 26 July 1995 laying down specific purity criteria concerning colours for use in foodstuffs. *Off. J. Eur. Commun.*, L226, 1–45.

Commission of the European Communities (1996). Regulation (EC) No. 2232/96 of the European Parliament and of the Council of 28 October 1996 laying down a Community Procedure for flavouring substances used or intended for use in or on foodstuffs. *Off. J. Eur. Commun.*, L299, 1–4.

Council of Europe (1992a). *Flavouring Substances and Natural Sources of Flavourings*, 4th edn, Vol. 1, *Chemically Defined Flavouring Substances*. Maisonneuve, Strasbourg.

Council of Europe (1992b). *Council of Europe Guidelines Concerning the Transmission of Flavour of Smoke to Food*. Council of Europe Press, Strasbourg.

Council of Europe (1994). *Council of Europe Guidelines for Flavouring Preparations Produced by Enzymatic or Microbiological Processes*. Council of Europe Press, Strasbourg.

Council of Europe (1995). *Council of Europe Guidelines for Safety Evaluation of Thermal Process Flavourings*. Council of Europe Press, Strasbourg.

Council of Europe (1998). *Council of Europe Guidelines for Flavouring Preparations Produced by Plant Tissue Culture*. Council of Europe Publishing, Strasbourg.

Food and Drug Administration (1982). *Toxicological Principles for the Safety Assessment of Direct Food Additives and Color Additives Used in Food*. Bureau of Foods, Washington, DC.

Food and Drug Administration (1993). Food Additives; Threshold of Regulation for substances used in food-contact articles. *Fed. Regist.*, **58**, 52719–52729.

Food and Drug Administration (1995). Food Additives; Threshold of Regulation for substances used in food-contact articles. *Fed. Regist.*, **60**, 36582–36596.

Ministry of Agriculture, Fisheries and Food (1995). *Flavourings in Food*. Food Surveillance Paper No. 48, HMSO, London.

World Health Organization (1987). *Principles for the Safety Assessment of Food Additives and Contaminants in Food. Environmental Health Criteria 70*. WHO, Geneva.

World Health Organization (1996). *Toxicological Evaluation of Certain Food Additives and Contaminants*. WHO Food Additives Series 35. WHO, Geneva.

World Health Organisation (1998). *Safety Evaluation of Certain Food Additives and Contaminants*. WHO Food Additives Series 40. WHO, Geneva.

Chapter 77

Regulatory Aspects and Strategy in Medical Device Safety Evaluation

Shayne C. Gad

CONTENTS

- Background
- History
- Regulatory Basis
- Toxicity Testing: Medical Devices
- Road Map to Testing
- References

BACKGROUND

In the USA, according to 201(h) of the Food, Drug and Cosmetic Act, a medical device is defined as an instrument, apparatus, implement, machine, contrivance, implant, *in vitro* reagent or other similar or related article, including a component, part, or accessory that is: recognized in the official *National Formulary*, or the *United States Pharmacopeia* (USP), or any supplement to them; intended for use in the diagnosis of disease or other condition, or in the cure, mitigation, treatment, or prevention of disease, in man or other animals, or intended to affect the structure or any function of the body or man or other animals, and which does not achieve any of its primary intended purposes through chemical action within or on the body of man or other animals, and which is not dependent upon being metabolized for the achievement of any of its principal intended purposes (CDRH, 1992).

Under this definition, devices might be considered as belonging to one of six categories: specialty devices, medical/surgical supplies, imaging systems, other equipment, *in vitro* diagnostics and health information systems (Wilkerson Group, 1995).

Specialty devices comprise disposable and long-term single-use products which are usually associated with a specific procedure and various types of implantable devices. These are usually technology-intensive and higher priced products which are used only in a specific procedure. Examples include pacemakers, heart valves, knee implants, laparoscopic endoscopes, hip implants, coronary angioplasty balloon catheters, intravenous (i.v.) pumps and cassettes, vascular grafts, stents and internal (surgical) staplers. These accounted for $10 billion in sales in 1993 in the USA.

Medical and surgical supplies include a broad range of commodity disposables and small reusable devices and instruments. These typically are lower technologically and in price, and enjoy broad use across a range of medical and surgical procedures. Items in this category include sutures, syringes and needles, gloves, i.v. administration sets, adhesive bandages, i.v. catheters, surgical packs, caps and gowns and surgical sponges. These accounted for $9.5 billion of US sales in 1993.

Imaging systems include all types of imaging equipment, contrast agents and films. Examples include X-ray, angiography, MRI (magnetic resonance imaging), CAT (computerized axial tomography) and nuclear and ultrasound systems plus the disposable film and contrast agents used in them. The imaging system category accounted for $9 billion of US sales during 1993.

The other equipment category includes non-imaging equipment systems such as patient monitoring machines, anaesthesia machines, critical care respirators, ECG (electrocardiogram) diagnostic systems and ventilators. In 1993, US sales for this category amounted to $3 billion.

In vitro diagnostics, also sometimes called simply diagnostics, are composed of chemical reagent and instrument systems used to evaluate patients' blood and other body fluids and tissues. Subsegments include clinical chemistry, haematology, microbiology, infectious disease immunology and other (cancer, etc.) immunodiagnostics. Diagnostics sales during 1993 were $6 billion in the USA.

The final category, health information systems, encompasses computer hardware and software used for clinical and laboratory purposes. However, those computer and software systems used exclusively for patient records and financial data processing are not included in this category or considered as medical devices. This category accounted for $500 million in US sales in 1993, but has undoubtedly grown rapidly since then.

HISTORY

As has previously been reviewed by Hutt (1989), the regulation of medical devices has followed a different history to that of drugs. Medical devices go back at least to the Egyptians and Etruscans. Problems with fraudulent devices in the USA date back to the late 1700s, although no legislative remedy was attempted until the 1900s. In fact, the legislative history of the 1906 Food and Drug Act contains no references to devices. Devices continued to be regulated under the postal fraud statutes. Such regulation was evidently ineffectual, as fraudulent devices flourished during this period. Starting in 1926, the Food and Drug Administration (FDA) monitored such devices and assisted the US Postal service in its regulatory actions. Medical devices were covered in the 1938 Act, but only in regard to adulteration and misbranding. Over the intervening years, various committees which examined medical device regulation consistently came to similar conclusions, that the FDA has inadequate authority and resources to regulate the medical device industry. As part of the agreement that resulted in passage of the 1962 amendments, however, all references to medical devices were deleted. The need and demand for increased regulation continued to grow. In 1967, President Lyndon Johnson supported the proposed Medical Device Safety Act, which nevertheless was not well received by Congress. In fact, no legislation pertaining to medical device safety was passed until 1976.

In 1969, at the request of President Richard Nixon, the Department of Health, Education and Welfare (HEW) established a Study Group in Medical Devices, also known as the Cooper Committee, because it was chaired by the Director of the National Heart and Lung Institute, Dr Theodore Cooper. Its report in 1970 concluded that a different regulatory approach was needed to deal with medical devices. This report initiated the chain of events that culminated in the Medical Device Amendment of 1976. In the interim, the Bureau of Medical Devices and Diagnostic Products was created in 1979. Remarkably, the 1976 Amendment retained the essential provisions of the Cooper Committee Report regarding inventory and classification of all medical devices by class: Class I (general controls), Class II (performance standards) or Class III (premarket approval). These classifications are discussed in greater detail later in this chapter. These remain the essential regulations applicable to medical devices. Both the Drug Price Competition and Patent Restoration Act of 1984 and the Orphan Drug Act of 1983 contained language that made the provisions of the laws applicable to medical devices but did not have provisions unique to medical devices. The recent perceptions, revelations and controversy surrounding silicone breast implants will probably cause additional changes in the regulation of devices.

As a consequence, 1978 brought guidelines for investigational device exemptions (IDEs, the equivalent of INDAs for drugs). These requirements, as will be seen later, effectively excluded a wide range of medical devices from regulation by establishing an exemption for those new or modified devices which are equivalent to existing devices. The passage of the Safe Medical Devices Act in 1990 made premarketing requirements and postmarketing surveillance more rigorous. The actual current guidelines for testing started with the USP guidance on biocompatability of plastics. A formal regulatory approach springs from the Tripartite Agreement, which is a joint intergovernmental agreement between the UK, Canada, and the USA (with France having joined later). After lengthy consideration, the FDA has announced acceptance of International Standards Organization (ISO) 10993 guidelines for testing (ASTM, 1990a; O'Grady, 1990; FAO, 1991; MAPI, 1992; Spizizen, 1992) under the rubric of harmonization. This is the second major trend operative in device regulation: the internationalization of the market place with accompanying efforts to harmonize regulations. Under the ICH (International Conference on Harmonization), great strides have been made in this area.

Independent of FDA initiatives, the USP has promulgated test methods and standards for various aspects of establishing the safety of drugs (such as the recent standards for inclusion of volatiles in formulated drug products), which were, in effect, regulations affecting the safety of drugs and devices. Most of the actual current guidelines for the conduct of non-clinical safety evaluations of medical devices have evolved from such quasi-agency actions [such as the USP's 1965 promulgation of biological tests for plastics and ongoing American National Standards Institute (ANSI) standard promulgation]. The same has been true of the other pharmacopoeias.

REGULATORY BASIS

Regulations: General Considerations for the USA

Regulations

The US federal regulations that govern the testing, manufacture and sale of medical devices are covered in Chapter 1, Title 21 of the Code of Federal Regulations (21 CFR). These comprise nine 6×8 inch volumes which stack 8 inches high. This title also covers foods, veterinary products, medical devices and cosmetics. As these topics will be discussed elsewhere in this book, this section briefly reviews those parts of 21 CFR that are applicable to medical devices (Chengelis *et al.*, 1995).

Of most interest to a toxicologist working in this arena is Chapter 1, Subchapter A (Parts 1–78), which cover general provisions, organization, etc. The good laboratory practices (GLPs) are codified in 21 CFR 58. The regulations applicable to medical devices are covered in Subchapter H, Parts 800–895 of 21 CFR. As discussed earlier, the term medical device covers a wide variety of products: contact lenses, hearing aids, intrauterine contraceptive devices, syringes, catheters, drip bags, orthopedic prostheses, etc. The current structure of the law was established by the Medical Device Amendment of 1976. Products on the market on the day the amendment was passed were assigned to one of three classes (I, II or III), based on the recommendation of advisory panels. Medical device classification procedure is described in Part 860. Class I products (the least risk laden) were those for which safety and effectiveness could be reasonably assured by general controls. Class II products were those for which a combination of general controls and performance standards were required reasonably to assure safety and effectiveness. Class III products were those for which general controls and performance standards were inadequate; these were required to go through a premarket approval process. All devices commercially distributed after May 28, 1976 ('preamendment Class III devices') which are not determined to be substantially equivalent to an existing marketed device are automatically categorized as Class III and require the submission of a PMA. It should be noted that these are classifications for regulatory purposes only and are distinct from the classification (HIMA/PHRMA) of product types (e.g. internal versus external) discussed elsewhere in this chapter. Kahan (1995) provides a detailed overview of what comprises general controls, performance standards, etc.

As with the subchapter on drugs, much of the subchapter on medical devices in the regulations concerns categorizations and specifies for a wide variety of devices. For a toxicologist involved in new product development, the parts of greatest interest are 812 and 814. As with drugs, devices must be shown to be safe and effective when used as intended, and data must be provided to demonstrate such claims. In order to conduct the appropriate clinical research to obtain these data, a sponsor applies to the Agency for an IDE, as described in 21 CFR 812. As stated in this section, 'an approved investigational device exemption (IDE) permits a device that would otherwise be required to comply with a performance standard or to have premarket approval to be shipped lawfully for the purpose of conducting investigations of that device'. Given the broad range of products that fall into the category of medical devices, the toxicological concerns are equally broad; testing requirements to support an IDE are vaguely mentioned in the law, even

by FDA standards. In this regard, the law simply requires that the IDE application must include a report of prior investigations which 'shall include reports of all prior clinical, animal and laboratory testing'. There is no absolute requirement for animal testing, only a requirement that such testing much be reported. There are, of course, standards and conventions to be followed in designing a safety package to support an IDE, and these are discussed in a subsequent section of this chapter.

In order to obtain a licence to market a device, a sponsor either submits a 510(k) premarket notification or applies for a Premarket Approval (PMA), as described in 21 CFR 814. Like an NDA, a PMA application is a very extensive and detailed document that must include, among other things, a summary of non-clinical laboratory studies submitted in the application 921 CFR 814.20(b)(3)(v)(A), in addition to a section containing results of the non-clinical laboratory studies with the device, including microbiological, toxicological, immunological, biocompatibility, stress, wear, shelf-life and other laboratory or animal tests as appropriate. As with drugs, these tests must be conducted in compliance with the GLP Regulations. Under the language of the law, a sponsor submits a PMA, which the FDA then 'files'. The filing of an application means that 'FDA has made a threshold determination that the application is sufficiently complete to permit substantive review.' Reasons for refusal to file are listed in 814.44(e), and include items such as an application that is not complete and has insufficient justification for the omission(s) present. The agency has 45 days from receipt of an application to notify the sponsor as to whether or not the application has been filed. The FDA has 180 days after filing of a complete PMA (21 CFR 814,40) to send the applicant an approval order, an 'approved' letter or a 'not approved' letter, or an order denying approval. An 'approval order' is self-explanatory and is issued if the agency finds no reason (as listed in 814.45) for denying approval. An 'approved' letter 814.44(e) means that the application substantially meets requirements, but some specific additional information is needed. A 'not approved' letter, 814.45(f), means that the application contains false statements of fact, does not comply with labelling guidelines or non-clinical laboratory studies were not conducted according to GLPs, etc. Essentially, an order denying approval means that the sponsor must do substantially more work and must submit a new application of PMA for the device in question. The 510(k) premarket approval submissions are less extensive than PMAs, but must still include appropriate preclinical safety data; 510(k)s are supposed to be approved in 90 days.

Actual review and approval times historically have been much longer than the statutory limits. For 1995, the average total review time for Class III products in the USA cleared by 510(k) was 579 days (versus 240 or less in the EU) (Gray Sheet, 1996a). For fiscal year 1996, overall average 510(k) review times (for an expected 5875 filings) is projected to be 137 days (with low risk exempted devices and refusals to file not being included in the totals or average). Average PMA review times are projected to be 250 days (Gray Sheet, 1996b). See also Chengelis *et al.* (1995) for more information on general regulatory considerations.

Good Laboratory Practices

The original promulgation of GLPs was by the US FDA in 1978 in response to a variety of cases which led the agency to conclude that some of the data that it had obtained in support of product approvals were not trustworthy. Subsequently, other regulatory agencies and authorities in the USA and across the world have either promulgated their own version of similar regulations or required adherence to the set generated by the FDA or another body. The EEC requirement for compliance with GLPs for safety tests has been reinforced in a modification of Directive 75/318/EEC (Regulatory Affairs Focus, 1966). The FDA last revised the GLP regulations in 1989 (Food and Drug Administration, 1989).

The GLPs require that all pivotal preclinical safety studies, that is, those which are used and required by regulation to make decisions as to the safety of the product (in our case, a device), are conducted under a well defined protocol utilizing procedures set forth in written standard operating procedures by trained (as established by documentation) personnel under the direction of a study director. All work must be reviewed by an independent Quality Assurance Unit (QAU). The regulations require rigorous attention to record keeping, but do not dictate how actual studies are designed or conducted in a technical sense (Gad and Taulbee, 1996).

Animal Welfare Act

Gone are the days when the pharmaceutical scientist could conduct whatever procedures or studies that were desired using experimental animals. The Animal Welfare Act (APHIS, 1989) (and its analogues in other countries) rightfully requires careful consideration of animal usage to ensure that research and testing uses as few animals as possible in as humane a manner as possible. As a start, all protocols must be reviewed by an Institutional Animal Care and Use Committee. Such review takes time, but should not serve to hinder good science. When designing a study or developing a new procedure or technique, the following points should be kept in mind:

■   Will the number of animals used be sufficient to provide the required data, yet not constitute excessive use? (Note: it ultimately does not reduce animal use to utilize too few animals to begin with and then have to repeat the study.)

■   Are the procedures employed the least invasive and traumatic available? This practice is not only required by regulations, but is also sound scientific practice, since any induced stress will produce a range of responses in test animals that can mask or confound the chemically induced effects.

Regulations Versus Law

A note of caution must be inserted here. The law (the document passed by Congress) and the regulations (the documents written by the regulatory authorities to enforce the laws) are separate documents. The sections in the law do not necessarily have numerical correspondence. For example, the regulations on the PMA process is described in 21 CFR 312, but the law describing the requirement for a PMA process is in Section 515 of the FDCA. Because the regulations rather than the laws themselves have a greater impact on toxicological practice, greater emphasis is placed on regulation in this chapter. For a complete review of FDA law, the reader is referred to the monographs by Food and Drug Law Institute in 1995.

Laws authorize the activities and responsibilities of the various federal agencies. All proposed laws before the US Congress are referred to committees for review and approval. The committees responsible for FDA oversight are summarized in **Table 1**. This table also highlights the fact that authorizations and appropriations (the funding necessary to execute authorizations) are handled by different committees. **Figure 1** presents the organization of the Center for Devices and Radiological Health (CDRH). As can has seen from this organizational structure, the categorization of devices for division review purposes is functionally based.

Table 1 Congressional committees responsible for FDA oversight

Authorization:	
Senate	All public health service agencies are under the jurisdiction of the Labor and Human Resources Committee
House	Most public health agencies are under the jurisdiction of the Health and the Environmental Subcommittee of the House Energy and Commerce Committee
Appropriation:	
Senate	Unlike most other public health agencies, the FDA is under the jurisdiction of the Agriculture, Rural Development and Related Agencies Subcommittee of the Senate Appropriations Committee
House	Under the jurisdiction of the Agriculture, Rural Development and Related Agencies Subcommittee of the House Appropriations Committee

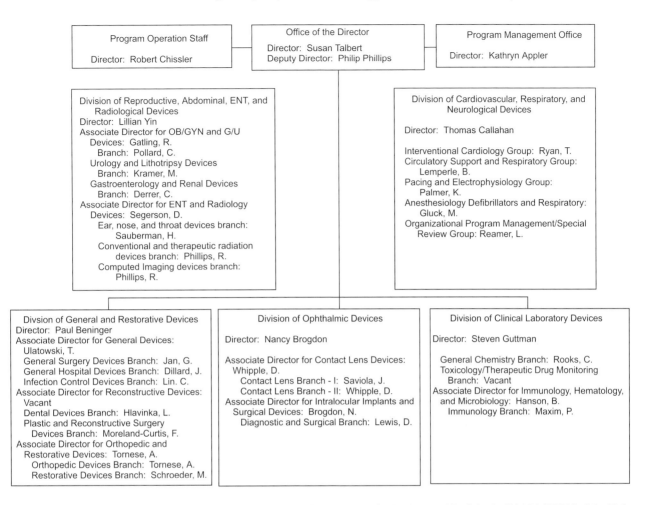

Figure 1 Organization of the Office of Device Evaluation (ODE) for the Center for Devices and Radiological Health (CDRH) of the FDA. Officials in place at the beginning of 1997 are identified by name. ODE evaluates submissions for new device approvals.

Organizations Regulating Drug and Device Safety in the USA

The agency formally charged with overseeing the safety of drugs and devices in the USA is the FDA. It is headed by a commissioner who reports to the Secretary of the Department of Health and Human Services (DHHS) and has a tremendous range of responsibilities. Medical devices are overseen by the CDRH, headed by a director. Drugs are overseen primarily by the Center for Drug Evaluation and Research (CDER) [although some therapeutic or health care entities are considered as biologically derived and therefore regulated by the Center for Biologic Evaluation and Research (CBER)]. There are also 'combination products' (part drug, part device) which may be regulated by either or both CDER/CBER and CDRH, depending on where the expertise is perceived to be in the FDA (CFR, 1992).

Most of the regulatory interaction of a toxicologist involved in assessing the biocompatability of devices is with the appropriate part of the CDRH, although for combination products the two centers charged with drugs or biologicals may also come into play. Within the CDRH there is a range of groups (called divisions) which focus on specific areas of use for devices (such as general and restorative devices; cardiovascular, respiratory and neurological devices; ophthalmic devices; reproductive, abdominal, ear, nose and throat and radiological devices; and clinical laboratory devices). Within each of these there are engineers, chemists, pharmacologists/toxicologists, statisticians and clinicians.

There is also at least one non-governmental body which must review and approve various aspects of devices, setting forth significant 'guidance' for the evaluation of safety of devices. This is the USP, and its responsibilities and guidelines are presented later in this chapter.

TOXICITY TESTING: MEDICAL DEVICES

In a statutory sense, any item promoted for a medical purpose which does not rely on chemical action to achieve its intended effect is a medical device (as discussed earlier). *In vitro* diagnostic tests are also regulated as medical devices. The regulation of devices under these definitions has had a different history than that of drugs—it has not been as strict and it has evolved at a slower rate. Also, requirements for safety evaluation of devices have not been as strict as those for drugs. The safety concerns are also somewhat different. Toxicological safety concerns for devices (as opposed to concerns of mechanical safety, such as disintegration of heart valves) are called biocompatibility concerns.

Medical devices are classified as being in three different classes and are regulated accordingly. Class III devices are subject to the greatest degree of regulation and include devices which are implanted in the body, support life, prevent health impairment or present an unreasonable risk of illness or injury. These are subject to premarketing approval. Class II and Class I devices are subject to lesser control, required only to comply with general controls and performance standards.

There are several governing schemes for dictating what testing must be done on new Class III devices in the general case, with each developed and proposed by a

Table 2 FDA device categories and suggested biological testing

Device categories	Body contact duration[a]	Irritation tests	Sensitization assay	Cytoxicity	Acute systemic toxicity	Haemocompatibility/haemolysis	Pyrogenicity (material-mediated)	Implantation tests	Mutagenicity (carcinogenicity)	Subchronic toxicity	Chronic toxicity	Carcinogenesis bioassay
						Short-term →			← Long-term			
Intact surface	A	×	×	×								
	B	×	×	×								
	C	×	×	×	×							
External devices:												
Breached or surface comprised	A	×	×	×	×	×						
	B	×	×	×	×	×				×		
	C	×	×	×	×	×		×	×	×	×	
Intact natural channels	A	×	×	×	×	×	×	×				
	B	×	×	×	×	×	×	×		×		
	C	×	×	×	×	×	×	×	×	×	×	×
Externally communicating devices:												
Blood path indirect	A	×	×	×	×	×	×	×	×			
	B	×	×	×	×	×	×	×	×	×		
	C	×	×	×	×	×	×	×	×	×	×	×
Blood path direct	A	×	×	×	×	×	×	×	×			
	B	×	×	×	×	×	×	×	×	×		
	C	×	×	×	×	×	×	×	×	×	×	×
Bone	A	×	×	×	×	×	×	×	×			
	B	×	×	×	×	×	×	×	×	×		
	C	×	×	×	×	×	×	×	×	×	×	×
Internal devices:												
Tissue and tissue fluids	A	×	×	×	×	×	×	×	×			
	B	×	×	×	×	×	×	×	×	×		
	C	×	×	×	×	×	×	×	×	×	×	×
Blood	A	×	×	×	×	×	×	×	×			
	B	×	×	×	×	×	×	×	×	×		
	C	×	×	×	×	×	×	×	×	×	×	×

1. For these devices with possible leachables or degradation products, e.g. absorbable surfaces, haemostatic agents, testing for pharmacokinetics may be required.
2. Reproductive and developmental toxicity tests may be required for certain materials used for specialized indications.
3. Considerations should be given to long-term biological tests where indicated in the table taking into account the nature and mobility of the ingredients in the materials used to fabricate the device.
[a] A, transient (≤ 5 min); B, Short-term (5 min–29 days); C, long-term (≥ 30 days).

different regulatory organization at different times over the last few years. ICH has attempted to harmonize these requirements so that different (or duplicate) testing would not need to be performed to gain device approval in different national markets. There are also specialized testing requirements for some device types such as contact lenses (CDRH, 1995a, b) and tampons (CDRH, 1995c).

As with drugs, all safety testing for devices must be conducted in conformity with GLPs. **Table 2** presents the existing FDA CDRH requirements for device characterization and testing. The exact nature of the test protocols is based on recommendations by USP, ISO and others. It should be noted that Class II devices, if new, are also subject to the Tripartite guidelines.

Additional concerns with devices are considerations of their processing after production. Recently, concerns have risen about the potential for allergies to develop to latex components. Concern has grown not only for natural rubber used in devices with systemic exposure (catheters, stoppers on syringes, etc.), but also for such devices which have been washed in fluids used to wash other items which contain latex. It is likely that all devices containing latex will soon have to be labelled as such.

Devices which have systemic exposure need to be sterilized. Radiation and heat can be used for some devices, but others cannot be sterilized by these methods. Ethylene oxide or other chemical sterilants must be used, raising concerns that residual sterilants may present problems. At the same time, devices with exposure to the fluid path must be demonstrated to be neither pyrogenic nor haemolytic in their final manufactured form.

■ The selection of material(s) to be used in device manufacture and its toxicological evaluation should initially take into account full characterization of the material, for example, formulation, known and suspected impurities and processing.

■ The material(s) of manufacture, the final product and possible leachable chemicals or degradation products should be considered for their relevance to the overall toxicological evaluation of the device.

■ Tests to be utilized in the toxicological evaluation should take into account the bioavailability of the bioactive material, i.e. nature, degree, frequency, duration and conditions of exposure of the device to the body. This principle may lead to the categorization of devices which would facilitate the selection of appropriate tests.

■ Any in vitro or in vivo experiments or tests must be conducted according to recognized good laboratory practices followed by evaluation by competent informed persons.

■ Full experimental data, complete to the extent that an independent conclusion could be made, should be available to the reviewing authority, if required.

■ Any change in chemical composition, manufacturing process, physical configuration or intended use

of the device must be evaluated with respect to possible changes in toxicological effects and the need for additional toxicity testing.

■ The toxicological evaluation performed in accordance with this guidance should be considered in conjunction with other information from other non-clinical tests, clinical studies and postmarket experiences for an overall safety assessment.

Device Categories: Definitions and Examples

Non-contact Devices

These are devices that do not come into contact with the patient's body directly or indirectly; examples include *in vitro* diagnostic devices.

External Devices

1. *Intact surfaces*. Devices that come into contact with intact external body surfaces only; examples include electrodes, external prostheses and monitors of various types.
2. *Breached or compromised surfaces*. Devices that come into contact with breached or otherwise compromised external body surfaces; examples include ulcer, burn and granulation tissue dressings or healing devices and occlusive patches.

Externally Communicating Devices

1. *Intact natural channels*. Devices communicating with intact natural channels; examples include contact lenses, urinary catheters, intravaginal and intraintestinal devices (sigmoidoscopes, colonoscopes, stomach tubes, gastroscopes), endotracheal tubes and bronchoscopes.
2. *Blood path, indirect*. Devices that come into contact with the blood path at one point and serve as a conduit for fluid entry into the vascular system; examples include solution administration sets, extension sets, transfer sets and blood administration sets.
3. *Blood path, direct*. Devices that come into contact with recirculating blood; examples include intravenous catheters, temporary pacemaker electrodes, oxygenators, extracorporeal oxygenator tubing and accessories and dialysers, dialysis tubing and accessories.

Internal Devices

1. *Bone*. Devices principally coming into contact with bone; examples include orthopaedic pins, plates, replacement joints, bone prostheses and cements.

2. *Tissue and tissue fluid.* Devices principally coming into contact with tissue and tissue fluid or mucus membranes where contact is prolonged; examples include pacemakers, drug supply devices, neuromuscular sensors and stimulators, replacement tendons, breast implants, cerebrospinal fluid drains, artificial larynx, vas deferens valves, ligation clips, tubal occlusion devices for female sterilization and intrauterine devices.

3. *Blood.* Devices principally coming into contact with blood; examples include permanent pacemaker electrodes, artificial arteriovenous fistulae, heart valves, vascular grafts, blood monitors, internal drug delivery catheters and ventricular assist pumps.

Biological Tests

In order to appreciate fully the biological testing needs (**Table 2**), a knowledge of the objectives of the specified biological tests is required. These can be considered as follows.

Sensitization assay. Estimates the potential for sensitization of a test material and/or the extracts of a material when used in an animal and/or human.

Irritation tests. Estimate the irritation potential of test materials and their extracts, using an appropriate site or implant tissue such as skin and mucous membrane in an animal model and/or human.

Cytotoxicity. With the use of cell culture techniques, this test determines the lysis of cells (cell death), the inhibition of cell growth and other toxic effects on cells caused by test materials and/or extracts from the materials.

Acute systemic toxicity. Estimates the harmful effects of either single or multiple exposures to test materials and/or extracts, in an animal model, during a period of less than 24 h.

Haematocompatibility. Evaluates any effects of blood contacting materials on haemolysis, thrombosis, plasma proteins enzymes, and the formed elements using an animal model.

Pyrogenicity, material-mediated. Evaluates the potential for material-mediated pyrogenicity of test materials and/or extracts.

Haemolysis. Determines the degree of red blood cell lysis and the separation of haemoglobin caused by test materials and/or extracts from the materials *in vitro*.

Implantation tests. Evaluate the local toxic effects on living tissue, at both the gross level and microscopic level, to a sample material that is surgically implanted into appropriate animal implant site or tissue, e.g. muscle, bone, for 7–90 days.

Mutagenicity (genotoxicity). The application of mammalian or non-mammalian cell culture techniques for the determination of gene mutations, changes in chromosome structure and number and other DNA or gene toxicities caused by test materials and/or extracts from materials.

Subchronic toxicity. The determination of harmful effects from multiple exposures to test materials and/or extracts during a period of 1 day up to 10% or less of the total life of the test animal (e.g. up to 90 days in rats).

Chronic toxicity. The determination of harmful effects from multiple exposures to test materials and/or extracts during a period of 10% to the total life of the test animal (e.g. over 90 days in rats).

Carcinogenesis bioassay. The determination of the tumorigenic potential of test materials and/or extracts from either single or multiple exposures, over a period of the total life (e.g. 2 years for rat, 18 months for mouse or 7 years for dog).

Pharmacokinetics. To determine the processes of absorption, distribution, biotransformation and elimination of toxic leachables and degradation products of test materials and/or extracts.

Reproductive and developmental toxicity. The evaluation of the potential effects of test materials and/or extracts on fertility, reproductive function and prenatal and early postnatal development.

The tests for leachables such as contaminants, additives, monomers and degradation products must be conducted by choosing appropriate solvent systems that will yield the maximum extraction of leachable materials to conduct biocompatibility testing.

The effects of sterilization on device materials and potential leachables, and also toxic by-products, as a consequence of sterilization should be considered. Therefore, testing should be performed on the final sterilized product or representative samples of the final sterilized product.

United States Pharmacopeial Testing

The earliest guidance on what testing was to be done on medical devices was that provided in the USP and other pharmacopoeias. Each of the major national pharmacopoeias offers somewhat different guidance. The test selection system for the USP (presented in **Table 3**), which classified plastics as Classes I–VI, is now obsolete and replaced in usage by the other guidelines presented here. However, the actual descriptions of test types, as provided in the USP (and presented in the appropriate chapters elsewhere in this book) are still very much in operation (USP, 1990).

There are British, European and Japanese pharmacopoeias, of which the last requires the most attention because of some special requirements that are still in operation if product approval is desired.

ISO Testing Requirements

The European Union has adopted a new set of testing guidelines for medical devices under the aegis of ISO

Table 3 Classification of plastics (USP XXII)

Plastic class[a]						Tests to be conducted			
I	II	III	IV	V	VI	Test material	Animal	Dose	Procedure[b]
×	×	×	×	×	×	Extract of sample in sodium chloride injection	Mouse	50 ml kg^{-1}	A (i.v.)
	×	×	×	×			Rabbit	0.2 ml per animal at each of 10 sites	B
×	×	×	×	×		Extract of sample in 1 in 20 solution of alcohol in sodium chloride injection	Mouse	50 ml kg^{-1}	A (i.v.)
×	×	×	×	×			Rabbit	0.2 ml per animal at each of 10 sites	
	×		×	×		Extract of sample in polyethylene glycol 400	Mouse	10 g kg^{-1}	A (i.p.)
		×	×	×			Rabbit	0.2 ml per animal at each of 10 sites	A (i.p.)
		×	×	×	×	Extract of sample in vegetable oil	Mouse	50 ml kg^{-1}	B
			×	×	×		Rabbit	0.2 ml per animal at each of 10 sites	
		×		×	×	Implant strips of sample	Rabbit	4 strips per animal	C

[a] Tests required for each class are indicated by × in appropriate rows.

[b] A (i.p.), systemic injection test (intraperitioneal); A (i.v.) systemic injection test (intravenous); B, intracutaneous; C, implantation test (intramuscular implantation).

The table lists the biological tests that might be applied in evaluating the safety of medical devices and/or polymers. This does not imply that all the tests listed under each category will be necessary or relevant in all cases. Tests for devices made of metals, ceramics, biological materials, etc., are not included here but are under consideration. Categorization of medical devices is based on body contact and contact duration.

(ISO, 1992; Gray Sheet, 1992). The ISO 10993 guidelines for testing provide a unified basis for international medical device biocompatibility evaluation, in terms of both test selection (as presented in **Tables 4 and 5**) and test design and interpretation. In 1996, the US FDA also announced that it would adhere to ISO 10993 standards for device biocompatability evaluation.

This international standard specifies methods of biological testing of medical and dental materials and devices and their evaluation with regard to their biocompatibility. Because of the many materials and devices used in these areas, the standard offers a guide for biological testing. Committees dealing with materials and devices must decide on tests and test series relevant to the respective materials and devices. It is the responsibility of the product committees to select adequate test methods for products. The standard contains animal tests, but tries to reduce those tests to the justifiable minimum. Relevant international and national regulations must be observed when animals are used.

ISO 10993 is based on existing national and international specifications, regulations and standards wherever possible. It is open to regular review whenever new research work is presented to improve the state of scientific knowledge.

Table 4 ISO initial evaluation tests

Device categories	Body contact duration[a]	Cytotoxicity	Sensitization	Irritation or Intracutaneous	Acute systemic toxicity	Subchronic toxicity	Mutagenicity	Pyrogenicity	Implantation	Haemocompatability
Surface devices:										
Skin	A	×	×	×						
	B	×	×	×						
	C	×	×	×						
Mucous membranes	A	×	×	×						
	B	×	×	×						
	C	×	×	×		×	×			
Breached surface	A	×	×	×						
	B	×	×	×						
	C	×	×	×		×	×			
Externally communicating:										
Blood path indirect	A	×	×	×				×		×
	B	×	×	×				×		×
	C	×	×		×	×	×	×		×
Tissue/bone communicating	A	×	×	×						
	B	×	×				×		×	
	C	×	×				×		×	
Internal devices:										
Circulating blood	A	×	×	×	×			×		×
	B	×	×	×	×		×	×		×
	C	×	×	×	×	×	×	×		×
Implant devices:										
Bone/tissue	A	×	×	×						
	B	×	×				×		×	
	C	×	×				×		×	
Blood	A	×	×	×	×			×	×	×
	B	×	×	×	×		×	×	×	×
	C	×	×	×	×	×	×	×	×	×

[a] A, limited exposure; B, prolonged or repeated exposure; C, permanent contact.

Table 5 ISO special evaluation tests

Device categories	Body contact duration[a]	Chronic toxicity	Carcinogenicity	Reproductive/developmental	Degradation
			Biological tests		
Surface devices:					
Skin	A				
	B				
	C				
Mucous membranes	A				
	B				
	C				
Breached surface	A				
	B				
	C				
Externally communicating:					
Blood path indirect	A				
	B				
	C	×	×		
Tissue/bone communicating	A				
	B				
	C		×		
Internal devices:					
Circulating blood	A				
	B				
	C	×	×		
Bone/tissue	A				
	B				
	C	×	×		
Blood	A				
	B				
	C	×	×		

[a] A, limited exposure; B, prolonged or repeated exposure; C, permanent contact (time limits to added)

Medical Device Directive Guideline

The EEC had adopted its own guidance, Council Directive 93/42/EEC, for manufacturers of medical devices (European Committee for Standardization, 1991; Gray Sheet, 1992). According to the preamble of the MD Directive, the classification rules are 'based on the vulnerability of the human body taking account of the potential risks associated with the technical design and Manufacture of the devices'. The classification rules are presented in Annex IX of the MD Directive. Implementation of the MD Directive requires that the classification rules are applied in accordance with the intended purpose, or most critical specified use, of a device. Should more than one rule apply, the strictest takes precedence.

Except for the special rules 13–18, which will probably not be combined with the active device rules, the classification rules contained in Annex IX distinguish between two categories of device: non-invasive and invasive, Both of these categories are further divided into four rules. Among non-invasive devices, distinction is made among:

■ Devices for channelling or storing substances for infusion, administration or introduction into the body;
■ Devices for the biological or chemical modification of liquids for infusion;
■ Devices that come into contact with injured skin;
■ All other non-invasive devices.

Invasive devices are divided into those that are introduced into natural body orifices and those that are surgically introduced into the body. Classification criteria of the surgically introduced devices include:

■ Duration (transient, short-term or long-term use);
■ Interaction (biological, chemical or ionizing radiation);
■ Location (heart, central circulatory or central nervous systems).

Four additional rules are stated for active medical devices, and within these a distinction is made among:

■ Devices used for therapy;
■ Devices for diagnosis;
■ Devices for the administration and/or removal of substances to and from the body;
■ All other active devices.

Classification criteria for medical devices are based on potential hazards, taking into account the:

■ Nature, density and site of energy application;
■ Substance involved;
■ Part of the body concerned;
■ Mode of application or immediate danger to the patient in respect to cardiac performance, respiration and/or central nervous system.

Reduction of non-active characteristics. By combining active and non-active characteristics, the following assumptions regarding active medical devices were made:

■ Only those non-active characteristics that would lead to a higher class were considered; therefore, all Class I characteristics of rules 1–8 were omitted.

■ Implantable and long-term surgically invasive devices (rule 8) that are also active should be covered by the Active Implantable Medical Device (AIMD) Directive 90/385/EEC (although definitions of 'implantable' in the AIMD and MD Directives are slightly different);

■ Connection to another active medical device, as described in rules 2 and 5, will not change the class of an active medical device;

■ Energy supplied in the form of ionizing radiation (rules 6 and 7) is sufficiently covered under rule 10;

■ Because surgically invasive active devices are not intended to be wholly or mainly absorbed by, or chemically changed in, the body (rules 6 and 7), these characteristics were omitted. Devices 'intended to administer medicines' (rules 6 and 7) are sufficiently covered under rule 11.

ROAD MAP TO TESTING

Determining what testing is required for the development and approval of a new medical device can be a complex issue. This is even more the case after the issue of when to perform necessary tests is factored in. Post-approval, one must determine what ongoing testing is required to ensure continued safety of the product. Understanding the complexities requires careful consideration of some key concepts.

Key Concepts

There are 10 major categories on consideration in evaluating and establishing the safety of a medical device, and in so doing defining what testing must be performed. These are listed in **Table 6**, and will each be considered in detail in this section.

Table 6 Key concepts in medical device safety assessment

1. Condition of use
2. Materials/components/products
3. Chemical and physical property considerations
4. Factors of influence
5. Prior knowledge
6. Types and uses of tests
7. Reasonable man
8. Qualification versus process control
9. Tiers of concern: consumers health care providers and manufacturing employees
10. Sterilization and cleanliness

Condition of Use

The starting point for evaluating the safety of a near (or potential) medical device (or material for use in devices)

must be understanding both how it is intended to be used (which governs the type of contact it will have with the end-use consumers, i.e. patients, and therefore the areas of potential risk and the applicable regulations) and how it is likely to be used (or misused).

Intended use starts with developing an objective statement of what purpose the device is to serve, and therefore how it is to be in contact with the patient [skin/body surface, only body cavity, indirectly with a fluid path (such as and most commonly the blood stream) within the body] and for how long there is to be patient contact. The categories for type of contact are drawn from the nation's regulatory guidelines presented earlier, but actual devices may fit in several categories. It is also important to know more details of the contact (such as what body cavity contact is with—mouth, nose, vagina, anus, etc.).

The duration of exposure in use should also be established. This should be the cumulative duration for any patient, and not just the single time/use duration (that is, if a device is to be used for 5 min per day each day for a week, it should be considered to have an approximately 35 min cumulative patient exposure). For most devices, the intended use for any one patient is a single time. However, if the device (say a glove) is used by a health care provider, over the course of a day, cumulative exposure can be extensive.

One must also consider unintended uses or expected abuses of the device. People may use devices in ways that are not planned, such as using elastic bandages to cover wounds. Such is especially (but not exclusively) the case for children and the elderly, who are more likely to be susceptible to adverse effects. It should also be kept in mind that, although many electronic devices (disposable gloves and syringes, for example) are intended to be single-use disposables, in poorer cultures this frequently may not be the case. One cannot guard against every—or even the most unusual—device usage, but one should exercise some consideration as to what the most likely misuses are.

Materials, Components and Products

What is actually sold for use by 'or on the end-use consumer (the patient)' is what is regulated by the various government agencies. This is the product, which must be evaluated for biocompatibility in conformance with applicable guidelines, in the form or forms (sterilized or unsterilized) that it is intended to be sold.

However, products are frequently composed of components. Simple examples are a disposable syringe (needle, barrel, plunger, lubricant and stopper) or a surgical prep set (scrub, disinfectant, razor, etc.). Changing a component can significantly alter the biocompatibility of a product. Also, certain components, by the nature of both their composition and exposure to patients, are more likely to present biocompatibility problems. An example is the common disposable plastic syringe, of which billions are used each year. For the syringe, the most likely problem component is the stopper—the flexible piece at the end of the plunger. The stopper is most commonly made of natural rubber, and has direct contact with fluids entering the body (and frequently a fluid path). This is the most common problem component for a syringe.

Components, of course, are manufactured from or composed of materials. Materials (polymers, elastomers, steel, etc.) are the fundamental starting point for development of a device, and are very frequently not produced by the device (or component) manufacturer, but are rather provided by an outside vendor.

Almost all biocompatability problems (the exceptions being due to sterility, sterilization and cleanliness) for devices are due to the materials used in a device. **Table 7** provides a concise list of material-based considerations for safety of a device.

Table 7 Raw material characterization

Chemical Characterization:
- List materials
- List potential extractables or leachables from materials
- Physicochemical tests, USP:
    water and propan-2-ol extracts
- International pharmacopoeial tests
- Infrared analysis:
    document polymer identification
- Chromatographic characterization:
    molecular weight distribution
    additive and/or extract analysis
- Trace metals
- Specific gravity
- Moisture content

Physical Characterization:
- Hardness
- Surface characterization
- Colour, opacity or haze
- Strength properties:
    tensile/elongation
    flexure
    compression
- Thermal analysis
- Viscosity, melting-point, refractive index

Biological characterization

Chemical and Physical Property Considerations

Engineers involved in the design and development of new medical devices are primarily concerned with the physical properties essential for the proper functioning of the device. Accordingly, the most important aspects of materials being used in device construction are its physical properties. Toxicologists and others responsible for device safety (the subject of this chapter) are primarily concerned with the chemical nature and properties of

materials used in devices, but must also be conversant with physical property considerations. For that reason, this section presents a primer on the chemical nature and chemical and physical properties of materials used in devices.

The majority of components of medical devices are constituted from a small number of categories of materials. The important categories of materials in device formulation and construction are the following: water, stainless steels, polymers, elastomers, silicones and natural fibres (cotton and wood pulp, primarily). Each of these needs to be considered in turn. Additionally, biologically derived materials are seeing increased utilization in devices (Kambric *et al.*, 1986), but are of such diverse nature that it is not currently possible to overview them adequately here.

There are interactions which occur between material used in a device and the organism ('host') with which it has contact. Device materials having systemic contact with a host ('biomaterials') may be degraded by the host by a number of chemical means which should be kept in mind when considering the use of any of the materials described in this section. These pathways of chemical degradation of biomaterials include:

- Hydrolysis (acid, base, neutral aqueous media);
- Oxidation (corrosion, chain cleavage);
- Thermolysis;
- Photo-oxidation;
- Specific enzyme-catalysed hydrolysis or oxidation;
- Attack by complex media (culture media, serum, blood, gastric juices, urinary fluids, phagocyte-containing fluid, etc.);
- Chain cleavage due to mechanical fracture.

Water

Water, in one way or another, is involved in the production of virtually every medical device. For many devices (particularly diagnostics), it is also incorporated into the device. Yet water tends to be invisible to many considering device biocompatability and safety.

Water's greatest uses are in cleaning and rinsing devices and their components. Purified water is obtained by distillation, ion-exchange treatment, reverse osmosis or other suitable processes. Such water is prepared from source material complying with the regulations of the US Environmental Protection Agency (US EPA) for drinking water. Water can be a problem in device safety and biocompatability, generally owing to the presence of things in it which do not comply with US EPA and other regulations (such as microorganisms, pesticides, organics, other pyrogens and heavy metals), and also contaminants from other devices or components which may have been previously rinsed in the water (such as latex from gloves or stoppers). Water is usually a source of problems in the production of devices and not in the development stage.

Metals

A variety of metals have significant use in medical devices, although, with the exception of stainless steel, their use in patient contacting situations is largely limited to implants. The uses are a reflection of the properties of the various metals, as summarized by Gad (1997).

Factors of influence

Actual decisions as to what testing is to be done are based on a complex set of reasons, some of which are particular to the company involved and some of which are generally applicable. The author labels these reasons as 'factors of influence', and believes that they can be summarized as belonging to the seven categories presented in **Table 8**. The first of these factors, regulatory requirements, was extensively covered in the first section. The others are discussed briefly here.

Table 8 Factors of influence on safety test selection

Regulatory requirements
Perceptions
Hazard identification
Risk assessment
Animal welfare concerns
Claims
Time and economics

Perceptions

It should be kept in mind that what people believe or perceive is as important as what is real. What materials are used, how a device is designed and what testing is done are significantly influenced by current public and health care provider beliefs. Concerns about and memories of silicones, latex, toxic shock syndrome, etc., may dictate more extensive testing than regulations. Beliefs can also influence device acceptance, such as the case of IUDs (intrauterine devices) as contraceptive devices after the publicity around the Dalkon Shield.

Hazard Identification

The most fundamental requirement in testing is to identify quickly (or eliminate the possibility of) any significant hazards, their services and how to eliminate or minimize them if they are present. Many of the tests used for medical devices are really designed to act as sensitive screens for hazards. They purposely maximize the potential to obtain a positive response (that is, they are very sensitive). Such tests share a number of common characteristics (see **Table 9**) and do not establish the relevance of such findings of hazard to real life device use.

Risk Assessment

The process of taking the results of toxicity and biocompatibility tests of literature findings and all other sources of information and then relating them to actual device use in the market place is risk assessment. The need to be able to perform a meaningful and convincing risk assessment may require additional tests which allow for the quantification of risk (which screens usually do not). Such tests are usually focused on a single, well defined end-point (such as mucosal irritation) as identified in a hazard identification test or screen, and have their own set of characteristics as summarized in **Table 9**. It should be stressed at this point that all substances (even water and green apples) are toxic at some dose. The real life hazard is when the dose at which harm may occur is within the realm of likely exposure. **Table 10** addresses the point of relative toxicity.

Table 9 Characteristics of screens and specific toxicity assay screens (Gad, 1994)

Screens:
  Assay for overt toxicity
  Macroscopic, qualitative data
  Dose not related to material application
  Limited definition of test substance
  Rapid
  Usually single exposure
  Small number of replicates
  No internal statistical validity
  Minimum false negatives and maximum false positives

Specific toxicity assays:
  Assay for no adverse effect level and toxic level
  Quantitative data
  Systematic observations on multiple end-points (health behaviour, nutrition, necroscopy, pathology, clinical chemistry, haematology, etc.)
  Specific data on strength, identity and purity of test material
  Short or long duration
  Quantitative extrapolation of safely allowed
  Single well defined end-point
  Formal internal statistical validity

Claims

Claims are what is said in labelling and advertising, and may be of either a positive (therapeutic or beneficial) or a negative (lack of an adverse effect) nature. The positive or efficacy claims are not usually the direct concern of the toxicologist, although it must be kept in mind that such claims both must be proved and can easily exceed the limits of the statutory definition of a device, turning the product into a drug or combination product.

Negative claims such as 'non-irritating' or 'hypoallergenic' also must be proved, and it is generally the responsibility of the product safety professional to provide proof. There are special tests for such claims.

Time and Economics

The final factors of influence or arbitrator of test conduct and timing are the requirements of the market place, the resources of the organization and the economic worth of the product.

Table 10 Classification of chemical hazards[a]

| Commonly used term | Routes of administration | | | | Probable lethal dose for man |
	Single oral dose, rats LD_{50}	Inhalation 4 h vapour exposure mortality 1/6–4/6 rats (ppm)	Single application to skin of rabbits LD_{50}	
Extremely toxic	$\leq 1\,mg\,kg^{-1}$	10	$\leqslant 5\,mg\,kg^{-1}$	A taste, a drop, 1 grain
Highly toxic	$1 - 50\,mg\,kg^{-1}$ [b]	10–100	5–$43\,mg\,kg^{-1}$	1 teaspoonful (4 ml)
Moderately toxic	50–$500\,mg\,kg^{-1}$	100–1000	44–$340\,mg\,kg^{-1}$	1 ounce (30 g)
Slightly toxic	0.5–$5\,g\,kg^{-1}$	1000–10000	0.35–$2.81\,g\,kg^{-1}$	1 pint (250 g)
Practically or non-toxic	5–$15\,g\,kg^{-1}$	10000–100000	$\geqslant 22.6\,g\,kg^{-1}$	> 1 quart or >1 l

[a] From Deichman and Gerard (1966) and Gad and Chengelis (1988).

[b] By law, those materials with oral LD_{50}s of 50 mg kg^{-1} or less in rats are classified as Class B poisons and must be labeled 'Poison' in the US. Class A poisons are defined not by testing, but rather by inclusion on a regulatorily mandated list (CFR 173, Section 173.326), as follows:

'S 173.326 Poison A.

(a) for the purpose of Parts 170–189 of this subchapter, extremely dangerous poison. Class A are poisonous gases or liquids of such nature that a very small amount of the gas, or vapour of the liquid, mixed with air is dangerous to life. This class includes the following: (1) Bromactone. (2) Cyanogen. (3) Cyanogen chloride containing less than 19% water. (4) Diphosgene. (5) Ethyldichloroarsine. (6) Hydrocyanic acid (see Note 1 of this paragraph). (7) [Reserved] (8) Methyldichlorarsine. (9) [Reserved] (10) Nitrogen peroxide (tetroxide). (11) [Reserved] (12) Phosgene (diphosgene). (13) Nitrogen tetroxide–nitric oxide mixtures containing up to 33.2% weight nitric oxide. Note 1: Diluted solutions of hydrocyanic acid of not exceeding 5% strength are classed as poisonous articles. Class B (see S 173–343)' (b) Poisonous gases or liquids, Class A as defined in paragraph (a) of this section, except as provided in S 173.331, must not be offered for transportation by rail express.

239 FR 18753, Dec. 29, 1964. Redesignated at 32 FR 5606, Apr. 5, 1967, and amended by:
Amdt. 173–94, 41 FR 16081, Apr. 15, 1976;
Amdt. 173–94A, 41 FR 40883, Sept. 20, 1976.

Plans for filings with regulatory agencies and for market launches are typically set before actual testing (or final stage development) is undertaken, as the need to be in the market place in a certain time frame is critical. Such timing and economic issues are beyond the scope of this chapter, but must be considered.

Prior Knowledge

The appropriate starting place for the safety assessment of any new chemical entity, particularly a potential new material for a medical device, is first to determine what is already known about the material and whether there are any close structural or pharmacological analogues (pharmacological analogues being agents with assumed similar pharmacological mechanisms). Such a determination requires complete access to the available literature. In using this information, one must keep in mind that there is both an initial requirement to build a data file or base and a need to update such a store on a regular basis. Updating a database requires not merely adding to what is already there, but also discarding out-of-date (i.e. now known to be incorrect) information and reviewing the entire structure for connections and organization.

The first step in any new literature review is to obtain as much of the following information as possible:

■ Correct chemical identity including molecular formula, Chemical Abstracts Service (CAS) Registry number, common synonyms, trade names and a structural diagram. Gosselin et al. (1984) and Ash

and Ash (1994, 1995) are excellent sources of information on existing commercial products and their components and uses.

■ Chemical composition (if a mixture) and major impurities.
■ Production and use information.
■ Chemical and physical properties (physical state, vapour pressure, pH, solubility, chemical reactivity, etc.)
■ Any structurally related chemical substances that are already on the market or in production.
■ Known or presumed biological properties.

Collection of the above information is not only important for hazard assessment (a high vapour pressure would indicate a high inhalation potential, and high and low pH would indicate a high irritation potential), but the prior identification of all intended use and exposure patterns may provide leads to alternative information sources; for example, drugs to be used as antineoplastics or antibiotics may already have extensive toxicological data obtainable from government or private sources. A great deal of the existing toxicity information (particularly information on acute toxicity) is not available in the published or electronic literature because of concerns about the proprietary nature of this information and the widespread opinion that it does not have enough intrinsic scholarly value to merit publication. This unavailability is unfortunate, as it leads to substantial replication of effort and expenditure of resources that could be better used elsewhere. It also means that an experienced toxicologist must use an informal search

Table 11 Published information sources for safety assessment

Title	Author, date
Annual Report on Carcinogens	National Toxicology Program, various
Burger's Medicinal Chemistry	Wolff, 1996
Carcinogenically Active Chemicals	Lewis, 1991
Catalog of Teratogenic Agents	Shepard, 1998
Chemical Hazards of the Workplace	Proctor and Hughes, 1978
Chemically Induced Birth Defects	Schardein, 1985
Clinical Toxicology of Commercial Products	Gosselin *et al.*, 1984
Contact Dermatitis	Cronin, 1980
Criteria Documents	NIOSH, various
Current Intelligence Bulletins	NIOSH, various
Dangerous Properties of Industrial Materials	Sax, 1985
Documentation of the Threshold Limit Values for Substances in Workroom Air	ACGIH, 1986
Handbook of Toxic and Hazardous Chemicals	Sittig, 1985
Hygienic Guide Series	AIHA, 1980
Hamilton and Hardy's Industrial Toxicology	Finkel, 1983
Medical Toxicology	Ellenhorn *et al.*, 1997
Merck Index	Budavari, 1989
NIOSH/OSHA Occupational Health Guidelines for Chemical Hazards	Mackison, 1981
Patty's Industrial Hygiene and Toxicology	Clayton and Clayton, 1981
Physician's Desk Reference	Barnhart, annual
Registry of Toxic Effects of Chemical Substances (RTECS)	NIOSH, 1984
Casarett and Doull's Toxicology: The Basic Science of Poisons	Klaassen, 1996
Toxicology of the Eye	Grant, 1993

of the unpublished literature of his colleagues as a supplement to searches of the published and electronic literature.

There are now numerous published texts that should be considered for use in literature-reviewing activities. An alphabetical listing of 23 of the more commonly used sources for safety assessment data is provided in **Table 11**. Obviously, this is not a complete listing and consists of only the general multi-purpose texts that have a wider range of applicability for toxicology. Texts dealing with specialized classes of agents (e.g. disinfectants) or with specific target organ toxicity (e.g. neurotoxins and teratogens) are generally beyond the scope of this text. Parker (1988) should be consulted for details on the use of these texts. Parker (1988), Wexler (1988) and Sidhu *et al.* (1989) should be consulted for more extensive listings of the literature and computerized databases.

Miscellaneous Reference Sources

There are some excellent published information sources covering some specific classes of chemicals, e.g. heavy metals, plastics, resins and petroleum hydrocarbons. The National Academy of Science series *Medical and Biologic Effects of Environment Pollutants* covers 10–15 substances considered to be environmental pollutants. *CRC Critical Reviews in Toxicology* is a well known journal that over the years has compiled over 20 volumes of extensive literature reviews of a wide variety of chemical substances. A photocopy of this journal's topical index will prevent one from overlooking information that may be contained in this important source. Trade organizations such as the Fragrance Industry Manufacturers Association and the Chemical Manufacturers Association have extensive toxicology databases from their research programmes that are readily available to toxicologists of member companies. Texts that deal with specific target organ toxicity, e.g. neurotoxicity, hepatotoxicity or haematotoxicity, often contain detailed information on a wide range of chemical structures. Published information sources such as the *Target of Organ Toxicity* series (Taylor & Francis, now halfway through revision) is an example of the types of publications that often contain important information on many industrial chemicals that may be useful either directly or by analogy. Upon discovery that the material that one is evaluating may possess target organ toxicity, a cursory review of these types of texts is warranted.

In the last decade and, for many toxicologists, the on-line literature search has changed from an occasional, sporadic activity to a semicontinuous need. Usually, non-toxicology-related search capabilities are already in place in many companies. Therefore, all that is needed is to expand the information source to include some of the databases that cover the types of toxicology information one desires. However, if no capabilities exist within an organization one can approach a university, a consultant or a private contract laboratory and utilize their on-line system at a reasonable rate. It is even possible to access most of these sources from home using a personal computer. The major available on-line databases are as follows:

A. National Library of Medicine.   The National Library of Medicine (NLM) information retrieval service contains the well known and frequently used Medline, Toxline and Cancerlit databases. Databases commonly used by toxicologists for acute data in the NLM service are the following:

1. Toxline (Toxicology Information Online) is a bibliographic database covering the pharmacological, biochemical, physiological, environmental and toxicological effects of drugs and other chemicals. It contains approximately 1.7 million citations, most of which are complete with abstract, index terms, and CAS Registry numbers. Toxline citations have publication dates from 1981 to the present. Older information is on Toxline 65 (pre-1965 to 1980).

2. Medline (Medical Information Online) is a database containing approximately 7 million references to biomedical journal articles published since 1966. These articles, usually with an English abstract, are

from over 3000 journals. Coverage of previous years (back to 1966) is provided by back files, searchable online, that total some 3.5 million references.

3. Toxnet (Toxicology Data Network) is a computerized network of toxicologically oriented data banks. Toxnet offers a sophisticated search and retrieval package that accesses the following three subfiles:

   a. Hazardous Substances Data Bank (HSDB) is a scientifically reviewed and edited data bank containing toxicological information enhanced with additional data related to the environment, emergency situations and regulatory issues. Data are derived from a variety of sources including government documents and special reports. This database contains records for over 4100 chemical substances.

   b. Toxicology Data Bank (TDB) is a peer-reviewed data bank focusing on toxicological and pharmacological data, environmental and occupational information, manufacturing and use data and chemical and physical properties. References have been extracted from a selected list of standard source documents.

   c. Chemical Carcinogenesis Research Information System (CCRIS) is a National Cancer Institute-sponsored database derived from both short- and long-term bioassays on 2379 chemical substances. Studies cover carcinogenicity, mutagenicity, promotion and cocarcinogenicity.

4. Registry of Toxic Effects of Chemical Substances (RTECS) is the NLM's on-line version of the National Institute for Occupational Safety and Health's (NIOSH) annual compilation of substances with toxic activity. The original collection of data was derived from the 1971 Toxic Substances Lists. RTECS data contain threshold limit values, aquatic toxicity ratings, air standards, National Toxicology Program carcinogenesis bioassay information and toxicological/carcinogenic review information. NIOSH is responsible for the file content in RTECS and for providing quarterly updates to NLM; RTECS currently covers toxicity data on more than 106 000 substances.

B. The Merck Index.   This is now available on-line for up-to-the minute access to new chemical entities.

Search Procedure

As mentioned earlier, chemical composition and identification information should already have been obtained before the chemical is searched for. With most information retrieval systems this is a relatively straightforward procedure. Citations on a given subject may be retrieved by entering the desired free text terms as they appear in titles, keywords and abstracts of articles. The search is then initiated by entering the CAS Registry number and/ or synonyms. If one is only interested in a specific target organ effect, e.g. carcinogenicity, or specific publication

years, searches can be limited to a finite number of abstracts before requesting a printout.

Often it is unnecessary to request a full printout (author, title, abstract). One may choose to review just the author and title listing before selecting the abstracts of interest. In the long run, this approach may save computer time, especially if the number of citations being searched is large.

Once one has reviewed the abstracts, the last step is to request photocopies of the articles of interest. Extreme caution should be used in making any final health hazard determination based solely on an abstract or non-primary literature source.

Monitoring Published Literature and Other Research in Progress

Although there are a few other publications offering similar services, the *Life Sciences* edition of *Current Contents* is the publication most widely used by toxicologists for monitoring the published literature. *Current Contents* monitors over 1180 major journals and provides a weekly listing by title and author. Selecting those journals one wishes to monitor is one means of selectively monitoring the major toxicology journals.

Another mechanism for monitoring research in progress is by reviewing abstracts presented at the annual meetings of professional societies such as the Society of Toxicology, Teratology Society, Environmental Mutagen Society and American College of Toxicology. These societies usually have their abstracts prepared in printed form; for example, the current *Toxicologist* contains over 1700 abstracts presented at the annual meeting. Copies of the titles and authors of these abstracts are usually listed in the societies, journals, which, in many cases, would be reproduced and could be reviewed through *Current Contents*.

Other Testing Considerations

Safety assessment tests used for medical devices can generally be considered as either hazard identification/ screens or special studies uniquely designed for specific problems or types of devices **(Table 9)**. The bulk of this chapter looks at how each of the significant types of such tests are performed and interpreted. Earlier in this chapter the author summarized the common varieties of available biocompatibility tests and their objectives, and also where in the text they are considered in detail.

Reasonable Man

The reasonable man is a concept in law which, though not universally applicable, still provides guidance as to what one can expect from those who use devices (and what, therefore, the limits are on uses for which the manufacturer of the device should be considered responsible for ensuring safety). The standard of reasonableness is obviously open to interpretation, but does provide a conceptual basis for determining which uses one must ensure a device is safe for (and for a precautionary label) and those which it is not. The 'test' employed in a legal sense is one of foreseeability, i.e. would a reasonable man in the defendant's position foresee a measurable risk to the plaintiff? (Madden, 1992).

Qualifications versus Process Control

Most of this chapter addresses testing from the point of view of what is done to quality a product—to get it access to the marketplace. Such testing is done, at a minimum, to meet specific regulatory requirements which one can

Table 11 Product and process validation

This is a series of qualification studies to demonstrate that manufacturing process controls are sufficient for preproduction quality assurance requirements and product specifications. Testing is performed to verify the effectiveness of such control and to evaluate the biological effects of processing aids added during manufacture.

Environmental control:
Environmental monitoring programme
Microorganism identification
Viable and non-viable particulate analysis

Manufacturing process control—initial qualification and ongoing control:
Raw material characterization (compare effects of process on characteristics determined in Phase I):
   infrared analysis
   cytotoxicity
   physicochemical tests (USP, JP, etc.)
Other materials characterization tests:
   bioburden testing
   process water system validation
Purified water monograph tests, USP
Water for injection monograph tests, USP:
   endotoxin concentrations (LAL testing)
   quality device cleaning processes
   package qualifications

Sterility:
Bioburden testing and organism identification
Biological indicator studies (sport count, D-value)
Sterilization cycle development
Sterilization cycle validation, plan for periodic revalidation
Dose determination studies (AAMI) plan for quarterly dose audits
Sterility tests
EO dissipation curve studies and assessment of user exposure levels (AAMI/ISO)
Package validation

Finished product qualification—single use or reusable:
Physical testing for function and performance stability
Chemical residues
Testing for bacterial endotoxins
   in vitro, limulus amoebocyte lysate (LAL)
   in vivo, rabbit pyrogen tests
Biocompatibility:
   cytotoxicity test
   haemocompatibility test
Special materials and device tests:
   chemistry tests
   microbiology tests
   toxicology tests
Non-viable particulate analysis
Label claim (instructions) for reusable devices:
   decontamination
   cleaning
   disinfection/sterilization
Other product specific testing
Shelf-life stability qualification:
   accelerated ageing studies
   real time ageing

Table 12 Routine testing

Release testing involves what is performed routinely to satisfy GMP and ISO requirements for finished product testing prior to the release of product for distribution. In addition, Phase IV includes testing that may be incorporated into the manufacturer's quality assurance audit programme by conducting periodic raw material and finished product testing in order to document that materials and product conform to specifications.

Release testing:
    Endotoxin concentration:
        Limulus amoebocyte lysate (LAL), USP
    Pyrogenicity:
        rabbit test, USP
    Safety test, USP:
        infusion/transfusion assemblies
    Sterility testing
    Microbial limit test, USP
    Cytotoxicity, USP/ISO
    Materials characterization

Periodic audit testing:
    Endotoxin concentration:
        limulus amoebocyte lysate (LAL), USP
    Pyrogenicity:
        rabbit test, USP
    Cytotoxicity:
        raw materials
        finished products
    In vitro haemolysis test for blood contract products
    EO residual testing
    Materials characterization
    Physical testing
    Particulate testing
    Bioburden testing

determine by consulting the appropriate guidelines. However, biocompatibility testing does not end once a product is approved for the market place. Rather, some form of testing must be conducted on an ongoing basis to ensure that the batches of product that enter the marketplace over time continue to be safe. The testing to be done to ensure this is generally specified in the device master file (DMF), but what tests are done and with what frequency are left to the judgment of the manufacturer (who is, however, charged in the GMPs with conducting an adequate programme of periodic testing to ensure the continued quality and safety of the product). Such testing is usually derived from the results of qualification testing and product and (manufacturing) process validation studies **(Table 11)**. Careful consideration and statistical analysis of these and the variables that are involved in the manufacturing process generally identify which biocompatibility tests best serve to identify when the product is not as it should be, either because the process is not under control (or there have been a series of small incremental changes which in summation have altered the process) or because changes in vendor supplied materials have occurred. A statistical analysis of the data will also clarify sampling strategies and required frequency of testing. This will lead to specification of a routine testing programme for lot release, most commonly utilizing the approaches shown in **Table 12**.

The DMF on plant manufacturing SOPs need to specify what happens when a lot fails routine or release testing. It is sometimes wise to have a conditional two-tier test scheme—an inexpensive but somewhat sensitive screening test (such as cytotoxicity) which is performed on some specified regular basis, and a second, more specific (and expensive) test which is conducted in those cases where a lot fails the screening test.

Tiers of Concern: Consumers, Health Care Providers and Manufacturing Employees

This chapter focuses primarily on the tests done to meet regulatory requirements for new product approval. Such requirements are intended to ensure the safety on the end-use consumer of devices, the patients. Knowing what the intended use and claims are for a product, it is generally easy to identify what routes, duration, and extent of 'exposure' or 'dosing' will be.

However, patients represent only the final tier of those who will be exposed to a device. There are (at least) two other tiers that we must consider. The others are the health care providers and those involved in actually producing and packaging the devices. Health care providers include nurses, doctors, laboratory technicians, pharmacists and public health workers. Although they do not use the devices on a daily basis, they will handle and apply or administer the products. As such, they will have different routes and durations of exposure which must be considered and evaluated for safety. Skin exposure in particular is likely to be more extensive.

Likewise, those involved in manufacturing and packaging the product will have significantly different exposures. For these individuals, we must also be concerned with exposure to materials used in device construction and formulation. Here, the potential for inhalation exposure is most likely.

Sterilization and Cleanliness

It goes without saying that microbial contamination of devices must be controlled and that appropriate steps must be taken to sterilize products and materials. The subject is addressed elsewhere in this volume in some detail. It should also be remembered, however, that the means of sterilization (ethylene oxide, radiation, chemical sterilization or steam) may affect device quality and also, in some cases, carry their own biocompatibility concerns. Here, residuals are the issue.

Finally, it must be stressed that cleanliness, in the sense of exclusion of foreign matter (even seemingly innocuous things such as lint and dust), is essential. If such foreign materials should gain entry to the body, they can trigger dangerous immune modulated responses (Turco and Davis, 1973). The FDA has specifically considered the problem of particles in medical devices from the perspective of physiological effects and provided guidance on the issue (Marlowe, 1980).

REFERENCES

ACGIH (1986). *Documentation of the Threshold Limit Values for Substances in Workroom Air*, 5th edn. American Conference of Governmental Industrial Hygienists, Cincinnati, OH.

AIHA (1980). *Hygienic Guide Series*, Vols I and II. American Industrial Hygiene Association, Akron, OH.

APHIS (1989). *Animal and Plant Health Inspection Service*. United States Department of Agriculture, *Fed. Regist.*, **54**, 36112–36163.

Ash, M. and Ash, I. (1994). *Cosmetic and Personal Care Additives, Electronic Handbook*. Gower, Brookfield, VT.

Ash, M. and Ash, I. (1995). *Food Additives, Electronic Handbook*. Gower, Brookfield, VT.

ASTM (1990a). *1990 Annual Book of ASTM Standards, Vol. 13.01, Medical Devices*. ASTM, Philadelphia, PA.

ASTM (1990b). Standardization in Europe: a success story. *ASTM Stand. News*, February, 38.

Barnhart, E. R. (1991). *Physician's Desk Reference*. Medical Economics, Oradell, NJ.

Budavari, S. (1989). *The Merck Index*, 11th edn. Merck, Rahway, NJ.

CDRH (1992). *Regulatory Requirements for Medical Devices: a Workshop Manual*. Center for Device and Radiological Health, HHS Publication FDA 92-4165. Food and Drug Administration, Washington, DC.

CDRH (1995a). *Premarket Notification (510(k)): Guidance Document for Contact Lens Car Products*. Center for Device and Radiological Health, Food and Drug Administration, Washington, DC.

CDRH (1995b). *Testing Guidelines for Class III Soft (Hydrophilic) Contact Lens Solutions*, Center for Device and Radiological Health, Food and Drug Administration, Washington, D.C.

CDRH (1995c). *Draft Guidance for the Content of Premarket Notifications for Menstrual Tampons*. Center for Device and Radiological Health, Food and Drug Administration, Washington, DC.

CFR (1992). FDA's policy statement concerning cooperative manufacturing arrangements for licensed biologics. *Fed. Regist.*, **57**, 55544.

Chengelis, C. P., Holson, J. F. and Gad, S. C. (1995). *Regulatory Toxicology*. Raven Press, New York.

Clayton, D. G. and Clayton, F. E. (1981). *Pattys Industrial Hygiene and Toxicology*, 3rd edn, Vols. 2A, 2B and 2C. Wiley, New York.

Cronin, E. (1980). *Contact Dermatitis*. Churchill Livingston, Edinburgh.

Deichman, W. and Gerard, H. (1966). *Toxicology of Drugs and Chemicals*. Academic Press, New York.

Ellenhorn, M. J., Schonwald, S., Ordog, G. and Wasserberger, J. (1997). *Medical Toxicology*, 2nd Edn. Elsevier, New York.

European Committee for Standardization (1991). *CEN Annual Report 1991*. European Committee for Standardization, Brussels.

FAO (1991). *Report of the FAO/WHO Conference on Food Standards, Chemicals in Food and Food Trade (in Cooperation with GATT)*, Vol. 1, FAO, Rome.

FDLI (1995). *Compilation of Food and Drug Laws*, Vols I and II. Food and Drug Law Institute, Washington, DC.

Finkel, A. J. (1983). *Hamilton and Hardy's Industrial Toxicology*, 4th edn. John Wright PSG, Boston.

Food and Drug Administration (1987). Good Laboratory Practice Regulations: Final Rule. *Fed. Regist.*, **52**, No. 172.

Gad, S. C. (1994). *In Vitro Toxicology*. Raven Press, New York.

Gad, S. C. (1997). *Safety Evaluation of Medical Devices*. Marcel Dekker, New York.

Gad, S. C. and Chengelis, C. P. (1988). *Acute Toxicology*. Telford Press, Caldwell, NJ.

Gad, S. C. and Taulbee, S. (1996). *Handbook of Data Recording, Maintenance and Management for the Biomedical Sciences*. CRC Press, Boca Raton, FL.

Goering, P. L. and Galloway, W. D. (1989). Toxicology of medical device material. *Fundam. Appl. Toxicol.*, **13**, 193–195.

Gosselin, R. E., Smith, R. P. and Hodge, H. C. (1984). *Clinical Toxicology of Commercial Products*, 5th edn. Williams and Wilkins, Baltimore.

Grant, W. M. (1993). *Toxicology of the Eye*, 4th edn. Charles C. Thomas, Springfield, IL.

Gray Sheet (1992). EC 'Medical Devices' Directive slated for adoption in mid-1993, EC Commission official says: CEN estimate development of 92 standards for Directive M-D-D-1 Reports. *The Gray Sheet*, October 12.

Gray Sheet (1996a). European Union Class III Device Approvals average 240 days or less, HIMA survey says: study release intended to bolster support for FDA reform legislation. *The Gray Sheet*, February 26, 7–8.

Gray Sheet (1996b). FDA 510(k) average review time for fiscal 1996 projected to be on par with FY 95 figure of 137 days: PMA average review time expected to drop to 250 days. *The Gray Sheet*, March 25.

Hutt, P. B. (1989). A history of government regulation and misbranding of medical devices. *Food Drug Cosmet Law J.*, **44**, (2), 99–117.

ISO (1992). *Biological Evaluation of Medical and Dental Materials and Devices*. ISO, Brussels.

Kahan, J. S. (1995). *Medical Devices—Obtaining FDA Market Clearance*. Parexel, Watham, MA.

Kambric, H. E., Muraboyoshi, S. and Nose, Y. (1986). Biomaterials in artificial organs. *Chem. Eng. News*, April 14, 30–48.

Klaassen, C. D. (1996). *Casarett and Doull's Toxicology*. McGraw-Hill, New York.

Lewis, R. J. (1991). *Carcinogenically Active Chemicals*. Van Nostrand Reinhold, New York.

Mackison, F. (1981). *Occupational Health Guidelines for Chemical Hazards*. Department of Health and Human Services, National Institute for Occupational Health and Safety/Occupational Safety and Health Administration (NIOSH)/Department of Labor (OSHA), DHHS no. 81–123, US Government Printing Office, Washington, DC.

Madden, M. S. (1992). *Toxic Torts Handbook*. Lewis, Boca Raton, FL.

MAPI (1992). The European Community's new approach to regulation of product standards and quality assurance (ISO 9000): what it means for US manufacturers, *MAPI Economic Report ET-218*, January.

Marlowe, D. E. (1980). *Particles in Medical Devices*. US Food and Drug Administration, National Technical Information Service (PB81-131625), US Department of Commerce, Springfield VA.

National Toxicology Program (1985). *Fourth Annual Report on Carcinogens*. Department of Health and Human Services, PB 85- 134633, US Government Printing Office, Washington, DC.

National Toxicology Program (1990) *Review of Current DHHS, DOE, and EPA Research Related to Toxicology*. Department of Health and Human Services, NTP-85-056, US Government Printing Office, Washington, DC.

National Institute for Occupational Safety and Health. *NIOSH Criteria for a Recommended Standard for Occupational Exposure to XXX*. Department of Health, Education and Welfare, Cincinnati, OH.

NIOSH (19XX). *Current Intelligence Bulletins*. National Institute for Occupational Safety and Health, Department of Health, Education and Welfare, Cincinnati, OH.

NIOSH (1984). *Registry of Toxic Effects of Chemical Substances*, 11th edn., Vols 1–3. National Institute for Occupational Safety and Health, Department of Health and Human Services, DHHS No. 83–107, 1983, and RTECS Supplement DHHS 84–101, Washington, DC.

O'Grady, J. (1990). Interview with Charles M. Ludolph. *ASTM Stand. News*, February, 26.

Parker, C. M. (1988). Available toxicology information sources and their use. In Gad, S. C. (Ed.), *Product Safety Evaluation Handbook*. Marcel Dekker, New York pp. 23–41.

Proctor, N. H. and Hughes, J. P. (1978). *Chemical Hazards of the Workplace*. J. B. Lippincott, Philadelphia, PA.

Regulatory Affairs Focus (1996). European update. *Regulatory Affairs Focus*, **1** (4), 8.

Sax, N. I. (1985). *Dangerous Properties of Industrial Materials*, 6th edn. Van Nostrand Reinhold, New York.

Schardein, J. L. (1985). *Chemically Induced Birth Defects*. Marcel Dekker, New York.

Shepard, T. H. (1998). *Catalog of Teratogenic Agents*, 9th edn. Johns Hopkins University Press, Baltimore.

Sidhu, K. S., Stewart, T. M. and Netton, E. W. (1989). Information sources and support networks in toxicology. *J. Am. Coll. Toxicol.*, **8**, 1011–1026.

Sittig, M. (1985). *Handbook of Toxic and Hazardous Chemicals*, 2nd edn. Noyes Publications, Park Ridge, NJ.

Spizizen, G. (1992). The ISO 9000 standards: creating a level playing field for international quality. *Nat. Productivity Rev.*, Summer.

Turco, S. and Davis, N. M. (1973). Clinical significance of particular matter: a review of the literature. *Hosp. Pharm.*, **8**, 137–40.

USP (1990). Biological tests—plastics. In *The United States Pharmacopeia, XXI Revision*. United States Pharmacopeial Convention, Rockville, MD, pp. 1235–1238.

Wexler, P. (1988). *Information Resources in Toxicology*, 2nd edn. Elsevier, New York.

Wilkerson Group (1995). *Forces Reshaping the Performance and Contribution of the US Medical Device Industry*. Health Industry Manufacturers Association, Washington, DC.

Wolff, M. E. (1996). *Burger's Medicinal Chemistry*. Wiley, New York.

PART NINE

ISSUES RELEVANT TO TOXICOLOGY

Chapter 78
Radiation Toxicology

Gerald E. Adams, Angela Wilson and Roy Hamlet

C O N T E N T S

INTRODUCTION

The Nature of Radiation Action

Ionizing radiation causes many different types of damage in mammalian systems. These include effects in both proliferative and non-proliferative tissues, the induction of genetic abnormalities that in some circumstances can be passed on to offspring and the induction of malignancy. The nature and severity of radiation-induced effects can vary with radiation type, the magnitude of the radiation dose and the period over which it is delivered, the age, sex and health status of the individual and, particularly, the degree of post-irradiation care that may be available.

The energies of radiation emanating from X-ray sets, many radionuclides and particle accelerators are usually vastly in excess of the chemical bonds that are present in all biological molecules. Following interactions between radiation and any molecule, simple or complex, electron ejection, or ionization, is the primary event. The time-scale is governed by various factors, but a quantum of gamma-radiation or a high-energy particle will pass through a small molecule and impart energy to it in times of the order of 10^{-17}s. The subsequent physical, chemical and biological processes are complex and occur over very different time-scales. For example, the onset of malignancy does not occur in many instances until 20 or even 30 years after irradiation.

It is often convenient, although not necessarily rigorous, to classify radiation action into physical, chemical, cellular and tissue effects.

The Physical and Chemical Stages

Radiation deposits energy in discrete packages in 'tracks' through the absorbing medium. The spatial distribution of energy deposition depends on the type of radiation, the composition of the medium and the energy of the radiation. The so-called densely ionizing radiations such as α-particles, neutrons and heavier particles, lose energy over much shorter distances than low linear energy transfer (LET) radiations such as X- or γ-rays. LET is a measure of the rate at which energy is imparted to the absorbing medium per unit distance of track length. The biological effectiveness of the former type is generally greater in inducing most types of biological effect, including malignancy. Particulate radiations, with the exception of neutrons, are absorbed over short distances, except at extremely high energies. Following primary ionizations, the secondary electrons, which are still highly energetic, lose energy by various collisional and other interactions, thereby producing other ions, excited molecules and molecular fragments.

The chemical stage of radiation action is mainly concerned with the formation, diffusion and eventual reaction of the molecular fragments and other unstable entities. Because of the high energy of the radiations relative to the normal bond energies in molecules, radiation is absorbed fairly non-selectively. This is not necessarily true in all cases, particularly in materials abundant in heavy atoms, but it is certainly a sound approximation in biological material. The 'principle of equipartition of energy' implies that, in cellular material, about 80% of the energy is initially deposited in the aqueous component. This is why so much attention has been given in the past to the study of the radiation chemistry of water, particularly aqueous solutions or mixtures containing various biological molecules. There is now abundant evidence that damage to such molecules, particularly the nucleic acids, caused by free radicals, contributes to loss or change of intracellular function following irradiation. The continuing problem, however, is to distinguish those processes that are relevant to the observed cellular response to radiation from those that are not.

The Cellular Stage

Various morphological changes in the cell can often be observed shortly after irradiation. Local protrusions of the plasma membrane follow within minutes of exposure to relatively high doses of radiation. These are followed within hours by other membrane changes, including an increase in permeability and loss of essential enzymes. However, the more important effects concerning the loss of, or changes in, cellular function that occur at much lower doses can only be observed much later. For clonogenic cells *in vitro*, loss of reproductive capacity is evident only when the cells fail to divide. Subcellular effects, such as mutation and the induction of aberrant chromosomes, can only be observed when sufficient cell divisions have taken place to permit analysis. Mammalian cells are often at their most sensitive during mitosis and early in G phase. Resistance is usually greatest during early S phase, although this is very dependent on radiation quality, i.e. the type of radiation.

Repair processes occur in irradiated cells both *in vitro* and *in vivo*. When radiation is delivered at a low dose rate or in a series of multiple fractions separated by several hours, the overall effect on cell kill is usually less than that for an acute dose of radiation. This phenomenon, more commonly seen with low LET radiation, is attributable to repair of sublethal injury. It is relevant to dose–response relationships for cell kill and various sublethal effects such as mutation and cell transformation. Repair processes of various kinds occur both *in vitro* and *in vivo* and are responsible for the reduced severity of some radiation injuries when the exposure is protracted.

Radiation dose to tissue is expressed in terms of the quantity of absorbed energy per unit mass. The SI unit is the gray (Gy), which is defined as 1 joule of absorbed energy per kilogram. The older unit, the rad, which is still in common use, is equivalent to 100 erg g^{-1} and is equal to 0.01 Gy. A dose of 1 Gy of X-rays will cause about 2×10^5 separate ionizations within the mammalian cell. Of these, about 1% occur in the genomic material and a major consequence of this is breakage of DNA strands. Of the many breaks that occur, almost all disappear within a few hours, probably by enzyme-mediated repair. Some breaks remain, however, probably as aligned double-strand breaks, and these are the major cause of loss of cell viability and also contribute to various types of sublethal injury. In many mammalian cells it is remarkable that, for this high dose of radiation, a substantial population of the cells retain a degree of reproductive capacity despite the large amount of chemical damage sustained by the cells. Much of the initial chemical damage caused by the radiation must therefore be of little consequence to the fate of the cell. It is likely that only a small part of the damage, caused perhaps by the fairly rare local deposition of energy close to critical molecular sites, is important.

The Tissue Stage

The response time of mammalian tissues to radiation varies widely, as do their sensitivities. The general finding *in vitro* that mammalian cells are at their most radiation sensitive during mitosis predicts that *in vivo* the mammalian fertilized egg cell (zygote) will be highly radiation sensitive and that tissues with high rates of cell turnover will also be particularly sensitive. Both predictions are correct. Rapidly proliferating stem cells of the intestinal epithelium and the haematopoietic system are highly sensitive and respond more rapidly than do less sensitive cells, such as those in the lung and the basal layer of the skin, which have lower proliferation rates. Cells that do not divide, or do so only after an appropriate stimulus, e.g. parenchymal cells of the liver, are even less sensitive. Cells that divide only during embryogenesis are the least sensitive.

In this chapter, the nature, origin and expressions of radiation injury are classified according to the organ in which it occurs, and particularly with regard to the stochastic or deterministic (non-stochastic) nature of the pathological response. [Note: the International Commission on Radiological Protection (ICRP) made the distinction between stochastic and non-stochastic effects (ICRP, 1977). ICRP more recently redefined non-stochastic effects as *Deterministic effects* and although the latter is used in this chapter, readers should be aware that the term non-stochastic is still current in some areas of the literature.] Stochastic effects are those for which the probability of an effect occurring, but not its severity, increases with radiation dose, without a threshold. In contrast, deterministic effects are those for which the severity of the effect depends on the magnitude of the dose, and for which a threshold dose exists, below which no detrimental effects are observable. The types of damage that result from injury to substantial populations of cells in tissues such as the eye, skin, lung, gonads, gastro-intestinal tract and haematopoietic system are considered to be deterministic. On the other hand, stochastic effects can result from injury to a single cell or to a small number of cells, and include the induction of various hereditary defects and most types of cancer.

A further distinction is often made between the somatic and hereditary effects of radiation. Somatic effects refer to those which are manifest in the exposed individual, and include both deterministic and stochastic effects. The hereditary effects of radiation are of a stochastic nature and are transmitted via germ cell damage. The effects may be expressed in the immediate offspring or in later generations. **Figure 1** (ICRP, 1984) illustrates the essential features of stochastic and deterministic effects.

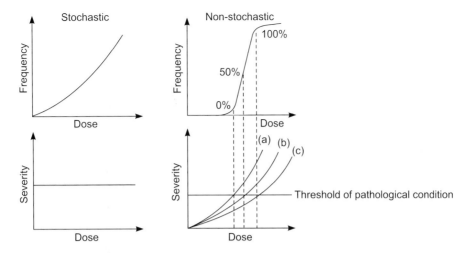

Figure 1 Dose–effect curves illustrating stochastic and deterministic (non-stochastic effects). The upper and lower plots on the right of the figure show how the frequency and severity of a given radiation injury of a deterministic type increase with radiation dose in a population of mixed susceptibilities (a, b and c). The severity increases most rapidly with dose in the most sensitive group (curve a) and reaches a level of clinical detectability at a dose lower than those for the other two subgroups (curves b and c). The upper and lower plots on the left illustrate that the frequency of a stochastic effect increases with radiation dose, but not the severity. Redrawn from ICRP (1984).

DETERMINISTIC EFFECTS

General

Deterministic radiation effects are due to radiation-induced cell killing with the accompanying disruption of functions for which the cells are responsible.

Cell death is most likely to occur when the irradiated cells attempt to resume dividing. This leads to a lack of replacement of mature cells which have been lost through natural senescence and death. For certain cell types, including lymphocytes and oocytes, radiation-induced cell deaths occur during interphase. In general, the rate at which cells divide, differentiate, age and are lost from a given tissue will influence the rapidity with which that tissue exhibits radiation damage. Those tissues containing actively dividing cells will tend to exhibit greater radiosensitivity than do those composed of fully differentiated cells with little or no mitotic activity.

The life-span of the comparatively radioresistant mature cells represents a further factor influencing the interval between irradiation and the time when damage becomes evident in tissues with well defined stem cell populations. In the case of fractionated or protracted exposures, stem cell division can partially compensate for cell killing and so reduce the effectiveness of the radiation.

Populations containing cells with a relatively short life-span, e.g. the gastro-intestinal mucosa, will exhibit radiation damage much more quickly than populations where the cell life-span is longer, e.g. blood cells of the circulatory system. On this basis, it is possible to distinguish between early effects, which may appear within a few weeks, depending on the pattern of exposure, and later effects, which do not appear until months or years after irradiation.

In those tissues which lack a well defined stem cell population and exhibit low cellular proliferations, radiation effects, although dose dependent, may not appear for some time. These tissues, e.g. the liver, where the turnover of parenchymal cells is low, have much less protection from the effects of radiation in the absence of an ability to compensate for cell killing through stem cell proliferation.

Other factors, besides the proliferative ability of cells in a given tissue, which may contribute to a reduction in the effects of irradiation, include tissue repopulation by surviving cells, the ability of differentiating, maturing and functioning cells to buffer stem cell damage, the ability of a tissue to undergo compensatory changes to maintain the supply of differentiated cells and the tissue's functional reserve capacity.

The severity and clinical expression of deterministic effects will differ, depending on whether an individual has received a partial or whole-body irradiation. Whole-body exposures at doses of between a few and tens of grays of acute irradiation, i.e. delivered over a short time interval, may result in the development of the haemato-poietic, gastro-intestinal or cerebral syndromes. Partial-body irradiation at sufficiently high doses may result in damage to self-renewing tissues, including the skin and skin adnexa, bone marrow, gastro-intestinal lining, testis and lens of the eye, and to other radiosensitive tissues, including the ovary, lung, central nervous system and kidney. Specific functioning in each of these tissues is impaired, owing to the radiation-induced loss of parenchymal cells. To some extent damage may persist even after repair and repopulation, due to the relative increase in connective tissue. This may lead to tissue fibrosis following the loss of parenchymal cells and associated functions.

In the following sections the deterministic effects resulting from whole and partial body irradiation are considered in detail. Subsequently the stochastic effects, namely radiation carcinogenesis and hereditary defects, are examined. The effects resulting from *in utero* irradiation are also discussed, although these are not easily classified as stochastic or deterministic.

Whole-body Irradiation

In man, death may occur within a few weeks following acute radiation exposure. The survival time and mode of death are dose dependent. A dose of 100 Gy can cause death from neurological damage within a few hours; 5–12 Gy can cause death from gastro-intestinal injury within a few days; and 2.5–5 Gy may cause death from irreversible damage to the haematopoietic system in several weeks. The prodromal syndrome (see below) develops shortly after irradiation, and precedes the onset of neurological, gastro-intestinal and haematopoietic syndromes. Although the exact cause of death in the neurological syndrome is uncertain, depletion of the stem cells in the critical self-renewing tissues of the gut epithelium and circulating blood cells causes death in the gastro-intestinal and haematopoietic syndromes, respectively. Differences in the population kinetics of the gut epithelium and haematopoietic system, and the amount of damage that can be tolerated by each before death, are responsible for differences in the doses at which death occurs and for the different times of onset.

The Prodromal Syndrome

The prodromal syndrome comprises the symptoms and signs that appear within 48 h of irradiation. It is mediated through the autonomic nervous system, and appears as gastro-intestinal and neuromuscular symptoms. After an acute dose of 4–5 Gy, the principal symptoms include anorexia, nausea, vomiting and fatigue. At higher doses the symptoms include diarrhoea, fever, sweating, listlessness, headache and apathy. Vomiting is infrequent at doses below 1 Gy. Prodromal symptoms may occur within an hour or so following irradiation, persist for a few days and then gradually diminish in intensity.

The Haematopoietic Syndrome

Uniform whole-body irradiation with 1–10 Gy of low-LET radiation causes damage to the haematopoietic system. Proliferating haematopoietic stem cells are highly radiosensitive and are sterilized by radiation, thereby reducing the body's supply of red and white cells and platelets. The full effect of the damage is not experienced until the number of circulating cells in the blood reaches a critical minimum value. In human bone marrow the total number of nucleated cells is reduced at day 1 by 10–20% after 1–2 Gy, by 25–30% after 3–4 Gy, by 50–60% after 5–7 Gy and by a maximum of 80–85% after 8–10 Gy. Resistant cells such as macrophages, stromal cells, cells of vascular epithelium and some mature granulocytes and eosinophils remain (IAEA, 1971).

The lymphocyte count is the most sensitive index of radiation injury in the blood; for a given dose, nadir levels are reached earlier than for other cell types. Lymphocytes undergo interphase death and their numbers decrease to about 50% of normal by 48 h following a dose of 1–2 Gy.

Neutrophils show an initial increase over the first few days after irradiation, then a dose-related fall. Between 10 and 15 days after a dose of 2–5 Gy, there is a second abortive rise due to recovering haematopoiesis from precursor cell populations, followed by a second decline to about day 25. This is due to a lack of recovery in the stem cell population. With doses greater than 5 Gy the second abortive rise does not occur. The time course for platelet loss is similar to that for granulocytes, but there is no second abortive rise. A decrease in platelet levels in the blood is associated with bleeding. Owing to the long lifespan of radioresistant red blood cells (109–127 days in man), anaemia results only when there has been substantial bleeding.

Figure 2 shows data from accident cases, depicting the average time courses for suppression and recovery of neutrophils, lymphocytes and platelets in man following irradiation.

Approximately 3 weeks after irradiation, symptoms including chills, fatigue, ulceration of the mouth and petechial haemorrhages of the skin develop as a result of the reduction in blood cell components. Infections and fever arise as a result of granulocyte depression and impairment of the immune system, while bleeding and possibly anaemia may develop from haemorrhage caused through platelet depression. Death, which is often caused by infection, will follow at this stage unless bone marrow regeneration has commenced. Where the radiation dose is less than 4–5 Gy, it is possible to treat the individual in response to specific symptoms, e.g. by administering antibiotics for infection until the immune system has fully recovered.

Humans develop signs of haematological damage and recover from it much more slowly than do other mammals. Peak incidence of death occurs at about 30 days after irradiation, although deaths may continue for up to 60 days. The 50% lethal dose or LD_{50} for man is therefore expressed as the $LD_{50/60}$ (i.e. the dose that causes 50% mortality within 60 days), in contrast to the $LD_{50/30}$ for most animal species, where the peak incidence of death occurs between 10 and 15 days after irradiation.

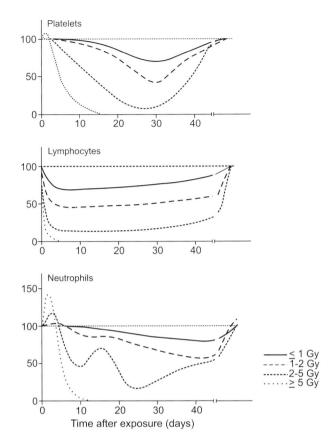

Figure 2 Schematic picture of average time courses for various cells in the blood after various doses of radiation in man. Curves derived from accident case data. Redrawn from UNSCEAR (1988).

The Gastro-intestinal Syndrome

A whole-body dose of 10 Gy or more of low LET radiation will produce the gastro-intestinal syndrome in most mammals, resulting in death 3–10 days later. Signs and symptoms follow those of the prodromal phase, and include nausea, vomiting, increased lethargy, prolonged diarrhoea, loss of appetite and loss of fluids and electrolytes. After a few days individuals show signs of dehydration, weight loss, gastric retention and decreased intestinal absorption, emaciation and complete exhaustion. There is a marked reduction in the leucocyte count, and haemorrhages and bacteraemia may occur, aggravating the injury and contributing to death. The symptoms and subsequent death are due to the radiation-induced damage to the epithelium lining the gastro-intestinal tract. A dose of about 10 Gy will sterilize a large proportion of the mitotic cells in the crypts of the intestinal mucosa. This arrests the continuous supply of new cells which normally move up the villi, differentiate to become functioning cells and eventually slough off. Sterilization of cells in the crypts prevents repopulation. After a few days, the villi begin to shrink and the intestinal lining is eventually denuded of villi.

The Neurological Syndrome

A radiation dose of more than about 100 Gy will cause death from cerebrovascular damage in most mammalian species within 2 days. The neurological syndrome is characterized by severe prodromal effects followed by transitory periods of depressed or enhanced motor activity. Severe nausea may occur within minutes, which is then followed by vomiting, disorientiation, loss of coordination and muscular movement, respiratory distress, diarrhoea, convulsive seizures, coma and eventually death.

The exact cause of death in the neurological syndrome is not fully understood. Although death is usually attributed to direct damage to the central nervous system, much higher doses are required to produce death if only the head is irradiated, which indicates that effects elsewhere in the body are also important. An increase in the fluid content of the brain due to leakage from small vessels creating a build-up of pressure inside the skull has been suggested as the cause of immediate death.

Effects from Partial Body Irradiation

Eye

The lens of the eye is one of the most radiosensitive tissues of the body. Exposure to ionizing radiation may cause a cataract, a term used to describe any detectable change in the normally transparent lens of the eye. This may range from tiny flecks in the lens to virtually complete opacification, causing blindness.

Radiation-induced cataracts arise through damage to the mitotic cells in the anterior epithelium of the lens. Under normal conditions these cells continue to proliferate throughout life and differentiate into lens fibres. Damage to the dividing cells results in abnormal lens fibres which are not translucent. These damaged cells and their breakdown products migrate posteriorly and accumulate beneath the capsule at the posterior pole of the lens, where they cause posterior displacement of the lens bow. If enough damaged cells accumulate, they become visible opthalmologically as a dot, usually situated at the posterior pole.

During the early stages, radiation-induced cataracts are unique in that, unlike other radiation-induced effects, they can be distinguished in most cases from cataracts resulting from other causes. As the cataract enlarges, small granules and vacuoles appear around it, and by the time the opacity is a few millimetres in diameter, it may have developed a clear centre and have assumed a doughnut shape. The radiation dose received will determine whether the cataract remains stationary or continues to progress. If the cataract progresses, it becomes indistinguishable from other types of cataract.

In humans, lens opacities may appear between 6 months and 35 years after irradiation. The latent period between irradiation and appearance of a cataract is dose related. At high doses, lens opacities develop within months, progress rapidly and produce vision-impairing cataracts. At lower doses the opacities develop more slowly, remain microscopic in size and cause no significant impairment of vision (Merriam *et al.*, 1972). A threshold dose of about 2 Gy of X-irradiation in a single exposure is required for the induction of minimally detectable lens opacities; larger doses are required with fractionated or protracted exposures (Merriam *et al.*, 1972). Compared with the lens, other parts of the eye are less radiosensitive.

Skin

The effect of radiation on the skin is dependent on various factors, including dose, the depth and area of skin irradiated and the anatomical location and its vascularity. It is also influenced by the age, hormonal status and genetic background of the irradiated individual. Within hours of irradiation, transitory erythema may occur, indicating capillary dilation brought about by the release of histamine-like substances from injured epithelial cells. Typically this persists for only a few hours. Two to four weeks later, one or more waves of deeper and more prolonged erythema usually appear. Thereafter, depending on the dose received, epilation, dry desquamation, moist desquamation and necrosis of the skin may occur.

The severity of the skin response is determined by the dose to the germinal cells in the basal layer of the epidermis. Since damage to these cells appears to be critical to the pathogenesis of erythema and desquamation, post-irradiation treatments using corticosteroids may decrease the severity of the desquamation reaction but will have no effect on erythema. In human skin, the threshold dose of X-or γ-rays required to produce erythema in a 10 cm^2 field ranges from 6–8 Gy for single, brief exposures to more than 30 Gy for highly fractionated or protracted exposures. Threshold doses for dry desquamation, moist desquamation and necrosis are higher, but also increase with fractionated or protracted exposures (Rubin and Casarett, 1968).

The effect of radiation-induced damage to the dermis appears later than it does to the epidermis or to the epidermal-associated hair follicles, principally because of the slower turnover of cell types in the dermis. The dermis contains connective tissue, sebaceous glands, muscle fibres, nerve plexuses and nerve fibres, sweat glands and blood vessels. The effects of high doses on blood vessels are visible as erythema and later as haemorrhages, which may appear as small (petechiae) or larger (purpura) lesions. The peak onset of purpura occurs 3–4 weeks after irradiation, and can be produced by doses of 4–6 Gy. Following high doses of radiation to the dermis, a second wave of erythema is produced as a result of damage to the deep dermal plexus of blood vessels.

Temporary epilation may result after a single brief exposure to 3–5 Gy of low-LET radiation and is most severe 2–3 weeks after irradiation. Permanent epilation

may occur after a single exposure to more than 7 Gy, or to 50–60 Gy fractionated over a period of weeks. Hair on the scalp is more sensitive than the beard or body hair.

Skin on the anterior aspect of the neck, antecubital and popliteal areas is most sensitive to radiation, followed by that on the anterior surfaces of extremities, the chest and abdomen. Thereafter, skin on the face (not strongly pigmented), the back and posterior surfaces of extremities, the face (strongly pigmented), the nape of the neck and the scalp are of decreasing sensitivity. Skin on the palms and soles is least sensitive to radiation.

The long-term effects of radiation on the skin, which develop months or years after exposure, include changes in pigmentation, atrophy of the epidermis, sweat glands, sebaceous glands and hair follicles, fibrosis of the dermis and increased susceptibility to trauma and chronic ulceration. These changes result in part from depletion of fibroblasts and in part from injury to blood vessels in the dermis. It is possible that the loss of epidermal cells may also contribute.

The Reproductive System

The germ cells of the ovary and testis are very radiosensitive and their irradiation impairs fertility in both sexes in a dose-dependent manner. In male mammals, spermatozoa are continuously produced in the seminiferous tubules of the testes. Spermatogonial stem cells divide to produce primary spermatocytes, which, in turn, give rise to secondary spermatocytes, spermatids and mature spermatozoa. In humans the development of mature sperm of spermatogonial stem cells takes about 10 weeks.

Spermatogonial stem cells are more radiosensitive than are postspermatogonial cell stages. The second and third stages of spermatogenesis, from preleptotene spermatocytes through to the spermatids, are not affected by doses of less than 3 Gy. After such doses, postspermatogonial cells mature and a normal sperm count can be maintained for approximately 46 days, the time period required for the development of spermatozoa from preleptotene spermatocytes. Thereafter, the sperm count will drop, approaching azoospermia by 10 weeks following a dose in excess of 1 Gy. Sterility will remain until the surviving 'stem' spermatogonia are able to repopulate the seminiferous tubules. In humans a dose of 2.5 Gy may cause temporary sterility for 1–2 years, and a dose of 6 Gy will often cause permanent sterility. The threshold dose for permanent sterility does not increase appreciably on fractionation of irradiation over days or even weeks.

The mature oocyte is the most radiosensitive germ cell stage in females. Exposure of both ovaries to an acute dose of more than 0.65–1.5 Gy can cause temporary sterility. With doses below 2–3 Gy, enough immature oocytes may survive to restore fertility. It has been estimated that the ovary can withstand 6–20 Gy of low-LET radiation in highly fractionated or protracted exposure regimes (Lushbaugh and Ricks, 1972; Lushbaugh and Casarett, 1976). The threshold dose for permanent sterility decreases with age, probably owing to the decrease in oocyte number with age.

An important consideration in germ cell irradiation is the potential increase in mutation incidence in the offspring. In general, irradiation of the female is less damaging than irradiation of the male with regard to the induction of mutations. This is due to the greater lethal radiosensitivity of mature oocytes, thereby decreasing the number of viable cells carrying mutations which could be passed to the offspring.

The genetic consequences of a given dose can be reduced if a time interval is allowed between irradiation and conception. This is due to the variation of radiation sensitivity with stage of germ cell development. In males, irradiation immediately prior to conception, so that mature sperm are irradiated, increases the senstivity to mutation induction. This is a direct consequence of the greater resistance of mature sperm cells to the lethal effects of radiation. If the time interval between irradiation and conception is longer, so that the sperm involved in fertilization are irradiated during an earlier developmental stage, then fewer mutations result.

The Digestive System

Radiation damage to the epithelial cells of the mucous membranes in the mouth and throat evokes inflammation and swelling, with ulceration and necrosis developing after high doses. Mucosal injury is greatest in the cheeks, soft palate and hypoglossal region, and less in the gums, hard palate, nose, posterior wall of the throat, tongue and larynx. Following doses of up to 10 Gy of low-LET radiation, the mucosal surfaces recover after 2–3 weeks. With doses of 10–20 Gy, extensive mucosal necrosis occurs after 4–5 days and recovery is much slower (1.5–2 months).

The salivary glands are radiosensitive but may recover even after high doses, provided that the dose is given in a fractionated regimen. Following 50–70 Gy of conventionally fractionated X-rays, the salivary glands undergo necrosis, atrophy and fibrosis, which result in reduced salivary flow (Rubin and Casarett, 1968). In humans there may be a loss of taste after doses as low as 2.4–4.0 Gy (Congar, 1973).

The glandular mucosa of the stomach, small intestine and colon respond more rapidly and tolerate less radiation in a single exposure than do the squamous cell mucosa of the oral cavity, pharynx, oesophagus and anus. Radiation damage to the germinal epithelium in the mucosa interferes with cell renewal and may cause ulceration and, possibly, denudation of the affected mucosae. Exposure of a large part of the intestine to an acute dose in excess of 10 Gy may lead to the induction of the rapidly fatal gastro-intestinal syndrome, as described earlier. With regard to long-term effects, fibrosis, stricture, intestinal perforation and fistula formation may develop months or years after exposure as complications arising from radiation injury to the gastro-intestinal tract (Rubin and Casarett, 1968).

Clinically, alimentary tract radiation damage following the use of radiation in anti-tumour therapy or pre-transplant total body irradiation is sufficiently severe to have generated a substantial literature. The complications generally relate to the onset of diarrhoea up to 4 weeks after irradiation and to the presence of fistulae and bleeding thereafter (Galland and Spencer, 1990; Hauer-Jensen, 1990; Coia et al., 1995; Spitzer, 1995). Many reports either describe the histopathology of the lesions or use a radiobiological assay for intestinal radiation injury. The pathological manifestations over a broad time-scale include inflammation, haemorrhage, ulceration, fibrosis, vascular distortion, necrosis and neoplasia (Busch, 1990). The radiobiological assay is based on radiation-induced DNA damage to cryptal proliferative cells, quantified by counting the number of surviving crypts or microcolonies per intestinal circumference in wax histology sections (Withers and Elkind, 1970). Although low doses produce no response in the dose–response curves, the method has been useful in determining the relative biological effectiveness of different types of radiation. Such data sets show that neutrons have a greater impact on crypt numbers than the corresponding doses of photons (Hornsey, 1970) and allow the effects of different types of heavy ion beam to be studied (Alpen et al., 1980; Fukutsu et al., 1997).

The clinico-pathological and crypt assay reports have been supplemented by investigations on other aspects of the mechanism of intestinal radiation response (Becciolini, 1987; Dubois et al., 1995), using a range of radiation schedules including those relevant to current treatment techniques, such as IORT (Schultz-Hector et al., 1996). Radiation has been reported to affect electrolyte transport (Gunter-Smith, 1989, 1995). The radiation-induced villous shape changes (Anderson and Withers, 1973), which must influence the functionally important absorptive process, do not have the same response characteristics as the decrease in crypt numbers (Carr et al., 1979), although villus-to-crypt feedback has been suggested (Saxena et al., 1991) and it has recently been shown that there may be signalling pathways between villous and cryptal epithelial cells (Coopersmith and Gordon, 1997). However, villous collapse may also be linked to structural features other than crypt depletion, such as alterations to smooth muscle (Carr et al., 1992). There are confirmatory reports of radiation-induced impairment in muscle metabolism, reduced contractile activity (Otterson and Summers, 1995), possible ulcer-associated changes in rectal distensibility (Tamou and Trott, 1995) and increased sensitivity in the cholinergic muscarinic system (Krantis et al., 1996).

The reports that radiation affects many cell types lead on to the finding that the responses of the different cell types are not standard but vary substantially (Carr et al.,

1991). Crypt-counting data will not, therefore, be informative in predicting responses of non-cryptal tissues or even changes in the constituent cryptal sub-populations, such as endocrine or cryptal goblet cells. There are various dose or time-dependent changes in the responses of the various cell types and sometimes substantial interindividual variations. Characteristic response profiles are seen for different types of radiation. There is a range of epithelial damage after all types of radiation. In addition, low LET radiation treatment may produce vascular effects as early as 6h after treatment (Carr et al., 1996). In contrast, radiation of higher LET than photons, such as neutrons or neon ions, produces more neuromuscular changes, although this effect is not maintained as LET is increased further (Carr et al., 1994). The fact that integrative tissues are included in the radiation response, as well as the cells responsible for the main functions of the organ, is confirmed by reports of the specific involvement of these cell types. These include neuroendocrine and/or neuronal cell responses (Hirschowitz and Rode, 1991; Otterson et al., 1995; Esposito et al., 1996, Griffiths et al., 1996; Linard et al., 1997). The radiation-induced decrease in neurally evoked electrolyte transport has been linked to mast cell depletion (McNaughton et al., 1994). Other connective tissue cells and vascular elements have also been implicated (Eriksson et al., 1983; Buell and Harding, 1989).

Work has been done on the molecular mechanisms involved in the radiation response (Pirollo et al., 1995) and there has been recent confirmation, at the molecular level, of the involvement of cells other than those of the proliferative compartment of the crypts. Links have been shown between TGF-β immunoreactivity and both mucosal barrier breakdown (Richter et al., 1996) and mast cell hyperplasia (Richter et al., 1997). A molecular approach has also been applied to crypt depletion. Sequential steps have been postulated whereby radiation-induced signals from villous epithelial cells may cause cryptal epithelium to induce p53 and influence apoptosis (Coopersmith and Gordon, 1997). Apoptotic elimination of intestinal cells (Henry and Potten, 1982; Potten, 1997) has itself been correlated with expression of clusterin mRNA (Arai et al., 1996), which may have a role in post-apoptotic tissue remodelling.

Complementary to these general mechanistic studies, there have been attempts to understand the role of radiation in sensitising tissues to other agents such as staphylococcal enterotoxin B (Aboud-Pirak et al., 1995). Factors associated with the protective effects of shielding (Vigneulle, 1995) or with adaptive mechanisms (Brennan et al., 1998) have also been studied. There has also been work on the use of external protocols to minimize the side-effects, such as the use of altered dietary status (Srinivasan and Dubois, 1995), radioprotectants (Hanson, 1995; Weiss et al., 1995) or vitamin supplements (Felemovicius et al., 1995). Finally, in addition to the many reports of the gastro-intestinal effects of external radiation sources, there is also literature on the uptake of ingested radioactive substances with implications for environmental concerns. The effects depend on the nature, form and half-life of the radionuclide and on the type and energy of the emissions produced (Harrison and Stather, 1996).

Of the parenchymatous organs of the digestive tract, the liver appears to have the lowest threshold for injury. Impaired liver function results from exposure of the whole organ to 30 Gy of conventionally fractionated therapeutic X-radiation. Changes which may include damage to centrilobular veins, with thrombosis and portal hypertension, may lead to hepatic failure, ascites and death (Kraut et al., 1972; Wharton et al., 1973). With partial irradiation of the liver, substantially larger doses can be tolerated.

The Respiratory System

The respiratory system can tolerate considerable localized radiation injury, as, for example, when a small part of a lung is heavily irradiated for therapeutic purposes. If, however, both lungs or a large proportion of lung tissue are irradiated with doses of greater than about 8 Gy, a fatal pneumonitis may develop after a latent period of 1–3 months. The earliest signs of radiation injury to the lungs are oedema and changes in blood circulation, which precede pneumonitis.

Individuals who survive the acute inflammatory phase of pneumonitis may later develop pulmonary fibrosis and cor pulmonale. With a whole-body dose of more than 8 Gy, bone marrow failure may occur before severe lung damage becomes evident. The target cell population responsible for pneumonitis after irradiation is unknown, but type II alveolar cells are implicated and vascular injury may be contributory (Travis and Tucker, 1986; De Saint-Georges et al., 1988).

In the case of the upper respiratory tract, including tissues of the nasopharynx, larynx, trachea and bronchi, doses in excess of 30 Gy in 2 Gy fractions are required to cause ulceration, atrophy and fibrosis (van den Brenk, 1971).

The Nervous System

Radiation-induced damage to the spinal cord, including demyelination and delayed necrosis of neurons in the white matter and damage to the fine vasculature, may develop between 6 months and 2 years after exposure (Rubin and Casarett, 1968). Typical neurological symptoms resulting from this damage include numbness, tingling, anaesthesia, paraesthesia, weakness and paralysis.

The brain is relatively resistant to radiation damage, with a dose of about 15 Gy required to produce deleterious effects. Necrosis of the brain, associated with demyelination and damage to cerebral vasculature, may occur within 1–3 years of receiving a dose of 55 Gy delivered over about 5 1/2 weeks to the whole brain, or about 65 Gy delivered over 6 1/2 weeks to a small part of the brain. This may lead to neurological symptoms and, in some cases, death. Many months after accidental or therapeutic irradiation in the range over 10 Gy, leukoencephalopathy, electroencephalographic changes and functional disturbances have been reported in humans, especially children. In addition, detectable morphological and physiological changes in children have been reported following a dose of 1–6 Gy (Ron *et al.*, 1982). With regard to the peripheral nervous system, damage may occur at doses above 60 Gy delivered in conventional fractionated radiotherapy regimens (Rubin and Casarett, 1968).

The Cardiovascular System

The heart is not a particularly radiosensitive organ, but a dose of 40 Gy, in conventionally fractionated radiotherapy, may cause myocardial degeneration, while a dose of more than 60 Gy to the entire heart may lead to death from pericardial effusion or constrictive pericarditis. If only a part of the heart is irradiated, tolerance is greater, but degenerative changes and fibrosis in the exposed tissues may occur following a dose of 60 Gy.

A dose of 40–60 Gy will cause changes in the blood vessels in all organs (Rubin and Casarett, 1968). Vascular permeability and blood flow will increase in the early phases of the response. Endothelial cell degeneration, thickening of the basement membrane and progressive sclerosis will follow within a few months. Blood vessels may undergo late changes, including focal endothelial proliferation, thickening of the wall, narrowing of the lumen and decrease in blood flow. It has been suggested that vascular damage may play a major role in most forms of late radiation-induced tissue injury (Law, 1981).

The Endocrine System

Endocrine glands, including the thyroid, parathyroid, adrenal and pituitary glands, have a low cell turnover rate in normal adults, and are therefore relatively radioresistant. If, however, these glands are in a growing and proliferative state, they will be more radiosensitive.

In children, irradiation of the thyroid gland by external γ-radiation or internally deposited radioiodine can lead to hypothyrodism and growth retardation (Conrad *et al.*, 1975). In adults thyroid damage with myxoedema has been reported to develop between 4 months and 3 years after fractionated X-ray therapy with doses of between 26 and 48 Gy for tumours in the neck (Markson and Flatman, 1965; Glatstein *et al.*, 1971).

The pituitary and adrenal glands are less radiosensitive than the thyroid; in adults threshold doses of conventionally fractionated irradiation of about 45 and 60 Gy, respectively, are required to depress permanently the functioning of these glands (Rubin and Casarett, 1968). The threshold for severe functional damage following irradiation of the entire adult thyroid gland is approximately 25–30 Gy fractionated over 30 days; at lower doses, subclinical damage may occur.

Although the female breast is relatively radioresistant during adult life, normal breast development may be impaired if doses of more than 10 Gy of conventionally fractionated X-irradiation are administered before puberty (Rubin and Casarett, 1968).

The Urinary Tract

Of the organs of the urinary tract, the kidneys are most radiosensitive, followed by the bladder and the ureters. The threshold dose for a fatal nephritis-like reaction in the kidneys, which can develop 6–12 months after irradiation, is estimated to be about 23 Gy of X-rays delivered in fractions of about 1 Gy over a 5-week period (Maier, 1972).

Radiation-induced renal injury involves degenerative changes in the fine vasculature of the kidney and in the epithelium of the nephron itself (Rubin and Casarett, 1968; Law, 1981). Histologically, degeneration and depopulation of the renal tubules can be detected in the kidney within 6–12 months after irradiation following doses of more than 10 Gy; with high doses depopulation may be permanent, with degenerative changes in the vasculature, if the individual survives for several years after irradiation, the kidneys shrink in size, the capsule thickens and adheres to the cortex and there will be cortical thinning and disorganization.

The bladder is less radiosensitive than the kidneys. With high doses complications, including cystitis, ulceration, fistula, fibrosis, contraction and urinary obstruction, may occur (Rubin and Casarett, 1968).

The Musculoskeletal System

Muscle, bone and cartilage are relatively resistant to the direct cytocidal actions of radiation. Early radiation damage in mature bone and cartilage is difficult to detect because of the paucity of cells, the abundance of matrix, the radioresistance of the matrix and the mature cells and the normally slow turnover rate of most of the matrix. The principal factor in radiation damage to these tissues is the injury to the fine vasculature supplying these structures. The degeneration and loss of dependent cells are secondary to interference with the blood supply, with changes in the matrix secondary to either of these changes. In the event of a large degree of vascular and cellular damage where there is degeneration and loss of many of the bone or cartilage cells, this will eventually be reflected in changes in the matrix, with the development of 'radiation osteitis' or 'radiation chrondritis'. Whether or not the devitalized bone or cartilage results in structural disintegration depends on the degree at which occlusion of fine vasculature and loss of parenchymal cells occurs, and on the occurrence of complicating factors such as infection or trauma.

In a proliferative state, as, for example, in growing children, or during the healing of fractures, cartilage and bone may exhibit a greater response to radiation than when in the mature state. In children a dose of 1 Gy may cause some growth retardation, depending on the age at irradiation and the exposure conditions (Tefft, 1972; Blot, 1975). With doses exceeding 20 Gy, administered in conventionally fractionated radiotherapy in childhood, skeletal changes, including scoliosis, kyphosis, slipped upper femoral epiphysis and exostosis, may occur.

In adults, mature cartilage will tolerate 40 Gy fractionated over 4 weeks or over 70 Gy fractionated over 10–12 weeks; mature bone will tolerate up to 65 Gy fractionated over 6–8 weeks (Parker, 1972). Although these doses may be tolerated by adult bone and cartilage without necrosis, these tissues may exhibit increased susceptibility to trauma in the long term (Rubin and Casarett, 1968).

Large radiation doses (500 Gy) are required to cause early necrosis of muscle which involves disruption of the fine vasculature and microcirculation, with increased capillary permeability, oedema and inflammation. At lower doses the acute oedematous and inflammatory response to vascular damage is more moderate and transient. However, the associated vascular damage and connective tissue reactions from acute interstitial oedema and inflammation may progress to cause delayed secondary degeneration, atrophy or necrosis and fibrosis of irradiated muscles.

STOCHASTIC EFFECTS

The acute or early effects of radiation as described above result mainly from cell killing. By contrast, some late effects of irradiation result from damage to surviving cells which is transmitted to their progeny. Damage to germ cells may result in a genetic mutation that is expressed in a later generation; in the case of somatic cells, the result may be cancer induction in the exposed individual. Cancer and the induction of hereditary damage represent the stochastic effects of irradiation and are regarded as the principal risk to health from low doses of radiation.

Radiation Carcinogenesis

Radiation is effective both as a carcinogen and in the treatment of cancer. The use of radiation in cancer therapy is based on its cell-killing ability, when administered in sufficiently large doses to replicating malignant cells. For cancer induction, sublethal doses of radiation are important.

Several general principles apply to the induction of tumours by radiation. As a carcinogen, radiation is unique in that it can cause cancer in almost every tissue of the body, and radiogenic cancers are indistinguishable from those cancers which arise naturally or as a result of other carcinogens. Leukaemia (except for chronic lym-

phatic leukaemia) is the most frequently induced cancer. Chronic lymphatic leukaemia, squamous cell carcinoma of the cervix and Hodgkin's lymphoma are not induced by radiation.

Prior to the appearance of an induced tumour there is a latency period, the length of which depends on the type of tumour, its growth rate and metastatic form. The latency period for leukaemia is 2–5 years, whereas for other tumours a period of 10 or more years is usual. There is also a delay before the initially 'transformed' cell or cells begin to divide to form a tumour, and there may be a further delay before the tumour assumes the 'malignant' characteristics of growth and spread. Radiation carcinogenesis is thought to be a multi-stage process involving initiation, promotion and progression.

Various factors influence the probability that an individual exposed to radiation will develop cancer. Current information suggests that sex has little or no effect on radiation carcinogenesis, while increasing age is associated with a decrease in radiation-induced tumours. Irradiation conditions, including the dose delivered, the time period over which the dose is received and the radiation quality, are also important. Genetic constitution may be influential. Other factors, such as the host's susceptibility, living habits and exposure to other toxic agents, may contribute to cancer development.

Populations exposed to moderate to high levels of radiation form the basis of radiation risk assessment and are fundamental to the development of models of radiation carcinogenesis in man. The most useful human data on the risk of radiation-induced cancer in terms of the length of time of follow-up and population size have been obtained from follow-up studies of the incidence of tumours in survivors of the atomic bombings at Hiroshima and Nagasaki in Japan during World War II, and from medically irradiated populations. Occupationally exposed individuals, e.g. certain groups of workers in the nuclear industry, also represent a potentially useful source of data, although as yet they have yielded little quantitative data on cancer risk estimates (Beral et al., 1985, 1988; Smith and Douglas, 1986).

The Life Span Study of the Japanese atomic bomb survivors represents the largest single study population examined for age and sex trends with a wide range of doses, and currently has a follow-up period of over 45 years (Shimizu et al., 1987, 1988). Of about 280 000 individuals who survived the bombings, 80 000 have been followed up, with about 24 000 deaths, 5000 of which were caused by cancer; some of these were in excess of the number expected and have therefore been attributed to radiation. For those survivors exposed as adults, almost the entire course of induced cancer is now known; however, for those exposed as children the picture is still incomplete.

Investigations of medically irradiated populations contributing useful information on the risk of radiation-induced cancer include the follow-up of over 14 000 ankylosing spondylitic patients given a single course of X-rays to ameliorate pain associated with the disease (Darby *et al.*, 1987), follow-up studies of patients irradiated as part of their treatment for cervical cancer (Boice *et al.*, 1988) or benign breast disease (Baral *et al.*, 1977) and follow-up of children irradiated for an enlarged thymus (Hempelmann *et al.*, 1975; Shore *et al.*, 1985) or for tinea capitus (scalp ringworm) (Ron *et al.*, 1988). In the ankylosing spondylitic patients, it has been shown that the relative risk for all neoplasms, other than leukaemia or colon cancer, more than 25 years after their first treatment, is lower than that in the earlier years (5–24.9 years after treatment) (Darby *et al.*, 1987). This is in contrast to the results of follow-up studies of the Japanese atomic bomb survivors (Darby *et al.*, 1985) and of patients irradiated as part of their treatment for cervical cancer (Boice *et al.*, 1985, 1988). In both instances the relative risk for all neoplasms (other than leukaemia and colon cancer) increased with time since exposure (Darby *et al.*, 1987).

As yet, no study population has been followed up for a long enough period to yield the lifetime incidence of cancers following irradiation. The overall risk for an exposed population must therefore be extrapolated over time, using models based on limited data. Two such projection models are used: an additive risk model and a relative risk model. The additive or absolute model postulates that the annual excess risk arises after a period of latency and then remains constant. In this case the risk from radiation appears to be additional to the natural incidence. The relative or multiplicative risk model postulates that the distribution of excess risk follows the same pattern as the time distribution of natural cancers, i.e. the excess (after latency) is given by a constant factor applied to the age-dependent incidence of natural cancers in the population. Because the natural incidence of cancer increases with increasing age, this model predicts a large number of radiation-induced cancers in old age. While it is not possible to distinguish between the two models for most cancers, for leukaemia and bone cancer (which have shorter latency periods) it has been established that these fit the absolute risk model.

Most of the data relating to human radiation carcinogenesis are derived from exposures at high doses and dose rates from which it is impossible to deduce the shape of the dose–response relationship, especially at low doses. Frequently the data are fitted to linear and linear-quadratic relationships. The former assumes that the excess cancer incidence is proportional to dose; the latter implies that at low doses cancer incidence is proportional to dose but that at high doses it is proportional to dose squared. In extrapolating the risk of cancer from high to low doses, the linear model implies that the risk per unit dose is the same at high and at low doses; the linear-quadratic model implies a smaller risk per unit dose at low doses. Because risk estimates are associated with a large degree of uncertainty, and are dependent on the choice of model used to extrapolate from high to low

doses, they should not be viewed as definitive, but as the best available estimates based on inadequate data. Despite the difficulties associated with estimating the risk of radiation-induced cancer, the number of fatal malignancies induced by sparsely ionizing radiation in the range of 1 Gy is reported to be of the order of 10^{-2} per sievert (Sv) (UNSCEAR, 1988).

Dose–response relationships for radiation-induced cancers vary, depending on the tumour type and the radiation quality. For low-LET radiations, the incidence of many types of cancer increases with increasing dose, up to a maximum, which usually occurs in the dose region 3–10 Gy. Thereafter, the cancer incidence decreases with increasing dose. The shape of the dose–response curve is the result of two phenomena: a dose-related increase in the proportion of normal cells transformed into a malignant state and a dose-related decrease in the probability that such cells may survive the radiation exposure. Both phenomena normally operate but to different degrees, depending on the dose and tumour type. The decreasing slope at high doses is attributed to the killing of the radiation-initiated cells from which tumours eventually arise.

For densely ionizing neutron irradiation, tumour induction in animals, in general, follows an almost linear curve at the lower end of the dose scale and exhibits little dose-rate dependence. For X- and γ-rays the dose–response relationships tend to be curvilinear and concave at low doses. Tumour induction is dose-rate dependent, in that a reduction in the dose rate, or fractionation of the dose, reduces the tumour yield.

Hereditary Effects

General

Radiation-induced hereditary effects may be dominant or recessive, appearing in the first or later generations, respectively, and may involve changes to a single gene or to the gross structure of a chromosome. A gene mutation involves a change in the structure of DNA and may involve the base composition, the sequence, or both. Chromosomal changes can involve the loss or addition of chromosomes, chromosome breakage and translocation.

Radiation-induced mutations represent an increase in the frequency of the same mutations that already occur spontaneously or naturally within a species. Since radiation-induced mutations are indistinguishable from those which occur naturally, large sample sizes are necessary to detect any increase in their frequency caused by radiation. Human data relating to the genetic effects of radiation are scarce, with the exception of the follow-up of survivors of the atomic bombings of Hiroshima and Nagasaki (Neel *et al.*, 1989). Estimation of genetic risk from radiation in humans is therefore based predominantly on animal data. It should be noted, however, that the results of *in vitro* studies of human cells, in conjunction with the limited evidence from Hiroshima and Nagasaki, suggest that humans are not especially sensitive to the induction of chromosome aberrations and gene mutations by radiation (Neel *et al.*, 1989). Genetic risk is estimated on the basis that the doses received are genetically significant, i.e. that they are received by individuals before or during the reproductive period.

In using the data from animal studies to make quantitative estimates of genetic risks in man, three important assumptions are made unless there is evidence to the contrary:

1. The amount of genetic damage induced by a given type of radiation under a given set of conditions is the same in human germ cells and in those of the test species used as the model.
2. The biological factors (e.g. sex, germ cell stage and age) and physical factors (e.g. radiation quality and dose rate) affect the magnitude of the damage in similar ways and to a similar extent in humans and in the experimental species from which extrapolations are made.
3. At low doses and at low dose rates of low-LET irradiation, there is a linear relationship between dose and the frequency of genetic effects.

The genetic risks from radiation can be estimated by either the direct method or the doubling dose method. The direct method estimates the incidence of genetic diseases resulting from mutations or chromosomal disorders as a function of dose, and ignores the natural rate of these diseases in a population. By contrast, the doubling dose method involves a comparison between the rate of radiation-induced genetic disorders and the spontaneous incidence of these diseases in the population, and is expressed in terms of the dose required to double the spontaneous incidence of gene or chromosomal disorders.

On the basis of animal experiments, which have shown an approximately linear increase in point mutations with radiation doses of 1–100 mGy, it is assumed that the increased irradiation of humans will result in a proportional increase in mutation frequency (Searle, 1989). Point-mutation frequencies of between 1 and 10 per million cells Gy^{-1} for human lymphoblasts (Grossovsky and Little, 1985; Konig and Kiefer, 1988), and less than 20 mutations per million cells Gy^{-1} for erythroblasts in atomic bomb survivors (Langlois *et al.*, 1987), have been reported.

Survivors of the atomic bombs have been studied for four genetic indicators: (1) abnormal outcome of pregnancy (stillbirth, major congenital defects or death during the first postnatal week); (2) childhood mortality; (3) sex chromosome abnormalities; (4) mutations resulting in electrophoretic variation in blood proteins (Schull *et al.*, 1981). For these four parameters, differences

between the children of proximally and distally exposed survivors were in the direction expected if a genetic effect did result from irradiation. However, none of the findings was statistically significant.

On the basis of mouse data (Russell and Russell, 1956; Russell, 1965), the doubling dose for low-rate exposure in humans was estimated by the Biological Effects of Ionizing Radiation (BEIR) III Committee of the US National Academy of Sciences (National Research Council, 1980) to be in the range of 0.5–2.5 Sv. The corresponding estimate in the 1986 UNSCEAR Report was 1 Gy (UNSCEAR, 1986).

Table 1 gives estimates of genetic damage, obtained according to the direct method. The estimates are expressed as the expected number per million of genetically abnormal children born in the first generation after irradiation, per 0.01 Gy of sparsely ionizing low dose rate irradiation (UNSCEAR, 1986, 1988).

The genetic effect of 0.01 Gy per generation of low-LET, low dose-rate irradiation in a population of 10^6 liveborn estimated by the doubling dose method is given in **Table 2**. These values have been derived assuming a doubling dose of 1 Gy.

Table 1 Risks of induction of genetic damage in man per 0.01 Gy at low dose rates of low-LET radiation, estimated using the direct method. From UNSCEAR (1986, 1988)

Risk associated with	Expected frequency per 10^6 of genetically abnormal children in the first generation after irradiation	
	Males	Females
Induced mutations having dominant effects	~10 to ~20	0 to ~9
Induced recessive mutations	0	0
Unbalanced products of induced reciprocal translocations	~1 to ~15	0 to ~5

Table 2 Effects of 0.01 Gy per generation of low-LET radiation at low dose rates on a population of 1 million liveborn, estimated using the doubling-dose method with an assumed doubling dose of 1 Gy. From UNSCEAR (1982, 1988)

Disorder	Current incidence per million offspring	Effect of 0.01 Gy per generation	
		First generation	Equilibrium
Autosomal dominant and X-linked diseases	10000	15	100
Autosomal recessive diseases	2500	Slight	Slow increase
Chromosomal diseases			
–structural anomalies	400	2.4	4
–numerical anomalies	3000	Probably very small	Probably very small
Irregularly inherited	90000	4.5	45
Total	105900	~22	~150

Preconceptual Irradiation and Cancer Induction

There is considerable experimental evidence of the induction of genetic abnormalities by preconceptual irradiation of either parent. Searle (1989, and references therein) has estimated that the risk factors for a mutation at a specific locus in F_1 mice after paternal irradiation is about 0.001% Gy^{-1}. From data such as these, UNSCEAR (1988) has estimated that the total genetic risk for all loci in F_1 and F2 humans after parental irradiation is about 0.3%. This is in line with risk estimates for general congenital malformations in the offspring of irradiated male mice (0.5% Gy^{-1}) (Nomura, 1982; Kirk and Lyon, 1984).

Interest in the induction of cancer-proneness by preconceptual irradiation was stimulated by the results of a reanalysis of the incidence of leukaemia in children living near the nuclear installation at Sellafield in the UK. Gardner et al. (1990) reported that the raised incidence appeared to be associated with paternal employment at the plant and the recorded doses of radiation received by the fathers during the periods of their employment. It was suggested that these doses, although low, may have increased the risk of leukaemia in the offspring. The implications of the hypothesis, which became known as the Gardner hypothesis, is that if the association is truly causal, then it would follow that the risk of cancer arising from irradiation of pre- or postmeiotic germ cells must be very high.

The risk factors calculated from the data of Gardner et al. (1990) depend upon the period of preconceptual exposure assumed to be important. These would be in the range of about 2% Gy^{-1} for a lifetime dose to about 20% Gy^{-1} for a 6-month dose. The problem arises in that risk factors of these magnitudes are vastly in excess of those normally expected for mutation at defined loci, as determined in radiation genetic studies in the laboratory. There are some experimental data, however, that are supportive. Nomura et al. (1982, 1983, 1986) have reported the induction of lung tumours and leukaemia after paternal irradiation in three strains of mice. The risk factors were found to be dose dependent and varied with mouse strain, the germ cell stage at the time of irradiation and the type of tumour induced. Some responses in the offspring were also noted for preconceptual irradiation of female mice. The risk factors of a few % Gy^{-1} found in some of the studies imply that, in these experimental systems, induced mutations leading to cancer induction occur at much higher frequencies than those normally found for other types of mutations arising from preconceptual irradiation. More recently, radiation genomic instability (see below) has also been invoked as a possible explanation for the Gardner hypothesis.

The Gardner study raised considerable concern both inside the nuclear industry and in the general public and the independent advisory committee to the UK Government, the Committee on Medical Aspects of Radiation in the Environment (COMARE) was asked for and gave interim advice to Government (*Hansard*, 2 April 1990). COMARE also made recommendations for further research. Two epidemiological and several biological studies were instigated as a result of these recommendations. One epidemiological study has been completed (Draper et al., 1997) and the results of this study do not support the Gardner hypothesis. An attempt to replicate the earlier work of Nomura using different mouse strains was also unsuccessful (Cattenach, 1995).

It was also suggested that the measured dose of external radiation may be a surrogate measure for internal exposure to radionuclides or to chemicals. The UK Health and Safety Executive commissioned a study to examine these suggestions (HSE, 1993, 1994). The HSE study found no association between exposure of workers to internal emitters and health effects in their offspring.

Genomic Instability

Exposure to ionizing radiation produces a number of biological consequences, including gene mutations, chromosome aberrations, cellular transformation and cell death. These effects have been attributed to radiation-induced DNA damage producing irreversible changes during DNA replication or during the processing of the damage by enzymatic repair processes. Accordingly, it has been widely accepted that most of these changes take place during the cell cycles immediately following exposure. However, there is a rapidly growing body of evidence that the progeny of cells exposed to ionizing radiation exhibit delayed mutational responses, including specific gene mutations (Pampfer and Streffer 1989; Chang and Little 1992; Harper et al., 1997) and chromosome aberrations (Kadim et al., 1992; Holmberg et al., 1993; Martins et al., 1993; Ponnaiya et al., 1997a, b). These responses, most effectively demonstrated as non-clonal mutations/aberrations in the clonal descendants of irradiated cells, are generally regarded as the consequences of a destabilization of the genome collectively termed radiation-induced genomic instability.

Radiation-induced chromosomal instability has been demonstrated in a variety of human and rodent cell types after exposures to radiations of both high and low linear energy transfer (LET). However, many studies have been of a single-cell type after exposure to low-LET radiation and no comparisons have been made with high-LET exposures (Marder et al., 1993; Durante et al., 1996). In some situations, radiation quality comparisons have been made and differences in the types of aberrations have been recorded (Little et al., 1997) or low-LET radiation has proved to be significantly less effective in inducing instability than high-LET radiation (Kadim et al., 1994, 1998). Genetic 'predisposition' has also been reported to be an important determinant of the expression of chromosomal instability with growing evidence that susceptibility is a genetically recessive characteristic (Kadim *et al.*, 1995; Watson *et al.*, 1997).

Almost all the studies of induced instability have used *in vitro* systems and the number of studies designed to assess instability *in vivo* are limited. However, the earliest report of the induction of chromosomal instability in normal cells is that of mouse zygote irradiation (Kadim *et al.*, 1992). In this study, skin fibroblast cultures obtained from foetuses derived from 2 Gy X-irradiated zygotes were found to have a 2–3-fold increase in the types of chromosome and chromatid breaks found as spontaneous aberrations in control animals. An example of chromosomal instability being expressed *in vivo* is provided by studies of the transplantation of irradiated mouse bone marrow in which chromosomal instability in haematopoietic cells of donor origin was recorded for up to a year after transplantation (Ponnaiya *et al.*, 1997a).

At present, the mechanism underlying the phenomenon of radiation-induced genomic instability is not understood (although free radicals have been implicated), nor is it clear whether there is a single mechanism for all end-points.

Effects of Prenatal Irradiation

Developmental harm to an individual exposed to radiation *in utero* is not easily classified as a stochastic or a deterministic effect. Irradiation of the developing embryo and foetus may result in death, malformation or growth retardation. The observed effect is dependent on the radiation dose, the dose rate and the gestational stage at which irradiation occurs. Prenatal irradiation effects are due to the fact that foetal tissues are continuously differentiating and growing, and foetal development follows a predetermined pathway; irradiation of the developing organism with the subsequent killing of embryonic or foetal cells at critical developmental stages can cause disruption in the normal complex sequence of events.

Gestation may be divided into three major stages: preimplantation, which extends from fertilization until the embryo attaches to the uterine wall; organogenesis, which represents the period during which the major organs are developed; and the foetal stage, during which growth of the preformed structures occurs. The relative duration of each of these periods, the length of the intrauterine life, and the state of differentiation or maturation of any one structure, with respect to the others, varies between different animal species. **Table 3** shows the appropriate beginning and end of the major developmental periods in man and in some of the commonly used laboratory mammals.

The preimplantation period is most sensitive to the lethal effects of radiation. Irradiation at this stage does not result in growth retardation, and few if any

Table 3 Approximate time of beginning and end of the major developmental periods (in days post-conception) in mammalian species. From UNSCEAR (1977)

Species	Preimplantation	Organogenesis	Foetal period
Hamster	0–5	6–12	13–16.5
Mouse	0–5	6–13	14–19.5
Rat	0–7	8–15	16–21.5
Rabbit	0–5	6–15	16–31.5
Guinea pig	0–8	9–25	26–63
Dog	0–17	18–30	31–63
Man	0–8	9–60	61–270

abnormalities are produced. If the irradiated preimplantation embryo survives, it will continue to grow and develop normally. At the preimplantation stage the embryo consists of a small cluster of cells, so that, if a few cells are killed by radiation, one or two cell divisions will rectify the damage. If, however, a larger number of cells are killed, the embryo will die and become resorbed.

Irradiation during organogenesis can induce congenital defects. In the mouse, a dose of 2 Gy during the period of maximum sensitivity can produce 100% malformations in the offspring at birth (Russell and Russell, 1954). although in man, radiation-induced malformations of structures other than the central nervous system are uncommon. This is probably related to the fact that the sensitive period for the induction of congenital malformations during organogenesis in humans represents a smaller fraction of the total period of gestation compared with that in small rodents. In humans, however, CNS development is occurring for much of the gestational period, which makes it a likely target for radiation-induced damage. Consequently, the principal effects of irradiation during the period of organogenesis in humans are microcephaly and mental retardation.

Embryos exposed to radiation in early organogenesis exhibit the most severe intrauterine growth retardation, from which there may be recovery later (i.e. temporary growth retardation). Irradiation in the foetal period leads to the greatest degree of permanent growth retardation.

Irradiation during the foetal period, which extends from about 14 days onward in the mouse and 6 weeks onward in man, can result in damage to the haematopoietic system, liver, kidney and developing gonads, the last affecting fertility. Higher radiation doses are required to cause lethality during the foetal stage than at earlier developmental stages. In man the most commonly reported effects of *in utero* irradiation are microcephaly, mental retardation and other central nervous system defects and growth retardation. Other effects, including spina bifida, deformities, alopecia of the scalp, divergent squint and blindness at birth, are also recognized (Murphy and Goldstein, 1930). **Table 4** summarizes the effects of radiation on the mammalian embryo and foetus.

Table 4 Radiation effects on the mammalian embryo and foetus. From Hall (1988)

State of gestation	Growth retardation	Death	Congenital malformations	
			General	Microcephaly and mental retardation in humans
Preimplantation	None	Embryonic death and resorption	None	None
Organogenesis	Temporary	Neonatal death	High risk	Very high risk
Foetal period	Permanent	LD$_{50}$ similar to that for adult	Less risk	High risk

Follow-up studies of individuals exposed *in utero* during the atomic bombings of Hiroshima and Nagasaki have shown that microcephaly can result from an air dose (Kerma) of 0.1–0.19 Gy. In addition, an increased incidence of severe mental retardation has been reported in atomic bomb survivors exposed *in utero* (Otake and Schull, 1984). A child was classified as severely mentally retarded when he/she was 'unable to perform simple calculations, to make simple conversation, to care for her/himself, or if he/she was completely unmanageable or has been institutionalized'. The probability of radiation-related severe mental retardation is essentially zero with exposure before 8 weeks after conception, is maximum with irradiation between 8 and 15 weeks and decreases between 16 and 25 weeks. After 25 weeks and for doses below 1 Gy, no case of severe mental retardation has been reported. On the assumption that the induction of the effect is linear with dose, the probability of induction per unit dose was estimated at 0.4 and 0.1 Gy^{-1} at 8–15 and 16–25 weeks after conception, respectively (Otake and Schull, 1984). The period of highest risk of severe mental retardation coincides with the period of most rapid proliferation of neuronal elements, and with the migration of neuroblast cells from the proliferative zones to the cerebral cortex. It is thought that severe mental retardation results from radiation interfering with this normal sequence of events.

Prenatal irradiation with diagnostic X-rays has also been associated with the subsequent development of leukaemia and other childhood malignancies (MacMahon, 1962; MacMahon and Hutchison, 1964; Stewart and Kneale, 1970). In the Oxford Childhood Cancer study, irradiated children received between one and five films, with a dose of 0.2–0.46 rad per film. While these studies have been interpreted as indicating that relatively low doses of radiation result in an increased incidence of cancer during the first 10–15 years of life, by a factor of 1.5–2.0, they do not prove that *in utero* irradiation caused the malignancies. It has been suggested that the irradiated mothers represent a select group whose children are more prone to cancer and that the irradiation is coincidental. The strongest evidence in support of a causal relationship between irradiation and childhood cancer is that provided by Mole (1974) in an analysis of the Oxford data relating to twins. Twins who were X-rayed more frequently than singletons were found to have a higher incidence of childhood cancer.

ACKNOWLEDGEMENTS

The authors thank Professor K. E. Carr of the Queen's University of Belfast and Professor E. Wright of the MRC Radiation and Genome Stability Unit for their contributions to the sections on the Digestive System and on Genomic Instability.

REFERENCES

Aboud-Pirak, E., Lubin, I., Pirak, M. E., Canaan, A., Lowell, G. H. and Reisner, Y. (1995). Lethally irradiated normal strains of mice radioprotected with SCID bone marrow develop sensitivity to low doses of staphylococcal enterotoxin B. *Immunol. Lett.*, **46**, 9–14.

Alpen, E. L., Powers-Risius, P. and McDonald, M. (1980). Survival of intestinal crypt cells after exposure to high Z, high-energy charged particles. *Radiat. Res.*, **83**, 677–687.

Anderson, J. H. and Withers, R. H. (1973). Scanning electron microscope studies of irradiated rat intestinal mucosa. *Scanning Electron Microsc.*, **3**, 566–572.

Arai, T., Kida, Y., Harmon, B. V. and Gobe, G. C. (1996). Expression and localisation of clusterin mRNA in the small and large intestine of the irradiated rat: its relationship with apoptosis. *Int. J. Radiat. Biol.*, **69**, 547–553.

Baral, E., Larsson, L. E. and Mattsson, B. (1977). Breast cancer following irradiation of the breast. *Cancer*, **40**, 2905–2910.

Becchiolini, A. (1987). Relative radiosensitivities of the small and large intestine. *Adv. Radiat. Biol.*, **12**, 83–128.

Beral, V., Inskip, H., Fraser, P., Booth, M., Coleman, D. and Rose, G. (1985). Mortality of employees of the United Kingdom Atomic Energy Authority, 1946–1979. *Br. Med. J.*, **291**, 440–447.

Beral, V., Fraser, P., Carpenter, L., Booth, M., Brown, A. and Rose, G. (1988). Mortality of employees of the Atomic Weapons Establishment 1951–82. *Br. Med. J.*, **297**, 757–770.

Blot, W. J. (1975). Growth and development following prenatal childhood exposure to atomic radiation. *J. Radiat. Res.*, **16** (Suppl.), 82–88.

Boice, J. D., Day, N. E., Anderson, A., *et al.* (1985). Second cancers following radiation treatment for cervical cancer. An international collaboration among cancer registries. *J. Natl. Cancer Inst.*, **74**, 955.

Boice, J. D., Engholm, G., Kleinerman, R. A., Blettner, M., Stovall, M., Lisco, H., Moloney, W. C., Austin, D. F., Bosch, A., Cookfair, D. L., Krementz, E. T., Latouret, H. B., Merrill, J. A., Peters, L. J., Schulz, M. D., Storm, H. H., Bjorkholm, E., Pettersson, F., Janine Bell, C. M., Coleman, M. P., Fraser, P., Neal, F. E., Prior, P., Won Choi, N., Gregory Hislop, T., Koch, M., Kreiger, N., Robb, D., Robson, D., Thomson, D. H., Lochumller, H., von Fournier, D., Frischkorn, R., Kjorstad, K. E., Rimpela, A., Pejovic, M.-H., Kirn, V. P., Stankusova, H., Berrino, F., Sigurdsson, K., Hutchison, G. B. and MacMahon, B. (1988). Radiation dose and second cancer risks in patients for cancer of the cervix. *Radiat. Res.*, **116**, 3–55.

Brennan, P. C., Carr, K. E., Seed, T. and McCullough, J. S. (1988). Acute and protracted radiation effects on small intestinal morphological parameters. *Int. J. Radiat. Biol.*, **73**, 691–698.

Buell, M. G. and Harding, R. K. (1989). Proinflammatory effects of local abdominal irradiation on rat gastrointestinal tract. *Dig. Dis. Sci.*, **34**, 390–399.

Busch, D. B. (1990). Pathology of the irradiated bowel. In Galland, R. B. and Spencer, J. (Eds), *Radiation Enteritis*. Edward Arnold, London, pp. 66–87.

Carr, K. E., Hamlet, R., Nias, A. H. W. and Watt, C. (1979). Lack of correlation between villus and crypt damage in irradiated mouse intestine. *Br. J. Radiol.*, **52**, 485–493.

Carr, K. E., McCullough, J. S., Nunn, S., Hume, S. P. and Nelson, A. C. (1991). Neutron and X-ray effects on small intestine summarised by using a mathematical model or paradigm. *Proc. R. Soc. London, Ser. B*, **243**, 187–194.

Carr, K. E., McCullough, J. S., Nelson, A. C., Hume, S. P., Nunn, S. and Kamel, H. M. H. (1992). Relationship between villous shape and mural structure in neutron irradiated small intestine. *Scanning Electron Microsc.*, **6**, 561–572.

Carr, K. E., McCullough, J. S., Brennan, P., Hayes, T. L., Ainsworth, E. J. and Nelson, A. C. (1994). Heavy ion induced changes in small intestinal parameters. *Adv. Space Res.*, **14**, 521–530.

Carr, K. E., Hume, S. P., Nelson, A. C., O'Shea, O., Hazzard, R. A. and McCullough, S. J. (1996). Morphological profiles of neutron and X-irradiated small intestine. *J. Radiat. Res.*, **37**, 38–48.

Cattanach, B. M., Patrick, G., Papworth, D., Goodhead, D. T., Hacker, T., Cobb, L. and Whitehill, E. (1995). Investigation of lung tumour induction in BALB/cJ mice following paternal X-irradiation. *Int. J. Radiat. Biol.*, **67**, 607–616.

Coia, L. R., Myerson, R. J. and Tepper, J. E. (1995). Late effects of radiation therapy on the gastrointestinal tract. *Int. J. Radiat. Oncol. Biol. Phys.*, **33**, 217–224.

Conard, R. A., Knudson, K. D., Dobyns, B. M., Meyer, L. M., *et al.* (1975). *A Twenty-year Review of Medical Findings in a Marshallese Population Accidentally Exposed to Radioactive Fallout*. Brookhaven National Laboratory, New York, BNL 50424.

Congar, A. D. (1973). Loss and recovery of taste acuity in patients irradiated to the oral cavity. *Radiat. Res.*, **53**, 338–347.

Coopersmith, C. M. and Gordon, J. I. (1997). Gamma-ray-induced apoptosis in transgenic mice with proliferative abnormalities in their intestinal epithelium: re-entry of villous enterocytes into the cell cycle does not affect their radioresistance but enhances the radiosensitivity of the crypt by inducing p53. *Oncogene*, **15**, 131–141.

Darby, S. C., Nakashima, E. and Kato, H. (1985). A parallel analysis of cancer mortality among atomic bomb survivors and patients with ankylosing spondylitis given X-ray therapy. *J. Natl. Cancer Inst.*, **72**, 1.

Darby, S. C., Doll, R., Gill, S. K. and Smith, P. G. (1987). Long term mortality after a single treatment course with X-rays in patients treated for ankylosing spondylitis. *Br. J. Cancer*, **55**, 179–190.

De Saint-Georges, L., Van Gorp, U. and Maisin, J. R. (1988). Response of mouse lung air-blood barrier to X-irradiation: ultrastructural and stereological analysis. *Scanning Microsc.*, **2/1**, 537–543.

Draper, G. J., Little, M. P., Sorahan, T., Kinlen, L. J., Bunch, K. J., Conquest, A. J., Kendall, G. M., Kneale, G. W., Lanchashire, R. J., Muirhead, C. R., O'Connor, C. M. and Vincent, T. J. (1997). Cancer in the offspring of radiation workers: a record linkage study. *Br. Med. J.*, **315**, 1181–1188.

Durante, M., Grossi, G. F. and Yang, T. C. (1996). Radiation-induced chromosomal instability in human mammary epithelial cells. *Adv. Space Res.*, **18**, 99–108.

Dubois, A., King, G. L. and Livengood, D. R. (1995). *Radiation and the Gastrointestinal Tract*. CRC Press, Boca Raton, FL.

Eriksson, B., Johnson, L. and Lundquist, P.-G. (1983). Ultrastructural aspects of capillary function in irradiated bowel. *Scand. J. Gastroenterol.*, **18**, 473–480.

Esposito, V., Linard, C., Maubert, C., Aigueperse, J. and Gourmerlon, P. (1996). Modulation of gut substance P after whole body irradiation. *Dig. Dis. Sci.*, **41**, 2070–2077.

Felemovicius, I., Bonsack, M. E., Baptista, M. L. and Delaney, J. P. (1995). Intestinal radioprotection by vitamin E (alpha-tocopherol). *Ann. Surg.*, **222**, 504–510.

Fukutsu, K., Kanai, T., Furasawa, Y. and Ando, K. (1997). Response of mouse intestine after single and fractionated irradiation with accelerated carbon ions with a spread-out Bragg peak. *Radiat. Res.*, **148**, 168–174.

Galland, R. G. and Spencer, J. (1990). *Radiation Enteritis*. Edward Arnold, London.

Gardner, M. J., Snee, M. P., Hall, A. J., Powell, C. A., Downes, S. and Terrell, J. D. (1990). Results of case-control study of leukaemia and lymphoma among young people near Sellafield nuclear plant in West Cumbria. *Br. Med. J.*, **300**, 423–429.

Glastein, E., McHardy-Young, S., Brast, N., Eltringham, J. G. and Kriss, J. P. (1971). Alterations in serum thyrotropin (TSH) and thyroid function following radiotherapy in patients with malignant lymphoma. *J. Clin. Endocrinol. Metab.*, **32**, 833–841

Griffiths, N. M., Francois, A., Dublineau, I., Lebrun, F., Joubert, C., Aigueperse, J. and Gourmelon, P. (1996). Exposure to either gamma or a mixed neutron/gamma field irradiation modifies vasoactive intestinal peptide receptor characteristics in membranes isolated from pig jejunum. *Int. J. Radiat. Biol.*, **70**, 361–370.

Grossovsky, A. J. and Little, J. B. (1985). Evidence for linear response for the induction of mutations in human cells by X-ray exposure below 10 rads. *Proc. Natl. Acad. Sci. USA*, **82**, 2092–2095.

Gunter-Smith, P. J. (1989). Ionising radiation affects active electrolyte transport by rabbit ileum. II. Correlation of alanine and theophyllene responses with morphology. *Radiat. Res.*, **117**, 419–432.

Gunter-Smith, P. J. (1995). The effect of radiation on intestinal electrolyte transport. In Dubois, A., King, G. L. and Livengood, D. R. (Eds), *Radiation and the Gastrointestinal Tract*. CRC Press, Boca Raton, FL, pp. 149–160.

Hall, E. J. (1988). *Radiobiology for the Radiologist*, 3rd edn. Lippincott, Philadelphia.

Hanson, W. R. (1995). Modification of radiation injury to the intestine by eicosanoids and thiol radioprotectors. In Dubois, A., King, G. L. and Livengood, D. R. (Eds), *Radiation and the Gastrointestinal Tract*. CRC Press, Boca Raton, FL, pp. 171–182.

Harper, K., Lorimore, S. A. and Wright, E. G. (1997). Delayed appearance of radiation-induced mutations at the Hprt locus in murine haemopoietic cells. *Exp. Hematol.*, **25**, 263–269.

Harrison, J. D. and Stather, J. W. (1996). Assessment of doses and effects from intakes of radioactive particles. *J. Anat.*, **189**, 521–530.

Hauer-Jensen, M. (1990). Late radiation injury of the small intestine. Clinical, pathophysiologic and radiobiologic aspects. A review. *Acta Oncol.*, **29**, 401–415.

Health and Safety Executive (1993). *HSE Investigation of Leukaemia and Other Cancers in the Children of Male Workers at Sellafield*. HSE, London.

Health and Safety Executive (1994). *HSE Investigation of Leukaemia and Other Cancers in the Children of Male Workers at Sellafield: Review of the Results Published in October 1993*. HSE, London.

Hempelmann, L. H., Hall, W. J., Phillips, M., Cooper, R. A. and Ames, W. R. (1975). Neoplasms in persons treated with x-rays in infancy: fourth survey in 20 years. *J. Natl. Cancer Inst.*, **55**, 519–530.

Hendry, J. H. and Potten, C. S. (1982). Intestinal radiosensitivity: a comparison for cell death assayed by apoptosis or by a loss of clonogenicity. *Int. J. Radiat. Biol.*, **42**, 621–628.

Hiroshowitz, I. and Rode, J. (1991). Changes in neurones, neuroendocrine cells and nerve fibres in lamina propria of irradiated bowel. *Virchows Arch. A, Pathol. Anat.*, **418**, 163–168.

Holmberg, K., Falt, S., Johansson, A. and Lambert, B. (1993). Chromosome aberrations and genomic instability in X-irradiated human T-lymphocyte cultures. *Mutat. Res.*, **286**, 321–330.

Holmberg, K., Meijer, A. E., Auer, G. and Lambert, B. (1995). Delayed chromosomal instability in human T-lymphocyte clones exposed to ionizing radiation. *Int. J. Radiat. Biol.*, **68**, 245–255.

Hornsey, S. (1970). The relative biological effectiveness of fast neutrons for intestinal damage. *Radiology*, **97**, 649–652.

International Atomic Energy Agency (IAEA) (1971). *Manual on Radiation Haematology*. IAEA, Vienna.

International Commission on Radiological Protection (ICRP) (1977). *Recommendations of the International Commission on Radiological Protection*. ICRP Publication No 26. Annals of the ICRP, Vol. 1, No. 3. Pergamon Press, Oxford.

International Commission on Radiological Protection (ICRP) (1984). *Nonstochastic Effects of Ionizing Radiation*. ICRP Publication No 41. Annals of the ICRP, Vol. 14, No 3. Pergamon Press, Oxford.

Kadhim, M. A., Macdonald, D. A., Goodhead, D. T., Lorimore, S. A., Marsden, S. J. and Wright, E. G. (1992). Transmission of chromosomal instability after plutonium α-particle irradiation. *Nature*, **355**, 738–740.

Kadhim, M. A., Lorimore, S. A., Hepburn, M. D., Goodhead, D. T., Buckle, V. J. and Wright, E. G. (1994). Alpha-particle-induced chromosomal instability in human bone marrow cells. *Lancet*, **344**, 987–988.

Kadhim, M. A., Lorimore, S. A., Townsend, K. M. S., Goodhead, D. T., Buckle, V. J. and Wright, E. G. (1995). Radiation-induced genomic instability: delayed cytogenetic aberrations and apoptosis in primary human bone marrow cells. *Int. J. Radiat. Biol.*, **67**, 287–293.

Kadhim, M. A., Marsden, S. J. and Wright, E. G. (1998). Radiation-induced chromosomal instability in human fibroblasts: temporal effects and the influence of radiation quality. *Int. J. Radiat. Biol.*, **73**, 143–148.

Kirk, K. M. and Lyon, M. F. (1984). Induction of congenital malformations in the offspring of male mice treated with x-rays at pre-meiotic and post-meiotic stages. *Mutat. Res.*, **125**, 75–85.

Konig, F. and Kiefer, J. (1988). Lack of dose rate effect for mutation induction by gamma-rays in human TK_6 cells. *Int. J. Radiat. Biol.*, **54**, 891–897.

Krantis, A., Rana, K. and Harding, R. K. (1996). The effects of gamma-radiation on intestinal motor activity and faecal pellet expulsion in the guinea pig. *Dig. Dis. Sci.*, **41**, 2307–2316.

Kraut, J. E., Bagshaw, M. A. and Glatstein, E. (1972). Hepatic effects of irradiation. *Front. Radiat. Ther. Oncol.*, **6**, 182–195.

Langlois, R. G., Bigbee, W. L. and Kyoizumi, S. (1987). Evidence of increased somatic cell mutations at the glycophorin A locus in atomic bomb survivors. *Science*, **236**, 445–448.

Law, M. F. (1981). Radiation-induced vascular injury and its relation to late effects in normal tissues. *Adv. Radiat. Biol.*, **9**, 37–73.

Linard, C., Griffiths, N. M., Esposito, V., Aigueperse, J. and Gourmelon, P. (1997). Changes in gut neurotensin and modified colonic motility following whole-body irradiation in the rat. *Int. J. Radiat. Biol.*, **71**, 581–588.

Little, J. B., Nagasawa, H., Pfenning, T. and Vetrovs, H. (1997). Radiation-induced genomic instability: delayed mutations and cytogenetic effects of X-rays and alpha-particles. *Radiat. Res.*, **148**, 299–307.

Lushbaugh, C. C. and Casarett, G. W. (1976). The effects of gonadal irradiation in clinical radiation therapy: a review. *Cancer*, **37**, 1111–1120.

Lushbaugh, C. C. and Ricks, R. C. (1972). Some cytokinetic and histopathologic considerations of irradiated male and female gonadal tissues, *Front. Radiat. Radiat. Ther. Oncol.*, **6**, 228–248.

MacMahon, B. (1962). Prenatal X-ray exposure and childhood cancer. *J. Natl. Cancer Inst.*, **28**, 1173–1191.

MacMahon, B. and Hutchison, G. B. (1964). Prenatal X-ray and childhood cancer: a review. *Acta Univ. Int. Contra Cancrum*, **20**, 1172–1174.

McNaughton, W. K., Leach, K. E., Prud'homme-Lalonde, L., Ho, W. and Sharkey, K. (1994). Ionising radiation reduces neurally-evoked electrolyte transport in rat ileum through a mast cell-dependent mechanism. *Gastroenterology*, **106**, 324–335.

Maier, J. G. (1972). Effects of radiations on kidney, bladder and prostate. *Front. Radiat. Ther. Oncol.*, **6**, 196–227.

Marder, B. A. and Morgan, W. F. (1993). Delayed chromosomal instability induced by DNA damage. *Mol. Cell. Biol.*, **13**, 6667–6677.

Markson, J. L. and Flatman, G. E. (1965). Myxoedema after deep X-ray therapy to the neck. *Br. Med. J.*, **1**, 1228–1230.

Martins, M. B., Sabatier, L., Ricoul, M., Pinton, A. and Dutrillaux, B. (1993). Specific chromosome instability induced by heavy ions: a step towards transformation of human fibroblasts. *Mutat. Res.*, **285**, 229–237.

Merriam, G. R., Szechter, A. and Focht, E. F. (1972). The effects of ionizing radiations on the eye. *Front. Radiat. Ther. Oncol.*, **6**, 346–385.

Mole, R. H. (1974). Antenatal irradiation and childhood cancer causation or coincidence. *Br. J. Cancer*, **30**, 199–208.

Murphy, D. P. and Goldstein, L. (1930). Micromelia in a child irradiated *in utero*. *Surg. Gynecol. Obstet.*, **50**, 79–80.

National Research Council (1980). Advisory Committee on the Biological Effects of Ionizing Radiation. BEIR III. National Academy of Sciences, Washington, DC.

Neel, J. V., Schull, W. J., Awa, A. A., Satoh, C., Otake, M., Kato, H. and Yoshimoto, Y. (1989). The genetic effects of atomic bombs: problems in extrapolating from somatic cell findings to risk for children. In Baverstock, K. F. and Stather, J. W. (Eds), *Low Dose Radiation*. Taylor and Francis, London, pp. 42–53.

Nomura, T. (1982). Parental exposure to x-rays and chemicals induces heritable tumours and anomalies in mice. *Nature*, **296**, 575–577.

Nomura, T. (1983). X-ray-induced germ-line mutation leading to tumours. *Mutat. Res.*, **121**, 59–65.

Nomura, T. (1986). Further studies on x-ray and chemically induced germ line alterations causing tumors and malformations in mice. In Ramel, C., Lambert, B. and Magnusson, J. (Eds), *Genetic Toxicology of Environment Chemicals. Part B: Genetic Effects and Applied Mutagenesis*. Alan R. Liss, New York, pp. 13–20.

Otake, M. and Schull, W. J. (1984). *In utero* exposure to A-bomb radiation and mental retardation: a reassessment. *Br. J. Radiol.*, **57**, 409–414.

Otterson, M. F. and Summers, R. W. (1995). Postirradiation alterations in small bowel motility. In Dubois, A., King, G. L. and Livengood, D. R. (Eds), *Radiation and the Gastrointestinal Tract*. CRC Press, Boca Raton, FL, pp. 77–88.

Otterson, M. F., Koch, T. R., Zhang, Z., Leming, S. C. and Moulder, J. E. (1995). Fractionated irradiation alters enteric neuroendocrine products. *Dig. Dis. Sci.*, **40**, 1691–1702.

Pampfer, S. and Streffer, C. (1989). Increased chromosome aberration levels in cells from mouse fetuses after zygote X-irradiation. *Int. J. Radiat. Biol.*, **55**, 85–92.

Parker, R. G. (1972). Tolerance of mature bone and cartilage in clinical radiation therapy. In Vaeth, J. M. (Ed.), *Frontiers of Radiation Therapy and Oncology*, Vol. 6. Karger, Basle, and University Park Press, Baltimore, pp. 312–331.

Pirollo, K. F., Lin, X., Hao, Z. M., Villegas, Z. and Chang, E. (1995). Molecular mechanisms of cellular radioresistance and radiosensitivity. In Dubois, A., King, G. L., and Livengood, D. R. (Eds), *Radiation and the Gastrointestinal Tract*. CRC Press, Boca Raton, FL, pp. 129–148.

Ponnaiya, B., Cornforth, M. N. and Ullrich, R. L. (1997a). Radiation-induced chromosomal instability in BALB/c and C57BL/6 mice. The difference is as clear as black and white. *Radiat. Res.*, **147**, 121–125.

Ponnaiya, B., Cornforth, M. N. and Ullrich, R. L. (1997b). Induction of chromosomal instability in human mammary cells by neutrons and gamma rays. *Radiat. Res.*, **147**, 288–294.

Potten, C. S. (1997). Epithelial cell growth and differentiation. II. Intestinal apoptosis. *Am. J. Physiol.*, **273**, G253–G257.

Richter, K. K., Langberg, C. W., Sung, C. C. and Hauer-Jensen, M. (1996). Association of transforming growth factor beta (TGF-beta) immunoreactivity with specific histopathologic lesions in subacute and chronic experimental radiation enteropathy. *Radiother. Oncol.*, **39**, 243–251.

Richter, K. K., Langberg, C. W., Sung, C. C. and Hauer-Jensen, M. (1997). Increased transforming growth factor (TGF-beta) immunoreactivity is independently associated with chronic injury in both consequential and primary radiation enteropathy. *Int. J. Radiat. Oncol. Biol. Phys.*, **39**, 187–195.

Ron, E., Modan, B., Floro, S., Harkedar, I. and Gurewitz, R. (1982). Mental function following scalp irradiation during childhood. *Am. J. Epidemiol.*, **116**, 149–160.

Ron, E., Modan, B. and Boice, J. D., Jr. (1988). Mortality after radiotherapy for ringworm of the scalp. *Am. J. Epidemiol.*, **127**, 13–25.

Rubin, P. and Casarett, G. W. (1968). *Clinical Radiation Pathology*, Vols I and II. Saunders, Philadelphia.

Russell, L. B. and Russell, W. L. (1954). An analysis of the changing radiation response of the developing mouse embryo. *J. Cell. Physiol.*, **43** (Suppl. 1), 103–149.

Russell, L. B. and Russell, W. L. (1956). The sensitivity of different stages in oogenesis to the radiation induction of dominant lethals and other changes in the mouse. In Mitchell, J. S., Holmes, B. E. and Smith, C. L. (Eds), *Progress in Radiobiology*. Oliver and Boyd, Edinburgh, pp. 187–192.

Russell, W. L. (1965). Studies in mammalian radiation genetics. *Nucleonics*, **23**, 53–56.

Saxena, S. K., Thompson, J. S., Crouse, D. A. and Sharp, J. G. (1991). Epithelial cell proliferation and uptake of radiolabelled urogastrone in the intestinal tissues following abdominal irradiation in the mouse. *Radiat. Res.*, **128**, 37–42.

Schull, W. L., Otake, M. and Neal, J. V. (1981). Genetic effects of the atomic bomb: a reappraisal. *Science*, **213**, 1220–1227.

Schultz-Hector, S., Brechenmacher, P., Dorr, W., Grab, J., Kallfass, E., Krimmel, K., Kummermehr, J., Sund, M., Wilkowski, R., Willich, N., Zaspel, J. and Kramling, H. J. (1996). Complications of combined intraoperative radiation (IORT) and external radiation (ERT) of the upper abdomen: an experimental model. *Radiat. Oncol.*, **38**, 205–314.

Searle, A. G. (1989). Evidence from mammalian studies on genetic effects of low level irradiation. In Baverstock, K. F. and Stather, J. W. (Eds), *Low Dose Radiation*. Taylor and Francis, London, pp. 123–138.

Shimizu, Y., Kato, H., Schull, W. J., Preston, D. L., Fujita, S. and Pierce, D. A. (1987). Life Span Study Report 11, Part I: *Comparison of Risk Coefficients for Site-specific Cancer Mortality Based on DS86 and T65DR Shielded Kerma and Organ Doses*. Hiroshima Radiation Effects Research Foundation, RERF TR12–87.

Shimizu, Y., Kato, H. and Schull, W. J. (1988). Life Span Study Report 11, Part II: *Cancer Mortality in the Years 1950–1985 Based on the Recently Revised Doses (DS86)*. Hiroshima Radiation Effects Research Foundation, RERF TR5–88.

Shore, R. E., Woodard, E., Hildreth, N., Dvoretsky, P., Hempelmann, L. and Pasternack, B. (1985). Thyroid tumors following thymus irradiation. *J. Natl. Cancer Inst.*, **74**, 1177–1184.

Smith, P. G. and Douglas, A. J. (1986). Mortality of workers at the Sellafield plant of British nuclear fuels. *Br. Med. J.*, **293**, 845–854.

Spitzer, T. R. (1995). Clinical aspects of radiation-induced alimentary tract injury. In Dubois, A., King, G. L. and Livengood, D. R. (Eds), *Radiation and the Gastrointestinal Tract*. CRC Press, Boca Raton, FL, pp. 3–20.

Srinivasan, V. and Dubois, A. (1995). Nutritional support of irradiated intestine. In Dubois, A., King, G. L. and Livengood, D. R. (Eds), *Radiation and the Gastrointestinal Tract*. CRC Press, Boca Raton, FL, pp. 201–214.

Stewart, A. and Kneale, G. W. (1970). Radiation dose effects in relation to obstetric X-rays and childhood cancers. *Lancet*, **i**, 1185–1188.

Tamou, S. and Trott, K. R. (1995). The effects of local X-irradiation on the distensibility of the rectum in rats. *Br. J. Radiol.*, **68**, 64–69.

Tefft, M. (1972). Radiation effect on growing bone and cartilage. *Front. Radiat. Ther. Oncol.*, **6**, 289–311.

Travis, E. L. and Tucker, S. L. (1986). The relationship between functional assays of radiation response in the lung and target cell depletion. *Br. J. Cancer*, **53** (Suppl. VII), 304–319.

UNSCEAR (1977). *Sources and Effects of Ionizing Radiation. Annex J: Developmental Effects of Irradiation* in utero. Effects of Atomic Radiation. United Nations, New York, pp. 655–710.

UNSCEAR (1982). *Sources and Biological Effects of Irradiation. Annex I: Genetic Effects of Irradiation*. United Nations Scientific Committee on the Effects of Atomic Radiation. United Nations, New York, pp. 425–569.

UNSCEAR (1986). *Genetic and Somatic Effects of Ionizing Radiation. Annex B: Dose–Response Relationships for Radiation-induced Cancer*. United Nations Scientific Committee on the Effects of Atomic Radiation. United Nations, New York, pp. 165–262.

UNSCEAR (1988). *Sources, Effects and Risks of Ionizing Radiation. Annex E: Genetic Hazards*, pp. 375–403. *Annex F: Radiation Carcinogenesis in Man*, pp. 405–543. *Annex G: Early Effects in Man of High Doses of Radiation*, pp. 545–612. United Nations Scientific Committee on the Effects of Atomic Radiation. United Nations, New York.

van der Brenk, H. A. S. (1971). Radiation effects on the pulmonary system. In Berdjis, C. C. (Ed.), *Pathology of Irradiation*. Williams and Wilkins, Baltimore, pp. 569–591.

Vigneulle, R. M. (1995). Nearby shielding influences survival of the irradiated intestine. In Dubois, A., King, G. L. and Livengood, D. R. (Eds) *Radiation and the Gastrointestinal Tract*. CRC Press, Boca Raton, FL, pp. 161–170.

Watson, G. E., Lorimore, S. A., Clutton, S. M., Kadhim, M. A. and Wright, E. G. (1997). Genetic factors influencing alpha-particle-induced chromosomal instability. *Int. J. Radiat. Biol.*, **71**, 497–503.

Weiss, J. F., Landauer, M. R., Gunter-Smith, P. and Hanson, W. R. (1995). Effect of radioprotective agents on survival after acute intestinal radiation injury. In Dubois, A., King, G. L. and Livengood, D. R. (Eds), *Radiation and the Gastrointestinal Tract*. CRC Press, Boca Raton, FL, pp. 183–200.

Whang, W. P. and Little, J. B. (1992). Persistently elevated frequency of spontaneous mutations in progeny of CHO clones surviving X irradiation: association with delayed reproductive death phenotype. *Mutat. Res.*, **270**, 191–199.

Wharton, J. T., Declos, L., Gallagher, S. and Smith, J. P. (1973). Radiation nephritis induced by abdominal irradiation with the cobalt-60 moving strip technique. *Am. J. Roentgenol.*, **117**, 73–80.

Withers, H. R. and Elkind, M. M. (1970). Microcolony survival assay for cells of mouse intestinal mucosa exposed to radiation. *Int. J. Radiat. Biol.*, **17**, 261–267.

SUGGESTED FURTHER READING

Baverstock, K. F. and Stather, J. W. (Eds) (1989). *Low Dose Radiation: Biological Bases of Risk Assessment*. Taylor and Francis, London.

Hall, E. J. (1988). *Radiobiology for the Radiologist*, 3rd edn. Lippincott, Philadelphia.

International Commission on Radiological Protection Publications. Pergamon Press, Oxford.

National Council on Radiation Protection and Measurements Reports. 7910 Woodmont Avenue, Bethesda, MD 20814, USA.

National Research Council Advisory Committee on the Biological Effects of Ionizing Radiation. BEIR Reports. National Academy Press, 2101 Constitution Avenue, NW, Washington, DC 20418, USA.

Steel, G. G. (ed.) (1989). *The Radiobiology of Human Cell and Tissues*. Taylor and Francis, London.

United Nations Scientific Committee on the Effects of Atomic Radiation. Reports to the General Assembly, with Annexes. United Nations, New York.

Chapter 79

Idiopathic Environmental Intolerances

Patricia J. Sparks

CONTENTS

INTRODUCTION AND CASE DEFINITION

Idiopathic environmental illness (IEI) is defined as an acquired disorder with multiple recurrent symptoms, associated with diverse environmental factors tolerated by the majority of people, and not explained by any known medical or psychiatric disorder [International Programme on Chemical Safety (UNEP–ILO–WHO) et al., 1996].

The name IEI supplants, and is more inclusive than, other terms such as multiple chemical sensitivity (MCS) syndrome and environmental illness (EI). The term IEI also attempts to address other of the numerous ever-shifting labels assigned to patients reporting symptoms they attribute to environmental exposure depending on the most recent hypothesis regarding aetiology.

A select panel convened by the World Health Organization [International Programme on Chemical Safety (UNEP–ILO–WHO et al., 1996] concluded that the labels MCS and EI should be replaced for several reasons. Use of the word 'sensitivity' in a diagnostic label can be construed as connoting an allergic or other idiosyncratic pathophysiological cause of these phenomena, and there is no scientific foundation for such causative explanations. Second, environmental intolerances other than chemicals have been described (such as electromagnetic fields). Third, the relationship between symptoms and putative exposures is unproved. Finally, neither MCS nor EI can be recognized as a clinically defined disease with generally accepted underlying pathophysiological mechanisms or validated criteria for diagnosis.

A widely cited definition for MCS, created by Cullen (1987) primarily for research purposes, characterizes MCS as 'a subjectively defined disorder acquired in relation to some documentable environmental exposure, with symptoms involving more than one organ system and elicited by exposures to chemicals that are demonstrable, but very low, and typically involving chemicals of widely varied structural classes and different mechanisms of toxicologic action. No widely available test of organ system function can explain symptoms, and there is no objective evidence of organ system damage or dysfunction'.

This definition attempts to distinguish IEI individuals from those reporting similar symptoms with other labels such as chronic fatigue syndrome or fibromyalgia; however, this definition is problematic. Major practical limitations include the subjectivity and non-specificity of the available information regarding the 'predictable' and 'demonstrable' attributes of the exposure–symptom relationship. Whereas these data might be most meaningfully established by double-blind and controlled exposure challenge testing, they are usually characterized solely on the basis of the patient's report (Sparks et al., 1994a, b). MCS is an illness in which the patient defines both the cause and manifestations of his or her own condition (Gots, 1995).

The term IEI will be used throughout this chapter to encompass those syndromes previously labelled as MCS or EI, in addition to other phenomena such as some variants of 'sick building syndrome'.

IEI must be distinguished from objectively defined illness and injury diagnoses, such as allergic rhinitis/sinusitis or asthma. In these conditions, objective findings are present during active disease, and the causal relationship of those findings to environmental exposure is more readily established. In clinical practice, however, there may be overlap between acute and chronic occupational or environmental illnesses, associated with objective signs of disease, and IEI.

PREVALENCE

It is difficult to assess the prevalence of a condition with a variable, subjectively defined case definition without validated objective findings. Although definitive population-based studies have not been published, the estimated prevalence of IEI ranges from 0.2 to 4% of the general population. Women represent 70–80% of the affected population (Bell *et al.*, 1994).

A survey of the self-reported (not validated medically) prevalence of allergy and chemical sensitivity in a rural population in eastern North Carolina found that chemical sensitivity was reported by 33% of individuals with 18.3% reporting symptoms from chemical sensitivity at least once or more each week; 3.9% of the population reported symptoms almost daily (Meggs *et al.*, 1996a). There is a report of varying severity of self-reported chemical odour intolerance in 15–30% of a young adult college student and active, retired, community elderly populations (Bell *et al.* 1993a, b).

A telephone survey performed by the California Department of Health (Agency for Toxic Substances and Disease Registry, 1996; Kreutzer, 1997) found that 6.3% of those surveyed had been given a diagnosis of EI or MCS and 15.9% considered themselves allergic or unusually sensitive to everyday chemicals such as household cleaners, paints, perfumes and soaps. About 3% considered themselves restricted in activities of daily living because of their sensitivities.

Many IEI patients (about 40%) report the onset of symptoms as being gradual with no specific exposure or event recalled. Across various studies the most prevalent symptoms have involved the central nervous system and respiratory and gastro-intestinal tract, although symptoms in any organ system have been reported and there is no consistent pattern of symptoms that distinguishes patients with IEI from those labeled with other diagnosis manifested primarily by subjective symptoms. Also, almost any environmental exposure has been described to precipitate symptoms. No single chemical exposure or psychosocial situation appears to have been more prevalent than any other in association with the onset of IEI (Fiedler and Kipen, 1997).

THEORIES OF AETIOLOGY OF IEI

A broad spectrum of individuals may be diagnosed with IEI. As most physicians see only a few of these patients, who are heterogeneous, caution is recommended in generalizing experience with one patient to others with this diagnosis.

There are four major views about the aetiology of this syndrome, although more than one of these proposed mechanisms are likely to be operating in different patients and there is some overlap among the views of

pathogenesis. (In this chapter we will discuss these theories in relation to low-level chemical exposures.) One view is that IEI is a primarily physical or toxicological reaction to multiple environmental chemical exposures. A second view is that IEI symptoms may be precipitated by low-level environmental exposures, but the underlying increased sensitivity is due primarily to psychophysiological factors or stress, such that IEI is primarily a behavioural phenomenon. A third view is that IEI is a misdiagnosis, and chemical exposure is not the cause of the symptoms. In this case, the symptoms may be due to misdiagnosed physical or psychological illness. The fourth view is that IEI is simply a culturally acquired belief system instilled by certain practitioners, the media or others in society; IEI is therefore the manifestation of culturally shaped illness behaviour. These four views are discussed in more detail below.

Physical/Toxicological Mechanisms

Assuming that symptoms in IEI may be caused by environmental exposure (predominately to synthetic chemicals), proposed mechanisms include immunological injury, oxidative injury, abnormalities of porphyrin metabolism, non-specific neurogenic inflammation of the respiratory tract and neurotoxicity.

Immunological Theories

The concept of 'allergy' has been invoked as a rationale for why IEI patients experience symptoms on exposure to various chemical substances at doses far lower than those associated with objective manifestations of toxicity in most similarly exposed individuals. Physician specialists in 'clinical ecology' have developed theories of allergic aetiology of environmental illness (Terr, 1989). Some (Miller, 1997) have proposed that IEI be characterized as an illness due to individual susceptibility in combination with chemical toxicity.

Various immunological mechanisms for IEI have been postulated based on case reports and clinical laboratory test data (Broughton and Thrasher, 1988; Thrasher *et al.*, 1989; Madison *et al.*, 1991; Vojdani *et al.*, 1992). Some reports have described alterations in T cell subsets, elevated or reduced helper/suppressor ratios, low titres of auto-antibodies, T lymphocyte activation or altered interleukin-1 or interleukin-2 levels in individuals who report low-level chemical exposures and various subjective symptoms. All but one study are case series or cross-sectional studies without control of preceding exposures or concurrent blind testing of controls. Across the case reports, however, there is no consistent pattern of test abnormalities or a consistent correlation of the reported findings with either specific chemical exposures or disease due to such exposures (Patterson *et al.*, 1987; Sparks *et al.*, 1990; Simon *et al.*, 1993, Salvaggio, 1996). Also, rarely are data presented for controls, nor are the controls known to be without low-level chemical exposures.

There are multiple problems with theories implicating a disturbance of the immune system as the cause of IEI (Sparks et al., 1994a; Salvaggio, 1996). There are inadequate or widely variable reference ranges for many of the tests used; several lack accepted and standardized laboratory protocols. There has been a lack of standardization of immunophenotyping using flow cytometry. Immune parameters may fluctuate with exposure to infectious agents, hormones or environmental stressors. The published research has often been performed by persons associated with commercial laboratories; other investigators have generally failed to replicate the reported findings.

In an outbreak of illness in aerospace workers (Sparks et al., 1990), a number of the workers had been evaluated with such immunological tests performed by one commercial laboratory. Retesting in a university-based immunology research laboratory showed that the previously reported IgE and IgG antibodies to formaldehyde were not detectable (Grammer et al., 1990).

Simon et al. (1993) performed a controlled and blind study of IEI clinic patients and controls selected from a musculoskeletal clinic population. There were no significant differences between cases and controls in the prevalence of 'positive' anti-tissue, auto-immune antibodies or anti-chemical antibodies, the average number of T-cell lymphocyte subsets (including TA1 cells) or the generation of interleukin-1 by in vitro cultured monocytes. Immunological assays generally have shown poor reproducibility during submission of duplicate samples to this commercial laboratory (on a limited number of split samples, the reliability of the laboratory was little better than chance), suggesting methodological problems also. Thus, the one controlled and blind cross-sectional evaluation of immune parameters in IEI patients that currently exists in the medical literature revealed no consistent pattern of abnormalities.

The proper interpretation of any laboratory test must rely on how well the test discriminates between patients with and without the disease, and what impact the test result has on clinical decision making (Vogt, 1991). No controlled and blind challenge studies have been published demonstrating a consistent pattern of alteration in immune parameters in IEI patients following chemical exposure, even with the patient serving as his or her own control. Even if immunological changes were to be subsequently confirmed, their role with regard to IEI is not clear. There has been no attempt to relate a particular set of symptoms and/or exposures to any specific alteration in function.

Toxic/Metabolic Theories

Another hypothesis is that IEI results from inflammatory mediators released by cell membranes. This process is thought to be initiated by toxic free radicals produced by offending chemical exposures. Vulnerability to IEI is postulated to be due to a deficiency of antioxidants (Levine and Reinhardt, 1983). There are few or no scientific data available to examine this theory.

A case series (Morton, 1995) has been collected in which individuals with IEI have been described as having hereditary coproporphyria, or other porphyrias, on the basis of a fundamentally flawed assay for erythrocyte coproporphyrinogen oxidase or other enzymes in blood, or small elevations of urinary coproporphyrin excretion in urine (which may be seen in a variety of conditions other than the porphyrias). There is no pathophysiological model that would explain a relationship between any of the porphyrias and IEI, nor have abnormalities of porphyrin metabolism been demonstrated in IEI patients compared with appropriate controls (Hahn and Bonkovsky, 1997; Daniell et al., 1997).

Theories of Non-specific Inflammation

Other investigators have postulated that IEI is related to altered function of the respiratory mucosa through amplification of the non-specific immune response to low-level irritants (Bascom, 1992; Meggs, 1997). It is postulated that this might be mediated through c-fibre neurons and the release by the airway epithelium of cytokines producing an acute local inflammatory response, or altered neuro-epithelial interaction. Sensory c-fibres may serve as both afferent and efferent nerves for neurogenic inflammation triggered by environmental irritants and may release various mediators, such substance P, capable of producing vasodialation, oedema and other manifestations of inflammation. Substance P is degraded by neutral endopeptidase (NEP), whose action is inhibited by environmental irritants such as cigarette smoke. It is postulated that depletion of NEP or other enzymes by irritant exposure might amplify the response to exposure to other irritants.

Studies of exposure to the organic vapour phase of environmental tobacco smoke (ETS) in rats have demonstrated vascular extravasation thought to occur from irritant stimulation of the c-fibre neurons (Lundberg et al., 1984). Vascular congestion may be the mechanism of increased nasal resistance observed in human subjects with self-reported sensitivity to ETS when challenged with brief high levels of tobacco smoke (Bascom et al., 1991). An increase in baseline nasal resistance in response to odours has been observed in patients with IEI when compared with controls (Doty et al., 1988).

One study (Meggs and Cleveland, 1993) described findings of oedema, excessive mucus, a cobblestone appearance of the posterior pharynx and base of the tongue, focal areas of blanched mucosa and mucosal injection in 10 IEI patients who underwent rhinolaryngoscopy. In a preliminary study of a small number of patients who developed IEI in temporal association with an irritant exposure, upper airway biopsies revealed defects in tight junctions, mucosal desquamation, glandular hyperplasia, lymphocytic infiltrates and peripheral nerve fibre proliferation (Meggs et al., 1996b). A model was proposed in which a positive feedback loop is set up between the inflammatory response to low-level irritants and the epithelial changes produced by the inflammation (Meggs, 1997).

Sensory nerve fibres that react to chemical irritants to produce inflammation are located beneath the epithelial cell layer. High-dose exposure to an irritant chemical can penetrate this barrier to trigger inflammation and damage the layer. When the epithelial barrier is lost, neurogenic inflammation may be triggered at lower doses. Ongoing inflammation continues to damage the epithelial barrier. A proliferation of nerve fibres would mean that there are more receptors for chemical irritants and more inflammatory mediators to be released. With epithelial damage, there is a lower threshold at which chemicals produce inflammation, and this inflammation, in turn, leads to ongoing loss of integrity of the epithelium (Meggs, 1997).

Neurogenic inflammation of the upper respiratory tract does not appear, however, to account for all the multiorgan system complaints in IEI patients, but might help explain some of them. It is possible for local inflammation to be associated with systemic symptoms, such as the fatigue and myalgia associated with viral infection of the upper respiratory tract. Mediators of inflammation, such as interleukins, may be released from the site of inflammation and affect distant sites. Meggs (1997) proposed the concept of neurogenic switching whereby it is possible that stimulation of respiratory receptors by airborne chemicals can lead to involvement of other organ systems. The concept of site switching is derived by analogy with food allergies which can trigger urticaria, rhinitis and asthma. He proposed that there are neuronal pathways from the site of stimulation in the upper airway through the central nervous system to other peripheral locations.

No well designed and controlled studies have been published which confirm a greater prevalence of objective parameters of non-specific upper airway inflammation in IEI patients, nor have any studies been done to test the hypothesis of neurogenic switching.

In most studies, a disproportionate number of patients with IEI are women (Fiedler and Kipen, 1997). It is possible that women have a different physiological response to men to low-level chemcial exposure. Most studies of the health effects of occupational exposure to chemicals have involved primarily men, and may not be readily applicable to IEI. It has been noted that women have a lower threshold for the perception of odour than do men (Doty et al., 1988). However, a lowered olfactory threshold was not more common in IEI patients than in controls. Other physiological and/or hormonal gender differences have not been studied in humans as they may relate to the IEI phenomenon.

Hummel et al. (1997) performed a double-blind experiment with 23 IEI subjects and healthy controls with regard to their responsiveness to room air and propanol-2 using measures of chemo-sensory event-related potentials and psychophysical measures of olfactory function. Exposure to propanol-2 did not lead to specific changes in olfactory function in IEI patients compared with controls. In contrast, the ability of IEI patients to identify and discriminate odours was lower compared with controls.

Neurotoxic Theories

Another popular theory of causation of IEI proposes a biological mechanism for the behavioural conditioning model described below. It has been proposed that chemical sensitivity may be a neural sensitization phenomenon: exposure to odours and respiratory irritants may precipitate physiological and psychological symptoms, due to interactions between the nervous (limbic) and endocrine systems (Bell et al., 1992; Sorg, 1996).

There are direct anatomical links between the olfactory nerve, the 'limbic system' (including portions of the hippocampus, amygdala, cingulate and subcallosal gyri) and the hypothalamus, which govern the parasympathetic and sympathetic nervous systems. Bell et al. (1993a) postulated that these rich neural interconnections may explain how odour or irritation of the respiratory tract indirectly produce symptoms referable to multiple organ systems.

Rodent studies (Gilbert, 1992) have demonstrated that single high-level or intermittent repeated low-level environmental chemical exposures cause limbic 'kindling' (e.g. the ability of a repeated, intermittent electrical or chemical stimulus that is initially incapable of producing a response eventually to induce seizure activity in later applications). Animal studies also demonstrate time-dependent sensitization, or amplification of subsequent responses to a chemical or novel and threatening psychological stimulus, by the passage of time between stimuli (Antelman et al., 1992).

Rodents pre-treated with formaldehyde inhalation demonstrated a significantly enhanced locomotor response to cocaine compared with controls, suggesting that specific limbic pathways may have been sensitized (Sorg et al., 1996).

It has been suggested (Bell et al., 1992, 1997; Sorg, 1996) that subconvulsive chemical kindling of the olfactory bulb, amygdala, piriform cortex and hippocampus, as well as time-dependent sensitization (TDS), are central nervous system mechanisms that could amplify reactivity and lower the threshold of response to low levels of inhaled chemicals, and could initiate persistent affective, cognitive and somatic symptomatology in some vulnerable individuals who may be genetically predisposed to affective spectrum disorders. It has been postulated that this neurological sensitization might occur with either a single, high-dose exposure to a chemical substance, followed by much smaller subtoxic levels of exposure to the same chemical, or with repeated lower dose exposures, as has been demonstrated in animals. It has been observed that time-dependent sensitization occurs more readily in female rats (Antelman, 1988), which is postulated to have relevance to the apparent preponderance of females among IEI patients (Bell et al., 1992).

Kindling and time-dependent sensitization have also been postulated to explain the initiation of psychiatric disorders such as depression (Post, 1992) and post-traumatic stress disorder (Pitman et al., 1993) in some individuals, independently of the IEI phenomenon.

Bell et al. (1997) emphasized that sensitization is distinct, although interactive with other psychological, learning and memory theories such as conditioning which may occur simultaneously.

There are, however, no experimental data in humans to support or refute the role of chemically induced kindling or TDS in producing IEI, or to determine whether the proposed mechanisms, if verified experimentally, would be specific to IEI patients. In addition, kindling occurs in animals in response to pharmacologically effective doses of drugs or other chemical substances rather than trace exposures. Finally, the proposed effects in humans may be indistinguishable from those that are behaviourally or cognitively mediated.

Central neurophysiological alterations consequent to exogenous chemical exposures might represent toxic injury or perhaps a maladaptive but reversible central nervous system response pattern, i.e. a form of behavioural conditioning. The treatment and lifestyle implications of these alternative response patterns are contradictory, since chemically induced injury would probably preclude further exposure to the suspect chemicals and would justify some physicians' recommendations for chemical avoidance. However, the latter response pattern might be amenable to readaptation through behavioural, cognitive, environmental or even pharmacological interventions, with the goal of progressive resumption of normal activity.

With regard to measurable neuropsychological parameters, Selner and Staudenmeyer (1992) reported that the EEG activity in IEI patients more closely resembled those of psychological patients than controls, but no controlled and blind studies have examined IEI patients exposed to various chemical substances to look for acute reproducible alterations of brain electrical activity.

There is limited peer-reviewed literature with regard to neurotoxicity and functional brain imaging. The studies that have been published have had poor study design, with lack of appropriate controls or validation of findings (Society of Nuclear Medicine Brain Imaging Council, 1996). No controlled and blind studies have demonstrated any patterns of abnormalities on brain imaging studies (such as SPECT or PET scans) that would distinguish IE patients from normals or individuals with primary psychiatric disorders.

It has been found (Simon et al., 1993; Fiedler and Kipen 1997) that IEI patients differed little from controls on selected measures of neurocognitive function, despite the high prevalence of complaints of cognitive dysfunction. There are no data to show that IEI patients demonstrate a consistent or specific pattern of neurocognitive deficits, at least in cross-sectional studies, and disturbances of memory and attention observed in some IEI patients may be a result of depression and/or anxiety.

Summary of Theories of Physical/Toxic Injury

Arguing against physical toxic injury as a cause of symptoms in IEI patients is the observation that the intensity of exposure to various chemical exposures does not match the prevalence of IEI symptoms, violating a basic tenet of toxicology: 'the dose makes the poison'. The relationship of IEI symptoms to environmental chemical exposures also does not appear to fit other established principles of toxicology. There is agreement among occupational health professionals that any natural or synthetic chemical exposure in sufficient doses may be harmful to specific organs of the body and can produce objectively measurable toxic effects. Causal relationships between toxic exposures and human disease generally are established by determining the strength of the association between exposure and the development of disease using epidemiological methods and toxicological animal models, dose–response relationships and the consistency and predictability of the clinical responses to specific chemical exposures in affected human subjects (Sullivan and Krieger, 1992). In IEI, all of these criteria are lacking.

IEI as a Behavioural Phenomenon

Behavioural Conditioning and Stress

Some investigators have proposed a behavioural conditioned response (CR) to odour (Bolla-Wilson et al., 1988), in which a strong-smelling chemical irritant causes a direct and unconditioned physical or psychophysiological response (UCR). Later, the same odour or irritant at a much lower concentration causes a conditioned response of the same symptoms. Through stimulus generalization, different odours or irritants become the precipitant for similar symptoms.

Siegel and Kreutzer (1997) noted that many toxic chemicals have distinctive odours and, thus, over-exposure to these chemicals, with irritant of toxic effects, could involve pairing of a distinctive olfactory cue with illness. (IEI patients rarely, if ever, develop their symptoms following exposure to odorless substances.) For patients who may have been exposed to an irritant in the context of distinctive environmental cues, after some number of pairings, the environment itself may elicit a conditioned irritant response.

Some individuals tend to produce highly specific physiological responses to many stressors, which has been termed 'individual response stereotypy' (Lehrer, 1997). Severe chemical exposure may act as an unconditioned stimulus producing one-trial learning of a conditioned neurophysiological response that may have a particular sensitizing effect upon individuals who are predisposed to stereotypical psychophysiological responsiveness, even before the exposure. Later, this same physiological response may generalize and be elicited by other substances. If actual or perceived exposure to chemicals is a psychological stressor among IEI patients, a stress-related autonomic reaction may occur (Lehrer, 1997).

Some specific symptoms can even be triggered by suggestion. In 1896, McKenzie noted that a patient who was allergic to roses displayed an asthma reaction when presented with an artificial rose. The visual features of the rose served as a CS for the allergic response. In the asthma literature, a number of studies have provided evidence that psychogenic asthma attacks can occur even when a person simply thinks that exposure to an asthma trigger has occurred (Isenverg et al., 1992). A double-blind placebo-controlled study on intranasal chemoreception in patients with IEI, in which chemosensory event-related potentials were used an objective measure of outcome, demonstrated that 20% of subjects responded regardless of the type of challenge, suggesting that these individuals were susceptible to non-specific experimental manipulation (Hummel, et al., 1997). Thus, some IEI patients may respond on the basis of belief that they have been exposed to something capable of eliciting symptoms, rather than conditioning.

Pavlovian conditioning does not entirely explain the wide array of symptoms presented by IEI patients. Also, in many cases of IEI there is no substantiated initial exposure event that would constitute the unconditioned stimulus. Staudenmayer et al. (1993a) demonstrated in double-blind placebo-controlled studies that conditioning alone cannot explain a 'chemical reaction'. When the unconditioned stimulus, usually an odour, is not detectable because it is either masked by another odour to which the patient shows tolerance, or is presented below olfactory and irritant thresholds, some patients still report having symptoms.

Jewett (1992) postulated that IEI may be a manifestation of the human response to stress. Whatever the initial precipitating event (whether it be psychological, loss of self esteem, fear of harm from chemical exposure or other physical illness), the individual experiencing stress may exhibit heightened sensitivity to odors or respiratory tract irritants.

Bell and co-workers performed a questionnaire survey of college students (Bell et al., 1993a) and community elderly volunteers participating in a longitudinal survey of bone density at a local hospital (Bell et al., 1993b). Extreme cacosmia was defined as a self-report of feeling ill on exposure to four or more of the following chemicals: pesticides, automobile exhaust, paint, new carpet or perfume. Both surveys revealed a fairly high prevalence of extreme cacosmia to multiple odours (15% and 17%, respectively). The extremely cacosmic subgroup of college students had higher anxiety and depression rating scores than did students who reported a lower degree of cacosmia. The extremely cacosmic elderly respondents reported higher ratings for anxiety and recent major life changes, but not depression. These findings support the theory that psychological stress may play a role in an individual's subjective sensitivity to odours from chemical exposure.

The perceived risk of harm associated with an odour has a great deal to do with one's psychophysiological reaction to the odor. Survey data have indicated that perceived risk from exposure was the most significant correlate of odour annoyance from factories with occasional emissions (McClelland et al., 1990). Dalton (1996) confirmed experimentally that there was a direct relationship between perceived risk and odour intensity. Variation in perception and intensity of odours can result from the explicit characterization given to the odour and gives support to the position that odour perception is both a sensory and cognitive function.

Other studies, including Dalton's (Dalton, 1996), have shown inhibition of olfactory adaptation and elevated olfactory sensitivity (hyperosmia) among individuals reporting high levels of anxiety or stress (Rovee et al., 1973; Schneider, 1974).

Odour-induced Anxiety

There are small case series reports in which organic solvents (Dager et al., 1987; Bolla-Wilson et al., 1988; Schusterman et al., 1988) or cocaine (Post et al., 1987) have precipitated panic attacks. Schusterman and Dager have proposed the descriptive designation of 'odour-triggered panic attacks or panic disorder' for cases in which one or more chemical odours trigger either typical or limited panic attacks. They postulate that odour produces annoyance and autonomic arousal, which then may be amplified in an individual with predisposing cognitive, personality or biological susceptibility (Schusterman and Dager, 1987).

Although there are limited data to support this contention, low-level exposure to irritants or odours may produce psychophysiological symptoms which, in some vulnerable individuals, may evolve into IEI. Psychophysiological symptoms occurred with very high prevalence in a group of aerospace workers (Sparks, 1990), most of whom had no significant past histories of psychiatric illness. The exposures to organic solvents and other chemicals were several standard deviations below the levels reported to be associated with toxic or irritant effects. Follow-up information on almost all the workers evaluated in this outbreak indicated that most workers experienced improvement in symptoms following removal of the offending chemical odour/irritant (phenol–formaldehyde composite material) from the plant, suggesting that some of the prevalent symptoms of depression and anxiety might have been induced by exposure to this material (although other contributing psychosocial factors were clearly operant in this situation) (Sparks, 1990).

Leznoff (1997) challenged 15 patients with IEI with trigger substances. Pre-and postchallenge pulmonary function tests and blood gases were measured. All of the patients whose symptoms were reproduced by the challenge (11 of 15) showed clinical evidence of acute hyperventilation with a rapid fall in pCO_2 and no change or rise in oxygen saturation. The symptoms and signs were consistent with an anxiety reaction with hyperventilation. This suggests that IEI is a manifestation of an anxiety syndrome triggered by the perception of an environmental insult with at least some symptoms induced by hyperventilation.

Leznoff (1997b) noted that one of the most common symptoms of IEI-impaired mentation is often described as 'brain fog', which may also be characteristic of acute hypocarbia which causes restriction of cerebral flow and decreased brain perfusion.

Binkley and Kutcher (1997) reported that patients referred to an allergy and clinical immunology service for evaluation of 'chemical sensitivity' were investigated to rule out underlying medical conditions including asthma as a cause of their symptoms. After a standardized psychiatric assessment had been performed, patients underwent single-blind intravenous infusion of a normal saline solution (placebo) and sodium lactate (which reproduces symptoms in individuals with underlying panic disorder). Four of the five patients met DSM-III-R diagnostic criteria for panic disorder along with other depressive and/or anxiety related disorders. All five patients with self-identified chemical sensitivity exhibited a positive symptomatic response to sodium lactate compared with placebo infusion.

Independent psychiatric assessment confirmed the diagnosis of panic disorder on the basis of DSM-III-R criteria in each of the five patients. The results suggest that IEI may have a neurobiological basis similar to, if not identical with, that of panic disorder. Although sodium lactate infusion is less sensitive than clinical assessment in identifying panic disorder, the results of the infusions are compelling because they are less likely than clinical assessments to be distorted by bias.

The concept of IEI as a type of phobic disturbance is compatible with the panic disorder hypothesis. Underlying panic disorder with conditioned phobic responses to 'chemical' triggers could account for the full clinical picture in at least a subset of patients with IEI. Through the mechanism of conditioned response, environmental 'toxins' could become psychologically linked with panic symptoms. This link, reinforced by caregivers, could result in increased anticipatory anxiety with a production and maintenance of panic attacks and phobic avoidance with reluctance to seek potentially helpful psychiatric treatments (Binkley and Kutcher, 1997).

IEI as Other Misdiagnosed Illnesses

It has been suggested that IEI is a misdiagnosis and chemical exposure is not the cause of the symptoms. In contrast, the patient's complaints may be due to a misdiagnosed physical or psychological illness. The likelihood of misdiagnosis may be furthered by conscious or subconscious attempts by the patient or physician to avoid a psychiatric diagnosis (Brodsky, 1987; Stewart, 1987; Terr, 1989; Black et al., 1990). Among proponents of the theory that primary psychiatric illness has been inappropriately attributed to environmental exposure, terms such as environmental somatization (Gothe et al., 1995) or toxic agoraphobia (Kurt, 1995) have been used.

In situations where a history of chemical exposure is obtained, the clinical ecologist or other physician may misinterpret symptoms of common psychiatric disorders as indicating the patient has IEI. Published case series (with varying case definitions) have reported an increased frequency of symptoms categorizable as depression, anxiety disorders, somatization, obsessive–compulsive and other personality disorders in persons diagnosed with IEI, as well as greater frequency of abnormal elevations on various subscales of the Minnesota Multiphasic Personality Inventory (Scottenfeld, 1987; Stewart, 1987; Terr, 1989; Simon et al., 1990; Black, 1993a).

Black et al. (1990) compared 26 subjects recruited from a community and clinic population with IEI with 46 age- and sex-matched general population controls. Twenty-three were given standardized psychiatric assessments including the Diagnostic Interview Schedule (DIS) and the Structured Interview for DSM-III-R Personality Disorders. Several self-report instruments were used to assess somatic concerns, hypochondriacal behaviour and past and current major depression. Some 65% of assessed subjects met criteria for mood, anxiety or somatiform disorders compared with 28% of the controls, a significant difference. Nearly three-quarters of the subjects met criteria for at least one personality disorder, compared with 28.3% of controls, also a statistically significant difference. Only three of the 23 subjects assessed were free of a major mental or personality disorder, certainly a higher prevalence than community controls. The authors concluded that most patients diagnosed with environmental illness have unrecognized emotional problems that were not being appropriately diagnosed and treated (Black, 1993b).

Staudenmayer *et al*. (1993b) have reported significantly higher rates of physical and sexual abuse among IEI patients.

The prevalence of somatization disorder among studies varies, depending on whether or not IEI is accepted as an organic explanation for physical symptoms. It is clear, however, that the studies overall demonstrate that IEI subjects relative to controls tend to report a larger number of physical symptoms and score higher on scales that reflect concerns with somatic sensations.

Because of the possibility that IEI itself might produce psychiatric symptoms, some investigators have tried to evaluate the presence of pre-existing symptoms of psychiatric illness in patients diagnosed with IEI (Simon *et al*., 1990, 1993). Among the group of aerospace plastics workers evaluated by Sparks *et al*. (1990), there was a subgroup of 13 who fit a case definition of IEI similar to Cullen's and who also had a history of decreased functional status due to their symptoms. The 13 workers with IEI scored significantly higher on measures of pre-existing somatization and psychopathology than did the other workers. A history of somatization and psychiatric morbidity predating workplace exposure to chemicals was the strongest predictor of IEI (Simon *et al*., 1990).

Terr (1989) found that the prior medical records of 90 patients diagnosed as having work-related IEI, and engaged in workers' compensation litigation, contained documented evidence of the same multiple symptoms for many years prior to the employment of concern in 56 (62%) of the cases.

Simon *et al*. (1993) evaluated psychological and other parameters in IEI, and included case and control groups from two defined clinic populations. Psychiatric assessment was performed using self-report measures and structured interviews, but including modifications to contrast dates of onset of any diagnosable psychological disorders and the study condition. Again, there was a greater prevalence of symptoms consistent with depression, anxiety and somatization in IEI cases than controls, who were patients from a musculoskeletal clinic without evidence of systemic disease.

In particular, although there was no apparent difference in the prevalence of pre-existing anxiety or depression, the prevalence of somatization symptom pattern among IEI patients *prior* to onset of IEI was significantly greater than in matched controls. While acknowledging that retrospective assessment has limited ability to discern temporal patterns of disease, the authors postulated that, among a substantial proportion of individuals who develop IEI, pre-existing psychological vulnerability plays a significant role in their development of the syndrome.

Even in the studies reporting an excess of psychiatric illness in IEI subjects there is a relatively small proportion of persons diagnosed with IEI who do not have histories of pre-existing (or concurrent) psychiatric disorders or abnormal elevations on self-report measures of psychological distress predating exposures of concern.

Bell *et al*. (1992) and others argue that (1) DSM-III-R diagnoses are simply a collection of symptoms and do not define aetiology, (2) identifying affective disorders in persons diagnosed with IEI does not establish their aetiological role, nor does it rule out other concomitant illnesses, and (3) the observation that psychiatric treatments improve symptoms in many (but not all) patients with IEI does not rule out neurotoxic or other causal mechanisms.

Finally, the finding of a higher prevalence of current psychiatric disorders in IEI patients does not exclude the possibility that some patients with IEI experienced odour-triggered panic attacks or other psychophysiological symptoms on exposure to low-level respiratory tract irritants as the precipitating event for their illness (Sparks, 1990). However, Staudenmayer (1996) maintains that panic disorder combined with conditioned phobic responses to 'chemical triggers' is neither necessary nor sufficient to explain the many psychological factors and psychiatric disorders that have been identified in this heterogeneous population. He maintains that the primary unifying psychological factor among these patients is their over-valued idea that factors in the physical environment are the source of their misery.

IEI as an Illness Belief System

Other professionals have postulated that, in many ways, IEI is a belief system. Promoted by clinical ecologists and those sympathetic to their views, and followed by medically unsophisticated lay persons, the belief is reinforced by referring patients to a network of similarly minded clinicians and establishing support groups, hotlines, journals and clinics to support and reinforce these beliefs. Some have called this phenomenon a medical subculture. According to this model, the group psychosocial dynamic amongst patients diagnosed with IEI facilitates and perpetuates rationalizations regarding the role of external and uncontrollable factors in their illness, rejects the concept that symptoms are not indicative of severe disease or may have psychological components that can be helped by behavioural or pharmacological treatments, and promotes the assumption of the patient as a victim, associated with assertive or adversarial interactions with conventional health care and disability systems (Brodsky, 1987).

It has been observed previously that IEI shares many features with other conditions such as chronic fatigue syndrome, fibromyalgia, neurasthenia or chronic post-viral syndrome, which encompass individuals with distress and functional disability characterized by few or no objective findings. It has been speculated that IEI is simply the most contemporary cultural expression of psychosomatic illness (Brodsky, 1987). In at least some patients, IEI may result from iatrogenic (physician-induced) hypochondriasis (Black, 1996).

Shorter (1992), a sociologist and historian, chronicles the connection between psychological distress and its expression as shaped by the patient's interaction with the physician and the prevailing culture. Psychosomatic symptoms become attached to a disease label by the establishment of parallels between common symptoms and conventionally accepted organic diseases. Conditions popularly believed to be difficult to detect or substantiate, and which are thought to have a cause of origin external to the patient, provide a template or point of reference. Subsequently, sympathetic physicians, patient support and advocacy groups and the media publicize the presumed aetiological association. Eventually this may result in an increase in symptom attribution, rather than an increase in actual organic illness. Physicians play an important role in shaping symptom expression by their patients (Shorter, 1992).

The public, understandably, has increasing concerns regarding environmental pollution and health effects of exposure to man-made chemicals. Employers and manufacturers have been asked to reduce noxious exposures and provide those exposed with detailed information regarding health risks. Patients and their primary care physicians, many of whom obtain their information regarding chemical hazards from the lay press, increasingly regard man-made chemicals of any kind as unacceptable threats to health (McCallum, 1991). Many physicians do not appear to apply accepted principles of pharmacology and toxicology to their assessment of health risk of environmental chemical exposures. For example, 38% of physicians surveyed by McCallum reported the belief that it was not how much of a chemical to which one was exposed that determined health risk but whether one was exposed at all (McCallum, 1991).

Gomez et al. (1996) postulated that if IEI represents psychosomatic illness modified by belief of environmental attribution, then methods for representing beliefs should show systematic differences between IEI and other populations including medical patients, and indeed, their research confirms this.

It is unlikely that the majority of IEI patients are simulating their symptoms, or that symptoms in most IEI patients result from suggestion or shaping on the part of the culture or their physicians, although the attribution of symptoms to environmental chemical exposure is probably due to these factors in some cases.

Summary of Theories of Pathogenesis

The available evidence shows that patients diagnosed with IEI are heterogeneous, and that more than one causal mechanism may be operative in different cases. It is possible that pre-existing or concurrent psychiatric illness, particular health belief models and psychological stress may produce a vulnerable group of individuals who then develop a sensitivity to odours or low-level chemical irritants that occurs as a result of one or more of the above-proposed mechanisms. None of the above views of aetiology of IEI is universally accepted on the basis of substantial scientific evidence and dogmatic adherence to any one of them is unwise as a basis for managing individual patients with an IEI diagnosis. The fact that there is no agreement upon any one aetiology for most patients with IEI does not prevent clinicians from helping affected patients with their symptoms.

EVALUATION, DIAGNOSIS AND TREATMENT

Understanding the phenomenon of IEI requires evaluation of pathophysiological, psychological and social factors using the biopsychosocial model of illness. The comprehensive biopsychosocial model (Engel, 1980) is a systems approach which conceptualizes an intimate mind–body connection; physical diseases have psychological and social correlates, and psychological illnesses have physical correlates. Illness should not be regarded as less 'real' because of the possibility that psychogenic mechanisms may play a major role in causation for many sufferers. The IEI patient's distress should never be dismissed with a statement that it is 'all in the head'.

Clinicians with different views about the pathogenesis of IEI still may agree on clinical management programmes aimed at symptom control and improved functional ability rather than 'cure' of IEI (Sparks et al., 1994b).

Diagnostic Evaluation

The History and Physical Examination

The keys to diagnosis and clinical management of the individual presenting with suspected or previously diagnosed IEI include a detailed exposure history, as well as a comprehensive medical and psychosocial evaluation of the patient (Sparks et al., 1994b). It is critical to rule out the presence of a physical disease caused by defined occupational or environmental factors. A pitfall to avoid is to diagnose inappropriately patients with well defined toxic or allergic disease or irritant injury, such as asthma, lead intoxication or sinusitis, with IEI, and thus possibly fail to provide appropriate treatment. There also may be some overlap of these conditions and IEI syndrome.

The clinical evaluation of IEI is challenging enough for the occupational and environmental physician specialist with formal training and experience in exposure assessment and clinical toxicology, and therefore may be extremely difficult for the primary care physician who usually is not trained to evaluate the clinical significance of the patient's exposure history. In most cases, consultation with a physician who is board-certified in occupational and environmental medicine or industrial toxicology should be obtained. The evaluation of a patient presenting with IEI may take several hours and it is necessary to allot sufficient time.

Industrial hygiene data regarding the patient's exposures should be obtained whenever possible. If the exposure occurred in the workplace, the relevant Material Safety Data Sheets should be obtained from the patient or employer. Many chemicals are well established potential causes of the symptoms that IEI patients describe (e.g. toluene diisocyanate and chest tightness, or headache and nausea from exposure to lead or organic solvents). Clearly, it is the physician's job to estimate the dose of environmental exposure, and to determine the probability that an individual patient's symptoms are due to a known toxic or irritant effect of exposure.

Some clinicians have suggested having the patient keep a symptom diary throughout the day, along with information regarding activities and environmental exposures. If, however, culturally and physician-shaped belief systems or misdiagnosed psychiatric or physical illness are operative, this could tend to reinforce the patient's perception of the relationship between symptoms and chemical exposures rather than other potential psychological stressors, for example. Hence this approach is probably not appropriate for many IEI patients, and there is a fine line between urging the patient to pay attention to the effect of various environmental exposures on their symptoms and promoting symptom attribution by suggestion.

It is essential that the physician rule out other non-environmental illness or disease in the differential diagnosis. The physician should take a detailed medical history regarding current and past illnesses, previous diagnostic evaluations and treatments and a possible historical pattern of many unexplained physical symptoms with onset early in adulthood or frequent utilization of medical care. Access to prior medical and psychiatric records and their thorough review are particularly important. Physical examination and laboratory evaluation should be sufficiently comprehensive to establish or rule out all other occupational and non-occupational disease conditions in the differential diagnosis.

Psychiatric evaluation of the individual diagnosed with IEI may be appropriate, given the high prevalence of co-existing or pre-existing psychiatric disorders in these patients. Unfortunately, most patients given a diagnosis of IEI resist the idea that psychological factors may play any aetiological role at all in their distress; however, this should not necessarily be interpreted that the patient has a primary psychiatric illness.

Table 1 Diagnostic evaluation for IEI

A. History
  Detailed exposure history (workplace and other environmental exposures)
  Industrial hygiene data (Material Safety Data Sheets, results of exposure monitoring, etc.)
  Current and past medical illnesses, and results of previous diagnostic work-ups and treatments
  Review of prior medical records
B. Physical examination
  Rule out other illnesses in the differential diagnosis
C. Consultation
  Occupational and environmental medicine specialist
  Psychiatrist
  Other specialists as appropriate to rule out other medical conditions in the differential diagnosis
D. Other
  Symptom diary
  Short-term removal from exposure

Source: Sparks *et al.*, 1994b.

The adamant rejection of psychological factors in symptom formation and expression by IEI patients is a challenge for the physician, but the important role of psychological stress in symptom severity should be discussed.

Recommendations regarding the evaluation are summarized in **Table 1**.

Diagnostic Testing in IEI

Since there is no established and widely available test to use to diagnose IEI, the physician must be extremely cautious about excessive or inappropriate testing or the misinterpretation of such tests. This may merely reinforce a detrimental pattern of illness behaviour (Sparks *et al.*, 1994b).

Diagnostic testing in patients expressing symptoms of IEI is necessary to rule out the presence of other environmental or non-environmental illness or treatable disease conditions in the differential diagnosis. For example, if the patient has prominent respiratory tract complaints, appropriate pulmonary function tests are needed, as a minimum, to rule out the presence of reactive airway disease. Biological monitoring might be used in some cases to assess exposure to specific chemical substances where there is known to be good correlation of the specific exposure with measured blood or urine levels and health effect (e.g. heavy metals). However, results of diagnostic tests should not be presumed to explain multi-organ symptoms. For example, if pulmonary function tests show airway reactivity, this does not explain central nervous system, gastro-intestinal, dermal, visual or other organ system complaints.

Also, subtle variations in physiological testing may be hard to distinguish from normal variability in a heterogeneous population, and caution is necessary so as not to overinterpret results as an explanation for the patient's symptoms. The patient should be informed that normal test results do not indicate that insufficient testing was done, but rather that evidence of organ system damage was not present (Weaver, 1996).

In some patients, hyperventilation may play a significant role in their symptoms. Observation of breathing rate and pattern, chemistry screening for hypophosphataemia or measurement of arterial blood gases may be indicated.

Definitive research on controlled challenge procedures is necessary before they can be recommended as useful tools for diagnosis (Staudenmayer et al., 1993a; Staudenmayer, 1996). The clinical use of environmental challenge units for diagnosing IEI remains controversial. The problems with this approach are that we usually do not know the actual level of environmental exposure causing symptoms, testing of substances having distinct odours or irritant properties cannot be done in a blind fashion and proper controls and objective measures of response that are relevant to the patient's symptoms are unavailable. Successfully blinded chemical challenges have reportedly resulted in both high false-positive and false-negative rates of response.

Quantitative EEG (QEEG), brain electrical activity mapping (BEAM), evoked potentials and positron emission tomography (PET) and single photon emission computed tomography (SPECT) scans, which measure regional blood flow or brain metabolic function, are procedures which have been misapplied in an effort to provide 'objective findings' for patients with IEI.

Any technique for investigating the CNS effects of low-level exposure to chemical substances should take place only in a research setting with proper controls to validate its clinical use as a diagnostic tool to confirm the presence of IEI (Nuwer, 1990; Society of Nuclear Medicine Brain Imaging Council, 1996).

At present, no form of immunological testing has been shown to be diagnostic of either exposure to specific chemicals or illness due to exposure in patients with IEI (Simon et al., 1993; Terr, 1993; Sparks et al., 1994a, Salvaggio, 1996). For example, low titres of antibodies to formaldehyde have not been correlated either with exposure or with disease due to exposure to formaldehyde. Non-traditional tests such as provocation–neutralization show no correlation with exposure or disease resulting from specific chemicals (Jewett et al., 1990; Council on Scientific Affairs, American Medical Association, 1992), and cannot be justified because of lack of evidence of symptom provocation by sub-neutralizing concentrations.

Some commercial laboratories offer measurements of parts per billion concentrations of various organic solvents or other exogenous chemicals in blood. Often the chemicals are reported to be present at concentrations in the range of error noise of mass spectrometric analysis

and have no clinical relevance. Unfortunately, some physicians have misinterpreted such measures as evidence of unusual chemical exposure and/or toxicity or as an explanation for the symptoms of IEI. Clinical misuse and misinterpretation of such testing is to be avoided.

Neuropsychological testing is dependent on patient cooperation and might be useful to rule out other conditions in the differential diagnosis, but currently does not reveal consistent or specific findings in IEI patients that may be used for diagnosis of this condition.

Finally, blood enzyme assays (corproporphyrin oxidase, for example), or slight increases in urinary coproporphyrin excretion, have been used inappropriately to diagnose various porphyrias or 'porphyrinopathies' in IEI. Such testing does not confirm the diagnosis of porphyria in these patients, the enzyme assays have numerous limitations and there is no scientific evidence supporting a causal link between any of the porphyrias and IEI (Daniell et al., 1997; Hahn and Bonkovsky, 1997).

Recommendations with regard to diagnostic testing in IEI patients are summarized in **Table 2**.

Reinforcement of illness behaviour by unjustifiably giving a patient the diagnosis of a disease due to toxic, immunological, metabolic or neurological mechanisms based on diagnostic testing that is clinically unsubstantiated or invalid may actually perpetuate illness, prolong disability and delay effective therapy.

Table 2 Diagnostic testing for IEI

No established diagnostic test for IEI
Done primarily to rule out other illnesses in the differential diagnosis
Results of test should not be presumed to explain multiorgan symptoms
The following tests are currently not validated for clinical use to confirm the diagnosis of IEI:
Environmental challenge testing (uncontrolled, unblinded)
Quantitative electroencephalography
Brain electrical activity mapping
Evoked potentials (brainstem, visual, sensory)
Position emission tomography scan
Single photon emission computed tomography scan
Immunological testing
Measurements of trace concentrations of volatile organic compounds or pesticides in blood (parts per billion)
Neuropsychological testing
Blood enzyme tests for porphyrias

Source: Sparks et al., 1994b.

Treatment

Even if the aetiologies of the symptoms in patients diagnosed with IEI are controversial and unknown in most patients, these individuals can still be helped with their symptoms. A non-judgmental approach to evaluation and treatment, based on the assumption that the patient's symptoms are 'real' and distressing regardless of the presence or absence of observable organic pathology is suggested (Haller, 1993, Sparks, 1994b). The physician may affirm the illness experience without affirming the attribution for it. The goal of therapy is control of symptoms, and success is not dependent upon a specific organic diagnoses or aetiology, but rather by the patient's improved understanding of the role of stress on his or her illness and the acquisition of skills for coping with the illness' impact on daily life (Sparks et al., 1994b).

A multidisciplinary and behavioural medicine approach similar to that taken in the treatment of chronic pain, chronic fatigue syndrome or fibromyalgia, which also may not have objective physical correlates, may help patients cope better with their symptoms (Institute of Medicine, 1987). The fundamental principle of behavioural approaches is symptom desensitization by gradually increasing exposure in an organized programme allowing for accommodation and increasing tolerance.

Any behavioural programme should also promote an overall increase in physical and social activity. There are few published reports related to such desensitization treatments for IEI, but clinical experience suggests that the efficacy of this approach warrants controlled study (Simon, 1992, Guglielmi et al., 1994; Amundsen et al., 1996). This approach assumes that an important contributing factor to the manifestation of IEI is primarily behavioural without associated objective or progressive physiological impairment, dysfunction and disease. Provocation chamber challenges under double-blind placebo-controlled conditions may have therapeutic value in selected patients (Staudenmayer, 1996) as part of this process.

Recently, researchers in Sweden (Andersson et al., 1996) found in a controlled study of 17 randomly assigned IEI patients (reporting sensitivity to electricity) that cognitive–behavioural therapy was effective in reducing self-reports of functional disability. Double-blind provocation tests also indicated that the IEI patients could not distinguish reliably between the presence or absence of the putative environmental cause of their symptoms.

Enhancing the patient's sense of control over workplace or home stressors, including environmental chemical exposures, is likely to be effective in managing symptoms. A variety of approaches to reducing stress in the IEI patient exist, and many do not involve treatment by a mental health professional or physician. These may include massage, physical therapy, prayer, meditation or regular exercise, for example.

Systematic changes in the organization of work may be needed to reduce organizational stress. Odours and exposure to volatile organic compounds in the workplace and home, which are perceived as irritating or noxious by the symptomatic individual, should be reduced and controlled as much as possible. This should be attempted even if levels of exposure are below government-mandated or recommended permissible exposure limits. It is necessary, although challenging, to balance the benefits of the above recommendations with the potential risks of a spiralling pattern of progressively severe environmental restrictions and loss of employment.

Importantly, treatment of co-existing psychiatric manifestations, such as depression and panic attacks, is likely to reduce symptoms and disability (Simon, 1992). Psychiatric treatments may be helpful in controlling symptoms regardless of aetiology. Even if specific immunological, neurophysiological or neurotoxic mechanisms are ultimately discovered to be operative in some patients with IEI, treatment of psychiatric symptoms may still be a most effective approach to palliation.

For those patients in which hyperventilation and anxiety may be playing a major role in their symptoms, instruction in techniques such as re-breathing into a paper bag are helpful. Some such patients have noted improvements in symptoms with the wearing of a respirator, which also increases the dead space and raises blood CO_2 (Leznoff, 1997b).

As most patients given a diagnosis of IEI resist the idea that psychological factors may play any role at all in their distress, it may be more helpful to co-manage such patients with a primary-care physician experienced in the diagnosis and treatment of depression, anxiety and somatiform disorders, rather than a psychiatrist. The goal of treatment at this time must be relief of symptoms, rather than expectation of cure (Simon, 1992; Sparks et al., 1994b).

Pharmacological treatment may be a helpful adjunct in relief of the psychophysiological symptoms that accompany chemical sensitivity such as depression and mood swings, chronic fatigue, difficulty sleeping and anxiety, regardless of the aetiology of those symptoms. Certainly, those who meet DSM-III-R criteria for major depression should be considered for a trial of antidepressant medication, but psychopharmacological drugs should be prescribed only as part of an overall treatment programme, ideally involving an expert in mental health. However, many patients with IEI report intolerance to relatively low doses of any medication or 'chemical' intervention, and this needs to be considered in initiating antidepressant therapy. In spite of these obvious challenges, the rewards from successfully uncovering and relieving depression, anxiety and mood swings justify the effort.

Those patients who deny that stress or psychological factors might play any role at all in their symptoms, and who perceive their locus of control outside themselves, probably cannot be helped by any of the above medical therapies.

Some IEI patients have attempted to pursue bizarre and costly treatments and may appear desperate as they seek unorthodox therapies such as sublingual neutralization or various 'detoxification' treatment programmes. While remaining non-judgmental about the patient's motivation to seek such therapies, it is the physician's responsibility to educate the patient about their lack of efficacy (American College of Physicians, 1989).

A definite medical recommendation for complete avoidance of chemical exposures is not indicated at this time. In fact, since there is no evidence for a cumulative toxic injury underlying IEI, recommendation for long-term avoidance of chemical exposures is contraindicated. It is also impossible to accomplish. One cannot readily remove the IEI patient from chemical exposures if the patient presents with an ever-changing list of exposures of concern which cannot be measured or tested and which result in unpredictable or individually determined responses. Without negating the patient's symptoms, reassurance should be given that IEI is not associated with signs of progressive disease, nor is it fatal.

Currently there are no data showing that long-term withdrawal from exposure produces an improvement in symptoms and there are some data that indicate that symptoms become worse (Terr, 1986). Since major lifestyle modifications frequently lead to substantial and deleterious consequences, such as loss of work and social support, which may exacerbate or produce depression and anxiety, the burden of proof rests with the proponents of avoidance that it is effective in reducing symptoms and is necessary to prevent toxic injury.

Finally, IEI has been recognized as a potentially disabling condition by some governmental agencies such as the Social Security Administration and the US Department of Housing and Urban Development. Political or social definitions of IEI as work-related or disabling, however, should not cloud the physician's judgment regarding the diagnosis, attribution and treatment of symptoms associated with IEI in the individual patient.

Recommendations for treatment are summarized in **Table 3**.

Table 3 Treatment recommendations for IEI

Treatment should be individualized but may include the following:
  Non-judgmental, supportive therapy
  Enhance patient's sense of control
  Reduce psychosocial stress and/or patient's response to stress
  Biofeedback, relaxation response
  Treatment of co-existing psychiatric illness
  Behavioural desensitization to low-level chemical exposures
  Pharmacological treatments to control symptoms
  Increase in physical and social activity
  Specific treatment for hyperventilation (paper bag, respirator)
  Treatment of other co-existing medical illnesses

Source: Sparks *et al.*, 1994b.

RESEARCH RECOMMENDATIONS

There is an ongoing problem in reliably and distinctively defining IEI for studies of pathogenesis. Any definition, however, should at a minimum consider circumstances of symptom onset in relationship to some demonstrable environmental exposure, otherwise there will be little to distinguish IEI from other illnesses such as chronic fatigue syndrome, or psychiatric diagnoses such as major depression or somatization disorder. A clear distinction should be made between IEI and other medical diagnoses that may be due to occupational exposure such as allergic rhinitis, contact dermatitis and acute solvent intoxication. Research is needed to determine the actual prevalence and incidence of IEI in various populations as well as changes over time (Sparks *et al.*, 1994a).

Because of the subjective nature of IEI, the consistency of response may only be reliably demonstrated by double-blind placebo-controlled challenge testing with multisystem monitoring and biomarkers that identify relevant pathology. Uncontrolled and unblinded challenge testing (i.e. removal from the offending chemicals and then re-challenge, after an appropriate interval with the outcome of interest being a clearing of symptoms with removal from the offending chemical and recurrence of symptoms upon re-challenge) has no defensible role in research and is too open for misinterpretation to be useful in forming a case definition for IEI either clinically or in research.

The various clinical presentations of IEI should be clearly defined, as different clusters of causal factors may be operating in each. For research, the definition of IEI must fit the stated aim of the investigation. One that specifically excludes individuals with pre-existing psychiatric disorders might facilitate the evaluation of IEI patients with regard to the effect of environmental exposure on well defined clinical outcomes.

Because IEI is expressed subjectively, proper scientific methods are mandatory in the evaluation of outcome measures of the effects of low-level chemical exposure. The use of a specially constructed environmental challenge chamber may be required for double-blind, placebo-controlled testing of specific outcome measures after low-level chemical exposure (Selner, 1996). The outcome measures may include subjective responses or objective measures consistent with the individual's subjective symptoms.

The theory that neurogenic inflammation plays a prominent role in the pathogenesis of IEI could be tested. This might include the measurement of inflammatory cells and mediators of neurogenic inflammation in nasal washings in IEI patients and controls following controlled and blinded low-level chemical exposures. Biopsies of nasal mucosa of IEI patients and controls following chemical exposure might be done to investigate the presence of inflammation. IEI patients should be compared with normal individuals, in addition to those with allergic rhinitis.

Future research should involve controlled and objective measurement of the possible neurophysiological effects of odour or respiratory tract irritation from low levels of volatile organic compounds and other respiratory irritants, perhaps using electrophysiological or radiological tools to measure acute or chronic alterations in CNS function. Research is also necessary to establish the diagnostic efficacy of such tools as brain electrical activity mapping, SPECT or PET scans in measuring changes in CNS function in IEI patients. At this time these tools (and other yet-to-be-discovered tests of neurological dysfunction) should be performed only by appropriately trained health professionals in a research setting using proper methodology and controls for investigation (Society of Nuclear Medicine Brain Imaging Council, 1996).

Previously discussed research has shown that patients with IEI have an illness characterized by a high prevalence of pre-existing and co-existing psychiatric disorders. An epidemiological community-based study might further define the sequencing of the development of psychiatric disorders and the onset of IEI. Prospective studies of chemically exposed groups could address whether psychiatric illness is a direct consequence of the syndrome, or aetiological by making one more vulnerable to the development of IEI from the psychophysiological effects of various chemical exposures and/or the adoption of illness belief systems.

Controlled clinical research is needed to determine the extent to which various psychiatric, behavioural and other treatments are effective in different categories of patients with IEI. Clarification of mechanisms of aetiology of this syndrome will also aid efforts at prevention.

A framework for establishing research directions and priorities in IEI has been proposed based on results that are valuable for risk-related decisions and that advance scientific knowledge and understanding, in addition to hypotheses that are both biologically plausible and readily testable (Dyer and Sexton, 1996). Other recommendations with regard to further research relevant to existing theories of pathogenesis may be found in a monograph on experimental approaches to IEI (National Institutes of Health, National Institute of Environmental Health Sciences, 1997).

SOCIAL AND POLITICAL IMPLICATIONS OF THE IEI PHENOMENA

The administrative recognition of IEI as an occupational or environmental illness may interfere with the objective study of this phenomenon as a clinical condition (Cullen, 1991; Gots, 1995). Recognition of this syndrome as an illness with potential to cause permanent disability could necessitate changes in health care coverage and delivery, awarding of workers' compensation benefits and the regulation of chemicals in the workplace and the environment. There are also social implications for the increasing human and economic cost of disability. Establishing whether IEI is due to a behavioural or psychological response to perceived chemical toxicity or to a toxic or pathophysiological effect of low-level exposure on organ systems is critical to these issues (Gots, 1996).

There is currently pressure to answer several questions of social policy regarding IEI. First, there is the issue of whether compensation should be awarded for a condition that relies entirely on a patient's report of subjective symptoms for diagnosis without an objective basis for confirming the diagnosis, rating its severity or even determining that it is due to environmental exposure.

Second is how the expanded recognition of the phenomenon of IEI would impact regulation and exposure control. Should employers attempt to reduce specific chemical exposures or to investigate organizational factors that may put an individual in a workplace at risk of expressing this type of illness? At this point, it is unclear whether controlling exposure to chemical substances far below levels associated with known toxic or irritant effects would have any positive impact on symptom expression or the natural history of IEI.

Third, there is the perceived need to regulate and control non-traditional unproven medical practices, such as those which have been promoted by clinical ecologists and other 'environmental physicians' to limit potentially dangerous or misleading practices and iatrogenic chronic disability.

Several medical societies and other organizations have issued position statements expressing concern about the IEI diagnoses, misuse of diagnostic procedures, use of inappropriate treatment modalities and the lack of scientific support for the alleged toxic effects of environmental (chemical) exposure in patients labelled with various IEI diagnoses. These have included the American Academy of Allergy and Clinical Immunology Executive Committee (1986), the American College of Physicians (1989), the American College of Occupational and Environmental Medicine, the Council on Scientific Affairs, American Medical Association (1992), the Ministry of Health of the Province of Ontario (1989) and the California Medical Association Scientific Board Task Force on Clinical Ecology (1986). The US National Academy of Sciences (1992), the World Health Organization (1996) and the International Society of Regulatory Toxicology and Pharmacology (1993) have held symposia on the subject. The American Council on Science and Health (1992) and the General Medical Council of Great Britain (1993) have published reports indicating the lack of scientific basis for the attribution of the IEI illness to environmental exposures.

This effort has angered many IEI patients, who view this as an attempt by mainstream medicine to negate the existence of IEI as an illness. Yet the controversy is not about whether IEI patients have 'real' versus simulated illness, but rather about whether the illness (which is accepted as present) is explained by toxicological versus behavioural effects of chemical exposure, or culturally shaped fear of environmental chemical exposure.

IEI has been primarily a politically defined illness. IEI appeals to the widespread fear of man-made chemicals in addition to the distrust that the public has of science, medicine technology and government (Gots, 1995). Society has a justifiable concern about the role that chemical pollution has had in environmental deterioration over the past century and the long-term implications of this for humans and other animal species.

Some believe or fear that the current controversy surrounding IEI is similar to that which existed several decades ago regarding asbestos-related lung disease and that medical science simply has not yet found a way to link environmental chemical exposure causally with the illness or to measure the impairment and disability of patients given an IEI diagnosis. Physicians who question or are agnostic about its relationship to workplace or environmental exposure, and those who have performed research to test the hypotheses of advocates of environmental attribution, have been targeted by hostile attack from IEI support groups or others with an economic stake in the outcome of the debate, in some cases even being removed from government jobs for the expression of their views (Deyo, 1997).

In the future, IEI may increasingly impact the total burden of chronic disability, much as low back pain and cumulative trauma disorders of the upper extremities do now. IEI patients make an average of 23 health care visits per year (Bell *et al.*, 1997). It would thus be appropriate to obtain the data necessary to define this condition and its relationship to environmental exposure medically, before medical science becomes increasingly irrelevant to the diagnosis, treatment and social policy decisions relating to IEI.

REFERENCES

Agency for Toxic Substances and Disease Registry (1996). *Evaluating individuals reporting sensitivities to multiple chemicals: final report*. US Department of Health and Human Services, Washington, DC.

American Academy of Allergy and Clinical Immunology Executive Committee (1981). Position statement: controversial techniques. *J. Allergy Clin. Immunol.*, **67**, 333.

American Academy of Allergy and Clinical Immunology Executive Committee (1986). Position statement: clinical ecology. *J. Allergy Clin. Immunol.*, **78**, 269–271.

American College of Occupational and Environmental Medicine (1993). ACOEM statement about distinctions among indoor air quality, MCS, and ETS [position statement]. *ACOEM Report* H5-H7.

American College of Physicians (1989). Position statement: clinical ecology. *Ann. Intern. Med.*, **111**, 168–178.

American Council on Science and Health (1993). Unproven 'allergies': an epidemic of nonsense.

American Medical Association (1992). Council on Scientific Affairs. Clinical ecology: council report. *JAMA*, **268**, 3465–70.

Amundsen, M. A., Hanson N. P., Bruce B. K., Lantz, T. D., Schwartz, M. S. and Lukach, B. M. (1996). Odor aversion or multiple chemical sensitivities: a name change and description of successful behavioral medicine treatment. *Regul. Toxicol. Pharmacol.*, **24**, S116–S118.

Andersson, B., Berg, M., Arnetz, B. B., Melin, L., Langlet and Liden S. (1996). A cognitive-behavioral treatment of patients suffering from 'electric hypersensitivity': subjective effects and reactions in a double-blind provocation study. *J. Occup. Environ. Med.*, **38**(8), 752–758.

Antelman, S. M. (1988). Time-dependent sensitization as the cornerstone for a new approach to pharmacotherapy: drugs as foreign/stressful stimuli. *Drug Dev. Res.*, **14**, 1–30.

Antelman, S. M., Kocan, D., Knopf, S., Edwards, D. J. and Cagguila, A. R. (1992). One brief exposure to a psychological stressor induces long-lasting, time-dependent sensitization of both the cataleptic and neurochemical responses to haloperidol. *Life Sci.*, **51**, 261–266.

Barrett, S. (1994). *MCS: Multiple Chemical Sensitivity*. American Council on Science and Health, New York.

Bascom, R. (1992). Multiple chemical sensitivity: a respiratory disorder? *Toxicol. Ind. Health*, **8**, 221–228.

Bascom, R., Kulle, T., Kagey-Sobotka, A. and Proud, D. (1991). Upper respiratory tract environmental tobacco smoke sensitivity. *Am. Rev. Respir. Dis.*, **143**, 1304–1311.

Bell, I. R., Miller, C. S. and Schwartz, G. E. (1992). An olfactory–limbic model of multiple chemical sensitivity syndrome: possible relationships to kindling and affective spectrum disorders. *Biol. Psychiatry*, **32**, 218–242.

Bell, I. R., Schwartz, G. E., Peterson, J. M. and Amend, D. (1993a). Self-reported illness from chemical odors in young adults without clinical syndromes or occupational exposures. *Arch. Environ. Health.*, **48**, 6–13.

Bell, I. R., Schwartz, G. E., Peterson, J. M., Amend, D. and Stini, W. A. (1993b). Possible time-dependent sensitization to xenobiotics: self-reported illness from chemical odors, foods, and opiate drugs in an older adult population. *Arch. Environ. Health.*, **48**(5), 315–327.

Bell, I. R., Schwartz, G. E., Peterson, J. M., Amend, D and Stini, W. A. (1994). Sensitization to early life stress and response to chemical odors in older adults. *Biol. Psychiatry*, **35**, 857–863.

Bell, I. R., Schwartz, G. E., Baldwin, C. M., Hardin, E. E., Limas, N. G., Klline, J. P., Patarca, R. and Song, Z. Y. (1997). Individual differences in neural sensitization and the role of context in illness from low-level environmental chemical exposures. *Environ. Health Perspect.*, **105**, Suppl. 2, 457–466.

Binkley, K. E. and Kutcher, S. (1997). Panic response to sodium lactate infusion in patients with multiple chemical sensitivity syndrome. *J. Allergy Clin. Immunol.*, **99**(4), 570–574.

Black, D. W., Rathe, A. and Goldstein, R. B. (1990). Environmental illness: a controlled study of 26 subjects with 20th century disease. *J. Am. Med. Assoc.*, **264**, 3166–3170.

Black, D. W., Rathe, A. and Goldstein, R. B. (1993a). Measures of distress in 26 'environmentally ill' subjects. *Psychosomatics*, **34**, 131–138.

Black, D. W. (1993b). Environmental illness and misdiagnosis—a growing problem. *Regul. Toxicol. Pharmacol.*, **18**, S23–S31.

Black, D. W. (1996). Iatrogenic (physician-induced) hypochondriasis: four patient examples of 'chemical sensitivity'. *Psychosomatics*, **37**, 390–393.

Board of the International Society of Regulatory Toxicology and Pharmacology. (1993). Report of the ISRTP Board. *Regul. Toxicol. Pharmacol.*, **18**, 79.

Bolla-Wilson, K., Wilson, R. J. and Bleecker, M. L. (1988). Conditioning of physical symptoms after neurotoxic exposure. *J. Occup. Med.*, **30**, 684–686.

Brodsky, C. M. (1983). 'Allergic to everything'; a medical subculture. *Psychosomatics*, **24**, 731–732, 734–736.

Brodsky, C. M. (1987). Multiple chemical sensitivities and other environmental illnesses: a psychiatrist's view. In Cullen, M. R. (Ed.), *Occupational Medicine: State of the Art Reviews*, Vol. 2. Hanley and Belvus, Philadelphia, pp. 695–704.

Broughton, A. and Thrasher, J. D. (1988). Antibodies and altered cell mediated immunity in formaldehyde exposed humans. *Common Toxicol.*, **2**, 155–174.

Buchwald, D. and Garrity, D. (1994). Comparison of patients with chronic fatigue syndrome, fibromyalgia, and multiple chemical sensitivities. *Arch. Intern. Med.*, **154**, 2049–2053.

California Medical Association Scientific Board Task Force on Clinical Ecology. (1986). Clinical ecology: a critical appraisal. *West. J. Med.*, **144**, 239–245.

Committee on Environmental Hypersensitivities (1985). *Report of the Ad Hoc Committee on Environmental Hypersensitivity Disorders*. Ministry of Health of the Province of Ontario, Toronto.

Council on Scientific Affairs, American Medical Association (1992). Clinical ecology. *J. Am. Med. Assoc.*, **268**, 3465–3467.

Cullen, M. R. (1987). The worker with multiple chemical sensitivities: an overview. In Cullen, M. R. (Ed.), *Occupational Medicine: State of the Art Reviews*, Vol. 2. Hanley and Belfus, Philadelphia, pp. 655–661.

Cullen, M. R. (1991). Multiple chemical sensitivities: development of public policy in the face of scientific uncertainty. *New Solutions*, **Fall**, 16–24.

Dager, S. R., Holland, J. P., Cowley, D. S. and Dunner, D. L. (1987). Panic disorder precipitated by exposure to organic solvents in the workplace. *Am. J. Psychiatry*, **144**, 1056–1058.

Dalton, P. (1996). Odor perception and beliefs about risks. *Chem. Senses*, **21**, 447–458.

Daniell, W. E., Stockbridge, H. L., Labbe, R. F., Woods, J. S., Anderson, K. E., Bissell, D. M., Bloomer, J. R., Ellefson, R. D., Moore, M. R., Pierach, C. A., Schreiber, W. E., Tefferi, A. and Frankllin, G. M. (1997). Environmental chemical exposures in disturbances of heme synthesis. *Environ. Health Perspect.*, **105**, Suppl. 1, 37–53.

Deyo, R. A. (1997). The messenger under attack—intimidation of researchers by special-interest groups. *N. Engl. J. Med.*, **336**(16), 1176–1179.

Doty, R., Deems, D. A., Frye, R. E., Pelberg, R. and Shapiro, A. (1988). Olfactory sensitivity, nasal resistance and autonomic function in patients with multiple chemical sensitivities. *Arch. Otolaryngol. Head Neck Surg.*, **114**, 1422–1427.

Dyer, R. S. and Sexton, K. (1996). What can research contribute to regulatory decisions about the health risks of multiple chemical sensitivity? *Regul. Toxicol. Pharmacol.*, **24**, S139–S151.

Engel, G. L. (1980). The clinical application of the biopsychosocial model. *Am. J. Psychiatry*, **137**, 535–544.

Fiedler, N., Kipen, H. M., DeLuca, J., Kelly-McNeil, K. and Natelson, B. (1996). A controlled comparison of multiple chemical sensitivity and chronic fatigue syndrome. *Psychosom. Med.*, **58**, 38–49.

Fiedler, N. and Kipen, H. (1997). Chemical sensitivity: the scientific literature. *Environ. Health. Perspect.*, **103**, Suppl. 2, 409–415.

Gilbert, M. E. (1992). Neurotoxicants and limbic kindling. In Isaacson, R. L. and Jensen, K. F. (Eds), *The Vulnerable Brain and Environmental risks. Vol. 1. Malnutrition and Hazard Assessment*. Plenum Press, New York.

Gomez, R. L., *et al.* (1996). Assessing beliefs about 'environmental illness/multiple chemical sensitivity'. *J. Health Psychol.*, **1**(1), 107–123.

Gothe C. J., Odont C. M., and Nilsson C. G. (1995). The environmental somatization syndrome. *Psychosomatics*, **36**(1), 1–11.

Gots, R. E. (1995). Multiple chemical sensitivities—public policy. *Clin. Toxicol.*, **33**(2), 111–113.

Gots, R. E. (1996). Multiple chemical sensitivities: distinguishing between psychogenic and toxicodynamic. *Regul. Toxicol. Pharmacol.*, **24**(1), S8–S15.

Grammer, L. C., Harris, K. E., Shaughnessy, M. A., Sparks, P., Ayars, G. H., Altman, L. C. and Patterson, R. (1990). Clinical and immunological revaluation of 37 workers exposed to gaseous formaldehyde. *J. Allergy Clin. Immunol.*, **86**, 177–181.

Guglielmi, R. S., Cox, D. J. and Spyker, D. A. (1994). Behavioral treatment of phobic avoidance in multiple chemical sensitivity. *J. Behav. Ther. Exp. Psychiatry*, **25**, 197–209.

Haller, E. (1993). Successful management of patients with 'multiple chemical sensitivities' on an inpatient psychiatric unit. *J. Clin. Psychiatry*, **54**, 196–199.

Hahn, M. and Bonkovsky, H. L. (1997). Multiple chemical sensitivity syndrome and porphyria. *Arch. Intern. Med.*, **157**, 281–285.

Hummel, T., Roscher, S., Jaumann, M. P. and Kobal, G. (1996). Intranasal chemoreception in patients with multiple chemical sensitivities: a double blind investigation. *Regul. Toxicol. Pharmacol.*, **24**, 579–586.

Hummel, T., *et al.* (1997). A double blind, randomized, controlled investigation of olfactory and trigeminal chemoreception in healthy controls and patients with multiple chemical sensitivities, before and after challenge with 2-propanol or room air. In preparation.

Institute of Medicine (1987). *Pain and Disability*. National Academy Press, Washington, DC, pp. 232–257.

International Programme on Chemical Safety (UNEP–ILO–WHO), *et al.* (1996). Conclusions and recommendations of a workshop on multiple chemical sensitivities (MCS). *Regul. Toxicol. Pharmacol.*, **24**, S188–S189.

International Society of Regulatory Toxicology and Pharmacology. (1993). ISRTP Board Conclusions. *Reg. Toxicol. Pharmacol.*, **18**, 79.

Isenberg, S. A., Lehrer, P. M. and Hochron, S. (1992). The effect of suggestion and emotional arousal on pulmonary function in asthma: a review. *Psychosom. Med.*, **54**, 192–216.

Jewett, D. L., Fein, G. and Greenberg, M. H. (1990). A double-blind study of symptom provocation to determine food sensitivity. *N. Engl. J. Med.*, **323**, 429–433.

Jewett, D. L. (1992). Research strategies for investigating multiple chemical sensitivity. *Toxicol. Ind. Health*, **8**, 175–179.

Kay, A. B. (1993). Alternative allergy and the General Medical Council. *Br. Med. J.*, **306**, 122–124.

Kreutzer, R. (1997). Personal communication.

Kurt, T. L. (1995). Multiple chemical sensitivities–a syndrome of pseudotoxicity manifest as exposure perceived symptoms. *Clin. Toxicol.*, **33**(2), 101–105.

Lehrer, P. (1997). Psychology hypotheses regarding multiple chemical sensitivity syndrome. *Environ. Health. Perspect.*, **105**, Suppl. 2, 479–483.

Levine, S. A. and Reinhardt, J. (1983). Biochemical pathology initiated by free radicals, oxidant chemicals and therapeutic drugs in the etiology of chemical hypersensitivity disease. *J. Orthomol. Psychiatry*, **12**, 166–183.

Leznoff, A. (1997a). Clinical aspects of allergic disease: provocation challenges in patients with multiple chemical sensitivity. *J. Allergy Clin. Immunol.*, **99**(4), 438–442.

Leznoff, A. (1997b). Personal communication.

Lundberg, J. M., Lundblad, L., Saria, A. and Anggard, A. (1984). Inhibition of cigarette smoke induced edema of the nasal mucosa by capsaicin pretreatment and a substance P antagonist. *Naunyn-Schmiedeberg's Arch. Pharmacol.*, **326**, 181–185.

Madison, R. E., Broughton, A. and Thrasher, J. D. (1991). Immunologic biomarkers associated with an acute exposure to exothermic byproducts of a urea–formaldehyde spill. *Environ. Health Perspect.*, **94**, 219–223.

McCallum, D. B. (1991). Physicians and environmental risk communications. *Health Environ. Digest*, **6**, 3–5.

McClelland, G. H., *et al.* (1990). The effects or risk beliefs on property values: a case study of a hazardous waste site. *Risk Anal.*, **10**, 485–497.

McKenzie, J. N. (1896). The production of the so-called 'rose cold' by means of an artificial rose. *Am. J. Med. Sci.*, **91**, 45–47.

Meggs, W. J. and Cleveland, C. H. (1993). Rhinolaryngoscopic examination of patients with the multiple chemical sensitivity syndrome. *Arch. Environ. Health.*, **48**, 14–18.

Meggs, W. J., Elsheik, T., Metzger, W. J., Albernaz, M. and Bloch, R. M. (1996a). Nasal pathology and ultrastructure in patients with chronic airway inflammation (RADS and RUDS) following an irritant exposure. *J. Toxicol. Clin. Toxicol.*, **34**, 383–396.

Meggs, W. J., Dunn, K. A., Bloch, R. M., Goodman, P. E. and Davidoff, A. L. (1996b). Prevalence and nature of allergy and chemical sensitivity in a general population. *Arch. Environ. Health.*, **51**, 275–282.

Meggs, W. J. (1997). Hypothesis for induction and propagation of chemical sensitivity based on biopsy studies. *Environ. Health Perspect.*, **105**, Suppl. 2, 473–478.

Miller, C. (1997). Toxicant-induced loss of tolerance on emerging theory of disease. *Environ. Health. Perspect.*, **105**, Suppl. 2, 445–453.

Morton, W. E. (1995). Redefinition of abnormal susceptibility to environmental chemicals. Presented at the Second International Congress on Hazardous Waste: Impact on Human and Ecological Health, Atlanta, Georgia.

National Institutes of Health, National Institute of Environmental Health Sciences (1997). Experimental approaches to chemical sensitivity: a monograph based on papers presented at the Workshop on Experimental Approaches to Chemical Sensitivity held September 20–22, 1995, in Princeton, NJ. *Environ. Health Perspect.*, **105**, Suppl. 2.

National Research Council. (1992). In the mind's eye: enhancing human performance. National Research Council, Washington, D. C.

National Research Council. (1992). Multiple chemical sensitivities. National Academy Press, Washington, D. C.

Nuwer, M. R. (1990). On the controversies about clinical use of EEG brain mapping. *Brain Topogr.*, **3**, 103–111.

Patterson, R., Dykewicz, M. S., Grammer, L. C., Pruzansky, J. J., Zeiss, C. R. and Harris, K. E. (1987). Formaldehyde reactions and the burden of proof. Editorial. *J. Allergy Clin. Immunol.*, **79**, 705–706.

Pitman, R. K., Orr, S. P. and Shalev, A. Y. (1993). Once bitten, twice shy: beyond the conditioning model of PTSD. *Biol. Psychiatry*, **33**, 145–146.

Post, R. M. *et al.* (1987). Chronic cocaine administration: sensitization and kindling effects. In Raskin, A. and Uhlenhath, E. H. (Eds.), *Cocaine: clinical and biobehavioral aspects*. Oxford University Press, New York.

Post, R. M. (1992). Transduction of psychosocial stress into the neurobiology of recurrent affective disorder. *Am. J. Psychiatry*, **149**, 999–1010.

Report of the Ad Hoc Committee on Environmental Hypersensitivity Disorders (1985). Ontario Ministry of Health, Toronto.

Rovee, C. K., Harris, S. L. and Yopp, R. (1973). Olfactory thresholds and level of anxiety. *Bull. Psychosom. Soc.*, **2**, 76–78.

Salvaggio J. E. (1996). Understanding clinical immunological testing in alleged chemically induced environmental illnesses. *Regul. Toxicol. Pharmacol.*, **24**(1), S16–S27.

Schneider, R. A. (1974). Newer insights into the role and modifications of olfaction in man through clinical studies. *Ann. N. Y. Acad. Sci.*, **237**, 217–223.

Scottenfeld, R. S. (1987). Workers with multiple chemical sensitivities: a psychiatric approach to diagnosis and treatment. In Cullen, M. R. (Ed.), *Occupational Medicine: State of the Art Reviews*, Vol. 2. Hanley and Belfus, Philadelphia, pp. 739–753.

Selner, J. C. (1996). Chamber challenges: the necessity of objective observation. *Regul. Toxicol. Pharmacol.*, **24**(1), S87–S95.

Selner, J. C. and Staudenmayer, H. (1992). Neuropsychophysiologic observations in patients presenting with environmental illness. *Toxicol. Ind. Health*, **8**, 145–155.

Shorter, E. (1992). *From Paralysis to Fatigue: a History of Psychosomatic Illness in the Modern Era*. Macmillan, New York, pp. 233–323.

Schusterman, D. J. and Dager, S. R. (1987). Prevention of psychological disability after occupational respiratory exposures. In Harber, P. and Balmes, J. R. (Eds), *Prevention of Pulmonary Disease. Occupational Medicine: State of the Art Reviews*, Vol. 6. Hanley and Belfus, Philadelphia, pp. 11–27.

Schusterman, D., Balmes, J. and Cone, J. (1988). Behavioral sensitization to irritants/odorants after acute overexposure. *J. Occup. Med.*, **30**, 565–567.

Siegel, S. and Kreutzer, R. (1997). Working Group Report 2: Pavlovian conditioning and multiple chemical sensitivity. *Environ. Health. Perspect.*, **105**, Suppl. 2, 521–526.

Simon, G. E., Katon, W. J. and Sparks, P. J. (1990). Allergic to life: psychological factors in environmental illness. *Am. J. Psychiatry*, **147**, 901–906.

Simon, G. E. (1992). Psychiatric treatment in MCS. *Toxicol. Ind. Health*, **8**, 221–228.

Simon, G. E., Daniell, W., Stockbridge, H., Claypoole, K. and Rosenstock, L. (1993). Immunologic, psychological and neuropsychological factors in multiple chemical sensitivity: a controlled study. *Ann. Intern. Med.*, **119**, 97–103.

Simon, G. E. (1994). Questions and answers #3. *Toxicol. Ind. Health*, **4/5**, 523–535.

Society of Nuclear Medicine Brain Imaging Council (1996). The ethical clinical practice of functional brain imaging. *J. Nucl. Med.*, **37**(7), 1256–1259

Sorg, B. A. (1996). Proposed animal neurosensitization model for multiple chemical sensitivity in studies with formalin. *Toxicology*, **111**, 135–145.

Sparks, P. J., Simon, G. E., Katon, W. J., Altman, L. C., Ayars, G. H. and Johnson, R. L. (1990a). An outbreak of illness among aerospace workers. *West. J. Med.*, **153**, 23–33.

Sparks, P. J. (1990b). The aerospace syndrome. Comment. *West. J. Med.*, **153**, 445.

Sparks, P. J., Daniell, W., Black, D. W., Kipen, H. M., Altman, L. C., Simon, G. E. and Terr, A. I. (1994a). Multiple chemical sensitivity syndrome: a clinical perspective. I. Case definition, case definition theories of pathogenesis and research needs. *J. Occup. Med.*, **36**(7), 718–730.

Sparks, P. J., Daniell, W., Black, D. W., Kipen, H. M., Altman, L. C., Simon, G. E. and Terr, A. I. (1994b). Multiple chemical sensitivity syndrome: a clinical perspective. II. Evaluation, diagnostic testing, treatment, and social considerations. *J. Occup. Med.*, **36**(7), 731–737.

Staudenmayer, H. and Selner, J. (1987). Post-traumatic stress syndrome (PTSS): escape in the environment. *J. Clin. Psychol.*, **43**, 156–157.

Staudenmayer, H. and Selner, J. C. (1990). Neuropsychophysiology during relaxation in generalized, universal 'allergic' reactivity to the environment: a comparison study. *J. Psychosom. Res.*, **34**(3), 259–270.

Staudenmayer, H., Selner, J. C. and Buhr, M. P. (1993a). Double-blind provocation chamber challenges in 20 patients presenting with 'multiple chemical sensitivity'. *Regul. Toxicol. Pharmacol.*, **18**, 44–53.

Staudenmayer, H., Selner, M. E., Selner, J. C. (1993b). Adult sequelae of childhood abuse presenting as environmental illness. *Ann. Allergy*, **71**, 538–546.

Staudenmayer, H. (1996). Clinical consequences of the EI/MCS 'diagnosis': two paths. *Regul. Toxicol. Pharmacol.*, **24**(1), S96–S110.

Stewart, D. E. (1987). Environmental hypersensitivity disorder, total allergy and 20th century disease: a critical review. *Can. Fam. Physician*, **33**, 405–409.

Sullivan, J. B. and Krieger, G. R. (1992). *Hazardous Materials Toxicology*. Williams and Wilkins, Baltimore.

Terr, A. I. (1986). Environmental illness: a clinical review of 50 cases. *Arch. Intern. Med.*, **146**, 145–149.

Terr, A. I. (1989). Clinical ecology in the workplace. *J. Occup. Med.*, **31**, 257–261.

Terr, A. I. (1993). Immunological issues in 'multiple chemical sensitivities'. *Regul. Toxicol. Pharmacol.*, **18**, 54–60.

Thrasher, J. D., Madison, R., Broughton, A. and Gard, Z. (1989). Building-related illness and antibodies to albumin conjugates of formaldehyde, toluene diisocyanate, and trimellitic anhydride. *Am. J. Ind. Med.*, **15**, 187–195.

Vogt R. D. (1991). Use of laboratory tests for immune biomarkers in environmental health studies concerned with exposure to indoor air pollutants. *Environ. Health Perspect.*, **25**, 85–91.

Vojdani A., Ghoneum, M. and Brautbar, N. (1992). Immune alteration associated with exposure to toxic chemicals. *Toxicol. Ind. Health*, **8**, 239–253.

Weaver, V. M. (1996). Medical management of the multiple chemical sensitivity patient. *Regul. Toxicol. Pharmacol.*, **24**(1), S111–S115.

Chapter 80
The Emerging Threat of Chemical and Biological Terrorism

Jeffrey D. Simon

C O N T E N T S

INTRODUCTION

Terrorism is a violent form of human behaviour that has existed throughout history. During the first century, the Jewish Zealots and Sicariis committed terrorist acts in their struggle against Roman rule in Palestine, while in the 11th century the Assassins, an Islamic sect, spread terror throughout Persia and Syria. In modern times, terrorists have come from all types of movements and groups, perpetrating their violence by hijacking and blowing up airplanes, setting off car and truck (lorry) bombs and seizing embassies.

Yet as traumatic as the world's experience with terrorism has been, it pales in comparison with what lies on the horizon: terrorists in possession of chemical and biological weapons. The release of the nerve agent sarin in the Tokyo subway system in 1995 by the Japanese cult Aum Shinrikyo (Supreme Truth), and an earlier attack by the same cult in the city of Matsumoto, are harbingers of the future course of terrorism. The twenty-first century will likely witness terrorists utilizing a variety of chemical and biological weapons against unsuspecting civilian populations.

There are many factors that distinguish chemical–biological (CB) terrorism from 'conventional' terrorism. The most significant is the potential for extraordinarily large numbers of casualties in CB terrorism. For the USA, the worst terrorist attack on American soil was the 1995 bombing of the Alfred P. Murrah Federal Building in Oklahoma City that claimed 168 lives. The worst international terrorist incident for the USA was the suicide truck bombing of the Marine barracks in Beirut in 1983 which claimed 241 US servicemen. Other countries have experienced terrorist incidents, both on their soil and in the international arena, that killed at times hun-

dreds of their citizens. But no nation has yet had to face the consequences of a major terrorist attack with chemical or biological weapons. The sarin attack in the Tokyo subway killed 12 people, but the death toll could have been much higher had the terrorists mixed a more potent batch of the nerve agent and had they used a better delivery method to release the sarin—Aum Shinrikyo members simply left punctured bottles of sarin in the subway trains. Chemical weapons could kill tens of thousands of people, while biological weapons could kill hundreds of thousands or even millions of people.

CB terrorism is also more difficult to prevent than conventional terrorism. Many different physical security measures have been put in place at airports, embassies, federal buildings and other high-risk facilities to protect against terrorists with conventional weapons. These include metal detectors, X-ray machines, plastic explosive detectors, bomb-resistant glass and fortified buildings. Yet while such measures can be effective in preventing terrorists with guns, knives and bombs from penetrating security, they would be useless in detecting a terrorist in possession of a chemical or biological agent.

Another factor that separates CB terrorism from conventional terrorism is the unique situation it presents for counterterrorist forces. A traditional hijacking or hostage situation can lead to a military rescue effort or some other type of operation against the terrorists. The risk of losing a few hostages during the rescue may be deemed worth taking in order to prevent further killings or other violent actions by the terrorists. But all this changes if instead of a bomb or an automatic weapon, the terrorists possess chemical or biological weapons. In that case there would be no room for error in the counter-terrorist strike. The terrorists could still release the chemical or biological agent seconds before they are captured or killed, which could have serious repercussions for nearby populated areas.

Terrorists in possession of chemical or biological agents also pose a threat to the national security of the target country. While conventional terrorism has often been portrayed by policymakers, politicians and the media as a national security threat, the reality is that for the most part governments can survive the periodic outbreaks of terrorist activity. But an entirely different situation exists with CB terrorism. A major terrorist incident with a chemical or biological agent would create a crisis unlike any the target country has ever experienced. Unless a government has prepared for the aftermath of such an attack, the survivability of the nation could be at stake.

Understanding this new age of terrorism, and preparing for it, should be a high priority for governments and public around the world. Among the key questions that need to be addressed are the following:

- What are the implications of recent trends in terrorism for the potential use of CB weapons by terrorists?
- What are the chemical and biological warfare agents likely to be used by terrorists?
- Which types of terrorist groups are more likely than others to use chemical and biological weapons?
- How should governments and public prepare for CB terrorist incidents?

RECENT TRENDS IN TERRORISM

Several recent trends in terrorism indicate that chemical and biological weapons will likely become a part of future terrorists' strategies. First, terrorists are committing more spectacular and violent attacks, thereby increasing the likelihood that they will eventually turn to CB weapons. Terrorist incidents have become more lethal in recent years, with several incidents causing large numbers of casualties. In July 1994, a car bomb exploded at a Jewish cultural centre in Buenos Aires, killing 86 people and wounding about 300 others. In January 1996, a truck bomb destroyed the Central Bank in Colombo, Sri Lanka, killing 90 civilians and injuring more than 1400 others. The 1995 Oklahoma City bombing that killed 168 people also injured 850 others. Terrorists escalate their violence when they perceive that the public and governments have become desensitized to the 'normal' flow of terrorism. By perpetrating a violent act that causes more casualties than previous attacks, terrorists are guaranteed widespread publicity for their cause and reaction from various parties. Since a major terrorist attack with a chemical or biological agent would probably cause more casualties than any previous terrorist incident, it would fit into the recent pattern of high-casualty incidents.

Even when a conventional terrorist attack fails to kill a large number of people, it can still elicit widespread reaction and fear among the public if it is a spectacular incident that represents a departure from previous attacks. The Islamic extremists who committed the 1993 World Trade Center bombing in New York City had hoped to kill many more people than the six who actually died in the blast. Their plan was for the car bomb that they set off in the underground parking garage of one of the twin towers to shear the support beams of the Trade Center, thereby toppling one of the towers into the other and killing tens of thousands of people. Although they failed in that attempt, the bombing nevertheless sent shock waves across America as people realized that the USA could not remain invulnerable to major terrorist attacks. Thus, even though their ultimate plan for mass fatalities had failed, they still succeeded in gaining worldwide attention by being the first terrorists to commit a major terrorist incident in one of America's most populated cities and against one of the world's most famous business and financial structures.

Similarly, the Oklahoma City bombing represented a departure from previous incidents in the USA since it was not a major, world-famous metropolis that the terrorists attacked, but rather a small city in the heartland of the country. Thus, even if convicted terrorist Timothy McVeigh had failed to kill a large number of people in that blast, he still would have succeeded in shocking the nation since a major terrorist attack had never happened before in Oklahoma City. Every town and city across the USA could now be considered to be a potential target for terrorism. Since no country has yet experienced a major terrorist attack with a biological weapon, and only Japan has experienced a major terrorist attack with a chemical weapon, the incentive is there for terrorists to use such weapons as a way of gaining instant attention and reaction.

Another trend that points to the future use of CB weapons by terrorists is the emergence of 'smarter' and more creative terrorists. Recent years have witnessed terrorists attempting more daring types of attacks that required a certain level of technical expertise. For example, the mastermind of the World Trade Center bombing, Ramzi Yousef, was also convicted for plotting to blow up 12 US airliners flying to the USA from Asia over a two-day period in 1995. Yousef and his conspirators had planned to place the bombs and the timing devices on the various airlines before their first stops in Asia, and then depart from the planes before they took off again for the USA. Yousef had learned how to make bombs from unsuspicious-looking types of objects that could easily pass through airport security. These included a digital wrist-watch that was modified to serve as a timer, and a plastic contact-lens solution bottle that was filled with liquid components for nitroglycerine. After his arrest in Pakistan and on the flight back to the USA, Yousef told federal agents that he had considered using poison gas to kill people at the World Trade Center, but decided against it because he believed it would be too costly.

The level of scientific expertise needed to develop CB weapons for terrorists is not that high, nor is the cost prohibitive. For those terrorists who lack the required scientific and medical knowledge to build a home-made CB weapon, they could recruit into their ranks those who do. Furthermore, a foreign government could easily train a terrorist group in the proper use of chemical and biological warfare agents, and also supply the group with the weapon. In addition, the information revolution, including the Internet, has produced voluminous material on CB weapons. The information and technology are there for all to take advantage of, including terrorists.

Biotechnology and genetic engineering have also made it both easier and 'safer' for terrorists to experiment with and handle biological agents. Recombinant DNA technology can lead to the creation of more potent biological agents than would be the case with traditional methods of processing such weapons. With biotechnology, it may be possible to make infectious microorganisms into biological agents that are environmentally stable—thereby improving their ability to be dispersed effectively upon a target. The new technology can also be used to develop novel biological agents for which a target country has no defences or vaccines. Furthermore, genetically engineered vaccines can be designed to protect a terrorist group when it uses a particular biological agent.

The prospect of terrorists around the world gaining access to chemical and biological weapons has also increased owing to the collapse of the Soviet Union, and with it the former communist government's tight control over its weapons arsenal. This opened the gates for the potential outflow of various weapons from that country. Nuclear, chemical and biological weapons could now be accessible to all types of extremist groups. There are also thousands of ex-Soviet nuclear scientists, weapons experts and microbiologists out of work and available to sell their expertise to the highest bidder.

The numerous ethnic–nationalist and religious conflicts that are brewing around the world are another trend that could hasten the day when terrorists begin routinely to use CB weapons. Long after the fighting ends there will still be bitter memories and hatreds among the various warring factions. Since it does not take much to form a terrorist cell to carry on the struggle, some of these cells may attempt to gain instant attention to their cause and revenge against their enemies by trying new forms of terrorism, including the use of chemical and biological weapons.

Finally, the risk of terrorists using weapons of mass destruction has increased because extremist groups have now seen the global fear that doomsday weapons can generate. The threat to unleash biological and chemical weapons by Saddam Hussein during the 1991 Persian Gulf War was the first signal to terrorists that exotic weapons could create a level of fear and anxiety unmatched in the history of terrorism. Televised pictures of US troops training in the Middle East in special protective suits that looked more like spaceman outfits than military uniforms, and reporters filing live stories wearing gas masks, all presented vivid pictures of the potential terror of chemical and biological weapons. The second signal was the world reaction and global publicity to the release of sarin in the Tokyo subway system. These will be lessons not lost on current and future terrorists.

CB WEAPONS LIKELY TO BE USED BY TERRORISTS

What, then, are the likely chemical and biological warfare agents to be used by terrorists?

In recent years, chemical and biological warfare agents, along with nuclear weapons, have been characterized as 'weapons of mass destruction'. This terminology evokes images of large and complex weapons in the hands of terrorists. However, chemical and biological warfare agents, and their delivery systems, can be small and not even look like a 'weapon'. For example, Aum Shinrikyo simply left several punctured containers of sarin on baggage racks or on the floor of five subway trains in its attack in Tokyo in March 1995. In an earlier attack in Matsumoto in June 1994, the cult simply sprayed sarin out of a nozzle device that was attached to a truck and used an electric heater to heat the liquid into a gaseous state for dispersal by an electrically powered fan (US Senate, 1995, p.23). The sarin was released within 30 feet of a dormitory where three judges who were hearing a land fraud case against the cult were staying. Biological warfare agents can also be delivered in ways in which it would not appear to be a 'weapon', such as by aerosol canisters, trucks or low-flying airplanes equipped with spray tanks, and in other simple devices

Chemical and biological agents are more likely to be used by terrorists than are nuclear weapons. One reason is that despite reports of lax security around nuclear weapon sites in the former Soviet Union, it would still be very difficult for terrorists to steal or acquire by clandestine means a nuclear weapon and then transport it without being detected. In addition, the technical expertise required for building or detonating a nuclear device is much higher than that for chemical or biological weapons. Furthermore, chemical and biological warfare agents are more readily available and cheaper to purchase and develop into weapons than are nuclear materials.

In terms of chemical warfare agents, they can be defined as 'poisons that incapacitate, injure or kill through their toxic effects on the skin, eyes, lungs, blood, nerves or other organs' (US Congress, 1993a, p. 3). Some chemical warfare agents can be lethal when vaporized and inhaled in amounts as small as a few milligrams. Chemical warfare agents include, among others, blistering agents such as mustard and lewisite, choking agents such as chlorine, phosgene and PFIB, blood agents such as cyanogen chloride and hydrogen cyanide and nerve agents such as tabun (GA), sarin (GB), soman (GD), GF and VX (US Congress, 1993a, p. 47; see Chapter 101).

Chemical agents have been used by terrorists and criminals in various product contamination cases. Several people died after taking Tylenol capsules laced with cyanide in the USA in 1982. Although nobody was ever caught and no demands ever made, police suspected that it was the work of a mentally ill person. The publicity surrounding the incident led to copycat episodes throughout the USA, with extortionists trying to blackmail a variety of companies with similar types of threats. Pharmaceutical firms had to introduce new forms of packaging for their products to alert consumers to potential tampering. In Japan, a group known as 'The Man With 21 Faces' demanded large sums of money from private Japanese companies after placing cyanide-laced candy and food in several stores. Tamil guerrillas in 1986 notified several Western embassies that they had put potassium cyanide in exported Sri Lankan tea. After extensive testing by the US Food and Drug Administration, no poison was reportedly found. However, in 1989, minute traces of cyanide were discovered in Chilean grapes by US inspectors after a threat was received by the US Embassy in Santiago. All Chilean fruit in the USA was subsequently quarantined and recalled, severely damaging the Chilean economy. Leftist terrorists were suspected of this incident. Palestinian terrorists in the past used the tactic of placing mercury in Israeli oranges in an effort to damage the Israeli economy.

Most of the cases of product contamination have resulted in minimal casualties. However, terrorists, criminals and mentally ill individuals have also threatened to use chemical weapons with the objective being to kill large numbers of people. In 1975, German terrorists reportedly stole canisters of mustard gas from US stockpiles in West Germany and threatened to use it on civilian populations. In the same year, German businessmen were arrested in Vienna for attempting sell the nerve agent tabun to Palestinian terrorists.

Since the number of casualties in a CB weapons attack is likely to be much higher than that in an attack with conventional weapons, all CB terrorist or criminal threats have to be taken very seriously by government authorities. Two cases involving criminals and chemical weapons illustrate this point. One occurred in Cyprus in the 1980s and the other in Los Angeles in the 1970s.

In March 1987, a letter was sent to the president of Cyprus, Spiros Kiprianou, signed by a man calling himself 'Commander Nemo of Force Majerius'. He threatened to disperse dioxin, a toxic chemical, over the Troodos mountains south of Nicosia unless he was paid $15 million. Commander Nemo claimed that the dioxin would be released by radio-controlled devices that were already in place and would be carried by wind over populated areas. Since the letter was in fluent English, Cypriot officials suspected it originated in London (Cyprus gained independence from Britain in 1960). The Cyprus chief of police, Frixos Yangou, went to London to collaborate with Scotland Yard. Owing to the potential for panic among the Cypriot public, the entire matter was kept secret until British police arrested four people in London in May 1987.

The first task for the Cypriot and British authorities was to determine if the threat was credible. The blackmail letter was extremely detailed, including scientific data on the ingredients Commander Nemo claimed he used to make the dioxin. In order to convince the authorities that the dioxin would be carried by wind from the mountains to populated areas, he invited them to try an experiment. He told them to burn a large number of tyres and watch as the black smoke drifted across populated areas. He warned them that a dioxin attack would be a thousand times worse. He cited the disaster at Seveso, Italy, where an explosion at a chemical factory in 1976 caused dioxin to escape. Several people near the plant suffered burns and sores on their skin, and large numbers of people complained of nervousness, fatigue and loss of appetite. Many animals were killed, and Italian authorities were forced to slaughter more than 80 000 domestic animals as a protective measure. Commander Nemo also mentioned the explosion at a chemical factory in Bhopal, India, and the nuclear reactor disaster at Chernobyl in the former Soviet Union, and warned that his attack would be much worse since Cyprus is a small island. He also pointed out that the economy of Cyprus is dependent on agriculture and therefore could not afford the damage that would be caused by the release of the dioxin. He further argued that Cyprus would not have the medical facilities and resources to deal with the human casualties of a dioxin attack.

British scientists analysed the balckmail letter and concluded that Commander Nemo could not make dioxin from the ingredients he listed. However, the letter was couched in enough scientific jargon that the scientists had to spend some time analysing its contents before dismissing the threat. Commander Nemo continued to contact the Cyprus government and was finally apprehended by Scotland Yard detectives when he went to the Cyprus High Commission office in London, posing as the 'scientific adviser' to Commander Nemo, to collect a passport and some money.

The extortionist turned out to be a 36-year-old British citizen of Cypriot origin, Panos Koupparis. Also arrested in London were his wife, who worked for the British High Commission, and two brothers, one of whom was a chemistry student at London's Polytechnic Institute. Koupparis's sister-in-law was arrested in Cyprus, but ordered to be released by a judge for lack of evidence. Police stated that they found documents and weapons in Koupparis's Cyprus apartment—he had an offshore company in Cyprus—which indicated he had planned a series of bombings on the island to convince the government that his dioxin threat was real. After the arrests, Scotland Yard issued a statement that although the dioxin plot was not the most practical method for causing widespread harm, it was still a viable threat. They pointed out, though, that the extortionists did not have the means to carry out their threat.

The aftermath of the Commander Nemo affair had Cyprus reeling. The public reaction was one of fear, concern and disbelief. One independent newspaper worried that the four people arrested were part of a larger 'criminal general staff of men of science'. The government was criticized by some opposition parties for keeping the whole affair secret when lives were potentially at stake, while others criticized them for taking the hoax too seriously. One opposition newspaper called the episode a 'fiasco', claiming the government was exploiting the situation for its own purposes and that the threat was 'devoid of any seriousness'. The ruling Democratic party newspaper defended the government's handling of the case, claiming that the extortionists had 'planned the crime of the century'. The Cyprus government spokesman said that 'the content of the threat and the nature of the blackmail were such that it would be [an] act of lack of responsibility for the government and the police to underestimate the affair, the more so that first assessments by British experts spoke of a realizable threat if the blackmailers had the necessary means'. The government and police also stated that steps had been taken to protect lives in case the threat was real.

The Commander Nemo incident was a very clever scheme by an individual criminal with psychological problems. Koupparis was under the care of two psychiatrists. But he was clever enough to hatch a plan that caused two governments to consult in secrecy, brought in top-level scientists to assess the threat and led to a mini-crisis for the Cyprus government in explaining their handling of the affair. Had the scientific data been more credible, and the terrorist's intentions more believable, the crisis would have been much worse for the government. Public revelations by Commander Nemo before he was caught, either through communications with newspapers or television stations, might well have cause great alarm and panic in Cyprus.

In another case where a mysterious person publicly threatened to launch a nerve gas attack, a city was held in fear until the criminal was caught. This occurred in Los Angeles during the summer of 1973. A group calling itself the 'Aliens of America', but which turned out to be just one individual, exploded a bomb at Los Angeles International Airport, killing three people and injuring several others. In a series of tape recordings that were sent to the media, the terrorist stated that the first bomb was marked with the letter 'A', which stood for 'airport', a

second bomb will be associated with the letter 'L', a third with the letter 'I', and so forth, 'until our name has been written on the face of this nation in blood'. The terrorist subsequently placed a bomb in a locker (letter 'L') at a downtown Los Angeles Greyhound Bus station, but decided to alert police to its location and the bomb was safely defused. The terrorist became known in the media as the 'Alphabet Bomber'. The terrorist stated that he was committing his acts of violence to protest unfair treatment of immigrants and other various causes. Among his demands were that all immigration and naturalization laws be declared unconstitutional.

The Alphabet Bomber threatened to escalate his violence to include the use of nerve gas attacks. In one of his communiques received on August 9, 1974, he stated that '[w]ithin two weeks from today, we shall vacuum test the first portion of our sarin nerve gas manufacturing facility, which shall be used to produce two tons of sarin, which in turn shall be used to destroy the entire US Capitol personnel'. An alarming headline appeared in the *Los Angeles Herald-Examiner* on August 15, with the following words: 'L.A. BOMBER PLEDGES GAS ATTACK'. The terrorist also claimed to have sent postcards to the nine US Supreme Court justices with toxic material placed in metal disks under the stamps. Postal authorities intercepted the cards when they became caught in the cancelling machine in a Palm Springs post office, but no toxic material was found in the metal disks.

Police finally arrested a mentally ill Yugoslav immigrant, Muharem Kurbegovic, for the bombing and bomb threats. He had been denied a permit to open a dance hall because of a prior arrest, and he felt that the justice system was persecuting himself and other immigrants. Kurbegovic was an engineer who was very bright and had an extensive knowledge of chemicals. An initial search of his apartment found live pipe bombs, explosive materials, books and manuals on germ and chemical warfare and a gas mask. Subsequent searches of his apartment found 25 pounds of sodium cyanide. The Alphabet Bomber case illustrates how a single individual could use the threat of chemical warfare terrorism to generate widespread fear and alarm. Kurbegovic was, in many respects, a criminal terrorist ahead of his time, since he was among the first criminals to threaten to use sarin gas, which was the nerve agent that Aum Shinrikyo used more than 20 years later in the Tokyo subway attack.

The use of sarin by Aum Shinrikyo has put that nerve gas at the top of the list of likely chemical warfare agents to be used by other terrorists. There has been enough publicity about that attack and enough information about sarin to make it an attractive CW agent for future terrorists. The religious cult went further than any other terrorist group or individual in its plans for using sarin. Whereas the Alphabet Bomber had threatened to develop and drop 2 tons of sarin on Washington, DC,

Aum Shinrikyo planned to produce 70 tons of sarin within 40 days of completion of a sarin production facility at their compound in Kamikuishiki, Japan. Some 20 kg of sarin were used by the cult in the June 1994 attack in Matsumoto. The cult also planned to spray sarin via a helicopter that the group had purchased (US Senate, 1995, p. 60). Also, as noted earlier, the death toll in the Tokyo subway attack would have been much higher had the chemical mixture and delivery system been different. There could have been tens of thousands of civilian casualties in the subway system, which moves over five million people a day (Ranger and Wiencek, 1997).

Terrorists are not limited to sarin in perpetrating chemical terrorism attacks. In fact, Aum Shinrikyo had conducted research into other nerve agents such as tabun (GA), soman (GF) and VX. The cult chose sarin because of the relative ease of producing that nerve agent and the ready availability of its precursors. However, Aum did produce VX for experimental purposes in the same laboratory where it manufactured sarin, but never went into full-scale production of VX. They did use small quantities of VX in at least two attacks on enemies of Aum. In one instance the victim was attacked in December 1994 while walking on an Osaka street and died 10 days later. Monoethylmethylphosphoric acid, a by-product of VX, was detected in the victim's blood serum. In another incident, the head of the 'Association of the Victims of Aum Shinrikyo' was sprayed with VX that was dispensed from a hyperdermic syringe. The victim survived the attack. Police also reportedly found as much as 8.5 kg of sodium cyanide in the hideout of a Aum Shinrikyo member. In addition, sodium cyanide was discovered in devices left in a Tokyo subway station in the months following the sarin attack. The devices were designed to generate highly toxic cyanide gas (US Senate, 1995, pp. 60–62).

Whereas chemical warfare agents have been used in a major terrorist attack—the 1995 sarin attack in the Tokyo subway—and have also been used by governments during wartime, biological warfare agents have not yet been used either during wartime or in a large-scale terrorist attack. However, the threat of terrorists or rogue states using such weapons in major incidents has increased dramatically in recent years.

Biological warfare agents involve 'the deliberate use of disease and natural poisons to incapacitate or kill people. Potential [biological warfare] agents include living microorganisms such as bacteria, rickettsia, fungi and viruses that cause infection resulting in incapacitation or death; and toxins, nonliving chemicals manufactured by bacteria, fungi, plants and animals' (US Congress, 1993b). Biological agents can be 'silent' killers, sometimes slowly working their way through their victims. Symptoms of a biological agent attack may not appear for hours or even days. Terrorists could thus unleash these agents without raising suspicions at the scene of the attack. The silent nature of biological weapons would

also give terrorists an advantage in penetrating security at airports and other facilities. A terrorist could walk right into a crowded terminal and release an agent or even place it along with a timed-release device in an unsuspecting passenger's baggage.

Bacillus anthracis, *Clostridium botulinum* and ricin are among the biological agents likely to be used by terrorists. *Bacillus anthracis*, which causes the deadly disease anthrax, is an attractive agent for terrorists since it is easy to produce in a laboratory in almost unlimited quantities and is environmentally stable—can resist degradation by environmental factors—when released in the atmosphere as anthrax spores. Terrorists can disperse anthrax spores in aerosols which may remain suspended for hours in certain weather conditions over populated areas (Franz *et al.*, 1997). They can be delivered by several means, including low-flying airplanes, crop dusters, spray cans or trucks, cars or boats equipped with spray tanks and releasing the agent upwind of populated areas. The biological agent can also be delivered by missiles or bombs, although the likelihood that the organisms will be destroyed in the explosion does not make this a viable delivery method. The now defunct Office of Technology Assessment of the US Congress estimated in 1993 that dispersal of 100 kg of anthrax spores from an airplane over Washington, DC, would kill between one and three million people (US Congress, 1993a, p. 54). A US Army experiment in the late 1960s demonstrated the vulnerability of the USA to a terrorist attack with a biological agent. The Army wanted to determine how a deadly biological agent could spread through the New York City subway system. They sprayed aerosol clouds of a non-lethal substitute for dry anthrax into the stations through sidewalk vents. They also tossed light bulbs containing the harmless agent from trains into the subway tunnels. The fake bacteria then spread to many other stations by the wind of the speeding trains. The group took measurements of the harmless bacteria and concluded that had the attack been real, several hundred thousand people would have been killed.

Clostridium botulinum produces the botulinum toxin, which causes botulism, and which is among the most poisonous of toxins known. In 1980, police raided a Red Army Faction apartment in Paris and reportedly found a miniature laboratory containing a culture medium of *Clostridium botulinum*. Police also found notes about bacteria-induced diseases in the apartment. More recently, Saddam Hussein was stockpiling *Clostridium botulinum*, *Bacillus anthracis* and other weapons of mass destruction prior to the 1991 Persian Gulf War. According to Dr Gordon C. Oehler, former Director of the CIA's Nonproliferation Center, Iraq filled more than 150 bombs and 50 warheads with biological warfare agents and dispersed these weapons to forward storage locations. Iraq also designed four aircraft drop tanks for biological agent spray operations. Each tank was designed to spray up to 2000 litres of anthrax on a target

(US Senate, 1995, p. 212). In addition, Aum Shinrikyo engaged in an intensive research and development programme for biological weapons. Japanese authorities believe that the cult produced botulinum toxin and may have produced *Bacillus anthracis* (US Senate, 1995, p. 62).

Ricin, which is a potent protein toxin derived from the bean of the castor plant (*Ricinus communis*), has been used in the past for selective assassination attempts. For example, in 1978, Bulgarian agents assassinated Georgi Markov, a Bulgarian emigré and writer for the British Broadcasting Company, by stabbing him in London with an umbrella-type weapon that contained ricin. A similar attack was made on the life of another Bulgarian emigré, Vladimir Kostove, in Paris that same year. Kostove survived when physicians were able to remove the pellet containing ricin from his body. More recently, four members of a small anti-government tax protest group known as the Patriot's Council manufactured ricin with the intent to use it in an assassination attempt. The men were convicted in Minnesota in 1995 for violating the Biological Weapons Anti-Terrorism Act of 1989. The group had planned to kill a deputy US marshal and a sheriff who had previously served papers on a Patriot's Council associate. The FBI reported that the amount of biological agent the group produced could have killed over 100 people if effectively delivered (US Department of Justice, 1995). Also, in 1995, a member of the white supremacist group Aryan Nations was arrested in Ohio for obtaining three vials of bubonic plague bacteria. The man had lied about owning a laboratory when he ordered the cultures of *Yersinia pestis* bacteria, which causes bubonic plague.

Prior to Aum Shinrikyo's attack in the Tokyo subway system, CB terrorism had involved relatively 'low-level' types of incidents. However, the Tokyo incident foreshadows a new age of terrorism where terrorists will be attracted to the very large number of casualties that CB weapons can cause. The question, therefore, is what types of terrorists or other criminal individuals are more likely than others to use such weapons.

TYPES OF TERRORIST GROUPS LIKELY TO USE CHEMICAL AND BIOLOGICAL WEAPONS

There are several factors that affect a terrorist group's decision to utilize chemical or biological weapons. The availability of the weapon is naturally a critical factor, for if the terrorists either cannot obtain the necessary chemical or biological agents—or believe they cannot—then they are not likely to consider using such weapons in an attack. And even if a terrorist group believed it could gain access to chemical or biological agents, they would also have to be convinced that they have effective dispersal means available to carry out a successful attack. While a bomb merely has to be detonated at the site of the target, a terrorist attack with CB agents will need to have efficient means for spreading the agent in order to achieve maximum effect. Aerial spraying produces a wider lethal area than an explosive bomb or missile warhead, and in the case of biological agents, as noted earlier, the explosion could kill the agent organisms (US Congress, 1993a, p. 48).

Although dispersing chemical or biological agents would be a more complicated process than simply detonating a bomb, it is still within the means of most terrorist groups. Chemical and biological agents are best dispersed as low-altitude aerosol clouds (US Congress, 1993a, p. 48). The aerosol release of chemical or biological agents could be accomplished by using low-flying airplanes or trucks equipped with spray tanks and releasing the agent upwind of populated areas, leaving aerosol canisters filled with the agent and timing devices in subways, airports, air-conditioning/heating systems in buildings or other crowded places, or directly contaminating bulk food supplies in restaurants, supermarkets or other places with a chemical or biological warfare agent. However, city water supplies in the USA would not be a likely target for a CB terrorist attack owing to the large amount of chemical or biological agent required to contaminate the water supply and the water purification procedures used by most cities (Simon, 1997).

Chemical and biological weapons could be readily obtained or manufactured by the determined terrorist. The precursors for many chemical and biological agents are available, and the scientific and medical knowledge necessary to manufacture such weapons is not that difficult to obtain. Several chemical and biological warfare agents can be produced either at home or in a small laboratory without sophisticated scientific knowledge.

Therefore, a terrorist group that wants to launch a CB attack will not face insurmountable obstacles. Most terrorist groups, however, will not be attracted to chemical or biological weapons, because the use of such weapons could create a backlash among the group's supporters. Ethnic–nationalist and revolutionary terrorist groups, such as the Irish Republican Army, the Basque separatist group ETA and others, depend upon the support—political, logistical and financial—of significant segments of the population. While their 'constituency' may not necessarily approve of the group's violent tactics, they nevertheless support the group's political objectives. However, that support could be eroded if such groups used weapons of mass destruction.

The terrorist groups and individuals that are likely to use chemical or biological weapons will probably exhibit the following characteristics:

■ A general, underfined constituency whose possible reaction to a CB weapons attack does not concern the terrorist group.

- A perception that conventional terrorist attacks are no longer effective and that a higher form of violence or a new technique is needed.
- A willingness to take risks by experimenting with and using unfamiliar weapons.

Among the terrorist groups that could be described as meeting the above criteria would be doomsday or millenarian cults, global revolutionary groups, neo-Nazis and white supremacist groups and right-wing anti-government militias. These types of terrorist groups have amorphous constituencies for which concern about a public backlash would not be likely to deter the use of chemical or biological weapons. They are also likely to view conventional terrorist tactics as insufficient to gain the attention and reaction they seek in furtherance of their various goals. Among the reasons cited for Aum Shinrikyo's sarin attack in the Tokyo subway was to set in motion a sequence of events that would eventually lead to Armageddon, a prediction that had been made by the cult's leader, Shoko Asahara. Another reported reason for the attack was to create a crisis in Japan that would preoccupy or topple the Japanese government and thereby prevent an anticipated raid by Japanese authorities on the cult's headquarters.

Religious extremists, state-sponsored groups and individual criminals are also candidates for using CB weapons. If a terrorist believes that acts of violence are not only politically but also morally justified, there is powerful incentive for any type of terrorist attack. The belief that one is rewarded in the afterlife for violence perpetrated on Earth encourages undertaking high-risk and high-casualty attacks. Groups that have the sponsorship of a foreign government would also be potential candidates for CB weapons since, as noted above, they could easily be provided with the necessary training, resources and weapons. The state sponsor would have to decide that a chemical or biological weapons attack by a terrorist group would accomplish the foreign government's objectives and not be traced back to the state sponsor. Further, those individual criminals with scientific or medical knowledge, and who are obsessed with revenge (the Alphabet Bomber) or lured by large amounts of money (Commander Nemo), would also be candidates for using or threatening to use CB weapons since such weapons would gain the immediate attention and possible reaction by the authorities.

PREPARING FOR CB TERRORIST INCIDENTS

There are two basic elements involved in fighting terrorism. One involves the measures that can be taken by governments, police, businesses and others to prevent terrorists from succeeding in their attacks. The second involves the countermeasures that can be taken after an incident has taken place to mitigate the consequences of the attack, capture the terrorists or retaliate against the terrorists or their state sponsors.

The threat of chemical and biological terrorism is changing the nature of both of these components in combating terrorism. It can no longer be assumed that what is effective in dealing with terrorists with conventional weapons will be effective in dealing with terrorists with CB weapons. As noted earlier, preventive measures such as metal detectors, X-ray machines, concrete barriers and surveillance cameras, which were designed to stop the terrorist attacks involving bombs and other conventional weapons, will not be able to stop the terrorist who is armed with a chemical or biological weapon. Similarly, post-attack response measures such as emergency rescue operations will now have to take into account the risk that first responders—firefighters, police officers, emergency medical personnel—could fall victim themselves to the chemical or biological agent as they try to aid those who were exposed initially to the attack. Also, as noted earlier, there can be no room for error in counter-terrorist operations against terrorists with CB weapons since the release of the chemical or biological agent by the terrorist as he is captured or killed could result in large-scale casualties if the counter-terrorist operation is taking place near a populated area.

In terms of trying to prevent CB terrorism, the most important factor will be good intelligence. Among the scientific and intelligence indicators that will need to be monitored to alert governments and public health officials to the possibility that a terrorist group or state sponsor is planning a chemical or biological weapons attack would be the following: recruitment of scientific or technical personnel into the group; development of chemical or biological agent productions facilities; acquisition of information on agent production and/or dispersal techniques; detection of agent dispersal equipment; procurement of stock cultures/raw materials and detection of bulk agents in storage or transportation; unexplained acquisition of vaccines, antibiotics or protective clothing; training of individuals in the handling of chemical or biological agents; training of individuals in offensive use of CB agents; and direct information from human sources that a group is developing, producing or acquiring CB agents.

Preventing terrorism, however, is an extremely difficult task. Despite all the elaborative preventive measures that have been employed over the years in the battle against conventional terrorism, there are still bombings, hijackings, kidnappings and other terrorist acts occurring daily around the world. There can never be perfect security or intelligence against conventional terrorism, and the same is true for CB terrorism.

Therefore, since it is likely that there will be major CB terrorist incidents in the future, it is important to place high priority in improving emergency responses to potential incidents. There will be more opportunity to save lives in the aftermath of a chemical or biological terrorist attack than in a conventional attack. Whereas most of the fatalities in a conventional bombing occur immediately or shortly after the incident (Mallonee et al., 1996), this is not the case with chemical or biological terrorism. There will still be time to save many lives through accurate diagnosis and speedy treatment. It is therefore crucial that hospitals and clinics have adequate supplies, or ways to obtain such supplies quickly, of antibiotics, antitoxins and other medicine to treat victims, and that medical personnel be trained to recognize the various symptoms of CB warfare agents (Simon, 1997).

Rescue workers who treated victims of Aum Shinrikyo's first sarin attack in Matsumoto in June 1994 did so without wearing gas masks or using decontamination procedures because they initially did not know what the victims were suffering from. It was not until a week later that the exact cause of the disaster became known. Several rescue workers were found to have mild symptoms of sarin gas poisoning. The emergency manual for mass disaster that rescue workers in Matsumoto had been trained under had no provisions for wearing gas masks and using decontamination procedures. Subsequently, a decontamination team for chemical weapons from the Japanese Self Defence Force was established as a procedure for situations where nerve gas is suspected. This team was used 7 months later when Aum Shinrikyo struck again in the Tokyo subway system (Okudera et al., 1997).

Steps are also being taken in the USA to improve the readiness of first responders to deal with chemical or biological terrorism. In 1995, President Clinton signed Presidential Decision Directive 39 (PDD-39), which broadly defines the lines of authority and emergency arrangements among federal agencies in case there is a terrorist act involving chemical, biological or nuclear weapons. In 1996, Congress created the Domestic Preparedness Program (DPP) under the Department of Defense (DOD) to help train first responders to recognize if a CB terrorist attack has taken place and to take appropriate measures to deal with it. For fiscal 1997 and 1998 at least $92 million has been appropriated for the programme, which includes special DOD teams 'training the trainers' in metropolitan areas throughout the USA (Paige, 1998).

An important part in preparing for CB terrorism will be dealing with the mental health of those involved in the rescue and treatment of victims. Police, firefighters and emergency medical personnel will be carrying out their tasks during a period of unprecedented crisis in the country. In addition to coping with the psychological stress of seeing potentially very large numbers of casualties, first responders and others will also have to take personal risks as they try to save lives. They might fear

that even with protective clothing and gas masks they still could fall victim themselves to the chemical or biological agent. Therefore, it is important that psychological stress-reducing techniques be established in all contingency plans for a CB terrorist attack.

One such technique is the Critical Incident Stress Debriefing (CISD) process, which is part of a broader crisis intervention programme known as the Critical Incident Stress Management (CISM). CISD and CISM are aimed at preventing or mitigating the development of adverse psychological reactions among first responders and other emergency and medical personnel. Through different types of psychological intervention techniques, CISD teams led by mental health professionals and including peer support personnel from the emergency services try to help medical personnel and emergency workers recover as quickly as possible from the stress associated with crises such as earthquakes, terrorist bombings, plane crashes and other tragedies. This process could be a major benefit to those whose job it will be to deal with the aftermath of a chemical or biological terrorist incident (Mitchell and Everly, 1995; Simon, 1997).

Since time is a critical factor in treating victims of either a chemical or biological terrorist attack, it would also be extremely helpful to have detection systems that could warn that an attack has occurred. Otherwise, the only indicator, in the case of a biological terrorist attack, would be the large number of victims appearing at hospitals and clinics complaining of various symptoms associated with the different diseases caused by biological warfare agents. Also, in the case of a chemical terrorist attack, while the sight of people collapsing within minutes of exposure or experiencing other violent reaction would be an obvious indicator that something has happened, the quicker it is known that chemical warfare agents have been released, and exactly what type of agent, the better are the chances for accurate diagnosis and proper treatment of victims.

Unfortunately, it may still be years before reliable CB detection systems are designed and implemented at potential target sites. The Presidential Advisory Committee on Gulf War Veterans' Illnesses revealed in an interim report in February 1996 that the military equipment used to detect chemical agents during the Persian Gulf war was inadequate and unreliable, and that there was no system to identify the release of biological agents. There is also the problem of where to place the detection systems once they become available. Since CB agents could be released virtually anywhere, including in shopping malls, subways and city streets, it may not be economically feasible to have early warning systems throughout the nation. There would also be the problem of needless public anxiety in the event of false alarms (Cole, 1996). Nevertheless, research needs to be continued in developing accurate CB agent detection systems since it is still unclear as to exactly what steps will, and will not, bear positive results in the future.

Progress has been made in designing scientific methods for determining if people have been exposed to organophosphate (OP) compounds such as nerve agents. In one recent study, a new method for retrospective detection of such exposure was reported (Polhuijs *et al.*, 1997). Serum samples from victims of both the Tokyo subway attack and the earlier incident in Matsumoto were tested with the new procedure. The procedure, which involves fluoride-induced reactivation of sarin-inhibited butyrylcholinesterase in human serum, could have applications in cases of suspected exposure to nerve agents during wartime or from terrorist attacks and in forensic cases against suspected terrorists that may have handled nerve agents (Polhuijs *et al.*, 1997).

Science, medicine and technology hold the most promise for reducing the risks of large numbers of casualties in the event of a chemical or biological terrorist attack. The better we are prepared to meet this threat, the less are the chances that terrorists will succeed in creating total chaos and panic throughout a country.

CONCLUSION

Following a failed attempt to assassinate Prime Minister Margaret Thatcher at the Conservative Party convention in Britain in 1984, the Irish Republican Army issued the following statement: 'Today we were unlucky, but remember, we only have to be lucky once. You will have to be lucky always'. That statement remains today the best description of the difficult task governments face in the endless battle against terrorism. We are living in an age where small groups, and even criminals or mentally unstable individuals, can gain access to chemical and biological weapons. Whether they build the weapons themselves, are supplied with them by a foreign government or gain possession of them by other means, the fact remains that the determined terrorist could wreak unimaginable suffering upon a country with a single attack.

Japan was 'lucky' on the morning of March 20, 1995, when Aum Shinrikyo's plan to kill tens of thousands of Tokyo subway riders failed owing to the poor quality of the sarin gas that they manufactured and the equally poor delivery system that they designed. Under different circumstances, the results could have been a catastrophe that no nation has yet experienced at the hands of terrorists.

The challenge in designing and implementing effective countermeasures to the terrorist threat regarding chemical and biological weapons will be among the most important tasks facing governments and societies in the twenty-first century. This will require a heightened awareness level about the threat and cooperation among the medical community, law enforcement, emergency services personnel, scientists, policymakers and the public. The consequences of a successful terrorist attack with CB weapons are so great that preparing for that day, particularly in how to deal with the aftermath of an attack, must become a high priority in countries around the world.

REFERENCES

Cole, L. (1996). Countering chem-bio terrorism: limited possibilities. *Polit. Life Sci.*, **15**, 196–198.

Franz, D., Jahrling, P., Friedlander, A., McClain, D., Hoover, D., Bryne, W., Pavlin, J., Christopher, G. and Eitzen, E. (1997). Clinical recognition and management of patients exposed to biological warfare agents. *J. Am. Med. Assoc.*, **278**, 399–411.

Mallonee, S., Shariat, S., Stennies, G., Waxweiler, R., Hogan, D. and Jordan, F. (1996). Physical injuries and fatalities resulting from the Oklahoma City bombing. *J. Am. Med. Assoc.*, **276**, 382–390.

Mitchell, J. T. and Everly, G. S. (1995). *Critical Incident Stress Debriefing: an Operations Manual for the Prevention of Traumatic Stress Among Emergency Services and Disaster Workers*, 2nd edn. Chevron Publishing, Ellicott City, MD.

Okudera, H., Morita, H., Iwashita, T., Shibata, T., Otagiri, T., Kobayashi, S. and Yanagisawa, N. (1997). Unexpected nerve gas exposure in the city of Matsumoto: report of rescue activity in the first sarin gas terrorism. *Am. J. Emerg. Med.*, **15**, 527–528.

Paige, S. (1998). At the eleventh hour. *Insight*, **14**, January 26, 8–10.

Polhuijs, M., Langenberg, J. and Benschop, P. (1997). New method for retrospective detection of exposure to organophosphorus anticholinesterases: application to alleged sarin victims of Japanese terrorists. *Toxicol. Appl. Pharmacol.*, **146**, 156–161.

Ranger, R. and Wiencek, D. (1997). *The Devil's Brews II: Weapons of Mass Destruction and International Security*. Bailrigg Memorandum 17. Centre for Defence and International Security Studies, Lancaster University, Lancaster, p. 28.

Simon, J. (1997). Biological terrorism: preparing to meet the threat. *J. Am. Med. Assoc.*, **278**, 428–430.

US Department of Justice (1995). *Terrorism in the United States: 1995*. Federal Bureau of Investigation, Terrorist Research and Analytical Center, National Security Division, Washington, DC, p. 6.

US Congress (1993a). Office of Technology Assessment. *Proliferation of Weapons of Mass Destruction: Assessing the Risks*. OTA-ISC-559. US Government Printing Office, Washington, DC.

US Congress (1993b). Office of Technology Assessment. *Technologies Underlying Weapons of Mass Destruction*. OTA-BP-ISC-115. US Government Printing Office, Washington, DC, p. 71.

US Senate (1995). *Global Proliferation of Weapons of Mass Destruction, Hearings Before the Permanent Subcommittee on Investigations of the Committee on Governmental Affairs*. US Senate, 104th Congress, 1st Session, Part 1, October 31 and November 1, 1995. US Government Printing Office, Washington, DC.

Chapter 81
Medical Device Toxicology

Randy D. White and Steven J. Hermansky

CONTENTS

HISTORICAL PERSPECTIVE

The use of medical devices dates to antiquity. The use of natural materials for medicinal purposes was first documented in the Egyptian papyrus and the writings of Susrata (Boretos and Eden, 1984). The treatment of wounds with silver and gold, including the implantation of these materials into the human body, was described more than 3000 years ago. More recent examples of the use of natural materials range from leather sculptures used to replace a lost ear or nose, goose trachea used as flexible, unkinkable tubing in the measurement of arterial pressure, and porcine heart valves used as replacements for defective human heart valves. Throughout history, it is apparent that the developers of medical devices were looking for materials with appropriate mechanical properties in the absence of adverse biological reaction.

Writings and archeological discoveries suggest that at least some patients invasively treated with early medical devices survived for some period of time after the procedure. Aside from experimental applications that were generally impractical, the successful medical use of materials with intimate tissue contact was limited until Lister described the use of aseptic techniques in the 1860s. Once the importance of infection control was better understood, the major focus of material use for medical purposes shifted from mere patient survival to understanding tissue response and implant rejection. As the use of medical devices derived from natural sources became more routine, the application of synthetic materials to address specific medical applications was evaluated.

Originally, the synthetic materials used for medical devices were created for military, industrial or commercial purposes. Common materials such as silk thread and metal alloys are examples of materials originally developed for alternative purposes and adopted for use in medical device applications. The availability of apparently inert synthetic materials, such as these, during and following World War II led to a rapid expansion of the development of medical devices. During this time, an almost endless catalogue of compounds became available nearly overnight and efforts were launched to screen these industrial materials to find appropriate candidates for clinical application. Initial selection of these new-found materials relied mostly on intuition based upon the intended industrial use of the material and its relationship to the perceived medical need. Examples of materials that were developed for non-medical applications during this time period, and that have become pivotal in modern medical device development, include stainless steel, titanium, silicone elastomers, epoxy resins, high-density polyethylene, polytetrafluoroethylene, polyurethane and polyvinyl chloride.

Upon discovery of groups of materials that appeared to be inert and stable in the biological environment, attention initially focused on cleanliness, sterility and mechanical performance. Once diverse materials were readily available, the fledgling medical device industry began to recognize the need for evaluating and regulating the safe use of materials for medical applications. As the science of biocompatibility (see definition below) developed, the focus of manufacturers, clinicians and, subsequently, regulatory agencies shifted considerably from material discovery to device development. Using the philosophy that a medical device must cause less adverse biological change than the malady it was intended to circumvent, the medical device industry moved forward. The modest beginnings of medical device science, which started as material discovery, have resulted in the development of a substantial, diverse and generally successful industry.

The medical progress made with materials is remarkable considering the limited knowledge of biological and physical mechanisms associated with material and tissue interaction. Indeed, even today the knowledge of these mechanisms is limited. Furthermore, since a considerable proportion of medical device development is driven by industrial research considered to be proprietary information, publication of scientific discoveries associated with tissue interaction with materials has been limited. Only recently has significant progress been made in understanding the local effects of material–tissue contact as well as the systemic response to chemical constituents of the materials that are bioavailable.

An example of a basic principle that is just beginning to be understood involves the material–tissue reaction in which macrophages and other cells (e.g. giant cells) accumulate at the implant interface. This reaction is termed the 'foreign body response' and the development of the response at the implant interface evolves as follows:

implant → monocytes → macrophages → giant cells → fibroblasts

However, the material–tissue interaction is actually much more complicated than suggested by this simplistic diagram. With the advancement of increasingly sensitive analytical chemistry capabilities, the role of intrinsic biochemistry in the systemic response of the body to an implanted material is being discovered. The previously assumed inertness of many materials is now being challenged (Sheftel, 1994). Now, not only are the obvious physical interactions known to exist, but also chemical and biochemical interactions of the body with a material are evident (Anderson, 1993; Ratner, 1993). Both physical and chemical influences on the local and systemic response are exemplified by the increased understanding of material-induced cytokine production (Corry et al., 1998; Girndt et al., 1998). The release of these mediators in response to materials and/or material-derived chemicals results in both adverse and beneficial changes to tissues (Gesualdo et al., 1998).

As indicated above, medical device development has evolved over time beginning with the simple emphasis on patient survival from basic maladies and injuries to the development of eloquent and sophisticated devices for the treatment of not only basic but also complex disorders and diseases. Today, the major areas of emphasis for medical device development are as follows: (1) characterization of physical and chemical properties of materials; (2) characterization of biological mechanisms with emphasis on local and systemic response from implants as well as chemicals that may diffuse or 'leach' into body fluids, tissues or therapeutic solutions; (3) synthesis of new materials with specific properties for durability, architectural influences, and chemical properties to decrease adverse effects and/or increase beneficial chemical availability. With the development of specifically formulated and designed materials, devices and supportive equipment, the magnitude of injury and disease intervention and prevention based upon the use of medical devices will continue to expand.

DEFINITIONS

Many definitions of medical devices exist. In general, the degree of intimacy in which materials make contact with living tissues has been the basis of defining materials and devices. A simple categorization of medical devices is whether the device is placed into the body tissues (that is, 'implantable'), generally by surgical means, for an extended time or if the device is placed on or near the surface of the body (that is, 'non-implantable'), generally by non-surgical means, for a brief or extended time. Another way to separate these classes is to consider implantable devices as those that need to be located inside the body for their intended use, whereas non-implantable medical devices are used external to the body. Non-implantable devices may directly contact the body or they may have 'indirect' contact such as when tubing connects the device and the body.

Because the definitions associated medical device industry continue to be variable, the following definitions are included in this chapter for clarification.

Medical device. Any instrument, apparatus, appliance, material or other article, including software, whether used alone or in combination, intended by the manufacturer for use by human beings solely or principally for the purpose of: diagnosis, prevention, monitoring or treatment; or alleviation of disease, injury or handicap; investigation, replacement or modification of the anatomy or of a physiological process; control of conception and that which does not achieve its principle intended action of the human body by pharmaceutical, immunological or metabolic means, by may be assisted in its function by such means (ISO 10993–1).

Biomedical material. A material that has direct or indirect patient contact (see below). A biomedical material (also termed a 'biomaterial') may be composed of any synthetic or natural rubber or fibre, polymeric or elastomeric formulation, alloy, ceramic, bonding agent, ink or other non-viable substance, including tissue rendered non-viable, used as a device or any part thereof. As defined above, not all medical devices are made of biomedical materials.

Direct contact. When the materials of a device are in intimate contact with the surface or tissues of the body—for example, the lead for a cardiac monitor that adheres directly to the skin or a blood dialysis chamber in which the blood of the patient leaves the body and enters the device.

Indirect contact. When the materials of a device do not contact the surface or tissues of the body but the materials of the device may influence the body—for example, the plastic components of an intravenous (i.v.) bag never directly contact the body, but a chemical that diffuses into the contents of the bag which are administered to a patient may illicit a biological response.

Biocompatibility (biological compatibility). The science of determining the suitability of a material for a proposed contact with biological tissues. Biocompatibility determinations should consider the intimacy of contact as well as duration of contact for the specific material. Therefore, a material that is considered to be 'biocompatible' for an application that is not invasive (a surface device) may not be considered biocompatible for an implantable device such as a replacement heart valve.

Combination product. A product comprised of two or more regulated components, e.g. drug–device, biological–device, drug–biological or drug–device–biological, that are physically, chemically or otherwise combined or mixed and produced as a single entity (21 CFR).

Finished product. Medical device in its 'as used' state (ISO 10993–1).

DEVICE VERSUS DRUG

The differences between devices and drugs may seem obvious owing to the difference in appearance. This difference can generally be diluted down to the simple fact that the biological effects of a drug are more or less independent of its physical form, while the physical form of a device usually defines its biological activity. In spite of this obvious difference, there are many similarities between the toxicological evaluation of chemicals (drugs) and devices. In both cases, the evaluation of local (site of administration) and systemic effects is necessary and similar health-related end-points need to be evaluated. For drugs or chemicals, the potential for adverse effects related to systemic exposure tends to be the focus of attention while the local effect of a device has historically been the focus of attention.

HISTORY OF MEDICAL DEVICE TESTING

As stated above, until recently (within the last 25 years), medical device developers based the selection of materials almost entirely on physical properties, and relied heavily on intuition with regard to biological compatibility. As experience was gained with synthetic and natural materials with potential medical device applications, adverse events were increasingly noted (Rubin and Yaremchuk, 1997). Therefore, regulatory agencies, and also the medical device industry, recognized that more than intuition was necessary for predicting which materials could be used safely (Gotman, 1997).

The explosive growth of the medical device industry also caused the US Food and Drug Administration (FDA) and international regulatory agencies to consider the safety of medical devices. To address the developing safety needs of the industry, efforts to establish a rationale for biological compatibility evaluation were initiated. With no precedence to follow, a set of tests designed by the US Pharmacopeia for classifying plastics using a series of biological tests was selected as a guidance (Northup, 1987). In 1976, the US Congress passed the Medical Device Amendments to the Food, Drug, and Cosmetic Act. The wording of this Act necessitated an emphasis on the critical nature of the end use of a medical device in the assessment of safety parameters. To facilitate rational evaluation while complying with the intent of this Act, various industry organizations drafted guidance documents outlining systematic testing schemes. In 1987, the FDA, in collaboration with Canada and Great Britain, drafted a guidance document known as the Tripartite Agreement. This document used a matrix approach to categorize a medical device and, therefore, identify the necessary safety evaluations that had to be successfully completed before the device could be marketed. The areas of toxicity to be evaluated were based on the duration and intimacy of body contact with the assumption that an increasing duration of more intimate body contact would indicate a more critical device. Therefore, the Tripartite Agreement was considered to comply with the intent of the Act. However, the Tripartite Agreement did not identify acceptable testing protocols. Therefore, the industry had to design these protocols based upon currently accepted toxicological testing methods adapted for materials.

The methods of the Tripartite Agreement in which a matrix approach is used to categorize the duration and intimacy of contact has formed the basis for all device testing to this time. From a safety perspective, this approach is considered to have been generally successful and the level of concern increases as the degree of intimate tissue contact increases (Pinchuk, 1994). Another area of focus for categorizing medical devices is based on whether the device has direct or indirect contact with biological tissues. As the science of biocompatibility expanded, so did the perceived needs of the testing to establish safety. Today, biocompatability considerations include inductive and inflammatory responses, general toxicity, specific organ toxicity, immunotoxicity, reproductive toxicity, genetic toxicity and carcinogenicity.

Recognition of the increasingly international aspects of the medical device industry led to the International Organization for Standardization (ISO) to establish a medical device guideline. Utilizing the matrix approach introduced by the Tripartite Agreement, ISO set forth a guidance in 1992. The primary document of this

Table 1 ISO 10993: Biological Evaluation of Medical Devices

Part	Title
1	Guidance on selection of tests
2	Animal welfare requirements
3	Tests for genotoxicity, carcinogenicity and reproductive toxicity
4	Selection of tests for interaction with blood
5	Tests for cytotoxicity: *in vitro* methods
6	Tests for local effects after implantation
7	Ethylene oxide sterilization residuals
8	Clinical investigation
9	Degradation of materials related to biological testing
10	Tests for irritation and sensitization
11	Tests for systemic toxicity
12	Sample preparation and reference materials
	The following draft documents are at various stages of preparation and approval. These titles have been included in this table to allow for an awareness of potential resources and to emphasize the dynamic nature of the ISO documents
13 (draft)	Identification and quantification of degradation products from polymers
14 (draft)	Identification and quantification of degradation products from ceramics
15 (draft)	Identification and quantification of degradation products from metals and alloys
16 (draft)	General guidance on toxicokinetic study design for degradation products and leachables
17 (draft)	Establishment of allowable limits for leachable substances
18 (draft)	Chemical characterization of materials
ISO/DIS 14155	Clinical investigation of medical devices
ISO/DIS 12891	Implants for surgery—retrieval and analysis of surgical implants

guidance, ISO 10993–1: Biological Evaluation of Medical Devices—Part 1: Guidance on Selection of Tests, along with the substitutive series of documents that describe acceptable protocols for testing, was formally adopted by the FDA, with modification, in 1995. Other parts of the ISO 10993 document describe specific testing methods or other aspects of safety evaluation. The title of other parts of the ISO 10993, available at the time this chapter was prepared, are shown in **Table 1**. The ISO 10993 guidance documents are dynamic and have subsequently replaced the Tripartite Agreement in the industry. These have become the standard for manufacturers desiring to market medical devices in Europe, Japan and the USA, in that the ISO 10993 guidance documents are dynamic modifications to existing documents and additions of new documents will occur as the industry and biomaterials science continue to evolve.

DETERMINING TESTING NEEDS

ISO Categorization

To aid in the determination of testing needs, the ISO standard 10993–1 document categorizes medical devices by the Nature of Body Contact: non-contact, surface-contacting (skin; mucosal membranes; and breached or compromised surfaces), external communicating (blood path, indirect; tissue/bone/dentris communicating and circulating blood), or implant devices, and by the dura-

tion of contact: limited exposure ($\leq$ 24 h), prolonged exposure ($\geq$ 24 h to 30 days), or permanent contact (> 30 days). Testing requirements increase as intimacy and duration of contact increase, and the ISO 10993–1 matrix for initial evaluation tests as modified by the FDA is shown in **Table 2**. Once the intimacy of contact and duration of contact categories have been determined, the required tests for biological evaluation can be identified. In general, the tests include: acute, subchronic and chronic toxicity; irritation to skin, eyes and mucosal surfaces; sensitization; haemocapatibility; genotoxicity; carcinogencity; effects on reproduction including developmental effects; and biodegradation. Depending on varying characteristics and intended use of the device and the nature of contact, additional tests for specific target organ toxicity such as immunotoxicity or neurotoxicity may be necessary. **Table 3** provides examples of medical devices according to body contact categories of ISO 10993–1.

An example of how to use the ISO 10993–1 guidance matrix is as follows. A haemoabsorbent is considered to be a direct contact device (via an externally communicating method) with circulating blood and prolonged (category B) contact duration. Following the ISO recommendations for this type of device, as indicated in the matrix shown in **Table 2**, the initial biological responses that should be considered are cytotoxicity, sensitization, intracutaneous reactivity, acute systemic toxicity, genotoxicity and haemocompatability. The recommendation from the FDA would be the same but would include

Table 2 Guidance for initial evaluation tests

Device category / Body contact		Contact duration[a]	Cytotoxicity	Sensitization	Irritation or intracutaneous reactivity	Systemic toxicity (acute)	Subchronic toxicity (subacute)	Genotoxicity	Implantation	Haemocompatibility	Chronic toxicity	Carcinogenicity	Reproductive/developmental	Biodegradation
Surface devices	Skin	A	X	X	X									
		B	X	X	X									
		C	X	X	X									
	Mucosal membranes	A	X	X	X									
		B	X	X	X	O	O		O					
		C	X	X	X	O	X	X	O			O		
	Breached or compromised surfaces	A	X	X	X	O								
		B	X	X	X	O	O		O					
		C	X	X	X	O	X	X	O			O		
External communicating devices	Blood path, indirect	A	X	X	X	X				X				
		B	X	X	X	X	O			X				
		C	X	X		X	X	X	O	X	X	X		
	Tissue/bone/dentine communicating[c]	A	X	X	X	O								
		B	X	X		O	O	X	X					
		C	X	X		O	O	X	X			O	X	
	Circulating blood	A	X	X	X	X		O[2]		X				
		B	X	X	X	X	O	X	O	X				
		C	X	X	X	X	X	X	O	X	X	X		
Implant devices	Tissue/bone	A	X	X	X	O								
		B	X	X		O	O	X	X					
		C	X	X		O	O	X	X			X	X	
	Blood	A	X	X	X	X			X	X				
		B	X	X	X	X	O	X	X	X				
		C	X	X	X	X	X	X	X	X	X	X		

[a] A, limited ($\leq$ 24h); B, Prolonged ($\geq$ 24h to 30 days); C, permanent (> 30 days)
[b] O = Additional tests which may be applicable per FDA.
[c] Tissue includes tissue fluids and subcutaneous species per FDA.
[d] For all devices used in extracorporial circuits per FDA.
Note—Each device shall be considered on its own merits.

consideration of subchronic toxicity. Although implantation is also suggested in the FDA modified matrix, the knowledgeable researcher would recognize that this test was not necessary for a haemodialyser as it is not an implantable device. Therefore, international regulatory agencies, including the FDA, may allow the researcher to alter the testing described by the matrix based upon sound scientific rationale. On the other hand, the FDA has indicated that tests not mandated by the ISO 10993 matrix may be necessary, based upon the end use of the device, prior to a device being marketed in the USA. Once ISO testing is identified as necessary, the actual tests suggested to satisfy these recommendations are then selected from those delineated in the ISO standards

10993–3, 10993–4, 10993–5, 10993–10 and 10993–11 (as shown in **Table 1**). Specific methods, and difficulties encountered with devices, are described later in this chapter.

In conjunction with ISO 10993–1, special standards for specific devices or categories of devices may be available for safety evaluation guidance. However, specific device testing, as designed by ISO 10993–1, are beyond the scope of this chapter. Therefore, the reader is referred to the ISO 10993–1 documentation for the availability and location of device-specific guidance documents.

Ultimately, the end use of the device and the materials used in its manufacture determine which tests may be

Table 3 Examples of medical devices for ISO 10993–1 body contact catagories

	Body contact category	Examples of devices
Surface devices	Skin	Electrodes
		Compression bandages
		Industrial gloves
		Surgical gowns
	Mucosal membrane	Nebulizers, repirators, inhalers
		Anaesthesiology masks and tubing
		Airway tubes
		Endotracheal tubes
		Urinary catheters
		Stomach tubes
		External feeding tubes
		Examination gloves
	Breached or compromised surface	Bandages, dressings
		Occlusive patches, tapes
External communicating devices	Tissue/bone/dentine communicating	Surgical drains
		Laparoscopes
		Arthroscopes
		Endoscopes
		Surgical gloves
	Blood path indirect	Extension sets
		Transfer sets
		Hypodermic needles
		Solution administration sets (tubing, spike, flashball, Y-connector)
		Autotransfusion sets
		Blood administration sets
	Circulating blood	Dialysis tubing
		Haemoadsorbents
		Haemodialysers
		Immunoadsorbents
		I.v. catheters
		Oxygenators, oxygenator tubing
Implant devices	Tissue/bone	Cements
		Cerebrospinal fluid drains
		Internal drug delivery port
		Orthopaedic joints, pins, plates, screws
		Pacemakers
		Dental implants
	Blood	AV fistulae
		Blood monitors
		Heart valves
		Vascular grafts
		Internal drug delivery catheter
		LVAD (left ventricular assist device)
		Permanent pacemaker electrodes
		Ventricular assist pump

appropriate. The ISO 10993 standard is not intended to be a definitive document to be followed by individuals not qualified in materials and/or safety assessment. Therefore, the establishment of the safety assessment plan for a device should be made by the appropriate professionals qualified by training and experience using interpretation and judgment when considering the factors relevant to the device or its materials, intended use of the same and current knowledge of the device and its materials provided by scientific literature and previous clinical experience (ANSI/AAMI, 1997).

As a note for the reader, packaging materials for drugs and biologics (although they are generally composed of materials similar to those used for constructing various medical devices) are not considered medical devices. Examples of packages that fall into this category include container closure systems for drug products, intravenous solution bags, blood component storage bags, and inhalation aerosol container closure systems. With regard to the safety assessment of packaging materials, consideration is especially important for components that may be in direct contact with the dosage form, but is important for any component from which substances may migrate into the dosage form such as inks or adhesives. The safety evaluation of packaging materials involves extraction studies to determine chemicals that may migrate into the dosage form and a toxicological evaluation of those substances. Guidance for safety evaluation of these materials and devices can be found in an FDA document (USDHHS, 1997).

Additional Classification of Devices

There are many ways of classifying devices. While the international community is moving towards the use of standardized systems that depend on the extent and duration of contact with the body, the FDA has established classifications for approximately 1700 different generic types of devices and grouped them into 16 medical specialties referred to as panels. Each of these generic types of devices is assigned to one of three regulatory classes based on the level of control the FDA considers to be necessary to assure the safety and effectiveness of the device. The three classes and the regulatory requirements that apply along with some examples are shown in **Table 4**.

Table 4 US FDA device classes and regulatory controls

1. Class I. General Controls (with or without exemptions)
   Examples
   - Oesophageal stethoscope
   - Stethoscope head
   - Manual stethoscope
   - Hearing aid (air-conduction)
   - Canes and crutches

2. Class II. General Controls and Special Controls (with or without exemptions)
   Examples
   - Mercury thermometer
   - Blood pressure cuff
   - Continuous flush catheter
   - Electronic stethoscope
   - Vascular clamp
   - Hearing aid (bone-conduction)
   - Condom

3. Class III. General Controls and Premarket Approval
   Examples
   - Pacemaker (implantable pulse generator)
   - Replacement heart valve
   - Implanted neuromuscular stimulator
   - Foetal scalp clip electrode

The class to which a device is assigned determines, among other things, the extent and nature of the safety/toxicology testing required for inclusion in the submission to the FDA for approval. Device classification depends on the intended use of the device and also upon indications for use. In addition, classification is risk based, that is, the risk the device poses to the patient and/or the user is a major factor in the class to which it is assigned. Class I includes devices with the lowest perceived risk and Class III includes those with the greatest perceived risk.

In some cases, a regulatory submission must be submitted to and approved by the FDA before a device can be marketed in the USA. This submission may either be a premarket notification [510(k)] or a premarket approval (PMA). The regulatory submission includes several sections such as intended use; indications for use; target population; design; materials; performance; sterility; biocompatibility; mechanical safety; chemical safety; anatomical sites; human factors; energy used and/or delivered; compatibility with the environment and other devices; where used; standards met; electrical safety; thermal safety; and radiation safety. A description of the specifics of regulatory submissions is well beyond the scope of this chapter but a general description may be of use to the toxicologist.

Premarket Notification [510(k)]

A premarket notification [510(k)] is a marketing application submitted to FDA to demonstrate that a medical device intended for marketing is as safe and as effective (that is, substantially equivalent) to a legally marketed device that was or is currently on the US market and that does not require premarket approval. Most devices on the market in the USA are Class II and, therefore, most devices are cleared for commercial distribution in the USA by the premarket notification [510(k)] process. Most Class I devices are exempt from the 510(k) requirement by regulation and most Class III devices require a premarket approval application (see below) prior to marketing in the USA.

An important aspect of the 510(k) process is the identification of the previously marketed, substantially equivalent device to which the proposed device will be compared. A claim of substantial equivalence does not mean that the devices must be identical. Substantial equivalence is established with respect to intended use, design, energy used or delivered, materials, performance, safety, effectiveness, labelling, biocompatibility, standards and other applicable characteristics.

The 510(k) application must include a discussion of the safety parameters of the proposed and substantially equivalent device. For devices which come into direct contact with the patient or user, an exact identification and composition of all materials that contact the patient should be provided and a statement regarding any material or manufacturing (processing and sterilization) differences from the substantially equivalent device should be stated. If the materials and manufacturing processes are not identical, or this information is not available for a predicate device, biocompatibility testing must be performed. Therefore, manufacturers will need to provide biocompatibility test results for any new materials when the new device is compared with a legally marketed device made of different materials. The FDA is currently using the ISO 10993 Biological Evaluation of Medical Devices in the evaluation of manufacturers' biomaterial testing programmes for medical devices.

Premarket Approval (PMA)

Premarket approval (PMA) is the process by the FDA to evaluate the safety and effectiveness of Class II devices for which a currently marketed, substantially equivalent device cannot be identified as well as most Class III devices. Class III is the most stringent regulatory category for medical devices and these are usually devices that support or sustain human life, are of substantial importance in preventing impairment of human health or which present a potential, unreasonable risk of illness or injury. Owing to the level of risk associated with Class III devices, the FDA has determined that the controls assigned to Class I and II devices alone are insufficient to ensure the safety and effectiveness of Class III devices. Therefore, each of these devices requires a more rigorous regulatory submission to obtain marketing clearance. The PMA process does not allow for comparison with a pre-existing device alone to substantiate safety and efficacy of a device. Therefore, each Class III device marketed in the USA must be individually shown by pre-clinical and clinical evaluations to be safe and effective.

Notified Bodies

In the European environment, medical devices are regulated through a legal framework that is defined in the Active Implantable Medical Device Directive and the Medical Device Directive. These Directives have been cooperatively reviewed and agreed upon by the 15 Member States that comprise the European Community. Under the control of these Directives, medical device manufacturers must qualify their proposed devices for marketing through a Notified Body. A Notified Body is a legally separate entity that has been appointed by a national government agency such as the UK Department of Trade and Industry as qualified to assess for approval the results of testing of a medical device for compliance with the Directives. A Competent Body is legally separate from Notified Bodies and testing laboratories. A

Competent Body is a person confirmed by a national government agency as qualified to review and assess for approval the results obtained by a testing programme. Competent Bodies are qualified to issue assessment certificates when a successful review of a technical file has been developed.

As in the USA, all implants in European Member States must meet certain essential requirements to ensure that they do not harm the patient, clinician or any third party. For most medical devices this will be indicated on the product or its packaging by a 'CE marking' coordinated and granted through the independent Notified Body. Medical devices are classified in proportion to the risk associated with their use. After placing a medical device on the market, the manufacturer must set up a system of post-market surveillance, including a vigilance procedure, to monitor medical device for performance including safety and efficacy. While, in theory, a CE marking obtained through a Notified Body associated with one of the Member States, an individual Member State always has the right to exercise a safeguard clause when a product appears to have had the CE marking incorrectly applied.

BIOCOMPATIBILITY TESTING

The Use of Extracts

Materials used in the manufacture of medical devices are generally cured plastics, rubber or silicone, metal, fabric or ceramics. These components either do not completely break down in a biological environment or break down at such a slow rate that biologically significant changes may be undetectable for many years (Pinchuk, 1994). A significant proportion of these materials is not bioavailable under conditions of normal use. However, the potential adverse effect of chemicals (contaminants, unreacted monomer, processing aids, etc.) that may be bioavailable (viz., leachable under biological conditions) should be evaluated. Total dissolution of the material using an aggressive solvent and or physical pulverization would not generally be relevant to the safety evaluation of these materials since this level of material destruction would never occur *in vivo*. Therefore, a rational approach to the safety evaluation of the bioavailable chemicals had to be devised.

Since the biological system in which these materials will be placed is a complex mixture of hydrophobic (nonpolar) and hydrophilic (polar) environments, incubating a material in both a hydrophobic solution (e.g. a vegetable oil) and a hydrophilic solution (e.g. saline) should provide a vehicle into which the bioavailable chemicals can diffuse. Hence these potentially bioavailable chemicals should be present in the solution after an appropriate incubation period. These chemicals, which have potential to diffuse away from the material when the material is in contact with a biological system, are often referred to as 'leachables'.

Unfortunately, neither science nor the product development cycle will allow the incubation period to approximate the actual time and exposure of use for a medical device (e.g. a chronically implanted device that may be implanted for 20 or more years in a patient cannot be incubated in an appropriate solution for 20 years before being evaluated for toxicity). Therefore, the prudent medical device manufacturer and regulatory agencies have utilized the physical laws of diffusion which state that a concentration equilibrium is reached in a dynamic system more rapidly at a higher temperature to maximize the departure of leachables from the solid matrix of the material. Thus, these leachable chemicals are 'extracted' from the material using higher temperatures and solutions that maximize the potential for their departure from the solid material. This extraction procedure that uses solutions at high incubation temperatures is then combined with a ratio of material to solution that is expected to exceed greatly that which would be encountered in a biological system. The resulting solution, rich in potential leachable materials, may now be used to predict potential adverse effects of the materials. Commonly used solutions, temperatures and ratios of extraction conditions are listed in **Table 5**. ISO 10993–12 provides guidance for preparation of extract samples suitable for biocompatibility testing.

Using generally standard toxicological methods for the detection of adverse effects in biological systems,

the solutions used to extract potential leachable compounds are evaluated for toxicity. Several complications, not encountered by routine toxicology, exist in this system. First, and most obviously, the need to extract both hydrophobic and hydrophilic leachable compounds yields two solutions of potentially toxic materials. Thus, the volume of testing is automatically doubled. Second, regardless of the attempts to concentrate the leachable chemicals within the solution during the extraction procedure, the final concentration of any single chemical will probably be low. Therefore, a considerably high dosing volume of the solution needs to be administered to test animals to successfully detect a potential toxic response to the material. Third, it is often difficult, sometimes seemingly impossible, to administer appropriately an extraction solution to an animal by an appropriate route in a necessary volume that will yield meaningful results for the risk assessment process. For example, the hydrophobic solution (e.g. vegetable oil) from a device that will be in direct contact with the blood cannot be directly injected into the bloodstream of an animal in an appropriate volume as this would, obviously, result in the immediate death of the test animal. Therefore, the hydrophobic solution must be administered to the animal using an alternative route of dosing. Clearly, the oral route of administration is inappropriate since the leachable materials will not encounter the first-pass metabolic capacity of the liver when they diffuse away from the material under the routine use of the device. Hence an intraperitoneal injec-

Table 5 Commonly used parameters for extraction

Examples of extraction media (solutions)
Polar liquid
  Water
  Saline
  Culture media without sera
Non-polar liquid
  Vegetable oil (e.g. cottonseed or sesame oil)
Additional extraction liquids
  Ethanol–saline (5% v/v)
  Polyethylene glycol 400 (diluted to physiological osmotic pressure)

Temperature/time conditions
  $37 \pm 1°C$ for $24 \pm 2h$
  $37 \pm 1°C$ for $72 \pm 2h$
  $50 \pm 2°C$ for $72 \pm 2h$
  $70 \pm 2°C$ for $24 \pm 2h$
  $121 \pm 2°C$ for $1.0 \pm 0.2h$

Extraction ratios

Thickness (mm)	Extraction ratio ($\pm 10\%$)	Examples of materials
≤ 0.5	$6\ cm^2\ ml^{-1}$	Metal; synthetic polymer; ceramic; film, sheet and tubing wall
> 0.5	$3\ cm^2\ ml^{-1}$	Metal; synthetic polymer; ceramic; tubing wall; slab; moulded items
≤ 1.0	$3\ cm^2\ ml^{-1}$	Elastomer
> 1.0	$1.25\ cm^2\ ml^{-1}$	Elastomer
Irregular	$0.1–0.2\ g\ ml^{-1}$	Pellets
	$6\ cm^2\ ml^{-1}$	Moulded parts

tion of the solution, although not a perfect model of exposure, may be used.

These adaptations to standard toxicological methods may significantly complicate the risk assessment process as compared with cosmetics, drugs and chemicals. The risk assessment process is, necessarily, at least one more level of uncertainty removed from the human exposure condition. In an attempt to maximize the detection of potential adverse effects of materials, the medical device industry has, using extracts of materials/devices, standardized several testing methods. Where possible, physical aliquots (i.e. implants) of the actual material are utilized in the biological testing system. However, much more often, implantation testing procedures are not easily adapted so that a physical piece of plastic, metal, fabric or other solid material can be used as the test article, thus requiring the use of extracts.

It is generally accepted that procedures used to sterilize biomaterials can change the physical characteristics of the material and it is now more widely accepted that sterilization procedures can also affect the biocompatibility of a material/device (Nair, 1995). Therefore, prior to initiating biocompatibility testing, the intended sterilization procedure(s) and specific conditions should be identified. The biomaterials or final device should be evaluated for biocompatibility after the test article has been sterilized according to the selected procedures. Multiple sterilization procedures may necessitate multiple evaluations for biocompatibility. A guidance document regarding sterilization procedures is ISO 10993–12.

Testing Methods

Cytotoxicity

The medical device industry is leading the way over all other industries in their requirements and dependence on *in vitro* methods, specifically cytotoxicity. To this end, assessment of cytotoxicity is considered for all medical device categories. The methods recommended for cytotoxicity testing are described in detail in various established guidelines (e.g. ISO 10993–5). With the use of cell culture techniques, this test evaluates the lysis of cells (cell death), the inhibition of cell growth and other effects caused by the material and/or extracts of the material. Cytotoxicity assays measure the local toxicity potential of medical device materials or extractives to isolated mammalian cells. Local effects are irritant in nature and are pertinent to those that occur at the site of primary contact between the biological system and the material. Cytotoxicity assays are often used as an initial biological screen for new plastic or silicone formulations and are also used to aid in the evaluation of biological effects of formulation, manufacturing and sterilization process changes.

The method by which the biomaterial is exposed to the cells, selection of control material and end-points evaluated in the testing can have a significant impact on the results and conclusions of the study (Tsuchiya, 1994; Hanks *et al.*, 1996). Appropriate experience of the laboratory and strict adherence to consistent procedures is necessary to ensure that the results obtained from cytotoxicity studies are useful in the risk assessment process.

Sensitization

Assessment of biomaterials for the potential to induce a sensitization response is suggested for all medical device categories owing to the potential morbidity that may be caused to a patient treated or implanted with a material that induces an allergic sensitization reaction (Danz, 1990; Warfvinge, 1994; Klinkmann *et al.*, 1996). The potential for both natural and synthetic materials to produce a sensitization reaction in humans is well known in medicine. However, the need for an immune sensitization test may not be necessary if acceptable preclinical data or published literature exist indicating a lack of sensitization potential. It is important, indeed it is a requirement of the Animal Welfare Act, that the researcher consider previously conducted preclinical data or published literature before initiating a study using animals (Schwindaman, 1994). Immune sensitization tests measure the potential for materials and/or medical devices to induce the immune system after repeated or prolonged exposure. There are several methods for determining immune sensitization. Currently, the two methods most commonly used are the maximization and closed patch methods as described in ISO 10993–10. Details of these assays are described in other chapters of this book. Other assays may be considered, such as the local lymph node assay (Kimber *et al.*, 1990). The selection of an appropriate assay and route of exposure should be made carefully so as to provide an accurate assessment of sensitization hazard of the material or device.

Skin Irritation (Topical and Intracutaneous Reactivity)

Assessment of the skin irritation potential of a material is recommended for most device categories (see **Table 2**). Skin irritation assays measure the local toxicity potential of a medical device material or extractives and are particularly useful in detecting irritants that are not rapidly detoxified or diluted after systemic administration. Local effects refer to those that occur at the site of first contact between the biological system and the toxicant. A stepwise approach to irritation testing is recommended, i.e. literature review, *in vitro* cytotoxicity assay followed by *in vivo* assays in animals. If assessment is not possible using this staged approach, then consideration should be given to non-invasive testing in humans.

Skin irritation evaluations can include test methods that are generally similar to those for standard toxicology evaluations of drugs and chemicals. These tests are conducted as would be expected by applying a piece of the material directly to the intact or abraded skin of the rabbit and scoring the treated site for signs of skin irritation (erythema and oedema). However, the local irritation of a biomaterial destined for incorporation into a device to be implanted into the body also needs to be evaluated. This can be done by directly implanting a piece of the material into the body of an animal (see below) or by injecting very small (0.2 ml) aliquots of the hydrophilic and hydrophobic extraction vehicles directly into the skin of a rabbit. The sites of injection are then observed for signs of skin irritation. This test, the intracutaneous test, is frequently used and is an indicator of the potential for an irritating chemical to leach from a biomaterial. Methods for intracutaneous reactivity assays have been summarized in regulatory documents (ISO 10993–11 and US Pharmacopeia).

Acute Systemic Toxicity

Consideration for acute toxicity is given for the device categories indicated in **Table 2**. Acute systemic toxicity assays estimate the potential for harmful effects of exposures (single or multiple during a period of less than 24 h) to materials and/or their extracts in an animal model. The animal models can be designed to evaluate effects following oral, intravenous, intraperitoneal and/or cutaneous exposure and focus on systemic effects (that is, effects at sites distant from the treatment site). The testing can, when appropriate, evaluate intact material but, owing to the difficulties associated with providing relevent doses of the materials to animals, hydrophilic and hydrophobic extraction vehicles obtained from the material are often evaluated in these studies. Acute systemic toxicity testing is typically not necessary for devices constructed of well known materials that are expected to contact only intact skin surfaces. Methods for acute systemic toxicity assays have been summarized in regulatory documents (ISO 10993–11 and US, European, or Japanese Pharmacopeia).

Haemocompatibility

Haemocompatibility is considered for all devices having indirect or direct blood contact (see **Table 2**). Haemocompatibility assays assess the potential for medical devices and/or their materials to affect the formed cellular elements of the blood or activate the coagulation and/or complement systems. The most frequently conducted haemocompatibility evaluation is an *in vitro* haemolysis method that measures the ability of a material, device or hydrophilic extract thereof to interact with the red blood cell membrane and cause lysis. The methods for this study have been standardized but refinements are continually being evaluated (Malinauskas, 1997). Haemolysis testing is frequently conducted using the blood obtained from laboratory animals but there is evidence that erythrocytes from species differ in cell fragility (Jikuya *et al.*, 1998). *In vitro* haemolysis testing may be sufficient for most materials and/or devices but additional testing (including *in vivo* studies) may be considered when *in vitro* studies are inconclusive. Such testing may focus on simulating the configuration, contact conditions and flow dynamics during clinical use. The guidance found in ISO 10993–4 may be useful in selecting haemocompatibility assays.

Implantation

The device categories considered for implantation evaluation are shown in **Table 2**. Implantation assays measure the local toxicity and irritation potential of materials and medical devices when in direct contact with living tissue. Depending on the intended use and animal species selected for testing, a sample of material is implanted in an animal for a period of 1–12 weeks for short-term evaluation or for a period of 12–104 weeks for long-term evaluation. The primary purpose of the implantation test is to evaluate the intrinsic properties of the material, not the configuration. Therefore, it is important that the shape of the implant should be such that configuration-induced trauma is minimized (that is, sharp edges and/or corners should be minimized).

The most frequent site for the test article to be implanted is a large muscle of the animal. The implantation technique can be by injection (using a large-gauge needle and plunger apparatus) or by surgery. In either case, the animal is anaesthetized prior to the implantation technique. Following the prescribed duration of exposure, the animal is euthanized and the sites are removed and examined macroscopically and, generally, microscopically. While some basic muscle implantation techniques require only macroscopic evaluation, a microscopic evaluation of the implantation site should be considered so that the cellular response can be better identified. Owing to the characteristic cellular reactions of a biological tissue to an implant, it is critical that the macroscopic and microscopic evaluations be conducted by experienced personnel.

Implantation studies can also be conducted by surgically implanting a material, materials, or a complete device into the target organ. Specifically designed studies are most appropriate for specialized devices that will contact specific organs such as the central nervous system, intraocular tissue or bones. In all cases, the macroscopic and histopathological response as a function of time is used to evaluate the biological response. ISO 10993–6 provides guidance for implantation testing.

Genotoxicity

Genotoxicity assays measure the potential for materials and/or medical devices to produce gene mutations, changes in chromosome structure, or other DNA or gene changes. Genotoxicity tests are used for materials or devices having direct tissue or fluid path contact for a duration of greater than 24 h. As with other end-points, a stepwise approach to genotoxicity testing is recommended, i.e. literature review, *in vitro* genotoxicity assays followed by *in vivo* assays in animals if the end-point has not been resolved. The tests should preferably evaluate the three categories of genotoxic effects: DNA effects, gene mutations and chromosomal aberrations. Additional details on genotoxic effects and testing methods can be found in other chapters of this book and will not be addressed further here (see Chapters 48 and 49). ISO 10993–3 provides guidance for genotoxicity testing.

Subchronic and Chronic Toxicity

Evaluations for subchronic toxicity and chronic toxicity should be considered for materials or devices having direct tissue contact for a duration of greater than 24 h and greater than 30 days, respectively. Chronic toxicity for medical devices is rarely appropriate and should be considered on a case-by-case basis. Subchronic and chronic toxicity studies are used to evaluate potential adverse effects that may develop as a result of the repeated or daily exposure to or dosing of a material, medical device or extract thereof. The principle goals of these studies are to identify and characterize any specific organ(s) affected by the test material after repeated exposure or administration. The study design and choice of laboratory animal species for subchronic and chronic testing will vary with the medical device, component materials, and end use of the device. Individually designed protocols to evaluate subchronic and/or chronic toxicity are generally necessary owing to the specialized and varied use of the medical devices. ISO 10993–11 provides guidance for tests for systemic toxicity.

Carcinogenicity

ISO 10993–1 indicates the device categories and contact duration that require consideration for carcinogenicity assessment. Carcinogenesis bioassays should be considered when results of the genotoxicity studies, implantation test and/or evidence in the literature indicate the potential for carcinogenicity. The duration and frequency of patient exposure to a material or device should be considered when evaluating the need for carcinogenicity testing. Care should be taken in selecting an appropriate animal model and study design that will provide an accurate assessment of carcinogenicity of the material or device. Studies to determine the tumorigenic potential of test materials or material extracts in an appropriate ani-

mal model are conducted over a period of the major portion of the life span (e.g. 2 years for rat, 18 months for mouse or 7 years for dog). Guidance for selection of an appropriate carcinogenicity assay may be obtained in ISO 10993–3.

CHEMICAL CHARACTERIZATION

The toxicologist associated with medical devices may have access to some data relating to the chemical characterization of device components. Currently, this term has no standardized definition in the medical device industry, but several sections of ISO 10993 are currently being prepared to provide guidance on this issue. However, a brief description of the widely varied definitions of 'chemical characterization' historically used within the industry may be of benefit to the toxicologist.

First, a very general form of chemical characterization has been used to describe the physical characteristics of the material such as hardness, opacity and heat stability. This form of chemical characterization has little value in the safety evaluation of a biomaterial but may have some utility in manufacturing controls.

Chemical characterization has also been used to define the description of the chemical constituents of a material. This degree of characterization does not account for reactive intermediates, changes in chemical composition of the final material caused by production modifications, contaminants or variability in raw materials.

A more toxicologically functional form of chemical characterization, and which is the current focus of ISO 10993, attempts to identify experimentally the chemical structure of the material along with any other chemical entities that may be a routine component of the material and that may be bioavailable under routine biological exposure conditions. While complete destruction of the polymeric matrix is possible using heat and/or aggressive solvents, the biological significance of identification of the resulting free chemicals is unclear since the biomaterial, with the exception of absorbable materials, will never encounter such conditions during routine use. Under these more biologically relevant conditions of chemical characterization, no attempt is made to denature the polymeric component(s) of the biomaterial using aggressive solvents, heating or biological degradation (enzymes). This chemical characterization of a biomaterial may include identification of chemicals derived directly from the biomaterial or secondary to the metabolism, hydrolysis, oxidation or other biological processes of chemicals within the biomaterial or that leach away from the device.

ISO guidance document 10993–16 is currently being prepared to address toxicokinetics. The effects of biological processes, including the tissue repair process on a biomaterial, can result in the creation of chemical entities not present at the time of initial use. These biodegradation products may have the potential to cause a toxic response that would not be anticipated in short-term biocompatibility tests. As experience is gained with biomaterials, improved information regarding the biodegradation of implanted materials is becoming available in the peer-reviewed literature (Stokes *et al.*, 1995).

The toxicological evaluation procedures used by much of the medical device industry currently focuses primarily on biocompatibility testing of raw materials and final devices using the *in vitro* and *in vivo* methods described above. The identification of individual chemical entities that may leach out of a device or its components is not always performed. While the lack of chemical identification of test articles would generally be considered unacceptable to the chemical and drug industries, the diversity and multitude of chemicals within a device that have the potential to be biologically available can be surprising. Indeed, the characterization of leachable materials from a device may yield from one to several different chemicals. Therefore, the cost associated with the chemical characterization of these leachable chemicals may be similarly large. For biocompatibility testing that does not require subchronic or chronic testing, minimal chemical characterization may suffice, whereas extensive chemical characterization may be used if longer term subchronic and chonic testing is required.

The continued, successful growth of the industry, including the development of increasingly complex, safe devices, requires the chemical characterization of, at least, the major bioavailable chemical entities. To this end, the ISO guidance documents 10993–13, –14 and –15 reflect standardized approaches to chemical characterization. Utilizing these guidelines allows for toxicity evaluation of leachables using procedures similar to the drug industry, a quantitative estimation of exposure potential and, therefore, quantitative risk assessment (addressed in ISO 10993–17). The FDA has prepared a draft guidance document based upon these procedures. Furthermore, many successful medical device companies throughout the world currently have broad, on-going chemical characterization programmes to aid in the evaluation of the risk assessment, efficacy, and manufacturing controls of their devices. As experience is gained with chemical characterization and quantitative risk assessment, the *in vitro* and *in vivo* biocompatibility testing requirements for well known and characterized materials will decrease. The resources conserved by this decrease in repetative biocompatibility testing may be available for the development of improved biomaterials and continued advancement of the medical device industry.

PARADIGM FOR ASSESSING POTENTIAL TOXICITY

Until recently, toxicological testing of medical devices relied essentially on screening tests evaluating the final device in its final sterilized form. In response to what was considered a lack of specific guidance in certain areas of medical device evaluation and, in an effort to conserve resources, the Health Industry Manufacturers Association (HIMA) developed a draft paradigm (see **Figure 1**) for the characterization and biocompatibility evaluation of materials intended for use in medical devices. This was presented to the FDA in 1994 to open a dialogue and serve as a basis of a collaborative effort between industry and regulators to develop a characterization paradigm. Since that time, this approach has gained international acceptance. At the time this chapter was written, the FDA had prepared a draft paradigm. When the final FDA paradigm is available, it should be considered rather than the HIMA paradigm.

The essence of this approach is that biocompatibility testing of materials and devices should be based on sound science and coordinated by using a screening paradigm. This paradigm should be used to define the level of testing required for a given material or device based on knowledge of the chemicals in the formulation of the final product, and their toxicological activity. In this paradigm, emphasis is placed on toxicological data, either generated by the sponsor or found in the open literature, for those chemicals which pose toxic risks associated with the biological effects of toxicological concern identified in the guidance found in ISO 10993–1 (see **Table 1**). Based on the potency and the level of expected human exposure to these chemicals, the safety of the device can be predicted. The paradigm to assist in selecting toxicity testing for 510 (k) submissions is shown in **Figure 2**. In addition, the FDA has prepared toxicology profiles for specific devices.

The practical use of the paradigm involves a tiered approach. A description of how this might work is as follows. To determine the expected human exposure to the chemicals from the device, either exhaustive extraction of the device or its consituent materials is performed. While the identification of chemicals is in progress, a cytotoxicity test could be conducted, in that it is a rapid, inexpensive assay and is a biological effect of concern for all device categories. Once the chemicals of expected exposure are identified, then a literature search is conducted focusing on the toxicological activity associated with the biological effects identified in ISO 10993–1 for the category of device. If the data available for these chemicals are insufficient to justify the expected exposure levels of these chemicals for all biological effects of concern, then biological testing would be required for those biological effects with insufficient data to predict acceptable risk.

RISK ASSESSMENT

Risk assessment can be defined as the characterization of the potential adverse effects of human exposure to a specific agent or substance. In all cases, the goal of risk

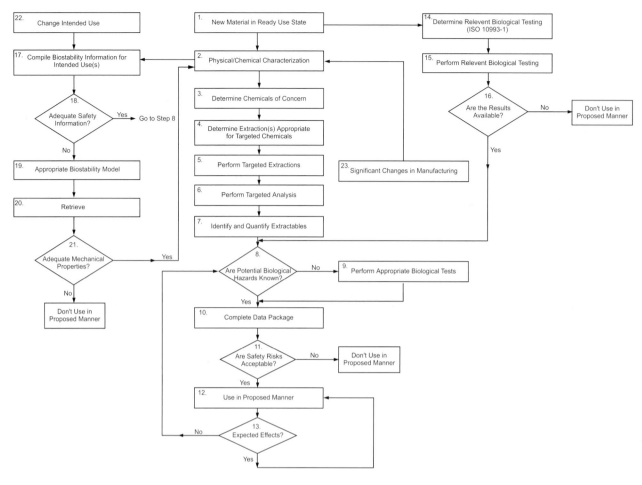

Figure 1 Material characterization/biocompatibility paradigm.

assessment is to establish safe exposure levels or determine the probability of harm. Detailed descriptions of the risk assessment process can be found in other chapters of this book and will not be described here. Briefly, the risk assessment process can be divided into four major steps **(Table 6)**. Owing to the chemical complexity of biomaterials, physical changes in materials following processing and sterilization, and the lack of establishment of a dose–response relationship for many toxicological end-points, several of the steps of risk assessment, specifically hazard identification and dose–response assessment, are poorly defined for most biomaterials. Historically, the medical device industry, therefore, established standardized 'pass' or 'fail' criteria to aid in the interpretation of many of the short-term biocompatibility tests that were described above. These criteria have been defined following years of experience with the testing procedures using many different materials. By establishing these standardized pass/fail criteria, the need for complex risk assessment procedures has generally been considered to be eliminated. Essentially, any biomaterial that does not meet the criteria to 'pass' one of the biocompatibility tests successfully has, in the past, not been used in the development of devices or has been used only

when the potentially adverse biological effect can be avoided.

As medical devices have become more complex and the industry has matured, the development of biomaterials and the understanding of their biological effects have also improved. Increasingly, the standard parameters of risk assessment shown in **Table 6** are becoming available in the open literature for some biomaterials (Szycher and Siciliano, 1991; Stokes *et al.*, 1995). To this end, standard risk assessment procedures are being used more frequently in the design and safety evaluation of medical devices. The ISO committees and the FDA are currently focusing on the development of guidance documents to improve the availability of sound scientific data for use in the risk assessment process. These data will include such end-points as bioavailability and biodegradation.

While biodegradation of a chemical is often part of the risk assessment process, and is always considered in the evaluation of drugs, this aspect of biomaterials is less frequently considered in the safety evaluation of medical devices. However, the biodegradation potential of several materials has been utilized in several specialized areas of medicine such as bioabsorbable sutures and/or impants (Piskin, 1995; Ashammakhi and Rokkanen,

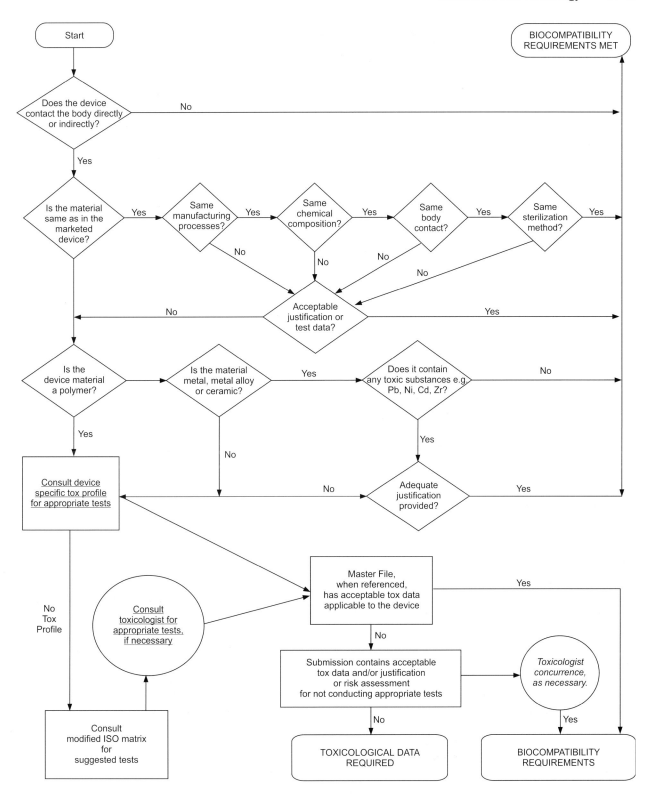

Figure 2 Biocompatibility flow chart for the selection of toxicity tests for 510(k)s.

1997; Cleland, 1998; Kissel *et al.*, 1997; Rokkanen, 1998). The total body dose of a biodegradable biomaterial following implantation can be fairly large with the variable duration of exposure. These issues complicate the risk assessment process but must be considered in the overall safety evaluation of these materials.

Finally, the once clear line between drugs and devices is rapidly blurring. The use of biomaterials to control the rate and/or location of drug delivery is a rapidly expanding area of research (Tanguay *et al.*, 1994; Bertrand *et al.*, 1998; Chang, 1998; Deshpande *et al.*, 1998; Vert *et al.*, 1998). The combination of drugs and biomaterials into a

Table 6 Four steps of risk assessment

Hazard identification
Dose–response assessment
Exposure assessment
Risk characterization

single therapeutic apparatus (ie. combination product) adds a new level of complexity to the risk assessment process. The potential physical and/or biological interaction of the drug with the device must be considered. As these combination therapeutic devices continue to develop, the overall safety evaluation of medical devices will also probably develop.

FUTURE AREAS FOR DEVELOPMENT

The use of medical devices is a rapidly growing and developing industry. Several regulatory agencies and international guidance committees are aggressively addressing the changes and growth. Several areas that are routinely addressed in the safety evaluation of drugs and chemicals are not as well addressed by the medical device industry. These include biodegradation and developmental and reproductive effects of biomaterials. Furthermore, the potential for environmental hazards associated with the production, use and disposal of medical devices will need to be addressed more extensively. As the industry grows and develops, the differences between safety evaluation procedures used by the medical device industry and the drug and chemical industries will decrease.

REFERENCES

Anderson, J. M. (1993). Mechanisms of inflamation and infection with implanted devices. *Cardiovasc. Pathol.*, **2**, 33S–41S.

ANSI/AAMI (1997). *10993–1: Biological Evaluation of Medical Devices—Part 1. Guidance on Selection of Tests.* Association for the Advancement of Medical Instrumentation, Arlington, Virginia.

Ashammakhi, N. and Rokkanen, P. (1997). Absorbable polyglycolide devices in trauma and bone surgery. *Biomaterials*, **18**, 3–9.

Bertrand, O. F., Sipehia, R., Mongrain, R., Rodes, J., Tardif, J. C., Bilodeau, L., Cote, G. and Bourassa, M. G. (1998). Biocompatibility aspects of new stent technology. *J. Am. Coll. Cardiol.*, **32**, 562–571.

Boretos, J. W. and Eden, M. (Eds) (1984). In *Contemporary Biomaterials: Material and Host Response, Clinical Applications, New Technology and Legal Aspects.* Noyes Publications, Park Ridge, NJ.

Chang, T. M. (1998). Pharmaceutical and therapeutic applications of artificial cells including microencapsulation. *Eur. J. Pharm. Biopharm.*, **45**, 3–8.

Cleland, J. L. (1998). Solvent evaporation processes for the production of controlled release biodegradable microsphere formulations for therapeutics and vaccines. *Biotechnol. Prog.*, **14**, 102–107.

Corry, D. C., DeLucia, A., III, Zhu, H., Radcliffe, R. R., Brevetti, G. R., El-Khatib, H., Vance, S. J., Moyer, B. R., Cotts, W. G. and Richenbacher, W. E. (1998). Time course of cytokine release and complement activation after implantation of the HeartMate left ventricular assist device. *ASAIO J.*, **44**, M347–M351.

Danz, W. (1990). Mobility implants: a review. *Adv. Ophth. Plast. Reconstr. Surg.*, **8**, 46–52.

Deshpande, A. A., Heller, J. and Gurny, R. (1998). Bioerodible polymers for ocular drug delivery. *Crit. Rev. Ther. Drug Carrier Syst.*, **15**, 381–420.

Gesualdo, L., Pertosa, G., Grandaliano, G. and Schena, F. P. (1998). Cytokines and bioincompatibility. *Nephrol. Dial. Transplant.*, **13**, 1622–1626.

Girndt, M., Sester, U., Kaul, H. and Kohler, H. (1998). Production of proinflammatory and regulatory monokines in hemodialysis patients shown at a single-cell level. *J. Am. Soc. Nephrol.*, **9**, 1689–1696.

Gotman, I. (1997). Characteristics of metals used in implants. *J. Endourol.*, **11**, 383–389.

Hanks, C. T., Wataha, J. C. and Sun, Z. (1996). *In vitro* models of biocompatibility: a review. *Dent. Mater.*, **12**, 186–193.

Jikuya, T., Tsutsui, T., Shigeta, O., Sankai, Y. and Mitsui, T. (1998). Species differences in erythrocyte mechanical fragility: comparison of human, bovine, and ovine cells. *ASAIO J.*, **44**, M452–M455.

Kimber, I., Hilton, J., and Botham, P. A. 1990. Identification of contact allergens using the murine local lymph node assay: comparisons with the Buehler occluded patch test in guinea pigs. *J. Appl. Toxicol.*, **10**, 173–180.

Kissel, T., Koneberg, R., Hilbert, A. K. and Hungerer, K. (1997). Microencapsulation of antigens using biodegradable polyesters: facts and phantasies. *Behring Inst. Mitt.*, **98**, 172–183.

Klinkmann, H., Grassmann, A. and Vienken, J. (1996). Dilemma of membrane biocompatibility and reuse. *Artif. Organs*, **20**, 426–432.

Malinauskas, R. A. (1997). Plasma hemoglobin measurement techniques for the *in vitro* evaluation of blood damage caused by medical devices. *Artif. Organs*, **21**, 1255–1267.

Nair, P. D. (1995). Currently practised sterilization methods—some inadvertent consequences. *J. Biomater. Appl.*, **10**, 121–135.

Northup, S. J. (1987). Strategies for biological testing of biomaterials. *J. Biomater. Appl.*, **2**, 132–148.

Pinchuk, L. (1994). A review of the biostability and carcinogenicity of polyurethanes in medicine and the new generation of 'biostable' polyurethanes. *J. Biomater. Sci. Polym. Ed.*, **6**, 225–267.

Piskin, E. (1995). Biodegradable polymers as biomaterials. *J. Biomater. Sci. Polym. Ed.*, **6**, 775–795.

Ratner, B. D. (1993). Characterization of biomaterial surfaces. *Cardiovasc. Pathol.*, **2**, 87S–100S.

Rokkanen P. U., 1998. Bioabsorbable fixation devices in orthopaedics and traumatology. *Ann. Chir. Gynaecol.*, **87**, 13–20.

Rubin, J. P. and Yaremchuk, M. J. (1997). Complications and toxicities of implantable biomaterials used in facial reconstructive and aesthetic surgery: a comprehensive review of the literature. *Plast. Reconstr. Surg.*, **100**, 1336–1353.

Schwindaman, D. (1994). Federal regulation of experimental animal use in the United States of America. *Rev. Sci. Technol.*, **13**, 247–260.

Sheftel, V. O. (1994). *Handbook of Toxic Properties of Monomers and Additives*. CRC Press, Lewis Publishers, New York.

Stokes, K., McVenes, R. and Anderson, J. M. (1995). Polyurethane elastomer biostability. *J. Biomater. Appl.*, **9**, 321–354.

Szycher, M. and Siciliano, A. A. (1991). An assessment of 2,4-TDA formation from surgitek polyurethane foam under simulated physiological conditions. *J. Biomater. Appl.*, **5**, 323–336.

Tanguay, J. F., Zidar, J. P., Phillips, H. R., III and Stack, R. S. (1994). Current status of biodegradable stents. *Cardiol. Clin.*, **12**, 699–713.

Tsuchiya, T. (1994). Studies on the standardization of cytotoxicity tests and new standard reference materials useful for evaluating the safety of biochemicals. *J. Biomater. Appl. 1994*, **9**, 138–157.

USDHHS (1997). *Guidance for Industry:* Submission of Documentation in Drug Applications for Container Closure Systems Used for the Packaging of Human Drugs and Biologics. US Department of Health and Human Services, Food and Drug Administration, Center for Drug Evaluation (CDER), Center for Biologics Evaluation and Research (CBER), Rockville, MD (Draft).

Vert, M., Schwach, G., Engel, R. and Coudane, J. (1998). Something new in the field of PLA/GA bioresorbable polymers? *J. Controlled Release*, **53**, 85–92.

Warfvinge, G. (1994). Screening tests for sensitization potential of dental materials. *J. Dent.*, **22**, Suppl. 2, S16–S20.

Chapter 82

Environmental Health Risk Assessment: Theory and Practice

Michael L. Gargas, Brent L. Finley, Dennis J. Paustenbach and Thomas F. Long

CONTENTS

INTRODUCTION

The assessment of risk has preoccupied man since our emergence as a thinking species. Broadly defined, risk assessment is any methodological approach that is used to predict the likelihood of an unwanted event in the presence of *uncertainty* (Carrington and Bolger, 1998). This can include such concerns as industrial explosions, workplace injuries, machine failure, natural disasters (e.g. earthquakes, tornadoes), impacts from voluntary choices (e.g. smoking, diet), diseases (e.g. cancer, birth defects, infection) and other potentially adverse outcomes (Paustenbach, 1995). For the majority of history, the focus has primarily been on risks of an economic, political or religious nature (Covello and Mumpower, 1985). Further, these risk assessments have typically relied on experiential and historical databases when attempting to estimate the outcome of a new endeavour. With enough information, the probability of an event, desired or undesired, can be estimated. However, without a fairly complete understanding of the system under consideration and sufficient information, the probability (or risk) of being wrong increases. Thus, today's understanding of insurance risks is based on actuarial tables derived and refined from years of life expectancy data, but the early history of the insurance industry is replete with failures as a result of improper understanding of the actual nature of the risks involved. Similarly, the probability of a technological failure is estimated from the results of repeated testing and practical experience over time. New technologies that have little history attempt to attract venture capital by promising greater financial reward in exchange for the uncertainty of success or other unknown risks. Health risk assessment was for many years simply a form of applied toxicology in which the experience of the workplace, accidental exposures, or clinical or animal testing was used in a very limited way to assess and avoid potential harm. Typically, this effort relied on avoiding damage from relatively high-dose exposures associated with work or the use of consumer products.

The Paradigm Shift

With the emergence of the environmental movement in the 1960s and 1970s, concern began to be expressed over the potential consequences of chronic low-level exposure to chemical and physical agents (Carson, 1962). Beginning with the infamous Delaney Clause of the 1950s, which required the elimination of compounds from the food supply shown to cause cancer in animals, this effort was largely a tyranny of simple answers in which adverse experimental outcomes often resulted in banning the compound from further use. Indeed, for many years, a single positive animal test of uncertain quality would typically be given greater weight than any number of negative studies of higher quality without regard to concepts of dose–response, mechanisms of toxicity or actual human exposure (Barr, 1988; Paustenbach, 1995). Since more than 400 of the 2000 or so chemicals routinely employed in industry have been labelled as carcinogens, the public demand for accountability and regulation led to the creation of the Environmental Protection Agency (US EPA), the Occupational Safety and Health Administration (OSHA), the Agency for Toxic Substances and Disease Registry (ATSDR) to focus on risks in the environment and workplace and a new regulatory agenda across the board. Throughout the 1970s and 1980s, a number of Federal laws were passed to address the presumed hazard posed by the presence of largely unregulated chemical residues in the air, water, soil and food supply of the nation (Rosenthal et al., 1992). These included the Resource Conservation and Recovery Act

(RCRA), Safe Drinking Water Act (SDWA), Clean Air Act (CAA), Clean Water Act, Toxic Substances Control Act (TSCA), the Comprehensive Environmental Response, Compensation and Liability Act (CERCLA or Superfund), and amendments to the Food, Drug and Cosmetics Act (FDCA) and the Federal Insecticide, Fungicide and Rodenticide Act (FIFRA). Whatever good intentions lay behind these initiatives, lacking was a clear understanding of what exposure to trace levels of chemical and physical agents actually meant to the human population and the environment. Despite years of study of the acute and chronic effect of relatively high doses of chemical and physical agents on experimental animals, and of accidental or occupational human exposure, neither the regulatory nor scientific communities possessed the intellectual tools or knowledge necessary to assess the significance of low-level exposure on a large scale. Suddenly there emerged a need for an entirely new kind of discipline (Cumming, 1981). From this need, the risk assessment culture that has become dominant in the regulation of environmental, occupational and other health hazards evolved. A number of historical perspectives on the development of risk assessment and the resultant lessons learned over the past 20 years are available (Friess, 1987; CRA, 1994; Paustenbach, 1995).

The Development of Risk Assessment

Health risk assessment as practised today involves combining toxicological data derived from animal experiments, or epidemiological studies, with information about exposure potential to determine the likelihood of an adverse outcome under given conditions of use. Toxicity is the inherent property of an agent to cause an adverse effect, if the dose (or concentration) is sufficient. Exposure is the frequency and duration of contact with the agent at a given concentration and is equivalent to the concept of dose. Thus, risk assessment relies on the fundamental concept of toxicology, the dose–response relationship. Risk differs from toxicity in that risk is the probability (or uncertainty) that, under given specific conditions of exposure, an adverse outcome will occur. Obviously, the degree of risk is influenced by both toxicity and exposure. A change in either parameter, or both, results in an equivalent change in the risk posed. A compound of relatively low toxicity but for which exposure is large (e.g. alcohol) may, therefore, pose a higher risk to an individual or population than a highly toxic compound to which there is little or no exposure (e.g. cyanide). While the goal of risk assessment is to integrate our knowledge about toxicity and exposure in a meaningful way to estimate the magnitude or absence of risk, an equally important, if usually unfulfilled, goal is to provide some insight into the uncertainty surrounding the process and the risk estimate. Over time, as information and understanding improves, the ability to estimate

risk should change, not because the risk itself necessarily is altered, but because the uncertainty around the estimate is reduced.

Although risk assessment in one form or another has been practised for about 50 years in the USA, primarily in the area of health physics, food or cosmetic safety, or medical products, it was not a systematic approach with well accepted techniques and practices (Lehmann and Fitzhugh, 1954). As previously noted, the need for a consistent, rational and transparent risk assessment policy to assess low-level exposures emerged along with the legislative mandates passed in the early 1980s (Kaplan and Garrick, 1981). The first formal description of the process, Risk Assessment in the Federal Government: Managing the Process (National Research Council, 1983), described and attempted to reconcile the risk assessment processes then in use by the US EPA, the Food and Drug Administration (FDA), the OSHA and the Consumer Product Safety Commission (CPSC). The methodology that ultimately emerged from this endeavour differed from the earlier risk assessment techniques by incorporating increasingly complex and quantitative dose–response modelling (Crump et al., 1976; Crump, 1980, 1996) and exposure assessment (US EPA, 1986b, 1988d, 1992a). Such risk assessment models allow a better estimation of the likelihood that a specific untoward event may occur over a wide range of doses.

Significantly, in addition to defining the risk assessment process, an attempt was also made to clarify the difference between risk assessment and risk management. While risk assessment is intended to be a largely objective, scientific pursuit to arrive at the best estimate of the potential hazard, risk management is the decision-making process that incorporates political, social, economic and engineering information with the outcome of the risk assessment to select the appropriate regulatory response to a potential health hazard (National Research Council, 1983). As such, this part of the process requires value judgements on such issues as risk acceptability and control costs (see **Figure 1**). Unfortunately, the large amount of uncertainty present in the risk assessment process as the result of necessarily employing assumptions in the place of knowledge also consciously and unconsciously introduces value judgements with the potential to warp the final product of the risk estimate (Burmaster and Lehr, 1991; Breyer, 1994; Finkel, 1995; Paustenbach, 1995; Wilson, 1995).

(How) Does Risk Assessment Work?

By the late 1980s, a risk assessment culture was thoroughly entrenched at the US EPA and other Federal agencies, and it was spreading through State environmental and health agencies (US EPA, 1989a; ATSDR, 1992; Rhomberg, 1997). Since formally defining the process, over 60 guidance documents (about 10 000 pages) have been written (primarily by the US EPA) on various aspects of risk assessment, including how risk assessments should be conducted and what data to use. These include guidelines on assessing the risk from carcinogens, mutagens, teratogens, male and female reproductive toxicants, conducting exposure assessments and addressing chemical mixtures (US EPA, 1986a–d, 1988a, b 1992a, 1996c). Additionally, efforts have been made to provide accepted, peer-reviewed toxicity criteria for carcinogens (i.e. cancer potency factors or CPFs) and non-carcinogens (i.e. reference doses or RfDs), data for exposure assessment, and methodological approaches to addressing various routes of exposure (US EPA, 1990, 1992b, 1996a, 1997b, 1998a). Armed with a consistent methodology and a variety of well funded mandates, the government was prepared to use risk assessment to help reduce or eliminate chronic environmental health risks. It was acknowledged by all involved that significant uncertainty in the process existed, but risk assessment was nonetheless believed to be the best and most logical approach to address the problem. The uncertainties were addressed by several layers of conservative, generally inflexible assumptions intended to protect sensitive members of the population under the theory that it was better to err on the side of protection when uncertainty existed. The end result has been that most risk assessments have, for the sake of public safety, often overestimated rather than underestimated the true risk (Maxim, 1989). Proponents also assumed that, as time went on, research would improve the quality of the risk assessments by replacing assumptions with information and reducing the uncertainties inherent in the process. While risk assessment has now become a pervasive process and a significant amount of research has been carried out in an attempt to improve the risk assessment process, in practice neither reduction of risk nor improvement in the quality of risk assessments has occurred very fast or very far. The question is, why?

One interpretation is that the developers of the risk assessment process failed to foresee two basic problems in their vision. First, the originators of the risk assessment process were scientists immersed in the theory and practice of toxicology and related disciplines. Today's risk assessment professional, in contrast, is not typically a toxicologist by training and, while most may understand the mechanics of risk assessment, the underlying philosophy of the process has been largely lost. In other words, risk assessors know how to do a 'risk assessment' and obtain a quantitative answer, but they often lack an appreciation of what the answer truly means. The process has simply become the goal rather than a means to illuminate uncertainty and prioritize decision-making and research. Many risk assessments have been reduced to little more than cookbook exercises that do little to assure the public that a critical evaluation of the situation and resultant decisions has been performed. For instance, the impact of risk assessment or risk-based regulations are regularly reported by the regulators and media as the number of cancers (or other diseases) caused by an activity or prevented by a control strategy. A US EPA scientist remarked at a professional meeting that implementation of a risk-based regulation had resulted in the saving of 1000 lives annually. While certainly an impressive statement, because of the uncertainty and conservatism in the process, the more reasonable interpretation (and one that is in keeping with Agency policy) is that no more than 1000 lives per year would be saved, almost certainly many less, and maybe zero. The difference in the two interpretations is significant in conveying both information and understanding of risk assessment. A more topical example is the US EPA report on environmental tobacco smoke (ETS), which boldly estimated that 3800 lung cancer deaths could be annually attributed to ETS (US EPA, 1990c). This estimate persists in a number of media, policy and advocacy forums despite several Science Advisory Board and independent reviews which found the risk estimates to be overstated and that the actual impact from ETS was far less. More recently, a member of the US EPA staff reported that 58 000 excess cancers were attributable to cumulative exposure to air toxins over a lifetime, without any caveat on the estimate being provided (Risk Policy Report, 1998).

The second problem arose from the understandable desire to standardize the risk assessment process in order to make the process both transparent and accessible to the public. This led to the codification of risk assessment methodologies, assumptions and risk acceptability by regulatory agencies, principally the US EPA. Inclusion of specific techniques and assumptions into environmental laws and regulations accomplished this standardization, but at the cost of reduced flexibility and an unwillingness or inability to keep pace with and incorporate new scientific information or understanding of risks. Thus, success in making the process consistent has resulted in a system often too rigid to characterize properly the true or most likely risks. Imposing such strictures on a young and evolving discipline has had a chilling effect on the development and incorporation of new information and approaches, as well as serving to introduce economic and social inefficiencies into the competition for scarce resources. Even though the toxicological criteria, risk assessment methodologies and assumptions employed are provided as guidance and are not legally mandated or necessarily correct, they are often treated as 'holy writ' by some risk assessors. Thus, a risk assessment that utilizes the best and most current information may be rejected because it does not conform to the expectations of reviewers who lack the ability (or time) critically to evaluate the information and its interpretation.

Risk management decisions based on such risk assessments have led over the years to remedial actions that were very costly in terms of both time and money. Aside from failing basic 'reality checks', the standard risk assessment has begun to diverge markedly from those produced using newer and arguably better information and approaches. Owing to the limited and delayed integration and utilization of innovative approaches to assessing risk that have emerged over the past 10 years, the costs of regulation and remediation are not balanced against the benefits to society. One of the purposes of this chapter is to demonstrate how new scientific advances can improve the risk assessment process and the decisions arising from it, and to encourage scientists to participate in the processing; first, by maintaining data stewardship to ensure that their work is interpreted and employed properly and, second, to become involved in the process by insisting that the best science be incorporated in the process (Clayson and Iverson, 1996; Finley and Paustenbach, 1997; SOT, 1998; Younes and Amoruso, 1998).

The Potential of Risk Assessment

The growth of risk assessment as a policy tool has been due in part to the public concerns over the perceived relationship between diseases, usually cancer, and chemical exposures, as well as the lack of governmental control or industrial stewardship that preceded the environmental movement of the 1960s and 1970s. Concurrently, industry, faced with new laws and increased regulatory vigilance, focused its goal (usually through the courts) on requiring an adequate and transparent approach to regulation that avoided (in theory) arbitrary and capricious regulatory mandates (Young, 1987). As a result, over the last 20 years, quantitative risk assessment (QRA) has developed into an accepted methodology for assessing environmental and occupational hazards in order to make balanced risk management decisions (AIHC, 1989; Paustenbach 1990, 1995, 1997). In fact, many of the current environmental regulations are now risk-based (Paustenbach, 1995). Occupational regulations are also moving in that direction (Paustenbach, 1990, 1997). Despite this regulatory reliance, risk assessment has also been roundly criticized from all quarters with industry claiming that it grossly overestimates risks, environmentalists claiming it provides a license to pollute, and others that it diverts attention and resources from other, equally important, societal needs. All critics are right to some extent (Finkel, 1989; Paustenbach, 1989c, 1993; Abelson 1992, 1993; Silbergeld, 1993; Tengs et al., 1995).

A few years ago, the National Research Council (NRC) evaluated the risk assessment process in accordance with provisions of the Clean Air Act Amendments of 1990 in a report entitled Science and Judgement in Risk Assessment (National Research Council, 1994). This report concluded that the '... overall approach to assessing risks is fundamentally sound despite often-heard criticisms, but the agency must more clearly establish the scientific and policy basis for its risk assessments and better describe the uncertainties in its estimates of risks'. The report includes 70 specific recommendations whereby the policies, practices and methods for risk assessment may be improved, in terms of both short-term refinements in methodologies and a long-term research agenda. The US EPA identified eight broad areas to begin implementing the NRC recommendations. These include improving: (1) risk assessment for hazardous air pollutants; (2) risk characterization; (3) the Integrated Risk Information System (IRIS); (4) cancer risk assessment guidelines; (5) assessment for non-cancer hazards; (6) multi-path and multi-source exposure assessments; (7) understanding of inter-individual susceptibility to chemicals; and (8) risk assessment tools in general (National research Council, 1994; US EPA, 1994c). State environmental and health agencies relying on risk assessment are also aware of the need to increase the amount and consistency of the science used in the process (CalEPA, 1998). It has also become important in recent years that, owing to integration of the world economy, the differences in the risk assessment approaches used by international regulatory authorities be reconciled and standardized (Paustenbach, 1995).

Despite its weaknesses and problems, risk assessment represents a clear advance over the previous 'ban it, reduce it or control it as much as possible' approach to regulation that previously dominated much of environmental decision making. Requiring the use of 'as low as reasonably achievable' (ALARA) or 'best available technology' (BAT) can obviously reduce exposure, but may be very costly without an arguably proportionate reduction of risk to society (Maxim, 1989; Burmaster and Lehr, 1991; Paustenbach, 1993; Breyer, 1994; Tengs et al., 1995). Similarly, a simple ban may not ensure a significant or even measurable risk reduction. Banning one risk can result in the introduction of another technology with uncertain, perhaps greater, risks and the financial sacrifice may be not be off-set by the gain to society in such circumstances. Recognizing the significance of this 'trickle down effect', it seems better to study, assess and manage the risks whenever possible. The tool of choice is risk assessment and it will continue to grow in its role in regulatory decision making. The question is, how well will it accomplish this?

In a recent Congress, approximately 15 major bills were introduced that required the use of risk assessment and cost–benefit analysis in environmental regulatory programs (Paustenbach, 1995; Barnard, 1996a, b; Crouch et al., 1997). Currently, about $200 billion is spent annually on environmental issues in the USA with an additional $400 billion spent on environmental issues in other countries each year (AIHC, 1989; Paustenbach, 1995). Since demands and expenditures for environmental protection are expected to continue well into the next century, it is critically important that competition for scarce resources be decided based on the best information and interpretation that science can provide. Performed consistently, and with continual improvement to reduce uncertainty, risk assessment holds the promise of providing public health and environmental protection based on a scientific, defensible rationale that gives risk managers, policy makers and society a range of options, each with specific cost–benefit information, on which to make reasoned decisions.

THE RISK ASSESSMENT PROCESS

Since the initial formulation of the risk assessment paradigm (National Research Council, 1983), risk assessments have been divided into four complementary steps: hazard identification; dose–response evaluation; exposure assessment; and risk characterization **(Figure 1)**. Hazard identification is the first and most recognizable step in risk assessment, particularly to a toxicologist. It asks the questions, what adverse effects can the agent in question cause, and what is the likelihood that they will occur in humans? The dose–response evaluation attempts to define the quantitative relationship between the dose of the agent and the biological response. Low-dose extrapolation models have been extensively employed at this step for the purpose of estimating carcinogenic risks. Exposure assessment estimates the magnitude and probability of intake from

various environmental media by any combination of oral, skin or inhalation exposures. As many as 20 or more exposure factors may need to be accounted for and included in an exposure assessment of most environmental issues. Exposure assessments of occupational hazards, however, typically are confined to skin and inhalation exposures (Paustenbach, 1990). The final step in the process, risk characterization, is arguably the most important as it summarizes and interprets the information developed during the previous steps and identifies the uncertainties in the risk assessment. **Figure 1** also demonstrates the desired relationship between applied research, risk assessment and risk management (National Research Council, 1983, 1994; OTA, 1993; NAS, 1994; Milloy, 1995). The remainder of this chapter examines the theory behind each of these steps, considers how risk assessment is carried out in practice and illustrates how applied scientific research can improve the process by reducing uncertainty (Finley and Paustenbach, 1997).

Hazard Identification

Hazard identification is a largely qualitative step which involves a description of the toxicity of the agent as influenced by its physical and chemical properties, and its environmental and biological fate and interactions.

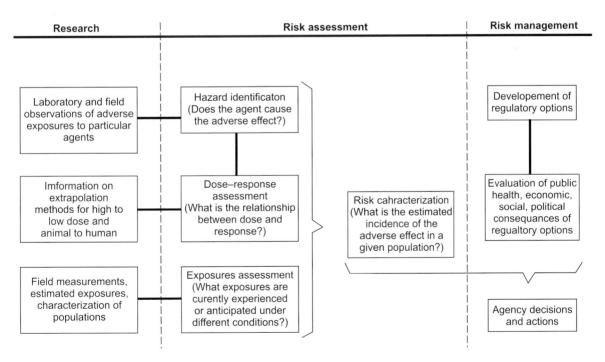

Figure 1   The risk assessment process consists of four inter-related steps: hazard identification, dose–response evaluation, exposure assessment and risk characterization. Risk assessments should be based on the best available science and be as free from value judgements and biases as possible. The results with appropriate description of the uncertainty involved is then provided to risk managers for decisions on actions required to reduce the risks, which include economic, political and other value judgements. The relationship between basic and applied research, risk assessment and risk management is also illustrated. The intent is that uncertainty be identified through the risk assessment process and, if critical to understanding the risks, research efforts would be devoted to reducing the uncertainty and improving the estimates of risk. Adapted from National Research Council (1983).

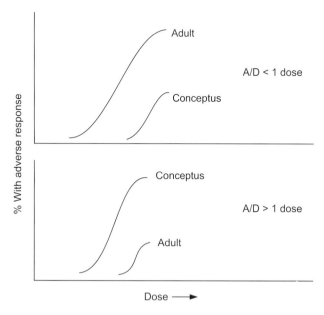

Figure 2 In consideration of developmental hazards, one useful approach is to examine the dose–response curves for both maternal and foetal toxicity to develop the A/D ratio (adult/developmental). A ratio of ≤ 1 suggests that the possibility of a developmental hazard existing is unlikely, whereas a ratio of ≥ 1 increases the likelihood that a compound poses a potential developmental hazard.

Such information will be critical in determining if the kinds of adverse effects known to be caused by a chemical or physical agent in one population group or experimental protocol are likely to occur in the exposed group of interest. It is clear that most chemical or physical agents will pose a human hazard at a high enough dose, but the effects at low levels, particularly for carcinogens, are still hotly debated. The risk assessor's responsibility at this stage in the process is to determine not only the type of adverse effects that an agent might cause, but also whether such effects are conceivable at doses which humans or wildlife could possibly receive. The criteria by which an agent is judged to pose a potentially significant threat to a target species involves consideration of at least six factors. These include the number of species affected, the relevance of the experimental route of exposure to that experienced by the target population (human or otherwise), the number and type of tumours in the case of carcinogens, the number of target organs and the severity of the effect in the case of non-carcinogens, the dose at which an effect is noted and the quantitative relationship between the dose and response, and the relevant mode of action (*e.g.* genotoxic, saturatable enzymatic pathways, cytotoxic) (Squires, 1981; Calabrese, 1983; Huff *et al.*, 1994; US EPA, 1996a). For developmental toxicants, the important issues in hazard identification are similar, but also include the relationship between the doses causing maternal toxicity and those affecting the offspring (Wang and Schwetz, 1987;

Hart *et al.*, 1988) **(Figure 2)**. The strength of causation from all available data sources ought to be examined in order to make this evaluation, although typically the most readily available and useful information is derived from animal studies. All information, negative and positive, should be reviewed in order to make the judgement about the type and degree of hazard posed by the agent in question. Hazards may also be selected on the basis of environmental mobility, frequency of detection, and environmental and biological persistence, in addition to toxicity (US EPA, 1989c; ATSDR, 1992).

Data Sources for Hazard Identification

The primary information source for hazard identification and dose–response assessment is the animal bioassay, usually long-term rodent tests (HHS, 1985; Taylor *et al.*, 1993). This is based on the proposition that, in properly designed and conducted tests, animals are assumed to predict the human response relatively accurately. This has certainly proved largely correct for purposes of clinical evaluation and acute toxicity testing, although there are important exceptions to this generalization (Ottoboni, 1991). It is less certain that chronic animal toxicity testing, specifically for carcinogens, is predictive for humans (Ames, 1987; Ames and Gold, 1990; Cohen, 1995; Ames *et al.*, 1996). Assumptions concerning the applicability of toxicity test conditions to human populations and exposures, and also the appropriateness of the (quantitative) extrapolation methods used, need to be clarified and understood in order to make reasoned and correct judgements (Andersen *et al.*, 1987a, 1995; National Research Council, 1994). Nonetheless, in an effort to be protective, unless there are data from human studies that refute specific findings in animal studies or biological arguments that allow some animal data to be rejected as irrelevant to humans (e.g. $\alpha_{2\mu}$-microglobulin mediated nephropathy in male rats), it is assumed that the human response may be inferred from animal responses (typically the most sensitive species) (Albert, 1994). The assumption that all forms of adverse reactions observed in animals could be mimicked in humans remains basically a conservative policy decision accepted for reasons of prudent public health policy or regulatory mandate (Paustenbach, 1995). However, the bulk of evidence indicates, and most professionals believe, that animal data alone are not sufficient to conclude that an agent will cause specific effects in humans exposed at a particular dose. It should be kept in mind that the concordance of positive or negative results between rats and mice, for instance, is only about 70%, and it is unlikely that the concordance between rodents and humans would be higher (Allen *et al.*, 1988; Lave *et al.*, 1988; Piegorsch *et al.*, 1992; Freedman *et al.*, 1993, 1996; Meijers *et al.*, 1997). Even when a positive response occurs in two species, it is not uncommon for there to be great variability (up to 10^7-fold) in potency of the carcinogenic response. It also should be kept in mind that although it is certainly true that all human carcinogens have caused cancer in at least one species of animal tested, all animal carcinogens have not been shown to be human carcinogens (Gaylor and Chen, 1986; Paustenbach, 1995; Haseman and Elwell, 1996). Some of the observed and critical species differences can be traced to differences in pharmacokinetics and metabolism. Certainly, when selecting an appropriate animal bioassay for use in hazard identification, the best study would be one that uses the relevant exposure pathway, an appropriate duration of exposure and adequate number of doses. Other common qualities of an adequate animal bioassay include a minimum of two species, testing in both sexes and an appropriate number of animals per dose. Positive results include increased number of tumours in a given organ or organs, the occurrence of rare tumours, earlier appearance of tumours, and increases in the total number of tumours (National Research Council, 1983; HHS, 1985; Barr, 1988; Paustenbach, 1995).

The main problem with interpreting the results of most animal bioassays is the dose levels employed in the testing. For example, it has become clear that most animal carcinogens will pose a human cancer risk at some dose; however, at the very low doses that typify most environmental exposures, the risk may be very small and perhaps zero (Abelson, 1993). Despite this, animals are usually tested at the maximally tolerated dose (MTD) and half MTD. The MTD is defined as the highest dose that does not cause a significant mortality in the test species or loss of body weight (potentially indicating a disruption of homeostasis). The highest doses are usually those associated with the tumour response and often these doses produce frank systemic toxicity (Zeise et al., 1984; Metzger et al., 1989; Goodman and Wilson, 1992; Krewski et al., 1993). One theory advanced to explain this is that the high doses tested result in cytotoxicity, which increase cell turnover markedly. Consequences of increased cell turnover include increased replication error, decreased time for repair and increased fixation of damage, leading to increased risk of altered cell lines and ultimately tumour (Ames and Gold, 1990; Gold, 1993; Ames et al., 1996). Even in the absence of increased cell turnover, there are questions about how relevant high doses are to the low-dose exposure that is the focus of concern. At high doses, the biological response of an organism may be significantly different as the result of saturatable metabolic pathways and repair mechanisms, as well as finite supplies of necessary co-factors. Additional problems include defining exactly what a tumour is (e.g. benign vs malignant, proliferative lesions vs frank tumours) and what the background incidence of tumour is in control animals. The extrapolation of the animal response to humans and the extrapolation of a 10–100% response rate in the animal study to the 0.0001% response rate that is of regulatory concern is problematic, but is the focus of the dose–response assessment of the agent, and some of these issues can be addressed at that point.

Other data sources are available, but generally serve a supplemental function to the animal bioassay data. In the first half of the twentieth century, data on worker exposures and health outcomes provided the basis for assessing risk and setting exposure limits (Irish, 1959). Epidemiological evidence provides the most convincing data for an association between an exposure and disease in the relevant species (man) (HHS, 1985), but is relatively uncommon and rarely fills a dominant role in hazard identification or subsequent risk assessment steps. There are three types of epidemiological studies: cross-sectional or ecological, cohort and case-control. These studies may be retrospective (backward-looking) or prospective (forward-looking) in design. Cross-sectional studies are basically hypothesis-generating studies that survey populations for excesses of disease and attempt to identify risk factors. These studies do not provide evidence of cause and effect and suffer from the 'ecological fallacy' (because two things are associated in time and space, this does not imply they are cause and effect). Cohort studies, either retrospective or prospective, are designed based on exposure to an agent. Individuals are classified according to exposure status and monitored for development of disease. In the case of chronic disease and prospective studies, the latency period may confound the proper interpretation of the results. In the case of retrospective studies, there is a risk of exposure misclassification. Case-control studies match individuals with disease to age-and sex-matched disease-free controls. The exposure histories of the two groups determine exposure differences and other consistent features. All case-control studies are retrospective by definition, but characteristically suffer from a lack of good exposure data.

Epidemiological studies typically suffer from a number of problems (HHS, 1985; Wyzga, 1988; Layard and Silvers, 1989; Federal Focus, 1996). The numbers of people studied are usually small, exposure measures are crude or absent, latency periods for chronic disease may not coincide with the study period, there may be multiple exposures or other uncontrolled confounders (e.g. smoking), variation in susceptibility (e.g. the healthy worker effect), various biases including selection, recall, and diagnostic biases and so forth. Additionally, the language of epidemiology is unfamiliar to most risk assessors, and uncertainty on study quality and interpretation may limit the use of such studies (Paustenbach, 1995).

The so-called Hill criteria are used to judge the significance of the findings of epidemiological studies (Hill, 1965). These include: (1) strength of association, (2) consistency of observations (i.e. reproducibility), (3) specificity (i.e. unique quality or quantity of response), (4) temporal relationship (i.e. exposure precedes disease), (5) dose–response, (6) biological plausibility and coherence, (7) verification and (8) analogy (biological extrapolation). A recent report, 'the London Principles', discusses the use of epidemiological data in risk assessment and provides recommendations for evaluating and incorporating epidemiologic data into risk assessment as well as designing future epidemiologic studies to improve their utility in risk assessment (Federal Focus, 1996).

Additional supporting information on potential hazards can also be derived from the results of structure–activity relationship (SAR) studies and short-term *in vivo* and *in vitro* studies (typically studies of genotoxicity) (HHS, 1985; Paustenbach, 1989a). Generally, these tests provide only qualitative information since there is no agreement on how to extrapolate such information quantitatively. SAR is based on the observation that compounds with similar effects often have similar structural features. This has served as an effective screening tool in medicinal chemistry and has been suggested as a means of prioritizing agents for more detailed toxicity studies. For instance, SAR was used as a key in developing toxicity equivalence factors (TEFs) for polychlorinated dioxins and furans based on induction of the Ah receptor (US EPA, 1989d, 1994a). It is difficult, however, to make reliable predictions across chemical classes and toxic end-points using a single biological response as indicated by the disappointing results of computerized SAR programs when compared with the results of long-term animal bioassays (Ashby and Tennant, 1994). Since a single, relatively minor chemical change can significantly alter toxicity (e.g. ethanol vs methanol), these assays should be interpreted with caution and never serve as the sole basis for hazard identification.

Short-term *in vitro* and *in vivo* tests can range from simple bacterial mutation tests such as the Ames assay to more complex whole animal studies involving altered liver foci or chromosomal breakage in dosed animals (Hayes, 1994). Although most such studies have been developed to determine the potential genetic toxicity and mutagenicity of agents tested, there are similar tests available for developmental and reproductive, immunotoxic and neurotoxic endpoints. While such studies can provide useful information on mechanism of action and are inexpensive and quick, the ability to make quantitative extrapolations from such results is limited. Validation of such assays requires a knowledge of the assay's sensitivity (identification of true positives), specificity (identification of true negatives) and predictive value for the end-point under consideration. The problem of false negatives and false positives may present substantial uncertainty in using such assays to identify hazards and, as a result, currently tend to relegate these assays to a role of supporting evidence.

Issues in Hazard Identification

Unfortunately, it is atypical for most risk assessments to characterize fully the potential hazard posed by an agent by carrying out an independent toxicological review of the agent in question. Instead, there is a widespread reliance on boilerplate language or cursory reviews designed by various government groups or agencies, some of which may be out of date. The circumstances of exposure are not often taken into account. Given the large amount of toxicological research conducted and published over the last decade, such a cursory approach offers the possibility that new and relevant data may be overlooked. This may result in an over - or underestimation of the potential hazard associated with a technology or pollution episode.

Equally important in the hazard identification process is the recognition that agents are not equipotent in their toxic actions and therefore should not be considered as posing equal hazards to humans or wildlife (Paustenbach, 1989b, 1995). For example, it has been convincingly demonstrated that carcinogens may vary by seven orders of magnitude or more in their potency (Gaylor and Chen, 1986; Paustenbach, 1995). Others are mutagenic (and potentially carcinogenic) at low doses while others clearly have little direct action on genetic material. For instance, the US EPA recently promulgated two separate toxicity criteria for the carcinogenicity of polychlorinated biphenyls (PCBs) based on the degree of chlorination and biological half-life. Lower chlorinated PCBs with shorter half-lives have a lower carcinogenic toxicity criteria than higher chlorinated PCBs with longer half-lives (US EPA, 1996d). The toxic equivalence factor (TEF) approach for polyhalogenated dioxins and furans (US EPA, 1989d, 1994a) is another example of the recognition that similar compounds may not pose similar risks. In this approach, the toxicity of environmental mixtures of these compounds is estimated that multiplying the concentration of each individual chemical by its TEF value (ranging from 1 for 2,3,7,8-TCDD to 0.001 for octachlorodioxin) to determine what the equivalent amount of 2,3,7,8-TCDD (the benchmark compound) would be when the weighted results are added together **(Table 1)**. A similar approach has been taken with polynuclear aromatic hydrocarbons (PAHs) (US EPA, 1993; Collins *et al.*, 1998) and PCBs (Ahlborg *et al.*, 1994), and suggested for non-carcinogenic effects, including developmental, reproductive and neurotoxicity. Others, however, have been critical of this approach as an appropriate way to assess the hazards of related compounds (Kimbrough, 1997, 1998; Putzrah, 1997). A hazard identification that simply lumps all carcinogens together (or toxicants with other end-points) without consideration of potency or target organs is inadequate for decision-making purposes. The role of the risk assessor at this point in the risk assessment process is to use the available data to make a judgement about the relative significance of the agents under consideration in terms of their potential to cause injury, perhaps with a mind to eliminating some agents from further consideration. Care must be taken, of course, since most exposure is not simply to a single agent and the possibilities of interactions must also be taken into account (Krewski *et al.*, 1989b; Calabrese, 1991;

Table 1 Recommended toxicity equivalency factors (TEFs) for chlorinated dioxins (CDDs) and furans (CDFs).

CDDs	TEF	CDFs	TEF
MonoCDDs	0	MonoCDFs	0
DiCDDs	0	DiCDFs	0
TriCDDs	0	TriCDFs	0
2,3,7,8-TCDD	1	2,3,7,8-TCDF	0.1
Other tetraCDDs	0	Other tetraCDFs	0
2,3,7,8-PentaCDD[a]	0.5	1,2,3,7,8-PentaCDF	0.1
		2,3,4,7,8-PentaCDF	0.5
Other pentaCDDs	0	Other pentaCDFs	0
2,3,7,8-HexaCDD	0.1	2,3,7,8-HexaCDF	0.1
Other hexaCDDs	0	Other hexaCDFs	0
2,3,7,8-HeptaCDD	0	2,3,7,8-HeptaCDF	0
Other heptaCDD	0	Other heptaCDF	0
OctaCDD	0	OctaCDF	0

[a] Any isomer that contains chlorine in the 2,3,7,8-positions.
Source: adapted from US EPA (1989d).

Auton, 1991; Krewski and Thomas, 1992; Pelekis and Krishnan, 1997; ACGIH, 1998a, b).

It has been considered prudent public health policy in the recent past to place the greatest weight on data that suggest that an agent may pose a hazard, and little weight on experimental data that suggest that the compound may not cause adverse effects at environmentally relevant exposures. Further, study quality may vary markedly and it has been a frequent criticism that more confidence has been placed on a study's results than is warranted by the study quality (Barr, 1988; Paustenbach, 1989b, 1995). In these circumstances, a single positive study of poor quality may carry more weight in deciding hazard than several negative studies of better quality. Regulatory agencies have now accepted in theory the notion that all data are not equivalent and that equal weight should not be given to studies of unequal quality. In the USA, the process by which an agent is determined to be 'more likely than not' to pose a human hazard is known as the 'weight-of-evidence' approach. This simply refers to the assemblage and review of all studies of approximately equal quality to determine if there is a consistent message about the type of effects that may occur. This 'weight-of-evidence' approach has been successfully employed with such diverse chemicals as *d*-limonene, formaldehyde, methylene chloride, chloroform and dioxin (Paustenbach, 1995). This approach represents an important policy shift from the earlier period (1960–80) when the study that produced the lowest 'no observed adverse effect level' (NOAEL) (or the highest risk) was automatically given the greatest weight. While the 'weight-of-evidence' approach has been embraced by regulatory agencies both within and outside the USA, it should be recognized that the practice began to be applied to hazard identification and risk assessment only recently, and even then not always consistently or completely. Older hazard identifications and risk

assessments may need to be re-evaluated using the 'weight-of-evidence'. The 'weight-of-evidence' is also applicable to the subsequent steps in the risk assessment process (e.g. dose–response evaluation, exposure assessment). Taking such an approach minimizes the possibility that scarce resources and time will be taken up to conduct additional toxicity studies merely to refute the results of one or two poorly conducted studies.

Additionally, it remains the case that toxicity criteria used in various risk assessment steps have typically been derived from a single critical study. The applicability of these studies to the exposure and response of the target species may be questionable in the light of the weight of evidence and newer data or alternative interpretations and should be reconsidered whenever possible. This is particularly important when the agent is an important contributor to estimated risk levels, and control would require significant expenditure of resources (Brown and Hoel, 1986; Spear *et al.*, 1991; Keenan *et al.*, 1991; Velazquez *et al.*, 1994).

Case Study in Hazard Identification: Speciation and Extractability

Barium was identified as a potential hazard at an industrial property based on its toxicity, soil concentrations and frequency of detection. Upon review, it was determined that the toxicity value was based on barium chloride, a highly soluble form of barium that can result in electrolyte imbalance and cardiac arrhythmia (ATSDR, 1991). The barium species in the site soil was predominantly barium sulphate. Evidence suggested that different compounds or species of a chemical might have significant differences in toxicity and hazard (Barltrop and Meeks, 1975; Hughes *et al.*, 1995). The problem for the risk assessor was to determine whether the hazard potential of the two barium compounds was equivalent.

A simple experiment was designed to provide the answer. Site soil was added to an oscillating flask containing simulated gastric juices maintained at body temperature for a period equivalent to that needed for a bolus dose to transit the gut. Following the extraction period, the amount of barium in solution was determined. It was found that only 5–20% of the barium sulphate in soil was extractable under simulated gastric conditions. From these results, the level of barium in soil would conservatively have to be five times higher to reach the level of concern. Based on this information, barium was eliminated as a potential hazard for this situation. Similar techniques have been employed in developing an understanding of chemical behaviour and its potential influence on toxicity and hazard (Davis et al., 1992, 1993, 1997; Freeman et al., 1992, 1995; Ruby et al., 1992; Paustenbach et al., 1997; Schoof and Nielsen, 1997). The obvious value in such work is that it can improve the information used in risk assessment rather quickly and at a relatively low cost.

Dose–Response Assessment

The dose–response assessment is the process of characterizing the quantitative relationship between the dose (or intake) of an agent and the resultant biological response (National Research Council, 1983, 1994). A variety of different techniques are used to assess the dose–response relationship and derive toxicity criteria (Table 2). The data used are typically derived from animal studies or, less frequently, from epidemiological studies. It is recognized by toxicologists that different dose–response relationships exist for an agent depending on

species and population tested, conditions of exposure, route of administration and end-point of concern (Calabrese, 1978a, b; Park and Snee, 1983; Krewski et al., 1989a; Kodell et al., 1991; Paustenbach et al., 1997c). This fact and its implications for risk assessment, however, may escape the risk managers and public if not adequately explained. With very rare exceptions, for any given agent and exposure, the severity and frequency of effect decrease with decreasing dose. In addition, the type of adverse effect will often change in relation to the dose and duration of exposure. For example, carbon monoxide at high doses rapidly produces coma and death. At lower doses, dizziness, confusion and incoherence result, while headaches and malaise may predominate at still lower doses. Exposure to background levels or just above are unlikely to cause noticeable symptoms in most individuals (Ottoboni, 1991). Clearly, information on the dose–response relationship and the critical effect is key to accurately assessing human risk. If the concern is neurotoxicity, the use of a toxicological that had irritation as its end-point is clearly inappropriate (Gaylor and Slikker, 1994). The basis for the selection of the key study or studies should be the end-point of concern. To the extent that the dose–response relationship is not well defined, uncertainty about the estimated risk at various doses will exist and, accordingly, the uncertainty will become greater as one attempts to predict response far below the doses tested. While the dose–response relationship is a fundamental concept in toxicology, developing the dose–response relationship in risk assessment usually requires two major steps: (1) an interpecies adjustment (animal to man) to account for differences in body weight, size, life span and basal metabolism; and (2) an extrapolation from the generally high doses used in typical toxico-

Table 2 General approaches to deriving toxicity criteria based on toxicological end-points

Approach	Methodology	Toxicological end-point
Threshold effects	NOAEL/LOAEL with uncertainty factors Benchmark dose with uncertainty factors	Irritation Non-cancer effects Epigenetic carcinogenic effects
Non-threshold effects	Linearized multistage model Other low-dose extrapolation models Benchmark dose with linear extrapolation	Reproductive effects Genotoxic carcinogenic effects
Pre-derived non-cancer values	Reference doses (RfDs) Reference concentrations (RfCs)	All non-carcinogenic effects except for irritation (see IRIS or HEAST)[a]
Pre-derived cancer values	Unit cancer risks (UCRs) Cancer potency factors (CPFs) Virtually safe doses (VSDs)	Carcinogenic effects (see IRIS or HEAST)
Pharmacokinetics	Physiologically based pharmacokinetic models (PBPK)	Target organ effects (including cancer)
Monte Carlo analysis	Combination of several approaches, data sets, or expert opinions	All effects

[a] IRIS, US EPA's Integrated Risk Information System, available on-line; HEAST, US EPA's Health Effects Assessment Summary Table, updated quarterly, available on paper.

logical testing to the low-dose range to which the general population is exposed. Some type of mathematical model is employed to estimate the likely response at doses below those tested since effects that occur at less than a 10% response rate cannot be reliably observed or measured (Food Safety Council, 1980; Krewski et al., 1989a; Holland and Sielken, 1991, 1993; ILSI, 1995). Both the extrapolation from animal to man and from high dose to low dose are among the most controversial steps in risk assessment and this methodology contains the largest amount of uncertainty in the process (Sielken, 1985, 1987, 1989; Paustenbach, 1989b, 1995).

Most risk assessors do not themselves derive the dose–response relationships and toxicity criteria used in their risk assessments. They rely instead on authoritative sources of information such as US EPA's Integrated Risk Information System (IRIS) or Health Effects Assessment Summary Tables (HEAST) (US EPA, 1997b, 1998a), which are available in paper form or through the Internet or on-line services such as TOX-NET. Other countries often rely on the same sources or, at times, they may develop their own toxicity criteria using similar or different data sources and extrapolation methodologies (e.g. the WHO International Program on Chemical Safety's Environmental Health Criteria series). This accounts for why multiple (and arguably valid) toxicity criteria for a compound such as dioxin can be found (Paustenbach, 1989b). The problem with these data sources is that the original effort may not have relied on the most appropriate toxicity information or extrapolation models, or the data upon which these values are based may have been supplanted by newer data that have not been incorporated into the regulatory database owing to time and/or resource constraints. One effort to consolidate, if not reconcile, the differences in available toxicity criteria is being conducted by Toxicological Excellence in Risk Assessment (TERA) in Cincinnati, Ohio, which is developing an on-line database of peer-reviewed toxicity criteria developed by various governmental entities (both US and world-wide), as well as those developed by private institutions, including industry and academia. This resource is accessible at www.tera.org.

The dose–response assessment also differs between carcinogens and non-carcinogens, based on assumptions regarding the presence or absence of a threshold and differing mechanisms of action. This has often created problems in comparing risks and making reasoned risk management decisions, and ought to be resolved (Bartell, 1996; Crump et al., 1997). It is recognized that most carcinogens will also produce non-carcinogenic effects, but, for virtually all chemicals, the doses needed to minimize the cancer hazard are so low that non-carcinogenic effects are not of concern. Therefore, the term 'non-carcinogenic' is itself strictly operational (i.e. a term useful for describing a situation rather than an inherent biological property of a compound). For example, it may be used equally correctly to describe either an agent that has not been shown to be carcinogenic in epidemiological or animal studies or a compound that has yet to be tested for its carcinogenic potential. The term 'non-carcinogen' is therefore used only for convenience and may be rendered moot by future research. Non-carcinogenic effects include such diverse response as sensory irritation, organ-specific damage or adverse reproductive outcomes. Non-carcinogens are assessed using a no observed adverse effect level or benchmark dose approach whereas carcinogenic dose–response assessment relies on a variety of statistical extrapolation models into the low-dose range (Gibb and Chen, 1986; Barton and Dass, 1996; Gibson et al., 1997; Ragas and Huijbregts, 1997; Ohanian, 1997). Each method has its own strengths and weaknesses and, at this juncture, one approach is not clearly superior to another in all circumstances.

Assessment of Non-Carcinogens

NOAEL Model

The assessment of non-carcinogens typically employs a simple approach in which a threshold, defined as a dose level below which no effect is observed, is assumed to exist (Shoaf, 1991; Amdur et al., 1995). For non-carcinogens, the highest dose for which no significant (in terms of biological and statistical significance) effect is seen, termed the no observed adverse effect level (NOAEL), is preferentially selected for extrapolation purposes. In the absence of a NOAEL, the lowest dose eliciting a response, referred to as the lowest observed adverse effect level (LOAEL), is used (Ottoboni, 1994). These values are dependent on the number of doses, the number animals tested at each dose and the background response rate in control animals. The NOAEL, however, is not necessarily a dose without risk. NOAELs based on toxicity testing providing continuous end-points average a 5% risk whereas quantal data reportedly have an associated risk of 10% or greater (Allen et al., 1994a, b; Faustman et al., 1994).

Once determined, the NOAEL (or LOAEL) is divided by a series of uncertainty and modifying factors to arrive at a reference dose (RfD) expressed in milligrams of agent per kilogram of body weight per day (Lehmann and Fitzhugh, 1954; Weil, 1972; Zielhuis and van der Kreek, 1979; Dourson and Stara, 1983; Dourson et al., 1985; Barnes and Dourson, 1988; Johnson, 1988). This dose is defined as the amount, with an uncertainty spanning perhaps an order of magnitude, that can be 'taken up' each day by the majority of the population without eliciting an adverse effect. The size of the uncertainty factor (UF) used to derive this dose is inversely related to the degree of comfort that the risk assessor has about the quality of the data in terms of its intended use: the protection of human health from chronic health effects (**Table 3**). A modifying factor (MF) can also be used to adjust the UF based on mechanistic or

Table 3 Criteria and guidelines for the application of uncertainty factors

Uncertainty	Magnitude	Comments
Interindividual variability	3–10	Accounts for variations in susceptibility among the human population (*i.e.* high-risk groups)
Interspecies variability	3–10	Accounts for uncertainty in extrapolating between species Applied in all cases where the NOAEL or LOAEL is derived from an animal study
Less than lifetime to lifetime (subchronic to chronic)	5–10	Accounts for uncertainty in extrapolating from subchronic (less than lifetime) to chronic (lifetime) exposures UF of 10 is applied to all studies 90 days or less in duration in rodents or 1/10 to 1/5 the lifespan of other species
LOAEL to NOAEL	5–10	Accounts for uncertainty in extrapolating downward from a LOAEL to a NOAEL

Source: adapted from Calabrese and Kenyon (1991).

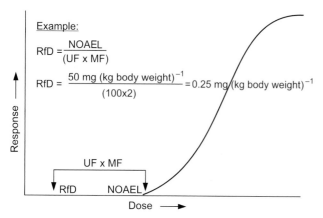

Figure 3 Among the most common approaches to the assessment of non-carcinogens is to determine a no observed adverse effect level (NOAEL) from an animal or human study and divide this value by uncertainty (UF) factors ranging from 10 to 1000 or more (depending on the level of confidence one has in the data) and possibly a modifying factor (MF) of between 1 and 10 (depending on the severity of effect among other things) to derive a reference dose (RfD), the dose to which the majority of the population can be exposed daily without risk of adverse effects. In this example, a NOAEL is identified and divided through by an appropriate UF (usually 100) to derive the RfD.

pharmacokinetic knowledge, severity of effect or relevance of the effect to humans. The approach is illustrated in the following equation (see also **Figure 3**):

$$RfD = \frac{NOEL}{UF \times MF}$$

The uncertainty factors are usually expressed in multiples of 10 based largely on convention (Barnes and Dourson, 1988; Johnson, 1988; Abdel-Rahman and Kadry, 1995; Naumann and Weideman, 1995; Kadry *et al.*, 1995; Dourson, 1996), although there have been a number of suggestions for improving the scientific underpinnings for the selection of uncertainty factors and the application of this technique (Krewski *et al.*, 1984; Lewis *et al.*, 1990; Calabrese and Gilbert, 1993; Clewell and Jarnot, 1994; Schwartz, 1995; Nair *et al.*, 1995; Calabrese and Baldwin, 1995; Cicmanec and Poirier, 1995; Jara-

bek, 1995; Dourson *et al.*, 1996; Dourson *et al.*, 1997; Kadry *et al.*, 1997; Naumann *et al.*, 1997; Price *et al.*, 1997; Swartout *et al.*, 1998).

Typically, a UF of 3–10 is used to adjust for intraspecies variability (i.e., individual susceptibility) (Bogen and Spear, 1987; Hattis *et al.*, 1987; Hattis and Silver, 1994; Dills *et al.*, 1994; Hattis and Barlow, 1996; Renwick and Lazaris, 1998). This is combined with a UF of 3–10 to account for interspecies differences (e.g. animal to man). Although rare, an RfD based on a human study could be based on a UF as low as 10 since such a study would presumably be in all ways directly relevant to the population and end-point of concern. The RfD for nitrate in drinking water is an example of a toxicological criterion based on human evidence and utilizes a UF of 10 alone. Since most toxicity criteria are derived from long-term animal studies, the most common UF is 100 (10 for human-to-human extrapolation multiplied by 10 for animal-to-man extrapolation). However, deficiencies or uncertainties in the toxicity data can result in a higher UF being used. For instance, in the absence of a NOAEL, a LOAEL may be used. In this case, an additional UF of 10 may be added to increase the overall UF to 1000. Similarly, if a short-term toxicity test is used in place of a long-term study, an additional UF of 10 may be employed (Nessel *et al.*, 1995; Kramer *et al.*, 1996; Pieters *et al.*, 1998). Generally, if the overall UF exceeds 10 000, the data are considered of questionable use for the protection of human health. When used, the MF selected is generally between 1 and 10, again based of relevance of the study to the target species, severity of effect and other considerations. For certain airborne agents, a similar approach is used to define a reference concentration (RfC) expressed in milligrams of agent per cubic metre of air (Jarabek *et al.*, 1990; US EPA, 1990a; Malsch *et al.*, 1994; Paustenbach, 1997).

As an example, consider a 1-year oral toxicity study in rats which provides a NOAEL of 100 mg kg^{-1} day^{-1}. The RfD in this case would be as follows:

$$RfD = \frac{100 \, mg \, (kg \, body \, weight)^{-1} \, day^{-1}}{10 \times 10} = 1 \, mg \, (kg \, body \, weight)^{-1} \, day^{-1}$$

In this case, the overall UF of 100 accounts for the inter-individual difference between humans (10) and species differences (10). In contrast, the RfD for a 30 day oral toxicity study in rats with a LOAEL of 100 mg kg^{-1} day^{-1} would be

$$\text{RfD} = \frac{100 \, \text{mg} \, (\text{kg body weight})^{-1} \text{day}^{-1}}{10 \times 10 \times 10 \times 10} = 0.01 \, \text{mg} \, (\text{kg body weight})^{-1} \text{day}^{-1}$$

The overall UF of 10 000 results from the inter-individual (10) and species (10) differences in combination with the use of a short-term test instead of a long-term test (10) and a LOAEL instead of a NOAEL (10). In general, a 10 000-fold uncertainty factor will provide an enormous margin of safety and it is rarely used.

The NOAEL approach to deriving RfDs can be criticized on several levels, including the fact that the NOAEL must by definition be one of the doses tested; otherwise a LOAEL is used as a default. The additional UF used in this instance may not off-set the increased dose level from which the RfD is derived. The NOAEL approach also does not utilize the slope of the dose–response curve and, therefore, important information about the toxicity and potency of the compound is not taken into account, nor is the actual nature of the adverse effect being measured taken into account in the evaluation of the data and derivation of the RfD. This may result in toxicity criteria being developed over a range of possible responses. Finally, it can be argued that the NOAEL approach rewards testing that produces less certain rather than more certain NOAEL values, since experimental data using few animals usually result in larger NOAELs and thus higher RfDs.

Benchmark Dose Model

An alternative approach to the NOAEL model relies on the benchmark dose approach to developing RfDs first suggested by Crump (1984) and Kimmel and Gaylor (1988) for assessing non-carcinogenic risks. This approach relies on modelling from the actual dose–response curve and determining a lower confidence bound for a dose at some specified response level (the benchmark dose or BMD) (Allen et al., 1998; Faustman, 1997; Fung et al., 1998). The BMD is usually selected at a response rate between 1 and 10% and a 95% lower confidence bound on the dose used to derive a conservative value **(Figure 4)**. The BMD rather than a NOEL is then used in combination with the same UFs and MFs used in the NOAEL approach, although a lower UF and MF (e.g. 3) may be employed because of increased confidence in the response gained by employing the slope of the dose–response curve and recognition of the experimental variability resulting from the use of the lower confidence bound on the dose (Barnes et al., 1995; Crump, 1995; Kavlock et al., 1996; Fung et al., 1998; Kalliomaa et al., 1998; Kimmel et al., 1995; Krewski and Zhu, 1995). The RfD in this case would be derived as follows:

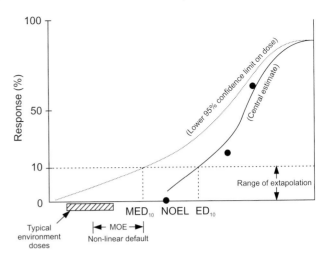

Figure 4   An alternative approach to the NOAEL method of deriving reference doses is the benchmark dose (BMD) method. In this approach, an effect level (usually between a 1 and 10% response rate) is identified from the dose–response curve (solid line) and a bounding estimate on that dose derived (dotted line). A bound on the dose evoking the response of interest is identified and this value is once again divided by appropriate uncertainty factors to derive a reference dose or concentration. In this example, the dose causing a 10% response is chosen (ED10) and a bounding estimate (dotted line) on this response is used to derive the minimum effective dose (MED10). The MED10 is then divided by an uncertainty factor to derive the RfD. In this case, the margin of exposure (MOE) is shown indicating where the MED10 is found in relation to the typical environmental exposure.

$$\text{RfD} = \frac{\text{BMD}}{\text{UF} \times \text{MF}}$$

Obvious advantages to the BMD approach over the NOAEL approach to deriving RfDs include the use of consistent response levels to derive the RfDs, incorporation of all the information presented by the dose–response curve, inclusion of potential variability through the use of confidence limits in the derivation of the RfD and avoiding the uncertainty caused by relying on extrapolated responses from low dose exposure (Crump, 1995; Gaylor, 1996; Price et al., 1996; Barnes et al., 1995; Kimmel et al., 1995; Krewski and Zhu, 1995). Guidance for the derivation of toxicity criteria using the BMD approach has been published by the US EPA (1996b). Both the strengths and weaknesses of the BMD approach have been reviewed (Crump, 1995; Murrell et al., 1998).

Case Study in Dose–Response Evaluation: Benchmark Dose Approach

The BMD approach to setting toxicity values can be illustrated by work done on chromium. Differences in the valence and physical form of chromium in the air suggest that the various forms of these compounds (tri- and hexavalent chromium) ought to be assessed differently (Finley et al., 1992). Malsch et al. (1994) reviewed the toxicological database for different forms (acidic mists and particulates) of trivalent (Cr^{III}) and hexavalent (Cr^{VI}) chromium to determine if information existed sufficient to use in a BMD-derived reference concentration (RfC). This review suggested that data meeting minimum quality and data requirement for the suitable BMD approach existed only for hexavalent chromium particulates in the work of Glaser et al. (1985, 1990), who exposed rats to hexavalent chromium particulates for differing periods of time. These requirements included: (1) appropriate aerosol characterization (e.g. chemical speciation known, particulate form identified, mass mean aerodynamic diameter and standard deviation reported) has been successfully applied to the reference concentration for chromium; (2) adequate exposure measures (e.g. dose groups defined, exposure via inhalation pathway, exposure duration known and two or more exposure groups identified); (3) appropriate end-point considerations (e.g. dose–response evident, non-cancer end-point, response data reported, mean and standard deviation reported and number of animals per dose known); and (4) adequate experimental design (e.g. confounders absent, controls present, appropriate statistics and good laboratory practices used). Based on these studies, continuous exposures of 90 days were evaluated for effects thought to be associated with toxicity: lung and spleen weight, lactate dehydrogenase (LDH) in broncheoalveolar lavage fluid (BALF), protein in BALF and albumin in BALF.

The BMD was defined as the 95% lower confidence limit (LCL) on the dose corresponding to a 10% relative change in the end-point under consideration in comparison with controls. Selection of a 10% response rate is appropriate since most mathematical models agree well in the range near the experimental doses used. This level is small enough that the BMD reflects the shape of the dose–response curve but large enough that the LCL does not depend to great extent on the model. A commercially available software program (TIIC; Clement International Group, Ruston, LA, USA) was used to determine the BMD (Howe, 1990). The BMD was subjected to appropriate adjustments and uncertainty factors to arrive at a reference concentration (RfC) using the following equation:

$$RfC = \frac{BMD \times RDDR}{UF_A \times UF_S \times UF_H}$$

where

RfC = inhalation reference concentration ($mg\ m^{-3}$)

BMD = benchmark dose (the lower 95% confidence limit on a 10% increase in response)

RDDR = regional deposited dose ratio for pharmacokinetic differences between species

UF_A = a threefold uncertainty factor to account for pharmacodynamic differences not covered by the RDDR

UF_S = a three fold uncertainty factor to account for subchronic to chronic exposures

UF_H = a 10-fold uncertainty factor to account for inter-individual members of a population

The term RDDR is a dosimetric adjustment factor that accounts for the fact that animals and humans do not receive the same doses in comparable respiratory tract areas when exposed to the same aerosol (Jarabek et al., 1990). In this case, the mass median aerodynamic diameter (MMAD) and standard deviations for the particulates were used to derive the RDDRs via US EPA guidance (US EPA, 1990a). Since the RDDRs only account for pharmacokinetic differences, an additional uncertainty factor of 3.16 (mid-point between 1 and 10 on a log scale) was used to account for other pharmacodynamic differences. The UF of 10 was used to account for the difference in the human populations and 3.16 to account for a less-then-lifetime exposure (90 days being equivalent to 12% of a rat lifespan). No UF was employed for the use of a LOAEL since the BMD by definition employs a low-effect dose. The overall UF for this effort was, therefore, 100 ($10 \times 3.16 \times 3.16$).

The presence of LDH in BALF was selected as the most sensitive indicator of toxicity since it is only found in extracellular fluid upon cell death and threefold increases have been associated with the development of lung pathology (e.g. fibrosis). A threefold increase in LDH in BALF was associated with a dose level of 400 $\mu g\ m^{-3}$ in the study of Glaser et al. (1990). The BMD identified in this study (16 $\mu g\ m^{-3}$) is 25-fold below this dose while the RfC derived (0.34 $\mu g\ m^{-3}$) is three orders of magnitude below this level. This RfC represents the lowest toxicity criteria based upon a known adverse effect, and is considered a conservative value since it represents the 95% LCL on a sensitive end-point with conservative UFs incorporated into it. Additionally, all RfCs derived from Glaser et al.'s data fell within a factor of four of one another (0.34–1.4 $\mu g\ m^{-3}$). Since RfCs/RfDs are defined as having an uncertainty spanning perhaps an order of magnitude, selection of the lowest RfC is appropriate. In comparison, an RfC for hexavalent chromium of 0.002 $\mu g\ m^{-3}$ was proposed by theb US EPA based on nasal mucosa atrophy in workers exposed to chromic acid mists and using an overall UF of 300 and an LOAEL of 2.0 $\mu g\ m^{-3}$. Since it is inappropriate to assess particulates and chromic acid mist toxicity in the same way, and the BMD RfC for hexavalent chromium particulates is based on a more sensitive indicator of toxicity than the LOAEL for chromic acid mists, the RfC of 0.34 $\mu g\ m^{-3}$ was proposed as an alternative to the US EPA's RfC for hexavalent chromium particulates (Malsch et al., 1994). The US EPA agreed and has incorporated this approach in the IRIS database (US EPA, 1998b).

Assessment of Carcinogens

A no-threshold assumption for carcinogens has been in place in the regulatory agenda for nearly four decades as a conservative, health-protective step (Park and Snee, 1983; Bailer *et al.*, 1988; Paustenbach, 1995; AIHC, 1989; Goldsmith and Kordysh, 1993; Gaylor, 1997; Cohen, 1998). In theory, any exposure to a carcinogen is assumed to carry a finite risk because a single molecule of the agent interacting with a single DNA molecule could cause damage sufficient to result ultimately in a tumour. In other words, no threshold is assumed to exist for carcinogens. However, because DNA is damaged thousands of times each day owing to routine biological processes, it is inappropriate to assume that any single mutation in itself will pose a tumour risk. Thresholds may well exist for some if not all classes of carcinogens since many appear to act through mechanisms that would require a threshold dose to be exceeded prior to initiation of the carcinogenic process (Butterworth and Slaga, 1987; Butterworth, 1990, 1993; Williams and Weisburger, 1991). Functionally, in the light of the fact that our diets are abundant with natural carcinogens, there must be a practical threshold below which we would consider exposures 'safe' (Ames, 1987, 1996; Ames *et al.*, 1987; Ames and Gold, 1993; Crawford and Wilson, 1996; Brown *et al.*, 1997; Calabrese and Baldwin, 1997; Bogen, 1997). In the past few years, there has been growing agreement among scientists that all carcinogens do not pose the same degree of hazard at all doses. This understanding has now been acknowledged in the risk assessment arena. This is reflected in the recent proposed revisions to the US EPA's carcinogen assessment guidelines (US EPA, 1996c; Farland and Tuxen, 1997), which acknowledges that many agents that are carcinogenic at high doses in animals may not pose a risk to humans exposed to much lower doses. In other words, there is a tacit agreement that thresholds for carcinogens exist, at least on a practical level.

Toxicity criteria for carcinogens are typically derived from the application of mathematical models to the results of high-dose animal testing (Crump *et al.*, 1976; Crump, 1980; Krewski *et al.*, 1984). Such models describe the expected quantitative relationship between risk and doses too small to resolve experimentally (*i.e.* environmentally relevant doses). The accuracy of the risk estimates at doses of interest is a function of how well the model describes the true, but unmeasurable, relationship between dose and risk at these levels. It is clear that low-dose extrapolation of carcinogens is the area of greatest uncertainty in the risk assessment of chemical and physical agents. We possess only a limited ability to estimate risks associated with environmental exposures from information derived from rodent bioassays. It is interesting to note that such rodent bioassays were originally intended only to provide qualitative information on potential human hazards, rather than a quantitative esti-

mate of that risk (Gold *et al.*, 1987, 1992; Paustenbach, 1995; Barr, 1998). The reasons are several: (1) the mechanisms of action for carcinogens (and other classes of toxicants for that matter) are not fully understood and, therefore, cannot be predicted accurately (Williams and Weisburger, 1991; Butterworth, 1993); (2) the high doses under which animal bioassays are conducted may not be relevant to the human exposure to doses thousands of times lower, and may produce effects that would not occur at environmentally relevant doses (Ames, 1987); (3) the species differences in absorption, distribution, metabolism and excretion may produce different responses and cannot be accounted for using the most current dose–response extrapolation models (Paustenbach, 1994, 1995); and (4) the delivered dose to the target organ in animals may be different and produce a different response in humans (Andersen *et al.*, 1987a).

As a result of these uncertainties, scientists must rely on models or theory to estimate the human response at doses often one thousandth of the lowest animal dose tested. Low-dose extrapolation models have become the backbone of the carcinogenic dose–response assessment process. A variety of such models (up to 15) exist and share a number of characteristics in common (Brown and Chui, 1989; Holland and Sielken, 1991, 1993; Gaylor *et al.*, 1994). The most commonly used models all fit the observed experimental data well, but diverge widely in the low-dose range where most human exposure takes place **(Figure 5)**. The difference in the best-fit predictions from the most conservative (i.e. one-hit) to the least sensitive (i.e. probit) may range over several orders of magnitude **(Table 4)**. The results of the modelling exercise will vary in a predictable manner because they rely on different mathematical equations for assessing the carcinogenic potency of an agent. To date, most regulatory decisions in the USA used to identify safe or acceptable levels of exposure to air, water or soil contaminants have been based on these statistical models rather than biologically based models. As in the hazard identification step, strict adherence to a single dose–response model as laid out in regulatory guidance (typical for most regulatory agencies) can result in such a constrained assessment of cancer potency that valuable biological information (that might alter the outcome of the analysis) is lost. Therefore, it is useful to use other models when assessing the dose–response relationship and compare the results. Significant variation in model output should prompt additional study to explain why the results vary. This evaluation in turn may shed new light on the risk and its significance to humans.

In general, because of the 'spread' in the various risk estimates from the various models **(Figure 5)**, and because science cannot determine which model is best suited to estimate cancer risk for a given agent and given exposure, most regulatory agencies default to the most conservative model that includes some measure of biology. The US EPA has, for a number of years, employed

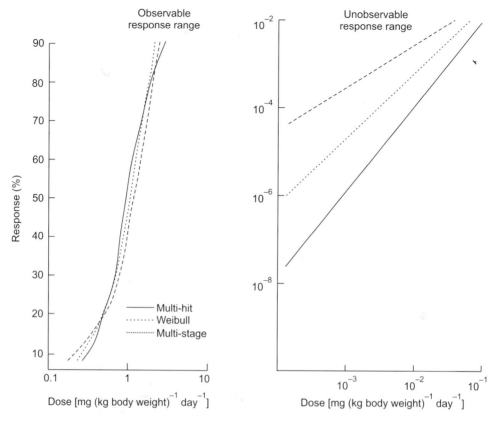

Figure 5   Cancer risk assessment relies on the use of mathematical models to extrapolate from the observed experimental range (left plot) to the unobservable environmental exposure range (right plot). All models tend to agree in the high-dose range, but may diverge widely in the low-dose range. As a result, the same risk level may be associated with a dose range spanning several orders of magnitude depending on which extrapolation models are used. The US EPA typically relies on linearized multistage (LMS) model as a default, one of the most conservative of the dose extrapolation models, although alternative models may be used if justified.

Table 4   The divergence in dose–response model best fit predictions at low doses[a]

Chloroform dose [mg (kg body weight)$^{-1}$]	Ratio of fitted multistage to fitted Weibull	Ratio of fitted multistage to fitted Probit
10	1.2	1.3
1	4.4	560
0.1	21	2900000
0.01	102	–
0.001	496	–

[a] The multistage model is employed by US EPA and is considered more conservative than the Weibull or Probit models
Source: adapted from Sielken (1987).

a linearized version of the multistage model (LMS), which is among the most conservative of the dose response extrapolation models (Crump *et al.*, 1976; Crump, 1980, 1996; Anderson, 1983; Crump and Houe, 1984; Brown and Chui, 1989). This model was first developed by Armitage and Doll (1957) based on the hypothesis that a series of ordered changes involving mutation, initiation, transformation and progression was necessary to produce a tumour. This idea was generalized by Crump *et al.* (1976) and Crump (1980) to the following equation used in the GLOBAL dose–response

computer programs utilized by the US EPA to develop their cancer risk assessments (Chen, 1993):

$$P(d) = 1 - \exp(-\lambda_0 + \lambda d_1 + \lambda d_2 + \ldots + \lambda_1 d^k)$$

where $P(d)$ represents the probability of disease (cancer). When the value of λ_1 is replaced with λ_1^* (the upper confidence bound of λ_1), a linearized multistage model in which the output is dominated by $(\lambda d^*)\, d$ in the low-dose range results.

Three types of carcinogenic toxicity criteria are derived from such modelling: cancer potency factors (CPFs), virtually safe doses (VSDs) and unit cancer risks (UCRs). CPFs are derived from the slope of the extrapolated dose response curve and are also referred to as cancer slope factors. The actual CPF is the 95% upper confidence bound on the best fit of the dose–response model (also referred to as the q_1^*) and is adopted as an extra measure of conservatism **(Figure 6)** (Wilson, 1991; Kodell and West, 1993). The difference between the best fit of the LMS model and the 95% upper bound confidence interval may be an additional six orders of magnitude **(Table 5)**. The larger the CPF, expressed in terms of (milligrams of agent per kilogram body weight per day)$^{-1}$, the more potent is the carcinogen. The unitless risk is

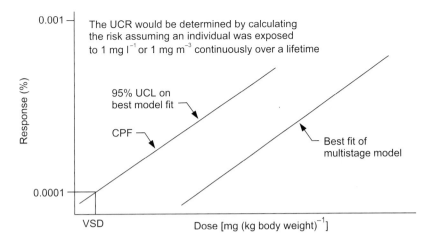

Figure 6 Once a model has been selected and the low–dose response has been modelled, the 95% upper bound on the estimated dose–response curve is generated. From the slope of this line, the cancer potency factor (CPF) is derived for use in calculating added cancer risk. The risk associated with exposure to one unit of an carcinogen per unit volume (1 mg l^{-1} or 1 mg m^{-3}) is known as the unit cancer risk (UCR). The dose [in mg (kg body weight)$^{-1}$ day^{-1}] associated with the acceptable risk level (i.e. 1 in 1 million or 1E-6) is known as the virtually safe dose (VSD). [1E-b = 1×10 exponential b].

Table 5 The divergence at low doses between the best fit of the dose–response model and the 95% upper confidence limit (UCL) on the best fit[a]

Formaldehyde dose (ppm)	Ratio of the 95% UCL to fitted multistage
5.6	2
2	41
1	368
0.5	3140
0.1	417000
0.01	423000000

[a] The 95% upper confidence limit on the best fit of the multistage model is used to ensure that risk is not underestimated.
Source: adapted from Sielken (1987).

calculated by multiplying the CPF by some measure of exposure (or dose) as follows:

$$\text{risk} = \text{CPF} \left[\text{ mg (kg body weight)}^{-1} \text{ day}^{-1}\right]^{-1}$$
$$\times \text{ exposure } \left[\text{mg (kg body weight)}^{-1} \text{ day}^{-1}\right]$$

The VSD can be easily identified by extrapolating from the acceptable risk level selected (e.g. 1×10^{-6}) to the dose [mg(kg body weight)$^{-1}$ day^{-1}] associated with it from the extrapolated dose–response curve. The UCR is the added cancer risk that results from a lifetime (70 year) exposure of a 70 kg human to a unit amount of a carcinogen (e.g. 1 μg per cubic metre of air or 1 μg per litre of water) **(Figure 6)**. Either the CPF or the VSD can be used to develop a UCR, and the UCR can be used to derive the CPF or the VSD through back-calculation.

Route-Specific Toxicity Criteria

It is recognized that the potential toxicity associated with an agent may vary with the route of exposure for both carcinogenic and non-carcinogenic responses (Gerrirty and Henry, 1990). For instance, hexavalent chromium is carcinogenic by inhalation but not by ingestion. Thus the US EPA has developed an inhalation CPF for hexavalent chromium, but no oral CPF. Likewise, inhalation of silver or cadmium causes lung effects whereas ingestion does not. Where data exist and a difference in response is evident, toxicity criteria for both inhalation and oral routes of exposure have been (or should be) promulgated. In the absence of appropriate toxicity criteria for a specific route of exposure (e.g. inhalation), toxicity criteria for another route (e.g. oral) have been substituted without adjustment. This obviously introduces an additional uncertainty into the evaluation. An exception to this practice is for dermal toxicity for which no specific toxicity criteria exist. Since skin contact is an important consideration in many risk assessment (CDHS, 1986; McDougal et al., 1990; McArthur, 1992; Paustenbach et al., 1992c; US EPA, 1992b; Fenske, 1993; CDTS, 1994; Mattie et al., 1994b; Michaud et al., 1994; Cherrie and Robertson, 1995; van Hemmen and Brouwer, 1995), this uncertainty has been addressed by adjusting existent toxicity criteria, usually oral RfDs or CPFs, using a literature-derived absorption factor (AF), which ranges from 1 to 100% (Poiger and Schlatter, 1980; Shu et al., 1988a, b; Owen, 1990; Paustenbach et al., 1998). In theory, this approach converts the applied dermal dose to an absorbed dose appropriate for use in risk assessment. For non-carcinogens, the adjustment is as follows:

$$\text{RfD}_{\text{dermal}} = \text{RfD}_{\text{oral}} \times \text{AF}$$

and for carcinogens:

$$\text{CPF}_{\text{dermal}} = \frac{\text{CPF}_{\text{oral}}}{AF}$$

Whether the theory behind this approach is correct is debatable. In practice, this approach together with certain assumptions regarding exposure often results in the dermal pathway becoming the predominant source of risk in spite of logic and experience. Obviously, a source of great uncertainty, development of specific dermal toxicity criteria or a validated methodology for deriving them from other routes of exposure should be a high research priority. One approach that holds some promise for route-to-route extrapolation is physiologically based pharmacokinetic (PBPK) modelling, discussed below (Andersen *et al.*, 1987a; Corley *et al.*, 1990; Clewell and Jamot, 1994; Reitz *et al.*, 1996).

Issues in Dose–Response Assessment

There are some notable controversies associated with low-dose modelling, particularly for carcinogens (Gaylor *et al.*, 1993; Hill and Hoover, 1997; Faustman, 1997; Farland and Tuxen, 1997). Unlike the early years of cancer theory and risk assessment, we are now aware that there are at least three and probably eight distinct classes of carcinogens (Butterworth, 1993; Paustenbach, 1995). These classes differ in a number of ways, and the appropriate methods for estimating associated cancer risks differ as such. The dose extrapolation method applied to low-level exposure to a cytotoxicant or promoter should be different to that used for an initiator or complete genotoxicant. Indeed, for those compounds in which high-dose exposure results in rapid cell turnover as a mechanism of tumorigenicity, a practical threshold dose is likely to exist (Ames *et al.*, 1987; Andersen *et al.*, 1991). For genotoxicants, on the other hand, evidence supports a non-threshold mechanism. An additional criticism of the current regulatory approach to low-dose modelling is that the predictions of the model employed (typically the LMS) are not responsive to the dose–response curve, a concept that should be anathema to every toxicologist. As demonstrated by Sielken (1987), the CPFs derived from even wildly different dose–response curves typically vary by no more than an order of magnitude. Consequently, it seems inappropriate to base important and costly regulatory decisions on the results of models that do not fully incorporate all information contained in the rodent bioassays

Alternative Dose–Response Models

As a consequence of these distinctions, the use of a model which produces linearity in the low-dose region of concern is arguably appropriate for both genotoxicants and ionizing radiation. However, compounds without direct action on DNA or biomolecules (promoters and cytotoxicants) would not be expected to have a linear dose–response curve, particularly at low levels. Data seem to suggest that many (but not all) carcinogens are very nonlinear at low doses and support the notion of a threshold

(Bailer *et al.*, 1988; Purchase and Auton, 1995; Wilson, 1997; Purchase, 1998). Forcing the use of an non-threshold model in such circumstances would provide conservative, although erroneous, estimates of risk. Such an approach is not only potentially wasteful of resources but also places scientific credibility at risk ('everything causes cancer'). While attitudes have begun to shift, as witnessed by the US EPA position that the LMS model is inappropriate for estimating cancer risks for a number of agents, including TCDD, thyroid tumorigens such as ethylenethiourea (ETU) and chloroform (Paustenbach, 1995; US EPA, 1996c; Farland and Tuxen, 1997), it should be noted that virtually all CPFs currently in use were derived from the LMS and, therefore, may be suspect. Since it is unlikely that many of these toxicity criteria will be revised in the near future, the risk assessor should carefully consider whether it can be justified to revisit these values independently.

The proposed revisions to the US EPA Carcinogen Guidelines (US EPA, 1996c) do make provisions for the use of alternative models in deriving CPFs, but the time, effort and cost in developing and justifying these alternative values may not be off-set by the savings in changes in regulatory action. Other innovative techniques have been proposed for the development of toxicity criteria involving the use of the whole toxicological database rather than a single end-point from a single bioassay or by statistical or probabilistic simulation of responses (Sielken, 1989; Shlyakhter *et al.*, 1992; Velazquez *et al.*, 1994; Evans *et al.*, 1994a, b; Sielken *et al.*, 1995; Cox, 1996).

Presentation of Risk Ranges

Additional steps can be taken by the risk assessor to improve the information value of the risk assessment. Typically, risk assessments only present the upper confidence limit on the calculated risks. As illustrated in **Table 5**, there is a large difference between the best fit of the LMS (or any) model in the low-dose range and the 95% upper confidence bound at the same dose. Although it has been suggested that the best fit of the model is unstable and, therefore, not useful in estimating risk, presenting both the best fit and the lower confidence limit estimates does provide useful information in terms of bounding the risk and demonstrating the degree of uncertainty associated with that risk estimate (Sielken, 1987, 1989; Paustenbach 1989b, 1995) **(Figure 7)**. In many cases presenting a single number as the risk provides a false sense of certainty, which results in unfortunate statements such as the number of lives saved by a particular regulation. Historically, most regulators and risk managers have been unaware of the breadth of equally plausible risk estimates. Risk managers and the public need to fully informed as to the breadth of the risk estimates and the uncertainties, and providing the bounding information is a means to this end. For

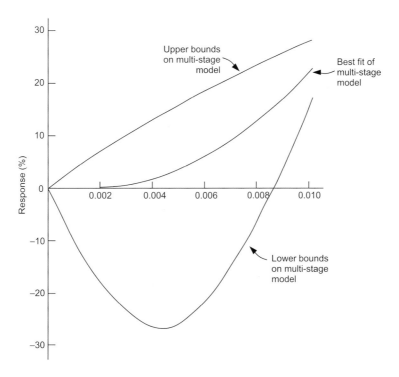

Figure 7 An illustration of the range of plausible risks using the bounding techniques inherent in the multi-stage model. In this case, the multistage model is applied to the results of a Chemical Industry Institute of Toxicology rodent bioassay of formaldehyde. Adapted from Sielken (1987).

instance, whereas the upper bound estimate on the exposure to chloroform is 1 in 10 000 (1E−4) using the LMS, the best fit of the model suggests that the risk is about 1 in 1 000 000 (1E−6) and the lower bound estimate is virtually zero (less than 1 in 10 000 000 or 1E−7). The plausible risk range in this instance is somewhere between 1 in 10 000 and zero, and is probably closer to zero given the weak nature of this carcinogen and the numerous conservatisms present in the risk assessment (Corley *et al.*, 1990). Even if required to use the results of a conservative model, the risk assessor can and should illustrate the conservatism in the model through graphical means and text. Hence the proper presentation of the chloroform risk example to managers, policy makers and the public is that the lifetime risk is no more than one additional cancer in 10 000 exposed individuals, probably much less, and perhaps zero (Paustenbach, 1995). It is the responsibility of the risk assessor to avoid focusing exclusively on upper bound risk estimates and ensure that the risk managers are presented with the full range of equally plausible risk estimates, as well as an interpretation of the meaning and uncertainty.

As stated above, there are other low-dose extrapolation models available to the risk assessor, most of which can be run on a personal computer (Sielken, 1989). Depending on the characteristics of the dose–response curve, the suspected mechanism of action and the pharmacokinetics at low doses, each model will yield plausible results (most of which are less conservative than the

LMS). The regulatory agencies are willing to entertain the results of alternate models if justified. Support for this flexibility, however, has been criticized on the basis of our imperfect understanding of carcinogenesis and less restrictive changes are often assumed to be a retreat from safety rather than a reduction in uncertainty, so taking this tack may be an uphill battle (Wilson, 1997). Because of the data requirements and probable negotiations required, use of alternative low-dose extrapolation models is probably not justified for risk assessments of limited scope (e.g. clean-up of a single industrial site), but the time and effort may be worth while if the agent commonly occurs, the regulation altered is broad-based or implementation is likely to be costly (e.g. national ambient air, water quality or occupational standards).

Physiologically Based Pharmacokinetic Modelling

Among the most promising developments toward improving the dose–response assessment is the use of physiologically based pharmacokinetic (PBPK) models (Andersen *et al.*, 1987a; NAS, 1987; Corley *et al.*, 1990; Leung, 1991; Clewell and Jamot, 1994; Leung and Paustenbach, 1995; Clewell, 1995; Clewell *et al.*, 1995; McDougal, 1996; Reitz *et al.*, 1996; Hays *et al.*, 1998). The technique allows the risk assessor to account quantitatively for the differences in the experimental species (typically a rodent) and the target species (typically a

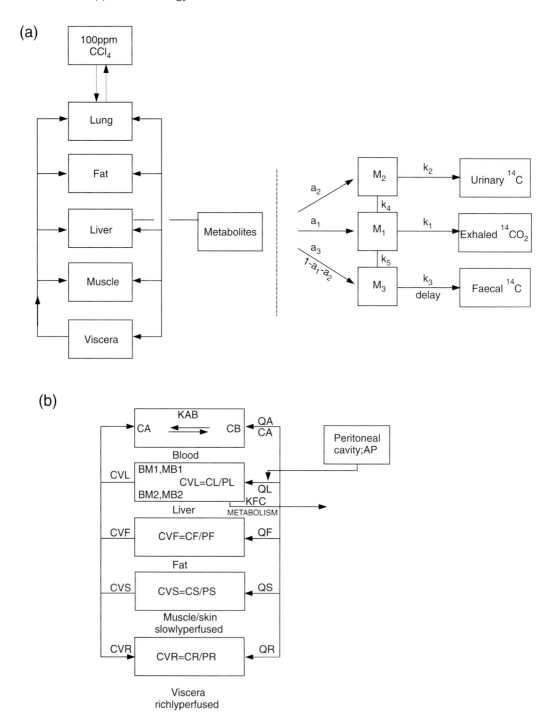

Figure 8 A schematic representation of a typical physiologically based pharmacokinetic (PBPK) model. **(a)** represents an inhalation model for volatiles (i.e. carbon tetrachloride) and **(b)** an IP exposure to an non-volatile chemical such as dioxin. The animal is divided into its relevant compartments and is validated using experimental data in combination with species-specific information on such items as blood flow, respiration rate, blood–tissue partition coefficients and metabolic rates. Once validated, the model can be used to predict target doses for other species and other routes of exposure. Adapted from Andersen *et al.* (1987a).

human). PBPK modelling divides the animal into relevant compartments and, using chemical and species-specific information, estimates the movement and behaviour of the chemical within the body **(Figure 8)**. In doing so, the model incorporates body weight, organ size, respiration rate, cardiac output and blood flow, blood and tissue partition coefficients, fat content, metabolic rates and products, mechanism of action and numerous other parameters (Watanabe and Bois, 1996). The model is then tested using experimental results separate from those used to define the parameters in order to validate its predictions (Gargas *et al.*, 1989; McDougal *et* *al.*, 1990; Mattie *et al.*, 1994a; Clewell *et al.*, 1995; Reitz *et al.*, 1996). Following the validation, the model can be used in a variety of ways including route-to-route extrapolation and scale-up from rats to humans. Complete confidence in the results of these models often requires reliance on untestable assumptions such as the amount of an unstable metabolite delivered to the target tissue (Spear *et al.*, 1991; Woodruff *et al.*, 1992; Hattis *et al.*, 1993; Clewell *et al.*, 1994), but this approach still represents a significant improvement in our ability to extrapolate from animal to man and from high doses to low doses, conduct route-to-route extrapolation, pertinent interindividual differences (e.g., age or gender) or address the issues posed by mixtures or exposure duration (Calabrese, 1986; NAS, 1987; Andersen *et al.*, 1989b; ILSI, 1992; Paustenbach, 1994; Tardiff *et al.*, 1995; Jarabek; 1995; Skrowronski *et al.*, 1997; Roy and Georgopoulos, 1998). Properly scaled data, estimates of delivered dose and inclusion of mechanism of action into PBPK models can regularly result in health-protective toxicity criteria that are 50–100-fold less conservative than those derived by less rigorous techniques. A number of PBPK models have been developed and validated for both carcinogens and non-carcinogens (Leung, 1991; Leung and Paustenbach, 1994; Paustenbach, 1994, 1995) and some have played a role in altering standards or toxicity criteria for compounds such as methylene chloride and vinyl chloride (Andersen *et al.*, 1987a; Reitz *et al.*, 1996; Bogen and Gold, 1997). The US EPA has recognized the potential for PBPK modelling both by providing guidance for the development and use of models (US EPA, 1989c) in addition to its acceptance of the results of some models in revising toxicity criteria (US EPA, 1996b).

Additionally, the US EPA has incorporated similar principles and concepts in its Integrated Uptake and Exposure Biokinetic Model (IUEBK) for estimating blood lead levels in children (US EPA, 1994b), although other PBPK models for lead such as that developed by O'Flaherty and co-workers are available and arguably provide estimates that are more responsive to the data (Polak *et al.*, 1996; Lakind, 1998). If the results of such a PBPK modelling exercise are accepted, the development and validation of these models may be costly and time consuming. Therefore, like the use of alternate dose–response models, the effort is probably only justified for issues of major national or economic import.

Scaling Factors

One step that the risk assessor can take without much effort is to determine how (or if) the toxicological data were 'scaled up' properly to predict human response. The simplifying assumption operating in most risk assessment is that the dose, expressed in equivalent terms of body weight or surface area [mg (kg body weight)$^{-1}$ day^{-1} or mg m^{-2} day^{-1}] will cause an equivalent response between species. These scaling factors are needed to account for species differences in body weight, size, life span and metabolism (Andersen *et al.*, 1987a, 1995; Allen *et al.*, 1988; Freedman and Zeisel, 1988; Travis and White, 1988; Travis *et al.*, 1990; Travis and Morris, 1992; Watanabe *et al.*, 1992). This approach may be reasonable for non-carcinogenic compounds with short half-lives, but is probably inaccurate for carcinogens. The response between animals and humans in chronic exposures is likely to be influenced by the biological half-lives, which are likely to be different for virtually each agent (and target organ). These differences will tend to vary predictably based on a body weight to surface area ratio or life span. Scaling may be a valid assumption for carcinogens requiring activation, but may be inaccurate for carcinogens that do not require activation. For example, the US EPA originally employed surface area scaling since that provided the most conservative risk estimates per unit of dose. The Food and Drug Administration (FDA), on the other hand, relied on body weight. This resulted in the two agencies having different risk estimates for the same compound based on the same study. More recently, regulatory agencies have agreed to surface area corrections using body weight to the 2/3 or 3/4 power to adjust for pharmacokinetic differences between rodents and humans (assuming no compelling information to the contrary) (US EPA, 1996c). The reliability of using surface area corrections to extrapolate equivalent doses between species will depend on the mechanism of toxic action and necessarily on the critical form of the dose (e.g. parent chemical or metabolite concentration at a target cell or organ). In most cases when a metabolite is the toxic moiety, surface area corrections do not seem to be necessary or appropriate (Andersen *et al.*, 1987a; Reitz *et al.*, 1996).

Other dose metrics (e.g. area under the blood-time curve, time above a particular tissue concentration, peak circulating blood concentration) may also be more appropriate for different compounds. For instance, for non-genotoxic compounds with long biological half-lives, the peak concentration in a tissue multiplied by the amount of time above that level will probably be the most appropriate dose metric (Aylward *et al.*, 1996). It is clear that one method cannot be used as the basis for interspecies extrapolation for the pantheon of adverse effects possible. It is likely that the most appropriate dose metric for scaling will depend on the mechanism of action, the specific effect(s) and the toxicokinetics of the agent in question. Significant research is needed to determine the correct scaling factor for different agents and different effects. Because of when they were derived, many of the toxicity criteria in common use today may not be properly scaled (either because of the scaling factor used or whether one was used at all). It would behove the risk assessor to confirm how these criteria were derived and make appropriate alterations where necessary.

Biologically Based Modelling

While the PBPK approach improves estimates of the doses reaching the target tissue, the biological response of that target tissue is not addressed by this model or the low-dose extrapolation models currently used (Golden et al., 1997). While these models can rank classes of carcinogens, they are statistical in nature and do not account for biology in their derivation. Hence they are unable to predict accurately types of tumour, time to onset, genotoxic potential or other aspects of cancer risk.

A class of models, the so-called biologically based models, has emerged that attempts to correct these shortcomings (Clayson and Iverson, 1996). Several of these models, exemplified by the Moolgavkar–Knudson–Venzon (MKV) model (Moolgavkar, 1986; Moolgavkar et al, 1988; Wilson, 1989; Dewanji et al., 1989; Heidenreich et al., 1997; Moolgavkar and Luebeck, 1990), exist and can be incorporated with a PBPK model to create a physiologically based pharmacodynamic (PBPD) model. The MKV model is a two-stage model in which two mutations are required for tumour production and the birth and death rates of cells are estimated via clonal expansion and neoplasm growth. Such a model allows not only a better estimate of the target dose, but also predicts how the target tissue will respond by accounting for the number of mutations or cell events required for malignancy and the role of target cell birth, repair and death in the accumulation of mutations. As such, the key requirement for these models is to have a quantitative description of how the agent affects these cellular processes. Currently such information is lacking for most compounds and so this modelling is of limited utility, but it holds great promise for the future and our understanding of low-dose biological interactions (Crump, 1996). Biologically based models for end-points other than cancer (e.g. developmental) are also being considered. Based on the US EPA's recent proposed revisions to the carcinogen assessment guidelines, it should be expected that a much greater weight will be placed on assessments that attempt to account quantitatively for biological phenomena associated with different carcinogens and their mechanism of action (US EPA, 1996a). The US EPA has already considered some biologically based modelling in its reassessment of dioxin and its receptor binding capacity (Andersen et al., 1993), although the Agency's use and acceptance of this type of modelling is neither uniform nor consistent as yet. For instance, it recently rejected (or ignored) a similar biologically based modelling approach for estimating chloroform risks. This latter action resulted in the Society of Toxicology protesting that the US EPA was ignoring the best science in estimating risk and developing regulations for this compound (SOT, 1998).

Epidemiology in Context

A final recommendation for risk assessors is not to ignore the epidemiological record (Paustenbach, 1995). While epidemiological evidence is routinely denigrated by risk assessors for a variety of reasons (e.g. numbers too small, exposure uncertain, multiple exposures, heterogenous population), it seems clear that there is information of value in these studies in improving our understanding and appreciation of risk estimates (Enterline, 1987; Fingerhut et al., 1991; Stayner and Bailer, 1993; Reitz et al., 1996). Total rejection of the epidemiological record out of hand is inappropriate and unwarranted since these studies can, at the very least, establish the degree of confidence that can be placed on the results of the low-dose extrapolation models (Scheuplein and Bowers, 1995; Valberg and Watson, 1996). Such studies certainly represent a high-dose exposure to the relevant species and whatever their statistical weakness (which may now be overcome by combining similar studies through meta-analysis), they can establish some degree of confidence in the results of the low-dose extrapolation models (Gross and Berg, 1995; Federal Focus, 1996; Paddle, 1997). For instance, although the risk assessment for ethylene dibromide (EDB) predicted an extraordinarily high occupational cancer risk for workers, no excess cancer rates were observed among these workers (Hertz-Picciotto et al., 1988). Similarly, polychlorinated biphenyls (PCBs) are the archetypal environmental carcinogen; however, repeated studies of worker populations exposed long-term to very high doses have failed to find any consistent pattern of cancer (or other health effects) in these workers (Kimbrough, 1995). Often epidemiological studies containing weaknesses can be combined with retrospective exposure assessments (Stewart and Herrick, 1991) to yield stronger estimates of potential human health risks than the statistical estimates produced from models of animal bioassays (Karch and Schneiderman, 1981; Layard and Silvers, 1989; Paustenbach, 1989b, 1995; Baxter et al., 1997. An example of this effort is furnished by the repeated analysis of cancer risk associated with benzene exposure among the Pliofilm worker cohort (Paustenbach et al., 1992d; Paxton et al., 1994a, b; Schnatter et al., 1996; Crump et al., 1997).

Case Study in Dose–Response Evaluation: PBPK Modelling

PBPK models represent the best hope for improving our understanding of the toxicity of low-dose exposure to chemical agents and for re-evaluating the results of previously developed toxicity criteria. The applicability and utility of this approach can be demonstrated using the example of vinyl chloride (Reitz et al., 1996). Vinyl chloride is an industrial monomer used in the production of plastic polymers [poly(vinyl chloride)] and is a breakdown product of chlorinated solvents such as trichloro-

Table 6 Comparison between cancer risks from doses predicted by a PBPK model for vinyl chloride and actual cases of cancer observed in vinyl chloride workers exposed at least 20 years

Vinyl chloride (ppm)	ppm-years	PBPK LADD[a]	Predicted cases (per 100 000) based on PBPK dose	Observed cases (per 100 000)
50	1000	6.7	376	6.2
100	2000	13.3	747	–
200	4000	26.1	1465	42.2
	8000	–	–	152.3
500	10000	53.4	2971	–
	15000	–	–	280
1000	20000	62.6	3476	–
2000	40000	72.1	3993	–

[a] LADD = lifetime added daily dose.
Source: adapted from Reitz *et al.* (1996).

ethylene in groundwater. Although vinyl chloride has low acute toxicity, it does cause liver tumours in rodents and is one of the rare compounds known to cause cancer in humans. Workers exposed to high levels of vinyl chloride developed angiosarcoma of the liver at a much higher rate than expected. The animal dose–response curve is flat above 1000 ppm, indicating a saturatable system.

A PBPK model for vinyl chloride will reduce, but not eliminate, the uncertainty associated with dose–response extrapolation and toxicity criteria derived. It can, however, provide a quantitative description of metabolic saturation, dose–route differences and species variability, ultimately leading to a more reliable estimate of risk based on the delivered rather the administered dose. The process began by parameterizing the model. Physiological constants were derived from the literature, partition coefficients were developed through a number of *in vitro* experiments, including vial equilibrium studies, and metabolic constants were measured via *in vivo* experiments. Once the model had been developed, it was validated by adjusting its predictions to independent *in vivo* data for rat, mouse and human experiments. Once validated, the PBPK model was used to extrapolate the risks between species (rats to mice; rats to humans), between doses or between routes of exposure. The PBPK model furnished the dose in terms of the average vinyl chloride metabolite produced per day per litre of liver tissue (Reitz *et al.*, 1996). This dose was extrapolated using the GLOBAL83 LMS model to provide a best fit and upper confidence bound estimate. This result was compared with the LMS model fitted to the top two doses as per standard US EPA protocol. The PBPK model estimates fitted the dose–response curve more consistently than that derived from the administered dose data **(Figure 9)**. The UCR for 1 μg of vinyl chloride per cubic metre of air was found to be 6×10^{-7} for the PBPK upper bound estimate and $806:5310^{-5}$ for the typical EPA upper bound estimate, a difference of approximately two orders of magnitude. The PBPK results suggest that the US EPA estimate is 150-fold too high, but are the results of the PBPK model adequately protective of human health?

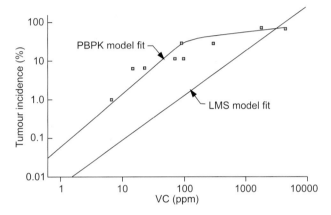

Figure 9 In this example, the validated PBPK model for vinyl chloride (VC) fits the experimental dose response data far better than the linearized multistage model upon which the US EPA makes its judgments on the potential cancer risks of various agents. (Reitz *et al.*, 1996).

There is epidemiological evidence from a vinyl chloride disease registry ($n = 14\,000$ workers) that can be used for comparison and model validation as suggested above **(Table 6)**. In this case, the validated PBPK model was found still to over-predict the observed tumour incidence by a factor of 10 at best. Therefore, the US EPA estimate would be considered at least 1500-fold overly conservative in predicting the actual cancer incidence arising from vinyl chloride exposure. The import of this effort indicates that the PBPK model reduces uncertainty around the risk estimate resulting in less conservative CPFs (and RfDs). Less conservative toxicity criteria result in higher allowable emission rates or clean-up levels, and consequently in a reduction of demands on scarce resources. This, however, takes place without sacrificing the desired public health and environmental protection. As a result of efforts such as this and other PBPK models for vinyl chloride, the US EPA is in the process of revising its cancer potency factor for vinyl chloride.

Exposure Assessment

Exposure assessment is the step that quantifies the intake of an agent as the result of contact with various environmental media (e.g. air, water, soil, food) (US EPA, 1986b, 1988c, 1992a; ATSDR, 1992). Exposure assessments can address past, current or future anticipated exposures, although uncertainties will compound when addressing questions on what might have happened or what will happen (Stewart and Herrick, 1991; Georgopoulos and Roy, 1994; Duan and Mage, 1997). Several factors influence the estimation of *absorbed* dose including the duration and route of exposure, bioavailability of an agent from the media in question, and the unique characteristics of the exposed populations. The duration of exposure is the period of time over which the exposure occurs: 'acute' refers to a single exposure, usually for less than a day; 'chronic' refers to exposures covering a substantial portion of the subject's lifetime (usually in excess of 10%); and intermediate exposures (between acute and chronic) are referred to as subchronic. Because of the number of possibilities for exposure that might exist for individuals in a population, this is typically developed as a series of hypothetical scenarios in a conceptual exposure model. For example, persons who live within 1 mile of an incinerator, children who trespass on hazardous waste sites, or persons who rely on home-grown produce, meat or milk for much of their food. These scenarios rely on often conservative assumptions about various types of exposure (e.g. soil or food ingestion, inhalation rate, ingestion of water or dermal contact with soil), populations at risk (e.g. children, adults, workers), and durations and frequency of exposure (e.g. lifetime or some fraction thereof). There are a large number of factors to consider when estimating exposure and it is a complicated process to understand and incorporate the fate and transport of agents in the environment. Concentration of an agent in the environment is essential in determining the magnitude of the absorbed dose. Such information is typically obtained from limited sampling or estimates from various fate and transport models. Modelling is most often relied on for contaminants transported in air or ground water, particularly when time or distances are important considerations. Because the distribution of contaminants, population size and make-up and behaviours may vary markedly in time and space, attempts to make the risk assessment as generalizable as possible can result in the use of highly conservative assumptions intended to be protective of the public health and the environment. The use of default assumptions and modelling results regarding exposure can introduce a significant amount of uncertainty into the risk assessment, and may introduce inaccuracies into the resultant regulatory decisions (Maxim, 1989; Paustenbach, 1989a, b, 1995; US EPA, 1989b; Barnard, 1995). Despite this, the exposure assessment step is the point in the process where the uncertainty can be reduced significantly by incorporat-

ing site and chemical-specific information whenever possible. In certain cases, the uptake of agents need not be estimated, but can be measured directly in a variety of biological tissues (Hattis, 1986; APHA, 1988; Beauchamp et al., 1992; McMillan et al., 1994; Schlenk, 1996).

The first step in the exposure assessment is qualitative: establishment of completed exposure pathways (US EPA, 1989b; ATSDR, 1992). A pathway is considered complete if there is: (1) a release source; (2) a transport mechanism; (3) a point of contact; and (4) a receptor. If any of the four components is missing, then exposure by that pathway is incomplete and should not be considered further in the risk assessment. For instance, a leaking gasoline tank (source) may lead to groundwater contamination (transport), but if downgradient populations (receptors) do not use groundwater wells (point of contact), then no drinking water exposure exists and this pathway is not relevant in the risk assessment.

It should be clear, however, that eliminating one pathway does not necessarily eliminate others. It is important that indirect exposure pathways be considered in the exposure assessment (Nessel et al., 1991; Travis and Blaylock, 1992; Magee and Smith, 1995; ILSI, 1998). In the previous example, while drinking water (a direct exposure) does not exist as a completed pathway, vapour emissions from the subsurface to indoor air (an indirect exposure) could be considered a completed pathway (Finley et al., 1996; Giardino and Andelman, 1996). Some of these indirect pathways may actually pose a greater exposure than related direct exposure pathways. For instance, the ingestion of particulate emissions deposited on soil and plants and subsequently eaten by grazing animals is a potentially important exposure pathway only recently considered in some risk assessments. Ingestion of meat and milk from these animals, depending on the agent and exposure, may pose risks as high as 500 times that of the direct inhalation risk (Stevens and Gerbec, 1988; Fries and Paustenbach, 1990; Paustenbach, 1995; Paustenbach et al., 1996; Price et al., 1996a).

One of the major failings in most exposure assessments is a failure to evaluate critically the exposure pathways and scenarios for both current and future use (Gargas and Long, 1997). This results in sites being inappropriately evaluated (e.g. an industrial property assessed as if it were residential). Such a review is important in order to avoid inappropriate expenditure of resources in pursuit of remediation that is not warranted.

Within each completed exposure pathway, a number of relevant exposure scenarios can be constructed. For example, groundwater may be used domestically for drinking and washing over extended periods by both adults and children, commercially for industrial uses with exposure limited to workers, as a source of irrigation for farming or gardening intermittently, or recreationally (e.g. filling the swimming pool). Each population has exposure variables unique to the pathway and scenario due to the different rates of intake, age, length of exposure and other physiological, behavioural and social factors. The differing contributions from each completed pathway (e.g. inhalation, ingestion or dermal contact with soil, groundwater, surface water, air or foodstuffs) in each exposure scenario (e.g. resident child, resident adult, worker, recreator, trespasser) are determined and summed to assess the overall exposure dose for that receptor (US EPA, 1989b; ATSDR, 1992).

The appropriate exposure scenarios are selected according to the populations exposed, the pathways involved and the behaviours that result in the exposures (Coad and Newhook, 1992). This comprises the conceptual exposure model as discussed. For instance, the resident child may be exposed to contaminants in drinking water and exterior soils through ingestion, inhalation and dermal contact while the working parent may be exposed to water at home and work, air in the workplace and fish from the local river, but no other source. Even when the same pathways are complete for the selected scenarios, the exposure variables for sub-populations may differ, resulting in significant variation in the final dose estimate (Scow et al., 1979; Beech, 1983; Jo et al., 1988; Byard, 1989; Paustenbach, 1989a, b, 1995; Richardson and Currie, 1993). Numerous methodologies for estimating uptake of environmental contaminants and addressing the uncertainty in those estimates have been proposed and refined in recent years (Fries and Paustenbach, 1990; McKone, 1991; McKone and Bogen, 1991, 1992; McKone and Daniels, 1991; Navidi and Luhrman, 1995; ILSI, 1998; Price et al., 1998).

Although variations abound depending on the specific needs and parameters that must be addressed in each exposure pathway and scenario, the basic calculation for estimating dose from an exposure takes the following form:

$$\text{dose} = \frac{\text{EC} \times \text{IR} \times \text{AF} \times \text{EF} \times \text{ED}}{\text{BW} \times \text{AT} \times 365 \frac{\text{days}}{\text{years}}}$$

where

dose = exposure intake, expressed in mg (kg body weight)$^{-1}$ day^{-1}

EC = the environmental concentration, expressed in units specific to the media analysed (e.g. mg kg^{-1} for soil or food, mg l^{-1} for water or mg m^{-3} for air)

IR = daily intake or contact rate, expressed in kg day^{-1} (soil or food), l day^{-1} (liquids), m^3 day^{-1} (air) or cm^2 day^{-1} (surface area exposure)

AF = absorption factor, expressed as per cent absorbed for solids (unitless) or mass absorbed per unit area per unit time for liquids (mg cm^{-2} min^{-1})

EF = exposure frequency expressed in days per year

ED = exposure duration expressed in years

BW = body weight expressed in kg

AT = averaging time; for evaluation of carcinogens, this value is set equal to 70 years; for evaluation of non-carcinogens, it is set equal to the actual duration of exposure.

The development of the quantitative exposure estimate (dose) requires the risk assessor to select the values for each variable for each completed pathway in each scenario. A number of standard assumptions are shown in **Table 7**. The choice and manipulation of these variables and the calculations become critical to the accurate expression of exposure and, ultimately, risk. Obviously, the more care is taken in selecting (or developing) population and site-specific exposure, the less uncertainty exists in the final dose estimate.

As an example of an exposure scenario evaluation, consider the determination of the dose from a long-term (30 year) exposure to dioxin-contaminated soil (Paustenbach et al., 1992b, 1996). In this case, the individual may be exposed as both a child and adult to an average soil concentration of 0.1 mg dioxin kg^{-1} soil.

Table 7 Some standard assumptions used in exposure assessment

Variable	Assumption[a]
Ingestion	
Drinking water	2 l day^{-1} (RME adult)
	1.4 l day^{-1} (adult, av.)
	1.0 l day^{-1} (child)
	0.1 l day^{-1} (incidental ingestion during swimming)
Soil	200 mg day^{-1} (child, av.)
	800 mg day^{-1} (child, 90th percentile)
Food	2000 g day^{-1} (adult, total)
Beef (home-grown)	44 g day^{-1} (av.)
100 g day^{-1} (all sources)	75 g day^{-1} (RME)
Dairy (home-grown)	160 g day^{-1} (av.)
400 g day^{-1} (all sources)	300 g day^{-1} (RME)
Fruit (home-grown)	28 g day^{-1} (av.)
140 g day^{-1} (all sources)	42 g day^{-1} (RME)
Vegetables (home-grown)	50 g day^{-1} (av.)
200 g day^{-1} (all sources)	80 g day^{-1} (RME)
Sport fish	30 g day^{-1} (av.)
	140 g day^{-1} (RME)
Inhalation	10 m^3 day^{-1} (av. 8 h shift.)
	20 m^3 day^{-1} (adult, av.)
	30 m^3 day^{-1} (RME)
Body weight	13.2 kg (2–5 yr)
	20.8 kg (6 yr)
	70 kg (adult, av.)
Lifespan	70 yr
Exposed skin area	0.2 m^2 (adult, av.)
	0.53 m^2 (adult, RME)
	1.94 m^2 (male bathing)
	1.69 m^2 (female bathing)
Showering	7 min (av.)
(5 min. shower uses 40 gallons)	12 min (90th percentile)
Residence time	9 yr (av.)
	30 yr (RME)

Source: US EPA (1996a).
[a] RME - Reasonable Maximally Exposure

Other variables used in this evaluation are either literature-derived, measured or modelled. The completed pathways for this soil exposure scenario include: (1) ingestion of soil; (2) dermal contact with soil; (3) inhalation of dust; and (4) ingestion of garden produce. The total scenario dose is represented by the sum of the doses from each completed pathway.

Soil Ingestion Dose

$$\text{dose} = \frac{EC_{soil} \times EF \times AF_O}{CF \times AT} \times \left(\frac{IR_A \times ED_A}{BW_A} + \frac{IR_C \times ED_C}{BW_C} \right)$$

where

A	=	adult
C	=	child
EC_{soil}	=	average dioxin concentration in soil (0.1 mg kg^{-1})
BW	=	body weight (15 kg, child; 70 kg, adult)
AT	=	averaging time (70 years or 25 550 days)
EF	=	exposure frequency (365 days per year)
ED	=	exposure duration (6 years, child; 24 years, adult; 30 years total)
AF_O	=	oral absorption factor (0.4 oral bioavailability)
IR	=	ingestion rate (100 mg day^{-1}, child; 50 mg day^{-1}, adult)
CF	=	conversion factor (10^6 mg kg^{-1})

hence

$$\text{dose} = \frac{(0.1 \text{ mg kg}^{-1}) \times (365 \text{ days}) \times (0.4)}{(10^6 \text{ mg kg}^{-1}) \times (25\,550 \text{ days})}$$
$$\times \left[\frac{(50 \text{ mg day}^{-1} \times (24 \text{ yr})}{(70 \text{ kg})} + \frac{(100 \text{ mg day}^{-1}) \times (6 \text{ yr})}{(15 \text{ kg})} \right]$$

In this example, the estimated dose from soil ingestion is 3.2×10^{-8} mg (kg body weight)$^{-1}$ day^{-1}

Dermal Contact Dose

$$\text{dose} = \frac{EC_{soil} \times EF \times AF_D \times Adh}{CF \times AT} \times \left(\frac{SA_A \times ED_A}{BW_A} + \frac{SA_C \times ED_C}{BW_C} \right)$$

where

A	=	adult
C	=	child
EC_{soil}	=	average dioxin concentration in soil (0.1 mg kg^{-1})
BW	=	body weight (15 kg, child; 70 kg, adult)
AT	=	averaging time (70 years or 25 550 days)
EF	=	exposure frequency (365 days per year)
ED	=	exposure duration (6 years, child; 24 years, adult; 30 years total)
AF_D	=	dermal absorption factor (0.01 dermal bioavailability)
SA	=	exposed skin surface area (2199 cm^2, child; 2836 cm^2, adult)

Adh = soil adherence factor (1.0 mg cm^{-2})
CF = conversion factor (10^6 mg kg^{-1})

Hence

$$\text{dose} = \frac{(0.1 \text{ mg kg}^{-1}) \times (365 \text{ days}) \times (0.01) \times (1.0 \text{ mg cm}^{-2})}{(10^6 \text{ mg kg}^{-1}) \times (25\,550 \text{ days})} \times$$
$$\left[\frac{(2836 \text{ cm}^2 \text{ day}^{-1}) \times (24 \text{ yr})}{(70 \text{ kg})} + \frac{(2199 \text{ cm}^2 \text{ day}^{-1}) \times (6 \text{ yr})}{(15 \text{ kg})} \right]$$

In this example, the estimated dose from dermal contact with soil is 1.8×10^{-8} mg (kg body weight)$^{-1}$day^{-1}

Dust Inhalation Dose

$$\text{dose} = \frac{EC_{soil} \times PC \times EF \times AF_I}{CF \times AT} \times \left(\frac{IR_A \times ED_A}{BW_A} + \frac{IR_C \times ED_C}{BW_C} \right)$$

where

A	=	adult
C	=	child
EC_{soil}	=	average dioxin concentration in soil (0.1 mg kg^{-1})
BW	=	body weight (15 kg, child; 70 kg, adult)
AT	=	averaging time (70 years or 25 550 days)
EF	=	exposure frequency (365 days per year)
ED	=	exposure duration (6 years, child; 24 years, adult; 30 years total)
AF_I	=	pulmonary absorption factor (1.0 inhalation bioavailability)
PC	=	particulate concentration (measured at 0.0008 mg m^{-3})
IR	=	breathing rate (10 m^3 day^{-1}, child; 20 m^3 day^{-1}, adult)
CF	=	conversion factor (10^6 mg kg^{-1})

Hence

$$\text{dose} = \frac{(0.1 \text{ mg kg}^{-1}) \times (0.0008 \text{ mg m}^{-3}) \times (365 \text{ days}) \times (1.0)}{(10^6 \text{ mg kg}^{-1}) \times (25\,550 \text{ days})} \times$$
$$\left[\frac{(20 \text{ m}^3 \text{ day}^{-1}) \times (24 \text{ yr})}{(70 \text{ kg})} + \frac{(10 \text{ m}^3 \text{ day}^{-1}) \times (6 \text{ yr})}{(15 \text{ kg})} \right]$$

In this example, the estimated dose from dust inhalation is 1.6×10^{-11} mg (kg body weight)$^{-1}$ day^{-1}

Produce Ingestion Dose

$$\text{dose} = \frac{EC_{soil} \times EF \times AF_O \times f_v \times k_v}{CF \times AT} \times \left(\frac{IR_A \times ED_A}{BW_A} + \frac{IR_C \times ED_C}{BW_C} \right)$$

where

A	=	adult
C	=	child
EC_{soil}	=	average dioxin concentration in soil (0.1 mg kg^{-1})
BW	=	body weight (15 kg, child; 70 kg, adult)
AT	=	averaging time (70 years or 25 550 days)

EF   =   exposure frequency (365 days per year)

ED   =   exposure duration (6 years, child; 24 years, adult; 30 years total)

AF_O =   oral absorption factor (0.4 oral bioavailability)

IR   =   produce ingestion rate (50 000 mg day^{-1})

f_v =   fraction of homegrown produce (0.38)

k_v =   soil to produce transfer coefficient (0.00145)

CF   =   conversion factor (10^{6}mg kg^{-1})

Hence

$$\text{dose} = \frac{(0.1 \text{ mg kg}^{-1}) \times (365 \text{ days}) \times (0.4) \times (0.38) \times (0.00145)}{(10^6 \text{ mg kg}^{-1}) \times (25\,550 \text{ days})} \times$$

$$\left[\frac{(50\,000 \text{ mg day}^{-1}) \times (24 \text{ yr})}{(70 \text{ kg})} + \frac{(50\,000 \text{ mg day}^{-1}) \times (6 \text{ yr})}{(15 \text{ kg})} \right]$$

In this example, the estimated dose from ingestion of contaminated produce is 1.2×10^{-7} mg (kg body weight)$^{-1}$ day^{-1}

The estimated dioxin dose from the soil pathway then becomes the sum of the four individual components making up this pathway: soil ingestion [3.2×10^{-8} mg (kg body weight)$^{-1}$ day^{-1}], dermal contact with soil [1.8×10^{-8} mg (kg body weight)$^{-1}$ day^{-1}], dust inhalation [1.6×10^{-11} mg (kg body weight)$^{-1}$ day^{-1}] and ingestion of contaminated produce [1.2×10^{-7} mg (kg body weight)$^{-1}$ day^{-1}], or 1.7×10^{-7} mg (kg body weight)$^{-1}$ day^{-1}. In this case, the exposure is dominated by the consumption of contaminated produce, which is based in turn on assumptions of the amount of produce consumed daily, the percentage that is from home gardens, the transfer rate of dioxin from soil to plant and the oral bioavailibility of dioxin to humans. Such assumptions will vary among different populations, different locations, different plants and soil types and different periods of time. The source and quality of assumptions will influence the results of the exposure assessment, and may warrant additional site or chemical-specific research to improve the estimates of dose. The most comprehensive source of exposure assumptions is the US EPA's *Exposure Factors Handbook* (US EPA, 1996a), although valuable information can be found in the health physics and biomedical literature and elsewhere (Snyder, 1975; AIHC, 1994; ILSI, 1998). Similar (or variant) formulae for assessing exposure and calculating dose can be found in a variety of sources (US EPA, 1989b; ATSDR, 1992; Derelanko, 1995).

Many past and some current risk assessments are characterized by the use of 'worst-case' scenarios dominated by the 'maximally exposed individual' (MEI) (Goldstein, 1989; Hawkins, 1991). This approach was first adopted in an attempt to be protective of public health and the environment. To accomplish this goal, conservative exposure values (usually the 95% upper confidence limit) were used in the estimate of exposure and dose. Because these were extreme values with a low probability

of being true individually, the combination of many such variables created estimates of exposure that defied belief, but was certainly protective by definition (Paustenbach, 1986; Maxim, 1989; AIHC, 1997; Cogliano, 1997; Beck and Cohen, 1997). Current regulatory and scientific guidelines recognize the inappropriateness of an MEI approach for all but screening level risk assessments (Paustenbach, 1989b, 1995; Paustenbach *et al.*, 1992b). In other words, if a worst-case scenario predicts an insignificant risk, then one can be reasonably assured that no real risk exists. The prediction of risk under such circumstances is not, however, evidence of a hazard, but calls for additional evaluation of the exposure. In this sense, risk assessment should be an iterative process; however, it rarely is in practice. Continually refining the risk assessment helps identify not only risk drivers, but also areas of uncertainty that would benefit from additional evaluation or research.

While it is agreed that it is inappropriate to rely on MEI-type evaluation of exposure and risk (also called reasonably maximal exposed or RME scenarios), it is also recognized that so-called 'reasonable' person assessments (also called most likely estimate or MLE scenarios) may fail to characterize certain segments of the population adequately (Smith, 1987; Richardson and Currie, 1993; Fitzgerald *et al.*, 1995; Edelman and Burmaster, 1997). The characterization of exposure to the majority (95%) of the population can be best represented by a combination of average and upper bound estimates of exposure under the notion that no single individual can achieve maximal values for all exposure variables simultaneously and continuously. At the same time, more emphasis is being placed on the recognizing that various groups have special exposure considerations (e.g. subsistence fishermen) that may need to be taken into account in the risk assessment (Murray and Burmaster, 1994; Ruffle *et al.*, 1994). One method of assessing highly or uniquely exposed populations in time or space is to employ 'micro-exposure' techniques where such populations exist and are of issue (Lioy *et al.*, 1992; Price *et al.*, 1996b).

While high-exposure groups must not be ignored, the initial focus of the risk assessment should always be on the exposure experienced by the majority of the population. For instance, a risk assessment based on an assumption that a person consumes 100 g of fish per day over the course of their lifetime (the 99th percentile) when the average fish consumption rate is 16 g per day should acknowledge that the dose for 99% of the population will be lower and probably much lower. It is suggested that risk assessors avoid this problem by describing the number of persons associated with each exposure level and also provide information on the upper and lower bounds of those exposure estimates and the associated risks (Paustenbach, 1995). Such information is crucial for managers and the public to appreciate the meaning of the risk assessment and make reasoned judgements as to the resources that should be devoted to addressing these risks (Johnson and Slovic, 1995; Mertz et al., 1998).

Issues in Exposure Assessment

A major responsibility for the risk assessor is to make their exposure assessments as realistic and site-specific as possible, and avoid compounding conservatisms that misrepresent the situation (Burmaster and Harris, 1993; Bogen, 1994b; Cullen, 1994; Barnard, 1995; Beck and Cohen, 1997). If at one time such conservatism was acceptable because knowledge was lacking, it is now a sign of technical weakness since much research in the area has been conducted in the past 10 years. For instance, although it is a standard assumption that an adult breathes at rate of 20 $m^3 day^{-1}$, research on the relation between breathing and metabolism suggests that this assumption may over- or underestimate breathing rates and hence exposure (Layton, 1993). Similarly, although 1.4 l day^{-1} is arguably an accurate representation of the average daily water intake by adults, it is known that in certain areas of the country or world the water intake is much higher (e.g. 3 l day^{-1}). Better population-or site-specific assumptions for these and other variables are available and ought to be incorporated into risk assessments in place of default assumptions whenever possible.

Multiplying together the 95% upper confidence limits of numerous exposure variables used in the exposure assessment does not necessarily result in a 95% upper confidence limit on the overall dose, but may result in a significantly more conservative estimate of exposure or dose (> 99% upper confidence limit), which again may ultimately misrepresent the true nature of the risk to the risk manager and the public (Cogliano, 1997). This kind of problem is typified by a screening analysis of risks associated with dioxin emissions from an incinerator (Nessel et al., 1991; Paustenbach, 1995). Using a child as the receptor, regulators assumed that the child resided very close to the plant in the downwind direction, ate exterior soil each day, ate fish from an adjoining pond, consumed water from the pond, food came from the family garden and livestock and milk from the family cow (Paustenbach et al., 1992a, 1996). All consumption and contact with contaminated media were at a very high level (95% percentile). Under these conditions, it is not surprising that risks in excess of 1 in 100 were predicted, but what value does such an assessment serve when all authorities recognize that such a person does not exist in reality. Unfortunately, these estimates are the ones typically reported by the media and embraced by opponents of both the specific projects and the risk assessment process as a whole. Such risk assessments serve no purpose, do little to identify true risk or illuminate uncertainties and do not reassure the public or policy makers that they are being protected or the right decisions are

being made (Barnard, 1995; Milloy, 1995; Sielken et al., 1995; Johnson and Slovic, 1995; Mertz et al., 1998; Younes and Amoruso, 1998).

Exposure assessment is the one area where the individual risk assessor can truly influence the process through either careful review of the literature, applied research or both. An example of the benefit of applied research in exposure assessment is furnished by our knowledge of soil ingestion in children (one of the major contributors to risk in many assessments) (Paustenbach, 1995; Johnson and Kissel, 1996). Since the first estimate of soil ingestion by children was published 15 years ago (Kimbrough et al., 1984), research on the topic has resulted in a refinement of this exposure variable, reducing it by two to three orders of magnitude (LaGoy, 1987; Calabrese et al., 1989, 1996; Calabrese and Stanek, 1991; Stanek and Calabrese, 1991, 1995a, b; Thompson and Burmaster, 1991). **Table 8** presents a historical view of the changes in soil ingestion estimates. Similar research on adults soil ingestion is needed due to the existence of unverified assumptions (Hawley, 1985; LaGoy, 1987; Proctor et al., 1997) or preliminary results (Calabrese et al., 1990) and is currently under way. A similar effort has been conducted to identify the most appropriate factor(s) to assess the adherence of soil to exposed skin for purposes of calculating systemic dermal uptake (Driver et al., 1989; Finley et al., 1994b; Mattie et al., 1994b; Sheppard and Evenden, 1994; Holmes et al., 1996; Kissel et al., 1996a, b; US EPA, 1996a; Finley and Scott, 1998). It is recognized that different soils adhere differently to different areas of the body and this information becomes important in refining risk assessments involving dermal exposure and absorption (Kissel et al., 1996a, b; Finley and Scott, 1998). The available studies on soil adherence provide sufficient data to generate point estimates of soil adherence, but their representativeness to the general population is uncertain. Recent efforts measuring adherence to different skin surfaces (e.g. hands, forearms, lower legs, feet and face) under different work and recreation conditions found that the adherence to hands alone varied over five orders of magnitude (Kissel et al., 1996b). Differences between pre- and post-activity adherence also indicated the episodic nature of dermal contact with the soil. Obviously additional research into the importance of dermal exposure with soil and other media is needed in order to make meaningful exposure estimates. This effort together with age-specific time–activity patterns (US EPA, 1996a; Dorre, 1997; Zartarian et al., 1995, 1997, 1998) and information on dermal absorption (modelled or measured), would be critical to reducing uncertainty in this area (McKone, 1990; Burmaster and Maxwell, 1991; McKone and Howd, 1992; Wilschut et al., 1995). More work remains to be done in this and other areas to refine the exposure variables used in this step.

It again becomes the risk assessor's job to identify and incorporate the best science in the exposure assessment

Table 8 Historical estimates of childhood soil ingestion rates used in health risk assessment (1984–96)

Source	Soil ingested (mg day^{-1})
Kimbrough *et al.* (1984)[a]	10000
Hawley (1985)	200
Paustenbach (1987)[b]	100
Binder *et al.* (1986)[c]	100–600
Clausing *et al.* (1987)[c]	100–1000
Van Wijnen *et al.* (1989)[c]	100–150
Calabrese *et al.* (1989)[c]	10–40
Davis *et al.* (1990)[c]	25–80
de Silva (1994)	4
Appling (personal communication, 1996)	10

[a] Childhood soil ingestion estimate developed for Times Beach Risk Assessment
[b] Alternate estimate for Times Beach childhood soil ingestion
[c] Quantitative tracer study of childhood soil ingestion

whenever feasible. In the above example, failure to embrace the best available soil ingestion data still results in ingestion risks from contaminated soils driving most risk assessments. This amounts to a risk management decision embedded in the risk assessment, contravening the intent of the NRC recommendation separating risk assessment and risk management. Hazard, however, is not always what it seems or what a risk assessment indicates. Interestingly, a number of remedial actions of soil contaminated with persistent compounds (e.g. lead, PCBs, DDT) resulted in no observable change in body burdens among exposed populations (Weitzman *et al.*, 1993; Kimbrough, 1995; US EPA, 1995b). This suggests that either the agents were not bioavailable enough to be absorbed in the first place, or that other unaccounted for sources of exposure exist. In this case, house dust may serve as a critical reservoir for indirect exposure from soil (Que Hee *et al.*, 1985; Lioy *et al.*, 1993; Roberts, *et al.*, 1993; Simcox *et al.*, 1995; Paustenbach *et al.*, 1997b) and failure to clean the house may result in continued exposure and risk through dust ingestion and inhalation despite an expensive and time-consuming remedial action (Thatcher and Layton, 1995; Lioy *et al.*, 1997; Trowbridge and Burmaster, 1997). In such cases, the simple expedient of paving or tilling soil and cleaning the house may be a more appropriate remedial action than a massive soil removal project.

Bioavailability

Other areas of applied research that can be employed in the exposure assessment process include an appreciation of bioavailability, speciation, chemical fate and the role of biological monitoring. As suggested above, bioavailability will become an increasing important aspect of the exposure assessment process (Hrudey *et al.*, 1996; Risk Policy Report, 1998b). Alexander (1995) has shown that a variety of organic chemicals in soil lose the ability to interact with biological receptors over time despite the fact that the chemical concentration in soil remains lar-

gely the same. The alteration in bioavailability extends across the various routes of exposure as well (Lucier *et al.*, 1986; Umbreit *et al.*, 1986a, b; Shu *et al.*, 1988a, b; Skrowronski *et al.*, 1988; Ruoff *et al.*, 1994). Inorganic compounds, even those posing potentially significant degrees of hazard (e.g. cyanide), react similarly (Davis *et al.*, 1993, 1997; Shifrin *et al.*, 1996). These losses in hazard potential are presumably due to (irreversible?) chemical interactions with soil constituents. **Table 9** indicates that the bioavailability of lead added to soil is immediately halved and that it is further reduced over time (Chaney *et al.*, 1984). This suggests that an assumption of 100% bioavailability of this compound (and others) from soil is erroneous, particularly if the issue is one of long-standing. It is also clear that the environmental media in which the compound occurs will also influence its uptake into the body (Ruoff *et al.*, 1994). The US EPA recognized this fact when it developed two RfDs for manganese depending on whether it occurred in solid matrices (e.g. food, soil) or water (US EPA, 1998a). One simple method to improve estimates of bioavailability is to conduct extractions under more biologically relevant conditions.

Bench-scale extraction experiments in simulated gastric fluids or sweat can be used to measure cheaply and accurately how readily environmental residues can be released from the media in which they occur (Ruby *et al.*, 1992; Horowitz and Finley, 1993). As with inhalation of vapours or ingestion of solutions, both the release and absorption rates of agents from an environmental matrix (e.g. soil) across biological membranes need to be incorporated into the risk assessment where such data are available, and generated where absent. This need is particularly important for assessing dermal exposure. The problem for materials in aqueous solutions is less problematic than from solid matrices (Leung and Paustenbach, 1994). For liquids, permeability constants expressed in terms of agent weight per unit area per unit time (mg cm^{-2} min^{-1}) have been developed for a number of agents and *in vivo* and *in vitro* techniques or

Table 9 Effect of matrix and ageing on the bioavailability of lead from soil[a]

Treatment		Tibial lead (ppm)[b]	Relative lead absorption
Lead acetate (ppm diet)	Soil lead (ppm)		
–	–	0.3 (0.3)	–
–	11.3	0	–
50	–	247 (10)	100
50	11.3	130 (30)	53
–	706	40 (6)	16
–	995	108 (26)	44
–	1080	37 (7.3)	15
–	1260	53.6 (7)	22
–	10420	173 (22)	70

[a] Lead acetate in the diet results in an increase in tibial lead whereas lead acetate mixed with soil is only 50% as well absorbed. Aged lead from garden soil must reach high levels before significant absorption occurs
[b] Standard deviation in parentheses.
Source: adapted from Chaney et al. (1984).

mathematical models exist to develop similar flux rates if needed (Bartek et al., 1972; Wester and Noonan, 1980; Guy et al., 1982; Frantz, 1990; Surber et al., 1990; Shatkin and Brown, 1991; Barber et al., 1992; McKone, 1993; Bogen, 1994a; Bogen et al., 1998). From soil, however, the typical approach in many risk assessments has been to assume a constant percentage absorbed from soil adhered to skin as a default. For volatiles, an absorption rate of 25% has been used whereas for semi-volatiles and inorganics, absorption rates of 10% and 1% have been used, respectively. Some experimental data for absorption are available for a few agents (e.g. PCBs, DDT, dioxin, benzo[a]pyrene), which suggests that a simple assumption of a constant percentage absorbed may over- or underestimate the dose depending on the agent, co-contaminants, soil type, exposure duration and similar considerations (Shu et al., 1988a; Skrowronski et al., 1988; Wester et al., 1993a, b). The impact of this default approach results in an instantaneous dermal dose being assumed regardless of whether the soil remains in contact with the skin for 1 min or 1 day. This assumption, together with the questionable route-to-route adjustment of toxicity criteria from oral to dermal previously discussed, results in the dermal absorption of agents from soil, which arguably should present a minor exposure and risk in most cases, being a major driver in the risk assessment of soil-bound contaminants. Additionally, the calculated dermal dose is generally intractable to changes in exposure assumptions that markedly alter doses from other routes of exposure (e.g. ingestion) since the absorption is assumed to occur instantaneously. However, a lag time, ranging from minutes to days, exists for pure chemicals and may be even more significant for soil-bound contaminants (Leung and Paustenbach, 1994). From an exposure standpoint, if the exposure duration is shorter than the lag time, it is unlikely that any significant systemic absorption occurs (Gargas et al., 1989). Models that incorporate the time factor (e.g. fugacity) are available (McKone, 1990; Bur-master and Maxwell, 1991; McKone and Howd, 1992; Phillips et al., 1993; Wilschut et al., 1995) and the development and use of such refined models ought to be encouraged. Further, research in the area of dermal absorption of soil-bound contaminants ought to be performed in order to improve both data and modelling approaches. The US EPA and other agencies provide some useful information and suggestions on assessing dermal absorption of contaminants (US EPA, 1992b; CDTS, 1994), although much of it is theory and practical applications or recommendations for risk assessment are limited.

Case Study in Exposure Assessment: Biomonitoring and Bioavailability

Owing to past disposal activities, a large number of residential properties are contaminated with hexavalent chromium and may present a risk to inhabitants (ESE, 1989; NJDEP, 1990; Fagliano et al., 1997). Air monitoring indicates no measurable chromium in ambient and indoor air, so soil and dust ingestion is the presumptive primary route of exposure (Falerios et al., 1992; Finley and Mayhall, 1994). Does the presence of high levels of hexavalent chromium in soil, therefore, pose a risk? A screening risk assessment indicates that an ingestion hazard exists; however, directed research indicates otherwise. Following informed consent, human volunteers consumed sterile soil containing high levels of hexavalent chromium over a 3-day period. Additionally, capsules containing hexavalent chromium at the RfD level were also consumed over an additional 3-day period. The 24 h urine output was collected over both dosing periods and urinary chromium levels were measured. As illustrated in **Figure 10**, consumption of chromium in soil resulted in no measurable increase in urinary chromium levels whereas consumption of chromium at RfD concentrations caused a significant elevation of chromium levels.

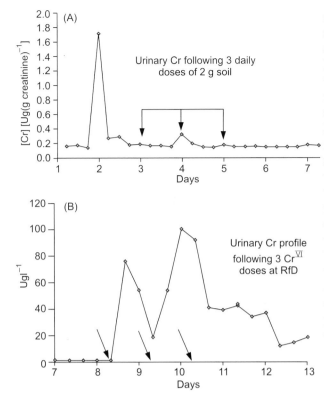

Figure 10 In order to determine if chromium (both hexavalent and trivalent) in soil was bioavailable and so presented a potential risk to individuals living on or near contaminated areas as suggested by a risk assessment, a two-pronged experiment was conducted. Adapted from Gargas *et al.* (1994) and Finley *et al.* (1996a). Sterilized soil containing high levels of chromium was ingested over three consecutive days by human volunteers and 24 h urine samples were collected and analysed for chromium. Additionally, hexavalent chromium at a concentration equivalent to the RfD was also ingested and a similar collection and analysis were performed. (A) represents the results of the soil ingestion experiment for a single individual and indicates that little or no impact on urinary chromium output was observed even when soil was known to be ingested; (B) represents the results of the ingestion of hexavalent chromium at the RfD level and suggests that even a 'safe' dose of hexavalent chromium has a clear impact on the urinary output of chromium. This suggests that any exposure to soil-bound chromium would have to be at substantially higher levels in order to pose a potential health risk.

These results suggest that no hazard is presented by hexavalent chromium in soil since little or no hexavalent chromium is apparently absorbed from whatever incidental soil ingestion occurs (Paustenbach *et al.*, 1991a, b; Sheehan *et al.*, 1991; Gargas *et al.*, 1994; Finley *et al.*, 1996; Paustenbach *et al.*, 1997d).

Case Study in Exposure Assessment: Controlled Human Testing

Hexavalent chromium is also known to cause allergic contact dermatitis (ACD) in sensitized individuals (Bur-

rows, 1983). Because of the presence of hexavalent chromium is soil, concern was expressed over a possible dermatological or allergic hazard to exposed individuals. Based on 1950s patch testing for establishing ACD threshold and an assumption of 100% bioavailability, regulators established a clean-up level for hexavalent chromium of 10 ppm (Bagdon, 1989; Bagdon and Hazen, 1991; NJDEP, 1992). Is this an appropriate remedial goal? Following informed consent, individuals already sensitized to hexavalent chromium were patch tested to identify the response threshold and determine the equivalent concentration in soil (Swann and Eschenroeder, 1983; Nethercott *et al.*, 1994). Additionally, the extractability of chromium from soil was determined using actual human sweat (Horowitz and Finley, 1993; Wainman *et al.*, 1994). This work established that the threshold for ACD in sensitized individuals was 0.089 μg of hexavalent chromium per square centimetre of skin **(Table 10)**. This was determined to be equivalent to 455 ppm of hexavalent chromium in soil. Further, less than 0.1% of hexavalent chromium was found to be extracted from soil by sweat. These findings suggest that hexavalent chromium levels in soil less than 10 000 ppm would be unlikely to result in ACD in exposed, sensitized individuals. Unsensitized individuals would be unlikely to have any dermatological response (Paustenbach *et al.*, 1992a; Horowitz and Finley, 1993). This type of work illustrates the utility of applied research in checking the reliability of risk assessments and presents a valid approach for deriving protective levels for non-cancer (e.g. allergic) hazards in soil or other media (Robinson *et al.*, 1989; Horowitz and Finley, 1994; Proctor *et al.*, 1998).

Table 10 Cumulative dermal response of 54 participants sensitized to hexavalent chromium (Cr^{VI}) to various concentrations of Cr^{VI} in an attempt to determine the elicitation threshold for allergic contact dermatitis (ACD)[a]

Cr^{VI} (μg cm^{-2})	Minimum elicitation threshold response (%)	Cumulative response (%)
0.018	1/54 (2)	1/54 (2)
0.088	4/54 (7)	5/54 (9)
0.18	5/54 (9)	10/54 (19)
0.88	22/54 (41)	32/54 (59)
4.4	22/54 (41)	54/54 (100)

[a] This information was subsequently used to assess the risk of ACD from soil contaminated with Cr^{VI}.
Source: adapted from Nethercott *et al.* (1994).

Chemical Fate

Risk assessors ought to incorporate, when possible, information on the fate of chemicals in the environment in their exposure estimates (Keith, 1988). Many organic compounds tend to degrade over time and may disappear from exposed surfaces relatively quickly or otherwise change (Paustenbach, 1989b; Alexander, 1995). As suggested above, inorganic compounds may also undergo changes in the environment over time that effects their fate (Chaney *et al.*, 1984; Shifrin *et al.*, 1996). Influencing factors include degradation by sunlight, soil and water, microbes, evaporation and chemical interactions. The resultant changes can dramatically alter the outcome of exposure assessments (Paustenbach, 1989b; Copeland *et al.*, 1993). For instance, most criticism of incinerators has focused on the inhalation risk of dioxin emitted from the stacks. As it turns out, the environmental half-life of dioxin (as a vapour) is only 90 min as a result of photolytic degradation. In contrast, the half-life for dioxin in soil or fly-ash is 50–500 years. The focus of the concern often turns out not to be the main risk issue when environmental fate is considered since levels and availability change over time (Paustenbach, 1995). Incorporation of half-life data into risk assessments can have substantial benefits to improving the understanding of the potential exposures and risks associated with a specific situation (Paustenbach, 1989b; Borgert *et al.*, 1995). In a similar manner, the risk from persistent contaminants (e.g. DDT) in fish has usually been assessed using the results from the analysis of raw fish fillets in combination with assumptions about the size and number of fish meals. The effects of cleaning and cooking on these residues are not typically considered, but have been shown to reduced substantially in many cases (i.e. 50% or greater) (Morgan *et al.*, 1997; Wilson *et al.*, 1998). Since many of these risk assessments form the basis of fish advisories or bans with potentially significant economic repercussions, there is obviously an important reason to make these estimates of exposure as accurate as possible. Additionally, since there are known health benefits to the consumption of fish, recommendations against eating fish based on a theoretical risk need to be rigorously defended.

Biomonitoring and Human Testing

Other methods of improving exposure estimates include incorporation of the results of biological monitoring (both human and ecological), human testing or human use surveys into risk assessment (Hattis, 1986; Henderson *et al.*, 1992; McMillan *et al.*, 1994; Hewitt *et al.*, 1995; Del Pup *et al.*, 1996; Engels and Vaughan, 1996; Hamar *et al.*, 1996; Holdsway, 1996; Schlenk, 1996; Timbrell, 1996; Wolfe, 1996). In the above example of fish advisories, the consumption rate is based on human use surveys although typically these are national surveys or surveys of specific populations, including subsistence fishermen (Roseberry and Currie, 1991; Richardson and Currie, 1993; Ebert *et al.*, 1994; Murray and Burmaster, 1994; Price *et al.*, 1994; Ruffle *et al.*, 1994; Fitzgerald *et al.*, 1995; Stern *et al.*, 1996; US EPA, 1996a; Hoover and Hill, 1997; Thomas *et al.*, 1997). The applicability of these data to estimates of local consumption

rates or different populations may be poor, as mentioned above. The techniques for conducting such surveys are well known and can be employed with a minimum of effort. Similar techniques can be effectively employed for the consumption of other foodstuffs or to assess other exposures that entail human use (e.g. recreational resources, showering time, gardening). Such efforts are critical to improving exposure assessments by reducing the reliance on default assumptions and preventing unnecessary expenditure of scarce resources. Directed human testing such as the ingestion of chromium-contaminated soil (Gargas *et al.*, 1994) or allergic challenge testing with hexavalent chromium (Nethercott *et al.*, 1994) are examples of this approach and, as described earlier, demonstrate that such testing has a place in fine tuning or validating exposure assessment. Similar studies of dermal absorption or pharmacokinetics of chromium have also been conducted with the goal of both improving exposure assumptions and checking the predictions made in exposure and risk assessment (Stern *et al.*, 1992; Wallace *et al.*, 1993, 1997; Kerger *et al.*, 1996; Corbett *et al.*, 1997; Finley and Paustenbach, 1997). Controlled short-term human testing at levels that are not of toxicological concern can still provide important information on pharmacokinetics that are necessary to validate PBPK models or confirm experimental observations in other species without placing anyone at risk (Maibach *et al.*, 1971; Jo *et al.*, 1988; McDougal *et al.*, 1990; Mraz and Nohova, 1992; Hamar *et al.*, 1996; Kezic *et al.*, 1997). Finally, biological monitoring of exposed populations can serve as a check of the predictions of exposure assessment (Kneip and Crable, 1988; Caudill and Pirkle, 1992; McMillan *et al.*, 1994). The ability to detect small amounts of exogenous chemicals in blood, fat, breath, hair, nails, urine or faeces can represent direct evidence of either recent or chronic exposure to agents and is a superior method for assessing possible health risks than the series of mathematical equations that dominate exposure and risk assessment. For instance, despite the prediction of high risks associated with soil-bound PCBs, over a dozen biomonitoring studies of populations exposed to PCBs in soil at levels as high as 13% have found no correlation between soil PCBs and PCB body burdens (Kimbrough, 1995). Similarly, studies of lead and chromium in residential soils have found little correlation between residues of these compounds in the environment and levels in biological tissues, despite conclusions to the contrary by risk assessments (Weitzman *et al.*, 1993; US EPA, 1995a; Finley and Paustenbach, 1997). In situations where reliable methods for biological monitoring of human or wildlife populations exist, consideration should be given to employing these techniques to improve the regulatory decisions required. Anderson *et al.* (1993) discussed the characteristics of a biological monitoring programme to provide useful information for exposure and risk assessment.

Consideration of Background

An equally difficult issue in making decisions about exposure involves the proper consideration and evaluation of the field data in terms of background occurrence, statistical analysis and analytical issues. Until recently, background levels of compounds identified as potential hazards were rarely considered in risk assessments. This is particularly relevant in the case of inorganic compounds which occur naturally in soils, sediments, water and food, but may also be important in consideration of synthetic organic compounds with multiple sources in the home, workplace or environment (Shacklette and Boerngen, 1984; US EPA, 1987; Abermathy and Poirier, 1997; Brown et al., 1997; Manca et al., 1997). Failure to consider background occurrence may result in inappropriate identification of exposures in a risk assessment and ultimately to inappropriate or unnecessary regulatory action (LaGoy and Schulz, 1993; Paustenbach, 1995; Smith et al., 1996). Statistical design and analysis of sampling data may also skew the results of the exposure assessment and ultimately the risk assessment as a whole. Environmental field sampling has generally been biased toward identifying problem areas. Hence stained soils, water with multi-coloured slicks, or sediments adjacent to outfalls are usually the source of data used to identify contamination and make judgements on potential hazards and exposures. Unfortunately, such bias may mis-characterize the extent and type of contamination and result most typically in an overestimation of risk associated with a site or facility. As noted in recent US EPA guidance for exposure assessment (US EPA, 1992a), inappropriate statistical analysis of environmental data represents one of the most easily corrected of the common errors in exposure analysis. Exposure assessment would benefit from the use of a random sampling programme of sufficient size to supplement data collected during field investigations. The theory and design of such sampling programmes are readily available (Gilbert, 1987; Keith, 1988, Dakins et al., 1996). Failing that, explicit consideration and recognition of the inherent bias in field sampling data could improve the qualitative and quantitative decisions at this stage of the risk assessment process and in subsequent steps.

Statistical and Analytical Issues

In the same vein, despite the use of very precise and reproducible analytical methods, the use of chemical concentrations to estimate exposure is fraught with uncertainty. Owing to resource availability, it has often been the case that a single round of analytical results or samples collected for other purposes (US EPA, 1989a) serves as input and the surrogate for long-term or lifetime exposure. As pointed out above, chemical concentrations vary over both time and space (Paustenbach, 1989b). To use, for instance, the (estimated) average

dose may seriously over- or underestimate the actual dose received over time. Additionally, the average dose may be less important in the biological scheme of things than peak exposures or exposures at specific times (i.e. developmental), and ought to be considered as such in the evaluation of exposure (Brown and Hoel, 1986; Kodell et al., 1987; Andersen et al., 1987b; Murdoch et al., 1992; Paustenbach, 1994; Verhagen et al., 1996). Techniques do exist for estimating long-term exposure from short-term data (Buck et al., 1995, 1997; Slob, 1996; Stanek et al., 1998), but the reliability of these estimates is uncertain. Similarly, a variety of mathematical or bench-scale models exist that have been used to estimate exposure in the absence of measurements or long-term monitoring data (Price et al., 1996b; Wilkes et al., 1996). As with any model, 'all are wrong, some are useful' (George Box), and risk assessors should carefully evaluate both mesoscale and microscale models and model outputs for relevance and accuracy. In such a case, additional measurements can and should serve as a useful and relatively inexpensive 'reality checks' on model results.

Equally important are the statistics used to analyse the field data. Environmental data are most often log-normally distributed. Under such conditions, a geometric average is generally assumed to be a better measure of central tendency of the data than the arithmetic mean (Crump, 1998). Despite this, the arithmetic mean (and the 95% upper confidence limit of the arithmetic mean) is typically used to identify environmental concentrations for use in exposure assessment. Since the advances in analytical chemistry have improved our ability to measure trace amounts of chemicals in different media and identify potential sources, less reliance should be placed on the use of mathematical models to predict the distribution of chemical and physical agents in the environment (Horwitz, 1984; Wenning and Erickson, 1994). Another issue revolves around how the analytical limit of detection (LOD) is addressed. An agent reported as not detected may be treated as a numerical zero, or occurring at the LOD or some fraction of the LOD, typically half, for purposes of calculating statistics. The manner in which censored data are assessed may affect the outcome of the risk assessment process (Helsel, 1990; Perkins et al., 1990; Travis and Land, 1990). For instance, analysis of highly contaminated samples or samples containing interfering substances may result in high LODs. Under such conditions and in the absence of additional analysis, assuming that non-detected compounds are present at half the LOD could result in the exposure assessment and subsequent risk assessment being driven by compounds that are not truly present in the environmental media. When such an approach is used on a site that may be only 2–10% contaminated (based on surface area), the predicted severity of the average level of contamination will be much higher than what actually occurs (Paustenbach, 1989b, 1995).

The practical result of these decisions can be illustrated by considering the following 11 data points resulting from analysis of field samples: not detected (ND), ND, ND, ND, ND, 5, 6, 6, 8, 55 and 500 ppm. The results are log-normally distributed, as expected. The LOD is 0.05 ppm and non-detected compounds are assumed to be present at half the LOD (0.025 ppm). Using these assumptions, the arithmetic mean of the data set is 52.7 ppm while the geometric mean is 1.3 ppm. The practical consequence of choosing one descriptor over the other may be to mis-identify or mis-characterize the dose and ultimately the risk and will influence regulatory decisions involving remediation and regulation.

Monte Carlo Analysis

Among the most promising and exciting techniques to emerge in the area of exposure assessment in recent years is the application of Monte Carlo or other probabilistic analyses to environmental health issues (Burmaster and Von Stackelberg, 1991; Thompson et al., 1992; Anderson and Yuhas, 1996; Burmaster, 1996; Richardson, 1996). Monte Carlo analysis has existed as an engineering analytical tool for many years, but the development of the personal computer and software (e.g. Crystal Ball [Desisioneering, Boulder, CO], @RISK [Palisades Corp., Newfield, NY]) has allowed its application to new areas of endeavour. As discussed above, a justified criticism of many exposure assessments has been a reliance on overly conservative assumptions about exposure and the problem of how to account properly for the highly exposed (but usually small) populations that do exist (Burmaster and Harris, 1993; Smith, 1994). It is self-evident that most of the variables used in the exposure assessment actually exist as ranges rather than single point values. For instance, the common assumption that adult body weight is 70 kg is replaced in Monte Carlo analysis by the appropriate distribution (i.e. normal) of body weights (including maximum, minimum, mean and standard deviation). Virtually every exposure variable, whether physiological, behavioural, environmental or chronological, can be replaced with a probability distribution (Glickman, 1986; Thompson and Burmaster, 1991; Israeli and Nelson, 1992; Murray and Burmaster, 1992; Taylor, 1993; Burmaster and Anderson, 1994; Finley et al., 1994a; Lee and Wright, 1994; Ruffle et al., 1994; Price et al., 1996b; Wilson et al., 1996; Burmaster and Huff, 1997; Burmaster and Thompson, 1997; Trowbridge and Burmaster, 1997; Allen et al., 1998; Burmaster 1998a,b; Frey and Rhodes, 1998; Funk et al., 1998; Price et al., 1998; Sedman et al., 1998). Since no population (or individual) is exposed to a single concentration, breathes, eats or drinks at a single rate or is exposed for the same length of time, it is not appropriate to assess them as such. To be protective, high values were employed, resulting in the problems of compounding conservatisms mentioned previously (Maxim, 1989; Burmaster and

Harris, 1993; Bogen, 1994b; Cullen, 1994; Beck and Cohen, 1997). The probabilistic analysis addresses the main deficiencies of the point estimate approach because it imparts much more information to the risk managers and the public, and uses all of the available data (Mertz et al., 1998). The range of values (i.e. the distribution) for all the variables used in an exposure assessment is determined (e.g. normal, log-normal, uniform, triangular) and combined into a 'distribution of distributions' (Figure 11). Due to the extrapolations involved and the assumptions made, the area of single greatest uncertainty in risk assessment is associated with the dose-response evaluations. It should also be clear that, in addition to exposure variables, the toxicologic data that form the basis of the toxicologic criteria (CPFs and RfDs) are also amenable to Monte Carlo-style analysis where a robust database exists (Sielken, 1989; Shlyakhter et al., 1992; Evans et al., 1994a, b; Velazquez et al., 1994; Sielken et al., 1995; Baird et al., 1996; Cox, 1996; Crouch, 1996a, b; Hill and Hoover, 1997; Sielken and Valdez-Flores, 1997; Boyce, 1998). As with exposure variables, the advantage to this approach is that it allows all the data to be used (and weighted appropriately where necessary), thus avoiding reliance on a single experiment or endpoint.

Instead of presenting a single point estimate of exposure and risk, Monte Carlo-style exposure assessments characterize a range of possible exposures and their likelihood of occurrence (Copeland et al., 1993, 1994; Finley and Paustenbach, 1994; Sielken et al., 1995). In addition, the factors that most affect the results, and their relationship to one another and the entire range of exposure, can easily be identified and explained. For instance, in a Monte Carlo analysis, the final outcome of the risk assessment may be expressed as 'the plausible increased cancer risks at the 50th, 95th and 99th percentiles of the exposed population are $1 \times 10^{-8}, 5 \times 10^{-7}$ and 1×10^{-6}, respectively'. Whereas the typical US EPA estimate of risk might rely on the 99th (or greater) percentile (owing to compounding conservatisms) and result in regulatory action, the Monte Carlo analysis suggests that the most likely estimate of risk (50th percentile) is well below the level of regulatory concern and even a conservative estimate (95th percentile) suggests no risk exists for the largest part of the population. For instance, the current US EPA point assumption for soil ingestion by children is typically 200 mg day^{-1} (US EPA, 1996a), despite the fact that the best scientific estimates suggest that it is probably between 10 and 20 mg day^{-1} for most children (Calabrese et al., 1989; Stanek and Calabrese, 1995b). The higher value is considered 'protective' and indeed it is, in the same way that simply banning an animal carcinogen is protective. Use of a probabilistic analysis of the soil ingestion data is illuminating in this regard (Figure 12). This information suggests that the best estimate for child soil ingestion is 16 mg day^{-1} and the 95th percentile ingestion rate is of the order of 100 mg day^{-1} (Finley and

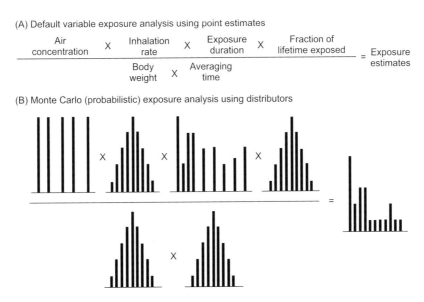

(A) Default variable exposure analysis using point estimates

(B) Monte Carlo (probabilistic) exposure analysis using distributors

Figure 11 Standard exposure assessments utilize point estimates of the different variables in the exposure equation (A). The use of a Monte Carlo approach to assessing exposure (B), however, allows all available information about the ranges of variables previously expressed as point values to be combined and expressed as a distribution of possible exposures with an estimate of their probability of occurrence. Such information is of greater value to the risk manager and the public in terms of understanding the meaning and uncertainty of a risk estimate. Additionally, it avoids the false precision often associated with presenting the risk as a single point estimate.

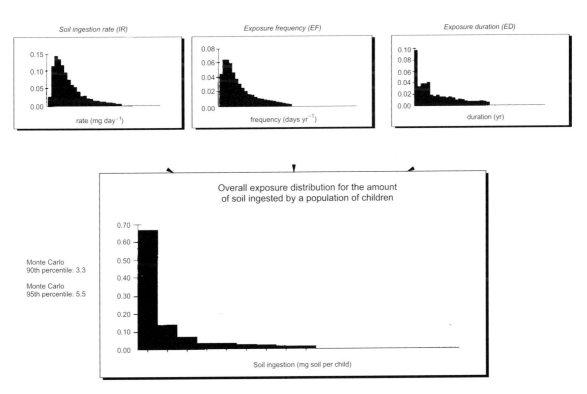

Figure 12 An example of the potential issues associated with consistent use of upper bound or worst case exposure variables can be illustrated in the following example. Using data collected on soil ingestion by children by Calabrese *et al.* (1989) and others, as well as estimates on the duration and frequency of exposure (US EPA, 1996a), a probability density function (PDF) for child soil ingestion is generated. Adapted from Finley *et al.* (1994a). Examination of the results indicates that the average consumption of soil by children is something else than 20 mg day^{-1} and the 95th percentile ingestion rate is slightly over 100 mg day^{-1}. Compare these results with the EPA default assumption of 200 mg day^{-1} for an average child's soil ingestion rate. Use of such a default is between 2 and 10 times more conservative than needed and if this same conservatism is repeated for other exposure (or toxicity) variables, the over-prediction of risk may be substantial. The use of probabilistic analysis may be useful in proving better estimates of exposure without any loss of protection to public health or the environment.

Paustenbach, 1994). Incorporating these values into risk assessment and expanding the risk characterization to include best and upper bound risks would improve the understanding and utility of these estimates without sacrificing protection.

Probabilistic analysis of this type has been recognized in regulatory guidance (US EPA, 1992a) and the US EPA's Risk Assessment Forum has published a document of principles for conducting Monte Carlo analysis (US EPA, 1997a). Like traditional exposure analysis, one problem with performing Monte Carlo analysis properly is having appropriate distributions for use in the analysis. A review of possible distributions (Finley et al., 1994a) and numerous other studies on individual variables have been published in the risk assessment literature (Finley et al., 1994a; Trowbridge and Burmaster, 1997; Burmaster 1998a, b; Sedman et al., 1998) and the impact on the distributions employed on the outcome has also been discussed (Smith et al., 1992; Mattis and Burmaster, 1994; Hoffman and Hammonds, 1994; Bukowski et al., 1995; Cooper et al., 1996; Haas, 1997; Hamed and Bedient, 1997). It should be pointed out that these techniques can be combined with other cutting edge methods (e.g. PBPK modeling) to reduce further the uncertainty in the estimates (Cronin et al., 1995; Simon, 1997). Information appropriate to probabilistic analysis can also be found or developed from other published sources. This or similar techniques should be employed whenever possible, both to ensure their acceptance in regulatory circles and to stimulate the needed research to improve the process.

Case Study in Exposure Assessment: Monte Carlo Analysis

As an example of the power of Monte Carlo analysis, the health protectiveness of drinking water standards (i.e. maximum contaminant limits or MCLs) was evaluated (Finley and Paustenbach, 1993, 1994). Concern has been raised that these regulatory limits are not sufficiently protective and certain Federal and State regulatory programmes (e.g. RCRA) are justified in requiring groundwater remediation to levels below that of drinking water standards as a result. To test this supposition, the plausible increased cancer risk at the MCLs was assessed using probabilistic analysis to examine exposure via tap-

water ingestion, dermal contact with water while showering, inhalation of indoor vapours and ingestion of produce irrigated with groundwater. Probability density functions for each exposure variable (e.g. water ingestion, skin surface area, fraction of exposed skin, showering time, inhalation rate, air exchange and water use rates, exposure time) were identified and used in the exposure equation to calculate dose and risk. A commercially available software package (@RISK) was used to conduct the Monte Carlo analysis (Palisade, 1990).

Table 11 represents the risk associated with exposure to water use at the current MCL level for four different contaminants and both the 50th and 95th percentiles of exposure as determined by probabilistic analysis. At the 50th percentile level ('the best estimate'), the risk ranges from 6×10^{-7} (tetrachloroethylene) to 9×10^{-6} (chloroform), while at the 95th percentile ('the upper bound risk'), these risks range from 4×10^{-6} (tetrachloroethylene) to 1.5×10^{-4} (chloroform). These values can be compared with the point estimate-type risks calculated for the MCLS which range from 7×10^{-6} (tetrachloroethylene) to 5.4×10^{-5} (vinyl chloride). For the 50th percentile (average) person, all calculated risks are within the range of 'acceptable' risks adopted by regulatory authorities for Superfund sites (1×10^{-4} to 1×10^{-7}). For the 95th percentile person (upper-bound), the risks are still mostly below the 1×10^{-4} benchmark risk level generally used to separate acceptable from unacceptable risks. For tetrachloroethylene, these results are 30 (50th percentile) to 3 (risk at the MCL) times below the RME risk of 2×10^{-5} developed by combining the 95th percentile values for each exposure variable using standard EPA risk assessment methodologies **(Figure 13)**. This point estimate is greater than the 99th percentile of risk and is consistent with Burmaster and Lehr (1991) statements regarding the conservatism of the RME approach. These results suggest that chemical residues in drinking water at the MCL levels will be health protective and that remedial goals based on *de minimis* requirement (1×10^{-6}) might be unnecessarily low and wasteful of resources.

In terms of the RME estimates, which often serve as the basis for regulatory decisions, several observations on the utility of probabilistic assessment can be made. First, exposure assessments that incorporate two to three

Table 11 Risks calculated for exposure to four halogenated solvents in water using probabilistic analysis at the MCL level and for 50th and 95th percentile exposure

Chemical	50th percentile risk	95th percentile risk	MCL risk
Tetrachloroethylene	0	0.000005	0.000007
Chloroform	0.000009	0.00014	0.000017
Bromoform	0.000002	0.000016	0.000023
Vinyl chloride	0.000005	0.000029	0.000054

Source: adapted from Finley and Paustenbach (1994b).

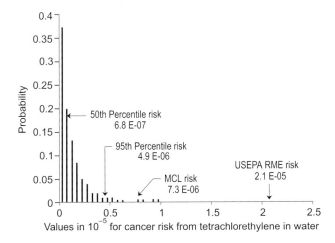

Figure 13 Combining a Monte Carlo analysis of both exposure and toxicity allows the likely distribution of risk to be completely displayed. Adapted from Finley and Paustenbach (1994). This includes the risk that results from the use US EPA-type of default point values (RME), all of which may typically use an upper 95% statistical bound (or higher) on a given variable. In this example, the US EPA RME risk is 2.1×10^{-5}, which implies that we are at least 95% certain the risk is no higher than 2 in 100 000 excess cancers over a lifetime. Since this exceeds the 1×10^{-6} nominal acceptable cancer risk, regulatory action is possible. The additional information from fully displaying the risk range and the probability associated with each risk allows the risk manager (or the public) to see that the risk to the majority of the population is most probably well below this level (4×10^{-8} or less).

direct exposure pathways usually show that the 95th percentile probabilistic estimates are three to five times below the traditional RME estimates. Second, for multi-pathway assessments that contain several indirect exposure pathways, the 95th percentile probabilistic estimates can be as much as an order of magnitude below the RME estimates. Third, when the number of distributions used in the exposure assessment is 10 or more, the difference between the 50th and 95th percentile estimates may be between 5 and 10. Finally, in such assessments, the difference between the RME estimates and the 95th percentile probabilistic estimates can be as high as 100. In the probabilistic approach to estimating exposure and risk, the complete range of potential risks can be illustrated along with the likelihood estimates and estimates of uncertainty associated with such risks. While the availability and confidence of distributions for exposure variables differ, risk assessors ought to take advantage of this and similar approaches in their risk assessments to advance and improve the process. Additionally, since the highest degree of uncertainty in risk assessment tends to be the CPFs, attention ought to be directed to applying probabilistic analysis to the development of toxicity criteria in a similar manner (Sielken, 1989; Shlyakhter et al., 1992; Evans et al., 1994a, b; Sielken et al., 1995).

Sensitivity Analysis

In addition to establishing the distribution of exposures and risks, probabilistic analysis can also be used to identify the variables that have the greatest impact on the estimates and illuminate the uncertainties associated with exposure variables through sensitivity analysis (Bogen and Spear, 1987; Iman and Helton, 1991; Shlyakhter, 1994; Robinson and Hurst, 1997; Rai and Krewski, 1998). This also provides some insight into the confidence that resides in the estimates of exposure and risk. This has two important results. First, it identifies the inputs that would benefit most from additional research to reduce uncertainty and improve the estimates of risk. Second, assuming a thorough assessment has been conducted, it is possible to phrase the results in more easily accessible terms such as 'the risk assessment of PCBs in small mouth bass is based on a large amount of high-quality, reliable data and we have high confidence in the risk estimates derived. The analysis has determined that 90% of the increased cancer risk could be eliminated through a ban on carp and catfish, but there is no appreciable reduction in risk from extending such a ban to bass and trout'. Such a description provides much more information to all stakeholders than a simple point estimate of risk based on a traditional exposure and risk assessment (Paustenbach, 1995).

If the most 'sensitive' exposure variables are based on limited or uncertain data, then the confidence in estimates is poor. Robust data sets, on the other hand, lead to increased confidence in the resulting estimates. In the above example (Finley and Paustenbach, 1993, 1994), sensitivity is defined as the ratio of the relative change in risk produced by a unit relative change in the exposure variables used. A Gaussian approximation (the product of the normalized sensitivity and the standard deviation of the distribution) was used to allow both sensitivity and uncertainty to be gauged. In this case, the true mean of each distribution was chosen as the baseline point value and the differential value for each variable was calculated by increasing this value by 10%. For each variable, the differential value was substituted, the risks were recalculated and the baseline value was replaced. Sensitivity was calculated using the following equation:

$$\text{sensitivity} = \frac{|\text{risk}_{\text{baseline}} - \text{risk}_{10\%}|}{|X_{\text{baseline}} - X_{10\%}|} \times [\sigma]$$

where X_{baseline} and $X_{10\%}$ are the baseline and differential values, respectively, for the variable X and σ is the standard deviation for the distribution of variable X.

The sensitivity of each variable relative to one another is assessed by summing the unitless sensitivity values and determining the relative percentage that each variable contributes to the total. **Table 12** indicates which variables are the most important in the probabilistic analysis for tetrachloroethylene. In this case, the most sensitive

Table 12 Results of sensitivity analysis for tetrachloroethylene exposure in household water

Exposure variable	Sensitivity (unitless)	Percentage rank
Shower exposure time	0.000004	55.0
Exposure duration	0.000001	20.0
Plant–soil partition factor	0	8.4
Water ingestion rate	0	4.6
Surface area of exposed skin	0	4.4
Body weight	0	3.8
Dermal permeability constant	0	1.8
Skin fraction contacting water	0	1.5

Source: adapted from Finley and Paustenbach (1994b).

exposure variables in household exposure to tapwater are exposure time in shower and exposure duration. Relatively small changes in these variables will result in relatively large changes in the risk estimates. Since these estimates are based on actual time–use studies and census information, this suggests that a high level of confidence can be placed on this estimate, particularly if site-specific data are being used. If the critical variables (in terms of sensitivity) were not based on robust data, this would suggest that the risk assessment could be improved by additional research on these exposure variables. It is interesting to point out that the form of the distribution chosen for the variables are less important than the validity of the data. When the empirical distribution of the tapwater ingestion rate from Ershow and Cantor (1989) was substituted with a log-normal distribution developed by Roseberry and Burmaster (1992), the resultant change in the risk estimates was less than 1%. In this case, the value of the sensitivity analysis is that it allows the input variables to be ranked in order of importance and confidence in the output established to a higher degree than previously possible. As pointed out by the EPA: 'Where possible, exposure assessors should report variability in exposures as numerical distributions and should characterize uncertainty as probability distributions. They need to identify clearly where they are using point estimates for 'bounding' potential exposure variables or estimates; these point estimates should not be misconstrued to represent, for example, the upper 95th percentile when information on the actual distribution is lacking. *Such explicit presentation of the data reduces the temptation to use the exposure assessment process for veiling policy judgements*' [italics added] (Graham et al., 1992).

Risk Characterization

Risk characterization is the final step in the risk assessment process and, to paraphrase Samuel Johnson, '... like a dog walking on its hind legs; it is rarely done well, but the wonder is that it is done at all'. In theory, risk characterization is a two-stage process. First, it entails combining the results of the dose–response and exposure assessment steps to form a quantitative estimate of the risk evaluated. Second, a detailed qualitative and, if possible, quantitative description of the uncertainties involved in the risk assessment should be provided. In practice, because this component requires the assessor to draw on numerous aspects of science and regulatory policy to describe properly whether a significant human health or ecological risk exists in a specific setting, a thorough risk characterization is often not completed. In other words, it is easier to calculate a number than explain what it means. Thus, the risk managers and the public may be left with a single numerical estimate of risk with an implied precision that does not truly exist (Meek, 1997; Risher and DeRosa, 1997).

The first stage of risk characterization is simply accomplished for both carcinogens and non-carcinogens. For carcinogens, the added risk is calculated by combining the dose estimate and CPF in a multiplicative fashion as follows:

$$\text{risk (unitless)} = \text{CPF} \left([\text{mg (kg body weight)}^{-1} \text{day}^{-1}]^{-1} \times \text{dose } [\text{mg (kg body weight)}^{-1} \text{day}^{-1}] \right)$$

The units cancel out and a unitless value representing an upper bound estimate on the added risk from a lifetime exposure remains. Risks from multiple carcinogens in a single pathway (e.g. all carcinogens found in drinking water) are assessed additively as are cancer risks from multiple pathways (e.g. total cancer risk from air, water, soil, and food).

For non-carcinogens, the risk is expressed by a hazard quotient (HQ) approach, which is calculated by dividing the dose estimate by the RfD (or RfC) such that the units again cancel out as follows:

$$\text{HQ} = \frac{\text{dose } [\text{mg (kg body weight)}^{-1} \text{day}^{-1}]}{\text{RfD } [\text{mg (kg bodyweight)}^{-1} \text{day}^{-1}]}$$

As with carcinogens, the non-cancer risk from exposure to multiple agents is addressed additively to form a hazard index (HI). As with cancer risks, HQ scores for each chemical in a pathway are added, and the non-cancer risks in all pathways in a given scenario are added together to get a total scenario HI. These values are then most often compared with an acceptable risk level.

For carcinogens, the most commonly cited acceptable or *de minimis* risk level is one additional cancer case per one million exposed individuals (1×10^{-6} or 1E–6) (Kelley and Cardon, 1991). This value representing a level of both voluntary and involuntary risk felt to be acceptable to the public at large (e.g. the risk of death due to lightning strikes or bee stings). In terms of practical application, an acceptable risk range of 1×10^{-4}–1×10^{-7} is often used to make decisions regarding remedial or regulatory action (US EPA, 1989b, 1995a; Habicht, 1992). The level of acceptable risk at this stage often becomes a judgement call and differs according to the regulatory authority and the circumstances of the risk assessed. For non-carcinogens, a hazard is not considered to exist if the HI remains below 1.0.

It should be clear that this approach to risk characterization is highly simplistic and ought to be confined to a screening-level type of analysis. Assuming that all carcinogens and non-carcinogens have additive effects implies that all compounds have the same target organs or mechanisms of action, that the interactions between compounds at trace levels are, in fact, additive and that the effects are of equal severeity (Cox, 1984; US EPA, 1986d; Seiler and Scott, 1987; Krewski *et al.*, 1989b; Krewski and Thomas, 1992; Kodell and Chen, 1994; Seed *et al.*, 1995; Gaylor and Chen, 1996; Krishnan *et al.*, 1997; Pohl *et al.*, 1997). If the results of a typically conservative analysis are below the *de minimis* risk levels of 1×10^{-6} (cancer) or 1.0 (non-cancer), one can be reasonably certain that no actual health risks exist. Risk estimates above the *de minimis* risk levels, however, cannot be taken of evidence of a risk because of the conservative assumptions inherent in most risk assessments. Providing these point estimates as the sole focus of the risk characterization creates a false impression of precision without an understanding of the uncertainty inherent in the process (Meek, 1997; Risher and DeRosa, 1997; Santos and McCallum, 1997). These risk estimates should never be treated or presented as predictions of future happenings or medical diagnoses, as often happens, but rather as decision-making tools for regulatory purposes (Gray, 1994).

To avoid misunderstanding the meaning of a risk assessment, it is important that the meaning of the estimates be presented properly. The cancer risk estimates that combine the results of a conservative exposure and dose–response assessment represent a plausible (and sometimes implausible) upper-bound estimate on that risk. Again, the proper interpretation of a cancer risk of a number such as 4×10^{-5} is not that there will be four additional cancer cases for every 100 000, but that there will be no more than four additional cases, probably fewer, and possibly zero. Left out of the risk characterization discussion is the fact that the nominal acceptable added risk of 1×10^{-6} does not, in fact, represent a significant public health issue. Even if accurate, such an increase represents a less than 0.0001% increase in the background rate of cancer. Society can demand and pay for this standard of protection if desired, but it is critical that both the public and risk managers be aware of the relative magnitude of various risks before committing resources in one direction or another. In this respect, it is interesting to note that if all carcinogens were regulated at the 1×10^{-6} level, the decrease in the annual cancer incidence in the USA would be negligible (probably far less than 1% of the annual cancer rate) (Doll and Peto, 1981; Gough, 1990; Paustenbach, 1995).

For non-carcinogens, an HI score above 1.0 is also not an indication of a hazard. Such an outcome indicates that either the dose of at least one agent exceeds its respective RfD, or that the sum of several acceptable (< 1.0) HQs together exceed 1.0. It must be kept in mind, however, that the RfDs used for comparison are originally derived from a dose that had little or no adverse effect (e.g. NOAEL, LOAEL or BMD) on a presumably sensitive end-point in test animals, which is then divided by a large UF (typically 100 or greater). Since these toxicity criteria include a substantial margin of safety in their derivation, an excursion above these values will rarely approach a level at which an adverse reaction is likely to occur. In situations where the HI is greater than 1.0, a more complete analysis should be conducted; specifically, the chemicals can be grouped into categories based on target organs affected or mechanisms of action. Primary target organs have been identified (Paustenbach, 1994; ACGIH, 1998b).

The consistent use of additivity of agents and pathways, particularly at RME levels, is also a questionable use of risk assessment, especially without explanation and further evaluation. In terms of toxicity, agents that act at the same target organ or through the same mechanism of action may act additively at low levels, although antagonistic or greater than additive response are also possible (Pohl *et al.*, 1997). Given the low levels of compounds generally encountered in the environment, it is often questionable if sufficient damage occurs at the target organ to make such interactions of any biological consequence in most cases (Kodell and Chen, 1994; Seed *et al.*, 1995). One of the major criticisms with most regulatory risk characterizations is their reliance on default assumptions and methodologies (AIHC, 1997). Such estimates are more plausible for some agents than others. As a result, the statement that these risk estimates represent a 'plausible upper bound' estimate of risk may provide reasonable estimates for some (arguably limited) compounds and exposures, but wild overestimates for many other situations. Generally most risk assessments assume a linear, no-threshold dose–

response relationship for carcinogens and some non-carcinogens (e.g. lead). However, for many, if not most, chemicals that are not direct mutagens such an assumption is likely to be inappropriate. For example, the calculated risk for a direct alkylating agent may indeed be close to the 'plausible upper bound' estimate, while the estimate for an non-mutagenic compound such as DDT may be an extreme over-estimate of the actual risk. In such circumstances, the two 'plausible upper bound' estimates that are generated through exactly the same process may have very different levels of scientific plausibility and this requires explanation. Thus, when applying a single standard to evaluating chemical or physical hazards without serious thought about individual characteristics, the amount of inherent conservatism in those estimates may vary by several orders of magnitude. Presentation of multiple estimates of risk will help avoid the trap of false precision referred to earlier, but it can also help combat false consistency by presenting all scientifically plausible choices and avoiding constant reliance on a single approach that may have applicability to only a limited number of compounds or exposures (Anderson and Yuhas, 1996). Equally important, since it is virtually impossible that a hypothetical receptor exposed at RME levels in one pathway can be exposed at RME levels in others, the representation of upper-bound risks as a sum of numerous RME exposures must generally be considered inappropriate (US EPA, 1986b, c, 1989b, 1992a).

Setting Acceptable Risk Levels

A variant of these same formulaic approaches can also be employed to set acceptable concentrations of agents in different environmental media through back-calculation for setting clean-up or 'safe' levels. Although this approach should be used with care since back-calculation can lead to erroneous results due to the assumptions and variability inherent in the risk equation (Mosleh and Bier, 1992; Burmaster and Bloomfield, 1995; Burmaster et al., 1995; Burmaster and Thompson, 1995; Ferson and Long, 1998). For instance, the acceptable concentration for an agent in soil based on soil ingestion could be derived by selecting the acceptable cancer risk level and solving the following equation for EC_{soil}:

$$ risk = \frac{CPF_O \times EC_{soil} \times EF \times AF_O}{CF \times AT} \times \left(\frac{IR_A \times ED_A}{BW_A} + \frac{IR_C \times ED_C}{BW_C} \right) $$

where:
- risk = acceptable cancer risk level $(1 \times 10^{-4}$ to $1 \times 10^{-7})$
- CPF_O = oral cancer potency factor
- A = adult
- C = child
- EC_{soil} = average concentration in soil

- BW = body weight (15 kg, child; 70 kg, adult)
- AT = averaging time (70 years or 25 550 days)
- EF = exposure frequency (365 days per year)
- ED = exposure duration (6 years, child; 24 years, adult; 30 years total)
- AF_O = oral absorption factor
- IR = ingestion rate (100 mg day^{-1}, child; 50 mg day^{-1}, adult)
- CF = conversion factor (10^6 mg kg^{-1})

Obviously, the risks from contaminated soil involve exposure pathways other than just soil ingestion (e.g. inhalation of dust, dermal contact with soil, ingestion of contaminated produce). Similar back-calculations are conducted for each completed exposure pathway and, since the total risk is cumulative for all completed pathways, the target concentration can be determined by combining the results of the relevant equations and solving as follows:

$$ EC_{soil} = \left[\sum_{i=1}^{n} \frac{1}{(EC_{soil})_i} \right]^{-1} $$

where i = pathways considered (e.g. soil ingestion, produce ingestion, dermal contact, dust inhalation), or

$$ (EC_{soil})_{all} = \left[\frac{1}{(EC_{soil})_{SI}} + \frac{1}{(EC_{soil})_{VI}} + \frac{1}{(EC_{soil})_{Inh}} + \frac{1}{(EC_{soil})_{Der}} \right] $$

where
- $(EC_{soil})_{all}$ = sum of the inverse of the acceptable soil concentration for completed pathways
- $(EC_{soil})_{SI, VI, Inh, Der}$ = acceptable soil concentrations for completed pathways (SI = soil ingestion, VI = produce ingestion, Der = dermal contact, Inh = dust inhalation)

Thus the soil (or other media) concentration for an agent at a given level of accepetable risk can be calculated, although the same problems inherent in developing point estimates exist in the development of such values.

Issues in Improving Risk Characterization

Risk characterization is potentially the most powerful stage in the risk assessment process, given its explanatory role in placing the results of the risk assessment in perspective (Paustenbach, 1995). The disclosure and open discussion of the basis and merits of the final risk estimates is referred to as 'transparency' and is critical for risk managers and the public to understand fully and appreciate the scientific plausibility or certainty associated with the estimate of risk (Lewis and Amoruso, 1997). Unfortunately, this potential is usually unrealized since most risk assessments are limited to the presentation of point estimates of the risk and stop short of discussing the assumptions and the uncertainties inherent in the process. This problem has been appreciated by the US EPA, which recognized that current practices in characterizing risk need to be improved in order to bring them more closely in line with the US EPA's stated policy (Habicht, 1992; US EPA, 1992a, 1995a) and the NRC and other recommendations (Finkel, 1991; CCSTG, 1993; National Research Council, 1994, 1996; US EPA, 1994c; CRARM, 1996). In addition to increasing explanation and reducing reliance on default assumptions, applications, proper use and inclusion of qualitative and quantitative uncertainty analysis was also specifically targeted for improvement (Mosleh and Bier, 1992; Ferson and Long, 1995, 1998; Cooper et al., 1996; Iman and Helton, 1997). In addition to allowing identification of the factor(s) that introduce the greatest uncertainties into the process, such techniques also can (and should) be employed to determine how effective or protective regulatory decisions or standards based on risk assessment have been. Additional research into important risk parameters and the cost-effectiveness of resultant decisions may further reduce the uncertainty involved and improve the process with substantial long-term savings in time and money (National Research Council, 1994; US EPA, 1994c; CalEPA, 1998; Younes and Sonich-Mullin, 1998).

A thorough risk characterization should include (where appropriate) a discussion of background concentrations of the agent in the environment and biological tissues, pharmacokinetic differences between experimental animals and the target species, the impact of the dose–response model used and that of potentially alternative models (e.g. PBPK or biologically based models), the effect of the specific exposure parameters employed, uncertainty and sensitivity analyses and other relevant factors influencing the magnitude of the risk estimate. A number of questions should be answered by the risk assessor in the risk characterization section as fully as possible. These include:

1. Are choice and impact of the data (environmental or toxicological) or dose-extrapolation model used in the risk assessment discussed, especially quantitatively?
2. Is an appropriate dose–response model (e.g. linear, no-threshold, or non-linear, threshold) used for the agent(s) in question?
3. Are all the adverse outcomes associated with agents of interest of equal severity and consequence, are the experimental results consistent across all species? Do the short-term results agree with those from long-term studies?
4. Is the animal model used relevant to human or the target species, is the dose expressed on a biologically relevant scale and are the high doses used experimentally relevant to low-dose exposure? Does the epidemiological record agree with the animal toxicology?
5. Have the relevant biological differences between species, and between the experimental and environmental routes of exposure, been taken into account?

6. Are the exposure patterns, frequencies and durations in experimental studies similar to those of the target species at risk?
7. Have the relevant exposures been completely identified in relation to routes, frequency, duration, dose levels and scenarios? Are the plausibility, source and impact of the conservative default assumptions used in the exposure assessment explicitly discussed in the risk characterization? Are exposures and risks stratified according to different populations that might be especially sensitive or highly exposed?
8. Are the plausibility and derivation of the 'upper bound' risks generated for multiple agents discussed in terms of their respective strengths and weaknesses? If uncertainty is described in terms of bounds on the risk, are the lower bounds and best estimate of that risk included in addition to the upper bound and their meaning and derivation described?
9. Are multiple estimates of risk provided to illustrate the entire risk range and the respective likelihood of occurrence to allow meaningful comparison of potential public health threats?
10. Is the stated risk inflated by relying on (repeated) single 'plausible' upper-bound estimates of exposure and toxicity? Are the actual best and 95th percentile estimates of the model provided in addition to 'worst-case' outputs?
11. Has the statistical variability in the sampling, exposure and experimental data been identified and properly assessed? Have uncertainty and sensitivity analyses been performed and incorporated into the risk characterization?
12. Have all assumptions, policy decisions, value judgements and uncertainties been clearly identified and discussed in terms of their impact on the outcome of the risk assessment? Are the risks characterized in an understandable and appropriate manner?
13. Is the risk assessment based on the most current and appropriate data and protocols? Are the risks based on site-specific and use-specific exposure scenarios that take into account current and future exposures?

Risk characterizations would be more useful for purposes of decision-making if they contained cost–benefit analyses (Breyer, 1994; Finkel, 1995; HGRMR, 1995; Barnard, 1996a, b; Crouch et al., 1997; Kopp et al., 1997). For each dollar, pound or euro spent, the public ought to be able to determine how much the risks are likely to be reduced for various sub-populations. This may be the primary reason for conducting such evaluations, and Monte Carlo analysis is a particularly valuable tool in this regard (Evans et al., 1994a, b; Sielken et al., 1995; Burmaster, 1996; Cox, 1996; Richardson, 1996; Sielken and Stevenson, 1997; Boyce, 1998; Swartout et al., 1998).

The hallmark of a high-quality risk characterization remains the thorough presentation and discussion of all relevant uncertainties (Lewis and Amoruso, 1997). Probabilistic techniques, such as Monte Carlo analysis, again have allowed quantitative, rather than qualitative, uncertainty analyses to be conducted and presented in an understandable manner. (Iman and Hetton, 1991; Molesh and Bier, 1992; Smith *et al.*, 1992; Hattis and Burmaster, 1994; Hoffman and Hammonds, 1994; Shlyakhter, 1994; Bogen, 1995; Ferson and Long, 1995, 1998; Bukowski *et al.*, 1997; Robinson and Hurst, 1997; Rai and Krewski, 1998). The key to these analyses is the inclusion of a statistical analysis of each parameter and the implication for the risk estimate for different segments of the population. A key trait in this respect is the accurate and unbiased discussion of the confidence in the risk estimates. For instance, the presentation of risk estimates as accurate predictions of cancer occurrence are erroneous and misleading when the uncertainty in dose–response models ensure they cannot be accurate predictors of the actual cancer risk. Risk estimates should be clearly presented as relative indicators of hazard used to illuminate uncertainties and prioritize issues for decision-making. The risk characterization offers numerous opportunities to fail in describing the true nature of the risk estimates to the audience. For instance, it is not unusual to see the hypothetical increase in cancer risk at 1×10^{-4} or even 1×10^{-6} depicted as a serious public health risk (Young, 1987; Maxim, 1989; Paustenbach, 1989a). If the public, media and risk managers have a clearer understanding of the source and proper interpretation of those numbers, the level of concern or outright panic (e.g. the Alar controversy) might be avoided and things placed in their proper perspective (Johnson and Slovic, 1995; Dudley and Gramm, 1997; McCallum and Santos, 1997; Santos and McCallum, 1997). The meaning of specific risk estimates now typically escapes policy makers and this situation must be corrected in order for resulting risk management decisions to be truly informed. For example, nearly all risk estimates generated by US regulatory agencies mention that these risks are upper bound estimates of the plausible risk, are unlikely to underestimate risk, and that the actual risk may be much lower and possibly zero. This caveat, however, is rarely fully explained and all but ignored in communication to the risk managers and the public, and ultimately in the risk-based decisions made. It is critical that the nature of the conservative procedures and models used and the likely overestimate of the risk resulting be properly and completely explained (Johnson and Slovic, 1995; Bartell, 1996; Carrington and Bolger, 1998; Felter and Dourson, 1998; Mertz *et al.*, 1998; Nakayachi, 1998)

For instance, the goal of all environmental standards (e.g. maximum contaminant levels or MCLs for drinking water) is to keep the maximum plausible cancer risk between 1×10^{-5} and 1×10^{-6} added lifetime risk (Fin-ley and Paustenbach, 1993, 1994). As a potential communication tool, it might be helpful to place these estimates in context with cancer rates as a whole. Since about 33% of all Americans living today will develop some form of cancer in their lifetime and approximately 25% will die of it (Doll and Peto, 1981), a 1×10^{-6} added risk is the equivalent of increasing the risk of death by 0.0001% if the risk estimate was completely accurate. Since it is an upper bound estimate, the true risk is much lower. These standards are therefore the functional, if not the actual, equivalent of no risk if met. This level of transparency in discussing uncertainty in risk estimates is necessary to ensure that appropriate decisions are made between competing risks and finite resources. For instance, is our money better spent addressing a theoretical cancer risk of 1×10^{-5} through air or water, or on basic research on treatment of cancer, childhood vaccination programmes or preventative medical care for the poor? Since the statistics for other public health concerns (e.g. disease incidence, accidents) or societal needs (e.g. infrastructure, defence, economic health) are not deliberately over-inflated, the risk characterization employed in discussing cancer (or other environmental or occupational risks) must go beyond the simple single point estimate to ensure meaningful comparisons (Tengs *et al.*, 1995). Only by making the meaning of the risk estimates and the uncertainty inherent in them plain can we be assured that efficient decisions regarding expenditure of resources are addressed.

Such improvements in the characterization of risks can benefit the risk assessment process and society in general. It will lead to a better understanding and realistic appreciation of the strengths and weaknesses of the process by regulators, policy makers, the media and the public. The ability to compare and rank health and environmental risks from chemicals and from other sources would also be improved. As a result, the scientific credibility of the risk assessment process is increased as scientists provide new data to reduce areas of uncertainty, see their work used in the risk assessment process and see their opinions and judgements reflected in the outcome of risk-based regulations and standards development. Finally, presentation of the full range of risk estimates and their validity will simply allow risk managers to make better and more consistent policy decisions (Rodricks *et al.*, 1987; Travis *et al.*, 1987; Mertz *et al.*, 1998). The improvements in risk characterization result in a 'full disclosure' policy for risk assessment in accordance with the NRC recommendations (National Research Council, 1994; US EPA, 1994c; Lewis and Amoruso, 1997).

Case Study in Risk Characterization: Consideration of Background Information

A screening level risk assessment recently completed of a former wood treatment facility found risks in excess of

1×10^{-4}, primarily as a result of ingestion and dermal contact of soil contaminated with polynuclear aromatic hydrocarbons (PAHs). The remedial decision based on this risk assessment called for large-scale soil removal and incineration at a cost in excess of 40 million dollars. In addition, neighbouring residents of the facility filed a 20 million dollar toxic tort alleging adverse health effects caused by the contamination and fear of future health impacts (i.e. cancerphobia). The characterization of the risk was confined to the presentation of the point estimate without discussion of the assumptions used, the uncertainties involved, and the meaning of the risk estimate.

A re-evaluation of the risk assessment was performed and the risks were more thoroughly and completely characterized. A review of the environmental data found that the contamination was indeed distributed log-normally and that the entire property was not contaminated. The geometric mean of the contamination was an order of magnitude below that of the arithmetic mean. Further, the concentration estimates were driven by a few hot spots located in remote areas of the property. The original risk assessment assumed no change in the environmental concentration over time despite information indicating that PAHs degrade over time or their bioavailability is reduced owing to chemical interactions with soil particles. Additionally, the exposure assumptions used were 'worst-case' conservative in terms of exposure frequency and duration, soil ingestion, dermal contact, absorption and so forth. An assumption was also made that all PAHs were carcinogenic and equipotent to that of benzo[a]pyrene (B[a]P).

The risk assessment was re-done using a Monte Carlo approach that incorporated the actual distribution of the contamination and exposure assumptions to generate both a best estimate and 95th percentile estimate of dose. Assumptions regarding the environmental half-lives of PAHs were incorporated into the assessment, in addition to an adjustment factor to account for the fact that only a portion of the property was contaminated. Finally, non-carcinogenic PAHs were eliminated from the risk assessment and the impact of carcinogenic PAHs was weighted according to their potency compared with B[a]P (US EPA, 1993). The results of this re-evaluation indicated that the 95th percentile risk was only slightly above the nominal acceptable risk of 1×10^{-6} while the best estimate was well below this value. As a results of this risk assessment, the remedial decision was altered to a limited removal of the hot spots. The risk characterization additionally presented the daily dose of PAHs received from exposure to site soils relative to the daily dose of PAHs expected to occur via the diet. PAHs in charbroiled meat have been measured (Creighton *et al.*, 1992; ATSDR, 1994). These residues have been measured as follows: B[a]P at 6–50 ppb, benz[a]anthracene at 1–31 ppb and chrysene at 1–25 ppb. These PAH levels were used in concert with the average daily consumption

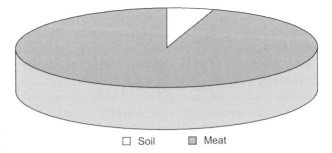

□ Soil   ■ Meat

Figure 14 Risk characterization can be done in a variety of ways to put the risk estimates in perspective. In this case, the polynuclear aromatic hydrocarbon (PAH) cancer risk from a contaminated soil situation was viewed as excessive by neighbours who sued for (future) damages. In order to place the risk assessment results into context, the daily dose of PAHs from the diet (specifically charbroiled meat) was determined. The average daily consumption of meat was combined with the percent age that is charbroiled and the average concentration of PAHs in such meat to estimate a daily dose. Since the dietary exposure to PAHs was estimated to be at least 25 times below the potential PAH dose from the site, the basis for the lawsuit collapsed and the case was settled out of court. Adapted from Copeland *et al.* (1993).

of meat (88 g day^{-1}), the percentage of meats that are charbroiled (25%) and an assumption of 50% absorbed. This comparative dose evaluation found that the PAH dose from soil was approximately 25 times lower than that received from the diet **(Figure 14)**. This evaluation in concert with the findings that the risks from the site were all within the acceptable risk range even under conservative assumptions resulted in a out-of-court settlement with the plaintiffs for under one million dollars (Copeland *et al.*, 1993).

CONCLUSION

The need for risk assessment is a function of the general smallness, uncertainty and other characteristics of the postulated risk of concern. Such risks would be readily apparent and easily measured if they were (1) large, (2) immediate in their consequences and (3) easily identifiable. The underlying justification for using risk assessment as a decision-making tool is that by performing it in a consistent manner, using the same techniques and assumptions, and providing a consistent interpretation of results, the degree of risk posed by various activities or agents will be accurately identified as they relate to one another. In other words, although the 'true' risks will rarely be known using such techniques, risk assessment can serve to rank and prioritize the risks for regulatory action (US EPA, 1990b). An advantage to standardizing the process and assumptions has been to make risk assessment 'transparent'. Anyone with a basic grounding in the terms and methodologies can understand and reproduce the logic and results, thus making the resultant decisions accessible to all stakeholders. Despite this strength, risk assessments conducted using the same environmental data, toxicity criteria and exposure assumptions may vary markedly in their final estimates and interpretations owing to the 'softness' of many assumptions, the conservative nature of the approach and particularly the insertion of value judgements by the risk assessor into the final product (Finkel, 1989; Paustenbach, 1989c; Barnard, 1995; Wilson, 1995; Barnard, 1996a, b).

Although risk assessment has become the basis for virtually all regulatory decisions involving environmental and health issues, the use of selected and biased sampling data, conservative default assumptions, conservatively derived toxicity criteria and inadequate characterization of the resultant risks have created an impression (largely correct in many cases) of risk assessment as misrepresenting the estimated risks and their significance. Part of the problem is that the regulatory mandates have created a mentality in which risk assessment has been reduced to a mechanical, cookbook exercise rather than a critical, evaluative tool. The science available for risk assessment has outstripped the regulatory practice and resulted in two different tracks being pursued (National Research Council, 1994; US EPA, 1994c; Milloy, 1995; CalEPA, 1998; Younes and Sonich-Mullin, 1998). The techniques of quantitative risk assessment first developed in the early 1980s were understandably conservative since they were created in the presence of much uncertainty and the immediate need for such a tool. However, many current practitioners forgot, or never learned, that risk assessment was intended to be technology-forcing and to take advantage of new information that could reduce the reliance on assumptions and the uncertainty in the process. Because such advances generally result in a lowering of the resultant risks calculated, attempts to incorporate such changes into the process met with regulatory resistance either because they conflicted with codified protocols or because the results were viewed as less protective of the public health and the environment. In fact, the risks never changed, only the information used in the risk assessment process.

In order to be responsive to societal needs, risk assessment must employ the best available science and most current techniques to reduce the uncertainty and improve the risk estimates (Graham et al., 1988; National Research Council, 1994, 1996; Milloy, 1995; Barnard, 1996a, b; Younes and Sonich-Mullin, 1998). These techniques include (1) a risk-based sampling plan to improve the dose and exposure estimates, (2) analysis of background levels in the environment and biological tissues, (3) incorporation of environmental half-lives, bioavailability and other factors that influence persistence, uptake and behaviour, (4) improvement in toxicity criteria by use of the most appropriate dose–response models and also other tools such as PBPK and

biologically based modeling, (5) use of site-specific exposure data that contain statistical variability information that is amenable to probabilistic (e.g. Monte Carlo) analysis, (6) explicit discussion of the uncertainty involved in the risk estimates, including sensitivity and uncertainty analyses, and identification of risks associated with various segments of the population and (7) inclusion of cost–benefit analyses so the public is aware of what the expenditure of resources is actually purchasing.

An appreciation for the need to identify clearly the uncertainties, the source of these uncertainties and the likely outcome of these uncertainties on the risk assessment suggests which information and experiments are needed to improve the estimates and reduce the uncertainties (Paustenbach, 1995). Beyond identifying data and methods to improve the risk assessment process, however, must come a commitment on the part of all stakeholders to adopt a cooperative attitude in improving the process to the maximum extent possible. Although some may believe that continued conservatism is necessary to protect the public health and environment, it is clear that incorporating science can improve risk assessments and decisions without sacrificing protection (Milloy, 1995; Hewitt et al., 1995; DelPup et al., 1996; Hamar et al., 1996; Reitz et al., 1996; Finley and Paustenbach, 1997; Younes and Sonich-Mullin, 1998). In this light, it is simply unethical to ignore advances that can serve to improve risk estimates by reducing uncertainty when the consequence is to re-direct scarce resources away from competing projects with measurable benefits (e.g. vaccination programmes, highway safety, basic research) to those for which the resultant benefits are far more uncertain (HGRMR, 1995; Johnson and Slovic, 1995; Tengs et al., 1995; Crouch et al., 1997; Kopp et al., 1997; McCallum and Santos, 1997; Mertz et al., 1998; Nakayachi, 1998). It will be how readily and rapidly science is incorporated into the process that will decide whether risk assessment evolves into a scientific discipline that positively aids difficult decisions or is ultimately relegated to a footnote in regulatory and social history.

ACKNOWLEDGEMENT

The authors acknowledge the valuable contribution of Vanessa Harvey in the completion of the manuscript.

REFERENCES

Abdel-Rahman, M. S. and Kadry, A. M. (1995). Studies on the use of uncertainty factors in deriving RfDs. *Human Ecol. Risk Assess.*, **1**, 614–624.

Abelson, P. H. (1992). Exaggerated carcinogenicity of chemicals. *Science*, **256**, 160.

Abelson, P. H. (1993). Health risk assessment. *Regul. Toxicol. Pharmacol.*, **17**, 219–223.

Abernathy, C. O. and Poirier, K. A. (1997). Uncertainties in the risk assessment of essential trace elements: the case of zinc. *Human Ecol. Risk Assess.*, **3**, 627–634.

ACGIH (1998a). *Threshold Limit Values for Chemical Substances and Physical Agents and Biological Exposure Indices for 1998–1999*. American Conference of Governmental Industrial Hygienists, Cincinnati, OH.

ACGIH (1998b). *Documentation of the Threshold Limit Values and Biological Exposure Indices*. American Conference of Governmental Industrial Hygienists, Cincinnati, OH.

Ahlborg, U. G., Becking, G. C., Birnbaum, L. S. *et al.* (1994). Toxic equivalency factors for dioxin-like PCBs. *Chemosphere*, **28**, 1049–1067.

AIHC (1989). *Presentation of Risk Assessments of Carcinogens*. American Industrial Health Council (AIHC), 20001 Pennsylvania Avenue NW, Suite 760. Washington, DC 20006.

AIHC (1994). *Exposure Factors Sourcebook*. American Industrial Health Council (AIHC), 20001 Pennsylvania Avenue NW, Suite 760. Washington, DC 20006.

AIHC (1997). *The role of toxicity default assumptions in risk assessment*. American Industrial Health Council (AIHC), 20001 Pennsylvania Avenue NW, Suite 760. Washington, DC 20006.

Albert, R. E. (1994). Carcinogen risk assessment in the US. *Crit. Rev. Toxicol.*, **24**, 75–85.

Alexander, M. (1995). How toxic are chemicals in soil? *Environ. Sci. Technol.*, **29**, 2713–2717.

Allen, B. C., Crump, K. S. and Shipp, A. M. (1988). Correlation between carcinogenic potency of chemicals in animals and humans. *Risk Anal.*, **8**, 531–544.

Allen, B. C., Kavlock, R. J., Kimmel, C. A. and Faustman, E. M. (1994a). Dose–response assessments for developmental toxicity II: comparison of generic benchmark dose estimates with NOAELs. *Fundam. Appl. Toxicol.*, **23**, 487–495.

Allen, B. C., Kavlock, R. J., Kimmel, C. A. and Faustman, E. M. (1994b). Dose–response assessments for developmental toxicity III: statistical models. *Fundam. Appl. Toxicol.*, **23**, 496–509.

Allen, B., Gentry, R., Shipp, A. and Van Landingham, C. (1998). Calculation of benchmark doses for reproductive and developmental toxicity observed after exposure to isopropanol. *Regul. Toxicol. Pharmacol.*, **28**, 38–44.

Allen, M. and Richardson, G. M. (1998). Probability density functions describing 24-hour inhalation rates for use in human health risk assessments. *Human Ecol. Risk Assess.*, **4**, 379–408.

Amdur, M. O., Doull, J. and Klaassen, C. K. (1995). *Casarett and Doull's Toxicology: The Basic Science of Poisons*, 5th edn. Pergamon Press, New York.

Ames, B. N. (1987). Six common errors relating to environmental pollution. *Regul. Toxicol. Pharmacol.*, **76**, 379–383.

Ames, B. N. (1996). The causes of aging and cancer: the misinterpretation of animal cancer tests. *Human Ecol. Risk Assess.*, **2**, 6–9.

Ames, B. N. and Gold, L. S. (1990). Too many rodent carcinogens: mitogenesis increases mutagenesis. *Science*, **249**, 970–971.

Ames, B. N. and Gold, L. S. (1993). Environmental pollution and cancer: some misconceptions. In Foster, K. R., Berstein, D. E. and Huber, P. W. (Eds.), *Phantom Risk: Scientific Inference and the Law*. MIT Press, Cambridge, MA.

Ames, B. N., Magaw, R. and Gold, L. S. (1987). Ranking possible carcinogenic hazards. *Science*, **236**, 271–273.

Ames, B. N., Gold, L. S. and Shigenaga, M. K. (1996). Cancer prevention, rodent high-dose cancer tests, and risk assessment. *Risk Anal.*, **16**, 613–617.

Ames, B. N. and Gold, L. S. (1997). Environmental pollution, pesticides, and the prevention of cancer: misconceptions. *FASEB Journal*, **11**, 1041–1052.

Andersen, M. E. (1991). Quantitative risk assessment and chemical carcinogens in occupational environments. *Appl. Ind. Hyg.*, **3**, 267–273.

Andersen, M. E., Clewell, H. J., Gargas, M. L., Smith, F. A. and Reitz, R. H. (1987a). Physiologically based pharmacokinetics and the risk assessment process for methylene chloride. *Toxicol. Appl. Pharmacol.*, **87**, 185–207.

Andersen, M. E., MacNaughton, M. G., Clewell, H. J. and Paustenbach, D. J. (1987b). Adjusting exposure limits for long and short exposure periods using a physiological pharmacokinetic model. *Am. Ind. Hyg. Assoc. J.*, **48**, 335–343.

Andersen, M. E., Clewell, H. J., Gargas, M. L., MacNaughton, M. G., Reitz, R. H., Nolan, R. J. and McKenna, M. J. (1991). Physiologically based pharmacokinetic modeling with dichloromethane, its metabolite, carbon monoxide, and blood carboxyhemoglobin in rats and humans. *Toxicol. Appl. Pharmacol.*, **108**, 14–27.

Andersen, M. E., Mills, J. J., Gargas, M. L., Kedderis, L., Birnbaum, L. S., Neubert, D. and Greenlee, W. F. (1993). Modeling receptor-mediated processes with dioxin: implications for pharmacokinetics and risk assessment. *Risk Anal.*, **13**, 25–35.

Andersen, M. E., Clewell, H. J. and Krishnan, K. (1995). Tissue dosimetry, pharmacokinetics modeling, and interspecies scaling factors. *Risk Anal.*, **15**, 533–537.

Anderson, E. (1983). Quantitative approaches in use to assess cancer risk. *Risk Anal.*, **3**, 277–295.

Anderson, P. D. and Yuhas, A. L. (1996). Improving risk management by characterizing reality: a benefit of probabilistic risk assessment. *Human Ecol. Risk Assess.*, **2**, 55–58.

Anderson, R. A., Colton, T., Doull, J., Marks, J. G., Smith, R. G., Bruce, G. M., Finley, B. L. and Paustenbach, D. J. (1993). Designing a biological monitoring program to assess community exposure to chromium: conclusions of an expert panel. *J. Toxicol. Environ. Health*, **40**, 555–583.

Armitage, P. and Doll, R. (1957). A two-stage theory of carcinogenesis in relation to the age distribution of human cancer. *Br. J. Cancer*, **11**, 161–169.

Ashby, J. and Tennant, R. W. (1994). Prediction of rodent carcinogenicity of 44 chemicals: results. *Mutagenesis*, **9**, 7–15.

ATSDR (1991). *Toxicological Profile for Barium*. Agency for Toxic Substances and Disease Registry US Department of Health and Human Services, Public Health Service, Atlanta, GA.

ATSDR (1992). *Public Health Assessment Guidance Manual*. Agency for Toxic Substances and Disease Registry. US Department of Health and Human Services, Public Health Service, Atlanta, GA.

ATSDR (1994). *Toxicological Profile for Polycyclic Aromatic Hydrocarbons (Update)*. Agency for Toxic Substances and Disease Registry. U. S. Department of Health and Human Services, Public Health Service, Atlanta, GA.

Auton, T. R. (1991). Joint risk from multiple compound exposures. *Risk Anal.*, **11**, 181–183.

Aylward, L. L., Hays, S. M., Karch, N. J. and Paustenbach, D. J. (1996). Evaluation of the relative susceptibility of animals and humans to the cancer hazard posed by 2,3,7,8-tetrachlorodibenzo-*p*-dioxin (TCDD) using internal measures of dose. *Environ. Sci. Technol.*, **30**, 3534–3543.

Bagdon, R. E. (1989). *Dermal Absorption to Selected Chemicals under Experimental and Human Exposure Conditions to Facilitate Risk Assessment and the Development of Standards for Soil. I. Chromium.* New Jersey Department of Environmental Protection, Trenton, NJ.

Bagdon, R. E. and Hazen, R. E. (1991). Skin permeation and cutaneous hypersensitivity as a basis for making risk assessments of chromium as a soil contaminant. *Environ. Health Perspect.*, **92**, 111–119.

Bailer, J. C., III, Crouch, E. A. C., Shaikh, R. and Spielgelman, D. (1988). One-hit models of carcinogenesis: conservative or not? *Risk Anal.*, **8**, 485–498.

Baird, S. J. S., Cohen, J. T., Graham, J. D., Shlyakhter, A. I. and Evans, J. S. (1996). Noncancer risk assessment: a probabilistic alternative to current practice. *Human Ecol. Risk Assess.*, **2**, 79–102.

Barber, E. D., Teetsel, N. M., Kolberg, K. F. and Guest, D. (1992). A comparative study of the rates of *in vitro* percutaneous absorption of eight chemicals using rat and human skin. *Fundam. Appl. Toxicol.*, **19**, 493–497.

Barltrop, D. and Meeks, F. (1975). Absorption of different lead compounds. *Postgrad. Med. J.*, **51**, 805–809.

Barnard, R. C. (1995). Risk assessment: the default conservatism controversy. *Regul. Toxicol. Pharmacol.*, **21**, 431–438.

Barnard, R. C. (1996a). Executive Order 12866: advantages and disadvantages of the Administration's new regulatory plan on risk, benefit, and cost. *Regul. Toxicol. Pharmacol.*, **23**, 178–182.

Barnard, R. C. (1996b). A new approach to risk assessment integrating scientific evaluation and economic assessment of costs and benefits. *Regul. Toxicol. Pharmacol.*, **24**, 121–125.

Barnes, D. G. and Dourson, M. (1988). Reference dose (RfD): description and use in health risk assessments. *Regul. Toxicol. Pharmacol.*, **8**, 471–486.

Barnes, D. G., Daston, G. P., Evans, J. S., Jarabek, A. M., Kavlock, R., J., Kimmel, C. A., Park, C. and Spitzer, H. L. (1995). Benchmark dose workshop: criteria for use of a benchmark dose to estimate a reference dose. *Regul. Toxicol. Pharmacol.*, **21**, 296–306.

Barr, J. (1988). Design and interpretation of bioassays for carcinogenicity. *Regul. Toxicol. Pharmacol.*, **7**, 422–426.

Bartek, M. J., LaBudde, J. A. and Maibach, H. I. (1972). Skin permeability *in vivo*: comparison in rat, rabbit, pig and man. *J. Invest. Dermatol.*, **58**, 114–123.

Bartell, S. M. (1996). Some thoughts concerning quotients, risks, and decision-making. *Human Ecol. Risk Assess.*, **2**, 25–29.

Barton, H. A. and Das, S. (1996). Alternatives for a risk assessment on chronic noncancer effects from oral exposure to trichloroethylene. *Regul. Toxicol. Pharmacol.*, **24**, 269–285.

Baxter, L. A., Finch, S. J., Lipfert, F. W. and Yu, Q. (1997). Comparing estimates of the effects of air pollution on human mortality obtained using different regression methodologies. *Risk Anal.*, **17**, 273–277.

Beauchamp, J. J., McCarthy, J., Rosenblatt, D. H. and Shugart, L. R. (1992). Statistical design for sampling and analysis of animal populations for chemical contamination. *Risk Anal.*, **12**, 233–237.

Beck, B. D. and Cohen J. T. (1997). Risk assessment for criteria pollutants vs. other non-carcinogens: the difference between implicit and explicit conservatism. *Human Ecol. Risk Assess.*, **3**, 617–626.

Beech, J. A. (1983). Estimated worst-case trihalomethane body burden of a child using a swimming pool. *Med. Hypoth.*, **6**, 303–307.

Binder, S., Sokal, D. and Maughan, D. (1986). Estimating the amount of soil ingested by young children through tracer elements. *Arch. Environ. Health*, **41**, 341–345.

Bogen, K. T. (1994a). Models based on steady-state *in vitro* dermal permeability data underestimate short-term *in vivo* exposures to organic chemicals in water. *J. Exp. Anal. Environ. Epidemiol.*, **4**, 457–476.

Bogen, K. T. (1994b). A note on compounded conservatisms. *Risk Anal.*, **14**, 379–382.

Bogen, K. T. (1995). Methods to approximate joint uncertainty and variability in risk. *Risk Anal.*, **15**, 411–419.

Bogen, K. T. (1997). Do U.S. county data disprove linear no-threshold predictions of lung cancer risk for residential radon? A preliminary assessment of biological plausibility. *Human Ecol. Risk Assess.*, **3**, 157–186.

Bogen, K. T. and Spear R. C. (1987). Integrating uncertainty and interindividual variability in environmental risk assessment. *Risk Anal.*, **7**, 427–435.

Bogen, K. T. and Gold, L. S. (1997). Trichloroethylene cancer risk: simplified calculation of pbpk-based mcls for cytotoxic endpoints. *Regul. Toxicol. Pharmacol.*, **25**, 26–42.

Bogen, K. T., Keating, G. A., Meissner, S. and Vogel, J. S. (1998). Initial uptake kinetics in human skin exposed to dilute aqueous trichloroethylene. *J. Exp. Anal. Environ. Epidemiol.*, **8**, 253–271.

Borgert, S. J., Roberts, S. M., Harbison, R. D. and James, R. C. (1995). Influence of soil half-life on risk assessment of carcinogens. *Regul. Toxicol. Pharmacol.*, **22**, 143–151.

Boyce, C. P. (1998). Comparison of approaches for developing distributions for carcinogenic potency factors. *Human Ecol. Risk Assess.*, **4**, 527–578.

Breyer, S. (1994). *Breaking the Vicious Circle: Toward Effective Risk Regulation.* Harvard Press, Boston, MA.

Brown, C. C. and Chui, K. C. (1989). Additive and multiplicative models and multistage carcinogenesis theory. *Risk Anal.*, **9**, 99–106.

Brown, K. G. and Hoel, D. G. (1986). Statistical modeling of animal bioassay data with variable dosing regimens: example – vinyl chloride. *Risk Anal.*, **6**, 155–166.

Brown, K. G., Guo, H.-R. and Greene, H. L. (1997). Uncertainty in the cancer risk at low doses of inorganic arsenic. *Human Ecol. Risk Assess.*, **3**, 351–362.

Buck, R. J., Hammerstrom, K. A. and Ryan, P. B. (1995). Estimating long-term exposures from short-term measurements. *J. Exp. Anal. Environ. Epidemiol.*, **5**, 359–374.

Buck, R. J., Hammerstrom, K. A. and Ryan, P. B. (1997). Bias in population estimates of long-term exposure from short-term measurements of individual exposure. *Risk Anal.*, **17**, 455–465.

Bukowski, J., Korn, L. and Wartenberg, D. (1995). Correlated inputs in quantitative risk assessment: the effects of distributional shape. *Risk Anal.*, **15**, 215–219.

Burmaster, D. E. (1998a). Lognormal distributions for skin area as a function of body weight. *Risk Anal.*, **18**, 27–32.

Burmaster, D. E. (1998b). A lognormal distribution for time spent showering. *Risk Anal.*, **18**, 33–36.

Burmaster, D. E. and Anderson, P. D. (1994). Principle of good practice for the use of Monte Carlo techniques in human health and ecological risk assessment. *Risk Anal.*, **14**, 477–491.

Burmaster, D. E. and Harris, R. H. (1993). The magnitude of compounding conservatisms in superfund risk assessments. *Risk Anal.*, **13**, 131–134.

Burmaster, D. E. and Lehr, J. H. (1991). It's time to make risk assessment a science. *Ground Water Monit. Rev.*, 1–3.

Burmaster, D. E. and Maxwell, N. I. (1991). Time and loading dependence in the McKone model for dermal uptake of organic chemicals from a soil matrix. *Risk Anal.*, **11**, 491–497.

Burmaster, D. E. and von Stackelberg, K. (1991). Using Monte Carlo simulations in public health risk assessments: estimating and presenting full distributions of risk. *J. Expos. Anal. Environ. Epidemiol.*, **1**, 491–521.

Burmaster, D. E., Lloyd, K. J. and Thompson, K. M. (1995). The need for new methods to backcalculate soil cleanup targets in interval and probabilistic cancer risk assessments. *Human Ecol. Risk Assess.*, **1**, 89–100.

Burmaster, D. E. and Thompson, K. M. (1995). Back-calculating cleanup targets in probabilistic risk assessments when the acceptability of cancer risk is defined under different risk management policies. *Human Ecol. Risk Assess.*, **1**, 101–120.

Burmaster, D. E. and Bloomfield, L. R. (1995). Mathematical properties of the risk equation when variability is present. *Human Ecol. Risk Assess.*, **2**, 348–355.

Burmaster, D. E. (1996). Benefits and costs of using probabilistic techniques in human health risk assessments – with an emphasis on site-specific risk assessments. *Human Ecol. Risk Assess.*, **2**, 35–43.

Burmaster, D. E. and Huff, D. A. (1997). Using lognormal distributions and lognormal probability plots in probabilistic risk assessments. *Human Ecol. Risk Assess.*, **3**, 223–234.

Burmaster, D. E. and Thompson, K. M. (1997). Estimating exposure point concentrations for surface soils for use in deterministic and probabilistic risk assessments. *Human Ecol. Risk Assess.*, **3**, 363–384.

Burrows, D. (1983). Adverse chromate reactions on the skin. In Burrows D. (Ed.), *Chromium: Metabolism and Toxicity*. pp. 137–163. CRC Press, Boca Raton, FL.

Butterworth, B. E. (1990). Consideration of both genotoxic and nongenotoxic mechanisms in predicting carcinogenic potential. *Mutat. Res.*, **239**, 117–132.

Butterworth, B. E. (1993). *A Review of Mechanisms of Carcinogenesis*. CRC Reviews. CRC Press, Boca Raton, FL.

Butterworth, B. E. and Slaga, T. (1987). *Nongenotoxic Mechanisms in Carcinogenesis*. Banbury Report 25. Cold Spring Harbor Laboratory Press, Cold Spring Harbor, NY.

Byard, J. (1989). Hazard assessment of 1,1,1-trichloroethane in groundwater. In Paustenbach, D. J. (Ed.), *The Risk Assessment of Environmental and Human Health Hazards: A Textbook of Case Studies*, pp. 331–344. J. Wiley, New York.

Calabrese, E. J. (1978a). *Methodologic Approaches to Deriving Environmental and Occupational Health Standards*. Wiley, New York.

Calabrese, E. J. (1978b). *Pollutants and High Risk Groups: the Biological Basis of Increased Human Susceptibility to Environmental and Occupational Pollutants*. Wiley, New York.

Calabrese, E. J. (1983). *Principles of Animal Extrapolation*. Wiley, New York.

Calabrese, E. J. (1986). *Age and Susceptibility to Toxic Substances*. John Wiley and Sons, New York.

Calabrese, E. J. (1991). *Multiple Chemical Interactions*. Lewis, Chelsea, MI.

Calabrese, E. J. and Gilbert, C. E. (1993). Lack of total independence of uncertainty factors (UF): implications for size of total uncertainty factor. *Regul. Toxicol. Pharmacol.*, **17**, 44–51.

Calabrese, E. and Kenyon, E. M. (1991). *Air Toxics and Risk Assessment*. Lewis, Ann Arbor, MI.

Calabrese, E. J. and Stanek E. J. (1991). A guide to interpreting soil ingestion studies. II. Qualitative and quantitative evidence of soil ingestion. *Regul. Toxicol. Pharmacol.*, **13**, 278–292.

Calabrese, E. J., Barnes, R., Stanek, E. J., Pastides, H., Gilbert, C. E., Veneman, P., Wang, X., Lasztity, A. and Kostecki, P. T. (1989). How much soil do young children ingest: an epidemiological study. *Regul. Toxicol. Pharmacol.*, **10**, 123–137.

Calabrese, E. J., Stanek, E. J., Gilbert C. E. and Barnes, R. M. (1990). Preliminary adult soil ingestion estimates: results of a pilot study. *Regul. Toxicol. Pharmacol.*, **12**, 88–95.

Calabrese, E. J. and Baldwin, L. A. (1995). A toxicological basis to derive generic interspecies uncertainty factors for application in human and ecological risk assessments. *Human Ecol. Risk Assess.*, **1**, 555–564.

Calabrese, E. J., Stanek, E. J. and Barnes, R. (1996). Methodology to estimate the amount and particle size of soil ingested by children: implications for exposure assessment at waste sites. *Regul. Toxicol. Pharmacol.*, **24**, 264–268.

Calabrese, E. J. and Baldwin, L. A. (1997). A quantitatively-based methodology for the evaluation of chemical hormesis. *Human Ecol. Risk Assess.*, **3**, 545–554.

CalEPA (1998). *Report on the Implementation of Governor Wilson's Executive Order W-137–96 to Improve the Science and Consistency of Risk Assessment in California*. California Environmental Protection Agency. The Office of Environmental Health Hazard Assessment, California Environmental Protection Agency, Sacramento, CA.

Carrington, C. D. and Bolger, P. M. (1998). Uncertainty and risk assessment. *Human Ecol. Risk Assess.*, **4**, 253–258.

Carson, R. (1962). *Silent Spring*. Houghton Mifflin, Boston.

Caudill, S. P. and Pirkle, J. L. (1992). Effects of measurement error on estimating biological half-life. *J. Exp. Anal. Environ. Epidemiol.*, **2**, 463–476.

CCSTG (1993). *Risk and the Environment, Improving Regulatory Decision Making*. Carnegie Commission on Science, Technology, and Government. The Carnegie Corporation, New York.

CDHS (1986). *The Development of Applied Action Levels for Soil Contact: a Scenario for the Exposure of Humans to Soil in a Residential Setting*. California Department of Health Services, Sacramento, CA.

CDTS (1994). *Guidance on Dermal Absorption Factors*. California Department of Toxic Substances Control. California Environmental Protection Agency, Sacramento, CA.

Chaney, R. L., Sterrett S. B. and Mielke, H. W. (1984). The potential for heavy metal exposure from urban gardens and soils. In Preer, J. R. (Ed.), *Proceedings of Symposium on Heavy Metals in Urban Gardens*. Agricultural Experimental Station, University of the District of Columbia, Washington, DC, pp. 37–44.

Chen, C. W. (1993). Armitage-Doll two stage model: implications and extension. *Risk Anal.*, **13**, 273–280.

Cherrie, J. W. and Robertson, A. (1995). Biologically relevant assessment of dermal exposure. *Ann Occup. Hyg.*, **39**, 387–392.

Cicmanec, J. L. and Poirier, K. A. (1995). Selected applications of reduced uncertainty factors in noncancer risk assessments. *Human Ecol. Risk Assess.*, **1**, 637–640.

Clayson, D. B. and Iverson, F. (1996). Cancer risk assessment at the crossroads: the need to turn to a biological approach. *Regul. Toxicol. Pharmacol.*, **24**, 45–59.

Clausing, P., Brunekreef, B. and Van Wijnen, J. H. (1987). A method for estimating soil ingestion in children. *Int. Arch. Occup. Environ. Health*, **59**, 73–82.

Clewell, H. J. (1995). The application of physiologically based pharmacokinetics modeling in human health risk assessment of hazardous substances. *Toxicol. Lett.*, **79**, 207–217.

Clewell, H. J., Lee, T. S. and Carpenter, R. L. (1994). Sensitivity of physiologically-based pharmacokinetics models to variation in model parameters: methylene chloride. *Risk Anal.*, **14**, 533–554.

Clewell, H. J. III and Jarnot, B. M. (1994). Incorporation of pharmacokinetics in noncancer risk assessment: example with chloropentafluorobenzene. *Risk Anal.*, **14**, 265–275.

Clewell, H. J., Gentry, P. R., Gearhart, J. M., Allen, B. C. and Andersen, M. E. (1995). Considering pharmacokinetics and mechanistic information in cancer risk assessments for environmental contaminants: examples with vinyl chloride and trichloroethylene. *Chemosphere*, **31**, 2561–2578.

Coad, S. and Newhook, R. C. (1992). PCP exposure for the Canadian general population: a multimedia analysis. *J. Exp. Anal. Environ. Epidemiol.*, **2**, 391–414.

Cogliano, V. J. (1997). Plausible upper bounds: are their sums plausible? *Risk Anal.*, **17**, 77–83.

Cohen, B. L. (1998). Test of the linear-no threshold theory. *Risk Anal.*, **18**, 229–230.

Cohen, S. M. (1995). Human relevance of animal carcinogenicity studies. *Regul. Toxicol. Pharmacol.*, **21**, 75–80.

Collins, J. F., Brown, J. P., Alexeeff, G. V. and Salmon, A. G. (1998). Potency equivalence factors for some polycyclic aromatic hydrocarbons and polycyclic aromatic hydrocarbon derivatives. *Regul. Toxicol. Pharmacol.*, **28**, 45–54.

Cooper, J. A., Ferson, S. and Ginzburg, L. (1996). Hybrid processing of stochastic and subjective uncertainty data. *Risk Anal.*, **16**, 785–792.

Corbett, G. E., Finley, B. L., Paustenbach, D. J. and Kerger, B. D. (1997). Systemic uptake of chromium in human volunteers following dermal contact with hexavalent chromium (22 MG/L). *J. Exp. Anal. Environ. Epidemiol.*, **7**, 179–190.

Copeland, T. L., Paustenbach, D. J., Harris, M. A. and Otani, J. (1993). Comparing the results of a Monte Carlo analysis with EPA's reasonable maximum exposed individual (RMEI): a case study of a former wood treatment site. *Regul. Toxicol. Pharmacol.*, **18**, 275–312.

Copeland, T. L., Holbrow, A. H., Otani, J. M., Connor, K. T. and Paustenbach, D. J., (1994). Use of probabilistic methods to understand the conservatism in California's approach to

assessing health risks posed by air contaminants. *J. Air Waste Manage. Assoc.*, **44**, 1399–1413.

Corley, R. A., Mendrala, A. L., Smith, F. A., Staats, D. A., Gargas, M. L., Conolly, R. B., Anderson, M. E. and Reitz, R. H. (1990). Development of a physiologically-based pharmacokinetic model for chloroform. *Toxicol. Appl. Pharmacol.*, **103**, 512–527.

Covello, V. T. and Mumpower, J. (1985). Risk analysis and management: a historical perspective. *Risk Anal.*, **5**, 103–120.

CRA (1994). *Historical Roots of Health Risk Assessment*. Center for Risk Analysis, Harvard University, Cambridge, MA.

Cox, L. A., Jr. (1984). Probability of causation and the attributable proportion of risk. *Risk Anal.*, **4**, 221–230.

Cox, L. A., Jr. (1996). More accurate dose-response estimation using Monte-Carlo uncertainty analysis: the data cube approach. *Human Ecol. Risk Assess.*, **2**, 150–174.

Crawford, M. and Wilson, R. (1996). Low-dose linearity: the rule or the exception? *Human Ecol. Risk Assess.*, **2**, 305–330.

Creighton, P. J., Greenberg, A. and Lioy, P. J. (1992). The effects of cooking methodology on benzo(a)pyrene exposure from 'home-cooked' bacon and hamburgers and 'fat-food chain' hamburgers. *J. Exp. Anal. Environ. Epidemiol.*, **2**, 27–44.

CRARM (1996). *Risk Assessment and Risk Management in Regulatory Decision-Making*. Commission on Risk Assessment and Risk Management. National Research Council, Washington, DC.

Cronin, W. J., Oswald, E. J., Shelley, M. L., Fisher, J. W. and Fleming, C. D. (1995). A trichloroethylene risk assessment using a Monte Carlo analysis of parameter uncertainty in conjunction with physiologically-based pharmacokinetic modeling. *Risk Anal.*, **15**, 555–566.

Crouch, E. A. C. (1996a). Uncertainty distributions for cancer potency factors: laboratory animal carcinogenicity and interspecies extrapolation. *Human Ecol. Risk Assess.*, **2**, 103–129.

Crouch, E. A. C. (1996b). Uncertainty distributions for cancer potency factors: combining epidemiological studies with laboratory bioassays – the example of acrylonitrile. *Human Ecol. Risk Assess.*, **2**, 130–149.

Crouch, E. A. C., Lester, R. A., Lash, T. L., Armstrong, S. R. and Green, L. C. (1997). Health risk assessments prepared per the risk assessment reforms under consideration in the U.S. Congress. *Human Ecol. Risk Assess.*, **3**, 713–777.

Crump, K. S. (1980). An improved procedure for low-dose carcinogenic risk assessment from animal data. *J. Environ. Pathol. Toxicol.*, **5**, 675–684.

Crump, K. S. (1984). A new method for determining allowable daily intakes. *Fundam. Appl. Toxicol.*, **4**, 854–871.

Crump, K. S. (1994). Risk of benzene-induced leukemia: a sensitivity analysis of the Pliofilm cohort with additional follow-up and new exposure estimates. *J. Toxicol. Environ. Health*, **42**, 2419–2421.

Crump, K. S. (1995). Calculation of benchmark doses from continuous data. *Risk Anal.*, **15**, 79–85.

Crump, K. S. (1996). The linearized multistage model and the future of quantitative risk assessment. *Hum. Exp. Toxicol.*, **15**, 787–798.

Crump, K. S. (1998). On summarizing group exposures in risk assessment: is an arithmetic mean or a geometric mean more appropriate? *Risk Anal.*, **18**, 293–297.

Crump, K. S., Hoel, D. G., Langley, C. H. and Peto, R. (1976). Fundamental carcinogenic processes and their implications for low dose risk assessment. *Cancer Res.*, **36**, 2973–2979.

Crump, K. S. and Howe, R. B. (1984). The multistage model with time-dependent dose pattern: applications to carcinogenic risk assessment. *Risk Anal.*, **4**, 163–175.

Crump, K. S., Clewell, H. J. and Andersen, M. E. (1997). Cancer and non-cancer risk assessment should be harmonized. *Human Ecol. Risk Assess.*, **3**, 495–500.

Cullen, A. C. (1994). Measures of compounding conservatism in probabilistic risk assessment. *Risk Anal.*, **14**, 389–393.

Cumming, R. B. (1981). Is risk assessment a science? *Risk Anal.*, **1**, 1–4.

Dakins, M. E., Toll, J. E., Small, M. J. and Brand, K. P. (1996). Risk-based environmental remediation: Bayesian Monte Carlo analysis and the expected value of sample information. *Risk Anal.*, **16**, 67–80.

Davis, A., Ruby, M. V. and Bergstrom, P. D. (1992). Bioavailability of arsenic and lead from the Butte, Montana, mining district. *Environ. Sci. Technol.*, **26**, 461–468.

Davis, A., Drexter, J. W., Ruby, M. V. and Nicholson, A. (1993). Micromineralogy of mine waste in relation to lead bioavailability, Butte, Montana. *Environ. Sci. Technol.*, **27**, 1415–1425.

Davis, A., Bloom, N. S. and Que Hee, S. S. (1997). The environmental geochemistry and bioaccessability of mercury in soils and sediments: a review. *Risk Anal.*, **17**, 557–569.

Davis, S., Waller, P., Buschom, R., Ballou, J. and White P. (1990). Quantitative estimates of soil ingestion in normal children between the ages of 2 and 7 years: population-based estimates using aluminum, silicon, and titanium as soil tracer elements. *Arch. Environ. Health*, **45**, 112–122.

Derelanko, M. A. (1995). Risk assessment. In Derelanko, M. J. and Hollinger, M. A., (Eds), *CRC Handbook of Toxicology*. CRC Press, Boca Raton, FL. pp. 591–676.

de Silva, P. E. (1994). How much soil do children ingest—a new approach. *Appl. Occup. Environ. Hyg.*, **9**, 40–43.

Del Pup, J., Kmiecik, J., Smith, S. and Reitman, F. (1996). Improvement in human health risk assessment utilizing site and chemical-specific information: a case study. *Toxicol.*, **113**, 346–350.

Dewanji, A., Venzon, D. J. and Moolgavkar, S. H. (1989). A stochastic two-stage model for cancer risk assessment. II. The number and size of premalignant clones. *Risk Anal.*, **9**, 179–187.

Dills, R. L., Ackerlund, W. S., Kalman, D. A. and Morgan, M. S. (1994). Inter-individual variability in blood/air partitioning of volatile organic compounds and correlations with blood chemistry. *J. Exp. Anal. Environ. Epidemiol.*, **4**, 229–245.

Doll, R. and Peto, R. (1981). The causes of cancer: quantitative estimates of avoidable risks of cancer in the United States today. *J. Natl. Cancer. Inst.*, **66**, 1191–1308.

Dorre, W. H. (1997). Time-activity patterns of some selected small groups as a basis for exposure estimation: a methodological study. *J. Exp. Anal. Environ. Epidemiol.*, **7**, 471–492.

Dourson, M. L. (1996). Uncertainty factors in noncancer risk assessment. *Regul. Toxicol. Pharmacol.*, **24**, 107.

Dourson, M. L. and Stara, J. F. (1983). Regulatory history and experimental support of uncertainty (safety) factors. *Regul. Toxicol. Pharmacol.*, **3**, 224–238.

Dourson, M. L., Herizberg, R. C., Hartung, R. and Blackburn, K. (1985). Novel methods for the estimation of acceptable daily intake. *Toxicol. Ind. Health*, **1**, 23–42.

Dourson, M. L., Felter, S. P. and Robinson, D. (1996). Evolution of science-based uncertainty factors in noncancer risk assessment. *Regul. Toxicol. Pharmacol.*, **24**, 108–119.

Dourson, M. L., Felter, S. P. and Robinson, D. (1997). Evolution of science-based uncertainty factors in noncancer risk assessment. *Human Ecol. Risk Assess.*, **3**, 579–590.

Driver, J. H., Konz, J. J. and Whitmyre, G. K. (1989). Soil adherence to human skin. *Bull. Environ. Contam. Toxicol.*, **17**, 1831–1850.

Duan, N. and Mage, D. T. (1997). Combination of direct and indirect approaches for exposure assessment. *J. Exp. Anal. Environ. Epidemiol.*, **7**, 439–470.

Dudley, S. E. and Gramm, W. L. (1997). EPA's ozone standard may harm public health and welfare. *Risk Anal.*, **17**, 403–406.

Ebert, E. S., Price, P. S. and Keenan, R. E. (1994). Selection of fish consumption estimates for use in the regulatory process. *J. Exp. Anal. Environ. Epidemiol.*, **4**, 373–394.

Edelmann, K. G. and Burmaster, D. E. (1997). Are all distributions with the same 95th percentile equally acceptable? *Human Ecol. Risk Assess.*, **3**, 235–355.

Engels, D. W. and Vaughan, D. S. (1996). Biomarkers, natural variability, and risk assessment: can they coexist?. *Human Ecol. Risk Assess.*, **2**, 257–262.

Enterline, P. E. (1987). A method for estimating lifetime cancer risks from limited epidemiologic data. *Risk Anal.*, **7**, 91–96.

Ershow, A. G. and Cantor, K. P. (1989). *Total Tapwater Intake in the United States: Population-Based Estimates of Quantities and Sources*. Life Sciences Research Office, Federation of American Societies for Experimental Biology, Bethesda, MD.

ESE (1989). *Remedial Investigation for Chromium Sites in Hudson County, New Jersey*. Environmental Science and Engineering. Prepared for the State of New Jersey, Department of Environmental Protection, Trenton, NJ.

Evans, J. S., Gray, G. M., Sielken R. L., Jr, Smith, A. E., Valdez-Flores, C. and Graham, J. D. (1994a). Use of probabilistic expert judgement in uncertainty analysis of carcinogenic potency. *Regul. Toxicol. Pharmacol.*, **20**, 15–36.

Evans, J. S., Graham, J. D., Gray, G. M. and Sielken R. L., Jr (1994b). A distributional approach to characterizing low-dose cancer risks. *Risk Anal.*, **14**, 25–33.

Fagliano, J. A., Savrin, J., Udasin, I. and Gochfeld, M. (1997). Community exposure and medical screening near chromium waste sites in New Jersey. *Regul. Toxicol. Pharmacol.*, **26**, S13–S22.

Falerios, M., Schild, K., Sheehan, P. and Paustenbach, D. J. (1992). Airborne concentrations of trivalent and hexavalent chromium from contaminated soils at unpaved and partially paved commercial/industrial sites. *J. Air Waste Manage. Assoc.*, **42**, 40–48.

Farland, W. H. and Tuxen, L. C. (1997). New directions in cancer risk assessment: accuracy, precision, credibility and uncertainty. *Human Ecol. Risk Assess.*, **3**, 667–672.

Faustman E. M., Allen, B. C., Kavlock, R. J. and Kimmel, C. A. (1994). Quantitative dose–response assessment of developmental toxicity I: characterization of data base and determination of NOAELs. *Fundam. Appl. Toxicol.*, **23**, 478–486.

Faustman, E. M. (1997). Review of non-cancer risk assessments: applications of benchmark dose methodologies. *Human Ecol. Risk Assess.*, **3**, 893–920.

Federal Focus (1996). *Principles for Evaluating Epidemiologic Data in Regulatory Risk Assessment*. Federal Focus, Washington, DC.

Felter, S. and Dourson, M. (1998). The inexact science of risk assessment (and implications for risk management?). *Human Ecol. Risk Assess.*, **4**, 245–252.

Fenske, R. A. (1993). Dermal exposure assessment techniques. *Ann. Occup. Hyg.*, **37**, 687–706.

Ferson, S. and Long, T. F. (1995). Conservative uncertainty propagation in environmental risk assessments. In Hughes, J. S., Biddinger, G. R. and Mones, E. (Eds.), *Environmental Toxicology and Risk Assessment: Vol. 3*. ASTM (American Society for Testing and Materials) Special Technical Publication 1218, Philadelphia.

Ferson, S. and Long, T. F. (1998). Deconvolution can reduce uncertainty in risk analyses. In Newman, M. and Strojan, C. (Eds.) *Risk Assessment: Measurement and Logic*. Ann Arbor Press, Ann Arbor, MI.

Fingerhut, M. A., Halperin, W. E., Marlow, D. A., Piacitelli, L. A., Honchar, P. A., Sweeney, M. H., Greife, A. L., Dill, P. A., Steenland, K. and Suruda, A. J. (1991). Cancer mortality in workers exposed to 2,3,7,8-tetrachlorodibenzo-*p*-dioxin. *N. Engl. J. Med.*, **324**, 212–218.

Finkel, A. M. (1989). Is risk assessment really 'too' conservative? Revising the revisionists. *Columbia J. Environ. Law*, **14**, 427–467.

Finkel, A. M. (1991). Edifying presentation of risk estimates: not as easy as it seems. *J. Policy Anal. Manage.*, **10**, 296–303.

Finkel, A. M. (1995). A second opinion on an economical misdiagnosis: the risky prescriptions of breaking the vicious circle. *N. Y. Univ. Law J.*, **3**, 295–381.

Finley, B. L. and Mayhall, D. A. (1994). Airborne concentrations of chromium due to contaminated interior building surfaces. *Appl. Occup. Environ. Hyg.*, **9**, 433–441.

Finley, B. L. and Paustenbach, D. J. (1994). The benefits of probabilistic exposure assessment: three case studies involving contaminated air, water, and soil. *Risk Anal.*, **14**, 53–73.

Finley, B. L. and Paustenbach, D. J. (1997). Using applied research to reduce uncertainty in health risk assessments: five case studies involving human exposure to chromium in soil and groundwater. *J. Soil Contam.*, **6**, 649–707.

Finley, B. L., Proctor, D. and Paustenbach, D. J. (1992). Inhalation reference concentrations for hexavalent and trivalent chromium. *Regul. Toxicol. Pharmacol.*, **16**, 161–176.

Finley, B. L. and Scott, P. (1998). Response to letter by Kissel. *Risk Anal.*, **18**, 9–12.

Finley, B. L., Scott, P. and Paustenbach, D. J. (1993). Evaluating the adequacy of maximum contaminant levels as health protective cleanup goals: an analysis based on Monte Carlo techniques. *Regul. Toxicol. Pharmacol.*, **18**, 438–455.

Finley, B. L., Proctor, D., Scott, P., Price, P., Harrington, N. and Paustenbach, D. J. (1994a). Recommended distributions for exposure factors frequently used in health risk assessments. *Risk Anal.*, **14**, 533–554.

Finley, B. L., Scott, P. K. and Mayhall, D. A. (1994b). Development of a standard soil-to-skin adherence probability density function for use in Monte Carlo analyses of dermal exposure. *Risk Anal.*, **14**, 555–569.

Finley, B. L., Scott, P. K., Norton, R. L., Gargas, M. L. and Paustenbach, D. J. (1996a). Urinary chromium concentrations in humans following ingestion of safe doses of hexavalent and trivalent chromium: implications for biomonitoring. *J. Toxicol. Environ. Health*, **48**, 101–121.

Fitzgerald, E. F., Hwang, S. -A., Brix, K. A., Bush, B., Cook, K. and Worswick, P. (1995). Fish PCB concentrations and consumption patterns among Mohawk women at Akwesasne. *J. Exp. Anal. Environ. Epidemiol.*, **5**, 1–20.

Food Safety Council (1980). Quantitative risk assessment. In *Food Safety Assessment*. Food Safety Council, Washington, DC.

Frantz, S. W. (1990). Instrumentation and methodology for *in vitro* skin diffusion Cells. In Kemppainen, B. W. and Reifenrath, W. G. (Eds), *Methods for Skin Absorption*. pp. 35–39. CRC Press, Boca Raton.

Freedman, D. A. and Zeisel, H. (1988). From mouse to man: the quantitative assessment of cancer risk. *Statist. Sci.*, **3**, 3–56.

Freedman, D. A., Gold, L. S. and Slone, T. H. (1993). How tautological are interspecies correlations of carcinogenic potencies? *Risk Anal.*, **13**, 265–373.

Freedman, D. A., Gold, L. S. and Lin, T. H. (1996). Concordance between rats and mice in bioassays for carcinogenesis. *Regul. Toxicol. Pharmacol.*, **23**, 225–232.

Freeman, G. B., Johnson, J. D., Killinger, J. M., Liao, S. C., Feder, P. I., Davis, A. O., Ruby, M. V., Chaney, R. L., Lovre, S. C. and Bergstrom, P. D. (1992). Relative bioavailability of lead from mining waste soils in rats. *Fundam. Appl. Toxicol.*, **19**, 388–398.

Freeman, G. B., Schoof, R. A., Ruby, M. V., Davis, A. O., Dill, J. A., Liao, S. C., Lapin, C. A. and Bergstrom, P. D. (1995). Bioavailability of arsenic in soil and house dust impacted by smelter activities following oral administration in cynomolgus monkeys. *Fundam. Appl. Toxicol.*, **28**, 215–222.

Frey, H. C. and Rhodes, D. S. (1998). Characterization and simulation of uncertainty frequency distributions: effects of distribution choice, variability, uncertainty, and parameter dependence. *Human Ecol. Risk Assess.*, **4**, 423–469.

Fries, G. F. and Paustenbach, D. J. (1990). Evaluation of potential transmission of 2,3,7,8-tetrachlorodibenzo-*p*-dioxin-contaminated incinerator emissions to humans via the food chain. *J. Toxicol. Environ. Health*, **29**, 1–43.

Friess, S. (1987). Risk assessment: historical perspectives. In *Drinking Water and Health*, Vol. 8. National Research Council, Washington, DC.

Fung, K. Y., Marro, L. and Krewski, D. (1998). A comparison of methods for estimating the benchmark dose based on overdispersed data from developmental toxicity studies. *Risk Anal.*, **18**, 329–341.

Funk, L. M., Sedman, R., Beals, J. A. J. and Fountain, R. (1998). Quantifying the distribution of inhalation exposure in human populations: 2. Distributions of time spent by adults, adolescents, and children at home, at work, and at school. *Risk Anal.*, **18**, 45–55.

Gargas, M. L. and Long, T. F. (1997). The role of risk assessment in redeveloping brownfield sites. In Davis, T. S. and Margolis, K. D. (Eds), *Brownfields: a Comprehensive Guide to Redeveloping Contaminated Properties*. American Bar Association, Chicago.

Gargas, M. L., Burgess, R. J., Voisaro, G. E., *et al.* (1989). Partition coefficients of low molecular weight volatile chemicals in various liquids and tissues. *Toxicol. Appl. Pharmacol.*, **98**, 87–99.

Gargas, M. L., Norton, R. L., Harris, M. A., Paustenbach, D. J. and Finley, B. L. (1994). Urinary excretion of chromium following ingestion of chromite-ore processing residues in humans: implications for biomonitoring. *Risk Anal.*, **14**, 1019–1024.

Gaylor, D. W. (1996). Quantalization of continuous data for benchmark dose estimation. *Regul. Toxicol. Pharmacol.*, **24**, 246–250.

Gaylor, D. W. (1997). Some current procedure and issues in cancer risk assessment. *Human Ecol. Risk Assess.*, **3**, 513–520.

Gaylor, D. W. and Chen, J. J. (1986). Relative potency of chemical carcinogens in rodents. *Risk Anal.*, **6**, 283–290.

Gaylor, D. W., Chen, J. J. and Sheehan, D. M. (1993). Uncertainty in cancer risk estimates. *Risk Anal.*, **13**, 149–153.

Gaylor, D. W., Kodell, R. L., Chen, J. J., Springer, J. A., Lorentzen, R. J. and Scheuplein, R. J. (1994). Point estimates of cancer risk at low doses. *Risk Anal.*, **14**, 843–849.

Gaylor, D. and Slikker, W., Jr. (1994). Modeling for risk assessment of neurotoxic effects. *Risk Anal.*, **14**, 333–337.

Gaylor, D. W. and Chen, J. J. (1996). A simple upper limit for the sum of risks of the components in a mixture. *Risk Anal.*, **16**, 395–398.

Georgopoulos, P. G. and Lioy, P. J. (1994). Conceptual and theoretical aspects of human exposure and dose assessment. *J. Exp. Anal. Environ. Epidemiol.*, **4**, 253–285.

Georgopoulos, P. G., Roy, A. and Gallo, M. A. (1994). Reconstruction of short-term multi-route exposure to volatile organic compounds using physiologically based pharmacokinetic models. *J. Exp. Anal. Environ. Epidemiol.*, **4**, 309–328.

Gerrity, T. R. and Henry, C. J. (eds.) (1990). *Principles of Route-to-Route Extrapolation for Risk Assessment*. Elsevier Science Publishing Co., New York.

Giardino, N. J. and Andelman, J. B. (1996). Characterization of the emissions of trichloroethylene, chloroform, and 1,2-dibromo-3-chloropropane in a full-size experimental shower. *J. Exp. Anal. Environ. Epidemiol.*, **6**, 413–424.

Gibb, H. J. and Chen, C. W. (1986). Multistage model interpretation of additive and multiplicative carcinogenic effects. *Risk Anal.*, **6**, 167–170.

Gibson, M. C., deMonsabert, S. M. and Orme-Zavaleta, J. (1997). Comparison of noncancer risk assessment approaches for use in deriving drinking water criteria. *Regul. Toxicol. Pharmacol.*, **26**, 243–255.

Gilbert, R. O. (1987). *Statistical Methods for Environmental Pollution Monitoring*. Van Nostrand Reinhold, New York.

Glaser, U., Hochrainer, D., Klöppel, H. and Kuhnen, H. (1985). Low level chromium (VI) inhalation effects on alveolar macrophages and immune functions in Wistar rats. *Arch. Toxicol.*, **57**, 250–256.

Glaser, U., Hochrainer, D. and Steinhoff, D. (1990). Investigation of irritating properties of inhaled Cr(VI) with possible influence on its carcinogenic action. In Seemayer, N. O. and Hadnagy, W. (Eds), *Environmental Hygiene II*. pp. 235–245. Springer, Berlin.

Glickman, T. S. (1986). A methodology for estimating time-of-day variations in the size of a population exposed to risk. *Risk Anal.*, **6**, 317–323.

Gold, L. W., Backman, G. M., Hooper, N. K. and Peto, R. (1987). Ranking the potential carcinogenic hazards to workers from exposures to chemicals that are tumorigenic in rodents. *Environ. Health Perspect.*, **76**, 211–219.

Gold, L. S. (1993). The importance of data on mechanism of carcinogenesis in efforts to predict low-dose human risk. *Risk Anal.*, **13**, 399–402.

Gold, L. S., Manley, N. B. and Ames, B. N. (1992). Extrapolation of carcinogenicity between species: qualitative and quantitative factors. *Risk Anal.*, **12**, 579–587.

Golden, R. J., Holm, S. E., Robinson, D. E., Julkunen, P. H. and Reese, E. A. (1997). Chloroform mode of action: implications for cancer risk assessment. *Regul. Toxicol. Pharmacol.*, **26**, 142–154.

Goldsmith, J. and Kordysh, E. (1993). Why dose-response relationships are often non-linear and some consequences. *J. Exp. Anal. Environ. Epidemiol.*, **3**, 259–276.

Goldstein, B. D. (1989). The maximally exposed individual. *Environ. Forum*, Nov.–Dec., 13–16.

Goodman, G. and Wilson, R. (1992). Comparison of the dependance of the TD50 on maximum tolerated dose for mutagens and nonmutagens. *Risk Anal.*, **12**, 525–534.

Gough, M. (1990). How much cancer can EPA regulate anyway? *Risk Anal.*, **10**, 1–6.

Graham, J. D., Green, L. and Roberts, M. J. (1988). *In Search of Safety: Chemicals and Cancer Risks*. Harvard University Press, Cambridge, MA.

Graham, J., Berry, M., Bryan, E. F., Callahan, M. A., Fan, A., Finley, B., Lynch, J., McKone, T., Ozkaynak, H., Sexton, K. and Walker, K. (1992). The Role of Exposure Databases in Risk Assessment. *Arch. Environ. Health*, **47**, 408–420.

Gray, G. M. (1994). Complete risk characterization. *Risk Perspect.*, **2**, 1–2.

Gross, A. J. and Berg, P. H. (1995). A meta-analytical approach examining the potential relationship between talc exposure and ovarian cancer. *J. Exp. Anal. Environ. Epidemiol.*, **5**, 181–196.

Guy, R. H., Hadgraft, J. and Maibach, H. I. (1982). A pharmacokinetic model for percutaneous absorption. *Int. J. Pharm.*, **11**, 119–129.

Haas, C. N. (1997). Importance of the distributional form in characterizing inputs to Monte Carlo risk assessments. *Risk Anal.*, **17**, 107–113.

Habicht, F. H. (1992). *Guidance on Risk Characterization for Risk Managers and Risk Assessors*. Memorandum on Behalf of the Agency's Risk Assessment Council, Deputy Administrator, EPA to Assistant and Regional Administrators, 26 February 1992. Risk Assessment Council, US EPA, Washington, DC.

Hamar, G. B., McGeehin, M. A., Phifer, B. L. and Ashley, D. L. (1996). Volatile organic compound testing of a population living near a hazardous waste site. *J. Exp. Anal. Environ. Epidemiol.*, **6**, 247–255.

Hamed, M. M. and Bedient, P. B. (1997). On the effect of probability distributions of input variables in public health risk assessment. *Risk Anal.*, **17**, 97–105.

Hart, W. L., Reynolds, R. C. and Krasavage, W. J., *et al.* (1988). Evaluation of developmental toxicity data: a discussion of some pertinent factors and a proposal. *Risk Anal.*, **8**, 59–70.

Haseman, J. K. and Elwell, M. R. (1996). Evaluation of false positive and false negative outcomes in NTP long-term rodent carcinogenicity studies. *Risk Anal.*, **16**, 813–819.

Hattis, D. B. (1986). The promise of molecular epidemiology for quantitative risk assessment. *Risk Anal.*, **6**, 181–194.

Hattis, D., Erdreich, L. and Ballew, M. (1987). Human variability in susceptibility to toxic chemicals – a preliminary analysis of pharmacokinetic data from normal volunteers. *Risk Anal.*, **7**, 415–425.

Hattis, D., White, P. and Koch, P. (1993). Uncertainties in pharmacokinetic modeling for perchloroethylene: II. Comparison of model predictions with data for a variety of different parameters. *Risk Anal.*, **13**, 5991–5610.

Hattis, D. and Burmaster, D. (1994). Assessment of variability and uncertainty distributions for practical risk analysis. *Risk Anal.*, **14**, 713–729.

Hattis, D. and Silver, K. (1994). Human interindividual variability – a major source of uncertainty in assessing risks for noncancer health effects. *Risk Anal.*, **14**, 421–432.

Hattis, D. and Barlow, K. (1996). Human interindividual variability in cancer risks – technical and management challenges. *Human Ecol. Risk Assess.*, **2**, 194–220.

Hawkins, N. C. (1991). Conservatism in maximally exposed individual predictive exposure assessments: a first cut analysis. *Regul. Toxicol. Pharmacol.*, **14**, 107–117.

Hawley, J. K. (1985). Assessment of health risk from exposure to contaminated soil. *Risk Anal.*, **5**, 289–302.

Hayes, W. A. (1994). *Principles and Methods of Toxicology*, 3rd edn. Raven Press, New York.

Heidenreich, W. F., Luebeck, E. G. and Moolgavkar, S. H. (1997). Some properties of the hazard function of the two-mutation clonal expansion model. *Risk Anal.*, **17**, 391–399.

Helsel, D. R. (1990). Less than obvious: statistical treatment of data below the detection limit. *Environ. Sci. Technol.*, **24**, 1766–1774.

Henderson, R. F., Bechtold, W. E. and Maples, K. R. (1992). Biological markers as measure of exposure. *J. Exp. Anal. Environ. Epidemiol.*, **2**, 1–14.

Hertz-Picciotto, I., Gravitz, N. and Neutra, R. (1988). How do cancer risks predicted from animal bioassays compare with the epidemiologic evidence? The case of ethylene dibromide. *Risk Anal.*, **8**, 205–213.

Hewitt, D. J., Millner, G. C., Nye, A. C., Webb, M. and Huss, R. G. (1995). Evaluation of residential exposure to arsenic in soil near a superfund site. *Human Ecol. Risk Assess.*, **1**, 323–335.

HGRMR (1995). Reform of risk regulation: achieving more protection at less cost. Harvard Group on Risk Management Reform. *Human Ecol. Risk Assess.*, **1**, 183–205.

HHS (1985). *Risk Assessment and Risk Management of Toxic Substances: a Report to the Secretary, Department of Health and Human Services*. Health and Human Services. DHHS Committee to Coordinate Environmental and Related Programs (CCERP), Washington, DC.

Hill, A. B. (1965). The environment and disease: association or causation. *Proc. R. Soc. Med.*, **58**, 295–300.

Hill, R. A. and Hoover, S. M. (1997). Importance of the dose-response model form in probabilistic risk assessment: a case study of health effects from methylmercury in fish. *Human Ecol. Risk Assess.*, **3**, 465–481.

Hoffman, F. O. and Hammands, J. S. (1994). Propagation of uncertainty in risk assessments: the need to distinguish between uncertainty due to lack of knowledge and uncertainty due to variability. *Risk Anal.*, **14**, 707–711.

Holdway, D. A. (1996). The role of biomarkers in risk assessment. *Human Ecol. Risk Assess.*, **2**, 263–267.

Holland, C. D. and Sielken, R. L., Jr (1991). *Cancer Modeling and Risk Assessment*. Texas Institute for Advancement of Chemical Technology, College Station, TX.

Holland, C. D. and Sielken, R. L., Jr (1993). *Quantitative Cancer Modeling and Risk Assessment*. Prentice Hall, Englewood Cliffs, NJ.

Holmes, K. K., Kissel, J. C. and Richter, K. Y. (1996). Investigation of the influence of oil on soil adherence to skin. *J. Soil Contam.*, **5**, 301–308.

Hoover, S. M. and Hill, R. A. (1997). Exposure of Aboriginals in British Columbia to methylmercury in freshwater fish: a comparison to reference doses and estimated thresholds. *Human Ecol. Risk Assess.*, **3**, 439–464.

Horowitz, S. B. and Finley, B. L. (1993). Using human sweat to extract chromium from chromite ore processing residue: applications to setting health-based cleanup levels. *J. Toxicol. Environ. Health*, **40**, 585–599.

Horowitz, S. B. and Finley, B. L. (1994). Setting health-protective soil concentrations for dermal contact allergens: a proposed methodology. *Regul. Toxicol. Pharmacol.*, **19**, 31–47.

Horwitz, W. (1984). Effects of scientific advances on the decision-making process: analytical chemistry. *Fundam. Appl. Toxicol.*, **4**, S309–S317.

Howe, R. B. (1990). *TIIC: A Computer Program to Compute a Reference Dose from Continuous Animal Toxicity Data Using the Benchmark Dose Method*. Clement International, Ruston, LA.

Hrudey, S. E., Chen, W. and Rousseaux, C. (1996). *Bioavailability*. CRC–Lewis Publishers, New York.

Huff, J., Haseman, J. and Rall, D. (1991). Scientific concepts, value, and significance of chemical carcinogenesis studies. *Annu. Rev. Pharmacol. Toxicol.*, **31**, 621–652.

Hughes, K., Meek, M. E., Newhook, R. and Chan, P. K. L. (1995). Speciation in health risk assessments of metals: evaluation of effects associated with forms present in the environment. *Regul. Toxicol. Pharmacol.*, **22**, 213–220.

Iman, R. L. and Helton, J. C. (1991). The repeatability of uncertainty and sensitivity analyses for complex probabilistic risk assessments. *Risk Anal.*, **11**, 591–606.

ILSI (1992). *Similarities and Differences Between Children and Adults: Implications for Risk Assessment*. Guzelian, P. S., Henry, C. J. and Olin, S. S. (Eds.). International Life Sciences Institute Press, Washington, DC.

ILSI (1995). *Low-Dose Extrapolation of Cancer Risks: Issues and Perspectives*. International Life Sciences Institute Press, Washington, DC.

ILSI (1998). *Aggregate exposure assessment: an ILSI Risk Science Institute Workshop report*. International Life Sciences Institute Press, Washington DC.

Irish, D. (1959). *Patty's Industrial Hygiene and Toxicology*, 2nd edn. Wiley-Interscience, New York.

Israeli, M. and Nelson, C. B. (1992). Distribution and expected time of residence for U. S. households. *Risk Anal.*, **12**, 65–72.

Jarabek, A. M., Menebe, M. G., Overton, J. H., Dourson, M. L. and Newton, G. J. (1990). The US Environmental Protection Agency's inhalation RfD methodology: risk assessment for air toxics. *Toxicol. Ind. Health*, **6**, 279–301.

Jarabek, A. M. (1995). Interspecies extrapolation based on mechanistic determinants of chemical disposition. *Human Ecol. Risk Assess.*, **1**, 641–662.

Jo, W. K., Weisel, C. P. and Lioy, P. J. (1988). Routes of chloroform exposure and body burden from showering with chlorinated tap water. *Risk Anal.*, **10**, 575–580.

Johnson, E. M. (1988). Cross-species extrapolations and the biologic basis for safety factor determination in developmental toxicology. *Regul. Toxicol. Pharmacol.*, **8**, 22–36.

Johnson, B. B. and Slovic, P. (1995). Presenting uncertainty in health risk assessment: initial studies on its effects on risk perception and trust. *Risk Anal.*, **15**, 485–494.

Johnson, J. E. and Kissel, J. C. (1996). Prevalence of dermal pathway dominance in risk assessment of contaminated soils: a survey of superfund risk assessments, 1989–1992. *Human Ecol. Risk Assess.*, **2**, 356–365.

Kadry, A. M., Skrowronski, G. A., Khodair, A. I. and Abdel-Rahman, M. S. (1995). Determining "safe" levels of exposure: the validity of the use of 10x safety factors. *Human Ecol. Risk Assess.*, **1**, 565–575.

Kadry, A. M., Suh, D. H. and Abdel-Rahman, M. S. (1997). Kinetic and dynamic data of analgesics and NSAIDS drugs reduce 10x uncertainty factors. *Human Ecol. Risk Assess.*, **3**, 567–578.

Kalliomaa, K., Haag-Gronlund, M. and Victorin, K. (1998). A new model function for continuous data sets in health risk assessment of chemicals using the benchmark dose concept. *Regul. Toxicol. Pharmacol.*, **27**, 98–106.

Kaplan, S. and Garrick, B. J. (1981). On the quantitative definition of risk. *Risk Anal.*, **1**, 11–28.

Karch, N. J. and Schneiderman, M. A. (1981). *Explaining the Urban Factor in Lung Cancer Mortality. A Report to the Natural Resources Defense Council.* Clement Associates, Washington, DC.

Kavlock, R. J., Schmid, J. E. and Setzer, R. W., Jr. (1996). A simulation study of the influence of study design on the estimation of benchmark doses for developmental toxicity. *Risk Anal.*, **16**, 199–409.

Keenan, R. E., Paustenbach, D. J., Wenning, R. and Parsons, A. (1991). Pathology re-evaluation of the Kociba *et al.* 1978 bioassay of 2,3,7,8-TCDD: implications for risk assessment. *J. Toxicol. Environ. Health*, **34**, 279–296.

Keith, L. H. (Ed.) (1988). *Principles of Environmental Sampling.* American Chemical Society, Washington, DC.

Kelley, K. E. and Cardon, N. C. (1991). The myth of 10^{-6} as a definition of acceptable risk (or, 'in pursuit of Superfund's Holy Grail'). *Presented at the 84th Annual Meeting Air and Waste Management Association*, Vancouver, BC, Canada, June 1991.

Kerger, B. D., Richter, R. O., Chute., S. M., Dodge, D. G., Overman, S. K., Liang, J., Finley, B. L. and Paustenbach, D. J. (1996). Refined exposure assessment for ingestion of tapwater contaminated with hexavalent chromium: consideration of exogenous and endogenous reducing agents. *J. Exp. Anal. Environ. Epidemiol.*, **6**, 163–179.

Kezic, S., Mahieu, K., Monster, A. C. and de Wolff, F. A. (1997). Dermal absorption of vapors and liquid 2-methoxyethanol and 2-ethoxyethanol in volunteers. *Occup. Environ. Med.*, **54**, 38–43.

Kimbrough, R. (1995). Polychlorinated biphenyls (PCBs) and human health: an update. *Crit. Rev. Toxicol.*, **25**, 133–163.

Kimbrough, R., Falk, H., Stehr, P. and Fries, G. (1984). Health implications of 2,3,7,8-TCDD contamination of residential soil. *J. Toxicol. Environ. Health*, **14**, 47–93.

Kimbrough, R. D. (1997/8). Selected other effects and TEFs. *Teratogen. Carcinogen. Mutagen.*, **17**, 265–273.

Kimmel, C. A. and Gaylor, D. W. (1988). Issues in qualitative and quantitative risk assessment for developmental toxicology. *Risk Anal.*, **8**, 15–20.

Kimmel, C. A., Kavlock, R. J., Allen, B. C. and Faustman, E. M. (1995). Benchmark dose concept applied to data from conventional developmental toxicity studies. *Toxicol. Lett.*, **82/88**, 549–554.

Kissel, J. C., Richter, K. Y. and Fenske, R. A. (1996a). Field measurement of dermal soil loading attributable to various activities: implications for exposure assessment. *Risk Anal.*, **16**, 115–125.

Kissel, J. C., Richter, K. Y. and Fenske, R. A. (1996b). Factors affecting soil adherence to skin in hand press trials. *Bull. Environ. Contam. Toxicol.*, **56**, 722–728.

Kneip, T. J. and Crable, J. V. (Eds) (1988). *Methods for Biological Monitoring.* American Public Health Association, Washington, DC.

Kodell, R. L., Gaylor, D. W. and Chen, J. J. (1987). Using average lifetime dose rate for intermittent exposures to carcinogens. *Risk Anal.*, **7**, 339–345.

Kodell, R. L. and Chen, J. J. (1994). Reducing conservatism in risk estimation for mixtures of carcinogens. *Risk Anal.*, **14**, 327–332.

Kodell, R. L., Howe, R. B., Chen, J. J. and Gaylor, D. W. (1991). Mathematical modeling of reproductive and developmental toxic effects for quantitative risk assessment. *Risk Anal.*, **11**, 583–590.

Kodell, R. L. and West, R. W. (1993). Upper confidence limits on excess risk for quantitative responses. *Risk Anal.*, **13**, 177–182.

Kopp, R., Krupnick, A. and Toman, M. (1997). Cost-benefit analysis and regulatory reform. *Human Ecol. Risk Assess.*, **3**, 787–852.

Kramer, H. J., van den Ham, W. A., Slob, W. and Pieters, M. N. (1996). Conversion factors estimating indicative chronic no-observed-adverse-effect levels from short-term toxicity data. *Regul. Toxicol. Pharmacol.*, **23**, 249–255.

Krewski, D. and Zhu, Y. (1995). A simple data transformation for estimation of benchmark doses in developmental toxicity experiments. *Risk Anal.*, **15**, 29–39.

Krewski, D., Brown, C. and Murdoch, D. (1984). Determining safe levels of exposure: safety factors or mathematical models. *Fundam. Appl. Toxicol.*, **4**, 383–394.

Krewski, D., Murdoch, D. and Withey, J. R. (1989a). Recent developments in carcinogenic risk assessment. *Health Phys.*, **57**, 313–325.

Krewski, D. and Thomas, R. D. (1992). Carcinogenic mixtures. *Risk Anal.*, **12**, 105–111.

Krewski, D., Gaylor, D. W., Soms, A. P. and Szyszkowicz, M. (1993). An overview of the report: correlation between carcinogenic potency and the maximum tolerated dose: implications for risk assessment. *Risk Anal.*, **13**, 383–397.

Krewski, D., Thorslund, T. and Withey, J. (1989b). Carcinogenic risk assessment of complex mixtures. *Toxicol. Ind. Health*, **5**, 851–867.

Krishnan, K., Paterson, J. and Williams, D. T. (1997). Health risk assessment of drinking water contaminants in Canada: the applicability of mixture risk assessment methods. *Regul. Toxicol. Pharmacol.*, **26**, 179–186.

LaGoy, P. K. (1987). Estimated soil ingestion rates for use in risk assessment. *Risk Anal.*, **7**, 355–360.

LaGoy, P. K. and Schulz, C. O. (1993). Background sampling: an example of the need for reasonableness in risk assessment. *Risk Anal.*, **13**, 483–484.

LaKind, J. S. (1998). Comparison of three models for predicting blood lead levels in children: episodic exposures to lead. *J. Exp. Anal. Environ. Epidemiol.*, **8**, 399–406.

Lave, L. B., Ennever, F., Rosenkranz, H. S. and Omenn, G. S. (1988). Information value of the rodent bioassay. *Nature*, **336**, 631–633.

Layard, M. W. and Silvers, A. (1989). Epidemiology in environmental risk assessment. In Paustenbach, D. J. (Ed.), *The Risk Assessment of Environmental Hazards: a Textbook of Case Studies*. pp. 157–173. Wiley, New York.

Layton, D. W. (1993). Metabolically consistent breathing rates for use in dose assessment. *Health Phys.*, **64**, 23–26.

Lee, R. C. and Wright, W. E. (1994). Development of human exposure factor distributions using maximum-entropy inference. *J. Exp. Anal. Environ. Epidemiol.*, **4**, 329–342.

Lehmann, A. J. and Fitzhugh, O. G. (1954). 100 fold margin of safety. *Q. Bull. Assoc. Food Drug Office US*, **18**, 33–35.

Leung, H. W. (1991). Development and utilization of physiologically based pharmacokinetic models for toxicological applications. *J. Toxicol. Environ. Health*, **32**, 247–267.

Leung, H. W. and Paustenbach, D. J. (1994). Techniques for estimating the percutaneous absorption of chemicals due to environmental and occupational exposure. *Appl. Occup. Environ. Hyg.*, **9**, 187–197.

Leung, H. W. and Paustenbach, D. J. (1995). Physiologically based pharmacokinetic and pharmacodynamic modeling in health risk assessment and characterization of hazardous substances. *Toxicol. Lett.*, **79**, 55–65.

Lewis, S. C., Lynch, J. R. and Nikiforov, A. I. (1990). A new approach to deriving community exposure guidelines from no observed effect levels. *Regul. Toxicol. Pharmacol.*, **11**, 314–330.

Lewis, S. C. and Amoruso, M. M. (1997). Perspective on flexibility, expert judgement, peer review, and transparency: critical elements of advanced risk assessment. *Human Ecol. Risk Assess.*, **3**, 655–658.

Lioy, P. J., Freeman, N. C. G., Wainman, T., Stern, A. H., Boesch, R., Howell, T. and Shupack, S. I. (1992). Microenvironmental analysis of residential exposure to chromium-laden wastes in and around New Jersey homes. *Risk Anal.*, **12**, 287–300.

Lioy, P. J., Wainman, T. and Weisel, C. (1993). A wipe sampler for the quantitative measurement of dust on smooth surfaces: laboratory performance studies. *J. Exp. Anal. Environ. Epidemiol.*, **3**, 315–320.

Lioy, P. J., Yiin, L. M., Adgate, J., Wiesel, C. and Rhodes, G. (1997). The effectiveness of home cleaning intervention strategy in reducing potential dust and lead exposures. *J. Exp. Anal. Environ. Epidemiol.*, **8**, 17–36.

Lucier, G. W., Rumbraugh, R. C., McCoy, Z., *et al.* (1986). Ingestion of soil contaminated with 2,3,7,8-tetrachlorodibenzo-p-dioxin (TCDD) alters hepatic enzyme activities in rats. *Fundam. Appl. Toxicol.*, **6**, 364–371.

Magee, B. and Smith, D. (1995). Risk assessment of dioxin congeners via plant uptake. *Human Ecol. Risk Assess.*, **1**, 249–282.

Maibach, H. I., Feldmann, R. J., Milby, T. H., *et al.* (1971). Regional variation in percutaneous penetration in man. *Arch. Environ. Health*, **23**, 208–211.

Malsch, P. A., Proctor, D. M. and Finley, B. L. (1994). Estimation of a chromium inhalation reference concentration using the benchmark dose method: a case study. *Regul. Toxicol. Pharmacol.*, **20**, 58–82.

Manca, D., Li-Muller, A. S. M. and Bell, R. W. (1997). Application of a predictive approach to estimate exposure of non-smoking urban sub-populations to background levels of benzene. *Human Ecol. Risk Assess.*, **3**, 415–438.

Mattie, D. R., Bates, G. D., Jepson, G. W., Fisher, J. W. and McDougal, J. N. (1994a). Determination of skin: air partition coefficients for volatile chemicals: experimental method and applications. *Fundam. Appl. Toxicol.*, **22**, 51–57.

Mattie, D. R., Grabau, J. H. and MacDougal, J. N. (1994b). Significance of the dermal route of exposure to risk assessment. *Risk Anal.*, **14**, 277–283.

Maxim, L. D. (1989). Problems associated with the use of conservative assumptions in exposure and risk analysis. In Paustenbach, D. J. (Ed.), *The Risk Assessment of Environmental and Human Health Hazards: a Textbook of Case Studies*. Wiley, New York.

McArthur, B. (1992). Dermal measurement and wipe sampling methods: a review. *Appl. Occup. Environ. Hyg.*, **7**, 599–606.

McCallum, D. B. and Santos, S. L. (1997). Comparative risk analysis for priority setting. *Human Ecol. Risk Assess.*, **3**, 1215–1234.

McDougal, J. N. (1996). Physiologically based pharmacokinetic modeling. In Marzulli, F. N. and Maibach, H. I. (Eds), *Dermatotoxicology*. pp. 37–60. Taylor and Francis, London.

McDougal, J. N., Jepson, G. W., Clewell, H. J., Gargas, M. L. and Andersen, M. E. (1990). Dermal Absorption of Organic Chemical Vapors in Rats and Humans. *Fundam. Appl. Toxicol.*, **14**, 299–308.

McKone, T. E. (1990). Dermal uptake of organic chemicals from a soil matrix. *Risk Anal.*, **10**, 407–419.

McKone, T. E. (1991). Human exposure to chemicals from multiple media and through multiple pathways: research overview and comments. Dermal uptake of organic chemicals from a soil matrix. *Risk Anal.*, **11**, 5–10.

McKone, T. E. and Bogen, K. T. (1991). Predicting the uncertainties in risk assessment. *Environ. Sci. Technol.*, **25**, 16–74.

McKone, T. E. and Bogen, K. T. (1992). Uncertainties in health risk assessment: an integrated case study based on tetrachloroethylene in California groundwater. *Regul. Toxicol. Pharmacol.*, **15**, 86–103.

McKone, T. E. and Daniels, J. L. (1991). Estimating human exposure through multiple pathways from air, water, and soil. *Regul. Toxicol. Pharmacol.*, **13**, 36–91.

McKone, T. E. and Howd, R. A. (1992). Estimating dermal uptake of nonionic organic chemicals from water and soil: I. unified fugacity-based models for risk assessment. *Risk Anal.*, **12**, 543–557.

McKone, T. E. (1993). Linking a PBPK model for chloroform with measured breath concentrations in showers: implications for dermal exposure models. *J. Exp. Anal. Environ. Epidemiol.*, **3**, 339–365.

McMillan, A., Whittemore, A. S., Silvers, A. and DiCiccio, Y. (1994). Use of biological markers in risk assessment. *Risk Anal.*, **14**, 807–813.

Meek, M. E. (1997). Perceived precision of risk estimates for carcinogenic versus non-neoplastic effects: implications for methodology. *Human Ecol. Risk Assess.*, **3**, 673–680.

Meijers, J. M. M., Swaen, G. M. H. and Bloemen, L. J. N. (1997). The predictive value of animal data in human cancer risk assessment. *Regul. Toxicol. Pharmacol.*, **25**, 94–102.

Mertz, C. K., Slovic, P. and Purchase, I. F. H. (1998). Judgements of chemical risks: comparisons among senior managers, toxicologists, and the public. *Risk Anal.*, **18**, 391–403.

Metzger, B., Crouch, E. and Wilson, R. (1989). On the relationship between carcinogenicity and acute toxicity. *Risk Anal.*, **9**, 169–177.

Michaud, J. M., Huntley, S. L., Sherer, R. A., *et al.* (1994). PCB and dioxin re-entry criteria for building surfaces and air. *J. Exp. Anal. Environ. Epidemiol.*, **4**, 197–227.

Milloy, S. J. (1995). *Science-Based Risk Assessment*. National Environmental Policy Institute, Washington, DC.

Moolgavkar, S. H. (1986). Carcinogenesis modeling: from molecular biology to epidemiology. *Annu. Rev. Publ. Health*, **7**, 151–169.

Moolgavkar, S. H. and Luebeck, G. (1990). Two-event model for carcinogenesis: biological, mathematical, and statistical considerations. *Risk Anal.*, **10**, 323–341.

Moolgavkar, S. H., Dewanji, A. and Venzon, D. J. (1988). A stochastic two-stage model for cancer risk assessment. I. The hazard function and the probability of tumor. *Risk Anal.*, **8**, 383–391.

Morgan, J. N., Berry, M. R. and Graves, R. L. (1997). Effects of commonly used cooking practices on total mercury concentration in fish and their impact on exposure assessments. *J. Exp. Anal. Environ. Epidemiol.*, **7**, 119–133.

Morgan, M. G. and Henrion, M. (1990). *Uncertainty: A Guide to Dealing with Uncertainty in Quantitative Risk and Policy Analysis*. Cambridge University Press, Cambridge.

Mosleh, A. and Bier, V. (1992). On decomposition and aggregation error in estimation: some basic principles and examples. *Risk Anal.*, **12**, 203–214.

Mraz, J. and Nohova, H. (1992). Percutaneous absorption of *N*,*N*-dimethylformamide in humans. *Int. Arch. Occup. Environ. Health*, **64**, 79–83.

Murdoch, D. J., Krewski, D. and Wargo, J. (1992). Cancer risk assessment with intermittent exposure. *Risk Anal.*, **12**, 569–578.

Murray, D. M. and Burmaster, D. E. (1992). Estimated distributions for total body surface area of men and women in the United States. *J. Exp. Anal. Environ. Epidemiol.*, **2**, 451–462.

Murray, D. M. and Burmaster, D. E. (1994). Estimated distributions for average daily consumption of total and self-caught fish for adults in Michigan angler households. *Risk Anal.*, **14**, 513–520.

Murrell, J. A., Portier, C. J. and Morris, R. W. (1998). Characterizing dose response I: critical assessment of the benchmark dose concept. *Risk Anal.*, **18**, 13–25.

Nair, R. S., Sherman, J. H., Stevens, M. W. and Johannsen, F. R. (1995). Selecting a more realistic uncertainty factor: reducing compounding effects of multiple uncertainties. *Human Ecol. Risk Assess.*, **1**, 576–589.

Nakayachi, K. (1998). How do people evaluate risk reduction when they are told zero risk is impossible? *Risk Anal.*, **18**, 235–242.

NAS (1987). Pharmacokinetics in risk assessment. In *Drinking Water and Health*, Vol. 8. National Academy of Sciences. National Academy Press, Washington, DC.

NAS (1994). *Science and Policy in Risk Assessment*. National Academy of Sciences. National Academy Press, Washington, DC, 1994.

National Research Council (1983). *Risk Assessment and Management in the Federal Government: Managing the Process*. National Academy Press, Washington, DC.

National Research Council (1994). *Science and Judgement in Risk Assessment*. National Academy Press, Washington, DC.

National Research Council (1996). *Understanding Risk: Informing Decisions in a Democratic Society*. National Academy Press, Washington, DC.

Naumann, B. D. and Weideman, P. A. (1995). Scientific basis for uncertainty factors used to establish occupational exposure limits for pharmaceutical active ingredients. *Human Ecol. Risk Assess.*, **1**, 590–613.

Naumann, B. D., Weideman, P. A., Dixit, R., Grossman, S. J., Shen, C. F. and Sargent, E. V. (1997). Use of toxicokinetic and toxicodynamic data to reduce uncertainties when setting occupational exposure limits for pharmaceuticals. *Human Ecol. Risk Assess.*, **3**, 555–566.

Navidi, W. and Lurmann, F. (1995). Measurement error in air pollution exposure assessment. *J. Exp. Anal. Environ. Epidemiol.*, **5**, 111–124.

Nessel, C. S., Butler, J. P., Post, G. B., Held, J. I., Gochfeld, M. and Gallo, M. A. (1991). Evaluation of the relative contribution of exposure routes in a health risk assessment of dioxin emissions from a municipal waste incinerator. *J. Exp. Anal. Environ. Epidemiol.*, **1**, 283–308.

Nessel, G. S., Lewis, S. C., Stauber, K. L. and Adgate, J. L. (1995). Subchronic to chronic exposure extrapolation: toxicologic evidence for a reduced uncertainty factor. *Human Ecol. Risk Assess.*, **1**, 516–522.

Nethercott, J., Paustenbach, D., Adams, R., Fowler, J., Morton, M. C., Taylor, J., Horowitz, B. and Finley, B. (1994). A study of chromium induced allergic contact dermatitis with 54 volunteers: implications for environmental risk assessment. *Occup. Environ. Med.*, **51**, 371–380.

NJDEP (1990). *Derivation of a Risk-Based Chromium Level in Soil Contaminated with Chromite-Ore Processing Residue in Hudson County*. New Jersey Department of Environmental Protection, Trenton, NJ.

NJDEP (1992). *Risk Assessment of the ACD Potential of Hexavalent Chromium in Contaminated Soil—Derivation of an Acceptable Soil Concentration*. New Jersey Department of Environmental Protection, Trenton, NJ.

OTA (1993). *Researching Health Risks*. Office of Technology Assessment. OTA-BBS-570. US Congress, Office of Technology Assessment, Washington, DC.

Ohanian, E. V. (1997). Improving noncancer risk assessments in regulatory decisions. *Human Ecol. Risk Assess.*, **3**, 591–598.

Ottoboni, M. A. (1991). *The Dose Makes the Poison: a Plain Language Guide to Toxicology*, 2nd edn. Van Nostrand Reinhold, New York.

Owen, B. A. (1990). Literature-derived absorption coefficients for 39 chemicals via oral and inhalation routes of exposure. *Regul. Toxicol. Pharmacol.*, **11**, 237–252.

Paddle, G. M. (1997). Metaanalysis as an epidemiological tool and its application to studies of chromium. *Regul. Toxicol. Pharmacol.*, **26**, S42–S49.

Palisade (1990). *@RISK (A Computer Program for Conducting Monte Carlo Analysis)*. Palisade Corp., Newfield, NY.

Park, C. N. and Snee, R. D. (1983). Quantitative risk assessment: state-of-the-art for carcinogenesis. *Fundam. Appl. Toxicol.*, **3**, 320–333.

Paustenbach, D. J. (1987). Assessing the potential environment and human health risks of contaminated soils. *Commun. Toxicol.*, **1**, 185–221.

Paustenbach, D. J. (1989a). A survey of environmental risk assessment. In Paustenbach, D. J. (Ed.), *The Risk Assessment of Environmental and Human Health Hazards: a Textbook of Case Studies*. pp. 27–124. Wiley, New York.

Paustenbach, D. J. (1989b). Health risk assessments: opportunities and pitfalls. *Columbia J. Environ. Law*, **14**, 379–410.

Paustenbach, D. J. (1989c). Shortcomings in the traditional practice of health risk assessments. *Columbia J. Environ. Law*, **14**, 411–427.

Paustenbach, D. J. (1990). Health risk assessment and the practice of industrial hygiene. *Am. Ind. Hyg. Assoc. J.*, **51**, 339–351.

Paustenbach, D. J. (1993). Jousting with environmental windmills. Letter to the Editor. *Risk Anal.*, **13**, 13–15.

Paustenbach, D. J. (1994). Occupational exposure limits, pharmacokinetics, and unusual work schedules. In: Harris, R. L., Cralley, L. J. and Cralley, L. V. (Eds), *Patty's Industrial Hygiene and Toxicology*, **3**, Part A, 191–348. Wiley, New York.

Paustenbach, D. J. (1995). The practice of health risk assessment in the United States (1975–1995): how the US and other countries can benefit from that experience. *Hum. Ecol. Risk Assess.*, **1**, 29–80.

Paustenbach, D. J. (1997). OSHA's program for updating the permissible exposure limits (PELs): can risk assessment help 'move the ball forward?'. *Harvard's Center Risk Anal. Risk Perspect.*, **5**, 1–6.

Paustenbach, D. J., Shu, H. P. and Murray, F. J. (1986). A critical examination of assumptions used in risk assessment of dioxin contaminated soil. *Regul. Toxicol. Pharmacol.*, **6**, 284–307.

Paustenbach, D. J., Clewell, H. J., Gargas, M. L. and Andersen, M. E. (1988). A physiologically-based pharmacokinetic model for carbon tetrachloride. *Toxicol. Appl. Pharmacol.*, **96**, 191–211.

Paustenbach, D. J., Meyer, D. M., Sheehan, P. J. and Lau, V. (1991a). An assessment and quantitative uncertainty analysis of the health risks to workers exposed to chromium contaminated soils. *Toxicol. Ind. Health*, **7**, 159–196.

Paustenbach, D. J., Rinehart, W. E. and Sheehan, P. J. (1991b). The health hazards posed by chromium-contaminated soils in residential and industrial areas: conclusions of an expert panel. *Regul. Toxicol. Pharmacol.*, **13**, 195–222.

Paustenbach, D. J., Sheehan, P. J., Paul, J. M., *et al.* (1992a). Review of the ACD hazard posed by chromium-contaminated soil: identifying a safe concentration. *J. Toxicol. Environ. Health*, **37**, 177–207.

Paustenbach, D. J., Wenning, R. J., Lau, V., Harrington, N. W., Rennix, D. K. and Parsons, A. H. (1992b). Recent developments on the hazards posed by 2,3,7,8-tetrachlorodibenzo-*p*-dioxin in soil: implications for setting risk-based cleanup levels at residential and industrial sites. *J. Toxicol. Environ. Health*, **36**, 103–149.

Paustenbach, D. J., Jernigan, J. D., Bass, R. D., Kalmes, R. and Scott, P. (1992c). A proposed approach to regulating contaminated soil: identify safe concentrations for seven of the most frequently encountered exposure scenarios. *Regul. Toxicol. Pharmacol.*, **16**, 21–56.

Paustenbach, D. J., Price, P. S., Bradshaw, R. D., Ollison, W., Peterson, D. and Blank, C. (1992d). Re-evaluation of benzene exposure for the Pliofilm workers (1939–1976). *J. Toxicol. Environ. Health*, **36**, 177–232.

Paustenbach, D. J., Shu, H. P. and Murray, F. S. (1996). A critical examination of assumptions used in risk assessment of dioxin-contaminated soil. *Regul. Toxicol. Pharmacol.*, **6**, 284–307.

Paustenbach, D. J., Bruce, G. M. and Chrostowski, P. (1997a). Current views on the oral bioavailability of mercury in soil: the impact on health risk assessments. *Risk Anal.*, **17**, 533–545.

Paustenbach, D. J., Finley, B. L. and Long, T. F. (1997b). The critical role of house dust in understanding the hazards posed by contaminated soils. *Int. J. Toxicol.*, **16**, 339–362.

Paustenbach, D. J., Alarie, T., Kulle, T., Schachter, N., Smith, R., Swenberg, J., Witschi, H. and Horowitz, S. B. (1997c). A recommended occupational exposure limit for formaldehyde based on irritation. *J. Toxicol. Environ. Health*, **50**, 101–148.

Paustenbach, D. J., Panko, J. M., Fredrick, M. M., Finley, B. L. and Proctor, D. M. (1997d). Urinary chromium as a biological marker of environmental exposure: what are the limitations? *Regul. Toxicol. Pharmacol.*, **26**, S23–S34.

Paustenbach, D. J., Leung, H. W. and Rothrock, J. (1998). Risk assessment and the practice of occupational dermatology. In Adams, R. (Ed.), *Occupational Skin Diseases*. Taylor and Francis, London, In Press.

Paxton, M. B., Churchill, V. M., Brett, S. M. and Rodricks, J. V. (1994). Leukemia risk associated with benzene exposure in the pliofilm cohort: I. Mortality update and exposure distribution. *Risk Anal.*, **14**, 147–153.

Paxton, M. B., Churchill, V. M., Brett, S. M. and Rodricks, J. V. (1994). Leukemia risk associated with benzene exposure in the pliofilm cohort: II. Risk estimates. *Risk Anal.*, **14**, 155–162.

Pelekis, M. and Krishnan, K. (1997). Assessing the relevance of rodent data on chemical interactions for health risk assessment purposes: a case study with dichloromethane-toluene mixture. *Regul. Toxicol. Pharmacol.*, **25**, 79–86.

Perkins, J. L., Cutter, G. N. and Cleveland, M. S. (1990). Estimating the mean, variance, and confidence limits from censored (< limit of detection), lognormally-distributed exposure data. *Am. Ind. Hyg. Assoc. J.*, **51**, 416–419.

Phillips, L. J., Fares, R. J. and Schweer, L. G. (1993). Distributions of total skin surface area to body weight ratios for use in dermal exposure assessments. *J. Exp. Anal. Environ. Epidemiol.*, **3**, 331–338.

Piegorsch, W. W., Carr, G. J., Portier, C. J. and Hoel, D. G. (1992). Concordance of carcinogenic response between rodent species: potency distributions and potential underestimation. *Risk Anal.*, **12**, 115–122.

Pieters, M. N., Kramer, H. J. and Slob, W. (1998). Evaluation of the uncertainty factor for subchronic-to-chronic extrapolation: statistical analysis of toxicity data. *Regul. Toxicol. Pharmacol.*, **27**, 108–111.

Pohl, H. R., Hansen, H. and Chou, C. -H. S. J. (1997). Public health guidance values for chemical mixtures: current practice and future directions. *Regul. Toxicol. Pharmacol.*, **26**, 322–329.

Poiger, H. and Schlatter, C. H. (1980). Influence of solvents and adsorbents on dermal and intestinal absorption of TCDD. *Food Cosmet. Toxicol.*, **18**, 477–481.

Polak, J., O'Flaherty, E. J., Freeman, G. B., Johnson, J. D., Liao, S. C. and Bergstrom, P. D. (1996). Evaluating lead bioavailability data by means of a physiologically based lead kinetic model. *Fundam. Appl. Toxicol.*, **29**, 63–70.

Price, B., Berner, T., Henrich, R. T., Stewart, J. M. and Moran, E. J. (1996). A benchmark concentration for carbon disulfide: analysis of the NIOSH carbon disulfide exposure database. *Reg Toxicol. Pharmacol.*, **24**, 171–176.

Price, P. S., Su, S. H. and Gray, M. N. (1994). The effect of sampling bias on estimates of angler consumption rates in creel surveys. *J. Exp. Anal. Environ. Epidemiol.*, **4**, 355–372.

Price, P. S., Su, S. H., Harrington, J. R. and Keenan, R. E. (1996a). Uncertainty and variation in indirect exposure assessments: an analysis of exposure to tetrachlorodibenzo-*p*-dioxin from a beef consumption pathway. *Risk Anal.*, **16**, 263–277.

Price, P. S., Curry, C. L., Goodrum, P. E., Gray, M. N., McCrodden, J. I., Harrington, N. W., Carlson-Lynch, H. and Keenan, R. E. (1996b). Monte Carlo modeling of time-dependent exposures using a microexposure event approach. *Risk Anal.*, **16**, 339–348.

Price, P. S., Keenan, R. E., Swartout, J. C., Gillis, C. A., Carlson-Lynch, H. and Dourson, M. L. (1997). An approach for modeling noncancer dose-responses with an emphasis on uncertainty. *Risk Anal.*, **17**, 427–437.

Price, P. S., Scott, P. K., Wilson, N. D. and Paustenbach, D. J. (1998). An empirical approach for deriving information on total duration of exposure from information on historical exposure. *Risk Anal.*, **18**, 611–619.

Proctor, D. M., Zak, M. A. and Finley, B. L. (1997). Resolving uncertainties associated with the construction worker soil ingestion rate: a proposal for risk-based remediation goals. *Human Ecol. Risk Assess.*, **3**, 299–304.

Proctor, D. M., Fredrick, M. M., Scott, P. K., Paustenbach, D. J. and Finley, B. L. (1998). The prevalence of chromium allergy in the United States and its implications for setting soil cleanup: a cost effectiveness case study. *Regul. Toxicol. Pharmacol.*, **28**, 27–37.

Purchase, I. F. H. and Auton, T. F. (1995). Thresholds in chemical carcinogenesis. *Regul. Toxicol. Pharmacol.*, **22**, 199–205.

Purchase, I. (1998). Threshold methods should be used in risk assessment for genotoxic carcinogens. *IUTOX Newsletter*, July 1998.

Putzrah, R. M. (1997). Estimating relative potency for receptor-mediated toxicity: reevaluating the toxic equivalence factor (TEF) model. *Regul. Toxicol. Pharmacol.*, **25**, 68–78.

Que Hee, S. S., Peace, B., Scott, C. S., *et al.* (1985). Evolution of efficient methods to sample lead sources, such as house dust and hand dust, in the homes of children. *Environ. Res.*, **38**, 77–95.

Ragas, A. M. J. and Huijbregts, M. A. J. (1997). Evaluating the coherence between environmental quality objectives and the acceptable or tolerable daily intake. *Regul. Toxicol. Pharmacol.*, **27**, 251–263.

Rai, S. N. and Kreski, D. (1998). Uncertainty and variability analysis in multiplicative risk models. *Risk Anal.*, **18**, 37–45.

Reitz, R. H., Gargas, M. L., Andersen, M. E., Provan, W. M. and Green, T. L. (1996). Predicting cancer risk from vinyl chloride with a physiologically based pharmacokinetic model. *Toxicol. Appl. Pharmacol.*, **137**, 253–267.

Renwick, A. G. and Lazarus, N. R. (1998). Human variability and noncancer risk assessment - an analysis of the default uncertainty factor. *Regul. Toxicol. Pharmacol.*, **27**, 3–20.

Rhomberg, L. R. (1997). A survey of methods for chemical risk assessment among Federal Regulatory Agencies. *Human Ecol. Risk Assess.*, **3**, 1029–1196.

Richardson, G. M. (1996). Deterministic versus probabilistic risk assessment: strengths and weaknesses in a regulatory context. *Human Ecol. Risk Assess.*, **2**, 44–53.

Richardson, G. M. and Currie, D. J. (1993). Estimating fish consumption rates for Ontario Amerindians. *J. Exp. Anal. Environ. Epidemiol.*, **3**, 23–38.

Risher, J. F. and DeRosa, C. T. (1997). The precision, use, and limitations of public health guidance values. *Human Ecol. Risk Assess.*, **3**, 681–700.

Roach, S. A. and Rappaport, S. M. (1990). But they are not thresholds: a critical analysis of the documentation of the threshold limit values. *Am. J. Ind. Med.*, **17**, 727–753.

Roberts, J. W., Budd, W. T., Chuang, J. and Lewis, R. G. (1993). *Chemical Contaminants in House Dust: Occurrences and Sources*. EPA/600/A-93/215. United States Environmental Protection Agency, Washington, DC.

Robinson, M. K., Stotts, J. and Danneman, P. J. (1989). A risk assessment process for allergic contact sensitization. *Food Chem. Toxicol.*, **27**, 479–489.

Robinson, R. B. and Hurst, B. T. (1997). Statistical quantification of the sources of variance in uncertainty analysis. *Risk Anal.*, **17**, 447–454.

Rodricks, J. V., Brett, S. M. and Wrenn, G. C. (1987). Significant risk decisions in Federal Regulatory Agencies. *Regul. Toxicol. Pharmacol.*, **7**, 307–320.

Roseberry, A. M. and Burmaster, D. E. (1991). A note: estimating exposure concentrations of lipophilic organic chemicals to humans via finfish. *J. Exp. Anal. Environ. Epidemiol.*, **1**, 513–521.

Roseberry, A. M. and Burmaster, D. E. (1992). Lognormal distributions for water intake by children and adults. *Risk Anal.*, **12**, 99–104.

Rosenthal, A., Gray, G. M. and Graham, J. D. (1992). Legislating acceptable cancer risk from exposure to toxic chemicals. *Ecol. Law. Qu.*, **190**, 269–362.

Roy, A. and Georgopoulos, G. (1998). Reconstructing week-long exposures to volatile organic compounds using physiologically based pharmacokinetic models. *J. Exp. Anal. Environ. Epidemiol.*, **8**, 407–422.

Ruby, M. V., Davis, A., Kempton, J. H., Drexter, J. W. and Bergstrom, P. D. (1992). Lead bioavailability under simulated gastric conditions. *Environ. Sci. Technol.*, **26**, 1242–1248.

Ruffle, B., Burmaster, D. E., Anderson, P. D. and Gordon, H. D. (1994). Lognormal distribution for fish consumption by the general U. S. population. *Risk Anal.*, **14**, 395–403.

Ruoff, W. L., Diamond, G. L., Velazquez, S. F., Stiteler, W. M. and Gefell, D. J. (1994). Bioavailability of cadmium in food and water: a case study on the derivation of relative bioavailability factors for inorganics and their relevance to the reference dose. *Regul. Toxicol. Pharmacol.*, **20**, 139–160.

Santos, S. L. and McCallum, D. B. (1997). Communicating to the public: using risk comparisons. *Human Ecol. Risk Assess.*, **3**, 1197–1214.

Scheuplein, R. J. and Bowers, J. C. (1995). Dioxin – an analysis of the major human studies: comparison with animal-based cancer risks. *Risk Anal.*, **15**, 319–333.

Schlenk, D. (1996). The role of biomarkers in risk assessment. *Human Ecol. Risk Assess.*, **2**, 251–256.

Schnatter, A. R., Nicolich, M. J. and Bird, M. G. (1996). Determination of leukemogenic benzene exposure concentrations: refined analysis of the pliofilm cohort. *Risk Anal.*, **16**, 833–839.

Schoof, R. A. and Nielsen, J. B. (1997). Evaluation of methods for assessing the oral bioavailability of inorganic mercury in soil. *Risk Anal.*, **17**, 545–555.

Schwartz, C. S. (1995). A semiquantitative method for selection of safety factors in establishing OELs for pharmaceutical compounds. *Human Ecol. Risk Assess.*, **1**, 527–543.

Scow, K., Wechsler, A. E., Stevens, J., *et al.* (1979). *Identification and Evaluation of Waterborne Routes of Exposure from Other than Food and Drinking Water*. EPA-440/4-79-016. US Environmental Protection Agency, Washington, DC.

Sedman, R., Funk, L. M. and Fountain, R. (1998). Distribution of residence duration in owner occupied housing. *J. Exp. Anal. Environ. Epidemiol.*, **8**, 51–57.

Seed, J., Brown, R. P., Olin, S. S. and Foran, J. A. (1995). Chemical mixtures: current risk assessment methodologies and future directions. *Regul. Toxicol. Pharmacol.*, **22**, 76–94.

Seiler, F. A. and Scott, B. R. (1987). Mixtures of toxic agents and attributable risk calculations. *Risk Anal.*, **7**, 81–90.

Shacklette, H. T. and Boerngen, J. G. (1984). *Element Concentrations in Soils and Other Surficial Materials of the Conterminous United States*. US Geological Survey Professional Paper No. 1270. US Government Printing Office, Washington, DC.

Shatkin, J. A. and Brown, H. S. (1991). Pharmacokinetics of the dermal route of exposure to volatile organic chemicals in water. A computer simulation model. *Environ. Res.*, **56**, 90–108.

Sheehan, P. J., Meyer, D. M., Sauer, M. M. and Paustenbach, D. J. (1991). Assessment of the human health risks posed by exposure to chromium-contaminated soils. *J. Toxicol. Environ. Health*, **32**, 161–201.

Sheppard, S. C. and Evenden, W. G. (1994). Contaminant enrichment and properties of soil adhering to skin. *J. Environ. Qual.*, **23**, 604–613.

Shifrin, N. S., Beck, B. D., Gauthier, T. D., Chapnick, S. D. and Goodman, G. (1996). Chemistry, toxicology, and human health risks of cyanide compounds in soils at former manufactured gas plant sites. *Regul. Toxicol. Pharmacol.*, **23**, 106–116.

Shlyakhter, A., Goodman, G. and Wilson, R. (1992). Monte Carlo simulation of rodent carcinogenicity bioassays. *Risk Anal.*, **12**, 73–82.

Shlyakhter, A. I. (1994). An improved framework for uncertainty analysis: accounting for unsuspected errors. *Risk Anal.*, **14**, 441–447.

Shoaf, C. R. (1991). Current assessment practices for noncancer end points. *Environ. Health Perspect.*, **95**, 111–119.

Shu, H. P., Teitelbaum, P., Webb, A. S., Marple, L., Brunck, B., Dei Rossie, D., Murray, F. J. and Paustenbach, D.

(1988a). Bioavailability of soil-bound TCDD: dermal bioavailability in the rat. *Fundam. Appl. Toxicol.*, **10**, 335–343.

Shu, H. P., Paustenbach, D., Murray, F. J., Marple, L., Brunck, B., Dei Rossie, D. and Teitelbaum, P. (1988b). Bioavailability of soil-bound TCDD: oral bioavailability in the rat. *Fundam. Appl. Toxicol.*, **10**, 648–654.

Sielken, R. L. (1985). Some issues in the quantitative modeling portion of cancer risk assessment. *Regul. Toxicol. Pharmacol.*, **5**, 175–181.

Sielken, R. L., Jr (1987). Cancer dose–response extrapolations. *Environ. Sci. Technol.*, **21**, 1033–1039.

Sielken, R. L., Jr (1989). Useful tools for evaluating and presenting more science in quantitative cancer risk assessments. *Toxic Subst. J.*, **9**, 353–404.

Sielken, R. L., Jr, Bretzlaff, R. S. and Stevenson, D. E. (1995). Challenges to default assumptions stimulate comprehensive realism as a new tier in quantitative cancer risk assessment. *Regul. Toxicol. Pharmacol.*, **21**, 270–280.

Sielken, R. L., Jr. and Valdez-Flores, C. (1996). Comprehensive realism's weight-of-evidence based distributional dose-response characterization. *Human Ecol. Risk Assess.*, **2**, 175–193.

Sielken, R. L., Jr. and Stevenson, D. E. (1997). Opportunities to improve quantitative risk assessment. *Human Ecol. Risk Assess.*, **3**, 479–490.

Silbergeld, E. K. (1993). Risk assessment: the perspective and experience of the US environmentalists. *Environ. Health Perspect.*, **101**, 100–104.

Simcox, N. J., Fenske, R. A., Wolz, S. A., Lee, I. -C. and Kalman, D. A. (1995). Pesticides in household dust and soil: exposure pathways for children of agricultural families. *Environ. Health Perspect.*, **103**, 1126–1135.

Simon, T. (1997). Combining physiologically based pharmacokinetic modeling with Monte Carlo simulation to derive an acute inhalation guidance value for trichloroethylene. *Regul. Toxicol. Pharmacol.*, **26**, 257–270.

Skrowronski, G. A., Turkall, R. M. and Abdel-Rahman, M. S. (1988). Soil absorption alters bioavailability of benzene in dermally exposed male rats. *Am. Ind. Hyg. Assoc. J.*, **49**, 506–511.

Skrowronski, G. A. and Abdel-Rahman, M. S. (1997). Interspecies comparison of kinetic data of chlorinated chemicals of potential relevance to risk assessment. *Human Ecol. Risk Assess.*, **3**, 635–654.

Slob, W. (1996). A comparison of two statistical approaches to estimate long-term exposure distributions from short-term measurements. *Risk Anal.*, **16**, 195–200.

Smith, A. E., Ryan, P. B. and Evans, J. S. (1992). The effect of neglecting correlations when propagating uncertainty and estimating population distribution of risk. *Risk Anal.*, **12**, 467–474.

Smith, A. H. (1987). Infant exposure assessment for breast milk dioxin and furans derived from waste incineration emissions. *Risk Anal.*, **7**, 347–354.

Smith, A. H., Sciortino, S., Goeden, H. and Wright, C. C. (1996). Consideration of background exposures in the management of hazardous waste sites: a new approach to risk assessment. *Risk Anal.*, **16**, 619–625.

Smith, R. L. (1994). Use of Monte Carlo simulation for human exposure at a Superfund site. *Risk Anal.*, **14**, 433–440.

Snyder, W. S. (1975). *Report of the Task Group on Reference Man*. International Commission on Radiological Protection, Publication No. 23. Pergamon Press, New York.

SOT (1998). *Chloroform Controversy*. Memorandum to the Membership, 4 August 1998. Society of Toxicology, Reston, VA.

Spear, R. C., Bois, F. Y., Woodruff, T. J., Auslander, D., Parker, J. and Selvin, S. (1991). Modeling benzene pharmacokinetics across three sets of animal data: parametric sensitivity and risk implications. *Risk Anal.*, **11**, 641–654.

Squires, R. (1981). Ranking animal carcinogens. *Science*, **214**, 877–880.

Stanek, E. J. and Calabrese, E. J. (1991). A guide to interpreting soil ingestion studies. I. Development of a model to estimate the soil ingestion detection level of soil ingestion studies. *Regul. Toxicol. Pharmacol.*, **13**, 263–277.

Stanek, E. J. and Calabrese, E. J. (1995a). Improved soil ingestion estimates for use in site evaluations using the best tracer method. *Hum. Ecol. Risk Assess.*, **1**, 133–157.

Stanek, E. J. and Calabrese, E. J. (1995b). Daily estimates of soil ingestion in children. *Environ. Health Perspect.*, **103**, 276–285.

Stanek, E. J. III, Calabrese, E. J. and Xu, L. (1998). A caution for Monte Carlo risk assessment of long term exposures based on short term exposure data. *Human Ecol. Risk Assess.*, **4**, 409–422.

Stayner, L. T. and Bailer, A. J. (1993). Comparing toxicologic and epidemiologic studies: methylene chloride – a case study. *Risk Anal.*, **13**, 667–674.

Stern, A. H., Freeman, N. C. G., Plesan, P., *et al.* (1992). Residential exposure to chromium waste—urine biological monitoring in conjunction with environmental exposure monitoring. *Environ. Res.*, **58**, 147–162.

Stern, A. H., Korn, L. R. and Ruppel, B. E. (1996). Estimation of fish consumption and methylmercury intake in the New Jersey population. *J. Exp. Anal. Environ. Epidemiol.*, **6**, 503–525.

Stevens, J. B. and Gerbec, E. N. (1988). Dioxin in the agricultural food chain. *Risk Anal.*, **8**, 329–335.

Stewart, P. A. and Herrick, R. F. (1991). Issues in performing retrospective exposure assessment. *Appl. Occup. Environ. Hyg.*, **6**, 280–289.

Surber, C., Wilhelm, K. P., Maibach, H. I., *et al.* (1990). Partitioning of chemicals into human stratum corneum: implications for risk assessment following dermal exposure. *Fundam. Appl. Toxicol.*, **15**, 99–107.

Swann, R. L. and Eschenroeder, A. (Eds) (1983). *Fate of Chemicals in the Environment*. ACS Symposium Series, Vol. 225. American Chemical Society, Washington, DC.

Swartout, J. S., Price, P. S., Dourson, M. L., Carlson-Lynch, H. L. and Keenan, R. E. (1998). A probabilistic framework for the reference dose (probabilistic RfD). *Risk Anal.*, **18**, 271–281.

Tardiff, R., Lapare, S., Charest-Tardif, G., Brodeur, J. and Krishnan, K. (1995). Physiologically-based pharmacokinetic modeling of a mixture of toluene and xylene in humans. *Risk Anal.*, **15**, 335–351.

Taylor, A. C. (1993). Using objective and subjective information to develop distributions for probabilistic exposure assessment. *J. Exp. Anal. Environ. Epidemiol.*, **3**, 285–298.

Taylor, A. C., Evans, J. S. and McKone, T. E. (1993). The value of animal test information in environmental control decisions. *Risk Anal.*, **13**, 403–412.

Tengs, T. O., Adams, M. E., Pliskin, J. S., Safran, D. G., Siegel, J. E., Weinstein, M. C. and Graham, J. D. (1995). Five-hundred life-saving interventions and their cost-effectiveness. *Risk Anal.*, **15**, 369–189.

Thatcher, T. L. and Layton, D. W. (1995). Deposition, resuspension, and penetration of particles within a residence. *Atmos. Environ.*, **29**, 1487–1497.

Thomas, K. W., Sheldon, L. S., Pellizzari, E. D., Handy, R. W., Roberds, J. M. and Berry, M. R. (1997). Testing duplicate diet sample collection methods for measuring personal dietary exposures to chemical contaminants. *J. Exp. Anal. Environ. Epidemiol.*, **7**, 17–36.

Thompson, K. M. and Burmaster, D. E. (1991). Parametric distribution of soil ingestion by children. *Risk Anal.*, **11**, 339–342.

Thompson, K. M., Burmaster, D. E. and Crouch, E. A. C. (1992). Monte Carlo techniques for quantitative uncertainty analysis in public health assessments. *Risk Anal.*, **12**, 53–63.

Timbrell, J. (1996). MRC/IEH workshop on the use of biomarkers in environmental exposure assessment, Leicester, UK, 30 November – 1 December. *Biomarkers*, **1**, 67–70.

Travis, C. C. and Land, M. L. (1990). Estimating the mean of data sets with nondetectable values. *Environ. Sci. Technol.*, **24**, 961–962.

Travis, C. C. and White, R. K. (1988). Interspecies scaling of toxicity data. *Risk Anal.*, **8**, 119–125.

Travis, C. C., Richter, S. A., Crouch, E. A. C., Wilson, R. and Klema, E. D. (1987). Cancer risk management: a review of 132 Federal regulatory decisions. *Environ. Sci. Technol.*, **21**, 415–420.

Travis, C. C., White, R. K. and Ward, R. C. (1990). Interspecies extrapolation of pharmacokinetics. *J. Theor. Biol.*, **142**, 285–304.

Travis, C. C. and Blaylock, B. P. (1992). Validation of terrestrial food chain. *J. Exp. Anal. Environ. Epidemiol.*, **2**, 221–240.

Travis, C. C. and Morris, J. M. (1992). Comment: on the use of 0.75 as an interspecies scaling factor. *Risk Anal.*, **12**, 311–314.

Trowbridge, P. R. and Burmaster, D. E. (1997). A parametric distribution for the fraction of outdoor soil in indoor dust. *J. Soil Contam.*, **6**, 161–168.

Umbreit, T. H., Hesse, E. J. and Gallo, M. A. (1986a). Acute toxicity of TCDD contaminated soil from an industrial site. *Science*, **232**, 497–499.

Umbreit, T. H., Hesse, E. J. and Gallo, M. A. (1986b). Comparative toxicity of TCDD contaminated soil from Times Beach, Missouri and Newark, New Jersey. *Chemosphere*, **15**, 2121–2124.

US EPA (1986a). Guidelines for carcinogen risk assessment. United States Environmental Protection Agency. *Fed. Regist.*, **51 CFR 2984 (185)**, 33992–34003.

US EPA (1986b). Guidelines for exposure assessment. United States Environmental Protection Agency. *Fed. Regist.*, **51 CFR 2984 (185)**, 34042–34054.

US EPA (1986c). Guidelines for health assessment of suspected developmental toxicants. United States Environmental Protection Agency. *Fed. Regist.*, **51 CFR 2984 (185)**, 33028–34041.

US EPA (1986d). Guidelines for health risk assessment of chemical mixtures. United States Environmental Protection Agency. *Fed. Regist.*, **51 CFR 2984 (185)**, 34014–34027.

US EPA (1987). *The Total Exposure Assessment Methodology (TEAM) Study. Summary and Analysis: Volume 1*. United States Environmental Protection Agency, Office of Acid Deposition, Environmental Monitoring and Quality Assurance. Research and Development. EPA/600/6-87/002a..

US EPA (1988a). Proposed guidelines for assessing male reproductive hazards. United States Environmental Protection Agency. *Fed. Regist.*, **53 (126)**, 24850–24869.

US EPA (1988b). Proposed guidelines for assessing female reproductive hazards. *Fed. Regist.*, United States Environmental Protection Agency. **53 (126)**, 24834–24847.

US EPA (1988c). *Superfund Exposure Assessment Manual*. Office of Remedial Response. EPA/540/1-88/001. United States Environmental Protection Agency, Washington, DC.

US EPA (1989a). *NATICH Database Report on State, Local, and EPA Air Toxics Activities*. EPA/450/3-89-29. United States Environmental Protection Agency, Washington, DC.

US EPA (1989b). *Risk Assessment Guidance for Superfund. I. Human Health Evaluation Manual (Part A). Interim Final*. Office of Emergency and Remedial Response. EPA/540/1-89/002. United States Environmental Protection Agency, Washington, DC.

US EPA (1989c). *Biological Data for Pharmacokinetic Modeling and Risk Assessment*. Office of Health and Environmental Assessment. EPA/600/3-90/019. United States Environmental Protection Agency, Washington, DC.

US EPA (1989d). *Interim Procedures for Estimating Risks Associated with Exposure to Mixtures of Chlorinated Dibenzo-p-dioxins and Dibenzofurans (CDDs and CDFs) and 1989 Update*. Risk Assessment Forum. EPA/625/3-89/016.

US EPA (1990a). *Interim Methods for Development of Inhalation Reference Doses*. Office of Health and Environmental Assessment. EPA/600/8-88/066F. United States Environmental Protection Agency, Washington, DC.

US EPA (1990b). *Reducing Risk: Setting Priorities and Strategies for Environmental Protection*. Science Advisory Board. United States Environmental Protection Agency, Washington, DC.

US EPA (1990c). *Health Effects of Passive Smoking: Assessment of Lung Cancer in Adults and Respiratory Disorders in Children*. Review Draft. Office of Health and Environmental Assessment. EPA/600/6-90/006A. United States Environmental Protection Agency, Washington, DC.

US EPA (1992a). Guidelines for exposure assessment. United States Environmental Protection Agency, *Fed. Regist.*, **57 (104)**, 22888–22938.

US EPA (1992b). *Dermal Exposure Assessments: Principles and Applications*. Exposure Assessment Group, Office of Health and Environmental Assessment. EPA/600/8-91/011B. United States Environmental Protection Agency, Washington, DC.

US EPA (1993). *Provisional Guidance for Quantitative Risk Assessment of Polycyclic Aromatic Hydrocarbons*. Office of Research and Development. EPA/600/R-93/089. United States Environmental Protection Agency, Washington, DC.

US EPA (1994a). *Estimating Exposure to Dioxin-Like Compounds*. Office of Health and Environmental Assessment, Exposure Assessment Group. United States Environmental Protection Agency, Washington, DC.

US EPA (1994b). *Guidance Manual for the Integrated Exposures Uptake Biokinetic Model for Lead in Children (ver. 0.99D)*. Office of Emergency and Remedial Response. EPA/540/P-93/081. United States Environmental Protection Agency, Washington, DC.

US EPA (1994c). *Memorandum to Carol Browner on "Science and Judgement in Risk Assessment," A Report by the National Research Council*. Sussman, R. M. and Goldman, Lr., United States Environmental Protection Agency, Science Policy Council. Washington, DC.

US EPA (1995a). *Guidance for Risk Characterization*. Science Policy Council. US Environmental Protection Agency, Washington, DC.

US EPA (1995b). *Urban Soil Lead Abatement Demonstration Project (Draft)*. United States Environmental Protection Agency. EPA/600/R-95/139. National Center for Environmental Assessment, Research Triangle Park, NC.

US EPA (1996a). *Exposure Factors Handbook. Volume I of III: General Factors—Review Draft*. Exposure Assessment Group, Office of Health and Environmental Assessment. EPA/600/P-95/002A. United States Environmental Protection Agency, Washington, DC.

US EPA (1996b). *Benchmark Dose Technical Guidance Document (External Review Draft)*. Risk Assessment Forum, Office of Research and Development. EPA/600/P-96/002A. United States Environmental Protection Agency, Washington, DC.

US EPA (1996c). *Proposed Guidelines for Carcinogen Risk Assessment*. Office of Research and Development. EPA/600/P-92/003C. United States Environmental Protection Agency, Washington, DC.

US EPA (1996d). *Polychlorinated Biphenyls. Integrated Risk Information System*. United States Environmental Protection Agency, Washington, DC.

US EPA (1997a). *Guiding Principles for Monte Carlo Analysis*. Risk Assessment Forum, Office of Research and Development. EPA/630/R-97/001. United States Environmental Protection Agency, Washington, DC.

US EPA (1997b). *Health Effects Assessment Summary Tables. FY97 Update*. Office of Emergency and Remedial Response. EPA/540/R-97/036. United States Environmental Protection Agency, Washington, DC.

US EPA (1998a). *Integrated Risk Information System*. United States Environmental Protection Agency, Washington, DC.

US EPA (1998b). *Chromium. Integrated Risk Information System*. United States Environmental Protection Agency, Washington, DC.

Valberg, P. A. and Watson, A. Y. (1996). Lung cancer rates in carbon-black workers are discordant with predictions from rat bioassay data. *Regul. Toxicol. Pharmacol.*, **24**, 155–170.

Van Hemmen, J. J. and Brouwer, D. H. (1995). Assessment of dermal exposure to chemicals. *Sci. Total Environ.*, **168**, 131–141.

Van Wijnen, J. H., Clausing, P. and Brunekreef, B. (1989). Estimated soil ingestion by children. *Environ. Res.*, **51**, 147–162.

Velazquez, S. F., McGinnis, P. M., Vater, S. T., Stiteler, W. S., Knauf, L. A. and Schoeny, R. S. (1994). Combination of cancer data in quantitative risk assessments: case study using bromodichloromethane. *Risk Anal.*, **14**, 285–292.

Verhagen, H., Feron, V. J. and van Vliet, P. W. (1996). Risk assessment of peak exposure to genotoxic carcinogens: summary of a report. *Human Ecol. Risk Assess.*, **2**, 275–276.

Wainman, T., Hazen, R. and Lioy, P. J. (1994). The extractability of Cr (VI) from contaminated soil in synthetic sweat. *J. Exp. Anal. Environ. Epidemiol.*, **4**, 171–182.

Wallace, L., Pellizzari, E. and Gordon, S. (1993). A linear model relating breath concentrations to environmental exposures: application to a chamber study of four volunteers exposed to volatile organic chemicals. *J. Exp. Anal. Environ. Epidemiol.*, **3**, 75–102.

Wallace, L., Nelson, W. C., Pellizzari, E. D. and Raymer, J. H. (1997). Uptake and decay of volatile organic chemicals at environmental concentrations: application of a four compartment model to a chamber study of five human subjects. *J. Exp. Anal. Environ. Epidemiol.*, **7**, 141–164.

Wang, R. and Schwetz, B. (1987). An evaluation system for ranking chemicals with teratogenic potential. *Teratogen. Carcinogen. Mutagen.*, **7**, 133–190.

Watanabe, K., Bois, F. Y. and Zeise, L. (1992). Interspecies extrapolation: a reexamination of acute toxicity data. *Risk Anal.*, **12**, 301–310.

Watanabe, K. H. and Bois, F. Y. (1996). Interspecies extrapolation of physiological pharmacokinetic parameter distributions. *Risk Anal.*, **16**, 741–754.

Weil, C. S. (1972). Statistics versus safety factors and scientific judgment in the evaluation of safety for man. *Toxicol. Appl. Pharmacol.*, **21**, 454–463.

Wenning, R. J. and Erickson, G. A. (1994). Interpretation and analysis of complex environmental data using chemometric methods. *Trends Anal. Chem.*, **13**, 446–457.

Weitzman, M., Aschengrau, A., Bellinger, D., Jones, R., Hamlin, J. S. and Beiser, A. (1993). Lead-contaminated soil abatement and urban children's blood lead levels. *J. Am. Med. Assoc.*, **269**, 1647–1654.

Wester, R. C. and Noonan, P. K. (1980). Relevance of animal models for percutaneous absorption. *Int. J. Pharmacol.*, **7**, 99–110.

Wester, R. C., Bucks, D. A. W. and Maibach, H. I. (1993a). Percutaneous absorption of contaminants from soil. In Wang, R. G. M., Knaak, J. B. and Maibach, H. I. (Eds), *Health Risk Assessment: Dermal and Inhalation Exposure and Absorption of Toxicants*. pp. 145–155. CRC Press, Boca Raton, FL.

Wester, R. C., Maibach, H. I. and Sedik, L. (1993b). Percutaneous absorption of pentachlorphenol from soil. *Fundam. Appl. Toxicol.*, **20**, 68–71.

Wilkes, C. R., Small, M. J., Davidson, C. I. and Andelman, J. B. (1996). Modeling the effects of water usage and cobehavior on inhalation exposures to contaminants volatilized from household water. *J. Exp. Anal. Environ. Epidemiol.*, **6**, 393–412.

Williams, G. M. and Weisburger, J. H. (1991). Chemical carcinogenesis. In Amdur, M. D., Doull, J. D. and Klaassen, C. D. (Eds), *Casarett and Doull's Toxicology: The Basic Science of Poisons*. pp. 127–200. Pergamon Press, New York.

Wilschut, A., Ten Berge, W. F., Robinson, P. J. and McKone, T. E. (1995). Estimating skin permeation. The validation of five mathematical skin permeation models. *Chemosphere*, **30**, 1275–1296.

Wilson, A. L., Colome, S. D., Tian, Y., Becker, E. W., Baker, P. E., Behrens, D. W., Billick, I. H. and Garrison, C. A. (1996). California residential air exchange rates and residence volumes. *J. Exp. Anal. Environ. Epidemiol.*, **6**, 311–326.

Wilson, J. D. (1989). Assessment of low exposure risk from carcinogens: implications of the Knudson–Moolgavkar two-critical mutation theory. In Travis, C. (Ed.), *Biologically Based Models for Cancer Risk Assessment*. pp. 275–288. Plenum Press, New York.

Wilson, J. D. (1991). A usually unrecognized source of bias in cancer risk estimation. *Risk Anal.*, **11**, 11–12.

Wilson, J. D. (1995). Letter to the Editor: Dueling Risk Assessors. *Risk Anal.*, **15**, 543–544.

Wilson, J. D. (1997). So carcinogens have thresholds: how do we decide what exposure levels should be considered safe? *Risk Anal.*, **17**, 1–4.

Wilson, N. D., Shear, N. D., Paustenbach, D. J. and Price, P. S. (1998). The effect of cooking practices on the concentration of DDT and PCB compounds in the edible tissue of fish. *J. Exp. Anal. Environ. Epidemiol.*, **8**, 423–440.

Wolfe, D. A. (1996). Insights on the utility of biomarkers for environmental assessment and monitoring. *Human Ecol. Risk Assess.*, **2**, 245–250.

Woodruff, T. J., Bois, F. Y., Auslander, D. and Spear, R. C. (1992). Structure and parameterization of pharmacokinetic models: their impact on model predictions. *Risk Anal.*, **12**, 189–202.

Wyzga, R. E. (1988). The role of epidemiology in risk assessments of carcinogens. *Adv. Mod. Environ. Toxicol.*, **15**, 189–208.

Younes, M. and Sonich-Mullin, C. (1998). Reducing imprecision in risk assessment – a plea for focused science. *Human Ecol. Risk Assess.*, **4**, 259–262.

Young, F. A. (1987). Risk assessment: the convergence of science and the law. *Regul. Toxicol. Pharmacol.*, **7**, 179–184.

Zatarian, V. G., Streicker, J., Rivera, A., Cornejo, C. S., Molina, S., Valadez, O. F. and Leckie, J. O. (1995). A pilot study to collect micro-activity data of two-to four year old farm labor children in Salinas Valley, California. *J. Exp. Anal. Environ. Epidemiol.*, **5**, 21–34.

Zartarian, V. G., Ferguson, A. C. and Leckie, J. O. (1997). Quantified dermal activity data from a four child pilot field study. *J. Exp. Anal. Environ. Epidemiol.*, **7**, 543–551.

Zartarian, V. G., Ferguson, A. C. and Leckie, J. O. (1998). Quantified mouthing activity data from a four child pilot field study. *J. Exp. Anal. Environ. Epidemiol.*, **8**, 543–553.

Zeise, L., Wilson, R. and Crouch, E. (1984). Use of acute toxicity to estimate carcinogenic risk. *Risk Anal.*, **4**, 187–200.

Zielhuis, R. L. and van der Kreek, F. W. (1979). Calculations of a safety factor in setting health based permissible levels. *Int. Arch. Occup. Environ. Health*, **42**, 203–215.

Chapter 83
Toxicology and Disasters*

H. Paul A. Illing

CONTENTS

- Introduction
- Theoretical Considerations
- Disasters and Serious Incidents Involving Toxicants
- Disaster Prevention and Mitigation
- Conclusion
- References

INTRODUCTION

Disasters (great or sudden misfortunes: *Concise Oxford Dictionary*, 1990) occur from time to time. Because they are portrayed and analysed extensively in the news media and subjected to careful examination in subsequent public enquiries, they become entrenched in everyone's mind. Unfortunately, the ideas on how to handle or prevent potential disaster situations occurring have often been developed from the lessons learnt through analysing previous disasters. In many cases, disasters can be avoided and the effects of accidents minimized by careful planning. In addition, by examining how to handle the consequences of an accident once it has occurred, it should be possible to mitigate the effects. It is these thoughts that have led to legislation aimed at considering the safety aspects of certain hazardous situations at an early stage in order to minimize the likelihood of their becoming disasters.

Disasters may be naturally occurring, as with earthquakes and volcanoes, or they may include the results of human activity, as with incidents involving food supplies or industrial plant. Some disasters are the consequences of a toxicant entering a biological system and creating a damaging perturbation to that system. These effects may be largely environmental (e.g. the consequences of an oil tanker spill in coastal waters) or they may affect human health, either directly (through ingestion of contaminated drinking water or inhalation of a toxicant as it is dispersed in air) or indirectly (e.g. via uptake, etc., into food species). Hence a knowledge of the effects of toxicants can be important when examining disasters and potential disaster situations.

In this chapter, concepts involved in planning to prevent disasters occurring are discussed first. This is followed by an evaluation of different types of disaster or serious incidents involving toxicants. Although purely environmental effects should not be ignored, the examples chosen are all associated with human health effects. Subsequently, approaches to the planning associated with preventing disasters due to toxicants and mitigating their effects are discussed.

THEORETICAL CONSIDERATIONS

Many of the concepts used in analysing major hazards and minimizing their potential for causing disasters have their origin in engineering concepts associated with the design of military equipment, aircraft and nuclear plant. As a consequence, different national and international organizations have developed definitions for aspects of this work and these definitions need examining, especially as difficulties can ensue if toxicologists and engineering-based risk assessors employ different interpretations of the same words. Although 'hazard' and 'risk' are interchangeable terms to the general public, they have separate meanings in the context of risk assessment, so their definitions will be examined carefully.

Hazard

Hazard is an intrinsic property of a substance or situation. The Royal Society Study Group on Risk Assessment (1992) defined hazard as 'a situation that could occur during the lifetime of a product, system or plant that has the potential for human injury, damage to property, damage to the environment or economic loss', and the Institution of Chemical Engineers called it 'a physical situation with a potential for human injury, damage to property, damage to the environment or some combination of these' (Jones, 1992). The 'Glossary for Chemists of Terms used in Toxicology' (IUPAC

* The views expressed in this chapter are those of the author and in no way commit any government body.

Recommendations; Duffus, 1993) called hazard the 'set of intrinsic properties of a substance, mixture of substances or a process involving substances that, under production, usage or disposal conditions, make it capable of causing adverse effects to organisms or the environment, dependent on the degree of exposure'. A chemical hazard was further defined by the Institution of Chemical Engineers (Jones, 1992) as 'a hazard involving chemicals or processes which may release its potential through fire, explosion, toxic or corrosion effects'. A major hazard is an imprecise term: the Royal Society Study Group called it 'a large scale hazard which may have severe consequences'; the Institution of Chemical Engineers used its narrower remit to call a major hazard 'an imprecise term for a large scale chemical hazard, especially one which may be released through an acute event', and thus excluded natural hazards and hazards from the use of nuclear power.

For chemicals or radiation to represent toxic hazards, they must be present in sufficient quantities to exert toxic effects on the individual. If they are to be major hazards, they must be present in quantities which, if released or dispersed, could result in effects being seen in many people.

Risk

Risk differs from hazard, as it involves a consideration of the probability or likelihood of a consequence occurring as well as what the consequence might be.

The Royal Society Study Group (1983) defined risk as 'the probability that a particular adverse event occurs during a stated period of time or results from a particular challenge'. The Institution of Chemical Engineers (1985; Jones, 1992) extended the statement to 'the likelihood of a specific undesired effect occurring within a specified time or in specified circumstances'. They go on to say that 'it may be either a frequency (the number of events occurring in unit time) or a probability (the probability of a specified event following a prior event), depending on circumstances'. If risk is quantified, it is a statistically based parameter.

Relationship Between Hazard and Risk

In engineering terms, the risk to the individual is obtained by identifying possible events associated with the release and dispersion of significant amounts of a toxic substance, and/or by analysing potential failure mechanisms which would allow the release to take place (Health and Safety Executive, 1989a, 1992; Department of the Environment, 1995). Likely frequencies and sizes of releases can then be calculated. The hazard is a quantitative statement of the exposure conditions associated with a specified level of harm ('harm criterion').

Risk is that associated with a failure occurring and includes identification of a geographic area for which, following dispersion, exposure matches or exceeds that harm criterion. In contrast, occupational and public health toxicologists and epidemiologists often think of risk in terms of likelihood of end effect occurring for a given level of exposure (the risk of end effect arising at the exposure level defined as the 'harm criterion'). To the engineering risk assessor, this is 'uncertainty in defining the hazard'. For the purposes of this chapter, risk will be taken as risk associated with the initiating event and dispersion pattern.

Individual and Societal (or Population) Risk

There are two principal types of risk which can arise from major hazards: individual risk and societal (or population) risk. The Health and Safety Executive (1988a, 1992) has called the individual risk associated with major industrial hazards 'the risk to any particular individual, either a worker or a member of the public'. A member of the public is considered to be 'either anybody living within a defined radius from the establishment or somebody following a particular pattern of life'. Societal risk was 'the risk to society as a whole, as represented, for example, by the chance of a large accident causing a

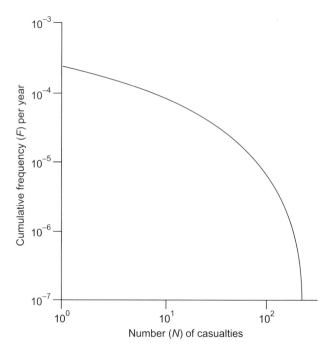

Figure 1 An *F–N* curve for societal risk. In assessing societal risk, a particular actuarial or estimated curve must be compared with a criterion curve. Actuarial curves (based on historic data) are usually only available for high-frequency–low-number events. Curves for low-frequency–high number events are normally estimated.

defined number of deaths and injuries'. It is expressed numerically as a frequency (F) that there will be a disaster harming more than a particular number of people (N) and the criteria for acceptability of a social risk can be aggregated in the form of an F–N curve (**Figure 1**). Although the individual risk remains the same for each person, the societal risk is governed also by the number of people likely to be affected. The individual risk of living 1 km from a major hazard (industrial or natural) remains the same irrespective of whether the hazard is located in an unpopulated area or in a city, but the societal risk is very different! The term population risk is used for environmental purposes, where usually it is the risk to the species, rather than to the individual organism, that matters.

Risk Assessment, Management and Communication

The concepts of hazard and risk are fundamental to analysing the causes of disasters and to preventing their recurrence. However, these concepts must be contained within a framework of analysis, management and communication if they are to be applied usefully to a given situation. In practice there is a multistage process involved in handling any hazard (**Figure 2**), and most of the people analysing and managing hazards from industrial plants have engineering or chemistry backgrounds. Their specialisms cover plant design and failure rates, event and fault tree analyses, dispersion modelling for releases of clouds of substances and rates of combustion,

etc., for explosions and burning gases (Lees, 1996; Wells, 1997). Geologists are often the principal people interested in the causes of natural disasters involving toxicants. These are 'overt' disasters where a clear point source can be identified readily.

Only when the substance released is a toxicant or is transformed into a toxicant will any toxicological input become important. This input will largely be in defining the hazard; it will be concerned with identifying whether the agents present are toxic, and defining the combination of exposure size and duration likely to produce a given toxic effect. Clinical toxicologists are also able to advise on the treatment of victims following an incident, i.e. they can have a role in the event of an incident occurring.

'Disseminated' disasters are those which only become apparent because of evidence of effect. Identifying the cause when the effect is ill-health may require persistent, painstaking research. If the suspected cause is non-infective, the investigation team will need the assistance of toxicologists in identifying the agent responsible.

Often risk can be managed in more than one way. The aim of risk management is to reduce the risk, both in terms of the frequency of an event and in terms of the nature of the potential consequences to an acceptable or tolerable level (see **Table 1** for definitions of acceptable and tolerable risk). This involves choices as to what chemical and physical agents are usable by society and in what circumstances. It involves selecting which processes to employ when manufacturing, using or disposing of these agents and their waste products. It also involves choices on where to site industrial plants (in the case of

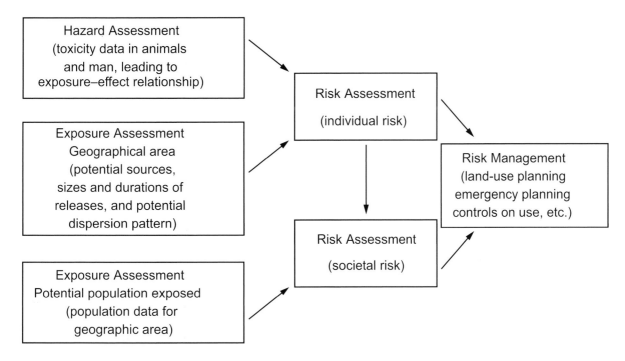

Figure 2 Block diagram illustrating the processes involved in risk assessment and risk management.

Table 1 Various aspects of risk, based on Royal Society Study Group (1983), Lovell (1986) and Health and Safety Executive (1988a, b)

Objective, actual or statistical risk	A statistically calculated risk evaluation
Perceived risk	The combined evaluation that is made by an individual of the likelihood of an adverse event occurring in the future and its consequences
Acceptable risk	An acceptable risk is one which, on objective criteria, should generally be regarded as not worth worrying about by those exposed to it
Tolerable risk	A tolerable risk is one which society is prepared to live with in order to have certain benefits
Accepted risk	People tend to accept the risks which they have experienced but are less prepared to accept new risks, even though, on 'objective' criteria, the risks are similarly acceptable. The new risk is regarded as worse
Voluntary and involuntary risk	Certain risks are accepted willingly by choice (e.g. in sport) by individuals but are not accepted (even by the same individuals) if they are unable to choose to accept the risk
Risk and benefit	Costs occur in reducing risks, either directly or indirectly. For example, many drugs used to treat cancers carry a significant risk that they will cause cancer in that patient at some future time; whooping cough vaccine may prevent severe illness and possible death in most recipients but can cause severe damage in a very few recipients. Risks to non-beneficiaries are regarded as worse than risks to beneficiaries

man-made hazards) and about methods of waste disposal, and whether to permit housing and other developments around major hazards. It is also concerned with examining how to handle the consequences of an untoward event at a particular site (emergency planning). What is an acceptable, or at least a tolerable, risk is a separate but interlinked problem, which depends on a number of factors. Some of these factors are listed in **Table 1**. Ultimately, government (on behalf of society) decides whether a societally regulated risk is generally acceptable or tolerable. Individuals or groups of individuals may attempt to vary the decision as it relates to their specific circumstances and perceptions. In the final analysis, risk acceptability revolves around political and personal decisions, although it is to be hoped that such decisions are based on scientific data.

Clear, effective and consistent communication between all parties is seen more and more as essential if risks are to be managed satisfactorily. This is a two-way process, and includes the technical specialist understanding the views of individuals and society as well as explaining his assessment to the general public.

DISASTERS AND SERIOUS INCIDENTS INVOLVING TOXICANTS

Many disasters are the result of major hazards fulfilling their potential for harm. They are part of a continuous spectrum of possible consequences which can arise from the accidental release of chemicals at a point source. These consequences range from minor difficulties through serious incidents until, in the worst cases, they become disasters. Most of these disasters are not due to toxicants. Their primary effects are physical in nature, and include crush injuries and burns. Other disasters may

be due to the ordinary exposure associated with covenanted releases of potential toxicants. This may be the result of failure to set and meet adequate exposure standards. Failure to set appropriate standards may be because the appropriate knowledge was not available or the criterion against which the knowledge was set was unsuitable. In either case the resulting standard can be inadequate. Alternatively, it may be because of some accidental or intentional deviation from the standard. A classification of disasters is given in **Table 2**. This classification is based on the type of event which caused the disaster or serious incident.

Health effects due to toxicants may result from inhalation or from absorption through skin or gastro-intestinal tract. Inhaled toxicants may be gases, liquids (aerosols, mists) or solids (dusts, fumes). Particle size is important when particulate material is inhaled since, if inhaled, a particle may be deposited in the lung alveoli or, as a result of the 'tracheo-bronchial escalator', it may be swallowed. An inhaled toxicant may cause injury to the lung, it may restrict the transfer of oxygen (asphyxiation), or it may act systemically in a particular organ (including skin). Skin and eye effects are often phenomena of surface contamination.

Gastrointestinal absorption may contribute to the overall toxicity of inhaled material. However, it is the main route of entry for those toxicants which are transmitted to man in food or drinking water.

Examples of different types of disaster or serious incident with the potential for disaster now follow.

Natural Disasters

Disasters due to natural causes include phenomena caused by the movement of the earth's crust and also as the consequences of abnormal weather. In general, these

Table 2 Classification of types of disasters involving toxic agents

Cause of disaster	Type	Example
Natural	Volcanic	Vesuvius, AD 79; Mount St Helens, 1980
	Non-volcanic	Lake Nyos, 1986
Man-made	Plant failures	Seveso, 1976; Bhopal, 1984; Chernobyl, 1986
	Fire	Manchester Airport, 1985; Kings Cross, 1987
	Food and drink adulteration	Ginger paralysis, 1930; toxic oil, 1981
	Accidental contamination	North Cornwall, 1988; Epping jaundice, 1966
	Environmental contamination	Minamata and Niigata, 1951–74
Interaction of man and nature	Shipping	mv Braer, 1993
	Mines and tunnels	Tokyo subway, 1995
	Waste disposal	Love Canal, 1960s; Minamata and Niigata, 1951–74

types of disasters cause injuries due to physical effects or disease due to infective organisms. Toxicants are rarely involved, and then usually secondarily (e.g. due to water contamination), except in the cases of volcanoes, and gas emission from lakes. Asphyxiation can be caused by emitted gases and irritant dusts, respiratory dysfunction, bronchial obstruction and pulmonary oedema.

Volcanoes

Volcanic eruption can be divided into two types— explosive and effusive. Each type may present different health hazards. In a volcanic eruption, magma (molten rock and associated dissolved gas below the earth's surface) is extruded to the surface. When it reaches the surface, it may appear as liquid (lava), fragments (pyroclastic debris) and exsolved gases. In effusive eruptions these flows are usually slow-moving, gas releases are steady and most of the limited amount of dust produced is non-respirable. Explosive eruptions tend to be more dangerous, the principal toxic hazards being hot ash released and gas emission. Volcanoes may change their nature from one type to the other.

The gas emitted by volcanoes is principally steam, but includes carbon dioxide, carbon monoxide, hydrogen sulphide, sulphur dioxide, hydrogen chloride and hydrogen. Plumes normally disperse by dilution in the atmosphere and are carried on the wind above human settlement. However, sulphur dioxide, hydrogen chloride or hydrogen fluoride may occasionally be present in sufficient quantities to contaminate air within settlements, water supplies and animal feedstuffs. Denser-than-air gases, principally carbon dioxide and hydrogen sulphide, can flow into valleys and low-lying basins and displace oxygen, giving rise to asphyxiation. A *nuée ardente* (a cinder cloud carrying trapped gases) can flow rapidly down slopes and may also endanger life.

Pyroclastic debris (tephra) and ash products vary in size. Blocks and bombs are large (over 64 mm), lapilli vary between 2 and 64 mm and cinders and ashes are smaller particles. Lapilli and ash, when released to the atmosphere, rise in a hot convection cloud which may be transmitted widely (several hundred kilometres) downwind. Eventually they fall to earth and blanket large areas. Finer particles are deposited further away. The particles have the ability to cause darkness during daylight hours. Ash products include respirable particles containing significant levels of crystalline silica (quartz and cristobolite). Volcanic ash can affect the respiratory tract and eyes. Severe tracheal injury, pulmonary oedema and bronchial obstruction can occur, leading to death from pulmonary injury or suffocation. Ash may also act as a respiratory tract and eye irritant. Irritation and inflammation of the upper and lower respiratory tract may persist if low-level chronic exposure occurs.

Lava is molten rock, the liquid product from the volcano. It is derived from the molten magma, but differs from it because the dissolved gases in the magma escape with the reduction of pressure which occurs as the material approaches the surface.

Debris flows occur when loose rock mixes with surface water or groundwater and flows as a mass of rock, mud and water.

This description of volcanoes is inevitably very short and much simplified. More detailed information can be found in Sheets and Grayson (1979) and Newhall and Fruchter (1986).

Vesuvius, Italy, AD 79

Perhaps one of the best-known historic volcanic eruptions is that of Vesuvius in Italy in AD 79. A contemporary description of the eruption and its effects on one victim was provided by Pliny the Younger in two 'letters' to Tacitus (Radice, 1969). More detailed information on the eruption and its consequences has been obtained during archaeological investigation of the sites at Pompeii and Herculaneum, both of which were buried in the eruption (Jashemski, 1979; Sigurdsson *et al.*, 1985).

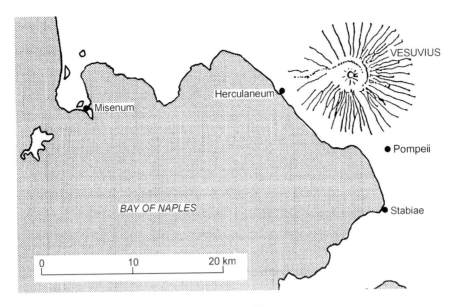

Figure 3 Sketch map of the Bay of Naples. Based on Jashemski (1979).

Vesuvius had been quiescent for many centuries before the eruption of AD 79. The first sign of its reawakening was an earthquake in AD 62 which damaged almost all the buildings in Pompeii. Then came the eruption of AD 79. There were three phases to this eruption. The first stage was expulsion of the vent plug on 24 August. This was followed by expulsion of ashes. There were six surges and pyroclastic flows during the last eruption.

Both Plinys were at Misenum when Vesuvius erupted, together with Pliny the Elder's sister (Pliny the Younger's mother). Pliny the Elder, who was in command of the Roman fleet at Misenum, gave instructions that a ship would be made ready so that he could investigate the phenomenon. However, by the time the ship got under way with the elder Pliny on board, he changed the mission to one of attempting to rescue the people living along the shore of the bay at the foot of Vesuvius (see **Figure 3**). Pompeii and Herculaneum were probably being buried at this time, the former from deposition of lapilli and ashes and the latter from a mud and tephra flow. Pliny found his mission impossible because of the falling debris near the shore, and eventually made port at Stabiae, where he stayed the night. During the night the courtyard of the house in which he was staying filled with ashes and debris. On the morning of 25 August it was still dark at Stabiae after dawn. Pliny the Elder went to the shore to investigate the possibility of escape by sea, and died. Pliny the Younger described the death as because 'the dense fumes choked his breathing by blocking his windpipe which was constitutionally weak and narrow and often inflamed'. In modern terms this might be described as asphyxiation.

The crew of the ship later successfully got away, and the younger Pliny and his mother were evacuated from Misenum on 25 August as ashes started falling there. Both survived. Although the 'letters' only describe ash and lapilli, there was also a lava flow on the north side of the volcano. The results of excavations at Pompeii suggest that at least 2000 people died. Most deaths were probably due to asphyxiation caused by inhaling the hot ash material in the first surge of the ash eruption, but some might have been due to thermal shock (Sigurdsson *et al.*, 1985). Presumably many more deaths went unrecorded.

Mount St Helens, USA, 1980

A much more recent volcanic eruption was that of Mount St Helens, in the Cascade range in the west of North America. Premonitory earthquakes started on 20 March and, towards the end of April, a bulge developed in an area to the north of the summit (Buist and Bernstein, 1986). On 18 May a major earthquake occurred, the roof of the bulge slid downhill and an explosive blast took place. Large quantities of ash, superheated steam and gas were released. There were five additional explosions over the following 5 months and ash falls accompanied four of these eruptions. The dispersion pattern is shown in **Figure 4**; the main land areas covered by the vented material lay in a north-easterly direction from the volcano.

There were 35 known deaths and at least 23 people missing without trace following the eruption (Baxter *et al.*, 1981, 1983; Buist and Bernstein, 1986). Asphyxiation was the cause of death in 18 of the 23 victims autopsied. Ash probably acted as an irritant to the respiratory tract and eye, causing tracheal injury, pulmonary oedema, and bronchial obstruction in those dying. The irritation of the respiratory tract continued as the result of chronic low-level exposure to ash, but there appeared

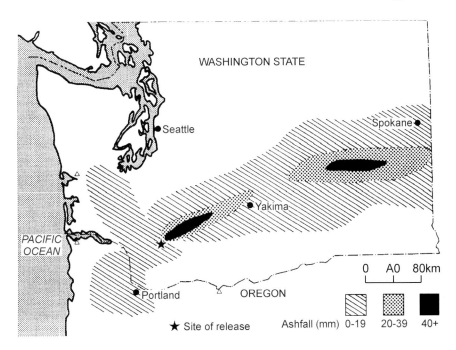

Figure 4 Sketch map of Washington State, showing deposition patterns of ash for the first three eruptions of Mount St Helens in 1980. The star indicates the position of the volcano. Based on Baxter *et al.* (1981).

to be few long-term sequelae. However, any potential pneumoconiotic effect from the single massive exposure to silica could not be detected within the short time-span since the eruption. Interview studies of patients with pre-existing chronic lung disease showed that the ashfall exacerbated the condition in these patients. There were dose-related increases in the prevalence of three psychiatric syndromes associated with disaster stress—generalized anxiety, major depression and post-traumatic stress. The duration of effect was related to the level of disaster stress suffered by the subject.

The toxic effects seen in the victims of the Mount St Helens eruption were largely those due to the nature of the ash deposited. Fortunately, the toxic gases that were emitted were vented to the atmosphere and diluted to non-toxic levels through dispersion.

Other Natural Disasters

Lake Nyos, Cameroon, West Africa, 1986

Volcanoes are not the only natural phenomenon which can cause major disasters due to toxic substances. On 21 August 1986 there was a catastrophic release of gas from Lake Nyos, Cameroon (Freeth and Kay, 1987; Kling *et al.*, 1987; Baxter *et al.*, 1989b). The cloud of gas was lethal at distances up to 10 km from the source. About 1700 people, 3000 cattle and many other animals died, mostly from asphyxiation. An earlier, smaller release from Lake Monoun, also in Cameroon, had resulted in 37 deaths, presumably from similar causes.

The generally accepted cause of the disaster is that, because of the geochemical and geophysical characteristics of the Cameroon rocks and the geological conditions in the Lake Nyos area, waters rich in carbon dioxide develop. The gas accumulated in the lake to near-saturating conditions. Although the trigger mechanism for the release is unknown, a small disturbance would have been sufficient to cause degassing in the form of a large release of the carbon dioxide The gas cloud produced was denser than air and dispersed through the river valleys. Simultaneously, a water surge resulted in the loss of about 200 000 t of water from the lake. That release was heard as a series of 'rumbling sounds' lasting 15–20 s, and one observer reported seeing a white cloud rise from the lake.

Many people lost consciousness rapidly and survivors woke 6–36 h after the event, weak and confused. Cutaneous erythema and bullae were present in about 19% of survivors treated in hospital. Very limited pathological investigations on those dying suggested that carbon dioxide was the toxicant, as it appeared that the potential toxicants, carbon monoxide, cyanide or hydrogen sulphide, were not relevant to the cause of death. Reports of the odour of sulphur compounds were probably a result of the sensory hallucination due to exposure to high levels of carbon dioxide.

This disaster was a consequence of the special geology of the area. Therefore, although a rare event, it does illustrate that natural disasters involving toxicants are not confined to volcanic releases.

Man-made Disasters

Plant Failures

Plant failures are a well known cause of major disasters. Those involving the release of toxic chemicals or radioactivity are relevant to toxicologists, and some examples are examined here. A much more comprehensive collection of case studies of the causes and consequences of chemical plant failure in major disasters, written from the chemical engineer/risk assessor's point of view, is given in Marshall (1987).

Seveso, Italy, 1976

An escape of toxic substances occurred at an industrial plant at Seveso, Italy, in 1976. The circumstances surrounding the escape and the potential health effects caused by the escape were investigated by a Parliamentary Commission of Enquiry (Orsini, 1977), and both the engineering and chemical aspects of the incident have been reviewed (Marshall, 1987; Skene *et al.*, 1989). The incident was important because of its influence on European Community legislation (the 'Seveso' Directive) concerned with major industrial chemical hazards.

The plant produced trichlorophenol by reaction of tetrachlorobenzene with sodium hydroxide (**Figure 5**). Following the reaction, the solvent (ethylene glycol–xylene) was partially vacuum distilled off by the end of shift, at which time the heating and agitation were switched off. Some 7.5 h later a safety plate on the reactor vessel burst and there was a consequent venting of the reaction mixture, including approximately 2–3 kg of the impurity dioxin (2,3,7,8-tetrachlorodibenzo-*p*-dioxin) to the atmosphere. Once in the atmosphere, the dioxin was spread over a wide area downwind of the plant and settled on fields and houses. Three major zones were identified according to the levels of dioxins present in the vegetation and soil (**Figure 6**). The resident populations in the zones were 733, 4800 and 22 000 people in the most contaminated, middle and least contaminated

areas, respectively. A medical surveillance programme was undertaken on these people.

Apart from burns arising directly from contact with the caustic reaction products, the other major effect was chloracne. This was reported some 6 weeks after the accident, with a frequency correlating approximately to the levels of dioxins in the soil. By the end of 1978 the chloracne had disappeared. Repeated-dose animal studies suggested that dioxin could cause porphyria and was hepatotoxic. In animal studies on reproductive effects, dioxin was a potent foetotoxin and teratogen. Hepatocarcinogenicity has also been established in animal studies. Therefore, these effects were examined in the follow-up to the single acute exposure at Seveso.

Studies on liver effects, including porphyria, in 700 children failed to identify significant illness, although two indicators of liver dysfunction, γ-glutamyl transferase and alanine aminotransferase, were slightly elevated in boys from the most contaminated zone.

A birth defects register was set up after the disaster. There were no birth defects that could be unequivocally linked to dioxin exposure among the limited number of births to residents of the high-exposure zone. In addition, although there were wide variations in the spontaneous abortion rate between zones, these could not be ascribed to dioxin. Examination of chromosomes in aborted tissue following artificially induced abortions suggested that there might have been a higher frequency of chromosomal aberrations in foetuses from mothers potentially exposed to dioxins, but it was not possible to establish whether these aberrations would have led to adverse reproductive outcomes.

Perhaps the greatest long-term worry from the Seveso incident was cancer. This has now been followed up for 10 years. There are no excesses of overall mortality or mortality due to all cancers (Bertazzi *et al.*, 1989; Bertazzi, 1991). Risks of deaths from certain individual cancers and from cardiovascular disease were elevated, but they could not be related to exposure patterns. Although restricted by the short observation time and

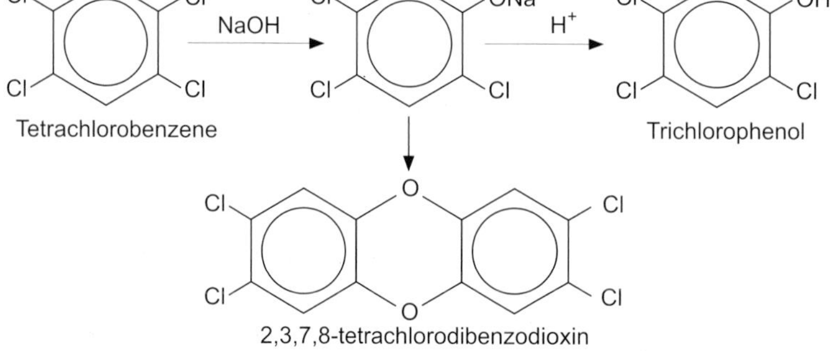

Figure 5 Reaction scheme for the formation of dioxin from tetrachlorobenzene. The condensation to form dioxin is a minor reaction compared with that of synthesizing trichlorophenol.

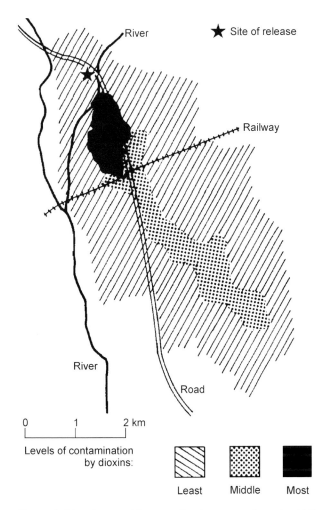

Figure 6 Sketch map of Seveso, showing areas of most, middle and least contamination by dioxin. Based on Marshall (1987).

the small numbers of deaths from certain causes, the study seems to suggest that there have not been the feared large increases in the overall numbers of deaths from cancer. A second study investigated occurrence (incidence) of cancer over the same period (Bertazzi *et al.*, 1993). A total of 14 cancers were seen in people from the most contaminated area, and this represented a relative risk for females of 1.0 and for males of 0.7. In the intermediate area, overall malignancy incidence was normal (females 36 cases, 95% confidence interval for relative risk 0.6–1.1; males 76 cases, 95% confidence intervals 0.9–1.4), although incidences of some cancers were elevated. A similar picture emerged in the lowest risk zone (relative risks for all malignancies 0.9 for both men and women, confidence intervals including the value of 1.0). Thus, overall, there was no indication of an increased risk of cancer.

The Seveso incident illustrates how an accidental release of a chemical may be perceived by the general public as a major disaster. So far, few, if any, human deaths have resulted from the single-dose exposure to dioxin. Those suffering chloracne or burns recovered.

Fears of large numbers of people being affected by potential long-term effects have not been confirmed. Nevertheless, the Seveso incident is important, as it raised the general awareness of the potential that there may be for ill-health following major plant failure.

Bhopal, India, 1984

Methyl isocyanate was a toxic substance responsible for a major disaster at Bhopal, India, in December 1984 at a factory manufacturing the pesticide carbaryl. The cause of the accident was the introduction of water into a storage tank containing methyl isocyanate. This resulted in the production of carbon dioxide:

$$CH_3NCO + H_2O \rightarrow CH_2NH_2 + CO_2 \qquad (1)$$

The combination of rising temperature due to a runaway exothermic reaction coupled with gas evolution led to a build-up of pressure which caused 30–35 t of methyl isocyanate to be vented to the atmosphere in a 2–3 h period (Marshall, 1987). The venting occurred during the night and the cloud dispersed over a densely populated area (**Figure 7**).

Estimates of the number of deaths which resulted from the release vary between 1700 and 5000, with up to 60 000 people being seriously injured (Bucher, 1987; Andersson, 1989). Survivors reported that the vapour cloud gave off considerable heat and had a pungent odour. Irritation, coughing and choking were early symptoms, and were followed by vomiting, defecation and urination, and panic, depression, agitation, apathy and convulsions. Although severe eye effects, including temporary blindness, were seen in many survivors, they did not persist (Andersson *et al.*, 1988). Initial lung effects (oedema, focal atelectasis) were probable causes of death and led, in survivors, to more persistent changes in lung function, and possible fibrosis and inflammation. Serial studies showed that some survivors improved, that there was no change in some and that some worsened. Liver and kidney function appeared to be normal in survivors (Bucher, 1987; Andersson *et al.*, 1988).

The Bhopal incident illustrates many important points. First, although the reasons for the water entering the methyl isocyanate tank were never clearly identified, the consequences were made substantially worse than they need have been because several of the design safety features had been rendered unusable and because there were substantial numbers of shanty houses right up to the factory fence. Also, there was a paucity of toxicological data on methyl isocyanate prior to the incident, which has now been rectified by undertaking substantial studies in animals as well as following up the victims (Bucher, 1987). At the time of the incident there was only one substantial published report on the toxicity of methyl isocyanate, and that was restricted to an animal study on the acute effects following a single exposure (Kimmerle and Eben, 1964).

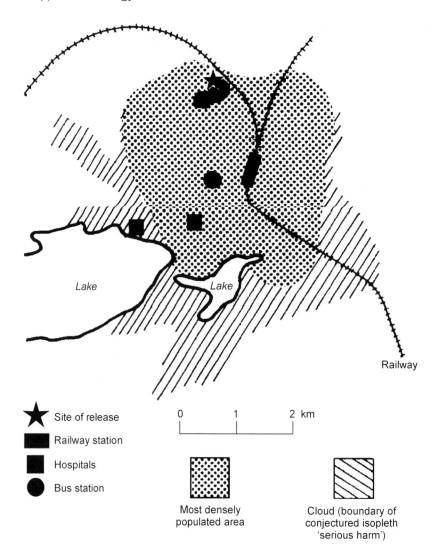

Figure 7 Sketch map of Bhopal, showing overlap between populated area and the approximate boundary for receiving serious harm from the vapour cloud. Based on Marshall (1987).

Chernobyl, Former USSR, 1986

Chernobyl, 80 km north of Kiev, Ukraine, was the site of probably the worst accident to have occurred at a nuclear plant.

In April 1986, a test was being conducted on a reactor during shut-down for routine maintenance (Henderson, 1987; Bertazzi, 1989; Wells, 1997). However, the planning of the test was poor and safety devices were deliberately switched off to allow the test to proceed. By the time it was realized that something was wrong, uranium oxide fuel elements in the upper part of the core had probably started to disintegrate because of the high temperatures. Explosions followed which released considerable quantities of radioactivity to the atmosphere, much of which was dispersed over the former Soviet Union and western and northern Europe.

By 1 year after the event only 31 people had died as a result of it. They died in the immediate aftermath of the accident, from acute radiation sickness. Although not apparent for the first 3 years after the accident, by the end of 1994 a clear increase in childhood thyroid cancers has been seen in children from the surrounding areas in Belarus and Ukraine (Likhtarev *et al.*, 1995; Stsjazhko *et al.*, 1995). For comparison, in 1981–85 there was 1 case (0.5 cases per million) of childhood thyroid cancer in the area (Gomel) in Belarus nearest Chernobyl. This increased to 21 (10.5) in 1986–89, and 143 (96.4) in the period 1991–94. In the Ukraine as a whole, incidence rates started to rise (from 0.63–0.72 cases per million) in 1989, with a peak of 4.24 in 1992 and a value of 3.70 for 1993 (the last year reported). These figures mask a much greater increase in the area of the Ukraine immediately surrounding Chernobyl, where incidences of 62.5 and 72.5 were recorded for the six and five cases found in the period 1990–92. No increase has been seen in countries outside the former USSR (Sali *et al.*, 1996). As data available cover only approximately 10 years since the incident, it is too early for there to be significant information concerning other cancers. However, there have been estimates that there might be a total of over 10 000 premature deaths due to cancers caused by the radioactivity, of which 35 might be in the UK, over the following 50 years (Henderson, 1987). This has to be set against the approximately 7 million anticipated deaths due to cancers in the UK alone over the same time.

The radioactivity from the accident was washed from the skies and entered food chains, notably in areas of high rainfall. In the UK this led to the banning of the sale for human consumption of sheepmeat from badly affected areas for over 1 year. Subsequent to the accident, the people in the area around Chernobyl were evacuated. They have not been allowed to return and the area is being converted to a national park where human activity, including farming, is banned.

This disaster is one in which future illness and premature deaths are the primary effects on man. It is this fear of the future effects of radiation which has made the nuclear industry so heavily regulated in comparison with other industries.

Fire

Thermal injuries, heat stress and physical trauma from collapsing structures are obvious problems in major fires. However, fire statistics indicate that deaths consequent on being overcome by smoke are the most common type of death (Committee on Fire Toxicology, 1986). Such deaths and incapacitations are due to the evolution of toxic combustion products. As toxicants are likely to be funnelled upwards and diluted to non-toxic levels in unconfined fires, major fire disasters usually occur in confined spaces when it is not possible to escape from the effects of the toxic combustion products.

Smoke includes all airborne products from the pyrolysis and combustion of materials (Committee on Fire Toxicology, 1986). Full oxidation of substances present in fires would result in products such as carbon dioxide, water (steam), nitrogen dioxide, sulphur dioxide and chlorine. However, complete combustion rarely occurs and other products such as carbon monoxide, soot (particles), hydrogen cyanide, hydrogen chloride, hydrogen fluoride, acrolein and other organic materials are often present. The toxicity of fires therefore arises from the evolution of smoke (including gases, dust/fume and aerosol) containing irritants and asphyxiants and, potentially, carcinogens. Those most at risk will normally be the fire-fighters in close proximity to the fire, and thus near enough to inhale undispersed toxic smoke and gases.

Potentially, risks from acute health effects of dispersed combustion products may occur in warehouse fires such as that at Brightside, Sheffield (Health and Safety Executive, 1985). Onlookers who were in close proximity to the fire may have acquired sore throats and chest symptoms due to effects from the fire. However, potential combustion product toxicants were dispersed to levels thought too dilute to pose a risk to the general population within very short distances. Asbestos roofing materials were dispersed widely in this fire, but the longer term health effects for people exposed to single doses of dispersed fire products were considered to be minimal.

Two examples of disasters in which the evolution of toxic combustion products from fires contributed significantly are given below. In both examples most of those who died were incapacitated by the effects of inhaling toxic smoke and gases in relatively confined spaces, and thus became unable to move to less polluted atmospheres.

Manchester Airport Crash, UK, 1985

One area where there is a potential for disasters due to toxic hazards is aircraft fires. An example of such a catastrophe was the Manchester Airport crash of 1985 (Air Accidents Investigation Branch, Department of Transport, 1989).

On 22 August 1985, a British Airtours Boeing 737 aircraft bound for Corfu was taking off from Manchester International Airport when the left engine suffered an uncontained failure which punctured a wing fuel tank access panel. The leaking fuel ignited and burnt as a large plume of fire trailing directly behind the engine. The crew abandoned take-off and cleared the runway by turning on to a taxiway as they stopped. A light wind carried the fire on to and around the rear fuselage (**Figure 8**). After the aircraft stopped, the hull was penetrated rapidly, and smoke and possibly flames entered through one of the cabin aft-doors which had just been opened. Fire subsequently developed inside the cabin and generated a dense black toxic/irritant smoke. Despite prompt attendance by the airport fire services the aircraft was destroyed and 55 people (53 passengers and two crew) died, one after 6 days in hospital. All those who died on board the aircraft had general congestion and oedema of the lungs with carbon particles in the air passages, consistent with inhalation of smoke. The cause of death was inhalation of smoke for 48 people and direct thermal injury (burns) for only six passengers.

Of those engulfed by smoke, only 38 (47%) survived. The survivors reported that a single breath of the cabin atmosphere was burning and painful, immediately causing choking. They experienced drowsiness and disorientation. Eight survivors actually collapsed, but recovered sufficiently to get out from the plane. Most of the deaths due to incapacitation might have been prevented if the people concerned had been protected from smoke or if external assistance had been more quickly available. All except one of the survivors of the immediate accident made their exit within 7 min of the aircraft stopping. The only survivor recovered by firemen was taken out after 33 min; he died 6 days later from severe pulmonary damage and associated pneumonia.

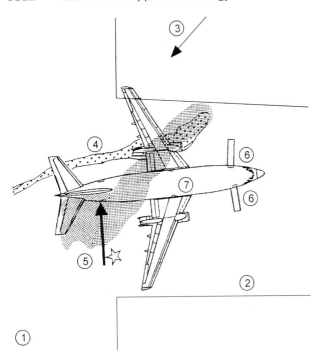

Figure 8 Sketch map to illustrate the position of the stopped plane in the Manchester Airport crash, 1985. 1, Main runway; 2, taxiway; 3, wind direction (wind speed 6 knots); 4, pool of jet fuel from punctured tank; 5, plume of fire/smoke from ignited fuel; 6, forward emergency doors (used to escape). Star indicates rear emergency door through which flames/smoke may have penetrated cabin. Based on data in Air Accidents Investigation Branch Report 8/88 (1989).

The thermal decomposition products of cabin materials included toxic irritant gases, such as carbon monoxide, hydrogen chloride and hydrogen cyanide. Some fluorinated materials (used as decorative films) yielded hydrogen fluoride. It was probably the combined effects of toxic combustion products which caused death. Elevated levels of carbon monoxide and cyanide and the metabolic product of cyanide, thiocyanate, were found in all except six of those dying on board the plane. Individually lethal levels of carbon monoxide were found in 13, and of cyanide in 21 of these people (nine had levels of both substances, either of which could have been lethal); for the remainder, the sum effects from the total amounts of toxic materials present probably caused death.

This aircraft accident is an example of a disaster where many of those who died might, in other circumstances, have been rescuable. One element that played a part in the disaster was disablement by the smoke from a fire in a confined space before exit from that space could be achieved. This has encouraged investigations into the potential for placing smoke-hoods of suitable design on aircraft for passenger use in this type of emergency, the investigation into possible 'in-cabin' firefighting systems and provision of low level lighting systems to indicate routes to fire exits.

Kings Cross (London) Underground Station, UK, 1987

Thirty-one people died and many more were injured in an escalator fire at Kings Cross Underground station. The fire took place in the evening at an extremely busy Underground station where four lines cross (**Figures 9** and **10**). Access to the three deep lines (Piccadilly, Victoria and Northern) is from the ticket hall below the main line station forecourt. The ticket hall is approached by subways from Kings Cross and St Pancras mainline stations and from street level. According to the Inquiry Report (Fennel, 1988), the fire started in the Piccadilly line escalator, among an accumulation of grease and detritus (dust, fibre and debris) on the running tracks, possibly as a result of a lighted match passing through the skirting board. This fire preheated the balustrades and decking, which were wooden. As a consequence of a 'trench' effect, the fire initially burnt cleanly and then produced dense, black smoke. 'Flashover' occurred as the fire erupted into the ticket hall. The deaths all occurred among people in the ticket hall at around the time 'flashover' occurred.

The inquiry did not pursue in detail the question of cause of death for the 31 people who died, but concluded

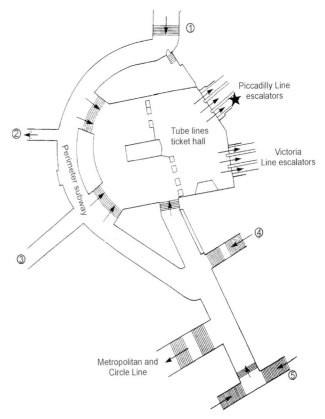

Figure 9 Sketch map of the layout of the subsurface ticket hall and subways at Kings Cross Underground station. 1, Entrance from Kings Cross mainline station; 2, entrance from St Pancras mainline station; 3, entrance from Pancras Road; 4 and 5, entrances from Euston Road. Star indicates escalator in which fire started. Based on Fennel (1988).

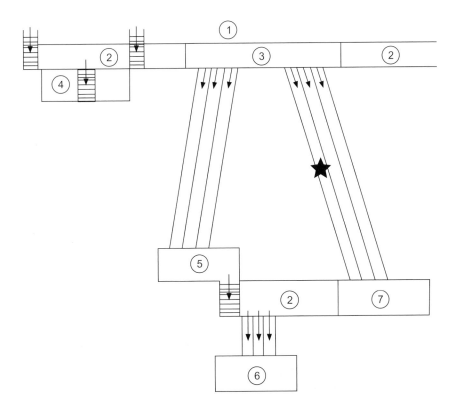

Figure 10 Sketch map of the levels of the components of Kings Cross Underground station. 1, Surface level (Kings Cross mainline station forecourt); 2, subways; 3, ticket hall; 4, Metropolitan and Circle Lines; 5, Victoria Line; 6, Northern Line; 7, Piccadilly Line. Star indicates escalator on which fire started.

that many deaths were due to the toxic effects of the smoke rather than to burns. In the report the Inspector says: 'After hearing expert evidence about the role of toxic gases in the fire and the findings of pathologists on post-mortem tests, I determined that the cause of death in individual cases could not be pursued any further in this investigation. On the evidence available to me no reliable assessment could be made of the relative importance of various materials present in the station to the production of toxic fire fumes or to the sources of toxic materials found in the bodies. Although separate statutory Coroner's Inquests were held, the Coroner decided not to take the matter further'.

A major part of the inquiry focused on the procedures by which London Underground dealt with escalator fires. It was clear that the Underground lacked an adequate approach to safety in terms of their attitudes to safety matters, their attention to staff training in safety and their equipment, and procedures to be used in emergencies. The lack of preparedness led to an emergency becoming a disaster.

Food and Drink

Mass poisonings due to contamination of food or drink may be considered disasters. Many episodes of this type of mass poisoning are the consequences of

bacterial or fungal contamination of foods consumed by the victims. If the causative agent is pathogenic, then health can suffer. However, a portion of such poisonings is due to the introduction of a chemical toxicant into the consumed material, either directly or via a food chain.

Because of the indirect way in which the contamination affects man, it can be difficult to demonstrate cause and effect. Ill-health may occur indirectly, in a species (man) remote from that (e.g. wheat) to which the toxicant was administered, possibly after transmission through a food chain (fed to farm animals, etc.) or directly (in bread). It may be some time before the toxicant accumulates sufficiently for the victim to exhibit symptoms of ill-health, or for the ill-health to be manifest following ingestion. Consequently, considerable detective work may be needed in order to identify the cause of ill-health, and on occasion it may never be properly characterized.

A series of examples of incidents involving contamination of food or water follow. Further examples can be found in Aldridge (1987).

Adulteration of Food or Drink

Adulteration (debasing by adding other or inferior substances: *Concise Oxford Dictionary*, 1990) of foodstuffs and deliberate poisonings by admixture in food have gone on from time immemorial. Adulteration for commercial reasons was rife in the eighteenth and nineteenth centuries (see Smullen, 1989). Bread from bakers often contained chalk, lime, lead salts or even bone to make it look white. Leaves of hawthorn, sloe or ash were used to dilute tea. With hindsight, several of these adulterants were toxic chemicals and may have had disastrous consequences for the recipients. Deliberate adulteration, when it occurs, is still capable of causing major disasters.

Ginger Paralysis, Mid-west and South-west USA, 1930.

During Prohibition in the USA, the Prohibition Bureau ruled that the USP fluid 'extract of ginger' was a non-potable beverage and its sale was not restricted. This beverage was an alcoholic extract of material from the ginger plant and was freely drunk. An adulterated 'fluid extract of ginger' entered circulation through dealers (non-pharmacists), mainly in Ohio and Tennessee early in 1930. Cases of paralysis started to occur in mid-February. Adult men were the principal victims and those showing symptoms seemed to do so some 10 days to 3 weeks after drinking the suspect ginger extract (Smith and Elvove, 1930). Ultimately some 50 000 people were affected (Morgan, 1982).

The paralysis first appeared as soreness of the muscles of the arms and legs, with occasional numbness in the fingers and toes. Foot and wrist drop and weakness of the fingers developed. The symptoms were found in distal parts of the limbs and were more marked in the feet and legs. This neuropathy was a primary axonopathy caused by demyelination and dying back from the distal end of the long nerves. In some cases recovery was very limited (Aldridge, 1987).

In a very detailed piece of work, the causative agent was identified chemically as tri-o-cresyl phosphate (**Figure 11**) (Smith, 1930; Smith and Elvove, 1930). Both the adulterated ginger extract and the presumed adulterant, tri-o-cresyl phosphate, were found to cause the symptoms of the neuropathy in calves, chickens and, to a much less marked degree, rabbits, but had little effect on monkeys or dogs following oral ingestion.

Toxic Oil Syndrome, Spain, 1981.

Toxic oil syndrome was a previously unknown disease syndrome which appeared in Spain in May 1981, principally in Madrid and the north-west provinces (World Health Organization, 1984; Aldridge, 1985, 1987). The epidemic was at its peak in mid-June and faded away thereafter. By March 1983, 340 deaths had occurred and over 20 000 cases had been recorded.

The disease developed in two phases. In the acute phase, a pleuropneumonia sufficient to cause respiratory distress and death in severe cases was present. This pleuropneumonia did not respond to antibiotic treatment and about 20% of survivors did not recover completely. A chronic phase of the disease, a sensorimotor peripheral neuropathy of variable appearance, developed, together with sclerodermal-like skin changes. There was little evidence of central nervous system involvement.

Although initially thought to be due to an infective agent, the syndrome was rapidly associated with the consumption of an oil sold for food use in 5 litre cans by itinerant salesmen. The oil was rapeseed oil, denatured with aniline, intended for industrial use. In most cases the oil had been re-refined, mixed with other seed oils, animal fats and poor-quality olive oil or chlorophyll, but in the cases of a small number of victims in the Seville area (well away from the main outbreak) the re-refined oil had not been further processed. The unsolved problem in toxic oil syndrome is the exact nature of the (presumed) chemical toxicant. Despite considerable effort aimed at its identification, the precise toxicant has not been identified.

Accidental Contamination

As opposed to deliberate addition of materials to foodstuffs or drinks, accidental addition of toxicants can also occur. If the toxicant is sufficiently effective and affects a large number of people, a major disaster could result.

Pollution of Drinking Water in North Cornwall, UK, 1988.

Mass intoxications, in theory at least, could occur due to contamination of drinking-water supplies. That this is not such a remote possibility was demonstrated in 1988, when the South West Water Authority found that a truck load (20 t) of alum (aluminium sulphate; **Figure 11**) had accidentally been released into the drinking-water supply to Camelford, a small town in Cornwall, and the surrounding district (Lowermoor Incident Health Advisory Group, 1989; 1991). The material was delivered into the treated water reservoir at Lowermoor Treatment Works. The pH of the water dropped below 5 and aluminium levels were raised to over 10 mg l^{-1}, considerably above the 0.2 mg l^{-1} set on aesthetic grounds (potential discolouration) in the European Community

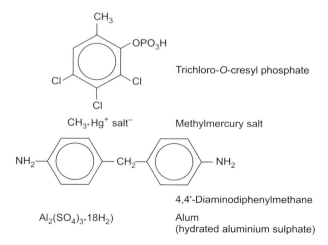

Figure 11 Structures of chemicals implicated in disasters mediated through food or water supplies.

Drinking Water Directive. Although initial advice from local sources suggested that little ill-health would occur, newspapers reported considerable acute health symptoms and speculated that there were potential long-term effects. The expert assessment was that the early symptoms of gastro-intestinal disturbances, rashes and mouth ulcers were probably due to the incident, but these would be short-lived. Up to 400 (out of a population of about 12 000) attributed continuing effects to the incident. Later complaints included joint and muscle pain, malaise, fatigue and memory problems. The 1991 report ascribed these symptoms to a heightened awareness provoked by the incident and subsequent events. Media coverage ascribed further symptoms, including shedding of toenails, to the incident, although these symptoms could not be confirmed from reliable sources. The expert committee concluded that there was no reason to predict any late consequences, but it could not categorically exclude them. Its recommendations included a follow-up study monitoring hospital discharges. This study of hospital discharge rates up to the fifth anniversary of the incident indicated a continuing significantly higher level of hospital admissions arising from the Camelford area, but, despite examining diagnoses by cause, the authors were unable to identify a statistical excess likely to be linked to aluminium exposure (Owen and Miles, 1995). There was a higher level of talipes in foetuses from mothers exposed to the aluminium sulphate (four cases, one control, $p = 0.01$), but, because of the low numbers involved (88 exposed mothers) and the likely general under-reporting of positional talipes, the importance of this finding is unclear. The only conclusion drawn was that there was no evidence from the study of major problems apparent at birth (Lowermoor Incident Health Advisory Group, 1991; Golding et al., 1991).

The incident is a sufficient reminder of the possibility of a disaster occurring as a result of contaminated water supplies. It also illustrates the difficulties which occur in allaying fears when the affected population receives initial advice which was, to quote the conclusions in the first report of the Advisory Group, 'contradictory, confusing and sometimes inappropriate', and when media reports claiming further health effects continue. The 1991 report suggests that many of the longer lasting symptoms and complaints arising from the Lowermoor incident would be expected as a consequence of the psychological reactions, and they cite evidence that, even when the victims concerned have suffered no direct physical damage, then worry, anxiety, depression and 'post-traumatic stress syndrome' may follow a major accident or disaster and can produce real mental and physical symptoms.

Contamination of Food During Storage—Epping Jaundice, UK, 1965.

Epping jaundice was an outbreak of jaundice which affected at least 84 people in the Epping area of London during February 1965 (Kopelman et al.,

1966a, b). It was traced to ingestion of wholemeal bread made from flour contaminated with 4,4-diaminodiphenylmethane (**Figure 11**). The chemical had spilled from a container on to the floor of a van which was carrying flour as well as chemicals.

In most of the cases, jaundice and liver enlargement were preceded by severe, intermittent pains in the upper abdomen and lower chest areas of the body. Normally, these pains were of acute onset (50 patients), but sometimes onset was insidious (27 patients). Of the 57 patients further investigated, most had raised serum bilirubin, alkaline phosphate and aspartate aminotransferase levels. Needle biopsies were performed on four patients within 3 weeks of the onset of symptoms; all showed considerable evidence of portal inflammation and bile duct cholestasis, and evidence of hepatocyte damage. The lesion was reproducible in mice given 4,4-diaminodiphenylmethane (Schoental, 1968). The patients slowly recovered over succeeding weeks.

The jaundice was the result of an accidental, undetected (until too late) contamination of a foodstuff because it was stored during delivery adjacent to chemicals which were insufficiently securely contained within the packaging. The chemicals were absorbed by the flour through the sacking and, following baking, were present in the bread.

Poisoning Due to Consumption of Foodstuff Not Intended for Human Consumption—Methylmercury Poisoning in Iraq, 1971–72.

An outbreak of organomercurial poisoning due to the consumption of treated grain by farmers and their families occurred in Iraq in 1971–72 (World Health Organization, 1976). There were 459 deaths and over 6000 further cases admitted to hospital.

Poisoning cases started to appear in hospitals in late December. Farming families only were affected, and the cause of the poisoning was identified as consumption of home-made bread, an important element of their diet, made from wheat treated with seed dressing. There was a latent period of up to 60 days from first consumption to the appearance of signs and symptoms of poisoning and in many cases consumption of contaminated grain ceased before the symptoms occurred.

Symptoms included speech disturbances, abnormal behaviour, loss of auditory and visual acuity, and ataxia. The severity varied from minimal effects to severe disability and death. Most of those showing only mild or moderate symptoms were symptom-free 2 years later, although symptoms were still present in severe cases. Mercury levels in hair were found to be good indicators of the dose of mercury received.

Organomercurials, such as the methylmercury (**Figure 11**) involved in this episode, are fungicides, the methylmercury being used as a seed dressing to prevent wheat bunt and other crop diseases. Grain dressed with methylmercury was distributed to farmers between mid-September and early December, 1971. Although much of the wheat had been consumed before a cause–effect relationship had been established, surplus treated grain was withdrawn to storehouses once the cause of the outbreak was known. The problem arose because wheat intended as seed for next year's crop was eaten by the farmers and their families rather than used for its intended function.

Environmental Pollution—Minamata and Niigata, Japan, 1951–74.

The examples of major disasters arising from toxic substances so far discussed arise from contamination of the foodstuff. It is also possible for contamination to arise indirectly as a result of an environmental pollutant entering a food chain. Two examples of this occurred in Japan, at Minamata and Niigata (Tsubaki and Irukayama, 1977).

Over the period 1951–74 there were over 700 recognized cases and 80 deaths due to 'Minamata disease', and over 2000 other people had applied for recognition as Minamata disease patients. The principal geographical areas affected were in two prefectures, Kumamoto and Kagoshima, which border Minamata Bay. The disease occurred mainly in fishermen and their families who consumed large quantities of locally caught fish containing high concentrations of mercury. The patients' nervous systems were affected, with symptoms of sensory, motor and visual involvement. Domestic cats (presumably also largely fed fish) exhibited similar clinical signs, and abnormal behaviour occurred among crows in the affected areas. Congenital effects also occurred.

The outbreak of poisoning at Niigata was first identified in 1965, with over 520 patients being identified by the end of 1974. The epidemic was also apparent in the domestic animal population.

In the Minamata outbreak, the effects were due to organically bound mercury present in sludges from industrial plant. The mercury was used as a catalyst. Mercury from the sludge or from the waste-water outlet entered food chains and was bioconcentrated in both shellfish and fish. These were eventually consumed by man. At Niigata, river fish from the lower reaches of the Agano river were the main foodstuff consumed which contained organic mercurial compounds. The source of the mercury was an industrial plant waste-water discharge containing low concentrations of mercury (**Figure 11**). Methylation took place in sediments and considerable bioconcentration occurred in the fish, as evidenced by the much higher levels of mercury in the fish when compared with the river water.

At both sites, consumption of contaminated fish had gone on for a considerable time before the causes of the disease were identified. This points to the great difficulties involved in deriving a cause–effect relationship when the effect is remote from the source of the causative agent.

Although the particular examples chosen to illustrate this effect related to human health, other species may be the final consumer in a food chain. The story of the

consequences of spraying persistent organochlorine insecticides, their bioconcentration in the food chain and their disastrous effects on raptor populations because the concentrations reached were sufficient to cause eggshell thinning and failure to reproduce effectively, summarized by Smith (1986), is well known.

Interactions of Man and Nature

This section includes a miscellaneous collection of disasters in which human activity and natural events have interacted. It includes disasters involving tide, current and weather, in addition to those due to human activity on (in) the land.

Shipping Disasters

The classic shipping disaster involving toxic effects is the spilling of oil from wrecked oil tankers. Most of the consequences are environmental, but there is also potential for indirect or direct effects on the human population.

Wreck of the mv Braer, Shetland Isles, Scotland, 1993

On 5 January 1993, the oil tanker mv Braer grounded in the Shetland Isles (off the north coast of Scotland) in bad weather (Ritchie and O'Sullivan, 1994; Topping et al., 1997; Whittle et al., 1997). The cargo of 8500 tonnes of a biodegradable light crude oil was released over the next 7 days. This oil was dispersed by the severe weather; dispersants were not used because of these weather conditions. Although the principal toxic effects were environmental, there was a potential human health problem arising from the food chain. The area contaminated was a fishing ground and it included several salmon farms. Because of potential human health problems, an exclusion order under the Food and Environment Protection Act 1985, banning the harvesting for market of fish, shellfish and farmed salmon from within a designated zone area around the wreck was made on 8 January. On 27 January, that zone was extended in order to ensure that all areas where contamination took place were included. **Figure 12** shows the approximate area covered by the zone. The order was lifted for fish on 23 April 1993, on crustaceans on 30 September 1994 and on molluscs in February 1995. The farmed salmon usually remain in sea cages for two winters. Both the 1991 and 1992 fish [date is year of transfer of the salmon smolts (young fish) to sea cages] were destroyed, but smolts transferred in early Spring 1993 were marketed.

The basis of the decision to allow marketing depended on analysis of polycyclic aromatic hydrocarbons present in the fish and taint analysis. Because no formal limits for acceptable levels of these contaminants in foodstuffs were available, the criteria chosen were:

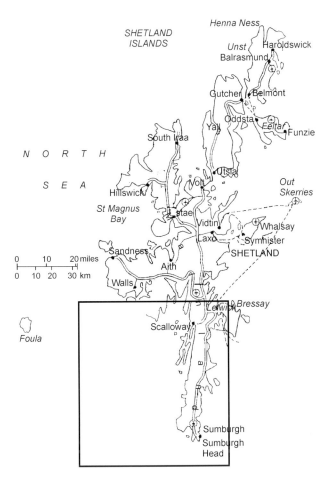

Figure 12 Map of Shetland Isles showing exclusion zone.

(1) fish and shellfish caught within the zone should not contain taint associated with crude oils and petroleum fractions; and
(2) concentrations of aliphatic and polycyclic aromatic hydrocarbons should fall within the background range of values for fish and shellfish from outside the exclusion zone.

This approach to the potential problem of contamination of the food chain was successful, in that it upheld the reputation of the Shetland Isles seafood industry, prevented entry of contaminated food into the chain and provided public reassurance concerning the wholesomeness of marketed fish and seafood. However, it did little to alleviate the direct environmental effects of the release of oil.

Mines and Tunnels

People have died as a result of lung cancer due to exposure to radon in mines or of pneumoconiosis caused by exposure to coal dust or silica, but the exposure to these agents was a consequence of inadequate working conditions rather than specific accidental exposures. Fire is a potential problem in mines and tunnels. For this reason, very strict precautions have been developed to prevent fires starting underground in coal mines in the UK. These have included testing and certifying machinery for use underground and strict prevention of miners taking potential ignition sources underground.

In general, toxicants are unlikely to be a primary cause of a specific mining disaster, as the conditions causing ill-health are unlikely to develop suddenly. Historically, it is possible that disasters due to asphyxiation or the release of toxic gases occurred. Canaries were taken underground to act as fail-safe biological monitors for these effects ('when the singing ceased . . .'). Nowadays forced ventilation makes these events extremely rare. However, disasters can occur in tunnels used by the public as a result of the deliberate release of toxic agents. The Kings Cross disaster, already examined, is a demonstration of the potential for disaster that can result from fire occurring in a confined space.

Terrorist Attack on the Tokyo Subway, 1995

The dramatic effects of deliberately releasing a toxic agent in a confined space were demonstrated in a terrorist attack in the Tokyo subway in 1995 (Masuda *et al.*, 1995; Nozaki and Aikawa, 1995; Nozaki *et al.*, 1995; Suzuki *et al.*, 1995). Sarin, an organophosphorus nerve agent, was released. Ten people died and over 5000 were poisoned by the attack. Classical symptoms of organophosphorus poisoning were exhibited. Atropine and pralidoxime iodide administration were the principal treatments employed. However, it was claimed that the atropine may have been of limited value as it is effective against muscarinic dominant responses, and sarin was thought to have produced principally nicotinic dominant responses.

Waste Disposal

Inadequately thought-out or poorly controlled disposal of wastes may cause disasters.

Love Canal, USA

Love Canal was a waste disposal site which contained municipal and chemical waste disposed of over a period of 30 years up to 1953. Homes were built on the site during the 1960s. Leaching became a problem in the late 1960s, when chemical odours were detected in basements. These were followed by fears of potential ill-health which led to considerable psychological stress. Dibenzofurans and dioxins were identified in the organic phases of leachates and were presumably derived from the disposal of waste products of the manufacture of chlorinated hydrocarbons. Animal studies, conducted on the organic phase of the leachate, indicated that there could be risks of immunotoxic, carcinogenic and teratogenic effects (Silkworth *et al.*, 1984, 1986, 1989a, b). Low birthweights have been found in the offspring of residents of Love Canal (Vianna and Polan, 1984).

Although follow-up was limited, no causal link has been established for exposure to chemicals and cancer in man (Janerich *et al.*, 1981) Nevertheless, serious social and psychological consequences have resulted from the use of the site for houses and the initial lack of understanding of the fears of residents concerning the toxic properties of the chemicals dumped at the site (Holden, 1980).

Minamata and Niigata

The mercury poisonings at Minamata and Niigata, already described, were caused by the disposal of industrial wastes in such a manner that the toxicant was concentrated to dangerous levels in a food chain in the aqueous environment.

Conclusions

Toxicants, whether derived from nature or the chemical plant, can cause disasters. Identifying the cause is relatively easy when the toxicant is airborne and the ill-health occurs during or shortly after exposure. It is usually more difficult if the effect is mediated via the food or water supply and/or if the effect is not immediately apparent. The former have been called 'overt' disasters and the latter 'dilute' disasters (Bertazzi, 1989). As 'dilute' implies some diminution of effect, it might be better to refer to the latter type of disaster as a 'disseminated' disaster.

In overt disasters due to airborne toxicants, there is usually a primary event such as volcanic eruption or a plant failure. This is followed by dispersal of the toxicant, which depends on the buoyancy of the material released and the meteorological conditions at the time of release. Any immediate dose received by man will depend on the level and duration of the exposure. Only very simple post-event preventative measures can be used to minimize the dose received. Although usually ill-health is immediate, long-term effects such as carcinogenicity could occur. However, they are difficult to link to a primary event and are chiefly known for releases of radioactivity. Toxic material can be deposited on to surfaces and ill-health due to the consequent continuing lower level exposures may be prevented by segregation (e.g. collection and containment of the contaminated material and/or banning public access to it).

Most known airborne toxicants involved in major disasters affect the respiratory tract. Irritation, asphyxiation (chemically induced by binding of toxicant or physically induced by blockage of the respiratory tract) and pulmonary oedema are common (Schwartz, 1987). Cancers are frequent effects of radiation. Other toxic effects may occur in organs away from the respiratory system, although this appears to be rare. When airborne, the toxicant reaches the lung and respiratory system first; consequently, they appear to be the most frequently affected organ systems.

When transport and dispersal of a toxicant are in water, then buoyancy, flow rates and ability to be taken up and released by sediment or biota become important determinants of the concentration present. Transport of toxic substances deposited on land depends, in large part, on the weather. In dry conditions, air dispersal of the material absorbed on particles is possible; in wet weather, dispersal will be along the same routes as those followed by the rain water. Soil adsorption and uptake by plants and animals may also occur. Water (or soil) borne toxic substances may affect human health as a result of direct intake as drinking water or via foodstuffs contaminated with the toxic substances. This type of dispersal may result in 'overt' disasters when the source is readily apparent, or in 'disseminated' disasters when the source of the toxic substance is not obvious.

'Disseminated' disasters are frequently more difficult to identify and they are often identified initially by end effect. Tracing the cause may take a considerable time, particularly as there may be a considerable time delay between exposure occurring and ill-health taking effect, and transfer between environmental compartments may occur. In consequence, withdrawal of the food, etc., containing the toxicant, although desirable, may not be possible until it is too late to be an effective post-event preventative measure.

One consistent complicating factor in major accidents and disasters is the possibility of psychological reactions being considered as physiological responses to exposure to a particular agent. Long-lasting consequences, including severe worry, anxiety, depression and 'post-traumatic syndrome', were identified following the Mount St Helens eruption and the Lowermoor incident. Although not toxicological responses *per se*, these effects can be real, distressing and disabling. In the absence of sufficient authoritative and accurate information, popular speculation generally favours the worst possible outcomes, however improbable. This is likely to worsen psychiatric consequences of the event and to complicate the emergency response. The provision of timely, accurate advice in an understandable form is one need that must be considered when examining how to handle the consequences of a serious incident.

DISASTER PREVENTION AND MITIGATION

One role of industry, individual governments and international organizations is to develop and implement procedures for preventing or minimizing the effects of potential or actual disasters. In most countries governments develop a series of legislative requirements in order to provide a framework of regulation within which to work. Rather than compare different national frameworks, this section will concentrate on conceptual approaches to handling the risks arising from major hazards.

Assessment of potential hazards and assessment and management of the likely consequences are the key elements in any process for dealing with major hazards. In the case of toxic hazards, one aspect of the hazard evaluation is an examination of the likely toxicity of the materials involved in the potentially disastrous situation, including the prediction of the amounts of toxic materials likely to cause these effects. Procedures can then be adopted for the assessment of the risks associated with the various uses. Interacting with, and dependent on, the risk assessment will be the approaches available by which the risks can be managed. These procedures of risk management differ fundamentally according to the type ('overt' or 'disseminated') of potential disaster envisaged.

Judging Risk

'Is it a risk?' is usually the first question asked when a potential hazard is being examined. Once the concept of risk has been explained, two questions will follow: 'what is the risk?' and 'is it acceptable/tolerable?' (see **Table 1** for definitions). This involves trying to define general criteria for acceptable or tolerable risk. These criteria should be based on societal judgements, but they are often taken by the technical expert on behalf of society as a whole. Once criteria for acceptability (tolerability) have been defined, a method is needed in order to compare the risk for the particular problem under study with the relevant criterion for acceptable risk. That method may be qualitative, of the form 'acceptable'/'non-acceptable', based on a judgement of the data available against broadly defined criteria. However, for many purposes, including much engineering-based risk assessment for initiating event, quantitative, numerical approaches are adopted. These numerical approaches are called quantified risk analyses. These quantitative analyses render decision-making easier, especially when choosing between options, as they give a clearer indication of the magnitude of a risk or of the relative risks for different options. However, because these decisions depend, in the final analysis, on societal judgements concerning acceptability, they may be unacceptable to certain individuals or groups within that society. Major reports on risk management and standard setting have emphasised that both communication between technical experts and key 'stakeholders' (acting on behalf of society) and transparency of decision taking process are essential if decisions taken on behalf of society are to be accepted by society (Presidential/Congressional Commission on Risk Assessment and Risk Management, 1997; Royal Commission on Environmental Pollution, 1998). Public (or 'stakeholder') involvement should be included in strategy formulation rather than solely in consultation on already drafted proposals, and may be conducted using 'focus groups', citizen juries, consensus conferences and deliberative polls as well as by more traditional means.

When considering the risk of an event leading to an end effect, a surrogate for that end effect, a 'dose' or exposure-time combination (a 'harm criterion') is often used. Uncertainty in the relationship between this surrogate and the end-effect (normally considered 'risk' by toxicologists and epidemiologists) is regarded, in this context, as uncertainty in defining the hazard.

Judging the acceptability of a human health harm criterion depends on three factors: the frequency level (the frequency with which the end effect is likely to occur), the definition of the biological effect (death, serious injury, etc.) and the status of the receiving individual (a 'normal' or a 'vulnerable' individual).

Judging environmental damage is more difficult as the importance of loss has to be considered in addition to the size of the effect. Descriptions of damage levels constituting a major disaster are therefore judgemental. One set of such end-effect criteria is that published by the UK Department of the Environment (1991). Generally loss of populations rather than loss of individuals is required when considering non-human species.

Framework for Risk Assessment

There are several levels of risk (either of initiating event or of end effect) that can be elaborated. At one level there is the 'trivial', 'negligible' or 'completely acceptable' risk. At the other extreme there is the 'intolerable' or 'unacceptable' risk. In between lies a range of risks which are tolerable under certain circumstances and/or provided they are minimized (**Figure 13**). In between the upper and lower bounds of acceptability lies a region where risks from known hazards should be reduced as far as is reasonably practicable. This means that the cost of reducing the risk should not be disproportionate to the level of risk encountered. A small reduction in an already low risk may not be justified if it is very expensive.

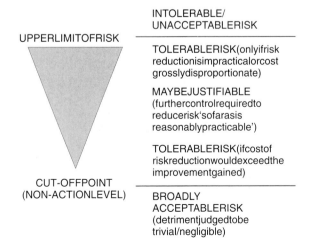

Figure 13 Diagram to illustrate the approach to risk evaluation for major hazards. Based on Royal Society Study Group (1983) and Health and Safety Executive (1988a).

Table 3 Comparisons of risk of death from various causes

Cause of death	Risk (as annual experience) (per year)	Year of statistic
Cancer	2.8×10^{-3}	1985
Industrial accidents to deep-sea fishermen (UK registered vessels)	8.8×10^{-4}	1984
All violent deaths	4.0×10^{-4}	1985
Industrial accidents during quarrying	3.0×10^{-4}	1985
Industrial accidents during coal extraction and manufacture of solid fuel	1.1×10^{-4}	1986–87
Road accidents	1.0×10^{-4}	1985
Industrial accidents in construction	9.2×10^{-5}	1986–87
Industrial accidents in agriculture	8.7×10^{-5}	1986–87
Industrial accidents in offices, shops, warehouses, etc.	4.5×10^{-6}	1985
Gas incidents	1.8×10^{-6}	1981–85
Lightning	1.0×10^{-7}	Average over several years

Data on deaths due to industrial accidents are based on accidents to the employee; data on deaths due to other causes are averaged over the general population. Based on Health and safety Executive (1988a).

Harm Criteria for 'Acceptable Risk'

When comparing risks, the risk of end-effect, and not of initiating event, is being examined. It is necessary to ensure that the particular end effect (usually 'death'; in reality foreshortening of life, often to the extent that death occurs during or shortly after the event occurring) for which the likelihood is being calculated is the same for all the likelihoods being examined, in terms of both the biological event and the type of recipient (usually a 'normal' individual). Criteria for assessing this 'risk of death' to the individual have been obtained by comparisons with everyday risks associated with various activities (Royal Society Study Group, 1983; Health and Safety Executive, 1988a, b, 1989a). For major hazards risk assessment, the acceptable 'risk of death' for exposure to the given agent has to be converted to a 'harm criterion' (exposure concentration–time relationship) for inclusion in the calculation of the overall risk arising from the initiating event.

A likelihood of about 1 in 10^6 per year that the exposure will result in the individual concerned dying from a given cause appears to be generally regarded in the UK as acceptable (Royal Society Study Group, 1983). This was justified by considering the death rates for different activities considered 'safe' (see **Table 3** for some comparative risks of 'death'). The 'risk of death' for workers in recognized dangerous occupations is of the order of 1 death per 10^3 per year, this is considered the highest bound of 'tolerable' risk for a lifetime risk. Any higher level is considered intolerable and unacceptable at all times. Because working in a 'risky' industry is, at least to some extent, voluntary, the individual risk just tolerable for a member of the general public living in the

neighbourhood of a hazard is considered to be 10-fold less (1 death per 10^4 per year) (Health and Safety Executive, 1989a). This is approximately the risk from death in a road traffic accident and slightly less than the risk of developing any form of cancer. All of these likelihood criteria relate to individual risk of end effect for the average individual.

A more conservative approach has been elaborated in The Netherlands (Versteeg, 1988). It depends on the frequency of deaths from natural causes and is based on the idea that industrial activity should not increase the background mortality by more than 1 per cent. An upper bound of 10^6 deaths per year has been derived, with a lower bound of 10^8 per year being considered trivial.

Although these types of numerical comparisons have been made for individual likelihoods associated with severe end effects, such as death, other end effects may be more important for evaluating the potential toxic effects of chemicals for disaster prevention and mitigation. Risks for events leading to more minor ill-health may be the evaluation required, and the risk may be societal (or population) risk. Although attempts have been made to consider what frequencies of end effect should be applied for many of these circumstances (e.g. Illing, 1991; Calman, 1996), consensus is absent.

'Overt' Disasters

Risk of the initiating event is the risk being examined. The aim of the risk assessment is therefore to examine the likelihood of events resulting in a release of a chemical or chemicals of a size and type that results in a harm criterion being exceeded in a given geographic location. Potential 'overt' disasters can be averted or minimized by a combination of land-use planning and emergency planning. Good land-use planning can minimize the potential of a release (a catastrophic failure of plant, etc.) leading to a disaster by restricting the size of any interaction of event and consequence. A hazardous process or a large store of hazardous material can be sited well away from large numbers of people (or, for environmental effects, away from important buildings or sensitive wildlife habitats). Potential developments involving significant numbers of members of the public can be sited away from natural or man-made major hazards.

There will remain a residue of risk after appropriate land-use planning has been achieved. Occasionally there will be the situation where inappropriate combinations of people and major hazards occurred prior to the time when the need for appropriate land-use planning became apparent. In addition, other considerations, such as a need for local employment, may mean that other factors were decisive when the planning decision was made. The consequences, should the event occur, can still be substantially reduced, provided that appropriate emergency planning has been undertaken. This includes both enabling potential victims to survive better prior to treatment and making available appropriate treatment sufficiently rapidly. It also involves protecting water and food supplies intended for human consumption.

Generally, owners (or intending owners) of potential major hazard installations will prepare 'safety cases' or 'safety assessments' for those sites. These often include assessments of the risks and consideration of the administrative and other arrangements for minimizing risks and for handling emergencies.

Land-use Planning

Although the effect of 'death' can be employed in relation to the harm criterion for human health effects and land-use planning, allowances need to be made for the uncertainties in developing the harm criterion for this effect for an individual within a population. Do we need the data for 5% dying or 95% dying? In addition, there may be serious, but sublethal, effects on health. These sublethal effects may be of great concern when handling toxic substances. In consequence, a broader concept, the 'dangerous dose', has also been employed. The dangerous dose is a description of the exposure conditions producing a level of toxicity (Health and Safety Executive, 1989a; Fairhurst and Turner, 1993):

(1) Severe distress will be caused to almost everyone.
(2) A substantial fraction will require medical attention.
(3) Some people are seriously injured and require prolonged treatment.
(4) Any highly susceptible people may be killed.

This type of criterion reflects that there is a range of individual ill-health effects and imprecision in the level of overall effect seen in the population.

The type of population being considered may also differ according to circumstances. Rather than examining the frequency of achieving a given biological effect in terms of the event occurring in an average individual in a 'normal' population, it may be that the consequence should be considered for an individual from a population containing a large number of particularly vulnerable (or susceptible) individuals.

If the biological effect being looked at changes, and the type of individual being examined is different, then the numerical value of any harm criterion ought also to be altered. When quoting a harm criterion it is therefore necessary also to mention the effect and the type of recipient.

Some arbitrary ratios have been enunciated for the relationships between the harm criterion for exposure conditions leading to 'death' and 'dangerous dose' in the same population (Health and Safety Executive, 1989a). The Health and Safety Executive has suggested that a likelihood of 1 in 10^6 per year for a dangerous dose corresponds to a likelihood of 3.3 in 10^7 per year for 'death'. Such a value will depend, in large measure, on the slope of the dose–response line. Comparisons for chlorine, ammonia, hydrogen fluoride and sulphur dioxide give the relationship:

$$\text{Dangerous dose} = \frac{\text{LD}_{50}}{2.57} \qquad (2)$$

(Franks et al., 1996)

A ratio of 3.3:1 is probably appropriate as a generalized, pragmatic assumption. Because risk is normally measured using logarithmic scales, this is a convenient value, as it represents a half-order of magnitude on such a scale.

A frequency of 3.3 in 10^7 per year for when there is a high proportion of 'highly susceptible' people receiving a 'dangerous close' has also been proposed in place of the 1 in 10^6 per year for an individual from a population containing a normal balance of 'highly susceptible' individuals (Health and Safety Executive, 1989a). The identity of the 'highly susceptible' people will depend on the effects seen, and the proportion will differ according to effect. Homes for the elderly, caring institutions and long-stay hospitals are considered to contain a high proportion of 'highly susceptible' people. However, the choice of the ratio of 3.3:1 (again, a half-order of magnitude) is a pragmatic decision. Although descriptive criteria as to what constitutes a major disaster to the environment have been developed for environmental incidents (Department of the Environment, 1991), these descriptions have not been related to predictive information. Thus judgement has to be substituted.

Emergency Planning

Emergency planning is essentially concerned with mitigating the consequences after an event has occurred. It involves both 'on-site' and 'off-site' planning and may cover immediate 'emergency' shutdown, responses of emergency services, the medical management of the immediate and long-term health effects, and the management of food and drinking water supplies and potential environmental effects (Murray, 1990; Home Office, 1994; OECD, 1994; Institution of Mechanical Engineers, 1995; Wells 1997). Such planning is concerned with a much wider range of biological effects than death. For immediate effects on human health, these include the 'severe health effect' (disability, requiring hospital treatment), and 'mild health effect' (discomfort or distress, detection or nuisance) (Baxter et al., 1989a; Illing, 1989). ECETOC has defined three 'emergency exposure indices' (essentially harm criteria) for airborne concentrations for exposures lasting up to a specified time (ECETOC, 1991). These are criteria below which direct toxic effects are unlikely to lead to one of death/permanent incapacity, disability or discomfort. Although hospital treatment may be essential for recovery from the severe health effects, it will usually have little influence in the case of milder effects (discomfort). It may also be necessary to consider longer term health effects, protection of food and drinking water supplies (by withdrawing affected foods and water from the supply chain), and possibly protection (if feasible) of the environment.

There is also a need to plan for an appropriately sized event. One proposal categorizes three types of release: small but likely accidents, severe but reasonably foreseeable events and large, unlikely events (Baxter et al., 1989a). If the severe, reasonably foreseeable event is chosen for planning purposes, then it should be possible to scale up or down the response for an individual event.

'Disseminated' Disasters

Essentially, 'disseminated' disasters should only occur as a result of failure of a regulatory system resulting in exposure to a toxicant. The risk should be that of the initiating event, the failure of the regulatory system. That failure may be because a new effect was uncovered by the disaster Alternatively, a known effect might have occurred because of non-adherence to existing regulatory requirements. The primary means of control has to be preventative, ensuring that, under normal conditions of exposure, the frequency of even minor ill-health is acceptably low. A sufficiently rigorous enforcement system is needed in order to ensure that failures of control which result in higher frequencies of ill-health or more severe ill-health effects do not occur. This type of approach is based on the conventional no effect level and safety factors, leading to such concepts as maximum 'acceptable daily intake' and 'occupational exposure limits' (Royal Society Study Group, 1983). Where carcino-

genic or other stochastic effects are concerned, the approach will be to minimize exposure as far as is reasonably practicable.

Determining Risk Levels

Determination of the risk levels associated with likely release sizes and dispersion patterns is required for overt hazards. There are essentially similar processes for determining risk levels for land-use planning and emergency planning (Health and Safety Executive, 1989a; ECETOC, 1991). The process can be divided into seven steps (Health and Safety Executive, 1989a):

(1) Identification of possible hazardous release events.
(2) Identification and analysis of the failure mechanisms which would allow a release.
(3) Estimation of rates and durations of the release.
(4) Estimation of the frequencies of releases using the analysis of failure mechanisms.
(5) Estimation of the injury consequences of releases, taking account of mitigating factors.
(6) Combination of the frequencies and consequences to determine the overall risk levels.
(7) Judgement of the significance of the risk levels (by comparison with appropriate criteria).

Although this process was described for land-use planning in the vicinity of major industrial hazards in the UK, it can also be used more generally. Essentially, it can be described as three elements—a description of a source, a model for looking at the dispersion of the substance, and a means of entering into the dispersion model parameters describing the conditions which will give a biological effect. Models have been developed for airborne dispersion, dispersion through surface and groundwaters and soils and sediments, and for dispersion through food chains.

The source term for inputting into the dispersion model can be obtained by 'fault tree' analysis of the frequency of events (failure rates), by 'event tree analysis' leading to an estimate of failure rates or by engineering judgement based on historical event frequency. The actual method(s) chosen will depend on the type of release being studied and the available data. The sizes and durations of the postulated/actual releases are also examined (Health and Safety Executive, 1989a). For land-use planning there is a continuum of event frequency and size of release. Usually, sets of release sizes and durations are selected from the continuum and assigned appropriate frequencies. However, for emergency planning the process can be simplified by using the 'severe, but reasonably foreseeable event' as the appropriate basis on which to plan (Baxter et al., 1989a). This event was exemplified as a large hole in or fracture of a liquid chlorine pipe, or of a road tanker delivery coupling at a chlorine installation. Scaling a response up or down should then be possible when an event actually occurs if the plan is sufficiently flexible.

The modelling then required is concerned with the dispersion of the toxic cloud in air or the toxic material through surface or groundwaters or in soils and sediments. Several models for airborne dispersion have been described (see McQuaid, 1989; Brighton *et al.*, 1994). In general, these models require a knowledge of the buoyant density of the cloud under different weather conditions. The dispersal conditions need to be combined with a function describing the combination of exposure concentration and time resulting in a defined frequency of a specified effect. For example, one concentration–time combination may be described as the 'dangerous dose' for land-use planning, while a different combination could be used for the outer boundary for 'discomfort' for emergency planning. When combined with the information on the source, the model is then used to calculate 'isopleths'. These are boundaries of areas within which, at a point time, the concentration–time combination of exposure to the toxic substance would exceed those expected to give the identified biological effect. An overall isopleth envelope can then be calculated for a given set of release conditions by combining the individual isopleths for each time point post-event. Similar approaches can be used for dispersion in river systems and for groundwater dispersion.

The information on the various isopleth envelopes for different types of release and meterological conditions, when combined using a knowledge of the frequencies with which these conditions occur, gives a generalized 'contour' for all source terms and dispersal conditions. This contour is a risk statement for individual risk for a person within the specified boundary. An estimate of societal risk can then be obtained if data on the distribution of people within the geographic area are input.

In view of the complexity of these systems, computer programs have been developed to carry out the calculations associated with the models. The aim of the toxicologist is to find appropriate information on which to base a function describing the concentration – time relationship for a particular biological effect or combination of effects.

Contribution of Human Health Toxicology to Hazard and Risk Assessment

The most likely direct hazards arising from a major accidental release of a toxic substance are the biological consequences of short-term exposure during dispersal of the toxicant. Longer term or delayed effects should be considered in addition to those more immediately apparent. Indirect consequences due to contamination of food or water supplies or to inhalation of dusts following settlement and subsequent disturbance are potentially important, but less immediate problems, and should be amenable to post-event measures aimed at preventing significant exposure.

The Data Available

In theory, at least, the ideal assessment of toxicity of a potential major hazard substance or agent would be based on accurate observations of the appropriate effect in humans. Reliable reports on severe effects in man are, fortunately, few, and mainly as a result of accidental exposure or exposure in wartime. Controversy often surrounds the exposure levels associated with such studies (Withers and Lees, 1987; Marshall, 1989) or the sources of the information (MHAP Toxicology Working Party, 1993). Results from studies on sublethal effects in man may be more plentiful. Nevertheless, the data on most substances are restricted to accidental exposures, often affecting only one or two people and rarely containing accurate exposure information. Except for radioactivity, human evidence concerning long-term effects of single exposures to most agents and substances is virtually non-existent. Further studies which require deliberate exposure of men (or women) to dangerous levels of a substance or agent are unethical.

As a consequence of the limited human data, heavy reliance has to be placed on animal and other experiments in attempting to predict the adverse effects in the human population. Often these animal data are confined to short-term effects (sometimes only lethality) following single exposures. For example, prior to Bhopal, the information available on the toxicity of methyl isocyanate was confined to a single published paper (Kimmerle and Eben, 1964) on short-term effects following acute exposure (Bucher, 1987). Also, many animal studies on the types of substances which might constitute major hazards were performed a long time ago and the data are, by modern standards, of poor quality.

In view of the very variable nature of the toxicity information, it is essential to evaluate this information critically and to understand the uncertainties introduced as a consequence of the nature and quality of the data (Illing, 1989; Marshall, 1989; ECETOC, 1991; Fairhurst and Turner, 1993). This means that assessments will normally be conducted using the original reports or published papers.

As the information may be required for quantitative risk analysis associated with an initiating event, where possible it will need to be described in numerical terms. Uncertainty has to be handled by sensitivity analysis. By inputting various potential values for particular effects into the risk assessments, it is possible to discover the differences that variation of the input parameter will have in terms of outcome, the areas of map covered by the contour envelope related to a particular risk value.

This sensitivity analysis is an essential part of the overall risk assessment

Usually there are few, if any, data on the immunological, carcinogenic or reproductive effects likely after single exposures to major hazard substances/agents. Indirect effects mediated through food chain uptake and bioconcentration, or disturbing settled material also need to be considered. If data are available, they should be evaluated. However, that evaluation will normally be descriptive as, except for the effects of radioactivity, there is currently no satisfactory way of obtaining the data in a form suitable for more quantitative approaches.

Problems of Extrapolation

The difficulties encountered in extrapolating from data in animals in evaluating the hazard to humans are similar whatever the nature of the hazard being examined. The ways in which these extrapolations can be carried out have been described in great detail elsewhere (Tardiff and Rodricks, 1987). Three principal problems—interspecies variation, population heterogeneity (interindividual variation) and route-to-route extrapolation—are particularly relevant when data for major hazard substances are being examined.

Interspecies variation in biological effects is an important area of uncertainty in the evaluation. In the absence of suitable alternatives the 'default option' is to use the most sensitive relevant species, i.e. after excluding those species for which mode of action or other data clearly suggest they are inappropriate models for humans. Toxicokinetic and toxicodynamic relationships between species, together with information on the relevant biochemical parameters in man, can lead to a better understanding of the relevance of results in a particular species for man, but are rarely available

Extrapolation between species is usually based on allometric scaling. As both lung surface area (for absorption) and body weight or body surface area (for effect) can both be scaled allometrically, such scaling is not relevant to inhalation studies.

In addition to interspecies variation, it is necessary to consider interindividual variation and the nature of the population being studied. Animal experiments, particularly those performed in recent years, have been conducted using animals specially bred to limit variations in response, and are usually young, healthy individuals. In many older studies much less closely defined animals were used. The general human population is more heterogeneous still, containing groups of individuals who must be considered 'highly susceptible' because of age, genetic constitution or disease state. These interindividual variations are a factor which adds to the uncertainty when extrapolating from animal studies to effects in man, or when extrapolating from a small sample to a large population.

Occasionally, toxicity data may be used which were obtained for a different route of exposure from that for which they are being assessed (Pepelco and Withey, 1985; Pepelco, 1987). For example, in the absence of sufficient inhalation data it may be possible, in some circumstances, to make use of oral data and to relate them to equivalent inhalation exposures. However, comparisons cannot be made if there are substantial differences in the toxicokinetics for the two routes. Often, effects on the lung are critical. These can be considered local effects, in which case it is not appropriate to extrapolate from oral data. Great caution is required when extrapolating data from studies using different routes of exposure.

Extrapolation of laboratory animal data to other, non-human species, although possible, is only done when there is a specific requirement.

Modelling the Toxicity Information

The best way of relating exposure level, duration and effect for quantitative risk assessment is probably based on toxicokinetic and toxicodynamic modelling, similar to that used for workplace exposure to inhaled gases and vapours. However, appropriate data are not usually available, so other, more pragmatic, approaches are adopted.

A generally available pragmatic approach is based on the need to obtain (1) a concentration–time relationship, usually based on the mid-point (LC_{50} or EC_{50}) of the effect(s) being examined and (2) an appropriate set of exposure conditions that are taken to result in a particular level of effect in the population (ECETOC, 1991; Fairhurst and Turner, 1993).

As the concentration–time (ct) relationships often have to be based on LC_{50} or EC_{50} data for various times (they are frequently the only data available), they normally refer to mid-point concentration, that where the effect is seen in 50% of the population. In general, the values have to be adjusted to yield the boundary between effects (disability with few immediate deaths for 'dangerous dose'; discomfort with few disabled in the case of defining zones where people needing hospital treatment are likely to be located). The dose response may also need to be adjusted to account for differences in the make-up of the populations being examined. It must be emphasized that any boundary will be approximate because of the nature of the data and the models being used.

In the early years of this century, studies on the acute inhalation toxicity for a limited number of gases yielded mortality data suggesting the following relationship:

$$ct = \text{constant} \qquad (3)$$

(Haber, 1924). This is usually known as the Haber rule. More recent observations have suggested a more general relationship:

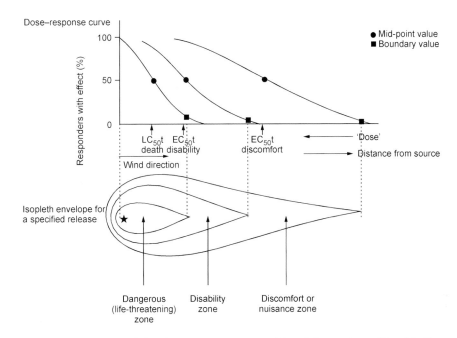

Figure 14 Diagram to illustrate the correlation between response and isopleth envelope. 'Dose' is the combined exposure concentration and duration function for the particular effect. The isopleth envelope described is that bounding the overall combination of concentrations and durations of exposure for a release, and can be built up from a series of isopleths describing the dispersion at different intervals after the start of the release. A combination of isopleth envelopes becomes a risk estimate when it incorporates the frequencies for different source and dispersion conditions.

$$c^n t = \text{constant} \qquad (4)$$

(ten Berg *et al.*, 1985; Klimisch *et al.*, 1987; Marshall, 1989). An alternative form of this equation, which can be used to plot data, is

$$n \log c = \log t + \text{constant} \qquad (5)$$

(this constant is the logarithmic value of the constant in Equation 4). Although a wide range of values for n have been cited, usually the value appears to be close to 1 or 2. Where it is possible, the relationship should be derived from experimental data, ideally from a single series of experiments in the same laboratory and using the same strain of animal. If data are combined from different laboratories and different strains or species, the relationship generated may represent interlaboratory or interspecies (or interstrain) variation, rather than a genuine concentration–time relationship.

Frequently there are insufficient data to verify the relationship and the 'default' value of $n = 1$ is used. It is probably adequate when extrapolating to longer times where it usually overestimates the consequences. However, the Haber rule could seriously underestimate the exposure if data are not available for shorter periods and extrapolation from longer exposure periods is undertaken. Because of underlying assumptions about 'steady-state' toxicokinetics inherent in any of these relationships, they are all likely to be overestimates at very short time intervals (say, less than 5 min) while

equilibration to some form of pseudo-steady state is taking place.

Usually it is also necessary to define the concentration–time combination for a boundary condition rather than for the mid-point value for an effect (**Figure 14**). Ideally this should be obtained from experimental data. Often it has to be derived from the slope of the dose–response curve. If data on the slope are not available, it may be possible to use equation 2 (see above), provided that the effects seen are reasonably similar to those used in deriving the equation, or the general rule of approximately 3.3.

A further reduction in concentration of approximately threefold has been suggested for transfer from a general healthy population to a population containing a high proportion of 'highly susceptible' people (see above). Thus, the slope of the dose–response curve depends on the type of population being studied (see **Figure 15**). In transferring from LC_{50} to an LC representing the boundary death–disability, it is necessary to consider population heterogeneity. The total change from an LC_{50} for a recent study using young, healthy adult inbred rats to the boundary death–disability for an outbred, poorly healthy mixed age and strain population of rats could be an order of magnitude (10-fold) or more. A similar order of magnitude change has been proposed in moving from the criterion of death in a normal human population to 'dangerous dose' for a population containing a large number of 'highly susceptible' people (Health and Safety Executive, 1989a; see above).

As an alternative to the approach to concentration–time relationships outlined above, it is sometimes possible to describe mathematically a line for the boundary conditions of the concentration–time relationship using scatter diagrams, showing all concentrations and times at which the effect occurred (**Figure 16**) (ECETOC, 1991). This approach normally requires access to more

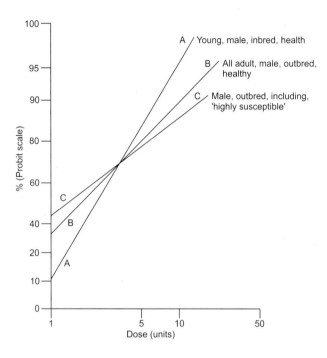

Figure 15 Diagram to illustrate hypothetical dose–response lines for different populations.

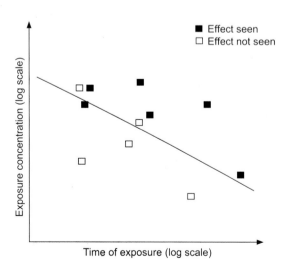

Figure 16 Idealized scatter diagram of hypothetical relationship for an exposure-time–concentration relationship for an effect. By plotting on logarithmic axes, the slope of the boundary line can be used to derive n. In the example shown the slope is $-n$ and $n = 2$.

detailed data, including, ideally, the results for individual animals. It also can suffer from problems relating to population heterogeneity and interspecies and interlaboratory variation.

Additional Points

Whatever information emerges from animal toxicity data must always be compared with any data that are available in the target species (humans). Those from the most sensitive species are normally chosen as representing a conservative approach.

The data are generally used predictively in order to describe the geographic areas where effects may occur or where the risk levels are associated with particular consequences. Best estimates are therefore usually considered preferable to more 'conservative' values based on the more severe confidence limit for the data. How closely defined the geographic areas affected by the risk analysis are when the toxicity data are limited in quality and quantity needs to be checked by uncertainty analysis in which the more extreme toxicity interpretations can be compared with the best estimate. Great accuracy is not required in view of the approximate nature of the overall evaluation.

Outcomes

The requirements from the overall assessment of the toxic risks are different for land-use planning and for emergency planning.

Land-use Planning

The outcome from a quantitative risk analysis is a risk statement based on a series of isopleth envelopes. This statement can be judged against pre-determined criteria to decide whether a risk is acceptable in pre-determined 'objective' terms. The risk assessor can recommend that no objection be raised to the proposed development or that the development should not go ahead. Acceptance by the general population may depend on different, often subjective, criteria. There is a political process associated with land use planning (in the UK, based on the local authority with access to a planning enquiry on behalf of central government) in order to allow expression of the objective and subjective opinions on the development. A decision has to be taken by the local authority councillors or a government minister on behalf of society as a whole.

Emergency Planning

In emergency planning, the aims include delineation of appropriate zones over which to provide public information on the type of hazard and on the protective measures that can be taken to ameliorate the likely damage. They also include delineating ways of tackling the problems likely to emerge post-event, guiding general emergency planning, search and rescue, planning for the medical needs of casualties, including setting permissible exposures for the people involved, planning for the protection of food and drinking water supplies and planning for (when possible) protection of the environment. Emergency planning and management is an important topic in its own right, and the ways in which emergencies are tackled can vary with the circumstances surrounding the site (Institution of Mechanical Engineers, 1995). For example, the management of an emergency on an oil rig will differ from that for a land-based chemical plant or nuclear reactor. The type of medical planning is also important and is discussed in greater detail elsewhere (Baxter *et al.*, 1989a; Murray, 1990; OECD, 1994).

CONCLUSION

Disasters can be caused when large amounts of toxicants interact with a (human) population and cause deleterious effects on that population. They can occur in many forms; some result from natural causes and many from man's efforts. Describing and understanding past disasters can be the first stage to preventing or ameliorating the effects of potential future disasters.

In general, sites which contain toxicants causing them to be classified as major hazards are so classified because of the amount of toxicant present, and also because of the toxicity of the substance. Unfortunately, both the evidence concerning the toxicity of many of these toxicants and the processes for managing the hazards and risks they pose are limited. Further work is needed to develop a proper database and good procedures on which to take decisions.

REFERENCES

Air Accidents Investigation Branch, Department of Transport (1989). *Report on the Accident to Boeing 737–236 Series 1, G-BGJL at Manchester International Airport on 22 August 1985*. Aircraft Accident Report 8/88. HMSO, London.

Aldridge, W. N. (1985). Toxic oil syndrome. *Hum. Toxicol.*, **4**, 231–235.

Aldridge, W. N. (1987). Toxic disasters with food contaminants. In Chambers, P. L. (Ed.), *Attitudes to Toxicology in the European Economic Community*. Wiley, Chichester.

Andersson, N. (1989). Long-term effects of methyl isocyanate. *Lancet*, **i**, 1259.

Andersson, N., Kerr Muir, M., Mehra, V. and Salmon, A. G. (1988). Exposure and response to methyl isocyanate: results of a community based survey in Bhopal. *Br. J. Ind. Med.*, **45**, 469–475.

Baxter, P. J., Ing, R., Falk, H. *et al.* (1981). Mount St. Helens eruptions, May 18 to June 12, 1980. An overview of the acute health impact. *J. Am. Med. Assoc.*, **246**, 2585–2589.

Baxter, P. J., Ing, R., Falk, H. and Plikaytas, B. (1983). Mount St. Helens eruptions: the acute respiratory effects of volcanic ash in a North American community. *Arch. Environ. Health*, **38**, 138–143.

Baxter, P. J., Davies, P. C. and Murray, V. (1989a). Medical planning for toxic releases into the community: the example of chlorine gas. *Br. J. Ind. Med.*, **46**, 277–285.

Baxter, P. J., Kapila, M. and Mfonfu, D. (1989b). Lake Nyos disaster, Cameroon, 1986: the medical effects of large scale emission of carbon dioxide. *Br. Med. J.*, **298**, 1437–1441.

Bertazzi, P. A. (1989). Industrial disasters and epidemiology. A review of recent experiences. *Scand. J. Work Environ. Health*, **15**, 85–100.

Bertazzi, P. A. (1991). Long term effects of chemical disasters. Lessons and results from Seveso. *Sci. Total Environ.*, **106**, 5–20.

Bertazzi, P. A., Zocchetti, C., Pesatori, A. C. *et al.* (1989). Ten year mortality study of the population involved in the Seveso incident in 1976. *Am J. Epidemiol.*, **129**, 1187–1200.

Bertazzi, P. A., Pesatori, A. C., Consonni, D. *et al.* (1993). Cancer incidence in a population accidentally exposed to 2,3,7,8-Tetrachlorodibenzo-*para*-dioxin. *Epidemiology*, **4**, 398–406.

Brighton, P. W. M., Byrne, A. J., Cleaver, P. R. *et al.* (1994). Comparison of heavy gas dispersion models for instantaneous releases. *J. Hazard. Mater.*, **36**, 193–208.

Bucher, J. R. (1987). Methyl isocyanate: a review of health effects research since Bhopal. *Fundam. Appl. Toxicol.*, **9**, 367–379.

Buist, A. S. and Bernstein, R. S. (Eds) (1986). Health effects of volcanos: an approach to evaluating the health effects of an environmental hazard. *Am. J. Publ. Health*, **76**, Suppl.

Calman, K. (1996). Cancer; Science and society and the communication of risk. *Br. Med. J.*, **313**, 799–802.

Committee on Fire Toxicology (1986). *Fire and Smoke: Understanding the Hazards*. National Academy Press, Washington, DC.

Department of the Environment (1991). *Interpretation of Major Accident to the Environment for the Purposes of the CIMAH Regulations*. Department of the Environment (Toxic Substances Division), London.

Department of the Environment (1995). *A Guide to Risk Assessment and Risk Management for Environmental Protection*. HMSO, London.

Duffus, J. H. (1993). Glossary for chemists of terms used in toxicology. (IUPAC Recommendations 1993). *Pure Appl. Chem.*, **65**, 2003–2122.

ECETOC (1991). *Emergency Exposure Indices for Industrial Chemicals. Technical Report No. 43*. European Chemical Industry Ecology and Toxicology Centre, Brussels.

Fairhurst, S. and Turner, R. M. (1993). Toxicological assessments in relation to major hazards. *J. Hazard. Mater.*, **33**, 215–227.

Fennel, D. (1988). *Investigation into the King's Cross Underground Fire*. HMSO, London.

Franks, A. P., Harpur, P. J. and Bilo, M. (1996). The relationship between risk of death and risk of dangerous dose for toxic substances. *J. Hazard. Mater.*, **51**, 11–34.

Freeth, S. J. and Kay, R. L. J. (1987). The Lake Nyos gas disaster. *Nature*, **325**, 104–105.

Golding, J., Rowland, A., Greenwood, R. and Lunt, P. (1991). Aluminium sulphate in water in North Cornwall and outcome of pregnancy. *Br. Med. J.*, **302**, 1175–1177.

Haber, F. (1924). *Funf Vortrage aus den Jahren 1920–1923*. Springer, Berlin.

Health and Safety Executive (1985). *The Brightside Lane Warehouse Fire*. HMSO, London.

Health and Safety Executive (1988a). *The Tolerability of Risk From Nuclear Power Stations*. HMSO, London.

Health and Safety Executive (1988b). *Comments Received on the Tolerability of Risk from Nuclear Power Stations*. HMSO, London.

Health and Safety Executive (1989a). *Risk Criteria for Land Use Planning in the Vicinity of Major Industrial Hazards*. HMSO, London.

Health and Safety Executive (1989b). *Quantified Risk Assessment: Its Input to Decision Making*. HMSO, London.

Health and Safety Executive (1992). *The Tolerability of Risk from Nuclear Power Stations*, 2nd edn. HMSO, London.

Health and Safety Executive. (1999). TOR Update.

Henderson, M. (1987). *Living with Risk: The British Medical Association Guide*. Wiley, Chichester, pp. 115–118.

Holden, C. (1980). Love Canal residents under stress. *Science*, **208**, 1242–1244.

Home Office (1994). *Dealing with Disasters*, 2nd edn. HMSO, London.

Illing, H. P. A. (1989). Assessment of toxicology for major hazards: some concepts and problems. *Hum. Toxicol.*, **8**, 369–374.

Illing, H. P. A. (1991). Possible risk considerations for toxic risk assessment. *Hum. Exp. Toxicol.*, **10**, 215–219.

Institution of Chemical Engineers Working Party (1985). *Nomenclature for Hazard and Risk Assessments in the Process Industries*. Institution of Chemical Engineers, Rugby.

Institution of Mechanical Engineers (1995). *Emergency Planning and Management*. Mechanical Engineering Publications, London.

Janerich, D. T., Burnett, W. S., Freck, W. *et al.* (1981). Cancer incidence in the Love Canal area. *Science*, **212**, 1404–1407.

Jashemski, W. P. (1979). Pompeii and Mount Vesuvius. In Sheets, P. D. and Grayson, D. K. (Eds), *Volcanic Activity and Human Ecology*. Academic Press, New York, pp. 587–622.

Jones, D. (1992), *Nomenclature for Hazard and Risk Assessment in the Process Industries*, 2nd edn. Institution of Chemical Engineers, Rugby.

Kimmerle, G. and Eben, A. (1964). Zur Toxicität von Methylisocyanat und desen quantitative Bestimmung in der Luft. *Arch. Toxicol.*, **20**, 235–241.

Klimisch, H. J., Bretz, R., Doe, J. E. and Purser, D. A. (1987). Classification of dangerous substances in the European Economic Community: a proposed revision of criteria for inhalation toxicity. *Regul. Toxicol. Pharmacol.*, **7**, 21–34.

Kling, G. W., Clark, M. A., Compton, H. R. *et al.* (1987). The 1986 Lake Nyos gas disaster in Cameroon, West Africa. *Science*, **236**, 169–174.

Kopelman, H., Robertson, M. H., Sanders, P. G. and Ash, I. (1966a). The Epping Jaundice. *Br. Med. J.*, **1**, 514–516.

Kopelman, H., Scheuer, P. J. and Williams, R. (1966b). The liver lesion of the Epping Jaundice. *Q. J. Med.*, **35**, 553–564.

Lees, F. P. (1996). *Loss Prevention in the Process Industries*. 2nd Edn. Butterworths Heinemann, London.

Likhtarev, I. A. Sobole, B. G., Kairo, I. A. *et al.* (1995). Thyroid cancer in the Ukraine. *Nature*, **375**, 365.

Lovell, D. P. (1986). Risk assessment—general principles. In Richardson, M. L. (Ed.), *Toxic Hazard Assessment of Chemicals*. Royal Society of Chemistry, London, pp. 207–222.

Lowermoor Incident Health Advisory Group (1989). *Water Pollution at Lowermoor, North Cornwall*. Cornwall and Isles of Scilly Health Authority, Truro.

Lowermoor Incident Health Advisory Group (1991). *Water Pollution at Lowermoor, North Cornwall. Second Report*. HMSO, London.

McQuaid, J. (1989). Dispersion of chemicals. In Bourdeau, P. and Green, G. (Eds), *Methods for Assessing and Reducing Injury from Chemical Accidents*. Wiley, Chichester, pp. 157–187.

Marshall, V. (1989). Prediction of human mortality from chemical accidents with special reference to the lethality of chlorine. *J. Hazard. Mater.*, **22**, 13–56.

Marshall, V. C. (1987). *Major Chemical Hazards*. Ellis Horwood, Chichester.

Masuda, N., Takatsu, M. Morinari, H., Ozawa, T. (1995). Sarin poisoning in Tokyo subway. *Lancet*, **345**, 1446.

MHAP Toxicology Working Party (1993). *Phosgene Toxicity*. Institution of Chemical Engineers, Rugby.

Morgan, J. P. (1982). The Jamaica ginger paralysis. *J. Am. Med. Assoc.*, **248**, 1864–1867.

Murray, V. (1990). *Major Chemical Disasters: Medical Aspects of Management*. International Congress and Symposium Series, No. 155. Royal Society of Medicine Services, London.

Newhall, C. G. and Fruchter, J. S. (1986). Volcanic activity: a review for health professionals. *Am. J. Publ. Health*, **76**, Suppl., 10–24.

Nozaki, H. and Aikawa, H. (1995). Sarin poisoning in Tokyo subway. *Lancet*, **345**, 1446–1447.

Nozaki, H., Aikawa, N., Shinozawa, Y., *et al.* (1995). Sarin. poisoning in Tokyo subway. *Lancet*, **345**, 980–981.

OECD (1994). *Health Aspects of Chemical Accidents. OECD Environmental Monograph, No. 81*. OECD, Paris.

Orsini, B. (1977). *Parliamentary Commission of Enquiry on the Escape of Toxic Substances on 10 July 1976 at the ICMESA Establishment and the Consequent Potential Dangers to Health and the Environment Due to Industrial Activity. Final Report*. English Translation. Health and Safety Executive, London.

Owen, P. J. and Miles, D. P. B. (1995). A review of hospital discharge rates in a population around Camelford in North Cornwall up to the fifth anniversary of an episode of aluminium sulphate absorption. *J. Publ. Health Med.*, **17**, 200–204.

Pepelco, W. E. (1987). Feasability of route extrapolation in risk assessment. *Br. J. Ind. Med.*, **44**, 649–657.

Pepelco, W. E. and Withey, J. R. (1985). Methods for route to route extrapolation. *Toxicol. Ind. Health*, **1**, 153–170.

Presidential/Congressional Commission on Risk Assessment and Risk Management. (1997). Framework for environmental risk assessment; final report. Washington, DC.

Radice, B. (translator) (1969). *Letters of the Younger Pliny*. Penguin Books, Harmondsworth.

Ritchie, W. and O'Sullivan, M. (1994). *The Environmental Impact of the Wreck of the Braer*. Scottish Office, Edinburgh.

Royal Commission on Environmental Pollution. (1998). Setting environmental standards. Twenty first report. Stationery Office, London.

Royal Society Study Group (1983). *Risk Assessment*. Royal Society, London.

Royal Society Study Group (1992). *Risk: Analysis Perception and Management*. Royal Society, London.

Sali, D., Cordis, E., Stanyik, L., *et al.* (1996). Cancer consequences after Chernobyl accident in Europe outside the former USSR: a review. *Int. J. Cancer*, **67**, 343–352.

Schoental, R. (1968). Carcinogenic and chronic effects of 4,4′–diaminodiphenylmethane. *Nature*, **219**, 1162–1163.

Schwartz, D. A. (1987). Acute inhalation injury. In Rosenstock, L. (Ed.), *Occupational Medicine: State of the Art Reviews—Lung Disease*. Hanley and Belfus, Philadelphia, pp. 297–318.

Sheets, P. D. and Grayson, D. K. (1979). *Volcanic Activity and Human Ecology*. Academic Press, New York.

Sigurdsson, H., Carey, S., Cornell, W. and Pescatore, T. (1985). The eruption of Vesuvius in AD 79. *Natl. Geogr. Res.*, **1**, 332–387.

Silkworth, J. B., McMartin, D. N., Rej, R. *et al.* (1984). Subchronic exposure of mice to Love Canal soil extracts. *Fundam. Appl. Toxicol.*, **4**, 231–239.

Silkworth, J. B., Tsumasonis, C., Briggs, R. G. *et al.* (1986). The effects of Love Canal soil extracts on maternal health and fetal development in rats. *Fundam. Appl. Toxicol.*, **7**, 471–485.

Silkworth, J. B., Cutler, D. S. Antrim, L. *et al.* (1989a). Teratology of 2,3,7,8-tetrachlorobenzo-*p*-dioxin in a complex environmental mixture from Love Canal. *Fundam. Appl. Toxicol.*, **13**, 1–15.

Silkworth, J. B., Cutler, D. S. and Sack, G. (1989b). Immunotoxicity of 2,3,7,8-tetrachlorodibenzo-*p*-dioxin in a complex environmental mixture from the Love Canal. *Fundam. Appl. Toxicol.*, **12**, 302–312.

Skene, S. A., Dewhurst, I. C. and Greenberg, M. (1989). Polychlorinated dibenzo-*p*-dioxins and polychlorodibenzofurans: the risks to human health. A review. *Hum. Toxicol.*, **8**, 173–203.

Smith, M. I. (1930). The pharmacological action of certain phenol esters, with special reference to the etiology of so-called ginger paralysis. *Pub. Health Rep.*, **45**, 2509–2524.

Smith, M. I. and Elvove, E. (1930). Pharmacological and chemical studies on the cause of so-called ginger paralysis. *Pub. Health Rep.*, **45**, 1703–1716.

Smith, S. (1986). Assessing the ecological and health effects of pollution. In Hester, R. E. (Ed.), *Understanding Our Environment*. Royal Society of Chemistry, London, pp. 226–290.

Smullen, I. (1989). Bread and bones. *Country Life*, **183**, 237.

Stsjazhko, V. A., Tsyb, A. F., Tronko, N. D., *et al.* (1995). Childhood cancers since the accident at Chernobyl. *Br. Med. J.*, **310**, 801.

Suzuki, T., Monita, H., Ono, K., *et al.* (1995). Sarin poisoning in Tokyo subway. *Lancet*, **345**, 980.

Tardiff, R. G. and Rodricks, J. V. (Eds) (1987). *Toxic Substances and Human Risk: Principles of Data Interpretation*. Plenum Press, New York.

ten Berg, W. F., Zwart, A. and Appelman, L. M. (1985). Concentration mortality response relationship for irritant and systemically acting gases and vapours. *J. Hazard. Mater.*, **13**, 301–309.

Topping, G., Davies, J. M., Mackies, P. R. and Moffat, C. F. (1997). The impact of the Braer spill on commercial fish and shellfish. In *The Impact of an Oil Spill in Turbulent Waters. The Braer*. Scottish Office, Edinburgh, pp. 121–143.

Tsubaki, T. and Irukayama, K. (1977). *Minimata Disease*. Kodansha/Elsevier, Tokyo.

Versteeg, M. F. (1988). External safety policy in the Netherlands: an approach to risk management. *J. Hazard. Mater.*, **17**, 215–222.

Vianna, N. J. and Polan, A. K. (1984). Incidence of low birth weight among Love Canal residents. *Science*, **226**, 1217–1219.

Wells, G. (1997). Major hazards and their management. Institution of Chemical Engineers, Rugby.

Whittle, K. J., Anderson, D. A., Mackie, P. R. *et al.* (1997). The impact of the Braer oil on caged salmon. In *The Impact of an Oil spill in Turbulent Waters. The Braer*. Scottish Office, Edinburgh, pp. 144–160.

Withers, R. M. J. and Lees, F. P. (1987). The assessment of major hazards: the lethal toxicity of chlorine. Part 3. C Doss checks. *J. Hazard. Mater.*, 15, 301–342.

World Health Organization (1976). Conference on intoxication due to alkyl-mercury treated seed. *Bull. World Health Org.*, **53**, Suppl.

World Health Organization (1984). *Toxic Oil Syndrome*. Report of WHO Meeting, Madrid, 21–25 March 1983. World Health Organization, Copenhagen.

Chapter 84
Biomarkers—An Overview

Catherine J. Waterfield and John A. Timbrell

C O N T E N T S

INTRODUCTION

Biological markers, or 'biomarkers', are both as old as Hippocrates, who diagnosed disease based on the colour of urine, and as new as the most recent advances in molecular biology (Goldstein, 1996). As with any scientific tool, it is common to define what the tool is and how it can be used. *Chambers English Dictionary* defines a marker as '. . . a memorial tablet (US); a tool for marking a position; a device for scoring'. This explains the current use of the word 'biomarker' in the context of living systems very well. Thus the field of 'biomarkers' aims to identify and validate markers in biological systems with (a) a sufficiently long half-life which will (b) locate *where* in a living system a change has been brought about and then (c) to *quantify* that change. Historically, the field has been concerned with the diagnosis of pre-existing conditions or disease states. However, a biomarker may also be predictive of disease, indicate the likely risk of disease, identify disease states and track the progress of the disease.

As our knowledge of mechanisms of toxicity increased, early diagnosis became more accessible and therefore more important. History has also taught us to be more aware of the hazards involved with exposure to foreign compounds with even very low levels of some compounds resulting in adverse effects, such as oestrogenic effects (e.g. DDT) (Fairbrother, 1994). This has prompted an interest in biomarkers of exposure and susceptibility as more compounds are released into the environment, increasing the risks of adverse effects to environmental pollutants and chemicals in combinations. It has also driven the development of analytical methods, including molecular biology, to greater levels of sensitivity and new methodologies for the detection of potential biomarkers. 'Ultimately they should serve to increase the cost-effectiveness of epidemiological studies, in the sense that, as a result of their use, more information is gained per unit cost' (Toniolo *et al.*, 1997a). Here we can include both time and the survival of the individual as 'costs'.

PRESENT STATUS OF BIOMARKERS

Today, most research into biomarkers is concerned with markers which will increase our ability to identify

- The long-term risks due to toxicant exposure, in particular to the risk of developing cancer; and
- Identify early markers of toxicity in the field of environmental or ecotoxicology (see McCarthy and Shugart, 1990; Huggett *et al.*, 1992; Peakall, 1992; Toniolo *et al.*, 1997b).

For the past 25 years, biomarkers have been used to identify biological changes due to toxic chemicals and, as part of an integrated approach, in the assessment of environmental health. In the future, many more biological markers predictive of long-term effects, such as chromosomal changes and DNA adducts, will be available, allowing risk assessment judgements to be made. In ecotoxicology, the techniques in biomonitoring populations have progressed from examining the exposure of sentinel species and population changes as biomarkers of pollution to include more specific markers of the health of individuals. The ultimate aim is to identify problems as early as possible, thus avoiding adverse effects on whole populations and communities. It is possible to identify biomarkers at all levels of biological organization (Fossi *et al.*, 1994) **(Figure 1)**, extending from the molecular or biochemical level to the physiology of the individual

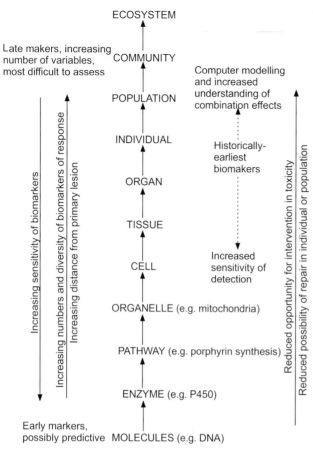

Figure 1 Biomarkers can be identified at all levels of biological organization. As systems become more complex, it becomes more difficult to relate biological changes to toxic effects at the primary target such as individual molecules. Adapted from Stegeman *et al.*, (1992) and Fossi *et al.*, (1994).

and ultimately to the level of populations. A goal in the use of biomarkers must be to identify adverse effects of chemical contaminants at the lowest level of biological organization, so avoiding toxicological problems at a later stage, which are both more difficult to identify and to correct. There is also a strong lobby in this field for selecting non-destructive biomarkers wherever possible (Fossi *et al.*, 1994; Timbrell *et al.*, 1994). In clinical situations there is also a drive to find totally non-invasive biomarkers.

DEFINING A BIOMARKER

A potential biomarker is any change which occurs in response to 'stressors' such as xenobiotics, disease states and physical changes in the environment, including alterations in temperature and salinity, which extend the adaptive responses of an organism beyond the normal range (Mayer *et al.*, 1992). The biomarkers of these responses or effects are likely to be as varied as the stressors themselves. Thus, it may be a measurable adap-

tive response such as the induction of 'heatshock' proteins triggered in response to raised temperatures (Burdon, 1986; Schlesinger, 1990) or a reduction in fecundity due to species overcrowding or environmental pollutants (Depledge, 1994; Depledge and Hopkin, 1995), or it could be the formation of a specific DNA adduct which provides specific information about the exposure of the organism to a chemical in the environment (Prevost *et al.*, 1996; Dubois *et al.*, 1997; Wild and Pisani, 1997). The use of DNA adducts as very sensitive biomarkers of 'effective dose' (unaccompanied by immediate, measurable effects in adaptive responses) requires that the original definition of a biomarker needs to be extended.

Ideally, biomarkers should be accessible (non-invasive), non-destructive and easy and cheap to measure.

The different types of biomarkers have been categorized by scientific bodies such as the US National Academy of Sciences Committee on Biological Markers (National Research Council, 1989) as

- Biomarkers of exposure;
- Biomarkers of response or effect; and
- Biomarkers of susceptibility.

These are the generally accepted categories by workers in the field (Timbrell *et al.*, 1994).

Figure 2 illustrates some possible biomarkers in an individual exposed to a chemical. If the compound is hepatotoxic as a result of metabolism to a reactive metabolite in the liver, there are various 'points' in the pathway, from the parent compound entering the body to the point where a pathological lesion can be identified and where biomarkers could provide valuable information about the exposure and effect of that toxin. The pathway will be modified by many variables such as the absorption, distribution and excretion of the compound and the metabolites as well as inter-individual differences in the susceptibility (i.e. metabolic capacity).

Monitoring the toxic effects of a paracetamol overdose can be used as an example of the use of various biomarkers. The following numbered points refer to those in **Figure 2**.

(1) Paracetamol.
(2) Measurement of the parent compound (*biomarker of exposure*).
(3) Metabolism of the parent compound to the reactive metabolite, *N*-acetyl-*p*-benzoquinone imine (NAPQI) by cytochrome P450 (CYP2E1, CYP3A4 and CYP1A2). NAPQI can react with glutathione to form a conjugate or be reduced back to paracetamol by GSH, both resulting in the removal of NAPQI. The levels of cytochrome P450 will determine the degree of metabolism to the toxic metabolite, and the amount of GSH present will determine the ability of the liver to detoxify the reactive metabolite. In this

BIOMARKERS

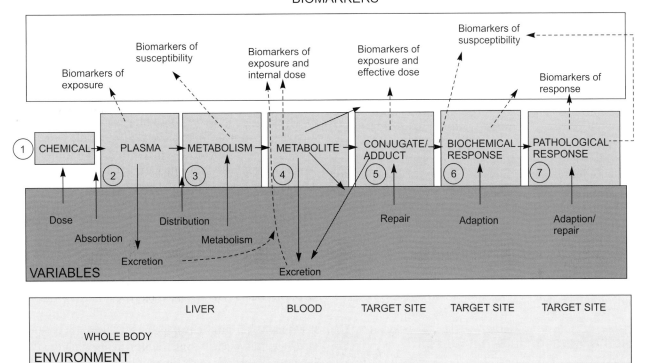

Figure 2 Identification of potential biomarkers in an individual exposed to a hepatotoxic compound. A number of variables must also be taken into account when biomarkers are measured. The compound paracetamol is used as an example of how various biomarkers could be used to determine the dose ingested and the extent of hepatotoxicity in a patient following an 'overdose'. For an explanation, see text; the numbered points in the text refer to the numbers on the diagram.

way *levels* of P450 and GSH are acting as *biomarkers of susceptibility*.

(4) The GSH metabolite of NAPQI (a mercapturic acid) can be measured in both the plasma and urine and is therefore a *biomarker of exposure*. The degree of conjugation with GSH could indicate the amount of GSH available, and thus act as another *biomarker of susceptibility*.

(5) The toxicity of paracetamol results from the alkylation of proteins by NAPQI, resulting in the formation of protein adducts which can be measured in the urine and plasma. As these are formed at the target site, their presence can be used as *biomarkers of both exposure and effective dose*.

(6) As a result of the paracetamol exposure various biochemical adaptations/responses will be initiated. These will include the initial depletion of GSH followed by a rebound in synthesis, an inhibition of protein synthesis (reducing both albumin and total protein in the serum) and reduced glyceraldehyde-3-phosphate dehydrogenase activity. These biochemical changes can be regarded as *biomarkers of response*.

(7) As a result of the alkylation of proteins, ion flux is impaired and water balance in cells is difficult to maintain, resulting in the hydropic degeneration of hepatocytes followed by necrosis. Depending on the

severity of the lesion, the presence of liver enzymes in the serum will be increased in addition to bile acids and bilirubin, and there may also be evidence of inflammation and repair as neutrophils and macrophages infiltrate the tissues. These pathological responses can be considered as *biomarkers of response*.

In many cases there is a continuum between biomarkers of exposure and effect. For example; the formation of carboxyhaemoglobin after exposure to carbon monoxide is the *effect* of that exposure, and the *amount* of carboxyhaemoglobin formed or breath carbon monoxide (which is in equilibrium with carboxyhaemoglobin) are directly related to the *exposure* (Goldstein, 1996). Similarly, a biomarker which could be classed as a biomarker of effect resulting from the direct chemical interaction between a cellular molecule such as DNA could also be considered to be a biomarker of exposure. However, most biomarkers will reflect primarily the exposure or the effect of that exposure. For example, the elevation of serum bilirubin is indicative of poor bile flow (cholestasis), which could be due to liver damage as a result of exposure to any one of a number of hepatotoxic compounds or the physical obstruction of bile flow by a gall stone, but it does not tell us which the culprit is (Zimmerman, 1978; Vore, 1991; Woodman, 1996).

BIOMARKERS OF EXPOSURE

Biomarkers of exposure can be divided into markers of

- Internal dose and
- Effective dose

(van Welie *et al.*, 1992; Coggon and Friesen, 1997; Timbrell, 1998). The former gives an indication of the occurrence and extent of exposure of the organism and thus the likely concentration of a parent compound or metabolite at the target site. The latter is an indication of the true extent of the exposure of what is believed to be the target molecule, structure or cell. Both markers of internal and effective dose are therefore preferable to measuring external levels of the compound in question, for example in the workplace, as they take into account the biological variations in absorption, metabolism and distribution of the compound in an individual.

Biomarkers of Internal Dose

Biomarkers of internal dose have been particularly useful in establishing the dose of a compound which has been absorbed in ecological studies, and in human studies when they provide information about long-term carcinogen exposure. Generally, they reflect recent exposure, although the half-life of the compound must be taken into account. For example, a useful marker in industrial settings is urinary methylhippuric acid (Inoue *et al.*, 1993; Huang *et al.*, 1994). This has a half-life of a few hours and is a biomarker of recent exposure to xylene. On the other hand, urinary cadmium, which is related to body burden, is a useful long-term biomarker of exposure to cadmium as it has an excretion half-life of more than 10 years (Ghezzi *et al.*, 1985). For practical reasons, the source of these biomarkers needs to be easily accessible, ideally present in urine, breath or possibly a blood sample. However, when a compound is accumulated in a particular tissue, as in the accumulation of DDT in adipose tissue, obtaining a tissue sample for analysis is more difficult. In this particular case the blood levels of the DDT metabolite DDE can be used to assess long-term exposure (Aguilar and Borrell, 1994). The accumulation of lead in bone and teeth is a measure of lead exposure. In this case, X-ray analysis can give information both about acute and chronic exposure (Goyer, 1986).

Biomarkers of Effective Dose

Chemicals can bind covalently to cellular macromolecules such as nucleic acids and proteins which may be the target molecule for that compound. These are called adducts' and can be measured in tissues or body fluids (van Welie *et al.*, 1992). The adduct may be specific for a particular carcinogen and can be used as a marker of effective dose since it has interacted with the target site. Owing to many inter-individual differences in the rate and route of the metabolism of a compound, and also the accessibility of the target, any measurement of the internal dose and effective dose will be different. Hence the effective dose at the target site is the preferred measurement to internal dose **(Figure 3)**.

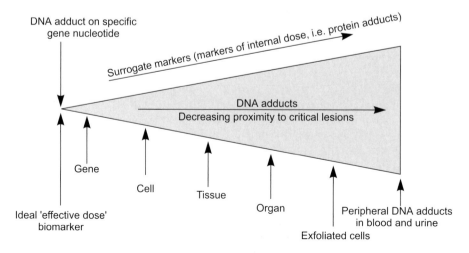

Figure 3 Measurement of DNA–carcinogen and protein–carcinogen adducts as markers of 'internal dose'. These can be measured in DNA or other tissues if there is insufficient material for analysis. The further the source is from the critical lesion, the more the extrapolation to the effective dose needs to be validated. Adapted from Wild and Pisani (1997).

Selective Adducts

If adducts are formed between the chemical and the target molecule, it is a clear indication that there has been exposure of that target. In this respect, reactive chemicals or metabolites which react with DNA are of particular interest and concern in relation to genotoxicity and therefore possible carcinogenicity (Shugart, 1994a, b; Shugart et al., 1992, Wild and Pisani, 1997). For example, protein and DNA adducts in blood are used as biomarkers of exposure to reactive alkylating agents such as the widely used industrial chemical styrene (Hemminki, 1997). These protein adducts are sometimes referred to as 'surrogate' markers of effective dose. DNA adducts, such as styrene oxide–O^6-guanine, have been detected in white blood cells of exposed workers and adducts such as N-(2-hydroxyethyl)valine have been detected in haemoglobin from hospital workers exposed to ethylene oxide (van Wylie et al., 1992). It is also possible to detect fragments of DNA adducts such as N^7-guanyl-aflatoxin B_1 in urine (Martin and Garner, 1977; Ross et al., 1992). These are a measure of effective dose of the carcinogen aflatoxin B_1, which can be found in the diet (Groopman et al., 1993).

Unfortunately, the amount of DNA available for analysis may be limited. However, protein adducts such as those associated with haemoglobin or albumin are normally more accessible and can give some idea of the duration of exposure as haemoglobin has a half-life of around 120 days and albumin around 20 days. Haemoglobin adducts have been used to investigate exposure of experimental animals to herbicides such as propanil (Maclure et al., 1996) and industrial workers to hexahydrophthalic anhydride (Jönsson et al., 1997). The disappearance of the adduct 4-aminobiphenyl–Hb in smokers who had stopped smoking has also been measured (Maclure et al., 1990). Paracetamol results in the formation of specific cellular protein adducts which can be detected in serum as a result of paracetamol-induced liver damage, the levels of which correlate well with the degree of liver damage (Roberts et al., 1991). Thus the internal exposure level can be measured and the effect predicted (**Figures 2 and 3**).

These DNA and protein adducts are therefore 'selective' or specific as they mark a specific exposure.

Aselective Adducts

There are 'aselective' biomarkers of DNA damage which indicate that covalent binding has taken place between DNA and another compound, but give no information about the structure of the adduct (van Welie et al., 1992). These include the ^{32}P-postlabelling assay, which is a widely used aselective biomarker for DNA adducts (Gupta and Randerath, 1988; Randerath et al., 1988) (**Figure 4**). The process requires the isolation of DNA and the enzymatic hydrolysis to 3′-monophosphates of both normal DNA nucleotides and adducts, which are subsequently separated. The nucleotides are then radiolabelled with ^{32}P at the 5′-position of the mononucleotide and the adducts and normal nucleotides are separated by chromatography. It is also possible to identify the products of oxidative DNA breakdown in urine such as 8-hydroxy-2′-deoxyguanosine and 5-hydroxymethyluracil, which have been proposed as general biomarkers of oxidative stress. However, the background DNA damage measured by this technique would appear to be higher than expected, probably owing to the oxidation of guanine during isolation, storage or hydrolysis of DNA when samples are prepared for HPLC. A more general marker of DNA damage is the detection of DNA strand breaks which are caused either directly or indirectly by toxic chemicals or by processing structural damage. The alkaline unwinding assay can estimate the increase in the level of breaks above the background resulting from exposure to environmental pollutants. DNA strand breaks can also be identified using gel electrophoresis applied to single cells using the 'comet assay'. The results suggest a lower detection rate for DNA strand breaks than HPLC measurement of oxidized bases, which is probably due to the simpler procedure involved (Collins et al., 1996).

The advantage of 'aselective' biomarkers of effective dose is that the structure of the potential toxicant does not have to be known. These also illustrate the overlap between biomarkers of exposure and effect as the toxicant in these cases is interacting and damaging the target molecule (**Table 1**).

BIOMARKERS OF EFFECT OR RESPONSE

Historically and in practical terms these biomarkers are those which have been used most widely and routinely. They can be grouped into different categories. Hence those markers which are the result of pathological damage could be considered separately from markers which indicate a metabolic lesion. Clinical or behavioural observations could also be considered as a separate type of biomarker. A metabolic lesion may or may not be the result of altered pathology; indeed, it may predict or precipitate a pathological lesion, making them potential 'early warning' markers such as elevated blood glucose levels in diabetic patients.

There is also growing interest in the use and identification of 'non-invasive biomarkers' (Fossi and Leonzio, 1994; Timbrell et al., 1994) rather than 'invasive biomarkers'. These allow more routine sampling in human studies and may overcome ethical issues, for example in screening children or monitoring endangered species. Thus biomarkers identified in urine, breath or saliva are potentially more useful than those measured in blood. Some examples of these are illustrated in **Table 1**.

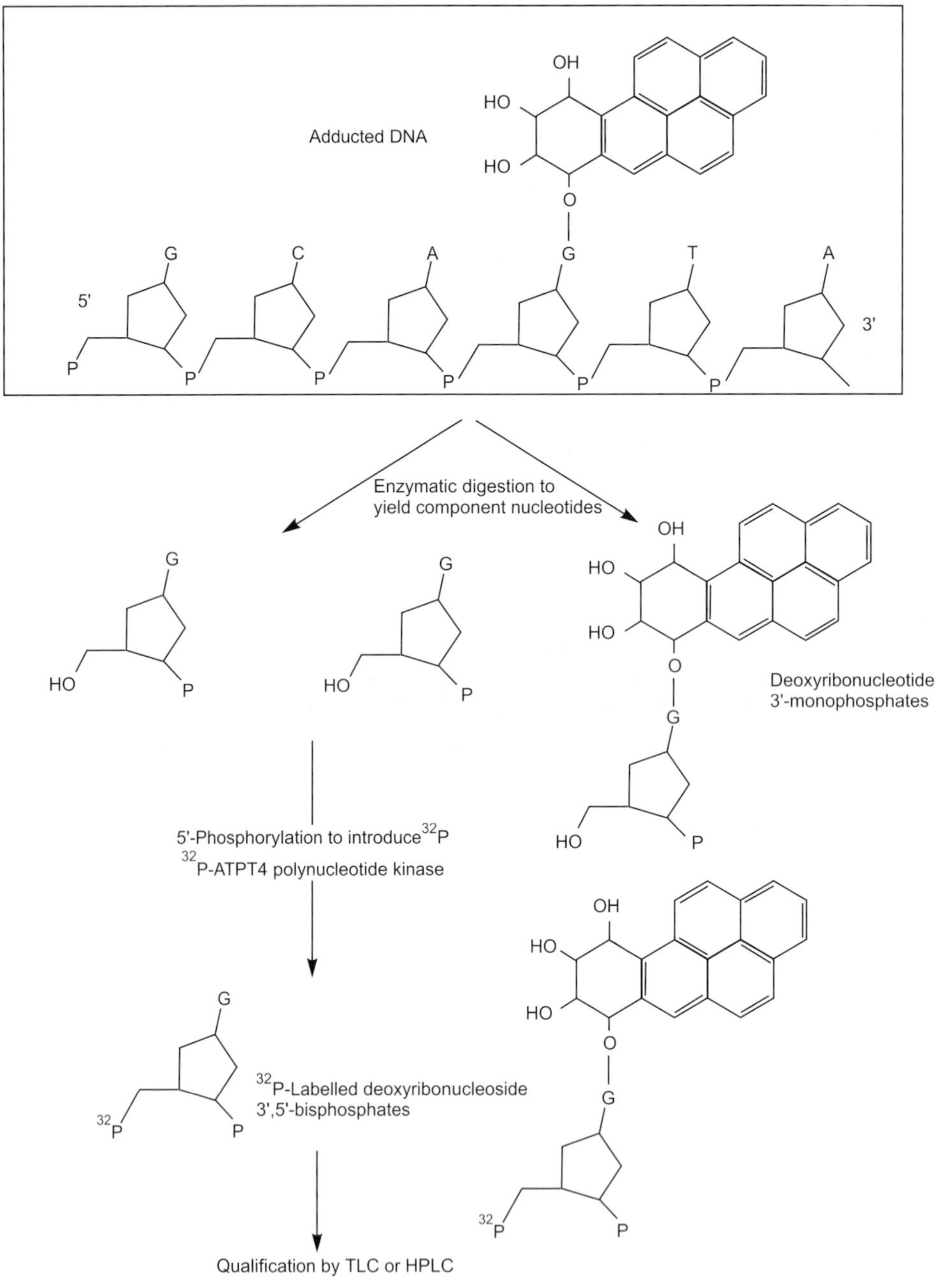

Figure 4 Schematic representation of the ^{32}P- postlabelling assay. TLC, thin-layer chromatography; HPLC, high-performance liquid chromatography.

Behaviour and Clinical Biomarkers

Some of the simplest biomarkers can be very important tools in biomonitoring (sometimes termed 'gross indices') as they may indicate more subtle or complex changes taking place in response to external stressors (Mayer *et al.*, 1992). Thus, monitoring changes in body weight, urinary output, food consumption and general behaviour or fecundity and population size may signify a change in the biochemistry or pathology of individual animals. These changes may be the first indications that there is a

problem in the environment. Similarly, in toxicology trials, the body weight of an animal can be a very sensitive measure of the adverse effects of a compound (Timbrell, 1991; Rhodes *et al.*, 1993; Timbrell *et al.*, 1994).

Pathology

Invasive markers of tissue damage cover an array of pathological techniques including gross pathology, organ weights and histopathology using light or electron

Table 1 Examples of different biomarkers illustrated with specific examples and examples of the stressor which may result in the biomarker changes

Type of biomarker	Biomarker	Specific example	Stressor
Exposure	DNA adducts	Styrene oxide-O^6 guanine	Styrene exposure
	Protein adduct	N^7-Guanyl-aflatoxin B_1	Dietary aflatoxin
	DNA fragments	7,8-Dihydro-8-oxoguanine	Reactive oxygen species
Exposure and effect (response)	Protein adducts	Carboxyhaemoglobin	CO inhalation
	Enzyme inhibition	Acetylcholinesterase inhibition	Organophosphates
	Urinary metabolites	Mercapturic acids	Buta-1,3 diene, allyl chloride
Effect (response)	Serum/plasma enzymes	AST (aspartate aminotransferase)	Xenobiotics causing necrosis
		LDH (lactate dehydrogenase)	Xenobiotics causing necrosis
		ALT (alanine aminotransferase)	Hepatotoxic compounds
		ALP (alkaline phosphatase)	Bile duct toxins
		CK or CPK (creatine kinase)	Heart/muscle toxins
	Serum/plasma biochemistry	Urea (changes)	Hepatotoxic and nephrotoxic compounds
		Protein (reduced, e.g. albumin)	Hepatotoxic compounds
		Bilirubin	Liver injury
	Clotting time	Prothrombin	Warfarin (rodenticide)
	Urinary metabolites	Glucose, raised creatinine, GSH conjugates	Pancreatic abnormalities, kidney damage
	Raised antioxidant levels	Liver glutathione	Reactive oxygen species
	Enzyme induction	P450 induction	Polycyclic aromatic hydrocarbons
	Stress proteins	hsp 60, hsp 70, hsp90	Cadmium, heat
	Protective proteins	Metallothionein	Heavy metals, e.g. cadmium
		Antibodies, e.g. IgG	Antigens
	Allergic response	Dermatitis	Nickel
	Histology	Chromosomal aberrations, micronuclei	Genotoxic agents
	Clinical observations	Heart rate, temperature, sleeping time	Barbiturates
	Population studies	Breeding patterns, migrations	Climate change
Susceptibility	Phenotype	Acetylator phenotype (NAT 2)	–
	Oncogenes	Dominant oncogenes (ras, mic)	–
		Recessive suppressor gene (p52)	–
	'Cancer' genes	Breast–ovary cancer gene (BRCA 1)	–

microscopy. Many of the changes observed can be correlated with biochemical changes. For example, the accumulation of triglycerides can be seen as well as measured biochemically. It is also possible to localize enzyme changes *in situ*, using immunohistochemistry (e.g. P450) and measure the enzyme activity biochemically. Changes in the biochemistry of tissues are also measured routinely, especially in toxicology studies. These may include glutathione levels (oxidized and reduced), lipid peroxidation and ATP levels as markers of oxidative stress (Hugget *et al.*, 1992; and Timbrell *et al.*, 1994).

Chromosomal aberrations can be identified microscopically, and there is good evidence that such changes can result in tumour formation (Tucker *et al.*, 1997a). Chromosomal abnormalities can also be identified in peripheral lymphocytes and may act as surrogate biomarkers of changes in other tissues. These abnormalities can be expressed as chromatid damage such as gaps and chromosomal rearrangements such as inversions, translocation and acentric fragments which can be observed in metaphase cells. Micronuclei are formed when acentric fragments lag at anaphase resulting in the separation of DNA fragments which can be seen in interphase cells; these are called 'micronuclei' (Bickman, 1994). Translocations between chromosomes can now be identified using *in situ* hybridization (FISH) with probes that can mark or 'paint' individual chromosomes with fluorochromes. By combining different fluorochromes together a range of colours can be produced which can identify all 24 chromosomes, one for each human chromosome, and therefore identify any recombinations between chromosomes (Tucker *et al.*, 1997b).

Clinical Chemistry/Pathology

Traditionally, body fluids have been a source of biochemical markers which are able to identify both the site and severity of a lesion within the organism. Thus, overt cellular damage or a biochemical lesion will usually be reflected in elevated serum levels of enzymes which have leaked from the damaged tissue and biochemical changes such as elevated bilirubin (Evans, 1996a). Markers may also be identified as changes in urinary and cerebrospinal fluid biochemistry. The sophistication and usefulness of these biomarkers can be enhanced by a knowledge of the levels of the enzymes in different tissues, their compartmentalization within the cell, their half-lives and the separation of the enzymes into different isoforms. For example, muscle cell damage will result in the enzyme creatine kinase leaking into the serum. It is a dimeric molecule which has been identified as existing in one of three forms, a 'brain type', a 'muscle type' and a 'heart type'. Identification of the particular isoenzyme in serum will indicate whether the injury is to heart or skeletal muscle. However the half-life of this enzyme is short (0.6 h in the rat) (Evans, 1996a) and diagnosis of

heart muscle damage would need to be verified by using measurements of other enzymes released as a result of myocardial damage, such as aspartate aminotransferase (AST) (half life 3.3–4.4 h) and the heart specific isoenzyme of lactate dehydrogenase (LDH). The pattern of enzyme release is discussed further in Chapter 88.

Enzymatic Changes: Inhibition/Induction

Changes in enzyme activity can be used as biomarkers of specific chemical exposure. For example, exposure to organophosphates will inhibit blood acetylcholinesterases and exposure to lead causes inhibition of serum aminoaevulinic acid dehydrase (Mayer *et al.*, 1992; Thompson and Walker, 1994). As these biomarkers are believed to be specific, the degree of enzyme inhibition has also been used as a biomarker of 'effective dose'.

The induction of specific enzymes, such as the cytochrome P450 isoenzymes, is an adaptive response to challenges from a wide variety of compounds including organochlorine compounds and polycyclic aromatic hydrocarbons. The induction of cytochome P450 requires an increase in protein synthesis and therefore implies a direct effect of a chemical at the gene level. The direct measurement requires tissues to be sampled, although urinary markers of cytochrome P450 activity, such as the excretion of D-glucaric acid in urine, can be used as a non-invasive marker (Melancon *et al.*, 1992). More recently, it has been shown that the constituents of breath are also a potential source of cytochrome P450-generated metabolites which could also be used as biomarkers (Mathews *et al.*, 1996).

Protein Synthesis

Other cellular proteins are increased in response to external stressors. These include the so-called 'heat-shock' proteins which were first identified as proteins which are rapidly synthesized (occurring in minutes to hours) in response to slight rises in temperature. They have since been found to result from altered gene expression in response to a variety of environmental stressors such as changes in salinity, teratogens, oxidative stress, chemical exposure and anoxia. These proteins include hsp90, hsp70 and hsp60 (also called chaperonin) and ubiquitin (Stegeman *et al.*, 1992). They appear to offer protection to molecules such as enzymes by stabilizing them, for example, by maintaining their tertiary structure. Similarly, metallothionein is a protein which is increased in organisms exposed to heavy metals such as cadmium. It acts as a protective agent, by binding the metal ions. As exposure to heavy metals induces the production of metallothionein it also acts as a marker of exposure to heavy metals.

The production of antibody proteins (total IgG, IgM and IgA serum levels) is also a response to exposure to antigens as well as very specific antigens (e.g. tetanus toxin or influenza virus). The identification of serum antibodies using antisera has been used as a biomarker of infectious diseases for many years. However, the recognition that xenobiotics can alter immune functions is a more recent development in the field of biomarkers (Weeks *et al.*, 1992; Descotes *et al.*, 1996). Thus compounds may interfere with immunocompetent cells either by suppressing their activity or stimulating a response, usually after the formation of a chemical–protein complex. Examples of compounds resulting in immune responses include nickel, *p*-phenylenediamine, penicillin and halothane (Timbrell, 1991).

Excretory Products

The ability to detect useful biomarkers non-invasively in urine samples in both animals and humans is an expanding area of current research. As already mentioned, Hippocrates knew the value of urine as a diagnostic tool and we know that the 'madness of King George' (George III) was probably due to porphyria because his urine was described as black. Today, urine analysis has been used very successfully to diagnose kidney dysfunction as the presence of kidney enzymes such as γ-glutamyl transferase and alkaline phosphatase in the urine appear to be early markers of nephrotoxicity.

There is also the potential to use urine analysis to identify liver injury. For example, urinary bilirubin and amino acids may be raised in response to cholestasis, although these do not appear to be very sensitive markers of liver damage.

A promising recent development in the identification of new biomarkers has come about through urine analysis using NMR spectroscopy (Nicholson and Wilson, 1989). This provides both structural and quantitative information about any molecules present containing protons or certain other nuclei and therefore offers the opportunity to identify both changes in endogenous metabolites and any metabolites resulting from the metabolism of xenobiotics. The technique has been particularly useful in identifying novel urinary markers of region specific toxicity in the kidney which are difficult to localize by conventional analysis of the enzymes released (Nicholson *et al.*, 1985; Anthony *et al.*, 1992). Although the equipment is expensive, the technique is non-selective. Thus any change found in a urine sample by NMR, in response to a toxic insult, can be investigated further as a potential biomarker by more conventional means (Sanins *et al.*, 1990; Waterfield *et al.*, 1993a, b). The technique is therefore able to identify biomarkers of exposure, such as the parent compound and the metabolites, and biochemical changes made in response to any toxicity. The data which are produced are non-selective and the methodology involved is unlikely to alter any of the compounds. Thus NMR is potentially a very power-

ful tool in that it can identify many biochemical changes simultaneously. The patterns of the metabolites can be used collectively in what is termed 'pattern recognition'.

DNA Damage and Gene Expression

Genotoxic chemicals may induce a cascade of genetic events. Structural alterations to DNA can be processed and subsequently expressed in mutant gene products. Finally, disease may result from the genetic damage. Detection and quantitation of the various events in this cascade have the potential to be employed as biomarkers of both exposure and effect in organisms exposed to genotoxic agents. These may be measured as

- Changes in DNA structure;
- DNA repair, either directly or indirectly;
- The production of mutations in the genome of the exposed organism.

(Shugart *et al.*, 1992)

Methods for measuring changes in DNA structure have been mentioned earlier, and include the ^{32}P postlabelling assay. Structural alterations to DNA, caused by toxic chemicals, are end-points or biomarkers of exposure. They are also biomarkers of an effect as the modified DNA may result in the expression of other cellular processes such as chromosomal aberrations and oncogene activation (Shugart *et al.*, 1992).

Tumour Genes and Tumour Markers

Changes in the genes involved in human carcinogenesis are better understood and alterations in these genes are now considered to be potential biomarkers of biological effect for certain cancers. One broad category of such cancer genes includes the dominant acting oncogenes, such as *ras* and *mic*, and the recessive tumour suppressor genes such as *p53* and *Rb*. These genes exert their effects as part of the biological pathway leading to tumorigenesis (Garte *et al.*, 1997). There is much evidence that environmental carcinogens (radiation, cigarette smoke) interact directly or indirectly with the structure and/or function of oncogenes and tumour suppressor genes. Any mutations or gene deletions at these targets will increase the risk of tumour formation. Thus, changes in these genes are aselective biomarkers both of exposure and direct effect of environmental carcinogens such as aflatoxin.

Tumour markers include many biological products related to the development and progression of neoplastic disease. These can be quantified and related to the burden or extent of the cancer. These include the serum carcinoembryonic antigen (CEA), α-fetoprotein (AFP) and prostate-specific antigen (PSA) (Sell, 1992).

More recently, interest has grown in the regulatory components of the cell cycle. Evidence suggests that certain cyclin genes may be involved in the regulation of tumour growth and development. The cyclin gene products (e.g. cyclins D1 and D3) have the potential to be biomarkers of abnormal cell growth (Montesano *et al.*, 1997; Wani *et al.*, 1997).

BIOMARKERS OF SUSCEPTIBILITY

Metabolism

The third category of biomarkers are factors which are likely to alter an organism's response to stressors such as toxic foreign compounds. Thus any variation in the response of an individual to identical exposures may represent some difference in susceptibility due either to the genetic make-up of the individual or to variables and environmental influences such as diet or the uptake and absorption of the xenobiotic. The most important source of variability is likely to be the metabolism of the compound by the organism, which may be genetically determined. A number of enzymes exhibit polymorphisms such as the ability to *N*-acetylate arylamines and *N*-hydroxylate heterocyclic arylamines (acetylator pheno-

type *NAT2*). In some cases, such as the null genotypes of glutathione *S*-transferases M1 (*GSTM1*) and T1 (*GSTT1*), the functional enzyme is completely missing (Seidegård and Ekström, 1997) **(Table 1)**.

Genotype

In several familial cancers, the presence of specific genes has been identified and can be considered as markers of susceptibility. Examples of these are the genes for familial breast–ovary cancer (*BRCA1*) and retinoblastoma (*RB1*) (Caporaso and Goldstein, 1997). An individual's sensitivity to genotoxic carcinogens could be associated, for example, with subtle polymorphisms influencing DNA repair processes, although such traits have not yet been found in the human population (Norppa, 1997).

AN INTEGRATED APPROACH

The principle of looking at a number of different biomarkers using NMR of body fluids is one which can be used with all other markers. Taken together, subtle

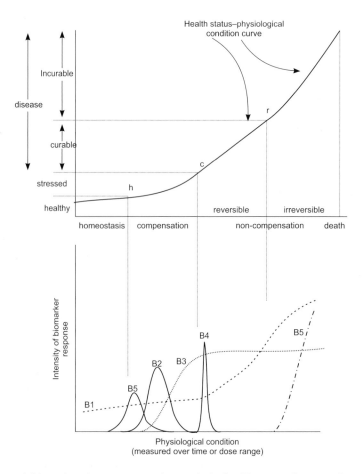

Figure 5 Hypothetical changes in biomarkers in response to changes in the health status of an organism exposed to increased doses of a toxicant or to a toxicant over time. For a full explanation, see the text. Redrawn and adapted from Depledge, M. H, *et al.* (1993), with permission.

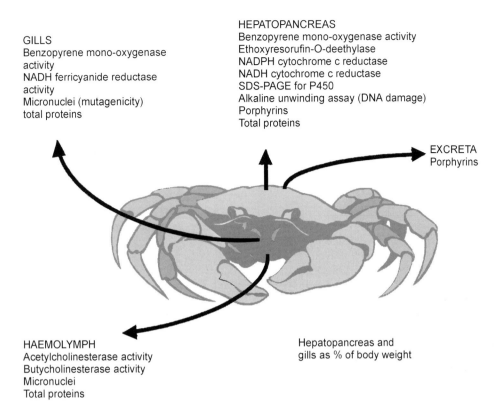

GILLS
Benzopyrene mono-oxygenase
activity
NADH ferricyanide reductase
activity
Micronuclei (mutagenicity)
total proteins

HEPATOPANCREAS
Benzopyrene mono-oxygenase activity
Ethoxyresorufin-O-deethylase
NADPH cytochrome c reductase
NADH cytochrome c reductase
SDS-PAGE for P450
Alkaline unwinding assay (DNA damage)
Porphyrins
Total proteins

EXCRETA
Porphyrins

HAEMOLYMPH
Acetylcholinesterase activity
Butycholinesterase activity
Micronuclei
Total proteins

Hepatopancreas and
gills as % of body weight

Figure 6 Biochemical metabolic and genotoxic biomarkers detected in different biological materials can provide an integrated approach to the use of biomarkers in assessing the effects of environmental contaminants. Adapted from Fossi *et al.* (1997).

quantitative changes can provide a more powerful tool for recognizing the development of pathological lesions. It is often the pattern of changes over time, such as the release of enzymes from the target organ into the serum, that is the clue to the lesion which may be present. If these data are collated with measurements of exposure and biological variation in the form of markers of susceptibility, an earlier diagnosis can be made. At the theoretical level, Depledge (1994) suggests that by following biomarkers over time, the multi-biomarker approach could be refined and extended, particularly in the environmental context. The approach is used in clinical situations where serum enzyme levels and serum biochemistry are monitored to follow the progression of a toxic insult. The proposed relationship between the hypothetical biomarker responses and the health and physical condition of the organism is illustrated in **Figure 5**.

The upper graph illustrates the physiological condition of a hypothetical organism exposed to pollutants. Although the organism may become stressed and show signs of disease, there is a period of time during which it can compensate for the toxic effects of the pollutants and may return to normal health, (c)–(r). Once the organism is no longer able to compensate for the toxic effects of pollutants (r), its health declines and the organism will die. During the deterioration in health status various physiological responses may be employed to compensate for the toxic effects of the pollutants. These would not

normally be evident during the period of homeostasis, although their appearance may be transitory (B5 and B2). Other biomarkers may gradually increase over the entire period (B1) whereas others may make only a brief appearance (B4). Levels of other biomarkers could become maximal during the compensatory period and remain at these levels once the organism is no longer able to compensate for the toxicity (B3). In the example cited here, the same biomarker appears twice, the second time signalling the irreversible state of the toxicity (B5). As any measurement of the different biomarkers will be a 'snapshot in time', it is important to measure as many markers as possible at the same time point. Thus, similar levels of B1 and B5 may indicate early toxicity, but if both levels are high and present with B3 it suggests that the organism will probably be unable to reverse its deteriorating physiological status, and will die. It would also be inadvisable to rely on the presence of B4 as an indicator of toxicity as its appearance is so short-lived. However, if it is found, this would be a clear warning that the organism has received a toxic insult but it is likely that the damage can be reversed. In theory then, these patterns could be used to assess where an organism lies on the health status or physiological condition curve.

The practical use of biomarkers which provide information about toxic effects at different levels of biological organization have been used in medicine for many years, but the use of a suite of biomarkers for providing early warning of long-term ecological effects is more recent (Depledge *et al.*, 1993; Depledge, 1994). Evaluation of the multi-response biomarker approach is currently being investigated in marine invertebrates. This has included investigations into the effects of the main contaminants in the Mediterranean (benzo[*a*]pyrene, polychlorobiphenyls and methylmercury) on biomarkers of effect in the crab *Carcinus aestuarii* **(Figure 6)**, (Fossi *et al.*, 1997) and in mullet taken from two eastern harbour sites in the Mediterranean (Karakoc *et al.*, 1997).

REFERENCES

Aguilar, A. and Borrell, A. (1994). Assessment of organochlorine pollutents in crustaceans by means of skin and hypodermic biopsies. In Fossi, M. C. and Leonzo, C. (Eds), *Nondestructive Biomarkers in Vertebrates*. Lewis Publishers (CRC Press), Boca Raton, FL, pp. 245–267.

Anthony, M. L., Gartland, K. P. R., Beddell, C. R., Lindon, J. C. and Nicholson, J. K. (1992). Cephaloridine-induced nephrotoxicity in the Fischer 344 rat: proton NMR spectroscopic studies of urine and plasma in relation to conventional histopathological assessments of nephronal damage. *Arch. Toxicol.*, **66**, 525–537.

Bickman, J. W. (1994). Genotoxic responses in blood detected by cytogenetic and cytomeric assays. In Fossi, M. C. and Leonzio, C. (Eds), *Nondestructive Biomarkers in Vertebrates*. Lewis Publishers (CRC Press), Boca Raton, FL, pp. 147–157.

Burdon, R. H. (1986). Heat shock and the heat shock proteins. *Biochem. J.*, **240**, 313–324.

Caporaso, N. and Goldstein, A. (1997). Issues involving biomarkers in the study of the genetics of human cancer. In Toniolo, P., Boffetta, P., Shucker, D. E. G., Rothman N., Hulka B. and Pearce, H. (Eds), *Application of Biomarkers in Cancer Epidemiology*. IARC Scientific Publications No. 142. IARC, Lyon, pp. 237–250.

Coggon, D. and Friesen, M. D. (1997). Markers of internal dose: chemical agents. In Toniolo, P., Boffetta, P., Shucker, D. E. G., Rothman, N., Hulka B. and Pearce, H. (Eds), *Application of Biomarkers in Cancer Epidemiology*. IARC Scientific Publications No. 142. IARC, Lyon, pp. 95–101.

Collins, A. R., Dušinská, M., Gedik, C. M. and Štětina, R. (1996). Oxidative damage to DNA: do we have a reliable biomarker? *Environ. Health Perspect.*, **104**, 465–469.

Depledge, M. H. (1994). The rational basis for the use of biomarkers as ecotoxicological tools. In Fossi, M. C. and Leonzo, C. (Eds), *Nondestructive Biomarkers in Vertebrates*. Lewis Publishers (CRC Press), Boca Raton, FL, pp. 271–295.

Depledge, M. H. Amaral-Mendes, J. J., Daniel, B., Halbrook, R. S., Kloepper-Sams, P. Moore, M. N. and Peakall, D. B. (1993). The conceptual basis of the biomarker approach. In Peakall, D. B. and Shugart L. R. (Eds), *Biomarker*. NATO ASI Series, Vol. H 68. Springer, Berlin, p. 19.

Depledge, M. H. and Hopkin, S. P. (1995). Methods to assess effects on brackish, estuarine, and near-costal water organisms. In Lindhurst, R. A., Bourdeau, P. and Tardiff, R. G. (Eds), *Methods to Assess the Effects of Chemicals on Ecosystems*. Wiley, New York, pp. 126–149.

Descotes, J., Nicolas, B., Vial, T. and Nicolas, J.-F. (1996). Biomarkers of immunotoxicity in man. *Biomarkers*, **1**, 77–80.

Dubois, M., Grosse, Y., Thomé, J. P., Kremers, P. and Pfohl-Leszkowicz A. (1997). Metabolic activation and DNA-adducts detection as biomarkers of chlorinated pesticide exposures. *Biomarkers*, **3**, 17–24.

Evans, G. O. (Ed.) (1996a). In *Animal Clinical Chemistry*. Taylor and Francis, London, pp. 59–70.

Evans, G. O. (Ed.) (1996b). Assessment of cardiotoxicity and myotoxicity. In *Animal Clinical Chemistry*. Taylor and Francis, London, pp. 147–154.

Fairbrother, A. (1994). Clinical biochemistry. In Fossi, M. C. and Leonzio, C. (Eds), *Nondestructive Biomarkers in Vertebrates*. Lewis Publishers (CRC Press), Boca Raton, FL, pp. 77–78.

Fossi, M. C., Savelli, C., Casini, S., Franchi, E., Mattei, N. and Corsi, I. (1997). Multi-response biomarker approach in the crab *Carcinus aestuarii* experimentally exposed to benzo(*a*)pyrene, polychlorobiphenyls and methyl-mercury. *Biomarkers*, **2**, 311–319.

Fossi, M. C., Leonzio, C. and Peakall, D. B. (1994). The use of nondestructive biomarkers in the hazzard assessments of vertebrate populations. In Fossi, M. C. and Leonzo, C. (Eds), *Nondestructive Biomarkers in Vertebrates*. Lewis Publishers (CRC Press), Boca Raton, FL, pp. 3–34.

Fossi, M. C. and Leonzio, C. (Eds) (1994). *Nondestructive Biomarkers in Vertebrates*. Lewis Publishers (CRC Press), Boca Raton, FL.

Garte, S., Zocchetti, C. and Toioli, E. (1997). Gene–environment interactions in the application of biomarkers of cancer susceptibility in epidemiology. In Toniolo, P., Boffetta, P., Shucker, D. E. G., Rothman N., Hulka B. and Pearce, H. (Eds), *Application of Biomarkers in Cancer Epidemiology*. IARC Scientific Publications No. 142. IARC, Lyon, pp. 251–264.

Ghezzi, I., Toffoletto, F., Sesana, G., Fagioli, M. G., Micheli, A., Di Silvestro, P., Zocchetti, C. and Alessio, L. (1985). Behaviour of biological indicators of cadmium in relation to occupational exposure. *Int. Arch. Occup. Environ. Health*, **55**, 133–140.

Goldstein, B. D. (1996). Biological markers and risk assessment. *Drug. Metab. Rev.*, **28**, 225–233.

Goyer, R. A. (1986). Toxic effects of metals. In Klaassen, C. D., Amdur, M. O. and Doull, J. (Eds), *Casarett and Doull's Toxicology, The Basic Science of Poisons*, 3rd edn. Macmillan, New York, pp. 582–635.

Groopman, J. D., Wild, C. P., Hasler, J., Junshi, C., Wogan, G. N. and Kensler, T. W. (1993). Molecular epidemiology of aflatoxin exposures: validation of aflatoxin-N^7-guanine levels in urine as a biomarker in experimental rat models and humans. *Environ. Health Perspect.*, **99**, 107–113.

Gupta, R. C. and Randerath, K. (1988). Analysis of DNA adducts by ^{32}P-labeling and thin layer chromatography. In Friedberg, E. and Hanawatt, P. H. (Eds). *DNA Repair*, Vol. 3. Marcel Dekker, New York, pp. 399–418.

Hemminki, K. (1997). DNA adducts and mutations in occupational and environmental biomonitoring. *Environ. Health Perspect.*, **105**, 823–827.

Huang, M. Y., Jin, C., Liu, Y. T., Qu, Q. S., Uchida, Y., Inoue, O., Nakatsuka, H., Wantanabe, T. and Ikeda, M. (1994).

Exposure of workers to a mixture of toluene and xylenes. I. Metabolism. *Occup. Environ. Med.*, **51**, 42–46.

Huggett, R. J., Kimerle, R. A., Mehrle, P. M., Jr, and Bergman, H. L. (Eds) (1992). *Biomarkers (Biochemical, Physiological, and Histological Markers of Anthropogenic Stress)*. SETAC Special Publications. Lewis Publishers, Boca Raton, FL.

Inoue, O., Seiji, K., Kawai, T., Wantanabe, T., Jin, C., Cai, S. X., Chen, Z., Qu, Q. S., Zhang, T. and Ikeda, M. (1993). Excretion of methylhippuric acids in the urine of workers exposed to a xylene mixture: comparison among three xylene isomers and toluene. *Int. Arch. Occup. Environ. Health*, **64**, 533–539.

Jönsson, B. A. G., Lindh, C. H. and Welinder, H. (1997). Haemoglobin adducts and specific immunoglobulin G in humans as biomarkers of exposure to hexahydrophthalic anhydride. *Biomarkers*, **2**, 239–246.

Karakoc, F. T., Hewer, A., Philips, D. H., Gaines, A. F. and Yuregir, G. (1997). Biomarkers of marine pollution observed in species of mullet living in two eastern Mediterranean harbours. *Biomarkers*, **2**, 303–309.

Maclure, G. Y. H., Freeman, J. P., Lay, J. O. and Hinson, J. A. (1996). Haemoglobin adducts as biomarkers of exposure to the herbicides propanil and fluometuron. *Biomarkers*, **1**, 136–140.

Maclure, M., Bryant, M. S. and Skipper, P. L. A. (1990). Decline of the hemoglobin adduct 4-aminobiphenyl during withdrawl from smoking. *Cancer Res.*, **50**, 181–184.

Martin, C. N. and Garner, R. C. (1977). Aflatoxin B-oxide generated by chemical or enzymic oxidation of aflatoxin B_1 causes guanine substitution in nucleic acids. *Nature*, **276**, 863–865.

Mathews, J. M., Raymer, J. H., VelEz, G. R. Garner, C. E. and Bucher, J. R. (1996). The influence of cytochrome P450 enzyme activity on the composition and quantity of volatile organics in expired breath. *Biomarkers*, **1**, 196–201.

Mayer, F. L., Versteeg D. J., McKee, M. J., Folmar, L. C., Graney, R. L., McCume, D. C. and Ratter, B. A. (1992). Physiological and nonspecific biomarkers. In Huggett, R. J., Kimerle, R. A., Mehrle, P. M., Jr, and Bergman, H. L. (Eds), *Biomarkers (Biochemical, Physiological, and Histological Markers of Anthropogenic Stress)*. SETAC Special Publications. Lewis Publishers, Boca Raton, FL, pp. 5–85.

McCarthy, J. F. and Shugart, L. R. (1990). *Biomarkers of Environmental Contamination*. Lewis Publishers, Boca Raton, FL.

Melancon, M. J., Alscher, R., Benson, W., Kruzynski, G., Lee, R. F., Sikka, H. C. and Spies R. B. (1992). Metabolic products as biomarkers. In Huggett, R. J., Kimerle, R. A., Mehrle, P. M., Jr, and Bergman, H. L. (Eds), *Biomarkers (Biochemical, Physiological, and Histological Markers of Anthropogenic Stress)*. SETAC Special Publications. Lewis Publishers, Boca Raton, FL, pp. 87–123.

Montesano, R., Hainaut, P. and Hall, J. (1997). The use of biomarkers to study pathogenesis and mechanisms of cancer: oesophagus and skin cancer as models. In Toniolo, P., Boffetta, P., Shucker, D. E. G., Rothman N., Hulka B. and Pearce, H. (Eds), *Application of Biomarkers in Cancer Epidemiology*. IARC Scientific Publications No. 142. IARC, Lyon, pp. 291–301.

National Research Council (1989). *Biological Markers in Reproductive Toxicology*. Committee on Biological Markers, National Academy Press, Washington, DC.

Nicholson, J. K. and Wilson, I. D. (1989). High resolution proton magnetic resonance spectroscopy of biological fluids. *Prog. Nucl. Magn. Reson. Spectrosc.*, **21**, 449–501.

Nicholson, J. K., Timbrell, J. A. and Sadler, P. J. (1985). Proton NMR spectra of urine as indicators of renal damage mercury-induced nephrotoxicity in rats. *Mol. Pharmacol.*, **27**, 644–651.

Norppa, H. (1997). Cytogenetic markers of susceptability: influence of polymorphic carcinogen-metabolising enzymes. *Environ. Health Perspect.*, **105**, 829–835.

Peakall, D. B. (1992). *Animal Biomarkers as Pollution Indicators*. Ecotoxicological Series 1. Chapman and Hall, London.

Prevost, V., Likhachev, A. J., Loktionova, N. A., Bartsch, H., Wild, C. P., Kazanova, O. I., Arkipov, A. I., Gershanovich, M. L. and Shuker, D. E. G. (1996). DNA base adducts in urine and white blood cells of cancer patients receiving combination chemotherapies which include *N*-methyl-*N*-nitro-surea. *Biomarkers*, **1**, 244–251.

Randerath, K., Reddy, M. and Gupta, R. C. (1988). Analysis of DNA adducts by ^{32}P-postlabeling analysis for DNA damage. *Proc. Natl. Acad. Sci. USA*, **78**, 6126–6129.

Rhodes, C., Thomas, M. and Athis, J. (1993). Principles of testing for acute toxic effects. In Ballantyne, B., Marrs, T. and Turner, P. (Eds), *General and Applied Toxicology*, Vol. 1. Stockton Press, New York and Macmillan, London, pp. 49–87.

Roberts, D. W., Bucci, T. J. Benson, R. W., Warbritton, A. R., McRae, T. A., Pumford, N. R. and Hinson, J. A. (1991). Immunohistochemical localization and quantifiction of the 3-(cystein-*S*-yl)acetaminophen hepatotoxicity. *Am. J. Pathol.*, **138**, 359–371.

Ross, R. K., Yuan, J. M., Yu, M. C., Wogan, G. N. Qian, G. S., Tu, J. T., Groopman, J. D., Gao, Y. T. and Henderson, B. E. (1992). Urinary aflatoxin biomarkers and risk of hepatocellular carcinoma. *Lancet*, **339**, 943–946.

Sanins, S. M., Nicholson, J. K., Elcombe, C. and Timbrell, J. A. (1990). Hepatotoxin-induced hypertaurinuria: a proton NMR study. *Arch. Toxicol.*, **64**, 407–411.

Schlesinger, M. J. (1990). Heat shock proteins. *J. Biol. Chem.*, **265**, 12111–12114.

Seidegård, J. and Ekström, G. (1997). The role of human glutathione transferases and epoxide hydrolases in the metabolism of xenobiotics. *Environ. Health Perspect.*, **105**, 791–799.

Sell, S. (1992). Cancer markers of the 1990s. In Sell, S. (Ed.), *Serological Cancer Markers*. Humana Press, Clifton, NJ, pp. 1–17.

Shugart, L. R. (1994a). Hemoglobin adducts. In Fossi, M. C. and Leonzo, C. (Eds), *Nondestructive Biomarkers in Vertebrates*. Lewis Publishers (CRC Press), Boca Raton, FL, pp. 159–168.

Shugart, L. R. (1994b). Genotoxic responses in blood. In Fossi, M. C. and Leonzo, C. (Eds), *Nondestructive Biomarkers in Vertebrates*. Lewis Publishers (CRC Press), Boca Raton, FL, pp. 131–145.

Shugart, L., Bickman, J. Jackin, G., McMohan, G., Ridley, W., Stein, J. and Steinert, S. (1992). DNA alterations. In Huggett, R. J., Kimerle, R. A., Mehrle, P. M., Jr, and Bergman, H. L. (Eds), *Biomarkers (Biochemical, Physiological, and Histological Markers of Anthropogenic Stress)*. SETAC Special Publications. Lewis Publishers, Boca Raton, FL, pp. 125–153.

Stegeman, J. J., Bronwer, M., DiGiulio, R. T. Förlin, L., Fowler, B. A., Sanders, B. M. and Van Veld, P. A. (1992). Molecular responses to environmental contamination: enzyme and protein as indicators of chemical exposure and effect. In Huggett, R. J., Kimerle, R. A., Mehrle, P. M., Jr, and Bergman, H. L. (Eds), *Biomarkers (Biochemical, Physiological, and Histological Markers of Anthropogenic Stress)*. SETAC Special Publications. Lewis Publishers, Boca Raton, FL, pp. 235–335.

Thompson, H. H. and Walker, C. H. (1994). Blood esterases as indicators of exposure to organophosphorus and carbamate insecticides. In, Fossi, M. C. and Leonzio, C. (Eds), *Nondestructive Biomarkers in Vertebrates*. Lewis Publishers (CRC Press), Boca Raton, FL, pp. 37–62.

Timbrell, J. A., Draper, R. P. and Waterfield, C. J. (1994). Biomarkers in toxicology. *Toxicol. Ecotoxicol. News*, **1**, 4–14.

Timbrell, J. A. (1998). Biomarkers in toxicology. *Toxicology*, **129**, 1–12.

Timbrell, J. A. (1991). *Principles of Biochemical Toxicology*, 2nd edn. Taylor and Francis, London.

Toniolo, P., Boffetta, P., Shucker, D. E. G., Rothman, N., Hulka, B. and Pearce, H. (Eds) (1997a). *Application of Biomarkers in Cancer Epidemiology*. IARC Scientific Publications No. 142. IARC, Lyon, pp. 1–18.

Toniolo, P., Boffetta, P., Shucker, D. E. G., Rothman, N., Hulka, B. and Pearce, H. (Eds) (1997b). *Application of Biomarkers in Cancer Epidemiology*. IARC Scientific Publications No. 142. IARC, Lyon.

Tucker, J. D., Eastmond, D. A. and Littlefield, L. G. (1997a). Cytogenetic endpoints as biological dosimeters and predictors of risk in epidemiological studies. In Toniolo, P., Boffetta, P., Shucker, D. E. G., Rothman N., Hulka B. and Pearce, H. (Eds), *Application of Biomarkers in Cancer Epidemiology*. IARC Scientific Publications No. 142. IARC, Lyon, pp. 185–200.

Tucker, J. D., Breveman, J. W., Briner, J. F., Eveleth, G. G., Langlois, R. G. and Moore, D. H., II (1997b). Persistence of radiation-induced translocations in rat peripheral blood determined by chromosome painting. *Environ. Mol. Mutagen.*, **30**, 264–272.

van Welie, R. T. H., van Dijck, R. G. J. M., Vermeulen, N. P. E. and van Sittert, N. J. (1992). Mercapturic acids, protein adducts and DNA adducts as biomarkers of electrophilic chemicals. *Crit. Rev. Toxicol.*, **22**, 271–306.

Vore, M. (1991). Mechanisms of cholestasis. In Meeks, R. S., Harrison, S. D. and Bull, R. J. (Eds), *Hepatotoxicology*. CRC Press, Boca Raton, FL, pp. 525–568.

Wani, G., Noyes, I., Milo, G. E. and D'Ambrosio, S. M. (1997). Expression of molecular biomarkers in primary breast tumours implanted into a surrogate host: increased levels of cyclins correlate with tumour expression. *Mol. Med.*, **3**, 273–283.

Waterfield, C. J., Turton, J. A., Scales, M. D. C. and Timbrell, J. A. (1993a). Investigations into the effects of various hepatotoxic compounds on urinary and liver taurine levels in rats. *Arch. Toxicol.*, **67**, 244–254.

Waterfield, C. J., Turton, J. A., Scales, M. D. C. and Timbrell, J. A. (1993b). Effects of various non-hepatotoxic compounds on urinary and liver taurine levels in rats. *Arch. Toxicol.*, **67**, 588–546.

Weeks, B. A., Anderson, D. P., DuFour, A. P. Fairbrother, A., Goren, A. J., Lahvis, J. P. and Perters, G. (1992). Immunological biomarkers to assess environmental stress. In Huggett, R. J., Kimerle, R. A., Mehrle, P. M., Jr, and Bergman, H. L. (Eds), *Biomarkers (Biochemical, Physiological, and Histological Markers of Anthropogenic Stress)*. SETAC Special Publications. Lewis Publishers, Boca Raton, FL, pp. 211–234.

Wild, C. P. and Pisani, P. (1997). Carcinogen–DNA and carcinogen–protein adducts in molecular epidemiology. In Toniolo, P., Boffetta, P., Shucker, D. E. G., Rothman, N., Hulka, B. and Pearce, H. (Eds), *Application of Biomarkers in Cancer Epidemiology*. IARC Scientific Publications No. 142. IARC, Lyon, pp. 143–158.

Woodman, D. D. (1996). Assessment of hepatotoxicity. In Evans, G. O. (Ed.), *Animal Clinical Chemistry*. Taylor and Francis, London, pp. 71–86.

Zimmerman, H. J. (1978). Indirect hepatotoxins—cholestatic. In *Hepatotoxicity: the Adverse Effects of Drugs and Other Chemicals on the Liver*. Appleton–Century–Crofts, New York.

Chapter 85
Biomarkers of Effect and Response

Catherine J. Waterfield

CONTENTS

INTRODUCTION

This chapter discusses biomarkers of effect and response. These are observable or measurable changes which take place as a result of adverse chemical interactions with an enzyme or other molecule in a biological system. The interaction could go on to produce a pathological lesion. Thus, they are markers showing that a potentially hazardous change has taken place in a biological system, usually caused by a chemical (**Figure 1**).

BEHAVIOURAL AND CLINICAL MARKERS OF TOXICITY

Gross Indices and Clinical Diagnosis in Clinical and Toxicology Trials

Many of the gross indices used as biomarkers in clinical diagnosis and toxicology studies are ones which have been used as long as disease has been diagnosed. They include changes in:

- Body weight (gain or loss);
- Food intake;
- Temperature;
- Breathing and heart rates;
- Skin/coat condition;
- Sleeping time;
- Urine output;
- Behaviour;
- Sexual changes (long term).

All these are sensitive biomarkers responding to a toxic insult at a lower level of molecular organization and therefore are useful empirical biomarkers (**Figure 1**, Chapter 3).

Pathology

Although gross pathology can provide information about organs or tissues which have been damaged in some way, it is unlikely that the pathological examination of an organism will be carried out without the inclusion of a histological examination of tissues, whether it is an animal in a drug trial or one taken from an environmental site of interest. The biochemistry of the organs and examination of blood samples are also likely to be part of the pathological examination. In this way, patterns of adverse effects can be identified and suggestions made about the probable target organ(s) of the chemical.

Organ Weights

Organ weights are normally expressed in one of three ways, as (a) absolute weight, (b) a percentage of the body weight or (c) a ratio of the organ weight to brain weight. The premise is that any change in an organ weight compared with unaffected/untreated animals will be detected as either (i) an increase in weight due to tissue damage and subsequent oedema, infiltration of fat or inflammatory cells such as macrophages or (ii) a reduction due to atrophy or loss of stored food reserve (i.e. liver glycogen).

Absolute weights are likely to vary as larger animals will simply have larger organs. Therefore, weights expressed as a percentage of body weight should compensate for this. However, an animal may lose body weight very rapidly if the toxicity of a compound reduces the animal's food intake, thus increasing the organ weight if expressed as a percentage of body weight. This

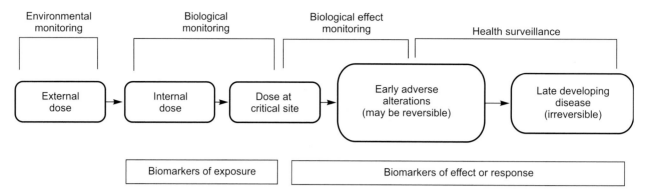

Figure 1 Biomarkers of effect or response may result from exposure to chemicals or other stressors. Modified from deZwart (1997).

is the reason for expressing the organ weight per gram brain weight. These measurements can also be biomarkers for subtle changes such as proliferation of the endoplasmic reticulum or glycogen loss. Any evidence of organ-specific effects could also be supported by histological examination of tissues and blood biochemistry.

Histopathology

Histological biomarkers are, by their nature, higher level responses to stressors. However, very subtle changes in both tissue morphology and biochemistry can be identified by using electron microscopy and histochemistry. Following a toxic insult, there may be generalized or specific biochemical disruption leading to physiological changes. At various stages following the physiological dysfunction cellular and tissue changes may be evident histologically. **Figure 2** illustrates a variety of techniques which can be used as biomarkers of physiological dysfunction resulting from a biochemical lesion (Hinton *et al.*, 1992).

(1) Adaptive responses such as the induction of enzymes can be visualized in tissue sections using specific antibodies to molecules of particular interest (immunohistochemistry).
(2) The rate of cell proliferation can be estimated using the incorporation of tritiated thymidine or bromodeoxyuridine given to the animal before taking the tissues.
(3) Individual proteins such as glycoproteins on the cell surfaces exposed during sectioning can be visualized by selective staining and the infiltration of macrophages as a result of cell death can be observed directly.
(4) Direct observations of cell damage or death, some of which can be very subtle changes such as apoptosis.
(5) Features of cellular adaptive responses such as mitochondrial swelling and proliferation of the endoplasmic reticulum.

(6, 7) Altered cell foci may be a very early marker of adenoma or carcinoma development such as the cervical intra-epithelial neoplasia or 'premalignant' changes which are screened for in a cervical smear.

However, histology requires a sound background knowledge of normal histopathology in addition to an appreciation of factors which can alter 'normal' tissue such as fixation artifacts, dietary and seasonal effects and the relative incidence of abnormalities within the normal or control population. Histology does, however, provide distinct advantages over some biochemical analysis. Whilst it is possible to identify marker enzymes and biochemical changes in organelles in tissue homogenates, it is not always possible to identify either the specific cell type or the location of cell type where the biochemical changes have taken place. Any histological changes can be confirmed with more cell-specific biochemical tests such as biliary function tests, for example, if histology indicates that there is damage to the bile ducts. A disadvantage is that these biomarkers are normally identified in only a few sections; the methods are invasive and very time consuming.

Clinical Chemistry/Pathology

Serum Enzymes

There are two important groups of enzymes that are used in clinical diagnosis:

- Those which are secreted for a specific prepose (e.g. coagulation enzymes); and
- Those released from damaged cells into the blood stream (Fairbrother, 1994).

Changes in serum enzymes and serum biochemistry resulting from tissue injury have been used for clinical diagnosis of disease in man and animals since 1927 and

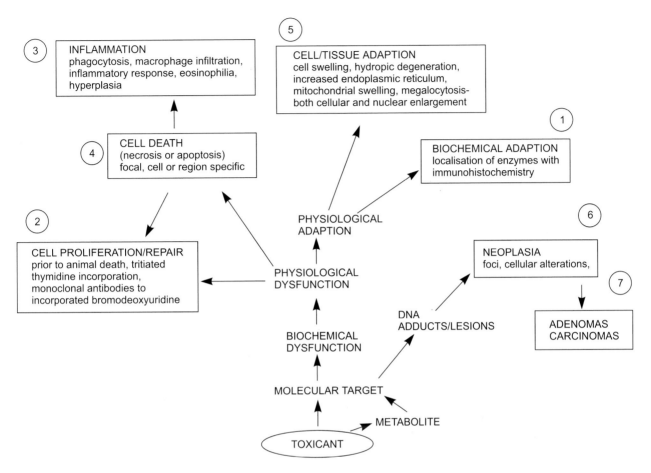

Figure 2 A variety of different histological techniques, some of which indicate very subtle changes, are available for identifying biomarkers of effect following a toxic insult. Adapted from Hinton *et al.* (1992).

routinely as biomarkers in toxicology studies (Kramer, 1989). Identifying the site of a lesion resulting in enzyme leakage relies on a knowledge of the tissue distribution of the different enzymes and the level at which they are normally found. To equate serum levels with the severity of a lesion, it is also necessary to know the half-life of the enzyme (degradation and excretion rate) and possibly the localization of the enzyme within the cell (i.e. cytosol, lysosome or mitochondria).

Figure 3 shows the different maximum serum elevations of four hepatic enzymes released into the bloodstream following a single oral dose of carbon tetrachloride to rats (0.25 ml kg^{-1}), which resulted in hepatocellular necrosis (Zimmerman, 1978). Although all the enzymes were elevated at 3 h when compared with control animals, the maximum elevation of each enzyme varied between 12 h (glutathione reductase) and 36 h (glutamate dehydrogenase). The differences in the time of release are partly due to the different distribution of the enzymes in the hepatocyte. Thus, aspartate aminotransferase (AST) is located in the cytoplasm, as is glutathione reductase (GR), alanine aminotransferase

(ALT) is present in both cytoplasm and mitochondria and glutamate dehydrogenase (GLDH) is located in mitochondria, resulting in the later release of this enzyme from damaged hepatocytes. What these graphs do not show is the degradation time of each of the enzymes, but clearly there will be a balance between this and the time of the release of the enzyme.

It is also important to know the distribution of the different enzymes in different tissues. The two enzymes AST and ALT are both found in high concentrations in the liver. However, both are also present in other tissues such as muscle, although muscle has proportionally higher amounts of AST than ALT. Thus, a high AST:ALT ratio in the blood *could* indicate that muscle rather than liver had been damaged (e.g. 8:1 rather than 3:1).

In the case of muscle injury, the muscle-specific cytosolic enzyme creatine phosphokinase (CPK) would be expected to be elevated, although it has a very short halflife **(Table 1)** (Evans, 1996). Heart and brain also contain CPK. However, this is a dimeric enzyme, containing the subunits B and M, which can be separated into three

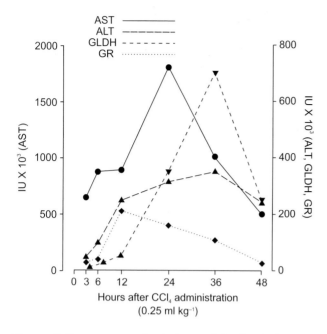

Figure 3 Serum enzyme levels in rats following dosing with carbon tetrachloride (CCl$_4$, 0.25 ml kg^{-1}). Redrawn from Zimmerman (1978).

Table 1 Plasma enzymes and their respective half-lives in three species

Enzyme	Range of estimates for enzyme half-life (h)		
	Dog	Rat	Man
Asparate aminotransferase (AST)	3.3–4.4	2.3	4–46
Alanine aminotransferase (ALT)	2.5–60.9	4.4	32–52
Creatine kinase (CK, total)	0.6–16.2	0.6	3.5–35
CK-MB (myocardial isoenzyme)	1.3–1.8	–	–
Lactate dehydrogenase (LDH, total)	1.6	–	40–114

From Evans (1996).

forms, 'muscle' enzyme (MM), 'brain' enzyme (BB) and that found in the heart (MB). Hence the sophistication of enzyme measurements can be improved by separating the enzyme activity into different isoenzymes. Lactate dehydrogenase (LDH) shows similar isomeric forms, LDH$_1$ and LDH$_2$ found in skeletal muscle and LDH-C$_4$ found in the testes.

The ratios of the different enzymes and the levels which are detected will vary widely between species and laboratories owing to species differences in tissue and organelle enzyme distribution and also the methodologies used in different laboratories. Hence, caution is needed when interpreting results.

Serum Biochemistry

Serum biochemistry will reflect changes in intermediates or end products of metabolism such as proteins and tri-glycerides. If the organ responsible for their production is injured, the biochemical profile of the serum will change.

Liver Injury

Many changes in serum biochemistry are associated with liver damage as the liver is the main site of intermediary metabolism. For example, an elevation of blood urea nitrogen indicates an increased rate of protein catabolism due to starvation, a high protein diet or a reduced rate of urinary excretion due to kidney malfunction. Plasma bilirubin is directly related to haem turnover, but will also be increased if bile flow is inhibited (cholestasis). Bile pigments can be measured in both blood and urine. However, these measurements are only of use in mammals as animals such as birds, amphibians and reptiles do not have sufficient biliverdin reductase activity to convert biliverdin to bilirubin.

Raised levels of both serum and urinary bile acids are indicative of cholestasis. The uptake, conjugation and biliary excretion of bile acids are usually very efficient, and most are cleared after a single pass through the liver. Therefore, any hepatocellular damage is very quickly reflected in raised serum levels of bile acids. Recent advances in high performance liquid chromatography (HPLC), radioimmunoassays and enzymatic methods have made these measurements easier and more sensitive. Individual serum bile acids, notably cholic, glycocholic and taurocholic acid, have been shown to be particularly sensitive markers of liver dysfunction (Bai *et al.*, 1992). Fat levels can be measured in both faecal material and blood. Reduced levels of serum triglycerides may indicate reduced transport of triglycerides from the liver and suggest fat accumulation in the liver. A reduction in serum proteins, both total and specific proteins, such as albumin, is found when the liver metabolism is compromised as the liver is the major source of serum proteins.

Testicular Injury

There is growing interest in serum markers which might help identify subtle changes which could contribute to problems in fertility. Recent studies have focused on the reproductive health of men in the general population as sperm counts appear to be becoming reduced. As semen samples are difficult to obtain, serum biomarkers of spermatogenesis are of major interest for population studies. Although follicle stimulating hormone (FSH) has been used as a marker of spermatogenesis and testicular function, some recent work suggests that serum inhibin B measured by an enzyme immunometric assay may offer some advantages, as FSH is also influenced by the hypothalamus (Jensen *et al.*, 1997).

Less specific testicular injury can sometimes be assessed by measuring changes in serum testosterone levels. Although the results from experimentally induced testicular injury tend to produce very variable results, a reduction in serum testosterone is usually indicative of damage to Leydig cells and the hormone status of the individual. Testosterone may be measured in serum at the same time as the testis-specific isozyme LDH-C4 which is released when mature spematozoa are damaged (Reader *et al.*, 1991). More recently, raised urine levels of the endogenous metabolite creatine have been identified as a biomarker of testicular injury and one which may also be more sensitive, (Timbrell *et al.*, 1994; Draper *et al.*, 1996; Traina *et al.*, 1997).

Bone Injury

Osteoporosis is another clinical problem which has received attention more recently. The use of biomarkers for identifying, and thereby treating the problem early, has prompted a search for more specific markers of bone formation and resorption. This has been monitored by measuring enzymes and other protein products in the urine, released by osteoblasts and osteoclasts, respectively. These include the bone isoenzyme of alkaline phosphatase, osteocalcin and the breakdown products of Type I collagen such as hydroxyproline. However, it has been suggested that megakaryocytes and peripheral blood platelets may contribute to serum osteocalcin levels (Thiede *et al.*, 1994) and hydroxyproline is not specific to bone collagen and is also derived from the diet. There is therefore interest in bone-specific collagen products for use as biomarkers such as galactosylhydroxylysine and the collagen cross-links pyridinoline and deoxypyridinoline. The pyridinolines and peptides derived from cross-linked regions in collagens appear to be the most promising markers of resorption and permit the quantitative evaluation of rates of bone resorption in man (Russell, 1997).

Lung Injury

Early lung injury is also difficult to identify. However, a Clara cell protein (CC16) is secreted in the respiratory tract by the non-ciliated Clara cells which are known for their vulnerability to toxic insults. This can be identified in bronchoalveolar lavage fluid and also in serum or sputum.

Studies on occupationally exposed workers and experimental animals indicate that the assay of CC16 in serum may be a sensitive and relatively specific biomarker for detecting early acute or chronic effects of toxicants on the tracheobronchial tree (Hermans and Bernard, 1996; Bernard and Hermans, 1997).

In order to maintain homeostasis, levels of serum minerals and electrolytes need to be balanced. Any changes in these can act as biomarkers for poor absorption (e.g. calcium) or of a hormone imbalance as the mechanisms involved in osmolyte regulation include aldosterone and arginine vasopressin (antidiuretic hormone) (York and Evans, 1996).

Analysis of Specific Data

This section discusses the integration of different pathological biomarker data to illustrate how it could be used to help identify the site of a toxic lesion. The clinical chemistry data are taken from rats of the same strain and sex (male), treated with well documented 'target organ-specific' toxins **(Table 2)**. The dose given was as a single injection and was calculated to result in injury to a specific target organ as indicated in the table. However, the serum enzyme levels and biochemistry were not always consistent with single organ damage. The data were obtained in the same laboratories.

Liver Injury

Liver injury was caused by carbon tetrachloride, thioacetamide, α-naphthyl isothiocyanate (ANIT) and galactosamine. The initial indication of liver injury is the increase in liver weight expressed as a percentage of body weight after carbon tetrachloride and ANIT treatment and the high levels of ALT and AST. In the case of carbon tetrachloride and thioacetamide, the ratio of these two enzymes is approximately 1:4, which is what might be expected. The ratio of these two enzymes after galactosamine and ANIT treatment is only 1:2, although the levels overall are higher, which suggests that the lesion may have been more severe. The plasma half-life of ALT is longer than that of AST **(Table 1)**, which may explain the lower serum concentration of AST than might have been expected following liver injury. The raised levels of ALP (an enzyme located in bile duct epithelial cells) indicate that three of the compounds probably resulted in bile duct damage which was most marked after treatment with ANIT. The bile duct damage was severe enough to cause cholestasis, resulting in a rise in bilirubin levels in the blood after both galactosamine and ANIT treatment. The toxicity of these compounds is progressive owing to the accumulation of bile. The low levels of serum triglycerides indicated that both carbon tetrachloride and galactosamine had affected transport of triglycerides from the liver. Indeed, histology confirmed that there was fat accumulation in these livers. There is also an indication that three of these hepatotoxic compounds caused kidney damage as the kidney weights expressed as a percentage of body weight were raised after thioacetamide, ANIT and galactosamine treatment. However, only in the case of thioacetamide was this confirmed both biochemically (raised serum creatinine and blood urea nitrogen and raised urinary protein) and histologically. Both ANIT and galactosamine had resulted in a marked reduction in food intake in the animals and therefore a loss of body weight, which artificially increases the kidney:body weight ratio.

Table 2 Various clinical and pathological observations made on rats treated with a variety of well documented toxins: the primary target organ for toxicity is indicated although other injuries are indicated by serum enzyme levels[a]

	Compound							
	Control	CCl₄	Thio	ANIT	Gal	Cd²⁺	Hg²⁺	TMPD
Main target organ at this dose		L	L	BD/L	L	T/K/L	K	SM
Dose (mg kg⁻¹)		3160	150	150	500	1.5	1.4	49
Liver (% b.w.)	3.85–4.66	5.9**↑	4.25	4.24*↑	3.40	4.16	3.67*↓	3.84
Kidney (2) (% b.w.)	0.71–0.76	0.76	1.03**↑	0.87**↑	0.83**↑	0.78	1.36***↑	0.84
Testes (2) (% b.w.)	0.96	–	–	–	–	0.92*↓	0.97	1.07*↑
Muscle (g) gastrocnemus	1.36	–	–	–	–	–	–	1.85***↑
Serum enzymes								
ALT (iu l⁻¹)	35–89	344*	442*	723**	4293*	86	52	1117*
AST (iu l⁻¹)	73–99	1219**	1735**	1501***	6479***	215	164	7174**
LDH (iu l⁻¹)	359	–	–	–	–	–	–	1095*
LDH₁₊₂ (iu l⁻¹)	14	–	–	–	–	–	–	301*
ALP (iu l⁻¹)	343–618	1007*	766	1508*	730**	173**↓	433	343*↓
CPK (total) (iu l⁻¹)	265	–	–	–	–	–	–	1255*
CPK (MM) (iu l⁻¹)	35	–	–	–	–	–	–	983*
HBDH (iu l⁻¹)	64	–	–	–	–	–	–	328*
Serum chemistry								
Total bilirubin (μ mol l⁻¹)	0.9–6.0	9.3	8.3*	177*	134***	1.5	8.7***	3.1
Creatinine (μ mol l⁻¹)	43–52	59	100*	35	48	44	359***	48
Blood urea nitrogen (mmol l⁻¹)	4.2–5.9	6.7	11.5*	5.8	5.1	5.6	43.4***	5.9
Cholesterol (mmol l⁻¹)	1.22–1.58	1.62	1.57	4.92	0.95	1.9	1.8	1.8
Triglycerides (mmol l⁻¹)	0.7–1.5	0.53**	0.84	0.7	0.43**	1.0	1.2	0.9
Albumin (g l⁻¹)	32.5–34.5	35	28	32	31	27**	30	25.8***

[a] ALT, alanine aminotransferase; AST, aspartate aminotransferase; LDH, lactate dehydrogenase; LDH₁₊₂, isoenzymes; may reflect heart damage; ALP, alkaline phosphatases; CPK, creatine kinase; MM, skeletal muscle isoenzyme; HBDH, α-hydroxybutyrate dehydrogenase; L, liver; BD, bile ducts; T, testes; K, kidney; SM, skeletal muscle; CCl4, carbon tetrachloride; thio, thioacetamide; ANIT, α-naphtyl isothiocyanate; Gal, galactosamine; TMPD, 2,3,5,6-tetra-p-phenylenediamine. Values are means (ranges shown for controls) for 4–5 animals. Significance:* p < 0.05;** p < 0.01;*** p < 0.001; treated data compared with 'same time/experiment' control. Data from Waterfield et al. (1991, 1993a,b).

Kidney Injury

Kidney injury is indicated following treatment with mercuric chloride. The kidney weights in these animals were increased and serum creatinine, blood urea nitrogen and urinary protein were raised. Treatment with this compound may also have had a toxic effect in the liver. Liver weight was reduced. However, this was probably due to a reduction in glycogen levels as these animals ate less. The results also indicated a reduction in protein synthesis as serum levels of albumin were low. These two factors may also have affected serum bilirubin levels, which were slightly raised. However, histological examination of the liver and normal levels of serum AST and ALT could not confirm liver injury.

Testicular Injury

Testicular injury is indicated after treating animals with cadmium chloride as the testes had become atrophied. The enzymes shown in **Table 2** did not indicate any other injury. However, testicular injury was confirmed by an increase in the testis-specific isoenzyme LDH-C4 in the serum, reduced serum testosterone and an increase in urinary creatine, as well as histological examination of the tissues.

Muscle Injury

Muscle injury due to xenobiotics is relatively uncommon, although ethanol myopathy is well characterized (Misulis *et al.*, 1993). However, compounds such as chloroquine, doxorubicin and some phenyldiamines (specifically the ring methylated forms) will produce a very specific muscle lesion. A characteristic of muscle damage is the raised level of creatine kinase in the serum, sometimes accompanied by myoglobinuria, which provides evidence of myoglobin breakdown (Shihabi, 1995).

In the example illustrated here, rats were treated with 2,3,5,6-tetra-*p*-phenylenediamine (TMPD). Serum levels of AST were raised but the increase in ALT was relatively less than would have been expected after liver injury, giving an ALT:AST ratio of 1:6. The raised levels of creatine kinase and the muscle-specific iso-enzyme (MM) in particular confirmed the muscle injury. However, the amount of damage to the muscles was more severe than indicated by the serum levels of these enzymes. The reason for this is probably the very short half-life of creatine kinase, as serum samples were taken 48 h after dosing and the maximum elevation of the enzyme may have been missed **(Table 1)**.

Since serum enzyme changes and some serum biochemical changes are the direct result of cell injury, they have tended to be biomarkers of higher level responses. However, serum enzyme analysis is a very valuable tool in identifying tissue injury both clinically and in experimental toxicology. Only a single blood sample needs to be taken for multiple enzyme and chemical analyses and when analysed together with gross pathology and histology a very specific diagnosis can be made.

URINARY BIOMARKERS

As urine can be obtained non-invasively and continuously, it provides an ideal source of biomarkers for kidney injury as well as metabolic perturbations indicating possible biochemical lesions else where in the body. The kidney controls the composition of normal plasma constituents by conserving or eliminating them from the blood. Any impairment in kidney function will inevitably result in the alteration of these functions and therefore the composition of the urine. For example, very little protein is normally present in the urine, and therefore an increase in urinary protein could indicate malfunction of the glomeruli. Similarly, the kidney is responsible for conserving glucose and maintaining acid–base, salt and water balances. Any change in these, including urinary volume, could be regarded as biomarkers of kidney malfunction. However, parameters such as these must be assessed in the light of dietary intake, as a high protein diet will reduce urinary pH and urinary volume will be dependent on fluid intake, sweating and excessive loss due to vomitus or diarrhoea. It is also possible to use urine as a source of biomarkers of metabolic disturbances and tissue injury in the whole body and to identify the products of oxidative damage and DNA adducts (see later, **Figure 8**). The same urine sample can also be analysed for xenobiotic metabolites which can be correlated with the metabolic findings.

Markers of Kidney Injury

Functional Assessment of Kidney

Renal clearance is often assessed by levels of urea and creatinine. As amino acids and glucose are reabsorbed in the proximal tubules when serum concentrations are low, any increase may be indicative of proximal tubule malfunction, as are changes in both Na^+ and K^+ (Stonard, 1987; Lock, 1993).

Kidney Enzymes

Overt cellular damage to the kidneys will result in enzyme leakage, just as it does from other tissues. However, in the case of the kidney, serum enzymes are of limited use as most will be lost into the lumen of the tubules. Hence urine is the source of kidney enzymes as a result of injury.

The enzymes which are most useful are those localized in the proximal tubule, which is also the region most

Table 3 Localization of renal tubular enzymes in the rat

Enzyme	Localization in the kidney[a]
Alanine aminopeptidase (AAP)	PST > PCT
Alkaline phosphatase (ALP)	PCT > PST > distal tubule
β-Galactosidase (GAL)	PST > PCT > distal tubule
γ-Glutamyl transferase (GGT)	PST > PCT > distal tubule
Lactate dehydrogenase (LDH)	Distal tubule > proximal tubule
N-Acetyl-β-D-glucosaminidase (NAG)	PCT > PST = distal tubule

[a] PST, proximal straight tubule; PCT, proximal convoluted tubule.
Adapted from Stonard (1996).

vulnerable to toxic injury **(Table 3)**. It is also possible to use the patterns of enzyme release to determine the site of injury within the nephron (Delacruz et al., 1997). Those enzymes located on the brush-border region of the proximal renal tubule (such as the amino peptidases, alkaline phosphatase and γ-glutamyl transferase) tend to be earlier markers of renal injury than other indices. Papillotoxic agents usually result in polyuria and a steady increase in urinary levels of N-acetyl-β-D-glucosaminidase, which may precede the appearance of other enzymes in the urine (Stonard, 1987, 1996).

Metabolic Urinary Biomarkers

Use of NMR Spectroscopy

High-resolution ^{1}H NMR spectroscopy has been used over the past 10 years to identify changes in the patterns of excretion of low molecular weight compounds in the urine as a result of organ damage and inborn errors of metabolism. The original work was focused on the effects of region-specific nephrotoxins. These result in patterns of glycosuria, amino aciduria and lactic aciduria following the exposure of rats to proximal tubular toxins, whereas papillary toxins cause early elevations of trimethylamine N-oxide and dimethylamine followed by the later elevation of urinary acetate, succinate and N,N-dimethylglycine (Bales et al., 1984; Iles et al., 1985; Nicholson et al., 1985; Gartland et al., 1988). The use of NMR spectroscopy to identify novel biomarkers has been made more sophisticated by the use of two-dimensional correlation spectroscopy (COSY), which allows the separation of overlapping resonances. The sensitivity of the technique has also advanced with the introduction of high-resolution 750 MHz NMR instruments. The complex patterns of endogenous small molecules which appear in the urine following changes in metabolism can be subjected to computer-based pattern recognition analysis. Different toxins and pathological conditions will result in different patterns, indicating both the mechanism of toxicity/

pathology and the probable organ(s) involved (Holmes et al., 1994).

The power of NMR spectroscopy has also been extended by combining it with HPLC. In this way, both abnormalities in endogenous metabolite excretion following drug treatment and metabolites of the drug itself can be identified. An example of the successful use of the technique is in cancer chemotherapy. When drugs such as ifosfamide (which is known to be nephrotoxic) are used, analysis of urine by NMR enables the progress of both the treatment and toxicity of the chemotherapeutic agent to be followed (Foxall et al., 1996). Urinary biomarkers have also been used following kidney transplantation to provide early warning of tissue rejection and/or kidney damage resulting from immunosuppressant drugs such as cyclosporin, both of which give different patterns of metabolites in the urine (J. K. Nicholson, personal communication).

Unfortunately, the use of NMR requires very specialized expertise and the instrumentation is very costly. However, as a result of the non-selective nature of NMR, a number of potential urinary biomarkers have been identified which can be measured by biochemical means **(Figure 4)**. These include urinary creatine, which is raised in experimental animals following testicular damage, and urinary taurine, which is increased following experimentally induced hepatic damage, including the induction of fatty liver and for which there are no urinary biomarkers (Timbrell et al., 1994, 1995; Draper et al., 1996). Both of these markers were identified by NMR as potential urinary markers as a result of the non-selective nature of the technique.

Urinary Taurine

Taurine is an end product of sulphur amino acid metabolism, primarily synthesized in the liver, where it is present in high concentrations (2–8 mM). The kidneys regulate the body pool of taurine and excess will be excreted in the urine (Huxtable, 1992).

Urinary taurine can be separated from other amino acids in urine using ion-exchange columns, then measured fluorimetrically after derivatization and separation by HPLC. In vivo studies in rats have shown that many compounds causing liver necrosis will raise levels of urinary taurine (e.g. after treatment with CCl_4 and thioacetamide; Waterfield et al., 1993a). Compounds which cause hepatic injury will also affect intermediary metabolism. If the changes in intermediary metabolism involve sulphur amino acids, taurine synthesis will also be affected. For example, a reduction in protein synthesis will increase taurine synthesis and excess taurine will overflow into the urine (e.g. after treatment with ethionine and cycloheximide). Conversely, an increase in the demand for cysteine by increasing either protein or glutathione synthesis will reduce urinary levels of

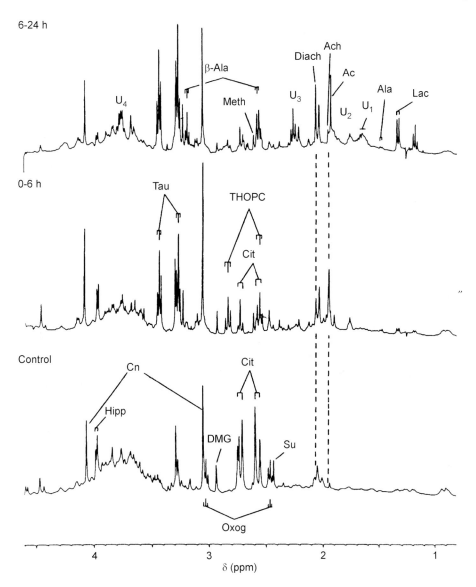

Figure 4 400 MHz proton NMR spectra of rat urine collected 24 h before and 0–6 and 6–24 h after dosing with hydrazine hydrate, showing both the metabolites of the parent compound and changes in endogenous metabolites which can be used as potential biomarkers of response. Abbreviations: Ach, acetylhydrazine; Diach, diacetylhydrazine; THOPC, 1,4,5,6-tetrahydro-6-oxopyridazinecarboxylic acid; Meth, methylamine; β-Ala, β-alanine; Lac, lactate; Ala, alanine; Ac, acetate; Su, succinate; Cit, citrate; Oxog, 2-oxoglutarate; DMG, dimethyglycine; Cn, creatinine; Tau, taurine; $U_1 - U_4$, unassigned resonances from hydrazine metabolites. From Sanins *et al.* (1990).

taurine (i.e. following treatment with clenbuterol or phorone).

A reduction in protein synthesis may also reduce the transport of triglycerides out of hepatocytes, which then accumulate in the cells; a common feature of hepatotoxic compounds. Consequently, liver injury and fatty liver (steatosis) often correlate with an increase in urinary taurine excretion. Thus, urinary taurine has the potential to be used as a non-invasive biomarker of hepatic injury and dysfunction, including triglyceride accumulation and changes in sulphur amino acid status (Timbrell and Waterfield, 1996; Waterfield *et al.*, 1993a, b, 1996).

Porphyrins

Haem and Porphyrin Synthesis

In the metabolic pathway responsible for producing haem, iron is incorporated into protoporphyrin in the mitochondrion **(Figure 5)**. The resulting haem molecules are then incorporated into the haem-containing proteins such as the haemoglobins, cytochromes and enzymes such as peroxidase and catalase. As the levels of haem regulate aminolaevulinic acid synthetase (ALA), any reduction in haem production removes the negative feedback and aminolaevulinic acid is synthesized unchecked

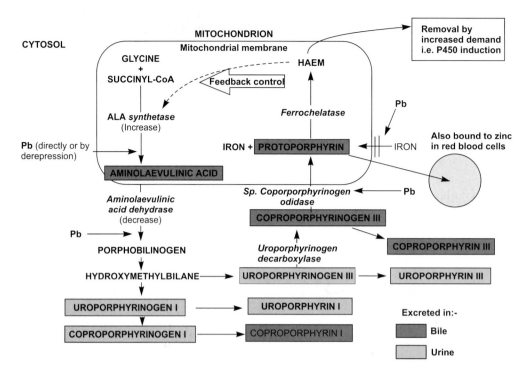

Figure 5 Metabolic pathway illustrating the steps where lead and excessive haem utilization may affect the pathway, resulting in the elevation of different prophyrins which are eliminated in the bile and urine, which can then be used as biomarkers.

(Andrew *et al.*, 1990). The uncontrolled production of aminolaevulinic acid will result in an excess production of porphyrins. These can be used as biochemical markers of disruption to the haem cycle. Uroporphyrinogen and uroporphyrin and also coproporphyrinogen are normally excreted into the urine, whereas coproporphyrin is eliminated almost completely in the bile, which will then appear in the faeces. Measuring porphyrins in faecal matter is complicated by the presence of haem breakdown products from the diet, e.g. from chlorophyll and haemoproteins of ingested food. The levels are also dependent on bile flow, which can be altered during liver injury. It is therefore more satisfactory to measure uroporphyrin and other carboxylated porphyrins and also aminolaevulinic acid and porphobilinogen in the urine if changes in porphyrins are to be used as biomarkers of disruption to this pathway (DeMatteis and Lim, 1994).

Porphyrin Excretion as a Biomarker

There are inborn errors in the haem pathway which result in the excretion of uroporphyrin I into the urine, which then darkens in the light. However, chemicals can also alter haem synthesis resulting in increased levels of porphyrins in both the urine and faeces. An increase in the demand for haem, for example following the alkylation of cytochrome P450 by ethylene, acetylene or related chemicals, increases urinary aminolaevulinic acid, as the control of ALA synthetase is removed and amino-

laevulinic acid is synthesized without check. This also results in an increase in haem precursors which exceed the capacity of the intermediary enzymes, resulting in their excretion into urine and bile.

Lead has a profound and well documented effect on haem synthesis, which is probably due to the sensitivity of sulphydryl (SH)-containing enzymes even to very low concentrations of lead (Piomelli, 1987; Amess, 1993). There are at least two steps in the pathway where lead interferes with the cycle. The first involves the activity of the enzyme D-aminolaevulinic acid dehydrase (ALAD), which is very susceptible to lead. The reduction in activity of this enzyme has been shown to correlate well with the degree of lead exposure. A direct consequence of the decreased activity results in a rise in aminolaevulinic acid, which can then be measured in the urine. The activity of ALAD can be measured in red blood cells where the enzyme appears to be the most sensitive.

Lead will also interfere with iron transport and another (SH)-rich enzyme, ferrochelatase, preventing the incorporation of iron into protoporphyrin. This results in an increase in protoporphyrin which then incorporates zinc non-enzymatically. The zinc protoporphyrin accumulates in red blood cells, the presence of which can be used as another marker of lead poisoning.

Other metals such as arsenic and mercury increase the excretion of coproporphyrin and other porphyrins, possibly by inhibiting uroporphyrinogen decarboxylase or coproporphyrinogen oxidase. Hexachlorobenzene and other polyhalogenated aromatic compounds and

2,3,7,8-tetrachlorodibenzo-*p*-dioxin (TCDD) will also result in the accumulation of uroporphyrin and other highly carboxylated porphyrins in liver and urine (Fowler *et al.*, 1987; Woods *et al.*, 1991).

Mercapturic Acids

Formation of Mercapturic Acids

Electrophilic compounds and intermediates can react with glutathione spontaneously or enzymatically, a reaction catalysed by glutathione *S*-transferases. This results in the formation of the glutathione conjugates in what is believed to be a multi-organ process **(Figure 6)**. Catabolism of the resulting glutathione *S*-conjugates produces the end products, mercapturic acids (*N*-acetyl-L-cystine *S*-conjugates), cysteine *S*-conjugates, mercaptoacetic acids and mercaptolactic acids. As the *S*-conjugates are excreted into the urine they can be used as biomarkers of exposure to specific electrophiles and also, since they are produced as a result of glutathione conjugation with reactive intermediates, they could also be regarded as biomarkers of effect or response.

Mercapturic Acids as Biomarkers

The half-life of most of the *S*-conjugates is relatively short and non-invasive repeated sampling of urine makes them particularly useful as biomarkers of recent exposure to potential toxicants. This has proved to be of value in monitoring industrial workplaces as many industrially used chemicals will form mercapturic acids, including ethylene oxide, which forms 2-hydroxyethyl mercaptoethanol, acrolein, which forms 3-hydroxypropylmercapturic acid, and methylformamides and methyl isocyanates, which result in the formation of *N*-methylcarbamoylmercapturic acids.

TISSUE ENZYME LEVELS

Enzyme Induction

Cytochrome P450 (Catalysing Phase I Reactions)

The induction of specific enzymes, such as the cytochrome P450 isoenzymes [mixed-function oxidase (MAO)], is an adaptive response to challenges with a wide variety of compounds including organochlorine compounds and polycyclic aromatic hydrocarbons and also endogenous compounds such as steroids and fatty acids. Thus, the induction of cytochrome P450 isoenzymes can be considered as a biomarker of effect or response.

Measuring cytochrome P450 can be carried out directly in tissues using

i. microsomal catalytic MAO activity using substrates such as ethoxyresorufin *O*-deethylase (EROD) activity and arylhydrocarbon (benzo[*a*]pyrene) hydroxylase (AHH) activity (Payne *et al.*, 1987);
ii. specific antibodies to cytochrome P450 (Stegeman, 1989);
iii. cDNA probes to detect messenger RNA (Heilmann *et al.*, 1988).

All three methods can detect the induction of cytochrome P450, although the activity of the enzyme may be masked if the compound or a metabolite subsequently inhibits or destroys the enzyme. There is also an increase in both time and cost in the methods from (i) to (iii). All three methods have been used successfully in experimental animals and humans and are being utilized increasingly to examine wild life, such as fish, for signs of environmental pollution.

The direct measurement of cytochrome P450 in tissues is invasive as it requires tissues to be sampled. However, surrogate markers such as the excretion of D-glucaric acid and the ratio of 6-*β*-hydroxycortisol to 17-hydroxycorticosteroid in urine can be used as non-invasive markers as they indicate cytochrome P450 *activity* (Ohnhaus and Park, 1979; Bienvenu *et al.*, 1991; Melancon *et al.*, 1992). However, it is now known that the 6-*β*-hydroxy-cortisol to 17-hydroxycorticosteroid ratio can also be altered by dietary factors, such as grape fruit (Seidegard *et al.*, 1998). More recently it has been shown that the constituents of breath are also a potential source of cytochrome P450-generated metabolites. Exposing rats to the cytochrome P450 inhibitor 1-aminobenzotriazole results in a marked increase in naturally occurring, low molecular weight, volatile organic compounds in the breath, with levels returning to normal when the enzyme activity returns (Mathews *et al.*, 1996). The induction of cytochrome P450 requires an increase in protein synthesis and therefore implies a direct or indirect effect of a toxin at the gene level.

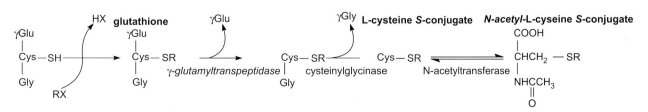

Figure 6 Formation of mercapturic acids following glutathione conjugation. Adapted from Van Welie *et al.* (1992).

Non-cytochrome P450 Enzyme Induction (Catalysing Phase II Reactions)

Glucuronosyl S-Transferases

The UDP-glucuronosyl S-transferases catalyse the transfer of the glucuronyl groups from uridine 5′-diphosphoglucuronate to many acceptors, including hydroxylated polycyclic aromatic hydrocarbons. Several forms exist in mammals, some of which appear to be inducible by xenobiotics **(Table 4)**. The possibility of using the induction of glucuronosyl S-transferases as biomarkers of effect to monitor environmental contamination in species such as fish has produced varied results (Stegeman et al., 1992).

Table 4 Induction of non-cytochrome P450 enzymes by different inducing agents

Enzyme	Inducing agent[a]
Glucuronosyl S-transferases	Pb, 3-MC, TCDD, PCBs
NADPH cytochrome P450 reductase	Pb, PCBs, isosasafrole
Epoxide hydrolases	Pb, 3-MC, Arochlor, isosafrole
Glutathione S-transferases	Pb, 3-MC, TCDD
Cytochrome b_5	2-Acetylaminofluorene, BHT
Catalase	Clofibrate, phthalates, paraquat
Carnitine acyl transferase	Clofibrate

[a] Pb, phenobarbital; BHT, butylated hydroxytoluene; 3-MC, 3-methylcholanthrene; TCDD, 2,3,7,8-tetrachlorodibenzdioxin; PCBs, polychlorinated biphenyls.

Glutathione S-Transferases

All eukaryotic species possess multiple cytosolic and membrane-bound glutathione transferases (GSTs) which catalyse the conjugation of various electrophilic compounds with glutathione (Sato et al., 1990; Daniel, 1993). The soluble GSTs also act as carrier proteins for lipophilic toxicants, increasing their availability to phase I enzymes (cytochrome P450s). By covalently binding electrophilic compounds, they reduce the likelihood of these compounds binding to other macromolecules (Stegeman et al., 1992). There are at least five classes or subfamilies of GSTs in mammals: alpha, mu, pi, sigma and theta. Many xenobiotics transcriptionally activate GST genes through their antioxidant responsive element (Hayes and Pulford, 1995). Classical inducers of drug metabolism such as phenobarbitone, polycyclic aromatic hydrocarbons and polychlorinated biphenyls are known to induce GSTs.

However, results using GSTs as biomarkers of pollutant exposure in investigations on mussels and fish from polluted estuary and river sites have been equivocal. An increase in total GST levels has been shown in mussels taken from polluted estuary sites, although this did not appear to be due to reactive oxygen species or changes in salinity as animals were transplanted from one site to another (Fitzpatrick et al., 1997). Another recent report demonstrated an increase in total GST activity in fish taken from polluted urban areas with a decrease in the activity of the pi class of GSTs. This suggested that there was inactivation of the enzyme due to the presence of lipohydroperoxides. In the same fish there was an increase in the mu class of GSTs, which are very active with several mutagens and DNA hydroperoxides (Lenártová et al., 1997).

Identification of the specific form of GST which is altered in an organism on exposure to xenobiotics or pollution would appear to make a far more powerful tool both as a marker of response but also potentially as markers of exposure to specific types of xenobiotics. Thus, the expression of some of the GST genes could act as biomarkers of oxidative stress. As individual GSTs may be active against specific classes of compounds such as carcinogens, antitumour drugs and environmental pollutants, their induction could be used as biomarkers for more specific substrates (Lenártová et al., 1997).

Epoxide Hydrolases

Epoxide hydrolases compete with the GSTs for epoxide substrates produced by the monooxygenase system. In mammals microsomal epoxide hydrolase is slightly inducible **(Table 4)**, but the cytosolic form does not appear to be. There is little evidence for an inducible form in aquatic species (Stegeman et al., 1992).

Enzyme Inhibition

Acetylcholinesterase (AChE)

Acetylcholinesterase (AChE) inhibition by organophosphorus and carbamate compounds (including nerve gas and pesticides) is well understood as the inhibition is linked directly with the mechanism of toxic action of these compounds. The measurement of AChE and other cholinesterases (ChE) such as butyrylcholinesterase and non-specific esterases such as carboxylesterases in blood has been established as a suitable marker of AChE activity in the brain (Walker and Thompson, 1991; Mayer et al., 1992; Thompson and Walker, 1994). In small mammals such as wood mice and shrews it would appear that measuring whole blood ChE as an indicator of brain AChE activity may be a superior measure as the inhibition of blood ChE activity remains for a longer period of time (Dell'Omo et al., 1996). The method also provides a less destructive method for sampling wild life and offers the possibility of re-sampling. The inhibition of AChE activity by tetraethyllead in vitro and in vivo has also been reported, and there has been a recent report of uranium inhibiting AChE activity in earthworms, molluscs and fish (Labort et al., 1996).

D-Aminolevulinic Acid Dehydrase (ALAD)

The dose-dependent inhibition of ALAD by lead can be shown in fish, birds and mammals. It appears that ALAD is inhibited before other signs of toxicity from lead become apparent, making this a sensitive early marker of the effect of lead exposure before overt lead toxicity is manifested (Haux *et al.*, 1986); see also haem synthesis above.

Biomarkers of Oxidative Stress

Oxidative Stress

Free radical damage is caused by highly reactive chemical species with unpaired electrons which are generated both endogenously and via xenobiotically mediated processes. Quantitatively, the most important biological free radicals are the superoxide free radical anion ($O_2^{\bullet-}$), the most reactive and damaging oxygen free radical, the hydroxyl radical ($^{\bullet}OH$) and hydrogen peroxide (H_2O_2) (Halliwell and Gutteridge, 1989; deZwart, 1997). Many cell components are targets for free radical attack, the key targets being proteins, phospholipids (producing highly reactive molecules such as aldehydes as a result of lipid peroxidation) and DNA. This can lead to enzyme malfunction, membrane damage and hydroxylation of DNA nucleotides which is implicated in mutagenesis and carcinogenesis **(Figure 7)**.

Although generated endogenously, there are many redox-active compounds, including quinones such as adriamycin, nitroaromatics, aromatic hydroxylamines, bipyridyls such as paraquat and some transition metal chelates, which can result in radical mediated injury. Metabolism of aromatic hydrocarbons can also result in the production of oxyradicals, both benzene and carbon tetrachloride being examples.

Products of Free Radical Damage

The potential clinical consequences of an increase in oxygen free radicals has made markers of oxidative stress an important area of biomarker research. The free radicals themselves could act as biomarkers of this toxic effect. However, the free radicals may not necessarily be specific for a particular toxicant and their highly reactive nature makes them hard to identify. Nevertheless, the products of free radical attack are more stable and can be measured as indirect evidence of free radical damage **(Figure 8)**.

Thus, the products of oxidative damage to nucleotides in DNA such as 8-hydroxy-deoxyguanosine (8-OH-dG) and thymidine glycol can be identified in human urine, where they are eliminated within 24 h with little or no further metabolism taking place. As 8-OH-dG is a product of DNA damage, the possibility also arises that this

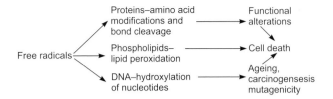

Figure 7 Free radical damage to macromolecules results in modifications to biomolecules and synthesis of small molecules which can be used as biomarkers of free radical damage.

could act as a potential cancer biomarker (Wild and Pisani, 1997). However, there has been some concern voiced over the apparent high frequency of these adducts appearing both in urine and as a direct result of DNA damage during the analysis. This may be the result of both increased oxidation of the DNA bases during the experimental work-up of DNA samples and possibly the breakdown products of DNA from dead kidney cells appearing in the urine (Collins *et al.*, 1996). Some of the short-chain alkanes derived from lipid peroxidation of cellular membranes can be identified in breath and include ethane, propane, *n*-butane and isopentane. Other lipid degradation products such as the aldehydes, *n*-alkenals and malondialdehyde have also been used extensively as indicators of lipid peroxidation, many in urine samples from experimental animals (deZwart *et al.*, 1997). More recently, prostaglandin-like compounds known as isoprostanes have been identified as products of free radical attack on arachidonic acid.

Besides identifying reactive radicals and their products, it is possible to measure the antioxidant status of the organism. The antioxidant defence systems could be divided into two categories

- Enzymatic antioxidant systems such as superoxide dismutase, catalase, peroxidases and glutathione reductase and
- Non-enzymatic oxidants such as vitamins E and A and glutathione (GSH), also measured as the ratio of reduced GSH to oxidized GSH (GSH: GSSG).

Oxidative or metabolic stress can also be measured under experimental conditions as an alteration in ATP levels or the ATP:ADP:AMP ratio.

Any changes in the levels of these enzymes, antioxidants or energy status are therefore indirect biomarkers of free radical generation and/or oxidative stress and therefore biomarkers of effect.

Antioxidant Enzymes

Superoxide Dismutase (SOD)

SODs are a highly inducible group of metalloenzymes which are present in all aerobic organisms, including

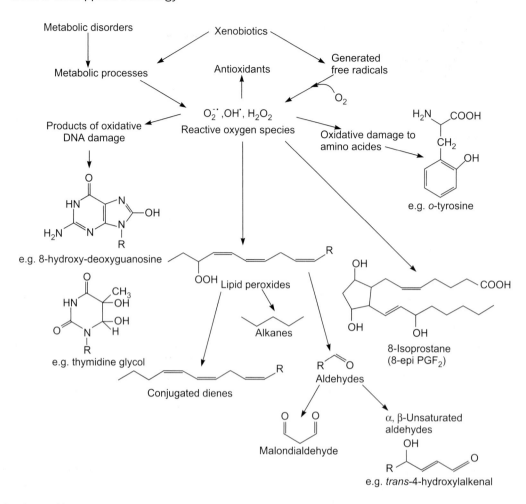

Figure 8 Products of free radical attack which can be identified in urine samples R = deoxyribose. Modified from deZwart (1997).

plants. The different forms are compartmentalized within the cell, which can be useful for determining the main site of oxidant activity. Thus mitochondrial SOD activity (MnSOD) can be distinguished from cytosolic SOD (CuZnSOD), which is inhibited by cyanide. Separating the different isoenzymes by electrophoresis also gives the opportunity for detecting the induction of specific isoforms.

Catalase (CAT)

CAT catalyses the decomposition of the H_2O_2 formed in peroxisomes and microbodies during fatty acid metabolism. Certain hypolipidaemic drugs and some phthalate esters used as plasticizers cause a marked increase in peroxisomes. This is turn increases fatty acid metabolism, resulting in a marked increase in H_2O_2 production. In rodents, these peroxisome proliferators are known to be non-genotoxic carcinogens. The induction in CAT may not be sufficient to remove the excess H_2O_2 generated. Therefore, the induction of CAT may have potential as a biomarker for excess H_2O_2 production. CAT is also found in erythrocytes, independent of peroxisomes. An increase in the activity in these cells is potentially

more useful as a marker of oxidative stress as the activity can be measured independently of fatty acid oxidation. As carnitine acetyl CoA transferase is another peroxisomal enzyme, an increase in peroxisomes will also result in an increase in this enzyme (Di Giuilio *et al.*, 1989).

Peroxidases

The group of enzymes which make up the peroxidases is very large and diverse. Selenium-dependent peroxidase reduces H_2O_2 using glutathione as the cofactor. Selenium-independent peroxidation is sometimes measured at the same time in toxicological investigations. This group of enzymes includes the glutathione *S*-transferase enzyme. The activity of the two enzymes can be distinguished from each other by using the two different substrates, H_2O_2 and *tert*-butylhydroperoxide.

Glutathione Reductase

Glutathione reductase is responsible for maintaining a high GSH:GSSG ratio, which means that it is not a direct antioxidant, but helps to maintain the antioxidant capacity of the cell. It also appears to be another inducible enzyme when there is an increase in the generation of oxidants in a cell. The measurement of this enzyme, in combination with the GSH:GSSG ratio, is important.

PROTEIN SYNTHESIS—SPECIALIZED PROTEINS

Heatshock Proteins

All organisms depend on correctly folded proteins for optimal function. Although a certain amount of spontaneous folding can occur in proteins, it is difficult to see how long polypeptide chains are able to do this in isolation from similar molecules which are often present at high concentrations. It has now been realized that the maintenance of protein secondary structure is largely due to the presence of the so-called 'heatshock' proteins or chaperones (Buchner, 1996). These were first identified in 1974 in *Drosophila* by Tissières *et al.*, as proteins which were induced by mild heat treatment. These proteins are expressed constitutively and are highly conserved through evolution. The main groups which are recognized are referred to by their apparent molecular weight and are hsp90, hsp70, hsp60 (chaperonin), a low molecular weight heat shock protein hsp20–30 and ubiquitin (an 8 kDa protein) (Aoki *et al.*, 1990; Blake *et al.*, 1990; Donati *et al.*, 1990).

The synthesis of heatshock proteins is increased dramatically when organisms are exposed to heat, salinity stress and anoxia. However, they also respond to xenobiotics including teratogens, hepatocarcinogens and chemicals resulting in oxidative stress. It is this response which makes them possible candidates as biomarkers (Martinus *et al.*, 1995). Several methods can be used to measure these proteins directly or indirectly:

- Metabolic labelling followed by autoradiography;
- cDNA probes to measure the mRNA coding for the protein;
- Immunohistochemistry.

Of the different groups of heatshock proteins, the hsp70 group are likely to be the most useful as biomarkers. Hsp72 and hsp73 are highly conserved and, although hsp73 synthesis is constitutive, it shows a rapid increase in the presence of environmental pollutants. On the other hand, hsp72 is not normally found but is rapidly induced in response to environmental stressors. Hence its presence will strongly indicate that the organism has been exposed to environmental stressors (de Pomerai, 1996).

Metallothioneins

Metallothioneins are low molecular weight (6000–12 000 Da), heat-stable proteins containing about 30% cysteine which are normally involved in the transport of metals such as zinc and copper around the body (Kammann *et al.*, 1997). The cysteinyl residues serve as ligands for metal chelation. They are ubiquitous in animals, plants and some eukaryotes and appear to occur as different isoforms (Stegeman *et al.*, 1992).

Although humans possess at least six forms of the protein, most animals have primarily one or two forms. The major role of metallothioneins in normal metabolism appears to be the homeostatic regulation of intracellular zinc and copper availability. By chelating excess heavy metal ions, metallathioneins act as protective proteins against the toxic effects of these metals. However, human metallothioneins are also known to be highly inducible proteins with the different isoforms being differentially regulated at the transcription level by heavy metals, glucocorticoid hormones and cytokines (peptide hormones such as interleukin I and interferon) (Waalkes and Goering, 1990). Although much of our understanding of the induction of metallothionein is the result of work in mammals, they have not been used routinely as biomarkers in mammalian species. The measurement of metallothionein concentration is not easy. It involves purification by gel filtration, followed by ion-exchange chromatography coupled with atomic absorption spectroscopy. It is also possible to identify metallothionein by ELISA, although the antibodies raised against metallothioneins may not provide information about which metal is bound to the protein (Hogstrand and Haux, 1990). This identification is important as different metals appear to induce different metallothioneins. In telecosts, the induction may also take place over a long period of time. For example, this may be as long as 3 weeks following exposure to Cd and the induction may not be more than a few-fold increase (Beyer *et al.*, 1997). However, it is the inducibility of metallothioneins by heavy metals which makes them an attractive and potential biomarker in ecological studies where levels of pollutant metal ions such as cadmium and mercury are of interest.

The half-life of the metal–metallothionein complex varies with the metal bound. Both Cu and Zn are lost when the metallothionein complex is degraded, but Cd remains bound to metallothionein in a steady state of biosynthesis and biodegradation. The Cd-bound metallothionein also appears to be concentrated in the kidneys, which may account for the selective toxicity of Cd in this organ. Other stressors are also known to affect metallothionein levels, such as growth, reproduction and tissue regeneration. There is still a need to investigate the sources of variability in metallothionein expression in the species where it is intended to use metallothionein as a biomarker of metal exposure.

BIOMARKERS AND ENVIRONMENTAL BIOMONITORING

As the impact of human activities on the environment becomes apparent and our ability to measure subtle changes in organisms has improved, the successful application of biomarker monitoring in the environment has grown in importance.

The interrelationships between fauna and flora in an ecosystem mean that any organism which is adversely affected by chronic toxicity is likely to impact on the other species in the same area. Thus, monitoring sensitive species, their numbers, breeding patterns and general health can provide early warnings of deterioration in environmental quality for other organisms in the area and possibly man. The condition of fish, birds or mammals is usually assessed by the hepatosomatic index (liver weight as a percentage of body weight) and gonadosomatic index (gonads as a percentage of body weight), fat and flesh condition and the overall appearance of the organism (Mayer *et al.*, 1992). These species could be called 'sentinel species'.

Flat fish are an example of a species used as sentinel species. As these live on the sea bed they are likely to be in close contact with any sediments containing chemical pollutants deposited around estuaries and costal ports. Specific examples of species which have been monitored for early molecular and cellular changes in the liver, which could indicate exposure to toxic chemicals include the North Sea dab (*Limanda limanda*) and mussel (*Mytilus edulis*) and the grey mullet (*Oedalechilus labeo* and *Lisa ramada*) from eastern Mediterranean harbours (Moore *et al.*, 1994; Fitzpatrick *et al.*, 1997; Karakoc *et al.*, 1997). The parameters which were measured as biomarkers in these species included glutathione peroxidase, glutathione reductase and glutathione *S*-transferase activity, all of which appeared to be raised in waters which were polluted. Levels of the antioxidant glutathione, however, were generally not altered.

At present, not enough is known about the time– and dose–response relationships of pollutants in these sentinel species to be able to use a suite of biomarkers reliably for monitoring environmental pollution in these organisms. This problem is, however, being addressed under controlled conditions by workers in the field. Thus, organisms have been exposed experimentally to a number of model pollutants such as the polycyclic aromatic hydrocarbon benzo[*a*]pyrene (BaP), the polychlorinated biphenyl 2,3,3′,4,4′,5-hexachlorobiphenyl (PCB-156) and heavy metals such as cadmium. Following exposure, biomarkers of response have been monitored, including glutathione *S*-transferase activity, metallothionein concentration and cytochrome P450 1A induction (Beyer *et al.*, 1997; Fitzpatrick *et al.*, 1997; Fossi *et al.*, 1997). The induction of cytochrome P4501A (CYP1A) has been reported to be very sensitive

to polycyclic aromatic hydrocarbon (PAHs) exposure (Beyer *et al.*, 1997 and Grosvik and Goksoyr, 1996). However, it is also important to understand the interactions between the different pollutants and the subsequent biomarker response. The responses may be different when more than one pollutant is present. For example, the induction of a particular cytochrome P450 isozyme by one pollutant may result in the altered metabolism of the second pollutant. Thus, the order in which the organisms are exposed to different pollutants may be important in determining which biomarkers of response are present. In this respect, Sandvik *et al.* (1997) have shown that the induction of CYP1A and hepatic metallothionein and glutathione *S*-transferase activity is affected differently in the European flounder (*Platichthys flesus* L.) when they are given cadmium, BaP and PCB-156, either in combination or separately.

Hence ecological studies underline the difficulties of applying clinical and laboratory knowledge of biomarkers in the field. Again, the successful use of biomarkers appears to rely on the use of patterns of biomarker changes, in time, in response to different doses and as a result of interactions between stressors.

REFERENCES

Amess, J. (1993). Haematotoxicology. In Ballantyne, B., Marrs, T. and Turner, P. (Eds), *General and Applied Toxicology*, Vol. 1. Stockton Press, New York and Macmillan, Basingstoke, pp. 839–867.

Andrew, T. L., Riley, P. G. and Dailey, H. A. (1990). Regulation of heme biosynthesis in higher animals. In Dailey, H. A. (Ed.), *Biosynthesis of Heme and Chlorophyls*. McGraw-Hill, New York, pp. 163–198.

Aoki, Y., Lipsky, M. M. and Fowler, B. A. (1990). Alteration in protein synthesis in primary cultures of rat proximal tubule epithelial cells by exposure to gallium, indium and arsenite. *Toxicol. Appl. Pharmacol.*, **106**, 462–468.

Bai, C.-L., Canfield, P. J. and Stacey, N. H. (1992). Individual serum bile acids as early indicators of carbon tetrachloride and chloroform induced liver injury. *Toxicology*, **75**, 221–234.

Bales, J. R., Higham, D. P., Howe, I., Nicholson, J. K. and Sadler, P. J. (1984). Use of high resolution proton nuclear magnetic resonance spectroscopy for rapid multi-component analysis of urine. *Clin. Chem.*, **30**, 426–432.

Bernard, A. and Hermans, C. (1997). Biomonitoring of early effects on the kidney or the lung. *Sci. Total Environ.*, **199**, 205–211.

Beyer, J., Sandvik, M., Skåre, J. U., Egaas, E., Hylland, K., Waagbo, R. and Goksoyr, A. (1997). Time-and dose-dependent biomarker responses in flounder (*Platichthys flesus* L.) Exposed to benzo[*a*]pyrene, 2,3,3′,4,4′,5-hexachlorobiphenyl (PCB-156) and cadmium. *Biomarkers*, **2**, 35–44.

Bienvenu, T., Rey, E., Pons, G., d'Athis, P. and Olive, G. (1991). A simple non-invasive procedure for the investigation of cytochrome P-450 IIIA dependent enzymes in humans. *Int. J. Pharmacol. Ther. Toxicol.*, **29**, 441–445.

Blake, M. J., Gershon, D., Fargnoli, J. and Holbrook, N. J. (1990). Discordant expression of heat shock protein mRNA in tissues of heat-stressed rats. *J. Biol. Chem.*, **265**, 15272–15279.

Buchner, J. (1996). Supervising the fold: functional principles of molecular chaperones. *FASEB J.*, **10**, 10–19.

Collins, A. R. Dušinská, M., Gedik, C. M. and Štětina, R. (1996). Oxidative damage to DNA: do we have a reliable biomarker? *Environ. Health Perspect.*, **104**, 465–469.

Daniel, V. (1993). Glutathione *S*-transferases: gene structure and regulation of expression. *CRC Crit. Rev. Biochem. Mol. Biol.*, **28**, 173–207.

Delacruz, L., Moret, M., Guastadisegni, C. and Bach, P. H. (1997). Urinary markers of nephrotoxicity following administration of 2-bromoethanamine hydrobromide: a comparison with hexachlorobutadiene. *Biomarkers*, **2**, 169–174.

Dell'Omo, G., Shore, R. F. and Fishwick, S. K. (1996). The relationships between brain, serum, and whole blood ChE activity in the wood mouse (*Apodemus sylvaticus*) and the common shrew (*Sorex araneus*) after acute sublethal exposure to dimethoate. *Biomarkers*, **1**, 202–207.

DeMatteis, F. and Lim, C. K. (1994). Porphyrins as 'nondestructive' indicators of exposure to environmental pollutants. In Fossi, M. C. and Leonzio, C. (Eds), *Nondestructive Biomarkers in Vertebrates*. Lewis Publishers (CRC Press), Boca Raton, FL, pp. 93–128.

de Pomerai, D. I. (1996). Heat-shock proteins as biomarkers of pollution. *Human Exp. Toxicol.*, **15**, 279–285.

deZwart, L. L. (1997). *Development of Non-invasive Biomarkers for Free Radical Induced Damage*. Thesis, Vrije Universiteit Amsterdam, Chapt. 1.

deZwart, L. L., Venhorst, J., Groot, M., Commandeur, J. N. M., Hermanns, R. C. A., Meerman, J. H. N., Van Baar, B. L. M. and Vermeulen, N. P. E. (1997). Simultaneous determination of eight lipid peroxidation degredation products in urine of rats treated with carbon tetrachloride with electron-capture detection. *J. Chromatogr. B*, **694**, 277–288.

Di Giuilio, R. T., Washburn, P. C., Wenning, R. J., Winston, G. W. and Jewell, C. S. (1989). Biochemical responses in aquatic animals: a review of determinants of oxidative stress. *Environ. Toxicol. Chem.*, **8**, 1103–1123.

Donati, Y. R. A., Slosman, D. O. and Polla, B. S. (1990). Oxidative injury and the heat shock response. *Biochem. Pharmacol.*, **40**, 2571–2577.

Draper, R. P., Creasy, D. M. and Timbrell, J. A. (1996). Comparison of urinary creatine with other biomarkers for the detection of 2-methoxyethanol-induced testicular damage. *Biomarkers*, **1**, 190–195.

Evans, G. O. (1996). General enzymology. In Evans, G. O. (Ed.), *Animal Clinical Chemistry*. Taylor and Francis, London, pp. 59–70.

Fairbrother A. (1994). Clinical biochemistry In Fossi, M. C. and Leonzio, C. (Eds), *Nondestructive Biomarkers in Vertebrates*. Lewis Publishers (CRC Press), Boca Raton, FL, pp. 63–89.

Fitzpatrick, P. O'Halloran J., Sheehan, D. and Walsh, A. R. (1997). Assessment of glutathione *S*-transferase and related proteins in the gill and digestive gland of *Mytilus edulis* (L.) as potential organic pollution biomarkers. *Biomarkers*, **2**, 51–56.

Fossi, M. C., Savelli, C., Casini, S., Franchi, E., Mattei, N. and Corsi, I. (1997). Multi-response biomarker approach in the crab *Carcinus aestuarii* experimentally exposed to benzo[a]-pyrene, polychlorinobiphenyles and methyl-mercury. *Biomarkers*. **2**, 311–319.

Fowler, B. A., Oskarsson, A. and Woods, J. S. (1987). Metal and metalloid-induced porphorinurias: relationships to cell unjury. *Ann. N. Y. Acad. Sci.*, **514**, 172–182.

Foxall, P. J., Lenz, E. M., Lindon, J. C., Neild, G. H., Wilson, I. D. and Nicholson, J. K. (1996). Nuclear magnetic resonance and high-performance liquid chromatography–nuclear magnetic resonance studies on the toxicity and metabolism of ifosfamide. *Ther. Drug Monit.*, **18**, 498–505.

Gartland, K. P. R., Bonner, F. W. and Nicholson, J. K. (1988). Investigations into the biochemical effects of region-specific nephrotoxins. *Mol. Pharmacol.*, **35**, 242–250.

Grosvik, B. E. and Goksoyr, A. (1996). Biomarker protein expression in primary cultures of salmon (*Salmo salar* L.) hepatocytes exposed to environmental pollutants. *Biomarkers*, **1**, 45–53.

Halliwell, B. and Gutteridge, J. M. C. (1989). *Free Radicals in Biology and Medicine*, 2nd edn. Clarendon Press, Oxford.

Haux, C., Larsson, A., Lithner, G. and Sjobeck, M.-L. (1986). A field study of physiological effects on fish in lead-contaminated Lakes. *Environ. Toxicol. Chem.*, **5**, 283–288.

Hayes, J. D. and Pulford, D. J. (1995). The glutathione *S*-transferase supergene family: regulation of GST and the contribution of the isoenzymes to cancer chemoprotection and drug resistance. *Crit. Rev. Biochem. Mol. Biol.*, **30**, 445–600.

Heilmann, L. J., Sheen, Y.-Y, Bigelow, S. W. and Nebert, D. W. (1988). Trout P4501A1: cDNA and deduced protein sequence expression in liver, and evolutionary significance. *DNA*, **7**, 379–387.

Hermans, C. and Bernard, A. (1996). Clara cell protein (CC16): characteristics and potential applications as biomarker of lung toxicity. *Biomarkers*, **1**, 3–8.

Hinton, D. E., Baumann, P. C., Garner, G. R., Hawkins, W. E., Hendricks, J. D. Murchelano, R. A. and Okihiro, M. S. (1992). Histopathologic biomarkers. In Huggett, R. J., Kimerle, R. A., Mehrle, P. M., Jr, and Bergman, H. L. (Eds), *Biomarkers: Biochemical, Physiological, and Histological Markers of Anthropogenic Stress*. Lewis Publishers, Boca Raton, FL, pp. 155–209.

Hogstrand, C. and Haux, C. (1990). A radioimmunoassay for perch (*Perca fluviatilis*) metallathionein. *Toxicol. Appl. Pharmacol.*, **103**, 56–65.

Holmes, E., Foxall, P. J., Neild, G. H., Brown, S. M., Beddell, C. R., Sweatman, B. C., Rahr, E., Lindon, J. C., Spraul, M, and Nicholson, J. K. (1994). Automatic data reduction and pattern recognition methods for analysis of ^{1}H nuclear magnetic resonance spectra of human urine from normal and pathological states. *Anal. Biochem.*, **220**, 284–296.

Huxtable, R. J. (1992). Physiological actions of taurine. *Physiol. Rev.*, **72**, 101–163.

Iles, R. A., Hind, A. J. and Chalmers, R. A. (1985). Use of proton nuclear magnetic resonance spectroscopy in detection and study of organic acidurias. *Clin. Chem.*, **31**, 1795–1801.

Jensen, T. K., Andersson, A. M., Hjollund, N. H., Scheike, T., Kolstad, H., Giwercman, A., Henriksen, T. B., Ernst, E., Bonde, J. P., Olsen, J., McNeilly, A., Groome, NP. and Skakkebaek, N. E. (1997). Inhibin B as a serum marker of spermatogenesis: correlation to differences in sperm concentration and follicle-stimulating hormone levels. A study of 349 Danish men. *J. Clin. Endocrinol. Metab.*, **82**, 4059–4063.

Kammann, U., Grymlas, J., Hein, W. and Steinhart, H. (1997). Metal-binding proteins in bream (*Abrimis brama* L.) caught in the River Elbe. *Biomarkers*, **2**, 125–129.

Karakoc, F. T., Hewer, A., Phillips, D. H., Gaines, A. F. and Yuregir, G. (1997). Biomarkers of marine pollution observed in species of mullet living in two eastern Mediterranean harbours. *Biomarkers*, **2**, 303–309.

Kramer, J. W. (1989). Clinical enzymology. In Kaneko, J. J. (Ed.), *Clinical Biochemistry of Domestic Animals*, 4th edn. Academic Press, San Diego, p. 338.

Labrot, F., Ribera, D., Denis, S. M. and Narbonne, J. F. (1996). *In vitro* and *in vivo* studies of potential biomarkers of lead and uranium contamination: lipid peroxidation, acetylcholinesterase, catalase and glutathione peroxidase activities in three non-mammalian species. *Biomarkers*, **1**, 21–28.

Lenártová, V., Holovská, K., Pedrajas, J.-R., Martinez-Lara, E., Peinado, J., López-Barea, J., Rosival, I. and Kosúth, P. (1997). Antioxidant and detoxifying fish enzymes as biomarkers of river pollution. *Biomarkers*, **2**, 247–252.

Lock, E. A. (1993). Responses of the kidney to toxic compounds. In Ballantyne, B., Marrs, T. and Turner, P. (Eds), *General and Applied Toxicology*, Vol. 1. Stockton Press, New York and Macmillan, Basingstoke, pp. 507–536.

Martinus, R. D., Ryan, M. T., Naylor, D. J., Herd, S. M. Hoogenraad, N. J. and Hoj, P. B. (1995). Role of chaperones in the biogenesis and maintenance of the mitochondrion. *FASEB J.* **9**, 371–378.

Mathews, J. M., Raymer, J. H., Velez, G. R., Garner, C. E. and Bucher, J. R. (1996). The influence of cytochrome P450 enzyme activity on the composition and quality of volatile organics in expired breath. *Biomarkers*, **1**, 196–201.

Mayer, F. L., Versteeg, D.J., McKee, M. J., FolMar, L. C., Graney, R. L., McCume, D. C. and Rattner, B. A. (1992). Physiological and nonspecific biomarkers. In Huggett, R. J., Kimerle, R. A., Mehrle, P. M., Jr, and Bergman, H. L. (Eds), *Biomarkers: Biochemical, Physiological, and Histological Markers of Anthropogenic Stress*. Lewis Publishers, Boca Raton, FL, pp. 5–85.

Melancon, M. J., Alscher, R., Benson, W., Kruzynski, G., Lee, R. F., Sikka, H. C. and Spies, R. B. (1992). Metabolic products as biomarker. In Huggett, R. J., Kimerle, R. A., Mehrle, P. M., Jr, and Bergman, H. L. (Eds), *Biomarkers: Biochemical, Physiological, and Histological Markers of Anthropogenic Stress*. Lewis Publishers, Boca Raton, FL, pp. 87–123.

Misulis, K. E., Clinton, M. E. and Dettbarn, W.-D. (1993). Toxicology of skeletal muscle. In Ballantyne B., Marrs, T. and Turner, P. (Eds), *General and Applied Toxicology*, Vol. 1. Stockton Press, New York and Macmillan, Basingstoke, pp. 715–742.

Moor, M., Köhler, A., Lowe, D. M. and Simpson, M. G. (1994). An integrated approach to cellular biomarkers in fish. In Fossi, M. C. and Leonzio, C. (Eds), *Nondestructive Biomarkers in Vertebrates*. Lewis Publisher (CRC Press), Boca Raton, FL, pp. 171–197.

Nicholson, J. K., Timbrell, J. A. and Sadler, P. J. (1985). Proton NMR spectra of urine as indicators of renal damage: mercury-induced nephrotoxicity in rats. *Mol. Pharmacol.*, **27**, 644–651.

Ohnhaus, E. E. and Park, B. K. (1979). Measurement of urinary 6β-hydroxycortisol excretion as an *in vivo* parameter in the clinical assessment of the microsomal enzyme inducing capacity of antipyrine, phenobarbitone and rifampicin. *Eur. J. Clin. Pharmacol.*, **13**, 139–145.

Payne, J. F., Fancey L. L., Rahimtula, A. D. and Porter, E. L. (1987). Review and perspective on the use of mied-function oxygenase enzymes in biological monitoring. *Comp. Biochem. Physiol.*, **86C**, 233–245.

Piomelli, S. (1987). Lead poisoning. In Nathan, D. G. and Garratty, G. (Eds), *Hematology of Infancy and Childhood*, 3rd edn. Saunders, Philadelphia, pp. 389–412.

Reader, C. S. J., Shingles, C. and Stonard, M. D. (1991). Acute testicular toxicity of 1,3-dinitrobenzene and ethylene glycol monomethyl ether in the rat: evaluation of biochemical effect markers and hormonal responses. *Fundam. Appl. Toxicol.*, **16**, 61–70.

Russell, R. G. (1997). The assessment of bone metabolism *in vivo* using biochemical approaches. *Horm. Metab. Res.*, **29**, 138–144.

Sandvik, M., Beyer, J., Goksoyr, A., Hylland, K., Egaas, E. and Skaare, U. (1997). Interaction of benzo[a]pyrene, 2,3,3′,4,4′,5-hexachlorobiphenyl (PCB-156) and cadmium on biomarker responses in flounder (*Platihthyf flasus* L.) *Biomarkers*, **2**, 153–160.

Sanins, S. M., Nicholson, J. K., Elcombe, C. and Timbrell, J. A. (1990). Hepatotoxin-induced hypertaurinuria: a proton NMR study. *Arch. Toxicol.*, **64**, 407–411.

Sato, K., Satoh, K., Hatayama, I., Tamai, K. and Sten, H. (1990). Glutathione S-transferases and (pre)neoplasia. In Hayes, J. D., Pickett, C. B. and Mantle, T. G. (Eds), *Glutathione S-transferases and Drug Resistance*, Taylor and Francis, London, pp. 389–398.

Seidegard, J., Dahlstrom, K. and Kullberg, A. (1998). Effect of grapefruit juice on urinary 6β-hydroxycortisol cortisol excretion. *Clin. Exp. Pharmacol. Physiol.* **25**, 379–381.

Shihabi, Z. K. (1995). Myoglobinuria detection by capillary electrophoresis. *J. Chromatogr. B*, **669**, 53–58.

Stegeman, J. J. (1989). Cytochrome P450 forms in fish: Catalytic, immunological and sequence similarities. *Xenobiotica*, **19**, 1093–1110.

Stegeman, J. J., Brouwer, M., Di Giulio, R. T., Förlin, Fowler, B. A., Sanders, B. M. and Van Veld, P. A. (1992). Enzyme and protein synthesis as indicators of contaminant exposure and effect. In Huggett, R. J., Kimerle, R. A., Mehrle, P. M., Jr, and Bergman, H. L. (Eds), *Biomarkers: Biochemical, Physiological, and Histological Markers of Anthropogenic Stress*. Lewis Publishers, Boca Raton, FL, pp. 235–335.

Stonard, M. D. (1987). Proteins, enzymes and cells in urine as indicators of the site of renal damage. In Bach, P. H. and Lock, E. A. (Eds), *Nephrotoxicity in the Experimental and Clinical Situation*, Vol. 2. Nijhoff, Lancaster, pp. 563–592.

Stonard, M. D. (1996). Assessment of nephrotoxicity. In Evans, G. O. (Ed.), *Animal Clinical Chemistry*. Taylor and Francis, London, pp. 87–96.

Thiede, M. A., Smock, S. L., Petersen, D. N., Grasser, W. A., Thompson, D. D. and Nishimoto, S. K. (1994). Presence of messenger ribonucleic acid encoding osteoclacin, a marker of bone turnover, in bone marrow megakaryocytes and peripheral blood platelets. *Endocrinology*, **135**, 929–937.

Thompson, H. M. and Walker, C. H. (1994). Blood esterases as indicators of exposure to organophosphorous and carbamate insecticides. In Fossi, M. C. and Leonzio, C. (Eds), *Nondestructive Biomarkers in Vertebrates*. Lewis Publishers (CRC Press), Boca Raton, FL, pp. 37–62.

Timbrell, J. A., Draper, R. and Waterfield, C. J. (1994). Biomarkers in toxicology–new uses for some old molecules? *TEN*, **1**, 4–14.

Timbrell, J. A., Waterfield, C. J. and Draper, R. P. (1995). Use of urinary taurine and creatine as biomarkers of organ dysfunction and metabolic perturbations. *Comp. Haematol. Int.*, **5**, 112–119.

Timbrell, J. A. and Waterfield, C. J. (1996). Changes in taurine as an indicator of hepatic dysfunction and biochemical perturbations: studies *in vivo* and *in vitro*. In Huxtable, R., Azuma, J., Nakagawa, M., Kuriyama, K. and Baba, A. (Eds), *Taurine 2: Basic and Clinical Aspects*. Plenum Press, New York, pp. 125–134.

Tissières, A., Mitchell, H.K. and Tracy, U. M. (1974). Protein synthesis in salivary glands of *Drosophila melanogaster* in relation to chromosome puffs. *J. Mol. Biol.*, **84**, 389–398.

Traina, M. E., Fazzi, P., Urbani, E. and Mantovani, A. (1997). Testicular creatine and urinary creatine–creatinine profiles in mice after the administration of the toxicant methoxyacetic acid. *Biomarkers*, **2**, 103–110.

Van Welie, R. T. H., Van Dijck, R. G. J. M., Vermeulen, N. P. E. and Van Sittert, N. J. (1992). Mercapturic acids, protein aducts, and DNA adducts as biomarkers of electrophilic chemicals. *Crit. Rev. Toxicol.*, **22**, 271–306.

Waalkes, M. P. and Goering, P. L. (1990). Metallathionein and other cadmium-binding proteins: recent developments. *Chem. Res. Toxicol.*, **3**, 281–288.

Walker, C. H. and Thompson, H. M. (1991). Phylogenetic distribution of cholinesterases and related esterases. In Mineau, P. (Ed.), *Cholinesterase-inhibiting Insecticides*. Elsevier, Amsterdam, pp. 1–18.

Waterfield, C. J., Turton, J.A., Scales, M. D. C. and Timbrell, J. A. (1991). Taurine, a possible marker of liver damage: a study of taurine excretion in carbon tetrachloride-treated rats. *Arch. Toxicol.*, **65**, 548–555.

Waterfield, C. J., Turton, J. A., Scales, M. D. C. and Timbrell, J. A. (1993a). Investigations into the effects of various hepatotoxic compounds on urinary and liver taurine levels in rats. *Arch. Toxicol.*, **67**, 244–254.

Waterfield, C. J., Turton, J. A., Scales, M. D. C. and Timbrell, J. A. (1993b). Investigations into the effects of various nonhepatotoxic compounds on urinary and liver taurine levels in rats. *Arch. Toxicol.*, **67**, 538–546.

Waterfield, C. J., Asker, D. S. and Timbrell, J. A. (1996). Does urinary taurine reflect changes in protein metabolism? A study with cycloheximide in rats. *Biomarkers*, **1**, 107–114.

Wild, C. P. and Pisani, P. (1997). Carcinogen–DNA and carcinogen–protein addcts in molecular epidemiology. In Toniolo, P., Boffetta, P., Shuker, D. E. G., Rothman, N., Hulka, B. and Pearce, N. (Eds), *Application of Biomarkers in Cancer Epidemiology*. IARC Scientific Publications No. 142. IARC, Lyon, pp. 143–158.

Woods, J. S., Bowers, M. A. and Davis, H. A. (1991). Urinary porphyrin profiles as biomarkers of trace metal exposure and toxicity: studies on urinary porphyrin excretion patterns in rats during prolonged exposure to methyl mercury. *Toxicol. Appl. Pharmacol.*, **110**, 464–476.

York, M. J. and Evans, G. O. (1996). Electrolyte and fluid balance. In Evans, G. O. (Ed), *Animal Clinical Chemistry*. Taylor and Francis, London, pp. 163–176.

Zimmerman, H. J. (1978). *Hepatotoxicity: the Adverse Effects of Drugs and Other Chemicals on the Liver*. Appleton–Century-Crofts, New York, p. 201.

Chapter 86
Biomarkers of Exposure and Susceptibility

Anthony P. DeCaprio

CONTENTS

INTRODUCTION

A wide variety of measurement tools have been developed with the goal of more accurately determining exposure and individual susceptibility to and effects of xenobiotics. These tools, collectively referred to as 'biomarkers' or 'biological markers', include a myriad of biological end-points, such as macromolecular (DNA and protein) adduct levels, enzyme activities and genetic polymorphisms (National Research Council, 1987, 1991; Henderson *et al.*, 1989; Marx, 1991; WHO, 1993; Albertini *et al.*, 1996; DeCaprio, 1997; Perera, 1997). While certain measurements that qualify as biomarkers (*e.g.* acetylcholinesterase inhibition, lead-induced blood changes) have been used for many years to indicate exposure, only recently have major efforts been conducted to develop, validate and utilize batteries of multiple biomarkers in human or animal studies (WHO, 1993).

In order for xenobiotic-induced toxicity to occur, a series of cellular and molecular events must take place. This concept is most developed in the field of carcinogenesis, where initiation, promotion and progression are widely recognized stages in cancer development (Harris, 1991). However, this scheme applies equally to non-cancer effects such as neurotoxicity and immunotoxicity (National Academy of Sciences, 1989a, b, 1992; WHO, 1993). When combined, these intermediate stages represent the toxicokinetics, toxicodynamics and mechanism of action of a given xenobiotic under specific exposure conditions. In the past, toxicological and epidemiological methods were not sufficiently sensitive to identify and characterize all of these events; they were instead considered part of a 'black box' **(Figure 1)** linking exposure and disease (Perera, 1987; Selikoff and Landrigan, 1992). Because of the lack of reproducible methods for measuring these events, they could not be easily employed

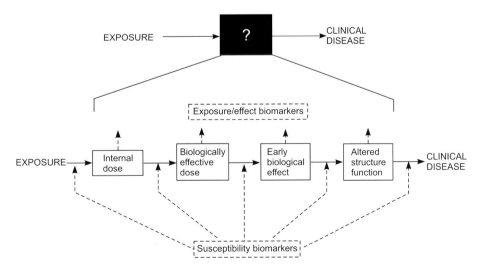

Figure 1 The biomarker paradigm linking exposure with disease and showing expansion of the classical epidemiological 'black box' to reveal discrete mechanistic stages. Reprinted with permission from *Environ. Sci. Technol.* (1997) **31**, pp. 1837–1848. Copyright 1997 American Chemical Society.

for predicting risk associated with exposure to xenobiotics.

The biomarker paradigm was first formalized in a 1987 report by the National Research Council (NRC) of the National Academy of Sciences (National Research Council, 1987). The NRC recognized that any or all of the events that occur sequentially between exposure to a xenobiotic and development of clinical disease might represent useful biomarkers. The report established three general classes of biomarkers, those for exposure, effect and susceptibility, and provided consensus definitions for each. It was recognized that classification of a particular end-point may involve some ambiguity and that the distinctions between sequential events in the biomarker pathway may frequently be blurred. The NRC report also emphasized that the link between exposure and disease is likely to be a continuum rather than a series of distinct events. The present chapter examines exposure and susceptibility biomarkers in the context of toxicological assessment in humans and animal models. Effect and response biomarkers are discussed in Chapter 85 and additional general issues are discussed in Chapter 84.

BIOMARKERS OF EXPOSURE

Introduction

Measurement of exposure to chemical substances under occupational, environmental or experimental scenarios has classically involved one of three general approaches: the determination of ambient levels of the substance of concern, the estimation of exposure through questionnaire data coupled with modelling procedures and the assumption of equivalency between applied dose and internal exposure (Sampson *et al.*, 1994). Although convenient, these measures are of variable accuracy, since they generally ignore important toxicokinetic and toxicodynamic factors that influence dose to the target site. Several categories of exposure biomarkers have evolved that theoretically address the shortcomings of and provide more relevant information than external dosimetric measures.

It has long been recognized that simple determination of ambient levels of xenobiotics in various media (air, water, food) does not always correlate with uptake into an organism. Consequently, one major use of exposure biomarkers is to define more accurately the amount of toxicant that has successfully crossed physiological barriers to enter the organism, i.e. the 'internal dose' **(Figure 2)**. When used in this manner, exposure biomarkers can reflect bioavailability and be influenced by numerous parameters such as route of exposure, physiological characteristics of the receptor and chemical characteristics of the xenobiotic (National Research Council, 1991). Exposure biomarkers have the

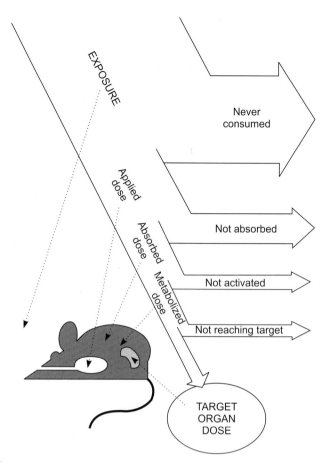

Figure 2 Representation of the relationships between ambient exposure and critical target dose and the progressive decrease in effective exposure due to various biological barriers. Source: *Low-Dose Extrapolation of Cancer Risks: Issues and Perspectives*, p. 188. Used with permission. © 1995 International Life Sciences Institute, Washington, DC, U.S.A.

advantage of providing an integrated measure of chemical uptake, a consideration that is important in the case of agents that exhibit large route-dependent differences in absorption.

The simplest indicator of internal dose is the blood concentration of a chemical agent measured at various times following exposure (Henderson *et al.*, 1989). Some disagreement exists as to whether these measurements are true biomarkers or are more appropriately considered under the older expression 'biomonitoring' (Naumann *et al.*, 1993). Regardless of the term used, blood levels do provide more relevant exposure information than can be obtained from the measurement of ambient levels. Determining xenobiotic metabolites in selected biological media represents a more sophisticated and relevant measure of internal dose, particularly if the metabolites are active or critical to the toxic effects seen. In addition, rapid metabolism of some xenobiotics can make the detection of the parent compound in body fluids virtually impossible. Measurement of metabolites in blood or urine can significantly extend the useful time frame of internal dose assessment following an acute exposure episode (Larsen, 1995). Urinary metabolites have been employed for many years as biological exposure indices (BEIs) for various agents in occupational exposure settings (Howe *et al.*, 1986; Schulte, 1991).

Simple measurement of concentrations of toxic substances in the blood, urine or other accessible body compartments does not always correlate with the level of toxicity present in the target organ or tissue. The concept of 'biologically effective dose' has evolved to reflect the fraction of total exposure that is directly associated with a given level of toxic effect (Perera and Weinstein, 1982). This fraction is almost always less than one. The fraction of absorbed dose that reaches the target tissue, the target macromolecule and finally the critical receptor site is determined by the toxicokinetics and physicochemical characteristics of the xenobiotic (Rhomberg, 1995). Markers of biologically effective dose are generally considered to include macromolecular reaction products (*i.e.* DNA and protein adducts), breakdown products of adducted DNA in urine and certain chromosomal alterations such as sister chromatid exchange (SCE) (National Research Council, 1987). There is some overlap in the assignment of these end-points to the various biomarker categories. For example, macromolecular adducts may also be used as internal dose markers, depending on their tissue source as compared to the ultimate target organ.

In general, blood protein adducts cannot be considered as effective dose biomarkers for carcinogens, since their source is seldom the actual target tissue for these carcinogens. Thus, blood protein adducts are most often used as 'surrogates' for dose to the relevant tissue or organ (Hemminki *et al.*, 1995). This problem applies even for DNA adducts, since in few if any reported instances has xenobiotic-induced adduction of a specific base within a particular DNA sequence in a target cell type been unequivocally linked to a specific clinical outcome in people (DeCaprio, 1997). Despite these concerns, many studies have shown good correlations between exposure markers in surrogate as compared to target tissues **(Figure 3)**. Chromosomal changes such as SCE can also be considered as a marker of early biologic effect (Albertini *et al.*, 1996) (see Chapter 49).

Types of Exposure Biomarkers

Several general classifications of exposure biomarkers have been recognized and explored (National Research Council, 1987; Sampson *et al.*, 1994). These vary greatly in specificity, sensitivity, temporal range of usefulness and technical feasibility. Major types of markers are discussed below.

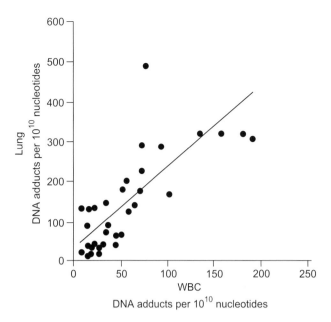

Figure 3 Concept of 'surrogate' marker of target dose, showing correlation between DNA adducts in white blood cells (surrogate tissue) compared with lung cells (target tissue) in lung cancer patients. Adapted from Christiani (1996), with permission.

Xenobiotics and Metabolites in Body Fluids

As mentioned previously, measurements of chemical substances and their metabolites in body fluids such as blood, plasma, serum and urine have been employed as biomarkers of internal exposure for decades. Examples of fields where they are commonly utilized include clinical toxicology (measurement of therapeutic and toxic levels of pharmaceutical agents), forensic toxicology (evaluation of exposure to poisons and substances of abuse) and occupational health (determination of compliance with occupational exposure standards and guidelines). Unless the target tissue is the sampled body fluid itself, none of these measurements can be considered as true markers of effective or critical dose. Nonetheless, many of them have been validated over the years and exhibit predictive value for assessing the potential for toxic effects in a particular target organ or system. The techniques employed for these determinations are extremely varied, and include physicochemical methods of separation and/or analysis (e.g. visible, UV, IR, atomic absorption, fluorescence and mass spectrometry, gas, liquid, and thin-layer chromatography and electrochemical methods). Details regarding biomonitoring of chemical agents can be found elsewhere in this book (Chapter 87) and in other general toxicology references.

Macromolecular Adducts

Much of toxicology, and in particular carcinogenesis, is based on the paradigm of the reactive xenobiotic, a

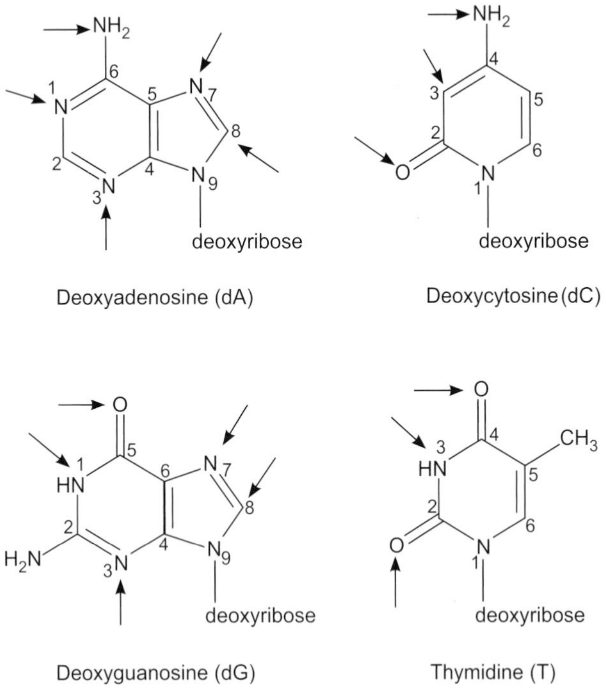

Figure 4 Nucleophilic adduction sites (arrows) for reactive xenobiotics in the four DNA bases. Not all sites are equally reactive with all xenobiotics. The phosphate moiety of the DNA chain (not shown) is also a potential reaction site.

parent compound, metabolite or short-lived intermediate that can combine covalently with macromolecules to cause damage, ultimately triggering cellular alterations, abnormal proliferation and/or death (Miller and Miller, 1981; Gillette, 1986). Both protein and DNA contain nucleophilic sites that are capable of reacting with elec-

trophilic xenobiotics to yield adducts (**Figures 4** and **5**). For DNA, up to 18 sites are potentially available for adduction, although modification at N-7 and N-3 of guanine and adenine, O-6 of guanine and O-2 and O-4 of guanine is most commonly encountered (Farmer and Sweetman, 1995). For proteins, reactive sites include thiol, amino (primary and secondary amine nitrogen), carboxyl and hydroxyl side-chains in addition to the N-terminal amino function, although the latter is often blocked in cellular proteins (Skipper and Tannenbaum, 1990). As with all nucleophiles, the relative rate and extent of reactivity of a given site will be governed by its electron density and polarizability (i.e. 'hard' vs 'soft' nucleophilic character) and by the nature of the electrophile (Swain and Scott, 1953; Pearson and Songstad, 1967). In addition, steric factors will influence the reactivity of specific protein sites, since some will be more or less accessible owing to the tertiary structure of a given protein. The theoretical aspects of protein adduction have been discussed in depth by various authors (Ehrenberg et al., 1983; Tannenbaum et al., 1993; Skipper, 1996), and the relationships between a xenobiotic, its metabolites and possible macromolecular adducts are summarized in **Figure 6**.

Much of the work leading to the current use of macromolecular adducts as exposure biomarkers was based upon earlier studies of endogenous nucleic acid and protein modification (Glazer, 1970; Lutz, 1979; Lawley, 1994). Methylation of RNA and DNA and post-translational modification of proteins were recognized for decades as being normal and necessary cellular processes, and methods were developed to characterize these phenomena. Research on cancer chemotherapeutic

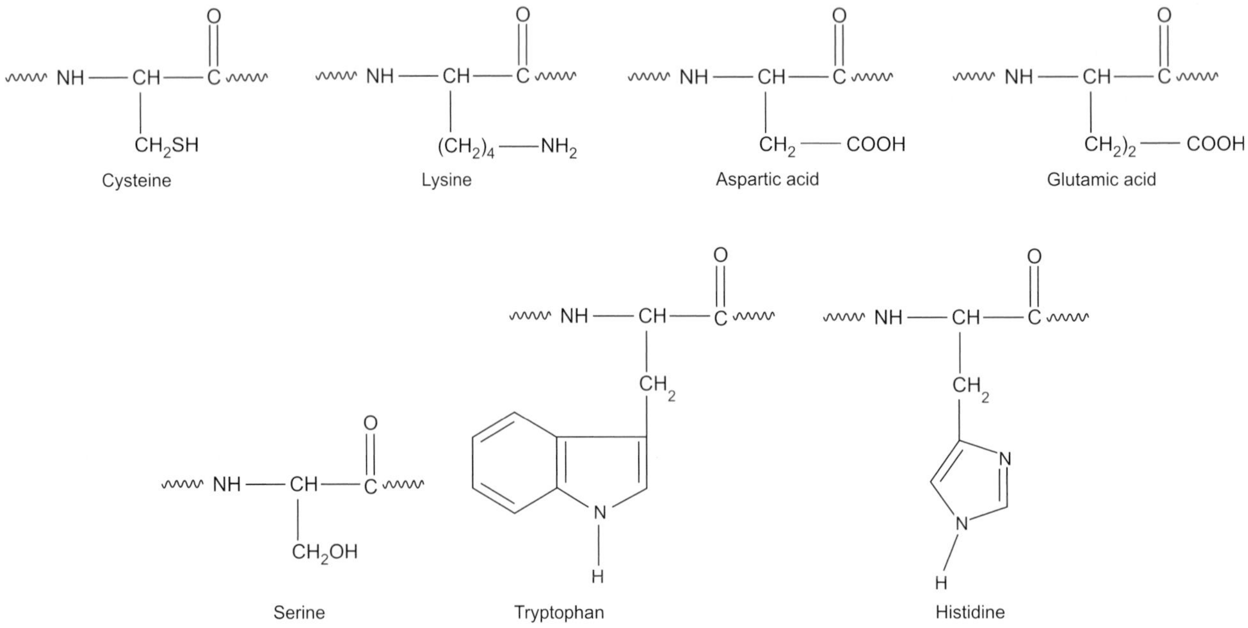

Figure 5 Major nucleophilic side-chains in protein potentially available for reaction with electrophilic xenobiotics. The free amino terminus (not shown) is also a highly reactive site in many proteins.

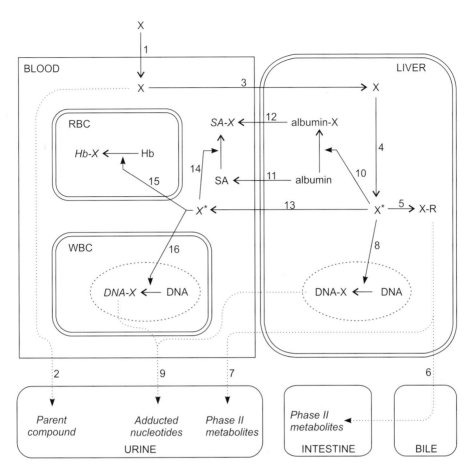

Figure 6 Schematic diagram illustrating the relationships between xenobiotic uptake, metabolism, macromolecular adduction and excretion as related to the measurement of biomarkers of exposure. Numbers indicate various biological processes for xenobiotic **X**, including absorption into blood from the ambient environment (**1**), urinary clearance of unchanged **X** (**2**), distribution of **X** to hepatocytes (**3**), Phase I (oxidative) metabolism to reactive metabolite **X*** (**4**), Phase II metabolism to form detoxified (usually) conjugates **X–R** (*e.g.* glucuronides, sulphates, glutathione conjugates) (**5**), excretion of conjugates from the hepatocyte via bile and faeces (**6**), excretion of conjugates from the hepatocyte via blood and urine (**7**), adduction of hepatocyte DNA by reactive metabolite (**8**), excretion of adducted nucleotides via urine following DNA repair or degradation processes (**9**), direct adduction of albumin within the liver by reactive metabolite (**10**), release of unadducted albumin into the blood from hepatocytes (**11**), release of adducted albumin into the blood from hepatocytes (**12**), release of reactive metabolite into the blood from hepatocytes (**13**), adduction of serum albumin (SA) by reactive metabolite in blood (**14**), adduction of haemoglobin (Hb) in RBCs by reactive metabolite in blood (**15**) and adduction of DNA in WBCs by reactive metabolite in blood (**16**). Derivatives shown in italics can serve as exposure biomarkers.

agents also revealed that many of these drugs were capable of chemically modifying DNA, and that this mechanism was likely to mediate some of their anticancer effects. Similarly, early studies indicated that protein modification by exogenous agents was not uncommon and that this process did not always lead to adverse effects in the organism.

Factors such as the half-life or life-span, relative abundance, ease of sampling and cellular vs extracellular localization strongly influence the choice of specific proteins as biological monitors (Skipper and Tannenbaum, 1990). The first use of protein adducts as exposure biomarkers was by Ehrenberg and co-workers, who proposed haemoglobin (Hb) as a monitor of internal dose of reactive alkenes and epoxides such as ethylene oxide (Osterman-Golkar *et al.*, 1976). It has since been

employed as an exposure monitor for a number of important chemicals (**Table 1**). One advantage in using Hb as a dosimeter is its relatively long lifetime in the bloodstream. The average lifespan of the red blood cell (RBC) in humans is 120 days, after which the cells are taken up by the liver and catabolized (Schnell, 1993). Once formed, Hb (or other protein) adducts are not removed or repaired, although a decreased lifespan for RBCs containing adducted Hb has occasionally been reported for certain chemicals (Carmella and Hecht, 1987). Consequently, Hb can act as a cumulative dosimeter for reactive xenobiotics, and chronic exposure conditions will result in a steady-state level of adducts dependent upon dose level (Henderson *et al.*, 1989; Fennell *et al.*, 1992). Other advantages of Hb as an exposure monitor include the large amounts available

Table 1 Reported human haemoglobin adduct levels for various xenobiotics

Chemical (type of exposure)	Adduct/analyte	Method	Adduct level (nmol g^{-1} haemoglobin)
N, N- Dimethylformamide (occupational)	3-Methyl-5-isopropylhydantoin	Hydrolysis; GC–MS	75–1000 (exposed) 4–12 (control)
Epichlorohydrin (occupational)	N- (2, 3-Dihydroxypropyl)valine	Modified Edman; GC–MS	0.020 (exposed smokers) 0.007 (exposed non-smokers) 0.013 (control smokers) 0.007 (control non-smokers)
Acetaminophen (drug overdose)	3-(Cystein-S-yl)acetaminophen	Immunoassay	100–4100
PAHs (occupational)	BPDE–Hb	Spectrofluorimetry	0.005–0.139
Ethylene oxide (occupational)	N- Hydroxyethylvaline	Modified Edman; GC–MS	5–20 (exposed) 0.1–0.5 (control smokers) 0.01–0.1 (control non-smokers)
Ethene (occupational)	N- Hydroxyethylvaline	Modified Edman; GC–MS	0.02
Propylene oxide (occupational)	N- Hydroxypropylvaline	Modified Edman; GC–MS	0.05–3.5 (exposed) < 0.02 (unexposed)
Acrylonitrile (smoking)	N- Cyanoethylvaline	Modified Edman; GC–MS	0.09
NNK (smoking)	4- Hydroxy-1-(3-pyridyl) butan-1-one	Hydrolysis; GC–MS	0.0015 (smokers) 0.0005 (non-smokers)
4-ABP (smoking)	4-ABP-cysteine	Hydrolysis; GC–MS	0.00025–0.0025 (smokers) 0.00005–0.0005 (non-smokers)
Acrylamide (occupational, smoking)	N- (2-Carbamoylethyl)valine	Modified Edman; GC–MS	9.5 (production workers) 0.054 (laboratory workers) 0.116 (smokers) 0.031 (non-smokers)
Butadiene (occupational)	N- (2,3,4-Trihydroxybutyl)valine	Modified Edman; GC–MS	0.010–0.014 (exposed) 0.002–0.003 (control)
Styrene (occupational)	2-Phenylethanol	Cleavage with Raney nickel, GC–MS	3.7–8.0 (exposed) 2.0–8.6 (control)

in human blood specimens and the relative ease of obtaining such samples.

The major drawback of Hb as an internal dosimeter concerns the need for reactive agents to be sufficiently long-lived and to have appropriate physicochemical characteristics to cross the RBC membrane. Serum albumin (SA) has been proposed as an alternative to Hb for adduct dosimetry. SA is synthesized in hepatocytes and released directly to the circulation, and albumin adducts have been employed as biomarkers of exposure to short-lived metabolites produced in the liver (Wild *et al.*, 1990, 1996; Bechtold *et al.*, 1992; Groopman *et al.*, 1992). The usefulness of SA adducts as exposure markers is limited by the relatively short lifetime of the protein in man (ca 20 days). Other proteins, including histones and collagen, have also been proposed as substrates to monitor *in vivo* exposure to reactive chemicals (Özbal *et al.*, 1994; Skipper *et al.*, 1994). To date, protein adduct biomarkers have been developed for many individual xenobiotics and for several major classes of occupational and environmental toxicants, including polycyclic aromatic hydrocarbons (PAHs), epoxides, aromatic amines,

nitrosamines and aflatoxins (Schnell, 1993; Wild and Pisani, 1998).

DNA adduction has also been extensively explored as a relevant class of exposure biomarker. Literally hundreds of DNA adducts have been structurally characterized over the past several decades, primarily as a consequence of *in vitro* experimentation and studies in experimental animals (Lutz, 1979; Hemminki *et al.*, 1994). Some of the more important of these are illustrated in **Figure 7**. In the early 1980s, the first explicit proposals were made for using DNA adducts as exposure biomarkers for carcinogens in human epidemiologic studies (Perera *et al.*, 1982; Sorsa *et al.*, 1982; Reddy *et al.*, 1984; Wogan and Gorelick, 1985). This work demonstrated, for example, a higher level of PAH–DNA adducts in lung tissue and white blood cell (WBC) DNA from lung cancer patients than in healthy controls, although no data were available for ambient PAH levels. This was followed by a series of studies to correlate PAH–DNA adducts (in addition to other exposure, effect and susceptibility biomarkers) with ambient levels in occupational and environmental exposure scenarios.

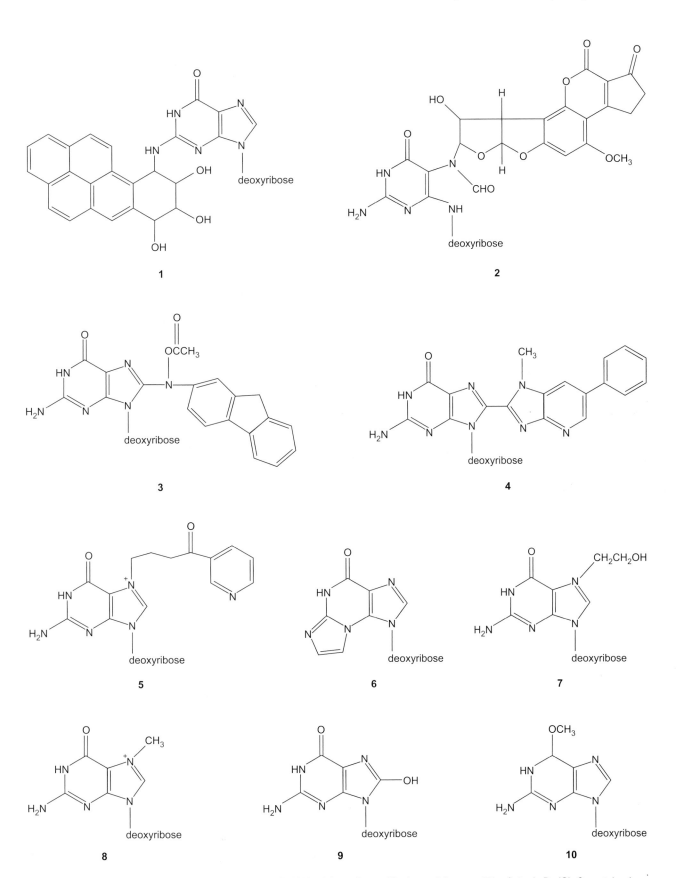

Figure 7 Structures of important deoxyguanosine (dG) DNA adducts formed by benzo[*a*]pyrene (**1**), aflatoxin B$_1$ (**2**), 2-acetylamino-fluorene (**3**), 2-amino-1-methyl-6-phenylimidazopyridine (PhIP) (**4**), NNK (**5**), vinyl chloride (**6**), ethylene oxide and ethene (**7**), various methylating agents (**8** and **10**) and oxidative stress (**9**). Many other structures are possible.

More recently, DNA adducts have been studied as exposure biomarkers for other environmental carcinogens, including aflatoxins, nitrosamines, aromatic amines and certain alkylating agents.

While the mechanistic justification for this approach is obvious (DNA is the target molecule; such adducts can initiate the carcinogenic process), there are numerous theoretical and technical factors that complicate this approach. For example, only rarely does a given carcinogen form a single, chemically distinct adduct with DNA; most reactive carcinogens produce multiple products. It therefore becomes critical to decide which adduct to quantitate as a relevant biomarker. Frequently, methodologies are not available for such specific determinations, and only data for total adduction can be generated. The source of DNA to be sampled will also affect the interpretability of adduct data. Typically, peripheral WBC DNA is utilized in human DNA adduct biomarker studies. However, subpopulations of WBCs differ greatly in their length of residence in the peripheral circulation, with granulocytes being the shortest lived and T-lymphocytes the longest. Significant differences in adduct levels between these cell types in individual people have been detected (Brescia et al., 1997). Rates of DNA repair processes may differ between cell types (Perera, 1996), indicating that WBC DNA may not always be an appropriate surrogate for target tissues of specific carcinogens. Finally, the total mass of DNA obtainable from a typical human blood sample is orders of magnitude less than the amount of Hb or SA available, generating a requirement for much higher sensitivity with DNA adduct measurement technologies.

Several methods are available for the quantitation of protein and DNA adducts as biomarkers for specific xenobiotic exposures. General methodologies for this purpose are complicated by certain technical issues, including whether to analyse the whole adducted macromolecule, hydrolysed samples (i.e. individual amino acids or nucleotides) or individual adducts, the extent of sample clean-up and separation procedures necessary prior to analysis and the analytical methodology to be employed. These are in turn influenced by the sensitivity and specificity required for a particular assay, which depend on the particular exposure scenario. For example, adduct biomarker measurements in an occupational cohort exposed to a single agent would benefit from high specificity, while screening of unknown adducts in a general population with presumed lower level exposure requires high sensitivity. Various methodologies for the quantitation of macromolecular adducts in biomarker studies are discussed below.

Physical Methods of Macromolecular Adduct Analysis

The earliest techniques of protein and DNA adduct analysis involved simple spectrophotometric analysis of blood or tissue samples for adducts that exhibit significant UV or visible light absorbance. Later technical evolution resulted in the initial separation of macromolecules or their cleavage products by techniques such as open column or high-performance liquid chromatography (HPLC), followed by spectrophotometric analysis of the eluates. Such methods are suited for adducts containing aromatic moieties such as PAHs and aromatic amines. While this approach can be appropriate for in vitro, high-dose animal and, in certain cases, occupational studies, its relatively low sensitivity has limited its application as a generic method for human exposure evaluation.

The use of spectrofluorimetry has resulted in order of magnitude increases in sensitivity over spectrophotometry in the detection of certain macromolecular adducts (Weston, 1993). In some cases, fluorescence-based adduct quantitation is of sufficient sensitivity to be employed in human environmental biomarker studies. One of these techniques, scanning synchronous fluorescence spectrophotometry (SFS), has been applied to the detection of both protein and DNA adducts of PAHs and aflatoxins in human and animal studies. Using SFS coupled with HPLC, PAH–DNA adduct levels as low as 1–3 per 10^8 base pairs can be detected (Dale and Garner, 1996). However, SFS is a fairly non-specific technique and is subject to interferences from other fluorescent compounds in the sample. Specificity can be improved by using fluorescence line narrowing spectrophotometry (FLNS), which can provide spectra characteristic of specific adducts (Jankowiak and Small, 1991).

More recently, mass spectrometry (MS) has become extremely important in the field of macromolecular adduct analysis. MS-based methods have the advantage of high specificity, since they can elucidate chemical structure and distinguish between related adducts in addition to providing quantitative information (Farmer and Sweetman, 1995). However, they are usually more labour intensive, require sophisticated instrumentation and often lack the sensitivity of other adduct measurement techniques. The last problem can be overcome to some degree by means of analyte derivatization prior to analysis (Halket, 1993).

Major advances have been made in MS-based techniques for protein adduct analysis. Early methods involved total acid (or base) hydrolysis of isolated globin, serum albumin or other protein followed by chromatographic separation and MS analysis of the modified amino acids. This technique was employed to analyse histidine adducts of ethylene oxide in Hb and S-phenylcysteine adducts formed by benzene exposure in occupational cohorts (Farmer et al., 1986; Bechtold et al., 1992). Although useful in laboratory and pilot studies, the technique is generally too labour intensive and insufficiently sensitive to be applied to larger population studies. In addition, many adducts are not stable under the harsh hydrolysis conditions employed, resulting in poor recovery and/or structural modification of the original adduct.

A milder alternative to this method involves total enzymatic hydrolysis, which uses proteases (at neutral or near-neutral conditions) such as pronase or proteinase-K to effect peptide bond cleavage. This has been successfully employed for both PAH and aflatoxin adduct analysis (Weston *et al.*, 1989; Sheabar *et al.*, 1993).

As an alternative to total protein hydrolysis, mild acid or base treatment has been employed to selectively cleave protein adducts formed by a variety of xenobiotics without destruction of the peptide bond itself (Farmer and Sweetman, 1995). The resulting free adducts can then be derivatized, separated and analysed by a variety of appropriate MS-based techniques, such as HPLC–MS, GC–MS with either electron impact (EI) or negative chemical ionization (NCI) and selected ion monitoring (SIM) or GC with tandem MS (GC–MS–MS). This approach has been employed extensively in the analysis of protein adducts formed by aromatic amines. For example, 4-aminobiphenyl (ABP), an industrially significant carcinogen that is also present in cigarette smoke, undergoes metabolism to an *N*-hydroxylamine and then to a nitrosoarene that subsequently reacts with protein cysteine (Cys) groups to form a sulphinamide adduct. Studies have shown that Cys-93 in the β-chain of human Hb is a major adduction site for the aromatic amines, while the tryptophan residue in human SA is also adducted (Bryant *et al.*, 1987; Farmer and Sweetman, 1995). Rat Hb contains a second highly reactive site at Cys-125 (Skipper and Tannenbaum, 1990). A typical assay involves isolation of Hb from a blood specimen, hydrolysis in 0.1 M NaOH to release the aromatic amine, purification by column chromatography or solid-phase extraction, derivatization (e.g. with pentafluoropropionic anhydride), separation by capillary GC and analysis by MS in the SIM mode. This method, along with the use of appropriate internal and calibration standards, permits quantitation with high reproducibility and sensitivity and has been employed in numerous human occupational and environmental exposure studies.

A similar approach has been employed for Hb adducts of the tobacco-specific nitrosamines *N'*-nitrosonornicotine (NNK) and 4-(methylnitrosamino)-1-(3-pyridyl) butan-1-one, which are metabolized to reactive α-hydroxy derivatives, and for PAHs, which are converted to reactive diol epoxides (Strickland *et al.*, 1993). The major protein reactive site for these metabolites appears to be the carboxyl groups of aspartic and glutamic acids, with the resultant formation of ester adducts, although histidine adduction also occurs with PAHs. Mild base hydrolysis of Hb or SA adducted by the nitrosamines releases 4-hydroxy-1-(3-pyridyl)butan-1-one, which may be readily quantitated by GC–MS. Mild acid hydrolysis of PAH-adducted Hb yields a variety of PAH tetrols, which, following extraction and purification, can be determined by HPLC with fluorescence detection. Alternatively, PAH tetrols can be purified by immunoaffinity chromatography, derivatized and analyzed by GC–MS with SIM. Unlike adducts formed by aromatic amines and nitrosamines, those formed by PAHs appear to be significantly less stable during protein isolation and purification, and great care must be taken to avoid low recovery.

One other major group of xenobiotics that form protein adducts isolatable by hydrolysis are the aflatoxins. Aflatoxins are a group of natural mycotoxins, many of which are carcinogenic in animal bioassays. Aflatoxin B$_1$ (AFB$_1$) is a known human carcinogen linked to high incidences of hepatocarcinoma in certain populations with high exposure to mouldy grains and other food products (Groopman *et al.*, 1994). In contrast to the previously discussed compounds, AFB$_1$ forms adducts primarily with lysine (amine) residues in SA, via reaction of the dialdehyde metabolite (Sabbioni, 1990). Such adducted lysine moieties can be recovered following enzymatic cleavage of the protein. Once recovered, AFB$_1$ adducts can be quantitated either by HPLC with fluorescence detection or by immunochemical techniques (discussed below).

A more recently developed, highly sensitive MS-based method for protein adduct determination, especially for alkylating agents, involves a modification of the Edman degradation technique for *N*-terminal amino acid analysis (Mowrer *et al.*, 1986; Törnqvist, 1991, 1994). In classical Edman degradation **(Figure 8A)**, amino acids are removed sequentially from the *N*-terminus by reaction of the amino group with phenyl isothiocyanate (PITC) in basic solution followed by cleavage of the peptide bond in anhydrous acid. The resulting phenylthiohydantoin (PTH) derivatives are then analysed by HPLC with UV detection. In the modified method, PITC is replaced by perfluorophenyl isothiocyanate (PFPITC) as the derivatizing agent **(Figure 8B)**. In addition, treatment is conducted under milder, slightly basic conditions. Under such conditions, the peptide bond of adducted amino acids is readily cleaved, whereas that of unadducted residues is stable, leading to an enrichment in free adducted amino acids in the solution. The resulting PFPTH residues are analysed qualitatively and quantitatively by GC–MS, with or without NCI, with very high sensitivity. Clean up by solid-phase extraction prior to GC–MS can also be employed to increase sensitivity further. The adducts are quantitated using SIM, with appropriate calibration and internal standards for particular species.

The *N*-terminal valine of Hb has been shown to be adducted by a number of reactive xenobiotics under *in vitro* and *in vivo* conditions, and the modified Edman assay has been applied in human studies to determine Hb adducts following occupational exposure to some of these compounds (Törnqvist, 1991). Major work has been conducted with ethylene oxide (EtO) as a model reactive xenobiotic (Fennell, 1996). EtO is a gas widely employed in sterilization of medical equipment in

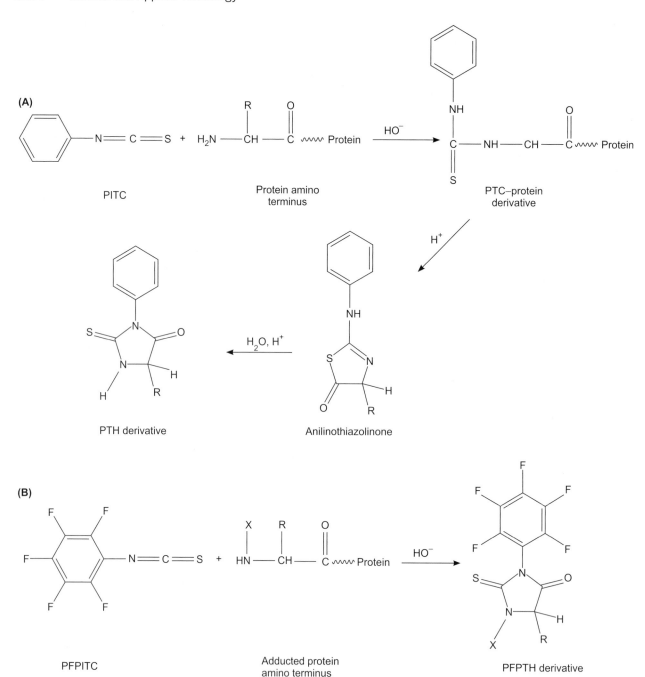

Figure 8 **(A)** Classical Edman degradation of proteins and **(B)** modified method for adducted *N*-terminal valine (or, potentially, other terminal amino acids) PITC, phenyl isothiocyanate; PTH, phenylthiohydantoin; PFPITC, perfluorophenyl isothiocyanate; PFPTH, perfluorophenylthiohydantoin.

hospitals and commercial settings. It is also present in cigarette smoke and as a metabolite of ethylene. EtO forms an *N*-(2-hydroxyethyl)valine (HOEtVal) derivative upon reaction with Hb. Background levels of HOEt-Val in unexposed persons (non-smokers) range from 10 to 100 pmol g^{-1} Hb, whereas smokers exhibit levels of 100–500 pmol g^{-1}. Occupational exposure at an ambient level of 1 ppm is associated with adduct levels as high as 2400 pmol g^{-1} Hb. Related studies have compared levels of Hb adducts of EtO with DNA adducts in various tissues, in order to validate the former as a surrogate marker for adduction at the DNA target site (Walker *et al.*, 1993). In addition to the extensive dataset for EtO, the modified Edman degradation method has been used to determine Hb adducts in human cohorts exposed to propylene oxide, ethene, acrylonitrile, butadiene, benzene, styrene, dimethyl sulphate, glycidyl ethers, dimethylformamide, epichlorohydrin and acrylamide. Application of the technique to proteins other than Hb or to xenobiotics forming bulkier adducts has not been reported.

MS-based methods for determining DNA adducts as exposure biomarkers are less well developed than those for protein adducts. Except for the analysis of adducted DNA bases excreted in urine (discussed below), MS-based techniques have not been applied nearly as extensively in human exposure biomarker studies, although they have been employed in *in vitro* and experimental animal studies (Strickland *et al.*, 1993; Farmer and Sweetman, 1995; Poirier and Weston, 1996). The reasons for this are primarily technical, as DNA is only available in microgram amounts from typical human samples compared with the milligram levels of Hb and SA obtainable. In addition, the nucleic acid components of DNA are less amenable to GC separation than are amino acids derived from proteins. Nevertheless, some progress in this area has been made, and continuing improvements in methodology and sensitivity are expected. The principles involved in DNA adduct analysis by MS are essentially the same as those for protein analysis: purification of the macromolecule, hydrolysis to yield either free adduct, adducted base or individual adducted nucleotides/nucleosides, extraction and clean-up of the sample, derivatization to enhance the volatility of the analyte, GC separation and MS-based analysis.

Most efforts involving human DNA adduct monitoring by spectrometric techniques have involved the determination of alkylated bases excreted in urine following enzymatically mediated base excision repair processes of adducted DNA (Shuker *et al.*, 1993). Such products include N^7- and O^6-alkylguanine and N^3-alkyladenine, which are formed as a result of exposure to alkylating xenobiotics such as nitrosamines and nitrosoureas and to complex mixtures such as tobacco smoke. N^7-Guanine adducts are particularly unstable and are excreted as a result of spontaneous depurination in addition to enzymatic cleavage. Methylated bases are also naturally present in urine, whereas the higher alkylated derivatives are not.

Although alkylated DNA bases in urine are not specific biomarkers of xenobiotic exposure and generally reflect only recent exposure, the low invasiveness of the method and the relatively straightforward analytical technique make this an attractive screening procedure for alkylating agents. Increases in the efficiency and sensitivity of this method have been accomplished by means of an immunoaffinity chromatography extraction step prior to GC–MS analysis. Such an approach has been employed to quantitate N^3-(2-hydroxyethyl)adenine adducts in rat urine following exposure to ethylene oxide, and in human urine as a result of exposure to an unknown dietary component (Walker *et al.*, 1992; Prevost *et al.*, 1993). Human exposure to AFB_1 has also been measured by means of urinary DNA adducts. The major adduct formed by AFB_1 is aflatoxin-N^7-guanine, which can be purified from urine by immunoaffinity chromatography, followed by HPLC separation and UV absorbance detection. Levels of the adduct have been shown to correlate with dietary intake of aflatoxin in highly exposed cohorts.

In contrast to urinary adducts, the determination by MS-based methods of DNA adducts in human WBC DNA has been limited (Weston *et al.*, 1989). At present, immunochemical and 'postlabelling' assays (described below) for WBC DNA adducts are considerably more sensitive and convenient to perform. However, as newer MS-based methods become more developed (Apruzzese and Vouros, 1998; Ranasinghe *et al.*, 1998), they will undoubtedly be employed for DNA adduct analysis in routine biomarker studies. Although such measurements do not strictly qualify as exposure biomarkers, a number of studies have examined DNA adducts by mass spectrometry in human surgical, biopsy and autopsy tissue samples. For example, correlations between tobacco-specific nitrosamine adducts to DNA in human lung and tracheobronchial tissue and individual smoking status have been demonstrated (Foiles *et al.*, 1991). Adducts were determined by mild acid hydrolysis of DNA followed by GC–MS analysis with NCI. In contrast, similar studies did not show a correlation between aromatic amine adducts in human lung DNA and exposure to cigarette smoke (Culp *et al.*, 1997).

Immunochemical Methods of Macromolecular Adduct Analysis

An additional tool for the detection and quantitation of macromolecular adducts is offered by antisera to individual or structurally related groups of xenobiotic adducts (Poirier, 1993; Strickland *et al.*, 1993; Hemminki *et al.*, 1995; Qu *et al.*, 1997). The principle for this methodology is simple: the macromolecular sample is incubated with primary antisera to an adduct in order to form immune complexes. These complexes are then detected and quantitated by measuring a radiolabel bound to the primary antisera or by incubation with a radioisotope-or colorimetric enzyme-labelled secondary antibody to the primary antisera. Both polyclonal and monoclonal antibodies have been developed for DNA and protein adducts in several assay types, including standard radioimmunoassay (RIA), enzyme-linked immunosorbent assay (ELISA) and ultrasensitive enzymatic radioimmunoassay (USERIA) (Strickland *et al.*, 1993). The last two methods are 10–100 times more sensitive than the older RIA technique for the detection of DNA adducts. In addition to their use in quantitation, these antisera can be employed in affinity-based methods for the separation and/or purification of specific adducts (or classes of adducts) from biological matrices such as urine.

Immunoassays for the detection and quantitation of macromolecular adducts can be sensitive, with ELISA and USERIA capable of detecting one adduct per 10^8 base pairs with a DNA sample of 50 μg. Considerable effort is required to produce and characterize the antisera needed for these assays, although once antisera are available, the assays are technically straightforward and do not require sophisticated instrumentation. Specificity is a critical issue for these assays, since antisera will differ in their affinity for adducts produced by a given xenobiotic. Immunoassays that employ antisera of lower specificity have the advantage of detecting a wider range of adducts in a single test, owing to cross-reactivity with multiple chemical structures. This is an important consideration for conducting screening studies in large cohorts. Alternatively, a high-specificity antiserum is important when quantitating specific adducts or when attempting to determine the confounding influence of complex exposures.

Extensive immunochemical measurement of DNA adducts in human blood and tissue samples as biomarkers of xenobiotic exposure has been performed for the PAHs. These compounds have been investigated as prototypical chemical carcinogens that are significant in both environmental and occupational settings. The most important carcinogenic PAHs are benzo[a]pyrene (BaP) and pyrene, which are the products of incomplete combustion of organic matter (Dellomo and Lauwerys, 1993). For BaP, metabolism by cytochrome P450 (CYP) 1A1 results in the formation of the reactive diolepoxide 7β, 8α-dihydroxy-9α,10α-epoxy-7,8,9,10-tetrahydro-benzo[a]pyrene (BPDE), which can adduct DNA, primarily at N^2-guanine (Beland and Poirier, 1989) (see **Figure 7**). Unrepaired BPDE–DNA adducts can produce mutations (primarily G–T transversions) that can ultimately result in tumour formation (Beland and Poirier, 1989).

Relevant biomarker studies using human WBC DNA in immunoassays have been reported for exposure to PAHs during smoking, consumption of charcoal broiled food, occupational scenarios (roofing, coke production, foundry work, electrode paste production) and as a result of air pollution in highly industrialized areas (Hemminki *et al.*, 1995; Angerer *et al.*, 1997). In general, these studies have indicated increased prevalence of BPDE–DNA adducts in occupational groups with PAH exposure, although clear relationships between ambient exposure and adduct level are not always present **(Figure 9A)**. Using immunoassay, DNA adduct levels range from undetectable to >400 adducts per 10^6 base pairs (Angerer *et al.*, 1997) in these cohorts. In addition, control subjects with detectable adducts tend to be smokers, and smoking generally results in increased adduct levels in exposed workers **(Figure 9B)**. These studies support the use of BPDE–DNA adducts as PAH exposure biomarkers but are generally not sufficient to establish clear dose–effect relationships. In addition, a large interindividual variation among exposed workers (and people in general; e.g. see **Figure 10**) is apparent (Perera, 1996). This variability is likely to reflect individual differences in PAH bioactivation and detoxification pathways, many of which may be genetically mediated. Immunochemical analysis has also been

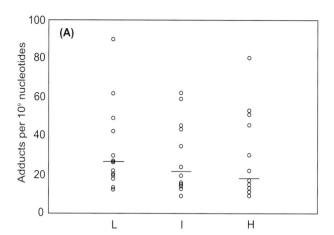

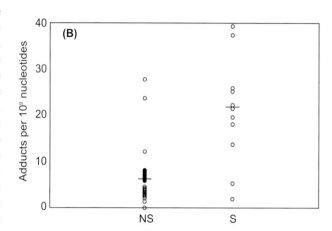

Figure 9 (A) PAH–DNA adducts in WBCs from electrode manufacturing workers with low (L), intermediate (I) and high (H) ambient PAH exposure. There is no clear dose–response relationship for DNA adducts for these individuals. **(B)** PAH–DNA adducts in WBCs from non-smokers (NS) and smokers (S), showing exposure-dependent relationship. Individual values (circles) and group means (bars) are indicated. Note the 10-fold higher overall adduct levels in occupationally exposed **(A)** compared with other **(B)** individuals. Reprinted from *Mutation Research*, **378**, Baan, R. A., *et al*. The use of benzo[a]pyrene diolepoxide-modified DNA standards for adduct quantification in ^{32}P-postlabeling to assess exposure to polycyclic aromatic hydrocarbons: application in a biomonitoring study, pp. 41–50. Copyright (1997), with permission from Elsevier Science.

used to detect DNA adducts of aromatic amines, certain chemotherapeutic agents, food-derived heterocyclic amines such as phenylimidazopyridine (PhIP), ethylene oxide and nitrosamines, although the great majority of these have not used blood cells as their source of DNA.

As discussed previously, antisera have been more generally employed for DNA adduct analysis, but a significant amount of data is also available for protein adducts. AFB_1–serum albumin adducts from experimental animals and humans have been quantitated by ELISA following enzymatic hydrolysis of the protein (Wild *et al.*, 1996). These studies employed synthetic AFB_1–lysine to generate calibration curves for quantitition of the

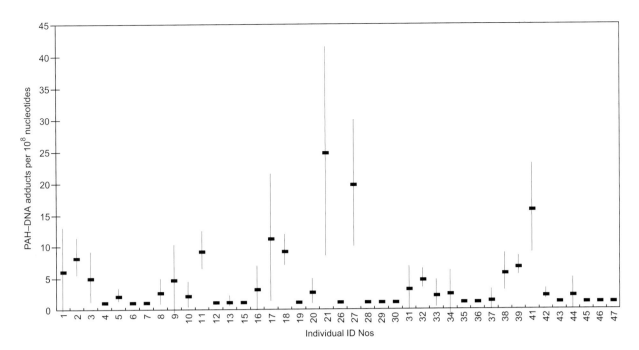

Figure 10 PAH–DNA adducts in WBCs from persons in the general population, showing both temporal (within-individual) and interindividual variability. For each person, the mean and SD of values for adducts determined every 3 weeks over a 15-week period are given. Points with no range are below the limit of detection. Reprinted with permission from Dickey, C., *et al., Risk Anal.* (1997), **17**, p. 652.

adduct. The results indicated that a given exposure to aflatoxin is associated with substantially higher adduct levels in humans than in several rodent species. In addition, good correlations were demonstrated between AFB_1–SA adducts and AFB_1–DNA adducts in liver of experimental animals. The studies suggested that the AFB_1–SA level was predictive of the relative carcinogenic potency of the chemical in animal species. Finally, chemoprotection experiments in rodents have shown that the administration of oltipraz, a substituted diethanolamine, reduces both the level of AFB_1–SA adducts and the incidence rate of hepatocellular carcinoma following exposure to aflatoxins (Kensler *et al.*, 1997). Similar studies are under way in human populations heavily exposed to aflatoxins.

Protein adducts of other reactive xenobiotics have also been examined immunochemically. A number of studies have utilized immunochemical approaches to determine PAH–protein adducts in humans and experimental animals. Sherson *et al.* (1990) measured PAH–SA adducts (by ELISA) in foundry workers and found significantly higher levels in smoking or non-smoking exposed workers (28 and 24 BaP equivalents per 100 μg of protein, respectively) compared with smoking or non-smoking controls (14 and 7 BaP equivalents per 100 μg of protein, respectively). In addition, a high interindividual variability was noted. Smaller increases in PAH–SA adducts over controls were reported in another study of roofers and foundry workers (Lee *et al.*, 1991). ELISA has also been employed to quantitate protein adducts in various tissues

from rats exposed to halogenated hydrocarbons such as trichloroethylene and to pharmaceutical agents such as acetaminophen (paracetarnd) (Hinson *et al.*, 1995; Halmes *et al.*, 1996).

^{32}P-Postlabelling Analysis of DNA Adducts

A highly sensitive and widely applicable assay for DNA adducts was developed in the early 1980s as an offshoot of methodology for determining endogenous covalent modification of RNA (Randerath and Randerath, 1993). These studies showed that a similar procedure could be employed for quantitating DNA adducts formed by various exogenous agents (including xenobiotics). The technique, known as '^{32}P-postlabelling analysis', has since become the predominant method for DNA adduct detection (Beach and Gupta, 1992; Gupta, 1993; Randerath and Randerath, 1994; Keith and Dirheimer, 1995). It has been applied as both a screening and a semiquantitative assay in exposure biomarker studies for hundreds of chemicals in both experimental and epidemiological studies.

As its name implies, the postlabelling method involves the detection of adducted DNA bases by attachment of an atom of radiolabelled phosphate (^{32}P or ^{33}P) to nucleotides after isolation and enzymatic cleavage of the DNA sample **(Figure 11)**. In the original version of the method (Randerath *et al.*, 1981), DNA is extracted and purified by treatment with RNAse A and proteinase-K, followed by enzymatic cleavage to 3'-nucleotide monophosphates with a mixture of spleen

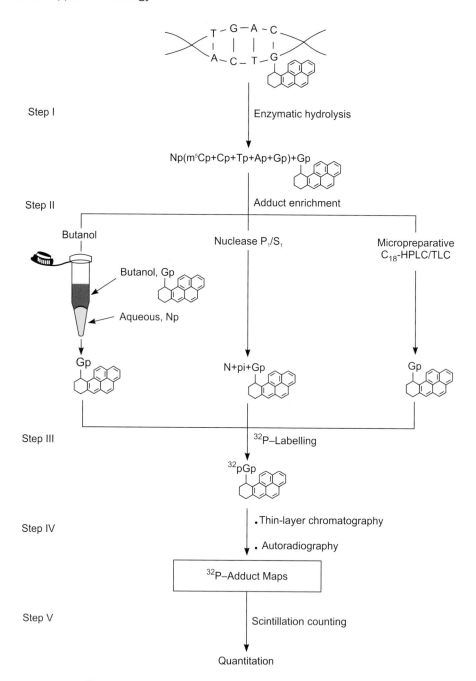

Figure 11 Schematic diagram of ^{32}P- postlabelling assay methodology with various DNA adduct enrichment options. Reprinted from Beach, A. C. and Gupta, R. C., *Carcinogenesis*, (1992), **13**, p. 1057 with permission from Oxford University Press.

phosphodiesterase and micrococcal nuclease. Both adducted and normal nucleosides are then phosphory-lated at the 5'-OH position with T4 polynucleotide kinase and an excess of high specific activity [$\gamma-^{32}$P]ATP. Labelled adducted nucleotides are separated from labelled normal nucleotides by means of TLC on a polyethyleneimine (PEI) substrate in multiple dimensions. Adducted nucleotides appear as distinct spots on the plate following autoradiography.

Numerous modifications of the original method have been made over the years to improve various parameters

of the assay and to increase selectivity for certain classes of adducts (Beach and Gupta, 1992; Keith and Dirhei-mer, 1995). One major change involved limiting the level of [$\gamma-^{32}$P]ATP used in the postlabelling reaction. This allowed an increase in the maximum quantity of DNA assayed from 1 to 10 μg, with a concomitant increase in sensitivity. The development of procedures to enrich the level of adducted nucleotides prior to ^{32}P labelling have produced further increases in sensitivity. Enrichment steps include butanol extraction, which separates hydro-phobic adducts from normal nucleotides, and nuclease

Table 2 Summary of methods for DNA adduct analysis[a]

Method	Sensitivity[b]	Sample size[c]	Advantages	Disadvantages
Physical				
Fluorescence–standard	100	1000	Relatively simple and rapid to conduct, minimal sample preparation	Large sample size, low sensitivity, limited to fluorescent adducts
Fluorescence—SFS	1–10	100	High sensitivity for specific adducts, minimal sample preparation	Specialized equipment, limited to fluorescent adducts
Fluorescence—FLNS	1–10	100–1000	High sensitivity for specific adducts, minimal sample preparation	Specialized equipment, limited to fluorescent adducts
GC-MS—EI/SIM	1–10	100–1000	High specificity	Large sample size, expensive set-up requirements, complex sample preparation
GC-MS—NCI	0.1–1	100	High specificity, sensitivity	Expensive set-up requirements, complex sample preparation
Electrochemical conductance	10–100	25–100	Relatively simple and rapid to conduct, high specificity, sensitivity	Not applicable for most types of adducts
Atomic absorption spectrometry	10–100	100–200	High specificity, sensitivity, minimal sample preparation	Useful primarily for metals, expensive set-up requirements
Immunoassay				
RIA	1	1000–10000	Relatively low cost, simple to conduct	Requires specific antisera, possible cross-reactivity, low sensitivity, large sample size
ELISA	1	50	Relatively low cost, simple to conduct, sensitive	Requires specific antisera, possible cross-reactivity
USERIA	1	50	Relatively low cost, simple to conduct, sensitive	Requires specific antisera, possible cross-reactivity
³²P-Postlabelling				
Standard	0.1–1	1	Relatively low cost, high sensitivity	Complex sample preparation, cannot accommodate large sample size, low specificity (without standards)
Nuclease P1 or butanol enhanced	0.01–0.1	10	Relatively low cost, very high sensitivity	Complex sample preparation, low specificity (without standards)

[a] Data from Weston (1993), Poirier and Weston (1996), Warren and Shields (1997) and Garner (1998).
[b] Lower limit of adducts detected per 10^8 base pairs.
[c] Typical sample size in μg DNA.

P_1 treatment, which preferentially cleaves the 3'-phosphate from normal, but not adducted, nucleotides. The resulting nucleosides are not substrates for T4 kinase and are therefore unlabelled and undetected. A typical assay will employ both enrichment options, as their overall selectivities are different. HPLC-based concentration of adducted nucleotides prior to labelling is also effective in increasing sensitivity. Most recently, a 'dinucleotide' variation of the assay that uses nuclease P_1 and prostatic acid phosphatase for the initial DNA cleavage and snake venom phosphodiesterase following ^{32}P labelling has been developed. This method theoretically avoids any interferences from labelling of normal nucleotides, thus reducing non-specific background labelling. Replacement of autoradiography with storage phosphor imaging as the ^{32}P detection system is also useful in increasing adduct detection sensitivity (Reichert et al., 1992).

Results from postlabelling assays fall into several categories of interpretation. The formation of new, unique adducts in DNA from exposed subjects is shown by the presence of distinct labelled spots on the chromatogram that are not present in control samples. Increased labelling intensity of spots from exposed vs unexposed subject DNA can reflect xenobiotic-induced enhancement of an adduction reaction that occurs at low levels in all individuals. The most common example of this is increased levels of 8-oxo-dG adducts, which are products of oxidative DNA damage (Möller and Hofer, 1997). A diffuse enhancement of labelling in the 'diagonal radioactive zone' (DRZ) of TLC plates is sometimes observed with exposures to complex mixtures such as cigarette smoke, and represents formation of multiple, poorly resolved adducted species (Beach and Gupta, 1992). Finally, exposure to certain xenobiotics is associated with decreased formation of 'I (i.e. indigenous) compounds', which are bulky DNA adducts present in normal individuals and which are thought to be functional DNA modifications important in growth (Randerath et al., 1993).

One major strength of the postlabelling method is its extreme sensitivity; as few as one adduct in 10^{10} base pairs, or < 1 adduct per human WBC genome, can be detected. This level of detection allows the method to be used as a screening assay in exposure biomarker studies in occupational cohorts and in the general population. A number of such studies have been published, in addition to extensive comparisons of ^{32}P-postlabelling results with other DNA adduct and exposure biomarker methodologies (Farmer et al., 1996; Angerer et al., 1997). Additional advantages are the ability to detect multiple adducted species in a single assay and its relative ease of performance. In contrast, the major drawback of the technique is the lack of qualitative information on adduct structure. Unlike spectrometric techniques, the method cannot be used to characterize unknown adducts, and absolute quantitation cannot be performed unless a labelled standard is available for the adduct of interest. Some progress has been made with the structural characterization of adducts recovered and purified from TLC plates by various chromatographic procedures. Finally, interpretation of postlabelling findings has been hampered to some extent by considerable interlaboratory variation in ^{32}P-postlabelling results (Phillips and Castegnaro, 1993). A comparison of the various methods for DNA adduct detection is given in **Table 2**.

BIOMARKERS OF SUSCEPTIBILITY

Toxicological research in experimental animals and humans over many years has revealed that individuals can often differ markedly in their qualitative and quantitative responses to chemical exposure (Marx, 1991; Perera, 1996, 1997; Preston, 1996; Barrett et al., 1997). Such interindividual differences can be genetically mediated or can be a result of some environmental stressor, disease process or other epigenetic factor. While these interindividual differences can complicate safety evaluation and risk assessment activities, they can also be usefully employed as biomarkers of individual susceptibility to xenobiotics (National Research Council, 1987). Many potential susceptibility biomarkers have been explored since this concept was first recognized.

Unlike the exposure markers discussed above, biomarkers of susceptibility do not represent stages along the dose–response mechanistic sequence, but instead represent conditions that alter the rate of transition between the stages or molecular events (National Research Council, 1987; Albertini et al., 1996). The kinetics of transition are often governed by specific enzymes or other gene products. Consequently, determination of relative enzyme activities or the presence or absence of other gene products are often employed as susceptibility biomarkers. Enzymes involved in xenobiotic metabolism can be particularly important in the overall mechanism of action of xenobiotics, and genetic polymorphism in metabolic enzymatic activity is a common basis for interindividual differences in toxicity (Albertini et al., 1996). For example, differences in Hb adduct data between individuals with similar ambient exposure to a chemical could be attributed to differences in metabolic activity. Alternatively, decreased DNA repair enzyme activity could result in increased mutation rates and enhanced tumour formation. Such polymorphisms can, in theory, be exploited as measures of individual susceptibility.

Several techniques are available for both genotypic and phenotypic analysis of genes and gene products for purposes of biomarker assessment (Barrett et al., 1997). Genotyping reveals the underlying gene complement and specific alleles for a given enzyme. In contrast, phenotyping also integrates the effects of environmental (epigenetic) influences on enzyme activity. While results from the two approaches are often in good agreement, occasionally poor correlations have led to disagreement regarding when each method is appropriate. Phenotyping can be performed by direct measurement of enzyme protein by immunochemical or other assays, quantitation of specific mRNA for the enzyme or determination of enzyme activity *in vitro* or *in vivo* by using known actual xenobiotics or surrogate (i.e. 'probe') substrates. Genotyping is done by means of Southern blot analysis of restriction fragment length polymorphisms (RFLPs) or, more recently, by amplification and analysis of relevant cDNA or mRNA sequences by polymerase chain reaction (PCR). Actual sequencing of genomic DNA can also provide information regarding polymorphic enzyme variants.

Xenobiotic Metabolizing Enzymes as Susceptibility Biomarkers

As extensively described in Chapter 5, the CYP enzyme system is responsible for oxidative (i.e. Phase I) metabolism of a multitude of xenobiotics and endogenous molecules, primarily in the liver but also in other tissues. Some of these oxidations result in detoxified and others bioactivated metabolites. Polymorphisms in CYPs 1A1, 1A2, 2C19, 2D6 and 2E1 activities in humans for various substrates have been reported (Vineis, 1995; Nebert *et al.*, 1996; Miller *et al.*, 1997; Guengerich and Shimada, 1998). CYP2D6, which metabolizes a number of drugs and xenobiotics, exhibits two distinct phenotypes in humans, respectively termed extensive and poor metabolizers. The extensive metabolizer phenotype has been correlated with increased lung (and other) cancer incidence in smokers and additional exposed cohorts, possibly due to enhanced bioactivation of the CYP2D6 substrate NNK. The *Msp*I and *Val/Val* polymorphisms of CYP1A1, which metabolizes PAHs, is also associated with increased lung cancer rates, particularly in Japanese smokers (Spivack *et al.*, 1997). This may be due to either heightened catalytic activity or enhanced inducibility of the mutant enzyme or structural gene, respectively. Elevated adduct levels have been noted in WBC DNA from individuals with CYP1A1 polymorphisms (Kaderlik and Kadlubar, 1995). Measurement of CYP1A2 activity is the basis of the 'caffeine breath test' and 'caffeine urinary metabolite ratio test' as possible susceptibility biomarker assays (Lambert *et al.*, 1990). These studies clearly indicate the promise of CYP gene polymorphisms as human xenobiotic susceptibility biomarkers.

Another important detoxification enzyme system with significant use in susceptibility studies is glutathione-*S*-transferase (GST), which catalyses the conjugation (*i.e.* Phase II metabolism) of the cellular thiol glutathione (GSH) with oxidized xenobiotics. Polymorphisms of the GST-M1, -M3, -P1 and -T1 genes have been

Table 3 Ethnic and geographic variation in GSTM-1 genotypes

Ethnic origin/geographic location	Frequency (%) of GSTM-1 'null' $(-/-)$ genotype
Pacific islander	> 90
Chinese	~ 60
Caucasian (European and North American)	40–55
Japanese	~ 50
African American	30–35
Indian subcontinent	33
West African (Nigeria)	20–25

demonstrated in humans (Nebert *et al.*, 1996; Miller *et al.*, 1997; Srám, 1998). For example, approximately 50% of the Caucasian population in the USA is of the 'null' $(-/-)$ genotype for GST-M1, due to inheritance of a homozygous gene deletion. The frequency of the null genotype in other populations and racial groups varies from 20 to 90% (**Table 3**). GST-M1 $(-/-)$ individuals have a decreased metabolic capability for GSH conjugation that would theoretically allow increased tissue levels of activated xenobiotics. This in turn could lead to increased DNA adduction and other damage and, ultimately, increased mutation rates. The null genotype and/or phenotype has been correlated in several studies with elevated susceptibility to lung, bladder and colon cancer, in addition to enhanced SCE and DNA adduction levels (Barrett *et al.*, 1997). Synergistic increases in cancer susceptibility have also been suggested in individuals with both GST-M1 $(-/-)$ and CYP1A1 *Val/Val* genotypes.

A third major group of xenobiotic metabolizing enzymes with significant polymorphism is the *N*-acetyltransferase (NAT) family (Feigelson *et al.*, 1996; Nebert *et al.*, 1996; Miller *et al.*, 1997). NAT1 and NAT2 are responsible, respectively, for *O*- and *N*-acetylation of aromatic amines, including the bladder carcinogen ABP. Both enzymes are polymorphic in humans, although the activity of the NAT2 enzyme appears to be 10-fold higher than NAT-1 for aromatic amine metabolism. Acetylation can be either activating or detoxifying depending upon the particular amine, toxicity endpoint and tissue examined. Individuals can be classed as either 'slow' or 'rapid' acetylator phenotype; slow acetylators are homozygous for the NAT2 *r* allele, whereas rapid acetylators are either heterozygous *rR* or homozygous *RR*. Slow acetylation phenotype varies from 10 to 90% in various populations. Unlike with GST-M1 polymorphisms, the correlation between cancer susceptibility and acetylator phenotype depends on which target organ is examined. For example, slow acetylator phenotype is correlated with excess incidence of bladder cancer, while the opposite is true for colorectal cancer. Increases in ABP–Hb adducts have been observed in slow as compared with rapid phenotypes, and elevated DNA adducts are associated with a specific NAT-1 polymorphism. These observations illustrate the complexities involved in interpreting the results of susceptibility biomarker studies using enzyme polymorphisms.

Other Biomarkers of Susceptibility

In addition to enzymes involved in biotransformation, other potential susceptibility biomarkers have been explored (or proposed) in human and animal studies. These include DNA repair enzyme activities, nuclear and cytoplasmic receptor protein levels, oncogenes and corresponding gene products, tumour suppressor genes and humoral and cellular immune system components.

Investigation of DNA repair enzyme status as a possible biomarker stems from the known involvement of defects and deficiencies in certain of these enzymes in inherited disorders such as xeroderma pigmentosum (Athas et al., 1991; Perera, 1996, 1997). For example, large (200–300-fold) interindividual variability in the activities of the repair enzyme O^6-alkyldeoxyguanine–DNA alkyltransferase and uracil DNA glycosylase are present in the human population. Decreased alkyltransferase activity has been found in lung cancer patients. Evidence for defects in enzymes involved in repair of UV light-induced DNA damage among individuals with breast and other cancers is also available. Newer assays have been developed that involve the determination of the overall DNA repair capacity (DRC) in WBCs as a potential indicator of susceptibility (Athas et al., 1991). In one such study, individuals with low DRC demonstrated a fivefold greater risk of skin cancer than a normal cohort.

Polymorphisms in nuclear and cytoplasmic receptor genes have been examined as possible susceptibility markers (Feigelson et al., 1996). For example, the aromatic hydrocarbon receptor (AhR) in mammalian cells binds a variety of xenobiotics, resulting in pleotropic activation of a number of genes, including that coding for CYP1A1. Interindividual differences in the affinity of the AhR for various ligands have been detected in humans, and ca 10% of the population has a high-affinity form of the receptor. This form is associated with heightened expression of the CYP1A1 and other genes, which has been suggested to correlate with increased susceptibility to cancer and other toxic effects. Other receptor polymorphisms that may correlate with susceptibility differences include those associated with various steroid-binding proteins.

Oncogenes and tumour suppressor genes encode cellular proteins involved with inter-and intracellular signalling, cell cycle control, mitosis, stress responses and a variety of other cellular 'housekeeping' functions. Their significance in carcinogenesis (idiopathic and/or chemically induced) has been extensively investigated over the past decade. The p53 tumour suppressor gene is one important example (Greenblatt et al., 1994; Lasky and Silbergeld, 1996; Preston, 1996). Inactivation of one of the p53 alleles (i.e. heterozygous genotype, $+/-$) in

humans is associated with greatly increased rates of tumorigenesis. Mice heterozygous for p53 are highly susceptible to chemically induced carcinogenesis. Polymorphisms in the ras oncogene family (e.g. the H-ras VTR allele) are also linked to high cancer incidence in human cohorts. Many other inherited cancer susceptibility genes have been elucidated, although it is not currently known which of these might predispose to chemically induced carcinogenesis. Nevertheless, genotypic and phenotypic analysis of such genes has been proposed for human susceptibility biomarker studies (Brandt-Rauf, 1988). Specific mutations and mutational spectra in oncogenes and tumour suppressor genes are often associated with exposure to specific carcinogens in animal studies. In addition, characteristic p53 mutations are frequently observed in several human tumour types (Lasky and Silbergeld, 1996). It is unclear, however, whether such mutations are related to increased susceptibility or are a consequence of the carcinogenic mechanism, and their use as susceptibility biomarkers is not yet established.

VALIDATION, INTERPRETATION AND ETHICAL ISSUES

Significant progress has been made in identifying and developing methodology for new potential exposure and susceptibility biomarkers for use in animal and human studies. Despite these advances, numerous issues must be resolved before a given marker can be employed for its intended purpose. Primary among these is the requirement for validation of the biomarker. Validation of a biomarker involves the characterization of parameters including biological and temporal relevance, sensitivity, specificity, technical feasibility, background rate and variability in the population, reproducibility and predictive value (National Research Council, 1987; Schulte and Mazzuckelli, 1991; Schulte and Talaska, 1995; Wahrendorf, 1995; WHO, 1995). The relative importance of each factor depends upon the intended use of the marker (i.e. for exposure, effect or susceptibility characterization). Validation is critical to the successful use of biomarker findings, since uncertainty in any of these parameters can lead to misinterpretation, misclassification and other errors and abuses.

For exposure biomarkers, a primary goal of validation is to determine the relationship between the measured end-point and both prior and subsequent events in the exposure–effect sequence, i.e. dose–response, toxicokinetic and toxicodynamic functions must be characterized (Schulte, 1989; Rhomberg, 1993; Schulte and Talaska, 1995). As an example, an Hb adduct considered for use as an exposure biomarker should exhibit a predictable relationship to the ambient level of the xenobiotic in the medium of concern. In addition, if used as a surrogate

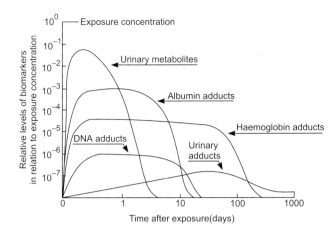

Figure 12 Useful temporal ranges for various exposure biomarkers following a hypothetical single exposure to a xenobiotic. Reprinted with permission from Henderson, R. F., *et al.*, (1989), *CRC Critical Reviews in Toxicology*, **20**, p. 78. Copyright CRC Press, Boca Raton, Florida.

for DNA adduction, then a reproducible correlation between Hb and DNA adducts must be demonstrated. Sensitivity and specificity are also critically important for exposure biomarker acceptability. Sensitivity reflects the ambient exposure level that can be detected by means of the biomarker. Highly sensitive markers are necessary to quantitate the low ambient levels typical of environmental exposures in advanced Western nations. Specificity is the probability that the biomarker is indicative of actual exposure to the specific xenobiotic that it is designed to detect. As discussed earlier, certain macromolecular adducts can be generated during exposure to a variety of chemical species and are therefore less specific than one unique to a single compound.

Temporal relevance strongly influence the design of studies employing exposure biomarkers (Henderson *et al.*, 1989; Fennell *et al.*, 1992; Nestmann *et al.*, 1996). Because of the 120-day lifespan of the human RBC, it is in theory possible, using Hb adducts, to detect an acute exposure that occurred 1 month, but not 4 months, in the past. Measurement of urinary metabolites or albumin adducts, markers that have a shorter temporal range, would not provide useful dosimetry at either time point. In contrast, continuing chronic exposure could be assessed using any of the three markers. Retrospective exposure assessment requires the use of a battery of markers with varying temporal ranges in order to provide maximum information about the time frame of the exposure event(s) **(Figure 12)**. The most challenging aspect of human exposure assessment involves characterizing either acute exposure occurring or chronic exposure ending more than 120 days in the past. Other than (possibly) measurement of unrepaired DNA adducts in long-lived cells, there are no available biomarkers for such prior exposure to non-persistent xenobiotics.

Unlike those for exposure, susceptibility biomarkers are, for the most part, quantal in nature, *i.e.* the marker is either present or not present in an individual. In addition, many susceptibility markers are present at birth and throughout an individual's lifetime. It is for this reason that genotyping can be widely employed for these biomarkers (Barrett *et al.*, 1997). Consequently, validation issues involving dose–response, temporal relevance and sensitivity are not as significant for susceptibility biomarkers as they are for markers of exposure. In contrast, biological relevance is critical to validation of markers of susceptibility. Biological relevance refers to the nature of the phenomenon being measured and its mechanistic involvement in the pathway from exposure to disease. Most, if not all, susceptibility biomarkers measure a molecular event directly involved in the mechanism of action of a xenobiotic, such as conversion to an active metabolite or lack of repair of a mutation-inducing DNA adduct. By definition, valid susceptibility biomarkers must also be predictive of increased risk for adverse health outcomes.

Other validation factors apply equally to both exposure and susceptibility biomarkers. Reasonable accessibility is important; invasive sampling procedures are generally unacceptable. Except for occasional tissue biopsies, samples for biomarker studies consist primarily of blood, urine, milk or other readily obtainable biological media. Since these are rarely target tissues for toxicological or carcinogenic effects, such studies are almost invariably conducted with surrogate biological materials. Reproducibility of biomarker results within and between laboratories is important, and is often difficult to achieve. Finally, cost and technical feasibility are important considerations in selection of appropriate biomarkers for applied studies.

The subject of the ethical use of biomarkers has received increasing attention in recent years (Schulte, 1992; Schulte and Sweeney, 1995; Barrett *et al.*, 1997; Schulte *et al.*, 1997). The issue is complex and involves concerns related to misinterpretation, misapplication and inappropriate release of biomarker data. Exposure biomarkers are designed to answer two basic questions: to what was an individual exposed and to how much was he or she exposed? Clear resolution of both questions requires qualitative and quantitative data with high specificity and sensitivity, in addition to understanding of the nature of 'background' chemical exposures. Ethical problems appear when the results of exposure screening studies are implied to reflect directly health risk rather than, simply, exposure. This may be particularly important once exposure biomarker data become more routinely used in sensitive situations such as toxic tort and environmental litigation proceedings (DeCaprio, 1997). Problems can also arise when claims are made, based upon biomarker data, for excessive chemical exposure in a particular cohort, particularly if the overall range of exposure in the general population is not well characterized. Finally, once exposure has been confirmed, clear and objective interpretation of the potential health significance (if any and if known) must be provided by physician, researcher or public health professional to the individuals involved.

The appropriate use of susceptibility biomarker data presents an even more serious dilemma than that for biomarkers of exposure (Soskolne, 1997). Careless or unethical treatment of susceptibility information can have far-reaching and adverse effects on an individual's personal and professional lives. There is great potential for misuse of data predicting enhanced individual susceptibility to xenobiotic-induced toxic effects by employers, insurance companies and other parties with financial interests in such information. At the very least, provisions for confidentiality and individual notification of susceptibility data are necessary. In addition, questions arise concerning the ethics of detecting (and reporting) increased risk of diseases for which no prevention or treatment options are available. Because of the sensitive nature and potential implications of susceptibility biomarker data, stringent validation and quality control requirements are of major importance (Aitio and Apostoli, 1995). Finally, a clear distinction between population and individual susceptibility must be recognized. Most susceptibility biomarker studies to date have examined factors related to elevated population or cohort risk; few markers have been sufficiently characterized and validated to allow the prediction of individual risk.

REFERENCES

Aitio, A. and Apostoli, P. (1995). Quality assurance in biomarker measurement. *Toxicol. Lett.*, **77**, 195–204.

Albertini, R. J., Nicklas, J. A. and O'Neill, J. P. (1996). Future research directions for evaluating human genetic and cancer risk from environmental exposures. *Environ. Health Perspect.*, **104**, 503–510.

Angerer, J., Mannschreck, C. and Gundel, J. (1997). Biological monitoring and biochemical effect monitoring of exposure to polycyclic aromatic hydrocarbons. *Int. Arch. Occup. Environ. Health*, **70**, 365–377.

Apruzzese, W. A. and Vouros, P. (1998). Analysis of DNA adducts by capillary methods coupled to mass spectrometry: a perspective. *J. Chromatogr.*, **794**, 97–108.

Athas, W. F., Hedayati, M. A., Matanoski, G. M., Farmer, E. R. and Grossman, L. (1991). Development and field-test validation of an assay for DNA repair in circulating human lymphocytes. *Cancer Res.*, **51**, 5786–5793.

Baan, R. A., Steenwinkel, M. J. S. T., Vanasten, S., Roggeband, R. and Vandelft, J. H. M. (1997). The use of benzo[a]-pyrene diol epoxide-modified DNA standards for adduct quantification in ^{32}P-postlabelling to assess exposure to polycyclic aromatic hydrocarbons: application in a biomonitoring study. *Mutat. Res.*, **378**, 41–50.

Barrett, J. C., Vainio, H., Peakall, D. and Goldstein, B. D. (1997). 12th Meeting of the Scientific Group on Methodologies for the Safety Evaluation of Chemicals—Susceptibility to Environmental Hazards. *Environ. Health Perspect.*, **105**, 699–737.

Beach, A. C. and Gupta, R. C. (1992). Human biomonitoring and the ^{32}P-postlabeling assay. *Carcinogenesis*, **13**, 1053–1074.

Bechtold, W. E., Willis, J. K., Sun, J. D., Griffith, W. C. and Reddy, T. V. (1992). Biological markers of exposure to benzene: *S*-phenylcysteine in albumin. *Carcinogenesis*, **13**, 1217–1220.

Beland, F. A. and Poirier, M. C. (1989). DNA adducts and carcinogenesis. In Sirica, A. E. (Ed.), *The Pathobiology of Neoplasia*. Plenum Press, New York, pp. 57–80.

Brandt-Rauf, P. W. (1988). New markers for monitoring occupational cancer: the example of oncogene proteins. *J. Occup. Med.*, **30**, 399–404.

Brescia, G., Foà, V., Viezzer, C., Celotti, L. and Assennato, G. (1997). Aromatic DNA adduct levels in human peripheral blood lymphocytes and total white blood cells by ^{32}P-post-labelling: need for validation. *Biomarkers*, **2**, 333–339.

Bryant, M. S., Skipper, P. L., Tannenbaum, S. R. and Maclure, M. (1987). Hemoglobin adducts of 4-aminobiphenyl in smokers and nonsmokers. *Cancer Res.*, **47**, 602–608.

Carmella, S. G. and Hecht, S. S. (1987). Formation of hemoglobin adducts upon treatment of F344 rats with the tobacco-specific nitrosamines 4-(methylnitrosamino)-1-(3-pyridyl)-1-butanone and *N'*-nitrosonornicotine. *Cancer Res.*, **47**, 2626–2630.

Christiani, D. C. (1996). Utilization of biomarker data for clinical and environmental intervention. *Environ. Health Perspect.*, **104**, 921–925.

Culp, S. J., Roberts, D. W., Talaska, G., Lang, N. P., Fu, P. F., Lay, J. O., Teitel, C. H., Snawder, J. E., Von Tungeln, L. S. and Kadlubar, F. F. (1997). Immunochemical, ^{32}P-postlabeling, and GC/MS detection of 4-aminobiphenyl–DNA adducts in human peripheral lung in relation to metabolic activation pathways involving pulmonary *N*-oxidation, conjugation, and peroxidation. *Mutat. Res.*, **378**, 97–112.

Dale, C. M. and Garner, R. C. (1996). Measurement of DNA adducts in humans after complex mixture exposure. *Food Chem. Toxicol.*, **34**, 905–919.

DeCaprio, A. P. (1997). Biomarkers: coming of age for environmental health and risk assessment. *Environ. Sci. Technol.*, **31**, 1837–1848.

Dellomo, M. and Lauwerys, R. R. (1993). Adducts to macromolecules in the biological monitoring of workers exposed to polycyclic aromatic hydrocarbons. *Crit. Rev. Toxicol.*, **23**, 111–126.

Dickey, C., Santella, R. M., Hattis, D., Tang, D. L., Hsu, Y. Z., Cooper, T., Young, T. L. and Perera, F. P. (1997). Variability in PAH–DNA adduct measurements in peripheral mononuclear cells: implications for quantitative cancer risk assessment. *Risk Anal.*, **17**, 649–656.

Ehrenberg, L., Moustacchi, E., Osterman-Golkar, S. and Ekman, G. (1983). Dosimetry of genotoxic agents and dose–response relationships of their effects. *Mutat. Res.*, **123**, 121–182.

Farmer, P. B. and Sweetman, G. M. A. (1995). Mass spectrometric detection of carcinogen adducts. *J. Mass Spectrom.*, **30**, 1369–1379.

Farmer, P. B., Bailey, E., Gorf, S. M., Törnqvist, M., Osterman-Golkar, S., Kautiainen, A. and Lewis-Enright, D. P. (1986). Monitoring human exposure to ethylene oxide by the determination of hemoglobin adducts using gas chromatography–mass spectrometry. *Carcinogenesis*, **7**, 637–640.

Farmer, P. B., Sepai, O., Lawrence, R., Autrup, H., Sabro Nielsen, P., Vestergård, A. B., Waters, R., Leuratti, C., Jones, N. J., Stone, J., Baan, R. A., van Delft, J. H. M., Steenwinkel, M. J. S. T., Kyrtopoulos, S. A., Souliotis, V. L., Theodorakopoulos, N., Bacalis, N. C., Natarajan, A. T., Tates, A. D., Haugen, A., Andreassen, Å., Ovrebo, S., Shuker, D. E. G., Amaning, K. S., Schouft, A., Ellul, A., Garner, R. C., Dingley, K. H., Abbondandolo, A., Merlo, F., Cole, J., Aldrich, K., Beare, D., Capulas, E., Rowley, G., Waugh, A. P. W., Povey, A. C., Haque, K., Kirsch-Volders, M., Van Hummelen, P. and Castelain. P. (1996). Biomonitoring human exposure to environmental carcinogenic chemicals. *Mutagenesis*, **11**, 363–381.

Feigelson, H. S., Ross, R. K., Yu, M. C., Coetzee, G. A., Reichardt, J. K. V. and Henderson, B. E. (1996). Genetic susceptibility to cancer from exogenous and endogenous exposures. *J. Cell. Biochem.*, **25S**, 15–22.

Fennell, T. R. (1996). Biomarkers of exposure and susceptibility: application to ethylene oxide. *CIIT Activities*, **16**, 1–8.

Fennell, T. R., Sumner, S. C. J. and Walker, V. E. (1992). A model for the formation and removal of hemoglobin adducts. *Cancer Epidemiol. Biomarkers Prev.*, **1**, 213–219.

Foiles, P. G., Akerkar, S. A., Carmella, S. G., Kagan, M., Stoner, G. D., Resau, J. H. and Hecht, S. S. (1991). Mass spectrometric analysis of tobacco-specific nitrosamine–DNA adducts in smokers and nonsmokers. *Chem. Res. Toxicol.*, **4**, 364–368.

Garner, R. C. (1998). The role of DNA adducts in chemical carcinogenesis. *Mutat. Res.*, **402**, 67–75.

Gillette, J. R. (1986). Significance of covalent binding of chemically reactive metabolites of foreign compounds to proteins and lipids. In Kocsis, J. J., Jollow, D. J., Witmer, C. M., Nelson, J. O. and Snyder, R. (Eds), *Biological Reactive Intermediates III*. Plenum Press, New York, pp. 63–82.

Glazer, A. N. (1970). Specific chemical modification of proteins. *Annu. Rev. Biochem.*, **39**, 101–130.

Greenblatt, M. S., Bennett, W. P., Hollstein, M. and Harris, C. C. (1994). Mutations in the *p53* tumor suppressor gene: clues to cancer etiology and molecular pathogenesis. *Cancer Res.*, **54**, 4855–4878.

Groopman, J. D., Dematos, P., Egner, P. A., Lovehunt, A. and Kensler, T. W. (1992). Molecular dosimetry of urinary aflatoxin-N7-guanine and serum aflatoxin albumin adducts predicts chemoprotection by 1,2-dithiole-3-thione in rats. *Carcinogenesis*, **13**, 101–106.

Groopman, J. D., Wogan, G. N., Roebuck, B. D. and Kensler, T. W. (1994). Molecular biomarkers for aflatoxins and their application to human cancer prevention. *Cancer Res.*, **54**, S1907–S1911.

Guengerich, F. P. and Shimada, T. (1998). Activation of procarcinogens by human cytochrome P450 enzymes. *Mutat. Res.*, **400**, 201–213.

Gupta, R. C. (1993). ^{32}P-Postlabelling analysis of bulky aromatic adducts. In Phillips, D. H., Castegnaro, M. and Bartsch, H. (Eds), *Postlabelling Methods for Detection of DNA Adducts*. International Agency for Research on Cancer, Lyon, pp. 11–23.

Halket, J. M. (1993). Derivatives for gas chromatography–mass spectrometry. In Blau, K. and Halket, J. M. (Eds),

Handbook of Derivatives for Chromatography. Wiley, New York, pp. 297–326.

Halmes, N. C., McMillan, D. C., Oatis, J. E. and Pumford, N. R. (1996). Immunochemical detection of protein adducts in mice treated with trichloroethylene. *Chem. Res. Toxicol.*, **9**, 451–456.

Harris, C. C. (1991). Chemical and physical carcinogenesis—advances and perspectives for the 1990s. *Cancer Res.*, **51**, S5023–S5044.

Hemminki, K., Dipple, A., Shuker, D. E. G., Kadlubar, F. F., Segerbäck, D. and Bartsch, H. (1994). *DNA Adducts: Identification and Biological Significance*. International Agency for Research on Cancer, Lyon.

Hemminki, K., Autrup, H. and Haugen, A. (1995). DNA and protein adducts. *Toxicology*, **101**, 41–53.

Henderson, R. F., Bechtold, W. E., Bond, J. A. and Sun, J. D. (1989). The use of biological markers in toxicology. *CRC Crit. Rev. Toxicol.*, **20**, 65–82.

Hinson, J. A., Pumford, N. R. and Roberts, D. W. (1995). Mechanisms of acetaminophen toxicity—immunochemical detection of drug–protein adducts. *Drug Metab. Rev.*, **27**, 73–92.

Howe, W., Stonard, M. D. and Woollen, B. H. (1986). The use of human biological measurements for safety evaluation in the chemical industry. In Worden, A., Parke, D. and Marks, J. (Eds), *The Future of Predictive Safety Evaluation*, Vol. 1. MTP Press, Boston, pp. 63–78.

Jankowiak, R. and Small, G. J. (1991). Fluorescence line narrowing—a high-resolution window on DNA and protein damage from chemical carcinogens. *Chem. Res. Toxicol.*, **4**, 256–269.

Kaderlik, K. R. and Kadlubar, F. F. (1995). Metabolic polymorphisms and carcinogen–DNA adduct formation in human populations. *Pharmacogenetics*, **5**, S108–S117.

Keith, G. and Dirheimer, G. (1995). Postlabeling: a sensitive method for studying DNA adducts and their role in carcinogenesis. *Curr. Opin. Biotechnol.*, **6**, 3–11.

Kensler, T. W., Gange, S. J., Egner, P. A., Dolan, P. M., Munoz, A., Groopman, J. D., Rogers, A. E. and Roebuck, B. D. (1997). Predictive value of molecular dosimetry: individual *versus* group effects of oltipraz on aflatoxin–albumin adducts and risk of liver cancer. *Cancer Epidemiol. Biomarkers Prev.*, **6**, 603–610.

Lambert, G. H., Schoeller, D. A., Humphrey, H. E., Kotake, A. N., Lietz, H., Campbell, M., Kalow, W., Spielberg, S. P. and Budd, M. (1990). The caffeine breath test and caffeine urinary metabolite ratios in the Michigan cohort exposed to polybrominated biphenyls: a preliminary study. *Environ. Health Perspect.*, **89**, 175–181.

Larsen, J. C. (1995). Levels of pollutants and their metabolites—exposures to organic substances. *Toxicology*, **101**, 11–27.

Lasky, T. and Silbergeld, E. (1996). *p53* Mutations associated with breast, colorectal, liver, lung, and ovarian cancers. *Environ. Health Perspect.*, **104**, 1324–1331.

Lawley, P. D. (1994). From fluorescence spectra to mutational spectra, a historical overview of DNA-reactive compounds. In Hemminki, K., Dipple, A., Shuker, D. E. G., Kadlubar, F. F., Segerbäck, D. and Bartsch, H. (Eds), *DNA Adducts: Identification and Biological Significance*. International Agency for Research on Cancer, Lyon, pp. 3–22.

Lee, B. M., Yin, B. Y., Herbert, R., Hemminki, K., Perera, F. P. and Santella, R. M. (1991). Immunologic measurement of polycyclic aromatic hydrocarbon–albumin adducts in foundry workers and roofers. *Scand. J. Work Environ. Health*, **17**, 190–194.

Lutz, W. K. (1979). *In vivo* covalent binding of organic chemicals to DNA as a quantitative indicator in the process of chemical carcinogenesis. *Mutat. Res.*, **65**, 289–356.

Marx, J. (1991). Zeroing in on individual cancer risk. *Science*, **253**, 612–616.

Miller, E. C. and Miller, J. A. (1981). Searches for ultimate chemical carcinogens and their reactions with cellular macromolecules. *Cancer*, **47**, 2327–2345.

Miller, M. S., McCarver, D. G., Bell, D. A., Eaton, D. L. and Goldstein, J. A. (1997). Genetic polymorphisms in human drug metabolic enzymes. *Fundam. Appl. Toxicol.*, **40**, 1–14.

Möller, L. and Hofer, T. (1997). [^{32}P]ATP mediates formation of 8-hydroxy-2′-deoxyguanosine from 2′-deoxyguanosine, a possible problem in the ^{32}P-postlabeling assay. *Carcinogenesis*, **18**, 2415–2419.

Mowrer, J., Törnqvist, M., Jensen, S. and Ehrenberg, L. (1986). Modified Edman degradation applied to hemoglobin for monitoring occupational exposure to alkylating agents. *Toxicol. Environ. Chem.*, **11**, 215–231.

National Academy of Sciences (1989a). *Biologic Markers in Reproductive Toxicology*. National Academy Press, Washington, DC.

National Academy of Sciences (1989b). *Biologic Markers in Pulmonary Toxicology*. National Academy Press, Washington, DC.

National Academy of Sciences (1992). *Biologic Markers in Immunotoxicology*. National Academy Press, Washington, DC.

National Research Council (1987). Biological markers in environmental health research. *Environ. Health Perspect.*, **74**, 3–9.

National Research Council (1991). Use of biological markers in assessing human exposure to airborne contaminants. In *Human Exposure Assessment for Airborne Pollutants*. National Academy of Sciences, National Academy Press, Washington, DC, pp. 115–142.

Naumann, C. H., Griffith, J., Blancato, J. N. and Aldrich, T. E. (1993). Biomarkers in environmental epidemiology. In Aldrich, T., Griffith, J. and Cooke, C. (Eds), *Environmental Epidemiology and Risk Assessment*. Van Nostrand Reinhold, New York, pp. 152–181.

Nebert, D. W., Mckinnon, R. A. and Puga, A. (1996). Human drug-metabolizing enzyme polymorphisms: effects on risk of toxicity and cancer. *DNA Cell Biol.*, **15**, 273–280.

Nestmann, E. R., Bryant, D. W. and Carr, C. J. (1996). Toxicological significance of DNA adducts. *Regul. Toxicol. Pharmacol.*, **24**, 9–18.

Osterman-Golkar, S., Ehrenberg, L., Segerbäck, D. and Hallstrom, I. (1976). Evaluation of genetic risks of alkylating agents. II. Haemoglobin as a dose monitor. *Mutat. Res.*, **34**, 1–10.

Özbal, C. C., Velic, I., Soohoo, C. K., Skipper, P. L. and Tannenbaum, S. R. (1994). Conservation of histone carcinogen adducts during replication: implications for long-term molecular dosimetry. *Cancer Res.*, **54**, 5599–5601.

Pearson, R. G. and Songstad, J. (1967). Application of the principle of hard and soft acids and bases to organic chemistry. *J. Am. Chem. Soc.*, **89**, 1827–1836.

Perera, F. P. (1987). Molecular cancer epidemiology: a new tool in cancer prevention. *J. Natl. Cancer Inst.*, **78**, 887–898.

Perera, F. P. (1996). Molecular epidemiology: insights into cancer susceptibility, risk assessment, and prevention. *J. Natl. Cancer Inst.*, **88**, 496–509.

Perera, F. P. (1997). Environment and cancer: who are susceptible? *Science*, **278**, 1068–1073.

Perera, F. P. and Weinstein, I. B. (1982). Molecular epidemiology and carcinogen–DNA adduct detection: new approaches to studies of human cancer causation. *J. Chron. Dis.*, **35**, 581–600.

Perera, F. P., Poirier, M. C., Yuspa, S. H., Nakayama, J., Jaretzki, A., Curnen, M. M., Knowles, D. M. and Weinstein, I. B. (1982). A pilot project in molecular cancer epidemiology: determination of benzo[*a*]pyrene–DNA adducts in animal and human tissues by immunoassays. *Carcinogenesis*, **3**, 1405–1410.

Phillips, D. H. and Castegnaro, M. (1993). Results of an interlaboratory trial of ^{32}P-postlabelling. In Phillips, D. H., Castegnaro, M. and Bartsch, H. (Eds), *Postlabelling Methods for Detection of DNA Adducts*. International Agency for Research on Cancer, Lyon, pp. 35–49.

Poirier, M. C. (1993). Antisera specific for carcinogen–DNA adducts and carcinogen-modified DNA: applications for detection of xenobiotics in biological samples. *Mutat. Res.*, **288**, 31–38.

Poirier, M. C. and Weston, A. (1996). Human DNA adduct measurements: state of the art. *Environ. Health Perspect.*, **104**, 883–893.

Preston, R. J. (1996). Genetic susceptibility and sensitivity to cancer. *CIIT Activities*, **18**, 1–8.

Prevost, V., Shuker, D. E. G., Friesen, M. D., Eberle, G., Rajewsky, M. F. and Bartsch, H. (1993). Immunoaffinity purification and gas chromatography–mass spectrometric quantification of 3-alkyladenines in urine: metabolism studies and basal excretion levels in man. *Carcinogenesis*, **14**, 199–204.

Qu, S. X., Bai, C. L. and Stacey, N. H. (1997). Determination of bulky DNA adducts in biomonitoring of carcinogenic chemical exposures: features and comparison of current techniques. *Biomarkers*, **2**, 3–16.

Ranasinghe, A., Scheller, N., Wu, K. Y., Upton, P. B. and Swenberg, J. A. (1998). Application of gas chromatography–electron capture negative chemical ionization high-resolution mass spectrometry for analysis of DNA and protein adducts. *Chem. Res. Toxicol.*, **11**, 520–526.

Randerath, K. and Randerath, E. (1993). Postlabelling methods—an historical review. In Phillips, D. H., Castegnaro, M. and Bartsch, H. (Eds), *Postlabelling Methods for Detection of DNA Adducts*. International Agency for Research on Cancer, Lyon, pp. 3–9.

Randerath, K. and Randerath, E. (1994). ^{32}P-Postlabeling methods for DNA adduct detection: overview and critical evaluation. *Drug Metab. Rev.*, **26**, 67–85.

Randerath, K., Reddy, M. V. and Gupta, R. C. (1981). ^{32}P-Labeling test for DNA damage. *Proc. Natl. Acad. Sci. USA*, **78**, 6126–6129.

Randerath, K., Li, D., Moorthy, B. and Randerath, E. (1993). I-compounds—endogenous DNA markers of nutritional status, ageing, tumour promotion and carcinogenesis. In Phillips, D. H., Castegnaro, M. and Bartsch, H. (Eds),

Postlabelling Methods for Detection of DNA Adducts. International Agency for Research on Cancer, Lyon, pp. 157–165.

Reddy, M. V., Gupta, R. C., Randerath, E. and Randerath, K. (1984). ³²P-Postlabeling test for covalent DNA binding of chemicals *in vivo*: application to a variety of aromatic carcinogens and methylating agents. *Carcinogenesis*, **5**, 231–243.

Reichert, W. L., Stein, J. E., French, B., Goodwin, P. and Varanasi, U. (1992). Storage phosphor imaging technique for detection and quantitation of DNA adducts measured by the ³²P-postlabeling assay. *Carcinogenesis*, **13**, 1475–1479.

Rhomberg, L. (1993). Use of biomarkers in quantitative risk assessment. In Travis, C. C. (Ed.), *Use of Biomarkers in Assessing Health and Environmental Impacts of Chemical Pollutants.* Plenum Press, New York, pp. 31–46.

Rhomberg, L. (1995). What constitutes 'dose'? (definitions). In Olin, S., Farland, W., Park, C., Rhomberg, L., Scheuplein, R., Starr, T. and Wilson, J. (Eds), *Low-Dose Extrapolation of Cancer Risks.* International Life Sciences Institute, Washington, DC, pp. 185–198.

Sabbioni, G. (1990). Chemical and physical properties of the major serum albumin adduct of aflatoxin B1 and their implications for the quantification in biological samples. *Chem.–Biol. Interact.*, **75**, 1–15.

Sampson, E. J., Needham, L. L., Pirkle, J. L., Hannon, W. H., Miller, D. T., Patterson, D. G., Bernert, J. T., Ashley, D. L., Hill, R. H., Gunter, E. W., Paschal, D. C., Spierto, F. W. and Rich, M. J. (1994). Technical and scientific developments in exposure marker methodology. *Clin. Chem.*, **40**, 1376–1384.

Schnell, F. C. (1993). Protein adduct-forming chemicals and molecular dosimetry: potential for environmental and occupational biomarkers. *Rev. Environ. Toxicol.*, **5**, 51–160.

Schulte, P. A. (1989). A conceptual framework for the validation and use of biologic markers. *Environ. Res.*, **48**, 129–144.

Schulte, P. A. (1991). Contribution of biological markers to occupational health. *Am. J. Ind. Med.*, **20**, 435–446.

Schulte, P. A. (1992). Biomarkers in epidemiology: scientific issues and ethical implications. *Environ. Health Perspect.*, **98**, 143–147.

Schulte, P. A. and Mazzuckelli, L. F. (1991). Validation of biological markers for quantitative risk assessment. *Environ. Health Perspect.*, **90**, 239–246.

Schulte, P. A. and Sweeney, M. H. (1995). Ethical considerations, confidentiality issues, rights of human subjects, and uses of monitoring data in research and regulation. *Environ. Health Perspect.*, **103**, 69–74.

Schulte, P. A. and Talaska, G. (1995). Validity criteria for the use of biological markers of exposure to chemical agents in environmental epidemiology. *Toxicology*, **101**, 73–88.

Schulte, P. A., Hunter, D. and Rothman, N. (1997). Ethical and social issues in the use of biomarkers in epidemiological research. In Toniolo, P., Boffetta, P., Shuker, D. E. G., Rothman, N., Hulka, B. and Pearce, N. (Eds), *Application of Biomarkers in Cancer Epidemiology.* International Agency for Research on Cancer, Lyon, pp. 313–318.

Selikoff, I. J. and Landrigan, P. J. (1992). The third epidemiological revolution. *Eur. J. Epidemiol.*, **8**, 625–626.

Sheabar, F. Z., Groopman, J. D. Qian, G. S. and Wogan, G. N. (1993). Quantitative analysis of aflatoxin–albumin adducts. *Carcinogenesis*, **14**, 1203–1208.

Sherson, D., Sabro, P., Sigsgaard, T., Johansen, F. and Autrup, H. (1990). Biological monitoring of foundry workers exposed to polycyclic aromatic hydrocarbons. *Br. J. Ind. Med.*, **47**, 448–453.

Shuker, D. E., Prevost, V., Friesen, M. D., Lin, D., Ohshima, H. and Bartsch, H. (1993). Urinary markers for measuring exposure to endogenous and exogenous alkylating agents and precursors. *Environ. Health Perspect.*, **99**, 33–37.

Skipper, P. L. (1996). Influence of tertiary structure on nucleophilic substitution reactions of proteins. *Chem. Res. Toxicol.*, **9**, 918–923.

Skipper, P. L. and Tannenbaum, S. R. (1990). Protein adducts in the molecular dosimetry of chemical carcinogens. *Carcinogenesis*, **11**, 507–518.

Skipper, P. L., Peng, X., Soohoo, C. K. and Tannenbaum, S. R. (1994). Protein adducts as biomarkers of human carcinogen exposure. *Drug Metab. Rev.*, **26**, 111–124.

Sorsa, M., Hemminki, K. and Vainio, H. (1982). Biologic monitoring of exposure to chemical mutagens in the occupational environment. *Teratog. Carcinog. Mutagen.*, **2**, 137–150.

Soskolne, C. L. (1997). Ethical, social, and legal issues surrounding studies of susceptible populations and individuals. *Environ. Health Perspect.*, **105**, 837–841.

Spivack, S. D., Fasco, M. J., Walker, V. E. and Kaminsky, L. S. (1997). The molecular epidemiology of lung cancer. *Crit. Rev. Toxicol.*, **27**, 319–365.

Srám, R. J. (1998). Effect of glutathione *S*-transferase M1 polymorphisms on biomarkers of exposure and effects. *Environ. Health Perspect.*, **106**, 231–239.

Strickland, P. T., Routledge, M. N. and Dipple, A. (1993). Methodologies for measuring carcinogen adducts in humans. *Cancer Epidemiol. Biomarkers Prev.*, **2**, 607–619.

Swain, C. G. and Scott, C. B. (1953). Quantitative correlation of relative rates. Comparison of hydroxide ion with other nucleophilic reagents toward alkyl halides, esters, epoxides and acyl halides. *J. Am. Chem. Soc.*, **75**, 141–147.

Tannenbaum, S. R., Skipper, P. L., Wishnok, J. S., Stillwell, W. G., Day, B. W. and Taghizadeh, K. (1993). Characterization of various classes of protein adducts. *Environ. Health Perspect.*, **99**, 51–55.

Törnqvist, M. (1991). The *N*-alkyl Edman method for haemoglobin adduct measurement: updating and applications to humans. In Garner, R. C., Farmer, P. B., Steel, G. T. and Wright, A. S. (Eds), *Human Carcinogen Exposure: Biomonitoring and Risk Assessment.* IRL Press, New York, pp. 411–419.

Törnqvist, M. (1994). Epoxide adducts to *N*-terminal valine of hemoglobin. *Methods Enzymol.*, **231B**, 650–657.

Vineis, P. (1995). Use of biomarkers in epidemiology. The example of metabolic susceptibility to cancer. *Toxicol. Lett.*, **77**, 163–168.

Wahrendorf, J. (1995). Design of studies for validation of biomarkers of exposure and their effective use in environmental epidemiology. *Toxicology*, **101**, 89–92.

Walker, V. E., Fennell, T. R., Upton, P. B., Skopek, T. R., Prevost, V., Shuker, D. E. and Swenberg, J. A. (1992). Molecular dosimetry of ethylene oxide: formation and persistence of 7-(2-hydroxyethyl)guanine in DNA following repeated exposures of rats and mice. *Cancer Res.*, **52**, 4328–4334.

Walker, V. E., Fennell, T. R., Upton, P. B., Macneela, J. P. and Swenberg, J. A. (1993). Molecular dosimetry of DNA and hemoglobin adducts in mice and rats exposed to ethylene oxide. *Environ. Health Perspect.*, **99**, 11–17.

Warren, A. J. and Shields, P. G. (1997). Molecular epidemiology: carcinogen–DNA adducts and genetic susceptibility. *Proc. Soc. Exp. Biol. Med.*, **216**, 172–180.

Weston, A. (1993). Physical methods for the detection of carcinogen–DNA adducts in humans. *Mutat. Res.*, **288**, 19–29.

Weston, A., Rowe, M. L., Manchester, D. A., Farmer, P. B., Mann, D. L. and Harris, C. C. (1989). Fluorescence and mass spectral evidence for the formation of benzo[*a*]pyrene anti-diol-epoxide–DNA and hemoglobin adducts in humans. *Carcinogenesis*, **10**, 251–257.

WHO (1993). *Biomarkers and Risk Assessment: Concepts and Principles*. World Health Organization, Geneva.

WHO (1995). Guiding principles for the use of biological markers in the assessment of human exposure to environmental factors: an integrative approach of epidemiology and toxicology. *Toxicology*, **101**, 1–10.

Wild, C. P. and Pisani, P. (1998). Carcinogen DNA and protein adducts as biomarkers of human exposure in environmental cancer epidemiology. *Cancer Detect. Prev.*, **22**, 273–283.

Wild, C. P., Jiang, Y. Z., Allen, S. J., Jansen, L. A. M., Hall, A. J. and Montesano, R. (1990). Aflatoxin–albumin adducts in human sera from different regions of the world. *Carcinogenesis*, **11**, 2271–2274.

Wild, C. P., Hasegawa, R., Barraud, L., Chutimataewin, S., Chapot, B., Ito, N. and Montesano, R. (1996). Aflatoxin-albumin adducts: a basis for comparative carcinogenesis between animals and humans. *Cancer Epidemiol. Biomarkers Prev.*, **5**, 179–189.

Wogan, G. N. and Gorelick, N. J. (1985). Chemical and biochemical dosimetry of exposure to genotoxic chemicals. *Environ. Health Perspect.*, **62**, 5–18.

ADDITIONAL RECOMMENDED READING

Chiarelli, M. P. and Lay, J. O. (1993). Mass spectrometry for the analysis of carcinogen–DNA adducts. *Mass Spectrom. Rev.*, **11**, 447–493.

Cohen, S. D., Pumford, N. R., Khairallah, E. A., Boekelheide, K., Pohl, L. R., Amouzadeh, H. R. and Hinson, J. A. (1997). Selective protein covalent binding and target organ toxicity. *Toxicol. Appl. Pharmacol.*, **143**, 1–12.

Colburn, W. A. (1997). Selecting and validating biologic markers for drug development. *J. Clin. Pharmacol.*, **37**, 355–362.

Ehrenberg, L., Granath, F. and Törnqvist, M. (1996). Macromolecule adducts as biomarkers of exposure to environmental mutagens in human populations. *Environ. Health Perspect.*, **104**, 423–428.

Finkel, A. M. (1995). A quantitative estimate of the variations in human susceptibility to cancer and its implications for risk management. In Olin, S., Farland, W., Park, C., Rhomberg, L., Scheuplein, R., Starr, T. and Wilson, J. (Eds), *Low-Dose Extrapolation of Cancer Risks*. International Life Sciences Institute, Washington, DC, pp. 297–328.

Gochfeld, M. (1998). Susceptibility biomarkers in the workplace: historical perspective. In Mendelsohn, M. L., Mohr, L. C. and Peeters, J. P. (Eds), *Biomarkers: Medical and Workplace Applications*. Joseph Henry Press, Washington, DC, pp. 3–22.

Hatch, M. and Thomas, D. (1993). Measurement issues in environmental epidemiology. *Environ. Health Perspect.*, **101**, 49–57.

McMichael, A. J. (1994). 'Molecular epidemiology': new pathway or new travelling companion? *Am. J. Epidemiol.*, **140**, 1–11.

National Research Council (1991). Biologic markers in studies of hazardous-waste sites. In *Environmental Epidemiology—Public Health and Hazardous Waste*. National Academy Press, Washington, DC, pp. 219–255.

National Research Council (1991). *Environmental Epidemiology*. National Academy Press, Washington, DC.

Perera, F. P. (1996). Uncovering new clues to cancer risk. *Sci. Am.*, **274**, 54–62.

Schulte, P. A. and Perera, F. P. (1993). *Molecular Epidemiology*. Academic Press, New York.

Vineis, P. and Porta, M. (1996). Causal thinking, biomarkers, and mechanisms of carcinogenesis. *J. Clin. Epidemiol.*, **49**, 951–956.

Zweig, F. M. (1998). Biomarkers in the courtroom. In Mendelsohn, M. L., Mohr, L. C., and Peeters, J. P. (Eds), *Biomarkers: Medical and Workplace Applications*. Joseph Henry Press, Washington, DC, pp. 407–414.

Chapter 87

Biological Monitoring in the Occupational Environment

Antero Aitio

C O N T E N T S

INTRODUCTION

Biological monitoring or biomonitoring means repetitive measurement of chemicals or their metabolites, usually in blood or urine, but sometimes in exhaled air or tissues, in order to assess the extent of exposure or the health risk it may induce. Sometimes an effect of the chemical may also be measured. The parameter being measured is called a biomarker (thus, biomarkers of exposure and of effect are discerned). Biomonitoring has long traditions: elevated urinary lead concentrations were reported among lead-exposed workers in the 1920s and the first evaluations of blood and urine lead determinations in diagnosis and occupational health care were published more than 60 years ago. At present, biomonitoring methods have been published for more than 100 individual chemicals or groups of related chemicals, but a reliable quantitative interpretation of the result can only be made for about 40 chemicals (**Table 1**). In several countries, biomonitoring has also been included in national legislation; it is also part of worker health protection in the European Union. In-depth reviews on biomonitoring are available [International Programme on Chemical Safety (IPCS), 1993; Lauwerys and Hoet, 1993; Aitio, 1994; Aitio et al., 1994; WHO, 1996a, b].

For most chemicals, industrial hygiene measurements are the best and often the only way of assessing exposure. However, in some instances biomonitoring may very effectively complement and be superior to industrial hygiene measurements. This is mainly because:

- ▦ Concentrations of chemicals in workplace air are seldom stable but fluctuate with time and are different in different locations.
- ▦ Workload dramatically changes the inhaled volume of air, and for many chemicals the amount absorbed is directly related to the amount inhaled. Exposure peaks often coincide with increased workloads caused by, e.g., the malfunctioning of a closed process.
- ▦ Absorption via routes other than inhalation is generally not related to concentrations of chemicals in the air.
- ▦ Personal working habits vary, and individuals may absorb different amounts of chemicals in apparently similar conditions.
- ▦ Protection afforded by masks varies depending on the individual who wears it and on the condition of the masks.
- ▦ Biomonitoring may help estimate the accumulation of chemicals in the body. This is especially important when exposure is not constant and continuous and the collection of representative samples of the air is therefore very difficult.

BIOMONITORING OF EXPOSURE AND OF EFFECT

Biomonitoring has traditionally been divided into two branches, biomonitoring of exposure and biomonitoring of effect. The former means measurement of the parent chemical or its metabolites in biological samples and the latter measurement of an effect of the chemical on the body which is ideally 'non-adverse' or 'reversible'.

Biomonitoring of Exposure

The term monitoring of exposure—like the equivalent 'biomarker of exposure'—is a misnomer, since the

Table 1 Biomonitoring action levels given by different organizations[a]

Exposure	Measured parameter	ACGIH	HSE	DFG	FIOH
Acetone	U—Acetone	60 mg/l[1,2]		80 mg/l[1]	
Organophosphate acetylcholinesterase inhibitors	E—Acetylcholinesterase	30% drop		30% drop[1,3]	30% drop
Acrylonitrile	B—Hb cyanoethylvaline adduct			420 μg/l[4]	
Aluminium	U—Al			200 μg/l[1]	6 μmol/l[5]
Aniline	U—p-Aminophenol B—Methaemoglobin U—Aniline	50 mg/g creat.[1] 1.5%		1 mg/l[1,3]	
Arsenic	U—As^{III} + As^V + MMA + DMA U—As^{III} + As^V	50 μg/g creat.[6]	230 μmol/mol creat.[7]		
Arsenic trioxide	U—As^{III} + As^V + MMA + DMA			130 μg/l[1,4]	0.07 μmol/l[1]
Benzene	U—Phenylmercapturic acid B—Benzene	25 μg/g creat.[1]		45 μg/g creat.[1,4] 5 μg/l[1,4]	0.2 μmol/l[8], 0.02 μmol/l[9] 40 μmol/l[10]
2-Butoxyethanol and 2-butoxyethyl acetate	U—Butoxyacetic acid		240 mmol/mol creat.[1]	100 mg/l[1]	
p-$tert$-Butylphenol	U—PTBP			2 mg/l[1]	2 mg/l[1]
Cadmium	U—Cd B—Cd	5 μg/g creat 5 μg/l	10 μmol/mol creat.	15 μg/l 15 μg/l	50 nmol/l 50 nmol/l
Carbon disulphide	U—TTCA	5 mg/g creat.[1]		8 mg/l[1]	2.0 mmol/mol creat.[10]
Carbon monoxide	Hb—COHb End-exhaled air—CO	3.5%[1] 20 ppm[1]		5%[1]	5%[1]
Carbon tetrachloride	B—CCl$_4$			70 μg/l[1,3]	
Chlorobenzene	U—4-Chlorocatechol	150 mg/g creat.[1]		300 mg/g creat.[1], 70 mg/g creat.[5]	
Chlorophenols	U—4-Chlorophenol U—Tri- + tetra- + pentachlorophenols	25 mg/g creat.[1]			2.0 μmol/l[10]
Chlorophenoxy acids	U—2,4-D + dichloroprop + MCPA + mecoprop				14 μmol/l[11]
Chromium (VI), water-soluble fume	U—Cr	10 μg/g creat.[12] 30 μg/g creat.[10]		40 μg/l[1,13]	0.6 μmol/l[1]

(Continued)

Table 1 *(Contd)*

Exposure	Measured parameter	ACGIH	HSE	DFG	FIOH
Chromium: alkalimetal chromates	B—Cr			17 g/l[3,13,4]	
	U—Cr			20 g/l[14]	0.1 mol/l[1]
Chromium (VI) oxide					
Cobalt	U—Cobalt	15 g/l[10]		60 g/l[4]	600 nmol/l[10]
	B—Cobalt	1 g/l[10]		5 g/l[4]	
Dichloromethane	Hb—COHb			5%[1]	5%[10]
	B—Dichloromethane			1 mg/l[1]	
N,N-Dimethylacetamide	U—N,N-Methylacetamide	30 mg/g creat[10]	100 mmol/mol creat[1]		
N,N-Dimethylformamide	U—N,N-Methylformamide	20 mg/g creat[12]		15 mg/l[1]	650 mol/l[1]
2-Ethoxyethanol and 2-ethoxyethyl acetate	U—2-Ethoxyacetic acid	100 mg/g creat[10]		50 mg/l[3,1]	
Ethylbenzene	U—Mandelic acid	1.5 g/g creat[10]			10 mmol/l[10]
Ethylene	B—Hb hydroxyethylvaline adduct			90 g/l[4]	
Ethylene oxide	B—Hb hydroxyethylvaline adduct			90 g/l[4]	
Ethylene glycol dinitrate	B—EGDN			0.3 g/l	
Fluorides	U—F	10 mg/g creat[1]		7 mg/g creat[1,14]	350 mol/l[1]
	U—F	3 mg/g creat[9]		4 mg/g creat[9,14]	200 mol/l[5]
Fluorotrichloromethane	B—Fluorotrichloromethane				100 nmol/l[10]
Formic acid	U—Formic acid				240 mmol/mol creat[11]
Furfural	U—Furoic acid	200 mg/g creat[1]			
Halothane	U—Trifluoroacetic acid			2.5 mg/l[3]	
Hexachlorobenzene	P/S—Hexachlorobenzene			150 g/l	
n-Hexane	U—Hexanedione	5 mg/g creat[1]		5 mg/l[1]	5 mol/l[1]
	U—Hexanedione 4,5-dihydroxy hexan-2-one				
Hydrazine	U—Hydrazine			380 g/g creat[14]	
	P—Hydrazine			340 g/l[4]	
Lead	B—Pb	30 g/100 ml	70 g/100 ml[15]	70 g/100 ml[16]	50 g/100 ml
	U—Pb	150 g/g creat		50 g/l[1]	
Lead, organic	U—Lead		40 g/g creat[10]		
Lindane	B—Lindane		10 g/l[1]	20 g/l[1]	
	P/S—Lindane		35 nmol/l[1]	25 g/l[1]	

(Continued)

Table 1 *(Contd)*

Exposure	Measured parameter	ACGIH	HSE	DFG	FIOH
Mercury	U—Hg, inorganic B—Hg, inorganic	35 μg/g creat.[9] 15 μg/l.[10]			
Mercury, inorganic	U—Hg B—Hg B—Hg		20 μmol/mol creat.	200 μg/l 50 μg/l 100 μg/l	250 nmol/l[17] 90 nmol/l
Mercury, organic	B—Hg				240 mmol/mol creat.[11]
Methanol	U—Methanol U—Formic acid	15 mg/l[1]		30 mg/l[1,3]	
Methaemoglobin inducers	B—Methaemoglobin	1.5% of haemoglobin.[18]			
Methyl butyl ketone	U—Hexanedione + 4,5-dihydroxy hexan-2-one			5 mg/l[1]	
Methylenebis (2-chloroaniline)	U—MOCA		15 μmol/mol creat.[1,7]		15 μmol/mol creat.[1]
Methylenedianiline	U—MDA		50 μmol/mol creat.[1,7,9]		50 μmol/mol creat.[1,9]
Methyl ethyl ketone	U—MEK	2 mg/l[1]		5 mg/l[1]	60 μmol/l[10]
Methyl isobutyl ketone	U—MIBK	2 mg/l[1]		3.5 mg/l[1]	
Nickel, soluble compounds	U—Nickel				1.3 μmol/l[10]
Nickel, insoluble[19]	U—Nickel	5 mg/g creat.[10]		45 μg/l[3,4]	
Nitrobenzene	U—pNitrophenol B—Methaemoglobin B—Aniline–Hb-conjugate	1.5% of haemoglobin		100 μg/l[3]	
Nitroglycerine	P/S—1,2-Glyceryl dinitrate P/S—1,3-Glyceryl dinitrate			0.5 mg/l[1] 0.5 mg/l[1]	
Organochlorine insecticides	P—Organochlorine compounds[20]				2.0 nmol/l[17]
Parathion	E—Acetylcholinesterase U—pNitrophenol	30% drop 0.5 mg/g creat.[1]		30% drop[1,3] 500 mg/l[3]	
Pentachlorophenol	U—PCP P—PCP	2 mg/g creat[11] 5 mg/l[1]			
Phenol	U—Phenol	250 mg/g creat[1]		300 mg/l[1]	3.2 mmol/l[1]
Propan-2-ol	U—Acetone B—Acetone			50 mg/l[1] 50 mg/l[1]	
Selenium	U—Se				1.25 μmol/l[10]

(Continued)

Table 1 *(Contd)*

Exposure	Measured parameter	ACGIH	HSE	DFG	FIOH
Styrene	U—Mandelic acid	800 mg/g creat.[1], 300 mg/g creat.[9]		400 mg/g creat.[1]	2.9 mmol/l[10]
	U—PGA	240 mg/g creat.[1], 100 mg/g creat.[9]		500 mg/g creat.[1]	1.2 mmol/l[11]
	U—Mandelic acid + PGA				
	B—Styrene	0.55 mg/l[1], 0.02 mg/l[9]			
Tetrachloroethylene	End-exhaled air—PER	5 ppm[11]			
	B—PER	0.5 mg/l[11]		1 mg/l[9]	6 μmol/l[11]
	U—Trichloroacetic acid	3.5 mg/l[10]			
Tetrahydrofuran	U—Tetrahydrofuran	8 mg/l[1,2]		8 mg/l[1]	
Toluene	B—Toluene	0.05 mg/l[11,2]		1.0 mg/l[1]	2.0 μmol/l[11]
	U—Hippuric acid	1.6 g/g creat.[1,2]		1.7 mg/l[1]	
	U—o-Cresol			3.0 mg/l[1,3]	
1,1,1-Trichloroethane	End-exhaled air—1,1,1-Trichloroethane	40 ppm[11]			
	B—1,1,1-Trichloroethane			550 μg/l[3,9]	2.0 μmol/l[11]
	B—Trichloroethanol	1 mg/l[10]			
	U—Trichloroethanol	30 mg/l[10]			
Trichloroethylene	U—TCA	100 mg/g creat.[6]	35 mmol/mol creat.[7]	100 mg/l[1,3]	360 μmol/l[10]
	B—Trichloroethanol	4 mg/l[10]		5 mg/l[1,3]	1 mmol/l[3]
	U—TCA + trichloroethanol	300 mg/g creat.[10]			
Trichlorofluoroethane	B—Trichlorofluoroethane				50 nmol/l[11]
Triethylamine	U—Triethylamine				0.85 mmol/l[10]
Vanadium pentoxide	U—Vanadium	50 μg/g creat.[10]		70 μg/g creat.[1,3]	600 nmol/l[10]
Vinyl chloride	U—Thiodiglycolic acid			2.4 mg/24 h[3,4]	
Xylenes	U—Methylhippuric acids	1.5 g/g creat.[1]		2 g/l[1]	10 mmol/l[1]
	B—Xylenes			1.5 mg/l[1]	

[a] ACGIH = American Conference for Government Industrial Hygienists [American Conference of Governmental Industrial Hygienists (ACGIH), 1997]; HSE = Health and Safety Executive (Wilson, 1996), UK; DFG = Deutsche Forschungsgemeinschaft [Deutsche Forschungsgemeinschaft (DFG), 1996], FIOH = Finnish Institute of Occupational Health (Ahlström, 1998). The status of the different reference values varies from legally binding statutes to unofficial guidelines. The reference values are given in units used in the original documents; for conversions, see Table 3. The volume-based concentrations from the Finnish Institute of Occupational Health refer to values corrected to a relative density of 1.024. Abbreviations: B = blood; P = plasma; S = serum; E = erythrocytes; Hb = haemoglobin; U = urine. Superscript numbers: 1 = end of shift; 2 = change intended in 1997; 3 = in continuous exposure, after several shifts, at the end of the exposure; 4 = exposure equivalent for carcinogenic chemicals (EKA); 5 = morning specimen after two free days; 6 = end of work week; 7 = benchmark value; 8 = 1 hr after end of exposure; 9 = prior to next shift; 10 = end of shift at end of work week; 11 = before the shift at end of work week; 12 = increase during shift; 13 = does not apply to exposure to welding fumes; 14 = also valid for hydrogen fluoride; 15 = 40 μg/100 ml for women of childbearing age; 16 = 30 μg/100 ml for women <40 years of age; 17 = morning specimen; 18 = during or end of shift; 19 = metallic nickel, nickel oxide, carbonate, sulphide, sulphide earths; 20 = sum of aldrin, dieldrin, endosulfan, heptachlor, lindane and methoxychlor.

purpose is not to measure exposure (contact of the body with the chemical) but the amount absorbed. The best studied biomonitoring methods make use of selective chemical methods; several non-selective methods have also been suggested (Vainio *et al.*, 1984; Clonfero *et al.*, 1990; Aringer *et al.*, 1991; Demarini *et al.*, 1997).

Selective methods are intended to measure exclusively the object of the biomonitoring. The selectivity depends on the analytical specificity and on the presence/relative importance of sources of the chemical other than the work environment.

Modern analytical techniques employing reasonably selective detection and efficient sample purification methods in combination are often very specific. However, specificity depends on the presence of disturbing chemicals and is therefore very dependent on the matrix: a method that is fully specific, e.g., in blood may be unspecific in urine.

The specificity of the parameter being measured with regard to the occupational exposure is an important consideration. For example, varying amounts of phenol, hippuric acid and cresols are derived from dietary components and are excreted in urine, and so are lead, mercury, cadmium and arsenic, among others. This makes it difficult to estimate occupational exposures to benzene, toluene or elements by biomonitoring. The significance of this non-occupational chemical source is inversely related to the level of occupational exposure: at high occupational exposure levels, urinary concentrations of the metabolites often accurately reflect the occupational exposure, whereas at low levels of occupational exposure metabolite levels tend not to be different from the background variation.

Biomonitoring measures the chemical irrespective of whether it is derived from the occupational or environmental exposure. From the point of view of the health risk, this is a marked strength of biomonitoring: the chemical has identical effects on the body independent of the source, and exposure from all sources is integrated by biomonitoring. However, from the point of view of prevention, this is a weakness: the source of the exposure has to be clarified by other means.

A further consideration for selectivity in biomonitoring is speciation: with the exception of arsenic and mercury, biomonitoring of elements has only been concerned with the analysis of the total amount of an element without separation into, e.g., valence states or noting the difference between ionized and non-ionized species. When the chemical has a systemic effect and only one species is present in the blood/urine (lead, mercury, cadmium, aluminium), this is not a problem, but for chemicals such as nickel and chromium compounds, where the important health effects are mainly local (skin, respiratory tract) and there are substantial differences in the toxicity and kinetics between different species of the element, this is an import limitation in biomonitoring **(Table 2)**.

Table 2 Relationship between concentrations of nickel and cobalt in the air and urine in different trades

Metal	Trade in which the metal used[a]	Concentration in air ($\mu g\ m^{-3}$)	Concentration in urine (nmol l^{-1})
Cobalt	Hard metal grinding	4.5	53–990
	Porcelain factory	0.1–1.4	10–95
	Chemical factory	0.02–0.57	120–2,220
	Smelter	0.1–3.2	126–2,110
Nickel	Buffers/polishers	26–48	70–54
	External grinders	1.6–3.0	92–41
	Arc welders	6.0–14.3	107–70
	Bench mechanics	52–94	208–232
	Electroplaters	0.8–0.9	179–138
	Nickel refinery workers	489–560	3780–3850

Adapted from Bernacki *et al.* (1978) and Hartung *et al.* (1983).
[a] The different trades represent exposures to different forms of the metals.

Macromolecule Adducts

During the last few years, analysis of macromolecule—protein or DNA—adducts has been extensively studied with the purpose of developing biomonitoring methods; polycyclic aromatic hydrocarbons and aromatic amines have been studied most extensively (Hemminki, 1992; Mumford *et al.*, 1993; Riffelmann *et al.*, 1995; Farmer *et al.*, 1996; Poirier and Weston, 1996). The idea is that the dose of the proximate carcinogen is measured at the target molecule (DNA adducts, or their surrogates = protein adducts), albeit not in the target cells, and this would reflect the health risk better than, e.g., the concentration of the parent chemical in the blood. The main problems with this approach are that usually no quantitative validation based on either health outcome or exposure is available and the techniques used are very sophisticated (expensive), and still tend to be working at their limit of detection. Some adduct analyses that are in routine use are listed in **Table 1**.

Biomonitoring of Mixed Exposures

Traditionally, biological monitoring is used for the evaluation of the uptake of a single chemical. To overcome the problem that the exposure may contain several or even many similar compounds, an indicator chemical may be selected for analysis. Apparently, the indicator chemical should behave in the organism in a fashion similar to the toxic components of the mixture. Additionally, one has to assume a stable composition for the mixture in order to be able to make any assessment of the risk. Biomonitoring of mixed exposures has been most extensively studied in the cases of polycyclic aromatic hydrocarbons and of tobacco smoke (Crawford *et al.*, 1994; Holiday *et al.*, 1995; Koyano *et al.*, 1996).

Polycyclic aromatic hydrocarbons (PAHs) usually appear in complex mixtures, and their main toxicological interest is their carcinogenic activity, which is most apparent in hydrocarbons with five or six aromatic rings, such as benzo [a]pyrene. Biomonitoring of PAHs has been mostly studied by determining 1-hydroxypyrene, a metabolite of pyrene, in the urine of exposed workers. Several studies have shown that the concentration of 1-hydroxypyrene is elevated in occupational PAH exposure, and also in smokers (vs non-smokers) (Kuljukka *et al.*, 1996; Nielsen *et al.*, 1996; Strickland *et al.*, 1996; Angerer *et al.*, 1997). The main problem with 1-hydroxypyrene measurements is that the toxicologically important PAHs are not measured, and the interpretation of the result is crucially dependent on the ratio of pyrene to the carcinogenic PAH in the airborne mixture. Passive smoking is being increasingly perceived as an occupational hazard, and biological monitoring methods to identify smoke-exposed people have been developed. Many parameters, including cyanide, thiocyanate, nicotine, cotinine, carbon monoxide and carboxyhaemoglobin, have been studied as means of biomonitoring tobacco smoke. All these show elevated levels in people who have been exposed to cigarette smoke or have smoked themselves. However, especially urinary thioethers, but in some occupational settings also blood carbon monoxide concentrations, are very unselective. Therefore, cotinine concentrations either in plasma or in urine seem to be the best choice at present.

Although some data exist on the relationship between the airborne concentration of PAHs and of pyrenol in the urine (Jongeneelen *et al.*, 1990; Jongeneelen, 1992), it seems that at present the interpretation of biomonitoring of mixed exposures by analyses of indicator chemicals is at best semiquantitative: exposed groups may be identified, but it is not possible to give either health-based or industrial hygiene-based biomonitoring action levels (see interpretation, below).

Assessment of Body/Organ Burden In Vivo

Most chemicals are distributed in several different compartments in the body. For several, a tissue or organ may present considerable concentrations, i.e. a chemical is stored there. Thus, for example, lipid-soluble solvents are accumulated in body fat, cadmium in the liver and kidneys and lead in the bones. Recently, methods have been developed to estimate directly the amount of the chemical at the site of accumulation. The most widely used methods are neutron activation measurement of cadmium and X-ray fluorescence spectrometry of lead and cadmium. *In vivo* methods have also been proposed for the determination of mercury, aluminium, iron and silicon (Landrigan and Todd, 1994; Nilsson, 1994; Todd and Chettle, 1994; Börjesson and Mattsson, 1995; Börjesson *et al.*, 1995, 1997; Nilsson *et al.*, 1995).

Neutron activation has been used to measure the cadmium content in the liver and kidneys, sites which show marked accumulation. The sensitivity of the assay depends on the dose of radiation used; levels occurring in the liver and kidneys of occupationally non-exposed adults may be measured; the accumulation of cadmium in the kidney of smokers has, for example, been well demonstrated and quantified using this technique. However, although neutron activation *in vivo* would be an effective tool in predicting the risk of kidney damage in cadmium exposure, it involves exposure to neutrons, which are still a rather unknown entity. The use of this method in routine biomonitoring would seem questionable.

X-ray fluorescence spectrometry has been used to measure the lead content of bones and also the content of cadmium in the kidney. If polarized X-rays are used, the sensitivity of the method for lead is at present sufficient to measure the lead concentrations in the bones of pre-school children. The radiation dose is very small, and only small volumes of tissue are irradiated. However, it seems that when a good history is available on the lead concentration in the blood, this reflects the effects of lead on neurophysiological/psychological parameters better than the content of lead in the tibia or calcaneus (Bleecker *et al.*, 1995, 1997; Kovala *et al.*, 1997; Hänninen *et al.*, 1998). Thus the main area of application for the determinations of lead in bone seems to be cases where such history is not available and there is a suspicion of lead-induced health impairment, that is, in diagnostics rather than in biomonitoring.

Kinetic Considerations and Sampling Strategies

In biological monitoring one may try to estimate the body burden of the chemical. An alternative approach is to ascertain the highest concentration attained in the body, especially in the target tissue. However, because the biological monitoring of chemicals with mainly acute toxicity cannot be preventive, this approach probably is not very rewarding.

The ease with which one can estimate the body burden of a chemical is very dependent on the kinetic properties of the chemical in the body. For chemicals with long half-times, such as lead, cadmium, and mercury, the concentration in the blood or urine reaches a plateau, which reflects the equilibrium between daily intake and excretion. In a stable exposure situation the daily variation of the concentration is small, and a fairly accurate picture of long-term exposure may be obtained from even single determinations of blood or urine levels.

The situation is different for chemicals with short half-times. First, the concentration, especially in the blood, changes rapidly with time, and the concentrations found reflect only very recent exposure. Very stringent standardization of the specimen collection time is needed in order to obtain meaningful results. Second, as the concentrations of the chemical in the workplace air tend to change, a single value may not reflect the average exposure accurately. Even if the working conditions are known, a single measurement gives only a rough idea of the most recent exposure. Hence one will have to do the monitoring frequently in order to obtain a representative picture of the amounts absorbed. In practice, it is not possible to monitor effectively chemicals with half-times shorter than a few hours. However, many chemicals have several successive half-times, reflecting their distribution in different compartments of the body. Thus, lipid-soluble organic solvents, which have a very short half-time (of the order of minutes only) in the blood and richly vascularized organs, accumulate in the fatty tissues and are slowly released after exposure has ceased. The fat stores thus function as integrators, and exposure over a whole day, or even several days, may be estimated from specimens collected approximately 16–18 h after the end of the exposure. At this point in time, the half-times of, e.g., lipid-soluble solvents are of the order of 10–20 h. Excretion in the urine also functions as an integrator or buffer for a chemical, and the half-times are generally longer than those found in the blood. Hence excretion of a metabolite in the urine is often a kinetically preferable alternative in biological monitoring.

Biomonitoring of Effects

Effect monitoring means that instead of the substance itself or a metabolite, an effect is measured. Monitoring of an early effect of the chemical would be ideal for the prevention of the adverse health effects of a chemical: it would take into account even the individual differences in susceptibility, not only in the amounts of the chemical taken up. In order to prevent adverse effects, the effect on which the monitoring is based should be reversible, non-adverse and predict the adverse effects.

Effects that are extensively used in biomonitoring programmes include plasma and blood cholinesterase activities, enzymes and intermediate metabolite levels of haemoglobin synthesis and proteins/enzymes in the urine.

Toxicological End-points

Analysis of acetylcholinesterase activity in the erythrocytes or that of pseudocholinesterase in the plasma of workers exposed to organophosphate (or carbamate) insecticides is well validated in the diagnosis and treatment of high exposure; however, the relationship between these enzyme activities and the symptoms is not equally close at low or moderate exposure levels. Where organophosphate poisoning is still common, cholinesterase inhibition remains the first choice of biomonitoring of organophosphorus pesticides (Gompertz and Verschoyle, 1996).

The best known example of effect monitoring is the assessment of exposure to lead by following its effects on the enzymes of haemoglobin synthesis, such as the 5-aminolaevulinate dehydratase or ferrochelatase, or the concentrations of different intermediates in this metabolic pathway, such as the protoporphyrin in erythrocytes or aminolaevulinate in the urine. Where the determination of lead can be performed reliably, these measures do not offer additional information in the biomonitoring of lead exposure: it has not been demonstrated that individuals who show changes in haemoglobin synthesis at lower than average lead exposure levels are exceptionally sensitive toward the effects of lead on the nervous system, which are the important effects of lead at present exposure levels. The situation is different if accurate blood lead analysis is not available; then the determination of erythrocyte protoporphyrin could be a cost-effective way of monitoring lead exposure: the instrumentation is inexpensive, contamination in sample collection is not a problem, the analysis is very simple and reasonable accuracy is easily achieved.

Urinary excretion of several proteins or other components leaking from different parts of the nephron correlate with long-term exposure to cadmium, and might be used for the biomonitoring of this nephrotoxic chemical. Among these, the most extensively studied are β_2-microglobulin and retinol-binding globulin (Roels et al., 1993). However, clearly elevated excretion of these markers in the urine is not reversible; it leads to indisputable kidney damage. Also, since the prediction of health effects from the urinary levels of cadmium is fairly reliable, it is not clear that the effect monitoring could give any further insight in the biomonitoring of cadmium. Again, the situation is different if the reliable determination of urinary cadmium is not available. In such circumstances, the determination of retinol binding globulin (β_2-microglobulin is notoriously unstable in acid urine) is an alternative worth considering, although it is fairly unspecific.

Genotoxic End-points

Most proven human carcinogens are clastogenic, i.e. they cause structural chromosomal aberrations (CA), micronuclei (MN) or sister chromatid exchanges (SCE), which can be detected microscopically. Several of these chemicals have been shown to cause cytogenetic damage in occupationally exposed people. There is therefore a rationale for biomonitoring of people exposed to genotoxic carcinogens by cytogenetic methods. There is also some epidemiological evidence that groups with elevated chromosomal aberration rates may have an increased risk of cancer (Hagmar et al., 1994; Forni, 1996). However, after exposure to chemicals, it is not known whether those individuals who show the highest frequencies of CA, MN or SCE are at a higher risk than average. Even on a group basis, no quantitative estimate of the cancer risk can be made. Neither can it be predicted what kind of cancer is to be expected. Hence the validation of cytogenetic monitoring as far as the health outcome is concerned is still limited. Cytogenetic monitoring has, however, been used successfully in the follow-up of groups of workers exposed to clastogenic chemicals and in the verification of the efficacy of protective measures introduced.

Specimens Used in Biological Monitoring

In principle, any tissue or body fluid could be used for biomonitoring analyses—and in research projects, the variety of tissues actually used has been fairly wide. However, for routine biomonitoring, the tissues must be easily accessible and the results must be interpretable—reference values must exist in order to identify exposed individuals and biomonitoring action levels must be available for the assessment of the magnitude of the risk/exposure. For these reasons, the only tissues that are normally used are blood and urine. Exhaled air is used to a limited extent, and most often gives information that is comparable to that from analyses of blood, but for most chemicals reproducible sample collection and storage are difficult. In environmental biological monitoring, where the main route of exposure is from the diet, hair and even nails have been used. However, in occupational settings, where the exposure is usually through the ambient air, these tissues are easily contaminated and the contamination-derived chemical cannot be distinguished analytically from the chemical that entered the hair or nails from inside the organism. Therefore, the use of hair and nails is of very limited value in occupational toxicology.

Concentration Units in Biomonitoring

From the toxicological point of view, the unit that is active in the body is the molecule. Therefore, the most logical way of expressing concentrations in biological fluids in biological monitoring would be molar units, which is also the recommendation of international organizations. Molar units are also directly related to the volumetric units of gaseous chemicals in the air (cm^3 m^{-3} or ppm). In biological monitoring there is a further reason to choose these units: the target of the measurement is often not a single and well defined chemical species, but rather a group of related metabolites, derived from the same basic chemical. This is the case, for example, for arsenic (As^{III}, As^V, methylarsonic acid, and dimethylarsinic acid being most often measured), phenol (free phenol, phenyl glucuronide and phenyl sulphate), styrene (mandelic and phenylglyoxylic acid), xylene (dimethylbenzoic acids and their conjugates with glycine and glucuronic acid) and pyrene (hydroxypyrene and its glucuronide). In these cases, the only way to indicate accurately the amounts measured is to give them in molar concentrations. However, in several countries the

Table 3 Conversion of mass-based results to molar units

Chemical	Molecular mass	μmol mg^{-1}
Acetone	58.08	17.22
Aluminium	26.98	37.06
4-Aminophenol	109.13	9.16
Aniline	93.13	10.74
Antimony	121.75	8.214
Arsenic	74.92	13.35
Benzene	78.11	12.80
2-Butoxyacetic acid	132.2	7.56
p-tert-Butylphenol	150.22	6.66
Cadmium	112.41	8.896
Carbon tetrachloride	153.82	6.50
Chlorocatechols	144.56	6.92
4-Chlorophenol	128.56	7.78
Chromium	52.00	19.23
Cobalt	58.93	16.97
Cresols	108.14	9.247
2,4-D	221.0	4.52
Dichlorprop	235.1	4.25
N, N-Dimethylacetamide	87.12	11.49
Ethoxyacetic acid	104.11	9.514
Ethyleneglycol dinitrate	152.06	82.92
Fluoride	19.0	52.64
Fluorotrichloromethane	137.37	7.28
Formic acid	46.03	21.72
Furoic acid	112.08	8.92
Glyceryl dinitrates	182.09	5.49
Hexachlorobenzene	284.78	3.51
Hexane-2,5-dione	114.15	8.759
Hippuric acid	179.18	5.580
Hydrazine	32.05	31.20
Lead	207.20	4.826[a]
Lindane	290.83	3.44
Mandelic acid	152.16	6.573
MCPA	200.6	4.99
Mecoprop	214.6	4.66
Mercury	200.59	4.985
Methanol	32.04	31.21
Methyl n-butyl ketone	100.16	9.98
Methylenebis (2-chloroaniline)	267.17	3.743
Methylenedianiline	198.3	5.04
Methyl ethyl ketone	72.11	13.87
N-Methylformamide	59.07	16.93
Methylhippuric acid	193.20	5.176
Methyl sobutyl ketone	100.16	9.98
Nickel	58.69	17.04
p-Nitrophenol	139.11	7.19
Pentachlorophenol	266.34	3.754
Phenol	94.11	10.63
Phenylglyoxylic acid	152.16	6.661
1-Pyrenol (1-Hydroxypyrene)	218.3	4.582
Selenium	78.96	12.67
Styrene	104.14	9.60
Tetrachloroethylene	165.82	6.030
Tetrachlorophenol	231.88	4.312
Thiocyanic acid	59.09	16.92
2-Thiothiazolidine-4-carboxylic acid	163.2	6.127
Toluene	92.13	10.85

(continued)

Table 3 (Contd)

Chemical	Molecular mass	μmol mg^{-1}
Trichloroacetic acid	163.39	6.120
1,1,1-Trichloroethane	133.4	7.495
Trichloroethanol	149.4	6.693
Trichlorofluoroethane	187.38	5.34
Trichlorophenol	197.44	5.064
Triethylamine	101.19	9.88
Trifluoroacetic acid	114.02	8.77
Vanadium	50.94	19.63
Xylenes	106.16	9.42

[a] The traditional unit for lead in blood is μg dl^{-1}; to convert to μmol l^{-1}, the figure is multiplied by 0.04826.

traditional mass-based units (mg l^{-1}, μg l^{-1}) remain in wide use. Molecular masses and conversion factors from mass-based to molar units for most widely used biomonitoring analyses are given in **Table 3**. In order to change mass-based, creatinine-corrected units (mg g^{-1} creatinine) to molar units (mmol mol^{-1} creatinine), the result should be divided by the molecular mass of the analyte and multiplied by the molecular mass of creatinine, 113.12.

SOURCES OF ERROR IN BIOLOGICAL MONITORING

All laboratory analyses are subject to error and biological monitoring is no exception. Biological monitoring shares the general problems of analytical work with tissue specimens, but has also other important specific sources of error.

The analytical error proper is beyond the scope of this chapter, but in many biological monitoring analyses the analytical techniques applied are demanding with respect to both the equipment involved and to the training and capabilities of the personnel.

Much variation is generated by physiological, kinetic and environmental factors that occur before the sample collection, and perhaps the largest errors are generated by contamination during specimen collection (Aitio and Järvisalo, 1984). All such errors must be handled by the health care personnel responsible for the sampling. The analysing laboratory can do little to avoid or detect them.

Physiological Variation

Body posture markedly affects the concentration of chemicals in the circulating blood. In the upright position water leaks from the blood vessels. Chemicals attached to cells or macromolecules show an apparent enrichment. In the recumbent position, the reverse takes place. The error thus generated may exceed 10% in a healthy person, but it may be many times higher in persons with various diseases. The same phenomenon is seen locally in the arm upon application of a tourniquet for specimen collection. The concentrations of many endogenous and even exogenous chemicals exhibit diurnal variations in body fluids, which are apparently independent of their intake. For example, concentrations of mercury in the urine are highest in the morning. The volume of urine excreted depends on the hydration state of the body. The effect of this variation on the concentration of different chemicals in the urine is largely unexplored. However, it is traditional to try to correct for the variation by standardizing the concentrations to a constant relative density (usually 1.018 or 1.024). The basis of correction chosen profoundly changes the figures obtained: correction to 1.024 gives values 33% higher than correction to 1.018. An alternative is correction to creatinine excretion, which remains stable irrespective of the hydration status, but is dependent on the body mass. Another alternative would be the use of timed urine specimens, e.g. 4-, 8- or even 24-h urine. This is not often achieved in routine biological monitoring. Which correction is best for each individual analysis is not always clear. Therefore, it is not surprising that the biomonitoring action levels given by different organizations differ in this respect. This also brings forth an important problem: there is no accurate mathematical relationship between data given in volumetric and creatinine-corrected units. It can be very roughly estimated that a concentration given in mg l^{-1} corresponds to approximately 0.5–1.0 mg g^{-1} creatinine.

The physiological variation has to be dealt with by rigorous standardization of the specimen collection. The sampling hour is to be standardized—preferably to the morning. This not only decreases the effect of diurnal variation, but also tends to decrease the effects of the preceding meal. The tested worker should avoid intensive physical stress for some hours before sampling. The subject should remain seated for 15 min before blood sampling. The tourniquet application time should be less than 1 min. Cigarette smoke contains, among other things, benzene, carbon monoxide, hydrogen cyanide and cadmium and hence is a significant source of error in the biological monitoring of at least these chemicals when there are smokers among the worker population.

Kinetic Variation

The concentration of an exogenous chemical is seldom stable in body fluids but shows an exposure-related fluctuation. The time of collecting the specimen, therefore, is a very important factor with regard to the concentration found; the interpretation depends crucially on the timing (Health and Safety Executive, 1992).

If a chemical is readily absorbed through the skin, this is usually regarded as a reason to prefer biological monitoring over air monitoring. However, when an analysis of the concentration in the blood of the chemical itself is used in biological monitoring, skin absorption may cause a substantial error. This is because the blood collected from a cubital vein does not represent the blood in the organism *in toto*, but rather a local concentration (Aitio *et al.*, 1984).

Contamination

The factors most likely to cause errors in specimen collection and storage include contamination, chemical deterioration, evaporation and precipitation and adsorption on vessel surfaces. Since the chemical natures of substances monitored differ widely, the relative importance of these processes also varies.

Contamination is by far the most important source of error in the analysis of trace elements. Contamination is a partial explanation to why, e.g., serum chromium values regarded as normal in non-exposed people in different studies (**Table 4**) have shown a precipitous fall in recent decades. A similar table can be given for many trace elements.

Contamination may come from the air in the workplace or the laboratory, from the worker's skin or clothes, from specimen containers, additives, reagents or from the analytical instrument.

Contamination from the workplace air causes the most dramatic analytical errors as the concentration of the chemical (organic or inorganic) in the dust tends to be very high. Dust is found also on the worker's clothes, as well as on the skin. Because proper cleaning of the skin is not easy, it is better to use only venous blood, not capillary blood, in trace element analysis.

The risk of contamination from the environment during specimen collection is greater for urine specimens than for blood specimens. Urine specimens should be collected in an uncontaminated area only, and only after the worker has taken a shower and changed clothes.

Nickel, chromium, manganese and cobalt may leach into blood from disposable stainless-steel needles. For the biological monitoring of these metals, blood samples should be collected through plastic cannulae—or, rather, urine should be used in the analyses since it also gives a better picture of the exposure to these metals.

Glass and plastics contain varying amounts of many trace elements and these may leach into water, urine and blood. It seems that no commercially produced container should be used for urine storage without prior cleaning by acid soaking. General-purpose evacuated tubes are a notorious source of, e.g., cadmium and lead, and probably also of other trace elements. Several manufacturers offer evacuated tubes specifically prepared for trace element analysis. For lead and cadmium determination, at least some of them are suitable; for less common trace element analyses, it still would seem preferable

Table 4 Evolution of the values regarded as normal average serum chromium concentrations in non-exposed humans

Year	Authors	Serum chromium (nmol l⁻¹)
1956	Monacelli *et al.*	3600
1966	Glinsman *et al.*	540
1972	Behne and Diehl	198
1972	Davidsohn and Secrest	97
1974	Pekarek *et al*	31
1974	Grafilage *et al.*	14
1978	Versieck *et al.*	3.1
1978	Kayne *et al.*	2.7
1983	Kumpulainen *et al.*	2.3
1984	Veillon *et al.*	2.1
1993	Brune *et al.*	1–3

Adapted from Kumpulainen *et al.* (1983), Veillon *et al.* (1984) and Brune *et al.* (1993).

to verify the absence of contamination by the element to be determined before using a new brand of evacuated tube.

INTERPRETATION OF BIOMONITORING DATA

Results from biomonitoring analyses are interpreted by comparing them with *reference limits* and *biomonitoring action levels*.

Reference Limits

Reference limits are the highest (usually 95th percentile) concentrations of the chemical observed in an occupationally non-exposed population which is similar in terms of ethnicity, sex, age and environmental exposure and also smoking and other social habits to the occupationally exposed population studied. For many industrial chemicals, the only source of the chemical is the occupational exposure and, therefore, the reference limit is equal to the limit of detection of the analytical method used. Concentrations higher than the reference limit indicate that the individual has been exposed at work, i.e. reference limits identify exposed individuals. They do not reflect the presence or magnitude of health risks. When biomonitoring results are available for more than one worker, identifying exposed groups should be done by a statistical comparison of the non-exposed and allegedly exposed groups. However, the distribution of the concentration levels in the non-exposed group is seldom available for the end user of the data and therefore such comparisons cannot be made. Because the results in biomonitoring often show a very skewed distribution, it may be assumed as a rule of thumb that if all workers in a group have a level of biomarker greater than half the reference limit, the group has been exposed at work.

Reference limits for chemicals for which the only source is the occupational exposure depend on the analytical method used. For other chemicals they vary from one geographical location to another (and may also depend on the analytical method, because of varying accuracy of the analysis). Moreover, changes may occur with time, as seen, for example, in the concentrations of lead in blood in several countries in the 1980s (Brody et al., 1994; Strömberg et al., 1995; Wietlisbach et al., 1995; Delves et al., 1996; Rodamilans et al., 1996; Torra et al., 1997). Smoking influences the concentrations of several exogenous chemicals in body fluids, such as carbon monoxide, benzene and cadmium. Hence, reference limits should be determined for each geographic area, taking into account concomitant environmental non-occupational exposures, and their accuracy should be verified from time to time.

Biomonitoring Action Levels

Biomonitoring action levels (BALs) (WHO, 1996a) are based on a judgement of what is an acceptable exposure. They are thus equivalent to standards and guidelines given for concentrations of chemicals in the work place air, i.e. occupational exposure limits (OELs). There are two ways in which a BAL may be developed: (1) from clinical, epidemiological and toxicological studies on the relationship between a measured concentration of a chemical/metabolite in body fluids and the health outcome (directly health-based BALs) or (2) from experience with good working practices.

Directly health-based BALs are ideally derived from long-term follow-up studies of workers exposed 8 h per day, 5 days per week, over their working lifetime as limits below which adverse effects on health have not been observed. Obviously, such values are not easy to obtain; best validated BALs are probably now available for lead, cadmium, mercury and carbon monoxide in blood and cadmium, fluoride and mercury in urine. Directly health-based BALs may change when further data accumulate. For example, the BALs for urinary and blood cadmium which have been used in most countries are based on the well defined measures of the nephrotoxicity of cadmium (Roels et al., 1993). The fact that cadmium is now considered to be a human carcinogen [International Agency for Research on Cancer (IARC), 1993] may well lead to changes in the BALs which are applicable to cadmium.

Another factor that very much affects the health-based BALs is the interpretation of what kind of change in the body is considered as harmful; for example, urinary concentrations of 6-ketoprostaglandin F_1 and sialic acid increase at urinary cadmium levels of 2, those of albumin and transferrin at 4 and those of, e.g., retinol-binding globulin, β_2-microglobulin, at 10 μmol mol^{-1} creatinine (Roels et al., 1993), and setting the action

level depends on which of these is considered as the relevant end-point.

The good working practice-derived BALs are usually derived mathematically from OELs concentration of the chemical/metabolite in the biological material that will occur in an average worker after an 8 hour exposure at the level of the OEL. Protection of health provided by the BALs derived from OELs thus depends on the appropriateness of the occupational exposure limit (a compromise between health protection and cost factors), the reliability of the estimate of the relationship between the occupational exposure limit and the BAL and the adequacy of the sampling strategy. It is important to realize that the uncertainty of the assessment of the relationship between OEL and BAL varies widely between different chemicals; for example, after exposure to styrene, the uncertainty is small for mandelic acid and phenylglyoxylic acid in urine (for which a large number of studies with concordant results have been published) but large for styrene itself in urine (for which few studies have been published) (Pekari et al., 1993).

An important problem with OEL-based BALs is that no single common BAL may be given for different compounds of an element: the relationship between airborne concentration of, e.g., readily water-soluble nickel compounds with urinary nickel concentration is very different from that for the practically insoluble nickel oxides and sulphides and metallic nickel (Sunderman et al., 1986). The same is true for, e.g., cobalt (Hartung et al., 1983) **(Table 2)** and chromium (Aitio et al., 1988).

For chemicals which are extensively absorbed through the skin, BALs cannot be derived from the OELs. In such cases, the only way of deriving a BAL is to determine the chemical/metabolite concentrations in biological specimens from exposed workers when good working practices are adhered to. Thus the BAL may, for example, be set at a value that 90% of the workplaces have actually achieved. This approach was introduced by the British Health and Safety Executive to set the BAL (called bench-mark value) for, e.g., methylenebis(2-chloroaniline) (MOCA) and methylenedianiline, and has since been used by others (Health and Safety Executive, 1993).

Biomonitoring Action Levels in Different Countries

Many countries and the European Union have more or less binding BALs for lead in blood. For biomonitoring other than lead, the most active countries in setting guidelines or limit values have been the USA (American Conference of Governmental Industrial Hygienists (ACGIH), Germany (Deutsche Forschungsgemeinschaft), Finland (Institute of Occupational Health) and the UK (Health and Safety Laboratory); sets of action levels have also been published in Switzerland, France and Poland. The ACGIH Biological Exposure

Indices (BEI) represent the levels of determinants which are most likely to be observed in specimens collected from a healthy worker who has been exposed to chemicals to the same extent as a worker with inhalation exposure to the threshold limit value (TLV) [American Conference of Governmental Industrial Hygienists (ACGIH), 1997]. In Germany, two sets of BALs are given, the first, the biological workplace chemical tolerance value [Biologischer Arbeitsstoff-Toleranz-Wert (BAT)], which, when regularly complied with, should usually protect the worker from adverse health effects. The second set, EKA values (Exposure equivalents for carcinogenic chemicals), are derived from the technical guidance limits for carcinogens at the workplace. The difference between EKA and BAT values is mainly due to the contention that no safe level can be given for a carcinogenic chemical. In the UK and Finland, guidance values are derived either from epidemiological clinical studies on exposed workers or from occupational exposure limits, or from good working practice, as benchmark values. BALs applied in these four countries are given in **Table 1**. It is important to note that the time of specimen collection may profoundly affect the numerical value of the BAL (see kinetic errors below).

ETHICAL ASPECTS IN BIOMONITORING

The first ethical question in biomonitoring is whether it is at all acceptable to use samples collected from a worker to judge if conditions at the workplace are acceptable, i.e., use the worker as a mobile sample collector. However, in this respect biological monitoring is only superficially different from collection of air samples using a personal sample collector (breathing zone samples). It is splitting hairs if a specimen collected from the air the worker is inhaling is considered different from the air he or she exhales or from blood that is in equilibrium with the air in pulmonary alveoli.

Biomonitoring produces data on an individual, and there is a need to use these data not only for the individual but also for fellow workers and the whole workplace, i.e. there is the ancient ethical dilemma of the rights of an individual *vs* those of the group. There may be an important conflict of interest between the need for workplace improvement and confidentiality of the individual data: the most expedient way to lower the average blood lead value in an enterprise is to fire all workers with high values—but on the other hand the employer has to know that there are 'too high' lead values and also in which tasks, i.e. in which workers, they occur. Confidentiality has also long-term importance, which is especially important now that all data tend to be registered on computers and may in principle become available to anyone: biomonitoring information on an individual may be used to discriminate against him/her in his/her later employment: employers may decide not to hire any-

one with a previous elevated blood lead level—or anyone with a documented previous non-exposure to lead. Thus biomonitoring data of an individual have to remain confidential for ever. Another type of confidentiality problem may arise especially in research-oriented biomonitoring laboratories: data published from small groups of enterprises may allow identification of the enterprises.

Accurate and honest risk communication is difficult: it should be made clear, what the significance of the reference limits and of the biomonitoring action levels is and whether the latter are health-based or good working habit-based. An important and difficult problem at present is the communication of the gaps of knowledge, so that gaps do not imply safety when it cannot be claimed, or a risk when one either does not exist or is not proved. Further, the important weakness of biomonitoring, absence of information on the source of exposure, has to be kept in mind.

The samples for biomonitoring analyses are open to misuse in that many other components may also be analysed from them, such as ethanol, drugs and HIV. In many headspace analyses of blood or urine for solvents, for example, ethanol will be measured automatically. It goes without saying that the workers have to be told what analyses will be performed, and the analysis must be limited to these items. When, which will happen in every laboratory, routine specimens are used for method development or reference value studies, the specimens must be coded and analysed blind.

The many sources of error that may occur in biomonitoring, together with the high costs often involved with workplace improvement, may make it tempting to transform biomonitoring into an endless series of postponements of action and follow-up of the situation. It is not unheard of that when considering which laboratory should perform obligatory biomonitoring analyses, the employer chooses the laboratory that reports the lowest values.

Above, it was indicated that elevated results in biomonitoring analyses should not be used against the worker. There is also another side of the coin, that is, malingering: if high levels of exposure—as determined by biological monitoring—are compensated in an inappropriate way (elevated wages for dirty or dangerous work, sick leave because of biomonitoring values in excess of action levels), it might become tempting for the worker to make sure that he or she is inadvertently exposed. This could be the case especially for chemicals with a short half-time: it is easy to make sure that on the day of the scheduled biomonitoring specimen collection the exposure is higher than usual.

Biomonitoring laboratories—like any commercial laboratories—work under economic pressures, and there is always the temptation to decrease costs where one is not automatically caught red-handed. Hence the laboratory may choose not to work out or keep up-to-date the reference values, or to invest in laboratory quality assurance (which may be very costly indeed in biomonitoring). In desperate situations it may happen that results are released that are more appealing than the

Table 5 Ethical responsibilities of the biomonitoring analytical laboratories and users of biomonitoring data

Biomonitoring laboratories
Analytical quality
Accuracy of reference values and action levels
Procedures for maintaining data confidentiality
Up-to-date knowledge of:
  chemical risks
  means of exposure assessment
  possibilities and limitations of biomonitoring methods
  continuous education and training of customers
Relative freedom of economic pressures

Users of biomonitoring data
Knowledge of sample collection and interpretation of
  biomonitoring
Responsible communication of results and interpretation
Use of individual data exclusively for the benefit of the individual
Prompt action for the improvement of the work place when
  needed
Selection of a responsible laboratory

true ones (see above), and in serious but less desperate situations the laboratory may advise biomonitoring analyses that are not really useful, excessive analyses or biomonitoring analyses when they are not the optimal approach for occupational exposure and risk assessment.

The ethical obligations of users of biomonitoring data **(Table 5)** therefore include knowledge (and application of this knowledge) on sample collection and interpretation of biological monitoring, responsible communication of the results and interpretation, use of individual data exclusively for the benefit of the worker and of his/her colleagues, prompt action for the improvement of the workplace when needed and selection of a high-quality and responsible laboratory. The ethical obligations of laboratories performing biomonitoring analyses include good and demonstrated analytical quality, provision of accurate and up-to-date reference values and action levels, procedures for maintaining data confidentiality, up-to-date knowledge of occupational chemical risks, of means of exposure assessment, of possibilities and limitations of different biomonitoring methods and continuous education and training of customers. It is apparent that these are easier to achieve if the laboratory has at least relative freedom from economic pressures.

REFERENCES

Ahlström, L. (Techn. ed.) (1998). Kemikaalialtistumisen biomonitorointi. Näytteenotto-ohjeet. Biomonitoring of chemical exposure: Guideline for sample collection (in Finnish). 5th ed. Institute of Occupational Health, Helsinki, 125pp.

Aitio, A. (1994). Biological monitoring today and tomorrow. *Scand. J. Work Environ. Health*, **20**, 46–58.

Aitio, A. and Järvisalo, J. (1984). Biological monitoring of occupational exposure to toxic chemicals. Collection, processing and storage of specimens. *Pure. Appl Chem.*, **56**, 549–566.

Aitio, A., Pekari, K. and Järvisalo, J. (1984). Skin absorption as a source of error in biological monitoring. *Scand. J. Work Environ. Health*, **10**, 317–320.

Aitio, A., Järvisalo, J., Kiilunen, M., Kalliomäki, P.-L. and Kalliomäki, K. (1988). Chromium. In Clarkson, T. W., Friberg, L., Nordberg, G. F. and Sager, P. R. (Eds), *Biological Monitoring of Toxic Metals*. Plenum Press, New York, pp. 369–382.

Aitio, A., Riihimäki, V., Liesivuori, J., Järvisalo, J. and Hernberg, S. (1994). Biologic monitoring. In Zenz, C., Dickerson, O. B. and J. Horvath, E. P. (Eds), *Occupational Medicine*, 3rd edn. Mosby Year Book, St Louis, MO, pp. 132–158.

American Conference of Governmental Industrial Hygienists (ACGIH) (1997). 1997 TLVs and BEIs. Threshold limit values (TLVs) for chemical substances and physical agents. Biological exposure indices. ACGIH, Cincinnati, OH.

Angerer, J., Mannschreck, C. and Gündel, J. (1997). Occupational exposure to polycyclic aromatic hydrocarbons in a graphite-electrode producing plant: biological monitoring of 1-hydroxypyrene and monohydroxylated metabolites of phenanthrene. *Int. Arch. Occup. Environ. Health*, **69**, 323–331.

Aringer, L., Löf, A. and Elinder, C.-G. (1991). The applicability of the measurement of urinary thioethers. A study of humans exposed to styrene during diet standardization. *Int. Arch. Occup. Environ. Health*, **63**, 341–346.

Bernacki, E. J., Parsons, G. E., Roy, B. R., Mikac-Devic, M., Kennedy, C. D. and Sunderman, F. W. J. (1978). Urine nickel concentrations in nickel-exposed workers. *Ann. Clin. Lab. Sci.*, **8**, 184–189.

Bleecker, M. L., McNeill, F. E., Lindgren, K. N., Masten, V. L. and Ford, D. P. (1995). Relationship between bone lead and other indices of lead exposure in smelter workers. *Toxicol. Lett.*, **77**, 241–248.

Bleecker, M. L., Lindgren, K. N., Tiburzi, M. J. and Ford, D. P. (1997). Curvilinear relationship between blood lead level and reaction time: differential association with blood lead fractions derived from exogenous and endogenous sources. *J. Occup. Environ. Med.*, **39**, 426–431.

Börjesson, J. and Mattsson, S. (1995). Toxicology; *in vivo* x-ray fluorescence for the assessment of heavy metal concentrations in man. *Appl. Radiat. Isot.*, **46**, 571–576.

Börjesson, J., Barregård, L., Sällsten, G., Schutz, A., Jonson, R., Alpsten, M. and Mattsson, S. (1995). *In vivo* XRF analysis of mercury: the relation between concentrations in the kidney and the urine. *Phys. Med. Biol.*, **40**, 413–426.

Börjesson, J., Gerhardsson, L., Schütz, A., Mattsson, S., Skerfving, S., and Österberg, K. (1997). *In vivo* measurements of lead in fingerbone in active and retired lead smelters. *Int. Arch. Occup. Environ. Health*, **69**, 97–105.

Brody, D. J., Pirkle, J. L., Kramer, R. A., Flegal, K. M., Matte, T. D., Gunter, E. W. and Paschal, D. C. (1994). Blood lead levels in the US population—Phase 1 of the third National

Health and Nutrition Examination Survey (NHANES III, 1988 to 1991). *J. Ann. Med. Assoc.*, **272**, 277–283.

Brune, D., Aitio, A., Nordberg, G., Vesterberg, O. and Gerhardsson, L. (1993). Normal concentrations of chromium in serum and urine—a TRACY project. *Scand. J. Work Environ. Health*, **19**, Suppl. 1, 39–44.

Clonfero, E., Jongeneelen, F., Zordan, M. and Levis, A. G. (1990). Biological monitoring of human exposure to coal tar. Urinary mutagenicity assays and analytical determination of polycyclic aromatic hydrocarbon metabolites in urine. In Vainio, H., Sorsa, M. and McMichael, A. J. (Eds), *Complex Mixtures and Cancer Risk*. IARC Scientific Publications, Vol. 104, International Agency for Research on Cancer, Lyon, pp. 215–222.

Crawford, F. G., Mayer, J., Santella, R. M., Cooper, T. B., Ottman, R., Tsai, W.-Y., Simon-Cereijido, G., Wang, M., Tang, D. and Perera, F. P. (1994). Biomarkers of environmental tobacco smoke in preschool children and their mothers. *J. Natl. Cancer Inst.*, **86**, 1398–1402.

Delves, H. T., Diaper, S. J., Oppert, S., Prescott-Clarke, P., Periam, J., Dong, W., Colhoun, H. and Gompertz, D. (1996). Blood lead concentrations in United Kingdom have fallen substantially since 1984. *Br. Med. J.*, **313**, 883–884.

Demarini, D. M., Brooks, L. R., Bhatnagar, V. K., Hayes, R. B., Eischen, B. T., Shelton, M. L., Zenser, T. V., Talaska, G., Kashyap, S. K., Dosemeci, M., Kashyap, R., Parikh, D. J., Lakshmi, V., Hsu, F., Davis, B. B., Jaeger, M. and Rothman, N. (1997). Urinary mutagenicity as a biomarker in workers exposed to benzidine: correlation with urinary metabolites and urothelial DNA adducts. *Carcinogenesis*, **18**, 981–988.

Deutsche Forschungsgemeinschaft (DFG) (1996). *MAK- und BAT-Werte-Liste 1996. Senatskommission zur Prüfung gesundheitsschädlicher Arbeitsstoffe*, 32nd edn. VCH, Weinheim.

Farmer, P. B., Sepai, O., Lawrence, R., Autrup, H., Nielsen, P. S., Vestergard, A. B., Waters, R., Leuratti, C., Jones, N. J., Stone, J., Baan, R. A., Vandelft, J. H. M., Steenwinkel, M. J. S. T., Kyrtopoulos, S. A., Souliotis, V. L., Theodorakopoulos, N., Bacalis, N. C., Natarajan, A. T., Tates, A. D., Haugen, A., Andreassen, A., Ovrebo, S., Shuker, D. E. G., Amaning, K. S., Schouft, A., Ellul, A., Garner, R. C., Dingley, K. H., Abbondandolo, A., Merlo, F., Cole, J., Aldrich, K., Beare, D., Capulas, E., Rowley, G., Waugh, A. P. W., Povey, A. C., Haque, K., Kirsch-Volders, M., Van Hummelen, P. and Castelain, P. (1996). Biomonitoring human exposure to environmental carcinogenic chemicals. *Mutagenesis*, **11**, 363–381.

Forni, A. (1996). Benzene-induced chromosome aberrations: a follow-up study. *Environ. Health Perspect.*, **104**, Suppl. 6, 1309–1312.

Gompertz, D., and Verschoyle, R. D. (1996). Organophosphorus pesticides. In *Guidelines on Biological Monitoring of Chemical Exposure at the Workplace*, Vol. 1. World Health Organization, Geneva, pp. 237–263.

Hagmar, L., Brogger, A., Hansteen, I.-L., Heim. S., Högstedt, B., Knudsen, L., Lambert, B., Linnainmaa, K., Mitelman, F., Nordenson, I., Reuterwall, C., Salomaa, S., Skerfving, S. and Sorsa, M. (1994). Cancer risk in humans predicted by increased levels of chromosomal aberrations in lymphocytes: Nordic Study Group on the Health Risk of Chromosome Damage. *Cancer Res.*, **54**, 2919–2922.

Hagmar, L., Bonassi, S., Stromberg, U., Brogger, A., Knudsen, L. E., Norppa, H. and Reuterwall, C. (1998a). Chromosomal aberrations in lymphocytes predict human cancer: a report from the European Study Group on Cytogenetic Biomarkers and Health (ESCH). *Cancer Res.*, **58**, 4117–4121.

Hagmar, L., Bonassi, S., Stromberg, U., Mikoczy, Z., Lando, C., Hansteen, I. L., Montagud, A. H., Knudsen, L., Norppa, H., Reuterwall, C., Tinnerberg, H., Brogger, A., Forni, A., Hogstedt, B., Lambert, B., Mitelman, F., Nordenson, I., Salomaa, S. and Skerfving, S. (1998b). Cancer predictive value of cytogenetic markers used in occupational health surveillance programs: a report from an ongoing study by the European Study Group on Cytogenetic Biomarkers and Health. *Mutat. Res.*, **405**, 171–178.

Hänninen, H., Aitio, A., Kovala, T., Luukkonen, R., Matikainen, E., Mannelin, T., Erkkilä, J. and Riihimäki, V. (1998). Occupational lead exposure and neuropsychological dysfunction. *Occup. Environ. Med.*, **55**, 202–209.

Hartung, M., Schaller, K.-H., Kentner, M., Weltle, D. and Valentin, H. (1983). Untersuchungen zur Cobalt-Belastung in verschiedenen Gewerbezweigen. *Arbeitsmed. Sozialmed. Präventivmed.*, **18**, 73–75.

Health and Safety Executive (1992). *Biological Monitoring for Chemical Exposures in the Workplace*. Guidance Note EH 56 from the Health and Safety Executive. HMSO, London.

Health and Safety Executive (1993). *Guidance on Laboratory Techniques in Occupational Medicine*, 6th edn. Health and Safety Executive, London.

Hemminki, K. (1992). Significance of DNA and protein adducts. In Vainio, H., Magee, P., McGregor, D. and McMichael, A. J. (Eds), *Mechanisms of Carcinogenesis in Risk Identification*. IARC Scientific Publications, Vol. 116. International Agency for Research on Cancer, Lyon, pp. 525–534.

Holiday, D. B., McLarty, J. W., Yanagihara, R. H., Riley, L. and Shepherd, S. B. (1995). Two biochemical markers effectively used to separate smokeless tobacco users from smokers and nonusers. *South. Med. J.*, **88**, 1107–1113.

International Agency for Research on Cancer (IARC) (1993). Cadmium and cadmium compounds. In *IARC Monographs on the Evaluation of Carcinogenic Risks to Humans. Vol. 58: Some Metals and Metal Compounds, and Occupational Exposures in the Glass Industry*. IARC, Lyon, pp. 119–237.

International Programme on Chemical Safety (IPCS). (1993). *Environmental Health Criteria, 155: Biomarkers and Risk Assessment: Concepts and Principles*. World Health Organization, Geneva.

Jongeneelen, F. J. (1992). Biological exposure limit for occupational exposure to coal tar pitch volatiles at cokeovens. *Int. Arch. Occup. Environ. Health*, **63**, 511–516.

Jongeneelen, F. J., van Leeuwen, F. E., Oosterink, S., Anzion, R. B. M., van der Loop, F., Bos, R. P. and van Veen, H. G. (1990). Ambient and biological monitoring of cokeoven workers: determinants of the internal dose of polycyclic aromatic hydrocarbons. *Br. J. Ind. Med.*, **47**, 454–461.

Kovala, T., Matikainen, E., Mannelin, T., Erkkilä, J., Riihimäki, V., Hänninen, H. and Aitio, A. (1997). Effects of low-level lead exposure on neurophysiological functions among lead battery workers. *Occup. Environ. Medi.*, **54**, 487–493.

Koyano, M., Oike, Y., Goto, S., Endo, O., Watanabe, I., Furuya, K. and Matsushita, H. (1996). Effect of smoking on urinary nicotine, cotinine and mutagenic activity. *Jpn. J. Toxicol. Environ. Health*, **42**, 263–267.

Kuljukka, T., Vaaranrinta, R., Veidebaum, T., Sorsa, M. and Peltonen, K. (1996). Exposure to PAH compounds among cokery workers in the oil shale industry. *Environ. Health Perspect.*, **104**, Suppl. 3, 539–541.

Kumpulainen, J., Lehto, J., Koivistoinen, P., Uusitupa, M. and Vuori, E. (1983). Determination of chromium in human milk, serum and urine by electrothermal atomic absorption spectrometry without preliminary ashing. *Sci. Total Environ.*, **31**, 71–80.

Landrigan, P. J. and Todd, A. C. (1994). Direct measurement of lead in bone—a promising biomarker. *J. Am. Med. Assoc.*, **271**, 239–240.

Lauwerys, R. R. and Hoet, P. (1993). *Industrial Chemical Exposure. Guidelines for Biological Monitoring*, 2nd edn. Lewis, Boca Raton, FL.

Mumford, J. L., Lee, X., Lewtas, J., Young, T. L. and Santella, R. M. (1993). DNA adducts as biomarkers for assessing exposure to polycyclic aromatic hydrocarbons in tissues from Xyan Wei women with high exposure to coal combustion emissions and high lung cancer mortality. *Environ. Health Perspect.*, **99**, 83–87.

Nielsen, P. S., Andreassen, A., Farmer, P. B., Øvrebø, S. and Autrup, H. (1996). Biomonitoring of diesel exhaust-exposed workers. DNA and hemoglobin adducts and urinary 1-hydroxypyrene as markers of exposure. *Toxicol. Lett.*, **86**, 27–37.

Nilsson, U. (1994). Quantitative *in vivo* elemental analysis using X-ray fluorescence and scattering techniques. Applications to cadmium, lead and bone mineral. PhD Dissertation, Lund University, Malmö.

Nilsson, U., Schütz, A., Skerfving, S. and Mattsson, S. (1995). Cadmium in kidneys in Swedes measured *in vivo* using X-ray fluorescence analysis. *Int. Arch. Occup. Environ. Health*, **67**, 405–411.

Pekari, K., Nylander-French, L., Pfäffli, P., Sorsa, M. and Aitio, A. (1993). Biological monitoring of exposure to styrene—assessment of different approaches. *J. Occup. Med. Toxicol.*, **2**, 115–126.

Poirier, M. C. and Weston, A. (1996). Human DNA adduct measurements: state of the art. *Environ. Health Perspect.*, **104**, Suppl. 5, 883–893.

Riffelmann, M., Müller, G., Schmieding, W., Popp, W. and Norpoth, K. (1995). Biomonitoring of urinary aromatic amines and arylamine hemoglobin adducts in exposed workers and nonexposed control persons. *Int. Arch. Occup. Environ. Health*, **68**, 36–43.

Rodamilans, M., Torra, M., To-Figueras, J., Corbella, J., López, B., Sánchez, C. and Mazzara, R. (1996). Effect of the reduction of petrol lead on blood lead levels of the population of Barcelona (Spain). *Bull. Environ. Contam. Toxicol.*, **56**, 717–721.

Roels, H., Bernard, A. M., Cárdenas, A., Buchet, J. P., Lauwerys, R. R., Hotter, G., Ramis, I., Mutti, A., Franchini, I., Buhdschuh, I., Stolte, H., De Broe, M. E., Nuyts, G. D., Taylor, S. A. and Price, R. G. (1993). Markers of early renal changes induced by industrial pollutants. III. Application to workers exposed to cadmium. *Br. J. Ind. Med.*, **50**, 37–48.

Strickland, P., Kang, D. and Sithisarankul, P. (1996). Polycyclic aromatic hydrocarbon metabolites in urine as biomarkers of exposure and effect. *Environ. Health Perspect.*, **104**, Suppl. 5, 927–932.

Strömberg, U., Schütz, A. and Skerfving, S. (1995). Substantial decrease of blood lead in Swedish children, 1978–94, associated with petrol lead. *Occup. Environ. Medi.*, **52**, 764–769.

Sunderman, F. W., Jr, Aitio, A., Morgan, L. G. and Norseth, T. (1986). Biological monitoring of nickel. *Toxicol. Ind. Health*, **2**, 17–78.

Todd, A. C. and Chettle, D. R. (1994). *In vivo* X-ray fluorescence of lead in bone–review and current issues. *Environ. Health Perspect.*, **102**, 172–177.

Torra, M., Rodamilans, M., Montero, F., Farré, C. and Corbella, J. (1997). Estudio de la exposición al plomo en la población de Barcelona: evolución cronológica entre 1984 y 1995. *Med. Clin.*, **108**, 601–603.

Vainio, H., Sorsa, M. and Falck, K. (1984). Bacterial urinary assay in monitoring exposure to mutagens and carcinogens. In Berlin, A., Draper, M., Hemminki, K. and Vainio, H. (Eds), *Monitoring Human Exposure to Carcinogenic and Mutagenic Agents*, vol. 59. International Agency for Research on Cancer, Lyon, pp. 247–258.

Veillon, C., Patterson, K. Y., and Bryden, N. A. (1984). Determination of chromium in human serum by electrothermal atomic absorption spectrometry. *Anal. Chim. Acta*, **164**, 67–76.

WHO (1996a). *Biological Monitoring of Chemical Exposure in the Workplace*, Vol. 1. World Health Organization, Geneva.

WHO (1996b). *Biological Monitoring of Chemical Exposure in the Workplace*, Vol. 2. World Health Organization, Geneva.

Wietlisbach, V., Rickenbach, M., Berode, M. and Guillemin, M. (1995). Time trend and determinants of blood lead levels in a Swiss population over a transition period (1984–1993) from leaded to unleaded gasoline use. *Environ. Res.*, **68**, 82–90.

Wilson, K. (Ed.) (1996). *Guidance on Laboratory Techniques in Occupational Medicine*, 7th edn. Health and Safety Laboratory, Sheffield.

Chapter 88
Toxicology and Implications of the Products of Combustion

James C. Norris and Bryan Ballantyne

C O N T E N T S

GENERAL CONSIDERATIONS

Combustion toxicology deals with the nature and potential adverse effects of products resulting from the heating or burning of materials; effects include local irritation, incapacitation, systemic toxicity and lethality. Although the major effort has been devoted to products generated in accidental fires, adverse effects may also result from exposure to products resulting from heating or burning materials in occupational and domestic situations. Two typical examples of illnesses from the inhalation exposure to the products resulting from heating polymers are meat wrapper 'allergy' and polyfume fever. The former affects some workers wrapping meat in poly(vinyl chloride) (PVC) film. The sources of exposure come from the hot wire cutting of the film from rolls (ca 105 °C), from heat sealing of the folded film ends, and from thermal fixing of an adhesive label to the wrapped product. The heating element temperature is around 200 °C (Levy, 1988). The major products from the hot wire cutting of PVC film include di-2-ethylhexyl phthalate and hydrogen chloride and those from thermal attachment of labels include dicyclohexyl phthalate, phthalic anhydride, dicyclohexyl ether and cyclohexyl benzoate (Levy et al., 1978; Vandevort and Brooks, 1979). Affected meat wrappers complain of cough, wheezing, shortness of breath, chest tightness and symptoms and signs due to irritation of the eye and throat. The spectrum of the illness should be interpreted as a complex response to emissions from all phases of the wrapping procedure (Andrasch et al., 1975). It is generally considered that exposure to the products from heating PVC in meat wrapping environ-

ments produces effects compatible with irritation of the eye and respiratory tract; in those with pre-existing asthma or chronic obstructional airways disease there may be an exacerbation of the condition. The effects produced accord with respiratory tract irritation and hyper-reactivity; the role of an immunological process (i.e. an asthmatic basis) is questionable (Brooks, 1983). It is possible that it is a reaction similar to that described as reactive airways dysfunction syndrome by Brooks et al. (1985).

Polyfume fever is an example of illness resulting from exposure to the pyrolysis products of polytetrafluoro-ethylene (PTFE) after contamination of cigarettes with the polymer in an occupational environment. Workers smoking cigarettes contaminated with PTFE subsequently develop an 'influenza-like syndrome', characterized by cough, tightness of the chest, a choking sensation and chills. There is characteristically a delay of several hours between exposure and the development of symptoms; recovery is complete within 12–48 h (Gantz, 1988). No long-term sequelae have been described. Thermal decomposition products up to 500 °C are principally the TFE monomer, but also perfluoropropene and other perfluoro compounds containing four or five carbon atoms. In the range 500–800 °C the major pyrolysis product is carbonyl fluoride (Hathaway et al., 1991).

In the USA there are approximately 6000 deaths each year due to fire, with a much larger number of non-lethal injuries (Alexeff and Packham, 1984; Gad, 1990a). Casualties occur during, or as a consequence of, exposure to a fire for various reasons, of which the following are more important:

- *Direct physical trauma*: e.g. resulting from structural collapse of buildings.
- *Flame and heat*: direct thermal injuries to skin and/or respiratory tract, or secondary complications from primary thermal injuries.
- *Oxygen depletion*: this may be a primary factor and/or enhance the toxicity of respirable chemicals in the fire atmosphere.
- *Factors hindering escape*: these may increase the likelihood of further exposure to flame, heat, oxygen depletion, and toxic materials in the atmosphere. Escape may be hindered by physical injury, obscuring smoke, prior use of alcohol or narcotic drugs, panic, the presence of peripheral sensory irritants, or depression of CNS function from specific materials in the atmosphere. It has been shown that alcoholic intoxication has been a significant factor in some fires and may have impeded escape. Thus, in one series of fire deaths in the UK, mainly occurring in dwellings, ethanol was present in the blood of most victims, and 59% of the adults had blood ethanol concentrations greater than 80 mg dl^{-1} or urine concentrations in excess of 107 mg dl^{-1}; the average blood ethanol concentration was 276 mg dl^{-1} (Harland and Wooley, 1979). In a study of fire deaths in Maryland, blood ethanol concentrations in excess of 150 mg dl^{-1} were found in 35% of victims (Radford *et al.*, 1976). The incapacitating effects of several chemicals, because of their effects on central nervous system or muscular function, are well appreciated. For example, with hydrogen cyanide vapour it is known that incapacitating effects can be produced rapidly. Purser *et al.* (1984), in a study of exposure of primates to HCN (102–156 ppm), found there was initial hyperventilation, with increased respiratory minute volume, followed by slow breathing, disturbance of consciousness, hypotonia and loss of reflexes. Post-exposure, there was rapid recovery. There was a linear relationship between exposure concentration and times to hyperventilation and signs of incapacitation. The slope of the relationship showed that doubling the concentration from 100 to 200 ppm reduced the time to incapacitation from 25 to 2 min. These findings emphasize that exposure to HCN in fire atmospheres could produce incapacitating effects such as muscle weakness, ataxia and dizziness. Behavioural impairment in smoke environments has been reviewed by Purser (1996).
- *Toxic substances in the atmosphere*: These may in gaseous, vapour or particulate form, being produced by the heating or burning of materials, or release from storage sites as a result of damage. These materials may produce local (skin, eye, respiratory tract) toxicity or adverse systemic effects if absorbed. Such effects may be acute or latent. Also, as for example with firefighters, the effect of repeated

exposure and the potential for cumulative and/or long-term effects needs to be considered.

According to the US Consumer Product Safety Commission, between 1970 and 1985, the total numbers of deaths from structural fires decreased from 5000 to 4000 per year, but the number of deaths attributable to smoke inhalation remained constant at around 3000 per year (USCPSC, 1988). Other estimates have indicated that about 30% of major burns victims have smoke inhalation injury, and for fatalities up to 80% may have had smoke inhalation (Bowes, 1976; Heimbach and Waeckerle, 1988; Haponik, 1993).

Smoke is a complex mixture of airborne solid and liquid particulates, vapours and gases, which are evolved when materials undergo vaporization or thermal decomposition. Thermal decomposition may be conveniently described under the following conditions:

- *Anaerobic pyrolysis*: thermal breakdown and chemical conversion of materials in a low oxygen environment.
- *Oxidative pyrolysis*: thermal breakdown and chemical conversion of materials in a normal oxygen environment but in the absence of flaming ('smouldering').
- *Flaming combustion*: thermal breakdown and chemical conversion of materials in a normal oxygen environment in the presence of flaming.

All these processes may be operating at the same time at different geographical regions in a fire, or one or other may be predominant. Pyrolysis is usually defined as the thermal degradation of a material at a temperature below the auto-ignition temperature. Flaming is the highly efficient burning of a material above the auto-ignition temperature in the presence of sufficient oxygen. Thermolysis is a generic term covering flaming, pyrolysis and smouldering.

The atmosphere in a fire is usually of extremely complex composition and, because of the constantly changing conditions during the progress of a fire, the chemical composition (both nature and concentration of materials) varies markedly at different stages of the fire. Also, the characteristics and hazards of one fire may be entirely different to that of another. The chemical composition of the atmosphere, and the concentrations of the individual constituents, depend on a large number of variable factors; the most important of these include:

- The nature of the materials available for heating or burning;
- Phase of the combustion process;
- The potential for chemical and/or physical interactions between materials present in the fire atmosphere;
- The potential for additive or synergistic toxic effects;

- Temperature;
- Air flow and oxygen availability.

A review of the European and North American literature suggests that some 50–75% of deaths which occur within a few hours of being involved in a fire are due to toxic effects of chemicals in the fire atmosphere. After about 12 h, the contribution of toxic effects to mortalities is considerably less. Over the past few decades, the contribution of toxic chemicals to mortalities and non-fatal casualties has increased. For example, in the UK during the period 1955–74, the total number of fire fatalities increased by 70%; whilst those due to burns and scalds fluctuated around 400–600 annually, those attributed to the effect of gas and smoke showed a steady increase (Ballantyne, 1981). The increasing hazard from toxic materials has also been shown by consideration of the total incidence of smoke casualties (i.e. fatal and non-fatal); there was a 600% increase over the 19-year period. In the USA there are approximately 6000 deaths annually due to fire, with smoke inhalation being responsible for about 80% of the fatalities (Alexeeff and Packham, 1984; Kaplan, 1988; Gad, 1990a). Also, the probability of death is increased for the fire victim having smoke inhalation and burns (Zawacki et al., 1977, 1979; Shirani et al., 1988). There are reasonable grounds to believe that the marked increase in smoke and gas casualties is due to the introduction of man-made materials for construction and furnishing. Combustion processes involving polymers result in the generation of a variety of lower molecular weight materials which may have significant irritant effects and acute and/or long-term systemic toxicity. The nature and relative amounts of toxic products from combustion of polymers vary with both the nature of the polymeric material and the conditions of burning. The range of toxicity possible is reflected in the following examples of typical products from polymer combustion: acetaldehyde, acrolein, phosgene, hydrogen cyanide, carbon monoxide, hydrogen chloride and vinyl chloride. It is of practical importance to note that the combustion products of some phosphorus-based fire retardants may present toxicological problems (Purser, 1992).

Lethalities resulting from inhalation of chemicals in a fire atmosphere may be due to local chemical injury to the respiratory tract and/or systemic toxicity following absorption of inhaled materials; the latter may include disturbance of biochemical mechanisms or transport processes, or tissue injury. Non-lethal adverse effects may be due to more restricted or less severe local respiratory tract injury or systemic toxicity. It should also be appreciated that inhaled smoke and fumes may contain products of incomplete combustion which continue to release heat following inhalation, resulting in thermal injury to the laryngeal and tracheobronchial mucosa and, with sufficient penetration, to the alveolar epithelium. These thermal injuries will complement any chemically induced respiratory tract injury (Zachria, 1972). Smoke inhalation may lead to pulmonary oedema, a factor in which there is increased permeability of the pulmonary microvasculature (Niemann et al., 1989). Studies of experimentally produced smoke inhalation injury in sheep showed that the primary, and dose-responsive, injury was acute cell membrane damage in the trachea and bronchi leading to oedema, progressive necrotic tracheobronchitis with pseudomembrane formation and obstruction of airways (Hubbard et al., 1991). Morphological changes occurring in the alveolar epithelium included intracellular oedema (Type I cells), changes in membrane-bound vacuoles (Type II cells) and interstitial oedema. Hales et al. (1988, 1992) postulated that acrolein may be a major component of smoke causing pulmonary oedema. In work with anaesthetized sheep, and using smoke from burning cotton, they found an acute increase in pulmonary vascular permeability, an increase in airways resistance and decreased PaO_2. A combined cyclo- and lipo-oxygenese inhibitor, BW-755C, prevented all those changes, whereas indomethacin, a cyclo-oxygenese inhibitor, prevented the increase in airways resistance but not the increase in microvascular permeability. They regard their studies as indicating that leukotrienes may have a role in producing cotton smoke-induced non-cardiogenic pulmonary oedema.

Although most emphasis has been devoted to the acute toxic effects of fire atmospheres, there is also a potential for long-term adverse effects particularly on repeated exposures. This is considered later in this chapter specifically under consideration of hazards of firefighting. The management of casualties from fires has been reviewed by Harrigan and Winograd (1994).

NATURE AND TOXICITY OF FIRE ATMOSPHERES

Thermal decomposition of a material may produce a wide range of lower molecular weight species of differing toxicity and irritancy. The number, nature and relative proportions of the products depend on the material burned and the conditions of the combustion process. This may be illustrated by considering the simple burning of wood in an enclosed space (Table 1). Carbon, hydrogen and sulphur are available as the common combustible elements. In the early phase of burning, sulphur dioxide, water and carbon dioxide are produced, together with some carbon monoxide. As oxygen becomes depleted and burning becomes slower, more carbon monoxide and sulphur dioxide are formed. With further decrease in oxygen availability, incomplete combustion occurs and hydrogen, methane, carbon monoxide and free carbon are produced. In the smouldering phase, hydrogen, methane, sulphur dioxide,

Table 1   Products of the burning of wood in an enclosed space and the influence of the stage of burning

| Factor | Burning stage[a] | | | |
	Free	Slowed	Incomplete Combustion	Smouldering
Oxygen (%)	20	17	15	<13
Temperature (°C)	40	205	370	550
Products	SO_2 +	SO_2 +	SO_2 + +	SO_2 + +
	H_2O + +	H_2O + +	H_2O + +	H_2O + +
	CO_2 + +	CO_2 + +	CO_2 + + +	CO_2 + + +
	CO +	CO +	CO + +	CO + + +
			H_2 +	H_2 +
			CH_4 +	CH_4 +
			Free C +	Free C + + +
			Smoke +	Smoke + + +

[a] The + designation = relative proportion of product.

Table 2   Examples of toxic and irritant chemicals that may be generated by combustion of commonly occurring materials

Material	Combustion products[a]	Reference
Poly(vinylchloride)	Hydrogen chloride	Dyer and Esh (1976)
	Carbon monoxide	Michal (1976)
Polyethylene	Formaldehyde	Morikawa (1976)
	Acrolein	
Polyacrylonitrile	Hydrogen cyanide	Morikawa (1978)
Polyurethane foams	Toluene diisocyanate	Wooley (1974)
	Hydrogen cyanide	Bowes (1974)
	Carbon monoxide	
Polytetrafluoroethylene	Hydrogen fluoride	Young et al. (1976)
	Carbonyl fluoride	

[a] These are not necessarily the only products generated, but are given to illustrate the more toxic materials. The relative amounts of materials generated depends on the conditions of heating.

carbon dioxide, carbon monoxide, free carbon and smoke are all produced. This single example indicates that as a fire progresses and the temperature increases, the available oxygen decreases (in enclosed spaces), toxic, irritant and flammable gases are produced and obscuring smoke is formed. Additionally, with combustion of wood, other irritant and toxic materials may be produced, e.g. formaldehyde, methanol, acetic acid and other organic irritants (DeKorver, 1976). Even in the apparently simple example of wood, a multiplicity of differing chemicals may be produced, e.g. combustion of Douglas fir produced more than 75 discrete chemicals in the smoke (Packham and Hartzell, 1981). Smoke is usually defined as a complex mixture of airborne solid and liquid particulates and gases produced when a material undergoes thermal decomposition (Kaplan, 1988). Smoke may be obscuring, contains smouldering particles which can produce thermal injury to the respiratory tract, and contains toxic and irritant material in gas or vapour form or absorbed on the surface of particulates.

As noted earlier, the widespread introduction of man-made polymeric materials into buildings and furnishings has been associated with a wider spectrum of toxicity than that produced from natural polymers (Alarie, 1985; Gad, 1990a). Products from the combustion of synthetic polymers may have a significant role in morbidity and mortality in fires (Ballantyne, 1981). At low temperatures (up to 400 °C) polymers decompose to give a range of complex products; at medium temperatures (400–700 °C) the complexity of products increases and complex organic species may develop; at high temperatures (> 700 °C) complex organic molecules are unstable and decompose (Ballantyne, 1989).

Examples of the differing highly toxic and irritant chemical species produced by the combustion of synthetic polymers are shown in **Table 2**. This table shows major toxic products, but it must be emphasized that, depending on the conditions of combustion, the number of chemical species produced by combustion of a specific polymer may be high. For example, PVC yields hydrogen chloride as a principal combustion product, but about 75 other organic compounds are generated (Wooley, 1971; Dyer and Esch, 1976). Combustion of polyethylene yielded 55 compounds and polypropylene yielded 56 compounds (Mitera and Michal, 1985). With polypropylene, the main thermal degradation products are

Table 3 Influence of various factors on the generation of thermolysis products from specific materials

Material	Variable	Observation	Reference
Polyurethane foam	Time	In the early stages both hydrogen cyanide and carbon monoxide produced; in the later stages only carbon monoxide	Bowes (1974)
Polyurethane foam	Temperature	Pyrolysis at 300 °C yields a polymeric smoke. At 800 °C smoke decomposes to N-containing materials, notably hydrogen cyanide, acetonitrile, acrylonitrile, pyridine and benzonitrile	Wooley (1972)
Polyethylene	Oxygen availability	Low-oxygen atmosphere (500–600 °C) gives high acrolein yield; high oxygen atmosphere (500–600 °C) gives low acrolein yield	Morikawa (1976)

formaldehyde, acetaldehyde, 2-methylacrolein, acetic acid and acetone (Frostling *et al.*, 1984). Nitrogen-containing polymers may yield hydrogen cyanide and various cyanogens.

The material inhaled as products of combustion, smoke, consists of solid and liquid particulates, vapours and gases. In general, the local injury from inhaled combustion products is of greater concern than thermal injury from the inhaled hot smoke. The upper airways dissipate heat, and most thermal injury is limited to the supraglottic airway (Bizovi and Leikin, 1995). The site and extent of injury will be determined by the nature and amounts of inhaled irritants and particulates. The histopathology of smoke inhalation has been well documented (Head, 1980; Haponik *et al.*, 1988). This includes hyperexpansion, atelectasis and congestion of the lung. Features such as focal intra-alveolar haemorrhage and pulmonary oedema may be superseded by infective changes (Hill, 1996).

Factors Influencing Combustion Products and Their Toxicological Effects

The specific chemical species, and their relative proportions, produced during the combustion processes are dependent on various environmental factors (**Table 3**). These factors may, additionally, quantitively modify the toxic response. The more important factors are summarized below.

Oxygen Availability

The availability of oxygen in the burning area may significantly affect the generation of combustion products. For example, at 500–600 °C polyethylene gives a high acrolein yield with low atmospheric oxygen, and a low acrolein yield when atmospheric oxygen is high (Morikawa, 1976). An example of the influence of oxygen availability on toxicity is illustrated in **Figure 1**, which demonstrates that for any given atmospheric carbon monoxide content, lethal toxicity increases with

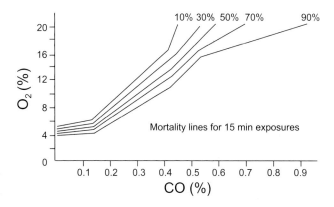

Figure 1 Mortality of male rats exposed for 15 min to atmospheres containing various proportions of oxygen and carbon monoxide. For any given carbon monoxide concentration, mortality increases with decreasing oxygen content. After Ballantyne (1981).

decreasing oxygen content. Clearly this is due, at least in part, to proportionately less oxygen being available to maintain vital process where oxygen transport is already compromised by carbon monoxide. This is also clearly relevant to practical fire situations, where carbon monoxide is ubiquitous and oxygen depletion common.

Temperature

The temperature in an area of burning or smouldering may significantly influence the products released into the atmosphere. For example, pyrolysis of polyurethane smoke at 300 °C yields polymeric smoke, but at 800 °C the smoke decomposes to N-containing materials, such as hydrogen cyanide, acetonitrile, acrylonitrile, pyridine and benzonitrile (Wooley, 1972). Several studies have shown that environmental temperature may influence toxicity. For example, Nomiyama *et al.* (1980) demonstrated an increase in acute toxicity for various organic solvents, heavy metals and agrochemicals at elevated environmental temperature. Sanders and Endecott (1991) showed, in laboratory rats, that incapacitation occurred earlier when exposure to carbon monoxide was combined with elevated temperature, compared with the effects of carbon monoxide or temperature alone.

INCAPACITATING FACTORS IN FIRES

Incapacitating effects are those which hinder escape from a fire by impairment of physical and/or mental functions. Clearly, obstacles, physical injury and dense smoke are physical factors which may impair mobility and escape. Hypoxia, discussed in the next section, may impair mental functions by a wide range of effects from impairment of judgement to loss of consciousness. Some substances encountered in fire atmospheres may be absorbed and affect central nervous system function and produce, for example, disturbance of consciousness, abnormalities of coordination, weakness and decreased reaction and responsiveness times; volatile organic solvents, carbon monoxide and hydrogen cyanide are all examples of materials which produce such effects. These considerations on the effect of hypoxia and absorbed chemicals on behaviour and judgement clearly not only apply to impairment of escape, but are also relevant to safe and effective performance by those occupationally involved in firefighting operations. Behavioural impairment in smoke environments has been reviewed by Purser (1996). The growing interest and recognition of the relevance of performance deficits has lead to the introduction of neurobehavioural toxicity testing as a component of some combustion toxicology procedures (Rossi et al., 1996).

Many materials of widely varying chemical nature which are released in a fire are peripheral sensory irritants. They are thus capable of inducing excess tear production, eye discomfort and blepharospasm. These ocular effects will clearly result in a disturbance of vision, and thus influence the performance of coordinated tasks and produce visual impairment (see Chapter 32).

HYPOXIA

Hypoxia is a condition in which there is a physiologically inadequate supply of oxygen to tissues or an impairment of the cellular utilization of oxygen. In the context of a fire, all of the following types of hypoxia may occur.

Hypoxic Hypoxia

This is present where there is a decrease in the arterial blood PO_2 resulting from inadequate availability of oxygen to blood in pulmonary alveolar capillaries. There is a reduction in the amount of O_2 in arterial blood, but no reduction in PaO_2. This may be a consequence of depletion of atmospheric oxygen in the inspired air, airways obstruction, lung injury sufficient

to reduce diffusing capacity, low tidal volume and increased dead space.

Anaemic Hypexia

This is present when there is a decreased oxygen-transporting capacity of the blood, as, for example, a reduced circulating erythrocyte mass. In a fire, anaemic hypoxia may occur from reduced haemoglobin oxygen-binding sites; this is frequently a result of carboxyhaemoglobin formation or the induction of methaemoglobinaemia.

Cytotoxic Hypoxia

This is a systemic effect where there is an interference with the utilization of oxygen by cells. A classical example is that of inhibition of cellular cytochrome oxidase activity by cyanide.

Hypoxia is a broad term referring to inadequate tissue supply or utilization of oxygen for any reason; hypoxaemia refers only to decreased carriage of oxygen in arterial blood (as in hypoxic and anaemic hypoxia). Although tissue O_2 supply is decreased in hypoxaemia, significant damage does not occur until arterial O_2 saturation falls to about 50% and PaO_2 falls to about 30 mmHg (Campbell et al., 1984). If of a sufficient degree, hypoxia may result in death. However, lesser degrees of hypoxia are also highly significant in fires because of the following possibilities:

- The development, sometimes insidious, of neurological abnormalities. These may include impaired coordination, impaired judgement, disturbance of consciousness ranging from drowsiness to coma and disorientation (Autian, 1976; Ganong, 1977). All these can clearly produce variable degrees of mental and/or physical incapacitation.
- Hypoxia may increase chemoreceptor activity, leading to an increase in the rate and depth of breathing. This could result in enhanced inhalation exposure to toxic materials in inspired air.
- Hypoxia may enhance the toxicity of some materials.

EXAMPLES OF COMMON MATERIALS IN FIRE ATMOSPHERES

Carbon Monoxide

Carbon monoxide is a major and ubiquitous component of fire atmospheres, often present at potentially lethal concentrations (Jankovic et al., 1991). Barnard (1979) measured carbon monoxide concentrations in 25 Los

Angeles fires and found that in 12% of fires the peak carbon monoxide was approximately 100 ppm; in 40% peak values were in the range 501–1000 ppm, 25% in the range 500–1000 and 23% approximately 1000 ppm; the highest concentration measured was 3000 ppm. A major factor in the toxicity of carbon monoxide is generally considered to be related to its high affinity for haemoglobin, being about 250 times that of oxygen. A sufficient exposure to carbon monoxide causes an anaemic hypoxia. An additional factor influencing the toxicity of carbon monoxide is the fact that the presence of carboxyhaemoglobin (COHb) causes a shift to the left of the oxygen–haemoglobin dissociation curve. As a consequence, there is an increased affinity of haemoglobin for oxygen, hence at any given PO_2 the release of oxygen will be reduced compared with conditions where COHb is not present (Ayres et al., 1973). Also, carbon monoxide inhibits cytochrome a_3; this will be a function of plasma carbon monoxide (Goldbaum et al., 1976; Goldbaum, 1977).

Interpretation of COHb values, particularly at lower concentrations, needs to be undertaken carefully because of the influence of environment (rural or urban) factors, and cigarette smoking on COHb concentrations (Ballantyne, 1981). Also, if dichloromethane is present, this may be endogenously converted to carbon monoxide (Hathaway et al., 1991). Additionally, if analysis for COHb is not performed promptly in appropriately stored containers, analytical artifact losses may occur (Chance et al., 1986; Levin et al., 1990). The majority of individuals exposed to fire atmospheres will have elevated concentrations of carboxyhaemoglobin, the degree of which depends on the time and exposure concentration. Low concentrations of carboxyhaemoglobin may indicate rapid death from trauma or extensive burning (Levin et al., 1990; Mayes, 1991; Mayes et al., 1992). In fires, and accidents involving fires, COHb measurements are of value in assessing the time between physical injury and death. For example, with aircraft accidents, if there is severe impact with subsequent fire, then those dying at impact will have low COHb concentrations. When there is less severe impact, or fire occurs before a crash, the COHb concentration may be higher in those who survive for a period. Clearly in such situations, the COHb concentrations need interpretation against other forensic information, e.g. inhaled smoke, pulmonary fat and bone marrow emboli (Blackmore, 1974). However, it should be noted that even though breathing continues after exposure to a fire, tracheal debris may not be present (Rogdt and Olving, 1996). Similar considerations apply to automobile crashes and fires. Wirthwein and Pless (1996) reviewed 28 fatalities involving fires in automobiles, and found that COHb concentrations ranged from < 10% to 92%. In 16 cases with COHb < 10% a collision occurred, and in 12 of these blunt trauma was sufficient to have caused death. In seven cases with no collision, six had COHb $\geqslant$ 47%. The authors concluded,

from a detailed review of the individual cases, that a COHb concentration > 30% strongly suggests inhalation of combustion products and the cause for death, but if COHb is < 20% a search for other causes of death should be made. When death is due solely to carbon monoxide poisoning, e.g. coal gas poisoning, the COHb concentrations stated to be compatible with death from acute carbon monoxide poisoning are usually in the range 50–60%. COHb concentrations measured in fire victims may show a wide range of values, some compatible with death from carbon monoxide poisoning, others significantly lower. For example, Harland and Wooley (1979) in a sample of 90 fire deaths found COHb >50% in half the cases; those above 50% had a mean value of 67% and those below had a mean of 18%. In interpreting lower concentrations of COHb in fatal cases, it should be remembered that hypoxia may enhance the toxicity of carbon monoxide, and that carbon monoxide toxicity may be an interactive factor in the presence of other toxic substances and physical and thermal trauma.

Maeda et al. (1996), in a review of cases and an evaluation of post mortem cases with a co-oximeter system, stated that with a COHb concentration $\geqslant$ 70% acute death fires may be explained by the immediate effects of CO poisoning; in the range COHb 30–70% there is CO poisoning combined with other factor(s); below COHb 30% other effects are the main cause of death. They noted that other oximetric findings, such as oxyhaemoglobin and reduced haemoglobin, may assist in determining the final balance of blood gases in fire victims. Patterns of COHb found in differing fires may reflect the circumstances of an individual specific fire. For example, in the MGM Grand Hotel fire, 51.3% of victims had COHb > 50%; in this fire most of the victims were found in areas remote from the conflagration (Birky et al., 1985). In contrast, in the DuPont Plaza Hotel fire in Puerto Rico, 80–85% of the victims had COHb <50%; in this fire the majority of victims were burned and found in the area of fire (Levin et al., 1990).

Exposure to sublethal concentrations of carbon monoxide may result in various potentially adverse health effects. Of notable importance are neurological and behavioural effects, which could hinder the performances of skilled tasks, or the recognition and escape from a critical situation. These include headache, dizziness, disturbance of vision, confusion, difficulties in coordination, decreased reaction time and drowsiness (Zarem et al., 1973; Stewart, 1974). Additionally, acute exposure to carbon monoxide may produce cardiac arrythmias, myocardial damage and circulatory failure (Stewart, 1974). Also, there may be aggravation of exercise-induced angina, decreased exercise tolerance, depression of the S–T segment in the ECG and increased vulnerability to ventricular fibrillation (Anderson et al., 1973; Aronow, 1976; DeBias et al., 1976).

The human foetus is particularly sensitive to carbon monoxide because of several differences from the adult.

Thus, under steady-state conditions, foetal COHb is around 10–15% greater than the corresponding maternal blood COHb. Additionally, the partial pressure of O_2 in foetal blood is lower, at 20–30 mmHg, compared with the adult value of 100 mmHg (Longo, 1976, 1977; McDiarmid et al., 1991). Furthermore, the foetal O_2–haemoglobin dissociation curve lies to the left of the adult curve, resulting in greater tissue hypoxia at equivalent COHb concentrations. It is also considered that the foetal half-life of elimination of CO is longer than in the mother (Margulies, 1986). Acute exposure to CO concentrations that are non-lethal to the mother have been associated with foetal loss (Muller and Graham, 1955; Goldstein, 1965) or permanent neurological sequelae in the foetus (Cramer, 1982). These factors need to be considered in relation to pregnant women exposed to fire atmospheres and the employment of women of child-bearing age in the fire services.

Since CO is ubiquitous in various types of fires, all accident victims associated with fires should have COHb determined on hospital admission and the immediate administration of 100% oxygen. Hyperbaric oxygen therapy enhances the elimination of CO, e.g. a half-life of 23 min at 3 atm compared with 60–90 min with 100% oxygen at 1 atm, and 240–320 min with room air (Reisdorff and Shah, 1993). Criteria for hyperbaric oxygen therapy in CO poisoning include the following (Harrigan and Winograd, 1994):

- COHb >25%;
- COHb >15% if cardiac disease present;
- ECG changes present;
- Metabolic acidosis with CO inhalation;
- PaO_2 <60 mmHg;
- Pregnant woman—symptomatic and/or COHb >15%;
- COHB >10% in a child.

Although coma is an undisputed indication for hyperbaric oxygen, investigations have not identified other circumstances which clearly indicate the need for this therapy (Tibbles and Perrotta, 1994; Ernst and Zibrak, 1998). As a consequence, the detailed suggested indications for hyperbaric oxygen in the treatment of CO poisoning vary with different authors. The following is a further list of indications for this form of treatment (Myers and Thom, 1994; Ernst and Zibrak, 1998):

- Coma;
- Any period of unconsciousness;
- Any abnormal score on the CO neuropsychological screening battery;
- COHb >40%;
- Pregnancy and COHb >15%;
- Signs of cardiac ischaemia or arrythmia;
- History of ischaemic heart disease and COHb >20%;
- Recurrent symptoms up to 3 weeks;

- Symptoms not resolving with normobaric O_2 after 4–6 h.

The pathophysiology and clinical features of CO poisoning in relation to combustion have been reviewed in detail by Shusterman (1993).

Hydrogen Cyanide

Any material containing carbon and nitrogen will liberate hydrogen cyanide (HCN) under appropriate combustion conditions. In addition, various cyanogens may be thermally generated, such as acrylonitrile, acetonitrile, adiponitrile, benzonitrile and propionitrile (Stark, 1974; Wooley, 1982). Cyanogens have also been detected in the blood of fire victims (Anderson et al., 1979). Polymeric materials are particularly notable sources of HCN, e.g. nylon (Purser and Woolley, 1983), polyacrylonitrile (Bertol et al., 1983), polyurethanes (Jellinek and Takada, 1977), urea–formaldehyde (Paabo et al., 1979) and melamine (Moss et al., 1951). Although some studies have shown that the evolution of HCN is proportional to the nitrogen content of polymeric materials (Morikawa, 1978), this is not a universal finding. For example, Bertol et al. (1983) found that proportionately more HCN (1500 ppm) was evolved from polyacrylonitrile (19.0% elemental nitrogen) than from wool (200 ppm; 14.3% elemental nitrogen). Also, Urhas and Kullik (1977) found that with pyrolysis temperatures in the range of 625–925 °C, the yield of HCN was inversely related to the nitrogen content of three fibres. Both temperature and oxygen availabilty influence the yield of HCN from a nitrogen-containing material. The general effect of temperature on HCN yield from nitrogen-containing polymers is shown in **Figure 2**. Under anaerobic conditions, high temperatures result in the generation of HCN, the yield of which increases with increasing temperature. In oxidizing atmospheres, HCN is evolved at lower temperatures, and as temperature increases so does HCN liberation, up to a maximum, and then decreases with further increase in temperature; a secondary rise in HCN may occur at even higher temperatures. Polyester and polyether flexible urethane foams decompose at relatively low temperature (200–300 °C) in inert atmospheres to produce a yellow smoke which is stable up to 800 °C; however, over the range 800–1000 °C there is decomposition yielding HCN, acetonitrile, benzonitrile and pyridine as the major nitrogen-containing products (Wooley, 1972). These and many other studies indicate that the evolution of HCN varies with temperature, oxygen availability, the chemical nature of the nitrogen-containing material, and the burning time. Although these variables will differ at any given time, practical estimates for HCN generation have been made. For example, Morikawa (1978) calculated that if nylon is burned at 950 °C under restricted air conditions, then only 1.5 g is necessary to raise the HCN concentration to

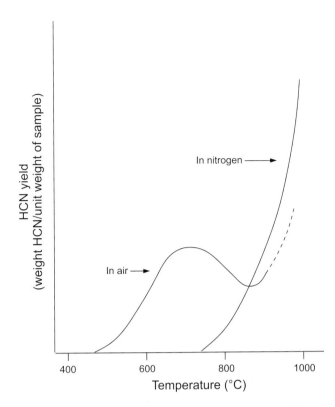

Figure 2 Graphical representation of HCN yields from nitrogen-containing polymers as a function of thermolysis temperature in oxidative and inert atmospheres. In air there is an initial increase in HCN yield followed by a decrease; a secondary increase in HCN yield may occur at higher temperatures. For anaerobic conditions the evolution of HCN begins at temperatures above those for oxidative conditions, and the yield increases with increasing temperature.

significance were measured. Purser *et al.* (1984) exposed primates to the combustion products from polyacrylonitrile, and a comparable group to HCN vapour. The pathophysiological effects were similar for the two groups: hyperventilation, loss of consciousness, bradycardia and cardiac arrythmias; following this, breathing was slowed and respiratory minute volume markedly decreased. For both groups there was a relationship between chamber HCN concentration and time to incapacitation. Blood cyanide concentrations in the polyacrylonitrile combustion group were similar to those in the HCN-alone group. Purser and Grimshaw (1984) exposed primates for 30 min to the products of pyrolysis of flexible polyurethane foam generated at 900 °C or oxidative thermal decomposition of rigid polyurethane foam at 600 °C. Signs included hyperventilation followed by loss of muscle tone and limb reflexes, and then loss of consciousness. Venous blood COHb at the end of the exposure period ranged from 17 to 28% and whole blood cyanide ranged from 1.9 to 2.3 μg ml^{-1}. They noted that the central nervous system effects could be extreme because the cytotoxic hypoxia, circulatory failure, and hyperventilation which may produce cerebral arterioconstriction due to the induced hypocapnia. Thomas and O'Flaherty (1979) demonstrated that the products of pyrolysis of polyurethane foam inhibited brain and heart cytochrome oxidase activity which was positively correlated with blood cyanide concentrations. These and many other studies involving exposure of animals to the products of combustion from various nitrogen-containing polymeric materials have shown that significant inhalation dosages of HCN may be received resulting in physical incapacitation, coma or lethality.

As with animal studies, there is a wealth of information suggesting that humans exposed to combustion products may have absorbed cyanide. The first detailed description of cyanide in the blood of fire victims was given by Wetherell (1966), who found cyanide in the blood of 39 of 53 individuals dying in fires; the average concentration was 0.65 μg ml^{-1} (range 0.17–2.20 μg ml^{-1}). Other representative studies are as follows. Hart *et al.* (1985) described five subjects with smoke inhalation who were comatose on admission to hospital; blood cyanide ranged from 0.35 to 3.9 μg ml^{-1} (average 1.62 μg ml^{-1}). The subject with the highest blood cyanide died 4 days after admission. In post-crash aeroplane fires, Mohler (1975) reported blood cyanide, in victims, having a range of 0.01–3.9 μg ml^{-1}. In some cases, increased cyanide concentrations clearly indicate death due to acute cyanide poisoning. For example, Tscuhiya (1977) described two persons found dead after a fire involving a polyurethane mattress; the blood cyanide concentrations were 7.2 and 23.0 μg ml^{-1}.

around 135 ppm in a 1 m^3 space. Extrapolating data from combustion studies, Bertol *et al.* (1983) calculated that a toxic concentration of HCN could be developed in an average sized room by the burning of 2 kg of polyacrylonitrile.

Many independent studies using laboratory animals have shown that when animals are exposed to combustion products, principally from nitrogen-containing polymers, then HCN may be generated in sufficient amounts to produce physical incapacitation or lethality. Yamamoto (1975) studied the acute toxicity of combustion products from various fibres and found that in rats exposed for up to 30 min signs of incapacitation developed most rapidly following exposure to polyacrylonitrile (<10 min). Blood removed after development of signs showed COHb concentrations were ca. 10% with polyacrylonitrile and wool, and in the range 20–40% for silk; blood cyanide concentrations ranged from 1.5 to 3.0 μg ml^{-1} for silk, 1.5–2.0 μg ml^{-1} for PAN and about 0.5 μg ml^{-1} for wool. Thus, under these conditions of exposure to the combustion products from silk and polyacrylonitrile, HCN was the major cause of incapacitation and blood cyanide concentrations of potentially lethal

Exposure to HCN vapour released in a fire can lead to muscle weakness, difficulty in coordination, physical incapacitation, a confusional state and partial or complete loss of consciousness. This clearly will impede escape from the area of a fire. The high concentration of cyanide measured in fire casualties has raised the question of the routine use of cyanide antidotes in cases of severe smoke inhalation (Daunderer, 1979; Hart *et al.*, 1985). Hydrogen cyanide as a product of combustion, and its significance, have been reviewed in detail by Ballantyne (1987).

TOXIC INTER-RELATIONSHIPS BETWEEN FIRE GAS COMPONENTS

As has been repeatedly stressed, the fire atmosphere is a continuously varying complex of numerous materials of differing chemical structure and differing toxicity. The acute and long-term hazards of many, but not all, individual components are known to varying extents. However, the influence of interactive factors on known toxicity and the potential for additional interactive toxicity is poorly understood. Nevertheless, studies have been conducted for a few binary chemical systems. Several illustrative examples are given below, which demonstrate that even with such simple binary systems the hazard may vary according to the relative proportions of the components.

Hydrogen Cyanide and Carbon Monoxide

Since carbon monoxide and HCN co-exist in a fire, this is a highly practical consideration, and has been discussed in detail by Ballantyne (1987). The investigational approaches have been variable and included mortality studies, measurements of blood cyanide and COHb, and assessment of physiological functions. Moss *et al.* (1951) found that simultaneous exposure to CO (2000 ppm) and HCN (10–20 ppm), both at individually sublethal concentrations, caused death. Smith *et al.* (1976) found that the times to death for rats exposed to an atmosphere containing 450 ppm HCN and 13 500 ppm CO (3.7 ± 0.4 SD min) was slightly longer than for a corresponding concentration of HCN alone (10.9 ± 2.0 SD min) or CO alone (5.8 ± 1.2 SD min). Norris *et al.* (1986) investigated the effect of a 3 min inhalation exposure of mice to CO (0.63–0.66%) on the lethal toxicity of intraperitoneal KCN [4–9 mg (kg body weight)$^{-1}$]. A significantly lower LD$_{50}$ for KCN [6.51 (6.04–7.00) mg (kg body weight)$^{-1}$] was found in CO-pretreated animals than in air-alone controls [7.90 (7.36–8.45) mg (kg body weight)$^{-1}$]. In further studies they found evidence for a synergism between CO and KCN. The authors suggested that this may have been the result of augmentation of the inhibition of cytochrome oxidase in the central nervous system.

Pitt *et al.*, (1979) investigated the effects of CO and HCN on cerebral circulation and metabolism in the dog.

When given together CO and HCN increased cerebral blood flow in an additive manner; however, a significant decrease in cerebral oxygen consumption occurred with combined exposure to CO and HCN, neither of which alone had an effect. Ballantyne (1984, 1987) investigated the effects of differing proportions of HCN and CO in the atmosphere on lethal toxicity and blood cyanide and COHb concentrations, and determined that the contribution of either substance to toxicity depends in their absolute and relative atmospheric concentrations. Thus, when there was a marked excess of CO, the presence of HCN lowered the lethal inhalation dosage for CO by a less than additive toxicity, i.e. HCN physiologically potentiated (by hyperventilation) the toxicity of CO. When there was excess CO with respect to HCN, but not sufficient to produce a clear biochemical evidence of death due to CO, then the blood picture indicated death not primarily due to CO or HCN. In these circumstances, because of the less than additive toxicity, it is likely that both are acting at a common target site, probably cytochrome oxidase. When CO and HCN are present in equal mass proportions, biochemical evidence indicates death due to acute cyanide poisoning.

Carbon Monoxide and Carbon Dioxide

Nelson *et al.* (1978) found that the 30 min lethal concentration of CO to rats was 6000 ppm, and was decreased to 2560 ppm in the presence of 1.44% CO_2. Redkey and Collison (1979) found more rapid times to death in rats exposed to 6000 ppm CO with 4.5% CO_2 (16.8 ± 0.6 min) compared with 6000 ppm alone. Levin *et al.* (1989), in detailed studies, found that above a certain concentration of CO (4100 ppm) some rats will die, and adding CO_2 has no influence. Below 2500 ppm CO the addition of CO_2 (up to 17.7%) is not sufficient to produce mortality. However, with a CO concentration range of 2500–4100 ppm (which produces few mortalities *per se*) CO_2 (>1.5%) will produce a higher level of mortality. They noted that CO and CO_2 act together by (1) increasing the rate of COHb formation, (2) producing severe acidosis which was greater than the metabolic acidosis from CO alone or respiratory acidosis from CO_2 alone, and (3) prolonging the recovery period from acidosis.

INVESTIGATION OF THE TOXICOLOGICAL HAZARDS OF FIRES

Investigation into, and assessment of, potential adverse health effects from the products of combustion are complex exercises because of the multiplicity of thermolysis products and the variability of factors affecting the qualitative and quantitative nature of the products and the biological responses to them. Therefore, in respect of most practical situations it is possible only to give an overview of the products likely to be present under given conditions of thermolysis, and a qualitative assessment of hazards. Although detailed studies have been carried out on some binary systems, allowing quantitative assessments of interactions to be made, the majority of studies have been conducted on combustion products. An overview of the various approaches to investigating toxicological hazards from fires is given below; details can be found in Gad (1990b) and Kaplan (1988).

Physicochemical Studies on Thermolysis Products

These laboratory studies are concerned with the analytical determination of the chemical nature and relative proportions of substances produced by thermolysis of materials under differing conditions. Ideally, the analyses should be conducted under the following conditions: simple heating, complete combustion, oxidative pyrolysis and anaerobic pyrolysis. It is thus necessary to subject materials to a range of temperatures in atmospheres of differing oxygen content, with the resultant effluent being analysed by appropriate instrumental procedures. In some instances, highly toxic materials may be generated over a narrow temperature range and, if a differential temperature study is not performed this may be missed. In addition to the influence of temperature and oxygen availability on the materials generated from combustion, it is important to study the nature of the materials generated as a function of time in the combustion phase since the pattern may change appreciably. A few examples are given in **Table 3** to illustrate the influence of variables on combustion products.

From a knowledge of the nature of the materials generated, under different conditions of combustion, it may be possible to give a hazard pattern for a given material providing that adequate information on toxicology is available. In some cases a major hazardous material may be identified from a large number of analytically detected substances produced by combustion of a specific material. For example, with PVC about 75 organic products have been detected on thermal decomposition, most being aliphatic or aromatic hydrocarbons (Wooley, 1971). However, a major product which begins to be liberated at 200–300 °C is hydrogen chloride, and it is estimated that 1 kg of PVC may yield about 400 g of hydrogen chloride on complete combustion. Hydrogen chloride causes sensory irritation of the eyes and respiratory tract, and in sufficient concentrations may cause inflammatory lesions in the respiratory tract. PVC combustion is recognized as a major hazard in fires involving modern buildings (Dyer and Esch, 1976).

The small-scale laboratory tests yield useful, although often preliminary, information on the nature of combustion products generated from specific materials under defined conditions, and allow a qualitative assessment of the hazards that may be encountered for a specific material in a fire. However, the majority of fires involve the burning of a multiplicity of materials including structural and furnishing components. In an attempt to obtain more reliable information it may be desirable to undertake large-scale experimental fires with appropriate instrumentation. Such tests are likely to be expensive and require careful planning, specifically with regard to sampling and analysis of the atmosphere. Guidance on the design of large-scale tests will clearly be obtained from preliminary small-scale laboratory combustion product studies.

Animal Exposure Studies

In the strictly physicochemical analytical approach to defining the nature and relative proportions of combustion products generated from specific materials, the likely hazard of the effluent smoke is determined by attempting to predict the probable combined toxicity of the constituents in the smoke from a knowledge of their individual toxicities. Such an approach may produce misleading predictions, since there is the possibility of chemical and toxicological interactions, including synergism. Attempts have therefore been made to determine the toxicity of smokes from specific material by exposing animals to the products of thermolysis and monitoring for adverse effects by standard and special procedures. Such tests readily lend themselves to observations on irritancy and acute toxicity. The former will give an index of potentially harassing and incapacitating properties of effluent smoke from the material, and the latter an indication of tissue injuring or potentially lethal adverse effects such as lung damage or neurobehavioural abnormalities. Such tests are frequently carried out with the smoke generated under differing conditions of atmospheric oxygen content and thermolysis temperature. For comparative purposes the findings are frequently referred to tests from the burning of a standard material, usually wood. Although such tests give useful information in themselves, they are particularly valuable when viewed in the light of studies on the analysis of combustion products generated under similar conditions. Thus, when interpreting laboratory data in an attempt to define possible hazards from combustion products of materials, it is highly desirable to have information on both the nature and relative proportions of combustion products and on their effects on experimental animals exposed to combustion products generated under similar conditions. Where appropriate facilities and expertise exist it is possible to combine analytical studies with animal exposure tests. Also, animal exposures have been performed in large-scale fire tests.

Problems may be encountered in defining the presence of novel or highly toxic materials, for several reasons; first, because of the multiplicity of materials generated, there may be limitations on the analytical capability and second, a knowledge of the toxicology of some materials generated is unknown. It therefore follows that animal studies may draw attention to the presence of highly toxic, or unsuspected, materials in a test atmosphere. This may be illustrated by investigations on a fire-retarded polyurethane foam. The products from non-flaming combustion of a trimethylolpropane-based rigid urethane foam fire retarded with an organo-phosphate, O,O-diethyl-N,N-bis(2-hydroxyethyl)amino-methyl phosphonate, were found to produce grand mal seizures in rats; similar effects were not observed when the foam was not fire retarded (Petajan *et al.*, 1974). Subsequent chemical analysis revealed the presence of 4-ethyl-1-phospha-2,6,7-trioxabicyclo[2.2.2] octane-1-oxide in the smoke (Voorhees *et al.*, 1975). This is a material of high acute toxicity (Kimmerle, 1976). Further work demonstrated no unusual toxicity when the flame-retarded polyurethane foam was either gradually or rapidly pyrolysed to 800 °C in the absence of air; however, convulsions were observed when the material was flash pyrolysed in the presence of an air flow (Hilando and Schneider, 1977). See Purser (1992) for a discussion of caged bicyclophosphorus esters in combustion processes.

Combustion Toxicity Apparatus

Several types of apparatus are currently available: the DIN 53–436 (a German standard), the radiant furnace (an ASTM draft standard) and the University of Pittsburgh (an ASTM draft standard and legislated in the State of New York). The selection of the apparatus will depend on the combustion conditions that are to be simulated. Some possible combustion conditions are smouldering, flaming, pre-flashover and post-flashover. These three types of apparatus have different capabilities for simulating these combustion conditions.

The DIN 53–438

The combustion device is a moving annular furnace encircling a quartz tube containing the test specimen. The intent of this design is to generate a consistent combustion environment for the time course of the experiment even though the animal exposure is dynamic. The furnace temperature is a fixed value during the experiment but that value can range between 100 and 900 °C. The animals are rats, and the exposure is head only. After the exposure, the animals are retained for a 2-week post-exposure period. Selection of the temperature can determine the combustion conditions of the test specimen for non-flaming or flaming mode.

The Radiant Furnace

The combustion device is a set of four quartz lamps designed to subject the test specimen to a heat flux density ranging from 2 to 7 kW m^{-2}. The animal exposure to the combustion products is static. The animals are rats, and the exposure is head only. The rats are observed for 2 weeks after exposure. The combustion conditions can be selected by changing the heat flux density and implementing the use of an piloted ignition source. Thus, non-flaming and flaming conditions can be investigated. The LC$_{50}$ value is expressed as mg l^{-1}min^{-1}. The methodology is an ASTM and NFPA standard.

The University of Pittsburgh

The combustion device is basically a muffle furnace. The test specimen is subjected to a ramping temperature of 20 °C min^{-1}. The animal exposure to the combustion products is dynamic. The animals are mice, and the exposure is head only. After the test specimen has lost 1% of its initial weight, the combustion products are presented to the animals, and 30 min later the exposure period is ended. For 10 min after the exposure period the animals are observed. The combustion conditions are the same for all test specimens. However, the test specimen can react differently to those conditions, thereby combusting in a non-flaming or flaming mode. The critical variable appears to be the weight of the specimen. The smaller weight specimens will not necessarily spontaneously flame, whereas larger weight specimens may spontaneously flame. Thus, more than one LC$_{50}$ value can be obtained for a test substance (Norris, 1990). The LC$_{50}$ value is expressed in grams. This is the weight of the test specimen placed in the furnace which is calculated to kill 50% of the animals. The State of New York legislated that certain building products be tested by this procedure and the results filed with the State before the products could be sold. New York City also uses this test for pass/fail criteria for some building materials.

Studies on Exposed Human Populations

Valuable and unique information may be obtained about the adverse effects of exposure to fire atmospheres and on the possible long-term hazards of recurrent exposures to fires, by appropriate investigations on the victims of fires and on firefighters. Major sources of information have been derived from post-mortem examination of fire victims, clinical, radiological and clinical chemistry examination of non-lethal fire victims, and routine medical and special epidemiological examination of firefighters. In the context of defining the requirement for respiratory and other protective equipment by firefighters based on the medical and epidemiological data, short-term repeated and chronic exposure situations as well as acute exposure all require consideration.

Toxic Hazard and Hazard Analysis

In 1986, the US National Institute of Building Sciences initiated a programme to develop a performance toxicity test to characterize building products. This performance test was developed so that it incorporated additional fire parameters, such as the LC_{50} value, time to ignition and mass loss rate. The concern was that regulation of products was to occur based solely on the LC_{50} values. Since a hazard analysis was not available, this was viewed as an interim step until the complete hazard analysis could be established (Norris, 1988).

The direction for the utilization of combustion toxicity data has been to enfold it into hazard analysis. These analyses include other fire performance parameters, such as time to ignition, flame spread and heat release rate. The fire scenario is also a part of these analyses. The National Institute of Standards and Technology has developed a hazard analysis called the HAZARD 1 Fire Hazard Assessment Method (Bukowski *et al.*, 1989).

CHEMICAL HAZARDS TO FIREFIGHTERS

Firefighting is one of the most hazardous of professions, having an associated high level of morbidity and mortality, with the most important health concerns being as follows:

- *Trauma*: notably from falling objects, in rescue situations and during close-in firefighting.
- *Thermal*: primary burns to the skin and respiratory tract and heat stress. The latter is a function of environmental temperature, insulating properties of protective clothing, and endogenous heat production from severe physical exertion compounded by the additional weight of equipment such as self-contained breathing apparatus.
- *Ergonomic*: the high energy costs of firefighting may clearly be interrelated with, and compounded with, other health concerns.
- *Psychological*: these are multiple in nature and include thoughts of personal security, victim rescue and loss, emotional scenes and heavy social responsibility (Guidotti and Clough, 1992).
- *Toxic chemicals*: sequential exposures to smoke and chemicals, often at high concentrations, which are known or suspected to produce acute and/or long-term health problems. An outline of this aspect of health concern is presented below; details are available in Guidotti and Clough (1992).

Firefighters are recurrently exposed to a large variety of materials that may cause acute, cumulative and/or chronic health problems; typical examples are carbon monoxide, hydrogen cyanide, sulphur dioxide, hydrogen chloride, phosgene, isocyanates, oxides of nitrogen, acrolein, acetaldehyde, asbestos, polycyclic aromatic hydrocarbons, benzene, methanol, methane, methylene, chloride and toluene (McDiarmid *et al.*, 1991; Guidotti and Clough, 1992; Aronson *et al.*, 1994). That such materials may be absorbed has been suggested by several studies. For example, that firefighters absorb hydrogen cyanide is indicated by increased serum thiocyanate (Levine and Radford, 1978). As expected, several studies have demonstrated that firefighters have increased blood COHb concentrations. Thus, Sammons and Coleman (1974) found a significant difference in COHb concentrations between non-smoking firemen (mean 5.0%, range 2.5–13.9%) and non-smoking controls (mean 2.3%, range 1.0–11.7%). Similarly, Radford and Levine (1976) found increased COHb concentrations in firemen after fighting a fire (4.53%) compared with unexposed controls (2.17%). Increased COHb concentrations were also found after firefighting by Loke *et al.* (1970) and Levy *et al.* (1976) **(Figure 3)**. Actual firefighter exposure in terms of exposure concentrations and/or dosage is usually unknown, but will vary between different fire situations and conditions. One estimate, for polycyclic aromatic hydrocarbons, was made during part of a firefighting exercise (Moen and Overebo, 1977). The participants gave urine samples 6–7 h after extinguishing burning diesel oil, and the samples were analysed for 1-hydroxypyrene by high-performance liquid chromatography. A small, but statistically significant, increase in urinary 1-hydroxypyrene was measured after the firefighting exercise. Because of the conditions and the personal protective equipment used, this may have represented an underestimate of actual exposure in real situations.

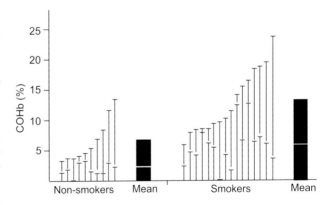

Figure 3 Increases in carboxyhaemoglobin concentration in firefighters following exposure to smoke. The lower bars represent COHb pre-exposure and the upper bars the increase in COHb post-exposure. Drawn from data in Levy *et al.* (1976) and Loke *et al.* (1970).

Firefighting carries a high mortality and morbidity for various reasons. Several epidemiological surveys have been undertaken with respect to general and specific causes of morbidity and mortality. Some major studies are as follows. In a study of Alberta firefighters, Guidotti (1993) did not find an association with heart or chronic pulmonary disease, but did find a possible association with occupational exposure for renal and ureteric cancer, and limited evidence for excess bladder, colon and rectal cancers. In a retrospective cohort study (1950–89) with 5995 subjects from six fire departments in the Toronto Metropolitan area, it was found (Aronson et al., 1994) that three specific causes of death had statistically significant excesses: brain tumours [standardized mortality rate (SMR) 201; 95% confidence interval 110–337], 'other' major neoplasms (SMR 238, 145–367), and aortic aneurysm (SMR 226; 136–354). Tornling et al., (1994) studied the incidences of mortality and cancer in Stockholm firefighters with at least 1 year of employment during the period 1931–83. They found overall mortality (1951–86, based on tracing of individuals) was lower than expected (SMR 82; 72–91) compared with local figures. Although the overall cancer incidence was equal to that expected (SMR 100), an excess of gastric cancer was noted (18 observed versus 9.37 expected; SMR 192). The results from various studies are somewhat inconsistent, as would be anticipated from the differing work conditions. However, in a review analysis of major publications up to 1995, Guidotti (1995) came to the following conclusions:

- Lung cancer—evidence for an association, but not sufficient for a general assumption of risk.
- Cardiovascular disease—no evidence for increased risk overall for heart disease.
- Aortic aneurysm—evidence incomplete.
- Genito-urinary cancer—evidence strong for an association and presumption of risk.
- Lympho-haematopoietic cancers—some evidence and a general presumption of risk, but requires case-by-case approach.
- Rectocolonic cancer—sufficient evidence to conclude an associating and not sufficiently strong to determine if there is a good presumption of risk.

Respiratory Disease

Several studies have shown that exposure to a fire atmosphere produces acute changes in pulmonary function and may be a factor in the development of chronic lung dysfunction. For example, Musk et al. (1979) studied acute changes in firefighters during routine duties and found an average decrease in FEV_1 (forced expiratory volume in 1 s) of 0.05 litres, which was related to subjectively assessed smoke exposure; decreases in FEV_1 of 0.1 liters or more were found in 30% of cases. Brandt-Rauf et

al. (1989) found that for firefighters not wearing respiratory protective equipment, there were statistically significant post-fire decrements in FEV_1 and FVC (forced vital capacity). Pre-and post-fire average FEV_1 values were 3.80 and 3.61 litres and FVC values were 5.03 and 4.81 litres, respectively ($n = 14$). Gu et al. (1996) studied acute respiratory effects in firefighters in a sustained store fire. Irritant effects were present in the eye and upper respiratory tract. Spirometry was conducted 2 days after the fire. They found that FEV_1 and FEV_1/FVC in smokers and FEV_1 in non-smokers were significantly less than in controls; there was no significant difference in average fire fighting times between smokers and non-smokers. Serra et al. (1996) examined pulmonary function in 92 firemen and compared the findings with a group of policemen (controls). They measured FVC, FEV_1, FEF (forced expiratory flow) at 75, 50 and 25% of the FVC, total lung capacity (TLC), residual volume (RV), functional residual capacity (FRC) and CO diffusion for alveolar–capillary integrity. They found the firemen to have significantly reduced FEV_1 (3.90 ± 0.50 SD versus controls at 4.04 ± 0.44; $p < 0.05$), FEV_1/FVC (80.07 ± 5.89 versus 83.89 ± 6.32; $p < 0.001$), FEF_{25} (1.58 ± 0.47 versus 1.99 ± 0.69; $p < 0.001$ and RV (1.57 ± 0.28 versus 1.76 ± 0.45; $p < 0.01$). Alveolar–capillary integrity (as evidenced by CO diffusion) was not different from the controls.

For cumulative effects, Peabody (1977) reported a decrease in pulmonary function for San Diego firefighters which was significantly greater than that of the general population. Peters et al. (1974), over a 2-year period, found that the rate of decline in pulmonary function, measured by FVC and FEV_1, was twice the expected rate; these changes were significantly related to frequency of exposure. A raised risk of emphysema was found in a mortality study by Demers et al. (1992). The importance of respiratory protective equipment was shown in a study by Tepper et al. (1991), who re-evaluated 632 Baltimore city firemen 6–10 years after baseline measurements, and found that in those who never wore a mask there was a 1.7 times greater decline than in mask wearers. NIOSH (1987) recommend a protection factor of 10 000 for the pressure-demand, self-contained breathing apparatus used by fire fighters.

Cardiovascular Disease

Firemen are exposed to carbon monoxide, carbon dioxide, acrolein, sulphur dioxide, organic solvents, noise, heat, and physical and emotional stress. It is therefore to be expected that they would be at increased risk from cardiovascular disease. Some epidemiological studies do not show an excess of cardiovascular disease or death from cardiovascular disease amongst firemen (Eliopulos et al., 1984; Sardinas et al., 1986; Beaumont et al., 1991; Demers et al., 1992; Guidotti, 1993; Deschamps et al.,

1995). Summarizing the available evidence, Guidotti (1992) stated that population-based mortality and disability surveillance studies suggest a relatively small but significant excess of disability, but not mortality, for non-malignant cardiovascular disease for firefighters. More targeted cohort and case-control studies do not support such an excess, but suggest a strong healthy worker effect (Howe et al., 1988; Aronson et al., 1994). However, some studies suggest an excess of coronary artery disease (Musk et al., 1978). Two studies have shown increased SMRs for circulatory diseases with increasing years of work (Vena and Fielder, 1987; Demers et al., 1992) and Aronson et al. (1994) showed an increase in aortic aneurysm.

Reproductive Hazards

Many of the chemicals that are found in a fire atmospheres have been associated with potential adverse reproductive effects (McDiarmid et al., 1991). In spite of this, little epidemiological evidence is available on the reproductive hazards of fire fighting. However, one study has indicated a possible excess of birth defects in children of firefighters (Olshan et al., 1990). Also, it has been noted that peak CO concentrations measured in fires could be immediately dangerous to an unprotected woman firefighter and her foetus (McDiarmid et al., 1991). There is a clear need for further investigation into the reproductive hazards of firefighting.

Carcinogenic Hazards

Several known or suspect carcinogens are present, to variable extents, in fire atmospheres, e.g. polycyclic aromatic hydrocarbons, acrylonitrile, vinyl chloride, asbestos, formaldehyde and PCBs. There are some inconsistences between various studies on the possible excess of cancers in firefighters. However, biological monitoring for genotoxic effects, including sister chromatid exchanges and polycyclic aromatic hydrocarbon–DNA adducts in peripheral blood, suggests a potential for carcinogenic effects (Liou et al., 1989). Particular sites for neoplasms, possibly occupationally related to firefighting, are buccal and pharyngeal (Mastromatteo, 1974), lung (Heyer et al., 1990), oesophagus (Beaumont et al., 1991), genito-urinary (Deschamps et al., 1995), colonorectal (Guidotti and Clough, 1992), brain (Howe and Burch, 1990; Demers et al., 1992; Aronson et al., 1994), lymphatic and leukaemia (Heyer et al., 1990; Demers et al., 1992). However, documentation for an association between lung cancer and occupational exposures is inconsistent. For example, a Danish study (Hansen, 1990) reported an SMR of 317 for older firefighters, but studies from San Francisco (Beaumont et al., 1991) and Buffalo (Vena and Fielder, 1987) showed no excess.

Cigarette smoking is a clear confounding factor (Liou et al., 1989), although according to one study the incidence of smoking amongst firemen is not excessive compared with other occupations (Gerace, 1990). The excesses of certain cancers may be the result of interaction of several factors, e.g. toxic substances, alcohol and smoking (Beaumont et al., 1991). Ford et al. (1992) suggest that the immunological detection of serum β-transforming growth factor-related proteins may be a possible biomarker for monitoring firefighters for potential development of cancer.

REFERENCES

Agnew, J., McDiarmid, M. A., Lees, P. S. J. and Duffy, R. (1991). Reproductive hazards of fire fighting. I. Non-chemical hazards. Am. J. Ind. Med., 19, 433–445.

Alarie, Y. (1985). The toxicity of smoke from polymeric materials during thermal decomposition. Annu. Rev. Pharmacol. Toxicol., 25, 325–347.

Alexeeff, G. and Packham, S. C. (1984). Evaluation of smoke toxicity using concentration–time products. J. Fire Sci., 2, 362.

Anderson, E. W., Andelman, R. J., Strauch, J. M., et al. (1973). Effect of low-level exposure on onset and duration of angina pectoris. Ann. Intern. Med., 79, 46–50.

Anderson, R. A., Thomson, I. and Harland, W. A. (1979). The importance of cyanide and organic nitriles in fire fatalities. Fire Mater., 3, 91–99.

Andrasch, R. H., Foster, F., Lawson, W. H., et al. (1975). Meat wrappers asthma: an appraisal of a new occupational syndrome. J. Allergy Clin. Immunol., 55, 130.

Aronow, W. S. (1976). Effect of cigarette smoking and of carbon monoxide on coronary heart disease. Chest, 70, 514–518.

Aronson, K. J., Tomlinson, G. A. and Smith, L. (1994). Mortality among fire fighters in Metropolitan Toronto. Am. J. Ind. Med., 26, 89–101.

Autian, J. (1976). Medical aspects of toxicity resulting from fire exposures. In Physiological and Toxicological Aspects of Combustion Products. National Research Council, National Academy of Science, Washington, DC, pp. 47–56.

Ayres, S. M., Giannelli, S. and Mueller, H. (1973). Carboxyhaemoglobin and the access to oxygen. Arch. Environ. Health, 216, 8–15.

Ballantyne, B. (1981). Inhalation hazards of fire. In Ballantyne, B. and Schwabe, P. H. (Eds), Respiratory Protection: Principles and Applications. Chapman and Hall, London, pp. 351–372.

Ballantyne, B. (1984). Relative toxicity of carbon monoxide and hydrogen cyanide in combined atmospheres. Toxicologist, 4, 69.

Ballantyne, B. (1987). Hydrogen cyanide as a product of combustions and a factor in morbidity and mortality from fires. In Ballantyne, B. and Marrs, T. C. (Eds), Clinical and Experimental Toxicology of Cyanides. Wright, Bristol, pp. 248–291.

Ballantyne, B. (1989). Toxicology. In Encyclopedia of Polymer Science and Engineering, Vol. 16. Wiley, New York, pp. 879–930.

Barnard, R. J. (1979). Coronary artery disease deaths in the Toronto Fire Department. *J. Occup. Med.*, **29**, 132–135.

Beaumont, J. J., Chu, G. S. T., Jones, J. R., *et al.* (1991). An epidemiological study of cancer and other causes of mortality in San Francisco firefighters. *Am. J. Ind. Health.*, **19**, 357–372.

Bertol, E., Mari, F., Orzalesi, G. and Volpato, I. (1983). Combustion products from various kinds of fibres: toxicologic hazards from smoke exposure. *Forensic Sci. Int.*, **22**, 111–116.

Birky, M. M., Malek, D. and Paabo, M. (1985). Study of biological specimens obtained from victims of MGM Grand Hotel fire. *J. Anal. Toxicol.*, **7**, 265–271.

Bizovi, K. E. and Leikin, J. D. (1995). Smoke inhalation among fire fighters. *Occup. Med. State Art Rev.*, **10**, 721–734.

Blackmore, D. J. (1974). Interpretation of carbon monoxide levels found at post-mortem. In Ballantyne, B. (Ed.), *Forensic Toxicology*. Wright, Bristol, pp. 99–113.

Bowes, P. C. (1974). Smoke and toxicity hazards of plastics in fire. *Ann. Occup. Hyg.*, **17**, 143–157.

Bowes, P. C. (1976). Casualities attributed to toxic gas and smoke at fires: a survey of statistics. *Med. Sci. Law*, **16**, 104–110.

Brandt-Rauf, P. W., Cosman, B., Fallon, L. F., Jr, *et al.* (1989). Health hazards of firefighters: acute pulmonary effects after toxic exposure. *Br. J. Ind. Med.*, **46**, 209–211.

Brooks, S. M. (1983). Bronchial asthma of occupational origin. In Rom, W. N. (Ed.), *Environmental and Occupational Medicine*. Little, Brown, Boston, pp. 242–243.

Brooks, S. M., Weiss, M. A. and Bernstein, I. L. (1985). Reactive airways dysfunction syndrome (RADS). *Chest*, **88**, 376–384.

Bukowski, R. M., Peacock, R. D., Jones, W. W. and Forney, C. L. (1989). *HAZARD 1—Fire Hazard Assessment Method. NIST Handbook*, No. 146 (3 volumes). National Institute of Standards and Technology, Washington, DC.

Burgess, J. L. and Crutchfield, C. D. (1995). Tucson fire fighter exposure to products of combustion: a risk assessment. *Appl. Occup. Environ. Hyg.*, **10**, 37–42.

Campbell, E. J. M., Dickinson, E. J., Slater, D. J. H., *et al.* (1984). *Clinical Physiology*. Blackwell, Oxford, pp. 116–118.

Chance, D. M., Goldbaum, L. R. and Lappas, N. T. (1986). Factors affecting the loss of carbon monoxide for stored blood samples. *J. Anal. Toxicol.*, **10**, 181–189.

Cramer, D. R. (1982). Fetal death due to accidental material carbon monoxide poisoning. *J. Toxicol. Clin. Toxicol.*, **19**, 297–301.

Daunderer, M. (1979). Fatal smoke inhalation of hydrogen cyanide from smouldering fires. *Fortschn. Med.*, **97**, 1401–1405.

DeBias, D. A., Banerjee, C. M., Birkhead, N. C., *et al.* (1976). Effect of carbon monoxide inhalation on ventricular fibrillation. *Arch. Environ. Health*, **31**, 42–46.

DeKorver, L. (1976). Smoke problems in urban fire control. In *Physiological and Toxicological Aspects of Combustion Products*. National Research Council, National Academy of Sciences, Washington, DC, pp. 4–10.

Demers, P. H., Heyes, N. J. and Rosenstock, L. (1992). Mortality among firefighters from three Northwestern United States Cities. *Br. J. Ind. Med.*, **49**, 664–670.

Deschamps, S., Momas, I. and Festy, B. (1995). Mortality amonst Paris fire-fighters. *Eur. J. Epidemiol.*, **11**, 643–646.

Dyer, R. F. and Esch, V. H. (1976). Polyvinyl chloride toxicity in fires. J. *Am. Med. Assoc.*, **235**, 393–397.

Eliopulos, E., Armstrong, B. K., Spickett, J. T. and Heyworth, F. (1984). Mortality of fire fighters in Western Australia. *Br. J. Ind. Med.*, **41**, 183–187.

Ernst, A. and Zibrak, J. D. (1998). Carbon monoxide poisoning. *N. Engl. J. Med.*, **339**, 1603–1608.

Ford, J., Smith, S., Luo, J. -C., *et al.* (1992). Serum growth factors and oncoproteins in firefighters. *Occup. Med.*, **42**, 39–42.

Frostling, H., Huff, A., Jacobsson, S., *et al.* (1984). Analytical, occupational and toxicologic aspects of the degradation products of polypropylene plastics. *Scand. J. Work Environ. Health*, **10**, 163–169.

Gad, S. C. (1990a). Introduction. In Gad, S. C. and Anderson, R. C. (Eds), *Combustion Toxicology*, CRC Press, Boca Raton, FL, Ch. 1, pp. 1–16.

Gad, S. C. (1990b). Combustion toxicity testing. In Gad, S. C. and Anderson, R. C. (Eds), *Combustion Toxicology*. CRC Press, Boca Raton, FL, Ch. 5, pp. 81–128.

Ganong, W. F. (1977). *Review of Medical Physiology*. Large Medical Publications, California. p. 511.

Gantz, N. M. (1988). Infectious agents. In Levy, B. S. and Wegman, D. H. (Eds), *Occupational Health*. Little Brown, Boston, pp. 281–295.

Gerace, T. A. (1990). Road to a smoke-free service for Florida: policies and progress. *J. Publ. Health Policy*, **11**, 206–217.

Goldbaum, L. R. (1977). Is carboxyhemoglobin concentration the indicator of carbon monoxide toxicity? *Legal Med. Ann.*, **176**, 165–170.

Goldbaum, L. R., Orellando, T. and Dergal, E. (1976). Mechanism of the toxic action of carbon monoxide. *Ann. Clin. Lab. Sci.*, **6**, 372–376.

Goldstein, D. P. (1965). Carbon monoxide poisoning in pregnancy. *Am. J. Obstet. Gynecol.*, **9**, 526–528.

Gu, T. -L., Liou, S.-H., Hsu, C.-H., Hsu, J.-C. and Wu, T.-N. (1996). Acute health hazards of fire fighters after fighting a department store fire. *Ind. Health*, **34**, 13–23.

Guidotti, T. L. (1992). Human factors in fire fighting: ergonomic-, cardiopulmonary-, and psychogenic stress-related issues. *Int. Arch. Occup. Environ. Health*, **64**, 1–12.

Guidotti, T. L. (1993). Mortality of urban fire fighters in Alberta, 1927–1987. *Am. J. Ind. Med.*, **23**, 921–940.

Guidotti, T. L. (1995). Occupational mortality among fire fighters: assessing the association. *J. Occup. Environ. Med.*, **37**, 1348–1356.

Guidotti, T. L. and Clough, V. M. (1992). Occupational health concerns of fire fighting. *Ann. Rev. Publ. Health*, **13**, 151–171.

Hales, C. A. Barkin, P. W., Jung, W., Trautman, E., Lamborghini, D., Herrig, N. and Burke, A. U. (1988). Synthetic smoke with acrolein but not HCl produces pulmonary edema. *J. Appl. Physiol.*, **64**, 1121–1133.

Hales, C. A., Musto, S. N., Janssens, S. P., Jung, W., Quinn, D. A. and Witten, M. (1992). Smoke aldehyde component influences pulmonary edema. *J. Appl. Physiol.*, **72**, 555–561.

Hales, C. A., Musto, S., Hutchison, W. O. and Mahoney, E. (1995). BW-775C diminishes smoke-induced pulmonary edema. *J. Appl. Physiol.*, **78**, 64–69.

Hansen, E. S. (1990). A cohort study on the mortality of firefighters. *Br. J. Ind. Med.*, **47**, 805–809.

Haponik, E. F. (1993). Clinical smoke inhalation injury: pulmonary effects. *Occup. Med. State Art Rev.*, **8**, 432–467.

Haponik, E. F., Cropo, R. O., Herdon, D. N., Traber, D. L., Hudson, L. and Moylan, J. (1988). Smoke inhalation. *Am. Rev. Resp. Dis.*, **4**, 1060–1063.

Harland, W. A. and Wooley, W. D. (1979). Fire fatality study—University of Glasgow. *Building Research Establishment Information Paper No. 18/79*. Fire Research Station, Borehamwood, Herts, UK.

Harrigan, R. and Winograd, S. (1994). Smoke inhalation injury and fire toxicology: evaluation and management. *Emerg. Med. Rep.*, **15**, 203–210.

Hart, G. B., Strauss, M. B., Lennon, P. A. and Whitcraft, D. D. (1985). Treatment of smoke inhalation by hyperbaric oxygen. *J. Emerg. Med.*, **3**, 211–215.

Hathaway, G. J., Proctor, W. H., Hughes, J. P. and Fishmann, M. C. (1991). *Chemical Hazards of the Workplace*, 3rd edn. Van Nostrand Reinhold, New York, pp. 393–395 and 485.

Head, J. M. (1980). Inhalation injury in burns. *Am. J. Surg.*, **139**, 508–512.

Heimbach, D. M. and Waeckerle, J. F. (1988). Inhalation injuries. *Ann. Emerg. Med.*, **17**, 1316–1320.

Heyer, N., Weiss, N. S., Demers, P. and Rosenstock, L. (1990). Cohort mortality study of fire fighters: 1945–1983. *Am. J. Ind. Med.*, **17**, 493–504.

Hilando, C. J. and Schneider, J. E. (1977). Toxicity studies of a polyurethane rigid foam. *J. Combust. Toxicol.*, **4**, 79–86.

Hill, I. R. (1996). Reactions to particles in smoke. *Toxicology*, **115**, 119–122.

Howe, G. R. and Burch, J. D. (1990). Fire fighting and risk of cancer: an assessment and overview of the epidemiologic evidence. *Am. J. Epidemiol.*, **132**, 1039–1050.

Howe, G. R., Chiarelli, A. M. and Lindsay, J. (1988). Components and modifiers of the healthy worker effect: evidence from three occupational cohorts and implications for industrial compensation. *Am. J. Epidemiol.*, **28**, 1364–1375.

Hubbard, G. B., Langinais, P. C., Shimazu, T., *et al.* (1991). The morphology of smoke inhalation injury in sheep. *J. Trauma*, **31**, 1477–1486.

Jankovic, J., Jones, W., Burkhart, J. and Noonan, G. (1991). Environmental study of firefighters. *Ann. Occup. Hyg.*, **35**, 581–602.

Jellinek, H. H. G., and Takada, K. (1977). Toxic gas evolution from polymers: evolutions of hydrogen cyanide from polyurethanes. *J. Polym. Sci.*, **15**, 2269–2288.

Kaplan, H. L. (1988). Evaluating the combustion hazards of combustion products. In Gad, S. C. (Ed.), *Product Safety Evaluation Handbook*. Marcel Dekker, New York, pp. 409–470.

Kimmerle, G. (1976). Toxicity of combustion products with particular reference to polyurethane. *Ann. Occup. Hyg.*, **19**, 269–273.

Kristensen, T. S. (1989). Cardiovascular disease and the work environment. A critical review of the epidemiologic literature on chemical factors. *Scand. J. Work Environ. Health*, **15**, 245–264.

Levin, B. C., Paato, M., Gurman, J. L., *et al.* (1989). Toxicologic interaction between carbon monoxide and carbon dioxide. *Toxicology*, **47**, 135–164.

Levin, B. C., Rechani, P. R., Gurman, J. L., *et al.* (1990). Analysis of carboxyhemoglobin and cyanide in blood from victims of the Dupont Plaza Hotel fire in Puerto Rico. *J. Fire Sci.*, **35**, 151–168.

Levine, S. and Radford, E. P. (1978). Occupational exposure to cyanide in Baltimore firefighters. *J. Occup. Med.*, **20**, 53–56.

Levy, A. L., Lum, G. and Abeles, F. J. (1976). Carbon monoxide in firemen before and after exposure to smoke. *Ann. Clin. Lab. Sci.*, **6**, 455–458.

Levy, S. A. (1988). An overview of occupational pulmonary disorders. In Zeng, C. (Ed.), *Occupational Medicine*, 2nd edn. Year Book Medical Publishing, Chicago. pp. 201–225.

Levy, S. A., Storey, J. D. and Plashko, B. E. (1978). Meat worker's asthma. *J. Occup. Med.*, **15**, 116–117.

Liou, S.-H., Jacobson-Kram, D. and Poirer, M. C., *et al.* (1989). Biological monitoring of firefighters: sister chromatid exchanges and polycyclic aromatic hydrocarbon–DNA adducts in peripheral blood cells. *Cancer Res.*, **49**, 4929–4935.

Locatelli, C., Candura, S. M., Maccarini, D., Butera, R. and Manzo, L. (1993). Carbon monoxide poisoning in fire victims. *Indoor Environ.*, **3**, 16–21.

Loke, J., Farmer, W. C., Mattham, R. A., *et al.* (1970). Carboxyhemoglobin levels in firefighters. *Lung*, **154**, 35–39.

Longo, L. D. (1976). Carbon monoxide effects on oxygenation of fetus in utero. *Science*, **194**, 523–525.

Longo, L. D. (1977). The biological effects of carbon monoxide on pregnant women, fetuses, and newborn infants. *Am. J. Obstet. Gynecol.*, **129**, 69–103.

Lowry, W. T., Juarez, L., Petts, C. S. and Roberts, B. (1985). Studies of toxic gas products during structural fires in the Dallas area. *J. Forensic Sci.*, **30**, 59–72.

Maeda, H., Fukita, K., Oritani, S., Nagai, O. and Zhn, B.-L. (1996). Evaluation of post-mortem oxymetry in fire victims. *Forensic Sci. Int.*, **81**, 201–209.

Margulies, S. L. (1986). Acute carbon monoxide poisoning during pregnancy. *Am. J. Emerg. Med.*, **4**, 516–519.

Mastromatteo, E. (1974). Mortality in city firemen. *Arch. Ind. Health.*, **20**, 1–7.

Mayes, R. W. (1991). The toxicological examination of victims of the British Air Tours Boeing 727 Accident at Manchester 1988. *J. Forensic Sci.*, **36**, 179–184.

Mayes, R., Levine, B. and Smith, M. L., *et al.* (1992). Toxicologic findings in the USS Iowa Disaster. *J. Forensic Sci.*, **37**, 1352–1357.

McDiarmid, M. A., Lees, P. S. J., Agnew, J., *et al.* (1991). Reproductive hazards of firefighting. II. Chemical hazards. *Am. J. Ind. Med.*, **19**, 447–472.

Michal, J. (1976). Toxicity of pyrolysis and combustion products of polyvinyl chloride. *Fire Mater.*, **1**, 57–62.

Mitera, J. and Michal, J. (1985). The combustion products of polymeric materials. 11. GC–MS analysis of the combustion products of polyethylene, polypropylene, polystyrene and polyamide. *Fire Mater.*, **9**, 11.

Moen, B. E. and Overebo, S. (1997). Assessment of exposure to polycyclic aromatic hydrocarbons during fire fighting by measurement of urinary 1-hydroxypyrene. *J. Occup. Environ. Med.*, **39**, 515–519.

Mohler, S. R. (1975). Air crash survival: injuries and evacuation hazards. *Aviation Space Environ. Med.*, **46**, 86–88.

Morikawa, T. (1976). Acrolein, formaldehyde, and volatile fatty acids from smouldering combustion. *J. Combust. Toxicol.*, **3**, 135–150.

Morikawa, T. (1978). Evaluation of hydrogen cyanide during combustion and pyrolysis. *J. Combust. Toxicol.*, **5**, 315–338.

Moss, R. H., Jackson, C. F. and Saberlick, J. (1951). Toxicity of carbon monoxide and hydrogen cyanide gas mixtures. *Arch. Ind. Hyg. Occup. Med.*, **4**, 53–60.

Muller, G. L. and Graham, S. (1955). Intrauterine death of the fetus due to accidental carbon monoxide poisoning. *N. Engl. J. Med.*, **252**, 1075–1078.

Musk, A. W., Morison, B. R., Peters, J. M. and Peters, R. K. (1978). Mortality among Boston firefighters, 1915–1975. *Br. J. Ind. Med.*, **35**, 104–108.

Musk, A. W., Smith, T. J., Peters, J. M. and McLaughlin, E. (1979). Pulmonary function in firefighters: acute changes in ventilatory capacity and their correlates. *Br. J. Ind. Med.*, **36**, 29–34.

Myers, R. A. M. and Thom, S. R. (1994). Carbon monoxide and cyanide poisoning. In Kindwall, E. P. (Ed.), *Hyperbaric Medicine Practice*. Best Publishing, Flagstaff, AZ, p. 47.

Nelson, G. L., Hixon, E. J. and Denine, E. P. (1978). Combustion product toxicity studies of burning plastics. *J. Combust. Toxicol.*, **5**, 222–238.

Niemann, G-F., Clark, W. R., Goyette, D., *et al.* (1989). Wood smoke inhalation increases pulmonary microvascular permeability. *Surgery*, **105**, 481–487.

NIOSH (1987). *NIOSH Respirator Decision Logic*. DHHS (NIOSH) Publication No. 87–108. National Institute for Occupational Safety and Health, Cincinnati, OH.

Nomiyama, K., Matsui, K. and Nomiyama, H. (1980). Environmental temperature, a factor modifying the acute toxicity of organic solvents, heavy metals, and agricultural chemicals. *Toxicol. Lett.*, **6**, 67–70.

Norris, J. C. (1988). National Institute of Building Sciences Toxicity Hazard Test. In *Proceedings of the Joint Meeting of the Fire Retardant Chemicals Association and the Society of Plastics Engineers*. Technomic Publishing, Lancaster, PA, pp. 146–155.

Norris, J. C. (1990). Investigation of the dual LC_{50} values of woods using the University of Pittsburgh combustion toxicity apparatus. *Stand. News STP*, **1082**, 57–71.

Norris, J. C., Moore, S. J. and Hume, A. S. (1986). Synergistic lethality induced by the combustion of carbon monoxide and cyanide. *Toxicology*, **40**, 121–129.

Olshan, A. F., Teschke, K. and Baird, P. A. (1990). Birth defect among offspring of firemen. *Am. J. Epidemiol.*, **131**, 312–321.

Paabo, M., Birky, M. M. and Womble, S. E. (1979). Analysis of hydrogen cyanide in fire environments. *J. Combust. Toxicol.*, **6**, 99–108.

Packham, S. C. and Hartzell, G. E. (1981). Fundamentals of combustion toxicology in fire hazard assessment. *J. Test Eval.*, **9**, 341.

Peabody, M. D. (1977). Pulmonary function and the firefighter. *J. Combust. Toxicol.*, **4**, 8–15.

Petajan, J. H., Voorhees, K. J., Packham, S. C., *et al.* (1974). Extreme toxicity from combustion products of a fire-retarded polyurethane foam. *Science*, **187**, 742–744.

Peters, J. M., Therrault, G. P., Fine, L. J. and Wegman, D. H. (1974). Chronic effects of fire fighting on pulmonary function. *N. Engl. J. Med.*, **291**, 1320–1322.

Pitt, B. R., Radford, E. P., Quartner, G. H., Traystman, R. J. (1979). Interaction of carbon monoxide and cyanide on cerebral circulation and metabolism. *Arch. Environ. Health.*, **34**, 354–359.

Purser, D. A. (1992). Combustion toxicology of anticholinesterases. In Ballantyne, B. and Marrs, T. C. (Eds), *Clinical and Experimental Toxicology of Organophosphates and Carbamates*. Butterworth-Heinemann, Oxford, pp. 386–395.

Purser, D. (1996). Behavioural impairment in smoke environments. *Toxicology*, **115**, 25–40.

Purser, D. A. and Grimshaw, P. (1984). The incapacitative effects of exposure to the thermal decomposition products of polyurethane foams. *Fire Mater.*, **8**, 10–16.

Purser, D. A. and Wooley, W. D. (1983). Biological studies of combustion atmospheres. *J. Fire Sci.*, **1**, 118–144.

Purser, D. A., Grimshaw, P. and Berrill, K. R. (1984). Intoxication of cyanide in fires: a study in monkeys using acrylonitrile. *Arch. Environ. Health.*, **39**, 394–400.

Radford, E. P. and Levine, M. S. (1976). Occupational exposure to carbon monoxide in Baltimore fire fighters. *J. Occup. Med.*, **18**, 628–632.

Radford, E. P., Pitt, B., Halpin, B., *et al.* (1976). Study in five deaths in Maryland, September 1971–January 1974. In *Physiological and Toxicological Aspects of Combustion Products*. National Research Council, National Academy of Science, Washington, DC, pp. 26–35.

Redkey, F. L. and Collison, H. A. (1979). Effect of oxygen and carbon dioxide in carbon monoxide toxicity. *J. Combust. Toxicol.*, **6**, 208–212.

Reisdorff, E. J. and Shah, S. M. (1993). Carbon monoxide poisoning: from crib to death to pickup trucks. *Emerg. Med. Rep.*, **14**, 182–190.

Rogdt, S. and Olving, J. H. (1996). Characteristics of fire victims in different sorts of fires. *Forensic Sci. Int.*, **77**, 93–99.

Rosenstock, L., Demers, P., Heyer, N. J. and Barnhart, S. (1990). Respiratory mortality among fire fighters. *Br. J. Ind. Med.*, **47**, 462–465.

Rossi, J., Ritchie, G. D., Macys, D. A. and Still, K. R. (1996). An overview of the development, validation, and application of immunobehavioural and neuromuscular toxicity assessment batteries: potential application to combustion toxicology. *Toxicology*, **115**, 107–117.

Sammons, J. H. and Coleman, R. L. (1974). Firefighters occupational exposure to carbon monoxide. *J. Occup. Med.*, **16**, 543–546.

Sanders, D. C. and Endecott, B. R. (1991). The effect of elevated temperature on carbon monoxide-induced incapacitation. *J. Fire Sci.*, **9**, 296–300.

Sardinas, A., Miller, J. W. and Hansen, H. (1986). Ischemic heart disease mortality of firemen and policemen. *Am. J. Publ. Health*, **76**, 1140–1141.

Serra, A., Mocci, F. and Randsccio, S. (1996). Pulmonary function in Sardinian fire fighters. *Am. J. Ind. Med.*, **30**, 78–82.

Shirani, K. Z., Puritt, B. A., McManus, W. F. and Mason, A. D. (1988). The influence inhalation injury and pneumonia on burn mortality. *Proc. Am. Burns Assoc.*, **18**, 131.

Shusterman, D. J. (1993). Clinical smoke inhalation injury. *Occup. Med. State Art Rev.*, **8**, 469–503.

Smith, P. W., Crane, C. R., Sanders, D. C., *et al.* (1976). Effect of carbon monoxide exposure to carbon monoxide and hydrogen cyanide. In *Physiological and Toxicological Aspects of Combustion Products*. National Research Council, National Academy of Science, Washington, DC, pp. 75–88.

Stark, G. W. V. (1974). *Smoke and Toxic Gases from Burning Plastics*. Building Research Establishment Current Paper 5/74. Building Research Establishment, Fire Research Station, Borehamwood, Herts, UK.

Stewart, R. D. (1974). The effect of carbon monoxide on man. *J. Combust. Toxicol.*, **1**, 167–176.

Symington, I. S., Anderson, R. A. and Thomson, I., *et al.* (1978). Cyanide exposure in fires. *Lancet*, July 8, 91–92.

Tepper, A., Comstock, G. W. and Levine, M. (1991). A longitudinal study of pulmonary function in firefighters. *Am. J. Ind. Med.*, **20**, 307–316.

Thomas, W. C. and O'Flaherty, E. J. (1979). Cytochrome a oxidase activity in tissues of rats exposed to polyurethane pyrolysis fumes. *Toxicol. Appl. Pharmacol.*, **49**, 463–472.

Tibbles, P. M. and Perrotta, P. L. (1994). Treatment of carbon monoxide poisoning: a critical review of human outcome studies comparing normobaric oxygen with hyperbaric oxygen. *Ann. Emerg. Med.*, **24**, 269–276.

Tscuhiya, Y. (1977). Significance of HCN generation in fire gases. *J. Combust. Toxicol.*, **3**, 363–370.

Tornling, G., Gustavsson, P. and Hogstedt, C. (1994). Mortality and cancer incidence in Stockholm fire fighters. *Am. J. Ind. Med.*, **25**, 219–228.

Urhas, E. and Kullik, E. (1977). Pyrolysis gas chromatographic analysis of some toxic compounds from nitrogen-containing fibres. *J. Chromatogr.*, **137**, 210–214.

USCPSC (1988). *Trends in Fire Deaths 1979–1985.* Directorate for Epidemiology, Division of Hazard Analysis, US Consumer Product Safety Commission, Washington, DC.

Vandevort, R. and Brooks, S. M. (1979). Polyvinyl chloride fibre decomposition products as an occupational illness. I. Environmental exposures and toxicology. *J. Occup. Med.*, **19**, 189.

Vena, J. E. and Fielder, R. C. (1987). Mortality of a municipal-worker cohort. IV. Firefighters. *Am. J. Ind. Med.*, **11**, 671–684.

Voorhees, K. J., Einhorn, I. N., Hileman, F. D. and Wojcik, C. H. (1975). The identification of a highly toxic bicyclophosphate in the combustion products of a fire-related urethane foam. *Polym. Lette.*, **13**, 293–297.

Wetherell, H. R. (1966). The occurrence of cyanide in blood of fire victims. *J. Forensic Sci.*, **11**, 167–172.

Wirthwein, D. P. and Pless, J. E. (1996). Carboxyhemoglobin levels in a series of automobile fires. *Am. J. Forensic Med. Pathol.*, **17**, 117–123.

Wooley, W. D. (1971). Decomposition products of PVC. *Br. Polym. J.*, **3**, 186–193.

Wooley, W. D. (1972). Nitrogen-containing products from the thermal decomposition of flexible polyurethane foam. *J. Combust. Toxicol.*, **1**, 259–267.

Wooley, W. D. (1974). The production of free tolylene diisocyanate (TDI) from the thermal decomposition of flexible polyurethane foam. *J. Combust. Toxicol.*, **1**, 259–276.

Wooley, W. D. (1982). Smoke and toxic gas productions from burning polymers. *J. Macromol. Sci. Chem.*, **A17**, 1–33.

Yamamoto, Y. (1975). Acute toxicity of the combustion products from various kinds of fibers. *Z. Rechtsmed.*, **77**, 11–26.

Young, W., Hilando, C. J., Kourtides, D. A. and Parker, D. S. (1976). A study of the toxicity of pyrolysis gases from synthetic polymers. *J. Combust. Toxicol.*, **3**, 157–165.

Zachria, B. A. (1972). Inhalation injuries in fires. In *Approach to Halogenated Fire Extinguishing Materials.* National Academy of Science, Washington, DC, pp. 42–52.

Zarem, H. A., Rattenberg, C. L. and Harmer, M. A. (1973). Carbon monoxide toxicity in human fire victims. *Arch. Surg.*, **107**, 851–853.

Zawacki, B. E., Jung, R. C., Joyce, J. and Rincon, E. (1977). Smoke, burns and the natural history of inhalation injury in fire victims. *Ann. Surg.*, **185**, 100–110.

Zawacki, B. E., Azen, S. P., Imbus, S. H. and Chang, Y. (1979). Multifactorial probit analysis of mortality in burned patients. *Ann. Surg.*, **189**, 1–10.

ADDITIONAL READING

Aseeva, R. M. and Zaikov, G. E. (1985). *Combustion of Polymer Materials.* Hanser, Munich.

Colloquium (1995). International Colloquium on Advances in Combustion Toxicology. *Toxicology*, **115**, 1–233.

Gad, S. C. and Andersen, R. C. (1990). *Combustion Toxicology.* CRC Press, Boca Raton, FL.

Orris, P., Melius, J. and Duffy, R. M. (1995). Firefighter's safety and health. *Occup. Med. State Art Rev.*, **10**, 691–883.

Shusterman, D. J. and Peterson, J. E. (1993). Combustion toxicology. *Occup. Med. State Art Rev.*, **8**, 415–672.

Chapter 89
Education of the Toxicologist

Robert Snyder

C O N T E N T S

INTRODUCTION

The idea that there can be training programmes for toxicologists bears within it the inherent concept that toxicology is a distinct scientific discipline. Among the biological sciences it has long been accepted that anatomy, biochemistry, physiology, microbiology, pathology and even pharmacology are distinct disciplines. Although the body of scientific effort in these areas justified disciplinary designation, the requirement for learning these sciences as part of professional medical education bolstered their claim to individuality. Toxicology came late to acceptance as a unique discipline, and in some quarters that concept is not yet accepted today. Nevertheless, the knowledge that chemicals can adversely affect biological organisms has been known for many centuries. We have been familiar with the concept of poisons from the death of Socrates, through Paracelsus and Lucretia Borgia. In the nineteenth century Orfila carried out the first scientifically based studies of toxicity and subsequently a number of great biologists, including Magendie, Bernard, Schmiedeberg and others, performed seminal research defining the effects of chemicals on biological systems, in the study of physiology and, later, pharmacology. Today, their work could legitimately be considered mechanistic studies on the toxicology of the chemicals they used.

The need for a formalized profession and separate discipline of toxicology arose primarily from several distinct sources in the USA. The Food, Drug and Cosmetics Act of 1938 demanded that prior to marketing a new drug the US Food and Drug Administration must be supplied with data from the manufacturer showing that when taken as directed the drug is 'safe'. While some side-effects may be observed, it must be demonstrated that no serious toxicity will occur through normal use of the drug. As a result, drug companies were forced to establish toxicology laboratories to evaluate their new products and to present the resultant data to the agency for approval before the drug could be marketed. The second milestone in the solidification of the discipline of toxicology came when the National Academy of Sciences/National Research Council established the Committee on Toxicology in 1947. The mandate of the Committee on Toxicology extends beyond foods and now covers the entire range of potentially toxic industrial and environmental chemicals. A third milestone derives from the formation of the Society of Toxicology, the first professional society in Toxicology, which dates from 1961–62. Finally, the establishment of a Toxicology Training Program by the National Institute of Environmental Health Sciences demonstrated that the discipline existed and that programs for toxicology training would be supported by the federal government because we needed people prepared to study the toxicology of a large range of chemicals.

Although the Society of Toxicology was founded in 1961–62, rapid expansion of training programmes in toxicology, except for a few pioneer programmes, began in the 1970 and accelerated growth continued into the 1980s. The impetus for the rapid expansion of toxicology training came from several sources. The growing awareness of the effects of chemicals in the workplace and in the environment at large resulted in the establishment of the National Institute of Environmental Health Sciences (NIEHS), the National Institute of Occupational Safety and Health, the Environmental Protection Agency and other federal agencies concerned with the impact of chemicals on health and the environment. These agencies required trained personnel to carry out their functions and created a demand for people which could only be accommodated by the development of new training programmes.

A stimulus of greater significance to the scholar resulted from a pattern of development of thought in the biological sciences which established an inevitability to the eventual coalescence of the discipline of toxicology. Toxicology is the study of the adverse effects of chemicals (and radiation) on biological systems. The study of adverse effects suggests that there must be a pre-existing understanding of normal biological functions before abnormal effects can be recognized and studied. The evolution of medical training in this country during the twentieth century led to the establishment of anatomy, physiology, biochemistry, pharmacology, microbiology, nutrition, immunology and pathology as the basic biomedical sciences. The accumulation of information on anatomy, which occurred over many centuries, led gradually, in the nineteenth century, to the development of physiology and then biochemistry. Pharmacology could not function as a separate discipline until the database in physiology and biochemistry, which utilized chemicals as tools to study biological functions, expanded to a critical level. Pathology was an expansion of anatomy which concentrated on a number of abnormal biological events, including effects of chemicals. Certainly, the development of new drugs required a full examination of their toxicological potential. Thus, after sufficient knowledge in the basic biomedical sciences was attained, and the practical examination of the potential toxic effects of chemicals became routine, the discipline of toxicology emerged.

Those involved in training graduate students in toxicology realize that their job is to launch the student into a lifetime of learning. The late Arnold J. Lehman of the US Food and Drug Administration is credited with stating that, 'You too can be a toxicologist in two easy lessons, each of ten years' (Gallo, 1996). In this discussion we will emphasize the training of graduate students and postdoctoral fellows. The average time required for formalized training is about 6–8 years as a graduate student and then as a postdoctoral fellow. The bulk of the remaining 20 years of training takes place as part of career development.

AIMS OF TOXICOLOGY TRAINING PROGRAMMES

The principal aim of any toxicology training programme is to offer a curriculum which will prepare the student to function at the highest possible level as a toxicologist. Although some toxicology training is available at the undergraduate level, the majority of toxicology training venues are in graduate schools. Each of the biomedical sciences can be approached at either the fundamental or the practical level and both approaches are needed by society. If we recognize that the toxicologist is a scientist and that scientific training requires both the assimilation of known information and research to help us learn more, then the training of toxicologists requires a series of courses plus an opportunity for the student to learn the principles of research by performing a research project. Some aspects of the curriculum may be devoted to applied research in toxicology, but the major effort should be in basic research, preferably at the mechanistic level, which will expand our fundamental understanding of the biological responses that underlie toxicology.

TOXICOLOGY TRAINING PROGRAMMES

Graduate training in toxicology is, of necessity, broad-based. Students must be exposed to the basic biomedical sciences and chemistry because these disciplines will be the tools of their trade regardless of where their career paths lead them. In the course of graduate training, students will become expert in their field of study and may develop other areas of expertise as their careers evolve. Although they need not be expert in the approaches of all of the biomedical disciplines, they must be sufficiently knowledgeable to know when to apply otherwise unfamiliar methodology necessary to solve specific problems. Consultation with specialists in other fields may be essential to complete the work, but the toxicologist must have sufficient knowledge to ask the proper question, to understand the results of such studie s and to involve the results in next stage of the work.

To ensure that programmes succeed in meeting their aims, there must be a faculty dedicated to graduate education. Often there is a Director for graduate education which may, or may not, be the department Chair. The Director, with the help of the faculty, administers the programme by overseeing recruitment of students, admissions, record keeping, progress towards the degree, examinations, grievances and the degree granting process. The Director is usually responsible for much of the fund-raising activities which go to support the students. Thus, obtaining teaching assistantships, externally supported fellowships, travel funds and other needs of the students falls in large measure on the shoulders of the Director. Finally, the Director is the direct conduit to higher university administration.

Perhaps of greatest importance is the necessity for the Director to ensure that students select laboratories of mentors where they can best proceed through the process of earning the degree. Usually this requires a meeting of the minds between mentor and student regarding the nature of the research project, but the issue of compatibility between the two protagonists should not be discounted. The mechanisms by which student–mentor relationships are established vary among programmes. They almost always involve a trial period in which the student spends a limited amount of time in the prospective mentor's laboratory to permit each to determine whether a successful research partnership can be established. Once a collective decision involving student, mentor and Director is made, the student relies on the mentor for advice on courses, research and career planning. Most mentors follow the careers of their students and stand ready to offer assistance long after they have left to develop their own careers. Senior Professors are often called upon by those seeking to fill a variety of positions in toxicology, at various levels. The Professor then has the opportunity to recommend former students to positions of advancement. The interplay is a two-way street: in some cases, former students having advanced in their careers, may find ways to help enhance the programmes from which they graduated through teaching, providing entrées to obtaining financial assistance, offering positions to more recent graduates, etc. The concept of the 'doctor father' in German Universities, which grew out of the citing of scientific lineages, exemplifies the lasting relationships that are possible between student and mentor.

PREREQUISITES TO GRADUATE TRAINING IN TOXICOLOGY

Those students best prepared to study toxicology at the graduate level will have earned a Bachelor's degree in chemistry or biology. In addition to introductory study in chemistry, the student will benefit from courses in analytical, organic and physical chemistry. A course in biochemistry is beneficial but can be taken at the graduate level. In biology a general introductory course followed by electives in areas such as comparative anatomy, histology and cell physiology would be helpful. Students are urged to study physics and mathematics in preparation for graduate school because of the rapid advances in application of these disciplines in modern toxicology.

REQUIRED GRADUATE COURSES

Although most curricula in toxicology require a basic course in general toxicology, it need not be the first course taken in graduate school. Most students require graduate level courses in physiology, biochemistry and molecular biology to succeed in toxicology. Many programmes require pathology, which would be most helpful if it could precede or run in parallel with the toxicology course. Programmes associated with institutions devoted to medical training often ask students to study pharmacology because of the areas of significant overlap between the two disciplines. Students planning a career in the drug industry should be required to study pharmacology. Other more relevant courses might substitute for students in non-medically related areas, e.g. students directed toward a career in environmental toxicology might include courses more directly related to their interests such as ecotoxicology. All students should be required to hone their communications skills by participation in seminar courses. Furthermore, they should be required to write papers aimed at evaluating and improving their skills in scientific writing. The area of biostatistics and experimental design and interpretation of results should be part of every graduate programme. Finally, the NIEHS has mandated that each programme offer a course in ethics as it applies to scientific research.

The most important course offering is the first course in general toxicology, which goes by a variety of names in various institutions and is required of all students. Among the subjects that it must cover to adequately introduce students to toxicology are:

1. A brief discussion of the history and scope of toxicology.
2. A discussion of general basic principles of toxicology.
3. Toxicodynamics, i.e. what does the chemical do to the body?
4. Toxicokinetics, i.e. how does the body deal with the chemical?
5. A survey of the effects of various chemicals.
6. A description of the specific toxic responses of various body organs.
7. Venues, i.e. toxicity observed in the home, workplace, environment, etc.
8. Applied toxicology: safety evaluation and risk assessment.
9. Mechanistic toxicology.

The extent to which any of these areas is covered will depend upon the time allotted to the course, the availability of advanced courses to cover any of the areas in detail, the interests of the faculty, etc. In every course in toxicology, however, there should be sufficient emphasis given to the Paracelsian admonition:

In all things there is a poison, and there is nothing without a poison. It depends only upon the dose whether a poison is a poison or not . . . (Jacobi, 1988).

ELECTIVE COURSES

The selection of elective courses will depend upon which courses are available in any given institution, but can generally be separated into those in toxicology versus those in allied disciplines. Many students opt to take advanced courses in chemistry or the biological sciences. Advanced courses in chemistry are many and varied. Course selection is often driven by the research project in which the student is engaged. In the biological sciences graduate students in toxicology should become familiar with microbiology, immunology and genetics.

Electives in toxicology depend upon the expertise of the faculty and may encompass such areas as neurotoxicology, pharmaco/toxicogenetics and pesticide toxicology, etc. Electives are also a mechanism for introducing students to the more applied areas of toxicology such as safety evaluation, risk assessment, public health and the environment, etc.

An important message for any student is that the best thing one can learn in graduate school is how to learn. Courses teach what is currently known, but cannot predict the future. Once the student has initiated an independent career, most learning will be self-stimulated and will not involve attending classes. To be sure there are many opportunities for formal continuing education. Both the Society of Toxicology and the American College of Toxicology offer continuing education courses at their annual meetings. Ultimately, however, most toxicologists should keep up with recent advances through their own efforts. Therefore, the value of time spent in classes, beyond learning the basics, and enough advanced information to permit the beginning of a research project, must be balanced against the value of time spent in the library and the laboratory.

QUALIFYING EXAMINATIONS

Advancement through graduate school is characterized by study and research on the part of the student and evaluation of the student via a variety of metrics. Courses require that students perform well on objective examinations, essay-type examinations or in the writing of research papers. Despite hurdling these barriers, in most programmes students must pass qualifying examinations. The requirements for the Master of Science and the Doctor of Philosophy degrees may be dissimilar. Thus, a single examination for the MS often suffices. For the PhD the process if usually more complex. Often there are two sets of examinations, written and oral. Some programmes use a comprehensive written examination at the end of the first year of graduate school to determine whether the student should continue. Some offer the comprehensive examination as a prelude to the oral examination to determine whether the student is prepared for the oral. Other programmes do not have written comprehensive examinations. There are a number of variations on this theme.

For many years students were required to pass one or more examinations in a foreign language, but that custom has become less popular as English has assumed a predominant position as the international language of science.

The oral examination is usually the point of decision with respect to whether or not the student becomes a candidate for the degree. There is more riding on the oral examination than on any other examination in the student's career. As a result, students study long and hard to prepare for the examination. Examination committees should inform students embarking on the candidacy process regarding faculty expectations. Toxicology is among the broadest of the biological sciences and each of the subdisciplines within toxicology deals with an extensive database. Furthermore, because of the breadth, much of the information that students should know comes from other areas such as biochemistry, physiology, pathology, etc. Hence the oral examination may become a free-for-all with faculty asking questions on subjects that range from a discussion of dose–response curves to estimating the weight of Saturn (the latter as an example of how a Professor once thought that a student's reasoning powers might best be measured.) A wise faculty will establish with the student the limits of required subject areas and will find a way to learn what they must from the student within the defined area.

There are many methods for defining the range of the oral examination, but one general form which can have many benefits for the students can be addressed here. In some universities students, with the advice of their mentors, submit to the Director, early in their graduate school careers, a list of, perhaps, 10 hypotheses, or propositions, which together define a broad area of toxicology, but results in some delimiting of the total range of information for which the student is responsible at the time of examination. An example might be 'The lethal effects of parathion can be explained solely on the basis of cholinesterase inhibition'. The student would then collect all of the information in the literature on this question and would defend or attack the proposition in a written paper which is presented to the members of the examination committee in advance of the examination for use as the basis of questioning. It has been demonstrated that 10 such papers prepared over a 2–3 year period offers the committee a chance to determine how well the information has been collected, evaluated and used in creative decision making by the candidate. The proposition method permits a narrowing of the range of areas on which the student will be questioned but permits the faculty to delve as deeply into the subject as seems warranted to make candidacy decisions.

Success in the oral examination is often difficult to attain for some students because of the significance of the examination to their future careers and perceived trauma they experience during the process. Often excellently prepared students fail to measure up to the expectations of the faculty because of nervousness or forgetfulness induced by the pressure-packed nature of the examination. To help prevent or to overcome the impact of emotions on examination performance, several approaches have been used. Often, graduate students within programmes offer a chance for candidates to participate in 'mock orals' in which their fellow students, or faculty members, act as the examining faculty and ask the questions they anticipate will be asked at the examination. If students appear to be in great difficulties during an examination the committee may decide to delay a decision and offer the candidate the option of completing the examination at a later date. The student is expected to complete the examination successfully at the continuation. Despite the recognized shortcomings of the oral examination system, it continues to play a significant role in graduate education both as a valuable mechanism for evaluating the qualifications of a student and for the sense of accomplishment engendered in the successful candidate.

THE RESEARCH EXPERIENCE

The essence of a PhD programme in toxicology is to train people to perform scholarly research. Although the requirements of many MS programmes can be met by having the student write a library-based paper without doing a research thesis, many others require a small-scale research project leading to a written thesis. For the PhD an extensive research project is required. The subject of the research is decided upon through discussions between the student and the mentor. Some students enter graduate school with the intention of working in a specific area of toxicology or with a specific mentor. The quality of the research training is in no way related to the area of toxicology in which the student works. Since most students select their mentor on the basis of compatibility, they naturally work in the area of interest to the mentor and many remain in this area long after they have completed their degrees and moved on.

The components of research training include an appreciation of the concept of a hypothesis and how hypotheses are developed, selecting an experiment model, use of appropriate controls, designing experiments to test the hypothesis, data evaluation, including biostatistics, and interpretation of the data. During the training of graduate students the mentor should provide opportunities for the student to sharpen those communication skills necessary to report the results of a research project. These would include writing of abstracts and research papers, oral presentation of results and preparation of posters showing the work for presentation at scientific meetings. The opportunity to meet with others working in the same field should be made available by sending the student to meetings of scholarly societies.

It is during the development of the dissertation that the student should be imbued with a concept of scholarship. The importance of gaining a complete understanding of the literature in the field under study before planning a full-scale project is of the utmost importance. Researchers often unknowingly perform studies which have been done previously and have already appeared in the literature. Students tend to rely on computerized databases for literature searches. Research performed prior to 1960–70 cannot be obtained from these sources. The conscientious student has no choice but to leave the safe confines of the laboratory and venture out into the challenging culture of the library and rummage around in the stacks for what may be valuable nuggets of otherwise lost information which could be of great value in the student's research.

Hypotheses derive from creative evaluation of existing literature and seminar presentations, discussions involving the mentor, discussions with other members of the research team in the laboratory and the performance of pilot experiments to indicate whether or not there is a reasonable chance that the project will succeed. Once the hypothesis is established, it is incumbent upon the student to develop an experimental design to challenge the hypothesis. Consultation with the mentor will enable the student to determine the feasibility of the planned studies. If the hypothesis is reasonable, it is necessary to ensure that it is technically possible to perform the experiments in the specific laboratory chosen for the research. Research costs, availability of necessary instrumentation and, where necessary, help from other people are issues that must be settled before a research project can begin. Assuming that these problems can be solved, the mentor must ask whether the student has selected a suitable problem. Is it sufficiently challenging to be worthy of the PhD upon completion? Can it be completed within approximately 4–5 years? The mentor must also consider the issues of costs, facilities and other people in the laboratory. These issues must be satisfactorily addressed to predict success in a graduate student thesis project.

In many universities, the mentor–student relationship is complemented by a thesis committee which follows the student through the process, meets with the student for regular updates, acts as a quality control mechanism, eventually decides when the project is completed and sits as the thesis defence committee. Outside reviewers are often asked to participate at some stage in the development of the thesis to act as impartial referees. An important job of the committee is to ensure that the student completes the thesis in as short a time as possible. Graduate disciplines often have cases of students who have been either improperly advised or insufficiently stimulated, who subsequently remain in graduate school for inordinately long times. The thesis committee is an important mechanism for maintaining an acceptable rate of progress toward the degree.

In toxicology, the aims of the specific piece of research may vary considerably. Until the early 1980s, most research in toxicology was aimed at describing the effects produced by chemicals administered via any of several routes to one or more species of animals. End-points such as lethality or pathology resulting from acute or subchronic treatments were common. With the emphasis placed on cancer prevention in the USA, the National Toxicology Program was developed specifically to expose animals to chemicals for a lifetime. After the death of the animals they were examined for signs of cancer. Chronic exposure studies of this type were less commonly performed in university laboratories because of the cost and the need for specialized personnel and facilities. Nevertheless shorter term carcinogenicity studies were performed in a number of laboratories.

The impetus towards maturation of toxicology as a discipline came from many sources but the emphasis by toxicologists on mechanisms of toxicity served to demonstrate that toxicology could contribute to the basic understanding of biological functions. The role of the metabolism of xenobiotic chemicals, especially the formation of biologically reactive intermediates, was a significant factor in developing thought in mechanistic toxicology. Studies of the interactions of chemicals with enzymes or nucleic acids and ensuing toxic effects led to a better understanding of structure – activity relationships and our ability to predict some types of toxic effects. Currently, many mechanistic studies revolve about the problems of mutagenicity, carcinogenicity, oxidative stress and mechanisms of cell death. All of these are being approached in university laboratories with the goal of understanding the underlying principles which lead to the production of adverse effects by chemicals on biological systems.

In any scholarly discipline, the ultimate measure of quality research is the contribution it makes to understanding of the most fundamental issues with which the discipline is concerned. Much productive science flows from the last reported observation. Occasionally new thoughts are injected into the scientific discourse by highly talented investigators. Quality research should shed new light on existing problems, open up new areas of investigation and present intellectual challenges which may not have previously existed. Graduate students play a significant role in the process. By sharing in the development of the hypothesis, performing the experiments and continually re-evaluating the results, new avenues emerge which benefit science but which also enrich the training of the student and help the student mature as a scientist. Participation in making significant observations stimulates the student in their maturation as scientists and helps them to develop their own successful careers as researchers.

Some students plan on careers that do not focus on laboratory research. There is a great need for toxicologists in regulatory agencies in federal and state government, in regulatory departments in industry, as consultants, in law firms and in a number of other occupations. Nevertheless, in any work as a toxicologist it will be important to review the results of both applied and basic research. Research training is the best way to prepare a student to read and understand the results of other researchers work. The more rigorous their research training, the better the job they can do in evaluating and criticizing research results as they apply to their specific problem.

STUDENT PRESENTATIONS

At each stage in the training of students in toxicology it is important that they learn how to communicate with their peers. Communications in science take many forms and training methods can also vary. Early in graduate education students should be asked to participate in exercises which will give them the opportunity to communicate in several ways. For example, the short paper form of delivery provides an excellent training ground. Many societies offer their members the chance to publish an abstract of their work in advance of a meeting and then present the work in a 10–15 min paper accompanied by slides to illustrate the data. This format makes for a good first-year course for graduate students. They may work on a topic, the data for which they may find in the literature, learn how to write an abstract, prepare appropriate slides and make their presentation to other students and faculty. In the course of this activity they will gain ease in making presentations before their peers, learn to write concise reports and become familiar with ways of presenting their data with slides. Learning how to make presentations in the classroom situation will help prepare them for presentations at scientific meetings.

When students go beyond the first year or two in graduate school, their seminar responsibility may take on a different form. The research that they are performing for inclusion in the thesis will progress from year to year and an annual update in the form of research reports that may require about 20–30 min provides a useful training tool. One approach is to have all advanced students present their progress reports in symposium format. It is an opportunity for a programme to have a day devoted to student presentations and attended by the entire faculty and invited guests. The students may be asked to prepare an extended abstract in advance to be given to the audience. The students will have benefitted by having prepared short presentations earlier in their careers and can make use of that experience in the symposium presentation.

The first presentation by a student at a society meeting these days is most likely to be a poster presentation. Here the student presents the results of thesis research in a series of panels mounted on a board that is approximately 4 × 6 feet. The poster usually contains an abstract of the work, a brief note on methodology, several panels on data and a summary statement. The poster is intended to generate discussion between the presenter and colleagues who stop to ask about the work as they stroll through the poster presentation area. Under these circumstances the student meets the questioner one-on-one rather than as a member of a large audience. These can be much more difficult interactions since they often require detailed information at the fingertips of the student. In some cases the poster sessions are followed by a discussion period where the essential information of the posters are briefly reported by the presenters. Thus, poster sessions and poster-discussion sessions present a challenge to the student which is different from that posed by the short platform presentation or the longer symposium presentation.

The most important type of communication is the written report intended for peer review. A published report will enter the literature and become available for reference in perpetuity. As a result, it is the most critically reviewed and criticized. Thus, during training the student should be prepared not only to perform the research project with excellence, but should also be trained to prepare a paper for publication at the highest possible level. The writing of the thesis, albeit a somewhat longer item of prose, should set the standard for the writing of papers which will emerge from the thesis work. Students who perform in exemplary fashion in the writing of papers may be asked to participate in the preparation of review articles. Reviews in excellent journals also undergo intensive review and serve as an important mechanism for deriving new ideas and research pathways based on compilation of reports from many sources. The authorship of a review article by a graduate student is unusual but if accomplished is an important step in developing a successful scientific career.

APPLIED TOXICOLOGY

Toxicology training as discussed above involves a series of classroom exercises and the completion of a basic research project. Many toxicologists trained in this way go on to a career in basic research for which they are well adapted. Many others enter careers in applied toxicology for which their university training did not prepare them directly. To be sure, learning how to understand and do science is critical for any career in toxicology. However, learning methods in areas of applied toxicology requires additional course work or on-the-job training. Many graduates move into positions, usually in industry, where they may be responsible for studies of safety eva-

luation. They must be thoroughly knowledgeable in all of the techniques of safety evaluation and must be prepared to manage and to perform these studies. Often large numbers of animals of different species are involved; animal welfare issues are of great significance; the studies may require different amounts of time, up to and including the life span of the animals; pathology studies go on after the animals' death; detailed reports must be prepared, often accompanied by recommendations for further action. While some of these problems may have been the subject of classroom discussion, and some similar types of studies may been included in the thesis project, generally, studies of these types are completely new to the recent graduate who is thrust into the role of safety evaluator in a company. Thus, both employee and employer must realize that advanced training in such studies, especially when the specific needs of the company must be met, is the responsibility of the company.

The processes that are termed risk assessment involve utilization of data gathered from many sources regarding the toxicology of chemicals to determine the risk to health of exposure to the chemicals at specific dose levels. Thus, toxicologists frequently become involved in the risk assessment process because of their training in the interpretation of the data produced in toxicology studies. The use of graphical techniques to analyse data leads biometricians to play an increasingly greater role in the interpretation of toxicological data. They have used their understanding of mathematical functions to influence the interpretation of data. Their input is particularly critical when extrapolation from observed data to results expected under other conditions must be made. Thus: what would be the result if the time of exposure, the dose and/or the species was different? The accuracy of these predictions depends upon the biology of the system, but the extrapolations are frequently driven by mathematics rather than by biology because we lack sufficient understanding of the underlying mechanisms and it is more convenient (and costs less) to fall back on mathematics than to do more experiments to verify the extrapolation. Regardless of the virtues or shortcomings of the process toxicologists are frequently involved in risk assessment. Some may have had classes in risk assessment, but these are insufficient to prepare them for performing such an exercise and to appreciate the responsibility entailed. This is another example of where on-the-job experience is essential.

There are training locations in forensic and clinical toxicology which are often separate from academic toxicology training programmes. Forensic laboratories are concerned with toxicological issues relating to legal matters. Their specialty is analytical chemistry. Among the most frequent calls upon these laboratories are to measure blood alcohol concentrations in samples from people involved in motor accidents. Measurements of body fluids or tissues are often made in questions of poisoning. The forensic toxicologist is usually associated with a government laboratory such as a city, county or state medical examiner. The FBI has one of the largest and most complete forensic laboratories in the USA. Forensic toxicologists are frequently called upon to provide testimony in court regarding their findings. There are relatively few sites for training in this field and there has for some time been a critical shortage of personnel with sufficient expertise to work in these laboratories.

Clinical toxicology is a medical specialty concerned with the detection and treatment of poisoning in people. Victims usually arrive in the emergency ward of a hospital in a state which suggests that they have either administered a poisonous level of a chemical or drug to themselves or have been poisoned by someone else. The clinical toxicologist must decide on the basis of whatever evidence is available, i.e. interview and observe the patient, have evidence of a container in which the material was found, physical examination, laboratory analyses, etc., and make decisions regarding treatment of the patient. The forensic laboratory plays an important role as a resource to which the clinician can turn to learn about the specific chemical, the dose, the blood level, etc. Since this is a medical specialty training is not usually performed in academic toxicology training centres, but as part of advanced medical training at the intern or resident level and board certification is available to those who wish to make a career as clinical toxicologists.

THE POSTDOCTORAL EXPERIENCE

Toxicology training does not end with the awarding of the PhD. Many graduates, upon completion of the degree, take positions in companies, in government agencies, with environmental groups, etc. In each of those venues they must undergo training to meet the specific needs of the job to meet the expectations of the employer. For those toxicologists who wish to enter a career in which research is a major component, most employers require postdoctoral training. The postdoctoral fellowship offers the trainee an opportunity to become a full-time researcher under the aegis of an experienced investigator. Postdoctoral mentors are selected by the trainee on the basis of the area of research in which they work and on the excellence of their productivity as scientists. Their laboratories may be in various departments or schools in universities, in research institutes or in government agencies. Popular locations for postdoctoral training in the USA include those institutions awarded NIEHS training grants, or laboratories within the various National Institutes of Health. A variety of research centres such as the Chemical Industry Institute of Toxicology in addition to a number of NIEHS Centres of Excellence, offer postdoctoral training opportunities. Additional opportunities can often be found in more specialized environments such as cancer research institutes or environmental health centres. In any of these locations the postdoctoral fellowship is intended to provide the fellows with the opportunity to demonstrate their scientific creativity and productivity in an environment in which they are totally devoted to research.

The postdoctoral experience begins with the selection of a specific problem, which in most laboratories is one of a group of problems in the same general area. In an active laboratory one often finds technicians, graduate students and postdoctoral fellows. Although each works on a separate problem, proximity leads to communication which helps all in the group. Learning techniques and approaches from each other enhances the total output of the laboratory. It is clear that the success of a laboratory is related to interaction of the various participants in a laboratory and the postdoctoral fellows usually take a leading role.

Ideally, a postdoctoral fellow should spend 2–3 years in training, at which point it is time to seek an independent position. At this point the postdoctoral fellows leave the safety, the support, the financial backing and the stipend paid by the mentor and must fend for themselves. Mentors usually help in securing positions for postdoctoral fellows, but a variety of placement services are available to assist the job-hunting process. Clearly, those fellows who have trained in highly respected laboratories and have been productive during the training period will have the upper hand in the job search. Upon securing a position beyond the postdoctoral level the toxicologist must now direct considerable effort toward securing research funding and developing an independent laboratory. It is the most challenging time in the career of toxicologists and success will in large measure depend upon the quality of training that they have enjoyed.

TRAINING IN COUNTRIES OTHER THAN THE USA

United Kingdom

An example of toxicology training in the UK is taken from the curriculum at the University of Surrey. Students at the University of Surrey have the opportunity to initiate their training in toxicology at the undergraduate level. Those students concentrating in biochemistry may elect to take courses in drug metabolism and pharmacokinetics, in mechanisms of toxicity, regulatory toxicology, pathology for toxicology, practical toxicopathology and forensic toxicology. Following the Bachelor's degree, students may enroll in the Master of Science in Toxicology programme. Progress toward the degree requires 338 h of lectures, 125 h of laboratory training and 400 h devoted to laboratory research on a dissertation project over a total of 44 weeks. The course includes tutorials and visits to industrial laboratories and utilizes a variety of assessment modes. The course work is varied, ranging from whole animal studies down to molecular biology in addition to regulatory affairs and safety evaluation. The student wishing to go on to the PhD registers for the Master of Philosophy, completes the course work and writes a report on the progress in a laboratory research project which is used to determine whether or not the student will be permitted to transfer to the doctoral programme. Upon approval of the report the student becomes a candidate for the PhD. The student continues the research project and upon completion (usually requiring a total of four years from the beginning of the studies at the Master's level) is awarded the PhD. The PhD at the University of Surrey is granted by the school or department without carrying the designation 'in Toxicology'.

Germany

Historically, toxicology in Germany has been closely associated with medical pharmacology. Toxicologists tend to be members of the German Society of Experimental and Clinical Pharmacology and Toxicology. In recent years, the Society has developed a mechanism by which individuals who hold doctorates in medicine, veterinary medicine, chemistry, biochemistry, biology, pharmacy or related disciplines can earn a certificate by which they are named 'Expert in Toxicology, DGPT'. The certificate is awarded on the basis of an examination. However, to be eligible to take the examination the applicant must have had at least 5 years of experience in a toxicology laboratory plus comprehensive knowledge in one area of toxicology, broad knowledge in two other areas of toxicology and basic knowledge in 15 areas of toxicology. They must submit three independent peer-reviewed papers or assessments of their professional skill. To meet the educational objectives of the programme, courses in specific areas of toxicology are offered in universities in Germany periodically. The courses run from 3 to 5 days. The areas covered by the courses include: animal welfare and techniques in animal experimentation; statistics and experimental design; principles of chemical and physical analysis in toxicology; pathological anatomy and histology of experimental animals; general principles of toxicology and target organ toxicology; drug metabolism and principles of toxicokinetics; principles of cellular and molecular biology and toxicology; chemical mutagenesis; chemical carcinogenesis; reproductive toxicology; immunotoxicology; epidemiology; ecotoxicology; and regulatory toxicology. The German approach, unlike the American approach, embodies both training and professional certification.

Although the formalities of earning the degree are somewhat different when comparing the American, the German and the British approach, the subject matter is largely the same. The German system carries with it the opportunity to board certification. In the USA most toxicologists can apply for and earn board certification from the American Board on Toxicology by passing an examination. For more senior toxicologists who have an established career and evidence of productivity and accomplishment, the Academy of Toxicological Sciences offers the opportunity of certification on the basis of peer review.

THE LITERATURE OF TOXICOLOGY

Toxicology training in all countries seems to involve the classical approaches which include classroom studies highlighted by lectures and discussions, practical laboratory experience and exercises in which students read literature and either write reports or present them orally. These are frequently termed seminars and are an essential part of toxicology training. Although it is important that the student can write well or make oral presentations which are clear and understandable, the basis of these reports is the literature which the student has read, assimilated and is prepared to offer as evidence of having learned the material.

The literature of toxicology over time reflects a parallel growing maturity of both the biomedical sciences and toxicology. Although much has been known about the descriptive toxicology of pure chemicals and mixtures since ancient times, it is only with the past few decades that important advances in our in-depth knowledge of mechanisms of toxicity have been uncovered. Much of that database can be accessed via online databases such those of the National Library of Medicine, i.e. Medline, Toxline, etc. Most studies published before the advent of databases must be accessed in library stacks or storage areas. Nevertheless, to gain full insight into a field of toxicology the student should trace the development of thought in that field back to its origins and build newly planned experiments on the basis of earlier work. A significant admonition worth offering to every new student is, 'Science did not begin the day you walked into the laboratory'.

TRAINING TOXICOLOGISTS FOR THE FUTURE

Unfortunately for people who plan structured curricula, changes in the science occur at rates faster than they can plan. Thus, within the past few decades the basic medical sciences have largely lost their distinctive boundaries in research. The result has been mergers of departments and changing modes of teaching the basic subjects. Since toxicologists have always had to deal with approaches to problems which crossed these classical boundaries, they are prepared to take advantage of changing curricula to the advantage of their students. Furthermore, with advances in the understanding of the molecular basis of physiological function, it is possible to apply the techniques generated by these exciting successes to the solution of toxicological problems. Toxicology has been called 'a borrowing science'. Scientists in any given discipline have always 'borrowed' techniques and approaches to research from each other. Borrowing of techniques from other disciplines was less common. In toxicology, however, it was the rule because there were few, if any, methods which were strictly tied to our discipline. Thus, in the current climate the disciplines have, to a large extent, merged and the toxicologist is quite at home in 'borrowing', e.g. the tools of the molecular biologist, for the solution of fundamental problems in toxicology. Thus the first, and most important, message related to the training of toxicologists in the future is that we must continue to teach students broadly and to be prepared to accept new ideas in science and apply them to understand mechanisms of toxicity, in addition to applying them to the process of safety evaluation.

Toxicology, and its sister science, pharmacology, have been termed the 'study of poisons'. Both toxicologists and pharmacologists are proud of that designation because the results of their studies have been a better understanding of how chemicals can cause damage to biological systems as studied by toxicologists and the development of new and better therapeutic agents by the pharmacologists. In many cases ground-breaking efforts in the nineteenth and early twentieth centuries were based on studying the effects of known poisons such as strychnine, eserine and nitrogen mustard. While the breakthroughs resulted in practical advances in the disciplines, they were accompanied by an increasing understanding, in these cases, of the physiology of the spinal chord, the mechanism of action of cholinesterase and certain aspects of the biology of cancer cells. Many other examples have shown that as we have extended knowledge in our own discipline we have made significant contributions to the study of biology. Thus, the training of students in toxicology should include ensuring that they understand the potentially greater significance of their results that may go beyond administering a given chemical to an animal in a given protocol followed by the observance of specific responses. The student should be aware that the responses observed are reflective of the underlying physiology of the animal and may shed light on those mechanisms. In the study of cancer, early workers had no trouble identifying tumours that resulted when they painted a solution containing any of several polycyclic aromatic hydrocarbons on the backs of mice. The mouse skin assay remains one approach to determining the carcinogenicity of chemicals. However, the study of how and why the tumours occurred, in studies where the chemical was a tool in the experiment, rather than the object of study, have led to a clearer understanding of the process of carcinogenesis.

As the biological sciences in general, and toxicology in particular, advance, new forms of technology are developed on a frequent basis. It is possible to gauge advances in the biological sciences associated with the development of tools such electrophysiology, the use of isotopes and their measurement, spectroscopy and chromatography in their various forms, application of immunological techniques and now flow cytometry and imaging systems and the computer. Toxicologists have always grasped at these innovations. In the training of toxicologists they should be made aware of advances in technology which will help them now, and to also be receptive to new technologies as they develop, since it is clear that they will develop and can represent significant improvements in our ability to find solutions to problems in toxicology. However, excellent scientific studies have been performed by toxicologists long before the advent of new hi-tech laboratory equipment became available. The training of toxicologists, while making use of new technologies, should concentrate on the knowledge base of toxicology, how to solve problems using the empirical approach and how to apply creative thought to the interpretation of data, the development of new hypotheses and the planning of new experiments to challenge our hypotheses.

REFERENCES

Gallo, M. A. (1996). History and scope of toxicology. In Klaassen, C. D., Amdur, M. O. and Doull, J. (Eds.), *Casarett & Doull, The Basic Science of Poisons*, 5th edn McGraw-Hill, New York, p. 9.

Jacobi, J. (Ed.) (1988). *Paracelsus, Selected Writings*. Princeton University Press, Princeton, NJ, p. 95.

Chapter 90
The Toxicologist and the Law

Arthur Furst and Daniel F. Reidy

C O N T E N T S

INTRODUCTION

At the present time, toxicologists are playing a pivotal role in many facets of our society. There are over a million chemicals in our environment; more are being introduced and few are being phased out. As a result, toxicologists are being called upon to be interpreters of the consequences of these exposures. Hence toxicologists must interact with many different units in our society, and most often with the legal system. Toxic torts are increasing, and in many cases, along with accidents, toxic problems dominate the courts. The judicial system relies on the toxicologist to make sense of the technical problems presented. The toxicologist must serve many different clients, and this can take many shapes. In the majority of cases, the toxicologist is likely to be retained by an attorney, either for the plaintiff or defendant, to be a consultant (non-testifying expert) or a potential expert witness. In some cases, a judge appoints his or her own expert. That expert is designated as 'the court-appointed expert'. No matter in what capacity the toxicologist serves as an expert witness, it is important for all parties concerned in a court case to appreciate that the toxicologist is not an advocate. His or her function is to render an unbiased opinion based on the 'facts of the case'.

The remainder of this chapter is written only from the toxicologist's perspective. To be effective, the toxicologist should be aware of the nature of the law, and what is expected if he or she becomes an expert witness. The expert witness must constantly rely on the lawyer who retains him or her for guidance on the legal aspects and protocol. At the same time, the toxicologist must also teach the lawyer how to deal with a toxicologist. The lawyer is an expert in the law; the toxicologist is the expert in the science. Each should not expect that the other is very knowledgeable in the other's profession. Teaching and learning go hand in hand.

Areas of Involvement

Besides being an expert witness, there are other times when a toxicologist interacts with different legal systems. Toxicologists are asked to testify at various government hearings and appear before legislative committees. Usually, this entails 'educating' the legislators on the scientific basis or implications of some pending law. Requests may come from members of Congress or Federal regulatory agencies such as the Environmental Protection Agency, Occupational Safety and Health Act, the Department of Energy, Federal Drug Administration, etc. Various State legislative bodies and regulatory agencies may also make similar requests. Besides testifying, the toxicologist may be asked to be on a task force or a committee, or be an advisor to some agency, either governmental or a non-profit organization, in developing policies and/or programme priorities.

Environmental groups often ask for the toxicologist's input for documents to be made public, or submitted to some government agency. If an environmental group initiates some legislation or opposes some, a toxicologist may be asked to endorse or to speak for or against the proposed bill.

Unique Contributions of Toxicologists as Experts

The expert witness has more responsibility than the *fact witness*, who can only testify on what he or she saw or experienced personally. The toxicologist, as an expert witness, is in a unique position to *interpret* the nature of adverse reactions after exposure to some 'toxic' agent. Toxicology, *per se*, must transcend any one scientific discipline. A modern toxicologist must be versed in chemical structure, and especially biochemistry as it pertains to activation or detoxification of a specific chemical. Biotransformations (or detoxification) encompass all aspects of biochemistry. The toxicologist must have a better than average knowledge of anatomy, physiology and pathological consequences due to exposure from an agent. Beyond this, a modern toxicologist is also knowledgeable in some mathematics, especially as it pertains to risk assessment.

Most toxicologists have a good knowledge of general toxicology as well as being a specialist in some sub-area such as carcinogenesis or teratology. Thus, the toxicologist, more than a physical or biological scientist, can present an entire picture of *exposure and response*. The toxicologist can reinforce the claim by a plaintiff that the damage claimed was the result of a specific exposure; or can give evidence to the contrary.

REASON FOR EXPERT WITNESS

In many court cases, especially those which involve toxic or potentially toxic materials, much information must be examined, and at times evaluated. Usually there are many facts which are agreed upon by all parties who are involved in litigation. There are some facts, however, that can be in dispute.

Some time prior to the trial, arbitration or a settlement conference, someone must evaluate the facts and come to some conclusion as to whether (for example) the exposure did or did not cause the damage claimed. Not every well educated scientist is permitted by law to give an interpretation of the facts. Only a *qualified expert witness* can perform the obligation of interpreting the facts and, above all, render an opinion.

Since an expert opinion is to be presented to the court, a court-accepted expert witness is needed to state that opinion and explain and justify the bases for that opinion.

Fact vs Expert Witness

Both the fact witness and the expert witness can perform a service in a dispute. The so-called fact, eye or lay witness can only testify on material that he or she personally experienced. That is, the fact witness can only testify on material that has been personally seen, felt or measured. The fact witness cannot discuss what others saw or said.

The court will not allow the fact witness to interpret the information.

The expert witness can also testify on the facts, but in addition is permitted to interpret them. The expert witness may, if the judge permits, discuss related materials. Permitted also are comments on the statements and the opinions of the other expert witnesses.

The major difference between the fact witness and the expert witness is that only the latter can render an opinion on the facts and can conclude that the damaged claimed is, or is not, related to the assumed exposure.

Real vs Junk Science

Toxic torts appear to be dominating the courts. To assist the court and the 'trier of facts' (the attorney), the toxicologist must rely upon both the scientific method and scientific theories. The toxicologist must be specific in explaining the bases of the opinion presented to the court. In the main, the opinion expostulated by the toxicologist may be crucial to the outcome of the trial. Of interest, however, is that the toxicologist does not win or lose a case; this is the domain of the attorney.

It is safe to say that conventional science is, by all means, the basis of the opinion given to the court

In contrast, many people, and in some cases even scientists who are not trained in the discipline of toxicology or even in some sub-classification of the discipline, will present testimony invoking unorthodox hypotheses. The expert witness must be prepared to give an objective evaluation of this unusual approach to the problem. Too often the unorthodox hypothesis presented as a theory can only be classified as *junk science* (junk science is best described as ideas without a scientific foundation, and these ideas are totally without merit).

Those who present this type of testimony often claim that their views are correct but are unfamiliar to the conventional scientist. 'Now, if the opposing scientist were educated, or with an open mind, he or she will recognize the real truth'. Often junk science is presented by an articulate proponent. Juries are hard pressed to separate junk science from the charismatic advocate.

Juries made up of lay persons are not usually aware of the difference between a hypothesis and a theory or a scientific law. They must sometimes be educated to the logical development; a hypothesis can come from an idea; a theory comes after the hypothesis has been around for a while and has been tested with most results in favour of the hypothesis. A scientific law comes only after a crucial experiment has been conducted successfully.

Newer Theories

As science continues to move at the present rapid pace, hypotheses will be made, modified and altered, or even dropped. New information may even modify the scientific laws that were considered the basis of our civilization. Advances can be expected in the science of genes and genetics and immunology. New approaches will be made in the protection of individuals from harmful effects of 'toxic' agents. Newer ideas will be forthcoming on the effect of diet and nutrition on these agents.

At all times the toxicologist must be alert to these changes. He or she must keep up with the latest theories in the best way he or she can. Certainly, prior to rendering an opinion, the expert must check the most recent literature. A decision must be made on the expert's evaluation of the validity and the applicability of this new information to the case under consideration. It is essential that the expert not be selective, and thus not screen out any information which does not strengthen the opinion given.

Naturally, the toxicologist must be objective at all times.

RESOURCES FOR THE EXPERT

Although the expert toxicologist can render an opinion, he or she must be able to rely upon valid information available in recognized publications, especially the biomedical literature. The toxicologist must be able to obtain copies of the *original* articles, that is, the scientific papers published by the person who did the work. Primary literature has much more meaning than secondary literature such as reviews or books, as the latter two cannot be considered as publications that report original studies.

The toxicologist can learn a great deal from the literature on the science of toxicology written for the attorney; legal treatises and law review articles are generally available in university and public law libraries.

Computer Searches

Many references can be retrieved from databases kept at the National Library of Medicine (Medlars). There are a few databases that are specific for the toxicologist, including TOXLINE and TOXBACK. The expert toxicologist must become familiar with these and with other specialized ones such as Cancerline, Pesticide Fact File and Registry of Toxic Effects of Chemical Substances (RTECS) to demonstrate that one is keeping up with developments and new information in the field. Many toxicologists are aware of at least of one commercial company which does literature searches for a fee. An example is Dialog; this sytem is now part of the Knight-Ridder Information Company (a source book is available from Knight-Ridder Information; e-mail: customer. @corp. dialog.com; web site: http://www.krinfo.com).

The Internet

The Internet system does contain, among other topics of interest to the toxicologist, information on toxicology *per se*. However, many people who enter material on the Web have a bias in favour of a pet 'theory'. Hence it is incumbent on the user to be critical and interpret any 'facts' obtained.

Marketing Self

How does the toxicologist–expert become known to prospective employers? A variety of professions are constantly seeking good unbiased experts in toxicology.

The toxicologist can use the Internet to good advantage for self-advertising. For example, a good home page gives the toxicologist an opportunity to present his or her background and expertise as he or she wishes. There are many other uses of the Internet for self-advertising or for making contact with a prospective client. A recent Web search using a term such as 'Legal Expert Witness' developed over one million hits.

Another way to advertise one's availability as an expert is through listing in published registers of expert witnesses, which typically appear in both printed form and on the Internet. Toxicologists who want their name and qualifications to be listed must contact the publishers. Copies of these registers can usually be found in a university or public law library, and are listed on the Internet. There is a fee for the listing and also for the use of the list.

There are also societies of testifying experts, which provide opportunities for networking and referrals, as well as standards of competence and good professional practice.

INTERACTION OF EXPERT WITH ATTORNEY

The attorney and the expert must be in constant contact. Each should notify the other concerning new pertinent material. Often a case will extend for over a year. Periodic conferences are necessary; this is especially important for the expert. If the meetings are infrequent, the attorney at the meetings should review the merits of the case to refresh the mind of the expert.

The attorney would be wise not to try to qualify the expert in more than one general and one specialty field. In light of the Daubert decisions, judges look for the specific area(s) in which the potential expert has actually done research or has written in the field prior to engagement as an expert in the specific case.

Techniques of Communication

One of the most sensitive aspects of the expert witness–lawyer relationship is how to deal with communication. Here the attorney must give exact instructions to the witness. Telephone communications are essential. In this modern day the communications can be through e-mail, although at present it is not clear whether e-mail communications might be considered as written material which must be shared with the opposing lawyer. Some attorneys do equate e-mail with a written letter, that must be shared. However, for the toxicologist, the axiom is 'never communicate with your lawyer in writing without explicit instruction to do so!'.

A number of dates are important. Too often the attorney fails to tell the expert to make a note and keep a record of these dates. These dates will, in all probability, be asked in court. An examples is, when was the expert appointed as such? If a lawyer engages the toxicologist as a non-testifying consultant, in this situation the attorney's Work Product Protection privilege comes into play. To be noted clearly is the exact date of when the toxicologist ceased to be a consultant and became a testifying expert. There are other important dates which will be noted in other sections.

Presenting the Toxicologist

Initially, the toxicologist must make clear to the lawyer what toxicology is and what toxicologists do and usually do not do. Second, the toxicologist must advise the lawyer on how to introduce and address a toxicologist in court. If the lawyer addresses the toxicologist as 'Dr' rather than 'Mr' or 'Ms (Mrs)', the judge and jury must be made to understand that the term doctor is not the sole possession of the medical profession. When members of the jury hear the term 'doctor', they picture the TV version of a person in a white coat with a stethoscope in the pocket or around the neck. If the lawyers fail to explain to a jury about the term 'doctor', the opposing lawyer will make every attempt to belittle the toxicologist, and hence make his or her testimony ineffective.

Is There Expert Liability?

There are no universal laws that protect the expert witness against a lawsuit. Different States have different laws against liability. Experts have been sued by their own lawyer; seldom is the expert sued by the opposing lawyer. Normally, experts are immune when answering a question under oath. However, when speaking outside the courtroom or when holding a press conference, or accepting an interview where the case is discussed, the expert is liable to be sued.

Experts have been sued if they have given false testimony. The best protection for the expert is at all times to tell the truth. In some cases, experts have been found liable when they take cases where they are not qualified, or have done an inadequate job of preparation.

QUALIFICATION OF THE EXPERT AFTER DAUBERT

The Frye Rule

Until June 1993, expert opinion based on a scientific technique was not admissible in a US Federal court and most State courts unless the technique was generally accepted as reliable in the relevant scientific community. This was the legal standard for admissibility of scientific expert opinion in the Federal courts for 70 years, stretching back to a law case called *Frye vs United States* decided in 1923, which dealt with a newly emerging scientific technique at the time, a primitive polygraph test for detecting stress associated with telling lies.

New technologies developed through research at the cutting edge of various fields were becoming available to scientists who wanted to use these new technologies in forming expert opinions when they were called as expert witnesses in court cases, and some parties and attorneys were increasingly chagrined to have what they thought was good science ruled out-of-bounds under the so-called Frye Rule, because these novel and cutting-edge scientific techniques were often ruled inadmissible in Federal courts as unreliable because they were not yet generally accepted by most scientists in the relevant field. In topical areas of environmental harm and toxic torts, pressure was building up for reform or at least modernization of the venerable Frye Rule.

Daubert and its Progeny

All this changed with the case called *Daubert vs Merrell Dow Pharmaceuticals (Daubert I)*. The case started off in a Federal district court in Southern California when the parents of two minor children sued a pharmaceutical company for damages associated with birth defects, claiming that the pregnant mother's ingestion of an anti-nausea prescription drug called Bendictin caused limb reduction birth defects. Before the matter ever got to a full-blown trial with live testimony, the drug company moved for summary judgment based on a scientific expert's affidavit that he had reviewed the published scientific literature on the subject and found that pregnant mothers' use of the drug Bendictin had not been shown to be a risk factor for human birth defects. As is typical in a toxic torts case, the plaintiffs' attorneys had lined up their own scientific experts, so they countered with affidavits opining that Bendectin can cause birth defects, basing their conclusion on various studies: *in vitro* laboratory studies, *in vivo* animal studies, chemical structure analyses and the re-analysis of previously published human statistical studies. The trial judge decided that the plaintiffs' expert opinions were inadmissible under the Frye Rule because their theories and methodologies were not generally accepted as reliable in the relevant scientific community.

The plaintiff parents filed an appeal in the 9th Circuit Court of Appeals, where a review panel of judges affirmed the District Court judge's decision that the plaintiffs' expert opinions were inadmissible. The 'sea change' occurred when the US Supreme Court reviewed the case, and replaced the 'general acceptance' Frye Rule with a more complex set of standards, as follows.

- ■ *Step 1. Reliability.* At the outset, the trial judge as 'gatekeeper' must determine whether the expert is proposing to testify to scientific knowledge that will help the trier of fact (jury or judge) to understand or determine a fact in issue. Several factors bear on this inquiry: (a) *Testability*: has the methodology been tested? (b) *Peer review*: has the methodology been submitted to the scrutiny of the scientific community through peer review and publication? (c) *Rate of error and standards*: what is the known or potential rate of error, and are there pertinent standards of operation? (d) *Degree of acceptance*: what is the degree of acceptance of the methodology within the relevant scientific community?
- ■ *Step 2. Relevance.* The trial judge must determine whether the theory or methodology and what it will yield 'fit' the issues involved in the legal dispute.

Since this seminal US Supreme Court decision in 1993, there have been hundreds of cases where the so-called 'Daubert Factors' have been applied in specific instances, and in most cases scientific experts at the cutting edge of science have been excluded from testifying. Trial judges became even more concerned about protecting juries from undue influence from 'experts for hire' with credentials as worthy scientists who were prepared to state opinions in court based on theories or methodologies which in effect were really 'junk science'.

When the Daubert case itself was sent back to the lower courts to be reconsidered in the light of the Daubert Factors, the 9th Circuit Court of Appeals stressed three additional factors as indicators of reliability: (1) whether the expert will testify about matters resulting from pre-existing research conducted independent of the litigation; (2) whether the expert can point to some objective source to show that he or she has followed the scientific method, such as the policy statement of a pro-

fessional association; and (3) whether the expert's methodology is used by at least a significant minority of scientists practicing in the field. This case, now known as *Daubert II*, is given great weight by courts throughout the USA in applying the Daubert principles in specific cases. The main significance of the Daubert I and Daubert II cases for toxicologists is that if these cases are applied too narrowly, it becomes difficult for newcomers to the field or even experienced toxicologists using newly emerging methodologies to qualify as expert witnesses in court.

Another case of major significance is the *Paoli Railroad Yard PCB Litigation*. This toxic torts case from Philadelphia which has unfolded over 10 years involved a complex battle of experts in which the admissibility of toxicological expert opinions on health effects of exposures to PCBs was addressed through extensive and exhaustive application of the Daubert Factors, yielding a virtual encyclopaedia of principles and practice tips for the toxicologist as expert witness.

Another PCB exposure case which has proved to be very significant is *Joiner vs General Electric*. A Federal judge in Georgia excluded from the trial experts who were prepared to testify that a city electrician's exposures in the workplace to PCBs caused or promoted his small cell cancer. The basis for the trial court's ruling was that the experts' work could not qualify as reliable under the principles of Daubert. The 11th Court of Appeal reversed this decision, in effect ruling that the trial judge had overstepped in his 'gatekeeper' role, going beyond a Daubert-type inquiry about the reliability of the experts' methodologies and delving into the worth of animal studies as such and the basic correctness of the opinions. In late 1997, the US Supreme Court upheld the trial judge and ruled that trial judges have great discretion in acting as 'gatekeepers' of scientific evidence and that this particular trial judge was justified in barring testimony based on studies of animals exposed to a toxin if the dosage exposure to animals in the laboratory is greater than that experienced by the human persons involved in the trial. This case had been closely watched by the scientific and legal communities to see if the Daubert principles would be modified in the direction of loosening up the limitations on scientific testimony, but the Supreme Court reaffirmed the value and force of Daubert-type analysis of the reliability of a scientific expert's theories and methodologies before allowing the expert's opinions to be presented to a jury.

For a toxicologist interested in being able to qualify as an expert witness in a US Federal court or in most of the States which have adopted the Daubert principles, it would be prudent to make sure that he or she has conducted research in the relevant field prior to being retained for the litigation, that the underlying theories and methodologies are testable by others and conform to standards set by government agencies or professional societies, and that the methodologies are used by at least a significant minority of scientists practicing in the relevant field.

THE EXPERT OPINION

One of the primary functions of an expert witness is to render an opinion. However, there are a number of details (unrelated to the actual opinion) which must be attended to. Here, too, many lawyers fail to impress upon the expert the importance of these apparent minor points. The judge and the opposing attorney will wish to know many or all of these details. Among these details are important dates. When did the expert came to the conclusion that an opinion can be rendered? The dates when drafts were made of the opinion and the date when the toxicologist made the final rendering of that opinion? The final opinion must be in writing, and should be clearly stated. A short review of the 'facts', as the expert understands them, should precede the opinion. The opinion should stand out, and then a section on the justification of that opinion should follow. The advice of the attorney is important here as to how long and how detailed this written report should be. The toxicologist must be careful of the true meanings of the words *probable* and *possible*.

For the written report, it is essential to clarify if this a preliminary draft or a final report. 'Preliminary' implies that more information will be added, or extensive revisions will be made or the report will be edited for clarification. A clear statement must be made that the conclusions in this report are solely that of the writer, and that there was no input from the engaging attorney or other parties. A suggested list of topics to be included is:

1. A brief summary.
2. A clear statement of the problem.
3. A clear statement of the 'facts' as you understand them.
4. What your assignment was.
5. What investigations you conducted.
6. What calculations were involved (if applicable).
7. Did you consult with other experts?
8. A clear statement of your opinion rendered.
9. What your limiting conditions and exclusions (if any) are.

IMPORTANCE OF THE DEPOSITION

If a toxicologist is designated an expert witness and is asked to render an opinion, the opposing attorney will no doubt take a deposition. For most toxicologists, having a deposition taken is a trying experience.

The deposition is usually taken in an office with the various attorneys present. Also present is a certified court reporter who administers the oath (of truth) and takes a verbatim record of the proceedings.

It is important for the expert to know that the testimony given in a deposition has the same legal binding force as testimony given in a courtroom. Since the opposing attorney is not trying to impress a jury, there usually are less theatrics or none at all. There are numerous reasons why a deposition is taken. The obvious ones are to give the opposing attorney an idea of what facts the expert witness knows and what the nature and direction of the opinion will be. Another reason for the deposition is that this can be a 'fishing expedition' which can lead to learning new facts. Also, this gives the opposing attorney an idea of how the expert witness thinks: how logically and clearly can the expert present his or her ideas? More subtle reasons for the deposition are for the opposing attorney to probe the weakness of the expert in the technique of delivery and, above all, to see how the expert behaves if provoked.

Since the expert witness will give the opposing attorney specific information, a fee is in order; the amount of the fee expected should be relayed to the opposing attorney by the expert's attorney. That fee should be paid just before or just after the deposition is given. If that is not the case, the expert should be told the exact date when the fee will be forthcoming. Some experts have refused to respond to the request for a deposition, even when a subpoena has been served, if the fee was not presented before the questioning started.

THE EXPERT IN THE COURTROOM

The expert must project at all times that he or she really is an expert. What must be kept in mind is that too often the lasting impression is of the demeanor and not the factual response to a question.

The Judge and the Jury

Some members of the jury (and, in some cases, the judge) have a preconceived idea of what a scientist is and what a scientist does. Many are influenced by the TV character; the scientist is either a naive character or an evil person. It is incumbent on the toxicologist when on the witness stand to project to the judge and jury that he or she is a thinking scientist without being prejudiced for or against a cause or the opposing subject or person.

In the courtroom, the only audience for the expert witness is the jury. Thus, when answering questions, the witness should start the answer looking at the asking attorney, then the witness should talk directly to the jury. Some attorneys have advised their experts not to talk directly to the jury. This may not be good advice, for eye contact with members of the jury goes a long way towards letting them know who is believable.

Occasionally, the witness should also look at the judge when answering a question. If the expert only looks at his or her lawyer, the jury may think he or she is looking for clues.

Testimony of the Expert

At all times, the expert, during the question–answer period, must use non-technical language. It can be assumed that members of the jury are at least high school graduates. They resent hearing technical jargon; they resent being spoken to as though they are morons.

Direct

Prior to testifying, the expert must review the answers he or she gave to the questions posed during the deposition. As during the deposition, the expert must take a few seconds to consider the question posed by the attorney retaining the expert or by the opposing attorney.

Indirect

At times the toxicologist cannot appear in court. It is permissible to present testimony by video tape. If the expert must use video tape, it must be recognized that video tapes are boring to many members of the jury. The expert should try to make the tape come alive. All speaking should be facing the camera, with head up and with the testifier leaning slightly forward. If charts are used, they should be simple and clear, and the lines and words should be large.

The attire should be dark, with no stark whites.

The tape can be most ineffective if the expert shows signs of nervousness, such as clearing throat constantly or pulling on one's ear, tapping fingers, chewing a pencil, looking down most of the time, speaking too quietly or using the same phrases over and over (example, 'you know', 'uh uh').

PROBLEMS ENCOUNTERED BY THE EXPERT

What is a Toxicologist?

What is the Educational Background?

Unlike chemists, physicists or physiologists or even pharmacologists, most older toxicologists do not have an advanced degree in toxicology. Until relatively recently, there was no specific degree in toxicology. The closest was a degree in some biological field with an emphasis on toxicology. Many board-certified toxicologists are considered toxicologists by virtue of their research or professional activities rather than formal training. This can be a problem when the attorney attempts to qualify the expert witness as a toxicologist.

How is a Toxicologist Different from an MD?

An MD degree is granted after the student completes a number of didactic courses, and also after the student has had experience in the clinic with some 'hands-on' training. No research is required as a rule for obtaining a medical degree. No matter from which field the toxicologist has come, a research project is a requirement.

Relation to Other Scientists

A toxicologist normally has a much broader training and experience than a chemist or a biologist. As mentioned, the toxicologist must be more than just familiar with a number of disciplines. The chemist need not be knowledgeable in physiology, the biologist need not be familiar with biochemistry; the toxicologist must be able to understand both.

Difficult Concepts to Present

Dose–Response

The general public usually relates a single physical or chemical insult to a definite pathological change. Many believe a single exposure to one fibre of asbestos which can penetrate a single cell will definitely induce any one of a variety of lung cancers.

The concept of dose–response is well accepted by toxicologists, but is not really known or accepted by the general public. It is essential for the expert witness to prepare a few examples of dose–response relationships. It is useful to practice the lay-person explanation a few times to sharpen up the way the concept is finally presented. Sometimes a simple diagram or graph will suffice. Of importance is that the graph must be both simple and large enough for all the jury members to see without straining.

Hormesis

A second difficult concept is the phenomenon of *hormesis*. In many cases (but not in 100% of the exposures) a very low dose of a toxic agent (a low dose can be quite variable) may result in a beneficial effect! A larger dose of the toxic agent will exhibit the normal toxicological response. Some examples are as follows.

Mice exposed to a small amount of whole body radiation live longer than the untreated controls. Mice exposed to larger dose of radiation develop many types of cancer and die long before the controls.

Chickens ingesting small amounts of arsenic in their food grow faster and bigger than the untreated controls.

Larger amounts of arsenic are poisonous and retard the growth of chickens.

Non-essential metals are considered toxic at high doses. Cadmium has no known biological function, yet at very low levels cadmium ions will stimulate some enzyme action and accelerate some cell growth. At high levels, cadmium inhibits enzyme action and kills cells.

Determination of Cause

Another difficult concept to present to the court is how to determine *cause*. The jury is most interested in the simple question, 'Did exposure to a specific agent *cause* the damage claimed?'. The answer to this question is not simple. In acute cases the damage can be observed very soon after the trauma. It is not necessary to theorize what happened if a cut on a bleeding finger is noted, or if there is a wound following a gun shot. However, to determine the cause of a pathological condition by some exposure to an agent that occurred weeks, months or years ago requires some reasoning and also some speculation.

Cause can be assigned to a bacterium for a specific disease. Koch's Postulates can be invoked here. Also, it is possible to inoculate an experimental animal with the bacterium in question. The same cannot be said of a chemical suspected of causing cancer. Humans cannot be ethically inoculated!

For cancer or birth defects, other disciplines must be consulted. Conclusions from a single discipline may not be sufficient to conclude *cause*. Juries may have heard an epidemiologist relate exposure to cause. They may have heard statements such as *causal relationships* or *causal association*. The toxicologist may reject the notion that epidemiological evidence can give us true causality.

It may be the toxicologist's task to spend a few moments on the meaning of confounding factors which must always be considered by the epidemiologist. In an early US Surgeon General's reports devoted to *criterion of judgment*, the term *causal factors* was used, not *cause*, *per se*.

Experimentally, it is easier to relate the effect of an agent on animals which are exposed to that agent. However, some judges have ruled against introducing information obtained from experiments. Much thought must be given before the toxicologist attempts to discuss the effects of any material on experimental animals. Although jurors may be open-minded on many ideas, some may have strong opinions against using animals. In the main, the opposing side will constantly remind the jury that animals live from two or three years whereas humans live three score years and ten.

If the judge does rule out evidence obtained from exposure of animals to the material under question, the toxicologist should make these points:

- Pathological effects are noted, either within a few hours or days. If cancer is the end-point, this may

take years. Rather than argue years of life of a human compared with years of life to a rodent, it is logical to argue in percentage of life span.
- Over the years, a great body of knowledge has been accumulated extrapolating the effect of a chemical on a human, and the effect of that chemical on a rodent. In the case of cancer, where identical routes of exposure have been tried, the following have induced identical types of cancer in both rodents and humans: β-naphthylamine, vinyl chloride and bischloroether.
- In some cases, the induction of a cancer in a rodent is in no way related to humans; for example, the zymbal gland in the rodent has no counterpart in humans.
- The development of the same pathological reaction in a number of different species gives more credence to the probability that the same pathology will be found in humans.

In the last analysis, there are no specific means to pinpoint what exactly caused a cancer in humans.

Opposing Opinion

Seldom do two experts differ on the facts of a case, but they may come to opposite opinions based on these facts. Since an opinion is just that, different conclusions can be expected at times. The toxicologist must give careful thought as to why the opposing expert does not agree. If possible, prior to the court trial the credentials of the opposing expert should be scanned and if possible the CV of the opposing expert should be obtained.

In the court, it is best to state openly that there is a disagreement. The testifying expert can give the following arguments if they are pertinent.

The expert can say the opponent overlooked some facts in the case. The opponent has not had sufficient experience in this particular area. There is a flaw in the opponent's logic.

At no time should the expert attack the opponent in a personal manner. This will rebound negatively against the person testifying. Avoid talking about the fees received by the opponent. Let the attorneys do that if they wish. It is best to say that you have some regard for your opponent, but disagree in this instance.

SELECTED REFERENCES

Cases

Daubert vs Merrill Dow Pharmaceuticals, 113 S. Ct. 2786 (1993) (Daubert I).

Daubert vs Merrill Dow Pharmaceuticals, 43 F. 3d 1311 (9th Cir. 1995) (Daubert II).

Frye vs United States, 293 F-1013 (D.C. Circuit 1923).

In re *Paoli R. R. Yard PCB Litigation*, 35 F. 3d 717 (3rd Cir. 1994).

Joiner vs General Electric, 864 F. Supp. 1310 (N.D. Georgia 1994); 78 F. 3d 524 (11th Cir. 1996);—S. Ct.—; (Case No. 96–188, December 15, 1997).

Publications

Cecil, J. S., Drew, C. E., Cordisco, M. and Miletich, P. P. (1994). *Reference Manual on Scientific Evidence*. Federal Judicial Center, Washington, DC.

Feder, H. A. (1991). *Succeeding as an Expert Witness*. Van Nostrand Reinhold, New York.

Furst, A. (1997). *The Toxicologist as Expert Witness*. Taylor and Francis, Bristol, PA

Chapter 91
Ethical, Moral and Professional Issues, Standards and Dilemmas in Toxicology

D. W. Vere

CONTENTS

WHAT ARE OUR DUTIES?

These are easy to state in abstract, but very difficult to work through in application. There seems to be wide agreement that our duties are beneficence (doing good, to others as well as to self), non-maleficence (avoiding harm), respect for autonomy or an individual's self-determining choices, and justice, which means perhaps equity rather than just equality of treatment of others. In addition, people should respect agreed formulations of good conduct, or codes ('deontology'), pay active attention to the possible or foreseeable consequences of what they are doing, to see that these will be beneficial to others (utilitarianism, consequentialism), and be truthful. Lastly, it helps to have a hierarchy (or pecking order) of 'goods'; this was Mills's only answer to Bentham's problem of whether it was better to be a contented pig or a discontented Socrates (Gillon, 1985). This seems as fine as 'liberty, fraternity, equality', until one tries to apply it all to toxicology.

THE TOXICOLOGICAL ENVIRONMENT OF ETHICAL DECISIONS

Why is there difficulty? Perhaps it is easiest to show the reasons if one compares toxicology with medicine, where ethics has been applied and debated for a very long time, and that not without difficulty. General awareness of ethics in toxicology seems to have been a more recent development. This seems odd, considering the extensive role of poisoners in former times; perhaps it reflects the fact that it is somewhat easier to kill someone by mis-applied medicine than by deliberate poisoning. In medicine, decisions are largely atomized to individual problems. A doctor, or a small group of medical people, discuss with one patient what may be their best treatment. Autonomy is well ventilated; beneficence for *that patient* is the aim. Issues of consequence do arise, but justice is considered little except where the provision of services to groups of patients are concerned, and there only very partially. But toxicology concerns groups, often very large groups, whether of people or of animals. The aim is risk avoidance or containment in general, not just for an individual. The difference between medical and toxicological ethics is seen in clearest relief with clinical trials, where risks to one and to all can be in conflict (Cancer Research Campaign Working Party in breast conservation, 1983). Are the pathological tests made in early phase I and II trials 'safeguards', or 'monitoring' the action of a new drug, or are they 'human toxicology' or tests on 'human guinea pigs'? They are, of course, in some senses, both, but the name one uses for them sets the minds of hearers towards sympathy or hostility, much as the same set of actions can be called those of a 'freedom fighter' or of a 'terrorist', depending on one's presuppositions.

This problem is seen very clearly when a chemical process benefits most while harming a few. Dry cleaning benefits everyone, but can cause liver damage to a tiny minority. The inverse is just as true. Signal benefits for some can cost all overmuch: cars and spray cans for the wealthy nations may have damaged the climate of the world. The geographical context of the toxicological problems can be much broader than those of medicine.

A similar dilemma exists over the time course of human actions: for most of medicine the time-course of effects does not transcend one life; in toxicology it may be short-lived, but can cover many generations or even reach permanence. This is well seen in the era of organohalogen insecticides and their effects, a story which seems likely to recur with dioxins and polyhalogenated biphenyls.

Perhaps the most obvious difference between the ethics of medicine and of toxicology resides in the part played by autonomy. In medicine the patient, or the experimental subject, is a person who can and should know about his or her own situation and express 'informed consent'. In toxicology the subjects of experiments, or of disaster, are animals; or if they are humans, those people may well be ignorant of the dangers about them, or are already the unwitting victims of them. So the whole atmosphere of ethical decision-making is different for these subjects from that in medicine. There is far more paternalism; for example, decisions are often made on behalf of the subjects, and often this is by those who already 'have an interest' in the outcome of the tests or procedures in question. There neither is, nor can be, 'informed consent' to chemical exposure, unless it be refusal to purchase, having read package warnings.

Last, the purview of toxicology is vastly wider than that of medicine. Medicine is about human illness, its remedies and prevention. Toxicology is about this in many ways, but it is also about natural pollutants, animal experiments, drugs in man's environment, weapons, microbiological toxins and hazards (when the toxin is chemical), pesticides and agrochemicals, sewerage and water treatment, biotechnology, radiation hazards and manufacturing pollutants.

Any of these aspects of toxicology can interact with others, so that it can be very hard even for experts to foresee the potential repercussions of a process, and to take responsible action about them. Because the public is often unaware of potential problems, unless they glare threateningly from media reports, there is great suspicion and vivid imagination, factors which may themselves impede helpful and satisfactory efforts to offset the feared ill-effects. So futile media debates about suspected toxicological hazards are almost daily events.

Since toxicological problems are so complex, they have an added dimension beyond the problems of many other subjects in that they can seldom be thought through once and for all; as time moves on, new aspects appear, and a second or third ethical assessment must be made. For example, it may be impossible at first to foresee how a toxin or metabolite may accumulate in animal tissues, or to collect sufficient instances of adverse effects to discover how often late manifestations of poisoning occur (such as carcinogenesis or teratogenesis). The usage of a product may change, and with it the toxicity profile; an example is the fact that chilled foods have probably always contained *Listeria* organisms, but it is only their newer methods of use which encourage *Listeria* to multiply and so to intoxicate. Every new productive process, be it a manufactured chemical, a drug or a food that is made, needs to be monitored at inception, during restricted trials, and after marketing.

WHAT ARE THE DIFFICULTIES OF BEING DUTIFUL?

No-one can reach decisions about something which they cannot define or measure. The toxicologist faces daunting problems already, for several reasons.

First, there is biostatistical uncertainty. The practical problems here are that experience with small numbers can rarely lead to conviction, whereas to obtain large numbers may require immense outlays of resource or time. Toxicological tests are often judged by their alpha probabilities; can a positive outcome of a test be claimed? But with smaller number tests the beta probability matters as much or more, if the result is to be 'we saw no evidence of the suspected effect'.

The next technical problem concerns the interpretation of tests: everyone naturally values expert opinions on histology, or the metabolic profile of a drug, or the likely risks of intoxication with stated plasma levels of a toxin. But how many experts does one need? Their disagreements are often wide once their number exceeds unity, yet many 'expert' committees are advised by a single pathologist, for example.

Then there is the vexed issue of when and how to warn if one thinks one has a signal. Thalidomide was a case in point: the first six cases of phocomelia were denied reporting space on evidential grounds; correctly in scientific terms, but wrongly in terms of the known eventual outcome. Even when a rigorous effort is made to achieve a significant noise-to-signal ratio, the data are often skewed by selection bias.

The next difficulty concerns the fact that many intoxicants merely amplify a natural but rare event. An example is failure of neural development in tadpoles, a rare spontaneous event whose frequency is amplified enormously, and in a dose-related manner, by calcium antagonist drugs. Hence, in such a human situation, no-one can point to one case and conclude that the drug did it; yet that is exactly what a court decided in the Mekdeci case in 1979, a decision reversed in 1981 (Smithells and Sheppard, 1978; *Current Problems*, 1981). Equally, one cannot look at an insignificant signal and conclude therefrom that the drug did not do it.

Last, there is the problem that a metabolite or a decomposition product may prove intensely toxic, perhaps only in certain situations. The net effect of these scientific and technical aspects of measure and detection is to obscure resolution of problems, so that ethical argument sways readily in either direction. Just as for smoking and lung cancer, it has proved immensely difficult to show an association between even expected toxicities and known toxins, a point demonstrated elegantly by a recent review of the human risks of dioxins and related compounds (Skene *et al.*, 1989).

As if science did not involve problems enough, ethics itself imports more into toxicological debate. Ethical decisions have to take account of the cost/harm versus gain/benefit ratios of any set of proposals. Who is to decide the hierarchy of values for any proposal? The problems are that interested parties differ inevitably in their value judgements; this is well seen in the question as to whether or not laboratory animals should suffer to test cosmetics. No doubt, cosmetic users want protection for themselves, and animal rights protesters for the animals. And may not the outcome depend as much on adjunctive issues as upon the main ones: Are alternative tests possible? Have they been sought? How much suffering is inflicted? These issues are compounded by the fact that some tests (e.g. the LD_{50} test) have been enjoined by regulators in situations where many others involved wanted to be rid of them. Sometimes things which could well be changed seem to roll on by sheer momentum (Walker and Dayan, 1986).

Animal testing is an especially thorny issue, well exposed by Rollin (1989), where the assumptions about animal pain made by many scientists in past years are questioned on common-sense logical grounds: if animals do not *perceive* pain, why do we use them to test analgesics? To argue that this is simply because their responses model well for analgesic effects in humans begs the whole question; it is simply a reductionist argument. We often use Occam's razor, and the simplest explanation has undoubted appeal; but how often is the simplest explanation shown to be the correct one in biology? The Occam postulate is a good test, but one which should always be tested, if only because it is so often wrong, and also because it has no necessary logical force in any single case. It is a useful initial postulate—no more.

The second ethical problem about animals is the question as to whether or not they differ from man, and if so, how? The infliction of suffering on animals, if we assume that they do suffer, in order to avoid human ills is justifiable only if we take them to be of a lower order, of less significance than, ourselves. ('You are of more value than many sparrows' [Matthew: 10, 26–31]). But even this is not to assert that animals are of *no* value; there still has to be a value judgement about *how much* suffering it is justifiable to inflict—hence our laws which regulate animal experimentation.

Similar ethical issues arise about resource allocation: How much is it right to pay volunteers for experiments? When is it necessary to halt development of an 'orphan' drug on grounds of market size? If a safe product has been found, how long should an older product remain on the market because major capital investment has gone into its production plant?

THE ETHICS OF TESTING

Testing for HIV infections has evoked many difficulties in this area; related issues arise for toxicological tests. These are a substantial concern of ethics committees when the tests are part of a research proposal, but most toxicological tests concern individuals and may not be part of research; these are not considered by ethics committees, but nevertheless give rise to the same problems. These problems include:

(i) The repercussions of a test upon the subject, or upon other persons including relatives.
(ii) The subject's prognosis, employment, insurance, compensation.
(iii) Consent for testing; rights in general, under law, and of minors or others of reduced capacity who may, or who should consent, or those who may have to assent and to be informed where consent is not informable or possible (e.g. the unconscious subject).
(iv) Who has a 'natural right' to know the test outcome?
(v) The likely errors inherent in testing; their repercussions upon (i) to (iii) above. What should be disclosed about these potential errors to the subject? What may be the implications of a false positive or negative result (i.e. the sensitivity and specificity of the test)?
(vi) Good laboratory and good clinical practice criteria. Standards.
(vii) The ethics of repeated testing.

In the present climate of autonomy, many request tests but may be unable to grasp the significance of their outcome. Counselling may be needed to prepare people to receive test results without making harmful consequent decisions.

The main ethical watershed involves (iii), consent for testing. If specimens are to be anonymized, as in much methodological research, then their donors should be told this and consent to use the specimen for research should be gained. They should be told that they cannot expect a result from the test. Even this is unnecessary where only the surplus part of a sample which is not needed for the donor's test is to be used. However, if the samples are to be donor annotated, very different ethical issues occur. The provisions of the Data Protection Act must be upheld, consent for research use is essential and confidentiality must be guaranteed explicitly. Also, the issue of what the subject may or may not expect as a test result must be considered; how, when and to whom it may be disclosed, with or without whose request, and whether counselling or other support may then be needed by the subject.

For examples of numerous different difficulties in these areas, it would be hard to find better than the drug testing programme of the Olympic Committee's Medical Commission (Editorial, 1992). Also, the Medical Research Council's Ethics Series are generally useful handbooks (Medical Research Council, 1991, 1992, 1993, 1994).

SCIENTIFIC MISCONDUCT AND PUBLICATION

Attention has focused principally upon fraud; the production and publication of data with deliberate intent to deceive, to gain an unjust advantage, to injure the rights or interests of others (Wells 1995, 1997). This includes plagiarism. The motives range from the obvious, financial or career gain, to pressure of overwork against publication or litigation deadlines.

However, there are more subtle faults and motives. Some believe in themselves so strongly that they resist vehemently the scrutiny of scientific critical detachment (Swan, 1989), leading to data publication by the media instead of submission to scientific review. Sometimes the problem is conceptual rationalism (the belief that data should be congruent with some received theory). Then data are selected for their conformity, only 'the best data' being published, whilst all sorts of reasons are used to reject other data which are equally reliable. This has many shades, which include subconscious data preference and failure to compare the current findings with other work. The motive may be simply wanting something to be true, or an effort to conceal former errors. However, it may not be deliberate deceit or malice, simply careless or sloppy work, The problems were summarized admirably by Kerr (1995).

In toxicology these flaws are serious, especially when judicial proceedings depend upon the findings as evidence, or where compensatable injury is under investigation. Then 'failed beneficence' is indistinguishable from direct 'maleficence' in its effect; justice is denied to those who cannot defend themselves against it. Numerous instances of flawed chemical and toxicological analyses in legal cases have appeared in recent years, including even banal faults such as failure to ensure that apparatus is not contaminated by the kind of substance for which the analysis is made.

Computer programs have been devised to signal potential cases of fraudulent data entry by detecting suspicious patterns within data. However, these will not be likely to detect single fraudulent entries (Wells, 1995). More reliable, if more arduous, methods include audit (data monitoring) and double data entry (O'Rourke, 1996). To guarantee that suspicious patterns are noted, and that those who may note them are not subjected to penalty, it is important for scientific departments to run Standard Operating Procedures and that everyone con-

cerned knows in advance that these will operate (Wells, 1997). Wells (1997) stated that 16 cases were referred to the UK General Medical Council between 1989 and 1997; in no case was the investigator exonerated.

Bias is not confined to authors; it can afflict reviewers and editors also. Refusal to publish work which does not fit established ideas, or which challenges a reviewer's own position, is also unethical. The problems of ethical issues in medical publication have been well reviewed by Riis (1995) and Stoker (1996). Journal reviewers and editors have a clear responsibility to refuse to publish data gained in unethical ways or which, in the case of human experiments, have not been submitted to ethical peer review.

One way to reduce the risk of scientific misconduct escaping attention is to set documented, generally agreed, standards for scientific work. These are now accepted across Europe and in many other countries as 'Good Laboratory Practice' (European Community, 1994) and 'Good Clinical Practice' (European Agency, 1997). The former includes animal research and the latter clinical trials, two fields where misconduct has been reported most frequently. These standards must be monitored internally and are widely used in the production of data for the regulatory authorities.

A more formal stage in the investigation of scientific integrity is the establishment of institutions for this purpose. The first of these was in Denmark (the Committee on Scientific Dishonesty) and similar bodies now exist in other Scandinavian countries, in Austria and in the USA, where the Office of Research Integrity had handled, up to 1996, some 27 cases of alleged or suspected misconduct (ORI, 1997). The UK possesses no body at this type, although well publicized procedures to notify suspected frand, and to protect the notifiers, are in place and have been used effectively in relation to laboratory work within the pharmaceutical industry (Wells, 1997). A more formal approach has been suggested (News, 1998).

WHAT CAN BE DONE?

First, a set of clear objectives ('goods') needs to be defined, without attempting to arrange them in any hierarchy. It must be good, other things being equal, to gain new knowledge, to create wealth, to prevent hazard, to conserve natural resources and to keep to codes which have been generally agreed, such as the Helsinki declaration on human experiment, and the various guidelines for 'good clinical practice', 'good laboratory practice' and 'good animal husbandry'. But even in their statement, it is at once clear that these 'goods' will at times conflict: it is obviously easy to create wealth while causing hazard, to gain knowledge by exploiting natural resources. It is possible to warn publicly to gain recognition, even when the evidence is inadequate, and to fail to warn when a warning is needed for fear of spreading needless alarm. So, some general conclusions emerge:

(1) It is essential to discover facts about all the envisageable aspects of a problem, and to consider their interactions and their likely repercussions on people, on animals and on the environment.

(2) This assessment must contain a hierarchy of value judgements, based upon the best knowledge available. This is the 'state of the art' justification for ethical judgements.

(3) The balance points must be found by considerations of 'natural justice'—not those of self or sectarian interest.

(4) It must never be assumed that a bit of good justifies a lot of evil: ends do not justify means.

(5) Given all goodwill, there will inevitably be mistakes, hurts and losses if there are to be any new things at all, as every mother knows.

So what? What can be done in practice? Obviously, where the public has interests, the public needs to be interested; but so often this is difficult because industry operates competitively (even within the same company!), and free sharing of information is impossible in this imperfect world. Regulatory authorities exist, and guarantee industrial confidence as essential to their very operation. They do seek to operate on a base of sound science, with members declaring personal interests, in strict confidence towards industry yet aiming at public safeguard. But these very safeguards exist because there is secrecy; hence, debate inevitably polarizes, becomes adversarial and frequently comes to appeal. This is the very opposite of wise, ethical judgement, but perhaps it is the best that can be done in a realm where competition generates secrecy rather than openness. But everyone, every company, every scientific group has the opportunity to consider what they are doing first, so that a regulatory hand need not interfere with what they are doing. Whether as regulator or regulated, no one can do better than his or her present knowledge will allow: the 'state of the art' has to be the determinant of fame or blame.

When mistakes or adversities occur, they should be compensated; how? Most scientists and doctors want 'no fault' indemnity; the problems are that governments will not fund the higher potential claims, and lawyers (who tend to be determinist and free from biostatistical qualms of any kind) want 'strict liability'. 'Strict liability' seems to secure exactly what it destroys, natural justice, because it is proof-, not hurt-, dependent (Laurence, 1989). It is also unscientific and irrational in the sense that its attributions of blame fall upon manufacturers in a biased way (Royal Commission on Civil Liability, 1974).

It is at this point that the discussion enters an unreal world, one might say a nightmare, in terms of something frighteningly unreal which nevertheless exists. This is the realm of public risk perception, the media presentation of matters toxicological and the impact of political decisions on such things. These issues cannot be presented here in detail; several points emerge in general. The most obvious is that distorted perceptions of risk, real or potential, will abound in the ethical environment of toxicological decisions. Whether deliberate or fear-driven, these distortions will not just go away. There is no point in being out raged rationally by them; they do not arise from evidenced grounds without bias, being reasoned from selected information. They are to do with people and their emotions. Often, they are linked to words or other fear cues. 'Nuclear' is an obvious example; it is interesting to reflect, while driving through a 'nuclear-free zone', how much radiation from natural and medical sources abounds within it. Many protesters at Chernobyl fallout must have enjoyed an equal burden sniffing the radon in a week's holiday in Cornwall. It was delightfully expressed in that misprint about 'the unclear threat'. But in the problem of public explanations and relations, suspicions and interpretations must always enter the ethical analysis.

The second point about public perceptions is that the amount of fear and noise evoked is greater when the perceived risk seems greater. Many scientists, engineers and policy-staters seem to expect public fears to retreat when a risk can be shown to be vanishingly small. This will not happen, since people are reacting to their perception of the risk size were the unthinkable to occur or were they the person affected. Three Mile Island is a case in point: the fact that the nuclear power plant was successfully shut down did not reassure those who envisaged what would have happened had it not been contained successfully.

A third generality is that public fears should not be countered by derision, however witty and factual these remarks may be. Destructive humour suggests insincerity and carelessness, and reaps its own reward.

Perhaps the greatest ethical burden concerns the clash between establishments and value judgements. Animal tests, causing some apparent suffering, became established, whether as a part of regulatory requirements or in the shape of an expensive laboratory process or plant of which they form an integral part. Then value perceptions changed. Which force will win, the changed perception or the money and effort enshrined in the established process?

This problem is exacerbated because one of the opposing forces is external, and the other internal to the company or institution involved. There may be no natural forum for debate between the two groups of proponents. Often this sort of ethical tension becomes prolonged until a flashover occurs, either through the media or even as physical violence.

Where there has to be uncertainty, what methods are open to help people to do their best? Those which are available are (1) analysis of decisions by ingredient factors, (2) peer review, (3) scale containment, (4) ongoing review and (5) risk analysis, in those cases where this can be done.

(1) Breaking a proposal down to identify all its ingredient factors guards against overlooking the vulnerable. It helps to consider:

(a) The impact severity of a potential hazard – that is, the product of intensity and range. The neglect of one abandoned caesium source in Brazil caused intense damage to a small number of those who handled it; ozone from photochemical smog causes some damage to large numbers of city dwellers; the human 'cost' of both kinds of hazard could be considered to be comparable.

(b) Vulnerable subgroups.

Sometimes these can be anticipated, as when the chemical cousins of known toxins are released into an environment. But biological mechanisms are subtle enough to outwit most such anticipations. Occasionally they succeed, as when it was foreseen by chemists that the drug alclofenac could yield an epoxide metabolite in man (Mercia et al., 1983). More often they are discovered as the result of release into human or animal populations, as with thalidomide. Even when an adverse effect can be anticipated quite strongly, minor chemical differences often decide whether or not it appears, and what its impact may be. For example, it is well known that a wide variety of inhibitors of 5-hydroxytryptamine uptake into neurons cause disorders of immunity in man. But these disorders vary from drug to drug. These inhibitors have such potential value in psychiatry that firms continue to prepare new compounds for human testing. The only way to discover their potential for immunological damage is to test them in man.

(2) Whatever the degree of likelihood of harm may be, it is an incontrovertible ethical onus on any experimenter or supplier of new chemical agents to try to anticipate toxic hazards and to seek expert opinion about potential risks. This leads naturally to the question of peer review. For new human experiments in medicine, all projects are referred to a research ethics committee. The problems with animal experiments are dealt with in the UK by a government inspectorate under the Animal Procedures Act. But this is concerned with limiting animal suffering and cruelty, not with the wider ethical questions which might arise from animal experiments. Pesticides and agrochemicals are regulated through a somewhat, but necessarily, cumbrous process (see Chapter 73): the Food and Agriculture Organization of the United Nations at Rome, and the World Health Organization Expert Group on pesticide residues in food, meet and publish recommendations on maximum residue limits, acceptable daily intakes and pesticide use practice ('good agricultural practice'). Evidence is also collected on continued evaluation of human exposure, including the results of volunteer testing. Most of the recommendations are based on animal tests for toxicity, mutagenicity

and growth to preformalized schedules. There are supervised trials of new agrochemicals and a review of toxicological databases. But all these digested facts issue as recommendations proposed for use by the member governments of the respective agencies. Important though they are, they cannot substitute effectively for local vigilance in manufacture, distribution and control in relation to the chemical environment, especially since not all governments are members of these agencies. Similarly, industrial safety is governed in the UK under the Factories Inspectorate, a system aimed to ensure conformity to safety regulations. None of these bodies can influence greatly either the broader ethical issues of chemical exposure or local decisions about the release of industrial chemicals. This has become very apparent with regard to toxic waste disposal, whether from hospital chimneys (burning polyvinyl chloride) or nitrate fertilizer in soil and river pollution. However good the regulations, they will not work without the local will to implement them, costly though that can often be.

(3) Another way to maximize safety and reduce risk is by scale containment. Exposures can be increased in a graded fashion so that, should adverse effects appear, they will be on a small scale and they can be studied. The problem here is that small-scale exposures seldom yield sufficient data to demonstrate an adverse effect unambiguously. As already shown with dioxins, a known and much studied group of toxins, even quite wide human exposure in accidents has so far failed to reveal definite long-term hazards (Skene et al., 1989). Planned exposures in critical experiments are not possible for ethical reasons; accidental exposures are usually too ill-defined and too riddled with litigation to yield clear scientific information.

(4) Ongoing review of successively wider releases of new chemical agents seems essential, but is almost impossible to achieve. For new drugs, successive stages of initial tests in healthy volunteers and clinical trials are reviewed by regulatory authorities, which may also require post-marketing surveillance (PMS) or 'monitored release' (MR) schemes. Unfortunately, PMS and MR often fail, although some have been successful in revealing new and unexpected toxicities. But such schemes cannot be mounted for industrial chemical exposures. In any case, it is often impossible to discriminate between natural disease and chemical toxicity; for example, a worker who becomes jaundiced after solvent exposure may have a problem which resists all efforts at firm diagnosis.

(5) Risk analyses can seldom be made. Risk ratios can be calculated only if all cells of a fourfold table can be denumerated; these are the numbers exposed and not exposed as columns, and the numbers with or without a defined adverse event as rows. These four totals are almost never all available. Partial analyses can be done using case controls and specialized statistical tests such as the Mantel–Haentzel procedure. But the work involved

is often substantial and the results debatable unless confirmed. All in all, risk analyses have contributed little to the detection and control of toxicological problems.

Again, the overriding problem in this difficult ethical area is the fact that most industrial development is competitive and so is secret until marketing occurs. The business of ethics is to act in prospect so as to maximize good and minimize harm, to one and to all. Its business is not detection and recrimination after some adverse event, although it is involved in securing justice for the victims. The law tends to be determinist, requiring proof of cause; justice for the victims of an accident of uncertain cause is therefore attained uncertainly, and involves costly hearings, enquiries or tribunals.

There are also four ethical paradoxes which bedevil any agreed policies. These are: (1) the value assessment of resources; (2) autonomous choice to accept risk – the 'self' or 'others' paradox; (3) differences between societies; (4) health versus survival.

Resource assessment. There is no easy way to decide the value of resources to any community or sector of a community. Natural resources are 'given', but are consumable. It may be our farmland against your climate when it comes to felling forests; this global example illustrates a problem which repeats endlessly upon lesser scales. The suggested solution is to live in balance with nature, to recycle, to return what has been taken. But this cannot be done with some toxic wastes; these can only be destroyed or stored, often at immense cost.

Choices, self and others. Chemical glues are necessary evils. I may resolve never to give them to children, but children may decide to take the risk of glue-sniffing. How paternalistic should a person, a company, a society be in seeking to protect those who accept the risk of self-harm? What is the balance of autonomy with deontology or consequentialism here. We accept risky sports: how much risk from intoxication should be accepted? Attitudes differ in bizarre ways towards various toxins: compare ethanol and nicotine with cannabis and amphetamine, counting deaths.

Differences between societies. There are enormous differences worldwide between societies about the amount of toxicological risk they will accept. Some of this relates obviously to the relative wealth of societies, some to the value set upon human life which their culture suggests or accepts. But the size of the differences between the protection afforded by various states to their citizens shows how impossible it is to state absolute values here. This is not to say that there is disagreement among peoples about what is or might be desirable, but there is enormous variation in the will and in the means to attain proper goals (Yudkin, 1978). Even within one society with decided health objectives in the United Kingdom, there are considerable regional differences in attainment of the agreed goals (DHSS, 1980). Griffin (1987) has reported remarkable variations in drug exposure and adverse reaction reporting rates between cultures.

Health versus survival. Good health and survival are not synonymous. There have been, and still are, times and places where the acceptance of a heavy toxicological burden is the price of survival. In some degree this happened in the industrial revolution in Britain: chronic bronchitis was the price and became known as 'the English disease' in mainland Europe. But this burden was accepted unwittingly; in many third world countries toxic industries are accepted deliberately as the only way to expand a weak economy, and widespread pollution has occurred as a result, often as a legacy for later generations.

CONCLUSIONS

In conclusion, it can be said that whereas it seems desirable for the same ethical considerations that apply to medicine to be used for toxicological work, there are often immense difficulties in so doing. These relate chiefly to the broader scope of toxicological work: animals as well as people, populations as well as individuals, and resource use on major scales. It also relates to the biostatistical uncertainty of prospective assessment of toxic hazard, and the difficulty of knowing when to warn. Because these problems exist, agreement is often reached on policies which benefit some but risk many, or which benefit soon but risk later, simply because it is so difficult to weigh the various risk probabilities prospectively. These risks vary differently in time and even well-informed and careful people may disagree strongly about the value judgements which should be made about each step of such complex processes. The central problem is that, if there is to be progress of any kind, there must be exploratory advance. These advances always carry risks, some foreseeable but some not. There will always be those whose vote is to try progress and take risk, and others who think it better to wait, and possibly not see. And biological systems are amazingly resilient in the face of threat; adaptive processes are remarkably strong. For this reason it is often the anticipated threats which prove to be unimportant and the unforeseeable which do most subtle damage. We can only seek to act responsibly, using the best current standards of due care, examining what has been done continuously for unforeseen hazards. Failure is to be seen chiefly in this last aspect, in the thorny but necessary process of public information and in the secrecy which is imposed upon innovation by the competitive nature of industry.

REFERENCES

Cancer Research Campaign Working Party in Breast Conservation (1983). Informed consent: ethical, legal and medical implications for doctors and patients who participate in randomised clinical trials. *Br. Med. J.*, **286**, 1117–1121.

Current Problems (1981). Data Sheet changes – Debendox. *Current Problems*, **6**, July 1981. Also *Daily Mirror*, Monday July 1984, p. 1; *Hospital Doctor*, June 16, 1983, p. 24.

Department of Health and Social Security (1980). *Inequalities in Health*. DHSS, London.

Editorial (1992). Olympic pseudoscience. A news editorial. *Bull. Med. Ethics*, **80**, 3–7.

European Agency for the Evaluation of Medicinal Products (1997). *Notes for Guidance on Good Clinical Practice*, (CPMP/ICH/135/95). European Agency for the Evaluation of Medicinal Products, London.

European Community (1994). *Good Laboratory Practice. European Community Directive. Rules Governing Medicinal Products in the European Union*, Vol. 1. HMSO, London.

Kerr, D.N.S. (1995). Fraud in science: time for a second look? *J. R. Coll. Physicians (London)*, **29**, 461.

Gillon, R. (1985). *Philosophical Medical Ethics*. Wiley, Chichester, pp. viii, 9–13.

Griffin, J. P. (1987). Differences between Protestant and Catholic religious ethics impinges on medical issues. *Int. Pharm. J.*, **1**, 145–148.

Laurence, D. R. (1989). Ethics and law in clinical pharmacology. *Br. J. Clin. Pharmacol.*, **27**, 718.

Medical Research Council (1991). *The Ethical Conduct of Research on Children*. Medical Research Council, London.

Medical Research Council, (1992). *Responsibility in Investigations on Human Participants and Material and on Personal Information*. Medical Research Council, London.

Medical Research Council, (1993). *Responsibility in the Use of Animals in Medical Research*. Medical Research Council, London.

Medical Research Council, (1994). *Responsibility in the Use of Personal Medical Information for Research. Principles and Guide to Practice*. Medical Research Council, London.

Mercia, M., Ponselet, F., de Meester, C., McGregor, D. B., Willins, M. J., Leonard, A. and Fabry, L. (1983). *In vitro* and *in vivo* studies on the potential mutagenicity of alclofenac, dihydroxyalclofenac and alclofenac epoxide. *J. Appl. Toxicol.*, **3**, 230–236.

News (1998). Editors call for misconduct watchdog. *Science*, **280**, 1685–1686.

ORI (1997). *ORI Newsletter*, **6**, 1–7. Office of Research Integrity, Washington, DC.

O'Rourke, K. (1996). Do low observed error rates lessen the need for study-specific data quality audits? *Controlled Clin. Trials*, **17**, 69–70.

Riis, P. (1995). Ethical issues in medical publishing. *Br. J. Urol.*, **76**, Suppl. 2, 1–4.

Rollin, B. (1989). *The Unheeded Cry: Animal Consciousness, Animal Pain and Science*. Oxford University Press, Oxford.

Royal Commission on Civil Liability (1974). *The First Circular of the Royal Commission on Civil Liability and Compensation for Personal Injury*, Para. 6, p. 2.

Skene, S. A., Dewhurst, I. C. and Greenberg, M. (1989). Polychlorinated dibenzo-*p*-dioxins and polychlorinated dibenzoxyfurans: the risks to human health. A review. *Hum. Toxicol.*, **8**, 173–203.

Smithells, R. W. and Sheppard, S. (1978). Teratogenicity testing in humans: a method demonstrating safety of Bendectin. *Teratology*, **17**, 31–35.

Stoker, D. (1996). Ethics in scientific publication—fraud, redundancy and errors. *Skel. Radiol.*, **25**, 205–206.

Swan, N. (1989). Presenting and dealing with scientific fraud in Australia. *Med. J. Aust.*, **150**, 169–170.

Walker, S. R. and Dayan, A. D. (1986). *Long-term Animal Studies, Their Predictive Value for Man.*, MTP, Lancaster.

Wells, F. O. (1995). Ethical issues in the pharmaceutical industry. *Br. J. Urol.*, **76**, Suppl. 2, 41–47.

Wells, F. O. (1997). Fraud and misconduct in medical research. *Br. J. Clin. Pharmacol.*, **43**, 3–7.

Yudkin, J. S. (1978). Provision of medicines in a developing country. *Lancet*, **1**, 810–812.

PART TEN
SPECIAL GROUPS OF SUBSTANCES

Chapter 92

Biotechnology: Safety Evaluation

John A. Thomas

CONTENTS

INTRODUCTION

History

Biotechnology has been used for centuries, but only recently has it become more complex in terms of the genetic manipulation of either plant or animal cells. Biotechnology may have various definitions, but classically it refers to techniques that change living organisms (or components of these organisms) to create or improve molecules for specific uses. Biotechnology has been used for centuries in making wine, cheese, yoghurt and bread and in the selective cross-breeding of both animals and plants—all leading to an enhancement of specific desirable traits. Only within the last two to three decades has biotechnology become an important source of new molecular moieties, including new drugs and recombinant hormones.

Applied genetics is basically the technology that involves the ability to manipulate, modify or otherwise 'engineer' genetic material. Through this technology it is possible to produce desired characteristics that have been the integral part of biotechnology (Liberman *et al.*, 1991). Genetic engineering also includes recombinant DNA technology. The contemporary era of biotechnology began about 25 years ago with the discovery of endonucleases or 'restriction enzymes' and their ability to 'cut-and-paste' segments of DNA. Such enzymes act as highly specific chemical scalpels, and hence can be used to obtain specific sequences of genetic material. Restriction enzymes recognize and can cut DNA at precise molecular locations. Recombinant DNA and similar genetic engineering procedures can lead to the transfer of genetic material from species to species.

Table 1 reveals several important events in biotechnology beginning with early fermentation techniques (e.g. antibiotics) to present-day recombinant DNA-derived products or materials. Such mileposts not only include important therapeutic proteins, but can also include environmental and agricultural improvements using these technologies. Notably, biotechnology has provided

Table 1 Selected events in biotechnology–biopharmaceutics

Year (approx.)	Milepost
1940	Commercial production of antibiotics
1953	Double helix structure of DNA discovered
1965	RNA used to break genetic code
1967	Automatic protein synthesizer developed
1967	Genetically engineered food introduced—potato
1970	Discovery of restriction enzymes (endonucleases)
1972	Splicing of viral DNA
1975	Discovery of monoclonal antibodies (hybridomas)
1976	First commercial company founded to develop recombinant DNA
1977	Expression of gene for human somatostatin
1978	Insulin produced using recombinant DNA
1978	Mammal-to-mammal gene transplants
1979	Human growth hormone and interferons reproduced
1979	Effect of recombinant BST on milk production in dairy cows
1980	Transgenic animals produced (mouse-to-mouse)
1982	Recombinant DNA animal vaccine
1982	Production of synthetic growth hormone
1983	Polymerase chain reaction (PCR) technique developed
1990	Clinical trials of human gene therapy
1993	Recombinant DNA erythropoietin
1993	Recombinant DNA blood coagulation factors
1995	Clinical use of recombinant FSH
1996	Cloning of adult mammal
1997	Plasmid DNA vaccines
1998	Further development of xenotransplants

an alternative source for many hormones that are used in endocrine replacement therapies.

There are numerous applications of these new biotechnologies. Hormone substitutes, nutritional supplements and improved food supplies are but a few general examples as to how this new biotechnology can impact the quality of life. The biotechnology industry consists of several segments, including therapeutics, diagnostics (e.g. monoclonal antibodies), agriculture and the environment. There is the potential to discover many new drug entities for the treatment of various diseases, and biotechnology will play a major role in the development of new and important diagnostic tests, therapeutic agents and vaccines.

Transgene Technologies

The advent of transgene technologies involving the transfer of a gene from one species to another has occurred along with other advances in recombinant DNA methodologies or genetic engineering. Specific laboratory mouse models for biomedical research, so-called designer mice (e.g. transgenic), are being used to study immune deficiencies, cancer and developmental biology (Goodnow, 1992; Grosveld and Kollias, 1992). Transgenic animals are produced by inserting a foreign gene into an embryo with this foreign gene subsequently becoming an integral part of the host animal's genetic material. Increasingly, there have been improvements in the techniques used for gene introduction into animals. Several techniques that have been used, including microinjections of DNA into the pronucleus, retroviral infection and embryonic stem cells which can be grown *in vitro* from explanted blastocysts. All of these techniques have been employed to create chimeric animals. It is now possible to use transgenic animals to study metabolic diseases such as diabetes mellitus, to understand better steroid receptor biochemistry and to elucidate renal and hepatic pathologies (Thomas and Thomas, 1993).

Transgenic animal models and genetically altered species have become increasingly important in the investigation of basic biochemical processes and in the development of biotherapeutics (Thomas and Thomas, 1993; Thomas, 1997). Many of these models are particularly useful in studying genetically related diseases (Tomlinson, 1992). Transgenic animals or animals engrafted with a retrovirus-derived expression vector are useful models to examine the effects of cytokines (Lubbert *et al.*, 1990). These transgene models have been very useful in studying the effects of continuous high levels of cytokines such as colony-stimulating factors (CSFs), granulocytes of interleukin (e.g. IL-2, IL-3, IL-6) and erythropoietin. Thus, these models are important in the pre-clinical safety evaluation of new biotherapeutics.

BIOPHARMACEUTICS

Introduction

The careful design of pre-clinical studies evolves around the end-use for the clinical indication of the biopharma-

ceutical (Cavagnaro, 1997). Optimization of the clinical development of biopharmaceuticals, usually proteinaceous materials, has depended upon pre-clinical protocols to assess their safety early in the discovery phase of the product development. A rational, science-based, flexible approach as been employed in the planning of pre-clinical pharmacology and toxicology studies (Cavagnaro, 1997). Such approaches have encompassed a case-by-case safety assessment of specific biotechnology-derived proteins and peptides. Peptides have emerged as high value-added biotherapeutics (Kelley, 1996). There are many peptide drugs in development, and they represent some of the same pre-clinical safety assessment challenges as more complex molecular entities such as proteins and glycoproteins.

The development of recombinant DNA technologies has allowed the pharmaceutical-related companies to synthesize large quantities of macromolecules in relatively pure form. Such technologies, often called scale-up technologies, have led to the production of therapeutic proteins including human insulin, human growth hormone, human tissue plasminogen activator (rtPA) and human erythropoietin. While hormone substitutes (e.g. insulin, HGH) represented an early entry in biopharmaceutics, several other classes of therapeutic agents have been produced or are otherwise undergoing development by the pharmaceutical industry. Since most of the early biopharmaceuticals were simple hormone replacement therapies (e.g. insulin, HGH), there was no need to undergo rigorous pre-clinical safety and efficacy studies such as those required for the interferons. During the last few years, several biopharmaceutical products have become available for various clinical indications **(Table 2)**. Human growth hormone (with or without methionine) (e.g. Genotropin, Bitropin and Norditropin) is now available for treating children with short statute or growth hormone deficiencies. New clinical indications have also been approved for some of the interferons (Intron-A for malignant melanoma; Roferon-A for chronic myelogenous leukemia). There has been more interest in the development of therapeutic agents than in the development of monoclonal antibody assays used for diagnostic agents. Blood coagulation factors and vaccines have been an important area of development. Undoubtedly, the regulatory approval for human growth hormone was accelerated by the discovery that some cadaveric human growth hormone was possibly contaminated by latent neural viruses responsible for Creutzfeld–Jacob disease.

Pre-clinical assessment of potential biotherapeutics destined for human medical therapies has brought forth the issue of immunogenicity between species. Macromolecules derived through biotechnology expectedly will challenge the immune system of the laboratory animal used for toxicological testing protocols. Despite some of these unique and early concerns, guidelines for the pre-clinical testing of high molecular weight biopharmaceu-

Table 2 Biopharmaceutics and clinical indications

Generic name	Trade name(s)	Classification	Indication(s)
Alteplase (rTPA)	Activase	Recombinant protein	Acute myocardial infarction Pulmonary embolism
Epoetin alfa (EPO)	Epogen Procrit	Recombinant protein	Anaemia of chronic renal failure Anaemia secondary to zidovudine treatment in HIV-infected patients
Antihaemophilic factor	Recombinant	Recombinant protein	Haemophilia A
Factor VIII	KoGENAte	Recombinant protein	Haemophilia A
Factor VIIIc	Monoclate-P	Recombinant protein	Haemophilia A
Factor IX	L-Nine SC	Recombinant protein	Haemophilia B
Filgrastim (G-CSF)	Neupogen	Recombinant protein	Neutropenia post-chemotherapy
Sargramostim	Leukine	Recombinant protein	Myeloid reconstitution after bone marrow transplantation
Interferon-α-2a	Roferon-A	Recombinant protein	Hairy cell leukaemia AIDS-related Kaposi's sarcoma
Interferon-α-2b	Intron-A	Recombinant protein	Hairy cell leukaemia, Kaposi's sarcoma, Hepatitis (non-A, non- B/C) *Condylomata acuminata*
Interferon-α-n3	Alferon N	Human	Genital warts
Interferon-β-1a	Avonex	Recombinant protein	Multiple sclerosis
Interferon-β-1b	Betaseron	Recombinant protein	Multiple sclerosis
Interferon-γ-1b	Actimmune	Recombinant protein	Chronic granulomatous disease
I-IGF-1	Myotropin	Recombinant protein	Amyotrophic lateral sclerosis (ALS)
Aldesleukin (IL-2)	Proleukin	Recombinant protein	Kidney cancer
Dornase-α-	Pulmozyme	Recombinant protein	Cystic fibrosis
Human insulin	Humulin	Recombinant protein	Diabetes mellitus
Somatrem (rMehGH)	Protropin	Recombinant protein	Growth hormone deficiency
Human FSH	Gonal-F	Recombinant protein	Infertility
Somatropin (rhGH)	Humatrope Nutrotropin	Recombinant protein	Growth hormone deficiency
Pegaspargase (PEG-L-asparaginase)	Oncaspar	Polyethylene glycol-modified protein	Acute lymphocytic leukaemia
Haemophilus B conjugate vaccine	HibTITER	Recombinant protein	Prophylaxis against *Haemophilus influenza*
Hepatitis B vaccine	Engeridx-B Recombivax HB	Recombinant protein	Prophylaxis against hepatitis B infection
Satumomab	OncoScint CR103	Monoclonal antibody	Colorectal cancer imaging
Satumomab	OncoScint OV103	Monoclonal antibody	Ovarian cancer imaging
Muromonab CD3 (OKT3)	Orthoceone (OKT3)	Monoclonal antibody	Acute allograft rejection

tics has proceeded and has generally been adopted by regulatory agencies. Not only has the advent of macromolecules represented a challenge to the design of toxicological protocols, but it has also led to challenges in the formulation and delivery of biopharmaceutics.

The New Biologies

Advances in the disciplines of genetics, immunology and molecular biology have provided a strong impetus for advances in biotechnology, and particularly in biopharmaceutics (Tomlinson, 1992). Advances in biotechnology-derived products could not have progressed to their current state had it not been for the coincidentally and independently developed technology of monoclonal antibodies. Recombinant DNA technologies and monoclonal antibody methodologies are two areas that are inseparably important to the development of new bio-

pharmaceutics. Monoclonal antibodies are very important in the identification, extraction and purification of most macromolecules.

The term molecular biology has come to signify particularly the biochemical study of nucleic acids, advanced by the discovery of a series of enzymes (viz. endonucleases) that allow specific manipulations of RNA and DNA. There are several new techniques or approaches used in molecular biology **(Table 3)** (Ausubel, 1995). The ability to manipulate the genetic material of a cell in order to modify gene expression has utilized a variety of techniques leading to new biopharmaceutics. Increasingly, a broad range of molecular biology techniques have become routine.

Major initiatives in recombinant DNA technologies have focused upon mammalian macromolecules, often peptides, for discovering therapeutically useful proteins. Mammalian biotechnology has advanced more rapidly than plant biotechnology, although the latter field

Table 3 Methodologies important to the new biologies

Recombinant DNA techniques
- Site-directed mutagenesis
- Single-strand conformational polymorphism (SSCP)
- Ligated gene fusions

Hybridoma technology
- Production of antibodies

Carbohydrate engineering

Novel instrumental techniques
- Polymerase chain reaction (PCR) and reverse transcription PCR (RT-PCR)
- Subtractive hybridization differential display
- Immunoblotting
- Confocal laser microscopy
- Fluorescence-activated cell sorting (FACS)
- Scanning tunnelling electron microscopy

Pulsed field electrophoresis

Northern blotting and solution hybridization

In situ hybridization

Southern blotting: gene deletions

Source: Demain (1991); Davis (1996).

promises to be very fast moving. Early successes witnessed the use of prokaryotic all systems (e.g. *E. coli*) capable of producing rather complex mammalian proteins (e.g. insulin). Subsequently, and with more advances in techniques employed in molecular biology, prokaryotic cell systems were found to be able to secrete even more complex proteins and glycoproteins (Tomlinson, 1992). Through improved methods of molecular characterization, it has been possible to create more complex and more highly purified molecular entities that possess therapeutic potential. Mammalian organisms possess a plethora of proteins that modulate many physiological processes.

Molecular biology, particularly through the use of polymerase chain reactions (PCR), has become very important in the discovery and production of recombinant proteins. Acting as a molecular 'photocopier', PCR has been employed extensively to amplify DNA sequences. Subsequently, the design of new biopharmaceutics can proceed with sufficient quantities of purified material in order to fulfil the amounts required for both pre-clinical and clinical protocols.

Most new biopharmaceutics usually must be administered parenterally. Proteins or large peptides are vulnerable to gastric degradation and loss of biological activity. There is considerable interest and the need to develop drug delivery systems for these macromolecules. Selective drug targeting is a characteristic that would be highly desirable. Advances have been made with some biopharmaceutics to modify their biological dispersion. Such approaches have included site-directed mutagenesis and hybrid site-specific proteins (Demain, 1991).

General Pharmacological Principles

Since the majority of recombinant substances are relatively large protein molecules **(Table 4)**, there are a number of physicochemical characteristics that must be considered in their pharmacological and toxicological evaluation **(Table 5)**. Generally, high molecular weight substances are very poorly absorbed by the oral route of administration. For example, either recombinant human insulin or recombinant human growth hormone (HGH) must be administered by a parenteral route of administration, thus by passing the proteotytic environment of the stomach. Because these recombinant products are usually proteins, glycoproteins or peptides, they are often antigenic and hence can provoke immune responses. Finally, blood aminopeptidases and other proteolytic enzymes often result in recombinant proteins having brief biological half-lives.

An early consideration in planning for the toxicological assessment of a prospective recombinant substance is the therapeutic use of the product **(Table 6)**. Diagnostic recombinant products (e.g. monoclonal antibody kits) are non-invasive and require less rigorous toxicological evaluation. Replacement products (i.e. hormones) such as insulin or HGH represent physiological supplements and hence reduce the likelihood of suprapharmacological levels causing side-effects. Also, the replacement of otherwise physiologically active substances minimizes the provocation of the immune system. Substances that require multiple injections in order to achieve a desired therapeutic effect (e.g. immunomodulators), particularly if they do not mimic a physiological mediator, are prone to alter the immune system.

Table 4 Selected rDNA-derived therapeutic products

Agent	Mol. wt (approx.)	Chemical composition
tPA(s)	25 000 – 100 000	Glycoprotein
Insulin	5 100	Protein
Erythropoietin	36 000	Glycoprotein
Interferon	17 000 – 25 000	Glycoproteins
HGH	21 500	Protein
Hepatitis B vaccine	Various sub-units	Glycoprotein
Factor VIII	> 1 000 000 (200 000–>3 000 000 sub-units)	Glycoprotein

Table 5 General pharmacological/toxicological characteristics of high molecular weight substances

- Poor oral absorption
- Usually protein or protein-like
- Often antigenic
- Brief biological half-life
- Provocation of immune response, causing reduced therapeutic effectiveness (i.e. resistance)

Table 6 rDNA derived protein—therapeutic use/purpose

- ■ Short-term/acute regimen
  - —Single injection (e.g. hepatitis B vaccine)
- ■ Intermediate regimen
  - —Multi-injections (e.g. tPA)
- ■ Prolonged administration
  - —Years (5–10) (e.g. HGH)
- ■ Lifetime replacement
  - —Hormonal and/or genetic (e.g. insulin, Factor VIII)

Table 7 Pre-test considerations for rDNA-derived proteins

■ Solubility	■ Acute vs chronic administration
■ Choice of vehicle	■ Species (small vs large animal)
■ Stability in solution	■ Dose ranging/standards
■ Route of administration	■ Comparison with prototype

Pre-test consideration for assessing the toxicology of recombinant substances requires host factors ranging from physicochemical properties to selecting the most suitable animal model **(Table 7)**. During the early discovery or advent of recombinant technologies, it was often difficult to secure sufficient amounts of the potential product and hence it was necessary to resort to *in vitro* test systems or small animals. Increasingly, gene amplification systems have been incorporated into the replication clones so that reasonably sufficient amounts of end-product are now available. With newer recombinant products, it has also not always been possible to identify a comparable prototype.

Some recombinant products have vastly different pharmacological profiles **(Table 8)**. While they may all be represented as protein substances, they have different onsets of action. The biological response may be very rapid (e.g. tPA) or it may require years (e.g. HGH) before its pharmacological efficacy is established. Some end-points used for either pharmacological or toxicological end-points may be very objective (e.g. blood clotting),

Table 8 Selected pharmacological properties of rDNA-derived agents

Agent	Pharmacological action	Onset	End-point
tPA	Clot dissolution	Rapid	Rapid (minutes)
Insulin	Hypoglyaemic	Rapid/ intermediate	Intermediate (minutes/ hours)
	Erythropoietin intermediate	Anti-anaemic Intermediate (days)	Rapid/ Interferon
	Immunomodulator	Rapid/ intermediate	Long (months/ years)
HGH	Protein anabolic	Intermediate	Long (years)

while still others may be less objective or even subjective (e.g. immunomodulators). Immunopharmacological agents or agents affecting the immune system may involve many complex biochemical interactions with lymphokines, cytokines, complement, kinins, autocoids and even neuropeptides (Pope, 1989).

Toxicological Testing and Drug Design

Proteins that are coincidentally used as drugs (or more appropriately hormones) have been used for many years. Animal-derived proteins (e.g. insulin—ovine, bovine and porcine) have been used therapeutically for several decades in the medical management of diabetes mellitus. Usually, patients receiving animal insulin possess titres of antibody, but seldom of either immunological significance or refractiveness to the hormone. Human proteins as drugs represent somewhat of a dilemma, in that these same substances become foreign proteins in the experimental animal. Thus species selection takes on an even greater significance in an effort to extrapolate to humans (Marafino *et al.*, 1988). The toxicological testing protocol of a recombinant product should contain both an immunological evaluation, i.e. safety, and a non-immunological evaluation, i.e. safety and efficacy **(Table 9)**. Immunogenicity testing may involve both *in vitro* and *in vivo* systems. The non-immunological evaluation is product specific and the animal testing strategy is focused upon the substance's therapeutic use. When the studies begin to examine the protein's biodistribution, it is usually necessary to have some means of measurement or identification. The development of a radioimmunoassay or a specific monoclonal antibody is often the only means for the product's detection. Alternatively, large protein molecules can be iodinated and hence afford some insight into their biodistribution, but usually not their metabolic fate. Target organ accumulation (or lack of) can be ascertained with iodinated protein, but may lack some degree of specificity.

Many new drug candidates, both recombinant and others, are being developed for the sole therapeutic purpose of affecting the immune system (Norbury, 1985). There is no uniform consensus of what constitutes a general battery of immunotoxicological procedures.

Table 9 Toxicological testing of rDNA-derived proteins

I. Immunological evaluation (safety)
- ■ Immunogenicity testing
  - *In vivo* (single vs multiple injection)
  - *In vitro*

II. Non-immunological evaluation (safety and efficacy)
- ■ Product specific
- ■ Pharmacologic/toxicologic profile
  - *In vitro* tests
  - *In vivo* tests (acute vs chronic)

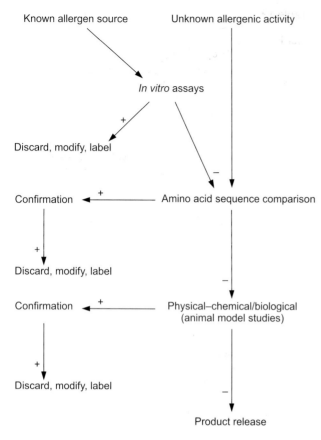

Figure 1 Testing recombinant proteins for their immunogenicity. Source: Lehrer *et al.* (1996).

The multiplicity of cell types that comprise the immune system precludes the use of a single test that evaluates all of the possible immunological changes. All immunological assays should be supplemented with routine clinical chemistries, haematology and histopathology. Potential allergenicity, including both immediate and delayed type hypersensitivity, should be included in the toxicological evaluation **(Figure 1)** (Lehrer *et al.*, 1996). A basic immunotoxicological profile should include

- Lymphoproliferation;
- Popliteal lymph node enlargement;
- Antibody response;
- Natural killer cells.

All of these assays represent a reasonable immunotoxicological profile. The National Toxicology Program (NTP) (Luster *et al.*, 1986) has proposed a two-tiered approach to determine immunotoxicity. Tier I, or screen, includes immunopathology, humoral-mediated immunity (IgM antibody plaques), cell-mediated immunity (T-cell response to mitogens) and non-specific immunity (natural killer cell activity). Tier II is more comprehensive and includes immunopathology (BT-cell response), humoral-mediated immunity (IgG antibody response), cell-mediated immunity (cytotoxic T-cell lysis of tumour

Table 10 Some safety considerations of biotechnologically derived products

Product-related impurities or variants
Genetic variants and mutants
Aggregated forms
Glycosylation patterns
Process-related impurities
Pyrogens
DNA and potential oncogenicity
Host cell-derived proteins
Viruses (human, simian, murine, bovine)

Source: Tomlinson (1992).

cells), non-specific immunity (macrophage function) and host resistance challenge modes (tumour cell, bacterial and viral systems).

Evaluating the 'safety' of drugs produced by biotechnology resembles the assessment of conventional new chemical entities (NCE), but with certain major differences in testing protocols (Zbinden, 1990; Dayan, 1995). Several aspects of the new biotechnologies represent a challenge to the classical pre-clinical safety and efficacy protocols. A host of safety considerations must be incorporated into the pre-clinical testing protocols **(Table 10)** (Tomlinson, 1992). The quality of each biotechnology-derived product necessitates careful control because of concern about immunogenic protein or peptides, endotoxins released by the harvesting of prokaryotic cell systems that secrete the product and other possible chemical contaminants emanating from the processing procedures. According to Zbinden (1990), there are at least three areas of concern regarding biotechnology-derived products: (1) toxicology issues pertaining to differences in pharmacodynamic properties, (2) 'intrinsic' toxicity, i.e. adverse effects due to the molecule itself and not a direct result of pharmacodynamic actions, and (3) 'biological' toxicity, responses resulting from the activation of a physiological mechanism (e.g. antigen–antibody reaction).

There are several toxicological or safety issues that form the basis of toxicity testing. There are safety issues pertaining to the intrinsic actions of the product itself and there are safety issues pertaining to the cellular system or process that lead to the production or secretion of the macromolecule (Thomas and Thomas, 1993; Dayan, 1995; Thomas, 1995). Product-related impurities or variants might include mutants, aggregated forms and aberrant glycosylation. Process-related impurities might include pyrogens, host-cell derived proteins, viruses and possibly prions (Jeffcoate, 1992). **Table 11** contains a summary of some of the more important aspects in evaluating the safety of potential biopharmaceutics (Dayan, 1995). Reliable cell systems, expressing the correct gene and ensuring its proper insertion along with any promoter are of fundamental importance. The secretion or presence of other bioactive moieties must always be a considered, and needs to be addressed through proper

Table 11 Selected guidelines for evaluating biopharmaceutics

Toxicological issues arising from the producing system

- Prokaryotic production system (recombinant DNA)
  Correct gene and promoter, stable expression, contaminating toxins, etc.
- Eukaryotic production system (recombinant DNA)
  Correct gene and promoter; stable expression, presence of antigens, other bioactive peptides, etc.
- Other
  Chemical modifications, infection-free animal vectors, etc.

Toxicological issues arising from the production process

- De- and re-naturation of protein(s)
- Presence of other bioactive molecules
- Presence of chemical residues
- Microbial contamination
  (e.g. endotoxins)

Toxicological issues arising from biopharmaceutics

- Pharmacodynamics
- Pharmacological and toxicological actions
- Immunological
- Other (e.g. live or attenuated vaccine)

Source: modified from Dayan (1995).

Table 12 Panel for detecting immune alterations

Tier I
Haematology (e.g. leukocyte counts)
Weights—body, spleen, thymus, kidney, liver
Cellularity—spleen, bone marrow
Histology of lymphoid organ
IgM antibody plaque-forming cells (PFCs)
Lymphocyte blastogenesis:
  T-cell mitogens (PHA, con A)
  T-cell (mixed leukocyte response, MLR)
  β-cell (lipopolysaccharide, LPS)
Natural killer (NK) cell activity

Tier II
Quantitation of splenic B and T lymphocytes
Lymphocytes (surface markers)
Enumeration of IgG antibody PFC response
Cytotoxic T lymphocyte (CTL)
Cytolysis or delayed hypersensitivity response (DHR)
Host resistance:
  Syngeneic tumour cells
  PYB6 sarcoma (tumour incidence)
  B16F10 melanoma (lung burden)
Bacterial models:
  Listeria monocytogenes (morbidity)
  Streptococcus species (morbidity)
Viral models:
  Influenza (morbidity)
Parasite models:
  Plasmodium yoelii (parasitaemia)

Source: condensed from Luster *et al.* (1992).

extraction and purification processes. Protein or peptide contaminants can produce both unwanted immunological and non-immunological actions. Clinical or standard toxicological protocols may not be relevant in attempting to characterize the pharmacodynamics of a macromolecule. Non-immunological testing is dependent on the products potential therapeutic use and, at a minimum, testing should include biodistribution, developmental and reproductive, and mutagenicity/oncogenicity assessments. It is very important that a panel for detecting possible immune alterations be an integral part of the toxicology testing protocol **(Table 12)**. The first tier consists of a screening panel which evaluates immunopathology, cell-mediated immunity and humoral immunity. Tier I should identify agents that may elicit an immune response. Those agents testing positive in Tier I are subsequently evaluated in more detail. Tier II seeks to evaluate the presence of any immunopathological effects.

Case Studies—Safety Evaluation

Insulin

Insulin was the first recombinant product to be approved by the US FDA for the treatment of diabetes mellitus (Galloway and Chance, 1983). Because mammalian insulins are simple proteins, prokaryotic cell systems could be employed. Insulin has been cloned from *E. coli* either by constructing a gene that produces proinsulin or by constructing a gene for the A-chain and a gene for the B-chain of the insulin molecule. In the latter cloning strategy, the A-chain and the B-chain are assembled chemically.

Insulin was a relatively easy recombinant product to produce because insulin's amino acid sequence was already established, and its safety and efficacy did not have to be subject to overly rigorous pharmacological or toxicological evaluation. Nevertheless, recombinant insulin underwent a fairly extensive battery of physicochemical and toxicological tests **(Table 13)**. This battery of physicochemical tests ensured molecular integrity and purity. Because prokaryotic systems were used, and because this necessitates harvesting the insulin from the *E. coli* by bursting its plasma membrane, it requires testing for endotoxins and/or pyrogens. In addition to these battery of tests **(Table 13)**, metabolic clearance rates of recombinant insulin labelled with radioactive iodine (^{125}I) were compared with ^{125}I-labelled porcine insulin. Thus, pre-clinical toxicological evaluation of recombinant insulin proceeded rapidly to clinical trials and approval by the US FDA.

Table 13 Evaluation tests for human insulin (rDNA)

USP rabbit hypoglycaemia assay
Insulin radioreceptor assay
In vitro bioassays
Insulin radioimmunoassay
Amino acid composition and sequence
HPLC fragment analysis
Polyacrylamide gel electrophoresis
HPLC—identity and purity
Absorption and circular dichroic spectra
Zinc insulin crystallization
X-ray diffraction analysis
Limulus test for endotoxin
USP rabbit pyrogen test
E. coli polypeptide radioimmunoassay

Human Growth Hormone (HGH) and Bovine Somatotropin

Unlike insulin, which was not in short supply for the treatment of diabetes, human growth hormone had to be obtained from limited sources of cadaveric pituitary glands prior to the advent of recombinant HGH. Similarly to insulin, the physiological actions of human growth hormones were known and hence it was perhaps not subjected to overly rigorous toxicological testing. Another factor that accelerated the cloning of both insulin and HGH was that the amino acid sequences had already been established for each hormone. Such information facilitated molecular confirmation and purity testing. However, HGH is a more complex molecule (Chawia *et al.*, 1983) than insulin and has a considerably higher molecular weight.

Initial efforts to clone rHGH resulted in an additional terminal amino acid, methionine. Subsequent safety and efficacy testing comparing methionine HGH with HGH failed to reveal any significant biological difference despite the presence of an additional amino aid.

Despite the established safety of human cadaveric GH, several safety and efficacy tests were required for regulatory agency approval of rHGH **(Table 14)**. The human pituitary dwarf responds only to monkey or human growth hormone. However, several animal species of GH will promote growth in the hypophysectomized rat. Hence this rat model has been used extensively in rHGH assessment.

Table 14 Summary for FDA basis for approving rHGH

- Provide lyophilized product
- Stability and purity (e.g. SDS, PAGE, NPLC)
- Absence of contaminants (*E. coli* proteins/peptides)
- Efficacy data (e.g. weight gain in rats)
- Comparison of natural vs rHGH
- Acute and subacute toxicity data (rats and monkeys)
- Immunotoxicology (e.g. autoantibodies)
- Clinical trials (4-year period)

Recombinant bovine somatotropin (rbSt) has been evaluated with respect to its safety and efficacy in lactating dairy cows (Marcek *et al.*, 1989). The advent of rbSt makes possible increased milk production. Toxicological assessments revealed this recombinant hormone not to be a teratogen nor have any side-effects on the neonate. It is not antigenic and has little effect upon blood chemistries and haematology.

Tissue Plasminogen Activator (tPA) and Blood Clotting Factors

tPA is an endogenous trypsin-like serine protease that is used clinically to lyse blood clots. There are both natural and recombinant 'clot busters'. The pharmacology and therapeutic use of this thrombolytic agent have been extensively reviewed (Collen *et al.*, 1989). rtPA is similar to, or identical with, the physiological plasminogen activators in blood. rtPA does not induce an antibody response and it is more fibrin-specific than most or all other known thrombolytic agents (Collen *et al.*, 1989).

Many safety and efficacy tests have been recommended for rtPA **(Table 15)**. Both rodent and non-rodent species are recommended and at dose projections of one, three and ten times that anticipated for clinical trials. Considerable efforts were devoted to establishing reliable and reproducible quantitative clot dissolution models in rabbits and in dogs. The use of ^{125}I-labelled fibrinogen as a means of monitoring clot dissolution aided in establishing the thrombolytic properties of rtPA (Cossum, 1989).

Blood clotting Factor VIII has been cloned, tested for its safety and efficacy and approved for clinical use. Likewise, Factor VIII:C (antihaemophilic factor) has been cloned and expressed. These complex glycoproteins are subjected to the same rigorous purity and stability assurances as other recombinant products. They do, however, necessitate special animal models to determine blood clotting efficacy. Special inbred colonies of dogs that exhibit genetically defective blood clotting disorders can be used to study the effectiveness of recombinant Factor VIII and Factor VIII:C (antihaemophilic factor). In both instances it is necessary to develop a specific monoclonal antibody (Mab) in order to measure these factors.

Table 15 Some recommended toxicity testing for tPA

- Acute toxicity (1, 3 and 10 × clinical dose) (4 species)
- Subchronic toxicity (rat, dog or monkey)
- Guinea pig maximization test
- Cardiopulmonary function in dogs (3 × clinical dose)
- Ames test
- Cytogenetic tests in rats (1, 3 and 10 × clinical dose)
- Peripheral vein—clot dissolution model (rabbit)
- Coronary artery—clot dissolution model (dog)
- Pharmacokinetic studies in rabbit (iodinated tPA)

Erythropoietin (EPO)

EPO is a hormone synthesized primarily by the kidney. It regulates the production of red blood cells by the erythroid marrow. Recombinant human erythropoietin (r-HuEPO) has been cloned and expressed in Chinese hamster ovary. r-HuEPO (Epogen) is used clinically to enhance the quality of life of anaemic patients (Winearls, 1989; Evans *et al.*, 1990). The most significant advance in the development of r-HuEPO was establishing a specific radioimmunoassay (RIA) for its detection. This RIA for EPO led to its isolation, fractionation and amino acid sequencing. Both a bioassay and eventually a Mab assay were required for it to be properly evaluated for safety and efficacy **(Table 16)**. Early bioassays for EPO often involved using the stimuli of anoxia in experimental animals (e.g. mice) for quantifying subsequent increases in red blood cells, but Mab assays have rendered this bioassays obsolete.

Table 16 Toxicological testing for erythropoietin (EPO)

- Purity (contaminants, pyrogenicity)
- Bioassay and Mab assay
- Acute toxicity (2 species)
- Subchronic toxicity (2 species)
- Antigenicity (guinea pig)
- Genotoxicity:
- Ames test
- Cytogenicity testing
- Pharmacokinetics

Interferons (INF)

The interferons (INFs) have been examined for anti-cancer and anti-infective properties. Animal models (e.g. Rhesus monkey) used to evaluate antimalarial and antiviral properties of human interferon gamma (HuINFg) and human interferon alpha 2 (HuINFα2) have proved useful in toxicological testing (Cossum, 1989). The chimpanzee is a better subhuman primate model than either the Rhesus or the Cynomolgus, but cost and limited availability preclude their widespread use for safety evaluation of rHuINFs. Several INFs (e.g. Roferon-A and Interon-A) are used clinically **(Table 2)**.

The pre-clinical testing and development of INFα2a (Roferon-A) involves a thorough and progressive battery of immunological and non-immunological evaluations (Trown *et al.*, 1986). Both acute and subchronic toxicity tests have been completed in several species including subhuman primates **(Table 17)**. Pre-clinical tests not only examined different species, but also various routes of administration were studied and local tolerance tests, dose ranging, reproductive assessment, and reversibility of INF-induced changes were recorded. Of four animal models examined, and after 2–13 weeks of INF administration, antibody titres were detected in the Cynomolgus monkey, the guinea pig and the rabbit. Other safety and efficacy evaluations for INF include:

- Antitumuor activity;
- *In vitro* antiproliferation studies;
- Inhibition of human tumour colony formation;
- Nude mouse studies;
- Pharmacokinetics (African green monkey).

Table 17 INF toxicity testing: acute and subchronic

Type of study	Study	Species	Route of administration	Length of treatment (weeks)
Acute parenteral toxicity	Single-dose	Mouse	i.m.	
			i.v.	
			s.c.	
		Rat	i.m.	
			i.v.	
			s.c.	
		Rabbit	i.m.	
			i.v.	
		Ferret	i.m.	
			s.c.	
	LD$_{50}$	Mouse	i.v.	
	Local tolerance	Rat	Venous irritation	
		Mouse	Venous irritation	
		Rabbit	Muscle irritation	
Subchronic toxicity		Squirrel monkey	i.m.	2
		Rhesus monkey	i.m.	4
		Mouse	i.m.	5
		Cynomolgus monkey	i.m.	13

Source: modified from Trown *et al.* (1986).

Unlike evaluating recombinant hormones (e.g. insulin, HGH), some information obtained from the pre-clinical testing of INF was less meaningful. Certain human proteins are species-restricted, but the fact that INFα2a is a protein that is antigenic in experimental animals may compromise toxicological end-points. Thus the development of neutralizing antibodies to INFα2a in laboratory animals may not only affect its antiviral and antitumour properties, but might also mask adverse effects produced by the recombinant product.

Lymphokines

There are a large number of lymphokines **(Table 18)** (Pope, 1989). Human IL-2 has undergone pre-clinical and clinical testing as an anticancer agent (Winkelhake and Gauny, 1990) **(Table 2)**. Initial testing of recombinant lymphokines involves various *in vitro* tests using both normal and neoplastic cell systems. Testing for antineoplastic activity involves both *in vitro* and *in vivo* tumour models. Some recombinant cytokines (G-CSF and GM-CSF) are clinically available and used for the treatment of bone marrow suppression associated with cancer therapy (Dozier, 1991) **(Table 2)**. These haematopoietic colony stimulating factors—granulocyte colony stimulating factor (G-CSF) and granulocyte–macrophage colony stimulating factor (GM-CSF)—act as chemical messengers between cells to stimulate the proliferation of blood cell precursors in bone marrow. These recombinant products promote full maturing and functionality of circulating blood cells. GM-CSF (e.g. Leukine, Prokine) is manufactured using yeast cells to express the GM-CSF gene. The Chinese hamster ovary cells and *E. coli* have also been used to express rGM-CSF.

Table 18 Selected list of biologically active lymphokines

Lymphokine	Major biological activity
IL-1	Enhanced IL-2 receptor expression on T-cells
IL-2	Enhanced T-cell proliferation
IL-3	Proliferation/differentiation of granulocytes, macrophages, etc.
IL-4	Stimulation of class II MHC antigen
IL-5	Differentiation of antigen-primed B-cells and cytotoxic cells
IL-6	Terminal differentiation of antigen-primed B-cells
IL-7	Growth and maturation of precursor B-cells
TNF	T-cell proliferation and lymphatic secretion
IFNg	Antiviral and antineoplastic activity

Source: modified from Pope (1989).

Growth Factors and Neurotrophic Factors

There are many cellular growth factors (Van Brunt and Klausner, 1988; Nimni, 1997). While their nomenclature is often confusing, they are perhaps best known by their initials, EGF (epidermal growth factor), FGF (fibroblast growth factor), PDGF (platelet-derived growth factor), TGF (alpha-and beta-transforming growth factors) and IGF (insulin growth factor). Therapeutic interest lies in their wound-healing properties. Some may stimulate endothelial cell growth (e.g. capillary growth), and growth of bone and connective tissue. Recombinant EGF has undergone clinical trials for healing corneal transplants and non-healing corneal defects. These growth factors are challenges for the toxicologist to ensure that these recombinant products are safe.

Toxicology protocols have been described for neurotrophic factors (Yaksh *et al.*, 1997). r-metHuBDNF (recombinant-methionyl human brain-derived neurotrophic factor) is a growth factor that may play a role in the therapy of certain trophic diseases of the central nervous system. As a potential recombinant product, it poses several challenges to the toxicologist, including a delivery system using lumbar intrathecal catheters. To assess the neurotrophic factor pharmacokinetics required the use of a dog with a backpack pump for continuous infusion. The toxicology protocol included drug kinetics, dose-ranging and safety studies and recovery studies. Ante-mortem observations may include neurological assessment, monitoring of cardiovascular function and CSF pressure measurements. Enzyme-linked immunosorbent assays (ELISAs) were developed for r-metHuBDNF to assist in determining its pharmacokinetics. The ELISA also assisted in determining the clearance profile of the neurotrophic factor from the CSF in the cisternal and lumbar space following bolus intrathecal infusions. Inulin can be used as a marker for extracellular space which aids in studying the neurotrophic factor's toxicokinetics (Yaksh *et al.*, 1997). The aforementioned case study represents a creative toxicological approach to determining the pre-clinical safety of a recombinant protein with CNS properties.

Regulatory

There are some difficulties in conceiving the applicable guidelines for the safety evaluation of biotechnology-derived products (Claude, 1992; Cohen-Haguenauer, 1996). Safety is highly dependent on the particular industrial process and on its quality control. Pharmaceutical companies and regulatory agencies responsible for public health must establish relevant and meaningful guidelines for the pre-clinical and clinical evaluation of new biopharmaceutics. When possible, there should be an effort to compare the new biopharmaceutics with a natural biological entity. Regulatory guidelines must be mindful of the importance of selecting an appropriate animal model.

Manufacturing procedures for biopharmaceutics are a very important part of the safety and regulatory process

Table 19 Aspects of regulatory importance

Source materials
  Genetically engineered microorganisms
  Transformed mammalian cell lines
  Hybridoma technology
Manufacture
  Clear production strategy and in-process controls
  Validation of virus inactivation and removal
Purification of final product
  Fraction and chromatographic procedures
  Affinity purification (e.g. Mab)
  Pasteurization
  Lyophilization
End-product quality
  Accurate and precise methods
  Rigorous specifications

Source: modified from Jeffcoate (1992).

Table 20 Regulatory aspects of biotechnology

Country	Regulatory Committee/Agency
Europe (EU)	Committee on Proprietary Medicinal Products (CPMP):
	Safety Working Party (SWP)
	Biotechnology Quality Working Party (BQWP)
	Operations Working Party (OWP)
	Council Directive 87.22 EEC:
	Concertation Procedure
	Notes for Guidance, e.g. pre-clinical safety (1987)
Japan (MHW)	Pharmaceutical Affairs Bureau (PAB)
	Central Pharmaceutical Affairs Council (CPAC):
	Committee on Drugs
	Committee on Antibiotic Drugs
	Committee on Blood Products
	National Institute of Hygienic Sciences:
	Notification No. 243 (1984)
	Notification No. 10 (1988)
USA (FDA)	Center for Drug Evaluation and Research (CDER)
	Center for Biologic Evaluation and Research (CBER)
	Public Health Services Act
	Food, Drug and Cosmetic Act:
	Federal Register: biotechnology notice (1984)
	Federal Register: regulation of biotechnology
	Product (class) oriented 'Points to Consider' (PTC)

Source: Bass *et al.* (1992); Thomas (1995); see also chapter 77.

(Jeffcoate, 1992; Federici, 1994). Certain aspects of the manufacturing process that convert the new biologicals into biopharmaceutics require attention by both manufacturers and regulatory agencies **(Table 19)**.

Biopharmaceutics are generally classified as biologicals by the regulatory agencies. Such a classification would ordinarily include 'any virus, therapeutic serum, toxin, antitoxin or analogous product applicable to the prevention, treatment or cure of diseases or injuries of man'. The quality control of biopharmaceutics engenders many of the same concepts as those applied to the analysis of conventional or low molecular weight pharmaceuticals.

In the USA, the FDA has the regulatory responsibility for approving genetically engineered products, particularly those that are to be used as either diagnostic or therapeutic agents. Various regulatory committees or agencies have been designated for ensuring the safety of recombinant products. The USDA and the US EPA are other regulatory agencies that become involved if the product is contained in a foodstuff or otherwise might pose an environmental concern **(Table 20)**. The Bureau of Biologicals of the FDA is generally responsible for approval of genetically engineered products. By definition, a biological product is 'any virus, therapeutic serum, toxin, antitoxin vaccine, blood, blood component or derivative, allergenic product, or analogous product ... applicable to the prevention, treatment or cure of diseases or injuries of man ...'. The FDA applies the same regulations and standards for a IND (Investigational New Drug) for a biological as it does for a drug. Good manufacturing practices (GMPs) apply to both biologicals and drugs (Miller and Young, 1988).

The approval of rDNA-derived products sometimes represents some unique criteria. It is possible that the recombinant's product may differ in molecular structure from that of the natural substance. Thus, certain human recombinant growth hormones contain an extra N-terminal amino acid (e.g. methionine). Conversely, bacterial-produced recombinant products may have the same amino acid sequence as the natural product, but the molecular stoichiometry might differ. It is not uncommon for large protein or protein-like molecules to fold or otherwise assume non-physiological conformational orientations. It is also possible for genetic variants of recombinant proteins to occur during fermentation processes leading to mutations in the gene's coding sequences. Similarly, fermentation processes may produce partial products or peptides that can potentially evoke toxicological responses. Documentation of biosynthetic agents through rDNA technology should fulfil requirements for documentation for new drugs produced by more conventional methodologies (Sjodia, 1988). The identity, purity and reproducible quality of the recombinant product must be established and documented. Toxicological or safety testing must be appropriately applied to batches of product.

Toxicity testing on recombinant products includes the customary clinical chemistry and histopathology. A sensitive and quantitative analysis of circulating antibodies is required. In fact, a highly specific monoclonal antibody (Mab) must be developed very early in order to monitor the biodistribution of the recombinant product,

Table 21 Phases in drug development

New drug			
Pre-clinical $\longrightarrow$	Clinical investigation $\longrightarrow$ (IND)	Marketing application $\longrightarrow$ (NDA)	Post-marketing
Biological product			
Pre-clinical $\longrightarrow$	Clinical investigation $\longrightarrow$ (IND)	Marketing application $\longrightarrow$ (PLA, ELA)	Post-marketing

for both pharmacokinetic and toxicokinetic information. Testing for immunotoxicity is important for FDA submissions for recombinant products. Whether the intended therapeutic use of the recombinant protein product involves a single administration or a multiple administration can affect the agents potential for immunogenicity.

The phases of drug development for a new drug and for a biologic product do not differ to any great extent (Esber, 1988) **(Table 21)**. These phases consist of the preclinical phase, a clinical investigational or IND phase, the marketing application and the post-marketing phase. The marketing application specified by US Federal Food, Drug and Cosmetic Act is the New Drug Application (NDA). For the biological product or recombinant, the licence application includes both the US Product License Application (PLA) and the establishment License Application (ELA). Whether a drug or a biological, the issues remain safety, purity, potency and efficacy. There is a pharmacological basis for the safety assessment of recombinant human proteins (Cossum, 1989). With the great variation and increasing complexities of recombinant proteins, it is probably the safest approach to adopt a case-by-case review of a particular product before it receives regulatory approval.

REFERENCES

Ausubel, F. M. (1995). *Current Protocols in Molecular Biology*. Wiley, New York.

Bass, R., Kleeberg, U., Schroder, H. and Scheibner, E. (1992). Current guidelines for the preclinical safety assessment of therapeutic proteins. *Toxicol. Lett.*, **64/65**, 339–347.

Cavagnaro, J. A. (1997). Considerations in the preclinical safety evaluation of biotechnology-derived products. In Sipes, I. G., McQueen, C. A. and Gandolfi, A. J. (Eds), *Comprehensive Toxicology. Toxicological Testing and Evaluation*, Vol. 2. Pergamon Press, Toronto, pp. 291–298.

Chawia, R. K., Parks, J. S. and Rudman, D. (1983). Structural variants of human growth hormone: biochemical, genetic, and clinical aspects. *Annu. Rev. Med.*, **34**, 519–547.

Claude, J. R. (1992). Difficulties in conceiving and applying guidelines for the safety evaluation of biotechnologically-produced drugs: some examples. *Toxicol. Lett.*, **64/65**, 349–355.

Cohen-Haguenauer, O. (1996). Safety and regulation at the leading edge of biomedical biotechnology. *Curr. Opini. Biotechnol.*, **7**, 265–272.

Collen, D., Lijnen, H. R., Todd, P. A. and Goa, K. (1989). Tissue-type plasminogen activator. *Drugs*, **38**, 346–388.

Cossum, P. A. (1989). Pharmacologic basis for the safety assessment of recombinant human proteins. *J. Am. Coll. Toxicol.*, **8**, 1133–1138.

Davis, J. R. E. (1996). Molecular biology techniques in endocrinology. *Clin. Mol. Endocrinol.*, **45**, 125–133.

Dayan, A. D. (1995). Safety evaluation of biological and biotechnology-derived medicines. *Toxicology*, **105**, 59–68.

Demain, A. L. (1991). An overview of biotechnology. *Occup. Med. State Art Rev.*, **6**, 157–168.

Dozier, N. (1991). Hematopoietic growth factors: focus on GM-CSF. *US Pharm.*, **16**, H1–H8.

Esber, E. C. (1988). Regulatory concerns for biologics: United States perspectives. In Marshak, D. R. and Liu, D. J. (Eds), *Banbury Report 29: Therapeutic Peptides and Proteins: Assessing the New Technologies*. Cold Spring Harbor Laboratory Press, Cold Spring Harbor, NY, pp. 265–273.

Evans, R. W., Rader, B., Manninen, D. L. and the Cooperative Multicenter EPO Clinical Trial Group (1990). The quality of life of hemodialysis recipients treated with recombinant human erythropoietin. *J. Am. Med. Assoc.*, **263**, 825–830.

Federici, M. M. (1994). The quality control of biotechnology products. *Int. Assoc. Biol. Stand.*, **22**, 151–159.

Galloway, J. A. and Chance, R. E. (1983). Human insulin rDNA: from rDNA through the FDA. In Lemberger, L. and Reidenberg, M. M. (Eds), *Proceedings of the Second World Conference on Clinical Pharmacology and Therapeutics*. American Society for Pharmacology and Experimental Therapeutics, Washington, DC, pp. 503–520.

Goodnow, C. C. (1992). Transgenic mice and analysis of β-cell tolerance. *Annu. Rev. Immunol.*, **10**, 489–518.

Grosveld, F. and Kollias, G. (1992). *Transgenic Animals*. Academic Press, San Diego.

Jeffcoate, S. L. (1992). New biotechnologies: challenges for the regulatory authorities. *J. Pharm. Pharmacol.*, **44**, Suppl. 1, 191–194.

Kelley, W. S. (1996). Therapeutic peptides: the devil is in the details. *Biotechnology*, **14**, 28–31.

Lehrer, S. B., Horner, W. E. and Reese, G. (1996). Why are some proteins allergenic? Implications for biotechnology. *Crit. Rev. Food Sci. Nutr.*, **36**, 553–564.

Liberman, D. F., Israeli, E. and Fink, R. (1991). Risk assessment of biological hazards. *Occup. Med. State Art Rev.*, **6**, 285–299.

Lubbert, M., Jonas, D. and Herrmann, F. (1990). Animal models for the biological effects of continuous high cytokine levels. *Blut*, **61**, 253–257.

Luster, M. I., Dean, J. H. and Moore, J. A. (1986). In Hayes, A. W. (Ed.), *Principles and Methods of Toxicology*. Raven Press, New York, pp. 561–586.

Luster, M. I., Portier, C., Pait, D. G., White, K. L., Jr, Gennings, C., Munson, A. E. and Rosenthal, G. J. (1992). Risk assessment in immunotoxicology; sensitivity and predictability of immune tests. *Fundam. Appl. Toxicol.*, **18**, 200–210.

Marafino, B. J., Young, J. D., Greenfield, I. L. and Kopplin, J. R. (1988). The appropriate toxicological testing of recombinant human proteins. In Marshak, D. R. and Darrell, T. L. (Eds), *Therapeutic Peptides and Proteins: Assessing the New Technologies*. Cold Spring Harbor Laboratory Press, Cold Spring Harbor, NY, pp. 175–187.

Marcek, J. M., Seaman, W. J. and Nappier, J. L. (1989). Effects of repeated high dose administration of recombinant bovine somatotropin in lactating dairy cows. *Vet. Hum. Toxicol.*, **31**, 455–460.

Miller, H. I. and Young, F. E. (1988). FDA and biotechnology: update 1989. *Biotechnology*, **6**, 1385–1392.

Nimni, M. E. (1997). Polypeptide growth factors: targeted delivery systems. *Biomaterials*, **18**, 1201–1225.

Norbury, K. C. (1985). Immunotoxicological evaluation: an overview. *J. Am. Coll. Toxicol.*, **4**, 279–290.

Pope, B. L. (1989). Immunopharmacology: a new frontier. *Can. J. Physiol. Pharmacol.*, **67**, 537–545.

Sjodia, L. (1988). Regulatory aspects of drugs produced by recombinant DNA technology. In Marshak, D. R. and Liu, D. J. (Eds), *Banbury Report 29: Therapeutic Peptides and Proteins: Assessing the New Technologies*. Cold Spring Harbor Laboratory Press, Cold Spring Harbor, NY, pp. 293–297.

Thomas, J. A. (1995). Recent developments and perspectives of biotechnology-derived products. *Toxicology*, **105**, 7–22.

Thomas, J. A. (1997). Use of animal models in biomedical research. In Sipes, I. G., McQueen, C. A. and Gandolfi, A. J. (Eds), *Comprehensive Toxicology. Toxicological Testing and Evaluation*, Vol. 2. Pergamon Press, Toronto, pp. 227–237.

Thomas, J. A. and Thomas, M. J. (1993). New biologies: their development, safety, and efficacy. In Thomas, J. A. and Myers, L. A. (Eds), *Biotechnology and Safety Assessment*, vol. 1. Raven Press, New York, pp. 1–22.

Tomlinson, E. (1992). Impact of the new biologies on the medical and pharmaceutical sciences. *J. Pharm. Pharmacol.*, **44**, 147–159.

Trown, P. W., Wills, R. J., and Kamm, J. J. (1986). The preclinical development of Roferon[R]-A. *Cancer*, **57**, 1648.

Van Brunt, J. and Klausner, A. (1988). Growth factors speed wound healing. *Biotechnology*, **6**, 25–30.

Winearls, C. G. (1989). Treatment of the anemia of chronic renal failure with recombinant human erythropoietin. *Drugs*, **38**, 342–345.

Winkelhake, J. L. and Gouny, S. S. (1990). Human recombinant interleukin-2 as an experimental therapeutic. *Pharmacol. Rev.*, **42**, 1–25.

Yaksh, T. L., Rathbun, M. L., Dragani, J. C., Malkmus, S., Bourdeau, A. R., Richter, P., Powell, H., Myers, R. R. and LeBel, C. P. (1997). Kinetic and safety studies on intrathecally infused recombinant-methionyl human brain-derived neurotrophic factor in dogs. *Fundam. Appl. Toxicol.*, **38**, 89–100.

Zbinden, G. (1990). Safety evaluation of biotechnology products. *Drug Saf.*, **5**, Suppl. 1, 58–64.

FURTHER READING

Brenner, M. K. (1995). Human somatic gene therapy: progress and problems. *J. Intern. Med.*, **237**, 229–239.

Crooke, S. T. (1992). Therapeutic applications of oligonucleotides. *Annu. Rev. Pharmacol. Toxicol.*, **32**, 329–376.

Henck, J. W., Hilbish, K. G., Serabian, M. A., *et al.* (1996). Reproductive toxicity testing of therapeutic biotechnology agents. *Teratology*, **53**, 185–195.

Lunel, J. (1995). Biotechnology regulations and guidelines in Europe. *Curr. Opin. Biotechnol.*, **6**, 267–272.

Mulligan, R. C. (1993). The basic science of gene therapy. *Science*, **260**, 926–932.

Ronneberger, H. (1990). Toxicological testing of monoclonal antibodies. *Dev. Biol. Stand.*, **71**, 185.

Steiner, J. and Dayan, A. D. (1994). Preclinical and clinical evaluation of products of biotechnology compared with conventional chemical entities. *J. Biotechnol. Healthcare*, **1**, 36–48.

Thomas, J. A. (Ed.) (1998). *Biotechnology and Safety Assessment*, 2nd edn. Taylor and Francis, Philadelphia, PA.

Vial, T. and Descotes, J. (1994). Clinical toxicity of the interferons. *Drug Saf.*, **10**, 115–150.

Chapter 93

Toxicology of Food and Food Additives

David M. Conning

CONTENTS

- Introduction
- Food Toxicology
- Toxicology of Food Additives
- References

INTRODUCTION

Since the 1850s, when the illegal adulteration of foodstuffs caused a public scandal, there has been legislation to control the use of non-nutritious chemicals in food. During this century, concomitant with the growth of food technology, food legislation has expanded to cover virtually every aspect of food manufacture and packaging, and has extended to regulate the residues in foodstuffs of the considerable number of chemicals used in agricultural production.

Such legislation, together with that devoted to medicines, has to a considerable extent paralleled the development of the technology, if not the science, of toxicology. As the scope of toxicology has enlarged, so has the amount of food law. In addition, the regulation of food chemicals has been undertaken by almost all national governments and the whole framework is now truly global in character. Given the international nature of trade, considerable efforts are made to ensure that national requirements do not conflict, thereby constituting barriers to trade.

Nutrition science has also demonstrated remarkable growth during the twentieth century, but for much of that time has concentrated almost exclusively on the study of dietary deficiency that results in disease. This has resulted in major advances in the knowledge and understanding of the roles of individual nutrients, although much remains to be accomplished in elucidating the biochemical detail. During this time, a few nutritionists have attempted to examine the influence of diet on health—that is, the attainment of optimal health and disease resistance as opposed to rectification of deficiency. Much of this work has been governed by an intuitive belief that the intensification of agricultural practice and the industrialization of food manufacture must diminish the nutritional value of foodstuffs.

The international comparisons of diet and heart disease, begun in 1947 (Keys, 1980), opened up a third line of development for nutrition science. This was the recognition that the excessive consumption of specified nutrients may be associated with certain conditions previously classified as age-related degenerative disease. By this time the concept of chronic toxicity had been identified by toxicology. Chronic toxicity is the induction of a disease process by the repeated administration of a small dose of a compound, over a long period of time. In most instances, but not all, the disease process itself is an age-related degenerative phenomenon, but the intensity is increased and the onset occurs earlier in the life-span, when the toxic compound is present. Usually a dose can be identified which does not influence the natural disease process or provoke other toxic responses.

In many respects the notion that a given nutrient consumed repeatedly to excess over many years can induce or enhance a chronic disease process is a precise replication of the concept of chronic toxicity, and has led to the recognition of food toxicology or nutrition toxicology as a complementary science to both toxicology and nutrition. In that this concept embraces the genetic basis for age-related degenerative diseases, the analogy is fairly close and could be a valuable adjunct in the study of disease mechanisms.

There are, however, other components of food which are toxic, the so-called natural toxicants. Until recent years these have been neglected as subjects of scientific study. With the present tendency towards a reduction in the use of agricultural chemicals, it is possible that natural toxicants, many of which constitute a plant's own defences against predators, will assume greater importance.

FOOD TOXICOLOGY

Nutrient Toxicity

Investigations of the relationship between diet and disease have concentrated in the main on two areas: (1) diet and vascular disease and (2) diet and malignant disease.

Diet and Vascular Disease

Vascular disease accounts for approximately 40% of deaths in the UK. Among males, 31% of deaths are due to coronary heart disease and 9% to cerebrovascular disease. The figures among females are 23% and 15%, respectively. The median age of deaths is around 75 years, but a third of the deaths from ischaemic heart disease in males occur before the age of 65 years (DHSS, 1984).

Coronary Heart Disease

Coronary heart disease (CHD) consists of two elements—arterial degeneration (atherosclerosis) of the coronary arteries, which is part of a generalized degeneration of the arterial system, and coronary thrombosis, resulting in myocardial ischaemic necrosis, which may be fatal. Studies of patients with the condition have revealed a number of shared characteristics, now designated 'predisposing risk factors'. The most consistent include age, hypertension, raised blood cholesterol concentration, maleness, cigarette smoking and family history. Other conditions that predispose to the disease are hyperlipidaemias, diabetes, obesity and lack of physical exercise.

Many of these factors may be assumed to raise the concentration of blood lipids, increase the myocardial burden and decrease the potential blood supply should the main supply be compromised. Women are protected until the menopause (unless hyperlipidaemia is present), but thereafter develop the same susceptibility as males.

Heavy cigarette smoking is associated with peripheral vascular disease, coronary heart disease and myocardial infarction, but the mechanism remains uncertain. It may be a combination of several factors, such as vasoconstriction, increased platelet adhesiveness and blood coagulation.

Studies of the effects of diet have concentrated on the causes of the elevated blood cholesterol and the induction of thrombosis.

Blood Cholesterol

The seminal cross-population studies of Ancel Keys (Keys, 1980) demonstrated that in males aged 40–59 years there was a direct association between the prevalence of CHD and serum cholesterol concentrations and a further association, though less striking, between blood cholesterol and the proportion of saturated fatty acids in the diet. This observation has been the basis of many national public health policies which attempt to achieve a reduced consumption of saturated fatty acids, mainly derived from animal fats, compensated by an increased consumption of polyunsaturated fatty acids, mainly derived from vegetable oils, to maintain the intake of adequate food energy.

Several large studies have attempted to decrease the incidence of CHD by reducing the blood concentrations of cholesterol through manipulations of the diet or the use of hypolipidaemic drugs. Such studies have not been strikingly successful. Although the prevalence of myocardial ischaemia has been slightly reduced in some instances, overall mortality has not been reduced. This may be because, in men over 65 years of age, there is an inverse relationship between mortality and blood cholesterol concentration (Kannel and Gordon, 1970).

The lipoprotein transport systems for serum cholesterol are known to be important in that low-density lipoprotein cholesterol (LDL) is strongly and directly associated with the risk of CHD, whereas high-density lipoprotein cholesterol (HDL) is inversely related, that is, HDL cholesterol has a protective effect.

Serum concentrations of LDL cholesterol are governed by the availability of the LDL receptors on cell surfaces, especially of the liver, and this availability is genetically controlled. The LDL receptors govern the access of blood cholesterol to the hepatic cells, where it is metabolized and excreted in the bile. HDL represents an additional transport mechanism that reduces the deposition of cholesterol in the arterial wall (Goldstein et al., 1983). Extreme reduction in the numbers of such receptors occurs in familial hypercholesterolaemia. The mechanism of action of saturated fatty acids in influencing LDL levels is not known, although it is now recognized that the most important fatty acids are C_{12} (lauric), C_{14} (myristic) and C_{16} (palmitic) acids. It is known also that monounsaturated fatty acids may be beneficial by causing an elevation of the circulating levels of HDL cholesterol.

Why LDL cholesterol exerts an adverse effect is not known, but is thought to be related to an oxidative damage that occurs as the LDL particle passes through the vascular endothelium. This damage, essentially to the protein moiety, renders the particle resistant to clearance by LDL receptors and toxic to macrophages which attempt to scavenge the particles. This causes the production of 'foamy' macrophages (that is, macrophages with accumulated fat), cellular disintegration and the possible release of growth factors which stimulate the proliferation of smooth muscle cells, another feature of the atheromatous lesion. Although highly speculative, this hypothesis has resulted in an analysis of the antioxidant protection known to be exercised in LDL particles by vitamin E and β-carotene, with the recognition that reduced dietary intake of vitamin E is an important additional 'risk factor' in CHD (Gey et al., 1987).

The possible role of antioxidants in preventing the adverse effects of high circulating levels of LDL cholesterol is compatible with experimental animal studies which have suggested that atheromatous lesions are mainly due to oxidized cholesterol or oxidized cholesterol esters.

In terms of toxicology, therefore, the problem is the nature of the change in LDL particles which renders them toxic to vascular endothelium or intima, resulting in the degenerative change that characterizes atherosclerosis;

and the mechanism by which this change is induced. Food components could be involved in several ways:

1. Heated fats might be a source of oxygen free radicals in the diet, although there is no means at present to measure the whole-body effect. In any case, food contains such a wide range of antioxidant compounds that it is unlikely that a specific food toxicity could be demonstrated.
2. High circulating levels of homocysteine increase the risk of CHD. The condition occurs in homocystinuria. Homocysteine is a reactive amino acid that promotes LDL oxidation and thrombosis. Whether lesser blood concentrations of homocysteine than those seen in the autosomal recessive condition would be as pathogenic is not known.
3. Although not directly related to LDL oxidation, there is evidence that the age-related increase in blood pressure commonly seen in Western populations is enhanced by excessive consumption of sodium, particularly as sodium chloride. This effect can be mitigated by an increased consumption of potassium. Hypertension is a risk factor for CHD, enhancing the damage to the arterial wall, presumably by mechanical trauma.

Thrombosis

Occlusion of a coronary artery by a thrombus is a common terminal event in CHD. It is likely that, before such a catastrophe, mural thrombi are formed on the damaged intima of diseased arteries and are incorporated into subendothelial plaques, thereby aggravating the condition. Considerations of the possible role of dietary components in this process have centred on the essential fatty acids (EFAs), linoleic and linolenic acid. These EFAs are known to be the precursors of the

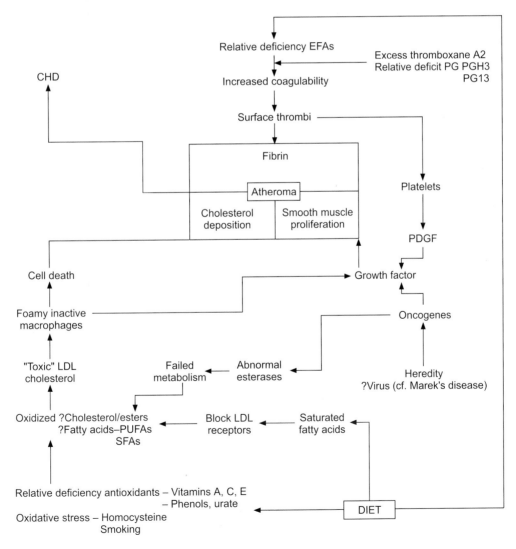

Figure 1 Scheme illustrating the possible interaction of a number of pathogenic factors in the development of atherosclerosis and coronary heart disease. CHD = coronary heart disease; PG = prostaglandin; PDGF = platelet-derived growth factor; LDL = low-density lipoprotein; PUFAs = polyunsaturated fatty acids; SFAs = saturated fatty acids; EFAs = essential fatty acids.

endoperoxides PGH2 and PGH3, which are converted, respectively, to prostaglandins and thromboxanes in vascular endothelium and platelets (Moncada and Vane, 1978). The hypothesis is that a dietary imbalance resulting in relative deficiency of synthesis of the linoleic pathway results in a relative excess of thromboxane A2, which promotes thrombosis. This hypothesis suggests that competition exists for the available cyclooxygenases, thereby influencing the final pathway.

It is known that a diet rich in marine products, with relatively high levels of eicosapentaenoic acid (EPA), causes a prolongation of the bleeding time and that even a moderate increase in fish consumption reduces CHD mortality (Kromhout et al., 1985). It has yet to be demonstrated that EPA and arachidonic acid compete for the available cyclooxygenase, or that the enzyme is limited in supply.

It is known that Factor VII activity is acutely increased after a high-fat meal and may be sustained at elevated levels by a high-fat diet. In these circumstances Factor VII is strongly correlated with CHD. Although no particular fatty acid is implicated, other studies have suggested that dietary stearic acid may increase the potential of platelets to aggregate. These findings await independent confirmation.

In conclusion, it is clear that atherosclerosis is a multifactorial disease and it is not possible at present to define the mechanism that explains the combined role of the known factors. The contemporary view **(Figure 1)** offers a scheme susceptible to experimental elucidation which may provide solutions in due course. In the meantime, it must be correct that public health policies seek to remove the risk factors known to be influenced by diet and lifestyle.

Diet and Cancer

Introduction

The belief that the diet is causally related to the burden of cancer in a community arises from the varying incidence of specific cancers in international comparisons of different populations consuming different patterns of foodstuffs. Such studies have been enhanced by case-control studies, studies of the changing incidences of cancer within populations undergoing changes in dietary intakes and, above all, by the study of cancer incidence in second-generation immigrants who adopt the lifestyle of their host country. Despite the many environmental factors that could be involved, it is now generally accepted that the diet is one of the most important. For excellent reviews of the evidence, see the joint publication by the World Cancer Research Fund and the American Institute for Cancer Research (1997) and the UK COMA report (DH, 1998).

It is still not known which elements of the diet, if any, can be regarded as carcinogenic and, given the nature of the cancerous process, it is highly doubtful that a single

entity will be incriminated. It is much more likely that dietary variation is associated with greater or lesser degrees of protection, although it remains possible that excessive consumption of some dietary components might be causally related to specific cancers.

Energy and Fat in Experimental Carcinogenesis

The study of the carcinogenicity of chemicals has had a central place in the development of toxicology as a science, and it has been known since 1941 that diet plays a very important role in modulating tumour incidence and tumour induction times (Lavik and Baumann, 1941). Since the demonstration that restriction of energy consumption reduced the incidence of spontaneous tumours in experimental animals and the susceptibility of skin to chemical carcinogenesis, this finding has been extended subsequently to a wide variety of experimental animals and tumour models. For example, the incidence of spontaneous mammary tumours in mice is greater in animals maintained on a high-fat diet than those on a low-fat or a carbohydrate-rich diet, even when the total energy consumption is identical. This observation, too, has been repeated in many studies, although the assumption that different diets have been isocaloric has depended on there being no significant changes in body weight or rate of weight gain rather than direct measurement. A confounding factor in many studies has been the failure to recognize that the available energy from fat may be much greater in experimental animals than the accepted figure for man and that this value varies according to the length of the fatty acid chain. Hence, depending on the type of fat used in the preparation of animal diets, the available energy may be greater than that computed. The use of body weight as a measure of energy consumption therefore requires much more precise measurement than has often been the case.

Further analysis of the roles of different types of fat has suggested that polyunsaturated fatty acids of the types found in vegetable oils (C_{16}–C_{20}) are much more active in promoting carcinogenesis than saturated fatty acids, although the longer chain polyunsaturated acids found in fish oils also show much less activity (Carroll and Khor, 1975).

These confusing findings were resolved to some extent when it was shown, subsequently, that the essential fatty acids may be the critical moiety in experimental mammary carcinogenesis. Tumour yield increases as the EFA content of the diet is increased, a maximum response being obtained with a dietary content of about 4%. Once this level is achieved, tumour yield may be further increased by the incorporation of greater percentages of fat, but the type of fat is not important. This would suggest that EFAs have an important role in experimental carcinogenesis which is enhanced by energy consumption. The nature of the specific role is uncertain (Ip et al., 1985). The position is further complicated by the finding that these properties of EFA may reside only with the linoleic series, which results in the synthesis of arachidonic acid, and that the linolenic series may actually be inhibitors of the carcinogenic process. It is known that eicosapentaenoic acids and decosahexaeonic acids inhibit arachidonic acid metabolism and it is possible that this is the important effect. Until more is known about the roles of prostaglandins, thromboxanes and leukotrienes, derivatives of arachidonic and eicosapentaenoic acids, in the carcinogenic process, no conclusions are possible.

Energy and Fat in Human Carcinogenesis

Epidemiological studies of human cancer in relation to dietary components are difficult on account of the virtual impossibility, in retrospective studies, of defining with any accuracy the precise consumption of nutrients for the many decades before the patient develops a tumour. Other confounding factors are insufficient dietary variance between cases and controls, failure to consider other factors such as smoking, the consumption of complex carbohydrates, dietary modification as a result of the presence of the disease itself and family history. Prospective studies would be expected to avoid most of these factors.

Plotting age-adjusted death rates for breast cancer against the putative intake of fat or energy-from-fat demonstrates a direct relationship with a high correlation coefficient, even though the quality of the dietary data from many countries is not good. A similar analysis reveals no relationship between death from breast cancer and the intake of polyunsaturated fatty acids.

The grossly obese demonstrate elevated mortality rates from cancer, mainly colorectal tumours in males and tumours of gall bladder, breast and uterus in females. The excess is not large.

Other studies have attempted to characterize the relationship between diet and the incidence of breast and colonic cancers by an analysis of religious sects or closed communities with strict dietary rules. In these studies the level of fat in the diet is assumed to equate with the amount of meat, since many communities control meat consumption, whereas none control fat consumption directly. Some studies have attempted to equate serum cholesterol measurements with the incidence of cancer, assuming cholesterol to be dependent on fat consumption. All of these studies have given inconsistent results that do not allow a clear correlation between dietary fat and the incidence of cancer to be made (Kinlen, 1987).

Meat

Several studies, both case-control and prospective, have shown a positive relationship between the consumption of red and processed meats and the incidence of breast and colorectal cancers. Some of these studies have demonstrated a dose–response relationship in terms of frequency of consumption. The relationship was not always statistically significant and in most the relative risk was small (Bingham, 1990).

Recognition that the aetiological agents may be nitrosamines or heterocyclic amines (see later) resulted in studies of the relationship between fried or 'broiled' red meat and the incidence of these cancers. Significant associations were found for breast cancer (Ronco et al., 1996) but, so far, not for colorectal cancer (Giovannucci et al., 1994).

No positive correlations have been reported between these cancers and the consumption of white meat or fish.

Non-starch Polysaccharides

The possible protective role of non-starch polysaccharides (NSP) against the induction of colonic cancer was suggested by a comparison of African and Western diets (Burkitt and Trowell, 1975). This has stimulated considerable research but very little in the way of consolidated findings. Many studies have been confounded by the failure to recognize that NSPs as a class includes compounds with very different biological effects, and the failure to compensate for the reduced energy content of diets high in NSP (BNF, 1990).

When properly controlled, there is no evidence at present that NSP has a significant influence on experimental or human colonic carcinogenesis, but in general most studies report a reduction in incidence with high NSP diets.

Carcinogens in Food

In addition to concepts relating the diet as a whole to the burden of cancer, a great effort has been made to identify carcinogenic compounds among the components of food. These studies have been handicapped by the difficult and laborious analytical procedures involved. In recent years the development of screening procedures for mutagenesis has resulted in a great increase in the number of compounds in food identified as having this capability and a search for evidence that public health is affected. No substantive evidence has yet been found but several studies have suggested that in due course it might become available.

Carcinogens in food may be (1) natural components, (2) compounds produced by food processing or (3) natural or synthetic contaminants.

1. *Naturally occuring carcinogens.* A number of compounds have been identified as experimental carcinogens. These include cycasin from the cycad nut, estiagole from tarragon, pyrrolizidine alkaloids from comfrey and safrole from oil of sassafras. In addition, many plants contain formaldehyde and benzene and several species of mushroom contain compounds that generate hydrazine and methylhydrazine. Each of these compounds occurs in some national diets but there is no evidence that they are associated with human disease and it is unlikely that such evidence will be forthcoming.

2. *Compounds produced by food processing.*

a. Polycyclic hydrocarbons. It has long been known that the pyrolysis of organic matter produces a range of polycyclic aromatic hydrocarbons (PAHs) and many of these have been shown to be experimental carcinogens. PAHs occur in food following preservation by smoking and cooking by frying or grilling, the latter particularly by open flame (broiling). Concentrations range up to $300 \mu g \ kg^{-1}$ in meat or fish but are much affected by temperature, fat content and food source (Larsen and Poulsen, 1987).

b. Heterocyclic amines. The discovery that extracts of the charred surface of broiled fish and meat exhibited potent mutagenic activity in bacterial screening procedures was rapidly followed by the identification of a number of heterocyclic amines as the culpable compounds. These have been shown to include compounds that are very active mutagens or clastogens and which readily form DNA adducts after intraperitoneal administration. Long-term feeding studies in rats and mice have shown them to be carcinogenic to many tissues at a dose around 15 mg (kg body weight)$^{-1}$ day^{-1}. The concentrations generated in meat and fish range up to $115 \mu g \ kg^{-1}$. The role of heterocyclic amines in human carcinogenesis has yet to be determined. Given the large difference between the carcinogenic dose and the levels of dietary exposure (1000–5000; Sugimura, 1986) it may be difficult to demonstrate a causal role.

c. Nitrosamines. N-Nitrosamines and N-nitrosamides may be formed in the human intestine by the reaction of amines derived from protein and exogenous nitrites or nitrites formed endogenously from nitrates by the action of the colonic microflora (MacFarlane *et al.*, 1995). High consumption of red meat may increase the concentrations of N-nitroso compounds detected in faeces (Bingham *et al.*, 1996); but this is not associated with DNA adduct formation. As yet, therefore, the association between a high consumption of red meat and increased incidence of colorectal cancer cannot be attributed to nitrosamine formation.

3. *Natural or synthetic contaminants.*

a. Natural contaminants. Interest centres almost exclusively on the mycotoxins, which are toxic metabolites of some moulds. Mould growth occurs on any stored agricultural produce or animal feedstuff, but especially ground nuts, tree nuts and cereals and particularly where storage conditions are warm and humid. Three species of mould are mainly concerned, *Aspergillus*, *Fusarium* and *Penicillium*. Each can produce a range of mycotoxins, several of which have been shown to be potent carcinogens in experimental animals. Aflatoxin B, for example, the product of *Aspergillus flavus*, is among the most potent of animal carcinogens.

Despite this, it has not been possible to prove that mycotoxins cause human cancer, though there is a close association between the prevalence of crop contamination with *Aspergillus* and the geographical distribution of liver cancer in Africa and Southern Asia. For this reason, aflatoxin B is regarded as a probable human carcinogen (IARC, 1993).

b. Synthetic carcinogens. Industrial economies generate and utilize many thousands of chemical compounds, including many designed specifically for use in food production and food processing. Any such chemical which is released into the environment may contaminate the food chain through uptake by crops and animals or through water contamination.

Serious attempts are made to regulate the concentrations of contaminants. By and large these have been very successful and there is no evidence that synthetic contaminants play a role in the aetiology of human cancer.

A possible exception was a group of polyhalogenated biphenyls and benzofurans used extensively as insulants in transformers and capacitors. These compounds, the use of which is now discontinued, resist biodegradation and therefore may accumulate in the food chain. Some are known experimental carcinogens and are regarded as possible human carcinogens on theoretical grounds. (IARC, 1997).

The Role of Antioxidants

Following the pioneering work of Miller and Miller (1966), the bioactivation of foreign compounds to yield electrophiles and radicals is now well established. If those reactive metabolites gain access to macromolecules such as enzyme proteins or nucleic acids, toxic damage may occur. In the case of DNA this could result, if unrepaired, in mutation which, in somatic cells, might produce cancer.

Since these ideas emerged in the 1960s, there have been a number of studies to examine the effect of dietary antioxidants on the incidence of human cancer. Most studies have concentrated on vitamin C, vitamin E and β-carotene, but more recently other carotenes have begun to be examined. The retrospective studies are hampered by the almost insurmountable difficulty of assessing nutrient intake and have depended on the habitual intake of fruit, vegetables and vegetable oils. Prospective studies also depend to a considerable extent on habitual food intake to achieve consistency. Better evaluation is obtained if serum levels can be measured, but the long-term preservation of antioxidants in serum samples may be unreliable.

Vitamin C. Studies of vitamin C have given equivocal results. Case-control studies have suggested a reduced dietary intake in subjects with cancer of the cervix, mouth, larynx and stomach, but not in cancers of the colon, bladder, prostate and breast. None of the correlations are large (odds ratio < 1.7). Animal studies in experimental carcinogenesis have shown variable results also, with different effects on tumours of different organs in the same study. Analysis of a large number of studies involving assessment of either vitamin C intake or fruit intake has suggested a probable inhibition of cancer incidence.

Vitamin E. The largest review study to date involved over 21 000 men in Finland, and showed that higher serum levels of vitamin E were correlated with lower risk of subsequently developing cancer. This was particularly evident in male smokers. A 3% reduction in serum levels was associated with a significant increase in the incidence of, although not death from, cancer, at the time of publication. In this study, the serum samples were stored at $-20°C$, which may not be adequate to preserve vitamin E concentrations (Knekt, 1991). Several animal studies have shown a strong inhibition of experimental carcinogenesis.

β-Carotene. Early studies failed to distinguish between vitamin A and β-carotene intake, but since the review by Peto *et al.* (1981), most have concentrated on β- and other carotenes. Most case-control studies have shown an inverse relationship between dietary intake or serum levels and cancer incidence and mortality. This is particularly striking for lung cancer, even in long-term smokers. More recently it has been suggested that better inverse correlations may be obtained with lycopene or with 9-*cis*-β-carotene. Nevertheless, in animal studies β-carotene has been shown to suppress experimental carcinogenesis with a number of carcinogenic agents and at a variety of sites.

Intervention in smokers utilizing supplements, however, has not supported the earlier findings, and indeed has resulted in increased incidence of lung cancer (ATBC, 1994). It is possible that the apparent beneficial effects of dietary β-carotene are due to some other component for which β-carotene is a marker, or that, to be effective, β-carotene must be present in adequate concentrations before cell transformation has occurred.

Selenium. Several studies have suggested that selenium intake is inversely related to cancer incidence, particularly in respect of cancers of breast, colon and prostate. Animal studies have also demonstrated an inhibitory effect. The selenium content in the diet, however, depends on soil content and bioavailability and may not be consistent in all geographical locations.

Uric Acid. Studies on the relationship between serum uric acid and total mortality have been negative. One study has examined the relationship with mortality from lung cancer and found a significant inverse relationship which persisted after adjustment for age and smoking habits.

Conclusion. Overall, it may be concluded that a low dietary intake of antioxidant micronutrients is associated with an increased incidence of cancers and, in particular, lung cancer. Given the range of compounds studied, it is likely that the effect is related to the antioxidant property and that the compounds studied cannot be regarded only as markers for some other, as yet unrecognized, dietary component. Furthermore, the

likely mechanism of action is based on a hypothesis for which there is considerable supporting evidence. Nevertheless, other dietary components, such as lycopene, may achieve much greater intake and tissue levels and have yet to be studied adequately.

Natural Toxicants

Plants produce a variety of toxic compounds as a defence against insect predators and fungal infections. The rate of production tends to be governed by the frequency of attack and, as a consequence of the widespread use of synthetic pesticides most agricultural produce contains only low concentrations. With the trend towards reducing the use of synthetic compounds because of concern about environmental contamination, it is likely that the natural toxicants will assume greater importance as potential hazards for consumers. Attempts to increase the concentrations of natural toxins by plant breeding programmes have occasionally resulted in illness among consumers of the products. It must be recognized, however, that there are very few plant toxins that have caused human illness when consumed as part of a normal diet, although, if the criteria used to assess the safety of synthetic substances were used to judge natural toxins, many more would be included as potential hazards.

Substances that have caused human disease as a result of excessive consumption or inadequate processing usually occur in the diet when food is otherwise not available.

Proteins

Phytohaemagglutinins occur predominantly in beans and are normally removed by soaking in water for several hours prior to thorough cooking. They cause agglutination and lysis of erythrocytes and some are cytotoxic to the intestinal mucosa.

Lathyrogens

Lathyrogens are unusual amino acids (diaminobutyric or diaminopropionic acid) and aminonitriles that cause amyotrophic lateral sclerosis of the spinal cord, resulting in spastic paralysis.

Glucosinolates

Glucosinolates are sulphur compounds metabolized to thiocyanates, isothiocyanates and cyclic thiocyanates, all of which inhibit thyroxine production, and may result in goitre.

Cyanogens

A number of glycosides yield hydrocyanic acid on hydrolysis. The glycosides occur in a variety of nuts and fruits but the most important are linamarin and lotaustralin, which occur in cassava root and lima beans. Normal processing releases and removes the HCN before consumption.

Toxicity that may result from the consumption of usual dietary components in normal amounts is unusual, but occurs with two components with sufficient regularity to be noted:

Honey

Honey produced by bees that have foraged rhododendron or azalea contains the complex substances andromedol and desacetylpieristoxin. These may cause cardiovascular collapse and acute peripheral neuropathies at very small dosage. Honey manufacturers take great care to ensure that their bees do not have access to such plants.

Potatoes

Potatoes produce the anticholinesterase glycoalkaloids α-solanine and α-chaconine. These compounds are heat resistant but occur at greatest concentrations in the green skins of immature potatoes. Poisoning is characterized by gastrointestinal symptoms and may be accompanied by central nervous depression (Whitaker and Feeney, 1973).

Protective Effects

There is increasing interest in the possibility that some plant constituents inhibit toxic processes such as carcinogenesis. Components such as polyphenolics (flavonoids, isoflavones, lignans and tannins) are antioxidants but also induce microsomal oxidases and conjugating enzyme systems. Glucosinolates (from brassicas) may also induce both phase I and phase II metabolic activity and this has been demonstrated in human studies (Vistisen et al., 1990; Bogaards et al., 1994). Diallyl sulphones (from onions, garlic and leeks) are thought to inhibit oxidases and exhibit anticarcinogenic activity in experimental models (Yang et al., 1992). Although there is some epidemiological evidence in support of a beneficial effect, the intakes required tend to be excessive. Nevertheless, this may prove to be a fruitful field of research.

TOXICOLOGY OF FOOD ADDITIVES

A food additive is defined here as a substance used to facilitate some part of the processing or manufacture of a foodstuff or deliberately added to a foodstuff to effect a particular characteristic. This definition excludes indirect additives derived from packaging and contaminants, including residues of agricultural chemicals.

Food additives may be classified according to their intended function. Although this does not necessarily coincide with their chemistry and therefore is not always directly pertinent to a study of toxicological properties, often such properties are related to the function rather than to the chemical structure and many additives are variants of a single structure, all having a similar function.

By far the most comprehensive surveys of the toxicology of food additives are those carried out by the Joint Expert Committee on Food Additives (JECFA) of the World Health Organization and the Food and Agriculture Organization of the United Nations. This committee has, over many years, reviewed toxicological data, both published and unpublished, on a large number of compounds, to determine the acceptable daily intake (ADI). The ADI is the maximum amount of substance, in milligrams per kilogram body weight (mg kg^{-1}), that may be consumed daily for a lifetime without adverse effect. It is usually derived by determining the maximum dosage without detectable effect in an assay of long-term toxicological feeding studies in a number (at least two) of animal species, divided by a safety factor of at least 100. This factor is said to encompass reduction by a factor of 10 to account for the difference in size between the human population and the test population of experimental animals, and by a factor of 10 to govern the variable sensitivity likely to be exhibited by man to the compound under test. It is clearly difficult to justify this derivation on scientific grounds and it has not been possible to test its efficacy in practice, but as a regulatory procedure it has served its purpose and is recognized as a convenient index by most authorities.

It may be noted in passing that the difficulty of assessing the efficacy of the ADI is due to the impossibility of determining the precise consumption of foods in which an additive is permitted and the concentration of the additive that is actually used. Such assessments have been attempted for food colours and flavours, and some dietary analyses have been undertaken for selected additives.

Where a number of compounds are used for the same purpose, they may be allocated a 'group ADI', which states the total permitted concentration of all the compounds in the group.

The Toxicology of Additives by Class (Table 1)

Acidity Regulators

Modification of acidity is an extremely important food manufacturing process having an influence on taste, texture and preservation. Many compounds are used for these purposes, most derived from simple organic acids, themselves natural body constituents, which exhibit little or no toxicity, except at overwhelming dosage.

Table 1 Classes of food additives

Class	Subclasses
Acidity regulator	Buffer, buffering agent, acid, base, alkali, pH-adjusting agent
Anticaking agent	Anticaking agent, drying agent, dusting powder, antistick agent
Antifoaming agent	
Antioxidant	Antioxidant, antioxidant synergist, sequestrant
Bulking agent	
Carbonating agent	
Clarifying agent	
Colour	Colour, colour adjunct, colour fixative, colour retention agent, colour stabilizer
Emulsifier	Emulsifier, plasticizer, dispersing agent, surface-active agent, surfactant
Enzyme preparation	
Flavour enhancer	
Flavouring agent	Flavouring agent, seasoning agent
Flour treatment agent	Bleaching agent, dough conditioner, flour improver
Foaming agent	Whipping agent, aerating agent
Freezant	
Gelling agent	
Glazing agent	Coating, sealing agent, polish, dusting agent, release agent, lubricant
Humectant	
Preservative	
Propellant	
Raising agent	
Solvent, carrier	
Solvent, extraction	
Stabilizer	
Sweetener	
Thickener	

A wide range of salts of phosphoric acid are accorded a group ADI of 70 mg kg^{-1} based on the dietary concentration that induces nephrocalcinosis in the rat. This effect, however, depends on the calcium: phosphate ratio in the diet, calcium deposition being more likely when the ratio falls below unity. Larger amounts of phosphate intake are permissible if the calcium intake is also high, and vice versa.

Fumaric acid and its sodium salt showed slightly increased mortality in the rat at a dietary concentration of 1.5% but not at 1.2%. Slight testicular atrophy was seen also. Tartaric acid and its sodium salt also showed no adverse effects at 1.2% in the diet of rats. The ADI for tartrates (30 mg kg^{-1} day^{-1}) is greater than that for the fumarates (6 mg kg^{-1} day^{-1}), because only 20% of ingested tartrate is absorbed.

Anticaking Agents

Phosphate compounds are again limited by the nephro-calcinosis that results from high dietary concentrations, but others, such as magnesium oxide or magnesium carbonate, various silicates and crystalline cellulose, show no toxicity by mouth.

Polydimethylsiloxane showed no toxicity at the highest dose administered (0.1%) and was excreted unchanged in the faeces.

The ferrocyanides are said to cause renal enlargement at 0.5% in the diet, with a minor degree of renal tubular damage.

Antifoaming Compounds

Propylene glycol alginate (also used as a thickener and an emulsifier) undergoes about 80% hydrolysis in the small intestine, releasing propylene glycol, which is absorbed. Residual propylene glycoalginate and the released alginic acid and salts are excreted unchanged in the faeces. Long-term feeding studies in rats and mice have shown no adverse effects at levels up to 5% in the diet.

Antioxidants

Antioxidants are an extremely important group of compounds, used extensively to prevent the oxidation of fats and oils in foods, thereby preventing rancidity during distribution and storage. The oxidation process is catalysed by trace metals such as iron and copper. Antioxidants as a class, therefore, include compounds which themselves act as oxygen receptors and compounds which chelate trace metals.

Electron transfer, the major mechanism whereby living cells generate energy, itself produces oxygen free radicals which, if uncontained, would prove lethal. Living tissues are equipped with potent antioxidant mechanisms dependent on compounds that acts as electron receptors or as metal chelators. These compounds are the so-called antioxidant vitamins, ascorbic acid (vitamin C) and α-tocopherol (vitamin E), and various salts of citric, tartaric and phosphoric acid. The vitamins and their derivatives are regarded as nutrients and have not been subjected to extensive toxicological analysis. Where limits on intake have been suggested, the limit is often dependent on the maximum dose administered in a particular study rather than that which produced a response.

Two groups of synthetic antioxidants, gallic acid esters and butylated hydroxytoluenes, warrant closer attention. Gallic acid esters (propyl, octyl and dodecyl) are used extensively. They can cause contact dermatitis. On ingestion, the gallates are hydrolysed, releasing the acid, which is absorbed. It is excreted unchanged in the urine or metabolized to 4-O-methylgallic acid and conjugated with glucuronic acid. In reproductive studies the gallates cause failure of the neonates to thrive at maternal dietary levels above 0.1%. This effect is abolished if the pups are fostered and is thus due to a product in the maternal milk. The effect is not seen with propyl gallate.

The butylated phenols butylated hydroxytoluene (BHT) and butylated hydroxyanisole (BHA) are two synthetic antioxidants that are very widely used, and not only in food products. The toxicology of these compounds has been studied in great detail over many years.

BHT is rapidly absorbed after ingestion, maximum tissue concentrations being achieved in 4 h in rats and mice. There is no evidence of tissue accumulation on repeated dosage but excretion is slow (half-life 7–10 days), probably owing to an enterohepatic circulation. In man absorption is rapid also but 50% of the dose is excreted in the urine in 24 h. The remainder is excreted more slowly, and this could indicate that biliary excretion with an enterohepatic circulation also occurs in humans.

In the experimental animal the main metabolite is BHT acid, both free and conjugated, whereas in man this is a minor metabolite. The main metabolite is benzofuran, excreted as a conjugate with glucuronic acid or mercapturic acid (Conning and Phillips, 1986).

Repeated exposure to BHT, by incorporation in the diet, results in liver enlargement and the induction of microsomal oxidases. The growth rate of animals is reduced and the life-span increased. No adverse effects occurred in reproductive studies. In one study an increased incidence of hepatic tumours occurred in animals surviving beyond 111 weeks (the control animals survived much less well) at a dose equivalent, on a body weight basis, to 250 mg kg^{-1} day^{-1}, but not at lower doses (25 and 10 mg kg^{-1} day^{-1}). The ADI is currently set at a maximum of 0.125 mg kg^{-1}.

BHA is absorbed after oral administration and excreted in the urine conjugated directly with glucuronic acid or sulphate. The half-life in man is 2–5 days. At small dosage, BHA may be excreted unconjugated and at high dosage there may be metabolism to a hydroquinone. BHA shows no adverse effects on reproduction. It has, however, been shown at high dosage to induce malignant tumours of the forestomach in several animal species that possess a forestomach. This effect occurs at dietary concentrations of 1% and 2% but not at 0.5%. The appearance of tumours is preceded by hyperplasia, which is slowly reversible if treatment is stopped (Ito et al., 1983).

These findings have resulted in further extensive studies of the roles of BHT and BHA as promoters of carcinogenesis, given that neither compound is genotoxic. Both have been shown, at high dosage, to promote tumours initiated by tissue-specific carcinogens and yet to inhibit carcinogenesis at low dosage. Similar studies with α-tocopherol, alone or with BHA and/or BHT, have consistently shown tumour inhibition.

It seems likely that at low dosage antioxidants reduce the likelihood of tumour formation, owing perhaps to a protective effect against free radical damage, but at high dosage, except for α-tocopherol, they may become oxygen donors and enhance the carcinogenic process.

Colours

Colouring materials are added to processed foodstuffs to restore or standardize colour. It is generally accepted that colour has an important role in making food attractive, but with advanced preservation techniques based on the rapid reduction of the temperature of cooked products, the need for added colour has become smaller. There is a general regulatory policy in the UK to reduce the use of colours except where the resultant product would be colourless, such as boiled sweets and other confectionery (Food Advisory Committee, 1987).

Colours used in food products may be classified in two groups—synthetic and natural. The synthetic colours can be produced to high specifications, whereas the natural colours are extracted and usually consist of mixtures. Some natural colours can be synthesized but this also usually results in mixtures that are nevertheless better characterized.

Synthetic Colours

Four main classes of compound are used.

Azo Dyes. These are compounds in which one or more azo groups (–N=N–) are present. They have been subjected to extensive toxicological study. They are, in general, poorly absorbed but the azo linkage is broken down by bacterial activity in the colon. The products are absorbed only to a minor extent and are usually excreted as glucuronide conjugates in the urine. The stimulus to bacterial metabolism of the large doses employed in toxicological studies commonly results in caecal hypertrophy. This may be associated, by mechanisms as yet unknown, with nephrocalcinosis in those experimental species susceptible to age-related nephrosclerosis such as the rat and mouse.

There have been a number of reports that azo dyes, in particular tartrazine, are associated with food intolerance. Food intolerance is characterized by a reproducible, unpleasant reaction to a food or food ingredient. It may give rise to many symptoms, the commonest being migrainous headaches, gastrointestinal disturbance or manifestation of an allergic reaction. Although commonly called 'food allergies', the demonstration of an immunological basis is rarely achieved. The condition occurs most commonly in children under the age of 5 years and usually does not persist beyond the age of 7 or 8 years, although a minority of adults may exhibit adverse reactions to specific food components.

Claims have been made that attention deficit disorder, commonly called hyperactivity, is due to food intolerance. This rare condition occurs in early childhood and is characterized by short attention span, disruptive behaviour, volatile temperament and underachievement in school. Studies of dietary causes have given conflicting results, but it is likely that a small minority of cases are the result of intolerance to some dietary items, which may include some food additives. Regrettably, the doses used to elicit responses have been much larger than would be obtained from food and drink, and the possibility of pseudoallergic (anaphylactoid) reactions cannot be excluded. The syndrome itself is difficult to diagnose without considerable experience, and there can be little doubt that it has been considerably overdiagnosed (Lessof, 1987).

Triphenylmethane Dyes.   In general, triphenylmethane dyes are poorly absorbed and long-term toxicity studies have shown no adverse effects.

Fluorescein Dyes.   Based on fluoran, the main example is erythrosine, a molecule in which iodine is incorporated. This has given rise to some concern in relation to thyroid function, in that in the rat, at high dosage, there is evidence of hypertrophy and hyperplasia of the thyroid gland with an accompanying increase of the serum concentrations of thyroxine and protein-bound iodine, and a reduction in serum triiodothyronine (T_3). Such findings suggest that erythrosine stimulates the release of thyroid stimulating hormone, possibly by inhibiting the conversion of thyroxine to T_3, thereby reducing the feedback mechanism. The effect does not occur at the concentrations experienced in food usage, which are about 1000 times less than the minimal effect dosage.

Sulphonated Indigo Dyes. Sulphonated indigo dyes are poorly absorbed and have demonstrated no adverse effects in several long-term toxicity studies.

Natural Colours

Natural colours are obtained from naturally occurring materials which may or may not be foods. Usually those derived from natural foods by physical means (pressing, filtration or aqueous extracts) are accepted for use in foods, although they have not been subjected to rigorous toxicological study. Such studies will be required if their use increases substantially. The main colours of this type are the riboflavins, cochineal carmine, the carotenes (with the exception of a carotenoid, canthoxanthin), the anthocyanins, chlorophyll and chlorophyllins and beetroot red. Directly extracted annatto, but not the solvent-extracted compound, is also included.

Of the naturally occurring compounds which are synthesized, caramel is by far the most important. It is very extensively used in cola drinks and beers. Caramels are formed when simple sugars are heated. The process involves dehydration and the formation of furans and furfuraldehyde, which then degrade and polymerize to form brown-coloured compounds. The precise chemistry is unknown. Pyrolysis may occur but can be prevented in the presence of ammonium salts, acids, alkalis or sulphates.

Industrially, a wide range of caramels are produced through the use of ammonia and ammonium sulphite. This has made the toxicological evaluation difficult. The position improved when the British Caramel Manufacturers Association specified six types of caramels (including starting materials) to which industrial use would be confined. This proposal was later modified by international industrial agreement and the modified proposal

has been accepted, provisionally, by the regulatory authorities.

Four main types of caramel have been specified:

Alkali compounds, made with sodium or potassium hydroxide.
Ammonia compounds, made with ammonia or ammonium hydroxide, carbonate, bicarbonate, phosphate or sulphate.
Sulphite compounds, made with sulphur dioxide, sulphurous acid, sodium or potassium sulphite or metabisulphite.
Ammonium sulphite compounds, made with ammonium sulphite or bisulphite; this group is classified in two strengths.

In each case the process must be specified. Burnt sugar caramels, used essentially as flavouring agents, are additional to these groups.

Although many studies have been undertaken with many caramels, the main finding has been caecal enlargement in the rat, not considered to be of toxicological significance. Other adverse effects have been attributed to imidazole contaminants at high dosage. With ammonia caramels, however, it was noted that rats developed lymphocytopenia, an effect enhanced by reduced dietary levels of vitamin B_6. It is thought that this effect is mainly due to the presence of a tetrahydroxybutyl imidazole (THI), although it cannot be excluded that other active compounds are present. It is not known whether this effect occurs in other species, such as man, or whether it has any functional significance. Work proceeds and, for the time being, the THI content of ammonia caramel is limited to 25 ppm.

As caramel colours represent 98% usage of all colours in foodstuffs, they are of considerable economic importance. More importantly, such widespread usage could have serious implications for public health if adverse effects occur in man. At present there is no evidence that this is the case (Food Advisory Committee, 1987).

Emulsifiers

Food manufacture involves to a considerable extent the mixing of ingredients, especially ingredients that are either fat- or water-soluble. Such mixing is greatly facilitated by the use of emulsifiers. These are usually chain-like molecules with a water-soluble group at one end and a fat-soluble group at the other. Additionally, the group includes some proteins and some simple salts of organic acids. Emulsifiers are almost invariably compounds and derivatives that occur naturally, the commonest being based on esters of fatty acids with glycerol or simple sugars. They have been extensively studied and generally are of low toxicity, the observed effects being associated with the physical consequences of very large dosage, such as bladder stones and altered calcium–phosphate balance. Many studies conducted at lower dosage in man have shown no adverse effects.

Flavours

Modern food processes employ flavouring materials very extensively. This has resulted in the development of a wide range of flavouring materials. At present about 6000 flavouring agents have been identified, of which about 3500 are in common use, many in complicated mixtures. It is a considerable technological challenge to develop for a particular foodstuff an identifiable and acceptable flavour from the large array of compounds that exist. Most flavouring compounds occur naturally, having been identified through the laborious extraction of prepared foods. Having been characterized, the compounds are often synthesized. These are the so-called 'nature-identical' compounds. Their manufacture allows adherence to tighter specifications than is possible with extracts of natural materials and, of course, improves their availability and reduces costs.

Flavour compounds are extremely potent, often eliciting a distinct flavour at molecular concentrations. As a consequence, although their use is widespread, the concentrations in food are very low indeed, and the amounts manufactured are small in comparison with foodstuffs themselves or industrial chemicals generally.

One result has been that very few of the compounds have been subjected to extensive toxicological testing, essentially because conventional toxicity studies are too insensitive to detect effects at the concentrations likely to be present in food, so that the resultant safety margins will be very large. An additional reason is that, for many flavouring substances, the amount of material required to mount a comprehensive toxicological analysis would be difficult to obtain (Food Additives and Contaminants Committee, 1976).

Flavouring substances are classified as follows:

Natural—compounds that are extracted from foodstuffs and spices and used directly. They consist of complex mixtures and are generally regarded as offering no hazard where their usage does not greatly exceed that which occurs naturally.

Nature-identical—compounds that have been characterized as part of a natural flavour complex and synthesized. They are regarded, for regulatory purposes, as new chemicals requiring toxicological evaluation. Many have been subjected to such studies and the rest will be when priorities have been agreed.

Artificial—wholly new compounds with flavouring characteristics. In the UK, four such compounds comprise the bulk of consumption, ethylvanillin, ethylmaltol, ethylmethylphenyl glycidate and butylbutyryl lactate. All have repeatedly given negative responses in a variety of toxicological studies. The average individual consumption of these compounds in the UK does not exceed $16 \, \mu g \, kg^{-1} \, day^{-1}$ for each compound.

It is likely that in due course the use of flavouring substances will diminish as preservation techniques based on quick freezing are developed, but for the forseeable future a substantial usage will remain, given the increasing popularity of processed foods and meals.

Flavour Enhancers

Flavour enhancers have the ability to intensify the flavour of cooked, processed foods without, at the concentrations used, adding flavour of their own. They have been in use for many centuries, although it is only in the last century or so that they have been chemically characterized. They are particularly popular with Japanese and Chinese cooks. The mode of action is not known but seems to involve both the taste buds and the tactile nerve endings in the buccal cavity, enhancing taste and imparting a satisfactory 'mouth feel'.

The compounds are salts of glutamic and guanylic acid and of the nucleotides inosinic and ribonucleic acid. As naturally occurring compounds, they are not associated with adverse toxicity, except at very high dosage.

The commonest compound in use is monosodium glutamate (MSG). Adult diets normally contain approximately 20 g of MSG daily, of which not more than 0.7 g is 'added'. Quantities as high as $45 \, g \, day^{-1}$ ($0.75 \, g \, kg^{-1} \, day^{-1}$) have been consumed without adverse effect. One animal study showed that neonatal mice given $0.5 \, g \, kg^{-1} \, day^{-1}$ by mouth developed hypothalamic lesions, although these did not occur when MSG was given subcutaneously. Human breast milk contains $21.6 \, mg \, dl^{-1}$ of free L-glutamate.

Some people claim to experience a variety of symptoms, such as tingling of the mouth and tongue and weakness of the limbs, after the consumption of food reputedly containing MSG, the so-called 'Chinese restaurant syndrome'. This effect has not been confirmed by double-blind clinical trials but it remains a possibility that some individuals exhibit an idiosyncratic sensitivity. The mechanism remains obscure.

Preservatives

In many respects, the history of mankind is characterized by the increasing ability to produce and preserve food. The origins of many preservation techniques, such as salting, pickling, acidification, smoking and dehydration, are lost in antiquity. Although many of these methods are still used today, food manufacture has latterly relied more on chemical expertise. Chemical preservation depends on the ability of certain compounds to inhibit microbial growth, thereby preventing microbiological spoilage of foodstuffs. At the concentrations used, preservatives are not bactericidal.

Most chemical preservatives are simple acids or their salts, and exert their effect through a reduction in pH. The commonest are benzoic, acetic, propionic and sorbic acids. Sulphites, nitrites and nitrates are also in common use. Another major group is the ethyl and propyl esters of p-hydroxybenzoic acid, valuable because they exert an antimicrobial effect across a wide range of pH values.

Each compound is effective against a limited range of microorganisms (bacteria, moulds, yeasts) in a particular type of foodstuff and tends to have been developed for that purpose, although there is a considerable overlap. Sorbic acid, for example, is used in chemically leavened baked goods, propionic and acetic acid in yeast-leavened baked goods, sulphites in wines and beers, benzoates and p-hydroxybenzoates in beverages, fruit juices, purées and pie fillings and nitrites and nitrates almost exclusively in meat products.

Benzoic Acid
Benzoic acid is conjugated in the liver and excreted in the urine as hippuric acid. This reaction was used for many years as a test of liver function in man. Absorption is rapid and excretion complete. The only adverse effects resulting from long-term administration at high dosage are gastric irritation and a possible disturbance of acid–base balance. Some individuals exhibit allergy to benzoates.

p-Hydroxybenzoic Acid Esters
p-Hydroxybenzoic acid esters are readily absorbed and metabolized in the liver. The main excretion product is p-hydroxybenzoic acid and its glucuronide conjugate. Hydroxyhippuric acid is also formed. Extensive studies in several species have shown only marginal effects on growth rate at high dosage. Some individuals may show allergic responses.

Sorbic Acid
Sorbic acid is readily absorbed and converted to the fully saturated caproic acid. It is then metabolized as any other fatty acid and is used as a source of energy. Extensive toxicity studies have revealed no adverse effects at 5% in the diet.

Sulphites
The sulphites are reactive chemicals and, in foods, tend to be bound to sugars and proteins. On absorption they are converted to sulphates. In in vitro studies, sulphite can bind to DNA, causing bacterial mutation. This effect has not been observed in mammalian systems. The only adverse effect seen in extensive toxicological studies has been a slight reduction in litter size or litter weight in three-generation reproduction studies.

Between 4 and 7% of severely asthmatic patients exhibit sensitivity to sulphur dioxide, which may be released from sulphite in acid media or on ingestion. This seems particularly the case where sulphites are used, in spray form, to preserve salads. The prevalence in all asthmatics is 1–2%. The mechanism is not known but is unlikely to be an immune effect. Hypersensitivity of bronchial receptors has been postulated.

Nitrates and Nitrites
Nitrates are readily absorbed and excreted unchanged, although a small percentage may be converted to nitrite. At high levels of intake this conversion may result in the formation of methaemoglobin. The ingestion of nitrite is, of course, much more likely to result in methaemoglobinaemia in neonates.

Nitrites can react with amines to produce volatile N-nitrosamines and with ureas amides, carbamates or guanidines to form N-nitrosamides. These reactions occur both endogenously and in response to exogenous nitrites. N-Nitrosamines and N-nitrosamides are potent animal carcinogens although, in practice, the former are much more stable and therefore more important. The role of N-nitrosamines in human carcinogenesis is not known. The major source of nitrites to man is derived from nitrates in the diet, mainly from vegetables and from water. The use of nitrites in food probably adds a negligible burden and, given its efficacy in controlling the growth of Clostridium botulinum and, hence, deadly botulism, its continued use is probably justified. Nevertheless, this is a field of very active research aimed at the quantification of N-nitroso compounds in order to gauge the carcinogenic hazard.

Sweeteners

Sucrose is a unique food in that it confers not only sweetness but also textural characteristics that are indispensable to certain products such as baked confectionery. However, its energy content (3.75 kcal g^{-1}) has led to its association with being overweight. There is a general cultural perception that being overweight is undesirable and a consequent requirement to reduce energy consumption. This has resulted in a search for compounds that possess similar characteristics to sucrose but with less energy content. None has been found, but two groups of compounds have been developed which approximate certain technical functions.

Bulk Sweeteners
Bulk sweeteners are polyhydric alcohols (polyols and sugar alcohols) and most of those in use in foodstuffs occur naturally. They are five-or six-carbon molecules essentially similar to the equivalent sugar, except that the aldehyde group or linkage is replaced by an alcohol group. They are of equivalent sweetness to sucrose and, in cooking, show several of the technical characteristics, such as effects on viscosity, crystallization and stability. They tend to be hygroscopic, and this, associated with their reduced absorption after ingestion, results in the

main toxicological hazard—the production of diarrhoea. Individuals vary in their susceptibility to this effect but, in general, ingestion of less than 20 g day^{-1} does not cause problems. In the experimental rat these compounds cause the caecal enlargement associated with bacterial fermentation, but no other effect. The reduced absorption confers a reduced energy contribution to the diet.

Intense Sweeteners

Intense sweeteners are chemical compounds that exhibit intense sweetness but contribute little or no energy to the diet. Their sweetness ranges from 30 to 2000 times the sweetness of sucrose, so that they are used in very small amounts. They have none of the technological characteristics of sugars or sugar alcohols.

Aspartame.   Aspartame is the methyl ester of phenylalanine and aspartic acid, and is approximately 180 times sweeter than sucrose. On ingestion, it is metabolized to the constituent amino acids and methanol. Very extensive toxicological studies in experimental animals and in man have not revealed adverse effects attributable to the compound. There is continuing discussion on the possible effects of of intakes of phenylalanine but as yet no definite effects have been consistently observed. In the UK, products containing aspartame must contain a statement warning to phenylketonurics of the possible presence of phenylalanine. The methyl ester undergoes hydrolysis in acid and aqueous products on storage, with the formation of a substituted piperazine. This too has been subjected to extensive study, with no adverse effects detected at acceptable dosage. The breakdown product is not sweet-tasting, so that extensive consumption is unlikely.

Cyclamic Acid, Sodium and Calcium Salts.   Cyclamic acid was used for many decades in combination with saccharin because it reduced the bitter aftertaste associated with the latter compound. Its regulatory approval was discontinued when it was claimed that a cyclamate–saccharin mixture caused bladder carcinoma in the rat, the putative agent being cyclohexylamine, a metabolite of cyclamate produced by bacterial fermentation in the gut. Subsequent study has demonstrated that neither cyclamate nor cyclohexylamine are carcinogenic or mutagenic but that the amine can cause testicular atrophy at high dosage in the rat. Humans vary in their ability to generate the amine and certainly cannot produce toxic amounts, given the likely concentrations of cyclamate in the diet. Nevertheless, the use of cyclamate remains severeley restricted in the UK and is not permitted in the USA.

Saccharin, Potassium, Sodium and Calcium salts.   Saccharin, discovered in 1879, has been used as an intense sweetener since the turn of the century. It is some 300 times sweeter than sucrose but is associated with a bitter aftertaste. For many years it was regarded as absolutely safe, being absorbed and excreted unchanged. A study of a cyclamate–saccharin mixture with added cyclohexyla-

mine claimed to detect a carcinogenic effect which was initially attributed to cyclamate. Subsequent studies with cyclamate failed to confirm this conclusion. Since then attention turned to saccharin, and innumerable investigations have been undertaken with this compound and its salts.

These studies have examined whether saccharin is a complete carcinogen or is a promoter of carcinogenesis initiated by primary carcinogens. The main findings which have been confirmed in repeated studies are as follows:

(1) Sodium saccharin induces bladder tumours in male (but not female) rats when administered for the lifetime of the animals at dietary concentrations of 5% and above, provided that the administration commences within 2 weeks of birth or is fed to the mother during pregnancy and is continued thereafter. It does not exhibit this effect in other species.
(2) Sodium saccharin is not mutagenic.
(3) Sodium saccharin at a dietary concentration of 5% will promote bladder tumours initiated by a known bladder carcinogen, N-butyl-N-(4-hydroxybutyl)-nitrosamine (BBN). This effect is shared with sodium ascorbate, sodium bicarbonate and sodium citrate. Several similar claims using other initiators or the implantation of pellets in the urinary bladder have not been confirmed by repeated experiments.
(4) Sodium saccharin, but not potassium and calcium saccharin or the free acid, at 5% in the diet induces epithelial hyperplasia in the urinary bladder of the rat.
(5) Sodium saccharin results in increased pH of rat urine. Studies employing 5% sodium cyclamate or sodium hippurate, which do not elevate urinary pH, have not resulted in the formation of bladder tumours.

The overall conclusion is that sodium saccharin is a bladder carcinogen for the male rat, provided that the compound is administered soon after birth and continued for a lifetime. The dose–response relationship is steep and suggests a threshold limit of 1% in the diet, equivalent, on a body weight basis, to 500 mg kg^{-1} day^{-1}. Potassium and calcium saccharin and the free acid are not associated with these effects. The current ADI of 2.5 mg kg^{-1} incorporates a 200-fold safety factor and applies to all forms of saccharin. Such an intake represents approximately 12 cans of a diet drink, sweetened with saccharin, per day (Munro, 1989).

REFERENCES

ATBC (1994). Alpha-Tocopherol, Beta-Carotene Cancer Prevention Study Group. The effect of vitamin E and beta-carotene on the incidence of lung cancer and other cancers in male smokers. *N. Engl. J. Med.*, **330**, 1029–1035.

Bingham, S. (1990). Diet and large bowel cancer, *J. Roy. Soc. Med.*, **83**, 420–422.

Bingham, S., Pignatelli, B., Pollock, J. H., Ellul, A., Malaveille, C., Gross, G., Runswick, S., Cummings, J. H., and O'Neill, J. K. (1996). Does increased formation of endogenous *N*-nitroso compounds in the human colon explain the association between red meat and colon cancer? *Carcinogenesis*, **17**, 515–523.

BNF (1990). British Nutrition Foundation's Task Force. *Report: Complex Carbohydrates in Foods*. Chapman and Hall, London.

Bogaards, J. J. P., Verhagen, H., Willems, M. I., Vanpoppel, G. and Vanbladeren, P. J. (1994). Consumption of Brussels sprouts results in elevated alpha-class glutathione-S-transferase levels in human blood plasma. *Carcinogenesis*, **15**, 1073–1075.

Burkitt, D. P. and Trowell, H. C. (1975). *Refined Carbohydrate Foods and Disease: Some Implications of Dietary Fibre*. Academic Press, London.

Carroll, K. K. and Khor, H. T. (1975). Dietary fat in relation to tumorigenesis. *Prog. Biochem. Pharmacol.*, **10**, 308–353.

Conning, D. M. and Phillips, J. C. (1986). Comparative metabolism of BHA, BHT and other phenolic antioxidants and its toxicological relevance. *Food Chem. Toxicol.*, **24**, 1145–1148.

Department of Health (1998). *Report on Health and Social Subjects No. 48. Nutritional Aspects of the Development of Cancer*. Stationery Office, London.

DHSS (1984). *Diet and Cardiovascular Disease*. Department of Health and Social Security Report on Health and Social Subjects 28. HMSO, London.

Food Additives and Contaminants Committee (1976). *Report on the Review of Flavourings in Food*. F.A.C./Rep./22, HMSO, London.

Food Advisory Committee (1987). *Final Report on the Review of the Colouring Matter in Food Regulations 1973*. F.A.C./Rep/4. HMSO, London.

Gey, K. F., Brubacher, G. B. and Stahelin, H. B. (1987). Plasma levels of antioxidant vitamins in relation to ischaemic heart disease and cancer. *Am. J. Clin. Nutr.*, **45**, 1368–1377.

Giovannucci, E., Rimm, E. B., Stampfer, M. J., Colditz, G. A., Ascherio, A. and Willett, W. C. (1994). *Cancer Res.*, **54**, 2390–2397.

Goldstein, J. L., Kita, T. and Brown, M. S. (1983). Lessons from an animal counterpart of familial hypercholesterolemia. *N. Engl. J. Med.*, **309**, 288–296.

IARC (1993). *Monographs on the Evaluation of Carcinogenic Risk of Chemicals to Humans. Vol. 56. Some Naturally Occurring Substances: Food items and Constituents, Heterocyclic Aromatic Amines and Mycotoxins*. International Agency for Research on Cancer, Lyon.

IARC (1997). *Monographs on the Evaluation of Carcinogenic Risks of Chemicals to Humans. Vol. 69. Polychlorinated Dibenzo-dioxins and Benzo-furans*. International Agency for Research on Cancer, Lyon.

Ip, C., Carter, C. A. and Ip, M. M. (1985). Requirement of essential fatty acid for mammary tumorigenesis in the rat. *Cancer Res.*, **45**, 1997–2001.

Ito, N., Fukushima, S., Hagiwara, A., Shibata, M. and Ogiso, Y. (1983). Carcinogenicity of butylated hydroxyanisole in F344 rats. *J. Natl. Cancer Inst.*, **70**, 343–349.

Kannel, W. B. and Gordon, T. (Eds) (1970). *Some Characteristics Related to the Incidence of Cardiovascular Disease and Death*. Framingham Study 16-Year Follow-up. US Government Printing Office, Washington, DC.

Keys, A. (1980). *Seven Countries. A Multivariate Analysis of Death and Coronary Disease*. Harvard University Press, Cambridge, MA.

Kinlen, L. J. (1987). Diet and cancer. In Cottrell, R. (Ed.), *Food and Health*. Parthenon, Carnforth, pp. 83–98.

Knekt, P. (1991). Role of vitamin E in the prophylaxis of cancer. *Am. Med.*, **23**, 3–12.

Kromhout, D., Bosschieter, E. B. and de Lezenne Coulander, C. (1985). The inverse relationship between fish consumption and 20-year mortality from coronary heart disease. *N. Engl. J. Med.*, **312**, 1205–1209.

Larsen, J. C. and Poulsen, E. (1987). Mutagens and carcinogens in heat-processed food. In Miller, K. (Ed.), *Toxicological Aspects of Food*. Elsevier Applied Science, Barking, pp. 205–252.

Lavik, P. S. and Baumann, C. A. (1941). Dietary fat and tumour formation. *Cancer Res.*, **1**, 181–187.

Lessof, M. M. (1987). Allergies to food additives. *J. Roy. Coll. Physicians*, **21**, 237–240.

MacFarlane, G. T., Gibson, G. R., Drasar, B. S. and Cummings, J. H. (1995). Metabolic significance of gut microflora. In Whitehead, R. (Ed.), *Gastrointestinal and Oesophageal Pathology*. Churchill Livingstone, London, pp. 249–273.

Miller, E. C. and Miller, J. A. (1996). Mechanisms of chemical carcinogenesis: nature of proximate carcinogens and interactions with macromolecules. *Pharmacol. Rev.*, **18**, 805–836.

Moncada, S. and Vane, J. R. (1978). Pharmacology and endogenous roles of prostaglandin endoperoxides, thromboxane A2 and prostacyclin. *Pharmacol. Rev.*, **30**, 293–331.

Munro, I. C. (1989). A case study: the safety evaluation of artificial sweeteners. In Taylor, S. L. and Scanlan, R. A. (Eds), *Food Toxicology: a Perspective on the Relative Risks*. Marcel Dekker, New York, pp. 151–168.

Peto, R., Doll, R., Buckley, J. D. and Sporn, M. B. (1981). Can dietary β-carotene materially reduce human cancer rates? *Nature*, **290**, 201–208.

Ronco, A., DeStefani, E., Mendilaharsu, M. and Denio-Pellegrini, H. (1996). Meat, fat and the risk of breast cancer: a case-control study from Uruguay. *Int. J. Cancer*, **65**, 328–331.

Sugimura, T. (1986). Past, present and future of mutagens in cooked foods. *Environ. Health Perspect.*, **67**, 5–10.

Vistisen, K., Loft, S. and Poulsen, H. E. (1990). Cytochrome P4501A2 activity in man measured by caffeine metabolism: effect of smoking, broccoli and exercise. In Witmer, C. H. (Ed.), *Advances in Experimental Medicine and Biology: Biological Reactive Intermediates IV*. Plenum Press, New York, pp. 407–411.

Whitaker, J. R. and Feeney, R. E. (1973). Enzyme inhibitors in food. In *Toxicants Occurring Naturally in Foods*. Committee on Food Protection, National Research Council, National Academy of Sciences, Washington, DC.

World Cancer Research Fund and American Institute for Cancer Research (1997). *Food, Nutrition and the Prevention of Cancer: a Global Perspective*. American Institute for Cancer Research, Washington, DC.

Yang, C. S., Brady, J. F. and Hong, J. (1992). Dietary effects of cytochromes P450, xenobiotic metabolism and toxicity. *FASEB J.*, **6**, 737–744.

Chapter 94
Toxicology of Pesticides

T. C. Marrs and I. Dewhurst

C O N T E N T S

INTRODUCTION

Pesticides are a group of substances with heterogeneous toxicity whose desired activity is the killing of unwanted living organisms, in a more or less specific manner. In order to review the toxicity of pesticides, some method of classification of them is needed. In this chapter, they are divided by class of action, into insecticides, fungicides, herbicides, molluscides and rodenticides, these groups being subdivided by chemical class. Some chemical classes have more than one type of pesticidal activity and therefore appear in more than one category, for example, the carbamates and organophosphates (OPs), which include insecticides, herbicides and fungicides, and the phosphides, used as both fumigants and rodenticides.

The very definition of pesticides may vary, particularly in relation to regulatory affairs. Some veterinary products, for example compounds used as ectoparasiticides on cattle, sheep and domestic pets, are regulated in many countries under different legislation than when the same active ingredients are used on arable commodities. Moreover, pesticide legislation often controls substances such as growth promoters and defoliants; some of these will be briefly discussed here.

There are a number of possible ways in which humans can be exposed to pesticides, thus the toxic effects of pesticides may have consequences for consumers of food as well as farmers and other applicators. Moreover, pesticides used domestically in wood preservation or as household insecticides may be important sources of exposure of the general public. Furthermore, pesticides may enter the water supply. These various routes of exposure may be isolated or may need to be considered in combination when assessing potential effects in humans. It should also be remembered that the more

acutely toxic pesticides have been used for suicide and murder.

The effects of pesticide residues in food and water probably cause the greatest public concern. However, reports of clinical poisoning by residues seem to be extremely rare, certainly by comparison with occupational intoxication. The reasons for this are complex, but may reflect a true rarity of poisoning or the fact that occupational poisonings are far more easily identified. Occupational intoxications would be expected to be more severe than food-borne poisonings, and the proximity of cause and effect in occupational poisoning certainly makes diagnosis easier. Food-borne pesticide intoxication, especially where clinical signs are non-specific or trivial, would probably pass unnoticed or may not be attributed to pesticides. This would be particularly likely where the signs and symptoms could be ascribed to a microbiological cause. Acute poisoning, where pesticides had been used in accordance with regulations, seems likely to be a very uncommon occurrence, if it occurs at all, at least in developed countries. The problem of consumers who consume high levels of some foodstuffs is taken into account when residue levels are pronounced to be toxicologically acceptable by comparison with the acceptable daily intake (ADI) or the more recently developed concept of the acute reference dose (ARfD). Bearing in mind that, as a minimum, a 100-fold safety factor is used in calculating ADIs and ARfDs from animal studies (WHO, 1990a), residues of some multiples of the maximum residue limit (MRL) would probably be necessary to produce acute poisoning. On the other hand, simultaneous exposure to more than one pesticide of the same type might occur, but it would seem improbable that extreme consumption, by itself, could give rise to pesticide poisoning. In fact, analysis of reported consumer poisonings by pesticides shows that most reported instances occur from:

(a) spillage of pesticides on to food during storage or transport;
(b) eating grain or seed potatoes treated with pesticides, where the food article was not intended for human consumption;
(c) improper application of pesticides or failure to observe harvest intervals.

The pesticides responsible have often been ones with low LD_{50}s [< 20mg (kg body weight)$^{-1}$], such as the insecticides endrin, parathion and aldicarb and the rodenticides thallium sulphate and sodium fluoride. Other pesticides that have produced morbidity by ingestion with food include organic mercury fungicides (Ferrer and Cabral, 1991).

Weighed against the disadvantages of pesticides that accrue from their toxic effects is the fact that insects and fungi are important sources of agricultural loss and give rise to much damage to buildings, particularly in those countries, such as the USA and Canada, where construction is often of wood. Furthermore, many insects carry diseases such as malaria and sleeping sickness, which in the absence of control measures may render land uninhabitable or agriculturally unusable: despite control measures, these diseases continue to be major sources of morbidity and mortality. Furthermore, fungal contamination of agricultural produce can give rise to such conditions as ergotism and aflatoxicosis.

The key to a successful pesticide is selective toxicity. An ideal pesticide will interfere with a biological system in the pest, which has no counterpart in non-target species: this is the advantage of the juvenile hormone analogue insecticides. In the case of agricultural insecticides, the pesticide should be toxic to insects, but less toxic to plants, to humans and to other non-target organisms. Thus the neuroactive insecticides exploit the relative accessibility of the insect nervous system to xenobiotics, when compared with humans, together with the lack of a nervous system in plants.

In this chapter it is not possible to give more than an outline of the toxicology of the main groups of pesticides, pointing out major problems which occur in regulation of the use of pesticides and allowable residues in food and the treatment of poisoning.

INSECTICIDES

Many insecticides affect the nervous system of insects and, since many have some activity against the mammalian nervous system, in man the neurotoxic effects of insecticides are often prominent. The main groups of insecticides are listed in **Table 1**.

Table 1 The main groups of pesticides.

Group	Subgroups	Examples
Organochlorines (OCs)		DDT
		Endrin
		Aldrin
		Dieldrin
		Endosulfan
		γ-Hexachlorocyclohexane (lindane)
Anticholinesterases	Organophosphates (OPs)	Malathion
		Fenitrothion
		Dichlorvos
		Diazinon
	Carbamates	Carbaryl
		Aldicarb
Pyrethrins and synthetic pyrethroids		Pyrethrum
		Permethrin
		Cypermethrin
		Flumethrin
Natural compounds, other than pyrethrins		Abamectin
		Ivermectin
		Rotenone
		Nicotine
Substances which interfere with systems specific to insects	Juvenile hormone analogues	Cyromazine
	Chitin synthesis inhibitors	Diflubenzuron
	Ecdysone agonists	Tebufenozide
Miscellaneous synthetic insecticides	Formamidine	Amitraz
	$GABA_A$ blocker	Fipronil

Organochlorines

This group was formerly of great importance and includes DDT, hexachlorocyclohexane (HCH), the cyclodienes, dieldrin, endrin and heptachlor, and toxaphene. However, the use of organochlorines (OCs) has, in recent years, been severely restricted in most countries. This has mainly been due to the persistence of OCs in the environment and wildlife and humans, rather than to their toxicity to mammals. Despite the fact that OCs are less used than formerly, their toxicology is still important because they continue to be present in the environment and because, in foodstuffs on sale in developed countries, residues, sometimes above international MRLs, continue to arise (Working Party on Pesticide Residues, 1997). OCs are excreted in breast milk (Siddiqui and Saxena, 1985) and their persistence is shown by the continuing presence of OCs in human milk, though usually at declining levels (Working Party on Pesticide Residues, 1992). One OC that is still used is lindane, the γ-isomer of HCH.

The most prominent effects of the OCs are those referable to the nervous system, where OCs have an effect on Na^+ channels. DDT produces tremor and incoordination in lower doses and convulsions in high doses, with a clear incremental dose response. By contrast, HCH and the cyclodienes may produce convulsions as the first sign of intoxication, as well as fever, by a central effect possibly linked to disturbances in GABA-mediated inhibitory neurotransmission (Abalis et al., 1986; Cole and Casida, 1986). OCs have been associated with a chronic toxicity syndrome, which includes apathy, headache, emotional lability, depression, confusion and irritability (Proudfoot, 1996).

OC poisoning is treated symptomatically and diazepam is usually used to deal with the convulsions.

Carcinogenic Effects of OCs

OCs may produce microsomal enzyme induction and characteristic histopathological changes in the livers of experimental animals (hepatocellular hypertrophy with accumulation of lipid). If administration is prolonged and at high enough doses, liver nodules may appear and tumours are seen in rodents. These tumors do not appear to be indicative of genotoxic carcinogenicity. In human populations OCs have been linked with non-Hodgkin's lymphoma (Axelson, 1987; Cantor et al., 1992) but where a link between non-Hodgkin's lymphoma and OC exposure has been observed, the association has been weak and some studies, e.g. by Rothman et al. (1997), have shown no such association. Some OCs have weak oestrogenic properties. The suggestion has been made that exposure to OCs is related to increased susceptibility to breast cancer (e.g. Høyer et al., 1998). Some epidemiological studies have shown a link between high fat levels of DDT/DDE and breast cancer and there

is a similar link between β-HCH and breast cancer. The studies linking DDT/DDE and breast cancer were summarized by Key and Reeves (1994), who concluded that it was unlikely that DDT increased the risk of breast cancer.

Lindane (γ-HCH)

Lindane is used as a wood preserver, in arable agriculture and in human and veterinary medicine as an ectoparasiticide. It is the γ-isomer of 1,2,3,4,5,6-hexachlorocyclohexane (HCH), which is sometimes known as benzene hexachloride. HCH has eight stereoisomers, of which the α-, β-and γ-isomers are the most important. Of these isomers, only lindane ($> 99\%$ γ-isomer) is still approved in the West, but in some countries preparations of lesser purity continue to be available and these contain other isomers. Lindane is less biologically persistent than DDT and, in rodents, the α- and β-isomers of HCH accumulate more readily than does lindane (Eichler et al., 1983). In addition to differences in pharmacokinetics between the isomers, there are qualitative differences in toxicology: thus the effect of lindane on the CNS is stimulatory, causing convulsions, whereas the α-and β-isomers have a depressant effect (Coper et al., 1951; van Asperen, 1954).

As with other OCs, lindane produces histopathological changes in the livers of experimental animals. The mutagenicity of lindane in vitro and in vivo has been reviewed and the preponderance of evidence is that the compound is not mutagenic (FAO/WHO, 1990). Over the years usage of lindane on arable crops and in veterinary medicine has become more and more restricted but its uses have long outlived those of DDT.

Anticholinesterases

Two groups of anticholinesterases, the organophosphates (OPs) and the carbamates, are widely used as agricultural insecticides and veterinary medicines (Marrs, 1996); in addition, some anticholinesterase OPs are used as human drugs, for example malathion in the treatment of headlice infestation and metrifonate (trichlorfon) in schistosomiasis (Aden-Abdi et al., 1990). Several carbamates are used in human medicine, for example pyridostigmine in myasthenia gravis. The anticholinesterases are often more acutely toxic than the OCs, although some OPs, especially the P = S phosphorothioates (see below), show low acute mammalian toxicity. The action is respectively to phosphorylate or carbamylate esterases, particularly the enzyme acetylcholinesterase, causing accumulation of the neurotransmitter, acetylcholine. A variety of cholinergic symptoms and clinical signs occur at parasympathetic effector sites, including bronchorrhoea, salivation, constriction of the pupil of the eye and abdominal colic. Sympathetic effects can also ensue, together with signs of central nervous system involvement, such as confusion and apprehension. Convulsions will occur in severe poisoning. Actions at the neuromuscular junction result in muscle fasciculation and later paralysis. The terminal event in fatal poisonings seems to be respiratory paralysis, which may be of central or peripheral origin, although with pesticidal OPs both will usually contribute. It is generally believed that, provided the patient survives (without suffering cerebral anoxia), the symptoms and clinical signs of the cholinergic syndrome of anticholinesterase poisoning are reversible. Moreover, histopathological changes, from the anticholinesterase effects of OPs and carbamates, are, *per se*, exiguous and, in acute lethal poisoning, specific pathological changes are usually not noteworthy. However, there is recognition that survival after high doses of OPs and perhaps also lower doses and after carbamate intoxication may result in long-term clinical and electrophysiological changes in the central nervous system.

It is often stated that the main difference between the OPs and the carbamates is that the former produce irreversible inhibition of acetylcholinesterase, whereas the latter produce reversible inhibition; this is only true in a relative sense. With certain exceptions (see below), reactivation of the dialkylphosphoryl–enzyme complexes produced by OP-induced inhibition of cholinesterases, is produced by hydrolysis, but the stability of the phosphorylated enzyme is generally greater than that of the carbamylated enzyme, so that carbamate poisoning is less long-lasting.

The numerous cholinesterases in the body show different intensities of sensitivity to inhibitors. Although by no means always the case, plasma cholinesterase is usually the cholinesterase most open to inhibition and it reactivates slowly (Skrinjarić-Spoljar *et al.*, 1973), so that this enzyme is a useful marker of exposure. However, correlation with cholinergic symptoms is poor, so that plasma cholinesterase inhibition can be taken as a marker of exposure and no more. Erythrocyte acetylcholinesterase inhibition often correlates better with cholinergic symptomatology, but reactivation can take place sufficiently quickly to interfere with the validity of blood tests, in both clinical and experimental situations, unless care is taken (FAO/WHO, 1993; Mason *et al.*, 1993). Reactivation can occur *ex vivo* in blood samples. The great sensitivity to inhibition and poor correlation with clinical cholinergic effects of inhibition of erythrocyte cholinesterase and, even more so, plasma cholinesterase have caused the Joint Meeting on Pesticide Residues (JMPR) to prefer inhibition of brain cholinesterase in the derivation of acceptable daily intakes (ADIs) for OPs (WHO, 1990a). It is uncertain if such an approach will cover the implications of peripherally mediated intoxication (Ligtenstein, 1984).

Organophosphates

OP anticholinesterases are esters of phosphoric, phosphonic or phosphorothioic or related acids. Their general formula is

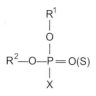

The R groups in pesticides are generally either both methyl groups or ethyl groups. The X or leaving group can be any one of large variety of moieties.

The OP pesticides have some similarities with the chemical warfare nerve agents, but these are often phosphonofluoridates. Many pesticidal OPs are phosphorothioates and those containing P = S groups such as malathion tend to be of lower acute mammalian toxicity than their corresponding phosphates and phosphonates. Thus paraoxon is much more toxic than parathion as is malaoxon compared to malathion. The reason for this is that the P = S phosphorothioates are inactive as anticholinesterases *in vitro* and only acquire toxicity after conversion of the P = S moiety to a P = O moiety, forming the oxon (WHO, 1986). Although OPs share their cholinergic symptomatology with the carbamates, the toxicology of OPs has certain features which do not resemble the effects of carbamates. These features are organophosphate-induced delayed polyneuropathy (OPIDP) and the so-called intermediate syndrome. Since the OP pesticides all have the same qualitative anticholinesterase action, and this property is responsible for their acute lethal toxicity, quantitative differences in toxicity are partly due to differences in absorption, distribution and metabolism. However, the rates of formation of the OP–acetylcholinesterase complex, of hydrolysis of this complex, and of the ageing reaction (see below) must also be considered.

Anticholinesterase Activity

Inactivation of cholinesterases by OPs involves a reaction in which the leaving group (X) is lost, producing a dialkylphosphoryl enzyme. Since most insecticides contain two methyl or two ethyl R groups, inactivation of cholinesterase produces a dimethoxyphosphorylated or a diethoxyphosphorylated enzyme and the kinetics of reactivation are the same for each derivative regardless of the structure of the leaving group of the OP. Reactivation of the dimethoxyphosphorylated enzyme will occur within a few hours and is considerably quicker than that of the diethoxy equivalent, whereas phosphorylated complexes containing one alkylthio group and one alkoxy group reactivate faster than those containing two alkoxy groups. By contrast, spontaneous reactivation of complexes containing larger R groups, e.g. isopropoxy and di-*sec*-butoxy, is slow or non-existent (WHO, 1986; Wilson *et al.*, 1992; Mason *et al.*, 1993), although large halogen-containing groups are an exception and seem to reactivate. With soman (pinacolyl methylphosphonofluoridate), a nerve agent that has as one of its R groups a pinacoloxy moiety, reactivation fails to occur but the mechanism is somewhat different: a further reaction takes place after dialkylphosphorylation of the enzyme in which the pinacolyl group is lost to leave a monoalkylphosphoryl enzyme. Such derivatives are refractory to oxime-induced reactivation and do not undergo spontaneous reactivation. With soman-inhibited enzyme the half-time for ageing is a few minutes. No pesticidal OP gives rise to a complex that ages at such a rate, but therapeutic failure with oximes has been attributed to ageing with certain pesticides (Glickman et al., 1984; Gyrd-Hansen and Kraul, 1984), and ageing half lives for dimethoxyphosphorylated cholinesterases are in the region of 2–9 h (Wilson et al., 1992).

Intermediate Syndrome

Senanayake and Karalliede (1987) reported a syndrome that followed therapy for and resolution of the cholinergic effects of OP intoxication. As the syndrome developed before the late effects of OPs, the authors called this syndrome the intermediate syndrome. Since 1987, other examples have been recorded, for instance that by Karademir et al. (1990), and this phenomenon is probably the same as the type II syndrome described by Wadia et al. (1987). The syndrome comprises a proximal limb paralysis starting 1–4 days after poisoning. The progression is not altered by atropine or oximes and, as the respiratory muscles are affected, respiratory support is necessary. A myopathy has been described post mortem in cases of human poisoning (de Rueck and Willems, 1975) and in experimental animals (Preusser, 1967; Wecker et al., 1978) and this may be related to the intermediate syndrome. The myopathy appears to be initiated by calcium accumulation in the region of the motor end-plate (Inns et al., 1990).

Organophosphate-induced Delayed Polyneuropathy (OPIDP)

OPIDP is a symmetrical sensory-motor axonopathy, tending to be most severe in the long axons, occurring 7–14 days after exposure. It is a polyneuropathy in that there are central and peripheral components. There is degeneration of axons and Schwann cell proliferation in the peripheral nervous system (Bouldin and Cavanagh, 1979a, b; Cavanagh, 1982), and also changes in the spinal cord and medulla oblongata (Barrett et al., 1985). Clinically, the most disabling feature is the paralysis of the legs which may result. Less severe cases exhibit a characteristic high-stepping gait, and some recovery may occur, but there is no specific treatment (Barrett et al., 1985). The initial event in the pathogenesis of the syndrome appears to be inhibition of neuropathy target esterase (NTE). This is followed by an ageing reaction similar to that described for soman with acetylcholinesterase above (Johnson, 1975). However, the structural requirements for inhibition of acetylcholinesterase and NTE are different, as shown by the fact that many OPs with powerful

anticholinesterase properties are devoid of ability to produce OPIDP. It should be noted that the nerve agents, which are powerful anticholinesterases, have little propensity to cause OPIDP (Gordon et al., 1983), whereas tri-o-cresyl phosphate, which has little anticholinesterase activity, is powerfully neuropathic.

Many regulatory authorities demand the use of tests to detect propensity for the development of OPIDP and this has resulted in the disappearance from the market of most OPs that are capable of producing OPIDP. The usual test that is carried out uses hens, because they are very susceptible to the syndrome. However, mice and rats also develop OPIDP (Veronesi et al., 1991) and the reported resistance of rodents to the development of OPIDP has been attributed to the use of young animals in studies (Moretto et al., 1992). Several OPs not in current use as pesticides produce OPIDP, including mipafox and diisopropyl phosphorofluoridate, and leptophos, also not currently used in most countries, have been consistently reported to produce OPIDP. There is some limited experimental and clinical evidence that a few OPs currently used in some countries can produced OPIDP, for example EPN, methamidophos, cyanofenphos and trichloronat (el-Sabae et al., 1981; Gallo and Lawryk, 1991).

Other Delayed Effects of OPs on the Nervous System.

The behavioural toxicity of anticholinesterases, inter alia OPs, has been reviewed (D'Mello, 1993). Since acute intoxication with OPs can cause major effects such as convulsions, respiratory failure and cardiac arrhythmias, all of which can result in anoxia, it is hardly surprising that major intoxication is sometimes associated with long-term CNS changes (Holmes and Gaon, 1956; Durham et al., 1965; Tabershaw and Cooper, 1966; Burchfiel et al., 1976; Korsak and Sato, 1977; Bartels and Friedel, 1979; Duffy et al., 1979; Hirshberg and Lerman, 1984; Savage et al., 1988). More debatable is whether long-term low-dose exposure produces delayed or chronic effects. Such an outome is biologically less plausible than delayed effects of acute exposure, but the two problems have frequently been conflated. Studies pertaining to long-term low-dose exposure, such as those by Ames et al. (1995), Stephens et al. (1995), Beach et al. (1996) and Fiedler et al. (1997) have been reviewed (e.g. Eyer, 1995; Steenland, 1996; IEH, 1998). Steenland (1996) concluded that studies had shown chronic subclinical effects in the central and peripheral nervous system in individuals previously poisoned by OPs but that the outcome after long-term low-level exposure was less consistent, although some studies had shown effects.

Other Effects of OPs

It should never be forgotten that OPs may have properties, some of which may be entirely independent of their anticholinesterase effects, including mutagenicity and carcinogenicity as well as organ-specific toxicity to the heart and kidney and other organs (Singer *et al.*, 1987; Baskin and Whitmer, 1992; Pimentel and Carrington da Costa, 1992; Wedin, 1992).

Treatment of OP Poisoning

The treatment of OP poisoning involves symptomatic treatment and the use of antidotes. Atropine, an anticholinergic compound, and an oxime enzyme reactivator such as pralidoxime chloride (2-PAM) or obidoxime is used (Bismuth *et al.*, 1992; Szinicz *et al.*, 1996), while convulsions and muscle fasciculation respond to diazepam (Johnson and Vale, 1992). The antidotal treatment is only effective against acute poisoning and specific treatment is not available for OPIDP or other long-term effects.

Carbamates

Carbamates are used as insecticides, herbicides and fungicides, but only the first group have marked anticholinesterase activity. Methiocarb (see below), an anticholinesterase, is used as a molluscicide.

The anticholinesterase carbamate pesticides are closely related to human drugs such as physostigmine and pyridostigmine. The general structure of most carbamate insecticides is as follows:

$$\begin{array}{cc} O & CH_3 \\ \| & | \\ R-O-C-NH \end{array}$$

In most cases, the R group is substituted a phenol or heterocycle, a notable exception being aldicarb, which is 2-methyl-2(methylthio)-propionaldehyde o-(methylcarbamoyl)oxime. Pirimicarb has two *N*-methyl groups.

In general, the carbamates produce toxicity similar to that of organophosphates, but less severe. A major difference is that carbamate-inhibited cholinesterases reactivate more rapidly than enzymes inhibited by OPs, with the result that the effects do not last as long in carbamate poisoning. Indeed, reactivation of carbamylated enzyme may be quick enough to render detection of cholinesterase depression difficult in both experimental animals and clinical situations. However, an insecticidal carbamate, aldicarb, is one of the few pesticides that has given rise to poisoning in consumers of treated food. Residues have occurred in cucumbers, watermelons, squashes and similar products sufficient to cause illness, in some cases severe. Outbreaks have occurred in the USA and Canada (Hall and Rumack, 1992) and in the Irish Republic (Department of Agriculture and Food, 1992). The reason for these problems is that aldicarb, in other respects a satisfactory pesticide, has a high mammalian toxicity, with an acute oral LD_{50} of about 1 mg (kg body weight)$^{-1}$. Atropine is effective in carbamate poisoning but oximes less so and there is some evidence that, with certain carbamates, oximes are harmful.

Pyrethroids (and Pyrethrins)

Pyrethrins are natural insecticides produced from, *inter alia*, pyrethrum, a plant of the Compositae group, and are esters of pyrethric or chrysanthemic acid. Pyrethrins are broken down and deactivated very readily in the environment, particularly by sunlight. The synthetic pyrethroids are structurally similar compounds rendered photostable by various substituent groups, such as chlorine, bromine or cyanide. Some of the newer ones bear a more distant structural relationship to the pyrethrins. Because of their low mammalian toxicity, high insecticidal potency and lack of persistence in the environment, the synthetic pyrethroids have achieved widespread usage in agriculture, as household insecticides and in wood preservation. Synthetic pyrethroids are also used in mosquito control (White, 1993). They have also been widely used on humans to treat such conditions as scabies. However, they are very toxic to aquatic organisms (Zitco *et al.*, 1979) and their lack of persistence can be a problem when used as wood preservatives. The advantageous properties of the synthetic pyrethroids result from the fact that they hydrolyse relatively easily, both in the mammalian body and in the environment. Consequently, bioaccumulation does not occur, nor do they persist in soils.

In general, by the oral route, the synthetic pyrethroids are of low acute toxicity, but this is not the case when they are administered to mammals parenterally when they are neurotoxic by virtue of their action upon voltage-dependent sodium channels (Vijverberg and van den Bercken, 1990; Vijverberg, 1994). As a result, there is often a large difference between the oral LD_{50} and that by parenteral routes. Despite the neurotoxicity of this group of compounds, underlying pathological changes in the nervous systems of animals exposed to pyrethroids are slight (Aldridge, 1990). Pyrethroids can be separated into two classes on the basis of the central neurotoxic syndrome that they produce by parenteral routes in experimental animals (Vijverberg, 1994). Type I synthetic pyrethroids, which include permethrin and resmethrin and also the components of natural pyrethrum, lack an α-cyano group and give rise to the T-syndrome. The T-syndrome is characterized by fine tremor, hypersensitivity to stimuli and aggressive sparring, progressing to coarse whole body tremor; this syndrome is similar to that produced by some of the OCs. Type II compounds, which include deltamethrin, flumethrin, cyfluthrin and γ-cypermethrin, have an α-cyano group and give rise to the CS-syndrome. The CS-syndrome consists of initial pawing and burrowing and later marked choreoathetosis, salivation, course tremor and convulsions (Aldridge, 1990; Joy, 1994). In addition to these central effects in experimental animals, pyrethroids cause peripheral nerve damage with functional impairment when administered repeatedly (Rose and Dewar, 1983). Axonal degeneration has been described, but generally at near lethal doses, and there is no evidence that pyrethroids can produce delayed neuropathy of the OP type (Aldridge, 1990).

Despite the findings in the central and peripheral nervous systems of animals, in humans the most prominent effect of the pyrethroids is to cause paraesthesia, mainly in the face, and there is little evidence of any permanent effects. Pruritis with blotchy erythema, itching, rhinorrhoea and lachrymation have also been described (Aldridge, 1990). Deltamethrin seems more potent and permethrin less so in producing these effects. Additionally, the pyrethroids are potent allergens and allergic rhinitis, asthma and extrinsic allergic alveolitis have been reported (Bismuth et al., 1987).

Specific treatment of the effects of synthetic pyrethroids is rarely necessary as systemic effects are very unusual in humans.

Insecticides of Biological Origin other than Pyrethrum

A number of insecticides are available that are of biological origin. The pyrethrins, discussed above with the synthetic pyrethroids, form one group. Of the others, only the avermectins and derris are at all widely used (see **Table 2**).

Table 2 Insecticides of natural origin

Group	Active ingredients
Avermectin group	Abamectin
	Ivermectin
Derris and similar insecticides	Rotenone
Cholinergic group	Nicotine
Pyrethrum	Pyrethrins

Avermectins

Abamectin is the common name for a mixture of avermectin B1a and B1b, macrocyclic lactone disaccharide antibiotics from *Streptomyces avermitilis*. Abamectin is an insecticide and acaricide used in crop protection and in veterinary medicine it is used as an anthelmintic. The dihydro derivative, ivermectin, is used to control nematodes and arthropods in animals and onchocerciasis in man (Wright, 1986) (see below). The insecticidal activity is based on action upon GABAergic nerve transmission; because mammals only have GABAergic synapses in the CNS, the mammalian blood/brain barrier ensures a degree of specificity. A notable feature of this group of compounds is their low LD_{50}s, the oral LD_{50} for abamectin in mice being 14–24 mg/kg and for ivermectin 25–40 mg/kg (Lankas and Gordon, 1989). Abamectin and ivermectin are neurotoxic, producing tremors, weakness and incoordination, and can induce malformations in off-

spring in teratological studies in CF-1 mice and in cultured embryos (Lankas and Gordon, 1989; FAO/WHO, 1993; Chaconas and Smoak, 1997). Ivermectin, used in human infestations with parasites, rarely gives rise to effects related to outcomes observed in animal toxicology studies: thus reported reactions (encephalopathy) to the use of ivermectin in infestation with *Onchocerca volvulus* were correlated with the load of microfilaria of *Loa loa*, and were probably not a direct toxic effect of ivermectin (Gardon et al., 1997). Both abamectin and ivermectin are non-genotoxic and almost certainly not carcinogenic (WHO, 1991, 1996; FAO/WHO, 1993).

Derris and Similar Insecticides

The other insecticide of biological origin that is very well known is rotenone, under the name derris. It acquired this name as the garden insecticide marketed under this name is derived from two Asiatic plants, *Derris eliptica* and *Derris mallaccensis*. Another plant, *Lonchocarpus utilis*, from South America, is a further source of an insecticide containing rotenone. Rotenone blocks mitochondrial electron transport and this is responsible for the toxic effects in mammals, including humans. It can also cause dermatitis. In severe human poisoning, the main effects that have been observed have been vomiting, depressed respiration and eventually apnoea (DeWilde et al., 1986).

Juvenile Hormone Analogues, Chitin Synthesis Inhibitors and Ecdysone Agonists

The attraction of these groups of insecticides is that they have no direct target organ or system in mammals. Examples are given in **Table 3**.

Table 3 Insecticides that interfere with insect growth and development

Group	Examples
Juvenile hormone analogues (insect growth regulators)	Methoprene
	Hydroprene
	Fenoxycarb
	Cyromazine
Chitin synthesis inhibitors	Diflubenzuron
Ecdysone agonists	Tebufenozide

Juvenile Hormone Analogues

The juvenile hormone analogues (insect growth regulators), which include hydroprene and methoprene, are esters of long-chain fatty acids and prevent metamorphosis to viable adults when applied to the larvae of insects. They are generally of low acute mammalian toxicity (oral LD_{50} ca 5 g kg^{-1}). They are usually non-teratogenic and non-genotoxic and are without endocrine activity in mammals (FAO/WHO, 1985; Ray, 1991). Methoprene caused changes such as bile duct proliferation in the livers of rats during a 2 year study (FAO/WHO, 1985). The carbamate fenoxycarb exerts most of its insecticidal activity as a juvenile hormone analogue and is of low mammalian toxicity (Evans, 1993; *Pesticide Manual*, 1994).

Chitin Synthesis Inhibitors

Chitin synthesis inhibitors, such as diflubenzuron, are also generally of low toxicity. These insecticides, which are benzoylphenylureas, act by interfering with the formation of the insect cuticle and the action is very specific, in that the compounds do not appear to inhibit hexosamine transferases, which are responsible for connective tissue glycosaminoglycan formation, in mammals (FAO/WHO, 1982; *Pesticide Manual*, 1994). A notable toxicological effect of diflubenzuron in experimental animals is to cause changes in haematological parameters, such as methaemoglobinaemia and sulphaemoglobinaemia, together with a fall in the red blood cell count and increased Heinz body formation. This probably results from the metabolism of the compound to, *inter alia*, 4-chloroaniline (FAO/WHO, 1982).

Ecdysone Agonists

Tebufenozide mimics the action of ecdysone by binding to its receptor and bringing about a lethal unsuccessful moult. It is of low toxicity to rodents but in experimental studies in laboratory animals it caused mild haemolytic anaemia. Methaemoglobinaemia is seen in mice. The compound is neither carcinogenic nor genotoxic (FAO/WHO, 1997)

Miscellaneous Synthetic Insecticides

Amitraz, a formamidine compound, has resulted in a number of intoxications (Aydin *et al.*, 1997). The main feature is central nervous system depression, which is accompanied by hypotension, hypothermia and bradycardia. Hyperglycaemia also occurs.

Fipronil, a malarial control agent, has a novel mode of action, acting on the $GABA_A$ receptor (FAO/WHO, 1998). At high doses in experimental animals, neurotoxicity is observed.

FUNGICIDES

The fungicides **(Table 4)** are a heterogeneous group of chemicals that defy convenient chemical classification; their action is often upon the cytoskeleton.

Table 4 The main groups of fungicides

Group	Sub-group	Examples
Metals	Inorganic	Copper sulphate (Bordeaux mixture) Mercurous chloride
	Organic	Organomercurials: Methylmercury sulphate
		Organotins: Tributyltin oxide Fentin
Carbamates	Dithiocarbamates	Methyl dithiocarbamates: Metam
		Dimethyl dithiocarbamates: Ferbam Ziram Thiram
		Ethylenebis dithiocarbamates: Maneb Zineb Mancozeb
	Benzimidazole carbamates and similar compounds	Benomyl Carbendazim Thiophanate Thiophanate-methyl Thiabendazole
	Other compounds similar to carbamates, e.g. dicarboximides	Iprodione

(continued)

Table 4 *(contd)*

Chloroalkyl thio compounds	Captan
	Folpet
	Captafol
Phenols and derivatives	Dinocap
	Pentachlorophenol
	Dichlorophen
	2-Phenylphenol
Hydantoins	Vinclozalin
Organophosphates	Pyrazophos
	Tolclofos-methyl
Azoles	Hexaconazole
	Penconazole
	Tebuconazole
	Cyproconazole
	Fenbuconazole
	Imazalil
Morpholines	Dodemorph
	Fenpropimorph
	Tridemorph
Miscellaneous	Quintozene
	Chlorothalonil
	Creosote
	Boron compounds

Metals

Inorganic Metallic Fungicides

Some of the first fungicides used in agriculture were neutralized copper sulphate preparations such as Bordeaux mixture. Compounds of mercury, both mercurous chloride (calomel) and mercuric chloride, have long been used as fungicides but have now been withdrawn in many countries owing to their toxicity and environmental concerns.

Organometallic compounds

Organometallic compounds are in general fairly toxic, many being neurotoxic. Trimethyltin and triethyltin are highly neurotoxic but not used as pesticides. Tributyltin oxide (TBTO) was, for a time, extensively used in wood preservatives and in anti-fouling paints on boats but its use has been considerably restricted some countries, e.g. the UK (Advisory Committee on Pesticides, 1990; Cavanagh and Nolan, 1994). Substances such as fentin (triphenyltin) and fenbutatin oxide, which are used in agriculture and horticulture, are poorly absorbed by mouth and are of low oral toxicity (FAO/WHO, 1992, 1993) and any neurotoxicity they possess is mild and non-specific (Bock, 1981; Manzo *et al.*, 1981). Organotins are immunotoxic; thus fentin causes lymphopenia and lymphocyte depletion of the spleen and thymus in experimental animals (FAO/WHO, 1992). The immuno-

toxicity of TBTO was reviewed extensively by the WHO (1990b).

Organic compounds of copper and zinc are also used as fungicides, especially as wood preservers.

Carbamate Fungicides and Thiabendazole

A number of carbamates, predominantly the dithiocarbamates and benzimidazole derivatives, possess fungicidal activity.

Dithiocarbamates

The dithiocarbamates include three main groups of fungicides, the methyl dithiocarbamate, metam, the dimethyl dithiocarbamates, ferbam, thiram and ziram and the ethylenebisdithiocarbamates (EBDCs), maneb, zineb and mancozeb, the last group being degraded to ethylenethiourea. All dithiocarbamates seem to have the potential to affect the thyroid, decreasing plasma thyroxine levels and increasing TSH levels.

The dimethyl dithiocarbamates ferbam, thiram and ziram contain the same core molecule together with iron in the case of ferbam and zinc in the case of ziram. Amongst their metabolites is carbon disulphide, which may account for hepatotoxicity. The dimethyl dithiocarbamates are generally not highly toxic, but they interact with alcohol in humans. In this context, it should be noted that the drug disulfiram (Antabuse), used to treat alcoholism, is the ethyl analogue of thiram (tetramethylthiuram disulphide). Both thiram and ziram but, on the basis of limited studies, apparently not ferbam have shown mutagenic potential in bacteria. Thiram and ziram are considered not to be mutagenic in mammalian systems *in vivo* (FAO/WHO, 1993, 1997).

Maneb is polymeric manganese ethylenebis(dithiocarbamate), zineb is the same compound with zinc replacing the manganese and mancozeb is a complex of the two. A notable feature of the EBDCs is that one of their metabolites is ethylenethiourea and this substance forms a major part of the residues to which consumers are exposed. The EBDCs reduce iodine uptake by the thyroid and repeated administration produces thyroid hyperplasia that is initially reversible and is associated with decreased plasma thyroxine and triiodothyronine levels; these effects are also observed in studies of ethylenethiourea (FAO/WHO, 1994). Prolonged dosage produces thyroid tumours in animals (FAO/WHO, 1994).

Benzimidazole Carbamates

The benzimidazole carbamates include benomyl and its hydrolysis product carbendazim, thiophanate and thiophanate-methyl. Thiabendazole, although not strictly a carbamate, shares many of the properties of the carbamate fungicides. The acute toxicity of carbamate fungicides of this type is usually low. Thus thiophanate has an oral LD_{50} of more than $5\,g\,kg^{-1}$ in rodents (Hashimoto *et al.*, 1970). Carbendazim and benomyl have detrimental effects on fertility of male rats (Carter and Laskey, 1982; Carter *et al.*, 1987) and these two fungicides have been shown to be embryotoxic and teratogenic, under experimental conditions; thus in rats, benomyl produces craniocerebral and ocular abnormalities (Kavlock *et al.*, 1982; Janardhan *et al.*, 1984; Cummings *et al.*, 1990; Hoogenboom *et al.*, 1991; FAO/WHO, 1996). Both carbendazim and benomyl have produced microphthalmia in certain experimental studies using high dose levels (FAO/WHO, 1996). With benomyl and carbendazim, a major area of concern has been the possibility of these two pesticides being spindle poisons and both pesticides cause numerical chromosomal changes *in vitro* and *in vivo* (Kirkhart, 1980; Albertini, 1989; Georgieva *et al.*, 1990; Pandita, 1988; FAO/WHO, 1996). Some of these effects may be related to the effects of benomyl and carbendazim upon microtubules and thus to the fungicidal effects, which are mediated through an effect in binding to fungal tubulin and preventing polymerization.

Other Compounds Similar to Carbamates

Iprodione is a dicarboximide of low acute toxicity. It is not genotoxic but in long-term studies high doses produced skin lesions in dogs and increased liver and testicular tumours in rodents. In dogs a reduced red blood cell count was seen with, in some studies, Heinz body formation (FAO/WHO, 1993, 1996). There are some reports that iprodione may disrupt androgen functions.

Chloroalkyl Thio-containing Fungicides

This group consists of captan, folpet and captofol, which are of low acute mammalian toxicity. However, because of the similarity of their molecules to thalidomide, there was considerable concern over their effect on reproductive and foetal development. The negative results of reproductive studies into the chloralkyl thio fungicides suggest that another part of the thalidomide molecule is responsible for the teratogenicity of that drug (Edwards *et al.*, 1991). There also have been concerns over the ability of some fungicides of this class to induce gastrointestinal tumours in experimental animals and captan and folpet are mutagenic *in vitro* but not *in vivo* (FAO/WHO, 1991, 1996).

Phenols

One of the most widely used wood preservers has been pentachlorophenol, which is a potent fungicide. Owing to concerns over its persistence and content of chlorinated dibenzo-*p*-dioxins, pentachlorophenol is now severely restricted in some parts of the world. Similar compounds include dinocap, which is an ester of an alkyl-substituted dinitrophenol and dinitro-*o*-cresol. The main toxic action of of this group of compounds in mammals is to cause uncoupling of oxidative phosphorylation and hyperthermia, with collapse and death at high dose. Liver and kidney involvement occurs in fatal human poisoning, while in experimental animals the onset of rigor mortis is notably fast after death. Some compounds of the phenol group of fungicides induce cataracts in experimental animals, e.g. dinocap (FAO/WHO, 1990).

Hydantoins

This group includes vinclozolin, which has been a cause of concern because of its reproductive toxicity (Advisory Committee on Pesticides, 1992). In a long-term study in rats, there was atrophy of the accessory sex glands and an increased incidence of Leydig cell tumours, and in multigeneration studies in the same species there was infertility in the males associated with feminization of the external genitalia. Changes have been observed in other species and it is likely that vinclozolin acts as an antiandrogen (FAO/WHO, 1996).

OPs

Pyrazophos, although an anticholinesterase OP, is used as a fungicide. It has anticholinesterase properties and, insofar as mammalian toxicity is concerned, has many features in common with OP insecticides (FAO/WHO, 1993). Tolclofos-methyl is an OP fungicide which has limited anticholinesterase properties and low toxicity (PSD, 1993).

Azoles

Fungicides of this group (the 'conazoles') inhibit sterol synthesis in fungi and they have some activity on steroid metabolism in animals. The toxicology of all members is rather similar, effects on the liver (hypertrophy and enzyme induction) being noted in subacute and long-term studies and, with some compounds, effects on the reproductive system such as delayed parturition, which are mild and do not appear adversely to affect reproductive performance. Anaemia is seen, for example, with hexaconazole. The compounds are mostly not carcinogenic, although Leydig cell tumours are sometimes observed and fenbuconazole produces effects on the thyroid, including tumours via effects on thyroxine metabolism (FAO/WHO, 1998). Fetotoxicity is seen at maternally toxic doses and, in some cases, e.g. tebuconazole and diniconazole, teratogenicity, although again generally only at maternally toxic doses (Advisory Committee on Pesticides, 1990, 1993).

Hexaconazole, a fairly typical triazole, produces effects on the female and male reproductive systems. From studies *in vitro*, it is believed that hexaconazole inhibits testosterone production. Nevertheless, reproductive parameters are not generally affected in multi-generation studies. This compound is not genotoxic and probably not carcinogenic, although the frequency of Leydig cell tumours appeared to be treatment related in rats (FAO/WHO, 1991). The compound is foetotoxic at maternally toxic doses but it is not teratogenic, although in a rabbit study there was reported to be some delayed ossification in rabbit foetuses. The toxicology of penconazole is similar; with this compound delayed ossification was observed more consistently than with hexaconazole (FAO/WHO, 1993). Cataracts were observed in the eyes of dogs fed tebuconazole (Advisory Committee on Pesticides, 1993). Imazalil was reported to have effects on the liver in a long-term rat study; furthermore, there was a decreased number of live births at the top dose in a multi-generation study (FAO/WHO, 1978, 1985). This fungicide is been used in humans and in veterinary medicine under the name enilconazole. It appears to have be well tolerated (Edwards *et al.*, 1991).

Table 5 The main groups of herbicides

Group	Sub-group	Examples
Inorganic		Sodium chlorate
Bipyridylium		Paraquat
		Diquat
Organic acid	Phenoxy	2,4-D
		2,4,5-T
		Mecoprop
		Fenoprop
	Other organic acids	Haloxyfop
		Dicamba
Substituted anilines		Alachlor
		Propachlor
		Propanil
Ureas and thioureas		Diuron
		Linuron
		Monolinuron
Nitriles		Ioxynil
		Bromoxynil
Triazines and triazoles	Triazines	Atrazine
		Simazine
	Triazoles	Amitrole
Organophosphates	Phosphonic acid derivatives	Glyphosate
	Phosphinic acid derivatives	Glufosinate

Morpholines

This group of fungicides has a similar action in fungi to the azoles. Dodemorph, fenpropimorph and tridemorph all inhibit the synthesis of ergosterol. They are of low acute toxicity, although tridemorph is reported to be teratogenic and foetotoxic in rodents (Barbiere and Ferioli, 1994).

Miscellaneous Fungicides

Chlorothalonil is a nitrile of low acute toxicity but severe irritant potential. There has been concern about findings from long-term rat and mice studies. In rats, there were gastric and renal changes, including renal epithelial hyperplasia, adenomas and carcinomas and forestomach hyperplasia and hyperkeratosis and gastric papillomas (FAO/WHO, 1991, 1993).

Creosote (coal-tar creosote), a widely used wood preserver in English-speaking countries, is a complex mixture, which contains quantities of various carcinogens and phenols. The amount of benzo[a]pyrene in some preparations has caused some concern and is subject to limits in a number of countries. However, it is likely that its irritancy reduces the potential of creosote for causing skin cancer and it probably presents little hazard to the public.

HERBICIDES

Herbicides are substances that kill plants and are of variable degrees of specificity. Examples are given in **Table 5**.

Inorganic Herbicides

Substances such as salt have, for many years, been used as non-selective herbicides and sodium chlorate continues to be used in this way. If ingested by humans, sodium chlorate produces immediate vomiting, abdominal pain and diarrhoea. A noteworthy feature is that acute poisoning with sodium chlorate produces methaemoglobinaemia and intravascular haemolysis may occur (Proudfoot, 1996).

Bipyridylium Herbicides

The two well known pesticides in this group are paraquat and diquat. The mechanism of action involves cyclic reduction–oxidation reactions producing reactive oxygen species and depletion of NADPH.

Paraquat

Paraquat is selectively toxic to the lungs, producing an acute alveolitis followed by fibrosis. Both type I and type II alveolar cells, and also the clara cells, are destroyed. Associated with this process, it has been noted that lung tissue accumulates paraquat by a saturable uptake process (Rose et al., 1974, 1976; Smith, 1982; Smith et al., 1990). In experimental animals, the main result of paraquat toxicity is histologically a proliferative pneumonitis with fibroblasts, alveolar oedema, perivascular and peribronchial oedema and accumulation of neutrophils and macrophages (Schoenberger et al., 1984). The precise histological changes observed in rats depend upon the dose of paraquat and time to death. In those dying early, haemorrhage and oedema are very prominent, while those dying later show greater evidence of fibrosis. These changes appear to occur largely independently of the route of administration of the paraquat and it should be noted that, in mice, similar histopathological findings have been observed after exposure to paraquat aerosol (Popenoe, 1979).

Poisoning with paraquat in man initially produces damage to the gastro-intestinal tract, including the mouth and pharynx, and to the liver and kidneys. Often partial recovery occurs and then from 10 days onwards, clinical signs and symptoms referable to the respiratory tract develop (Higenbottam et al., 1979; Schuster et al., 1981). Death occurs normally from respiratory failure. There is no effective treatment for paraquat-induced lung damage and the only effective measures involve prevention of absorption of the herbicide from the gastro-intestinal tract.

Diquat

Diquat poisoning differs from paraquat poisoning in that renal effects are more prominent and lung changes generally do not occur, because diquat does not have the nitrogen atoms in the correct spatial positions to permit active uptake by the lung. Cataractogenesis has been observed in long-term experimental animal studies, but not in humans (FAO/WHO, 1994). In man death in overdose is caused by renal failure (Vanholder et al., 1981).

Organic Acid Herbicides

Phenoxy Herbicides

The phenoxy herbicides, which are widely used to destroy broad-leaved weeds, are chemical analogues of plant growth hormones (auxins) of the indoleacetic acid type, and are used for the selective control of broad-leaved plants in monocotyledenous crops. Herbicides of this type have no hormonal action in animals. The phenoxy herbicides include 2,4-D, 2,4,5-T, mecoprop and fenoprop. Similar compounds are used as rooting powders (i.e. they stimulate rooting of cuttings). One herbicide of the group, 2,4,5-T, has come under a cloud as result of contamination with 2,3,7,8-tetrachlorodibenzo-p-dioxin, levels of which are now subject to strict limits. The whole group has attracted some suspicion because of certain epidemiological studies linking non-Hodgkin's lymphoma and soft tissue sarcoma with herbicide manufacture or application. 2,4,5-T is rarely used nowadays, but 2,4-D is extensively used as a selective pesticide on lawns and on monocotyledonous crops.

2,4-D

2,4-D is a moderately toxic compound with $LD_{50}s > 400$ mg (kg body weight)$^{-1}$ in subacute and chronic studies in experimental animals changes were found in the kidneys and sometimes the liver. Mutagenicity tests on 2,4-D have produced somewhat contradictory results (Pilinskaya, 1974; Zetterberg et al., 1977), so that the IARC (1977) concluded that results on mutagenicity and carcinogenicity were inadequate for a proper evaluation. However, it seems unlikely that pure 2,4-D is mutagenic. In man, large doses are necessary to produce major toxic effects, which include alterations in consciousness, muscle fasciculation, vomiting and convulsions. Gross overdose produces stupor, muscle hypotonia and coma, which may be prolonged; metabolic acidosis, hypotension and pulmonary oedema may occur (Ecobichon, 1994; Proudfoot, 1996). There is some evidence that alkaline diuresis is beneficial in 2,4-D poisoning and also with mecoprop.

2,4,5-T

2,4,5-T is not much used in Western countries any more. The toxicology is similar to that of 2,4-D; however, human case reports must be studied in the context of the content of TCDD of the material. At high dose levels, 2,4,5-T is reported to be teratogenic to rats and mice but not rabbits, monkeys and sheep (FAO/WHO, 1980).

Other Phenoxy Herbicides

The main target organs for fenoprop in experimental animals are the liver and kidneys (USEPA, 1988) and the material is not carcinogenic. The animal toxicology of mecoprop is very similar (PSD, 1994). A case of combined 2,4-D and mecoprop poisoning was reported by Kerr et al. (1997). The main symptoms featured were gastro-intestinal effects, hypotension, coma, muscle weakness, hyperthermia and tachycardia.

Other Organic Acid Herbicides

The toxicology of haloxyfop is notable for the production of liver tumours; these are observed in mice and are associated with peroxisome proliferation (FAO/WHO, 1996). Dicamba is a herbicide of low acute toxicity and

the few poisoning cases observed in humans have been complicated by ingestion of phenoxy herbicides at the same time. In animals, muscular spasms and dyspnea occur in acute studies, whilst in long-term studies, organ-specific effects are few (Stevens and Sumner, 1991). Dicamba is reported to lead to peroxisome proliferation (Espandiari et al., 1998).

Substituted Anilines

These are used as herbicides and include alachlor, propachlor and propanil. Some herbicides of this group have the general property of causing methaemoglobinaemia, as do many other aniline derivatives (Kiese, 1970). The probable mechanism of the methaemoglobinaemia is N-hydroxylation to the corresponding hydroxylamine, which then takes part in an intra-erythrocytic cycle with the corresponding nitroso derivative at the same time generating methaemoglobin. If this is the mechanism, for propanil the proximate methaemoglobin former would be N-hydroxy-3,4-dichloroaniline (McMillan et al., 1990). In the case of propachlor, which is a teritary amine, it would seem unlikely that the above mechanism would operate and rat data suggest that this is indeed the case (Panshina, 1973). However, it must be remembered that the rat is not a good experimental animal for demonstrating methaemoglobinaemia (Calabrese, 1983) and the dog is considered a more appropriate model for man. In addition to causing methaemoglobinaemia, propanil causes reduced red cell survival (McMillan et al., 1991).

Alachlor

Alachlor, like other substituted aniline herbicides is not a substance of high acute toxicity (Pesticide Manual, 1994). The substance is carcinogenic in rodents, producing posterior nasal and stomach tumours, possibly by a non-genotoxic mechanism (Berry, 1988).

Ureas and Thioureas

The herbicidal ureas, such as diuron, linuron and monolinuron, are of low acute toxicity. They appear to interfere with photosynthesis in plants. In man, they cause methaemoglobinaemia, intravacular haemolysis and haemoglobinuria (Proudfoot, 1996).

Nitriles

The nitrile herbicides include ioxynil and bromoxynil and they may act as toxicants partly by uncoupling oxidative phosphorylation and as inhibitors of oxidative phosphorylation (Stevens and Sumner, 1991; Proudfoot, 1996).

Triazines and Triazoles

Atrazine and simazine are triazines, while amitrole is a closely related triazole; they are a very widely used group of herbicides which inhibit photosynthesis. These compounds are of low toxicity and the effects of ingestion by humans are non-specific. In rats, mice and sheep, amitrole has effects upon the thyroid (hyperplastic changes) (FAO/WHO, 1994).

OP Herbicides

Two organophosphates, both of which have a low or non-existent ability to produce cholinesterase depression, are used as herbicides. Glyphosate (N-phosphonomethylglycine) is an inhibitor of amino acid synthesis in plants. In mammals it appears to be very non-toxic, with LD_{50}s in the $5\,g\,kg^{-1}$ range (Atkinson 1985). In general this appears to be true in humans, where studies have usually shown that high doses are necessary to produce fatality. However, the lethal dose in humans seems somewhat variable, some patients surviving doses which were fatal in others. Massive overdose of glyphosate produces gastric irritation, hypotension and pulmonary insufficiency, for which other constituents of the formulation may be to blame (Talbot *et al.*, 1991). Damage to the larynx can occur following respiratory aspiration (Hung *et al.*, 1997). Glufosinate ammonium is a non-selective phosphinic acid herbicide that acts as an inhibitor of glutamine synthetase in plants. It has some inhibitory action on glutamine synthetase in experimental animals, especially in the kidney (FAO/WHO, 1992). A range of genetically modified crops with resistance to glyphosate and glufosinate ammonium are being developed.

Defoliants and Desiccants

A number of substances are used as defoliants and desiccants in agriculture. Sulphuric acid is widely used to destroy potato haulms. S,S,S-Tributyl phosphorotrithioate (DEF) and S,S,S-tributyl phosphorotrithioite (merphos) are OPs used as cotton defoliants, since they produce leaf abscission. A notable feature of the toxicity of DEF and merphos is that in hens they produce OPIDP (Baron and Johnson, 1964).

MOLLUSCICIDES

Certain pesticides are used to kill slugs and snails. One of the more noteworthy is metaldehyde. This commonly causes mild poisoning when ingested by children and sometimes more severe poisoning in pet animals. Severe intoxication with metaldehyde is primarily due to its breakdown to acetaldehyde and is characterized by convulsions, hyperpyrexia and metabolic acidosis

(Proudfoot, 1996). Methiocarb is a molluscicide with cholinesterase-inhibiting properties (FAO/WHO, 1999).

RODENTICIDES

Anticoagulant Rodenticides

Many rodenticides are anticoagulants and include warfarin and newer substances such as brodifacoum, bromadialone and chlorophacinone. The main differences between warfarin and the newer compounds is the increased single dose toxicity and persistence of anticoagulant action. The mechanism of action of the coumarin group is inhibition of the synthesis of blood-clotting factors VII, IX and X, the vitamin K dependent ones. Poisoning in humans is similar to that seen in the rodents and usually follows ingestion. Spontaneous haemorrhages occur from the nose, into the skin and into internal organs. The prothrombin time is prolonged. Oral vitamin K_1 (phytomenadione) can be used as an antidote or alternatively, in extreme cases, transfusion of fresh frozen plasma or blood may be indicated.

Non-anticoagulant Rodenticides

α-Chloralose

α-Chloralose causes hypersalvation, increased muscle tone, hyperreflexia, opisthotonus and convulsions. Rhabdomyolysis is a possible complication and coma may occur.

Phosphides

These are used as fumigants in grain stores etc. and as rat poisons. Zinc and aluminium phosphide both give rise to phosphine on combination with stomach acid or moist air. Phosphine is very toxic by inhalation, producing local irritation to mucous membranes, together with hepatic effects and reductions in the red blood cell count. By the oral route the phosphides affect the liver and cause convulsions in experimental animals. In humans, exposure to phosphine causes coughing, dyspnoea, tight chest, headache, giddiness and retrosternal pain; pulmonary oedema, with resultant cyanosis, may be seen. Ingestion of metallic phosphides causes nausea, vomiting, hypotension and shock (Proudfoot, 1996). The mechanism of the poisoning is unclear. There is some evidence for inhibition of cholinesterase in cases of human poisoning; thus Rastogi *et al.* (1990) found that plasma cholinesterase was decreased in patients poisoned by aluminium phosphide by the oral route. Brain cholinesterase was not affected. Plasma cholinesterase inhibition did not appear to influence prognosis and aminotransferase estimation did not suggest liver disease, so that a hepatic origin for the decreased cholinesterase activity seems unlikely.

TOXICITY OF COMBINATIONS OF PESTICIDES

There has been some concern as to the possibility of deleterious effects from multiple pesticides exposure, either as residues in food or at the workplace. The former seems unlikely to be much of a problem acutely, except where exposure is to pesticides with substantial acute toxicity, e.g. OPs and carbamates. The workplace is more of a problem, raising the question of the safety of tank mixing of pesticides and other sources of combined exposure. Frequently data on a particular combination are scanty and general principles are necessary for predictive purposes. The possible types of toxicological interaction between two pesticides are (1) additive, (2) synergistic and (3) antagonistic. Often, compounds with the same toxic effects act additively, whereas in the case of pesticides with different toxic effects the combined effect is less than additive. If toxic effects were only determined by actions at receptors, this would probably always be the case. However, one also has to consider alteration by one pesticide of the pharmacokinetics or metabolism of the other and as a result interactions may be exceedingly complex. Thus, in combination, the acute toxicity of OCs is usually additive, although potentiation and antagonism can occur. With pairs consisting of one OP and one OC, the same is true (Keplinger and Deichmann, 1967). It has been shown that some pairs of OPs exhibit greater than additive toxic effects when administered together (Dubois, 1961). Because of the predictive difficulty, experimental approaches have been proposed (GIFAP, 1988). The question of the possible consequences of long-term exposure to a cocktail of pesticides remains unanswered and, indeed, may be unanswerable.

The views expressed in this chapter are those of the authors and do not necessarily reflect the views of any UK Government Department.

REFERENCES

Abalis, I. M., Eldefrawi, M. E. and Eldefrawi, A. T. (1986). Effect of insecticides on GABA-induced chloride influx into rat brain microsacs. *J. Toxicol. Environ. Health*, **18**, 13–23.

Aden-Abdi, Y., Villén, T., Ericsson, Ö., Gustafsson, L. L. and Dahl-Puustinen, M.-L. (1990). Metrifonate in healthy volunteers: interrelationship between pharmacokinetic properties, cholinesterase inhibition and side-effects. *Bull. World Health Org.*, **68**, 731–736.

Advisory Committee on Pesticides (1990). *Annual Report 1989*. HMSO, London.

Advisory Committee on Pesticides (1992). *Annual Report 1991*. HMSO, London.

Advisory Committee on Pesticides (1993). *Annual Report 1992*. HMSO, London.

Albertini, S. (1989). Influence of different factors on the induction of chromosome malsegregation in *Saccharomyces cerevisiae* D61.M by Bavistan and assessment of its genotoxic property in the Ames test and in the *Saccharomyces cerevisiae* D7. *Mutat. Res.* **216**, 327–340.

Aldridge, W. N. (1990). An assessment of the toxicological properties of pyrethroids and their neurotoxicity. *Crit. Rev. Toxicol.*, **21**, 89–103.

Ames, R. G., Steenland, K., Jenkins, B., Chrislip, D. and Russo, J. (1995). Chronic neurological sequelae to cholinesterase inhibition among pesticide applicators. *Arch. Environ. Health*, **50**, 440–444.

Atkinson, D. (1985). Toxicological properties of glyphosate, a summary. In Grossbard, E. and Atkinson, D. (Eds), *The Herbicide Glyphosate*. Butterworths, London, pp. 127–133.

Axelson, O. (1987). Pesticides and cancer risks in agriculture. *Med. Oncol. Tumor Pharmacother.*, **4**, 207–217.

Aydin, K., Kurtoğlu, S., Poyrazoğlu, M. H., Üzüm, K., Üstünba, H. B. and Hallaç, I. K. (1997). Amitraz poisoning in children: clinical and laboratory findings of eight cases. *Hum. Exp. Toxicol.*, **16**, 680–682.

Barbiere, F. and Ferioli, A. (1994). Morpholine derivatives. *Toxicology*, **91**, 83–86.

Baron, R. L. and Johnson, C. H. (1964). Neurological disruption produced in hens by two organophosphorus esters. *Br. J. Pharmacol.*, **23**, 295–304.

Barrett, D. S., Oehme, F. W. and Kruckenberg, S. M. (1985). A review of organophosphorus ester-induced delayed neurotoxicity. *Vet. Hum. Toxicol.*, **27**, 22–37.

Bartels, M. and Friedel, B. (1979). Langandauernde EEG-Veränderung bei einer E 605-Vergiftung. *Z. EEG-EMG*, **10**, 22–24.

Baskin, S. I. and Whitmer, M. P. (1992). Cardiac effects of anticholinesterases. In Ballantyne, B. and Marrs, T. C. (Eds.), *Clinical and Experimental Toxicology of Organophosphates and Carbamates*. Butterworth–Heinemann, Oxford, pp. 135–144.

Beach, J. R., Spurgeon, A., Stephens, R., Heafield, T., Calvert, I. A., Levy, L. S. and Harrington, J. M. (1996). Abnormalities on neurological examination among sheep farmers exposed to organophosphorous pesticides. *Occup. Environ. Med.*, **53**, 520–525.

Berry, C. L. (1988). The no-effect level and optimal use of toxicity data. *Regul. Toxicol. Pharmacol.*, **8**, 385–388.

Bismuth, C., Baud, F. J., Conso, F., Fréjaville, J. P. and Garnier, R. (1987). *Toxicologie Clinique*, 4th Edn. Flammarion, Paris, p. 424.

Bismuth, C., Inns, R. H. and Marrs, T. C. (1992). Efficacy, toxicity and clinical use of oximes in anticholinesterase poisoning. In Ballantyne, B. and Marrs, T. C. (Eds), *Clinical and Experimental Toxicology of Organophosphates and Carbamates*. Butterworth–Heinemann, Oxford, pp. 555–577.

Bock, R. (1981). Triphenyltin compounds and their degradation products. *Residues Rev.*, **79**, 1–270.

Bouldin, T. W. and Cavanagh, J. B. (1979a). Organophosphorus neuropathy I. A teased fiber study of the spatio-temporal spread of axonal degeneration. *Am. J. Pathol.*, **94**, 241–252.

Bouldin, T. W. and Cavanagh, J. B. (1979b). Organophosphorus neuropathy II. A fine structural study of the early stages of anonal degeneration. *Am. J. Pathol.*, **94**, 253–270.

Burchfiel, J. L., Duffy, F. H. and Sim, van M. (1976). Persistent effects of sarin and dieldrin upon the primate electroencephalogram, *Toxicol. Appl. Pharmacol.*, **35**, 365–379.

Calabrese, E. J. (1983). *The Principles of Animal Extrapolation.* Wiley, New York, pp. 307–320.

Cantor, K. P., Blair, A., Everett, G., Gibson, R., Burmeister, L. F., Brown, L. M., Schuman, L. and Dick, F. R. (1992). Pesticides and other agricultural risk factors for non-Hodgkin's lymphoma among men in Iowa and Minnesota. *Cancer Res.*, **52**, 2447–2455.

Carter, S. D. and Laskey, J. W. (1982). Effect of benomyl on reproduction in the male rat. *Toxicol. Lett.*, **11**, 87–94.

Carter, S. D., Hess, R. A. and Laskey, J. W. (1987). The fungicide methyl 2-benzimidazole carbamate causes infertility in male Sprague–Dawley rats. *Biol. Reprod.*, **37**, 709–717.

Cavanagh, J. B. (1982). Mechanisms of axon degeneration in three toxic 'neuropathies': organophosphorus, acrylamide and hexacarbon compared. In Smith, W. T. and Cavanagh, J. B. (Eds), *Recent Advances in Neuropathology*, Vol. 2. Churchill–Livingstone, Edinburgh, pp. 213–241.

Cavanagh, J. B. and Nolan, C. C. (1994). The neurotoxicity of organolead and organotin compounds: In de Wolff, F. (Ed.), *Handbook of Clinical Neurology*, Vol. 64. Elsevier, Amsterdam, pp. 129–150.

Chaconas, L. E. and Smoak, I. W. (1997). Dysmorphic effects of ivomec in mouse embryos *in vitro. Toxic Subst. Mech.*, **16**, 195–207.

Cole, L. M. and Casida, J. E. (1986). Polychlorocycloalkane insecticide-induced convulsions in mice in relation to disruption of the GABA-regulated chloride ionophore. *Life Sci.*, **39**, 1855–1862.

Coper, H., Herken, H. and Klempau, I. (1951). On the pharmacology and toxicology of chlorinated cyclohexane. *Naunyn-Schmiedebergs Arch. Exp. Pathol. Pharmakol.*, **212**, 463–479.

Cummings, A. M., Harris, S. T. and Rehnberg, G. L. (1990). Effects of methyl benzimidazole carbamate during early pregnancy in the rat. *Fundam. Appl. Toxicol.*, **15**, 528–535.

Department of Agriculture and Food (1992). *Press Release 117/92.* Government Information Services, Dublin.

de Rueck, J. and Willems, J. (1975). Acute parathion poisoning: myopathic changes in the diaphragm. *J. Neurol.*, **208**, 309–314.

DeWilde, A. -R., Heyndrickx, A. and Carton, D. (1986). A case of fatal rotenone poisoning in a child. *J. Forensic Sci.*, **31**, 1492–1498.

D'Mello, G. D. (1993). Behavioural toxicity of anticholinesterases in humans and animals—a review. *Hum. Exp. Toxicol.*, **12**, 3–7.

Dubois, K. P. (1961). Potentiation of the toxicity of organophosphorus compounds. In Metcalf, R. L. (Ed.), *Advances in Pest Control Research*, Vol. 4. Interscience New York, pp. 117–151.

Duffy, F. H., Burchfiel, J. L., Bartels, P. H., Gaon, M. and Sim, van M. (1979). Long-term effects of an organophosphate upon the human electroencephalogram. *Toxicol. Appl. Pharmacology*, 47, 161–176.

Durham, W. F., Wolfe, H. R. and Quinby, G. E. (1965). Organophosphorus insecticides and mental alertness. *Arch. Environ. Health*, **10**, 55–66.

Ecobichon, D. J. (1994). Herbicides. In Ecobichon, D. J. and Joy, R. M. (Eds), *Pesticides and Neurological Diseases.* CRC Press, Boca Raton, FL, pp. 353–360.

Edwards, R., Ferry, D. G. and Temple, W. A. (1991). Fungicides and related compounds. In Hayes, W. J. and Laws, E. R. (Eds), *Handbook of Pesticide Toxicology.* Academic Press, San Diego, pp. 1409–1470.

Eichler, D., Haupt, W. and Paul, W. (1983). Comparative study on the distribution of α-and γ- hexachlorocyclohexane in the rat with particular reference to the problem of isomerization. *Xenobiotica*, **13**, 639–647.

el-Sebae, A. H., Soliman, S. A., Ahmed, N. S. and Curley, A. (1981). Biochemical interaction of six OP delayed neurotoxicants with several neurotargets. *J. Environ. Sci. Health*, **816**, 465–474.

Espandiari, P., Ludewig, G. and Roberston, L. W. (1998). Activation of hepatic NF-KB by the herbicide dicamba in female and male rats. *Toxicologist*, **42**, 153–154.

Evans, R. G. (1993). Developmental and reproductive effects of the insect growth regulator, fenoxycarb, against the oriental cockroach *Blatta orientalis* L. In Wildey, K. B. and Robinson, W. H. (Eds), *Proceedings of the 1st International Conference on Insect Pests in the Urban Environment.* Organizing Committee, Cambridge, pp. 81–85.

Eyer, P. (1995). Neuropsychopathological changes by organophosphorus compounds—a review. *Hum. Exp. Toxicol.*, **14**, 857–864.

FAO/WHO (1978). *FAO Plant Production and Protection Paper 10 Sup. Pesticide Residues in Food: 1977 Evaluations.* The Monographs Data and Recommendations of the Joint Meeting of the FAO Panel of Experts on Pesticide Residues in Food and the Environment and the WHO Expert Group on Pesticide Residues, Geneva, 6–15th December 1977. Food and Agricultural Organization of the United Nations, Rome.

FAO/WHO (1980). *FAO Plant Production and Protection Paper 20 Sup. Pesticide Residues in food: 1979 Evaluations.* The Monographs Data and Recommendations of the Joint Meeting of the FAO Panel of Experts on Pesticide Residues in Food and the Environment and the WHO Expert Group on Pesticide Residues, Geneva, 3rd–12th December 1979. Food and Agricultural Organization of the United Nations, Rome.

FAO/WHO (1982). *FAO Plant Production Paper 42. Pesticide Residues in Food: 1981 Evaluations.* Data and Recommendations of the Joint Meeting of the FAO Panel of Experts on Pesticide Residues in Food and the Environment and the WHO Expert Group on Pesticide Residues, Geneva, 23rd November–2nd December 1981. Food and Agricultural Organization of the United Nations, Rome.

FAO/WHO (1985). *Pesticide Residues in Food—1984. Evaluations.* Joint Meeting Proceedings, Rome, 24th September–3rd October 1984. Food and Agricultural Organization of the United Nations, Rome and World Health Organization, Geneva.

FAO/WHO (1990). *FAO Plant Production and Protection Paper 100/2. Pesticide Residues in Food—1989. Evaluations 1989. Part II, Toxicology.* Food and Agriculture Organization of the United Nations, Rome.

FAO/WHO (1991). *Pesticide Residues in Food. Toxicology Evaluations.* Joint Meeting Proceedings, Rome, 17th–26th September 1990. Food and Agricultural Organization of the United Nations, Rome and World Health Organization, Geneva.

FAO/WHO (1992). *Pesticide Residues in Food. Toxicology Evaluations.* Joint FAO/WHO Meeting on Pesticide Residues, Geneva, 16th–25th September 1991. World Health Organization, Geneva.

FAO/WHO (1993). *Pesticide Residues in Food. Toxicology Evaluations.* Joint Meeting Proceedings, Rome, 20th September–1st October 1992. World Health Organization, Geneva.

FAO/WHO (1994). *Pesticide Residues in Food—1993. Evaluations. Part II, Toxicology.* Joint FAO/WHO Meeting on Pesticide Residues, Geneva, 20–29th September 1993. World Health Organization, Geneva.

FAO/WHO (1996). *Pesticide Residues in Food—1995. Evaluations 1995. Part II, Toxicology.* Joint FAO/WHO Meeting on Pesticide Residues, Geneva, 18–27th September 1995. World Health Organization, Geneva.

FAO/WHO (1997). *Pesticide Residues in Food—1996. Evaluations 1996. Part II, Toxicological.* Joint Meeting of the FAO Panel of Experts and the WHO Core Assessment Group, Rome, 16th–26th September 1996. World Health Organization, Geneva.

FAO/WHO (1998). *Pesticide Residues in Food—1997. Evaluations 1997. Part II, Toxicological.* Joint Meeting of the FAO Panel of Experts and the WHO Core Assessment Group, Lyon, 22nd September–1st October 1997. World Health Organization, Geneva.

FAO/WHO (1999). Pesticide residues in food - 1998. Evaluations, 1998. Part II toxicological. Joint meeting of the FAO Panel of Experts and the WHO Core Assessment Group, Rome, 22nd September–3rd October, 1998. World Health Organization, Geneva.

Ferrer, A. and Cabral, R. (1991). Toxic epidemics caused by alimentary exposure to pesticides: a review. *Food Addit. Contam.*, **8**, 755–776.

Fiedler, N., Kipen, H., Kelly-McNeil, K. and Fenske, R. (1997). Long-term use of organophosphates and neuropsychological performance. *Am. J. Ind. Med.*, **32**, 487–496.

Gallo, M. A. and Lawryk, N. J. (1991). Organic phosphorus pesticides. In Hayes, W. J. and Laws, E. R. (Eds), *Handbook of Pesticide Toxicology.* Academic Press, San Diego, pp. 917–1090.

Gardon, J., Gardon-Wendel, N., Demanga-Ngangue, N., Kamgno, J., Chippaux, J.-P. and Boussinesq, M. (1997). Serious reactions after mass treatment of onchocerciasis with ivermectin in an area endemic for *Loa loa* infection. *Lancet*, **350**, 18–22.

Georgieva, V., Vachkova, R., Tzoneva, R. and Kappas, A. (1990). Genotoxic activity of benomyl in different test systems. *Environ. Mol. Mutagen.*, **16**, 32–36.

GIFAP (1988). *GIFAP Position Paper on Toxicology of Crop Protection Products in Combination.* Groupement International des Associations Nationales de Fabricants de Produits Agrochimiques, Brussels.

Glickman, A. H., Wing, K. D. and Casida, J. E. (1984). Profenofos insecticide bioactivation in relation to antidote action and the stereospecificity of anticholinesterase inhibi-

tion, reactivation and aging. *Toxicol. Appl. Pharmacol.*, **73**, 16–22.

Gordon, J. J., Inns, R. I., Johnson, M. K., Leadbeater, L., Maidment, M. P., Upshall, D. G., Cooper, G. H. and Rickard, R. L. (1983). The delayed neuropathic effects of nerve agents and some other organophosphorus compounds. *Arch. Toxicol.*, **52**, 71–82.

Gyrd-Hansen, N. and Kraul, I. (1984). Obidoxime reactivation of organophosphate inhibited cholinesterase activity in pigs. *Acta Vet. Scand.*, **25**, 86–95.

Hall, A. H. and Rumack, B. H. (1992). Incidence, presentation and therapeutic attitues to anticholinesterase poisoning in the USA. In Ballantyne, B. and Marrs, T. C. (Eds), *Clinical and Experimental Toxicology of Organophosphates and Carbamates.* Butterworth–Heinemann, Oxford, pp. 471–493.

Hashimoto, Y., Makita, T., Mori, T., Nishibe, T., Noguchi, T., Tsuboi, S. and Ohtu, G. (1970). Toxicological evaluations of thiophanate. (I) Acute and subacute toxicity of a new fungicide, thiophanate (active ingredient of NF-35), 1,2-bis-(ethoxycarbonyl-thioureido)benzene. *Pharmacometrics*, **4**, 5–21.

Higenbottam, T., Crome, P., Parkinson, C. and Nunn, J. (1979). Further clinical observations on the pulmonary effects of paraquat ingestion. *Thorax*, **34**, 161–165.

Hirshberg, A. and Lerman, Y. (1984). Clinical problems in organophosphate poisoning: the use of a computerized information system. *Fundam. Appl. Toxicol.*, **4**, S209–S214.

Holmes, J. H. and Gaon, M. D. (1956). Observations on acute and multiple exposure to anticholinesterase agents. *Trans. Am. Clin. Chem. Assoc.*, **68**, 86–103.

Hoogenboom, E. R., Ransdell, J. F., Ellis, W. G., Kavlock, R. J. and Zeman, F. J. (1991). Effects on the rat eye of maternal benomyl exposure and protein malnutrition. *Curr. Eye Res.*, **7**, 601–612.

Høyer, A. P., Grandjean, P., Jørgensen, T., Brock, J. W. and Hartvig, H. B. (1998). Organochlorine exposure and risk of breast cancer. *Lancet*, **352**, 1816–1820.

Hung, D.-Z., Deng, J.-F. and Wu, T.-C. (1997). Layrngeal survey in glyphosate intoxication: a pathophysiological investigation. *Hum. Exp. Toxicol.*, **16**, 596–599.

IARC (1977). *IARC Monographs on the Evaluation of the Carcinogenic Risk of Chemicals to Man: Some Fumigants, the Herbicides 2,4-D and 2,4,5-T, Chlorinated Dibenzo-dioxins and Miscellaneous Industrial Chemicals*, Vol. 15. IARC, Lyon.

IEH (1998). *Organophosphorus Agents: an Evaluation of Putative Chronic Effects in Humans.* Institute for Environment and Health, Leicester.

Inns, R. H., Tuckwell, N. J., Bright, J. E. and Marrs, T. C. (1990). Histochemical demonstration of calcium accumulation in muscle fibres after experimental organophosphate poisoning. *Hum. Exp. Toxicol.*, **9**, 245–250.

Janardhan, A., Sattur, P. B. and Sisodia, P. (1984). Teratogenicity of methyl benzimidazole carbamate in rats and rabbits. *Bull. Environ. Contam. Toxicol.*, **33**, 257–263.

Johnson, M. K. (1975). Organophosphorus esters causing delayed neurotoxic effects. *Arch. Toxicol.*, **34**, 259–288.

Johnson, M. K. and Vale, J. A. (1992). Clinical management of acute organophsophate poisoning: an overview. In Ballantyne, B. and Marrs, T. C. (Eds), *Clinical and Experimental Toxicology of Organophosphates and Carbamates.* Butterworth–Heinemann, Oxford, pp. 528–542.

Joy, R. M. (1994). Pyrethrins and pyrethroid insecticides. In Ecobichon, D. J. and Joy, R. M. (Eds), *Pesticides and Neurological Diseases*, 2nd edn. ed CRC Press, Boca Raton, FL, pp. 291–312.

Karademir, M., Ertürk, F. and Koçak, R. (1990). Two cases of organophosphate poisoning with development of intermediate syndrome. *Hum. Exp. Toxicol.*, **9**, 187–189.

Kavlock, R. J., Chernoff, N., Gray, L. E., Gray, J. A. and Whitehouse, D. (1982). Teratogenic effects of benomyl in the Wistar rat and CD-1 mouse, with emphasis on the route of administration. *Toxicol. Appl. Pharmacol.*, **62**, 44–54.

Keplinger, M. L. and Deichmann, W. B. (1967). Acute toxicity of combinations of pesticides. *Toxicol. Appl. Pharmacol.*, **10**, 586–595.

Kerr, J. R., Ferguson, W. P. and Archbold, P. (1997). Severe intoxication following ingestion of 2,4-D and MCPP. *Intensive Care Med.*, **23**, 356–357.

Key, T. and Reeves, G. (1994). Organochlorines in the environment and breast cancer. *Br. Med. J.*, **308**, 1520–1521.

Kiese, M. (1970). Drug-induced ferrihemoglobinemia. *Hum. Genet.*, **9**, 220–223.

Kirkhart, B. (1980). *Micronucleus Test on Benomyl Test Substance was not Benomyl but MBC*. US EPA Report LSU 7553–19. Environmental Protection Agency, Washington, DC.

Korsak, R. J. and Sato, M. M. (1977). Effects of chronic organophosphate pesticide exposure on the central nervous system. *Clin. Toxicol.*, **11**, 83–95.

Lankas, G. R. and Gordon, L. R. (1989). Toxicology. In Campbell, W. C. (Ed.), *Ivermectin and Abamectin*. Springer, New York, pp. 89–112.

Ligtenstein, D. A. (1984). On the synergism of the cholinesterase reactivating bispyridinium oxime HI-6 and atropine in the treatment of organophosphate intoxications in the rat. *MD Thesis*, Rijksuniversiteit te Leiden, Leiden.

Manzo, L., Richelini, P., Sabbione, E., Pietra, R., Bono, F. and Guardia, L. (1981). Poisoning by triphenyltin acetate: report of two cases and determination of tin in blood and urine by neutron activation analysis. *Clin. Toxicol.*, **18**, 1343–1353.

Marrs, T. C. (1996). Organophosphate anticholinesterase poisoning. *Toxic Subst. Mech.*, **15**, 357–388.

Mason, H., Waine, E., Stevenson, A. and Wilson, H. K. (1993). Aging and spontaneous reactivation of human plasma cholinesterase activity after inhibition by organophosphorus pesticides. *Hum. Exp. Toxicol.*, **12**, 497–503.

McMillan, D. C., McRae, T. A. and Hinson, J. A. (1990). Propanil-induced methemoglobinemia and hemoglobin binding in the rat. *Toxicol. Appl. Pharmacol.*, **105**, 530–507.

McMillan, D. C., Bradshaw, T. P., Hinson, J. A. and Jollow, D. J. (1991). Role of metabolites in propanil-induced hemolytic anemia. *Toxicol. Appl. Pharmacol.*, **110**, 70–78.

Moretto, A., Capodicasa, E. and Lotti, M. (1992). Clinical expression of organophosphate-induced delayed neuropathy in rats. *Toxicol. Lett.*, **63**, 97–102.

Pandita, T. K. (1988). Assessment of the mutagenic potential of a fungicide Bavistan using multiple assays. *Mutat. Res.*, **204**, 627–643.

Panshina, T. N. (1973). Ramrod. In Medved, L. M. (Ed.), *Gigiena Primeninia Toksikologia Pesticidov Klinica Otravlenni*, Medizina, Leningrad (now St Petersburg), pp. 301–303.

Pesticide Manual (1994). 10th edn. British Crop Protection Council, Farnham, and Royal Society of Chemistry, Cambridge.

Pilinskaya, M. A. (1974). Cytogenetic effects of the herbicide 2,4-D on human and animal chromosomes. *Tsitol. Genet.*, **8**, 202–206.

Pimentel, J. M. and Carrington da Costa, R. B. (1992). Effects of organophosphates on the heart. In Ballantyne, B. and Marrs, T. C. (Eds), *Clinical and Experimental Toxicology of Organophosphates and Carbamates*. Butterworth–Heinemann, Oxford, pp. 145–148.

Popenoe, D. (1979). Effects of paraquat aerosol in the mouse lung. *Arch. Pathol. Lab. Med.*, **103**, 331–334.

Preusser, H.-J. (1967). Die Ultrastructur der motorischen Endplatte im Zwerchfell der Ratte und Veränderungen nach Inhibierung der Acetylcholinesterase. *Z. Zellforsch.*, **80**, 436–457.

Proudfoot, A. (1996). *Pesticide Poisoning: Notes for the Guidance of Medical Practitioners*. HMSO, London.

PSD (1993). *Evaluation of Fully Approved or Provisionally Approved Products. Evaluation of Tolclofos-methyl*. Pesticides Safety Directorate, York.

PSD (1994). *Evaluation of Fully Approved or Provisionally Approved Products. Evaluation of Mecoprop*. Pesticides Safety Directorate, York.

Rastogi, P., Raman, R. and Rastogi, V. K. (1990). Serum cholinesterase and brain acetylcholinesterase activity in aluminium phosphipe poisoning. *Med. Sci. Res.*, **18**, 783–784.

Ray, D. E. (1991). Pesticides derived from plants and other organisms. In Hayes, W. J. and Laws, E. R. (Eds), *Handbook of Pesticide Toxicology*. Academic Press, San Diego, pp. 585–636.

Rose, G. P. and Dewar, A. J. (1983). Intoxication with four synthetic pyrethroids fails to show any correlation between neuromuscular dysfunction and neurobiochemiocal abnormalities in rats. *Arch. Toxicol.*, **53**, 297.

Rose, M. S., Smith, L. L. and Wyatt, I. (1974). Evidence for the energy dependent accumulation of paraquat into rat lung. *Nature*, **252**, 314–315.

Rose, M. S., Lock, E. A., Smith, L. L. and Wyatt, I. (1976). Paraquat accumulation: tissue and species specificity, *Biochem. Pharmacol.*, **24**, 419–423.

Rothman, N., Cantor, K. P., Blair, A., Bush, D., Brock, J. W., Helzlsouer, K., Zahm, S. H., Needham, L. L., Pearson, G. R., Hoover, R. N., Comstock, G. W. and Strickland, P. T. (1997). A nested case-control study of non-Hodgkin lymphoma and serum organochlorine residues. *Lancet*, **350**, 240–244.

Savage, E. P., Keefe, T. J., Mounce, L. M., Heaton, R. K., Lewis, J. A. and Burcar, P. J. (1988). Chronic neurological sequelae of acute organophosphate pesticide poisoning. *Arch. Environ. Health*, **43**, 38–45.

Schoenberger, C. I., Rennard, S. I., Bitterman, P. B., Fukuda, Y., Ferrans, V. J. and Crystal, R. G. (1984). Paraquat-induced pumonary fibrosis. *Am. Rev. Respir. Dis.*, **129**, 168–173.

Schuster, R., Erkelenz, I. and von Romatowski, H.-J. (1981). Frühbild der Lungenfibrose nach Zytostatika and Paraquatintoxikation. *Röntgen Bl.*, **34**, 338–341.

Senanayake, N. and Karalliedde, I. (1987). Neurotoxic effect of organophosphorus insecticides: an intermediate syndrome. *N. Engl. J. Med.*, **316**, 761–763.

Siddiqui, M. K. J. and Saxena, M. C. (1985). Placenta and milk as excretory routes of lipophilic pesticides in women. *Hum. Toxicol.*, **4**, 249–254.

Singer, A. W., Jaax, N. K., Graham, J. S. and McLeod, C. G. (1987). Cardiomyopathy in soman and sarin intoxicated rats. *Toxicol. Lett.*, **36**, 243–249.

Skrinjarić-Spoljar, M., Simeon, V. and Reiner, E. (1973). Spontaneous reactivation and aging of dimethylphosphorylated acetylcholinesterase and cholinesterase. *Biochim. Biophys. Acta*, **315**, 363–369.

Smith, L. L. (1982). The identification of an accumulation system for diamines and polyamines into the lung and its relevence to paraquat toxicity. *Arch. Toxicol.*, Suppl. 5, 1–14.

Smith, L. L., Lewis, C., Wyatt, I. and Cohen, G. M. (1990). The importance of epithelial uptake systems in lung toxicity. In Volans, G. N., Sims, J., Sullivan, F. M. and Turner, P. (Eds), *Basic Science in Toxicology: Proceedings of the Vth International Congress of Toxicology, Brighton, England, 16th–21st July, 1989*. Taylor and Francis, London, pp. 233–241.

Steenland, K. (1996). Chronic neurological effects of organophosphate pesticides. *Br. Med. J.*, **312**, 1312–1313.

Stephens, R., Spurgeon, A., Calvert, I. A., Beach, J., Levy, L. S., Berry, H. and Harrington, J. M. (1995). Neuropsychological effects of long-term exposure to organophosphates in sheep dip. *Lancet*, **345**, 1135–1139.

Stevens, J. T. and Sumner, D. D. (1991). Herbicides. In Hayes, W. J. and Laws, E. R. (Eds), *Handbook of Pesticide Toxicology*. Academic Press, San Diego, pp. 1317–1408.

Szinicz, L., Eyer, P. and Klimmek, R. (1996). *Role of Oximes in the Treatment of Anticholinesterase Agent Poisoning*. Spectrum Akademischer Verlag, Heidelberg.

Tabershaw, I. R. and Cooper, W. C. (1966). Sequelae of acute organic phosphate poisoning. *J. Occup. Med.*, **8**, 5–20.

Talbot, A. R., Shiaw, M.-H., Huang, J.-S. *et al.* (1991). Acute poisoning with glyphosate-surfactant herbicide ('Roundup'): a review of 93 cases. *Hum. Exp. Toxicol.*, **10**, 1–8.

USEPA (1988). *Review of Environmental Contamination and Toxicology*, Vol. 104. Springer, New York.

van Asperen, K. (1954). Interaction of the isomers of benzene hexachloride in mice. *Arch. Int. Pharmacodyn. Ther.*, **99**, 368–377.

Vanholder, R., Colardyn, F., de Rueck, J., Praet, M., Lameire, N. and Ringoir, S. (1981). Diquat intoxication: report of two cases and review of the literature. *Am. J. Med.*, **70**, 1267–1271.

Veronesi, B., Padilla, S., Blackmon, K. and Pope, C. (1991). Murine susceptibility to organophosphate-induced peripheral neuropathy (OPIDN). *Toxicol. Appl. Pharmacol.*, **107**, 311–324.

Vijverberg, H. P. M. (1994). Pyrthroid insecticides. In de Wolff, F. (Ed.), *Handbook of Clinical Neurology, Vol. 64, Intoxications of the Nervous System, Part 1*. Elsevier, Amsterdam, pp. 211–222.

Vijverberg, H. P. M. and van den Bercken, J. (1990). Neurotoxicological effects and the mode of action of pyrethroid insecticides. *Crit. Rev. Toxicol.*, **21**, 105–126.

Wadia, R. S., Chitra, S., Amin, R. B., Kiwalkar, R. S. and Sardesai, H. V. (1987). Electrophysiological studies in organophosphate poisoning. *J. Neurol. Neurosurg. Psychiatry*, **50**, 1442–1448.

Wecker, L., Kiauta, T. and Dettbarn, W.-D. (1978). Relationship between acetylcholinesterase inhibition and the development of a myopathy. *J. Pharmacol. Exp. Ther.*, **206**, 97–104.

Wedin, G. P. (1992). Nephrotoxicity of anticholinesterases. In Ballantyne, B. and Marrs, T. C. (Eds), *Clinical and Experimental Toxicology of Organophosphates and Carbamates*. Butterworth–Heinemann, Oxford, pp. 195–202.

White, G. B. (1993). Optimization of pyrethroid impregnated mosquito nets. In Wildey, K. B. and Robinson, W. H. (Eds), *Proceedings of the 1st International Conference on Insect Pests in the Urban Environment, Cambridge England*. Organizing Committee of the International Conference on Insect Pests in the Urban Environment, Cambridge, pp. 117–118.

WHO (1986). *Environmental Health Criteria 63. Organophosphorus Insecticides: a General Introduction*. World Health Organization, Geneva, p. 78.

WHO (1990a). *Environmental Health Criteria 104. Principles for the Toxicological Assessment of Pesticide Residues in Food*. World Health Organization, Geneva.

WHO (1990b). *Environmental Health Criteria 110. Tributyltin Compounds*. World Health Organization, Geneva.

WHO (1991). *Toxicological Evaluation of Certain Veterinary Drug Residues in Food. 36th Meeting of the Joint FAO/WHO Expert Committee on Food Additives (JECFA), Rome, 5–14th February, 1990. WHO Food Additives Series, No. 27*. World Health Organization, Geneva.

WHO (1996). *Evaluation of Certain Veterinary Drug Residues in Food. 45th Meeting of the Joint FAO/WHO Expert Committee on Food Additives (JECFA), Geneva, 6–15th June, 1996. WHO Technical Report Series, No. 864*. World Health Organization, Geneva.

Wilson, B. H., Hooper, M. J., Hansen, M. E. and Nieberg, P. S. (1992). Reactivation of organophosphorus inhibited AChE with oxime. In Chambers, J. E. and Levi, P. E. (Eds), *Organophosphates: Chemistry, Fate and Effects*. Academic Press, New York, pp. 107–137.

Working Party on Pesticide Residues (1992). *Report 1991*. Stationery Office, London.

Working Party on Pesticide Residues (1997). *Report 1996*. MAFF Publications, London.

Wright, D. J. (1986). Biological activity and mode of action of avermectins. In Ford, M. G., Lunt, G. G., Reay, R. C. and Usherwood, P. N. R. (Eds), *Neuropharmacology of Pesticide Action*. Ellis Horwood, Chichester, pp. 174–202.

Zetterberg, G., Busk, L., Elovson, R., Starec-Nordenhammer, I. and Ryttman, H. (1977). The influence of pH on the effects of 2, 4-D (2,4-dichlorophenoxyacetic acid, Na salt) on *Saccharomyces cerevisiae* and *Salmonella typhimurium*. *Mutat. Res.*, **42**, 3–18.

Zitko, V., McLeese, D. W., Metcalfe, C. D. and Carson, W. G. (1979). Toxicity of permethrin, decamethrin, and related pyrethroids to salmon and lobster. *Bull. Environ. Contam. Toxicol.*, **21**, 336–343.

ADDITIONAL READING

Ballantyne, B. and Marrs, T. C. (1992). *Clinical and Experimental Toxicology of Organophosphates and Carbamates*. Butterworth–Heinemann, Oxford.

Ecobichon, D. J. and Joy, R. M. (1993). *Pesticides and Neurological Diseases*. CRC Press, Boca Raton, FL.

FAO/WHO (series). *Pesticide residues in Food—Evaluations—Toxicology*. Joint FAO/WHO Meeting on Pesticide Residues. World Health Organization, Geneva.

Hayes, W. J. and Laws, E. R. (1991). *Handbook of Pesticide Toxicology*. Academic Press, San Diego.

WHO (series). *Environmental Health Criteria*. World Health Organization, Geneva.

Chapter 95

The Rubber and Plastics Industries and Their Chemicals

Bo Holmberg

CONTENTS

- Introduction
- The Rubber Industry
- The Plastics Industry
- References

INTRODUCTION

The polymer industry produces elastomers and manufactures plastic or rubber goods from resins or elastomers. During the manufacture chemicals are added and mixed in. The procedure may involve thermic processes, hardening or vulcanization. The process is associated with a complex and dynamic chemical exposure panorama, varying with different formulas.

The prevention of health risks in the polymer industry, particularly the rubber industry and some plastic industries, cannot solely be dealt with chemical by chemical: the health hazards are associated with complex exposures and all types of exposures have to be controlled.

In addition, for many additives, the toxicology has been very little investigated and research interest has been focused on the more commonly used chemicals. Hygienic research has only during later years dealt with detailed analyses of chemicals in workroom air mainly in the rubber industry, both of degassed monomers and additives and of newly formed chemicals ('by-products'). Many additives are used in the form of technical products, with impurities, and others are used as less defined chemicals (polymerizates or prepolymerizates).

THE RUBBER INDUSTRY

The rubber industry produces rubber goods (IARC, 1982a; Enwald, 1984) from elastomers ('raw rubber') by adding additives. Elastomers and additives are weighed. The material then undergoes mixing, milling, calendering, extrusion, moulding, sometimes manual building (e.g. tyres) and subsequent curing (vulcanization), inspection and storage.

Besides natural rubber (NR), synthetic rubbers are commonly used as elastomers (IARC, 1982a). The synthetic elastomers can be isoprene 'rubber' (IR), acrylonitrile–butadiene (ANBR), styrene–butadiene (SBR), butyl (IIR), ethylene–propylene (EPM, EPDM) or polybutadiene rubber (BR). Rubber goods for special purposes are solvent-resistant rubbers (nitrile rubber, polychloroprenes, polyurethanes) and heat-resistant rubbers (e.g. silicones, polyacrylates and fluoroelastomers).

A great number of chemicals are used in the rubber industry and each different rubber material may have a different formula. Several hundred additives (Holmberg and Sjöström, 1980; Nutt, 1984; Fishbein, 1991) may be used. The additives are usually classified (**Table 1**) according to their function in the process and each functional class may consist of chemically very different substances. Some chemicals may also have more than one function.

Rubber workers are exposed by skin contact and by inhalation to dust, gases and vapours (Kromhout *et al.*, 1994; Kromhout and Heedereick, 1995) varying with job station in an industry and between industries. The weighing and mixing departments have the greatest exposure to additives. In recent years, improved industrial hygiene has been obtained in some work areas by the introduction of closed systems and automatic weighing. Additives may also be compounded into a rubber mixture from masterbatch preparations, i.e. by using additives premixed in larger amounts in a polymer 'dough', which can be cut and mixed in. This technique reduces exposure to dusty additives.

Many additives may later in the process have partly reacted with the polymer or are locked in. Volatile compounds may be degassed, particularly during heated steps. The temperature during the mixing process is between 90 and 180 °C and during milling, extrusion and calendering between 65 and 80 °C. Even if relatively non-toxic chemicals have been added, new and more harmful substances may be formed. In the vulcanization process, the temperature is much elevated (100–200 °C

Table 1 Examples of additives used in rubber compounding

Function	Substance	Purpose
Curing agents	Sulphur, sulphur donors (thiram, morpholine disulphide, dithiocarbamates, dithiophosphates), selenium, tellurium, organic peroxides	Cross-linking of polymer chains
Accelerators	Amines, ETU, thiurams, diphenylguanidine, dithiocarbamates	Shortening the curing time
Activators	Metal (Zn, Pb, Mg) oxides and organic salts, triethanolamine, glycols	Making accelerators more effective
Retarders	Salicylic acid, cyclohexylthiophthalimide, sulphonamides, nitroso compounds	Controlling curing process
Antidegradants	p-Phenylenediamine, phenols, naphthylamines, quinolines, BHT	Inhibits ageing process and UV degradation
Processing aids	Mineral oils, vegetable oils, phthalates, organic phosphates, thiol derivatives, phenolic compounds	Softening substance mixture
Reinforcing agents	Carbon black, synthetic silicones	Increasing abrasion resistance, strengthening
Fillers, diluents	Clays, carbonates, mineral oils	Volume expansion without changing polymer characteristics
Blowing agents	Azobisformamide, benzene sulphonhydrazide	Producing foam rubber by gas formation
Mould-release agents	Stearates, mineral oils, DEHP, TCP	To promote removal of rubber from mould and curing pans
Pigments/dyestuffs	TiO_2, CdS, Cr_2O_3	Colouring
Bonding agents	Resorcinol, hexamethylene tetramine, isocyanates	Facilitates binding to metal and textiles
Antitack agents	Stearates, talc	Prevents adhesion of rubber sheets
Solvents	Trichloroethylene, methyl ethyl ketone, methylene chloride, toluene, xylene, dimethylformamide, tetrahydrofuran	
Flame retardants	As_2O_3, decabromodiphenyl oxide	

for 20–60 min). This results in a cross-reaction between the curing agents and the polymer chains. In the curing fumes, many biologically active compounds are found, e.g. with irritating, mutagenic and carcinogenic effects.

The health hazards in the rubber goods manufacture are dependent on the total exposure. This means that both added and newly formed chemicals and evaporated residual monomers from the elastomer contribute to the risk. A great number of additional 'new' chemicals have been analysed in workroom air as 'by-products' (IARC, 1982a), formed in the process.

Tyre curing fumes have been known to be associated with respiratory diseases, and have therefore been focused upon in a number of scientific studies. Their chemical components have been identified in some hygienic studies. In particular, degassed additives and solvents have been looked for in the workroom air (IARC, 1982a). Some toxicity studies have characterized the effects of mixed exposures, showing, e.g., that curing fumes (Hedenstedt *et al.*, 1981) contain mutagenic and carcinogenic components.

Some *N*-nitroso compounds (IARC, 1982a; Spiegelhalder and Preussman, 1982) have been found in workroom air. Some of these compounds are more or less potent animal carcinogens and contribute to the human risk. Carcinogenic nitrosoamines may be formed from amines and thiurams in the rubber material from added non-carcinogenic nitrosoamines via transnitrosation processes.

Occupational Hazards in the Rubber Industry

A number of health effects, apart from cancer, have been observed in the rubber industry.

Effects on skin from rubber chemicals are well known in the manufacture of rubber goods (Cronin, 1980; IARC, 1982a) and have also been observed among users of rubber goods. A great number of additives are considered allergenic. Among them, mercaptobenzothiazole, thiuram compounds, dithiocarbamates, *N*-phenylnaphthylamine, dithiodimorpholine and *p*-phenylenediamine and related compounds are important sensitizers among the accelerators and antioxidants. Dermatitic reactions have also been reported from these groups of chemicals.

Irritating gases, dust and fumes may be emitted during certain process steps. An increased incidence of respiratory disease has been reported among tyre workers (Noweir *et al.*, 1972; Fine and Peters, 1976a–d) particularly among vulcanizers. Bronchitis, lung function disturbances, and chronic obstructive disease occur among rubber workers (Gamble *et al.*, 1976; McMichael *et al.*, 1976; Weeks *et al.*, 1981).

Long-term health effects (IARC, 1982a) have been observed in the rubber industry for decades. In fact, the rubber industry has a place in the history of the detection of occupational cancer. As early as 1954, a great number of cases of bladder cancers had been observed. The responsible hazardous compounds (mainly β-naphthylamine and similar compounds) (Fox and Collier, 1976; Parkes *et al.*, 1982) were then largely eliminated in many countries and the number of bladder cancers was reduced.

A vast number of epidemiological studies have since been performed in many countries (IARC, 1982a; Sullivan *et al.*, 1992). The literature contains both case reports (older literature) and case control and retrospective cohort studies. In many cases, as for the bicyclic aromatic amines mentioned above, specific chemicals have been suspected to be associated with specific tumour sites. However, in most studies the total emissions and work as a rubber worker were found to be associated with cancer risks without further specification as to individual chemicals. In some cases, the total scientific evaluation has been able to correlate specific tumours with a specific job function.

An overall evaluation (IARC, 1982a, 1987n) of epidemiological studies stated that urinary bladder tumours are associated with aromatic amine exposure and leukaemia with solvent or, more specifically, benzene exposure. Work with compounding, mixing and milling is associated with increased risks of stomach and lung cancer and tyre building (being partly manual work) with skin cancer. Other tumours occurring as elevated risks in some studies are colon and prostate cancer and lymphomas. Small increases in tumours of the brain, thyroid, pancreas and oesophagus appear in some studies. The latency time for occupational cancer is commonly decades and recent improvements in occupational hygiene in the rubber industry may take a number of additional years to be totally effective.

Some individual additives in the rubber industry have been investigated for their potential mutagenicity (Rannug *et al.*, 1984) in bacterial test systems. Not surprisingly, many accelerators, antioxidants, retarders and curing agents induce point mutations. Also, vulcanization gases, produced in the laboratory, are strong mutagens (Hedenstedt *et al.*, 1981) in *in vitro* systems, the activity depending on the composition of the additive mixture and elastomer formula. Workers in rubber plants have been investigated for genotoxicity (Sorsa *et al.*, 1982b; Sasadiek, 1993). In particular weighing and mixing workers showed chromosomal aberrations, especially sister chromatid exchanges. Urinary excretion of an oxidative DNA adduct (8-hydroxydeoxyguanosine) has been observed among rubber workers (Tagesson *et al.*, 1993), indicating a recent exposure to genotoxic compounds. In other studies, the urine mutagenicity was investigated (Sorsa *et al.*, 1982a, 1983). Weighers, mixers and vulcanizers excrete mutagenic metabolites in their urine.

Individual Chemicals

Monomers

Some residual monomers present in the elastomer may be degassed during the manufacture of rubber goods. In workroom atmosphere, e.g. acrylonitrile, styrene, chloroprene, isoprene and butadiene have been identified in small amounts.

Buta-1,3-diene (Sorsa *et al.*, 1993) is a multipotential carcinogen to rodents (Melnick *et al.*, 1993; Bond *et al.*, 1996) and produces haemangiosarcomas in the heart, liver adenomas and carcinomas, mammary tumours and thymic lymphomas in mice (Melnick *et al.*, 1990; IARC, 1992). In rats (Owen and Gleister, 1990), it produces pancreatic tumours, mammary tumours, testicular tumours, Zymbal gland tumours and tumours of the uterus. Butadiene is genotoxic and mutagenic and is metabolized to one monoepoxide and one diepoxide. Epidemiological studies of butadiene-exposed workers in the chemical industry suggest increased risks of lymphosarcoma, reticulosarcoma and leukaemias (Landrigan, 1990; Ott, 1990).

Isoprene is similar to butadiene in its toxic properties, although less studied (Taalman, 1996). It is biotransformed to epoxides and particularly the diepoxide is mutagenic in bacteria and produces tumours in rats and mice. Isoprene is less potent than butadiene.

Chloroprene (2-chlorobuta-1,3-diene) is a monomer for neoprene rubber. Exposure to chloroprene was associated with alopecia, CNS depression and liver injury after past high exposures (IARC, 1979a). Those effects are related to exposures, particularly during the monomer or elastomer synthesis.

Chloroprene produces mutations and is chemically related to butadiene. Therefore, it has been investigated for possible carcinogenic activity (IARC, 1987a). Chloroprene exposure causes chromosomal aberrations in peripheral lymphocytes among workers. A number of long-term bioassays of chloroprene were inadequate for an evaluation (IARC, 1987a) of its carcinogenicity.

For many additives used in the rubber industry, the toxicology, particularly as regards data relevant to long-term exposure, is unknown. In this section, selected chemicals are described with emphasis on those with some toxicological information.

Vulcanization (Curing) Agents

Curing agents are added to the rubber mixture to stabilize the polymers by cross-linking. At least two dozen different curing agents are regularly in use. Organic peroxides, phenolic resins and organometallic and sulphur compounds are used as vulcanizers. The sulphur-containing substances give off sulphur in the rubber process.

Sulphur, tellurium, selenium, organic selenium and tellurium compounds are common vulcanization agents. Tellurium and selenium, and their salts, are toxic. Exposure to tellurium causes a metallic taste. Tellurium and selenium are biotransformed to dimethyl telluride and dimethyl selenide. Such tellurides and selenides are volatile and will be exhaled with a distinct garlic odour. Selenium (Högberg *et al.*, 1987) is anticarcinogenic (Schrauzer, 1992) at low doses, owing to its involvement in enzymes which detoxify oxygen radicals. It is cytotoxic and carcinogenic in animals at higher doses (IARC, 1975). Selenium has been found in the blood of workers in a tyre repair shop (Sanchez-Ocampo *et al.*, 1996).

Other common vulcanization agents include dicumyl peroxide, di-*tert*-butyl peroxide and *tert*-butylcumyl peroxide. Peroxides are often irritating to the skin, eyes, and throat and are suspected mutagens and carcinogens, although their long-term toxicity is unknown. Butyl peroxide is a tumour promoter in mouse skin (Slaga *et al.*, 1981).

Accelerators

Many vulcanization agents may also function as accelerators, such as thiuram compounds, e.g. tetramethylthiuram disulphide (thiram, TMTD), tetraethylthiuram disulphide (disulfiram, TETD, 'antabus') and tetramethylthiuram monosulphide (TMTM). Dithiocarbamates, such as zinc dimethyl dithiocarbamate (ziram), the diethylcarbamates and their corresponding tellurium, cadmium and copper compounds are also used as accelerators, as is ethylenethiourea (ETU). All these compounds may cause sensitization. Most dithiocarbamates and dithiocarbamides are also mutagenic in bacterial test systems.

Both thiram and ziram are also used as fungicides. There is inadequate evidence for evaluating thiram as a carcinogen (IARC, 1991a). In one experimental study (Shukla *et al.*, 1996), thiram acted as an initiator and a promoter of skin tumours in mice. In another recent study, no such activity was revealed (George and Kuttan, 1995). Ziram causes thyroid carcinomas in the male rat (IARC, 1991b). Both compounds are weak mutagens (Franekic *et al.*, 1994).

Already in 1948, TETD was shown to cause alarming reactions on peroral intake in connection with or before alcohol ingestion: sensation of heat in the face, flushing in the face and neck, palpitations, increased heart rate, dyspnea, hyperventilation and nausea. This was due to the inhibition by disulfiram of aldehyde dehydrogenase and other acetaldehyde-metabolizing enzymes. It also inhibits dopamine-β-oxidase (Goldstein, 1983). These adverse reactions of disulfiram are much less pronounced among rubber workers who have experienced a too high exposure. Some mild signs on alcohol intolerance may, however, appear after manual handling or inhalation of disulfiram, other thiurams and dithiocarbamates.

ETU is weakly mutagenic (Dearfield, 1994) and carcinogenic to rats of both sexes (IARC, 1987d; Houeto *et al.*, 1995), causing thyroid tumours and thyroid follicular cell hyperplasia. In mice, it produces liver tumours. ETU may act via a tumour-promoting mechanism. Disturbances in thyroid function occur in the rat at low doses of ETU (Nebbia and Fink-Gremmels, 1996). ETU also causes developmental abnormalities in the rat (Saillenfait *et al.*, 1991).

Di-*n*-butylamine is a secondary amine and is irritating. It may be nitrosated in the presence of nitroso compounds and is transformed to the carcinogenic dibutylnitrosoamine (IARC, 1978a; Nicholson, 1992).

By substituting certain secondary amines for benzothiazolesulphenamides (Wacker *et al.*, 1991) as accelerators, a much lower degree of nitrosation and associated mutagenic potency is obtained.

Hexamethylenetetramine (HMT) is used also as a food additive and in drugs. HMT is decomposed to formaldehyde and is irritating.

Guanidine derivatives and most thiazoles are irritating agents. Commonly used guanidines among the accelerators are N, N'-diphenylguanidine, N, N'-di-o-tolylguanidine and o-tolyl diguanide. A much used thiazole is 2-mercaptobenzothiazole (2-MBT).

Activators

Activators are processing agents used for activating the accelerators. Many inorganic and organic compounds are used, such as zinc, magnesium, lead and cadmium oxides and stearates, triethanolamine, diethylene glycol and polyethylene glycol.

Retarders

Retarders are added as processing agents to the rubber mixture during handling to inhibit uncontrolled vulcanization. N-Nitrosodiphenylamine, N-methyl-N,4-dinitrosoaniline, phthalic anhydride and salicylic acid are common retarders. Phthalic anhydride is a strong irritant and causes respiratory symptoms, asthma and lung function disturbances (Nielsen *et al.*, 1991; Taylor, 1992).

Among the nitrosoamines are found potent animal carcinogens. Many nitrosoamines (Nicholson, 1992) are present in tobacco smoke, food, drinks, and different types of industries, including the rubber industry. The carcinogenic nitrosoamines may not be used as additives in the rubber industry today, but some non-carcinogenic nitrosoamines are used, which may undergo transnitrosation reactions with certain other additives, producing carcinogenic by-products, such as *N*-nitrosodimethylamine. This substance has been identified in the air in the tyre production plant (Rogaczewska and Ligocka, 1994; Rogaczewska and Wroblewska-Jakubowska, 1996) and in the salt curing area (Reh and Fajen, 1996).

Antioxidants

Antioxidants and antiozonants retard oxidation and ageing of the rubber product. They include *N,N'*-diphenyl-*p*-phenylenediamine (DPPD), phenyl-*α*-naphthylamine (PAN) and phenyl-*β*-naphthylamine (PBN). PBN biotransforms to *β*-naphthylamine, which is an established human carcinogen (IARC, 1987e), and has been found in the urine of workers exposed to PBN (IARC, 1978b). Phenylenediamines are suspect carcinogens.

Other common antioxidants include 4,4'-methylenediamine (DDM, MDA) and quinolines such as 6-ethoxy-1,2-dihydro-2,2,4-trimethylquinoline (EDT) and 2,2,4-trimethyl-2-dihydroquinoline (TDHQ) and its polymers. 2,6-Di-*tert*-butyl-*p*-cresol (butylated hydroxytoluene, BHT) has some use as an antioxidant. It is otherwise used in the food industry and is anticarcinogenic (Williams and Iatropoulos, 1996) and tumour promoting, the latter at higher doses (Thompson *et al.*, 1991; Malkinson *et al.*, 1997).

Reinforcing Agents

Reinforcing agents are used to expand the volume of the rubber and to strengthen the material. Clays, carbonates and silica may be used as fillers/reinforcers. A common, efficient and high-volume reinforcing agent in rubber manufacture is carbon black. Two types are available: furnace black and channel black, the former containing more polycyclic aromatic hydrocarbons (PAHs). Carbon black is extremely dusty and contaminates whole mixing and milling areas when handled. The carcinogenicity of carbon black has been evaluated (IARC, 1987f, 1996) and data have been found to be inadequate for an assessment of human risk, although carbon black and extracts of carbon black are animal carcinogens.

Extenders

Extenders reduce the amount of elastomer needed in the manufacture of rubber goods. Extenders may also function as processing aids, reinforcers or plasticizers. High-boiling mineral oil distillates or tar products are common extenders and they may be a source of PAH (benzo[*a*]pyrene, benz[*a*]anthracene, dibenz[*a,h*]anthracene, dibenzo[*a,i*]pyrene) emissions to the workplace atmosphere.

Blowing Agents

Blowing agents produces a porous product ('foamed rubber'). They are decomposed during warm process steps, giving off gases. Blowing agents include *N,N'*-dinitrosopentamethylenetetramine, benzene sulphohydrazide, 1,1'-azobisformamide and benzoic acid. Most of these compounds are irritating and may give off irritating decomposition products during the process.

Mould Release Agents

Mould release agents are used to facilitate the detachment of the rubber goods after moulding. Common release agents are various resins, Cd, Zn, Pb and Mg stearates, sebacates, adipates, mineral oil, diethylhexyl phthalate (DEHP) and dibutyl phthalate. Diethylene glycol or the more toxic tri-*m*-cresyl phosphate or tri-*p*-cresyl phosphate may also be used.

Antitack Agents

Antitacking agents inhibit the adhesion of the rubber sheets during handling. Lead, cadmium and zinc stearates are used. Most of these compounds have been very little studied in terms of toxicity, although they are expected to have similar characteristics to the inorganic salts.

Talc is a very common antitacking agent. This is a high volume material and is powdered in great amounts on rubber sheets. Some qualities of talc may contain asbestos-like fibres. Some studies indicate a mesothelioma risk in the talc mining and milling industry owing to the fibre content (IARC, 1987g) of certain qualities of talk.

Colourants

As colourants for rubber products, different metallic salts are used. Among them are fairly inert substances such as titanium oxide and iron oxide, but more toxic compounds, e.g. chromium oxide, lead chromate and cadmium sulphide, may also be used. Cadmium (IARC, 1976) and chromium (IARC, 1990a) and their salts are carcinogenic and lead salts may cause lead intoxication. Chromates may be irritating. Rubber tyres obtain their black colour from their high content of the reinforcer carbon black.

Solvents

Many organic solvents are used in the rubber industry for dissolving additives and for softening the rubber material during processing. In heated process steps, the solvents evaporate. A great number of different solvents may be used, such as dimethylformamide, tetrahydrofuran, white spirit, 1,1,1-trichloroethane, trichloroethylene, methylene chloride, butanol, methyl ethyl ketone, methyl isobutyl ketone, 1,4-dioxane, benzene, xylene and toluene.

1,4-Dioxane is an animal carcinogen, producing liver tumours in rats and guinea pigs and gall bladder tumours in guinea pigs. In perorally dosed mice, nasal tumours occurred (IARC, 1987h). Benzene has been very much used in the rubber industry and may still be used in some countries, in spite of its documented leukaemogenic risk (IARC, 1987i). The long-term bioassay data on 1,1,1-trichloroethane do not permit an evaluation as to its possible carcinogenicity (IARC, 1979b). Trichloroethylene is an experimental carcinogen causing renal cell tumours, testicular tumours, liver tumours and lung tumours in mice. In rats, renal and testicular cell tumours were observed. Epidemiological data suggest increased incidences of liver and biliary tract cancer and lymphomas (IARC, 1995b).

Flame Retardants

Antimony trioxide is a flame retardant in the rubber industry. It is irritant to the eyes, nose and throat in the rat (Newton *et al.*, 1994).

Decabromodiphenyl oxide is used as a flame retardant in ABS rubbers. It produces hepatocellular adenomas in both sexes of the rat on peroral administration and acinar cell adenomas of the pancreas and mononuclear cell leukaemia in males (IARC, 1990b).

Latex

The latex industry uses rubber material in dispersed liquid form and the compounding is followed by dipping, drying and subsequent curing. Latex products include gloves, balloons, teats and contraceptives. Specific latex chemicals are used (IARC, 1982a), such as dispersion agents (e.g. 2-naphthalene sulphonate reacted with formaldehyde), emulsifiers, coagulators (calcium chloride, calcium or zinc nitrate), in addition to the common curing agents, accelerators, antioxidants, etc. Specific exposures during latex handling may involve ammonia, formaldehyde, hydrogen chloride, chlorine and curing fumes, all of which are irritating.

THE PLASTICS INDUSTRY

Plastics are divided into two major types (Martinmaa, 1984a): the thermosetting plastics and the thermoplastics (**Table 2**). The thermosets may be decomposed or lose their characteristics when heated. The thermoplastics do

Table 2 Nomenclature and uses of plastics

Class	Type	Uses
Thermoplastics	Polyethylene (PE)	Films, sheets, food bags, packages
	Polypropylene (PP)	Home furnishings, carpets, pipes
	Poly(vinyl chloride) (PVC)	Floorings, cable insulation, films, table cloths, artificial 'leather'
	Poly(vinylidene chloride) (PVDC)	Films, laminates, food packages, textiles
	Polystyrene plastics (PS)	Packaging, insulation (foamed PS), baby rattles, spoons, forks, knives
	Poly(methyl methacrylate) (PMMA) (Plexiglas)	Windows, houseware, bathtubs
	Polyamides (PA) (nylon)	Textiles, carpets, films, medical ware
	Polycarbonates (PC) (Makrolon)	Safety helmets, bottles, doors, windows
	Polyfluorocarbons (PTFE) (Teflon)	Heat insulation
Thermosets	Unsaturated polyesters (UP)	Building construction, vehicles, appliances, boats
	Epoxy (EP) resins	Coatings, laminates, composites, floorings, adhesives
	Polyurethanes (PUR)	Coatings, adhesives, fibres, foams, mattresses, cushions, insulation
	Aminoplasts (UF, MF) (Melamine)	Laminates, bonding materials, wet strengthening. UF: insulants (foams), housings for electrical apparatus, lavatory seats. MF: buttons, plates, cups, ladles
	Phenol–formaldehyde (PF)	Adhesives, coatings, laminates

not. At least 50 plastic types are of major commercial interest. There are, moreover, many technical qualities and plastic materials designed for special purposes. All plastics are made from monomers polymerized by addition of 'catalysts' or by temperature treatment. Plastics may be produced by process industries, but for some purposes the use is connected with manual mixing of raw materials at the work site (e.g. epoxy).

As with the rubber industry, the plastics industry requires the use of a great number of added chemicals. These additives may be divided into 14 major classes (Fishbein, 1984), with many different chemicals, such as stabilizers, fillers, ultraviolet light absorbers, flame retardants, colourants, solvents, blowing agents and polymerization enhancers ('initiators', 'catalysts', 'hardeners'). In many instances new compounds are introduced for technical and commercial reasons. The toxicology of the majority of compounds is little known.

Polyethylene (PE) and Polypropylene Plastics (PP)

These plastics are used for the manufacture of films, sheets and layered packaging materials (PE) and of fibres and moulded goods (PP). PE manufacture involves handling of additives such as antioxidants, slip additives, antistatics and silica.

Ethylene (IARC, 1994a) is biotransformed to the mutagenic and carcinogenic ethylene oxide. Experimental and epidemiological data do not permit an evaluation of the carcinogenicity of ethylene. The same applies to propylene (IARC, 1994b), which is biotransformed to propylene oxide.

Poly(vinyl Chloride)

Poly(vinyl chloride) (PVC) is a very important plastic family in modern society. It consists of the homopolymer from the vinyl chloride monomer (VCM), or of copolymers between VCM and vinylidene chloride, ethylene, propylene or vinyl acetate (Holmberg, 1984a). PVC resin is formed from vinyl chloride (VC), which is a colourless gas. Residual VCM migrates from plastics, e.g. from food packages, and is of health concern. Before the 1970s VCM had also been used as a propellant for deodorants, hair sprays, insecticides, polishes and window cleaners.

The most important monomer in the series of homopolymers and coplymers is VCM. It was previously recognized (Holmberg and Molina, 1974) only to be slightly hazardous, possessing anaesthetic and some hepatotoxic properties. This was before its carcinogenicity was revealed in the early 1970s. PVC autoclave workers could, however, in some studies exhibit with acroosteolysis, Raynaud's phenomenon or scleroderma (Holmberg and Molina, 1974) due to high exposures.

Vinyl chloride is mutagenic in a number of bacterial test systems (Giri, 1995). It is biotransformed to an epoxide and gives an adduct binding to macromolecules. VCM produces chromosomal abberrations and chromosomal injuries (IARC, 1987j). Its genotoxic properties strongly support a carcinogenic effect.

The first observation of the carcinogenicity of VCM was made in 1971 (Viola et al., 1971). They showed that 30 000 ppm of VCM could be carcinogenic to rats in multiple sites. This exposure level was far above that of environmental concern and the finding was thus generally ignored. After a couple of years the general observation was confirmed, expanded and modified for rats, mice and hamsters in 1973 and 1974 (Maltoni and Lefemine, 1975). It was subsequently also shown to be active towards rodents at exposure levels equal to those of historical interest (Maltoni et al., 1984a). In the animal experiments tumours occurred in many different organs and the most important were liver haemangiosarcomas.

Maltoni and co-workers' first report on liver haemangiosarcoma in rodents inspired Creech and Johnson (1974) to scrutinize observations in a PVC plant. They reported three cases from one plant. The new data led to a scientific meeting in New York in 1974, where the toxicity of VCM was reviewed (Selikoff and Hammond, 1975), together with a great number of cancer cases among workmen. Among these cases were a couple of liver haemangiosarcomas in Sweden (Byrén and Holmberg, 1975) among a total work force of 771 workers in one plant, established in the 1940s. Later, several tens of case reports have been published in the Western world, not including those cases occurring in regular epidemiologal cohort studies. In addition, there are probably a large number of unpublished liver haemangiosarcomas (such as four additional cases in Sweden).

Creech and Johnson (1974) showed that haemangiosarcoma of the liver could be associated with VCM exposure also in man. Indeed, the findings of the carcinogenicity in animals before human observations and the fact that the very specific and very rare histological type of tumour occurred in animals and humans changed (Maltoni, 1975) the then dominant paradigm of risk assessment of carcinogenic chemicals, which said that animal data are of little value for assessing human risk.

Haemangiosarcomas of the liver (Doll, 1988; Simonato et al., 1991) and other liver tumour types were found to be elevated among PVC workers in a large number of epidemiological studies and case reports around the world (IARC, 1987j). Increased frequencies of lung tumors, brain tumors, malignancies of the lymphatic and haematopoietic system and skin melanomas were also observed (IARC, 1987j; Falk, 1992; Lundberg et al., 1993; Nicholson et al., 1984; Storetvedt Heldaas et al., 1984). In the PVC processing industry, which produces PVC goods from the resins, small amounts of residual VCM are emitted into the plant atmosphere. The processing industries have not showed a consistent over-risk of cancer (Chiazze et al., 1977; Molina et al., 1981), probably owing to low exposures. Two cases of liver haemangiosarcomas among extruders in one study (Maltoni et al., 1984b) suggest, however, that a liver cancer risk may also be of some concern in the processing industry. In one study (Molina et al., 1981), an increased risk of ischaemic heart disease was found.

VA is carcinogenic and produces nasal cavity tumours of the rat (IARC, 1995a); it is rapidly transformed to the carcinogenic acetaldehyde (IARC, 1985; 1987l). Both VA and acetaldehyde are genotoxic to human and mammalian cells.

Poly(methyl Methacrylate) (PMMA)

Poly(methyl methacrylate) (PMMA, Plexiglas) is an acrylic plastic (Holmberg, 1984b). PMMA is used for glazing, signs, sanitary ware, instrument panels and protective goggles. It is also used as a bone cement and in dentistry. Methyl methacrylate (MMA) polymerizes in water and contains an inhibitor, e.g. hydroquinone, to protect against spontaneous polymerization.

The toxicology of MMA has been reviewed (IARC, 1994c). MMA is irritating to the eyes, skin and airways and is a sensitizer. The most important systemic effect is the CNS effect. Skin absorption may cause disturbances in peripheral nerve function, experienced as coldness and numbness in the fingers. This is associated with a reduction in nerve conduction velocity. Manual handling of MMA is often responsible.

Polyesters

The monomer for polyester plastics is styrene (vinylbenzene). It is used in large quantities by spraying and hand rolling (lamination) of styrene-modified polyester plastics. For the production of boats, swimming pools, containers, etc., it is reinforced with fibreglass.

Fibreglass-reinforced polyester manufacture starts with mixing of styrene monomer with catalysts (e.g. methyl ethyl ketone peroxide or benzoyl peroxide), a hardener (e.g. cobalt naphthenate), anhydrides (phthalic anhydride or isophthalic anhydride, maleic anhydride) and glycols (propylene glycol or diethylene glycol). Acetone is used as a solvent for cleaning. The polyester plastic is commonly reinforced with fibreglass, which may be manually built on the so-called gel coat or sprayed on together with styrene.

Styrene (Sorsa et al., 1993) is absorbed by inhalation and via the skin. It is soluble in blood and distributed to other tissues. It has been found to be stored in fat tissue (Engström et al., 1978). Styrene can be demonstrated in fat tissue a couple of weeks after exposure and is thus accumulated. The biotransformation via styrene oxide leads to terminal metabolites (including mandelic acid) which can be analysed in the urine.

Styrene is irritating and affects the respiratory tract, and causes CNS effects (Edling et al., 1993; Pahwa and Kalra, 1993) and peripheral nerve injury (IARC, 1994d).

Chromosomal aberrations (Barale, 1991; Artuso et al., 1995) were found among plastic boat builders. Increases in SCE (Andersson et al., 1980) and single strand breaks (IARC, 1994d) in peripheral lymphocytes have also been reported in several studies. Styrene is genotoxic, via the adduct binding of its metabolite, styrene oxide, to DNA (Byfält Nordqvist et al, 1985). In the reinforced plastics industry, styrene adducts with haemoglobin were also determined (Hemminki and Vodicka, 1995; Yeowell-O'Connell et al., 1996) as an early indicator on a cancer risk.

Epidemiological studies on cancer risks of styrene-exposed workers may have not shown (Coggon, 1994; IARC, 1994d) an increased risk. However, it has not yet been possible to define a sufficiently large number of highly exposed workers for a sufficiently long time. Also, the fact that many styrene exposures occur in small boat factories contributes to the difficulty in collecting large groups of workmen to study.

An increased risk of leukaemia in the Danish reinforced plastics industry (Kolstad et al., 1995) was, however, recently found among workers employed during the time periods when exposures were particularly high. Animal studies have been difficult to assess, although one study (Conti et al., 1988) in particular showed dose-dependent frequencies of mammary tumours in rats. The IARC (IARC, 1994d) classified the animal data as showing *limited evidence* of styrene carcinogenicity. There is *sufficient evidence* for animal carcinogenicity of its metabolite, styrene oxide (SO). The genotoxicity and carcinogenicity of SO influenced the overall classification of styrene itself.

Central nervous system defects were observed (Holmberg, 1977) among children, whose mothers had been exposed to styrene. Styrene crosses the placenta (Lindbohm, 1993) and the question of whether styrene constitutes a reproductive hazard in the industry is still open. Increased rates of spontaneous abortions have been suggested (Hemminki et al., 1984) among workers in reinforced plastic workshops.

Styrene is a monomer also in polystyrene plastics, e.g. expanded (foamed) polystyrene, used for a variety of products. Monomeric styrene may migrate from food packages into foods and beverages.

Epoxy Thermosets

Epoxy resins are formed by reaction between an epoxy compound, such as epichlorohydrin, and a bifunctional alcohol, such as bisphenol A (Martinmaa, 1984b). Other epoxy monomers include 2,2-bis(p-2,3-epoxypropxyl)-phenylpropane used together with butane-1,4-diol diglycidyl ether. Monomers are activated by curing to give the final product. Amines are used as curing agents, e.g. triethylamine, diethylenetriamine, p-phenylenediamine and N-(3-dimethylaminopropyl) propylene-1,3-diamine. Diaminodiphenyl sulfone and acid anhydrides, such as pyromellitic dianhydride and hexylhydrophthalic anhydride, are other hardeners. Monomers, hardeners and polymers may all cause skin injuries and may be allergenic. The monomers are generally more or less biologically reactive (Hemminki and Vainio, 1984) and thus suspected to be mutagenic and carcinogenic. Epichlorohydrin and bisphenol A form adducts with DNA.

Epichlorohydrin is irritating, genotoxic and mutagenic (Giri, 1997) and induces forestomach tumours and nasal cavity tumours in the rat (IARC, 1987b). It is a tumour initiator in the skin in mice, produces local tumours in mice after sucutaneous injection, and enhances lung tumour frequencies in mice after intraperitoneal injections. Epidemiological information is not conclusive as regards a possibly increased risk for malignancies among occupationally exposed people. However, recent studies suggest (Barbone *et al.*, 1994) that resin plant workers exposed to epichlorohydrin have an increased risk of central nervous system neoplasms and of leukaemias (Enterline *et al.*, 1990).

4,4′-Methylenedianiline (MDA) is used as a hardener for epoxy resins. MDA is carcinogenic to experimental animals (IARC, 1986a), producing hepatocellular carcinomas in mice and thyroid carcinomas in rats, suggesting the involvement of multiple biological mechanisms. One report (Liss and Guirguis, 1994) describes cases of jaundice and one case of bladder cancer among workmen intoxicated by MDA.

Polyurethanes

The aromatic amine 4′-methylenebis(2-chloroaniline) (MOCA) is used as a hardening agent for goods and surface coatings made from polyurethane elastomers. It is taken up via the skin (Linch *et al.*, 1971) and as an aerosol via the lungs.

MOCA is carcinogenic to laboratory animals. It is a multipotential carcinogen, producing tumours of the lung, liver, thyroid, mammary gland and Zymbal gland. The tumour site depends on the dose, route of administration and species (IARC, 1987k; McQueen and Williams, 1990). Dogs develop tumours in the urinary bladder. The same organ has been predicted to be the affected after long-term human exposure, as MOCA is chemically related to benzidine. Benzidine is an established urinary bladder carcinogen for humans. MCA binds to DNA in blood and a couple of cases of bladder papillomas have been noted (McQueen and Williams, 1990).

Isocyanates consist of a number of different isocyanates and prepolymerizates, such as toluene diisocyanate (TDI), naphthalene diisocyanate, methylene diphenyldiisocyanate (MDI), triphenylmethane triisocyanate and polyurethane prepolymers (Rosenberg, 1984).

TDI causes irritation of the eyes, respiratory tract and skin. It can lead to serious bronchitis and pulmonary oedema. Exposure to TDI has produced asthma-like effects even in individuals who are not sensitized (Butcher *et al.*, 1993) and decreases in the pulmonary function (Wegman *et al.*, 1974). Some people may become sensitized to TDI even after long and very low exposures (Vandenplas *et al.*, 1993).

2,4-TDI is quickly hydrolysed to toluene-2,4-diamine and 2,6-TDT to toluene-2,6-diamine. Both diamines are mutagenic in bacterial test systems and a mixture of the two TDIs is carcinogenic (IARC, 1986b), causing multiple tumours in rats and mice. Epidemiological studies of polyurethane foam industry workers exposed to TDI and MDI (Hagmar *et al.*, 1993a, b) showed non-signific-

antly elevated risks of rectal cancer, Hodgkin's lymphoma and prostate cancer. MDI is mutagenic and biotransformed to the carcinogenic methylenediamine.

Polyacrylamides (PA)

Polyacrylamides have a wide use as dispersants and binders in paints, particularly in water-based paints. They may also be used as thickeners in cosmetic preparations. PA is used as a flocculating agent in waste water treatment in mineral processing and as a soil stabilizer. It is used as a water repellant and to prevent shrinking in the textile industry. Polyacrylamides are synthesized from the monomer acrylamide (AM) and derivatives (e.g. *N*-methylolacrylamide).

AM (Guirguis, 1992) is neurotoxic to the central nervous system and to peripheral nerves, causing tingling of fingers and lower limbs, coldness, ataxia and sensory changes (Calleman *et al.*, 1994; LoPachin and Lehning, 1994). The neurotoxic effects are related to duration of exposure to AM, as studied by determinations of DNA adducts in rats (Crofton *et al.*, 1996). AM is carcinogenic in animals (IARC, 1986c), producing lung tumours in the mouse and multiple tumours in the rat. Occupationally exposed men possess AM adducts with haemoglobin (Bergmark *et al.*, 1993; Bergmark, 1997), suggesting a cancer risk.

Acrylonitrile Fibers and Rubbers

Acrylonitrile (vinyl cyanide, AN) is used in the manufacture of many types of copolymers, including acrylonitrile–butadiene–styrene and styrene–acrylonitrile elastomers. Acrylonitrile (AN) is embryotoxic, teratogenic, genotoxic and mutagenic (IARC, 1987c; Guirguis, 1992). In rats of both sexes, tumours occur in the forestomach, brain or Zymbal gland after oral administration or inhalation. An overall assessment (Rothman, 1994) of epidemiological studies of acrylonitrile-exposed workers did not show an increase in the cancer risk.

Plastic Additives

Also in the production of plastics a number of different additives may be needed in order to provide the desired technical characteristics. Many individual additives are exchanged for new ones depending on technical and commercial requirements. A great number of additives have little known toxicology, except for their acute toxic properties. The additives can be divided into many groups, named after their function in the material.

Inorganic gases are used as *blowing agents* for producing foam plastics, e.g. nitrogen and carbon dioxide. Hydrogen peroxide may be used for producing oxygen that causes the foaming. Organic chemicals, which can be easily evaporated, have also been used, e.g. heptane, pentane, methylene chloride and dichlorodifluoromethane. Organic substances that decompose easily are also used, e.g. azo compounds, phthalimides and dinitropentamethylenetetramine. Azodicarbonamide, used in polyethylene and polypropylene processing, causes asthma (Slovak, 1984).

Plasticizers include mineral oils, adipates, phthalates, sebacates, oleates and stearates. Common plasticizers are di-*n*-butyl phthalate (DBP), di(2-ethylhexyl) phthalate (DEHP) and di(2-ethylhexyl) adipate (DEHA), used both in the rubber industry and in the PVC industry. Plastizicers in, e.g., blood bags and food packages can migrate from the PVC into blood or food and be of some concern as a health risk.

DBP is used as both a plasticizer and a solvent. It possesses testicular toxicity in rats, affecting the Sertoli cells, probably via its metabolite mono-*n*-butyl phthalate. In a multigenerational study (Wine *et al.*, 1997), Sprague–Dawley rats showed reproduction disturbances and endocrine-mediated effects on reproductive development.

DEHP is a liver-cell peroxisome proliferator (Rao and Reddy, 1991; WHO, 1992), causing hepatocellular tumours in rodents (IARC, 1982b; Huber *et al.*, 1996) and renal injuries (Woodward, 1990). Recent studies suggest that DEHP is teratogenic and spermatotoxic in rodents and causes testicular damage (Oishi, 1993; Siddiqui and Sristava, 1992), and acts as a hormone (endocrine) disruptor by interacting with oestradiol and ovulation (Thomas and Thomas, 1992; Davis *et al.*, 1994; Parmar *et al.*, 1995). Metabolites of DEHP have been found in the urine of PVC workers (Dirven *et al.*, 1993).

As a substitute for DEHP, trimellitic anhydride (TMA) is used in the PVC industry. It may cause irritation in the respiratory tract, rhinitis or asthma (Sale *et al.*, 1981; Zeiss *et al.*, 1983; Fraser *et al.*, 1995). Plasticizers used in the PVC industry include alkylsulphonic esters, arylphosphates, chloroalkanes (see *flame retardants*, below), qlycerol, polyglycols, and epoxidized soy bean oil.

As *hardeners* in the plastics industry, perbenzoates and certain organic peroxides are often used. Benzoyl peroxide and dicumyl peroxide are used in the manufacture of polyester and polyethylene plastics. All peroxides are irritants and cytotoxic. Benzoyl peroxide promotes skin tumour development in the mouse (Slaga *et al.*, 1981). It is cytotoxic and causes skin irritation (Spoo *et al.*, 1992), but also induces DNA injuries (Hazlewood and Davies, 1996), via the formation of free radicals (Binder *et al.*, 1995).

Stabilizers are used to stabilize the plastic polymer towards ageing. Organotin compounds, lead and cadmium stearates, and inorganic lead salts have been used (Fishbein, 1984).

UV absorbers protect against ultraviolet light, which degrades, e.g., PVC. A great number of chemicals

belonging to different groups, such as benzophenones, benzotriazoles, salicylates and acrylates, may be found here (Fishbein, 1984).

Fillers increase hardness and mechanical strength and are also used in large amounts to reduce manufacturing costs. They may also improve electrical properties, ultraviolet light resistance, processing characteristics or dimensional stability. They include many particulate materials, such as zinc oxide, calcium oxide, barium oxide, silica, kaolin, mica and talc. Fibrous materials are also used, such as glass, polyamide fibre (nylon), cellulose fibres and even asbestos.

Flame retardants (Fishbein, 1984) can be inorganic substances or halogenated organic compounds, such as chlorinated and brominated organic compounds, or phosphate esters, such as tris(chloroalkyl) phosphate esters. An important brominated flame retardant is tris(2,3-dibromopropyl) phosphate (Tris-BP). Other flame retardants include tetrabromobisphenol A used for epoxy plastics, brominated polyols for polyurethanes and ethylene bis(tetrabromo)isophthalimide used for polyethylene products. Tris(chloroalkyl) phosphate esters are used for polyurethane. Antimony trioxide and aluminium hydroxide are inorganic flame retardants used for PVC, polyethylene and poly(vinyl acetate).

Tris-BP (IARC, 1987m; WHO, 1995) administered by peroral dosing produces stomach tumours and lung tumours in both sexes of mice and liver tumours in females and kidney tumours in males. In rats, kidney tumours are found in both sexes. Tris-BP is gonadotoxic in male laboratory animals even after skin application (Osterberg *et al.*, 1977).

Chloroalkanes (CP) have been much used in the PVC cable industry and in other plastic materials for electrical equipment because it inhibits flammability. It is produced with varying lengths of the carbon chain and with varying degrees of chlorination.

CPs with an average length of 12 carbons and 60% chlorination produces hepatocellular tumours in mice (IARC, 1990d) of both sexes on peroral administration, and follicular cell tumours of the thyroid of females. In rats, it increased the incidence of hepatocellular tumours in both sexes and of follicular cell tumours of the thyroid in females, in addition to mononuclear cell leukaemia in males.

CPs with an average length of 23 carbon atoms and 43% chlorination increased the incidence of malignant lymphomas (IARC, 1990d) in male mice. In rats, adrenal tumours were produced in females.

Decabromodiphenyl oxide is used as a flame retardant in both thermoplastic and thermoset resins (polystyrene, polyester moulding, polypropylene, nylon, PVC). For toxicological information, see under The Rubber Industry.

Chlorendic acid is found as an intermediate in polyester resin manufacture for products for the electrical industry. It also acts as a flame retardant and is used as such in polyurethane foams. Chlorendic acid is carcinogenic (IARC, 1990c) to mice on peroral administration, producing liver tumours in males and lung tumours in females. In rats, liver tumours occur in both sexes and lung and pancreatic tumours in male rats.

Both inorganic and organic pigments are used as *colourants* in plastic materials (Fishbein, 1984). A number of chromium, cadmium and lead compounds may be used. Titanium dioxide and molybdate orange (a mixture of lead chromate, molybdate and sulphate) may also be used. Among the organic colourants are the phthalocyanines and quinacridones, and also some azo compounds (e.g. the carcinogenic *p*-aminoazobenzene). In some countries, the carcinogenic benzidine and benzidine-related compounds are still in use.

Foamed plastics are obtained by using *blowing agents*. Commonly used are organic substances which decompose at high temperature, giving off gases, such as the supposedly biologically highly reactive azobisisobutyronitrile, azobisformamide or oxybisbenzenesulphonyl hydrazides (Fishbein, 1984). Many of these compounds have not been much studied. For foaming of polyurethane, trichloromonofluoromethane (FC 11) or difluoromonochloromethane (FC 22) have been used. Owing to environmental concerns, these halogenated hydrocarbons have been replaced by nitrogen and nitrogen oxides.

A great number of *solvents* are used in the plastics industry. Acetone is a high-volume solvent used in styrene polyester manufacture. Other solvents include industrial gasoline, low aliphatic alcohols, esters, glycol ethers, ketones and nitroalkanes. Glycidyl ethers are important solvents (and also retardants) in epoxy resin systems.

Optical brighteners are used as fluorescent whitening agents in PVC and polystyrene. Derivatives of naphthotriazoles and coumarins are used to a certain extent (Fishbein, 1984).

Antistatics (Fishbein, 1984) dissipate electrostatic charge. The major chemical groups include amines, quaternary ammonium salts, organic phosphates, polyethylene glycols and metal salts (e.g. stannous chloride).

In order to start the polymerization reaction, a small amount of *initiators* may be added (Fishbein, 1984). Among them, many different organic peroxides, such as benzoyl peroxide, butyl peroxide, decanoyl peroxide and dilauryl peroxide, are used for PVC plastics. Peroxides are generally considered to be irritating. Some organometallic compounds may also be used as initiators.

REFERENCES

Andersson, H. C., Tranberg, E. A., Uggla, A. H. and Zetterberg, G. (1980). Chromosomal aberrations and sister chromatid exchanges in lymphocytes of men occupationally exposed to styrene in a plastic-boat factory. *Mutat. Res.*, **73**, 387–401.

Artuso, M., Angotzi, G., Bonassi, S., Bonatti, S., De Ferrari, M., Gargano, D., Lastrucci, L., Miligi, L., Sbrana, C. and Abbondanolo, A. (1995). Cytogenetic biomonitoring of styrene-exposed plastic boat builders. *Arch. Environ. Contam. Toxicol.*, **29**, 270–274.

Barale, R. (1991). The genetic toxicology of styrene and styrene oxide. *Mutat. Res.*, **257**, 107–126.

Barbone, F., Delzell, E., Austin, H. and Cole, P. (1994). Exposure to epichlorohydrin and central nervous system neoplasms at a resin and dye manufacturing plant. *Arch. Environ. Health*, **49**, 355–358.

Bergmark, E. (1997). Hemoglobin adducts of acrylamide and acrylonitrile in laboratory workers, smokers and nonsmokers. *Chem. Res. Toxicol.*, **10**, 78–84.

Bergmark, E., Calleman, C. J., He, F. and Costa, L. G. (1993). Determination of hemoglobin adducts in humans occupationally exposed to acrylamide. *Toxicol. Appl. Pharmacol.*, **120**, 45–54.

Binder, R. L., Aardema, M. J. and Thompson, E. D. (1995). Benzoyl peroxide: review of experimental carcinogenesis and human safety data. *Prog. Clin. Biol. Res.*, **391**, 245–294.

Bond, J. A., Himmelstein, M. W. and Medinsky, M. A. (1996). The use of toxicologic data in mechanistic risk assessment: 1,3-butadiene as a case study. *Int. Arch. Occup. Environ. Health*, **68**, 415–420.

Butcher, B. T., Mapp, C. E. and Fabbri, L. M. (1993). Polyisocyanates and their prepolymers. In Bernstein, I. L., Chan-Yeung, M., Malo, J. L. and Bernstein, D.-I. (Eds), *Asthma in the Workplace*. Marcel Dekker, New York, pp. 415–437.

Byfält Nordqvist, M., Löf, A., Osterman-Golkar, S. and Walles, S. A. S. (1985). Covalent binding of styrene and styrene-7,8-oxide to plasma proteins, hemoglobin and DNA in the mouse. *Chem.-Biol. Interact.*, **55**, 63–73.

Byrén, D. and Holmberg, B. (1975). Two possible cases of angiosarcoma of the liver in a group of Swedish vinyl chloride–polyvinyl chloride workers. *Ann. N. Y. Acad. Sci.*, **246**, 249–250.

Calleman, C. J., Wu, Y., He, F., Tian, G., Bergmark, E., Zhang, S., Deng, H., Wang, Y., Crofton, K. M. and Fennell, T. (1994). Relationship between biomarkers of exposure and neurological effects in a group of workers exposed to acrylamide. *Toxicol. Appl. Pharmacol.*, **126**, 361–371.

Chiazze, L., Nichols, W. E. and Wong, O. (1977). Mortality among employees of PVC fabricators. *J. Occup. Med.*, **9**, 623–628.

Coggon, D. (1994). Epidemiological studies of styrene-exposed populations. *Crit. Rev. Toxicol.*, **24**, Suppl., 107–115.

Conti, B., Maltoni, C., Perino, G. and Ciliberti, A. (1988). Long-term carcinogenicity bioassays on styrene administered by inhalation, ingestion and injection and styrene oxide administered by injection in Sprague–Dawley rats, and *para*-methylstyrene administered by ingestion in Sprague–Dawley rats and Swiss mice. *Ann. N. Y. Acad. Sci.*, **534**, 203–234.

Creech, J. L. and Johnson, M. N. (1974). Angiosarcoma of the liver in the manufacture of polyvinyl chloride. *J. Occup. Med.*, **16**, 150–151.

Crofton, K. M., Padilla, S., Tilson, H. A., Anthony, D. C., Raymer, J. H. and MacPhail, R. C. (1996). The impact of dose rate on the neurotoxicity of acrylamide: the interaction of administered dose, target tissue concentrations, tissue damage, and functional effects. *Toxicol. Appl. Pharmacol.*, **139**, 163–176.

Cronin, E. (1980). *Contact Dermatitis*. Churchill Livingstone, Edinburgh.

Davis, B. J., Maronpot, R. R. and Heindel, J. J. (1994). Di-(2-ethylhexyl) phthalate suppresses estradiol and ovulation in cycling rats. *Toxicol. Appl. Pharmacol.*, **128**, 216–233.

Dearfield, K. L. (1994). Ethylene thiourea (ETU). A review of the genetic toxicity studies. *Mutat. Res.*, **317**, 111–132.

Dirven, H. A. A. M., van den Broek, P. H. H., Arebds, A. M. M., Nordkamp, H. H., de Lepper A. J. G. M., Henderson, P. T. and Jongeneelen, F. J. (1993). Metabolites of the plasticizer di(2-ethylhexyl) phthalate in urine samples of workers in the polyvinylchloride processing industry. *Int. Arch. Occup. Environ. Health*, **64**, 549–554.

Doll, R. (1988). Effects of exposure to vinyl chloride. An assessment of the evidence. *Scand. J. Work Environ. Health*, **14**, 61–78.

Edling, C., Anundi, H., Johanson, G. and Nilsson, K. (1993). Increase in neuropsychiatric symptoms after occupational exposure to low levels of styrene. *Br. J. Ind. Med.*, **50**, 843–850.

Engström, J., Bjurström, R., Åstrand, I. and Övrum, P. (1978). Uptake, distribution and elimination of styrene in man. *Scand. J. Work Environ. Health*, **4**, 315–323.

Enterline, P. E., Henderson, V. and Marsh, G. (1990). Mortality of workers potentially exposed to epichlorohydrin. *Br. J. Ind. Med.*, **47**, 269–276.

Enwald, E. (1984). Production and processing of synthetic elastomers. *Prog. Clin. Biol. Res.*, **141**, 397–405.

Falk, H. (1992). Vinyl chloride and polyvinyl chloride. In Rom, W. M. (Ed.). *Environmental and Occupational Medicine*. Little, Brown, Boston, 911–920.

Fine, L. and Peters, J. (1976a). Respiratory morbidity in rubber workers: I. Prevalence of respiratory morbidity symptoms and disease in curing workers. *Arch. Environ. Health*, **31**, 5–9.

Fine, L. and Peters, J. (1976b). Respiratory morbidity in rubber workers: II. Pulmonary function in curing workers. *Arch. Environ. Health*, **31**, 10–14.

Fine, L. and Peters, J. (1976c). Respiratory morbidity in rubber workers: III. Respiratory morbidity in processing workers. *Arch. Environ. Health*, **31**, 136–140.

Fine, L. and Peters, J. (1976d). Respiratory morbidity in rubber workers: IV. Respiratory morbidity in talc workers. *Arch. Environ. Health*, **31**, 195–200.

Fishbein, L. (1984). Additives in synthetic polymers. *Prog. Clin. Biol. Res.*, **141**, 19–42.

Fishbein, L. (1991). Chemicals used in the rubber industry. *Sci. Total Environ.*, **101**, 33–43.

Fox, A. J. and Collier, P. F. (1976). A survey of occupational cancer in the rubber and cablemaking industries: analysis of deaths occurring in 1972–74. *Br. J. Ind. Med.*, **33**, 249–264.

Franekic, J., Bratulic, N., Pavlica, M. and Papes, D. (1994). Genotoxicity of dithiocarbamates and their metabolites. *Mutat. Res.*, **325**, 65–74.

Fraser, D. G., Regal, J. F. and Arndt, M. L. (1995). Trimellitic anhydride-induced allergic response in the lung: role of the complement system in cellular changes. *J. Pharmacol. Exp. Ther.*, **273**, 793–801.

Gamble, J. F., McMichael, A. J., Williams, T. and Battigelli, M. (1976). Respiratory function and symptoms: an environmental epidemiologic study of rubber workers

exposed to a phenol–formaldehyde type resin. *Am. Ind. Hyg. Assoc. J.*, **37**, 499–513.

George, J. and Kuttan, R. (1995). Studies on clastogenic and carcinogenic potency of tetramethyl thiuram disulphide. *Cancer Lett.*, **6**, 213–216.

Giri, A. K. (1995). Genetic toxicology of vinyl chloride. *Mutat. Res.*, **339**, 1–14.

Giri, A. K. (1997). Genetic toxicology of epichlorohydrin: a review. *Mutat. Res.*, **386**, 25–38.

Goldstein, D. B. (1983). *Pharmacology of Alcohol*. Oxford University Press, Oxford.

Guirguis, S. (1992). Acrylamide and acrylonitrile. In Rom, W. N. (Ed.). *Environmental and Occupational Medicine*. Brown, Boston, pp. 947–953.

Hagmar, L., Strömberg, U., Welinder, H. and Mikoczy, Z. (1993a). Incidence of cancer and exposure to toluene diisocyanate and methylene diphenyldiisocyanate: a cohort based case-referent study in the polyurethane foam manufacturing industry. *Br. J. Ind. Med.*, **50**, 1003–1007.

Hagmar, L., Welinder, H. and Mikoczy, Z. (1993b). Cancer incidence and mortality in the Swedish polyurethane foam manufacturing industry. *Br. J. Ind. Med.*, **50**, 537–543.

Hazlewood, C. and Davies, M. J. (1996). Benzoyl peroxide-induced damage to DNA and its components: direct evidence for the generation of base adducts, sugar radicals, and strand breaks. *Arch. Biochem. Biophys.*, **332**, 79–91.

Hedenstedt, A., Rannug, U., Ramel, C. and Wachtmeister, C. A. (1981). Mutagenicity of rubber vulcanization gases in *Salmonella typhimurium*. *J. Toxicol. Environ. Health*, **8**, 805–814.

Hemminki, K. and Vainio, H. (1984). Genotoxicity of epoxides and epoxy compounds. *Prog. Clin. Biol. Res.*, **141**, 373–384.

Hemminki, K. and Vodicka, P. (1995). Styrene: from characterisation of DNA adducts to application in styrene-exposed lamination workers. *Toxicol. Lett.*, **77**, 153–161.

Hemminki, K., Lindbohm, M.-L., Hemminki, T. and Vainio, H. (1984). Reproductive hazards and plastic industry. *Prog. Clin. Biol. Res.*, **141**, 79–87.

Högberg, J., Alexander, J., Thomassen, Y. and Aaseth, J. (1987). Selenium. In Seiler, H. G. and Sigel, H. (Eds), *Handbook of Toxicity of Inorganic Compounds*. Marcel Dekker, New York, pp. 581–594.

Holmberg, B. (1984a). The toxicology of monomers in the polyvinyl plastic series. *Prog. Clin. Biol. Res.*, **141**, 99–112.

Holmberg, B. (1984b). The production and use of some thermoplastics and their chemical occupational hazards. *Prog. Clin. Biol. Res.*, **141**, 319–334.

Holmberg, B. and Molina, G. (1974). The industrial toxicology of vinyl chloride. A review. *Work Environ. Health*, **11**, 138–144.

Holmberg, B. and Sjöström, B. (1980). Toxicological aspects of chemical hazards in the rubber industry. *J. Toxicol. Environ. Health*, **6**, 1201–1209.

Holmberg, P. C. (1977). Central nervous defects in two children of mothers exposed to chemicals in the reinforced plastics industry—chance or a causal relation? *Scand. J. Work Environ. Health*, **3**, 212–214.

Houeto, P., Bindoula, G. and Hoffman, J. R. (1995). Ethylenebisdithiocarbamates and ethylenethiourea: possible human health hazards. *Environ. Health Perspect.*, **103**, 568–573.

Huber, W. W., Grasl-Kaupp, B. and Schulte-Hermann, R. (1996). Hepatocarcinogenic potential of di(2-ethylhexyl) phthalate in rodents and its implications on human risk. *Crit. Rev. Toxicol.*, **26**, 365–481.

IARC (1975). *IARC Monographs on the Evaluation of the Carcinogenic Risk of Chemicals to Man. Vol. 9. Some Aziridines, N-, S- and O-Mustards and Selenium.* International Agency for Research on Cancer, WHO, Lyon, pp. 245–260.

IARC (1976). *IARC Monographs on the Evaluation of the Carcinogenic risk of Chemicals to Man. Vol. 11. Cadmium, Nickel, Some Epoxides, Miscellaneous Industrial Chemicals and General Considerations on Volatile Anaesthetics.* International Agency for Research on Cancer, WHO, Lyon, pp. 36–74.

IARC (1978a). *IARC Monographs on the Evaluation of the Carcinogenic Risk of Chemicals to Man. Vol. 17. Some N-Nitroso Compounds.* International Agency for Research on Cancer, WHO, Lyon, pp. 55–75.

IARC (1978b). *IARC Monographs on the Evaluation of the Carcinogenic Risk of Chemicals to Man. Vol. 16. Some Aromatic Amines and Related Nitro Compounds, Hair Dyes, Colouring Agents and Miscellaneous Industrial Chemicals.* International Agency for Research on Cancer, WHO, Lyon, pp. 325–341.

IARC (1979a). *IARC Monographs on the Evaluation of the Carcinogenic Risk of Chemicals to Humans. Vol. 19. Some Monomers, Plastics and Synthetic Elastomers and Acrolein.* International Agency for Research on Cancer, WHO, Lyon, pp. 131–156.

IARC (1979b). *IARC Monographs on the Evaluation of the Carcinogenic Risk of Chemicals to Humans. Vol. 20. Some Halogenated Hydrocarbons.* International Agency for Research on Cancer, WHO, Lyon, pp. 515–531.

IARC (1982a). *IARC Monographs on the Evaluation of the Carcinogenic Risk of Chemicals to Humans. Vol. 28. The Rubber Industry.* International Agency for Research on Cancer, WHO, Lyon.

IARC (1982b). *IARC Monographs on the Evaluation of the Carcinogenic Risk of Chemicals to Humans. Vol. 29. Some Industrial Chemicals and Dyestuffs.* International Agency for Research on Cancer, WHO, Lyon, pp. 269–294.

IARC (1985). *IARC Monographs on the Evaluation of the Carcinogenic Risk of Chemicals to Humans. Vol. 36. Allyl Compounds, Aldehydes, Epoxides and Peroxides.* International Agency for Research on Cancer, WHO, Lyon, pp. 101–132.

IARC (1986a). *IARC Monographs on the Evaluation of the Carcinogenic Risk of Chemicals to Humans. Vol. 39. Some Chemicals Used in Plastics and Elastomers.* International Agency for Research on Cancer, WHO, Lyon, pp. 347–365.

IARC (1986b). *IARC Monographs on the Evaluation of the Carcinogenic Risk of Chemicals to Humans. Vol. 39. Some Chemicals Used in Plastics and Elastomers.* International Agency for Research on Cancer, WHO, Lyon, pp. 287–323.

IARC (1986c). *IARC Monographs on the Evaluation of the Carcinogenic Risk of Chemicals to Humans. Vol. 39. Some Chemicals Used in Plastics and Elastomers.* International Agency for Research on Cancer, WHO, Lyon, pp. 41–66.

IARC (1987a). *IARC Monographs on the Evaluation of Carcinogenic Risks to Humans. Suppl. 7. Overall Evaluations of Carcinogenicity: an Updating of IARC Monographs Volumes 1 to 42.* International Agency for Research on Cancer, WHO, Lyon, p. 160.

IARC (1987b). *IARC Monographs on the Evaluation of Carcinogenic Risks to Humans. Suppl. 7. Overall Evaluations of Carcinogenicity: an Updating of IARC Monographs Volumes 1 to 42.* International Agency for Research on Cancer, WHO, Lyon, pp. 202–203.

IARC (1987c). *IARC Monographs on the Evaluation of Carcinogenic Risks to Humans. Suppl. 7. Overall Evaluations of Carcinogenicity: an Updating of IARC Monographs Volumes 1 to 42.* International Agency for Research on Cancer, WHO, Lyon, pp. 79–80.

IARC (1987d). *IARC Monographs on the Evaluation of Carcinogenic Risks to Humans. Suppl. 7. Overall Evaluations of Carcinogenicity: an Updating of IARC Monographs Volumes 1 to 42.* International Agency for Research on Cancer, WHO, Lyon, pp. 207–208.

IARC (1987e). *IARC Monographs on the Evaluation of Carcinogenic Risks to Humans. Suppl. 7. Overall Evaluations of Carcinogenicity: an Updating of IARC Monographs Volumes 1 to 42.* International Agency for Research on Cancer, WHO, Lyon, pp. 261–263.

IARC (1987f). *IARC Monographs on the Evaluation of Carcinogenic Risks to Humans. Suppl. 7. Overall Evaluations of Carcinogenicity: an Updating of IARC Monographs Volumes 1 to 42.* International Agency for Research on Cancer, WHO, Lyon, pp. 142–143.

IARC (1987g). *IARC Monographs on the Evaluation of Carcinogenic Risks to Humans. Suppl. 7. Overall Evaluations of Carcinogenicity: an Updating of IARC Monographs Volumes 1 to 42.* International Agency for Research on Cancer, WHO, Lyon, pp. 349–350.

IARC (1987h). *IARC Monographs on the Evaluation of Carcinogenic Risks to Humans. Suppl. 7. Overall Evaluations of Carcinogenicity: an Updating of IARC Monographs Volumes 1 to 42.* International Agency for Research on Cancer, WHO, Lyon, p. 201.

IARC (1987i). *IARC Monographs on the Evaluation of Carcinogenic Risks to Humans. Suppl. 7. Overall Evaluations of Carcinogenicity: an Updating of IARC Monographs Volumes 1 to 42.* International Agency for Research on Cancer, WHO, Lyon, pp. 120–122.

IARC (1987j). *IARC Monographs on the Evaluation of Carcinogenic Risks to Humans. Suppl. 7. Overall Evaluations of Carcinogenicity: an Updating of IARC Monographs Volumes 1 to 42.* International Agency for Research on Cancer, WHO, Lyon, pp. 373–376.

IARC (1987k). *IARC Monographs on the Evaluation of Carcinogenic Risks to Humans. Suppl. 7. Overall Evaluations of Carcinogenicity: an Updating of IARC Monographs Volumes 1 to 42.* International Agency for Research on Cancer, WHO, Lyon, pp. 246–247.

IARC (1987l). *IARC Monographs on the Evaluation of Carcinogenic Risks to Humans. Suppl. 7. Overall Evaluations of Carcinogenicity: an Updating of IARC Monographs Volumes 1 to 42.* International Agency for Research on Cancer, WHO, Lyon, pp. 77–78.

IARC (1987m). *IARC Monographs on the Evaluation of Carcinogenic Risks to Humans. Suppl. 7. Overall Evaluations of Carcinogenicity: an Updating of IARC Monographs Volumes 1 to 42.* International Agency for Research on Cancer, WHO, Lyon, pp. 369–370.

IARC (1987n). *IARC Monographs on the Evaluation of Carcinogenic Risks to Humans. Suppl. 7. Overall Evaluations of*

Carcinogenicity: an Updating of IARC Monographs Volumes 1 to 42. International Agency for Research on Cancer, WHO, Lyon, pp. 332–334.

IARC (1990a). *IARC Monographs on the Evaluation of Carcinogenic Risks to Humans. Vol. 49. Chromium, Nickel and Welding*. International Agency for Research on Cancer, WHO, Lyon, pp. 49–256.

IARC (1990b). *IARC Monographs on the Evaluation of Carcinogenic Risks to Humans. Vol. 48. Some Flame Retardants and Textile Chemicals, and Exposures in the Textile Manufacturing Industry*. International Agency for Research on Cancer, WHO, Lyon, pp. 73–84.

IARC (1990c). *IARC Monographs on the Evaluation of Carcinogenic Risks to Humans. Vol. 48. Some Flame Retardants and Textile Chemicals, and Exposures in the Textile Manufacturing Industry*. International Agency for Research on Cancer, WHO, Lyon, pp. 45–53.

IARC (1990d). *IARC Monographs on the Evaluation of Carcinogenic Risks to Humans. Vol. 48. Some Flame Retardants and Textile Chemicals, and Exposures in the Textile Manufacturing Industry*. International Agency for Research on Cancer, WHO, Lyon, pp. 55–72.

IARC (1991a). *IARC Monographs on the Evaluation of Carcinogenic Risks to Humans. Vol. 53. Occupational Exposures in Insecticide Application and Some Pesticides*. International Agency for Research on Cancer, WHO, Lyon, pp. 403–422.

IARC (1991b). *IARC Monographs on the Evaluation of Carcinogenic Risks to Humans. Vol. 53. Occupational Exposures in Insecticide Application and Some Pesticides*. International Agency for Research on Cancer, WHO, Lyon, pp. 423–438.

IARC (1992). *IARC Monographs on the Evaluation of Carcinogenic Risks to Humans. Vol. 54. Occupational Exposures to Mists and Vapours from Strong inorganic acids; and Other Industrial Chemicals*. International Agency for Research on Cancer, WHO, Lyon, pp. 237–285.

IARC (1994a). *IARC Monographs on the Evaluation of Carcinogenic Risks to Humans. Vol. 60. Some Industrial Chemicals*. International Agency for Research on Cancer, WHO, Lyon, pp. 45–71.

IARC (1994b). *IARC Monographs on the Evaluation of Carcinogenic Risks to Humans. Vol. 60. Some Industrial Chemicals*. International Agency for Research on Cancer, WHO, Lyon, pp. 161–180.

IARC (1994c). *IARC Monographs on the Evaluation of Carcinogenic Risks to Humans. Vol. 60. Some Industrial Chemicals*. International Agency for Research on Cancer, World Health Organization, Lyon, pp. 445–474.

IARC (1994d). *IARC Monographs on the Evaluation of Carcinogenic Risks to Humans. Vol. 60. Some Industrial Chemicals*. International Agency for Research on Cancer, WHO, Lyon, pp. 233–320.

IARC (1995a). *IARC Monographs on the Evaluation of Carcinogenic Risks to Humans. Vol. 63. Dry Cleaning, Some Chlorinated Solvents and Other Industrial Chemicals*. International Agency for Research on Cancer, WHO, Lyon, pp. 443–465.

IARC (1995b). *IARC Monographs on the Evaluation of Carcinogenic Risks to Humans. Vol. 63. Dry Cleaning, Some Chlorinated Solvents and Other Industrial Chemicals*. International Agency for Research on Cancer, WHO, Lyon, pp. 75–158.

IARC (1996). *IARC Monographs on the Evaluation of Carcinogenic Risks to Humans. Vol. 65. Printing Processes and Printing Inks, Carbon Black and Some Nitroso Compounds*. International Agency for Research on Cancer, WHO, Lyon, pp. 149–262.

Kolstad, H. A., Lynge, E., Olsen, J. and Breum, N. (1995). Incidence of lymphohematopoietic malignancies among styrene-exposed workers of the reinforced plastics industry. *Scand. J. Work Environ. Health*, **20**, 272–278.

Kromhout, H. and Heedereick, D. (1995). Occupational epidemiology in the rubber industry: implications of exposure variability. *Am. J. Ind. Med.*, **27**, 171–185.

Kromhout, H., Swuste, P. and Boleij, J. S. (1994). Empirical modeling of chemical exposure in the rubber manufacturing industry. *Ann. Occup. Hyg.*, **38**, 3–22.

Landrigan, P. J. (1990). Critical assessment of epidemiologic studies on the human carcinogenicity of 1,3-butadiene. *Environ. Health Perspect.*, **86**, 143–148.

Linch, A. L., O'Connor, G. B., Barnes, J. R., Killian, A. S. and Neeld, W. E. (1971). Methylene-bis-*ortho*-chloroaniline (MOCA): evaluation of hazards and exposure control. *Am. Ind. Hyg. Assoc. J.*, **32**, 802–819.

Lindbohm, M. L. (1993). Effects of styrene on the reproductive health of women: a review. In Sorsa, M., Peltonen, K., Vainio, H. and Hemminki, K. (Eds), *IARC Scientific Publications, No. 127. Butadiene and Styrene: Assessment of Health Hazards*. International Agency for Research on Cancer, WHO, Lyon, pp. 163–169.

Liss, G. M. and Guirguis, S. S. (1994). Follow-up of a group of workers intoxicated with 4,4′-methylenedinailine. *Am. J. Ind. Med.*, **26**, 117–124.

LoPachin, R. M. and Lehning, E. J. (1994). Acrylamide-induced distal axon degeneration: a proposed mechanism of action. *Neurotoxicology*, **14**, 247–260.

Lundberg, I., Gustavsson, A., Holmberg, B., Molina, G. and Westerholm, P. (1993). Mortality and cancer incidence among PVC-processing workers in Sweden. *Am. J. Ind. Med.*, **23**, 313–319.

Malkinson, A. M., Koski, K. M., Evans, W. A. and Festing, M. F. (1997). Butylated hydroxytoluene exposure is necessary to induce lung tumors in BALB mice treated with 3-methylcholanthrene. *Cancer Res.*, **57**, 2832–2834.

Maltoni, C. (1975). The value of predictive experimental bioassay in occupational and environmental carcinogenesis. *Ambio*, **4**, 18–23.

Maltoni, C. and Lefemine, G. (1975). Carcinogenicity bioassays of vinyl chloride: current results. *Ann. N. Y. Acad. Sci.*, **246**, 195–218.

Maltoni, C., Lefemine, G., Ciliberti, A., Cotti, G. and Carretti, D. (1984a). Experimental research of vinyl chloride carcinogenesis. In Maltoni, C. and Mehlman, M. (Eds), *Archives of Research on Industrial Carcinogenesis*, Vol **2**. Princeton Scientific Publishing, Princeton, NJ.

Maltoni, C., Clini, C., Vicini, F. and Masina, A. (1984b). Two cases of liver angiosarcoma among polyvinyl chloride extruders of an Italian factory producing PVC bags and other containers. *Am. J. Ind. Med.*, **5**, 297–302.

Martinmaa, J. M. (1984a). Synthetic polymers, main classes of plastics and their current uses. *Prog. Clin. Biol. Res.*, **141**, 3–10.

Martinmaa, J. M. (1984b). Production and manufacture of epoxy thermosets. *Prog. Clin. Biol. Res.*, **141**, 365–372.

McMichael, A. J., Gerber, W. S., Gamble, F. F. and Lednar, W. M. (1976). Chronic respiratory symptoms and job type within the rubber industry. *J. Occup. Med.*, **18**, 611–617.

McQueen, C. A., and Williams, G. M. (1990). Review of the genoxocity and carcinogenicity of 4, 4′-methylene-dianiline and 4,4′-methylene-bis-2-chloroaniline. *Mutat. Res.*, **239**, 133–142.

Melnick, R. L., Huff, J. E., Roycroft, J. H., Chou, B. J. and Miller, R. A. (1990). Inhalation toxicology and carcinogenicity of 1,3-butadiene in B6C3F1 mice following 65 weeks of exposure. *Environ. Health Perspect.*, **86**, 27–36.

Melnick, R. L., Shackelford, C. C. and Huff, J. (1993). Carcinogenicity of 1,3-butadiene. *Environ. Health Perspect.*, **100**, 227–236.

Molina, G., Holmberg, B., Elofsson, S., Holmlund, L., Maasing, R. and Westerholm, P. (1981). Mortality and cancer rates among workers in the Swedish PVC processing industry. *Environ. Health Perspect.*, **41**, 145–151.

Nebbia, C. and Fink-Gremmels, J. (1996). Acute effects of low doses of zineb and ethylenethiourea on thyroid function in the male rat. *Bull. Environ. Contam. Toxicol.*, **56**, 847–852.

Newton, P. E., Bolte, H. F., Daly, I. W., Pillsbury, B. D., Terrill, J. B., Drew, R. T., Ben-Dyke, R., Sheldon, A. W. and Rubin, L. F. (1994). Subchronic and chronic inhalation toxicity of antimony trioxide in the rat. *Fundam. Appl. Toxicol.*, **22**, 561–576.

Nicholson, W. J. (1992). Nitrosoamines. In Rom, W. N. (Ed.), *Environmental and Occupational Medicine*. Little, Brown, Boston, pp. 955–965.

Nicholson, W. J., Henneberger, P. K. and Seidman, H. (1984). Occupational hazards in the VC–PVC production industry. *Prog. Clin. Biol. Res.*, **141**, 155–175.

Nielsen, J., Bensryd, I., Alquist, H., Welinder, H., Alexandersson, R. and Skerfving, S. (1991). Serum Ig and lung function in workers exposed to phthalic anhydride. *Int. Arch. Occup. Environ. Health*, **63**, 199–204.

Noweir, M. H., El-Dakhakhny, A. A. and Osman, H. A. (1972). Exposure to chemical agents in rubber industry. *J. Egypt. Publ. Health Assoc.*, **47**, 182–201.

Nutt, A. R. (1984). *Toxic Hazards of Rubber Chemicals*. Elsevier, London.

Oishi, S. (1993). Strain differences in susceptibility to di-2-ethylhexyl phthalate induced testicular atrophy in mice. *Toxicol. Lett.*, **66**, 47–52.

Osterberg, R. E., Bierbower, G. W. and Hehir, R. M. (1977). Renal and testicular damage following dermal application of the flame retardant tris(2,3-dibromopropyl) phosphate. *J. Toxicol. Environ. Health*, **3**, 979–987.

Ott, M. G. (1990). Assessment of 1,3-butadiene epidemiology studies. *Environ. Health Perspect.*, **86**, 135–141.

Owen, P. E. and Gleister, J. R. (1990). Inhalation toxicity and carcinogenicity of 1,3-butadiene in Sprague–Dawley rats. *Environ. Health Perspect.*, **86**, 19–25.

Pahwa, R. and Kalra, J. (1993). A critical review of the neurotoxicity of styrene in humans. *Vet. Hum. Toxicol.*, **35**, 516–520.

Parkes, H. G., Veys, C. A., Waterhouse, J. A. H. and Peters, A. (1982). Cancer mortality in the British rubber industry. *Br. J. Ind. Med.*, **39**, 209–220.

Parmar, D., Srivastava, S. P., Singh, G. B. and Seth, P. K. (1995). Testicular toxicity of di(2-ethylhexyl) phthalate in developing rats. *Vet. Hum. Toxicol.*, **37**, 310–313.

Rannug, A., Rannug, U. and Ramel, C. (1984). Genotoxic effects of additives in synthetic elastomers with special consideration to the mechanism of action of thiurames and dithiocarbamates. *Prog. Clin. Biol. Res.*, **141**, 407–419.

Rao, M. S. and Reddy, J. K. (1991). An overview of peroxisome-induced hepatocarcinogenesis. *Environ. Health Perspect.*, **93**, 205–209.

Reh, B. D. and Fajen, J. M. (1996). Worker exposure to nitrosamines in a rubber vehicle sealing plant. *Am. Ind. Hyg. Assoc.*, **57**, 918–923.

Rogaczewska, T. and Ligocka, D. (1994). Occupational exposure to coal tar pitch volatiles, benzo(a)pyrene and dust in tyre production. *Int. J. Occup. Med. Environ. Health*, **7**, 379–386.

Rogaczewska, T. and Wroblewska-Jakubowska, K. (1996). Occupational exposure to N-nitrosamines in the production of automobile tyres. *Med. Pract.*, **47**, 569–576.

Rosenberg, C. (1984). Production and uses of polyurethanes (including thermodegradation). *Prog. Clin. Biol. Res.*, **141**, 337–346.

Rothman, K. J. (1994). Cancer occurrence among workers exposed to acrylonitrile. *Scand. J. Work Environ. Health*, **20**, 313–321.

Saillenfait, A. M., Sabate, J. P., and Langonne, J. (1991). Difference in the developmental toxocity of ethylenethiourea and three N,N-substituted thiourea derivatives in rats. *Fundam. Appl. Toxicol.*, **17**, 399–408.

Sale, S. R., Roach, D. E., Zeiss, C. R. and Patterson, R. (1981). Clinical and immunologic correlations in trimellitic anhydride airway syndromes. *J. Allergy Clin. Immunol.*, **68**, 188–193.

Sanchez-Ocampo, A., Torres-Perez, J. and Jimenez Reyes, M. (1996). Selenium levels in the serum of workers at a rubber tire repair shop. *Am. Ind. Hyg. Assoc. J.*, **57**, 72–75.

Sasadiek, M. (1993). Sister-chromatid exchanges and cell cycle kinetics in the lymphocytes of workers occupationally exposed to a chemical mixture in the tyre industry. *Mutat. Res.*, **302**, 197–200.

Schrauzer, G. N. (1992). Selenium. Mechanistic aspects of anticarcinogenic action. *Biol. Trace Elem. Res.*, **33**, 51–62.

Selikoff, I. J. and Hammond, E. J. (1975). Toxicity of vinyl chloride–polyvinyl chloride. *Ann. N. Y. Acad. Sci.*, **246**, 1–337.

Shukla, Y., Baqar, S. M. and Mehrotra, N. K. (1996). Carcinogenic and cocarcinogenic studies of thiram in mouse skin. *Food Chem. Toxicol.*, **34**, 283–289.

Siddiqui, A. and Sristava, S. P. (1992). Effect of di(2-ethylhexyl) phthalate administration on rat sperm count and sperm metabolic enzymes. *Bull. Environ. Contam. Toxicol.*, **48**, 115–119.

Simonato, L., Abbé, K., Andersen, A., Comba, P., Engholm, G., Ferro, G., Hagmar, L., Langård, S., Lundberg, I., Pirastu, R., Thomas, P., Winkelmann, R. and Saracci, R. (1991). A collaborative study of cancer incidence and mortality among vinyl chloride workers. *Scand. J. Work Environ. Health*, **17**, 59–69.

Slaga, T. J., Klein-Szanto, A. J. P., Triplett, L. L. and Yotti, L. P. (1981). Skin tumor-promoting activity of benzoyl peroxide, a widely used free radical-generating compound. *Science*, **213**, 1023–1025.

Slovak, A. J. M. (1984). Occupational hazards of polyethylene and polypropylene processing. *Prog. Clin. Biol. Res.*, **141**, 313–318.

Sorsa, M., Falck, K. and Vainio, H. (1982a). Detection of worker exposure to mutagens in the rubber industry by use of the urinary mutagenicity assay. In Sugimura, T., Kondo, S. and Takebe, H. (Eds), *Environmental Mutagens and Carcinogens*. University of Tokyo Press, Tokyo, pp. 321–329.

Sorsa, M., Mäki-Paakkanen, J. and Vainio, H. (1982b). Identification of mutagen exposure in the rubber industry by sister chromatid exchange method. *Cytogenet. Cell Genet.*, **33**, 68–73.

Sorsa, M., Falck, K., Mäki-Paakkanen, J. and Vainio, H. (1983). Genotoxic hazards in the rubber industry. *Scand. J. Work Environ. Health*, **9**, 103–107.

Sorsa, M., Peltonen, K., Vainio, H. and Hemminki, K. (Eds) (1993). *IARC Scientific Publications, No. 127. Butadiene and Styrene: Assessment of Health Hazards*. International Agency for Research on Cancer, WHO, Lyon.

Spiegelhalder, B. and Preussmann, R. (1982). Nitrosamines and rubber. In Bartsch, H., O'Neill, I. K., Castegnaro, M. and Okada, M. (Eds.), *IARC Scientific Publications, No. 41. N-Nitroso Compounds: Occurrence and Biological Effects*. International Agency for Research on Cancer, WHO, Lyon, pp. 231–243.

Spoo, J. W., Rogers, R.-A. and Monteiro-Riviere, N. A. (1992). Effects of formaldehyde, DMSO, benzoyl peroxide and laurylsulfate on isolated perfused porcine skin. *In Vitro Toxicol.*, **5**, 251–260.

Storetvedt Heldaas, S., Langard, S. L. and Andersen, A. (1984). Incidence of cancer among vinyl chloride and polyvinyl chloride workers. *Br. J. Ind. Med.*, **41**, 25–30.

Sullivan, J. B., Van Ert, M. and Lewis, R. (1992). Chemical hazards in the tire and rubber industry. In Sullivan, J. B. and Krieger, G. R. (Eds), *Hazardous Materials Toxicology, Clinical Principles of Environmental Health*. Williams and Wilkins, Baltimore, pp. 516–532.

Taalman, R. D. (1996). Isoprene: background and issues. *Toxicology*, **113**, 242–246.

Tagesson, C., Chabiuk, D., Axelson, O., Baranski, B., Palus, J. and Wyszynska, K. (1993). Increased urinary excretion of the oxidative adduct 8-hydroxydeoxyguanosine as a possible early indicator of occupational cancer hazards in the asbestos, rubber, and azo-dye industry. *Pol. J. Occup. Med. Environ. Health*, **6**, 357–368.

Taylor, A. J. N. (1992). Acid anhydrides. *Clin. Exp. Allergy*, **21**, Suppl. 1, 234–240.

Thomas, J. A. and Thomas, M. J. (1992). Biological effects of di-(2-ethylhexyl) phthalate and other phthalic acid esters. *Crit. Rev. Toxicol.*, **13**, 283–317.

Thompson, J. A., Bolton, J. L. and Malkinson, A. M. (1991). Relationship between the metabolism of butylated hydroxy-toluene (BHT) and lung tumor promotion in mice. *Exp. Lung Res.*, **17**, 439–453.

Vandenplas, O., Carter, A., Ghezzo, H., Cloutier, Y. and Malo, J.-L. (1993). Response to isocyanates: effect of concentration, duration of exposure, and dose. *Am. Rev. Respir. Dis.*, **147**, 1287–1290.

Viola, P. L., Bigotti, A. and Caputo, A. (1971). Oncogenic response of rat skin, lungs and bones to vinyl chloride. *Cancer Res.*, **31**, 516–522.

Wacker, C.-D., Spiegelhalder, B. and Preusmann, R. (1991). New sulfenamide accelerators derived from safe amines for the rubber and tyre industry. In O'Neill, I. K., Chen, J. and Bartsch, H. (Eds), *IARC Scientific Publications, No. 105, Relevance to Human Cancer of N-Nitroso Compounds, Tobacco Smoke and Mycotoxins*. International Agency for Research on Cancer, WHO, Lyon, pp. 592–594.

Weeks, J. L., Peters, J. M. and Monson, R. R., (1981). Screening for occupational health hazards in the rubber industry. Part II; Health hazards in the curing department. *Am. J. Ind. Med.*, **2**, 143–151.

Wegman, D. H., Pagnotto, L. D., Fine, L. J. and Peters, J. M. (1974). A dose response relationship in TDI workers. *J. Occup. Med.*, **16**, 258–260.

WHO (1992). *Environmental Health Criteria, Vol. 131. Diethyl hexyl phthalate*. World Health Organization, Geneva, pp. 1–142.

WHO (1995). *Environmental Health Criteria, Vol. 173. Tris (2,3-dibromopropyl) Phosphate and Bis(2,3-dibromopropyl) Phosphate*. World Health Organization, Geneva, pp. 1–129.

Williams, G. M. and Iatropoulos, M. J. (1996). Inhibition of the hepatocarcinogenicity of aflatoxin B1 in rats by low levels of the phenolic antioxidants butylated hydroxyanisols and butylated hydroxytoluene. *Cancer Lett.*, **104**, 49–53.

Wine, R. N., Li, L.-H., Hommel Barnes, L., Gulati, D. K. and Chapin, R. E. (1997). Reproductive toxicity of di-n-butyl phthalate in a continuous breeding protocol in Sprague–Dawley rats. *Environ. Health Perspect.*, **105**, 102–107.

Woodward, K. N. (1990). Phthalate esters. Cystic kidney disease in animals and possible effects on human health: a review. *Hum. Exp. Toxicol.*, **9**, 397–401.

Yeowell-O'Connell, K., Jin, Z. and Rappaport, S. M. (1996). Determination of albumin and hemoglobin adducts of workers exposed to styrene and styrene oxide. *Cancer Epidemiol.*, **5**, 205–215.

Zeiss, C. R., Wolkonsky, P., Chacon R., Tuntland, P. A., Levitz, D., Prunzansky, J. J. and Patterson, R. (1983). Syndromes in workers exposed to trimellitic anhydride—a longitudinal clinical and immunologic study. *Ann. Intern. Med.*, **98**, 8–12.

Chapter 96
Organic Solvents

Hanna Tähti, Lisbeth Aasmoe and Tore Syversen

CONTENTS

GENERAL PRINCIPLES

Organic solvents are a group of organic compounds with low molecular weight. They share properties such as lipophilicity and volatility, although some of them are also hydrophilic or less volatile. The vapour pressure of organic solvents at room temperature is usually high enough for them to represent an inhalation hazard. Organic solvents have been used in large and increasing quantities during the last 50 years in a variety of industrial settings (see, e.g., Chapter 87 on biological indicators in the occupational environment and Chapter 95 on chemicals used in the plastics and rubber industry). A wide variety of organic solvents are also used in consumer products.

Exposure

In general, inhalation and skin absorption represent the most significant routes of exposure to organic solvents. The uptake of vapour by inhalation is a simple physical process; the molecules diffuse from the alveolar space into the blood, where they dissolve. The solvent molecules partition between two media: between air and blood during the absorptive phase, and between blood and other tissues during the distribution phase. The more soluble a vapour is in the blood, the more of it will be absorbed into the blood during each respiratory cycle. The amount of vapour taken up by various tissues depends on the affinity of the organic solvent for each tissue. Thus, the rate of the absorption of organic solvents in the lungs and their distribution to various tissues are variable and depend on the blood–gas and fat–blood partition coefficients, respectively (Fiserova-Bergerova, 1985; Sato and Nakajima, 1987). Hydropho-

bic solvents have relatively small blood–gas partition coefficients and their fat–blood partition coefficients are much larger than unity. Hydrophilic solvents have blood–gas partition coefficients larger than 200 and fat–blood partition coefficients much smaller than unity (Fiserova-Bergerova, 1985). Differences in the uptake and distribution of various organic solvents have been shown to be, predominantly, a result of differences in their solubilities.

It is well known that physical activity during exposure may influence the uptake of an inhaled solvent. The pulmonary uptake of many organic solvents in working individuals is much larger than that in resting individuals, provided that the diffusion of the solvent from the alveolar space into the blood is not rate-limiting (Åstrand, 1983; Fiserova-Bergerova, 1985).

Intentional inhalation of volatile organic compounds is well known (Giovacchini, 1985; Flanagan and Ives, 1994). The abuse of a volatile substance (glue sniffing, inhalant abuse, solvent abuse) has been reported from most parts of the world. Small doses can lead to euphoria, delusions and hallucinations. Higher doses may produce life-threatening effects such as convulsions and coma. Death may ensue indirectly, e.g. after aspiration of vomit or from direct cardiac or CNS toxicity. Chronic abuse of toluene- containing products and of chlorinated solvents such as 1,1,1-trichloroethane can produce severe organ damage, especially in the liver, kidneys and brain. Prolonged use may be fatal.

Percutaneous absorption of solvents is generally considered to be of minor importance compared with pulmonary uptake. However, several solvents can be absorbed through the skin, depending on their physical and chemical properties (Nakaaki et al., 1980; Kezic et al., 1997; Brooke et al., 1998). The degree of uptake also depends upon exposure conditions, being proportional to time and the amount of skin surface exposed. Hydrophobic solvents of low molecular weight permeate the skin better than those of high molecular weight or hydrophilic solvents. Solvents that damage the skin will affect the skin integrity and this may enhance the percutaneous absorption of the agent. The glycol ethers 2-methoxyethanol and 2-ethoxyethanol are readily absorbed through the skin, and skin contact of both forearms and hands for 15 min may cause a body uptake exceeding the uptake by inhalation for 8 h that at the occupational exposure limit value (Kezic et al., 1997).

The multiplicity of hydrocarbon structures suggests that the number of molecules that can be constructed from the combination of carbon and hydrogen with oxygen, halogens, nitrogen, etc., is virtually limitless. However, organic compounds can be grouped into a few classes. There are several functional groups of frequent occurrence: alkenes, alcohols, aldehydes, ketones, acids, ethers, halogens and esters. Organic solvents are classified according to these functional groups, and this classification makes it easier to predict and understand the toxic effects caused by the solvents.

Toxic Effects of Organic Solvents

The common effects of most solvents include anaesthetic effects on the CNS and irritation of mucous membranes and tissues. These are the dominant signs of short-term exposure at a high concentration. Distinct from general effects are the specific toxic effects of solvents. They are often related to the metabolism of the solvent. Although normally associated with detoxification, metabolism can sometimes result in the formation of reactive metabolites that may cause cellular damage. The specific toxic effects are often not caused by the parent compound, but rather by the metabolites created by this metabolic activation.

Effects on the Nervous System

CNS-depressant Activity
It has been well established that organic solvents when inhaled at high concentrations show suppressive effects on the CNS. The effect is related to the brain concentration of the solvent (Papper and Kitz, 1963; Lowe, 1972; Eger, 1974; Tichy, 1983). There is no simple relation between the partition coefficient and the chemical structure or molecular weight which could help us to predict uptake or effects of the solvent in the nervous system (Sato and Nakajima, 1987). The length of the narcosis induced by organic solvents correlates well with their octanol–water partition coefficients (Wasserkort and Koller, 1997). A linear relationship between the 50% effective dose (ED_{50}) and the olive oil–water partition coefficients for 20 different narcotics have been reported (Miller et al., 1972). As a broad generalization, the CNS-

depressant activity of an organic compound correlates with its lipid solubility.

Aliphatic, alicyclic and aromatic hydrocarbons have in common the ability to interact with biological membranes (Engelke et al., 1996). This interaction has been thought to cause changes in neural membranes, which then cause the CNS-depressant effect. According to the 'lipid theory', the anaesthetic potency of inhalation anaesthetics and the CNS-depressant effects of organic solvents are related to their lipophilicity and to their effects on the lipid bilayer (Seeman, 1972). Organic solvents readily pass the blood–brain barrier and distribute into the lipid membranes of the neural cells, where they can affect neural membrane target proteins (Franks and Lieb, 1978; Korpela and Tähti, 1988; Edelfors and Ravn-Jonsen, 1992; Tähti et al., 1992; Naskali et al., 1993). The CNS-depressant effect is greatly enhanced by halogenation and to a lesser extent by alcoholic functional groups (James, 1985; Sato and Nakajima, 1987). For years it has been emphasized that many organic solvents have effects similar to anaesthetics, and indeed for good reasons, since several halogenated solvents are the systemic anaesthetic agents of choice in surgery. Trichloroethylene, diethyl ether and chloroform have been used for clinical anaesthesia. Today, halogenated solvents such as sevoflurane, isoflurane and halothane are commonly used as anaesthetics.

Neurotoxic Effects
Adverse effects may be found at various sites in the CNS and the peripheral nervous system (PNS). Prolonged exposure to aromatic hydrocarbons can cause permanent damage to the CNS (Hein et al., 1990), while long-term exposure to n-hexane is associated with the development of peripheral neuropathy (Bachmann et al., 1993). It has been proposed that repeated acute exposures to low levels of organic solvents can cause permanent damage in the CNS. It is therefore important to clarify the mechanisms of solvent neurotoxicity and to find appropriate and sensitive methods for detecting even subtle signs of deleterious effects.

The mechanisms of the CNS toxicity of solvents are not known. Generally it has not been possible to identify specific sites of toxic effects in the CNS. Chronic heavy exposures to, e.g., toluene cause multifocal disorders including cerebral, cerebellar and brain stem atrophy (Ikeda and Tsukagoshi, 1990). At low occupational exposure levels, organic solvents can cause many different symptoms of CNS origin: fatigue, anxiety, irritability, headache, weakness, depression, neurobehavioural changes and impairment of cognitive performance (Milanovic et al., 1990; Evans and Balster, 1991; Hakkola, 1994; Kishi et al., 1995). Also, temporal epileptic seizures have been found as a result of occupational exposure to solvents (Jacobsen et al., 1994). The molecular mechanisms underlying these diverse actions are unknown. Repeated acute exposures to low levels of organic solvents can, if they last for several years, cause permanent changes in the CNS. Occupational exposure to organic solvents for a period of 5 years or more have been shown to increase the risk of persistent memory difficulties and to decrease the ability to concentrate (Hein *et al.*, 1990).

Solvents with an aromatic structure are believed to localize in hydrophobic pockets in the membrane protein or simply to be concentrated at the protein–lipid interface, whereas *n*-hexane molecules are localized at the bilayer midplane without causing any change in membrane fluidity or enzyme activity (Engelke *et al.*, 1992). The accumulation of organic solvents in neural cell membranes produces bilayer disorder (Engelke *et al.*, 1992, 1996). The disorder in the phospholipid bilayer can indirectly affect the function of membrane enzymes (Edelfors and Ravn-Jonsen, 1992; Engelke *et al.*, 1992). The physical/chemical activity relationship has been found important for the effects of organic solvents on synaptosomal membrane Na^+/K^+-ATPase activity and membrane fluidity (Naskali *et al.*, 1993; Tanii *et al.*, 1994). They reported that partitioning of solvents into the lipid bilayer changes the membrane fluidity and leads to the inhibition of membrane-bound enzymes.

The mechanism of PNS toxicity caused by *n*-hexane is related to its metabolite hexane-2,5-dione **(Figure 1)**, which causes peripheral neuropathy (Ruff *et al.*, 1981). This metabolite causes neurofilament-filled swellings of the distal axons **(Figure 2)**. The neurotoxicity of methyl *n*-butyl ketone (MBK) is caused by the same toxic metabolite, 2,5-hexanedione. MBK is roughly 12 times more toxic in the PNS than *n*-hexane. In MBK neuropathy, swellings have also been found in the cerebellar white matter of the CNS and in the distal optic nerve, causing spastic gait and impairments of vision and memory respectively (Bos *et al.*, 1991). The long ascending and descending tracts of the spinal cord are also particularly vulnerable. Carbon disulphide causes similar axonal damage to that produced by the metabolite of *n*-hexane. The accumulation of neurofilaments has been shown to be the result of protein cross-linking of cytoskeletal components in the axon matrix (Graham *et al.*, 1995). The PNS seems to be the most sensitive target for *n*-hexane, whereas aromatic hydrocarbons (e.g. toluene) mainly cause CNS toxicity. Long-term *n*-hexane exposure in rats causes significant changes in the PNS but fails to reveal any significant changes in the CNS as measured by specific marker proteins (neuron-specific enolase, creatine kinase-B and beta-S100). In the CNS these marker proteins fail to reveal any significant changes after long-term *n*-hexane exposure, whereas chronic exposure of rats to toluene causes significant changes in these parameters in the CNS (Huang *et al.*, 1992, 1993).

Occupational exposures to low levels of organic solvents for several years have caused various CNS effects, such as impairment of short-term memory and changes in personality (Mikkelsen, 1997). Long-term

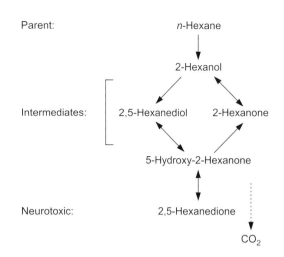

Figure 1 Biotransformation of *n*-hexane. Formation of the neurotoxic metabolite hexane-2,5-dione

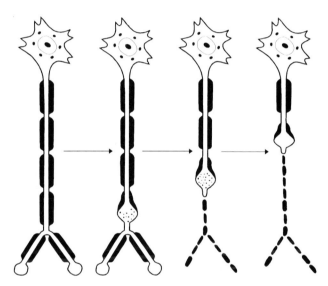

Figure 2 Mechanism of *n*-hexane-induced peripheral neurotoxicity. The axonal swellings are caused by the metabolite 2,5-hexanedione. Because of the axonal swelling there is no transport from the neuronal cell body to the peripheral part behind the swelling, and this part degenerates

occupational exposure to solvents may cause a neurotoxic syndrome commonly known as chronic toxic encephalopathy. Symptoms related to chronic toxic encephalopathy are impairment of memory and learning skills, increased irritability, tiredness, sleeping problems and changes in personality (Ng *et al.*, 1990; Mikkelsen, 1997). Epidemiological studies on occupational solvent exposures have shown impairment in short-term memory and in psychomotor function (Baker, 1994). In cross-sectional studies, differences between exposed and unexposed workers have been most commonly seen in performance tests of memory function and particularly in short-term memory ability (Moen *et al.*, 1990; Bleecker *et al.*, 1991; Hänninen *et al.*, 1991). The performance in associate learning tasks and in memory span has especially been reduced in solvent-exposed workers. In most epidemiological studies, a dose–response relationship has also been demonstrated. In heavily exposed workers the neurobehavioural deficits are similar to those seen in persons with pronounced neurobehavioural dysfunction due to solvent abuse (Baker, 1994). Follow-up studies have shown that after removal from solvent exposure, persistent deficits can be observed in persons with severe initial impairment (Gregersen, 1988; Edling et al., 1990).

In electrophysiological studies on solvent-exposed workers, some changes in electroencephalography consistent with diffuse cortical dysfunction have been found (Orbaek et al., 1988). Impairments in posture control mechanisms (Niklasson et al., 1997), colour vision (Mergler and Blain, 1987) and olfactory functions (Schwarz et al., 1990) have also been associated with the neurotoxic syndrome caused by chronic exposure to organic solvents.

Irritation of Mucous Membranes and Tissues

Irritation is a physiological response to chemical or physical stimuli. Depending on dose, most organic molecules have some irritant properties such as stinging, irritation, burning, prickling, freshness or tingling (Cometto-Muniz and Cain, 1992). Irritation may damage the skin, lungs or eyes. If certain functional groups are added to an organic molecule, the irritant properties of the chemical will increase. Examples are amines and acids which will add corrosive properties to the molecule. Aldehydes and ketones can produce narcosis, but this effect is usually prevented because the vapours are irritating to the eyes and respiratory tract at low concentrations (James, 1985). It has been shown that the irritation thresholds decrease logarithmically with carbon chain length for a homologous series of ketones, secondary and tertiary alcohols, acetates, aldehydes and alkylbenzenes (Cometto-Muniz and Cain, 1991, 1994; Cometto-Muniz et al., 1998). Eye irritation thresholds and nasal pungency thresholds were well below the odour threshold (Cometto-Muniz and Cain, 1995). However, irrespective of molecular size or chemical functional group, threshold of nasal pungency is achieved at a fairly constant percentage of vapour saturation, which implies an important role for a physical rather than chemical interaction with nasal mucosa (Cometto-Muniz and Cain, 1993). Thus, irritation of mucous membranes is probably related to the size of the organic molecule, rather than the structure of the molecule.

Metabolism

The metabolism of solvents can be divided into two parts, phase I and phase II. Phase I is characterized by oxidation, reduction and hydrolysis while phase II reactions involve conjugation. The products of phase I

reactions are often more reactive and toxic than the parent compound, while phase II reactions are usually true detoxification reactions. Metabolizing enzymes are widely distributed throughout the body, although the liver is the major metabolic organ. Several solvents are hepatotoxic owing to their activation to toxic intermediates or metabolites in the liver (Sipes and Gandolfi, 1982). Many of the haloalkanes and haloalkenes appear to have similar toxic effects in liver and kidney (Dekant et al., 1989; Kitchin and Brown, 1989). The hepatotoxic and carcinogenic effects of haloalkanes and haloalkenes are generally thought to be due to reactive metabolites rather than the parent molecule. Free radical intermediates are involved in the toxicity through mechanisms including lipid peroxidation, covalent binding and cofactor depletion (Cheeseman et al., 1985).

Metabolism of ethylene glycol is a key factor in understanding the specific toxic effects caused by this solvent. It is metabolized by alcohol dehydrogenase to glycolaldehyde and further to glycolic acid. Glycolic acid is oxidized to oxalic acid by glycolic acid oxidase (Gessner et al., 1960; von Wartburg et al., 1964; Liao and Richardson, 1973). The oxalate formation may cause acute renal tubular necrosis through the formation of insoluble oxalate crystals in the kidney (Gabow et al., 1986; Turk et al., 1986). The lethal dose of ethylene glycol is reported to be approximately 100 ml in an adult. Alcohol dehydrogenase catalyses oxidation of ethanol, and ethanol can be used as a antidote in ethylene glycol intoxication as it will prevent the production of oxalic acid (Jacobsen and McMartin, 1986). Specific toxic effects of several other solvents, e.g. benzene, styrene, n-hexane, glycol ethers and methanol, are also due to the production of toxic metabolites, and are discussed elsewhere in this chapter.

Enzyme Induction

A number of solvents may induce xenobiotic metabolizing enzymes, e.g. CYP2E1 (Conney, 1968; Nebert et al., 1978). This enzyme catalyses the metabolism of a large number of solvents including ethanol. As a socially accepted toxin, ethanol is consumed in large quantities compared with other solvents. Ethanol is known to inhibit drug metabolism acutely, and to stimulate xenobiotic metabolism through enzyme induction when administered repeatedly. Thus the effects of ethanol on the metabolism of other solvents are complex, depending on the timing and frequency of ethanol intake. It has been shown that chronic ethanol administration induces CYP2E1. Thus, in regular drinkers, elimination of solvent metabolites appears to be faster compared with nondrinkers, presumably caused by enzyme induction (Cherry, 1993). In addition to a faster elimination of solvents, chronic ethanol intake may lead to a faster and more pronounced formation of metabolites, and therefore increased risk of adverse effects due to the production of toxic metabolites. It has been shown that alcoholics have an increased susceptibility to solvents such as carbon tetrachloride and benzene (Morimoto et al., 1993; Ronis et al., 1996; Lindros, 1997). During fire extinguishing, seven workers were exposed to high concentrations of carbon tetrachloride. However, only two workers with a high ethanol intake developed hepatotoxicity and nephrotoxicity (Manno et al., 1996).

It has been shown that even a single dose of benzene, toluene or m-xylene may induce the activity of CYP2E1 significantly, and thereby enhance metabolism of other solvents (Kim and Kim, 1996). Methyl ethyl ketone pretreatment induced rat liver cytochrome P450 and increased the formation of the toxic metabolite hexane-2,5-dione in rat liver (Mortensen et al., 1998). Exposure to small aromatic hydrocarbons indicates that the addition of methyl groups to the aromatic ring affects the inductive capacity of different CYP isoenzymes (Pathiratne et al., 1986; Backes et al., 1993; Gut et al., 1993; Yuan et al., 1995; Wang et al., 1996). Sex differences in enzyme induction have been observed. Ethylbenzene treatment induced CYP2B1 and CYP2B2 to a greater extent in male than in female rats, and CYP2E1 only in female rats (Sequeira et al., 1992). Several studies indicated no induction of hepatic alcohol dehydrogenase following treatment with ethanol (Gillion et al., 1985; Guthrie et al., 1990; Singh and Pandey, 1991; Aasmoe and Aarbakke, 1999). The glycol ethers 2-methoxyethanol and 2-ethoxyethanol induced liver alcohol dehydrogenase in male rats only while no induction was observed in female rats (Aasmoe and Aarbakke, 1999).

However, induction is not always reflected in increased in vivo metabolism. If the hepatic blood flow rather that the enzyme activity rate-limits the metabolism of a solvent, enzyme induction may not affect the kinetics of the solvent. Thus, the blood flow limits the extent of solvent metabolism, and enzyme induction has little effect on metabolism when exposure concentration is low. Metabolism of, e.g., trichloroethylene and xylene is rate-limited by hepatic blood flow. In humans, enzyme induction resulted in increased metabolism of trichloroethylene only at high exposure concentration (Sato, 1993). Ethanol consumption increased the metabolism of xylene about five-fold in rats only at high exposure concentrations (Kaneko et al., 1993).

Solvent Mixtures

A thorough review on the toxicology of exposure to mixtures is given in Chapter 14 (Toxicology of Chemical Mixtures).

CNS Effects

Cross-sectional epidemiological studies have supported the hypothesis that occupational low-level, long-term exposure to solvent mixtures may cause adverse CNS effects (Tähti, 1984; Triebig et al., 1992; Hakkola, 1994; Hogstedt, 1994). They have demonstrated significant dose–response relations between exposure, mental symptoms and neurobehavioural performance. Occupational solvent exposure may be the cause of mental and cognitive impairment that can become chronic. In complex exposures, the adverse CNS effects seem to occur at exposure levels well below the accepted threshold limit values (Mikkelsen, 1997).

Metabolic Interactions

Organic solvents are more commonly used as mixtures than as individual chemicals. The mixtures mostly include a wide variety of compounds, such as alcohols, ketones, and aliphatic and aromatic hydrocarbons. Thus the metabolism, and hence the toxicity, of one solvent may be modified by other solvents.

The effect of ethanol on metabolism of organic solvents has been shown to be complex (Sato et al., 1981). In high concentrations ethanol may act like an inhibitor. Concurrent exposure to alcohol and solvents may reduce the clearance of other solvents and the result is prolonged internal dose of the solvent (Cherry, 1993). However, an acute dose of ethanol increased the metabolism of toluene and trichloroethylene in rat liver, and ethanol may enhance the hepatic metabolism of these solvents (Sato et al., 1981). Ethanol has impaired the metabolic clearance of m-xylene, causing raised xylene blood concentration and decreased excretion of methylhippuric acid (Riihimäki et al., 1982). Some people appear to be more susceptible to combined ethanol–xylene exposure and may develop nausea and dermal flush (Riihimäki et al., 1982).

Co-exposure to hexane and toluene decreased hexane neurotoxicity and urinary excretion of hexane metabolites in rats (Takeuchi et al., 1993). Methyl ethyl ketone inhibited the in vitro metabolism of n-hexane in a noncompetitive pattern, and decreased the levels of the toxic metabolite hexane-2,5-dione (Mortensen et al., 1998). Concomitant treatment of rats with a non-hepatotoxic dose of dichloromethane potentiated the hepatotoxicity of carbon tetrachloride (Kim, 1997). Several investigators have demonstrated that co-administration of toluene with benzene protects animals from benzene-induced haematotoxicity (Ikeda et al., 1972; Andrews et al., 1977; Sato and Nakajima, 1979; Tunek et al., 1982). However, such interactions are exhibited only at high concentrations.

Several kinetic studies have been conducted with volunteers and demonstrated similar metabolic interactions in humans (Engström et al., 1984; Wallen et al., 1985; Liira et al., 1988). In male workers exposed to benzene and toluene, the metabolism of both solvents was depressed, indicating a mutual suppression of metabolism between benzene and toluene (Inoue et al., 1988). Co-exposure to xylene (100 ppm) and methyl ethyl ketone (200 ppm) in humans resulted in reduced xylene metabolism (Liira *et al.*, 1988). However, the combined exposure did not cause any change in methyl ethyl ketone metabolism. In humans, metabolic interaction took place when the subjects were exposed to a combination of 95 ppm toluene and 80 ppm xylene, whereas no interaction was detected after exposure to a combination of 50 ppm toluene and 40 ppm xylene (Tardif *et al.*, 1991). Benzene and toluene competitively inhibit each other's metabolism (Sato, 1993). Male workers exposed to a mixture of solvents including toluene (18 ppm), methyl ethyl ketone (16 ppm), isopropyl alcohol (7 ppm) and ethyl acetate (9 ppm) (Ukai *et al.*, 1994) showed no signs or symptoms that suggested anything other than irritation effects due to toluene exposure. There was no evidence to suggest any modifications of toluene toxicity or metabolism due to co-exposure. The results indicate that metabolic interaction depends on the solvents and the level of exposure.

Gasoline (petrol) is a complex mixture of aromatic and aliphatic chemicals. The same enzyme that is responsible for the metabolism of benzene also metabolizes many components of gasoline. Studies at the Chemical Industry Institute of Toxicology (CIIT) have shown that the interactive effect of a complex mixture such as benzene in gasoline may only occur at saturating concentrations of these chemical mixtures. At lower and environmentally relevant concentrations, however, these interactions become negligible (Bond *et al.*, 1997). 1,2,4-Trimethylbenzene (1,2,4-TMB) mainly occurs in petroleum products, and in man it has been shown that the metabolism of 1,2,4-TMB is inhibited after exposure to white spirit compared with exposure to 1,2,4-TMB alone (Jarnberg *et al.*, 1997). It appears that components in white spirit inhibit metabolism of 1,2,4-TMB.

ALIPHATIC SOLVENTS

Aliphatic hydrocarbons are open-chain carbon-containing chemicals derived from crude oil. This group can be divided into three subgroups. Alkanes or paraffins (C_nH_{2n+2}) are saturated hydrocarbons. Alkenes or olefins (C_nH_{2n}) contain one or more double bonds. Alkynes or acetylenes (C_nH_{2n-2}) contain one or more triple bonds.

Aliphatic hydrocarbons containing four or less carbon atoms are gases (e.g. methane, ethane, butane, 1,3-butadiene and acetylene). Compounds with a 16-carbon atom chain or longer are solids at room temperature. Aliphatic hydrocarbons containing 5–16 carbon atoms are liquids. C_5–C_8 compounds are very volatile solvents. Gasoline is a complex mixture of liquid hydrocarbons.

Aliphatic hydrocarbons are found in fuels (natural gas, gasoline [petrol], kerosene [paraffin]), propellants, solvents, dyes, inks, plastics and coatings, dry cleaning agents and chemical intermediates. Aliphatic volatile alkanes (e.g. pentane, hexane, heptane, octane and non-

ane) are CNS depressants in high concentrations. They may also irritate the mucous membrane and the respiratory tract, in addition to causing drying of the skin that may develop into dermatitis. Alkenes, unsaturated aliphatic solvents, are toxicologically very similar to alkanes.

Alkanes and Alkenes

Industrial applications of *n*-hexane include a variety of uses, e.g. in solvents and thinners in the rubber, food and pharmaceutical industries, as a glue in shoes, in tape and cleaning agents, and in the chemical production of polypropylene and polyethylene. *n*-Hexane is usually mixed with other aliphatic hydrocarbons and toluene for its primary industrial uses as a solvent.

About 15% of inhaled *n*-hexane vapour is absorbed. Large quantities (50–60%) of *n*-hexane are expired by the lungs after vapour exposure. The remaining *n*-hexane is biotransformed by the cytochrome P450 mixed-function oxidase system to 2-hexanol. 2-hexanol is subsequently oxidized to 2,5-hexanediol, 2-hydroxy-5-hexanone, 2-hexanone and 2,5-hexanedione (see **Figure 1**). The metabolites of *n*-hexane are more neurotoxic than the parent compound. The neurotoxic potency of *n*-hexane and some of its metabolites are (in ascending order) *n*-hexane <2-hexanone <2,5-hexanediol < 2,5-hexanedione. *n*-hexane is known to cause peripheral neuropathies following long-term occupational exposures.

Short-term, high-dose *n*-hexane exposure can cause narcotic effects with headache and nausea at 1500 ppm, and confusion and dizziness at 5000 ppm within a few minutes (Jorgensen and Cohr, 1981).

Long-term exposure to *n*-hexane and other liquid aliphatic hydrocarbons that undergo biotransformation to γ-diketones can cause peripheral axonal damage (peripheral axonopathy) (Ruff *et al.*, 1981; Cavanagh, 1982; Bachmann *et al.*, 1993; Graham *et al.*, 1995). This toxic effect of *n*-hexane is based on the toxic biotransformation product 2,5-hexanedione **(Figure 1)**. The toxic mechanism appears to be that 2,5-hexanedione can bind and subsequently cross-link neurofilaments (Abou-Donia *et al.*, 1988; Graham *et al.*, 1995). The γ-diketone 2,5-hexanedione has been proposed to react with lysine amino groups of neurofilaments to form pyrrole rings, which can interact with other proteins (DeCaprio, 1987). Neurofilaments accumulate above the nodes of Ranvier and form giant axonal swellings characteristic of γ-diketone-induced neurotoxicity. Neurofilament cross-linking has been demonstrated both *in vitro* and *in vivo*. Although more than one mechanism may be operating, the following cascade of events seems to be supported by present knowledge: *n*-hexane is metabolized to 2,5-hexanedione, which causes decreased kinase-mediated phosphorylation of neurofilament proteins. This leads to a breakdown of the cytoskeletal matrix and dissociation of neurofilament proteins. Accumulated neurofilaments can then react with 2,5-hexanedione to form cross-linked neurofilaments, which results in giant axonal swellings and distal axonopathy **(Figure 2)**. Based on studies with specific marker proteins for both the central and peripheral nervous systems, long-term n-hexane exposure in rats has shown changes in the PNS but not significant changes in the CNS (Huang *et al.*, 1992, 1993). The PNS seems to be the most sensitive target for n-hexane, whereas toluene mainly causes CNS toxicity (Tähti *et al.*, 1997). Toluene has been shown to inhibit hexane metabolism and decrease its neurotoxicity (Takeuchi *et al.*, 1993).

Owing to the double bond in the carbon chain, alkenes, e.g. hexane and heptene, will not produce similar toxic metabolites to those of n-hexane. Thus, they have not been shown to cause peripheral axonopathy.

Some other solvents, e.g. methyl ethyl ketone (MEK), methyl n-butyl ketone (MBK) and carbon disulphide (CS$_2$), can also cause peripheral neuropathy. The neurotoxicity of MEK and MBK is caused by the same toxic metobolite, 2,5-hexanedione. MBK is roughly 12 times more potent than n-hexane (Bos *et al.*, 1991). In MBK neuropathy, swellings have also been found in the cerebellar white matter in the CNS and in the distal optic nerve, causing spastic gait and impairments of vision and memory respectively (Bos *et al.*, 1991). The long ascending and descending tracts of the spinal cord are also particularly vulnerable. Carbon disulphide itself causes neurofilament-filled swellings of the distal axons, as does the metabolite of n-hexane (Graham *et al.*, 1995).

Chlorinated Aliphatic Solvents

Chlorinated aliphatic hydrocarbons have been widely used as solvents, dry cleaning agents, aerosol propellants and as starting points in the chemical industry. Exposure to chlorinated aliphatic solvents can cause CNS depression and, in chronic exposure, permanent damage such as impaired memory, concentration difficulties and personality changes (Stevens and Forster, 1993). In experimental animals chlorinated solvents have also been shown to cause CNS depression (Honma, 1990). Many of these solvents have been used as inhalation anaesthetics.

Carbon Tetrachloride (Tetrachloromethane, Perchloromethane)

Carbon tetrachloride (CCl$_4$) is a well known hepatotoxic solvent (Kefalas and Stacey, 1991). Its use has been declining, and it has been replaced by less toxic chlorinated solvents such as trichloroethylene, methylchloroform (1,1,1-trichloroethane) and perchloroethylene (tetrachloroethylene) **(Table 1)**. However, it is still used, mainly in the chemical manufacture of fluorocarbon refrigerants, solvents and aerosol propellants.

Table 1 Structures, molecular weights and oil–water partition coefficients of selected solvents

Solvent	Structure	MW[a]	PC[b]
Benzene		78	177
Toluene	–CH$_3$	92	659
Styrene	–CH = CH$_2$	104	1168
o-Xylene	CH$_3$ / CH$_3$	106	1318
Ethylbenzene	–CH$_2$ – CH$_3$	106	2243
Cyclohexane		84	2754
n-Hexane		86	8710
Carbon tetrachloride	Cl–C–Cl (Cl, Cl)	154	631
1,1,1-Trichloroethane	Cl–C–C–H (Cl H, Cl H)	133	309
Trichloroethylene	Cl₂C=CHCl	131	263

[a] Molecular weight.
[b] Oil–water partition coefficients according to Leo *et al.* (1971).

Carbon tetrachloride is well absorbed by the lungs and gastro-intestinal tract. Percutaneous absorption can also occur. CCl$_4$ is concentrated in fatty tissues. The main excretion route (50–80%) is via the lungs as the unchanged compound. Dechlorination occurs in the liver microsomal cytochrome P450 system, and the formation of free radicals may cause lipid peroxidation and subsequent hepatocellular damage. Only a small part of the dose (4%) is excreted as carbon dioxide via the lungs or kidney.

Acute exposure to CCl$_4$ causes CNS depression followed by hepatic and renal dysfunction. The mechanisms of its CNS effects are still not completely clear. However, it has been demonstrated that exposure to acute high doses of CCl$_4$ leads to the same kinds of CNS effects as acute exposure to other organic solvents, e.g. headache, dizziness, blurred vision and constricted visual field (Stevens and Forster, 1993).

The cerebellum is particularly sensitive to CCl$_4$ actions. Bilateral visual field constriction, optic atrophy and amblyopia (reduced vision) characterize its effects on the optic system. Alcoholics are especially sensitive to CNS effects. Death results from respiratory depression or from dysrhythmias (Hyatt and Salmons, 1952).

The liver toxicity is based on the formation of free radicals in the biotransformation reactions. The dechlorination of CCl_4 produces phosgene and trichloromethyl free radical, which is subsequently metabolized to chloroform and carbon dioxide, as well as hexachloroethane. Free radicals can attack proteins and destroy membranes by affecting membrane lipids and producing lipid peroxidation (Sáez et al., 1987). Hepatotoxicity caused by CCl_4 is characterized by acute fatty degeneration of the liver, leading to hepatic necrosis. There are also theories that toxic liver cell death could be associated with alterations of Ca^{2+} homeostasis due to CCl_4 (Rechnagel, 1983). CCl_4 inhibits the ability of microsomes to sequester Ca^{2+} but does not prevent the influx of extracellular Ca^{2+}. The release of Ca^{2+} into the cytosol will result in a number of regulatory alterations (Rechnagel, 1983), which can lead to triglyceride accumulation in the cell. Calcium channel blockers have been shown to protect against CCl_4-induced liver toxicity (Romero et al., 1994). CCl_4 has been considered a potential carcinogen. It has produced hepatocellular carcinomas in hamsters and hepatomas in mice and rats. The data on humans are inadequate to link CCl_4 to liver cancer. CCl_4 can also produce renal damage via acute tubular necrosis.

Chloroform (Trichloromethane, Methenyl Trichloride)

Chloroform ($CHCl_3$) is now restricted to industrial uses as a solvent or a chemical intermediate. In 1847 it was introduced as a general anaesthetic because it was less volatile and not as flammable as diethyl ether. Its use as an anaesthetic was banned early in this century. The industrial use of chloroform is also very restricted, because it will cause liver cancer in experimental animals. Chloroform is a potent CNS depressant that produces a variety of symptoms, e.g. nausea, headache and coma, which appear soon after exposure (Schroder, 1965).

Chloroform is rapidly absorbed via the lungs and gastro-intestinal tract, the peak blood concentration developing in 1 h. A considerable amount (17–67%) is expired by the lungs. In the liver, cytochrome P450 enzymes dechlorinate chloroform by oxidation to trichloromethanol, which spontaneously dehydrochlorinates to phosgene. Phosgene can react with water to form carbon dioxide or bind covalently to cellular macromolecules. It produces hepatotoxicity characterized by fatty infiltration and necrosis (Larson et al., 1993).

Chronic oral exposure to chloroform has caused hepatocellular tumours in mice and kidney tumours in rats (Byron et al., 1994). However, Jorgenson et al., (1985) could not find any tumours in mice liver after chloroform administration in drinking water. The studies of Larson and et al., (1993) showed that chloroform administered in corn oil by gavage caused hyperplasia in mouse liver and in rat kidney. Chloroform-induced mouse liver cancer may be secondary to events associated with induced cytolethality and cell proliferation (Butterworth et al., 1998). Chloroform is an example of a non-genotoxic–cytotoxic carcinogen. Chloroform-induced cytotoxic effects (necrosis, inflammation and regenerative cell proliferation) can start the carcinogenic process and enhance endogenous and exogenous mutagenic activity (Butterworth et al., 1998). The possible carcinogenicity of chloroform has been of particular concern, because the process of municipal water purification by chlorination results in the formation of trace amounts of disinfection by-products such as trichloromethanes. Chloroform is often the most prevalent by-product in the chlorination process.

Chloroform may cause renal toxicity 24–48 h after exposure, and it is characterized by proteinuria. Like most chlorinated hydrocarbons, chloroform sensitizes the myocardium to endogenous catecheolamines.

Trichloroethylene

Trichloroethylene (TRI) ($CHCl = CCl_2$) has been widely used in metal degreasing, dry cleaning, chemical synthesis and as a cleaning agent in households. It was also used as a non-flammable narcotic in the early 1900s. TRI occasionally produces euphoria, and consequently it has been abused for that purpose. In cases of solvent abuse (glue sniffing), TRI has caused fatal accidents due to overdose, and perhaps through the induction of ventricular fibrillation.

TRI is readily absorbed into the body through the lung and gastro-intestinal mucosa. Elimination of TRI involves two major processes: pulmonary excretion of unchanged TRI and relatively rapid hepatic biotransformation to urinary metabolites. The major end metabolites of TRI are trichloroethanol, trichloroethanol glucuronide and trichloroacetic acid. Reactive intermediates can be produced in the biotransformation process: TRI epoxide, dichloroacetic acid, dichlorovinylcysteine, dichloroacetyl chloride and chloroform. The liver toxicity studied in animal models is dependent on the metabolism to trichloroacetic acid and dichloroacetic acid, although the possible role of TRI epoxide cannot be ruled out.

The acute toxic effects of TRI are CNS depression, visual disturbances, mental confusion, fatigue and nausea. In experimental studies, effects on myelin formation in the hippocampus of developing rats have been found (Isaacson and Taylor, 1989). TRI can cause changes in the lipid composition in the brain tissue. According to biochemical studies, it has caused changes in the proportion of the long-chain polyunsaturated fatty acids of ethanolamine phosphoglyceride in rat brain after subchronic and chronic exposures (Kyrklund et al., 1986). The changes in membrane fatty acid composition could modulate brain functions. The reduction in myelin could in part be responsible for the behavioral effects observed in TRI exposure (Isaacson and Taylor, 1989). TRI can also cause arrhythmias through sensitizing the heart to catecholamines, and pulmonary oedema if the exposure is severe. Compared with carbon tetrachloride and chloroform, TRI is a weak hepatotoxin. Hepatocellular carcinoma has been found in mice after large doses of TRI (Kimbrough *et al.*, 1985).

Epidemiological studies have presented only limited evidence for the carcinogenicity of TRI in humans (Kaneko *et al.*, 1997). A cohort study of 2050 male and 1924 female workers indicated an excess of cancers in the CNS and increased risk of multiple myeloma among TRI-exposed workers. However, the overall cancer incidence within the cohort was similar to that of the Finnish population as a whole (Anttila *et al.*, 1995).

Tetrachloroethylene

Tetrachloroethylene or perchloroethylene ($CCl_2 = CCl_2$) is used particularly in dry cleaning and degreasing. The toxicity of tetrachloroethylene resembles that of trichloroethylene. It has caused loss of myelin-enriched lipids, which might indicate a persistent loss of myelin membranes (Kyrklund *et al.*, 1990). According to studies with experimental animals, tetrachloroethylene may cause liver cancer (Kyrklund *et al.*, 1990). A cohort study of dry-cleaning workers exposed mainly to tetrachloroethylene has confirmed an increased risk of oesophageal, intestinal, pancreatic and bladder cancers (Ruder *et al.*, 1994).

1,1,1-Trichloroethane

Trichloroethane (CH_3CCl_3) is also known as methylchloroform. It has been considered to be a more or less non-toxic organic solvent with many industrial and household applications. Its relative low acute toxicity is mainly a consequence of the low blood–gas partition coefficient compared with other chlorinated solvents. Owing to the low blood solubility, the uptake of trichloroethane is low. The principal effect is CNS depression and high doses can sensitize the heart to the effects of catecholamines and thus cause arrhythmia. Trichloroethane can only cause changes in the fatty acid pattern in the rat brain at high concentrations (Kyrklund and Haglid, 1990).

ALICYCLIC SOLVENTS

These colourless liquid solvents are saturated or unsaturated hydrocarbons in which three or more carbon atoms join to form rings. They include cycloalkenes, cycloalkanes and naphthenes. They are present in petroleum solvents and are used in the manufacture of organic chemicals. Alicyclic hydrocarbons show similar effects to aliphatic hydrocarbons but have a greater depressive or anaesthetic effect on the CNS. Alicyclic solvents with low molecular weight, such as cyclopropane, have been used as anaesthetics. The larger compounds, e.g. cyclohexane, cannot be used as narcotics because the safety margin

between the narcotic dose and the lethal dose is very narrow. Cyclohexane does not change the neural membrane fluidity to the same extent as aromatic hydrocarbons (Engelke *et al.*, 1996).

AROMATIC HYDROCARBONS

Benzene

Benzene has mainly been used in chemical processes as a raw material and as a solvent in rubbers and glues. It is also used in the synthesis of ethylbenzene, styrene, cumene, phenolic resins, ketones and various dyes. However, in most industrial products, benzene has been replaced by other organic solvents because of its myelotoxicity and since it can cause aplastic anaemia and leukaemia (Vigliani and Forni, 1976; Infante *et al.*, 1977). Benzene is a natural constituent of gasoline (petrol) at concentrations of up to 5% and thus becomes a constituent of gasoline fumes and automobile exhaust. Tobacco smoke also contains benzene. Benzene is one of the components of volatile organic compounds (VOCs) in the city air, and its concentration is monitored in many cities. Workplace exposures to benzene are limited but both occupational and environmental exposures to benzene still occur (Hricko, 1994; Tompa *et al.*, 1994).

Benzene is metabolized in the liver to phenols by the cytochrome P450 mixed function oxidase system (**Figure 3**). Benzene epoxide is its most toxic metabolite and may be responsible for benzene-induced haematological abnormalities. The conjugation products with glutathione form phenylmercapturic acid, which is excreted in the urine (Schlosser *et al.*, 1998).

Acute exposure to benzene results in CNS effects, characterized by euphoria, headache, nausea and ataxia. These symptoms may progress to a change in gait, convulsions and coma. Acute exposure to benzene may cause arrhythmias due to myocardial sensitization to endogenous catecholamines (Snyder and Kocsis, 1975).

Chronic occupational exposure of humans to benzene can lead to bone-marrow damage, which may be manifested as anaemia, leukopenia and thrombocytopenia. Benzene has been found to induce leukaemia in humans (Snyder and Kalf, 1994). The carcinogenicity of benzene is supported by the chromosomal aberrations found in the peripheral blood lymphocytes of exposed workers (Tompa *et al.*, 1994). No ability of benzene to induce leukaemia has been shown in rats and mice (Snyder *et al.*, 1978). Even though it has been shown that metabolism plays a role in benzene toxicity, and that benzene can interfere with DNA, the exact mechanism of benzene-induced leukaemia is not known. Only recently was benzene oxide shown to be a product in the oxidative microsomal metabolism of benzene in mice, rats and humans (Schlosser *et al.*, 1998). Benzene oxide may be an important link between benzene and leukaemia.

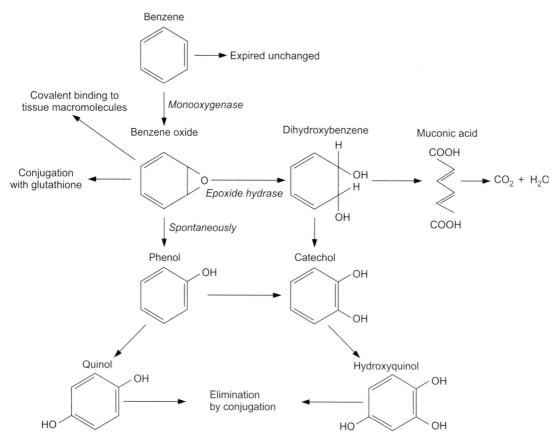

Figure 3 Biotransformation of benzene. The intermediate metabolite benzene oxide (epoxide) is reactive. Glutathione conjugation is very important when removing the reactive metabolite via formation of phenylmercapturic acid

Toluene

Toluene (methylbenzene) is used as a solvent for paints, lacquers, thinners, coatings, glues and cleaning agents. It is also used in the production of other chemicals and in the pharmaceutical industry. The important exposure route is by inhalation, but it is also slowly absorbed through the skin.

The biological half-life of toluene ranges from several hours for white adipose tissue to a few minutes in highly perfused organs (Pyykkö *et al.*, 1977). After inhalation exposure of rats to toluene, the distribution to various tissues is very rapid. Toluene accumulates in white adipose tissue, from which the elimination is slow compared with other tissues (Pyykkö *et al.*, 1977). Approximately 18% of the absorbed toluene is expired unchanged via the lungs, and only 0.06% is eliminated unchanged in the urine. Toluene is metabolized via cytochrome P450 to benzyl alcohol, which is further oxidized via alcohol and aldehyde dehydrogenase to benzaldehyde and benzoic acid, respectively (Pyykkö, 1983). Benzoic acid conjugates with glycine to form hippuric acid, which is excreted in the urine **(Figure 4)**. Some other solvents (e.g. *n*-hexane, benzene, styrene, xylene and trichloroethylene) can inhibit toluene biotransformation (Sato and Nakajima, 1979; Tähti, 1984; Liira *et al.*, 1988). A competitive

metabolic inhibition is the plausible mechanism of this toxicokinetic interaction between the individual solvents. Toluene causes induction of microsomal liver enzymes at relatively low concentrations (Pyykkö, 1983). Toluene has neither carcinogenic nor mutagenic potency. Kidney damage has been reported in sniffers of glues that may have contained toluene and other solvents.

The CNS is sensitive to the effects of toluene. Acute exposure to toluene causes CNS depression including symptoms such as drowsiness, tiredness, headache, dizziness, and nausea. The anaesthetic effect of toluene, like other CNS-depressant solvents, is thought to be based on its ability to disturb the lipid–protein interaction in neural membranes (Engelke *et al.*, 1992, 1996). Owing to their lipid solubilities, solvents incorporate readily into neural membranes **(Figure 5)**. Solvent molecules can bind to hydrophobic parts in the membrane integral proteins and disturb the ion balance in the membrane (Naskali *et al.*, 1993). Exposure for a short time to very high concentrations of toluene (10 000–30 000 ppm) produces unconsciousness and anaesthesia. Long-term inhalation of toluene by abusers is known to cause multifocal neurological disorders characterized by ataxia, tremors and emotional lability, and also cerebral, cerebellar and brain stem atrophy (King *et al.*, 1985; Ikeda and

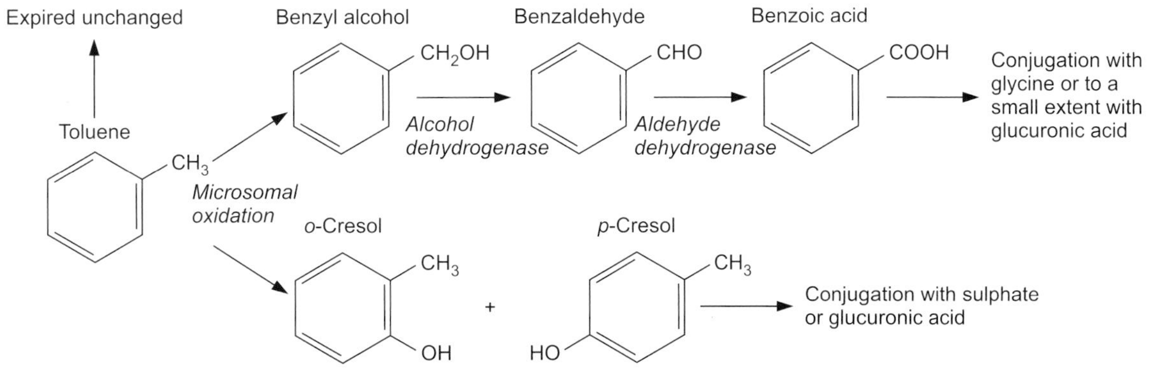

Expired unchanged   Benzyl alcohol   Benzaldehyde   Benzoic acid

Toluene   Microsomal oxidation   Alcohol dehydrogenase   Aldehyde dehydrogenase   Conjugation with glycine or to a small extent with glucuronic acid

o-Cresol   +   p-Cresol   Conjugation with sulphate or glucuronic acid

Figure 4 Biotransformation of toluene. The main metabolite in urine is hippuric acid

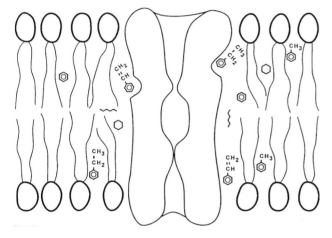

Figure 5 Schematic representation of the incorporation and location of solvent molecules in the neural membrane. Solvent molecules are drawn to approximately the same scale as the membrane molecules. Solvent molecules can bind into the hydrophobic pockets in the integral proteins [enzymes, e.g. (Na^+, K^+)-ATPase] and disturb the ion balance across the membrane

Tsukagoshi, 1990). The acute effect of toluene has been described in controlled conditions in exposure chambers at dose levels which are possible at work places. According to such studies, toluene can cause impairment of visual function (Dick *et al.*, 1984) and vestibular functions (Hydén *et al.*, 1983).

Experimental studies have shown some evidence that toluene can cause irreversible effects on noradrenaline, dopamine and 5-hydroxytryptamine mechanisms in various brain regions in rats (Ladefoged *et al.*, 1991) and in peripheral sympathetic ganglia (Alho *et al.*, 1986). Several case histories have demonstrated a consistent pattern of neurological damage in individuals repeatedly inhaling toluene at high concentrations because of its euphoric properties (Fornazzari *et al.*, 1983; Spencer and Schaumburg, 1985; Rosenberg *et al.*, 1988). There is evidence for an increased risk of neuropsychiatric disorders and behavioural disturbances after chronic toluene intoxications (Kishi *et al.*, 1995).

Xylene

There are three isomers (*ortho*, *meta* and *para*) of xylene (dimethylbenzene) in the commercial product, *meta* being the major isomer. Xylene is one of the most common solvents in paints and varnishes and it commonly also occurs in glues and printing inks. Furthermore, xylene is used as a solvent in the rubber and leather industries and in histological laboratories (Riihimäki *et al.*, 1979). It is also used in the chemical manufacture of insecticides, synthetic fibres, plastics and enamel. Xylenes are widely used to replace benzene as a solvent.

Xylene is rapidly absorbed through the lungs and approximately 65% of an inhaled dose is retained by the lung. It is also absorbed through the gastro-intestinal tract and the skin. Only 3–6% of the absorbed xylene is exhaled via the lungs. Most of the remaining xylene is oxidized to methylbenzoic acid, which is conjugated with glycine to form methylhippuric acid. Only 2% of the absorbed xylene is excreted in urine as xylenols (Riihimäki *et al.*, 1979).

The acute toxicity of xylene is greater than that of toluene, although the symptoms are similar. The major effect of xylene is depression of the CNS, resulting in lightheadedness, nausea, headache and ataxia at low doses. High exposure to xylene produces confusion, respiratory depression and coma. It causes conjunctivitis, nasal irritation, sore throat and respiratory irritation. Xylenes have been shown to induce microsomal enzymes in the liver, although their hepatotoxicity is considered to be low. Concentrations as high as 10 000 ppm produce a reversible and mild increase in hepatic aminotransferase activity and reversible renal failure. Like other aromatic solvents, xylenes may also cause skin and eye irritation.

Styrene

More than 50% of the world's production of benzene is used in the manufacture of styrene (vinylbenzene). Styrene materials account for 20% of all plastic production, e.g. polystyrene, resins and polyesters.

Styrene is readily absorbed via the lungs and gastro-intestinal tract, and also to some extent via the skin. Styrene is metabolized to mandelic acid (70%) and phenylglyoxylic acid (30%), which are excreted in the urine. It is also metabolized to styrene oxide, which is more toxic than the parent compound (Mendrala et al., 1993). Hippuric acid is also excreted in the urine following exposure to styrene, and it has been used for biological monitoring of occupational exposure (see Chapter 87 on biological monitoring in the occupational environment for further details).

The major effect of styrene is on the CNS (Pahwa and Kaira, 1993; Naskali et al., 1994, Pierce et al., 1998). In addition to CNS depression, styrene also causes mucosal irritation. Symptoms include eye irritation as well as nasal and respiratory tract irritation. Chronic exposure has also resulted in peripheral neuropathy characterized by decreased peripheral nerve conduction velocities.

Styrene is an indirect genotoxic agent, which requires metabolic activation to an epoxide in order to bind covalently to DNA. Styrene 7,8-oxide, the active metabolite of styrene, is a carcinogen in rodents and has been shown to be genotoxic in most in vitro test systems. Styrene has been found to be weakly genotoxic in the assay for sister chromatid exchange, especially in mice. Cytogenetic damage has been reported in many studies of workers, mainly from the reinforced plastics industry, where ambient concentrations of styrene have been high (Norppa and Sorsa, 1993).

ALCOHOLS

Methanol

Methanol (CH_3OH) is used as a solvent, an antifreeze agent and as a component of car windscreen washer fluid. It is also used in the production of stains, enamels and photographic films.

Recent plans to use methanol as a fuel, or as a component in gasoline, may increase the probability of exposures to methanol. Inhalation and skin absorption are the most important entry routes of methanol in occupational exposure. Ingested methanol is absorbed from the gastro-intestinal tract almost totally (Liesivuori and Savolainen, 1991). The first step in the metabolic pathway of methanol is oxidation to formaldehyde. In humans, alcohol dehydrogenase (ADH) is the enzyme that catalyses this reaction. The resultant formaldehyde is spontaneously hydrated to methanediol, which is further metabolized by ADH to formic acid (Liesivuori and Savolainen, 1991). The urinary formic acid can be used in biological monitoring of methanol exposure in the work place (Liesivuori and Savolainen, 1987). The effects caused by methanol exposure are dizziness, nausea and vomiting, various types of visual disturbances, headache and metabolic acidosis. At high doses methanol can cause permanent blindness, because of serious damage to the retina. (Liesivuori and Savolainen, 1991; Eells et al., 1996). Methanol poisoning is characterized by severe metabolic acidosis, which can inhibit cellular respiration and hasten cellular failure. Progressive acidosis will also induce circulatory and respiratory failure. This leads to tissue hypoxia and lactic acid production, both of which further increase the acid load (Jacobsen and McMartin, 1986). The toxic effects of formic acid are due to an inhibition of cytochrome oxidase complex at the terminal end of the respiratory chain in the mitochondria, which leads to hypoxia. In addition to the optic nerve and retina, other organs (brain, heart, kidney) with a high rate of oxygen consumption are possible targets. Oral ingestion of methanol as a single moderate to large dose [0.4–1 g (kg body weight)$^{-1}$] may cause blindness. Other common clinical manifestations of methanol poisoning in humans include CNS depression, weakness, headache and vomiting (McMartin et al., 1980). The symptoms of methanol poisoning may be delayed for up to 24 h owing to methanol oxidation to formic acid. The elimination of formic acid from the body is slow. In human methanol poisonings, the half-life of formic acid is about 20 h (Shahangian et al., 1984; Shahangian and Ash, 1986). The treatment of methanol poisoning includes administration of ethanol and folic acid. The ethanol will compete for ADH and thus reduce formate production, while the folic acid will enhance formate oxidation to carbon dioxide (Becker, 1983). Dialysis and alkalinization of urine have been used to increase the elimination of formic acid (Liesivuori and Savolainen, 1991).

Ethanol

Ethanol (CH_3CH_2OH) is used in the chemical industry and in the production of cosmetics and drugs. Exposure to ethanol by inhalation is rare in industry. Chronic alcohol consumption causes significant CNS toxicity characterized by cerebellar atrophy and dilatation of cerebral ventricles. Harper and Kril (1990) have proposed a model for alcohol-induced brain damage. It includes loss of dendritic arbour and shrinkage of the neuronal body. These changes are potentially reversible and occur in many brain regions. The second phase is neuronal death, which is irreversible and has been demonstrated primarily in the frontal cortex.

A serious consequence of ethanol consumption is its multiple effects on the developing embryo and foetus (Pratt, 1982). Foetal alcohol syndrome occurs in the children of approximately 10% of women who drink heavily during pregnancy (Sokol et al., 1986). Recent studies have indicated that a possible explanation for the toxic effects is the enhanced production of acetaldehyde in placenta and foetus due to induction of CYP2E1 (Carpenter et al., 1996, 1997; Boutelet-Bochan et al., 1997; Rasheed et al., 1997). One reason for the interindividual variations is that induction varies among heavy drinkers, and may be genetically controlled (Rasheed *et al.*, 1997).

Isopropanol

Isopropanol [isopropyl alcohol, $CH_3CH(OH)CH_3$] is used in industry as a solvent and disinfectant and as a rubbing alcohol (70% propan-2-ol) in the home. Isopropyl alcohol is metabolized via alcohol dehydrogenase to acetone, which is eliminated through the kidney and the lung. Acetone is further oxidized to acetic acid, formic acid and CO_2 (Daniel *et al.*, 1981).

Exposure to high concentrations of isopropyl alcohol causes CNS and cardiovascular depression, and lower concentrations can cause mild irritation of the eyes. Isopropyl alcohol exerts its primary effect on the CNS in both humans and laboratory animals, showing a more potent narcotic effect than ethanol (Daniel *et al.*, 1981). In industrial use, no toxic effects have been reported. It is the second most ingested alcohol after ethanol (Litovitz *et al.*, 1985) and has caused poisonings in connection with heavy drinking (Rich *et al.*, 1990)

TOXIC EFFECTS OF GLYCOL ETHERS

The acute toxicity of the glycol ethers is low. Until 15 years ago, the focus regarding these solvents was on the toxicity to the CNS and haematopoietic systems, blood, liver and kidneys. In recent years, attention has also been focused on the effects on reproduction and foetal development. Several animal studies have shown that 2-methoxyethanol (2-ME) and 2-ethoxyethanol (2-EE) have teratogenic and spermatotoxic effects (Nagano *et al.*, 1981; Lamb *et al.*, 1985). Workers exposed to 2-ME and 2-EE were found to have lower sperm counts than non-exposed workers (Welch *et al.*, 1988; Ratcliffe *et al.*, 1989). A case control study among patients at a clinic for reproductive disorders showed an association between a diagnosis of impaired fertility and exposure to glycol ethers (Veulemans *et al.*, 1993). Several studies of female workers have shown an increased risk of spontaneous abortions, subfertility, and congenital malformations due to glycol ether exposure (Beaumont *et al.*, 1995, Swan *et al.*, 1995; Correa *et al.*, 1996; Cordier *et al.*, 1997). The metabolism of glycol ethers is a key factor in understanding the biological interactions and structure–activity relationships of these compounds. The adverse effects have been attributed to the corresponding alkoxyacetic acid metabolites of the glycol ethers, methoxyacetic acid and ethoxyacetic acid, respectively (Miller *et al.*, 1982; Foster *et al.*, 1983; Brown *et al.*, 1984; Moss *et al.*, 1985)

The structure–activity relationships for the reproductive and developmental toxicity of methoxyacetic acid and ethoxyacetic acid have been studied. Shorter alkyl-chain glycol ethers produce greater embryotoxicity than those having a longer chain (Nelson *et al.*, 1984). Alkoxyacetic acids added to post-implantation rat embryo cultures increase the incidence of abnormalities in a dose-and structure-related manner, methoxyacetic acid being more effective than ethoxyacetic acid (Rawlings *et al.*, 1985). Ethoxyacetic acid has been shown to produce less severe testicular toxicity than methoxyacetic acid both *in vivo* and *in vitro* in the rat (Foster *et al.*, 1987). On a molar basis, 2-EE produces less severe toxic effects than 2-ME (Wess, 1992).

Little is known about the biochemical mechanisms that induce the embryotoxicity and testicular toxicity of 2-ME and 2-EE, and the possible contribution from the alkoxyacetic acid metabolites. Several studies in rats and mice have indicated that methoxyacetic acid undergoes further metabolism, and that the metabolites could be responsible for developmental and testicular toxicity (Welsch *et al.*, 1987; Mebus and Welsch, 1989; Mebus *et al.*, 1989, 1992; Sumner and Fennel, 1993). The developing embryo and late-stage spermatocytes both undergo rapid nucleic acid biosynthesis. Methoxyacetic acid or a product of its metabolism can influence common biochemical pathways by affecting the availability of one-carbon units, thus causing depression of purine and pyrimidine biosynthesis (Mebus and Welsch, 1989; Mebus *et al.*, 1992; Sumner *et al.*, 1992). Alterations in the availability of these precursors might be expected to affect DNA and/or RNA synthesis and thereby influence normal cellular proliferation and differentiation. Recent studies indicate that 2-ME induces spermatocyte apoptosis in rat and guinea pigs (Brinkworth *et al.*, 1995; Ku *et al.*, 1995; Wine *et al.*, 1997). It has been shown that MAA induces cell death of spermatocytes in both rat and human seminiferous tubules in the same dose ranges (Li *et al.*, 1996). MAA has been shown to increase progesterone production in rat and human luteinized granulosa cell, and this may probably result in reduced fertility due to a disturbed menstrual cycle (Almekinder *et al.*, 1997).

FUTURE CHALLENGES

The wide use of organic solvents in industry will also present an important occupational health risk in the future. In particular, epidemiological studies will be needed to study the effects of long-term exposure to low levels of organic solvents. This will require advanced neuropsychological test methods to detect impairment in CNS functions. However, it will be equally important to uncover the underlying mechanisms of these effects.

During the last decade, some sophisticated experimental techniques have been developed for studies of CN functions in experimental animal models (Vorhees, 1987; Vorhees *et al.*, 1991; Stanton and Freeman, 1994). However, extrapolation of behavioural data from animals to humans may be difficult and possibly misleading.

Epidemiological studies have shown that long-term exposures to specific solvents (benzene, trichloroethylene, tetrachloroethylene and carbon tetrachloride) may increase the cancer risks. Occupational exposure to mixtures of solvents in paints has consistently been associated with a 40% increased risk of lung cancer (Lynge et al., 1997). However, addressing these questions becomes ever more demanding when we consider that most long-term exposures are to mixtures rather than to single chemicals at any one time. The effects are difficult to detect and often we do not know even what kind of effects to look for.

REFERENCES

Aasmoe, L. and Aarbakke, J. (1999). Sex dependent induction of alcohol dehydrogenase activity in rats. Biochem. Pharmacol., in press.

Abou-Donia, M. B. and Lapadula, D. M. (1988). Cytoskeletal proteins as targets for organophosphorus compound and aliphatic hydrocarbon-induced neurotoxicity. Toxicology, 49, 469–477.

Alho, H., Tähti, H., Koistinaho, J. and Hervonen, A. (1986). The effect of toulene inhalation exposure on catheclamine contents in rat sympathetic neurons. Med. Biol., 64, 285–288.

Almekinder, J. L., Lennard, D. E., Walmer, D. K. and Davis, B. J. (1997). Toxicity of methoxyacetic acid in cultured human luteal cells. Fundam. Appl. Toxicol., 38, 191–194.

Andrews, L. S., Lee, E. W., Witmer, C. M., Kocsis, J. J. and Sbyder, R. (1977). Effects of toluene on the metabolism, disposition and hemopoietic toxicity of [3H]benzene. Biochem. Pharmacol., 26, 293–300.

Anttila, A., Pukkala, E., Sallmen, M., Hernberg, S. and Hemminki, K. (1995). Cancer incidence among Finnish workers exposed to halogenated hydrocarbons. J. Occup. Environ. Med., 37, 797–806.

Åstrand, I. (1983). Effect of physical exercise on uptake, distribution and elimination of vapors in man. In Fiserova, V. (Ed.), Modelling of Inhalation Exposure to Vapors: Uptake, Distribution and Elimination. CRC Press, Boca Raton, FL, Vol. 2, pp. 107–133.

Bachmann, M. O., De Beer, Z. and Myers, J. E. (1993). n-Hexane neurotoxicity in metal can manufacturing workers. Occup. Med., 43, 149–154.

Backes, W. L., Sequeira, D. J., Cawley, G. F. and Eyer, C. S. (1993). Relationship between hydrocarbon structure and induction of P450: effects on protein levels and enzyme activities. Xenobiotica, 23, 1353–1366.

Baker, E. L. (1994). A review of recent research on health effects of human occupational exposure to organic solvents. A critical review. J. Occup. Med., 36, 1079–1092.

Beaumont, J. J., Swan, S. H., Hammond, S. K., Samuels, S. J., Green, R. S., Hallock, M. F., Dominguez, C., Boyd, P. and Schenker, M. B. (1995). Historical cohort investigation of spontaneous abortion in the semiconductor health study: epidemiological methods and analyses of risk in fabrication overall and in fabrication work groups. Am. J. Ind. Med., 28, 735–750.

Becker, C. E. (1983). Methanol poisoning. J. Emerg. Med., 1, 51–58.

Bleecker, M. L., Bolla, K. I., Agnew, J., Schwartz, B. S. and Ford, D. P. (1991). Dose-related subclinical neurobehavioral effects of chronic exposure to low levels of organic solvents. Am. J. Ind. Med., 19, 715–728.

Bond, J. A., Leavens, T. L., Seaton, M. J. and Medinsky, M. A. (1997). Predicting the toxicity of chemical mixtures based on knowledge of individual components. CIIT Activities, 17 (12), 1–7.

Bos, P. M. J., de Mik, G. and Bragt, P. C. (1991). Critical review of the toxicity of methyl n-butyl ketone: risk from occupational exposure. Am. J. Ind. Med., 20, 175–194.

Boutelet-Bochan, H., Huang, Y. and Juchau, M. R. (1997). Expression of CYP2E1 during embryogenesis and fetogenesis in human cephalic tissues: implications for the fetal alcohol syndrome. Biochem. Biophys. Res. Commun., 238, 443–447.

Brinkworth, M. H., Weinbauer, G. F., Schlatt, S. and Nieschlag, E. (1995). Identification of male germ cells undergoing apoptosis in adult rats. J. Reprod. Fertil., 105, 25–33.

Brooke, I., Cocker, J., Delic, J. I., Payne, M., Gregg, N. C. and Dyne, D. (1998). Dermal uptake of solvents from the vapour phase: an experimental study in humans. Ann. Occup. Hyg., 42, 531–540.

Brown, N. A., Holt, D. and Webb, M. (1984). The teratogenicity of methoxyacetic acid in the rat. Toxicol. Lett., 22, 93–100.

Butterworth, B. E., Kedderis, G. L. and Conolly, R. B. (1998). The chloroform cancer risk assessment: a mirror of scientific understanding. CIIT Activities, 18 (4), 1–10.

Byron, E., Butterworth, J. L., Larson, J. L., Conolly, R. B., Borghoff, S. J., Kedderis, G. L. and Wolf, D. C. (1994). Risk assessment issues associated with chloroform-induced mouse liver tumors. CIIT Activities, 14 (2), 1–7.

Carpenter, S. P., Lasker, J. M. and Raucy, J. L. (1996). Expression, induction, and catalytic activity of the ethanol-inducible cytochromes P450 (CYP2E1) in human fetal liver and hepatocytes. Mol. Pharmacol., 49, 260–268.

Carpenter, S. P., Savage, D. D., Schultz, E. D. and Raycy, J. L. (1997). Ethanol-mediated transplacental induction of CYP2E1 in fetal rat liver. J. Pharmacol. Exp. Ther., 282, 1028–1036.

Cavanagh, J. B. (1982). The pattem of recovery of axons in the nervous system of rats following 2,5-hexanediol intoxication: a question of rheology. Neuropathol. Appl. Neurobiol., 8, 19–34.

Cheeseman, K. H., Albano, E. F., Tomasi, A. and Slater, T. F. (1985). Biochemical studies on the metabolic activation of halogenated alkanes. Environ. Health Perspect., 64, 85–101.

Cherry, N. (1993). Neurobehavioural effects of solvents: the role of alcohol. Environ. Res., 62, 155–158.

Cometto-Muniz, J. E. and Cain, W. S. (1991). Nasal pungency, odor, and eye irritation thresholds for homologous acetates. Pharmacol. Biochem. Behav., 39, 983–989.

Cometto-Muniz, J. E. and Cain, W. S. (1992). Sensory irritation. Relation to indoor air pollution. Ann. N. Y. Acad. Sci., 30, 137–151.

Cometto-Muniz, J. E. and Cain, W. S. (1993). Efficacy of volatile organic compounds in evoking nasal pungency and odor. Arch. Environ. Health, 48, 309–314.

Cometto-Muniz, J. E. and Cain, W. S. (1994). Sensory reactions of nasal pungency and odor to volatile organic compounds: the alkylbenzenes. *Am. Ind. Hyg. Assoc. J.*, **55**, 811–817.

Cometto-Muniz, J. E. and Cain, W. S. (1995). Relative sensitivity of the ocular trigeminal, nasal trigeminal and olfactory systems to airborne chemicals. *Chem. Senses*, **20**, 191–198.

Cometto-Muniz, J. E., Cain, W. S. and Abraham, M. H. (1998). Nasal pungency and odor of homologous aldehydes and carboxylic acids. *Exp. Brain Res.*, **118**, 180–188.

Conney, A. H. (1968). Pharmacological implications of microsomal enzyme induction. *Pharmacol. Rev.*, **19**, 317–353.

Cordier, S., Bergeret, A., Goujard, J., Ha, M.-C., Aymé, S., Bianchi, F., Calzolari, E., De Walle, H. E. K., Knill-Jones, R., Candela, S., Dale, I., Dananché, B., de Vigan, C., Fevotte, J., Kiel, G. and Mandereau, L. (1997). Congenital malformations and maternal occupational exposure to glycol ethers. *Epidemiology*, **8**, 355–363.

Correa, A., Gray, R. H., Cohen, R., Rothman, N., Shah, F., Seacat, H. and Corn, M. (1996). Ethylene glycol ethers and risks of spontaneous abortion and subfertility. *Am. J. Epidemiol.*, **143**, 707–716.

Daniel, D. R., McAnally, B. H. and Garriott, J. C. (1981). Isopropyl alcohol metabolism after acute intoxication in humans. *J. Anal. Toxicol.*, **5**, 110–112.

DeCaprio, A. P. (1987). n-Hexane neurotoxicity: a mechanism involving pyrrole adduct formation in axonal cytoskeletal protein. *Neurotoxicology*, **8**, 195–210.

Dekant, W., Vamvakas, S. and Anders, M. W. (1989). Bioactivation of nephrotoxic haloalkenes by glutathion conjugation: formation of toxic and mutagenic intermediates by cysteine conjugate beta-lyase. *Drug Metab. Rev.*, **20**, 43–83.

Dick, R. B., Setzer, J. V., Wait, R., Hayden, M. B., Taylor, B. J., Tolos, B. and Putz-Anderson, V. (1984). V. Effects of acute exposure of toluene and methyl ethyl ketone on psychomotor performance. *Int. Arch. Occup. Environ. Health*, **54**, 91–109.

Edelfors, S. and Ravn-Jonsen, A. (1992). Effect of organic solvents on nervous cell membrane as measured by changes in the (Ca^{2+}/Mg^{2+}) ATPase activity and fluidity of synaptosomal membrane. *Pharmacol. Toxicol.*, **70**, 181–187.

Edling, C., Ekberg, K., Ahlborg, G., Jr, Alexandersson, R., Barregard, L., Ekenvall, L., Nilsson, L. and Svensson, B. G. (1990). Long-term follow up of workers exposed to solvents. *Br. J. Ind. Med.*, **47**, 75–82.

Eells, J. T., Salzman, M. M., Lewandowski, M. F. and Murray, T. G. (1996). Formate induced alterations in retinal function in methanol-intoxicated rats. *Toxicol. Appl. Pharmacol.*, **140**, 58–69.

Eger, E. I. (1974). *Anesthetic Uptake and Action*. Williams and Wilkins, Baltimore, MD.

Engelke, M., Diehl, H. and Tähti, H. (1992). Effects of toluene and n-hexane on rat synaptosomal membrane fluidity and integral enzyme activities. *Pharmacol. Toxicol.*, **71**, 343–347.

Engelke, M., Tähti, H. and Vaalavirta, L. (1996). Perturbation of artificial and biological membranes by organic compounds of aliphatic, alicyclic and aromatic structure. *Toxicol. In Vitro*, **10**, 111–115.

Engström, K., Riihimäki, V. and Laine, A. (1984). Urinary disposition of ethylbenzene and m-xylene in man following separate and combined exposure. *Int. Arch. Occup. Health*, **54**, 355–363.

Evans, E. B. and Balster, R. L. (1991). CNS depressant effects of volatile organic solvents. *Neurosci. Biobehav. Rev.*, **15**, 233–241.

Fiserova-Bergerova, V. (1985). Toxicokinetics of organic solvents. *Scand. J. Work Environ. Health*, **11**, Suppl. 1, 7–21.

Flanagan, R. J. and Ives, R. J. (1994). Volatile substance abuse. *Bull. Narcot.*, **46**, 49–78.

Fornazzari, L., Wilkinson, D. A., Kapur, B. M. and Carlen, P. L. (1983). Cerebellar, cortical and functional impairment in toluene abusers. *Acta Neurol. Scand.*, **67**, 319–329.

Foster, P. M. D., Creasy, D. M., Foster, J. R., Thomas, L. V., Cook, M. W. and Gangolli, S. D. (1983). Testicular toxicity of ethylene glycol monomethyl and monoethyl ethers in the rat. *Toxicol. Appl. Pharmacol.*, **69**, 385–399.

Foster, P. M. D., Lloyd, S. C. and Blackburn, D. M. (1987). Comparison of the in vivo and in vitro testicular effects produced by methoxy-, ethoxy- and N-butoxyacetic acids in the rat. *Toxicology*, **43**, 17–30.

Franks, N. P. and Lieb, W. R. (1978). Where do general anaesthetics act? *Nature*, **274**, 339–342.

Gabow, P. A., Clay, K., Sullivan, J. B. (1986). Organic acids in ethylene glycol intoxication. *Ann. Intern. Med.*, **105**, 16–20.

Gessner, G. F., Parke, D. V. and Williams, R. T. (1960). Studies in detoxication. *Biochem. J.*, **74**, 1–5.

Gillion, R. B., Crow, K. E., Batt, R. D. and Hardman, M. J. (1985). Effects of ethanol treatment and castration on liver alcohol dehydrogenase activity. *Alcohol*, **2**, 39–41.

Giovacchini, R. P. (1985). Abusing the volatile organic chemicals. *Regul. Toxicol. Pharmacol.*, **5**, 18–37.

Graham, D. G., Amarnath, V., Valentine, W. M., Pyle, S. J. and Douglas, C. A. (1995). Pathogenetic studies of hexane and carbon disulfide neurotoxicity. *Crit. Rev. Toxicol.*, **25**, 91–112.

Gregersen, P. (1988). Neurotoxic effects of organic solvents in exposed workers: two controlled follow-up studies after 5.5 and 10.6 years. *Am. J. Ind. Med.*, **14**, 681–701.

Gut, I., Terelius, Y., Frantik, E., Linhart, I., Soucek, P., Filipcova, B. and Kluckova, H. (1993). Exposure to various benzene derivatives differently induces cytochrome P450 2B1 and P450 2E1 in rat liver. *Arch. Toxicol.*, **67**, 237–243.

Guthrie, G. D., Myers, K. J., Gesser, E. J., White, G. W. and Koehl, J. R. (1990). Alcohol as a nutrient: interactions between ethanol and carbohydrate. *Alcohol Clin. Exp. Res.*, **14**, 17–22.

Hakkola, M. (1994). Neuropsychological symptoms among tanker drivers with exposure to solvents. *Occup. Med.*, **44**, 243–246.

Hänninen, H., Antti-Poika, M., Juntunen, J. and Koskenvuo, M. (1991). Exposure to organic solvents and neuropsychological dysfunction: a study on monozygotic twins. *Br. J. Ind. Med.*, **48**, 18–25.

Harper, C. G. and Kril, J. J. (1990). Neuropathology of alcoholism. *Alcohol*, **25**, 207–216.

Hein, H. O., Suadicani, P. and Gyntelberg, F. (1990). Mixed solvent exposure and cerebral symptoms among active and retired workers. An epidemiological investigation of 3387 men aged 53–75 years. *Acta Neurol. Scand.*, **81**, 97–102.

Hogstedt, C. (1994). Has the Scandinavian solvent syndrome controversy been solved? *Scand. J. Work Environ. Health*, **20**, 59–64.

Honma, T. (1990). Effects of trichloroethylene, 1,1,1-trichloroethane and carbon tetrachloride on plasma lipoproteins of rats. *Ind. Health*, **28**, 159–174.

Hricko, A. (1994). Rings of controversy around benzene. *Environ. Health Perspect.*, **102**, 276–281.

Huang, J., Shibata, E., Kato, K., Asaeda, N. and Takeuchi, Y. (1992). Chronic exposure to *n*-hexane changes in nerve-specific marker proteins in the distal peripheral nerve of rat. *Hum. Exp. Toxicol.*, **11**, 323–327.

Huang, J., Kato, K., Shibata, E., Asaeda, N. and Takeuchi, Y. (1993). Nerve specific marker proteins as indicators of organic solvent neurotoxicity. *Environ. Res.*, **63**, 82–87.

Hyatt, A. V. and Salmons, J. A. (1952). Carbon tetrachloride poisoning. *AMA Arch. Ind. Hyg.*, **6**, 74–82.

Hydén, D., Larsby, B., Andersson, H., Ökvist, L. M., Liedgren, S. L. C. and Tham, R. (1983). Impairment of visuo-vestibular interaction in humans exposed to toluene. *Oto-Rhino-Laryngol.*, **45**, 262–269.

Ikeda, M. and Tsukagoshi, H. (1990). Encephalopathy due to toluene sniffing. *Eur. Neurol.*, **30**, 347–349.

Ikeda, M., Ohtsuji, H. and Immura, T. (1972). *In vivo* suppression of benzene and styrene oxidation by coadministered toluene and effects of phenobarbital. *Xenobiotica*, **2**, 101–106.

Infante, P. E., Rinsky, R. A., Wagoner, J. K. and Young, R. J. (1977). Leukemia in benzene workers. *Lancet*, **ii**, 76–78.

Inoue, O., Seiji, K., Watanabe, T., Kasahara, M., Nakatsuka, H., Yin, S. N., Li, G. L., Cai, S. X., Jin, C. and Ikeda, M. (1988). Mutual metabolic suppression between benzene and toluene in man. *Int. Arch. Occup. Environ. Health.*, **60**, 15–20.

Isaacson, L. G. and Taylor, D. H. (1989). Maternal exposure to 1,1,2-trichloroethylene affects myelin in the hippocampal formation of the developing rat. *Brain Res.*, **488**, 403–407.

Jacobsen, D. and McMartin, K. E. (1986). Methanol and ethylene glycol poisonings: mechanisms of toxicity, clinical source, diagnosis and treatment. *Med. Toxicol.*, **1**, 309–334.

Jacobsen, M., Baelum, J. and Bonde, J. P. (1994). Temporal epileptic seizures and occupational exposure to solvents. *Occup. Environ. Med.*, **51**, 429–430.

James, R. C. (1985). The toxic effects of organic solvents. In Williams, P. L. and Burson, J. L. (Eds), *Industrial Toxicology*. Van Nostrand Reinhold, New York, pp. 230–259.

Jarnberg, J., Johanson, G., Lof, A. and Stahlbom, B. (1997). Inhalation toxicokinetics of 1,2,4-trimethylbenzene in volunteers: comparisons between exposure to white spirit and 1,2,4-trimethylbenzene alone. *Sci. Total Environ.*, **199**, 65–71.

Jorgensen, N. K. and Cohr, K. H. (1981). *n*-Hexane and its toxicologic effects: a review. *Scand. J. Work Environ. Health*, **7**, 157–168.

Jorgenson, T. A., Meierhenry, E. F., Rushbrook, C. J., Bull, R. J. and Robinson, M. (1985). Carcinogenicity of chloroform in drinking water to male Osborne–Mendel rats and female B6C3F₁ mice. *Fundam. Appl. Toxicol.*, **5**, 760–769.

Kaneko, T., Wang, P. Y. and Sato, A. (1993). Enzyme induction by ethanol consumption affects the pharmacokinetics of inhaled *m*-xylene only at high levels of exposure. *Arch. Toxicol.*, **67**, 473–477.

Kaneko, T., Wang, P. Y. and Sato, A. (1997). Assessment of the health effects of trichloroethylene. *Ind. Health*, **35**, 301–324.

Kefalas, V. and Stacey, N. H. (1991). Potentiating effects of chlorinated hydrocarbons on carbon tetrachloride toxicity in isolated rat hepatocytes and plasma membranes. *Toxicol. Appl. Pharmacol.*, **109**, 171–179.

Kezic, S., Mahieu, K., Monster, A. C. and de Wolff, F. A. (1997). Dermal absorption of vaporous and liquid 2-methoxyethanol and 2-ethoxyethanol in volunteers. *Occup. Environ. Med.*, **54**, 38–43.

Kim, Y. C. (1997). Dichlormethane potentiation of carbon tetrachloride hepatotoxicity in rats. *Fundam. Appl. Toxicol.*, **35**, 138–141.

Kim, S. K. and Kim, Y. C. (1996). Effects of a single administration of benzene, toluene or *m*-xylene on carboxyhaemoglobin elevation and metabolism of dichloromethane in rats. *J. Appl. Toxicol.*, **16**, 437–444.

Kimbrough, R. D., Mitchell, F. L. and Hovic, V. N. (1985). Trichloroethylene: an update. *J. Toxicol. Environ. Health*, **15**, 369–383.

King, G. I., Jacobs, R. E. and White, S. H. (1985). Hexane dissolved in dioleoyllecithin bilayers has a partial molar volume of approximately zero. *Biochemistry*, **24**, 4637–4645.

Kishi, R., Harabuchi, I., Katakura, Y., Ikeda, T. and Miyake, H. (1995). Neurobehavioral effects of chronic occupational exposure to organic solvents among Japanese industrial painters. *Environ. Res.*, **62**, 303–313.

Kitchin, K. T. and Brown, J. L. (1989). Biochemical effects of three carcinogenic chlorinated methanes in rat liver. *Teratog. Carcinog. Mutagen.*, **9**, 61–69.

Korpela, M. and Tähti, H. (1988). Human and rat erythrocyte membranes as a model for studying the effects of organic solvents on membrane-bound acetylcholinesterase *in vitro*. *Toxicol In Vitro*, **2**, 135–139.

Ku, W. W., Wine, R. N., Chae, B. Y., Ghanayem, B. I. and Chapin, R. E. (1995). Spermatocyte toxicity of 2-methoxyethanol (ME) in rats and guinea pigs: evidence for the induction of apoptosis. *Toxicol. Appl. Pharmacol.*, **134**, 100–110.

Kyrklund, T. and Haglid, K. G. (1990). Exposure of rats to high concentrations of 1,1,1-trichloroethane and its effects on brain lipid and fatty acid compositions. *Pharmacol. Toxicol.*, **67**, 384–386.

Kyrklund, T., Kjellstrand, P. and Haglid, K. G. (1986). Fatty acid changes in rat brain ethanolamine phosphoglycerides during and following chronic exposure to trichloroethylene. *Toxicol. Appl. Pharmacol.*, **85**, 145–153.

Kyrklund, T., Kjellstrand, P. and Haglid, K. G. (1990). Long-term exposure of rats to perchloroethylene, with and without a post-exposure solvent-free recovery period: effects on brain lipids. *Toxicol. Lett.*, **52**, 279–285.

Ladefoged, O., Strange, P., Moller, A., Lam, H., Ostergaard, G., Larsen, J.-J. and Arlien-Soborg, P. (1991). Irreversible effects in rats of toluene (inhalation) exposure for six months. *Pharmacol. Toxicol.*, **68**, 384–390.

Lamb, J. C., Maronpot, R. R., Gulati, D. K., Russell, V. S., Hommel-Barnes, L. and Sabharwal, P. S. (1985). Reproductive and developmental toxicity of ethylene glycol in the mouse. *Toxicol. Appl. Pharmacol.*, **81**, 100–112.

Larson, J. L., Wolf, D. C. and Butterworth, B. E. (1993). The acute hepatotoxic and nephrotoxic effects of chloroform in male F 344 rats and female B6C3F₁ mice. *Fundam. Appl. Toxicol.*, **20**, 302–315.

Leo, A., Hansch, C. and Elkins, D. (1971). Partition coefficients and their uses. *Chem. Rev.*, **71**, 525–559.

Li, L. -H., Wine, R. N. and Chapin, R. E. (1996). 2-methoxyacetic acid (MAA)-induced spermatocyte apoptosis in human and rat testes: an *in vitro* comparison. *J. Androl.*, **17**, 538–549.

Liao, L. L. and Richardson, K. E. (1973). The inhibition of oxalate biosynthesis in isolated perfused rat liver by

DL-phenyllactate and *n*-heptanoate. *Arch. Biochem. Biophys.*, **154**, 68–75.

Liesivuori, J. and Savolainen, H. (1987). Urinary formic acid as an indicator of occupational exposure to formic acid and methanol. *Am. Ind. Hyg. Assoc. J.*, **48**, 32–34.

Liesivuori, J. and Savolainen, H. (1991). Methanol and formic acid toxicity: biochemical mechanisms. *Pharmacol. Toxicol.*, **69**, 157–163.

Liira, J., Riihimaki, V., Engstrom, K. and Pfaffli, P. (1988). Coexposure of man to *m*-xylene and methyl ethyl ketone. Kinetics and metabolism. *Scand. J. Work Environ. Health*, **15**, 322–327.

Lindros, K. O. (1997). Zonation of cytochrome P450 expression, drug metabolism and toxicity in liver. *Gen. Pharmacol.*, **28**, 191–196.

Litovitz, T. L., Normann, S. A., and Veltri, J. C. (1985). 1985 Annual Report of the American Association of Poison Control Centers National Data Collection System. *Am. J. Emerg. Med.*, **4**, 427–458.

Lowe, H. J. (1972). *Dose-regulated Penthrane methoxyflurane anesthesia.* Abbott Laboratories, Chigago.

Lynge, E., Anttila, A. and Hemminki, K. (1997). Organic solvents and cancer. *Cancer Causes Control*, **8**, 406–419.

Manno, M., Rezzadore, M., Grossi, M. and Sbrana, C. (1996). Potentiation of occupational carbon tetrachloride toxicity by ethanol abuse. *Hum. Exp. Toxicol.*, **15**, 294–300.

McMartin, K. E., Ambre, J. J. and Tephly, T. R. (1980). Methanol poisoning in human subjects: role of formic acid accumulation in the metabolic acidosis. *Am. J. Med.*, **68**, 414–418.

Mebus, C. A. and Welsch, F. (1989). The possible role of one-carbon moieties in 2-methoxyethanol and 2-methoxyacetic acid-induced developmental toxicity. *Toxicol. Appl. Pharmacol.*, **99**, 98–109.

Mebus, C. A., Welsch, F. and Working, P. K. (1989). Attenuation of 2-methoxyethanol-induced testicular toxicity in the rat by simple physiological compounds. *Toxicol. Appl. Pharmacol.*, **99**, 110–121.

Mebus, C. A., Clarke, D. O., Stedman, D. B. and Welsch, F. (1992). 2-Methoxyethanol metabolism in pregnant CD-1 mice and embryos. *Toxicol. Appl. Pharmacol.*, **112**, 87–94.

Mendrala, A. L., Langvardt, P. W., Nitschke, K. D., Quast, J. F. and Nolan, R. J. (1993). *In vitro* kinetics of styrene and styrene oxide metabolism in rat mouse, and human. *Arch. Toxicol.*, **67**, 18–27.

Mergler, D. and Blain, L. (1987). Assessing color vision loss among solvent-exposed workers. *Am. J. Ind. Med.*, **12**, 195–203.

Mikkelsen, S. (1997). Epidemiological update on solvent neurotoxicity. *Environ. Res.*, **73**, 101–112.

Milanovic, L., Spilich, G., Vucinic, G., Knezevic, S., Ribaric, B. and Mubrin, Z. (1990). Effects of occupational exposure to organic solvents upon cognitive performance. *Neurotoxicol. Teratol.*, **12**, 657–660.

Miller, K. W., Paton, W. D. M., Smith, E. B. and Smith, R. A. (1972). Physiochemical approaches to the mode of action of general anesthetics. *Anesthesiology*, **36**, 339–351.

Miller, R. R., Carreon, R. E., Young, J. T. and McKenna, M. J. (1982). Toxicity of methoxyacetic acid in rats. *Fundam. Appl. Toxicol.*, **2**, 158–160.

Moen, B. E., Kyvik, K. R., Engelsen, B. A. and Riise, T. (1990). Cerebrospinal fluid proteins and free amino acids in patients with solvent induced chronic toxic encephalopathy and health controls. *Br. J. Ind. Med.*, **47**, 277–280.

Morimoto, M., Hagbjork, A. -L. and Nanji, A. A. (1993). Role of cytochrome P4502E1 in alcoholic liver disease pathogenesis. *Alcohol*, **10**, 459–464.

Mortensen, B., Zahlsen, K. and Nilsen, O. G. (1998). Metabolic interaction of *n*-hexane and methyl ethyl ketone *in vitro* in a head space rat liver S9 vial equilibration system. *Pharmacol. Toxicol.*, **82**, 67–73.

Moss, E. J., Thomas, L. V., Cook, M. W., Walters, D. G., Foster, P. M. D., Creasy, D. M. and Gray, T. J. B. (1985). The role of metabolism in 2-methoxyethanol-induced testicular toxicity. *Toxicol. Appl. Pharmacol.*, **79**, 480–489.

Nagano, K., Nakayama, E., Oobayashi, H., Yamada, T., Adachi, H., Nishizawa, T., Ozawa, H., Nakaichi, M., Okuda, H., Minami, K. and Yamazaki, K. (1981). Embryotoxic effects of ethylene glycol monomethyl ether in mice. *Toxicology*, **20**, 335–343.

Nakaaki, K., Fukabori, S. and Tada, O. (1980). An experimental study on percutaneous absorption of some organic solvents. *J. Sci. Labour*, **56** (12, Part II), 1–9.

Naskali, L., Engelke, M., Tähti, H. and Diehl, H. (1993). The effects of selected organic solvents on rat synaptosomal membrane fluidity and integral enzyme activities. *Neurosci. Res. Commun.*, **13**, 27–35.

Naskali, L., Oksanen, H. and Tähti, H. (1994). Astrocytes as targets for CNS effects of organic solvents *in vitro*. *Neurotoxicology*, **15**, 609–612.

Nebert, D. W., Atlas, S. A., Guenthner, T. M. and Kuori, R. E. (1978). In Ts'o, P. O. P. and Gelboin, H. V. (Eds), *Polycyclic Hydrocarbons and Cancer*. Academic Press, New York, p. 345.

Nelson, B. K., Brightwell, W. S., Setzer, J. V. and O'Donohue, T. L. (1984). Reproductive toxicity of the industrial solvent 2-ethoxyethanol in rats and interactive effects of ethanol. *Environ. Health Perspect.*, **57**, 255–259.

Ng, T. P., Ong, S. G., Lam, V. K. and Jones, G. M. (1990). Neurobehavioral effects of industrial mixed solvent exposure in Chinese printing and paint workers. *Neurotoxicol. Teratol.*, **12**, 661–664.

Niklasson, M., Moller, C., Odkvist, L. M., Ekberg, K., Flodin, U., Dige, N. and Skoldestig, A. (1997). Are deficits in the equilibrium system relevant to the clinical investigation of solvent-induced neurotoxicity? *Scand. J. Work Occup. Health*, **23**, 206–213.

Norppa, H. and Sorsa, M. (1993). Genetic toxicity of 1,3-butadiene and styrene. *IARC Scientific Publication.*, No. **127**, pp. 185–193. International Agency for Research on Cancer, Lyon.

Orbaek, P., Rosen, I. and Svensson, K. (1988). Electroneurographic findings in patients with solvent induced central nervous system dysfunction. *Br. J. Ind. Med.*, **45**, 409–414.

Pahwa, R. and Kaira, J. (1993). A critical review of the neurotoxicity of styrene in humans. *Vet. Hum. Toxicol.*, **35**, 516–520.

Papper, E. M. and Kitz, R. J. (Eds) (1963). *Uptake and Distribution of Anesthetic Agents*. McGraw-Hill, New York.

Pathiratne, A., Puyear, R. L. and Brammer, J. D. (1986). A comparative study of the effects of benzene, toluene, and xylenes on their *in vitro* metabolism and drug-metabolizing enzymes in rat liver. *Toxicol. Appl. Pharmacol.*, **82**, 272–280.

Pierce, C. H., Becker, C. E., Tozer, T. N., Owen, D. J. and So, Y. (1998). Modeling the acute neurotoxicity of styrene. *J. Occup. Environ. Med.*, **40**, 230–240.

Pyykkö, K. (1983). Time-course of effects of toluene on microsomal enzymes in rat liver, kidney and lung during and after inhalation exposure. *Chem.–Biol. Interact.*, **44**, 299–310.

Pyykkö, K., Tähti, H. and Vapaatalo, H. (1977). Toluene concentrations in various tissues of rats after inhalation and oral administration. *Arch. Toxicol.*, **38**, 169–176.

Pratt, O. E. (1982). Alcohol and the developing fetus. *Br. Med. Bull.*, **38**, 48–53.

Rasheed, A., Hines, R. N. and McCarver-May, D. G. (1997). Variation in induction of human placental CYP2E1: possible role in susceptibility to fetal alcohol syndrome. *Toxicol. Appl. Pharmacol.*, **144**, 396–400.

Ratcliffe, J. M., Schrader, S. M., Clapp, D. E., Halperin, W. E., Turner, T. W. and Hornung, R. W. (1989). Semen quality in workers exposed to 2-ethoxyethanol. *Br. J. Ind. Med.*, **46**, 399–406.

Rawlings, S. J., Shuker, D. E. G., Webb, M. and Brown, N. A. (1985). The teratogenic potential of alkoxy acids in postimplantation rat embryo culture: structure–activity relationships. *Toxicol. Lett.*, **28**, 49–58.

Rechnagel, R. O. (1983). A new direction in the study of carbon tetrachloride hepatotoxicity. *Life Sci.*, **33**, 401–408.

Rich, J., Scheife, R. T., Katz, N. and Caplan, L. R. (1990). Isopropyl alcohol intoxication. *Arch. Neurol.*, **47**, 322–324.

Riihimäki, V., Pfäffli, P. and Savolainen, K. (1979). Kinetics of *m*-xylene in man. Influence of intermittent physical exercise and changing environmental concentrations on kinetics. *Scand. J. Work Environ. Health*, **5**, 232–248.

Riihimäki, V., Savolainen, K., Pfäffli, P., Pekari, K., Sippel, H. W. and Laine, A. (1982). Metabolic interaction between *m*-xylene and ethanol. *Arch. Toxicol.*, **49**, 253–263.

Romero, G., Lasheras, B., Sainz-Suberviola, L. and Cenarruzabeitia, E. (1994). Protective effect of calcium channel blockers in carbon tetrachloride-induced liver toxicity. *Life Sci.*, **55**, 981–990.

Ronis, M. J. J., Lindros, K. O. and Ingelman-Sundberg, M. (1996). The CYP2E subfamily. In Joannides, C. (Ed.), *Cytochromes P450: Metabolic and Toxicological Aspects*. CRC Press, Boca Raton, FL.

Rosenberg, N. L. M. C., Pitz, M. C., Filley, C. M., Davis, K. A. and Schaumburg, H. H. (1988). Central nervous system effects of chronic toluene abuse—clinical, brainstem evoked response and magnetic resonance imaging studies. *Neurotoxicol. Teratol.*, **10**, 488–495.

Ruder, A. M., Ward, E. M. and Brown, D. P. (1994). Cancer mortality in female and male dry-cleaning workers. *J. Occup. Med.*, **36**, 867–874.

Ruff, R. L., Petito, C. K. and Acheson, L. S. (1981). Neuropathy associated with chronic low level exposure to *n*-hexane. *Clin. Toxicol.*, **18**, 515–519.

Sáez, J. C., Bennett, M. V. L. and Sray, D. C. (1987). Carbon tetrachloride at hepatotoxic levels blocks reversibly gap junctions between rat hepatocytes. *Science*, **230**, 967–968.

Sato, A. (1993). Confounding factors in biological monitoring of exposure to organic solvents. *Int. Arch. Occup. Environ. Health*, **65**, S61–S67.

Sato, A. and Nakajima, T. (1979). Dose-dependent metabolic interaction between benzene and toluene *in vivo* and *in vitro*. *Toxicol. Appl. Pharmacol.*, **48**, 249–256.

Sato, A. and Nakajima, T. (1987). Pharmacokinetics of organic solvent vapors in relation to their toxicity. *Scand. J. Work Environ. Health*, **13**, 81–93.

Sato, A., Nakajima, T. and Koyama, Y. (1981). Dose-related effects of a single dose of ethanol on the metabolism in rat liver of some aromatic and chlorinated hydrocarbons. *Toxicol. Appl. Pharmacol.*, **60**, 8–15.

Schlosser, P. M., Kedderis, G. L., Lovern, M. R. and Turner, M. J. (1998). Identification of benzene oxide: the missing link in benzene metabolism. *CIIT Activities*, **18** (2), 1–7.

Schroder, H. G. (1965). Acute and delayed chloroform poisoning. *Br. J. Anaesth.*, **37**, 972–975.

Schwartz, B. S., Ford, D. P., Bolla, K. I., Agnew, J., Rothman, N. and Bleeker, M. L. (1990). Solvent-associated decrements in olfactory functions in paint manufacturing workers. *Am. J. Ind. Med.*, **18**, 697–706.

Seeman, P. (1972). The membrane actions of anesthetics and tranquilizers. *Pharmacol. Rev.*, **24**, 513–655.

Sequeria, D. J., Eyer, C. S., Cawley, G. F., Nick, T. G. and Backes, W. L. (1992). Ethylbenzene-mediated enduction of cytochrome P450 isoenzymes in male and female rats. *Biochem. Pharmacol.*, **44**, 1171–1182.

Shahangian, S. and Ash, K. O. (1986). Formic and lactic acidosis in a fatal case of methanol intoxication. *Clin. Chem.*, **32**, 395–397.

Shahangian, S., Robinson, V. L. and Jennison, T. A. (1984). Formate concentration in a case of methanol ingestion. *Clin. Chem.*, **30**, 1413–1414.

Singh, S. K. and Pandey, R. S. (1991). Ethanol potentiates *in vivo* hepatotoxicity of endosulfan in adult male rats. *Indian J. Exp. Biol.*, **29**, 1035–1038.

Sipes, I. G. and Gandolfi, A. J. (1982). Role of reactive intermediates in halothane associated liver injury. In Snyder, R., Parke, D. V., Kocsis, J. J. *et al.* (Eds), *Biological Reactive Intermediates. Chemical Mechanisms and Biological Effects.* Plenum Press, New York, vol. 2, pp. 603–618.

Snyder, R. and Kalf, G. F. (1994). A perspective on benzene leukemogenesis. *CRC Crit. Rev. Toxicol.*, **24**, 177–209.

Snyder, R. and Kocsis, J. J. (1975). Current concepts of chronic benzene toxicity. *CRC Crit. Rev. Toxicol.*, **3**, 265–288.

Snyder, R., Lee, E. W. and Kocsis, J. J. (1978). Binding of labeled benzene metabolites to mouse liver and bone marrow. *Res. Commun. Chem. Pathol. Pharmacol.*, **20**, 191–194.

Sokol, R., Ager, J., Martier, S., Debanne, S., Ernhart, C., Kuzma, J. and Miller, S. I. (1986). Significant determinants of susceptibility to alcohol teratogenicity. *Ann. N. Y. Acad. Sci.*, **477**, 87–102.

Spencer, P. S. and Schaumberg, H. H. (1985). Organic solvent neurotoxicity. Facts and research needs. *Scand. J. Work Environ. Health*, **11**, Suppl. 1, 53–60.

Stanton, M. E. and Freeman, J. H. (1994). Eyeblink conditioning in the infant rat: an animal model of learning in developmental neurotoxicology. *Environ. Health Perspect.*, **102**, 131–139.

Stevens, H., and Forster, F. M. (1993). Effects of carbon tetrachloride on the nervous system. *Arch. Neurol. Psychiatry*, **70**, 653–659.

Sumner, S. C. J. and Fennell, T. R. (1993). A possible mechanism for the formation of $^{14}CO_2$ via 2-methoxyacetic acid in mice exposed to ^{14}C-labeled 2-methoxyethanol. *Toxicol. Appl. Pharmacol.*, **120**, 162–164.

Sumner, S. C. J., Stedman, D. B., Clarke, D. O., Welsch, F. and Fennell, T. R. (1992). Characterization of urinary metabolites from [1,2-methoxy-^{13}C]-2-methoxyethanol in mice using ^{13}C nuclear magnetic resonance spectroscopy. *Chem. Res. Toxicol.*, 5, 553–560.

Swan, S., Beaumont, J. J., Hammond, S. K., VonBehren, J., Green, R. S., Hallock, M. F., Woskie, S. R., Hines, C. J. and Schenker, M. B. (1995). Historical cohort study of spontaneous abortion among fabrication workers in the semiconductor health study: agent-level analysis. *Am. J. Ind. Med.*, 28, 751–769.

Tähti, H. (1984). Combined effects of organic solvents. A review. In Manninen, O. (Ed.), *Combined Effects of Environmental Factors, Proceedings of the First International Conference on the Combined Effects of Environmental Factors, Tampere, Finland*. Central Printing House, Tampere, pp. 413–429.

Tähti, H., Hyppönen, S., Oksanen, H. and Korpela, M. (1992). Evaluation of the effects of organic solvents and solvent mixtures on cell membrane integral proteins *in vitro*. *In Vitro Toxicol.*, 5, 1–6.

Tähti, H., Engelke, M. and Vaalavirta L. (1997). Mechanisms and models of neurotoxicity of *n*-hexane and related solvents. *Arch. Toxicol.*, 19, Suppl., 337–345.

Takeuchi, Y., Hisanaga, N., Ono, Y., Shibata, E., Saito, I. and Iwata, M. (1993). Modification of metabolism and neurotoxicity of hexane by co-exposure of toluene. *Int. Arch. Occup. Environ. Health*, 65, S227–S230.

Tanii, H., Huang, J., Ohyashiki, T. and Hashimoto, K. (1994). Physical–chemical–activity relationship of organic solvents: effects on Na$^+$K$^+$-ATPase activity and membrane fluidity in mouse synaptosomes. *Neurotoxicol. Teratol.*, 16, 575–582.

Tardif, R., Laparé, S., Plaa, G. L. and Brodeur, J. (1991). Effects of simultaneous exposure to toluene and xylene on their respective biological indices in humans. *Int. Arch. Occup. Environ. Health*, 63, 279–284.

Tichy, M. (1983). Prediction of adverse activities from physical and chemical properties of vapors and gases (QSAR analysis). In Fiserova, V. (Ed.), *Modelling of Inhalation Exposure to Vapours: Uptake Distribution and Elimination*. CRC Press, Boca Raton, FL, Vol. 2, pp. 3–35.

Tompa, A., Major, J. and Jakab, M. G. (1994). Monitoring of benzene-exposed workers for genotoxic effects of benzene: improved-working-condition-related decrease in the frequencies of chromosomal aberrations in peripheral blood lymphocytes. *Mutat. Res.*, 304, 159–165.

Triebig, G., Barocka, A., Erbguth, F., Höll, R., Lang, C., Lehrl, S., Rechlin, T., Weidenhammer, W. and Weltle, D. (1992). Neurotoxicity of solvent mixtures in spray painters. II. Neurologic, psychiatric, psychological, and neuroradiologic findings. *Int. Arch. Occup. Environ. Health*, 64, 361–372.

Tunek, A., Hogstedt, B. and Olofsson, T. (1982). Mechanism of benzene toxicity. Effects of benzene and benzene metabolites on bone marrow cellularity, number of granulopoietic stem cells and frequency of micronuclei in mice. *Chem.–Biol. Interact.*, 39, 129–138.

Turk, J., Morrell, L. and Avioli, L. V. (1986). Ethylene glycol intoxication. *Arch. Intern. Med.*, 146, 1601–1603.

Ukai, H., Takada, S., Inui, S., Imai, Y., Kawai, T., Shimbo, S. and Ikeda, M. (1994). Occupational exposure to solvent mixtures—effects on health and metabolism. *Occup. Environ. Med.*, 51, 523–529.

Veulemans, H., Steeno, O., Masschelein, R. and Groeseneken, D. (1993). Exposure to ethylene glycol ethers and spermatogenic disorders in man: a case-control study. *Br. J. Ind. Med.*, 50, 71–78.

Vigliani, E. C. and Forni, A. (1976). Benzene and leukemia. *N. Engl. J. Med.*, 11, 122–127.

von Wartburg, J. P., Bethuen, J. L. and Vallee, B. L. (1964). Human liver alcohol dehydrogenase. Kinetic and physico-chemical properties. *Biochemistry*, 3, 1775–1782.

Vorhees, C. V. (1987). Reliability, sensitivity and validity of behavioral indices of neurotoxicity. *Neurotoxicol. Teratol.*, 9, 445–464.

Vorhees, C. V., Weisenburger, W. P., Ascuff-Smith, K. D. and Minck, R. D. (1991). An analysis of factors influencing complex water-maze learning in rats: effects of task complexity, path order and escape assistance on performance following prenatal exposure to phenytoin. *Neurotoxicol. Teratol.*, 13, 213–222.

Wallen, M., Holm, S., and Nordqvist, M. B. (1985). Coexposure to toluene and *p*-xylene in man: uptake and elimination. *Br. J. Ind. Med.*, 42, 111–116.

Wang, R. S., Nakajima, T., Tsurute, H. and Honma, T. (1996). Effects of exposure to four organic solvents on hepatic cyrochrome P450 isoenzymes in rat. *Chem.–Biol. Interact.*, 99, 239–252.

Wasserkort, R. and Koller, T. (1997). Screening effects of volatile organic compounds using *Drosophilia melanogaster*. *J. Appl. Toxicol.*, 17, 119–125.

Welch, L. S., Schrader, S. M., Turner, T. W. and Cullen, M. R. (1988). Effects of exposure to ethylene glycol ethers on shipyard painters: II. Male reproduction. *Am. J. Ind. Med.*, 14, 509–526.

Welsch, F., Sleet, R. B. and Greene, J. A. (1987). Attenuation of 2-methoxyethanol and methoxyacetic acid-induced digit malformations in mice by simple physiological compounds: Implications for the role of further metabolism of methoxyacetic acid in developmental toxicity. *J. Biochem. Toxicol.*, 2, 225–240.

Wess, J. A. (1992). Reproductive toxicity of ethylene glycol monomethyl ether, ethylene glycol monoethyl ether and their acetates. *Scand. J. Work Environ. Health*, 18, Suppl. 2, 43–45.

Wine, R. N., Ku, W. W., Li, L. -H. and Chapin, R. E. (1997). Cyclophilin A is present in rat germ cells and is associated with spermatocyte apoptosis. *Biol. Reprod.*, 56, 439–446.

Yuan, W., White, T. B., White, J. W., Strobel, H. W. and Backes, W. L. (1995). Relationship between hydrocarbon structure and induction of P450: effect on RNA levels. *Xenobiotica*, 25, 9–16.

Chapter 97

Metal Toxicology

Lennart Dock and Marie Vahter

CONTENTS

INTRODUCTION

About three-quarters of all known chemical elements are *metals*, generally characterized by high electrical and thermal conductivity, malleability, ductility and a high reflectivity of light. Aluminium (Al), iron (Fe), calcium (Ca), sodium (Na), potassium (K) and magnesium (Mg) are the most abundant metals in the Earth's crust. Only a few metals, such as copper (Cu), gold (Au), platinum (Pt) and silver (Ag), are found in the free state, while the majority of metals are found in the form of complexes with other elements. Most metals are crystalline solids in their pure form, with a relatively simple crystal structure distinguished by a close packing of atoms and a high degree of symmetry. Metal atoms usually contain less than half the full number of valence electrons and combine with non-metals, such as oxygen and sulphur, which generally have more than half the maximum number electrons in their outermost shell. The chemical reactivity of native metals vary, from the highly reactive lithium (Li), Na and K, to Au, Ag and Pt, which have very low chemical reactivity.

Metalloids have chemical properties intermediate between those of typical metals and non-metals. The group includes boron (B), silicon (Si), germanium (Ge), arsenic (As), antimony (Sb), selenium (Se) and tellurium (Te). Most of these elements have important commercial applications in transistors and other semiconductor devices, ceramics, solar batteries and certain polymers.

Heavy metals is an expression often used for elements, not necessarily 'true' metals, with a specific gravity exceeding 5 mg ml^{-1}. Several toxic elements, such as As, Sb, cadmium (Cd), mercury (Hg), lead (Pb), uranium (U) and bismuth (Bi), are often included in this group.

Alloys are metallic substances, solid compounds or solutions, that are composed of two or more elements, usually themselves metals. The value of certain alloys, such as brass (copper and zinc) and bronze (copper and tin), was discovered in ancient times. Today, the alloy steels are of primary importance. These contain significant amounts of elements other than iron and carbon, such as chromium, nickel, molybdenum, tungsten and vanadium. *Amalgams* are alloys of mercury and one or more other metals. An amalgam of silver and tin, with minor amounts of copper and zinc, is frequently used in dentistry. Amalgamation of precious elements, such as silver and gold, is a common practice in small-scale mining (De Lacerda and Salomons, 1998). Fine particles of silver and gold can be recovered by agitating their ores with mercury and allowing the resultant pasty or liquid amalgam to settle. The mercury is distilled off and the precious metal is isolated as a residue.

Trace elements usually classified as essential to man are iodine, iron, zinc, copper, manganese, selenium, molybdenum and cobalt (WHO, 1996). The uptake and utilization of essential trace elements are under physiological control and a well balanced diet is usually adequate in order to maintain trace element homeostasis. However, deficiencies in the gastro-intestinal uptake of elements or certain inborn errors of metabolism can result in disease due to sustained trace element imbalance (Lentner, 1986). For some essential trace elements, excess intake may be associated with adverse health effects, and the difference between essential and toxic intake levels may be small (Nord, 1995). Several other trace elements, notably arsenic, cadmium, lead and mercury, have no known function in the human body. Exposure to these elements may cause immediate as well as delayed adverse health effects, eventually developing into permanent impairment of essential bodily functions.

A full coverage of all aspects on metal toxicology is a daunting task and well beyond the purpose of this review, the focus of which is mainly on the chronic toxicity of non-essential trace elements, while some other elements are discussed more briefly.

NON-ESSENTIAL TRACE ELEMENTS OF MAJOR TOXICOLOGICAL CONCERN

Arsenic (As)

The name arsenic is derived from the Latin word *arsenicum* and the Greek word *arsenikon* (yellow orpiment). It can also be traced to the Arabic word, *Az-zernikh*, meaning the orpiment from zerni-zar, the Persian word for gold (Hammond, 1995). Elemental arsenic is a steel grey, very brittle, crystalline, semimetallic solid. Arsenic tarnishes in air and is rapidly oxidized to arsenous oxide (As_2O_3) when heated.

Arsenic in nature is mainly found bound to sulphur, most commonly as arsenopyrite (FeAsS) and orpiment or arsenic sulphide (As_2S_3). The sulphides are degraded to arsenates during weathering. The red or orange mineral realgar (As_2S_2) is another important ore of arsenic. Realgar is typically a minor constituent of ore veins in association with orpiment, to which it disintegrates on prolonged exposure to light. When arsenopyrite is heated, the arsenic sublimes, leaving ferrous sulphide. Orpiment was used as a pigment by Middle Eastern artists but gained little attention from Western artists until the eighteenth century, when artificial arsenic trisulphide started to be produced. However, owing to its high toxicity it was soon abandoned, except for the very fine grade King's yellow, which was used until cadmium yellow (principally cadmium sulphide) became available. As_2O_3 is mainly obtained as a by-product in the production of lead and copper.

Arsenic is used in bronzing and pyrotechnics, for hardening and improving the sphericity of shot and in the production of glass and ceramics. Various arsenic compounds (both inorganic and methylated arsenic acids) are used as agricultural insecticides, herbicides and defoliants. In combination with copper and chromium, arsenic is used for preservation of wood. A recent application is the use of arsenic as a doping agent in solid-state devices such as transistors. Gallium arsenide is used as a laser material to convert electricity directly into coherent light.

Arsenic has a long history of use in medicine, especially before the introduction of modern antibiotics. Recently, it has gained renewed interest in the treatment of cancer, especially leukaemia (Shen *et al.*, 1997).

The WHO guideline value for arsenic in drinking water is 10 μg l^{-1} (WHO, 1993), although it is recognized that this level may lead to arsenic intake levels corresponding to excess lifetime skin cancer risks of 6×10^{-4}. A concentration of arsenic in air of 1 μgm^{-3} has been estimated to be associated with a lifetime cancer risk of 3×10^{-3} (WHO, 1987).

Uptake, Metabolism and Excretion

Environmental arsenic is mainly in the pentavalent form. Trivalent arsenic may be found where reducing conditions prevail, such as in deep groundwater wells. Drinking water usually contains less than a few micrograms of arsenic per litre, but substantially higher levels, more than 1000 μg l^{-1}, can be found in wells in regions were the bedrock is rich in arsenic-containing minerals.

Soluble forms of arsenic are efficiently (70–90%) absorbed in the gastro-intestinal tract and distributed to other organs. Pulmonary absorption of soluble forms of arsenic, such as arsenic trioxide, is rapid while less soluble forms, such as lead arsenate and calcium arsenate, may reside in the lower airways and be absorbed during a prolonged period of time (Marafante and Vahter, 1987).

The pentavalent form of arsenic is metabolically reduced and methylated in a sequence of reaction catalysed by methyltransferase(s) with *S*-adenosylmethionine as cofactor and with glutathione as the reductant (Vahter and Marafante, 1988). About 50–60% of ingested arsenic is excreted within 1 week. The main excretion products found in human urine are inorganic arsenic, monomethylarsonic acid (MMA) and dimethylarsinic acid (DMA) in the proportions 10–20, 10–15 and 60–80%, respectively (Vahter and Marafante, 1988). Recently (Vahter *et al.*, 1995a), a population with a very low urinary MMA excretion was identified, suggesting polymorphism in human As methylation. MMA and DMA are less reactive than inorganic arsenic, especially As(III), with tissue constituents, and readily excreted in the urine. The biological half-time of ingested inorganic arsenic is about 4 days (Tam *et al.*, 1979; Buchet *et al.*, 1981). Following ingestion of MMA or DMA, about 75% of the dose is excreted in the urine within 4 days (Buchet *et al.*, 1981; Marafante *et al.*, 1987).

There are major differences in arsenic methylation between animal species. Whereas most rodents seem to be highly efficient in methylating arsenic, no methylated arsenic metabolites were detected in marmoset monkeys and chimpanzees exposed to inorganic arsenic (Vahter and Marafante, 1985; Vahter *et al.*, 1995b). Arsenite methyltransferase activity has been detected *in vitro* in liver from rabbit, rat, mouse, hamster, pigeon and rhesus monkeys (Zakharyan *et al.*, 1995; Aposhian, 1997), but not in liver from marmoset monkey, tamarin monkey, squirrel monkey, chimpanzee and guinea pig (Zakharyan *et al.*, 1996; Healy *et al.*, 1997). Gel electrophoresis of rabbit liver proteins showed that methylation of both arsenite and monomethylarsonic acid was associated with a single protein band. However, it is not clear if the two arsenic methylation reactions are catalysed by the same protein

Inorganic arsenic is bound to SH groups (Cullen and Reimer, 1989), and especially the bonds with vicinal SH groups are strong, e.g. with keratin in hair, nails and skin, and these tissues generally show the highest concentrations of arsenic (Vahter *et al.*, 1982). Tissues with the longest retention time of arsenic following exposure to DMA are the lungs, thyroid and the lens of the eye (Vahter *et al.*, 1984). Animal studies have shown that arsenic is transferred to the foetus across the placental barrier (Hood *et al.*, 1988), but there is a lack of human data.

Toxicity

Soluble inorganic arsenic salts are highly toxic. The lethal dose of ingested arsenic trioxide is about 1–3 mg (kg body weight)$^{-1}$ in adults while even lower exposure levels, 1–4 mg day^{-1}, have caused serious health effects, including fatalities, in small children (WHO, 1981). The Morinaga incident, where arsenic-contaminated powdered milk was fed to children, affected 12 000 Japanese children and 130 fatalities were recorded (Yamashita *et al.*, 1972). Symptoms of arsenic intoxication include nausea, headache and severe abdominal pain due to damage to the gastro-intestinal mucous membranes, violent vomiting and diarrhoea caused by paralysis of the capillary control in the intestinal tract. Eventually the gastro-intestinal epithelium may be sloughed off, followed by a decrease in blood volume, decreased blood pressure, disturbed heart action, failure of vital cardiovascular and brain functions and death. The massive loss of water may lead to renal failure and anuria. Acute arsenic intoxication may also lead to a general paralysis of the capillaries, acute excitability of the brain and death through general paralysis. Non-fatal acute intoxications may result in damage to the peripheral nervous system, manifested as sensory loss, and due to axonal degeneration. Other symptoms include anaemia and leukopenia, fever, anorexia, hepatomegaly and melanosis.

Inhalation of arsenic cause respiratory tract symptoms, such as rhinitis, laryngitis and bronchitis (Ishinishi *et al.*, 1977; Landrigan, 1981; Nemery, 1990). At high exposure levels, hyperplasia and atrophy in the respiratory tract and perforation of the nasal septum have been reported (Pinto and McGill, 1953; Lundgren, 1954).

Subchronic and chronic exposure to inorganic arsenic have been associated with a reduction in nerve conduction velocity (Blom *et al.*, 1985; Lagerkvist and Zetterlund, 1994) and hepatic injury (Lander *et al.*, 1975). Peripheral vascular damage has been observed among people exposed to arsenic in drinking water in Taiwan and Chile (Tseng, 1977). The disease may develop into gangrene of the lower extremities ('blackfoot disease') and the effect appears to be associated with the cumulative dose of arsenic through drinking water. Ingestion of arsenic induces characteristic changes in skin pigmentation. Areas of hyper- and hypopigmentation are frequently seen on the neck, chest and back. Palmoplantar and papular hyperkeratosis are other dermal manifesta-

tions, and these may eventually develop into malignant lesions.

Changes in the urinary excretion pattern of porphyrins have been observed in populations exposed to high levels of arsenic in drinking water. A reduction in coproporphyrin III excretion with a concomitant reduction in the coproporphyrin III/I ratio and a reduced excretion of uroporphyrin were reported (Garcia-Vargas *et al.*, 1994).

Arsine (AsH$_3$) is another highly toxic form of arsenic. Arsine cause severe haemolytic anaemia followed by acute renal failure (Klimecki and Carter, 1995). Toxicity is observed at exposure levels below 10 ppm. Haemolysis occurs after fixation of arsine in a non-volatile form by haemoglobin (Hatlelid *et al.*, 1996; Winski *et al.*, 1997). Haemolysis requires the presence of oxygen and it has been suggested that elemental arsenic is the active haemolytic species, or the arsenic dihydride intermediate. Another possibility is the generation of hydrogen peroxide during arsenic oxidation, in combination with inhibition of catalase.

Animal experiments have shown that high exposure to arsenic compounds during foetal development results in malformations of the brain, urogenital organs, skeleton and eyes (Ferm and Hanlon, 1985; Golub, 1994). Human data on reproductive or developmental toxicity due to arsenic exposure are lacking.

Carcinogenicity and Genotoxicity

An increased incidence of cancers in people exposed to arsenic was already observed in the early nineteenth century. Initially, these observations were made on lung cancers among smelter workers and miners followed by reports on an elevated incidence of skin cancers in patients using arsenical medications (IARC, 1980; Wang and Rossman, 1996). The association between ingestion of arsenic and the development of skin cancers has been confirmed by studies in areas where drinking water contains high concentrations of arsenic (Tseng *et al.*, 1968; Tseng, 1977). Various forms of arsenic-related skin cancers have been described, including basal cell carcinomas and squamous cell carcinomas (Shannon and Strayer, 1989). The former are usually only locally invasive, whereas the latter may metastasize to other tissues. The cancers generally occur as multiple lesions, not particularly on skin areas exposed to sunlight. More recently, an increase in mortality ratios for several internal cancers (bladder, liver, lung, kidney) have been observed in arsenic-exposed populations (Bates *et al.*, 1992; Chen *et al.*, 1992; Chiou *et al.*, 1995; Smith *et al.*, 1995).

Animal experiments have generally failed in demonstrating cancer causation due to arsenic exposure alone, although intratracheal administration of arsenic compounds has been shown to induce tumours in hamsters and rats under some conditions (Pershagen *et al.*, 1984; Pershagen and Björklund, 1985; Yamamoto *et al.*, 1987).

The relevance of these results for the human exposure situation is disputed. It is possible that arsenic mainly works as a co-carcinogen, a tumour promoter or as a tumour progressor under complex human exposure situation which are difficult to simulate in animal studies. Other contributing factors are the more efficient methylation of arsenic in most rodents (Vahter, 1994a) and the induced tolerance to arsenic seen in cells from rodent species (Wang and Rossman, 1993). Human cells are generally more susceptible to arsenic and similar induction of tolerance is not seen (Rossman *et al.*, 1997).

Arsenic has yielded mainly negative results in mutagenicity bioassays whereas positive results in tests for gene amplification, chromosome aberrations, sister chromatid exchanges, and DNA repair inhibition have been achieved (Barrett *et al.*, 1989). Although negative on its own, arsenic has been shown to be comutagenic in the presence of UV light and chemical mutagens. The reason may be that arsenic interferes with DNA repair systems, thus enhancing the persistence of modified DNA bases and increasing the likelihood of inaccurate DNA replication. The fact that arsenic is a potent inducer of gene expression and gene amplification (Lee *et al.*, 1988) may also be relevant in the cancer process.

Mechanism of Action

The underlying mechanisms for the different biochemical effects observed in response to arsenic may be associated with the high affinity of trivalent arsenic, the principal toxic form, for thiols, especially vicinal thiols. The thiol groups may be found on the same protein or on different proteins in close proximity. Although the number of proteins with vicinal thiols is small, this feature is common in the zinc fingers found in DNA binding proteins and transcription factors and some DNA repair enzymes (Coleman, 1992). A number of enzymes and cofactors contains essential thiols and these can be modified through arsenic binding. The modification can sometimes be reversed by mono- or dithiols. Arsenic impairs cellular respiration through interaction with mitochondrial enzymes, such as succinic dehydrogenase, and cofactors such as dihydrolipoic acid.

Exposure Assessment

Human exposure to arsenic can be monitored through the analysis of blood, urine and hair samples. Urinary arsenic levels are mainly used for assessment of recent exposure. In order to interpret urinary arsenic concentration data correctly it is important to distinguish between inorganic arsenic, including the methylated metabolites, and organic forms of arsenic, mainly arsenobetaine (Vahter, 1994b). The latter compound is found in high concentrations in crustaceans and certain species of fish (Edmonds and Francesconi, 1987) but is generally considered to be of little toxicological significance. However, consumption of fish and other marine organisms may increase the level of dimethylarsenic in urine (Vahter, 1986; Arbouine and Wilson, 1992; Buchet *et al.*, 1994). Speciation of arsenic in blood is more complex than speciation analysis of urinary samples. In situations of chronic inorganic arsenic exposure, e.g. via drinking water, there is a good correlation between the levels of arsenic in blood and urine. Inorganic arsenic, particularly the trivalent form, is tightly bound to sulphydryl groups in keratin, allowing the use of hair samples for exposure assessment. Segments of hair can be utilised for temporal analysis of arsenic exposure, although the risk for external contamination of the samples has to be recognized (Peters *et al.*, 1984; Poklis and Saady, 1990).

Cadmium (Cd)

The Latin word *cadmia* and the Greek word *kadmeia* are ancient names for calamine (zinc carbonate) and the element was discovered by Stromeyer in 1817 from an impurity in zinc carbonate (Hammond, 1995). Cadmium most often occurs in small quantities associated with zinc ores and almost all cadmium is obtained as a by-product during processing of zinc, copper and lead ores. The element is a soft, bluish-white metal which is easily cut with a knife and shows many similarities with zinc. Cadmium is mainly used in electroplating but also in certain alloys with low melting-points and in bearing alloys with low coefficients of friction and great fatigue resistance. It is also used in many types of solder and in Ni–Cd batteries. Cadmium sulphide is used as a yellow pigment.

In the general population, the diet is the main source of exposure to cadmium. Less than 5% of the total cadmium uptake can be attributed to inhalation (Vahter *et al.*, 1991). Food items which often contain high concentrations of cadmium include liver, kidney, shellfish, certain mushrooms and grain. A significant source of exposure to cadmium is cigarette smoke (Friberg *et al.*, 1974; Kuhnert *et al.*, 1988) and smokers generally show higher tissue concentrations of cadmium than non-smokers (Vahter, 1982).

The WHO guideline value for cadmium in drinking water is $3 \ \mu g \ l^{-1}$ (WHO, 1993). In assessing health risks due to airborne cadmium, the WHO has stated that an increase in existing cadmium levels in rural areas (<1–5 $ng \ m^{-3}$) and in urban areas without agricultural activities and in industrialized areas (10–20 $ng \ m^{-3}$) should not be permitted (WHO, 1987).

Uptake, Metabolism and Excretion

Depending on the size and solubility of the inhaled particles, the pulmonary absorption may be as high as 50% (WHO, 1992). The gastro-intestinal absorption of cadmium is much lower, in general only a few per cent.

However, subjects with iron deficiency (depleted iron stores) may absorb considerably more (Berglund et al., 1994). On the other hand, dietary factors such as fibres may decrease cadmium absorption. Gastro-intestinal uptake of cadmium occurs mainly in the proximal part of the duodenum (Sorensen et al., 1993).

Experimental studies have indicated that cadmium, following absorption, is bound to albumin and other high molecular weight proteins in the blood plasma. Most cadmium in blood is however found within the red blood cells. In the liver, cadmium binds to metal-lothionein (MT), a low molecular weight protein (6.5–7.0 kDa) that is induced by cadmium and other metals, such as zinc and copper. Each MT molecule can bind seven atoms of cadmium.

Recent experimental data indicate that ingested dietary cadmium may be bound to MT directly in the intestinal mucosa prior to uptake (Elsenhans et al., 1997). One part may be sequestered for several days and eliminated in faeces following desquamation of the mucosal cells. Ingested Cd–MT is absorbed as such. The absorbed Cd–MT complex is transported in the blood mainly to the kidneys (Groten et al., 1992). Women generally show higher concentrations of cadmium in blood, urine and kidneys than men, mainly owing to a higher rate of absorption as a consequence of low iron stores (Järup et al., 1998).

Experimental studies have shown that cadmium binds to the inner mitochondrial membrane of hepatocytes, which can lead to collapse of the membrane potential, depolarization and cell death (Muller, 1986; Liu and Liun, 1990; Martel et al., 1990). The mechanism may involve inhibition of enzymes of the citric acid cycle or the respiratory chain or by perturbation of mitochondrial calcium homeostasis. Glutathione-dependent biliary excretion of cadmium has been shown in animal experiments (Sugawara et al., 1996).

The Cd–MT complex is filtered through the renal glomeruli and reabsorbed in the S1 and S2 segments of the proximal tubules, where it accumulates (Nordberg et al., 1985). The complex is degraded by lysosomal activity in the tubular cells, releasing the free cadmium intracellularly, which induces renal MT synthesis. The biological half-time of cadmium in the kidney is in the order of decades. The kidney cortex contains the highest concentration of cadmium.

Cadmium may reach the embryo during early gestation, before the formation of the placenta. Once formed, the placental barrier excludes most cadmium from the foetus. Disturbances in placental function (nutrient transport, reduced blood flow, necrosis) due to cadmium toxicity may result in secondary foetal damage (Eisenmann and Miller, 1996).

Toxicity

Renal toxicity due to occupational exposure to cadmium was first described by Friberg (1948). The kidney is the critical organ on long-term cadmium exposure and the proximal tubuli are primarily affected. At a later stage, irreversible glomerular effects occur. Initially, the tubular damage results in an increased urinary output of several low molecular weight proteins such as β_2-microglobulin (MW 11.8 kDa), retinol-binding protein (21 kDa) and α_1-microglobulin (33 kDa), in addition to glucose and amino acids, due to impaired reabsorption in the proximal tubuli. Renal cell damage may result from lysosomal degradation of Cd–MT with liberation of free cadmium. Toxicity may also occur if the renal capacity for metallothionein synthesis and hence cadmium sequestration, is exceeded.

Recent data (Buchet et al., 1990; Järup et al., 1998) indicate that renal toxicity is induced at lower cadmium exposure levels than previously thought (WHO, 1992). Consequently, recommendations on human exposure limits (currently 7 μg Cd (kg body weight)$^{-1}$ week^{-1}; WHO, 1989) may have to be revised.

Inhalation of Cd may cause metal fume fever, which may be fatal in cases where oedema develops (WHO, 1992). Chronic exposure at lower exposure levels may cause chronic obstructive lung disease.

Itai-itai disease, which primarily affected post-menopausal women with multiple childbirths in the Jinzu River basin in Toyama Prefecture in Japan, is characterized by multiple bone fractures caused by the slightest external pressure and skeletal deformations (WHO, 1992; Nogawa and Kido, 1996). Radiological examinations of bone in patients showed osteomalacia and decalcification, and urine analysis generally showed an increased excretion of amino acids and proteins, including metallothionein, β_2-microglobulin, retinol-binding protein and lysozyme, in addition to glucose, calcium and cadmium. Pathological findings include osteomalacia, osteoporosis and renal tubular damage. The kidney concentration of cadmium has been found to be lower in patients than in controls, which may be due to the advanced kidney damage, resulting in increased urinary excretion of cadmium.

The Jinzu River, used for irrigation of rice field in the itai-itai endemic area, had carried cadmium from the Kamioka mine upstream. Cadmium was absorbed by rice which was subsequently, consumed, resulting in high exposure to cadmium. Studies established dose–response relationships between cadmium concentrations in rice, village rice consumption and the prevalence of renal effects, monitored as proteinuria and glucosuria. Cadmium-induced bone damage may be related to disturbances in vitamin D and parathyroid hormone metabolism (Kjellström, 1986).

Carcinogenicity and Genotoxicity

Cadmium was recently designated a human carcinogen (Group 1) by the IARC (1993). Occupational exposure to cadmium has been associated with lung tumours, and animal data include the lung as a target tissue for cadmium carcinogenicity. However, lung cancer causation due to cadmium exposure alone has recently been questioned, partly through a re-analysis of existing data (Sorahan *et al.*, 1995; Sorahan and Lancashire, 1997; Järup *et al.*, 1998). Other cancers are also suspected to be influenced by cadmium, notably prostate tumours, but the data are so far not considered convincing. The complex aetiology of prostatic cancer makes an association with a single factor difficult.

Animal experiments have shown that cadmium can produce tumours in multiple organs, including lungs, prostate and testis, and that dietary zinc can modulate the toxicity and carcinogenicity of cadmium (Takenaka *et al.*, 1983; Nordberg, 1993; Waalkes and Rehm, 1994a). Although generally protective, zinc can facilitate cadmium carcinogenesis in the prostate, probably through protection of the testes with ensuing maintenance of androgen production (Waalkes and Rehm, 1992). The rat is more sensitive than the hamster or the mouse to cadmium-induced pulmonary carcinogenesis after inhalation exposure. The basis for the differences in cadmium susceptibility between species, and also between strains within a species, is unclear (Waalkes and Rehm, 1994b).

The sensitivity to cadmium carcinogenicity may be linked to metallothionein expression and induction (Coogan *et al.*, 1994). The rat ventral prostate is highly susceptible to cadmium carcinogenicity whereas the dorsal prostate is a non-target site. Metallothionein gene expression is absent in the rat ventral prostate, while the dorsal prostate show constitutive and androgen-inducible expression (Ghatak *et al.*, 1996; Tohyama *et al.*, 1996).

Hypotheses to explain the genotoxicity of cadmium include an direct interaction with chromatin to induce strand breaks, cross-links or conformational changes; inhibition of DNA repair proteins; and catalysis of redox reactions generating DNA-reactive free radicals (Waalkes and Misra, 1996). All three hypotheses are supported by published experimental data, although dose levels and target cell characteristics have to be considered when the studies are evaluated in a human risk assessment scenario.

Mechanism of Action

The precise mechanism whereby cadmium exerts its toxic effect is unknown. However, as cadmium has a high affinity for thiols, the mechanism is likely to involve cadmium–thiol interactions. Cadmium may also interfere with calcium, for instance in the formation of bone. A model for cadmium-induced nephrotoxicity was recently presented by Nordberg (1996). Tubular toxicity is induced when the lysosomal degradation of MT with bound cadmium exceeds the rate of MT synthesis. Free cadmium will damage cellular membranes and inhibit calcium uptake and transport, resulting in an increased urinary excretion of calcium and proteins.

Exposure Assessment

Blood cadmium generally reflects the current exposure. However, the concentration of cadmium in blood is also influenced by the total body burden (Berglund *et al.*, 1994). If the exposure is discontinued, the blood cadmium concentration decreases fairly rapidly, with a half-time of 2–3 months (Elinder *et al.*, 1994). The influence of accumulated cadmium on the blood cadmium concentration leads to an increase in blood cadmium with age.

The concentration of cadmium in urine is mainly influenced by the body burden, and cadmium in urine is proportional to the concentration in the kidneys. However, tubular damage will increase the urinary output of cadmium in addition to proteins. Non-smokers generally have urinary cadmium concentrations below 1 μg l^{-1}, slowly increasing with age in parallel with the accumulation of cadmium in the kidney. It should be noted that in cases of tubular kidney damage, the normal reabsorption of Cd–MT decreases, and the excretion of cadmium in urine increases (Järup *et al.*, 1998). However, in the long run, both the concentrations of cadmium in kidney and urine will decrease, while the tubular damage remains.

Concentrations of cadmium in kidney cortex can be measured in samples obtained at autopsies, or *in vivo* by X-ray fluorescence spectrometry or neutron activation analysis (Nilsson and Skerfving, 1993). Whereas *in vivo* methods may be used for any population group, and may be used to follow individuals over time, the autopsy cases generally consist of 'victims of sudden and accidental death' in order to avoid effects of long-term diseases on kidney cadmium, and may not be representative of the general population.

Lead (Pb)

The chemical symbol Pb is derived from the Latin word for lead, *plumbum*. Lead has been known since antiquity, and is mentioned in *Exodus*. The alchemists believed lead to be the oldest metal and associated it with the planet Saturn (Hammond, 1995).

Lead is mainly obtained from the mineral galena (PbS). The pure element is a bluish-white metal of bright lustre. It is very soft, highly malleable, ductile and a poor conductor of electricity. Lead is very resistant to corrosion and has been used for water transport and in drainage systems since the Roman period. Large quantities of lead are used in storage batteries and significant amounts are also used for cable covering and ammunition. Alkyl-lead is still used as a gasoline additive, although several countries have largely abandoned the use of lead as an additive. Most of the alkyllead in gasoline is decomposed to inorganic lead during combustion. Lead is used as a radiation shield around X-ray equipment and nuclear reactors.

Basic lead carbonate and other lead compounds are used in paints, although less frequently nowadays owing to the health hazards associated with lead exposure. Lead oxide is used for crystal glass manufacture. Lead salts such as lead arsenate were previously used as insecticides.

Exposure to lead via inhalation may occur in certain occupational environments. The addition of alkyl lead compounds to gasoline is also a source of lead exposure via inhalation. The general population is mainly exposed to lead from food, either the food items themselves or through contamination of food stored in containers partly made of lead, such as soldered cans, or pottery glazed or painted with lead (Vahter et al., 1991; Rojas-Lopez et al., 1994; Romieu et al., 1995). Lead released from water pipes containing lead may contaminate drinking water. Lead-containing pigments in paint may contaminate soil and house dust and be a source of exposure, particularly during infancy and early childhood. High exposure, especially of children, has been observed due to glazing of tiles with lead obtained through the recycling of batteries (Vahter et al., 1997).

The WHO guideline value for lead in drinking water is $10 \mu g \, l^{-1}$ (WHO, 1993). An annual mean guideline value of $0.5-1.0 \mu g \, Pb \, m^{-3}$ of air has been proposed by the WHO (1987).

Uptake, Metabolism and Excretion

Inhaled particles of sufficiently small size ($< 5 \mu m$) are retained in the alveolar tract while larger particles are deposited in the upper airways and may be swallowed. The respiratory absorption of lead from inhaled particles may vary between 20 and 50% depending on the particle size (WHO, 1987; Skerfving, 1993; Elinder et al., 1994). Ingested soluble lead is absorbed in the gastro-intestinal tract, and children generally have a higher rate of absorption (up to 50% of ingested lead) than adults (about 10%). Dermal uptake of inorganic lead is generally low. Lead is absorbed in the blood plasma and transferred to the red blood cells. About 99% of lead in blood is present in the erythrocytes, manily bound to δ-aminolaevulinic acid dehydratase (Skerfving, 1993).

Lead has been shown to interact with the calcium-dependent second messengers calmodulin and protein kinase C (reviewed by Goldstein, 1993). Based on studies on the transport of lead into ghost erythrocytes and adrenal medullary cells, it has been postulated that cellular uptake of lead occur via Ca^{2+} channels and/or by a mechanism involving the anion (HCO_3^- / Cl^-) transport exchange system (Simons, 1984, 1986; Simons and Pocok, 1987).

A major part (about 90%) of the total body burden of lead is found in the skeleton, and the skeleton thus represents an endogenous source of lead exposure (O'Flaherty, 1993; Skerfving et al., 1993). Lead is found in both trabecular (about 10%) and cortical bone. Skeletal disease, menopause and pregnancy are conditions that may result in elevated lead exposure levels due to the mobilisation of stored lead (Silbergeld et al., 1993; Berlin et al., 1995). Lead is also incorporated in teeth.

Lead crosses the blood–brain and blood–placenta barriers. Carotid perfusion studies on rats suggested that lead in blood enters the brain as the free ion or as a closely related inorganic complex (Deane and Bradbury, 1990). The concentration of lead in cord blood at term is only slightly lower than in maternal blood (Eisenmann and Miller, 1996). The concentration of lead in the placenta varies, but the placenta does not appear to accumulate lead. Foetal exposure to lead has been shown to affect neurobehavioural parameters in children and also EEG profiles and hearing thresholds (Mushak et al., 1989).

Cessation of occupational lead exposure results in a decrease in blood-lead levels, which has been described with a three-compartment exponential model (Nilsson et al., 1991). The first component has a half-time of about one month while the second component probably reflects trabecular bone and has a half-time of about one year. The third and slowest component probably reflects cortical bone and has a half-time of about 13 years. However, substantial interindividual differences in kinetics have been observed. Excretion of lead occurs via urine and faeces.

The intracellular distribution of lead may be regulated by low molecular weight proteins with a high binding affinity for lead. Such proteins have been isolated from rat, monkey and human tissues, including kidney and brain, and have been suggested to play a role in mediating lead toxicity (Fowler and DuVal, 1991; Fowler et al., 1993; Quintanilla-Vega et al., 1995).

Toxicity

The toxicity of lead has been recognized since antiquity. Early interest in occupational health hazards associated with lead exposure has in more recent times given way to public health concern due to chronic exposure of sensitive population, notably children, to lead. Lead and its compounds primarily affect the central and peripheral nervous systems, and the developing nervous system is the most sensitive target organ system.

Signs of acute alkyl lead intoxication are irritability, insomnia, anorexia, nausea, tremor, cramps, delirium and coma (Skerfving, 1993). Severe inorganic lead intoxication may result in encephalopathy with symptoms such as ataxia, coma and convulsions. Morphological changes within the brain include diffuse cerebral oedema, swelling and proliferation of endothelial cells, focal necrosis and astrocyte proliferation in grey and white matter. Lower lead exposure levels mainly result in subjective symptoms such as fatigue, impaired concentration, memory loss, insomnia and irritability. Lead also affects auditory, visual and motor functions. Acute lead exposure may damage the proximal tubuli of the kidney causing proteinuria. Prolonged heavy lead exposure may result in interstitial nephritis, with interstitial fibrosis, tubular atrophy and arteriosclerotic changes. Colic, diarrhoea, cramps, nausea and loss of appetite are gastro-intestinal symptoms of lead intoxication. Acute exposure to high levels of lead can cause haemolytic anaemia as a result of increased erythrocyte plasma membrane fragility which is accompanied by inhibition of Na^+/K^+-dependent ATPases. High exposure to lead may result in the precipitation of lead sulphide in the gingiva ('lead lines').

Various psychometric and behavioural tests have been used in order to assess lead-induced neurotoxicity. A reduction in peripheral nerve conduction velocity have been observed in patients without obvious clinical signs. Peripheral neuropathy primarily affects the large myelinated nerve fibres, with demyelination and axonal degeneration. In vitro studies on cultured neurons suggest that lead primarily inhibits myelination and neurite initiation. The biochemical mechanism is unclear but may involve interactions with calcium and disturbance of calcium-mediated functions rather than a direct effect on the cytoskeleton.

Children are at particular risk to the neurotoxic properties of lead owing to their greater absorption of ingested lead, an immature blood–brain barrier and a nervous system still under development (WHO, 1995). In 1943, Byers and Lord reported that low-dose lead exposure, without overt clinical manifestations of intoxication, could induce persistent neurological damage. Prospective studies of children using cognitive testing in combination with early childhood lead exposure analysis and extensive information on socio-economic variables established associations between lead exposure in early life and decrements in IQ scores (Needleman et al., 1979). The pioneering work by Needleman et al. (1979) was followed by several other studies of similar design and the combined results have been evaluated by meta-analysis (Schwartz, 1993).

Infants and very young children are typically tested using the Bayley Scales of Infant Development (Mental Development Index, MDI) while older children are assessed using the McCarthy Scales of Child Development or Wechsler Intelligence Scale for Children-Revised (WISC-R). In recent years several longitudinal studies on children have been conducted (Needleman, 1996). These studies primarily address three major issues: (1) verification on cognitive impairment based on alterations in IQ scores or similar indices; (2) differentiating the contribution of lead exposure from other factors, such as socio-economic status and hereditary factors;

and (3) to define the dose–effect relationship. Bellinger et al. (1992) noted a decrease in cognitive function, evaluated using the WISC-R test, at blood lead levels of 40–140 μg l^{-1}. Impairment of cognitive and behavioural function is also seen in adult populations occupationally exposed to lead, albeit at higher blood lead concentrations than in children (Stollery et al., 1991).

There is no defined threshold for the neurotoxicity of lead. The CDC has identified a blood lead level of 100 μg l^{-1} as a level of concern (CDC, 1991), based on multiple studies on associations between blood lead levels and decrements in IQ scores in groups of children, assessed by standardized tests on neurobehavioural development, such as the MDI and the McCarthy scale. A blood lead level of 100 μg l^{-1} corresponds to a daily lead intake of about 60 μg in children. The third US National Health and Nutrition Examination Survey (NHANES III) conducted in 1988–91 indicated that 8.9% of the American children 1–5 years of age exceeded the level of concern for lead exposure, a substantial decline since the previous study.

Lead inhibits the biosynthesis of haem at several points through interaction with key enzymes, particularly δ-aminolaevulinic acid dehydratase (ALAD) and ferrochelatase (Woods, 1996). ALAD catalyses the first and rate-limiting step in the haem biosynthetic pathway and is inactivated through the displacement of zinc by lead at a thiol-mediated binding site (Goering, 1993). In non-erythropoietic tissues haem is mainly incorporated in cytochromes and other enzymes and participates in various oxidative processes vital for cellular respiration, xenobiotic metabolism and antioxidant defence. Disruption of the haem biosynthetic pathway may consequently have multiple effects on cellular function. Genetic polymorphism in ALAD has been described (Wetmur, 1994). One form of the encoded protein was shown to have a higher affinity for lead which resulted in higher blood lead levels in individuals carrying this gene variant. Thus, ALAD genotype may be a factor to consider when lead exposure assessments are based on blood-lead levels, although conflicting data have also been presented (Bergdahl et al., 1997a; Sithisarankul et al., 1997).

Individuals homozygous for ALAD deficiency show clinical symptoms similar to acute intermittent porphyria, whereas heterozygotes generally are free of symptoms but are more vulnerable to increased blood lead levels (Doss et al., 1982, 1983; Batlle et al., 1987).

Lead increases the fragility and reduces the lifespan of circulating erythrocytes which may be linked to inhibition of Na^+, K^+-ATPase and erythrocyte pyrimidine 5-nucleotidase and changes in membrane proteins (Hernberg and Nikkanen, 1970; Paglia et al., 1975; Raghavan et al., 1981; Ichiba and Tomokuni, 1990).

Lead has been shown to impair renal mitochondrial function and haem biosynthesis (Fowler et al., 1987; Woods, 1996). In addition, renal gene expression is modulated by lead (Mistry et al., 1985).

Exposure Assessment

Whole blood, plasma, bone and teeth are examples of biological specimens that have been utilized for the assessment of human lead exposure. Techniques for determining lead in bone *in vivo* by X-ray fluorescence spectrometry have recently become available (Nilsson and Skerfving, 1993). These techniques could be utilized in epidemiological studies (Skerfving *et al.*, 1993). Although blood is an imperfect indicator of lead levels in critical target tissues (i.e. brain), it is the most widely used total exposure indicator. Lead binds mainly to the erythrocytes, but as these tend to become saturated, non-linear relationships between lead in blood and uptake and between metabolic and toxic effects and lead in blood have been observed (Skerfving *et al.*, 1993; Bergdahl *et al.*, 1997b).

The concentrations of lead in umbilical cord blood and in the dentine of shed teeth have been used as indices of foetal and childhood lead exposure. The levels in dentine gives an integrated measure of exposure during teeth mineralization while blood levels reflect current exposure.

Seasonal variations in blood-lead levels have been observed in small children (Johnson *et al.*, 1996), probably reflecting an increased exposure to environmental lead during the summer months in temperate climates. However, it has also been suggested (Moon, 1994) that the increase is due to the increased synthesis of vitamin D and associated higher uptake of lead.

Several studies in different countries have shown that the average blood-lead level has decreased dramatically in parallel with the introduction and increased use of unleaded gasoline (Strömberg *et al.*, 1995).

Mercury (Hg)

The name of the element stems from the name of the planet Mercury (Hammond, 1995). The chemical symbol for mercury (Hg) is derived from the Latin word *hydrargyrum* ('liquid silver'). Mercury was known to the ancient Chinese and Hindus and has been found in Egyptian tombs from 1500 BC. Mercury is the only common metal that is liquid at ordinary temperatures and only rarely occurs free in nature. The chief mercury mineral is cinnabar, HgS. The metal is obtained by heating HgS in a current of air and by condensing the vapour. Mercury is a heavy, silvery white metal which easily forms alloys (amalgams) with other metals, notably gold, silver and tin. The metal is used in thermometers, barometers, diffusion pumps and other instruments. It is also used in mercury-vapour lamps and electronic apparatus, such as switches, in pesticides, mercury cells for caustic soda and chlorine production, in dental amalgams, antifouling paint, batteries and catalysts. The most important salts are mercuric chloride, mercurous chloride (calomel),

mercury fulminate (as detonator in explosives) and mercuric sulphide (vermillion, a paint pigment). Organic mercury compounds (alkyl and aryl compounds) have been used as herbicides and fungicides.

The use of metallic mercury for the amalgamation of gold in small-scale mining operations has recently been recognized as an environmental health problem in several regions around the world, such as the Amazon Basin (Palheta and Taylor, 1995; De Lacerda and Salomons, 1998). The acute health risks to the miners when the mercury is driven off by heating and the larger scale problem of environmental contamination by mercury and biologically formed methylmercury are matters of concern. Owing to the long residence time of mercury vapour in the atmosphere, regional use of mercury may result in global distribution and environmental problems far from the source of mercury release (Fitzgerald and Clarkson, 1991).

The main form of mercury of environmental concern is methylmercury. Methylmercury may be formed through methylation of inorganic mercury by microorganisms in aqueous environments (Jensen and Jernelöv, 1969). Methylmercury is enriched in the aquatic food chain and the mercury concentration in predatory fish and whales may exceed 1 mg kg^{-1}, while fish from unpolluted waters contain less than 0.05 mg kg^{-1}. The high concentration of mercury in certain species of fish is a public health concern in fish-eating communities. Large-scale poisonings have also occurred due to consumption of seed grain treated with methylmercury compounds (Bakir *et al.*, 1973). Primary risk groups are pregnant and nursing women, owing to the susceptibility of the developing nervous system of the foetus and infant to the toxicity of methylmercury.

Methylmercury was first recognized as an environmental health problem after the Minamata epidemic disaster (Hamada and Osame, 1996). Mercury compounds present in the effluent from an acetaldehyde factory were discharged into Minamata Bay, causing intoxication in the fishing communities. The first case was reported in 1954 and by the end of November 1993 2256 cases had been officially recorded. About 10 years after the Minamata poisoning a similar incident occurred in Niigata, although this time waste water was discharged into a river, restricting the number of persons affected. The main source of methylmercury exposure in both cases was contaminated fish. The health risks associated with the consumption of methylmercury-contaminated fish have been the subject of several national and international reviews (Berglund *et al.*, 1971; WHO, 1990a).

The WHO guideline value for mercury in drinking water is 1 μg l^{-1} (WHO, 1993). No ambient air quality guideline value for mercury has been proposed, although 1 μg m^{-3} as an annual average, irrespective of chemical form, is considered to offer adequate protection against health effects (WHO, 1987). The high concentrations of methylmercury in certain species of predatory fish have led to the issue of dietary recommendations for pregnant and nursing women in some countries.

Uptake, Metabolism and Excretion—Inorganic Mercury

Gastro-intestinal absorption of metallic mercury is minimal ($< 0.01\%$ in rats), while about 80% of inhaled mercury vapour is absorbed in the lungs (WHO, 1991b). Elemental mercury vapour is dissolved in the blood and distributed to other organs. Oxidation of elemental mercury to divalent mercury is rapid and catalysed by catalase in the red blood cells. Before oxidation, mercury vapour can penetrate the blood–brain barrier and induce damage within the brain subsequent to oxidation. Foetal exposure to mercury vapour released from dental amalgam have been demonstrated both in animal experiments (Vimy et al., 1990) and in humans (Drasch et al., 1994; Lutz et al., 1996).

Less than 10% of the ingested amount of inorganic mercury salts is absorbed in the gastro-intestinal tract, although absorption may be higher in children. The distribution of divalent mercury between red blood cells and plasma is roughly equal (WHO, 1991b). Inorganic mercury in plasma is probably bound to proteins and low molecular weight thiols (Lau and Sarkar, 1979; Zalups and Barfuss, 1995a, b). The kinetics of mercury in blood have been investigated in human volunteers following short-term exposure to mercury vapour. The first phase of inorganic mercury elimination from blood had a half-time of about 2–4 days and the second phase had a half-time of approximately 2–6 weeks (WHO, 1991b; Barregård et al., 1992). In contrast to mercury vapour, only a small fraction of divalent mercury penetrates the blood–brain and blood–placenta barriers (Khayat and Dencker, 1982; WHO, 1991b). However, a high proportion of inorganic mercury has been found in the brains of humans chronically exposed to methylmercury (Friberg and Mottet, 1989) and in monkeys administered methylmercury by oral dosage for several months (Vahter et al., 1994). The high proportion of inorganic mercury in these animals indicates demethylation of methylmercury within the brain.

The hepatic uptake of inorganic divalent mercury is independent of temperature and does not appear to involve thiol-dependent transport or calcium channels (Blazka and Shaikh, 1991, 1992). Within the hepatocyte, both inorganic mercury and methylmercury readily react with intracellular thiols such as glutathione (GSH) but also bind to metallothionein. Although the major part of hepatocyte GSH (about 90%) is localized in the cytosol, the mitochondrial GSH pool appears more critical for cell viability.

Inorganic mercury is mainly deposited in the kidney, which also is the critical organ following ingestion of inorganic mercury salts. Inorganic mercury is taken up by the proximal tubule and mercury also accumulates along the proximal tubule after exposure to organic forms of mercury (Zalups, 1991; Zalups and Barfuss, 1993). Excretion of inorganic mercury occurs mainly by the urinary route.

Toxicity

Brief exposure to high concentrations ($> 2\,\mathrm{mg\,m^{-3}}$) of mercury vapour may cause acute pneumonitis, chest pain, dyspnea and paroxysmal cough and chronic symptoms such as nervousness, irritability, lack of ambition and loss of sexual (McFarland and Reigel, 1978). Lower concentrations ($> 0.1\,\mathrm{mg\,m^{-3}}$ daily) may result in loss of appetite, weight loss, tremor, abnormal emotionality, salivation, gingivitis and proteinuria (Smith et al., 1970; Miller et al., 1975). Urinary mercury levels of about 100 $\mu\mathrm{g\,g^{-1}}$ creatinine, corresponding to air concentrations of $> 80\mu\mathrm{g\,m^{-3}}$, may increase the risk of neurological symptoms (tremor, erethism) of mercury intoxication and also kidney damage, manifested as proteinuria. Lower exposure levels ($25–80\ \mu\mathrm{g\,m^{-3}}$, corresponding to $30–100\ \mu$ $\mathrm{Hg\,g^{-1}}$ creatinine) may cause more subtle neurological effects, such as tremor and decreased nerve conduction velocity, and also diffuse subjective symptoms (fatigue, irritability, loss of appetite). Ingestion of mercuric compounds may cause gastro-enteritis, gastro-intestinal ulceration, haemorrhage and acute tubular necrosis. Prolonged dermal exposure to mercurials have been shown to cause 'pink disease', characterized by irritability, weight loss, painful extremities, rash and photophobia (WHO, 1991b).

Uptake, Metabolism and Excretion—Methylmercury

Several organic mercury compounds may cause toxic effects. Phenylmercury and methoxyethylmercury are rapidly degraded, mainly in the liver, to form inorganic mercury. Dimethylmercury is a neurotoxic and highly volatile organic mercury compound that easily penetrates the skin. However, the organic mercury compound that is usually considered to be of greatest toxicological interest is methylmercury. Methylmercury is rapidly and efficiently ($> 90\%$) absorbed in the gastro-intestinal tract and evenly distributed to other tissues within 4 days, although maximum levels in brain are attained after 5–6 days (Kershaw et al., 1980; WHO, 1990a). The major part of methylmercury in blood is found in the red blood cells. The erythrocyte-to-plasma ratio of methylmercury is about 20 in man (Kershaw et al., 1980) but over 100 in rats, probably owing to strong binding to haemoglobin cysteine residues in the latter species (Naganuma et al., 1980; Doi, 1990). The brain-to-blood ratio of mercury after prolonged methyl-mercury exposure varies considerably between animal species, and is usually lower in non-primate animals than in monkeys and humans (Omata et al., 1986; WHO, 1990a).

The daily elimination rate of methylmercury is about 1% of the total body burden. The biological half-time in blood and the whole body has been described by a single compartment and estimated as 40–70 days (WHO, 1990a).

Methylmercury crosses the placental barrier, which results in foetal exposure (WHO, 1990a). Animal experiments have shown that mercury is more evenly distributed in the foetus than in the dam following maternal methylmercury administration (Dock et al., 1994). Methylmercury is also excreted in milk, resulting in infant exposure during the sucking period (Amin-Zaki et al., 1981; Grandjean et al., 1994a, b)

In adult humans and other mammals, ingested methylmercury is primarily excreted in the faeces as inorganic Hg following demethylation in the liver and intestines (WHO, 1990a). Animal experiments conducted on rats (Thomas et al., 1982, 1988), mice (Doherty et al., 1977; Rowland et al., 1983; Shi et al., 1990), hamsters (Dock et al., 1995; Nordenhäll et al., 1995) and monkeys (Lok, 1983) have shown that the rate of methylmercury excretion during the neonatal period is very low. The increased rate of excretion after weaning has been attributed to changes in the intestinal microflora (Rowland et al., 1983), an increased biliary glutathione excretion, with concomitant increased excretion of methylmercury and inorganic mercury (Ballatori and Clarkson, 1985), and a decreased intestinal reabsorption of inorganic Hg (Kostial et al., 1983).

Toxicity

Signs of methylmercury toxicity becomes evident after a latency period in the order of 2–5 weeks. Methylmercury primarily affects the central nervous system and the foetus and the infant child are more sensitive than the adult (Choi, 1989). Methylmercury affects the sensory, visual and auditory cerebral functions and the cerebellar (co-ordination) capacity. Paraesthesia is an early symptom followed by constriction of the visual field, deafness, dysarthria and ataxia. In severe cases, seizures, coma and death will follow. Some of the effects are partly reversible, depending on the compensatory capacity of the nervous system.

Both the central and peripheral nervous system are affected by methylmercury. Within the brain, several distinct regions are affected by focal damage. Pathological lesions are primarily found in calcarine cortices, dorsal root ganglia and cerebellum, and correlate well with the clinical signs of intoxication (constriction of visual field, sensory disturbance and cerebellar ataxia).

In prenatally exposed children, cerebral palsy characterized by microcephaly, hyper reflexia and gross motor and mental impairment have been observed. In most cases the mothers were asymptomatic or had only mild symptoms which largely disappeared. The main clinical features in affected children were retardation of physical and mental development. In contrast to what is seen in the adult brain, the damage is more uniform. The possibility of a threshold for foetal methylmercury toxicity has been widely discussed. Using data from the exposed populations in Japan and Iraq and other available data, it was calculated that a maternal hair mercury concentration of 10–20 μg g^{-1} during pregnancy implies a 5% risk of adverse effects in the offspring (Cox et al., 1989; WHO, 1991a). However, it cannot be excluded that subtle effects may be detected by psychological or behavioural tests at even lower exposure levels.

Mechanism of Toxicity

Metallothionein has a high binding affinity for inorganic mercury whereas organic mercury compounds are bound to a considerably lesser degree. Owing to the high affinity of inorganic mercury and methylmercury for thiols, it is highly probable that mercury is primarily found as a thiol ligand in tissues and fluids. The cellular uptake and excretion of mercury compounds are therefore likely to involve thiol transport systems. Conjugates of GSH that are released into the bile are degraded by the sequential action of γ-glutamyltransferase and dipeptidase to glutamate, glycine and cysteine S-conjugates. The degradation of mercury–GSH conjugates is determined by the activities of the participating enzymes in the liver, bile and kidney. Substantial species differences in the renal-to-hepatic ratio of γ-glutamyltransferase activity suggest that the thiol complex of mercury that enters renal circulation will differ among species.

Uptake of mercury may occur through endocytosis of albumin-bound mercury or via uptake of a mercury–thiol complex. Inhibition of γ-glutamyltransferase has been shown to reduce the renal concentration of mercury administered as inorganic mercury or methylmercury, suggesting that this enzyme plays an important part in the mechanism of renal uptake of mercury. Other studies have shown that the urinary output of GSH and mercury increases when γ-glutamyltransferase activity is inhibited.

Mercuric chloride causes uncoupling and depolarization in isolated mitochondria. Divalent inorganic mercury also perturbs calcium homeostasis in hepatocytes. An increase in cytosolic free calcium may be due to an increased influx of calcium ions across the plasma membrane or a release of free calcium from intracellular stores.

Methylmercury inhibits neuronal migration and mitotic activity in the central nervous system (Mottet et al., 1997). The higher vulnerability of the foetus and child may partly be due to differences in the blood–brain barrier (BBB). The development of the tight junctions of the BBB may not be complete at the time of birth, and the foetus may also have systems for transport across the BBB not operational in adults. Also, some parts of the brain, notably the hypothalamus, have an incomplete BBB. In order to support the brain with essential nutrients such as vitamins, ions, amino acids and glucose, a number of specific carrier systems have been developed. These carrier systems may also govern the uptake of neurotoxic metals, such as mercury, lead and aluminium. Uptake of methylmercury is probably mediated by the neutral amino acid transport system (Aschner and Clarkson, 1987, 1988; Aschner and Aschner, 1990; Kajiwara et al., 1996). Methylmercury is taken up as an L-cysteine complex, a structural analogue of methionine. The uptake is inhibited by free L-methionine and by 2-aminobicyclo[2,2,1] heptane-2-carboxylic acid, a specific inhibitor of the L-amino acid transporter.

The permeability of the BBB can be modulated by inflammatory mediators and also by toxic agents. A direct action on the BBB integrity will result in influx of plasma into the brain parenchyma and ensuing oedema. Alterations of the specific transport systems could lead to transient or permanent deprivation of vital nutrients. The BBB integrity may also be influenced secondary to action on glial or neuronal function.

The finer details of the mechanism of methylmercury-induced changes in cognitive function and the health risk to children at low levels of maternal methylmercury exposure remains to be elucidated. Another important issue is the extent to which cognitive deficits detected at an early age can be compensated for during later development.

Exposure Assessment

Hair, blood and urine samples have been used to monitor mercury exposure (WHO, 1990a, 1991b; Elinder et al., 1994). Urine and blood are specimens frequently used in the assessment of inorganic mercury exposure, while methylmercury exposure is preferentially monitored through analysis of hair. When blood samples are used for mercury exposure analysis it is important to distinguish between inorganic mercury and methylmercury. Inorganic mercury show an equal distribution between red blood cells and plasma whereas methylmercury preferentially binds to the red blood cells. Hence plasma samples are to be preferred for the assessment of inorganic mercury exposure. Differentiation between inorganic mercury and methylmercury can be achieved by speciation analysis using selective extraction or reduction techniques and ion-exchange, gas or liquid chromatography.

Temporal analysis of methylmercury exposure is possible, utilizing the fact that hair grows at approximately 1 cm per month (Cox et al., 1989). The blood-to-hair ratio of methylmercury in man is about 1:250, although individual differences are considerable (WHO, 1990a).

TOXICOLOGICAL ASPECTS ON SOME OTHER TRACE ELEMENTS

Aluminium (Al)

Alum was used by the Greeks and Romans as an astringent in medicine and as a mordant in dyeing. The metal was isolated by Wohler in 1827. The element was named aluminium, derived from the Latin words *alumen* or *alum*, in the early nineteenth century, although the American Chemical Society has used the name aluminum in their publications since 1925. The element is mainly obtained from the mineral bauxite. Aluminum and aluminium alloys are appreciated owing to their strength and lightness and they have found a multitude of applications, including the manufacture of cooking utensils, aircrafts and rockets (WHO, 1997). Natural aluminium minerals are also used for water purification and aluminium salts have found use in antacids and antiperspirants.

The concentration of dissolved aluminium in natural freshwater is usually low (1–50 μg l^{-1}) but considerably higher in acidic water (500–1000 μg l^{-1}) (WHO, 1997). Waters affected by acids from mining operations may show even higher concentrations of dissolved aluminium.

Non-occupational human exposure to aluminium occurs mainly via food and is usually less than 15 mg day^{-1}. The use of aluminium-containing antacids and buffered analgesics may result in intake levels that are two or three orders of magnitude higher. Although the uptake of aluminium from these sources is very low, it may be enhanced by citrate.

Toxicity

The intake of aluminium in the form of antacids, although exceeding the normal dietary intake levels by two or three orders of magnitude, has not been associated with adverse health effects (WHO, 1997). The gastro-intestinal uptake of aluminium is generally very low but can be enhanced in the presence of citrate. Aluminium is a potential neurotoxic agents in humans (WHO, 1997). Cases of encephalopathy have been recorded in patients receiving dialysis treatment for renal failure (Rozas et al., 1978a, b; Platts and Anastassiades, 1981). The dialysis fluids used contained high concentrations of aluminium, usually above 200 μg l^{-1}. The pathogenic role of aluminium in the onset and progression of Alzheimer's disease is controversial and not supported by available data (Savory et al., 1996; WHO, 1997). Occupational exposure to aluminium compounds has been associated with pulmonary fibrosis and irritant-induced asthma (Dinman, 1988; O'Donnell et al., 1989; Kongerud, 1992; WHO, 1997). However, the exposure situations are usually complex and involve other compounds that may contribute to the observed effects.

Beryllium (Be)

The name of the element can be derived from the Greek words *beryllos* and *beryl*. Beryllium was discovered as the oxide by Vauquelin in 1798 and the metal was independently isolated in 1828 by Wohler and Bussy. Aquamarine and emerald are precious forms of the mineral beryl.

Toxicity

Exposure to beryllium is primarily an occupational health problem. Massive exposure ($> 100 \mu g \, m^{-3}$) to airborne beryllium causes acute beryllium disease, characterized by chemical pneumonitis, which may be fatal (WHO, 1990b). Long-term exposure to lower concentrations of beryllium may cause chronic beryllium disease, a form of granulomatous interstitial pneumonitis with symptoms including dyspnea, cough and reduced pulmonary function (Rossman, 1996). The disease may have an immunological component. Recently, it was proposed that a genetic modification of the major histocompatibility complex allele HLA-DPB1 may be used as a biomarker of susceptibility to chronic beryllium disease (Richeldi *et al.*, 1993).

Carcinogenicity

The International Agency for Research on Cancer has found sufficient evidence for the carcinogenicity of beryllium and beryllium compounds in humans and experimental animals to classify beryllium as carcinogenic to humans (IARC, 1993).

Bismuth (Bi)

The name originates from the German *Weisse Masse* (white mass), later transformed to *Wisuth* and *Bisemutum*. The element was confused with lead and tin in early times but shown to be distinct from lead in 1753 by Claude Geoffrey the Younger.

Bismuth is found in nature as the pure element and the oxide (Bi_2O_3) and sulphide (Bi_2S_3) and is mainly used in alloys but also as a pigment in cosmetic preparations (Fowler and Vouk, 1986; Bradley *et al.*, 1989). Bismuth salts have been used medicinally in the treatment of gastric ulcers (bismuth subcitrate) and diarrhoea (bismuth subsalicylate) (Arduino and DuPont, 1993).

Uptake, Metabolism and Excretion

The uptake of bismuth from ingested salts is generally low. The bioavailability of ingested bismuth subnitrate (6.3 g Bi), subcitrate (0.9 g Bi) and subgallate (0.5 g Bi) was estimated to be less then 0.2% (Thomas *et al.*, 1987). Benet (1991) estimated the gastro-intestinal absorption of bismuth from ingested bismuth subcitrate to be 0.2–0.3%.

The total absorption of bismuth within 8 days after a single oral dose of bismuth subsalicylate was estimated to be 0.003% (Bierer, 1990). Absorbed bismuth is mainly excreted in urine (Slikkerveer and de Wolff, 1989).

The blood level of bismuth is usually below 10 $\mu g \, l^{-1}$ (Thomas *et al.*, 1987; Thomas, 1991) and the highest tissue levels are found in the kidney (Slikkerveer and de Wolff, 1989). Bismuth has been shown to bind to a low molecular weight protein, distinct from metallothionein, in the kidney (Piotrowski and Szymanska, 1976; Szymanska and Piotrowski, 1980). Bismuth-containing inclusion bodies have been detected in renal tissue and may explain the high retention of Bi in the kidney (Beaver and Burr, 1963; Fowler and Goyer, 1975).

Toxicity

Reports on bismuth toxicity in humans are mainly found in connection with its therapeutic use. Nephropathies, encephalopathy, arthrosis, damage to the oral epithelium (gingivitis, stomatitis) and melanosis have been observed in patients treated with Bi-containing preparations (Bradley *et al.*, 1989; Slikkerveer and de Wolff, 1989). The effects depended on the type of preparations used.

During the mid-1970s, reports from France (Buge *et al.*, 1974; Martin-Bouyer *et al.*, 1980) and Australia (Burns *et al.*, 1974; Lowe, 1974; Robertson, 1974) showed a form of bismuth-associated encephalopathy of unknown aetiology. The clinical symptoms described in both countries (confusion, tremor, motor disturbances) were similar and developed after prolonged therapy (from 4 weeks to 30 years) with high doses (0.7–20 g day^{-1}) of mainly bismuth subnitrate (France) and bismuth subgallate (Australia) (Serfontein and Mekel, 1979). The effects were often reversible and disappeared after cessation of Bi therapy, although fatalities were also reported. In a review of 63 cases of bismuth-associated encephalopathy, blood bismuth levels of 170–2850 $\mu g \, l^{-1}$ were reported among the patients (Hillemand *et al.*, 1977). An epidemiological study saw no correlation between encephalopathy and age, type of bismuth compound administered, dose or length of treatment (Martin-Bouyer *et al.*, 1980). Constipation was more prevalent as a therapeutic indication among the encephalopathy patients, whereas diarrhoea and colon disease were more frequent among the controls (bismuth therapy without encephalopathy). The data suggested that the intestinal microflora may be of importance for the absorption of bismuth.

Chromium (Cr)

Chromium takes its name from the Greek word for colour, *chroma*. The element was discovered by Vauquelin in 1797.

Essentiality

Trivalent chromium [Cr(III)] is considered to be an essential trace element (Andersson, 1989; Mertz, 1992; Cohen, 1993), although this has recently been questioned (Nord 1995). In contrast, the hexavalent form of chromium (Cr(VI)) is generally regarded as highly toxic (WHO, 1988). For the purpose of this review, only Cr(VI) will be dealt with in the following.

Toxicity

Major sources of chromium exposure are chromated steel, cement, leathergoods and welding fumes. Chromium is a cause of occupational allergic contact dermatitis and the trivalent form of chromium [Cr(III)] is considered to be the sensitizing agent. Hexavalent chromium may be released from chromium metal by the corrosive action of sweat and penetrate the skin. Cr(VI) is subsequently reduced to Cr(III). Inhalation of corrosive Cr(VI) compounds may lead to ulceration and perforation of the nasal septum.

Carcinogenicity and Genotoxicity

Chromium has been associated with human tumours of the respiratory and nasal tracts since the late nineteenth century (IARC, 1980, 1990; WHO, 1988; Klein, 1996). The major occupational health hazard related to chromium exposure is encountered by chromate production workers, due to the inhalation of chromate particulates and dust. Other occupational settings where chromate exposure is prevalent are pigment manufacturing and the metallurgical industry with metal grinding, welding, etc. A positive correlation between increased concentration of chromium in lung tissue and chromium-induced lung cancers has been observed. Chromium accumulates primarily in the upper lobes.

Animal bioassays have demonstrated that Cr(VI) but not Cr(III) is carcinogenic (IARC, 1990). Chromium-induced tumours are mainly found at the primary site of exposure. The lack of distant site tumours is most likely due to chromium chemistry. Reduction of Cr(VI) to the trivalent form of chromium is accompanied by a substantial reduction in bioavailability. Trivalent chromium cannot be readily transported across cellular membranes. Experimentally, the slightly soluble hexavalent chromium salts are most effective in inducing tumours, while chromium metal or trivalent chromium compounds have rarely found to be tumourigenic, regardless of route of exposure.

Hexavalent chromium oxyanion is believed to be taken up by cells via the sulphate anion transport system. Hexavalent chromium is reduced intracellularly to Cr(III) via Cr(V) and Cr(IV) intermediates (Wetterhahn and Hamilton, 1989). These intermediates may exist as short-lived organic ligands. Hexavalent chromium pro-duce DNA strand breaks, DNA–DNA and DNA–protein cross-links and modified nucleotides, such as 8-hydroxyguanine, indicative of oxygen radical formation (Wetterhahn et al., 1989; Aiyar et al., 1991; Costa, 1991). However, these reactions are not formed in cell-free systems in the absence of reducing agents and the notion today is that the highly reactive intermediates formed during cellular Cr(VI) reduction are primarily responsible for the genotoxicity (Klein, 1996). Cellular reducing agents that may be of importance for Cr(VI) reduction includes ascorbate and sulphydryl compounds such as cysteine and glutathione (Borges et al., 1991; Standeven and Wetterhahn, 1992; Kortenkamp and O'Brien, 1994; Stearns et al., 1994). Although hydroxyl, cysteinyl and thionyl radicals may be formed during the reduction of Cr(VI), it is not known if these intermediates are of relevance in chromium-induced carcinogenesis (Wetterhahn et al., 1989; Standeven and Wetterhahn, 1991; Cohen et al., 1993).

Hexavalent chromium compounds have been tested for mutagenicity in many mammalian and bacterial test systems and generally found to give positive results (IARC, 1990). Trivalent chromium compounds are generally inactive in mutagenicity tests although positive results in Salmonella have been achieved when Cr(III) was complexed with organic ligands such as 2,2'-bipyridyl or 1,10-phenanthroline.

Chromium have been shown to inhibit inducible gene expression which may be linked to the formation of persistent DNA-adducts or cross-links (Wetterhahn et al., 1989).

Chromium is highly clastogenic and several studies suggest that human cells are more sensitive than rodent cells to chromosomal damage. Chromosomal damage and DNA strand breaks were reduced in mammalian cells in the presence of the antioxidants ascorbate and vitamin E. Chromate also disrupts chromosome segregation in dividing cells, resulting in aneuploidy and micronuclei. Cytogenetic studies of chromate workers and welders, exposed to chromium-containing fumes, have shown an increase in sister chromatid exchange and chromosome aberrations in peripheral lymphocytes (Stella et al., 1982; Popp et al., 1991; Jelmert et al., 1994).

Nickel (Ni)

The name of the element is derived from the German word Kupfernickel meaning 'Old Nick's (= Satan's) copper'. Nickel was discovered by Cronstedt in 1751.

Toxicity

Exposure to nickel and its salts is regarded as one of the most common causes of human skin sensitization and allergic contact dermatitis (WHO, 1991a). Dermal exposure to nickel may occur through jewellery, wrist watches with metal backs, coins and jeans buttons. The prime cause of nickel sensitization is ear piercing in combination with nickel-containing jewellery (Liden, 1992). The risk of sensitization has led to the adoption of nickel release limits for jewellery and other metal objects in close skin contact. It has been shown that exposure to nickel generates nickel-specific T-lymphocytes (Sinigaglia et al., 1985), probably mediated by nickel interaction with the major histocompatibility class II–peptide complex (Sinigaglia, 1994)

Carcinogenicity and Genotoxicity

The carcinogenicity of nickel was first recognized in the 1930s when an excess prevalence of lung and nasal cancers was found in nickel refinery workers (IARC, 1990). Nickel exposure through inhalation is mainly confined to industrial settings, whereas the general population is exposed to nickel by dermal contact. Numerous experimental studies have documented that nickel is an animal carcinogen, and water-insoluble salts, such as crystalline nickel sulphide and subsulphide, are the most potent compounds (Kasprzak, 1992). Water-soluble nickel salts do not enter cells, whereas crystalline nickel subsulphide is rapidly phagocytized. Dissolution of the nickel particles within the cell could lead to a high concentration of intracellular nickel. Nickel appears to damage selectively the genetically inactive heterochromatin, and the damage may involve cross-linking of oxidized amino acids to DNA (Conway and Costa, 1989; Klein and Costa, 1997). Nickel also affects DNA methylation, which may be relevant for gene regulation.

Although inhalation of nickel compounds is associated with lung and nasal tract tumours, the nature of the active compound(s) has not been elucidated. Oxides and sulphides of nickel are likely candidates, whereas exposure to nickel metal does not seem to be associated with an excess cancer risk. Inhalation of metallic metal may contribute to the development of 'hard metal' respiratory disease. Nasal irritation, damage to the nasal mucosa and perforation of the nasal septum are other effects reported due to nickel aerosol exposure.

Gallium (Ga)

The name stems from the Latin word for France, *Gallia*. The element was predicted and described by Mendeleev but discovered and isolated by Lecoq de Boisbaudran in 1875.

Radioactive gallium (^{67}Ga) is used clinically as a radiotracer in minute concentrations ng (kg body weight)$^{-1}$. Gallium concentrates in tumours and inflammatory tissue and ^{67}Ga and gallium nitrate have found therapeutic applications in the treatment of certain tumours (Jonkhoff et al., 1995). Nephrotoxicity in man has been noted at dose levels of Ga above 750 mg m^{-2}

surface area (20 mg [kg body weight]$^{-1}$) (Krakoff et al., 1979).

Gallium arsenide (GaAs) is finding increasing use in high-speed semiconductors. Experimental animal studies have shown that GaAs particles administered to hamsters are dissolved into the component elements and induce specific biochemical responses in renal tissue and cells, such as a chemical-specific porphyrinuria (Webb et al., 1984; Bakewell et al., 1988; Goering et al., 1988). GaAs treatment also produces morphological damage to renal mitochondria (Goering et al., 1988). Studies by Conner et al. (1993) demonstrated a GaAs-specific proteinuria pattern associated with gallium-and arsenite-specific changes in renal proximal tubule cell gene expression patterns (Aoki et al., 1990).

Indium (In)

The name of the element alludes to the brilliant indigo line in its spectrum. Indium is used in alloys and solders and in the electronics industry for the production of semiconductors. It has also found medical applications as a radiotracer (^{111}In) and antitumour agent.

Indium has been reported to produce teratogenic effects in the pregnant hamster at intravenous doses below 1 mg kg^{-1} (Ferm and Carpenter, 1970).

It accumulates in renal tissue (Yamauchi et al., 1992) and renal ALAD activity is inhibited following administration of InCl$_3$ in vivo (Woods and Fowler, 1983). Similar results were obtained when particles of InAs was administered by subcutaneous injection (Conner et al., 1995). Particles of indium arsenide (InAs) administered to hamsters subcutaneously are dissolved into the component elements and induce specific biochemical responses in renal tissue and cells (Yamauchi et al., 1992). Recent studies by Conner et al., (1995) have demonstrated that subchronic exposure to InAs produces a chemical-specific porphyrinuria.

A number of gene products are induced in primary cultures of renal proximal tubule cells exposed to InCl$_3$, including proteins with molecular weights similar to the 60, 70 and 90 kDa stress proteins (Aoki et al., 1990). Induction of these gene products have also been observed in hamsters administered InAs in vivo (Conner et al., 1993).

TOXICITY OF ESSENTIAL TRACE ELEMENTS

Essential trace elements are elements required in trace quantities for the proper functioning of cells and organisms. If the physiological requirements are not met, clinical signs of deficiency may develop. Deficiency usually results from an inadequate dietary intake of the essential trace elements. However, deficiency may also be a secondary phenomenon related to genetic factors (inborn errors of metabolism), interactions between dietary components, drugs and other chemicals which may limit trace element uptake and utilization, or the result of disease. Essential trace element deficiencies are usually a greater public health problem than excessive intake (intoxications).

Cobalt (Co)

Cobalt was isolated by the Swedish chemist Georg Brandt in the middle of the eighteenth century, although compounds containing cobalt were used already in ancient Egypt. *Kobold* was a name applied during the sixteenth century to ores eventually found to be toxic, arsenic-bearing cobalt ores.

Cobalt is essential to humans in the form of cyanocobalamin (vitamin B$_{12}$) (Lentner, 1986). Cobalamins function in rearrangement (adenosylcobalamin) and methyl transfer (methylcobalamin) reactions. Vitamin B$_{12}$ is essential for the production of red blood cells.

Toxicity

Intoxications (cardiomyopathies) due to its use as foam stabilizer in beer were described by Bonenfant et al., (1967). Inhalation of cobalt-containing dust may cause respiratory irritation and 'hard-metal' pneumoconiosis, developing into interstitial fibrosis.

Copper (Cu)

The element was discovered in prehistoric times and has its name from the island of Cyprus (Latin: *cuprum*). Copper is an essential trace element and necessary for the functioning of several enzymes involved in electron transfer (cytochrome oxidase), free radical defence (catalase, superoxide dismutase) and melanin formation (tyrosinase). Copper is also essential for the utilization of iron and formation of haemoglobin.

Uptake, Metabolism and Excretion

About 50% of dietary copper is absorbed into the blood and bound to serum albumin. Most copper in plasma is bound to ceruloplasmin, a copper-transporting protein important for the excretion of copper from the liver to the blood. However, most hepatic copper (80%) is excreted into the bile.

Toxicity

Intoxication by copper salts results in vomiting, hypertension, coma and death. Excess hepatic copper cause hepatitis leading to cirrhosis, hepatic failure and ultimately death. The liver shows pericentral necrosis. Copper may initiate lipid peroxidation through hydroxyl radical formation in a mechanism analogous to the Haber–Weiss cycle (Hanna and Mason, 1992; Stohs and Bagchi, 1995; Britton, 1996).

Inborn Errors of Copper Metabolism

Wilson disease is an autosomal recessive disorder of copper transport characterized by impaired incorporation of copper into ceruloplasmin and inhibited biliary copper excretion, initially resulting in hepatic accumulation of copper, later progressing to increased concentrations of copper in other organs such as the central nervous system, eyes and kidneys (Kodama, 1996). Symptoms of liver injury usually develops at the age of 4 or 5 years or later. The progress of the disease is followed by an increase in serum copper levels due to release of hepatic copper. The disease gene, located on chromosome 13q14.3, has been cloned and sequenced and found to encode a copper-transporting ATPase (Petrukhin et al., 1993, 1994; Tanzi et al., 1993; Thomas et al., 1995; Schilsky, 1996).

Indian childhood cirrhosis is a disease that has been associated with excess dietary copper intake through the use of cooking utensils made of brass, but genetic factors may also be involved (Scheinberg and Sternlieb, 1996).

Menkes disease, which is inherited as a X-linked recessive trait, is the result of a defective copper-transporting ATPase (Yamaguchi et al., 1996; Vulpe and Packman, 1995), closely related to the Wilson disease gene product (Tanzi et al., 1993). Clinical features of the disease include cerebral degeneration, mental and physical disorders and 'steel-wool' hair. The disease usually leads to death in early childhood.

Iron (Fe)

The chemical name stems from the Latin word *ferrum*. The use of iron is prehistoric and the element is mentioned in *Genesis*: Tubal-Cain, seven generations from Adam, was 'an instructor of every artefact in brass and iron' (Hammond, 1995). The most common ore is magnetite (Fe$_2$O$_3$). Carbon steel is an alloy of iron with carbon, and alloy steels are carbon steels with additives such as nickel, chromium and vanadium.

Uptake, Metabolism and Excretion

Iron deficiency is the most common single nutritional deficiency. Some foodstuffs, e.g. wheat flour, may be fortified with iron in order to enhance the dietary intake of iron. The uptake of iron occurs mainly in the upper part of the small intestine (duodenum and jejunum) and is regulated by the requirement of the body. Haem iron is absorbed intact via specific receptors and the iron is split from haem in the enterocytes by haem oxidase. The uptake of iron, primarily non-haem iron, is affected by dietary factors which may enhance (ascorbic acid) or decrease (tannins, fibres, calcium) the uptake.

More than 99% of iron in plasma is bound to transferrin, a glycoprotein with a molecular weight of 83 kDa. The transferrin–iron complex is bound to the transferrin receptor in the plasma membrane and taken up by endocytosis (Nieminen and Lemasters, 1996). Iron dissociates from the transferrin–receptor complex within the endosomal vesicle and can subsequently reach other cellular compartments. The transferrin–receptor complex recycles to the plasma membrane followed by release of transferrin back into the circulation.

Intracellular iron is stored as ferritin. Each ferritin complex consists of 24 subunits, with a combined molecular weight of 450 kDa, and can store 4500 atoms of iron. Ferric iron can be released from ferritin by reducing agents. Ferritin is degraded to haemosiderin, which accumulates in lysosomes. Most iron released during tissue and haemoglobin degradation is reutilized.

Iron is essential for oxygen transport, cellular respiration and the function of many enzymes involved in electron transport.

Toxicity

Iron is an essential element but intoxications may occur, particularly in children, due to ingestion of iron supplements. Acute symptoms include vomiting, diarrhoea, abdominal pain and gastro-intestinal haemorrhage. Later effects are circulatory collapse, periportal hepatic necrosis and renal failure. Primary haemochromatosis is a disease with autosomal recessive inheritance characterized by an increased absorption of iron in the gastro-intestinal tract resulting in chronic iron overload, hepatic portal fibrosis and ultimately cirrhosis. The defect has been localized to chromosome 6 closely linked to the HLA locus (Lombard et al., 1990). Redox cycling of iron may lead to hydroxyl radical formation and lipid peroxidation, which have been implicted as crucial events in iron toxicity.

Selenium (Se)

The name is derived from the word *selene*, the Greek name for moon. Selenium was discovered by Berzelius in 1817 (Hammond, 1995). The element was associated with tellurium, named after *Tellus*, the Earth. Selenium is obtained from by-products during refining of copper and in sulphuric acid production. The content of selenium in crops, the main human source of exposure, largely depends on the selenium content of the soil, which varies substantially around the world (Jackson, 1988). An average normative daily requirement of selenium of about 0.4μg (kg body weight)$^{-1}$ for adults has been calculated by the WHO (1996).

Uptake, Metabolism and Excretion

Selenate, selenite and selenomethionine are effectively absorbed in the gastro-intestinal tract. Selenium is reduced to selenide in a glutathione-dependent reaction before incorporation into amino acids (selenocysteine and selenomethionine). Selenium is excreted as methylated derivatives in the urine. Selenium-dependent glutathione peroxidase (GSH-Px) is important for the antioxidant defence. Red blood cell or platelet GSH-Px seem to reach a saturation level when the plasma selenium level reaches 100–120 μg l^{-1}, corresponding to an intake of 60–120 μg Se day^{-1}. Selenium also inhibits the toxicity of other elements such as arsenic, cadmium and mercury.

Deficiency

Negative health effects may occur at selenium intake levels below 20 μg day^{-1}. An endemic form of cardiopathy (Keshan disease) that occurs in the Keshan district of China has been associated with severe selenium deficiency (serum levels below 10 μg l^{-1}, corresponding to intake levels below 10 μg day^{-1}, especially in children and young women) (Chen et al., 1980). It is not clear if other factors (nutrition, infections) contribute to the disease.

Toxicity

A number of toxic manifestations due to acute or chronic exposure to selenium have been demonstrated in animals and man. Negative health signs (brittle hair and nails, prolonged plasma prothrombin time, skin lesions and changes in perpheral nerves) have been observed at daily intake levels exceeding 750–850 μg Se (Yang et al., 1989a, b). The mechanism(s) remain unclear, although several hypotheses including disturbances in sulphur metabolism, glutathione depletion and redox cycling of selenium metabolites have been presented. Based primarily on the studies performed in a seleniferous region in China (Yang and Zhou, 1994; Yang et al., 1989a, b), a maximum safe dietary selenium intake of 400 μg day^{-1} for adults has been suggested by the WHO (1996).

Carcinogenicity

Selenium compounds have been shown to inhibit tumour development in animal experiments. The underlying mechanism is unknown and it is uncertain if the results are applicable to man. Adequately performed epidemiological studies on the relationship between selenium status and cancer incidence in humans are lacking.

Exposure Assessment

Selenium levels in blood, plasma and urine can be used to monitor exposure. Concentrations of selenium in hair and nail clippings have also been used.

Zinc (Zn)

Zinc was used in alloys centuries before it was identified as an element. Metallic zinc was produced in thirteenth century India. The metal was rediscovered in Europe by Maggraf in 1746.

Zinc is required as a cofactor for a great number of enzymes catalysing the metabolism of proteins and nucleic acids and has also been shown to play an important role in a variety of eukaryotic transcription factors (Vallee and Auld, 1990; Coleman, 1992). Zinc deficiency causes growth retardation and delayed sexual maturation (Prasad, 1983). Teratogenic effects due to Zn deficiency have been demonstrated in animal experiments and effects in humans are also suspected (Keen, 1996).

Toxicity

Signs of toxicity due to excessive Zn intake include irritation of the gastro-intestinal epithelium, diarrhoea, vomiting and secondary copper deficiency. Inhalation of zinc oxide fumes may cause metal fume fever, characterized by attacks of chills and fever, nausea, dyspnea and fatigue. The underlying mechanism has not been identified (Gordon et al., 1992; Gordon and Fine, 1993).

SOME MECHANISTIC ASPECTS OF METAL TOXICOLOGY

Several mechanisms whereby toxic metals exert their effects are possible (Snow, 1992; Sanders et al., 1996). Metals may bind to thiol groups in catalytic or binding domains of enzymes, thereby inhibiting their activity. Toxic metals may also displace essential metals needed for the catalytic function of enzymes. The displacement may lead to conformational changes of the protein and disruption of electron transport. Inactivation of enzymes involved in DNA repair may result in genotoxic effects. Inorganic mercury, methylmercury and lead have been shown to inhibit the calcium channels of mammalian neurones. This may lead to substantial effects on cellular events that are calcium dependent, such as second messengers, enzyme activities and transmitter and hormone release. Metal ions can stimulate the production of oxygen free radicals, especially metals whose electronic configuration is altered under physiological conditions such as iron (Fe^{2+}–Fe^{3+}) and copper (Cu^+–Cu^{2+}). The generation of reactive oxygen species has been proposed to a contributing factor in chromium- and nickel-induced carcinogenesis (Cohen et al., 1993; Huang et al., 1994). Generation of free radicals may lead to modification of amino acids, nucleic acids and lipids. Metals may cause impairment of the antioxidant defence system, either through interaction with protective thiols (e.g. arsenic, mercury) or through their role as essential parts of antioxidant enzymes, such as selenium in glutathione peroxidase.

It is highly unlikely that a single general mechanism is sufficient to explain the various toxic effects observed as a result of metal exposure. The following sections briefly discuss some research areas currently being explored in order to further our knowledge of the mechanisms of metal toxicity.

Heat Shock Proteins and Metallothionein

The stress protein response is a cellular defence mechanism activated by physical stressors such as UV light, hyperthermia and anoxia in addition to chemicals, including certain metals (Taketani et al., 1988; Keyse and Tyrrell, 1989; Goering et al., 1992, 1993; Liu et al., 1996). This adaptive response confers increased cellular resistance to subsequent exposure to these agents or conditions. The induction of protein damage has been proposed to be a triggering event in the cellular stress protein response. The function of the stress proteins has not been fully elucidated. A 32 kDa stress protein (hsp32) has been identified as the haem oxygenase isozyme 1 (HO-1) (Maines, 1988; Keyse and Tyrell, 1989). This enzyme catalyse the oxidation of 5-hydroxyhaem to biliverdin in the degradation of haem. The 90 kDa stress protein (hsp90) is the glucocorticoid receptor-binding protein (Sanchez et al., 1985). Two stress proteins are members of the highly conserved hsp70 family. The larger of the two (73 kDa) is often referred to as the heat shock cognate protein (hsc70) since its synthesis is constitutive. The smaller protein (72 kDa) is highly inducible in response to environmental stressors. The 72 kDa stress protein (hsp70) has been shown to play a protective role in mediating cell killing following heat shock (Riabowol et al., 1988; Beckman and Welch, 1990). The function of hsp70 may be to salvage damaged proteins by solubilization or renaturing, or to facilitate their removal from the cell. Studies by Welch (1990) have shown redistribution of hsp70 to the periphery of cells during recovery from arsenite-induced stress, suggesting that this protein may chaperone damaged proteins which cannot be refolded to the cell membrane for extrusion from the cell.

The heat-inducible genes are activated through binding of a heat-shock factor (HSF) to a heat-shock element (HSE) of the gene. One class of HSF (HSF1) binds to HSE as a response to environmental stress, e.g. heat shock, oxidative stress or metal exposure. Another class

(HSF2) is regulated by physiological factors such as developmental stage and hormones. It has been shown that the presence of damaged proteins is a condition that triggers the induction of cellular stress proteins. It has been proposed that the function of the induced stress proteins is to refold damaged proteins or increase the rate of their degradation (Hightower, 1991). Some of the stress proteins are present under normal conditions and act as chaperones to facilitate the folding, assembly and distribution of newly synthesized proteins. The protective function of stress proteins may be due not only to an increased synthesis but also to intracellular translocation to sites susceptible to damage. Cytoplasmic stress protein 70 has been shown to move into the nucleus in response to heat shock and interact with the nucleolus (Edwards et al., 1991). During recovery, the protein returns to the cytoplasm. The intracellular localization of the stress protein depends on the stressor and may be associated with critical sites of cellular injury. The induction of stress proteins among tissues depends on the stressor and is generally most pronounced in target tissues.

Cells or tissues that are challenged by chemical or physical stress acquire a tolerance to subsequent similar stress conditions. A strong correlation between acquired tolerance and the induction of stress proteins has been shown.

Metallothionein (MT) is a low molecular weight (6–7 kDa) protein containing a large amount of cysteinyl residues. MT has a high affinity for metals and is inducible. Metallothioneins are divided into three classes based on primary structure and mode of synthesis. All vertebrates studied to date contain the Class I MTs. These proteins consists of 61 amino acids, lacks aromatic amino acids and have about 30% cysteinyl residues, arranged as Cys–X–X–Cys, Cys–X–Cys and Cys–Cys in the primary sequence (Hamer, 1986). MT binds several metals, the relative binding affinity being $Hg^{2+} > Ag^+ > Cu^+ > Cd^{2+} > Zn^{2+}$. Each molecule of MT binds 7–12 metal atoms via the cysteine thiol groups located in two domains and the stoichiometry and coordination geometry are metal-specific. For instance, the α-domain contains 11 cysteines and can bind four atoms of cadmium or zinc or five or six atoms of copper whereas the β-domain can bind three atoms of cadmium or zinc or six atoms of copper to its nine cysteine residues.

The Class I MTs occurs in at least four isoforms, MT-I to MT-IV. MT-I and MT-II appear to be functionally equivalent and similarly regulated, whereas MT-III and MT-IV are distinctly different. MT-III and MT-IV have been isolated from neuronal and stratified squamous epithelium, respectively (Uchida et al., 1991; Palmiter et al., 1992; Quaife et al., 1994). The synthesis of MT can be induced by various metals, including cadmium, mercury, copper and zinc. The induction is regulated by specific metal regulatory elements (MRE) located in the 5′ flanking region of the gene (Hamer, 1986; Andrews, 1990). Gene transcription probably depends on the interaction between the MREs and metal-binding transcription factors. However, the details of mammalian MT gene expression have not been elucidated. It is also known that apart from metals, a number of other factors also regulate MT gene expression, including glucocorticoid hormones and growth factors.

The physiological role of MT is probably to act as an inducible buffer for essential zinc and copper. However, studies using MT-I and MT-II knock-out mice seem to indicate that these genes are not essential for normal growth and differentiation, although the animals were more susceptible to cadmium hepatotoxicity (Michalska and Choo, 1993; Masters et al., 1994).

MT gene expression has been demonstrated in mouse preimplantation embryos (Andrews et al., 1991). In foetal mouse and rat liver, MT protein levels increase throughout late gestation but a drop is observed postnatally although the level of MT mRNA remains high, suggesting post-translational control of MT gene expression. In the pregnant rat, a decrease in hepatic MT mRNA level during gestation days 16–21 is followed by a sharp peak in the expression of MT at the time of parturition (Andersen et al., 1983). This is followed by a decline and a sustained level, lower than that of nulliparous rat, during lactation. On the other hand, in the pregnant mouse, hepatic MT mRNA is increased during late gestation and further increased during the sucking period (Daston et al., 1992).

It has been suggested that the major function of MT during foetal development is to act as a Zn storage protein. Maternal Zn deficiency has been shown to regulate the expression of MT in the offspring of rats (Gallant and Cherian, 1986).

Studies on mammalian cell lines have shown that amplification of the MT genes increase cellular resistance to toxic metals. Similar protection is offered by increased rate of MT synthesis.

Cytoskeletal Effects

Toxic elements can affect the cytoskeleton either directly, through binding to the amino acids of the tubulin proteins, or indirectly, by changing the intracellular environment, such as ion homeostasis, necessary for proper cytoskeletal function.

Some of the effects observed in response to mercury toxicity may to some extent be explained by interactions with cellular microtubules. The assembly of tubulin into microtubules is highly dependent on free sulphydryl groups. Oxidation or covalent modification of only a few of these is sufficient to inhibit microtubule assembly. Both inorganic mercury and methylmercury have been shown to inhibit tubulin dimer polymerization into microtubules and to disassemble microtubules. Vogel et al. (1989) showed that methylmercury binding to only two of 15 sulphydryl sites was sufficient to inhibit microtubule assembly. Microtubules of the mitotic spindle are particularly sensitive to methylmercury. During neuronal development, the microtubules become increasingly resistant to methylmercury.

Some metals and alkylmetal compounds have been shown to elevate markedly the level of the intermediate filament glial fibrillary acidic protein in astrocytes. The implication of this response in metal neurotoxicity is unclear.

Changes in the actin microfilaments, the smallest of the fibrillar proteins that make up the cytoskeleton, have also been implicated in metal neurotoxicity although the dynamic nature of the microfilaments has hampered experimental investigations.

Haem and Porphyrin Metabolism

The formation and degradation of haem has been shown to be modulated by metals in a number of ways, recently reviewed by Woods (1996). Toxic elements may inhibit different steps in the haem biosynthetic pathway through interaction with specific enzymes, either as ions (mercaptide bond formation) or as porphyrin chelates. The elements may also enhance the rate of haem degradation through induction of haem oxygenase. Perturbation of organelle membranes may lead to functional disturbance of membrane-associated enzymes. Certain elements can induce oxidant stress causing oxidation of reduced porphyrins, and the intracellular levels of GSH and other thiols can be down-regulated through oxidation or metal–thiol complex formation.

Bone Formation and Resorption

Osteomalacia (defective bone mineralization) and osteoporosis (demineralization of bone) are conditions that have been shown to be influenced by exposure to metals. Osteoporosis is common in postmenopausal women owing to the decrease in oestrogen levels. Nutritional and lifestyle factors may also contribute.

The mineral portion of bone is made up of hydroxyapaite $[Ca_{10}(PO_4)_6(OH)_2]$. More than 99.9% of total body Ca is stored in bone, and the bone-to-plasma ratio is 3400. Other essential metals vital for bone formation and osteoblast function are Mg, Zn, Mn and Cu.

Lead is known to be stored in bone, and this has been utilized for historical monitoring of lead exposure (Coleman, 1985). Over 95% of the total body burden of Pb is found in bone, with a bone-to-plasma ratio of 3600. Lead present during the foetal and early postnatal periods has been shown to inhibit bone growth. Lead stored in bone may act as an internal source of exposure, particularly in postmenopausal women.

Cadmium may cause skeletal damage by inhibition of bone formation, enhancing Ca release from bone, inhibiting renal tubular reabsorption of bone salts and inhibiting vitamin D metabolism.

Vitamin D_3 (cholecalciferol) is a ring cleavage product of 7-dehydrocholesterol produced in the skin by the action of ultraviolet light (DeLuca and Schnoes, 1983). Vitamin D_3 is metabolized to the 25-hydroxy derivative by calciol 25-monooxygenase in the liver. This metabolite is then activated to 1α,25-dihydroxyvitamin D (calcitriol) by the enzyme calcidiol 1-monooxygenase localized in the renal tubule mitochondria. Metabolism of ergocalciferol (vitamin D_2), derived from the diet, seems to proceed along the same line. Calcitriol is important for calcium uptake and transport and for bone mineralization. Lead has been shown to inhibit renal bioactivation of 25-hydroxycholecalciferol (Sauk and Somerman, 1991).

Chelation Therapy

A number of chelating agents have been developed in order to facilitate metal excretion in cases of intoxications and for therapeutic use in patients with genetic disorders affecting metal uptake, accumulation and excretion (reviewed by Aposhian et al., 1995; Goyer et al., 1995; Angle, 1996). Several of these are dithiol compounds utilizing the fact that many toxic metals are highly reactive towards vicinal thiols. The ideal chelator is water soluble, resistant to biodegradation, able to reach the target organs and sites of metal storage and forms biologically inactive complexes that are rapidly excreted. The chelator should also have a low affinity for essential metals.

BAL (British AntiLewisite; 2,3-mercaptopropanol) was developed as an antidote to arsenical war gases such as lewisite [dichloro(2-chlorovinyl)arsine] during World War I. It is a potentially toxic drug which is insoluble in water and has to be administered through injection. BAL has been used in the treatment of lead and inorganic mercury intoxications. BAL increase the renal concentration of cadmium and should not be used for treatment of cadmium intoxication.

Sodium 2,3-dimercaptopropanesulphonate (DMPS) and meso-2,3-dimercaptosuccinic acid (DMSA) are water-soluble and less toxic derivatives of BAL. DMPS and DMSA have been used in order to increase the rate of lead excretion in children and the rate of inorganic mercury excretion in occupationally exposed persons such as dental personnel. These compounds are also preferentially used for the treatment of arsenic intoxication. $CaNa_2$ EDTA, alone or in combination with DMSA or BAL, has been used in the treatment of lead poisoning, although $CaNa_2$ EDTA treatment alone has been shown to increase brain lead concentrations (Smith and Flegal, 1992; Maiorino et al., 1993; Flora et al., 1995). Early therapy with sulphydryl compounds (DMPS, DMSA) is essential for removing methylmercury from the blood. D-Penicillamine is used in the treatment of Wilson's disease. As hypersensitivity reactions due to treatment are common, trientine is an alternative chelator. Desferrioxamine is the only available and approved of iron chelator.

Although chelators are effective in reducing the levels of metals in body fluids, less is known about their actions in specific tissues and cells and to what extent they can be applied in order to enhance the reversal of functional impairments due to metal exposure (Goyer *et al.*, 1995).

REFERENCES

Aiyar, J., Berkovits, H. J., Floyd, R. A. and Wetterhahn, K. E. (1991). Reaction of chromium (VI) with glutathione or with hydrogen peroxide: identification of reactive intermediates and their role in chromium (VI)-induced DNA damage. *Environ. Health Perspect.*, **92**, 53–62.

Amin-Zaki, L., Majeed, M. A., Greenwood, M. R., Elhassani, S. B., Clarksson, T. W. and Doherty, R. A. (1981). Methylmercury poisoning in the Iraqi suckling infant: a longitudinal study over five years. *J. Appl. Toxicol.*, **1**, 210–214.

Andersen, R. D., Piletz, J. E., Birren, B. W. and Herschman, H. R. (1983). Levels of metallothionein messenger RNA in foetal, neonatal and maternal rat liver. *Eur. J. Biochem.*, **131**, 497–500.

Andersson, R. A. (1989). Essentiality of chromium in humans. *Sci. Total Environ.*, **86**, 75–81.

Andrews, G. K. (1990). Regulation of metallothionein gene expression. *Prog. Food Nutr. Sci.*, **14**, 193–258.

Andrews, G. K., Huet-Hudson, Y. M., Paria, B. C., McMaster, M. T., and Dey, S. K. (1991). Metallothionein gene expression and metal regulation during preimplantation mouse embryo development (MT mRNA during early development). *Dev. Biol.*, **145**, 13–27.

Angle, C. R. (1996). Chelation therapies for metal intoxication. In: Chang, L. W., (Ed.), *Toxicology of Metals*. CRC Press, Boca Raton, FL, pp. 487–504.

Aoki, Y., Lipsky, M. M. and Fowler, B. A. (1990). Alteration in protein synthesis in primary cultures of rat kidney proximal tubule epithelial cells by exposure to gallium, indium, and arsenite. *Toxicol. Appl. Pharmacol.*, **106**, 462–468.

Aposhian, H. V. (1997). Enzymatic methylation of arsenic species and other new approaches to arsenic toxicity. *Annu. Rev. Pharmacol. Toxicol.*, **37**, 397–419.

Aposhian, H. V., Maiorino, R. M., Gonzalez-Ramirez, D, Zuniga-Charles, M., Xu, Z., Hurlbut, K. M., Junco-Munoz, P., Dart, R. C. and Aposhian, M. M. (1995). Mobilization of heavy metals by newer, therapeutically useful chelating agents. *Toxicology*, **97**, 23–38.

Arbouine, M. W. and Wilson, H. K. (1992). The effect of seafood consumption on the assessment of occupational exposure to arsenic by urinary arsenic speciation measurements. *J. Trace Elem. Electrolyt. Health Dis.*, **6**, 153–160.

Arduino, R. C. and DuPont, H. L. (1993). Travellers' diarrhoea. *Ballière's Clin. Gastroenterol.*, **7**, 365–385.

Aschner, M. and Aschner, J. L. (1990). Mercury neurotoxicity: mechanisms of blood–brain barrier transport. *Neurosci. Biobehav. Rev.*, **14**, 169–176.

Aschner, M. and Clarkson, T. W. (1987). Mercury-203 distribution in pregnant and nonpregnant rats following systemic infusions with thiol-containing amino acids. *Teratology*, **36**, 321–328.

Aschner, M. and Clarkson, T. W. (1988). Distribution of mercury-203 in pregnant rats and their fetuses following systemic infusions with thiol-containing amino acids and glutathione during late gestation. *Teratology*, **38**, 145–155.

Bakewell, W. E., Jr., Goering, P. L., Moorman, M. P. and Fowler, B. A. (1988). Arsine and gallium arsenide-induced alterations in heme metabolism. *Toxicologist*, **8**, 20.

Bakir, F., Damluji, S. F., Amin-Zaki, L., Murtadha, M., Khalidi, A., al-Rawi, N. Y., Tikriti, S., Dahahir, H. I., Clarkson, T. W., Smith, J. C. and Doherty, R. A. (1973). Methylmercury poisoning in Iraq. *Science*, **181**, 230–241.

Ballatori, N. and Clarkson, T. W. (1985). Biliary secretion of gluthatione and of gluthatione-metal complexes. *Fundam. Appl. Toxicol.*, **5**, 816–831.

Barregård, L., Sallsten, G., Schutz, A., Attewell, R., Skerfving, S. and Jarvholm, B. (1992). Kinetics of mercury in blood and urine after brief occupational exposure. *Arch. Environ. Health*, **47**, 176–184.

Barrett, J. C., Lamb, P. W., Wang, T. C. and Lee, T. C. (1989). Mechanisms of arsenic-induced cell transformation. *Biol. Trace Elem. Res.*, **21**, 421–429.

Bates, M. N., Smith, A. H. and Hopenhayn-Rich, C. (1992). Arsenic ingestion and internal cancers: a review. *Am. J. Epidemiol.*, **135**, 462–476.

Batlle, A. M., Del, C., Fukuda, H., Parera, V. E., Wider, E. and Stella, A. M. (1987) In inherited porphyrias, lead intoxication is a toxogenetic disorder. *Int. J. Biochem.*, **19**, 717–720.

Beaver, D. L. and Burr, R. E. (1963). Bismuth inclusions in the human kidney. *Arch. Pathol.*, **76**, 89–94.

Beckman, M. and Welch, W. J. (1990). Interaction of Hsp 70 with newly synthesized proteins: implications for protein folding and assembly. *Science*, **248**, 850–854.

Bellinger, D. C., Stiles, K. M. and Needleman, H. L. (1992). Low-level lead exposure, intelligence and academic achievement: a long-term follow-up study. *Pediatrics*, **90**, 855–861.

Benet, L. Z. (1991). Safety and pharmacokinetics: colloidal bismuth subcitrate. *Scand. J. Gastroenterol., Suppl.*, **185**, 29–35.

Bergdahl, I. A., Gerhardsson, L., Schutz, A., Desnick, R. J., Wetmur, J. G. and Skerfving, S. (1997a). Delta-aminolevulinic acid dehydratase polymorphism: influence on lead levels and kidney function in humans. *Arch. Environ. Health*, **52**, 91–96.

Bergdahl, I. A., Schutz, A., Gerhardsson, L., Jensen, A. and Skerfving, S. (1997b). Lead concentrations in human plasma, urine and whole blood. *Scand. J. Work Environ. Health*, **23**, 359–363.

Berglund, F., Berlin, M., Birke, G., von Euler, U., Friberg, L., Holmstedt, B., Jonsson, E., Ramel, C., Skerfving, S., Swensson, Å. and Tejning, S. (1971). Methyl mercury in fish: a toxicologic–epidemiologic evaluation of risks. Report from an expert group. *Nord. Hyg. Tidskr.* Suppl. 4, 364 pp.

Berglund, M., Åkesson, A., Nermell, B. and Vahter, M. (1994). Intestinal absorption of dietary cadmium in women is dependent on body iron stores and fiber intake. *Environ. Health Perspect.*, **102**, 1058–1066.

Berlin, K., Gerhardsson, L., Borjesson, J., Lindh, E., Lundstrom, N., Schutz, A., Skerfving, S. and Edling, C. (1995).

Lead intoxication caused by skeletal disease. *Scand. J. Work Environ. Health*, **21**, 296–300.

Bierer, D. W. (1990). Bismuth subsalicylate: history, chemistry and safety. *Rev. Infect. Dis.*, **12**, Suppl. 1, S3–S8.

Blazka, M. E. and Shaikh, Z. A. (1991). Differences in cadmium and mercury uptakes by hepatocytes: role of calcium channels. *Toxicol. Appl. Pharmacol.*, **110**, 355–363.

Blazka, M. E. and Shaikh, Z. A. (1992). Cadmium and mercury accumulation in rat hepatocytes: interactions with other metal ions. *Toxicol. Appl. Pharmacol.*, **113**, 118–125.

Blom, S., Lagerkvist, B. and Linderholm, H. (1985). Arsenic exposure to smelter workers. Clinical and neurophysiological studies. *Scand. J. Work Environ. Health*, **11**, 265–269.

Bonenfant, J. L., Miller, G. and Roy, P. E. (1967). Quebec beer-drinkers' cardiomyopathy: pathological studies. *Can. Med. Assoc. J.*, **97**, 910–916.

Borges, K. M., Boswell, J. S., Liebross, R. H. and Wetterhahn, K. E. (1991). Activation of chromium (VI) by thiols results in chromium (V) formation, chromium binding to DNA and altered DNA conformation. *Carcinogenesis*, **12**, 551–561.

Bradley, B., Singleton, M. and Li Wan Po, A. (1989). Bismuth toxicity—a reassessment, *J. Clin. Pharmacol. Ther.*, **14**, 423–441.

Britton, R. S. (1996). Metal-induced hepatotoxicity. *Sem. Liver Dis.*, **16**, 3–12.

Buchet, J. P., Lauwerys, R. and Roels, H. (1981). Comparison of the urinary excretion of arsenic metabolites after a single oral dose of sodium arsenite, monomethylarsonate, or dimethylarsinate in man. *Int. Arch. Occup. Environ. Health.*, **48**, 71–79.

Buchet, J. P., Lauwerys, R., Roels, H., Bernard, A., Bruaux, P., Claeys, F., Ducoffre, G., de Plaen, P., Staessen, J., Amery, A., Lijnen, P., Thijs, L., Rondia, D., Sartor, F., Saint Remy, A. and Nick, L. (1990). Renal effects of cadmium body burden of the general population. *Lancet*, **336**, 699–702.

Buchet, J. P., Pauwels, J. and Lauwerys, R. (1994). Assessment of exposure to inorganic arsenic following ingestion of marine organisms by volunteers. *Environ. Res.*, **66**, 44–51.

Buge, A., Rancurel, G., Poisson, M., Gazengel, J., Dechy, C., Fressinaud, C. and Emile, J. (1974). 20 observations d'encéphalopathies aiguës avec myoclonies au cours de traitements oraux par les sels de bismuth. *Ann. Med. Interne*, **125**, 877–888.

Burns, R., Thomas, D. W. and Barron, V. J. (1974). Reversible encephalopathy possibly associated with bismuth subgallate ingestion, *Br. Med. J.*, **1**, 220–223.

Byers, R. K. and Lord, E. E. (1943). Late effects of lead poisoning on mental development. *Am. J. Dis. Child.*, **66**, 471–494.

CDC (1991). *Centers for Disease Control: Preventing Lead Poisoning in Young Children*. US Public Health Service, US Department of Health and Human Services, Atlanta, GA.

Chen, X., Yang, G., Chen, J., Chen, X., Wen, Z. and Ge, K. (1980). Studies on the relations of selenium and Keshan disease. *Biol. Trace Elem. Res.*, **2**, 91–107.

Chen, C. J., Chen, C. W., Wu, M. M. and Kuo, T. L. (1992). Cancer potential in liver, lung, bladder and kidney due to ingested inorganic arsenic in drinking water. *Br. J. Cancer*, **66**, 888–892.

Chiou, H. Y., Hsueh, Y. M., Liaw, K. F., Horng, S. F., Chiang, M. H., Pu, Y. S., Lin, J. S., Huang, C. H. and Chen, C. J. (1995). Incidence of internal cancers and ingested inorganic arsenic: a seven-year follow-up study in Taiwan. *Cancer Res.*, **55**, 1296–1300.

Choi, B. H., (1989). The effects of methylmercury on the developing brain. *Prog. Neurobiol.*, **32**, 447–470.

Cohen, M. D., Kargacin, B., Klein, C. B. and Costa, M. (1993). Mechanisms of chromium carcinogenicity and toxicity. *Crit. Rev. Toxicol.*, **23**, 255–281.

Coleman, D. O. (1985). Human remains. In *Histoical Monitoring*, MARC Report No. 31, Monitoring and Assessment Research Centre, University of London, London, pp. 281–315.

Coleman, J. E. (1992). Zinc proteins: enzymes, storage proteins, transcription factors, and replication proteins. *Annu. Rev. Biochem.*, **61**, 897–946.

Conner, E. A., Yamauchi, H., Fowler, B. A. and Akkerman, M. (1993). Biological indicators for monitoring exposure/toxicity from III–V semiconductors. *J. Exposure Anal. Environ. Epidemiol.*, **3**, 431–440.

Conner, E. A., Yamauchi, H. and Fowler, B. A. (1995). Alterations in the heme biosynthetic pathway from the III–V semiconductor metal, indium arsenide (InAs). *Chem.–Biol. Interact.*, **14**, 273–285.

Conway, K. and Costa, M. (1989). The involvement of heterochromatic damage in nickel-induced transformation. *Biol. Trace Elem. Res.*, **21**, 437–444.

Coogan, T. P., Shiraishi, N. and Waalkes, M. P. (1994). Apparent quiescence of the metallothionein gene in the rat ventral prostate: association with cadmium-induced prostate tumors in rats. *Environ. Health Perspect.*, **102**, Suppl. 3, 137–9.

Costa, M. (1991). DNA–protein complexes induced by chromate and other carcinogens. *Environ. Health Perspect.*, **92**, 45–52.

Cox, C., Clarkson, T. W., Marsh, D. O., Amin-Zaki, L., Tikriti, S. and Myers, G. G. (1989). Dose–response analysis of infants prenatally exposed to methyl mercury: an application of a single compartment model to single-strand hair analysis. *Environ. Res.*, **49**, 318–332.

Cullen, W. R. and Reimer, K. J. (1989). Arsenic speciation in the environment. *Chem. Rev.*, **89**, 713–764.

Daston, G. P., Overmann, G. J., Lehman-McKeeman, L. D., Taubeneck, M. W., Rogers, J. M. and Keen, C. L. (1992). Changes in hepatic metallothionein (MT) mRNA and protein levels during prequency and lactation in the mouse. *Teratology*, **45**, 501–502.

Deane, R. and Bradbury, M. W. (1990). Transport of lead-203 at the blood–brain barrier during short cerebrovascular perfusion with saline in the rat. *J. Neurochem.*, **54**, 905–914.

De Lacerda, L. D. and Salomons, W. (1998). *Mercury from Gold and Silver mining: A Chemical Time Bomb?* Springer, New York.

DeLuca, H. F. and Schnoes, H. K. (1983). Vitamin D: recent advances. *Annu. Rev. Biochem.*, **52**, 411–439.

Dinman, B. D. (1988). Alumina-related pulmonary disease. *J. Occup. Med.*, **30**, 328–335.

Dock, L., Rissanen, R. L. and Vahter, M. (1994). Demethylation and placental transfer of methyl mercury in the pregnant hamster. *Toxicology*, **94**, 131–142.

Dock, L., Rissanen, R. L. and Vahter, M. (1995). Metabolism of mercury in hamster pups administered a single dose of ^{203}Hg-labeled methyl mercury. *Pharmacol. Toxicol.*, **76**, 80–84.

Doherty, R. A., Gates, A. H. and Landry, T. D. (1977). Methyl-mercury excretion: developmental changes in mouse and man. *Pediatr. Res.*, **11**, 416.

Doi, R. (1990). Individual difference of methylmercury metabolism in animals and its significance in methylmercury toxicity. In Suzuki, T., Imura, N. and Clarkson, T. W. (Eds), *Advances in Mercury Toxicology*. Plenum Press, New York, pp. 77–98.

Doss, M., Schneider, J., Von Tiepermann, R. and Brandt, A. (1982). New type of acute porphyria with porphobilinogen synthase (delta-aminolevulinic acid dehydratase) defect in the homozygous state. *Clin. Biochem.*, **15**, 52–55.

Doss, M., Tiepermann, R. V. and Schneider, J. (1983). Porpho-bilinogen-synthase (delta-aminolevulinic acid dehydratase) deficiency in bone marrow cells of two patients with porphobilinogen-synthase defect acute porphyria. *Klin. Wochenschr.*, **61**, 699–702.

Drasch, G., Schupp, I., Hofl, H., Reinke, R. and Roider, G. (1994). Mercury burden of human fetal and infant tissues. *Eur. J. Pediatr.*, **153**, 607–610.

Edmonds, J. S. and Francesconi, K. A. (1987). Transformations of arsenic in the marine environment. *Experientia*, **43**, 553–557.

Edwards, M. J., Marks, R., Dykes, P. J., Merrett, V. R., Morgan, H. E. and O'Donovan, M. R. (1991). Heat shock proteins in cultured human keratinocytes and fibroblasts. *J. Invest. Dermatol.*, **96**, 392–396.

Eisenmann, C. J. and Miller, R. K. (1996). Placental transport, metabolism, and toxicity of metals. In Chang, L. W. (Ed.), *Toxicology of Metals*. CRC Press, Boca Raton, FL., pp. 1003–1026.

Elinder, C-G., Friberg, L., Kjellström, T., Nordberg, G. and Oberdoerster, G. (1994). *Biological Monitoring of Metals*. WHO/EHG/94.2. World Health Organization, Geneva.

Elsenhans, B., Strugala, G. J. and Schafer, S. G. (1997). Small-intestinal absorption of cadmium and the significance of mucosal metallothionein. *Hum. Exp. Toxicol.*, **16**, 429–434.

Ferm, V. H. and Carpenter, S. J. (1970). Teratogenic and embryopathic effects of indium, gallium, and germanium. *Toxicol. Appl. Pharmacol.* **16**, 166–170.

Ferm, V. H. and Hanlon, D. P. (1985). Constant rate exposure of pregnant hamsters to arsenate during early gestation. *Environ. Res.*, **37**, 425–432.

Fitzgerald, W. F. and Clarkson, T. W. (1991). Mercury and monomethylmercury: present and future concerns. *Environ. Health Perspect.*, **96**, 159–166.

Flora, S. J., Bhattacharya, R. and Vijayaraghavan, R. (1995). Combined therapeutic potential of *meso*-2,3-dimercaptosuc-cinic acid and calcium disodium edetate on the mobilization and distribution of lead in experimental lead intoxication in rats. *Fundam. Appl. Toxicol.*, **25**, 233–240.

Fowler, B. A. and DuVal, G. (1991). Effects of lead on the kidney: roles of high-affinity lead-binding proteins. *Environ. Health Perspect.*, **91**, 77–80.

Fowler, B. A. and Goyer, R. A. (1975). Bismuth localization within nuclear inclusions by X-ray microanalysis. *J. Histo-chem. Cytochem.*, **23**, 722–726.

Fowler, B. A. and Vouk, V. B. (1986). Bismuth. In Friberg, L., Nordberg, G. F. and Vouk, V. B. (Eds), *Handbook on the Toxicology of Metals*, Vol. II. Elsevier, Amsterdam, pp. 117–129.

Fowler, B. A., Oskarsson, A. and Woods, J. S. (1987). Metal- and metalloid-induced porphyrinurias. Relationships to cell injury. *Ann. N. Y. Acad Sci.*, **514**, 172–182.

Fowler, B. A., Kahng, M. W., Smith, D. R., Conner, E. A. and Laughlin, N. K. (1993). Implications of lead binding proteins for risk assessment of lead exposure. *J. Exp. Anal. Environ. Epidemiol.*, **3**, 441–448.

Friberg, L. (1948). Proteinuria and kidney injury among workmen exposed to cadmium and nickel dust. *J. Ind. Hyg. Toxicol.*, **30**, 32–36.

Friberg, L. and Mottet, N. K. (1989). Accumulation of methylmercury and inorganic mercury in the brain. *Biol. Trace Elem. Res.*, **21**, 201–206.

Friberg, L., Piscator, M., Nordberg, G., and Kjellström, T. (1974). *Cadmium in the Environment*, 2nd edn. CRC Press, Cleveland, OH.

Gallant, K. R. and Cherian, M. G. (1986). Influence of maternal mineral deficiency on the hepatic metallothionein and zinc in newborn rats. *Biochem. Cell Biol.*, **64**, 8–12.

Garcia-Vargas, G. G., Del, Razo, L. M., Cebrian, M. E., Albores, A., Ostrosky-Wegman, P., Montero, R., Gonse-batt, M. E., Lim, C. K. and De Matteis, F. (1994). Altered urinary prophyrin excretion in a human population chronically exposed to arsenic in Mexico. *Hum. Exp. Toxicol.*, **13**, 839–847.

Ghatak, S., Oliveria, P., Kaplan, P. and Ho, S. M. (1996). Expression and regulation of metallothionein mRNA levels in the prostates of noble rats: lack of expression in the ventral prostate and regulation by sex hormones in the dorsolateral prostate. *Prostate*, **29**, 91–100.

Goering, P. L. (1993). Lead–protein interactions as a basis for lead toxicity. *Neurotoxicology*, **14**, 45–60.

Goering, P. L., Maronpot, R. R. and Fowler, B. A. (1988). Effect of intratracheal administration of gallium arsenide administration of L-aminolevulinic acid dehydratase in rats: relationship to urinary excretion of aminolevulinic acid. *Toxicol. Appl. Pharmacol.*, **92**, 179–193.

Goering, P. L., Fisher, B. R., Chaudhary, P. P. and Dick, C. A. (1992). Relationship between stress protein induction in rat kidney by mercuric chloride and nephrotoxicity. *Toxicol. Appl. Pharmacol.*, **113**, 184–191.

Goering, P. L., Fisher, B. R. and Kish, C. L. (1993). Stress protein synthesis induced in rat liver by cadmium precedes hepatotoxicity. *Toxicol. Appl. Pharmacol.*, **122**, 139–148.

Goldstein, G. W. (1993). Evidence that lead acts as a calcium substitute in second messenger metabolism. *Neurotoxicology*, **14**, 97–101.

Golub, M. S. (1994). Maternal toxicity and the identification of inorganic arsenic as a developmental toxicant. *Reprod. Toxicol.*, **8**, 283–295.

Gordon, T. and Fine, J. M. (1993). Metal fume fever. *Occup. Med.*, **8**, 504–517.

Gordon, T., Chen, L. C., Fine, J. M., Schlesinger, R. B., Su, W. Y., Kimmel, T. A. and Amdur, M. O. (1992). Pulmonary effects of inhaled zinc oxide in human subjects, guinea pigs, rats, and rabbits. *Am. Ind. Hyg. Assoc. J.*, **53**, 503–509.

Goyer, R. A., Cherian, M. G., Jones, M. M. and Reigart, J. R. (1995). Role of chelating agents for prevention, intervention, and treatment of exposures to toxic metals. *Environ. Health Perspect*, **103**, 1048–1052.

Grandjean, P., Jorgensen, P. J. and Weihe, P. (1994a). Human milk as a source of methylmercury exposure in infants. *Environ. Health Perspect.*, **102**, 74–77.

Grandjean, P., Weihe, P. and Nielsen, J. B. (1994b). Methylmercury: significance of intrauterine and postnatal exposures. *Clin. Chem.*, **40**, 1395–1400.

Groten, J. P., Luten, J. B. and van Bladeren, P. J. (1992). Dietary iron lowers the intestinal uptake of cadmium-metallothionein in rats. *Eur. J. Pharmacol.*, **228**, 23–28.

Hamada, R. and Osame, M. (1996). Minamata disease and other mercury syndromes. In Chang, L. W. (Ed.), *Toxicology of Metals*. CRC Press, Boca Raton, FL, pp. 337–351.

Hamer, D. H. (1986). Metallothionein. *Annu. Rev. Biochem.*, **55**, 913–951.

Hammond, C. R. (1995). The elements. In Lide, D. R. (Ed.), *Handbook of Chemistry and Physics*, 76th edn. CRC Press, Boca Raton, FL, Sect. 4, pp. 4–1–4–34.

Hanna, P. M. and Mason, R. P. (1992). Direct evidence for inhibition of free radical formation from Cu(I) and hydrogen peroxide by glutathione and other potential ligands using the EPR spin-trapping technique. *Arch. Biochem. Biophys.*, **295**, 205–213.

Hatlelid, K. M., Brailsford, C. and Carter, D. E. (1996). Reactions of arsine with hemoglobin. *J. Toxicol. Environ. Health.*, **47**, 145–57.

Healy, S. M., Zakharyan, R. A. and Aposhian, H. V. (1997) Enzymatic methylation of arsenic compounds: IV. *In vitro* and *in vivo* deficiency of the methylation of arsenite and monomethylarsonic acid in the guinea pig. *Mutat. Res.*, **386**, 229–239.

Hernberg, S. and Nikkanen, J. (1970). Enzyme inhibition by lead under normal urban conditions. *Lancet*, **i**, 63–64.

Hightower, L. E. (1991). Heat shock, stress proteins, chaperones, and proteotoxicity. *Cell*, **66**, 191–197.

Hillemand, P., Pallière, M., Laquais, B. and Bouvet, P. (1977). Traitement bismuthique et bismuthémie. Sem. Hop. Paris, **53**, 1663–1669.

Hood, R. D., Vedel, G. C., Zaworotko, M. J., Tatum, F. M. and Meeks, R. G. (1988). Uptake, distribution, and metabolism of trivalent arsenic in the pregnant mouse. *J. Toxicol. Environ. Health*, **25**, 423–434.

Huang, X., Zhuang, Z., Frenkel, K., Klein, C. B. and Costa, M. (1994). The role of nickel and nickel-mediated reactive oxygen species in the mechanism of nickel carcinogenesis. *Environ. Health Perspect.*, **102**, Suppl. 3, 281–284.

IARC (1980). *IARC Monographs on the Evaluation of Carcinogenic Risk to Humans. Vol. 23. Some Metals and Metallic Compounds*. International Agency for Research on Cancer, Lyon.

IARC (1990). *IARC Monographs on the Evaluation of Carcinogenic Risk to Humans, Vol. 49. Chromium, Nickel and Welding*. International Agency for Research on Cancer, Lyon.

IARC (1993). *IARC Monographs on the Evaluation of Carcinogenic Risk to Humans. Vol. 58. Beryllium, Cadmium, Mercury, and Exposures in the Glass Manufacturing Industry*. International Agency for Research on Cancer, Lyon.

Ichiba, M. and Tomokuni, K. (1990). Studies on erythrocyte pyrimidine 5′-nucleotidase (P5N) test and its evaluation in workers occupationally exposed to lead. *Int. Arch. Occup. Environ. Health*, **62**, 305–310.

Ishinishi, N., Kodama, Y., Nobutomo, K., Inamasu, T., Kunitake, E. and Suenaga, Y. (1977). Outbreak of chronic arsenic poisoning among retired workers from an arsenic mine in Japan. *Environ. Health Perspect.*, **19**, 121–125.

Ivankovic, S., Eisenbrand, G. and Preussmann, R. (1979). Lung carcinoma induction in BD rats after a single intratracheal instillation of an arsenic-containing pesticide mixture formerly used in vineyards. *Int. J. Cancer*, **24**, 786–788.

Jackson, M. L. (1988). Selenium: geochemical distribution and associations with human heart and cancer death rates and longevity in China and the United States. *Biol. Trace Elem. Res.*, **15**, 13–21.

Järup, L., Berglund, M., Elinder, C. G., Nordberg, G. and Vahter, M. (1998). Health effects of cadmium exposure—a review of the literature and a risk estimate. *Scand. J. Work Environ. Health.*, **24**, Suppl. 1, 1–51.

Jelmert, O., Hansteen, I. L. and Langard, S. (1994). Chromosome damage in lymphocytes of stainless steel welders related to past and current exposure to manual metal arc welding fumes. *Mutat. Res.*, **320**, 223–233.

Jensen, S. and Jernelöv, A. (1969). Biological methylation of mercury in aquatic organisms. *Nature*, **223**, 753–754.

Johnson, D. L., McDade, K. and Griffith, D. (1996). Seasonal variation in paediatric lead levels in Syracuse, N. Y., USA. *Environ. Geochem. Health*, **18**, 81–88.

Jonkhoff, A. R., Huijgens, P. C., Versteegh, R. T., van Lingen, A., Ossenkoppele, G. J., Drager, A. M. and Teule, G. J. (1995). Radiotoxicity of 67-gallium on myeloid leukemic blasts. *Leukemia Res.*, **19**, 169–174.

Kajiwara, Y., Yasutake, A., Adachi, T. and Hirayama, K. (1996). Methylmercury transport across the placenta via neutral amino acid carrier. *Arch. Toxicol.*, **70**, 310–314.

Kasprzak, K. S. (1992). Animal studies: an overview. In Nieboer, E. and Nriagu, J. O. (Eds), *Nickel and Human Health*. Wiley, New York, pp. 387–420.

Keen, C. L. (1996). Teratogenic effects of essential trace elements: deficiencies and excesses. In Chang, L. W. (Ed.), *Toxicology of Metals*. CRC Press, Boca Raton, FL, pp. 977–1001.

Kershaw, T. G., Clarkson, T. W. and Dhahir, P. H. (1980). The relationship between blood levels and dose of methylmercury in man. *Arch. Environ. Health*, **35**, 28–36.

Keyse, S. M. and Tyrrell, R. M. (1989). Heme oxygenase is the major 32-kDa stress protein induced in human skin fibroblasts by UVA radiation, hydrogen peroxide, and sodium arsenite. *Proc. Natl. Acad. Sci. USA*, **86**, 99–103.

Khayat, A. and Dencker, L. (1982). Fetal uptake and distribution of metallic mercury vapor in the mouse: influence of ethanol and aminotriazole. *Int. J. Biol. Res. Pregn.*, **3**, 38–46.

Kjellström, T. (1986). Effects on bone, on vitamin D., and calcium metabolism. In Friberg, L., Elinder, C.-G., Kjellström, T. and Nordberg, G. F. (Eds), *Cadmium and Health: A Toxicological and Epidemiological Appraisal*, Vol. II. CRC Press, Boca Raton, FL, pp. 111–158.

Klein, C. B. (1996). Carcinogenicity and genotoxicity of chromium. In Chang, L. W. (Ed.), *Toxicology of Metals*. CRC Press, Boca Raton, FL, pp. 205–219.

Klein, C. B. and Costa, M. (1997). DNA methylation, heterochromatin and epigenetic carcinogens. *Mutat. Res.*, **386**, 163–180.

Klimecki, W. T. and Carter, D. E. (1995). Arsine toxicity: chemical and mechanistic implications. *J. Toxicol. Environ. Health*, **46**, 399–409.

Kodama, H. (1996). Genetic disorders of copper metabolism. In Chang, L. W. (Ed.) *Toxicology of Metals*. CRC Press, Boca Raton, FL, pp. 371–386.

Kongerud, J. (1992). Respiratory disorders in aluminium potroom workers. *Med. Lavoro*, **83**, 414–417.

Kortenkamp, A. and O'Brien, P. (1994). The generation of DNA single-strand breaks during the reduction of chromate by ascorbic acid and/or glutathione *in vitro*. *Environ. Health Perspect.*, **102**, Suppl. 3, 237–241.

Kostial, K., Simonovic, I., Rabar, I., Blanusa, M. and Landeka, M. (1983). Age and intestinal retention of mercury and cadmium in rats. *Environ. Res.*, **31**, 111–115.

Krakoff, I. H., Newman, R. A. and Goldberg, R. S. (1979). Clinical toxicologic and pharmacologic studies of gallium nitrate. *Cancer*, **44**, 1722–1727.

Kuhnert, B. R., Kuhnert, P. M. and Zarlingo, T. J. (1988). Associations between placental cadmium and zinc and age and parity in pregnant women who smoke. *Obstet. Gynecol.*, **71**, 67–70.

Lagerkvist, B. J. and Zetterlund, B. (1994). Assessment of exposure to arsenic among smelter workers: a five-year follow-up. *Am. J. Ind. Med.*, **25**, 477–488.

Lander, J. J., Stanley, R. J., Sumner, H. W., Boswell, D. C. and Aach, R. D. (1975). Angiosarcoma of the liver associated with Fowler's solution (potassium arsenite). *Gastroenterology*, **68**, 1582–1586.

Landrigan, P. J. (1981). Arsenic—state of the art. *Am. J. Ind. Med.*, **2**, 5–14.

Lau, S. and Sarkar, B. (1979). Inorganic mercury(II)-binding components in normal human blood serum. *J. Toxicol. Environ. Health*, **5**, 907–916.

Lee, T. C., Tanaka, N., Lamb, P. W., Gilmer, T. M. and Barrett, J. C. (1988). Induction of gene amplification by arsenic. *Science*, **241**, 79–81.

Lentner, C. (Ed.) (1986). *Geigy Scientific Tables, Vol. 4: Biochemistry, Metabolism of Xenobiotics, Inborn Errors of Metabolism, Pharmacogenetics and Ecogenetics*. Ciba-Geigy, Basle.

Liden, C. (1992). Nickel in jewellery and associated products. *Contact Dermatitis*, **26**, 73–75.

Liu, J., Squibb, K. S., Akkerman, M., Nordberg, G. F., Lipsky, M. and Fowler, B. A. (1996). Cytotoxicity, zinc protection, and stress protein induction in rat proximal tubule cells exposed to cadmium chloride in primary cell culture. *Renal Failure*, **18**, 867–882.

Liu, R. M. and Liun, Y. G. (1990). Effects of cadmium on the energy metabolism of isolated hepatocytes: its relationship with the nonviability of isolated hepatocytes caused by cadmium. *Biomed. Environ. Sci.*, **3**, 251–261.

Lombard, M., Bomford, A. B., Polson, R. J., Bellingham, A. J. and Williams, R. (1990). Differential expression of transferrin receptor in duodenal mucosa in iron overload. Evidence for a site-specific defect in genetic hemochromatosis. *Gastroenterology*, **98**, 976–984.

Lok, E. (1983). The effect of weaning on blood, hair, fecal and urinary mercury after chronic ingestion of methylmercuric chloride by infant monkeys. *Toxicol. Lett.*, **15**, 147–152.

Lowe, D. J. (1974). Adverse affects of bismuth subgallate. A further report from the Australian Drug Evaluation Committee. *Med. J. Aust.*, 664–666.

Lundgren, K. D. (1954). Damages in the respiratory organs of workers in a smeltery. *Nord. Hyg. Tidskr.*, **3**, 66–82.

Lutz, E., Lind, B., Herin, P., Krakau, I., Bui, T. H. and Vahter, M. (1996). Concentrations of mercury, cadmium and lead in brain and kidney of second trimester fetuses and infants. *J. Trace Elem. Med. Biol.*, **10**, 61–67.

Maines, M. D. (1988). Heme oxygenase: function, multiplicity, regulatory mechanisms, and clinical applications *FASEB J.*, **2**, 2557–2568.

Maiorino, R. M., Aposhian, M. M., Xu, Z. F., Li, Y., Polt, R. L. and Aposhian, H. V. (1993). Determination and metabolism of dithiol chelating agents. XV. The *meso*-2,3-dimercaptosuccinic acid–cysteine (1:2) mixed disulfide, a major urinary metabolite of DMSA in the human, increases the urinary excretion of lead in the rat. *J. Pharmacol. Exp. Ther.*, **267**, 1221–1226.

Marafante, E. and Vahter, M. (1987). Solubility, retention, and metabolism of intratracheally and orally administered inorganic arsenic compounds in the hamster. *Environ. Res.*, **42**, 72–82.

Marafante, E., Vahter, M., Norin, H., Envall, J., Sandström, M., Christakopoulos, A. and Ryhage, R. (1987). Biotransformation of dimethylarsinic acid in mouse, hamster and man. *J. Appl. Toxicol.*, **7**, 111–117.

Martel, J., Marion, M. and Denizeau, F. (1990). Effect of cadmium on membrane potential in isolated rat hepatocytes. *Toxicology*, **60**, 161–172.

Martin-Bouyer, G., Foulon, G., Guerbois, H. and Barin, C. (1980). Aspects épidémiologiques des encéphalopathies après administration de bismuth par voie orale. *Thérapie*, **35**, 307–313.

Masters, B. A., Kelly, E. J., Quaife, C. J., Brinster, R. L. and Palmiter, R. D. (1994). Targeted disruption of metallothionein I and II genes increases sensitivity to cadmium. *Proc. Natl. Acad. Sci. USA*, **91**, 584–588.

McFarland, R. B. and Reigel, H. (1978). Chronic mercury poisoning from a single brief exposure. *J. Occup. Med.*, **20**, 532–534.

Mertz, W. (1992). Chromium: history and nutritional importance. *Biol. Trace Elem. Res.*, **32**, 3–8.

Michalska, A. E. and Choo, K. H. (1993). Targeting and germline transmission of a null mutation at the metallothionein I and II loci in mouse. *Proc. Natl. Acad. Sci. USA*, **90**, 8088–8092.

Miller, J. M., Chaffin, D. B. and Smith, R. G. (1975). Subclinical psychomotor and neuromuscular changes in workers exposed to inorganic mercury. *Am. Ind. Hyg. Assoc. J.*, **36**, 725–733.

Mistry, P., Lucier, G. W. and Fowler, B. A. (1985). High-affinity lead binding proteins in rat kidney cytosol mediate cell-free nuclear translocation of lead. *J. Pharmacol. Exp. Ther.*, **232**, 462–469.

Moon, J. (1994). The role of vitamin D in toxic metal absorption: a review. *J. Am. Coll. Nutr.*, **13**, 559–569.

Mottet, N. K., Vahter, M. E., Charleston, J. S. and Friberg, L. T. (1997). Metabolism of methylmercury in the brain and its toxicological significance. In Sigel, A. and Sigel, H. (Eds), *Metal ions in Biological Systems*, Vol. 34. Marcel Dekker, New York, pp. 371–403.

Muller, L. (1986). Consequences of cadmium toxicity in rat hepatocytes: mitochondrial dysfunction and lipid peroxidation. *Toxicology*, **40**, 285–295.

Mushak, P., Davis, J. M., Crocetti, A. F. and Grant, L. D. (1989). Prenatal and postnatal effects of low-level lead exposure: integrated summary of a report to the US Congress on childhood lead poisoning. *Environ. Res.*, **50**, 11–36.

Naganuma, A., Koyama, Y. and Imura, N. (1980). Behavior of methylmercury in mammalian erythrocytes. *Toxicol. Appl. Pharmacol.*, **54**, 405–410.

Needleman, H. L. (1996). Current status of childhood lead exposure at low dose. In Chang, L. W. (Ed.), *Toxicology of Metals*. CRC Press, Boca Raton, FL, pp. 405–413.

Needleman, H. L., Gunnoe, C., Leviton, A., Reed, R., Peresie, H., Maher, C. and Barrett, P. (1979). Deficits in psychologic and classroom performance of children with elevated dentine lead levels. *N. Engl. J. Med.*, **300**, 689–695.

Nemery, B. (1990). Metal toxicity and the respiratory tract. *Eur. Resp. J.*, **3**, 202–219.

Nieminen, A.-L. and Lemasters, J. J. (1996). Hepatic injury by metal accumulation. In Chang, L. W. (Ed.), *Toxicology of Metals*. CRC Press, Boca Raton, FL, pp. 887–899.

Nilsson, U. and Skerfving, S. (1993). *In vivo* x-ray fluorescence measurements of cadmium and lead. *Scand. J. Work Environ. Health*, **19**, Suppl. 1, 54–58.

Nilsson, U., Attewell, R., Christoffersson, J. O., Schutz, A., Ahlgren, L., Skerfving, S. and Mattsson, S. (1991). Kinetics of lead in bone and blood after end of occupational exposure. *Pharmacol. Toxicol.*, **68**, 477–484.

Nogawa, K. and Kido, T. (1996). Itai-Itai disease and health effects of cadmium. In Chang, L. W. (Ed.), *Toxicology of Metals*. CRC Press, Boca Raton, FL, pp. 353–369.

Nord (1995). *Risk Evaluation of Essential Trace Elements—Essential Versus Toxic Levels of Intake*. Nord 1995:18. Nordic Council of Ministers, Copenhagen.

Nordberg, G. F. (1993). Cadmium carcinogenesis and its relationship to other health effects in humans. *Scand. J. Work Environ. Health*, **19**, Suppl. 1, 104–107.

Nordberg, G. F. (1996). Current issues in low-dose cadmium toxicology: nephrotoxicity and carcinogenicity. *Environ. Sci.*, **4**, 133–147.

Nordberg, G. F., Kjellström, T. and Nordberg, M. (1985). Kinetics and metabolism. In Friberg, L., Elinder, C.-G., Kjellström, T. and Friberg, L. (Eds), *Cadmium and Health: a Toxicological and Epidemiological Appraisal. Vol I. Exposure, Dose and Metabolism*. CRC Press, Boca Raton, FL, pp. 103–178.

Nordenhäll, K., Dock, L. and Vahter, M. (1995). Transplacental and lactational exposure to mercury in hamster pups after maternal administration of methyl mercury in late gestation. *Pharmacol. Toxicol.*, **77**, 130–135.

O'Donnell, T. V., Welford, B. and Coleman, E. D. (1989). Potroom asthma: New Zealand experience and follow-up. *Am. J. Ind. Med.*, **15**, 43–49.

O'Flaherty, E. J. (1993). Physiologically based models for bone-seeking elements. IV. Kinetics of lead disposition in humans. *Toxicol. Appl. Pharmacol.*, **118**, 16–29.

Omata, S., Kasama, H., Kasegawa, H., Hasegawa, K., Ozaki, K. and Sugano, H. (1986). Species difference between rat and hamster in tissue accumulation of mercury after administration of methylmercury. *Arch. Toxicol.*, **59**, 249–254.

Paglia, D. E., Valentine, W. N. and Dahlgren, J. G. (1975). Effects of low-level lead exposure on pyrimidine 5'-nucleotidase and other erythrocyte enzymes. Possible role of pyrimidine 5'-nucleotidase in the pathogenesis of lead-induced anemia. *J. Clin. Invest.*, **56**, 1164–1169.

Palheta, D. and Taylor, A. (1995). Mercury in environmental and biological samples from a gold mining area in the Amazon region of Brazil. *Sci. Total Environ.*, **168**, 63–69.

Palmiter, R. D., Findley, S. D., Whitmore, T. E. and Durnam, D. M. (1992). MT-III, a brain-specific member of the metallothionein gene family. *Proc. Natl. Acad. Sci. USA*, **89**, 6333–6337.

Pershagen, G. and Björklund, N. E. (1985). On the pulmonary tumorigenicity of arsenic trisulfide and calcium arsenate in hamsters. *Cancer Lett.*, **27**, 99–104.

Pershagen, G., Nordberg, G. and Björklund, N. E. (1984). Carcinomas of the respiratory tract in hamsters given arsenic trioxide and/or benzo[a]pyrene by the pulmonary route. *Environ. Res.*, **34**, 227–241.

Peters, H. A., Croft, W. A., Woolson, E. A., Darcey, B. A. and Olson, M. A. (1984). Seasonal arsenic exposure from burning chromium-copper-arsenate-treated wood. *J. Am. Med. Assoc.*, **251**, 2393–2396.

Petrukhin, K., Fischer, S. G., Pirastu, M., Tanzi, R. E., Chernov, I., Devoto, M., Brzustowicz, L. M., Cayanis, E., Vitale, E., Russo, J. J., *et al.* (1993). Mapping, cloning and genetic characterization of the region containing the Wilson disease gene. *Nature Genet.*, **5**, 338–343.

Petrukhin, K., Lutsenko, S., Chernov, I., Ross, B. M., Kaplan, J. H. and Gilliam, T. C. (1994). Characterization of the Wilson disease gene encoding a P-type copper transporting ATPase: genomic organization, alternative splicing, and structure/function predictions. *Hum. Mol. Genet.*, **3**, 1647–1656.

Pinto, S. S. and McGill, C. M. (1953). Arsenic trioxide esposure in industry. *Ind. Med. Surg.*, **22**, 281–287.

Piotrowski, J. K. and Szymanska, J. A. (1976). Influence of certain metals on the level of metallothionein-like proteins in the liver and kidneys of rats. *J. Toxicol. Environ. Health*, **1**, 991–1002.

Platts, M. M. and Anastassiades, E. (1981). Dialysis encephalopathy: precipitating factors and improvement in prognosis. *Clin. Nephrol.*, **15**, 223–228.

Poklis, A. and Saady, J. J. (1990). Arsenic poisoning: acute or chronic? Suicide or murder? *Am. J. Forensic Med. Pathol.*, **11**, 226–232.

Popp, W., Vahrenholz, C., Schmieding, W., Krewet, E. and Norpoth, K. (1991). Investigations of the frequency of DNA strand breakage and cross-linking and of sister chromatid exchange in the lymphocytes of electric welders exposed to chromium- and nickel-containing fumes. *Int. Arch. Occup. Environ. Health*, **63**, 115–120.

Prasad, A. S. (1983) Human zinc deficiency. In Sarkar, B. (Ed.), *Biological Aspects of Metals and Metal-related Disease*. Raven Press, New York, pp. 107–119.

Quaife, C. J., Findley, S. D., Erickson, J. C., Froelick, G. J., Kelly, E. J., Zambrowicz, B. P. and Palmiter, R. D. (1994). Induction of a new metallothionein isoform (MT-IV) occurs during differentiation of stratified squamous epithelia. *Biochemistry*, **33**, 7250–7259.

Quintanilla-Vega, B., Smith, D. R., Kahng, M. W., Hernandez, J. M., Albores, A. and Fowler, B. A. (1995). Lead-binding proteins in brain tissue of environmentally lead-exposed humans. *Chem. –Biol. Interact.*, **98**, 193–209.

Raghavan, S. R., Culver, B. D. and Gonick, H. C. (1981). Erythrocyte lead-binding protein after occupational exposure. II. Influence on lead inhibition of membrane Na$^+$, K$^+$

adenosinetriphosphatase. *J. Toxicol. Environ. Health*, **7**, 561–568.

Riabowol, K. T., Mizzem, A. L. and Welch, W. J. (1988). Heat shock is lethal to fibroblasts microinjected with antibodies against Hsp 70. *Science*, **242**, 433–436.

Richeldi, L., Sorrentino, R. and Saltini, C. (1993). HLA-DPB1 glutamate 69: a genetic marker of beryllium disease. *Science*, **262**, 242–244.

Robertson, J. F. (1974). Mental illness or metal illness? *Med. J. Aust.*, 887–888.

Rojas-Lopez, M., Santos-Burgoa, C., Rios, C., Hernandez-Avila, M. and Romieu, I. (1994). Use of lead-glazed ceramics is the main factor associated to high lead in blood levels in two Mexican rural communities. *J. Toxicol. Environ. Health*, **42**, 45–52.

Romieu, I., Carreon, T., Lopez, L., Palazuelos, E., Rios, C., Manuel, Y. and Hernandez-Avila, M. (1995). Environmental urban lead exposure and blood lead levels in children of Mexico City. *Environ. Health Perspect.*, **103**, 1036–1040.

Rossman, M. D. (1996). Chronic beryllium disease: diagnosis and management. *Environ. Health Perspect.*, **104**, Suppl. 5, 945–947.

Rossman, T. G., Goncharova, E. I., Rajah, T. and Wang, Z. (1997). Human cells lack the inducible tolerance to arsenite seen in hamster cells. *Mutat. Res.*, **386**, 307–314.

Rowland, I. R., Robinson, R. D., Doherty, R. A. and Landry, T. D. (1983). Are developmental changes in methylmercury metabolism and excretion mediated by the intestinal microflora? In Clarkson, T. W., Nordberg, G. F. and Sager, P. R., (Eds), *Reproductive and Development Toxicity of Metals*. Plenum Press, New York, pp. 745–758.

Rozas, V. V., Port, F. K. and Rutt, W. M. (1978a). Progressive dialysis encephalopathy from dialysate aluminum. *Arch. Int. Med.*, **138**, 1375–1377.

Rozas, V. V., Port, F. K. and Easterling, R. E. (1978b). An outbreak of dialysis dementia due to aluminum in the dialysate. *J. Dialysis*, **2**, 459–470.

Sanchez, E. R., Toft, D. O., Schlesinger, M. J. and Pratt, W. B. (1985). Evidence that the 90-kDa phosphoprotein associated with the untransformed L-cell glucocorticoid receptor is a murine heat shock protein. *J. Biol. Chem.*, **260**, 12398–12401.

Sanders, B. M., Goering, P. L. and Jenkins, K. (1996). The role of general and metal-specific cellular responses in protection and repair of metal-induced damage: stress proteins and metallothioneins. In Chang, L. W. (Ed.), *Toxicology of Metals*. CRC Press, Boca Raton, Fl, pp. 165–187.

Sauk, J. J. and Somerman, M. J. (1991). Physiology of bone: mineral compartment proteins as candidates for environmental perturbation by lead. *Environ. Health Perspect.*, **91**, 9–16.

Savory J., Exley, C., Forbes, W. F., Huang, Y., Joshi, J. G., Kruck, T., McLachlan, D. R. and Wakayama, I. (1996). Can the controversy of the role of aluminum in Alzheimer's disease be resolved? What are the suggested approaches to this controversy and methodological issues to be considered? *J. Toxicol. Environ. Health*, **48**, 615–635.

Scheinberg, I. H. and Sternlieb, I. (1996). Wilson disease and idiopathic copper toxicosis. *Am. J. Clin. Nutr.*, **63**, 842S–845S.

Schilsky, M. L. (1996). Wilson disease: genetic basis of copper toxicity and natural history. *Sem. Liver Dis.*, **16**, 83–95.

Schwartz, J. (1993). Beyond LOEL's, *p* values, and vote counting: methods for looking at the shapes and strengths of associations. *Neurotoxicology.*, **14**, 237–246.

Serfontein, W. J. and Mekel, R. (1979). Bismuth toxicity in man – II. Review of bismuth blood and urine levels in patients after administration of therapeutic bismuth formulations in relation to the problem of bismuth toxicity in man. *Res. Commun. Chem. Pathol. Pharmacol.*, **26**, 391–411.

Shannon, R. L. and Strayer, D. S. (1989). Arsenic-induced skin toxicity. *Hum. Toxicol.*, **8**, 99–104.

Shen, Z. X., Chen, G. Q., Ni, J. H., Li, X. S., Xiong, S. M., Qiu, Q. Y., Zhu, J., Tang, W., Sun, G. L., Yang, K. Q., Chen, Y., Zhou, L., Fang, Z. W., Wang, Y. T., Ma, J., Zhang, P., Zhang, T. D., Chen, S. J., Chen, Z. and Wang, Z. Y. (1997). Use of arsenic trioxide (As_2O_3) in the treatment of acute promyelocytic leukemia (APL): II. Clinical efficacy and pharmacokinetics in relapsed patients. *Blood*, **89**, 3354–3360.

Shi, C., Lane, A. T. and Clarkson, T. W. (1990). Uptake of mercury by the hair of methylmercury-treated newborn mice. *Environ. Res.*, **51**, 170–181.

Silbergeld, E. K., Sauk, J., Somerman, M., Todd, A., McNeill, F., Fowler, B., Fontaine, A. and van Buren, J. (1993). Lead in bone: storage site, exposure source, and target organ. *Neurotoxicology*, **14**, 225–236.

Simons, T. J. (1984). Active transport of lead by human red blood cells. *FEBS Lett.*, **172**, 250–254.

Simons, T. J. (1986). The role of anion transport in the passive movement of lead across the human red cell membrane. *J. Physiol.*, **378**, 287–312.

Simons, T. J. and Pocock, G. (1987). Lead enters bovine adrenal medullary cells through calcium channels. *J. Neurochem.*, **48**, 383–389.

Sinigaglia, F. (1994). The molecular basis of metal recognition by T cells. *J. Invest. Dermatol.*, **102**, 398–401.

Sinigaglia, F., Scheidegger, D., Garotta, G., Scheper, R., Pletscher, M. and Lanzavecchia, A. (1985). Isolation and characterization of Ni-specific T cell clones from patients with Ni-contact dermatitis. *J. Immunol.*, **135**, 3929–3932.

Sithisarankul, P., Schwartz, B. S., Lee, B. K., Kelsey, K. T. and Strickland, P. T. (1997). Aminolevulinic acid dehydratase genotype mediates plasma levels of the neurotoxin, 5-aminolevulinic acid, in lead-exposed workers. *Am. J. Ind. Med.*, **32**, 15–20.

Skerfving, S. (1993). *Inorganic Lead*. In Criteria Documents from the Nordic Expert Group. Beije, B. and Lundberg, P. (eds). Nordic Council of Ministers, Gothenberg, Sweden. Arbete and Hälsa, **1**, 125–237.

Skerfving, S., Nilsson, U., Schutz, A. and Gerhardsson, L. (1993). Biological monitoring of inorganic lead. *Scand. J. Work Environ. Health*, **19**, Suppl. 1, 59–64.

Slikkerveer, A. and de Wolff, F. A. (1989). Pharmacokinetics and toxicity of bismuth compounds. *Med. Toxicol. Adverse Drug Exp.*, **4**, 303–323.

Smith, A. H., Biggs, M. L., Hopenhayn-Rich, C. and Kalman, D. (1995). Arsenic risk assessment. *Environ. Health Perspect.*, **103**, 13–17.

Smith, D. R. and Flegal, A. R. (1992). Stable isotopic tracers of lead mobilized by DMSA chelation in low lead-exposed rats. *Toxicol. Appl. Pharmacol.*, **116**, 85–91.

Smith, R. G., Vorwald, A. J., Patil, L. S. and Mooney, T. F., Jr. (1970). Effects of exposure to mercury in the manufacture of chlorine. *Am. Ind. Hyg. Assoc. J.*, **31**, 687–700.

Snow, E. T. (1992). Metal carcinogenesis: mechanistic implications. *Pharmacol. Ther.*, **53**, 31–65.

Sorahan, T. and Lancashire, R. J. (1997). Lung cancer mortality in a cohort of workers employed at a cadmium recovery plant in the United States: an analysis with detailed job histories. *Occup. Environ. Med.*, **54**, 194–201.

Sorahan, T., Lister, A., Gilthorpe, M. S. and Harrington, J. M. (1995). Mortality of copper cadmium alloy workers with special reference to lung cancer and non-malignant diseases of the respiratory system, 1946–92. *Occup. Environ. Med.*, **52**, 804–812.

Sorensen, J. A., Nielsen, J. B. and Andersen, O. (1993). Identification of the gastrointestinal absorption site for cadmium chloride *in vivo*. *Pharmacol. Toxicol.*, **73**, 169–73.

Standeven, A. M. and Wetterhahn, K. E. (1991). Is there a role for reactive oxygen species in the mechanism of chromium (VI) carcinogenesis? *Chem. Res. Toxicol.*, **4**, 616–625.

Standeven, A. M. and Wetterhahn, K. E. (1992). Ascorbate is the principal reductant of chromium (VI) in rat lung ultrafiltrates and cytosols, and mediates chromium-DNA binding *in vitro*. *Carcinogenesis*, **13**, 1319–1324.

Stearns, D. M., Courtney, K. D., Giangrande, P. H., Phieffer, L. S. and Wetterhahn, K. E. (1994). Chromium(VI) reduction by ascorbate: role of reactive intermediates in DNA damage *in vitro*. *Environ. Health Perspect.*, **102**, Suppl. 3, 21–25.

Stella, M., Montaldi, A., Rossi, R., Rossi, G. and Levis, A. G. (1982). Clastogenic effects of chromium on human lymphocytes *in vitro* and *in vivo*. *Mutat. Res.*, **101**, 151–64.

Stohs, S. J. and Bagchi, D. (1995). Oxidative mechanisms in the toxicity of metal ions. *Free Rad. Biol. Med.*, **18**, 321–336.

Stollery, B. T., Broadbent, D. E., Banks, H. A. and Lee, W. R. (1991). Short term prospective study of cognitive functioning in lead workers. *Br. J. Ind. Med.*, **48**, 739–749.

Strömberg, U., Schutz, A. and Skerfving, S. (1995). Substantial decrease of blood lead in Swedish children, 1978–94, associated with petrol lead. *Occup. Environ. Med.*, **52**, 764–769.

Sugawara, N., Lai, Y. R., Arizono, K. and Ariyoshi, T. (1996). Biliary excretion of exogenous cadmium, and endogenous copper and zinc in the Eisai hyperbilirubinuric (EHB) rat with a near absence of biliary glutathione. *Toxicology*, **112**, 87–94.

Szymanska, J. A. and Piotrowski, J. K. (1980). Studies to identify the low molecular weight bismuth-binding proteins in rat kidney. *Biochem. Pharmacol.*, **29**, 2913–2918.

Takenaka, S., Oldiges, H., Konig, H., Hochrainer, D. and Oberdorster, G. (1983). Carcinogenicity of cadmium chloride aerosols in W. rats. *J. Natl. Cancer Inst.*, **70**, 367–373.

Taketani, S., Kohno, H., Yoshinaga, T. and Tokunaga, R. (1988). Induction of heme oxygenase in rat hepatoma cells by exposure to heavy metals and hyperthermia. *Biochem. Int.*, **17**, 665–672.

Tam, G. K., Charbonneau, S. M., Bryce, F., Pomroy, C. and Sandi, E. (1979). Metabolism of inorganic arsenic (74As) in humans following oral ingestion. *Toxicol. Appl. Pharmacol.*, **50**, 319–322.

Tanzi, R. E., Petrukhin, K., Chernov, I., Pellequer, J. L., Wasco, W., Ross, B., Romano, D. M., Parano, E., Pavone, L., Brzustowicz, L. M., *et al.* (1993). The Wilson disease gene is a copper transporting ATPase with homology to the Menkes disease gene. *Nature Genet.*, **5**, 344–350.

Thomas, D. J., Fisher, H. L., Hall, I. L. and Mushak, P. (1982). Effects of age and sex on retention of mercury by methyl mercury-treated rats. *Toxicol. Appl. Pharmacol.*, **62**, 445–454.

Thomas, D. J., Fisher, H. L., Sumler, M. R., Hall, I. L. and Mushak, P. (1988). Distribution and retention of organic and inorganic mercury in methyl mercury-treated neonatal rats. *Environ. Res.*, **47**, 59–71.

Thomas, D. W. (1991). Bismuth. In Merian, E. (Ed.), *Metals and Their Compounds in the Environment*. VCH, Weinheim, pp. 789–801.

Thomas, D. W., Hartley, T. F., Coyle, P. and Sobecki, S. (1987). Bismuth. In Seiler, H. G., Sigel, H. and Sigel, A. (Eds), *Handbook on Toxicity of Inorganic Compounds*. Marcel Dekker, New York, pp. 115–127.

Thomas, G. R., Forbes, J. R., Roberts, E. A., Walshe, J. M. and Cox, D. W. (1995). The Wilson disease gene: spectrum of mutations and their consequences. *Nature Genet.*, **9**, 210–217.

Tohyama, C., Suzuki, J. S., Homma, S., Karasawa, M., Kuroki, T., Nishimura, H. and Nishimura, N. (1996). Testosterone-dependent induction of metallothionein in genital organs of male rats. *Biochem. J.*, **317**, 97–102.

Tseng, W.-P. (1977). Effects and dose – response relationships of skin cancer and Blackfoot disease with arsenic. *Environ. Health Perspect.*, **19**, 109–119.

Tseng, W-P., Chu, H. M., How, S. W., Fong, J. M., Lin, C. S. and Yeh, S. (1968). Prevalence of skin cancer in an endemic area of chronic arsenicism in Taiwan. *J. Natl. Cancer Inst.*, **40**, 453–463.

Uchida, Y., Takio, K., Titani, K., Ihara, Y. and Tomonaga, M. (1991). The growth inhibitory factor that is deficient in the Alzheimer's disease brain is a 68 amimo acid metallothionein-like protein. *Neuron*, **7**, 337–347.

Vahter, M. (Ed.) (1982). *Assessment of Human Exposure to Lead and Cadmium Through Biological Monitoring*. National Swedish Institute of Environmental Medicine and Department of Environmental Hygiene, Karolinska Institute, Stockholm. Report prepared for the United Nations Environment Programme and the World Health Organization.

Vahter, M. (1986). Environmental and occupational exposure to inorganic arsenic. *Acta Pharmacol. Toxicol.*, **59**, Suppl. 7, 31–34.

Vahter, M. (1994a). Species differences in the metabolism of arsenic compounds. *Appl. Organomet. Chem.*, **8**, 175–182.

Vahter, M. (1994b). What are the chemical forms of arsenic in urine, and what can they tell us about exposure? *Clin. Chem.*, **40**, 679–680.

Vahter, M. and Marafante, E. (1985). Reduction and binding of arsenate in marmoset monkeys. *Arch. Toxicol.*, **57**, 119–24.

Vahter, M. and Marafante, E. (1988). *In vivo* methylation and detoxication of arsenic. In Craig, P. J. and Glockling, F. (Eds) *The Biological Alkylation of Heavy Elements*. Royal Society of Chemistry, London, pp. 105–119.

Vahter, M., Marafante, E., Lindgren, A. and Dencker, L. (1982). Tissue distribution and subcellular binding of arsenic in marmoset monkeys after injection of 74 As-arsenite. *Arch. Toxicol.*, **51**, 65–77.

Vahter, M., Marafante, E. and Dencker, L. (1984). Tissue distribution and retention of 74 As-dimethylarsinic acid in mice and rats. *Arch. Environ. Contam. Toxicol.*, **13**, 259–264.

Vahter, M., Berglund, M., Slorach, S., Friberg, L., Saric, M., Zheng, X. Q. and Fujita, M. (1991). Methods for integrated exposure monitoring of lead and cadmium. *Environ. Res.*, **56**, 78–89.

Vahter, M., Mottet, N. K., Friberg, L., Lind, B., Shen, D. D. and Burbacher, T. (1994). Speciation of mercury in the primate blood and brain following long-term exposure to methyl mercury. *Toxicol. Appl. Pharmacol.*, **124**, 221–229.

Vahter, M., Concha, G., Nermell, B., Nilsson, R., Dulout, F. and Natarajan, A. T. (1995a). A unique metabolism of inorganic arsenic in native Andean women. *Eur. J. Pharmacol.*, **293**, 455–462.

Vahter, M., Couch, R., Nermell, B. and Nilsson, R. (1995b). Lack of methylation of inorganic arsenic in the chimpanzee. *Toxicol. Appl. Pharmacol.*, **133**, 262–268.

Vahter, M., Counter, S. A., Laurell, G., Buchanan, L. H., Ortega, F., Schütz, A. and Skerfving, S. (1997). Extensive lead exposure in children living in an area in Ecuador with production of lead-glazed tiles. *Int. Arch. Occup. Environ. Health.*, **70**, 282–286.

Vallee, B. L. and Auld, D. S. (1990). Zinc coordination, function, and structure of zinc enzymes and other proteins. *Biochemistry*, **29**, 5647–5659.

Vimy, M. J., Takahashi, Y. and Lorscheider, F. L. (1990). Maternal – fetal distribution of mercury (203 Hg) released from dental amalgam fillings. *Am. J. Physiol.*, **258**, R939–R945.

Vulpe, C. D. and Packman, S. (1995). Cellular copper transport. *Annu. Rev. Nutr.*, **15**, 293–322.

Vogel, D. G., Margolis, R. L. and Mottet, N. K. (1989). Analysis of methyl mercury binding sites on tubulin subunits and microtubules. *Pharmacol. Toxicol.*, **64**, 196–201.

Waalkes, M. P. and Misra, R. R. (1996). Cadmium carcinogenicity and genotoxicity. In Chang, L. W. (Ed.), *Toxicology of Metals*. CRC Press, Boca Raton, Fl, pp. 231–243.

Waalkes, M. P. and Rehm, S. (1992). Carcinogenicity of oral cadmium in the male Wistar (WF/NCr) rat: effect of chronic dietary zinc deficiency. *Fundam. Appl. Toxicol.*, **19**, 512–520.

Waalkes, M. P. and Rehm, S. (1994a). Cadmium and prostate cancer. *J. Toxicol. Environ. Health*, **43**, 251–269.

Waalkes, M. P. and Rehm, S. (1994b). Chronic toxic and carcinogenic effects of cadmium chloride in male DBA/2NCr and NFS/NCr mice: strain-dependent association with tumors of the hematopoietic system, injection site, liver, and lung. *Fundam. Appl. Toxicol.*, **23**, 21–31.

Wang, Z. and Rossman, T. G. (1993). Stable and inducible arsenite resistance in Chinese hamster cells. *Toxicol. Appl. Pharmacol.*, **118**, 80–86.

Wang, Z. and Rossman, T. G. (1996). Arsenic carcinogenicity and genotoxicity. In Chang, L. W. (Ed.), *Toxicology of Metals*. CRC Press, Boca Raton, Fl. pp. 221–229.

Webb, D. R., Sipes, I. G. and Carter, D. E. (1984) *In vitro* solubility and *in vivo* toxicity of gallium arsenide. *Toxicol. Appl. Pharmacol.*, **76**, 96–104.

Welch, W. J. (1990). The mammalian stress response: cell physiology and biochemistry of stress proteins. In Moromoto, R., Tissieres, A. and Georgopoulos, C. (Eds). *The Role of the Stress Response in Biology and Disease*. Cold Spring Harbor Laboratory Press, Cold Spring Harbor, NY.

Wetmur, J. G. (1994). Influence of the common human delta-aminolevulinate dehydratase polymorphism on lead body burden. *Environ. Health Perspect.*, **102**, Suppl. 3, 215–219.

Wetterhahn, K. E. and Hamilton, J. W. (1989). Molecular basis of hexavalent chromium carcinogenicity: effect on gene expression. *Sci. Total Environ.*, **86**, 113–129.

Wetterhahn, K. E., Hamilton, J. W., Aiyar, J., Borges, K. M. and Floyd, R. (1989). Mechanism of chromium (VI) carcinogenesis. Reactive intermediates and effect on gene expression. *Biol. Trace Elem. Res.*, **21**, 405–411.

WHO (1981). *Environmental Health Criteria 18: Arsenic.* World Health Organization, Geneva.

WHO (1987). *Air Quality Guidelines for Europe.* WHO Regional Publications, European Series, No. 23. World Health Organization Regional Office for Europe, Copenhagen.

WHO (1988). *Environmental Health Criteria 61: Chromium.* World Health Organization, Geneva.

WHO (1989). Cadmium. In *Evaluation of Certain Food Additives and Contaminants. Thirty-third Report of the Joint FAO/WHO Expert Committee on Food Additives.* WHO Technical Report Series, No. 776. World Health Organization, Geneva, pp. 28–31.

WHO (1990a). *Environmental Health Criteria 101: Methylmercury.* World Health Organization, Geneva.

WHO (1990b). *Environmental Health Criteria 106: Beryllium.* World Health Organization, Geneva.

WHO (1991a). *Environmental Health Criteria 108: Nickel.* World Health Organization, Geneva.

WHO (1991b). *Environmental Health Criteria 118: Inorganic Mercury.* World Health Organization, Geneva.

WHO (1992). *Environmental Health Criteria 134: Cadmium.* World Health Organization, Geneva.

WHO (1993). *Guidelines for Drinking-water Quality.* World Health Organization, Geneva.

WHO (1995). *Environmental Health Criteria 165: Inorganic Lead.* World Health Organization, Geneva.

WHO (1996). *Trace Elements in Human Nutrition and Health.* World Health Organization, Geneva.

Winski, S. L., Barber, D. S., Rael, L. T. and Carter, D. E. (1997). Sequence of toxic events in arsine-induced hemolysis in vitro: implications for the mechanism of toxicity in human erythrocytes. *Fundam. Appl. Toxicol.*, **38**, 123–128.

Woods, J. S. (1996). Effects of metals on the hematopoietic system and heme metabolism. In Chang, L. W. (Ed.), *Toxicology of Metals*. CRC Press, Boca Raton, Fl. pp. 939–958.

Woods, J. S. and Fowler, B. A. (1983). Selective inhibition of delta-aminolevulinic acid dehydratase by indium chloride in rat kidney: biochemical and ultrastructural studies. *Exp. Mol. Pathol.*, **36**, 306–315.

Yamaguchi, Y., Heiny, M. E., Suzuki, M. and Gitlin, J. D. (1996). Biochemical characterization and intracellular localization of the Menkes disease protein. *Proc. Natl. Acad. Sci. USA.*, **93**, 14030–14035.

Yamamoto, A., Hisanaga, A. and Ishinishi, N. (1987). Tumorigenicity of inorganic arsenic compounds following intratracheal instillations to the lungs of hamsters. *Int. J. Cancer*, **40**, 220–223.

Yamashita, N., Doi, M., Nishio, M., Hojo, H. and Tanaka, M. (1972). Recent observations of Kyoto children poisoned by arsenic tainted 'Morinaga Dry Milk'. *Jpn. J. Hyg.*, **27**, 364–399 (in Japanese).

Yamauchi, H., Takahashi, K., Yamamura, Y. and Fowler, B. A. (1992). Metabolism of subcutaneously administered indium arsenide in the hamster. *Toxicol. Appl. Pharmacol.*, **116**, 66–70.

Yang, G. and Zhou, R. (1994). Further observations on the human maximum safe dietary selenium intake in a seleniferous area of China. *J. Trace Elem. Electrolyt. Health Dis.*, **8**, 159–165.

Yang, G., Zhou, R., Yin, S., Gu, L., Yan, B., Liu, Y., Liu, Y. and Li, X. (1989a). Studies of safe maximal daily dietary selenium intake in a seleniferous area in China. I. Selenium intake and tissue selenium levels of the inhabitants. *J. Trace Elem. Electrolyt. Health Dis.*, **3**, 77–87.

Yang, G., Yin, S., Zhou, R., Gu, L., Yan, B., Liu, Y. and Liu, Y. (1989b). Studies of safe maximal daily dietary selenium intake in a seleniferous area in China. II. Relation between Se-intake and the manifestation of clinical signs and certain biochemical alterations in blood and urine. *J. Trace Elem. Electrolyt. Health Dis.*, **3**, 123–130.

Zakharyan, R., Wu, Y., Bogdan, G. M. and Aposhian, H. V. (1995). Enzymatic methylation of arsenic compounds: assay, partial purification, and properties of arsenite methyltransferase and monomethylarsonic acid methyltransferase of rabbit liver. *Chem. Res. Toxicol.*, **8**, 1029–1038.

Zakharyan, R. A., Wildfang, E., Aposhian, H. V. (1996). Enzymatic methylation of arsenic compounds. III. The marmoset and tamarin, but not the rhesus, monkeys are deficient in methyltransferases that methylate inorganic arsenic. *Toxicol. Appl. Pharmacol.*, **140**, 77–84.

Zalups, R. K. (1991). Method for studying the *in vivo* accumulation of inorganic mercury in segments of the nephron in the kidneys of rats treated with mercuric chloride. *J. Pharmacol. Methods.*, **26**, 89–104.

Zalups, R. K. and Barfuss, D. W. (1993). Transport and toxicity of methylmercury along the proximal tubule of the rabbit. *Toxicol. Appl. Pharmacol.*, **121**, 176–185.

Zalups, R. K. and Barfuss, D. W. (1995a). Accumulation and handling of inorganic mercury in the kidney after coadministration with glutathione. *J. Toxicol. Environ. Health*, **44**, 385–399.

Zalups, R. K. and Barfuss, D. W. (1995b). Renal disposition of mercury in rats after intravenous injection of inorganic mercury and cysteine. *J. Toxicol. Environ. Health.*, **44**, 401–413.

Chapter 98
Toxicology of Chemical Warfare Agents

Robert L. Maynard

C O N T E N T S

HISTORICAL INTRODUCTION

Throughout history humans have sought more effective means of killing and disabling their fellow men. Stones, clubs, spears, bows and arrows, gunpowder, muskets, rifles, high explosives, machine-guns, tanks, warplanes, rockets and nuclear weapons comprise an apparently unending catalogue of increasing military sophistication designed for the destruction of one's enemies while exposing one's forces to decreasing risk. Accompanying this development of military hardware, the effects of which are based on the physical disruption of men or materials, has been a very much less marked development of chemical means of attack. Some chemicals have been used as a means of killing and others as a means of incapacitating. Recently, attempts have been made to stem the development of chemical weapons but it is a sad reflection on the world that in 1999 more countries than ever have acquired, or are in the process of acquiring, the means to wage a chemical war.

Chemical weapons probably began with smoke and flame, and the hurling of various concoctions of pitch and sulphur (Greek Fire) dates from classical times. Irritant smokes were described by Plutarch, hypnotic substances by the Scottish historian Buchanan, compounds allegedly capable of producing incessant diarrhoea by classical Greek authors (SIPRI, 1971) and preparations containing the saliva of rabid dogs by Leonardo da Vinci (1452–1519) (Reprint Society, 1938).

At the time these authors were writing, chemistry and chemical technology were in their infancy, and the chem-ical weapons developed had probably only a marginal effect on the outcome of battles or wars. However, during the mediaeval period the widespread use of poisons acquired, rightly, an evil reputation and the use of such compounds came to be despised by military men. The use of poisons was seen as running counter to the tenets of chivalrous conduct and this view has persisted and lies close to the root of the objections raised during the twentieth century to the use of chemical weapons (Haldane, 1925).

At the end of the nineteenth century, the first international convention to address, among other topics, chemical warfare was held. This, the First Hague Convention (1899), led to a wide-ranging prohibition of the use of chemicals in war: 'The contracting powers agree to abstain from the use of all projectiles the sole object of which is the diffusion of asphyxiating or deleterious gases' (Prentiss, 1937).

Despite this prohibition, chemical warfare was used on a large scale during World War I, some 113 000 tons of chemical weapons being used in all (Prentiss, 1937). Lefebure (1921) reported that on 9 March 1918 German forces fired some 200 000 mustard gas shells. This resulted in many casualties but compared with the total casualties produced during World War I the number of casualties from chemical warfare was low. This is shown in **Table 1** (Prentiss, 1937).

From the figures given in this table, a number of deductions can be made: (1) the proportion of deaths attributable to chemical warfare during World War I was low; (2) the ratio of dead to injured among those

Table 1 Chemical warfare and other casualties during World War I

Country	Battle casualties due to gas			Total battle deaths	Total wounds including battle deaths
	Non-fatal	Deaths	Total		
Russia	419 340	56 000	475 340	1 416 700	6 366 700
France	182 000	8 000	190 000	1 131 500	5 397 500
British Empire	180 597	8 109	188 706	585 533	2 590 509
Italy	55 373	4 627	60 000	541 500	1 488 500
USA	71 345	1 462	72 807	52 842	272 138
Germany	191 000	9 000	2 00 000	1 478 000	5 694 058
Austria/Hungary	97 000	3 000	1 00 000	1 000 000	4 620 000
Other	9 000	1 000	10 000	6 84 436	1 580 318
Total	1 205 655	91 198	1 296 853	6 890 511	28 009 723

Wounded due to chemical warfare as percentage of all wounded (including fatalities): 4.63%.
Deaths due to chemical warfare as percentage of total chemical warfare injured: 7.03%.
Deaths due to chemical warfare as percentage of all deaths: 1.32%.
UK forces deaths due to chemical warfare as percentage of total UK forces deaths: 4.3%.
Source: after Prentiss (1937).

affected by chemical warfare was very low; (3) ill-prepared forces, e.g. Russian troops on the Eastern Front, suffered badly. These observations have been examined in detail elsewhere (Maynard, 1988) and have been adduced by some as evidence of the efficacy of chemical warfare and by others as evidence of its inefficacy. Space here does not permit an examination of these interpretations.

After World War I, a widespread campaign to ban chemical warfare was mounted and the Geneva Protocol, promulgated in 1925, encapsulated widely held opinion. However, during the Italian campaign in Ethiopia (1935–36), Italian troops used mustard gas on a large scale against unprotected native forces (SIPRI, 1971). Many casualties were produced. During the late 1930s, fear that fascist countries might use chemical warfare on a substantial scale during a future war led to the incorporation of anti-gas drills into Air Raid Precautions (ARP) in the UK and the issue of gas masks to all troops and civilians. These fears were not demonstrated to have been justified during World War II despite the production of large quantities of chemical warfare munitions by both sides. Germany's reluctance to use chemical weapons has never been satisfactorily explained, particularly as she had what many might have considered a great advantage in having synthesized the very toxic nerve agents which were unknown to the Allied Powers. The discovery of large stocks of these compounds, the acquisition of the means of production by the USSR, and the worsening state of international relations led to the expansion of research into chemical warfare in both the UK and USA during the years following World War II.

The UK's programme of research, designed to produce chemical weapons, sometimes described as 'offensive research' (in contrast to work on antidotes and means of protection: 'defensive research'), was halted

permanently in 1956 with the decommissioning of the nerve agent production plant at the Chemical Defence Establishment out-station at Nancekuke in Cornwall. Production of nerve agents continued in the USA until 1969 and began again in 1981 in order to produce the components of the so called 'binary weapon system' (Meselson and Perry Robinson, 1980). Production in the USSR probably continued in parallel with that in the USA.

Accusations of use have been common since World War II. Those of their use by Egyptian forces in Yemen (1963–67) seem better supported than many others. US forces used defoliants and irritants on a large scale during the war in Vietnam. That this represented a use of chemical warfare has been strenuously denied by US sources and the view that the use of CS (2-chlorobenzylidene malononitrile) tear-gas, which had been sanctioned for use in the USA against rioting civilians, could not be regarded as an exercise in chemical warfare has been voiced.

Iraq, during the Iran–Iraq war in the early and mid-1980s, used chemical weapons on a large scale, mustard gas and probably the nerve agent tabun being used (United Nations Reports, 1984, 1986, 1987). Many casualties resulted, and in one particularly distressing incident, at Halabja, some 5000 civilians were killed. Death from chemical warfare on this scale had not been known since the gas cloud attacks of 1915 and attracted international condemnation.

Among less well known accusations are the use of 'Yellow Rain' in South East Asia (Seagrave, 1981) and the use of 'knock down agents' and 'black body agents' by USSR forces in Afghanistan. During 1988, reports that Libya had constructed a chemical warfare production plant appeared in the press. This report fuelled fears that terrorists might gain access to chemical weapons, and events in Japan have shown that terrorists are capable of deploying such weapons. Nevertheless, major steps were taken by both the USA and the USSR towards a verifiable ban on chemical weapons in 1988; on the other hand, expansion of the capacity to wage chemical warfare has continued in a number of other countries.

There is little evidence that chemical weapons were used during the Gulf War, although the production of such weapons by Iraq is not doubted. US and UK troops were provided with pyridostigmine as a pre-treatment against nerve agent attack (see below).

A detailed account of the subjects considered in this chapter may be found in the author's recent publication, *Chemical Warfare Agents: Toxicology and Treatment* (Marrs *et al.*, 1996).

CONCEPTS OF USE OF CHEMICAL WEAPONS

It is often assumed that chemical weapons would be used during a war to kill as many of the opposing forces as possible. This is fallacious and misrepresents the professed purpose of modern warfare. Modern warfare is, it is generally agreed, waged to compel governments to amend their actions and not to annihilate populations (Fotion and Elfstrom, 1986). It is a fact of military experience that the weapon systems which produce many casualties are likely to be more effective than systems which produce fatalities. Casualties require evacuation and nursing care and may sap morale. Because of this, chemical weapons would more likely be used to incapacitate than to kill. Some established chemical weapons such as mustard gas are rather ineffective as regards killing (the death rate in mustard casualties during World War I was about 2%) although particularly effective as incapacitants (Haldane, 1925).

Chemical weapons can be effectively defended against by the use of protective clothing, including a respirator, gloves, boots and special over-garments. Prophylactic drugs play a much less important part in providing protection. Physical protection inevitably carries the penalty of impaired performance and commanders might be loath to institute such measures. Indeed, aggressors might consider the use of, or the expression of willingness to use, chemical warfare as successful if they forced their opponents into protective clothing. Because of this, a policy of intelligent avoidance of contaminated areas would be likely to be observed. This has led to the development of the concept of use of chemical warfare agents as agents of 'ground denial' rather than as deliberate producers of casualties. Such an effect could well be exploited by an aggressor by attacks on centres of strategic and tactical importance, some 'behind the lines'. Such a use would inevitably lead to the exposure of civilians, probably less well trained and protected than

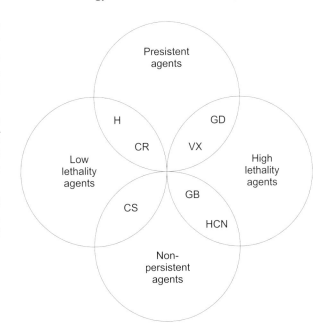

Figure 1 Categories of chemical warfare agents.

members of the Armed Forces, and the production of many civilian casualties. Lethal chemical warfare compounds could be used in high concentrations to permit the rapid breakthrough by well protected troops through strongly defended points.

These concepts of use permit a number of categories of chemical warfare agent to be defined (see **Figure 1**). Only a few well known chemical warfare agents have been included in **Figure 1**. Other compounds such as lewisite could well appear in more than one category. CS has been included as a non-persistent agent on the grounds of its rapid hydrolysis in contact with water.

It should be remembered that military concepts of use could well vary from area to area and reports of the use of specific chemical warfare agents may prove very difficult to understand unless details of the operational scenario are available.

Much of the thinking or doctrine as regards the use of chemical warfare agents was developed during periods of East–West tension when a war between NATO and Warsaw Pact forces was a possibility. Such a threat has now passed and the thinking is beginning to look dated.

STANDARD CLASSIFICATION OF CHEMICAL WARFARE AGENTS

A number of different classifications of chemical warfare agents have been devised. Two broad systems, 'medical' and 'service', are in general use and are compared in **Table 2** (HMSO, 1972). Both of these systems would be regarded today as outmoded by many experts. Several of the compounds listed in the table, e.g. LSD (lysergic acid diethylamide) and DM (10-chloro-5,

Table 2 Standard classifications of chemical warfare agents

Medical classification	Service classification
(1) Agents liable to be met in warfare	
Nerve agents (G and V)	Lethal agents (nerve)
Lung-damaging agents (phosgene and chlorine)	Lethal agents (choking)
Vesicant agents (sulphur mustard, lewisite, etc.)	Damaging agents (blister)
Psychotomimetic agents (LSD, BZ: 3-quinuclidinyl benzilate)	Incapacitating agents (mental)
Miscellaneous agents	
Cyanide	Lethal agents (blood)
Arsine	
Herbicides	–
(2) Agents liable to be met in riot control and/or war	
Sensory irritants CS and CR	Riot control agents
Vomiting agents, e.g. DM	Incapacitating agents (physical)

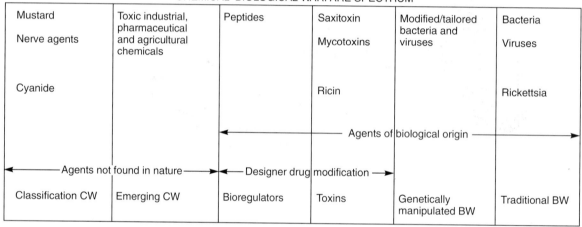

CHEMICAL–BIOLOGICAL WARFARE SPECTRUM

CW = chemical warfare; BW = biological warfare.   Source: after Pearson (1988).

Figure 2 Chemical–biological warfare spectrum.

10-dihydrophenarsazine), are no longer seen as likely to be used in war and chlorine and arsine are very unlikely to be used.

The possible means of production of chemical weapons have also changed in recent years as genetic engineering and the production of complex molecules on a large scale by cultures of bacteria and yeasts have been developed. Today, chemical weapons form a spectrum ranging from the classical chemical weapons, such as nerve agents and mustard gas, to the classical biological agents, such as the anthrax bacillus or the smallpox virus. Between the two extremes are compounds originally discovered as natural products, e.g. bacterial toxins, and which were classified as biological weapons, but which are in fact more or less well characterized chemical substances. The chemical–biological warfare spectrum is shown in **Figure 2** (Pearson, 1988). Useful though this classification is, it is likely that the simple military classification will remain in widespread use as it lends itself to

use in training and defining standard means of dealing with casualties.

GENERAL MANAGEMENT OF CHEMICAL WARFARE CASUALTIES

Few civilian doctors have any experience of the management of chemical warfare casualties; indeed, few military doctors in Western countries have ever seen a chemical warfare casualty. If casualties are to be well cared for and the carers not to be placed at risk, a number of key points must be borne in mind:

1. Early treatment of casualties is essential.
2. Attendants must be adequately protected from contamination.
3. Decontamination of casualties is the priority once life-saving measures, including the establishment of

adequate ventilation and the administration of antidotes, have been undertaken. Fullers' earth is an excellent decontaminant for liquid agents. Any source of water will suffice as a means of removing liquid agents from the eyes. Dilute solutions of bleach may also be used for decontamination. Care must be taken that such decontaminants are not allowed into the casualty's eyes.

4. Casualties should be moved as soon as possible after decontamination into a clean environment where clinicians may work under conditions with which they are familiar. Defence of this environment must be absolute.

5. Casualties will range from the mildly affected to the moribund and the rules of triage must be rigorously applied if optimal use is to be made of clinical resources.

6. Early identification of the agent responsible for the poisoning will be of great value to the clinician and every effort should be made to use such detectors and monitors as are available.

7. Some casualties will require intensive nursing and should be moved along evacuation routes as quickly as possible.

VESICANT COMPOUNDS

Vesicant compounds were introduced as chemical warfare agents on 12 July 1917 when German forces used sulphur mustard at Ypres (Prentiss, 1937). Mustard gas became the most effective chemical warfare agent used during World War I, 14 000 British casualties being produced during the first 3 months of use and 120 000 by the end of the war (HMSO, 1923). This efficacy earned for mustard gas the sobriquet 'King of the Battle Gases' but, despite this, it carried only a low lethality. This low lethality, of the order of 2%, was one of the points which convinced Haldane (1925) of the desirability of chemical warfare as compared with conventional warfare.

Physicochemical Properties of Mustard Gas

'Mustard gas' is an unfortunate misnomer as the compound which at room temperature gives off vapour and smells of mustard, garlic or leeks, is a liquid with a boiling point of 217 °C. Sulphur mustard is often referred to as HS (Hun Stoff) or more commonly as HD. The nitrogen mustards are referred to as HN1, HN2 and HN3. The formulae and some of the characteristics of the mustards are shown in **Table 3**.

Sulphur mustard is poorly miscible with water but on mixing hydrolysis takes place, leading to the production of thiodiglycol and hydrochloric acid **(Figure 3)**. The low miscibility and solubility of sulphur mustard in water leads to lengthy persistence of the compound in the field, particularly if protected from wind and rain. Sulphur mustard vapour passes quickly through clothing, although properly designed, modern military protective clothing provides good protection. Sulphur mustard in the liquid state passes quickly through ordinary surgical rubber gloves and heavy gloves made of butyl rubber should be worn when decontaminating casualties. The standard issue UK military respirator provides excellent protection against mustard gas vapour.

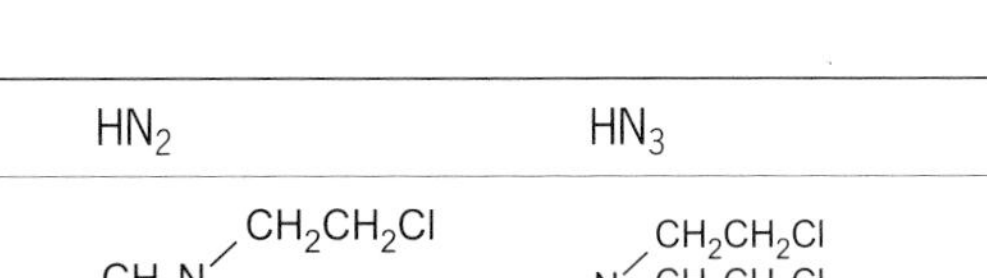

Figure 3 Hydrolysis of sulphur mustard.

Table 3 Physicochemical characteristics of mustard vesicants

Characteristic	H	HN$_1$	HN$_2$	HN$_3$
Formula	$S\begin{cases} CH_2CH_2Cl \\ CH_2CH_2Cl \end{cases}$	$C_2H_5N\begin{cases} CH_2CH_2Cl \\ CH_2CH_2Cl \end{cases}$	$CH_3N\begin{cases} CH_2CH_2Cl \\ CH_2CH_2Cl \end{cases}$	$N\begin{cases} CH_2CH_2Cl \\ CH_2CH_2Cl \\ CH_2CH_2Cl \end{cases}$
Appearance	Yellowish, oily liquid	←———— Colourless or yellowish oily liquids ————→		
M.P.(°C)	14	−34	−60	−4
B.P.(°C)	217	85	75	138
S.G.	1.27	1.09	1.15	1.24
V.P. (mmHg)				
10°C	0.032	0.0773	0.130	0.00272
25°C	0.112	0.2500	0.427	0.01090
40°C	0.346	0.7220	1.250	0.03820
Odour	Mustard-like, garlic, leek or horseradish-like		Soapy or fishy	

Absorption of Sulphur Mustard

Sulphur mustard, as a liquid or vapour, is lipid soluble and is absorbed across the skin. Renshaw (1946) demonstrated that 80% of a sample of sulphur mustard placed on the uncovered skin evaporated. Cameron et al. (1946) demonstrated, in rabbits, that some 80% of inhaled vapour was absorbed in the nose. Clinical experience suggests that the majority of inhaled sulphur mustard is absorbed in the upper airways.

Toxicity of Sulphur Mustard

The toxicity of sulphur mustard as an incapacitating agent is militarily of much greater importance than its capacity to kill in terms of LD_{50}, and compared with the nerve agents, sulphur mustard is a comparatively non-toxic compound. Intravenous LD_{50} figures include rat 3.3 mg kg^{-1} and mice 8.6 mg kg^{-1} (Anslow et al., 1948). Much more important are the effects of exposures to differing concentration/time products (Ct products). These are listed in **Table 4**.

Figure 4 shows the interdependence of concentration and time in defining the effects of mustard gas vapour.

Mechanism of Action of Sulphur Mustard

Sulphur mustard is an alkylating agent and a detailed account of the mode of action of such compounds will be found in Chapter 50 and in the works of Goodman and Gilman (1980) and Fox and Scott (1980). Both sulphur mustard and the various nitrogen mustards are bifunctional alkylating agents possessing two side-chains capable of undergoing cyclization. Cross-linking of guanine in nucleic acids results from this property. Cross-linked guanine molecules are shown in **Figure 5**.

Binding of the ethylenesulphonium ion (sulphur mustard) or the ethylimmonium ion (nitrogen mustard) to DNA produces a range of effects including:

- Alkylated guanine residues tend to form base pairs with thymine rather than with cytosine, leading to coding errors and hence inaccurate protein synthesis.
- Damaged guanine residues may be excised from the DNA molecule.
- A pair of guanine residues may become cross-linked as shown in **Figure 5**. This is considered by some as the most serious effect of alkylating agents on DNA (Rink and Hopkins, 1995).

Repair to DNA may take place as long as damage is not too widespread. Juarez-Salinas et al. (1979) reported the polymerization of NAD under the influence of the poly (ADP ribose) polymerase enzyme as part of the DNA repair process. Papirmeister et al. (1984a, b) suggested that the reduction in the cellular levels of NAD following DNA repair could lead to cell death.

Early work by Dixon (1946) suggested a correlation between skin injury and inhibition of glycolysis. Although the effects of alkyating agents such as mustard

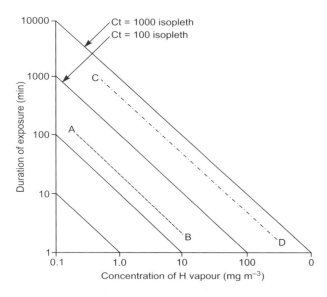

Figure 4 Effects of sulphur mustard vapour on humans. Lines AB and CD are offered as guides to early eye effects (AB: $Ct = 20$ mg min m^{-3}) and skin burns of significance (CD: $Ct = 500$ mg min m^{-3}). Because of uncertainty regarding the $Ct =$ constant relationship, extrapolation to extremes of time and concentration will be inaccurate.

Table 4 Effects of sulphur mustard vapour on humans

Exposure dose (mg min m^{-3})	Effects[a]
20–50	Onset of eye effects
70	Mild reddening of the eyes—tearing
100	Partial incapacitation from eye effects
100–400	Erythema of skin
200	Total incapacitation from eye effects
200–1000	Skin burns produced
750–10 000	Severe incapacitation from skin effects

[a] The effects of sulphur mustard vapour on the skin are very dependent on ambient temperature and the range shown for skin burns encompasses the effects of decreasing ambient temperature from 80 to 50 °F.

Figure 5 Cross-linking of guanine residues by sulphur mustard.

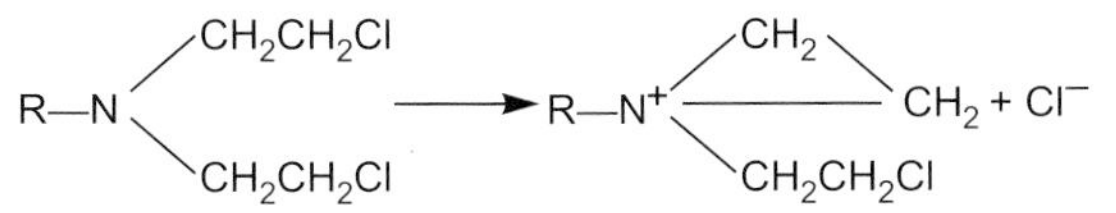

$$R-N \underset{CH_2CH_2Cl}{\overset{CH_2CH_2Cl}{<}} \longrightarrow R-N^+ \underset{CH_2CH_2Cl}{\overset{CH_2}{<}|CH_2 + Cl^-}$$

Figure 6 Formation of a quaternary ammonium compound.

on nucleic acids are usually stressed, it should be recalled that they also alkylate a wide range of other cellular components and enzymes. Membrane proteins at both the plasmalemma and the surfaces of intracellular organelles are liable to alkylation.

Despite this apparent understanding of how the alkylating agents act, no clear explanation of how mustard produces blisters is yet available. Miskin and Reich (1980) proposed increased protease synthesis and release after mustard-induced damage to cells. Release of such enzymes would be expected to set up an inflammatory response and would explain some of the effects of sulphur mustard. Acute inflammation does not, however, usually lead to blistering. Studies by Lindsay and Rice (1995, 1996) have suggested that laminin is a target for protease activation at the dermal–epidermal junction. Experiments in Yucatan mini-pigs showed that sulphur mustard induced micro-blister formation at this site. Damage to laminin was not accompanied by damage to Type IV collagen. Monteiro-Riviere and Inman (1995) have undertaken similar studies and have shown that the precise site of separation of the dermal–epidermal junction is beneath the hemidesmosomes in the upper part of the lamina lucida of the basal lamina.

The cholinomimetic effects of nitrogen mustard may be explained by cyclization leading to the formation of a quaternary ammonium compound (**Figure 6**).

Histopathology of the Skin Effects of Sulphur Mustard

Extensive experimental work was undertaken during World War I to discover the effects of sulphur mustard

on human skin. This work has been reported in detail by Ireland (1926).

Volunteer studies were undertaken, involving exposure of personnel to various concentrations of sulphur mustard; in some instances biopsies of damaged skin were taken. In one study small quantities (0.0004 ml drops) of sulphur mustard were placed on the skin. Small blisters were produced. The evolution of the lesions was followed by a timed series of biopsies.

Early vacuolation of the deeper layers of the epidermis was reported, as were nuclear changes in the stratum granulosum. Capillary dilation and leucocyte diapedesis were also noted. These changes were established some 30 min after exposure. Later separation at the dermal–epidermal junction occurred with liquefaction of the epidermis near the centre of the lesion. Epithelial cells of hair follicles and sweat glands were also affected. These changes were maximally developed by 18 h after exposure. Necrosis was followed by formation of an eschar by 72 h, sloughing by 4–6 days, a pigmented scar being present by 19 days.

Histochemical studies by Vogt *et al.* (1984) have confirmed the above and, furthermore, have demonstrated two phases of increased capillary permeability. Papirmeister (1984a, b) has undertaken detailed studies using athymic human skin-xenografted mice and has extended the above descriptions to the ultrastructural level. His papers should be consulted for details. Damage to the extracelullar matrix has been studied at the electron microscopic level by Chauhan *et al.* (1995).

Histopathology of the Effects of Sulphur and Nitrogen Mustard on the Eyes

These effects were investigated in detail by Mann (1948), who divided the compounds into two groups. These are described in **Table 5**. Note that the division does not correspond to the usual classification: sulphur mustard/ nitrogen mustard.

Table 5 Mann's classification of mustards by effects on the eye

	'Mustard gas group'	'Nitrogen mustard group'
Compounds	Sulphur mustard and HN_3	HN_1 and HN_2
Latent period	Present, may be some hours	Absent
Limits of early damage	Cornea and conjunctiva main site of damage	Rapid penetration to anterior chamber, pupil contracts and ciliary body releases a cellular exudate within 1 h of exposure
Later effects	Petechial haemorrhages Iridocyclitis rare	Haemorrhage Iridocyclitis common Intraocular haemorrhages often seen
Resolution	Usually complete	Permanent damage likely

Source: modified from Mann (1948).

Histopathology of the Effects of Mustard Gas on the Respiratory Tract

Several reports are available (Warthin and Weller, 1919; HMSO, 1923; Vedder, 1925; Ireland, 1926). These effects are largely confined to the conducting airways, with damage being particularly marked in the larger airways. The pseudostratified ciliated columnar epithelium becomes necrotic and sloughs; haemorrhages and inflammatory changes occur in the lamina propria and a false, diphtheritic membrane of sloughed cells, blood and exudate is formed. In severe cases damage to the submucosa and other layers of the airway wall may occur. Surface repair is by squamous metaplasia and complete restoration of a normal ciliated epithelium is suspected to be slow.

In the deeper lung, damage is usually less marked, although severe exposure can produce haemorrhagic pulmonary oedema. During World War I this was clearly recorded at post mortem and found to be most marked in the alveoli adjacent to conducting airways. Repair of damage at the alveolar level involves initial organization of the exudate and its subsequent removal by macrophages. Extensive fibrotic changes following exposure to mustard gas have not been demonstrated.

The findings described above have been confirmed in rats by Anderson *et al.* (1996). In addition to the already described effects, damage to bronchus-associated lymphatic tissue (BALT) and chondrocytes was reported. Examination of interalveolar septae with the electron microscope revealed peri-vascular oedema, although extensive pulmonary oedema was not reported.

Histopathology of the Effects of Mustard Gas on Bone Marrow

Alkylating agents in general have profound effects on rapidly dividing tissues and damage to the cells of the bone marrow produces an aplastic anaemia (Smith, 1986). The granulocyte series is first affected followed by the megakaryocytes and finally the erythropoietic series. In mustard gas casualties the peripheral white cell count has been observed to begin to fall on about the fourth day post-exposure after an initial post-exposure rise.

Symptoms and Signs of Exposure to Mustard Gas

The following is based on the accounts for Vedder (1925) and Warthin and Weller (1919) and the author's observations of Iranian casualties during 1985 and 1986. The comprehensive review of Willems (1989) should be consulted for further details. The symptoms and signs are listed in **Table 6**.

Clinical Investigations

Blood should be taken for estimation for thiodiglycol. Regular chest X-rays and standard haematological investigations are clearly indicated. Pulmonary function testing should be undertaken in all whose respiratory problems appear to be resolving particularly slowly.

Table 6 Symptoms and signs of exposure to mustard gas

Time post-exposure	Symptoms and signs
20–60 min	Nausea, retching and eye smarting have all been reported. More commonly a latent period of up to an hour occurs and was clearly recorded at first hand by Adolph Hitler from experience in 1918 (Hitler, 1925)
2–6 h	Inflammation of the eyes occurs with intense and burning eye pain. Lachrymation, blepharospasm, photophobia and rhinorrhoea appear; the face becomes reddened and the voice hoarse
6–24 h	Blisters develop on skin exposed to vapour or liquid. The blisters are delicate and are often rubbed off by the patient turning in bed. Blisters are not *per se* painful although if they occur over flexure lines at joints, pain may be produced on moving. The warm areas of the body are particularly liable to blistering with the axillae, inguinal folds, perineum and genitalia being badly affected. In contrast, the palms and soles appear to invariably escape blistering
24–48 h	Blistering becomes more marked and fresh crops of blisters appear. Coughing develops and sloughed tissue is expectorated. Intense itching of the skin may occur and frequently prevents sleep. Darkening of the skin, due to an increase of melanin in the basal layer of the epidermis, occurs and areas of dark brown or black hyperpigmentation are produced. Eye effects are maximal at this time and patients may be temporarily blinded
48 h–6 weeks	Blisters heal slowly and healing areas of skin are sensitive and secondary blistering may be produced by friction. Peeling of areas of hyperpigmentation to leave areas of hypopigmentation occurs and a striking piebald appearance may be produced. The eye problems resolve slowly and persistent roughening of the cornea may be observed
6 weeks–6 months	Many patients will have recovered by 6 weeks although in some the process takes much longer. A state of functional neurosis was described during World War I with depression and continuous eye problems. Persistent lachrymation and photophobia represent a particularly difficult problem

Management of Mustard Gas Casualties

As already stated, casualty management divides into two parts.

First Aid

Casualties should be moved quickly from the source of contamination by adequately protected attendants and decontaminated thoroughly with fullers' earth. Washing of the skin with kerosene to remove liquid contamination was strongly advocated by Vedder (1925), but if undertaken should be continued for 30 min.

Medical Management

There is no specific therapy for mustard gas lesions and no antidote has been demonstrated to be clinically effective in removing mustard from the body. Despite this, considerable amelioration of the effects may be achieved and secondary infection prevented.

Management of Skin Lesions

Large blisters should be aspirated aseptically as they are likely to be broken accidentally. Blister fluid is not harmful despite the oft repeated assertion that it contains free mustard and may cause damage to attendants. That blister fluid is harmless was conclusively demonstrated in volunteer studies by Sulzberger (1943). After aspiration blisters should be covered with sterile dry dressings. Treatment by exposure seems to be as effective as by wet dressings and demands less nursing care. A variety of ointments have been used in cases of mustard gas burns although none has been shown to enhance their rate of healing. Silver sulphadiazine cream (Flamazine) has been widely used and is useful in preventing secondary infection.

Severe itching and pain from damaged skin have been reported and in some cases narcotic analgesics have been used. This is probably unnecessary in the majority of cases and a milder analgesic combined with a sedative would be more appropriate therapy.

Most mustard gas burns are superficial or partial thickness burns. Deeper burns are occasionally seen and for these skin grafting should be considered as this may increase the rate of healing. Work by Rice (P. Rice, 1993, personal communication) has shown that in animal models light abrasion of mustard-damaged skin enhances the rate of healing.

Management of Eye Lesions

Early decontamination of liquid splashes in the eye is essential as a delay of more than a few minutes may make later decontamination ineffective and allow serious damage to occur (HMSO, 1972). For damaged eyes the following are recommended:

- Daily saline irrigations.
- The use of petroleum jelly on the follicular margins to prevent sticking.
- Chloramphenicol eye drops to prevent infection.
- Mydriatics, e.g. hyoscine drops, to prevent iridolenticular adhesions and to reduce pain caused by spasm of the ciliary muscle.
- It has been suggested that if eye pain is particularly severe, local anaesthetic drops should be used, amethocaine hydrochloride being recommended. Ophthalmological opinion should be sought before local anaesthetic or corticosteroid drops are used.
- Potassium ascorbate (10%) and sodium citrate (10%) drops 'alternately, each once an hour, i.e. half hourly drops, for 14 h or the waking day', are also recommended.
- Dark glasses to alleviate photophobia.
- Perhaps most important of all: constant reassurance that blindness will not be produced and that recovery *will* occur, albeit slowly.

Management of Lesions of the Respiratory Tract

Antibiotic cover is recommended if the respiratory effects are more than very mild. Codeine linctus is of value in preventing coughing at night. Mucolytics including acetylcysteine have been used in some cases although evidence of their efficacy is lacking. Calvet *et al.* (1996) have reported that betamethasone, given from 7–14 days post-exposure to sulphur mustard, enhanced regeneration of the airway epithelium. No clinical trials of glucocorticoids in mustard gas injuries of the respiratory tract have been reported, but this is a potentially important finding. In cases of very severe respiratory damage a chemical pneumonitis may be produced and may demand intensive care. Respiratory physicians and anaesthetists should be consulted if evidence of deteriorating respiratory function appears.

Management of Depression of the Bone Marrow

Until recently, no treatment has been available to restore the damaged bone marrow. However, the recent introduction of granulocyte colony stimulating factor (GCSF) has led to the hope that this might be useful in such cases.

Prognosis of Mustard Gas Casualties

Most mustard gas casualties recover fully. In a small proportion of cases, late-onset corneal problems producing blindness occur (Mann, 1948). Sulphur mustard is a recognized carcinogen and a study in Japanese mustard gas factory workers demonstrated an increase in the incidence of cancer (Yamada, 1963). The risk of cancer occurring as a result of a single exposure to sulphur mustard is exceedingly low.

LEWISITE (2-chlorovinyldichloroarsine)

Lewisite, developed as a chemical warfare agent in 1918 by Lee Lewis, has never been proven to have been used in war. Despite this, it has acquired a reputation as an agent of likely great effectiveness and lethality. In fact this is unlikely to be true. In the early 1920s Lewisite was considered as a compound likely to produce more severe effects than mustard gas and was nick-named 'The Dew of Death'. It has retained its place in the standard lists of chemical warfare agents although often as a mixture with sulphur mustard, the Lewisite lowering the freezing point of the mustard and making it more effective under cold conditions. Fears that Lewisite might be used during World War II prompted the work of Peters, Thompson and Stocken (Peters *et al.*, 1945; Peters, 1948, 1953) and led to the development of the chelating agent dimercaprol or British Anti-Lewisite (BAL). The view that Lewisite is unlikely to be used in war has limited interest in the compound and only a short account of its effects and the recommended management of those effects will be provided.

Physicochemical Properties of Lewisite

These are shown in **Table 7**. Unlike sulphur mustard, Lewisite decomposes rapidly on contact with water or even in a 'damp atmosphere' (Sartori, 1939). The reaction taking place is shown in **Figure 7**.

Table 7 Physicochemical characteristics of Lewisite

Formula	$CICH=CHAsCl_2$
M.W.	207.32
M.P. (°C)	−13
B.P. (°C)	190
V.P. (mmHg)	
0 °C	0.087
10 °C	0.196
20 °C	0.394
40 °C	1.467
S.G.	
0 °C	1.9200
10 °C	1.9027
30 °C	1.8682
Appearance	A colourless oily liquid. Impure samples may be blue–black in colour and smell, faintly, of geraniums

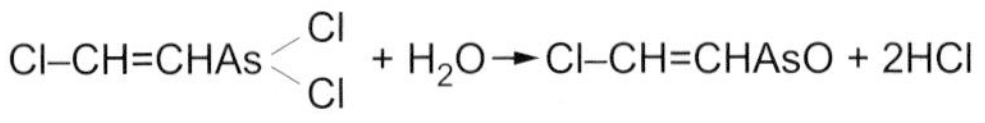

Figure 7 Hydrolysis of Lewisite.

Absorption of Lewisite

Lewisite is absorbed rapidly through the skin and mucous membranes. Its distribution in the body follows that of other arsenical compounds.

Toxicity of Lewisite

Lewisite has a much higher systemic toxicity than sulphur mustard and 0.5 ml allowed to remain on the skin would be expected to produce severe poisoning; 2.0 ml allowed to remain in contact with the skin has been said to represent a lethal dose in humans (Vedder, 1925). Because of its systemic toxicity, few volunteers have been exposed to Lewisite and data available regarding the effects of vapour on the skin are scanty. It is the author's impression that Lewisite vapour is more toxic to the skin and eyes than mustard gas vapour and the effects could be expected at lower concentrations.

Mechanism of Action of Lewisite

Peters *et al.* (1945) demonstrated that Lewisite attacked the pyruvate dehydrogenase system by combining with the coenzyme lipoic acid to form a cyclic compound **(Figure 8)**. The essential and ubiquitous nature of lipoic acid accounts for the widespread effects of Lewisite on the body. Interestingly, as in the case of sulphur mustard, the exact link between the primary biochemical effect of Lewisite and the production of blisters remains unknown. It should be recalled that other arsenical compounds such as sodium arsenite are not vesicants.

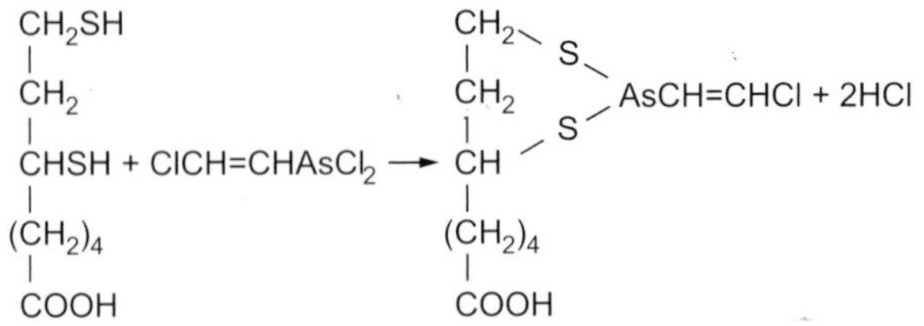

Figure 8 Reaction between Lewisite and lipoic acid.

Effects of Lewisite on Humans

Both in terms of histopathology and general patterns of symptoms and signs, it is believed that Lewisite would produce effects similar to those described above for mustard gas. However, certain important differences exist and instead of repeating much of the above only these will be considered:

■ Exposure of the eyes to Lewisite vapour is immediately painful and the damage produced is likely to be more severe than that produced by mustard gas vapour. Liquid contamination of the eyes is particularly painful, dangerous and demands immediate treatment.

■ Skin blisters produced by Lewisite appear more quickly post-exposure than those produced by mustard gas (Friedenwald and Hughes, 1948).

■ The inflammatory response associated with Lewisite lesions is likely to be more severe than that associated with mustard lesions.

■ Healing of Lewisite-induced skin lesions is likely to be more rapid than of those occurring as a result of exposure to sulphur mustard. Hunter (1978) described a case of blistering following exposure of another vesicant arsenical compound, phenyldichloroarsine, and reported that the skin lesions healed by the tenth day.

■ The collapse of the bone marrow seen in severe cases of mustard gas poisoning would not be expected after exposure to Lewisite. Goyer (1986), however, has pointed out that large doses of arsenical compounds can lead to leukopenia.

Clinical Investigations

Blood and urine should be analysed for arsenic. Under military conditions analysis should certainly be undertaken as information regarding the identity of chemical weapons used on the battle field might be of tactical importance.

Management of Lewisite Casualties

First Aid

This is as described for mustard gas.

Medical Treatment

Perhaps the most cheering difference between Lewisite and sulphur mustard is that specific therapy is available for the former but not for the latter.

Dimercaprol (BAL) binds the arsenical groups of Lewisite and produces a harmless complex. BAL competes avidly with binding sites in the body for arsenic and removes arsenic from them. BAL is available in a form suitable for injection and is used as such in the treatment of poisoning by a range of heavy metal compounds. Dose regimens for the management of arsenical poisoning

vary from author to author, the following being given in *Martindale* (Reynolds, 1989): 400–800 mg on first day of treatment, 200–400 mg on second and third days of treatment, 100–200 mg on fourth and subsequent days of treatment, all administered as divided doses.

For an alternative regimen, the HMSO publication *Medical Manual of Defence Against Chemical Agents* (HMSO, 1972) should be consulted. It is unlikely that one would need to continue treatment for more than about 14 days.

Marked reactions may be produced by the injection of BAL including tachycardia, nausea, vomiting, headache and sweating. Individual doses should not exceed 3 mg kg^{-1} and an interval of at least 4 h should separate these doses.

BAL may also be prepared as an ointment or as eye drops. Both preparations contain 5–10% dimercaprol. BAL ointment should not be used in conjunction with silver sulphadiazine (Flamazine) as chelation of silver will occur.

Recently, newer chelating agents have been proposed as replacements for BAL in the management of poisoning. The work of Graziano *et al.* (1978), Lenz *et al.* (1981), Aposhian *et al.* (1982, 1984) and Inns and Rice (1993) should be consulted for details. Despite the apparent advantages of some of the newer compounds in the treatment of systematic arsenic poisoning in experimental animals, it should be remembered that the high lipid solubility of BAL will probably lead to the ointment retaining its place in the management of Lewisite burns.

Prognosis of Lewisite Casualties

Given that adequate, early decontamination followed by the administration of BAL is undertaken, the prognosis should be good.

In war, eye splashes with liquid Lewisite would, fortunately, be expected to be rare but if such did occur the difficulties of immediate decontamination under battlefield conditions could lead to serious eye damage.

NERVE AGENTS

Nerve agents, produced first in Germany during the late 1930s, are often described as second-generation chemical weapons to distinguish them from those developed during World War I. Schrader synthesized the first nerve agent, tabun, in late 1936 or 1937. Sarin followed later in 1937 and soman in 1944. Tabun was stockpiled in Germany on a large scale, 12 000 tons being stored by 1945. Sarin was produced on a smaller scale with some 600 tons being available by 1945. Tabun, sarin and soman are usually referred to by the abbreviations GA, GB and GD, respectively. Other G agents exist, including GE and GF. During the 1950s, another group of nerve agents was developed and stockpiled in large quantities. These were the more toxic V agents, including VE, VM and VX (Tammelin, 1957). Of these, only VX has become well known. The history of the development of the nerve agents has been presented in some detail by Holmstedt (1963).

Physicochemical Properties of Nerve Agents

These are shown in **Table 8**.

Exposure to chemical warfare agents, including nerve agents, may occur during or as a result of destruction of military stockpiles. This problem has been considered by Watson et al. (1992). Care should be taken in re-entering areas potentially contaminated by the non-volatile agent VX. Nerve agents are hydrolysed by water. Khordagui (1996) has calculated that the half-life of G agents in seawater should be of the order of a few hours or less.

Military Use of Nerve Agents

Nerve agents may be disseminated on the battlefield by a variety of means and may be encountered as a vapour, liquid or artificially thickened liquid in the case of GD. GB is a comparatively volatile compound and presents a severe vapour hazard when encountered in the liquid state. VX, on the other hand, is a compound of very low volatility and presents little vapour hazard. The standard UK military respirator provides excellent protection against the effects of nerve agent vapour.

Use of Nerve Agents by Terrorists

In 1995, GB was used in an attack on the public in a Tokyo subway: several deaths and 5000 cases of poison-

ing resulted (Masuda et al., 1995). Some 10 weeks before the GB attack, three individuals were attacked with VX by the same terrorist group (Nozaki, et al., 1995). The publications associated with these attacks provide details of the symptomatology of such cases of poisoning and insights into the efficacy of standard treatment. (US Public Health Service, 1996). Interestingly (see below), the clinicians caring for the casualties found pupil diameter to be a reliable guide in assessing the effects of treatment with atropine. There has been evidence of sequelae in some of those exposed to GB in Tokyo and in a similar incident in Matsumoto (Marata et al., 1997; Sekijima et al., 1997).

Toxicity of Nerve Agents

Nerve agents are probably the most toxic compounds yet produced on a large scale. Many studies of their toxicity have been undertaken using animal models and a very wide range of LD_{50} values are known. A small selection of these values are shown in the **Table 9**. Fortunately, the number of accidental exposures of people to nerve agents has been small and, in consequence, information on the lethal doses of the compounds in humans is scarce. Many volunteers have, however, been exposed to low concentrations of nerve agents and the effects of such exposures are well understood. An account by Maynard and Beswick (1992) should be consulted for details. **Table 10** gives some indication of the approximate lethal toxicity figures for nerve agents in humans.

Absorption of Nerve Agents

Nerve agents in the liquid form are absorbed rapidly across the unbroken skin and mucous membranes. Vapour is not absorbed across the skin in significant

Table 8 Physicochemical properties of nerve agents[a]

Characteristic	Tabun GA	Sarin GB	Soman GD	GF	VX
Formula	CH₃CH₂O, O, P, (CH₃)₂N, CN	CH₃, CH₃CHO, O, P, CH₃, F	CH₂, (CH₃)₃C.CHO, O, P, CH₃, F	CH₂—CH₂, OH, CH₂, C, O, CH₂—CH₂, P, CH₃, F	CH₃CH₂O, O, P, CH₃, S(CH₂)₂N, CH(CH₃)₂, CH(CH₃)₂
M.W.	162.3	140.1	182.18	180.14	267.36
S.G. (20 °C)	1.073	1.0887	1.022	1.133	1.0083
M.P. (°C)	−49	−56	−80	−12	−20
B.P. (°C)	246	147	167	–	300
V.P. (mm Hg)					
0 °C	0.004	0.52	0.044	0.006	
10 °C	0.013	1.07	0.11	0.017	
20 °C	0.036	2.10	0.27	0.044	0.00044
30 °C	0.094	3.93	0.61	0.104	
40 °C	0.23	7.1	–	0.234	
50 °C	0.56	12.3	2.60	0.501	

[a] GA = ethyl N-dimethylphosphoramidocyanidate; GB = isopropyl methylphosphonofluoridate; GD = 1,2,2-trimethylpropyl methylphosphonofluoridate; GF = cyclohexyl methylphosphonofluoridate; VX = O-ethyl S-[2-(diisopropylamino)ethyl]methylphosphonothioate.
Source: from Maynard and Beswick (1992).

amounts, although it is absorbed across the cornea in sufficient quantities to produce miosis as a local effect. Absorption of vapour by the lung is rapid and more than 80% of inhaled agent is absorbed. This important point should be borne in mind whenever the $L(Ct)_{50}$ figure for a volatile nerve agent is quoted. During exercise, respiratory minute volume is increased but the absorption of the high percentage of the inhaled vapour is maintained. The $L(Ct)_{50}$ for GB in resting humans is approximately 100 mg min m^{-3}. On exercise, producing a fivefold increase in minute volume, this value could fall to 20 mg min m^{-3}.

Mechanism of Action of Nerve Agents

Nerve agents are organophosphorus anticholinesterases (anti-AChEs) and exert their toxic effects by long-lasting inhibition of acetylcholinesterase (AChE) at sites of activity of acetylcholine (ACh) in the body. The action of anticholinesterase compounds is discussed at length in Chapter 94 and by Koelle (1963), Taylor (1980), Murphy (1986), and will not be considered here. One point should, however, be borne in mind: many organophosphorus compounds undergo a reaction generally known as 'ageing' after they have combined with AChE (Fleisher and Harris, 1965). The rate at which this reaction occurs varies with the anti-AChE and is particularly rapid in the case of GD. Ligtenstein (1984) has compiled data illustrating this point (see **Table 11**).

The values given in **Table 11** should not, of course, be taken as representative of the half-lives of ageing of the nerve agents at human synaptic or neuromuscular junctions and are shown only for the purposes of comparing the rates of ageing of different agent–enzyme complexes. Differences in rates of ageing are important as regards

the treatment of nerve agent poisoning with oximes (see below).

Clinical Effects of Nerve Agents

The clinical effects of nerve agents may be deduced by recalling the sites of action of ACh in the body (Koelle, 1975). In addition to acting at autonomic ganglia, peripheral parasympathetic terminals and the neuromuscular junction, it should be recalled that ACh also plays an important role in transmission within the CNS.

The symptoms and signs of anti-AChE poisoning are described in Chapter 94 and will not be described in detail here. **Table 12** shows the symptoms and signs of nerve agent poisoning in terms of short-term exposure and AChE depression. The effects of systemic exposure leading to similar degrees of depression of AChE are also shown.

Information from volunteer studies on the effects of nerve agents relates only to comparatively short-duration exposures and, in the main, to exposures to concentration–time profiles of less than 30 mg min m^{-3}. It will be noted that considerable variations in the expected degrees of depression of AChE are indicated in **Table 12**. This is important and all workers have stressed the considerable variation in the effects observed in different individuals at identical levels of AChE depression. This point will be returned to in the next section.

Clinical Investigations

Measurements of whole blood, erythrocyte and plasma cholinesterase activities are often undertaken in cases of

Table 9 Toxicity of nerve agents[a]

Species	Route	Term	Units	GA	GB	GD	VX
Rat	Inhalation	$L(Ct)_{50}$	mg m^{-3} per 10 min	304[1]	150[2]	–	–
	Intravenous	LD$_{50}$	μg kg^{-1}	66[1]	39[3]	44.5[4]	–
	Subcutaneous	LD$_{50}$	μg kg^{-1}	193[5]	103[6]	75[7]	12[5]
Mouse	Inhalation	$L(Ct)_{50}$	mg m^{-3} per 30 min	15[1]	5[8]	1[8]	–
	Intravenous	LD$_{50}$	μg kg^{-1}	150[1]	113[9]	35[10]	–
	Subcutaneous	LD$_{50}$	μg kg^{-1}	250[11]	60[8]	40[8]	22[11]
Guinea pig	Inhalation	$L(Ct)_{50}$	mg m^{-3} per 2 min	393[1]	128[12]	–	–
	Subcutaneous	LD$_{50}$	μg kg^{-1}	–	30[13]	24[14]	8.4[15]

[a] Source: [1] Gates and Renshaw (1946); [2] Rengstorff (1985); [3] Fleisher (1963); [4] Pazdernik *et al.* (1983); [5] Jovanovic (1983); [6] Brimblecombe *et al.* (1970); [7] Boskovic *et al.* (1984); [8] Lohs (1960); [9] Schoene and Oldiges (1973); [10] Brezenoff *et al.* (1984); [11] Maksimovic *et al.* (1980); [12] Bright *et al.* (1991); [13] Coleman *et al.* (1968); [14] Gordon and Leadbeater (1977); [15] Leblic *et al.* (1984).

Table 10 Estimated values for toxicity of nerve agents in humans

Species	Route	Term	Units	GA	GB	GD	VX
Human	Inhalation	$L(Ct)_{50}$	mg min m^{-3}	150	70–100	40–60	–
	Intravenous	LD$_{50}$	mg kg^{-1}	0.08	0.01	0.025	0.007
	Percutaneous	LD$_{50}$	mg kg^{-1}	–	–	–	0.142

Table 11 Ageing of organophosphorus–AChE complexes

Nerve agent	Enzyme[a]	Ageing half-life	Reference
GA	BEA	46 h	De-Jong and Wolring (1978)
GB	BEA	12 h	Benschop and Keijer (1966)
GD	BEA	4 min	De-Jong and Wolring (1980)
VX	BEA	> 12 days	De-Jong (1983)

[a] BEA = bovine erythrocyte acetylcholinesterase.
Source: modified from Ligtenstein (1984)

Table 12 Signs and symptoms of nerve agent poisoning

Short-term Ct (mg min m^{-3})	AChE inhibition (%) ($\pm$ SD)	Symptoms and signs	
		Vapour exposure	Systemic exposure (eyes protected)
2	?	Incipient miosis, ? slight headache	Nil
5	20 ± 10	Miosis, headache, rhinorrhoea, eye pain, injection of conjunctivae, tightness of chest	? Tightness of chest
5–15	$20–50 \pm 10$	Eye signs maximal, bronchospasm in some	Symptoms in some, ? bronchospasm
15	50 ± 10	Effects as above but more severe	Wheezing, salivation, nausea, vomiting, miosis, local sweating, muscle fasciculation in cases of skin contamination
40	80 ± 10	As above but more severe with weakness, involuntary micturition and defaecation, paralysis and convulsions	
100	100	Respiratory failure. Death	

organophosphorus compound poisoning. Plasma contains butyrylcholinesterase and red cells contain acetylcholinesterase. It is often assumed that a measurement of the level of active, i.e. uninhibited, red cell cholinesterase will provide an accurate reflection of levels of AChE at synaptic and neuromuscular junctions and thus reflect the severity of the poisoning which the patient has sustained. This is not so. Willems (1989) studied the patterns of cholinesterase depression in 53 cases of poisoning by organophosphorus insecticides and showed there was a poor correlation between clinical severity of poisoning and the extent of enzyme depression. It is difficult to imagine that a better relationship would exist in cases of nerve agent poisoning.

Management of Nerve Agent Poisoning

First Aid

Casualties should be removed from risk of further contamination and decontaminated by adequately protected and trained attendants. Contaminated clothing should be removed as quickly as possible, taking care not to transfer liquid from the casualty's clothing to his skin. If protective clothing has been worn then this should be decontaminated with fullers' earth or a dilute solution of bleach before being removed. Under battlefield conditions, clean areas occupied by staff not wearing respirators and protective clothing must be protected at all costs. Monitoring equipment should be used to confirm adequate decontamination before casualties are transferred into these clean areas. One of the most serious consequences of nerve agent poisoning is respiratory failure produced by inhibition of the medullary centres. If respiration can be maintained while the drugs discussed below are administered, then the casualty's chances of recovery will be much enhanced. Under battlefield conditions the artificial ventilation of casualties presents formidable problems. 'Ambu' style bags (protected by suitable rubber coverings and equipped with adequate filters) and oro-pharyngeal airways can reduce these problems.

Medical Treatment

Drug therapy for nerve agent poisoning, as for poisoning by other anti-AChE compounds, is divided into three types: (1) cholinolytics such as atropine, (2) reactivators of the inhibited AChE: oximes and (3) anticonvulsants, e.g. diazepam or other benzodiazepines. To these should be added oxygen, which may be needed in cases of respiratory failure. The use of oxygen will not be considered further here.

In addition to the above, research has been undertaken to try to provide drugs which, if taken in advance of exposure to nerve agents, would reduce the effects of the exposure and make the treatment of poisoning resulting from that exposure the more effective. It was noted in the late 1940s that cats given the carbamate physostigmine became comparatively resistant to the effects of other anti-AChE compounds (Gilman and Cattell, 1948). It was suggested that the combination of a proportion of the available AChE with the carbamate would prevent subsequent combination of the enzyme with the organophosphorus compound and, furthermore, that the carbamate-combined enzyme would, later, spontaneously reactivate and provide the body with a supply of normal uninhibited enzyme. This hypothesis is now generally accepted. A great deal of work has been done in developing the carbamate pyridostigmine bromide for use in this way and Inns and Leadbeater (1983) summed up work on the efficacy of pre-treatment, combined with the treatment detailed above, in cases of GD poisoning in guinea pigs. **Table 13** shows some of the results obtained.

This research has been most successfully prosecuted in the UK and all UK forces are issued with pyridostigmine bromide tablets (30 mg three times daily) for use should the risk of exposure to nerve agents be deemed significant. Pyridiostigmine bromide was take by UK, US and some other forces during the Gulf War (1991). Sharabi *et al.* (1991) reported that non-specific side-effects including dry mouth, general malaise, fatigue and weakness were experienced. Nausea, abdominal pain, frequency of micturition and rhinorrhoea were infrequent. Side-effects tended to appear during the first few hours following each dose and then resolved. Interestingly, no correlation between acetylcholinesterase inhibition and symptoms was detected. Keeler *et al.* (1991) reported a study of 41 650 soldiers who took pyridostigmine bromide, in the dose described above, for between 1 and 7 days. About half of the study group reported side-effects including increased flatus, abdominal cramps, soft stools and urinary urgency. About 1% of soldiers 'believed their symptoms required medical attention' but in less than 0.1

% were the side-effects so severe as to require withdrawal of pyridostigmine. It was concluded that military efficiency was not impaired by taking the drug.

Cholinolytics

Atropine is the drug of choice and should be given intramuscularly or preferably intravenously, in aliquots of 2 mg, as soon as possible after poisoning. To enable servicemen to self-administer atropine and in some cases oxime, a wide variety of autoinjection devices have been developed commercially. Most contain 2 mg of atropine per injection and permit injection through clothing. Speed of administration as soon as the first signs of poisoning are detected is critical as the progress of symptoms and signs may be very rapid. It is essential, therefore, that servicemen should be well trained in the recognition of the early signs of poisoning and in the use of the autoinjection devices. As in cases of poisoning by other organophosphorus compounds, large total doses of atropine are often said to be likely to be needed. However, in casualties surviving to reach hospital it is unlikely that the heroic doses of atropine reported by some who were managing cases of organophosphorus pesticide poisoning would be required.

The dangers of atropine overdose should always be borne in mind:

- Drying of bronchial secretions making them tenacious and difficult to remove; the careful use of suction may be required.
- Large doses of atropine may induce arrhythmias, particularly if the myocardium is hypoxic as a result of respiratory failure.
- Bladder dysfunction may necessitate catheterization.

Atropine drops are sometimes recommended for the relief of visual impairment and eye pain caused by contraction of the iris and spasm of the ciliary muscle. Atropine drops may be expected to relieve the eye pain to some extent but seem to do little to improve vision. The combination of mydriasis and impairment of accommodation seems to produce at least as severe an impairment of vision as the miosis produced by exposure to the

Table 13 Effectiveness of oximes and bispyridinium compounds against soman poisoning in guinea pigs receiving various supporting drug treatments. Pyridostigmine (0.32 μ mol kg^{-1} im) was injected 30 min before challenge with soman (sc). One minute after poisoning P2S (130 μ mol kg^{-1}) was injected im with atropine (50 μ mol kg^{-1}). Diazepam (25 μ mol kg^{-1}) was given as a separate im injection

Compound	Protective ratio (95% confidence limits)			
	Atropine	Atropine, diazepam	Pyridostigmine, atropine	Pyridostigmine, atropine, diazepam
–	1.5 (1.2–1.9)	2.2 (1.8–2.7)	5.2 (4.1–6.6)	8.7 (5.7–14)
P2S	1.7 (1.5–1.9)	2.5 (1.9–3.1)	6.8 (5.4–8.5)	14 (10–19)

Source: modified from Inns and Leadbeater (1983).

nerve agent. The use of oxime, instead of atropine, eye drops has been suggested but not widely adopted. It has already been noted that in the Tokyo subway incident, atropine eye drops were found to be helpful in those with mild poisoning (Nozaki *et al.*, 1995).

Oximes

The oximes, developed in the 1950s (Wilson and Ginsburg, 1955; Wagner-Jauregg, 1956) represented a major step forward in the treatment of nerve agent poisoning. Hydroxylamine was the first compound demonstrated to be capable of reactivating the AChE–nerve agent complex. More effective oximes followed and the work of Davies and Green (1956, 1959) and others led to the development of pralidoxime methanesulphonate (pralidoxime mesylate or P2S). This compound and other pralidoxime salts have maintained their place as the oximes of choice in the treatment of organophosphorus poisoning in many countries. P2S is included in the autoinjection device issued to the UK Armed Forces. A number of studies have shown that oximes may act by blocking ion channels and thus not only by reactivating inhibited acetylcholinesterase (Tattersall, 1993; Alkondon *et al.* 1988; van Helden *et al.* 1991; Szinicz, 1996). That oximes show some effectiveness in animals poisoned by soman (GD), in which the nerve agent–enzyme complex ages rapidly, may be explained by these direct effects.

The two oximes in clinical use are pralidoxime (as various salts), which is a monopyridinium oxime, and obidoxime (Toxogonin), a bis-pyridinium oxime. Pralidoxime chloride is used in the USA while the methanesulphonate (P2S) is used in the UK; its chemical structure is shown in **Figure 9**. Obidoxime is used in Germany, while a number of other bispyridinium oximes have been developed including the series of oximes referred to as the Hagedorn, or H, oximes (Oldiges and Schoene, 1970). The structures of some of the better known compounds are shown in **Figure 10**.

If P2S is used it should be given intramuscularly, as soon as possible after poisoning, or better by slow intravenous injection, at a dose of 30 mg kg^{-1}. The dose should be repeated at 15 min intervals to a total dose of 2 or possibly 4 g. It should be remembered that very little experience of management of nerve agent casualties has been accumulated. Oximes should be administered carefully and a close watch kept on the patient's condition. Side-effects include headache, disturbances of vision and

muscular weakness and care should be taken to monitor the patient's condition before and after the administration of oxime to permit differentiation between the signs of deepening organophosphorus toxicity and the side-effects of therapy. If given too quickly, bronchospasm and laryngospasm may occur. The use of an intravenous infusion of 2 g of P2S in 250 ml of normal (0.9%) saline delivered over 30 min has also been recommended. Ligtenstein (1984) has made a strong case for the continuation of the use of oximes beyond the often suggested limit of a day or two.

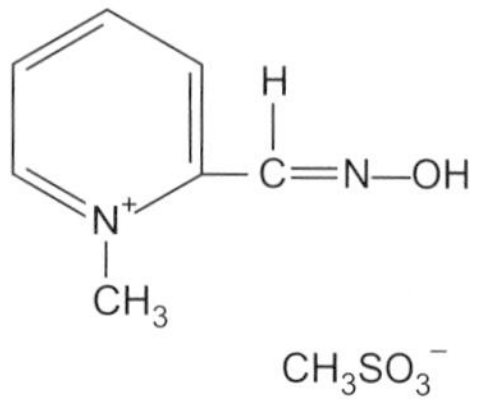

The choice of oxime, if more than one is available, may be difficult. The following points should be recalled:

- Pralidoxime (PAM) salts are probably still the most widely available oximes.
- PAM is likely to be markedly more effective in cases of GB and VX poisoning than in cases of GA and GD poisoning.
- Although obidoxime (Toxogonin) (3–6 mg kg^{-1} iv 4 hourly) is likely to be effective in cases of GA, GB and VX (but not GD) poisoning, cases of liver damage following its use have been reported.
- The Hagedorn oximes such as HI6 and HGG12 have been shown to be effective in GD poisoning in some animal models but are less effective than had been hoped in GA poisoning (Wolthuis and Kepner, 1978; Harris *et al.*, 1981; Clement, 1981, 1982a, b; Clement and Lockwood, 1982; Kassa, 1998). Studies by Kassa and Bajgar (1995) have shown that HI6 is a better antidote than obidoxime in rats poisoned with GF.
- The more recently developed Hagedorn oximes HLö7 and pyrimidoxime are effective in both GA and GD poisoning in some animal models (Eyer *et al.*, 1989; Clement *et al.*, 1992; Eyer *et al.*, 1992; Lundy *et al.*, 1992).
- In general, the Hagedorn oximes are unstable in solution and demand more complex autoinjection devices than the conventional oximes (Eyer *et al.*, 1989). Göransson-Nyberg *et al.* (1995) reported a study of the efficacy of a new binary autoinjector containing 500 mg of HI6 and 2 mg of atropine sulphate in pigs poisoned with soman (GD). The combination proved effective in opposing a lethal dose of soman (9 μg kg^{-1} iv every 20 min). The autoinjection device contained two chambers: mixing was initiated prior to injection.

In addition to the above, it should be recalled that atropine and oximes are synergistic in their effects and the administration of atropine and oxime has been shown to raise the LD$_{50}$ of some nerve agents in animal models by a factor of more than 20 (Inns and Leadbeater, 1983). GD remains a major problem and the publications of Wolthuis and Kepner (1978), Wolthuis *et al.* (1981) and Clement (1981, 1982a, b) should be consulted for

Figure 9 Pralidoxime methanesulphonate (P2S).

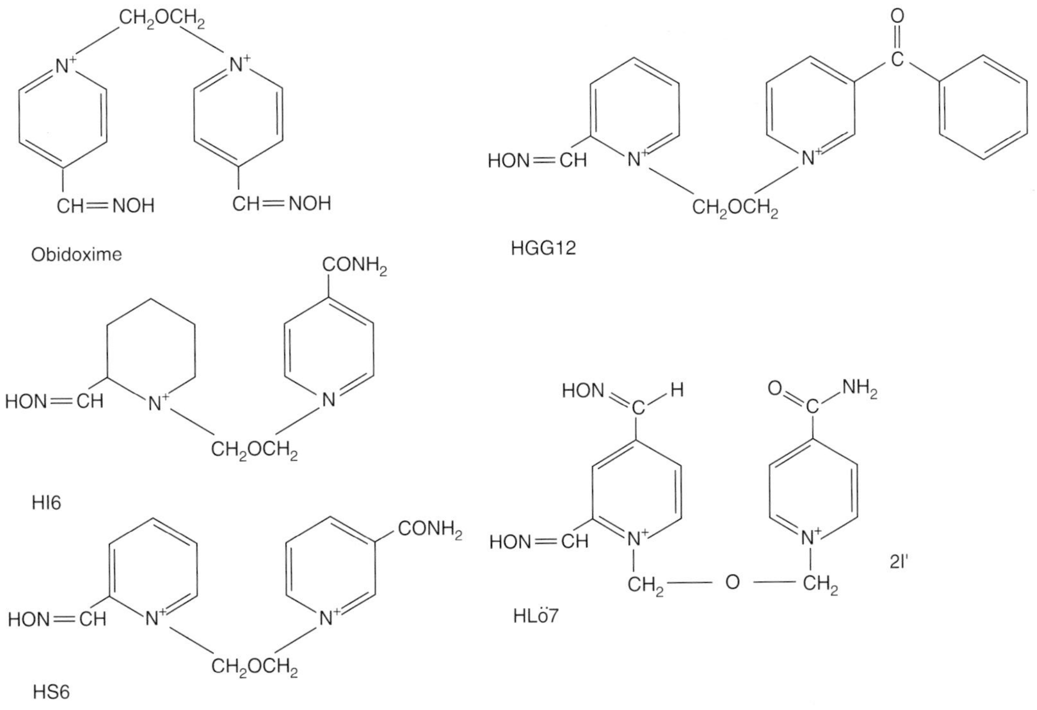

Figure 10 Structures of some of the better known oximes.

details of the intractability of poisoning with GD and for arguments regarding the use of H oximes.

Anticonvulsants

Diazepam has come to be regarded as a valuable addition to the combination of atropine and oxime in the management of nerve agent poisoning. Nerve agent poisoning, and particularly poisoning with GD in monkeys, is often complicated by convulsions and the control of these convulsions with diazepam has been shown to enhance the likelihood of survival (Lipp, 1972, 1973). A number of theories have been put forward to explain this effect, including the suggestion that diazepam may prevent the rise in cyclic GMP levels observed in the CNS of animals suffering GD-induced convulsions (Lundy and Magor, 1978). Recent work has, however, cast doubt on this theory (Liu *et al.*, 1988).

Diazepam should be given in a dose of 5 mg orally, intramuscularly or, better, intravenously. Diazepam is not suitable for combination in solution with atropine and P2S but a recently developed lysine–diazepam conjugate is. This has been incorporated in the autoinjection devices issued to the UK Armed Forces.

Prognosis of Nerve Agent Casualties

Animal studies have suggested that the combination of the pre-treatment and treatment described above would probably be effective in cases of nerve agent poisoning. It is, however, difficult to extrapolate from such work to the case of the soldier poisoned on the battlefield at a considerable distance from medical attention. For those casualties who have self-administered one or perhaps more of their autoinjection devices but who are slipping deeper into the effects of the nerve agent, the prognosis can hardly be other than poor. Those who sustain a dose of nerve agent sufficient to produce respiratory failure are unlikely to survive. It is believed that self-administration of therapy will delay the onset of symptoms and signs of nerve agent poisoning and make it more likely that the poisoned man will survive and reach medical attention.

Long-term Effects of Nerve Agent Poisoning

It is well known that organophosphorus compounds can produce permanent damage to the nervous system. These effects, thought to be dependent on the combination of the organophosphate with the enzyme known as neuropathy target esterase (NTE), have been studied in detail by Johnson and commented on in Chapters 33 and 94. Studies in animal models have demonstrated that the nerve agents are capable of producing these effects, but only when administered to animals protected by the prior administration of atropine and oxime, in doses many times in excess of their LD_{50}s. It is likely that a soldier who survives nerve agent poisoning on the battlefield will not have been exposed to a dose of nerve agent capable of inducing neuropathy.

Since the Gulf War, a great deal of publicity has been given to the so-called 'Gulf War Syndrome'. A very wide range of psychological and physical effects have been reported in soldiers who fought in the campaign. It seems clear that veterans of the campaign have a higher self-reported prevalence of medical and psychiatric conditions than other personnel who did not see active service in the Gulf. Whether such effects are causally linked to exposure to pre-treatment against nerve agent poisoning, perhaps in combination with immunization schedules, remains unknown. The reader should consult the excellent series of papers published in 1997 (Iowa Persian Gulf Study Group, 1997; Haley and Kurt, 1997; Haley *et al.*, 1997a, b). Hyams *et al.* (1996) have pointed out that outbreaks of difficult-to-explain symptoms have been seen after every major war since the US Civil War and that many questions remain unanswered regarding these 'war syndromes'.

PULMONARY OEDEMA-INDUCING COMPOUNDS

During World War I, the chemical warfare compounds with the highest lethality were those which induced pulmonary oedema, and included chlorine and phosgene. Phosgene was first used by German forces on 19 December 1915 and soon acquired a reputation as a dangerous compound: 85% of deaths resulting from exposure to chemical warfare compounds during World War I were caused by phosgene (HMSO, 1972). Despite this, well protected troops using modern respirators should not be placed at serious risk as a result of exposure to these compounds, and little development of pulmonary oedema-producing compounds for use as chemical warfare agents has taken place since World War I. During World War I great efforts to develop other pulmonary-damaging compounds were made and a large number of compounds were used, albeit sometimes on a comparatively small scale. Accounts dating from the 1920s should be consulted for details of these compounds. Among accounts generally available, that of Prentiss (1937) is particularly detailed and reliable.

During World War I, phosgene acquired a particularly evil reputation as it was soon realized that men who had inhaled a potentially lethal dose of the compound might show few symptoms and signs during the first few hours following exposure (Vedder, 1925). Early diagnosis was therefore difficult. It was further noted that men in the symptomless latent period could collapse with florid pulmonary oedema if exposed to physical stress (HMSO, 1923). It will be appreciated that the sensible clinical advice to rest all those thought to have been exposed, for 24–48 h, preferably in bed, was ill-received by commanders in the field.

While phosgene might not present a severe toxicological risk to modern troops, it is not detected by the various detectors and monitors in general military use, and troops thought to be at risk would be forced to don respirators and accept the concomitant drop in their performance.

Phosgene is produced in large quantities in peacetime by the chemical industry and cases of industrial accidents occur from time to time. The general effects of lung-damaging compounds have been described in Chapters 30 and 37 and only those aspects of the toxicology of phosgene of chemical warfare importance are mentioned here.

Physicochemical Properties of Phosgene

These are given in **Table 14**.

Table 14 Physicochemical properties of phosgene

Formula	$COCl_2$
M.W.	99
M.P. (°C)	−118
B.P. (°C)	8.2
Vapour density	3.5
V.P. (mm Hg)	
−13.7 °C	335
−10 °C	365
0 °C	555
8.2 °C	760
Odour	Stifling odour of new-mown hay

Likely Mode of Exposure

Phosgene is rapidly dispersed by wind and is regarded as an agent of short persistence likely to be used only in surprise attacks. It may, however, linger in cellars, tunnels and hollows as it is heavier than air. Lefebure (1921) described experiments undertaken during World War I in an attempt to convert phosgene into a more persistent compound by impregnating porous powders with the gas. These experiments do not seem to have been successful.

Absorption of Phosgene

Phosgene is not absorbed to a significant extent through the skin; it is, of course, absorbed by the lung. Nash and Pattle (1971) studied the reaction of phosgene with water at moist surfaces and concluded that the rate of hydrolysis would render penetration by phosgene of more than 'a few tens of microns' unlikely.

Toxicity of Phosgene

The toxicity of phosgene has been widely studied, and **Table 15** shows the range of toxicity encountered in differ-

Table 15 Toxicity of phosgene

Species	Route	Term	Units	Value	Source
Rat	Inhalation	LC_{50}	mg m^{-3} per 30 min	1400	NTIS[a]
Mouse	Inhalation	LC_{50}	mg m^{-3} per 30 min	1800	NTIS
Dog	Inhalation	LC_{50}	mg m^{-3} per 20 min	4200	NTIS
Monkey	Inhalation	LC_{50}	mg m^{-3} per 1 min	600	NTIS
Rabbit	Inhalation	LC_{50}	mg m^{-3} per 30 min	1000	NTIS
Rat	Inhalation	LC_{LO}	ppm per 30 min	50	NIOSH[b]
Dog	Inhalation	LC_{LO}	ppm per 30 min	80	NIOSH
Rat	Inhalation	100% mortality	ppm per 20 min	37	

[a] NTIS = National Technical Information Service.
[b] NIOSH = National Institute for Occupational Safety and Health.
The values quoted are often described in toxicological databases as LC_{50} values, e.g. the LC_{50} of phosgene for a 30 min exposure in mice is 1800 mg m^{-3}. Attempts to convert such values to $L(Ct)_{50}$ values by simple multiplication should be avoided as it is known that the $L(Ct)_{50}$ of phosgene is time dependent. It will be noted that as the duration of the exposure is increased the $L(Ct)_{50}$ value rises. This has also been noted by Ballantyne (1987) for hydrogen cyanide. A widely quoted statement of the toxicity of phosgene to humans is '50 ppm may be rapidly fatal (for phosgene 1ppm = 4.419 mg m^{-3} at STP). See Table 16.

ent species. As in the case of nerve agents, $L(Ct)_{50}$ is dependent on the respiratory state and will fall with exertion.

Mechanism of Action of Phosgene

Despite its long history, the exact mechanism of action of phosgene remains obscure. The hypothesis that phosgene acts by combining with water and forming hydrochloric acid (Winternitz, 1920; Vedder, 1925), which then produces tissue damage, was challenged by the work of Nash and Pattle (1971). These authors showed that the 'maximum concentration of acid in a blood–air barrier of thickness 1 μm in contact with 25 ppm of phosgene is 7×10^{-10} M, which is negligible. Buffering by tissue constituents would prevent any significant change in pH'. At high concentrations it was accepted that the formation of hydrochloric acid might play a role.

Potts et al. (1949) proposed that phosgene combined with the amino groups of proteins to form diamides **(Figure 11)**. Diller (1978) proposed a series of reactions to explain the combination of phosgene with a wider range of chemical groups **(Figure 12)**. Frosolono and Pawlowski (1977) studied the biochemical changes produced by phosgene in various lung fractions prepared from rats exposed to close to an $L(Ct)_{50}$ of phosgene. A number of enzymes showed decreased activity but the data did not allow a distinction to be drawn between reduction in enzyme activity as a result of direct inhibition and that resulting from loss from damaged cells.

In addition to the above, efforts have been made to produce a pathophysiological hypothesis to explain the production of pulmonary oedema. Phosgene clearly damages the blood–air barrier in the lung and allows the leak of fluid from the pulmonary capillaries. At first this leak may be contained by increased flow in the pulmonary lymphatic system but later an increase in fluid in the connective tissue spaces occurs and finally fluid spills over into the alveoli. This sequence, the

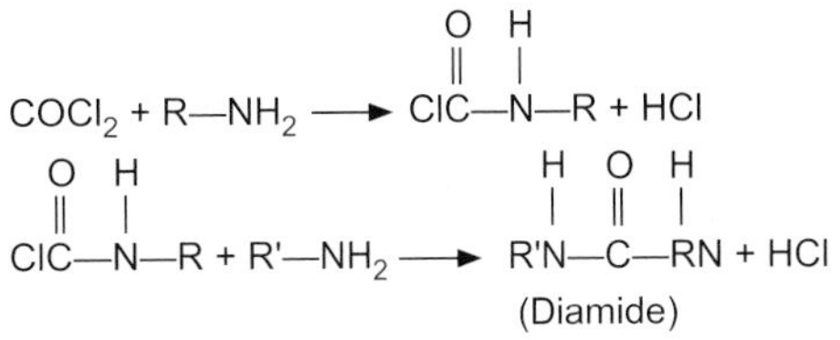

Figure 11 Formation of diamides.

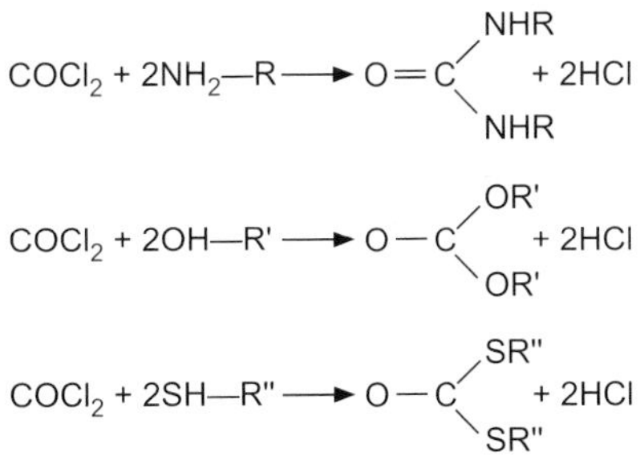

Figure 12 Reactions to explain the combination of phosgene with a wider range of chemical groups.

Table 16 Variations in lethal index of phosgene with duration of exposure (dogs)

Time of exposure (min)	Minimum lethal dose (mg l^{-1})	Lethal index (mg min m^{-3})
2	2.00	4000
5	1.10	5500
10	0.55	6500
15	0.46	6900
20	0.37	7400
25	0.30	7500
30	0.27	8100
45	0.20	9000
60	0.17	10200
75	0.16	12000

After Prentiss (1937).

standard pattern of 'permeability' as compared with 'hydrostatic' pulmonary oedema, has been most competently reviewed by Staub (1974), Robin (1979) and Teplitz (1979) and is discussed at greater length in Chapter 26. Some authors, including Ivanhoe and Meyers (1964) and Everet and Overholt (1968), have suggested that phosgene could lead to massive reflex vasoconstriction and the production of oedema as in neurogenic pulmonary oedema (NPE). In this condition a sudden redistribution of blood from the systemic to the pulmonary circulation is believed to occur, producing damage to the pulmonary capillary endothelium. The damage is believed to be such that, even when intravascular pressures have returned to normal, a leak of fluid continues. That phosgene acts by this mechanism seems unlikely as the extraordinary systemic hypertension recorded in cases of neurogenic pulmonary oedema has not been observed in animal models of phosgene poisoning.

It should be understood that the exact mechanism by which phosgene causes an increase in pulmonary capillary permeability is not known. Pulmonary capillaries possess a complete endothelium, the cells being joined by tight junctions. It is often assumed that compounds such as phosgene produce some loosening of these junctions, although the changes involved at the ultrastructural level are ill-understood. It would be particularly interesting to know whether phosgene produces any change in the pattern of strands of particles, revealed upon the p-face of the cell membrane by freeze–fracture techniques, which appear to be important in the structure of the tight junction.

Histopathology of Phosgene-induced Lung Damage

The light microscopic appearances of phosgene-damaged lungs were accurately described by Winternitz in 1920. Since then many studies have been carried out, Pawlowski and Frosolono's work (1977) at the ultrastructural level being particularly valuable. The sequence of changes they described is as follows:

- The epithelium of the terminal bronchiole appeared to be first affected. Intracellular vesiculation of ciliated epithelial cells and Clara cells was observed. These effects appeared very soon after exposure.
- An increase in the amount of extracellular fluid visible in the interalveolar septa was noted.
- Frank oedema of cells of the interalveolar septa was observed.
- Swelling of type II alveolar cells was noted.
- Type I alveolar cells showed areas of focal disruption.
- Interalveolar septa became widely distended with fluid.

- Oedema fluid appeared in alveolar spaces.

Oedema fluid in phosgene-induced lung damage is protein-rich and, by light microscopy, classically eosinophilic. Damage to type II alveolar cells is interesting, although a clear demonstration of a decline in surfactant production in phosgene-induced oedema is lacking. It is known, however, that by lowering the surface tension of the lining film of the alveoli, surfactant may reduce the forces acting to move fluid out of pulmonary capillaries (Pattle, 1965). Damage to cells which produce surfactant would then be expected to enhance the likelihood of alveolar oedema.

Symptoms and Signs of Phosgene Exposure

Because of the extensive use of phosgene during World War I, many detailed accounts of its effects on humans are available, Vedder (1925) and Ireland (1926) providing particularly valuable accounts. Accidental exposures occur and Seidelim (1961), Fruhman (1974), Diller (1978) and Bradley and Unger (1982) have also provided accounts.

Some authors describe eye irritation, coughing, lacrimation, choking and a feeling of tightness of the chest as early symptoms and signs of phosgene exposure. Doubtless these do occur in some patients, but it was clearly demonstrated during World War I that an absence of such effects did not preclude serious and sometimes lethal exposure.

The hallmark of phosgene poisoning has been recognized to be the occurrence of a latent period intervening between exposure and the onset of the symptoms and signs of pulmonary oedema. This period may range from 30 min to 24 h depending, in part, on the severity of the exposure. During this period it is notoriously difficult to distinguish the mildly exposed from the severely exposed.

Once the latent period is over, dyspnoea, a painful cough and cyanosis appear rapidly. Increasing quantities of initially whitish but later pink fluid are expectorated, a marked efflux of fluid, the 'champignon d'écume', sometimes appearing just before death. The cause of death is usually cardiac failure and circulatory collapse caused by hypoxia.

A World War I description of a chemist dying some hours after a brief exposure to a high concentration of phosgene during a laboratory accident gives the clinical picture:

His condition now rapidly deteriorated. Every fit of coughing brought up large quantities of clear, yellowish, frothy fluid of which about 80 ounces (2272 ml) were expectorated in one and a half hours. His face became of a grey, ashen colour, never purple, though the pulse remained fairly strong. He died at 6.50 pm without any great struggle for breath. The symptoms of irritation were very slight at the onset; there was then a delay of at least four hours and the final development of serious oedema up to death took little more than an hour though the patient was continually rested in bed.

(Vedder, 1925)

Management of Phosgene Poisoning

First Aid

Casualties should be removed from risk of further exposure by suitably protected attendants. Because phosgene would not be encountered in the liquid state, decontamination with fullers' earth or a dilute solution of bleach is unnecessary.

Medical Treatment

The management of phosgene poisoning is the management of permeability pulmonary oedema. No anti-phosgene drug of any proven value has been discovered, although hexamethylenetetramine is discussed briefly below. Steroids, antibiotics, bronchodilators, respiratory stimulants and cardiac stimulants have all been suggested, although none has received universal support. Two measures are, however, generally agreed:

Rest
All persons thought to have been exposed to phosgene should be confined to bed. It was demonstrated repeatedly during World War I that exertion during the latent period following exposure to phosgene could precipitate acute and fatal pulmonary oedema.

Oxygen
Patients unable to maintain an adequate arterial oxygen tension when breathing air should be given supplementary oxygen. This was stressed during World War I by Haldane (1917) and Barcroft (1920) when experience in the management of phosgene poisoning was unrivalled.

Of measures not commanding universal support the following should be considered:

Corticosteroids
Arguments both for and against the use of steroids in pulmonary oedema have been plentiful for some years and have been considered by Everett and Overholt (1968), Diller (1978) and Bradley and Unger (1982). Everett and Overholt reported the successful use of glucocorticoids and, Diller also supported their use, although Bradley and Unger found the evidence for their efficacy unconvincing. It is known that inflamm-atory changes are likely to occur in lung tissue damaged by phosgene and that these changes involve the release of mediators which are likely to increase capillary permeability and therefore worsen the oedema. That such release can be prevented by the prophylactic administration of corticosteroids seems likely; that such release can be reduced significantly, once initiated, remains doubtful. Some clinicians, perhaps the majority, have felt that the lack of serious side-effects usually associated with the short-term administration of large doses of corticosteroids and the seriousness of permeability pulmonary oedema justify the use of these drugs. Others have felt that the lack of clear evidence of efficacy should preclude their use. In some military manuals (HMSO, 1987), the use of a large single dose of corticosteroid as soon as possible after exposure has been advocated. Pritchard (1996) has discussed the question of the use of steroids in high-permeability oedema.

Antibiotics
The provision of antibiotic cover in phosgene poisoning has been supported by both Everett and Overholt (1968) and Diller (1978). During World War I, the absence of antibiotics made pneumonia a feared complication of lung damage arising as a result of exposure to a variety of chemical warfare compounds. Selgrade et al. (1995) showed that exposure to phosgene impaired the capacity of mice to deal with an inhalation challenge with bacteria. This was ascribed to impairment of macrophage and natural killer cell activity. The choice of antibiotics is wide, penicillin G, amoxycillin and chloramphenicol all having been recommended.

Of measures not receiving wide support, only one will be considered:

Hexamethylenetetramine (Hexamine, Methanamine, HMT)
Hexamine is used prophylactically as an antimicrobial drug in cases of recurrent urinary tract infections. It has been demonstrated to be of value, in animal models, if given before exposure to phosgene. Stavrakis (1971) argued that hexamine was also of value if given post-exposure in cases of phosgene poisoning and recommended the administration of 20 ml of a 20% solution, intravenously, as soon as possible after exposure. Diller (1978) reviewed the use of hexamine and concluded that there was no firm evidence to support the view that hexamine is of value if given after poisoning.

Sciuto et al. (1995, 1996) investigated the use of N-acetylcysteine (NAC) and dibutyryl cyclic AMP (DBcAMP) in phosgene poisoning. Post-exposure intratracheal administration of NAC in isolated perfused rabbit lung was shown to reduce the formation of oxidized glutathione and a number of markers of lipid peroxidation which was shown to be induced by exposure to phosgene. Similarly, DBcAMP acted as an antioxidant.

No clinical studies of the efficacy of these methods of treatment are yet available.

As in all cases of permeability pulmonary oedema, the administration of intravenous fluids should be approached with great caution.

Long-term Effects of Phosgene Poisoning

Chronic bronchitis and emphysema have been reported as a consequence of exposure to phosgene (Cucinell, 1974). Chronic pneumonitis has been reported in rats exposed to phosgene (Gross et al., 1965).

HYDROGEN CYANIDE

Of the poisons known to the general public, cyanide, arsenic and strychnine are perhaps the best known and it is often assumed that cyanide would be a dangerous chemical warfare agent. Despite this, hydrogen cyanide has been little used as a chemical warfare agent and its physicochemical and toxicological characteristics make it unsuitable for such use on any other than a fairly small scale. It has, however, been used as a means of judicial execution and was used for the large-scale murder of prisoners in German concentration camps during World War II.

Only France used hydrogen cyanide as a chemical warfare agent during World War I, the first use of hydrogen cyanide shells being on the Somme on 1 July 1916 (Prentiss, 1937). German respirators offered poor protection against hydrogen cyanide, although this was quickly remedied and hydrogen cyanide lost most of its advantages over the alternative lethal compound, phosgene. It will be recalled that phosgene has a density equal to 3.5 times that of air but that hydrogen cyanide is less dense than air. Rapid dispersion of hydrogen cyanide greatly reduced its value as a chemical warfare agent. Prentiss (1937) commented: 'Because of its extreme volatility and the fact that the vapours are lighter than air, it is almost impossible to establish a lethal concentration of hydrocyanic acid in the field and this is particularly true when the gas is put over in artillery shells'. Few authorities today believe that hydrogen cyanide would be used on a large scale as a chemical warfare agent although it has retained its place in military chemical warfare handbooks on the grounds that successful use, at high concentration, on selected targets could probably be achieved.

In view of the above, the discussion of hydrogen cyanide as a chemical warfare agent will be limited; a discussion of the antidotal management of cases of poisoning can be found in Chapter 20.

Physicochemical Characteristics of Hydrogen Cyanide

These are shown in **Table 17**. Below 26 °C, hydrogen cyanide occurs as a colourless to yellowish brown liquid. In its usual slightly impure state it is unstable, although it is said to be stable when highly purified. On standing, polymerization takes place and the compound may present an explosive hazard. The risk of explosion may be much reduced by the addition of a small quantity of an inorganic acid, e.g. phosphoric acid. Prentiss (1937) commented: 'Anhydrous hydrocyanic acid is extremely unstable and is quickly decomposed with the formation of a black resinous mass'. This tendency to decomposition led to difficulties with munitions and Sartori (1939) commented: 'Even in the anhydrous condition it cannot be kept long as it gradually decomposes, occasionally with explosive force. Filled in projectiles it soon becomes harmless'. Hydrogen cyanide smells of almonds, although not all individuals are able to detect the odour. The capacity to detect hydrogen cyanide rapidly wanes on exposure owing to failure of cells of the olfactory mucosa.

Table 17 Physicochemical properties of hydrogen cyanide

Formula	HCN
M.W.	27.02
Vapour density	$0.93 \times$ that of air
B.P. (760 mm Hg) (°C)	26
M.P. (°C)	-14
V.P. (mm Hg)	
-10 °C	165
0 °C	256
20 °C	600
26 °C	757

Absorption of Hydrogen Cyanide

Hydrogen cyanide vapour is readily absorbed across the lung but to only an insignificant extent across the skin.

Toxicity of Hydrogen Cyanide

The $L(Ct)_{50}$ value for hydrogen cyanide in humans is not known with any accuracy. It is, however, known that the $L(Ct)_{50}$ value is likely to be very time dependent. This is shown by the estimates of human toxicity given in **Table 18**. The variation in $L(Ct)_{50}$ with time is believed to relate to the detoxification of cyanide, by enzymatic conversion to thiocyanate (Ballantyne, 1987). Ballantyne and Schwabe (1981) have shown the variation in graphical form **(Figure 13)**.

Further guidance on the estimated toxicity of hydrogen cyanide may be gained from **Table 19**.

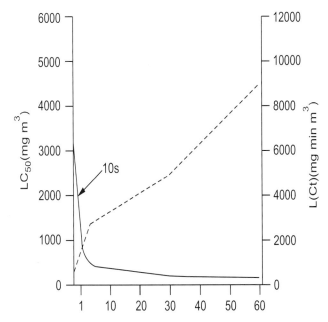

Figure 13 Acute lethal inhalation toxicity of hydrogen cyanide vapour. Solid line, LC_{50} of hydrogen cyanide (mg m^{-3}). Dashed line, corresponding $L(Ct)_{50}$ values (mg min m^{-3}). From Ballantyne and Schwabe (1981). Reproduced with the permission of the authors.

Table 18 Estimated toxicity of hydrogen cyanide in humans

Duration of exposure	Concentration (C) (mg m^{-3})	$L(Ct)_{50}$ (mg min m^{-3})
15 s	2400	660
1 min	1000	1000
10 min	200	2000
15 min	133	4000

Table 19 Estimated toxicity of hydrogen cyanide in humans

Toxic effects	Concentration (mg m^{-3})
Mild symptoms on inhalation for many hours	24–48
Maximum tolerance limit for 1 h	50–60
Hazardous to life on inhalation for 30–60 min	112–150
Death in 5–10 min	240–360
Death in 5 min	420
Death after several breaths	1000

Symptoms and Signs of Hydrogen Cyanide Poisoning

It is often assumed that exposure to a given concentration of hydrogen cyanide produces either sudden death or very few ill-effects. In military circles this is often summed up by the observation that the use of hydrogen cyanide leaves 'the quick and the dead' but no incapacitated or partly incapacitated individuals. This is incorrect. Work in animal models (D'Mello, 1987) has shown that exposure to sublethal doses of hydrogen cyanide can produce incapacitation. Dizziness and nausea have been recorded in people exposed to sub-lethal quantities of hydrogen cyanide, the effects lasting for some hours.

At lethal concentrations, collapse and death are rapid. Vedder (1925) has provided the following description:

"In an atmosphere containing a lethal concentration the odour of bitter almonds is noticed. This is followed rapidly by a sensation of constriction of the throat, giddiness, confusion and indistinct sight. The head feels as though the temples were gripped in a vice and there may be pain at the back of the neck, pain in the chest with palpitation and laboured respiration. Unconsciousness occurs and the man drops. From this moment if the subject remains in an atmosphere of hydrocyanic acid for more than two or three minutes death almost always ensues, after a brief period of convulsions followed by failure of respiration."

Management of Hydrogen Cyanide Poisoning

Here only a few points of relevance to battlefield casualties will be made:

- The usual points regarding the rapid removal of casualties from the risk of further contamination should be noted.
- Decontamination of casualties is unnecessary unless the clothing is contaminated with liquid hydrogen cyanide. This is very unlikely.
- All forms of treatment currently available demand intravenous administration. This will probably be impossible on the battlefield.
- Bearing the last point in mind, it is likely that casualties who reach aid-posts will be incapacitated by sublethal doses of hydrogen cyanide. Given that adequately trained medical orderlies, nursing staff or medical staff are available, antidotal therapy should be used. When deciding which therapy to recommend it should be borne in mind that the exact diagnosis of the cause of collapse may, under battlefield conditions, be difficult and treatment known to produce severe side-effects if given to casualties who have, in fact, not been exposed to hydrogen cyanide should perhaps be avoided.

Prophylaxis in Hydrogen Cyanide Poisoning

There are a number of antidotes to cyanide, which are highly effective in experimental animals and humans, where the antidotes can be used rapidly enough. These include sodium nitrite, sodium thiosulphate, dicobalt edetate and 4-dimethylaminophenol (Meredith *et al.*, 1993).

It is generally accepted that treatment of casualties suffering from hydrogen cyanide poisoning, under battlefield conditions, will be difficult and often unsuccessful. Because of this, attempts to provide a measure of pharmacological protection against the effects of hydrogen cyanide have been made. The conversion of a fraction of haemoglobin to methaemoglobin, thus providing a ready-made binding site for the cyanide, has been a favoured line of research and in 1948 Gilman and Cattell reported studies undertaken during World War II in America. *p*-Aminopropiophenone was found to be the best compound tested for the production of methaemoglobinaemia and oral doses of 2.0 mg kg^{-1} were given to volunteers. This produced a methaemoglobinaemia of some 20–30%. This was maintained by repeated dosing over 7 days without ill-effects, although 'at the end of this period there were observed the beginnings of a haemolytic anaemia'. Methaemoglobin levels of up to 15% were not found to interfere with exercise at light work loads. Animal work was reported to have shown that such levels of methaemoglobin (15%) would have provided protection against 10 lethal doses of hydrogen cyanide. On the battlefield, recalling the difficulty likely to be experienced in establishing a lethal concentration of cyanide, such a level of protection would be very valuable. Bright (1987) confirmed the above results in dogs, although the issue of *p*-aminopropiophenone to troops for use in anticipation of an attack with hydrogen cyanide has, as far as is known, not been undertaken by any country.

LESSER CHEMICAL WARFARE AGENTS

In addition to the compounds described above, many other substances have been considered, although in the main rejected, as possible chemical warfare agents. During World War I dozens, probably hundreds, of compounds were examined and during World War II several hundred mustard derivatives and variants were synthesized. The large number of compounds in this group which *could* be used in war makes any detailed consideration of individual compounds impossible. Instead, a few comments will be made on some older compounds of interest and on the riot control agents which could be encountered during modern warfare.

Early Irritant Compounds

Smoke from fires, used since classical times to discommode forces defending strong positions, exerted its effects by producing choking and eye irritation. In the early twentieth century, the Paris police force used grenades containing ethyl bromoacetate against rioters and it has been alleged that some of the police involved, later conscripted into the French Army, used the same grenades against German forces. The use of ethyl bromoacetate seems to have been taken up by the French and was also studied in London at Imperial College (the military abbreviation for ethyl bromoacetate, SK, is said to stand for South Kensington, the location of Imperial College). German workers also studied irritants and on 27 October 1914, at Neuve-Chapelle, HE shells containing lead balls embedded in the irritant *o*-dianisidine chlorosulphonate were deployed (SIPRI, 1971). This incident was followed by the use of other compounds, including xylyl bromide, chloroacetone, benzyl bromide and iodide, ethyl and methyl chlorosulphonate, 2-chloracetophenone and bromobenzyl cyanide. Prentiss (1937) held the last compound to be the most powerful irritant introduced during the war. In addition to the lacrimators, more toxic irritant smokes were developed. These included diphenylchlorarsine (DA), chlorodihydrophenarsazine (DM or Adamsite) and diphenylcyanarsine (DC).

These compounds were described as vomiting agents and in addition to producing nausea and vomiting, produced acute pain in the nose, uncontrollable sneezing, coughing, eye pain and lacrimation (HMSO, 1972). The marked sneezing led to these compounds being termed sternutators (Latin *sternuto*, sneezing). Of these compounds, only Adamsite has survived to modern use and has been used as a riot control agent, although not in the UK.

Other arsenical compounds developed during World War I included methyl-, ethyl- and phenyldichloroarsine, collectively known as 'The Dicks' (HMSO, 1972). These were vesicant compounds of considerable toxicity and were developed in an attempt to find a 'faster acting mustard gas' which would incapacitate casualties on contact. Attempts were also made to develop compounds combining irritancy with the lethality of hydrogen cyanide. Cyanogen bromide and chloride were produced, both effective irritants, capable of killing. Despite this, neither proved a very successful chemical warfare agent (Prentiss, 1937).

Modern Riot Control Compounds

The development of modern riot control compounds has been dominated by the perceived desirability of developing a compound with the following characteristics:

- Rapid incapacitating effect even when used against highly motivated individuals.
- Insignificant toxicity even to the very young or the very elderly bystander.
- Capacity for easy dissemination.
- Capacity for easy decontamination.
- Long shelf-life.
- Low cost.

It will be appreciated that these are difficult criteria to meet in full. At first glance the first two criteria listed might appear likely to be mutually exclusive and yet each is met remarkably well by compounds such as CS (2-chlorobenzylidene malononitrile) and CR (dibenz [b,f]-1,4-oxazepine) discussed below.

A detailed review of those compounds which might be considered for use today in riot control has been provided by Ballantyne (1977) and much of the present account has been based on his work. Information on the individual compounds is given in **Table 20**.

Dangers Associated with Exposure to Riot Control Compounds

Despite the low toxicity of these compounds exposure is not entirely without risk. The following points should be borne in mind:

- Exposure to levels much in excess of those anticipated, for example in a closed room, might produce significant toxic effects. CN (2-chloroacetophenone) in large doses may produce corneal damage, particularly if the compound enters the eye in the form of powder. Five deaths due to the pulmonary damage following exposure to high concentrations of CN in enclosed spaces have been reported (Gonzales et al., 1954; Stein and Kirwan, 1964). Exposure to high concentrations of riot control agents can occur as a result of use of personal protection devices. These are illegal in the UK but incidents involving their use are not uncommon. In 1995, Wheeler and Murray reported that 354 calls to the National Poisons Information Service (London) regarding CS had been received. Advice on management has been provided by Gray (1995).

- Exposure to irritants may produce transient although significant elevations of blood pressure. These have generally been regarded as not likely to do harm in healthy individuals, although those suffering from hypertension, aneurysms or myocardial disease might be placed at some risk (Ballantyne et al., 1976).

- Hysteria and panic may be produced by exposure to irritants particularly if the means of escape from exposure are blocked. Secondary injuries may be produced by stampeding crowds.

- Each of the compounds listed in **Table 20**, with the exception of CR, can produce contact sensitization (Rothberg, 1970; Holland and White, 1972).

Management of Casualties Exposed to Riot Control Agents

As for all other compounds discussed in this chapter, removal of casualties from the risk of further

Table 20 Riot control agents

Compound	Formula	Toxicometrics				V.P. 20 °C (mm Hg)	Water solubility (20 °C)	Onset of effects	Recovery
		L(Ct)$_{50}$ rat (pure compound) (mg min m^{-3})	L(Ct)$_{50}$ human (estimated) (mg min m^{-3})	TC$_{50}$ human eyes (mg m^{-3})	IC$_{50}$ human (mg m^{-3})				
DM		3700–12 710	11 000–35 000	–	25–220	2×10^{-13}	Insoluble	Delayed for some hours	1–2 h
CN		3700–18 800	8500–25 000	0.3	20–50	5.4×10^{-3}	4.4×10^{-3}	At once	20 min
CS		88 480	25 000–150 000	4×10^{-3}	3.6	3.4×10^{-5}	2.0×10^{-4} (rapid hydrolysis)	At once	20 min; erythema for up to 24 h
CR		> 425 000	>100 000	4×10^{-3}	0.7	5.9×10^{-5}	3.5×10^{-4}	At once	20 min; erythema for up to 1 h

contamination by adequately protected attendants is of first priority. Contaminated clothing should be removed and placed in polythene bags: CS and CR are notorious for spreading during decontamination of casualties. Lacrimation, blepharospasm, blepharoconjunctivitis and eye pain disappear quickly after removal from an irritant cloud. The effects on the eyes may be initially so distressing that casualties may require a great deal of reassurance that permanent eye damage has not been produced. The eyes should be kept open and those who have been regularly exposed to CS advise standing with the eyes open 'facing the wind'. Irrigation of the conjuctival sacs with 0.9% saline brings rapid, although in the author's personal experience, sometimes temporary, relief.

Skin should be decontaminated with soap and water. In the case of CS, hydrolysis occurs quickly and decontamination is rapidly accomplished. Showering is often advised but it should be remembered that CR and to a lesser extent CS may be washed out of the hair and produce secondary contamination of the eyes. Erythema generally subsides without treatment, although primary contact dermatitis may require treatment with corticosteroid ointment.

ALLEGED CHEMICAL WARFARE AGENTS

One of the commonest misconceptions regarding chemical warfare is represented by the view that compounds of great toxicity must, *ipso facto*, be likely effective chemical warfare agents. This view is so commonly put that it may be worth noting that in assessing the potential of a compound as a putative chemical warfare agent a number of factors have to be considered of which acute toxicity is only one and probably not the most important. These criteria include:

- Ease of manufacture in large quantities. Chemical warfare waged on a small scale during a major war is unlikely to produce significant results. It is sometimes argued that assassinations have been carried out using small quantities of highly toxic compounds. This is true, but assassination should not be confused with chemical warfare.
- The conditions of storage of the compound should not be demanding and the compound should not deteriorate on storage.
- The compound should be easy to disperse using inexpensive munitions and should not be destroyed by the dispersal system. The compound should be active in the form in which it is likely to be encountered by the opposing forces: a compound active only by the intravenous route would be an unsatisfactory chemical warfare agent.

- On the whole, compounds producing severe and care-demanding incapacitation are more effective chemical warfare agents than those which are inevitably lethal.
- It should be possible to protect one's own forces against the effects of the chosen compound without excessive expense or loss of efficiency.
- The compound should offer advantages when compared with already available compounds which meet the above criteria.

A rigorous application of these criteria will serve to remove many substances from accounts which purport to list possible or probable chemical warfare agents. In assessing the *probability* that a compound would be used as a chemical warfare agent the question, *Why should this compound be chosen?* should always be asked rather than the question, *Could this compound be used as a chemical warfare agent?*

A considerable range of exotic compounds have been examined as potential chemical warfare agents: batrachotoxin, tetrodotoxin, saxitoxin, palytoxin, botulinus toxin, staphylococcal enterotoxin B, ricin and abrin have all been examined in detail. Ricin was used to assassinate G. Markow in 1978. Figures are not available for the toxicity of staphylococcal enterotoxin B when absorbed by inhalation, although it is felt the compound would be significantly more toxic when administered in this way than by ingestion (Mattix *et al.*, 1995).

During the early 1980s, considerable attention was paid to toxins of fungal origin: mycotoxins. It was alleged that a group of mycotoxins known as trichothecenes had been used in South-East Asia. The compounds on which attention centred were T2 toxin (*Merck Index*, 1989a) and nivalenol (*Merck Index*, 1989b).

T2 is a caustic skin irritant which may cause dizziness, nausea, vomiting, diarrhoea and haemorrhage. The LD_{50} of T2 toxin (oral, rat) is 4.0 mg kg^{-1}. Nivalenol, also known to be capable of producing similar effects, has an LD_{50} (ip, mice) of 40 μg kg^{-1}. Further discussion of the toxicity of these compounds may be found in the work of Tatsuno (1968), Marasas *et al.* (1969), Wade (1981) and Rosen and Rosen (1982). Irrefutable evidence that these compounds were deliberately used as chemical warfare agents, is, however, lacking. During the Soviet occupation of Afghanistan it was alleged that Soviet forces had used chemical warfare agents against rebel tribesmen. No clear identification of the compounds alleged to have been used has appeared and the effects reported—the induction of unconsciousness with recovery with few ill-effects an hour or so later and the production of blackened and very rapidly decaying bodies—have been hard to explain.

In examining reports of alleged uses of chemical warfare agents, factors such as the likely naivity of observers, deliberate attempts to mislead and the more common causes of death in war should be borne in mind. Before dismissing such reports, however, it should also be remembered that small-scale use of chemicals on an *ad hoc* basis might occur during a war waged by poorly disciplined forces.

All the compounds considered thus far have been characterized as likely to have effects on humans. If the definition of chemical warfare is widened a little and the attack on food production resources or woodland, which provides hiding places for troops, is included then a number of herbicidal compounds could also be considered. Such compounds may be *per se* toxic to humans or, in the forms deployed, contain toxic contaminants. During the Vietnam War American forces used large quantities of herbicides, including the phenoxyacetates 2,4-D and 2,4,5-T, some preparations being contaminated with TCDD (tetrachlorodibenzodioxin). The mixture was often referred to as Agent Orange (Young *et al.*, 1978). Exposure to the mixture has been alleged, though not proven, to have produced long-term effects in both Vietnamese and American veterans. Details of the toxic effects of herbicides may be found in Chapter 97.

CONCLUSIONS

Chemical warfare has a long history, although only in the twentieth century has it been developed as a means of waging war on a large scale. Since the late 1980s moves to ban the production and stockpiling of chemical weapons were made and may yet prove completely successful between countries involved in these negotiations. During the revision of this chapter, the US Senate has again been discussing a ban on chemical weapons (April 1997). It should, be recalled however, that treaties have been violated in the past and that a number of countries currently believed to have acquired or to be acquiring chemical weapons are not involved in treaty negotiations. It seems, therefore, that although the risk of chemical warfare has diminished during the past decade, such a risk still exists.

BIBLIOGRAPHY

In addition to the sources identified in the text, a particular series of books deserve mention: *The Problem of Chemical and Biological Warfare*, Vols 1–6, published by the Stockholm International Peace Research Institute (SIPRI), 1971–75. ISBN numbers: 91-85114-10-3, -16-2, -17-0, -11-1, -13-8, -18-9. This invaluable work contains a wealth of information on all aspects of chemical warfare.

REFERENCES

Alkondon, M., Rao, K. S. and Albuquerque, E. X. (1988). Acetylcholinesterase reactivators modify the functional properties of the nicotinic acetylcholine receptor ion channel. *J. Pharmacol. Exp. Ther.*, **245**, 543–556.

Anderson, D. R., Yourick, J. J., Moeller, R. B., Petrali, J. P., Young, D. and Byers, S. L. (1996). Pathologic changes in rat lungs following acute sulfur mustard inhalation. *Inhalation Toxicol.*, **8**, 285–297.

Anslow, W. P., Karnofsky, D. A., val-Jager, B. and Smith, H. W. (1948). Intravenous, subcutaneous and cutaneous toxicity of bis (β-chloroethyl) sulphide (mustard gas) and various derivatives. *J. Pharmacol. Exp. Ther.*, **93**, 1–9.

Aposhian, H. V., Mershon, M. M., Brinkley, F. B., Hsu, C. A. and Hackley, B. E. (1982). Anti-Lewisite activity and stability of *meso*-dimercaptosuccinic acid and 2,3-dimercapto-1-propanesulfonic acid. *Life Sci.*, **31**, 2149–2156.

Aposhian, H. V., Carter, D. E., Hoover, T. D., Hsu, C. A., Maiorino, R. M. and Stine, E. (1984). DMSA, DMPS and DMPA as arsenic antidotes. *Fundam. Appl. Toxicol.*, **4**, S58–S70.

Ballantyne, B. (1977). Riot control agents: biomedical and health aspects of the use of chemicals in civil disturbances. *The Medical Annual*. Wright, Bristol, pp. 7–41.

Ballantyne, B. (1987). Toxicology of cyanides. In Ballantyne, B. and Marrs, T. C. *Clinical and Experimental Toxicology of Cyanides*. Wright, Bristol. pp. 41–126.

Ballantyne, B. and Schwabe, P. H. (1981). *Respiratory Protection: Principles and Applications*. Chapman and Hall, London, p. 113.

Ballantyne, B., Gall, D. and Robson, D. C. (1976). Effects on man of drenching with dilute solutions of *o*-chlorobenzylidine malononitrile (CS) and dibenz(*b,f*)-1:4-oxazepine (CR). *Med. Sci. Law*, **16**, 159–170.

Barcroft, J. (1920). Discussion on the therapeutic uses of oxygen. *Proc. R. Soc. Med. London*, Section on Therapeutics and Pharmacology, **xiii**, 59.

Benschop, A. P. and Keijer, J. H. (1966). The correlation between aging of phosphylated cholinesterases and unimolecular solvolysis of related reference compounds. *PML Report*. Prins Mauritz Laboratory TNO, Rijswick, The Netherlands.

Bosković, B., Kovacević, V. and Jovanovic, D. (1984). 2-PAM chloride HI6 and HGG-12 in soman and tabun poisoning. *Fundam. Appl. Toxicol.*, **4**, S106–S115.

Bradley, B. L. and Unger, K. M. (1982). Phosgene inhalation, a case report. *Tex. Med.*, **78**, 51–53.

Brezenoff, H. E., McGee, J. and Knight, V. (1984). The hypertensive response to soman and its relation to brain acetylcholinesterase inhibition. *Acta Pharmacol. Toxicol.*, **55**, 270–277.

Bright, J. E. (1987). A prophylaxis for cyanide poisoning. In Ballantyne, B. and Marrs, T. C. (Eds), *Clinical and Experimental Toxicology of Cyanides*. Wright, Bristol, pp. 359–382

Bright, F. E., Inns, R. H., Tuckwell, N. J., Griffiths, G. D. and Marrs, T. C. (1991). A histochemical study of changes observed in the mouse diaphragm after organophosphate poisoning. *Hum. Exp. Toxicol.*, **10**, 9–14.

Brimblecombe, R. W., Green, D. M., Stratton, J. A. and Thompson, P. B. (1970). The protective actions of some anticholinergic drugs in sarin poisoning. *Br. J. Pharmacol.*, **39**, 822–830.

British Medical Association and The Royal Pharmaceutical Society of Great Britain (1989). *British National Formulary*, No. 18, September. BMA and Pharmaceutical Press, London

Calvet, J. H., Coste, A., Levame, M., Harf, A., Macquin-Mavier, I. and Escudier, E. (1996). Airway epithelial damage induced by sulfur mustard in guinea pigs, effects of glucocorticoids. *Hum. Exp. Toxicol.*, **15**, 964–971.

Cameron, G. R., Gaddum, J. H. and Short, R. H. D. (1946). The absorption of war gases by the nose. *J. Pathol.*, **58**, 449–457.

Chauhan, R. S., Murthy, L. V. R. and Pant, S. C. (1995). Electron microscopic study of guinea pig skin exposed to sulphur mustard. *Bull. Environ. Contam. Toxicol.*, **55**, 50–57.

Clement, J. G. (1981). Toxicology and pharmacology of bispyridinium oximes. Insight into the mechanism of action vs soman poisoning *in vivo*. *Fundam. Appl. Toxicol.*, **1**, 193–202.

Clement, J. G. (1982a). HI-6: reactivation of central and peripheral acetylcholinesterase following inhibition by soman, sarin and tabun *in vivo* in the rat. *Biochem. Pharmacol.*, **31**, 1283–1287.

Clement, J. G. (1982b). Plasma aliesterase—a possible depot for soman (pinacolyl-methylphosphonofluoridate) in the mouse. *Biochem. Pharmacol.*, **31**, 4085–4088.

Clement, J. G. and Lockwood, P. A. (1982). HI-6, an oxime which is an effective antidote in soman poisoning: a structure activity study. *Toxicol. Appl. Pharmacol.*, **64**, 140–146.

Clement, J. G., Sansen, A. S. and Boulet, C. A. (1992). Efficacy of HLö-7 and pyrimidoxime as antidotes of nerve agent poisoning in mice. *Arch. Toxicol.*, **66**, 216–219.

Coleman, I. W., Patton, G. E. and Bannard, R. A. (1968). Cholinolytics in the treatment of anticholinesterase poisoning V. The effectiveness of Parpanit with oximes in the treatment of organophosphorus poisoning. *Can. J. Physiol. Pharmacol.*, **46**, 109–117.

Cucinell, S. A. (1974). Review of the toxicity of long-term phosgene exposure. *Arch. Environ. Health*, **28**, 272–275.

Davies, D. R. and Green, A. L. (1956). The kinetics of reactivation by oximes of cholinesterase inhibited by organophosphorus compounds. *Biochem. J.*, **63**, 529–535.

Davies, D. R. and Green, A. L. (1959). 2-Hydroxyiminoethyl-*N*-methylpyridine methanesulphonate and atropine in the treatment of severe organophosphorus poisoning. *Br. J. Pharmacol.*, **14**, 5–8.

De-Jong, L. P. A. (1983). Personal communication to Ligtenstein, D.

De-Jong, L. P. A. and Wolring, G. Z. (1978). Effect of 1-(AR) alkyl-2-hydroxyiminomethylpyridinium salts on reactivation and ageing of acetylcholinesterase inhibited by diethylphosphoramide-cyanidate (Tabun). *Biochem. Pharmacol.*, **27**, 2229–2235.

De-Jong, L. P. A. and Wolring, G. Z. (1980). Reactivation of acetylcholinesterase inhibited by 1,2,2′-trimethylpropyl-methyl-phosphonofluoridate (Soman) with HI6 and related oximes. *Biochem. Pharmacol.*, **29**, 2379–2387.

Diller, W. F. (1978). Medical phosgene problems and their possible solution. *J. Occup. Med.*, **20**, 189–193.

Dixon, H. (1946). Biochemical research on CW agents. *Nature*, **158**, 432–438.

D'Mello, G. D. (1987). Neuropathological and behavioural sequelae of acute cyanide toxicosis in animal species. In Ballantyne, B. and Marrs, T. C. (Eds), *Clinical and Experimental Toxicology of Cyanides*. Wright, Bristol, pp. 156–183.

Everett, E. D. and Overholt, E. L. (1968). Phosgene poisoning. *J. Am. Med. Assoc.*, **205**, 103–105.

Eyer, P., Ladstetter, B., Schafer, W. and Sonnenbichler, J. (1989). Studies on the stability and decomposition of the

Hagedorn oxime HLö-7 in aqueous solution. *Arch. Toxicol.*, **63**, 59–67.

Eyer, P., Hagedorn, I., Klimmek, R., Lippstreu, P., Löffler, M., Oldiges, H., Spöhrer, U., Steidl, I., Szinicz, L. and Worek, F. (1992). HLö 7 dimethanesulfonate, a potent bispyridinium-dioxime against anticholinesterases. *Arch. Toxicol.*, **66**, 603–621.

Fleisher, J. H. (1963). Effects of *p*-nitrophenyl phosphonate (EPN) on the toxicity of isopropyl methyl phosphonofluoridate (GB). *J. Pharmacol. Exp. Ther.*, **139**, 390.

Fleisher, J. H. and Harris, L. W. (1965). Dealkylation as a mechanism for ageing of cholinesterase after poisoning with pinacolyl methylphosphonofluoridate. *Biochem. Pharmacol.*, **14**, 641–650.

Fotion, H. and Elfstrom, G. (1986). *Military Ethics*. Routledge and Kegan Paul, London.

Fox, M. and Scott, D. (1980). The genetic toxicology of nitrogen and sulphur mustard. *Mutat. Res.*, **75**, 131–168.

Friedenwald, J. S. and Hughes, W. F. (1948). The effects of toxic chemical agents on the eye and their treatment. In Andrus, E. C. *et al.* (Eds), *Advances in Military Medicine*, Vol. II. Little Brown, Boston, Ch. XXXIX.

Frosolono, M. F. and Pawlowski, R. (1977). Effect of phosgene on rat lungs after single high level exposure 1. Biochemical alterations. *Arch. Environ. Health*, **32**, 271–277.

Fruhman, G. (1974). Vorkommen und Behandlung des Lungenödems nach Inhalation von Reizgas. *Med. Klin.*, **69**, 22–26.

Gates, M. and Renshaw, B. C. (1946). Fluorophosphates and other phosphorus containing compounds. In *Summary Technical Report of Division 9*, Vol. I, Parts I and II. NTIS PB 158508. Office of Scientific Research and Development, Washington, DC, pp. 131–155.

Gilman, A. and Cattell, M. (1948). Systemic agents: action and treatment. In Andrus, E. C. *et al.* (Eds), *Advances in Military Medicine*, Vol. 2. Little Brown, Boston, pp. 546–564.

Gonzales, T. A., Vance, M., Helpern, M. and Umberger, C. J. (1954). *Legal Medicine*. Appleton-Century Crofts, New York.

Goodman, L. S. and Gilman, A. (1980). *The Pharmacological Basis of Therapeutics*, 6th edn. Macmillan, London and Billière Tindall, New York.

Göransson-Nyberg, A., Cassel, G., Jeneskog, T., Karlsson, L., Larson, R., Lundström, M. and Persson, S.-Å. Treatment of organophosphate poisoning in pigs: antidote administration by a new binary autoinjector. (1995). *Arch. Toxicol.*, **70**, 20–27.

Gordan, J. J. and Leadbeater, L. (1977). The prophylactic use of 1-methyl-2-hydroxyiminomethylpyridinium methanesulfonate (P2S) in the treatment of organophosphate poisoning. *Toxicol. Appl. Pharmacol.*, **40**, 109–114.

Goyer, R. A. (1986). Toxic effects of metals. In Klaassen, C. D., Amdur, M. O. and Doull, J. (Eds), *Casarett and Doull's Toxicology: the Basic Science of Poisons*, 3rd edn. Macmillan, New York, pp. 582–635.

Gray, P. J. (1995). Treating CS gas injuries to the eye [Letter]. *Br. Med. J.*, **311**, 871.

Graziano, J. H., Cuccia, D. and Friedheim, E. (1978). The pharmacology of 2, 3-dimercaptosuccinic acid and its potential use in arsenic poisoning. *J. Pharmacol. Exp. Ther.*, **207**, 1051–1055.

Gross, P., Rinehart, W. E. and Hatch, T. (1965). Chronic pneumonitis caused by phosgene. *Arch. Environ. Health*, **10**, 768–775.

Haldane, J. B. S. (1925). *Callinicus: a Defence of Chemical Warfare*. Kegan Paul, French, Trubner, London.

Haldane, J. S. (1917). The therapeutic administration of oxygen. *Br. Med. J.*, **1**, 181.

Haley, R. W. and Kurt, T. L. (1997). Self-reported exposure to neurotoxic chemical combinations in the Gulf War. A cross-sectional epidemiologic study. *J. Am. Med. Assoc.*, **277**, 231–237.

Haley, R. W., Kurt, T. L. and Horn, J. (1997a). Is there a Gulf War Syndrome? Searching for syndromes by factor analysis of symptoms. *J. Am. Med. Assoc.*, **277**, 215–222.

Haley, R. W., Horn, J., Roland, P. S., Bryan, W. W., Van Ness, P. C., Bonte, F. J., Devous, M. D., Mathews, D., Fleckenstein, J. L., Wians, F. H., Wolfe, G. I. and Kurt, T. L. (1997b). Evaluation of neurologic function in Gulf War veterans. A blinded case-control study. *J. Am. Med. Assoc.*, **277**, 223–230.

Harris, L. W., Stitcher, D. L. and Heyl, W. C. (1981). Protection and induced reactivation of cholinesterase by HS-6 in rabbits exposed to soman. *Life Sci.*, **29**, 1747–1753.

Hitler, A. (1925). *Mein Kampf*, Vol. I.

HMSO (1923). *History of the Great War: Medical Services [Diseases of the War]*, Vol. II. HMSO, London.

HMSO (1972, 1987). *Medical Manual of Defence Against Chemical Agents*. JSP312. HMSO, London.

Holland, P. and White, R. G. (1972). The cutaneous reactions produced by *o*-chlorobenzylidine malononitrile and ω-chloracetophenone when applied directly to the skin of human subjects. *Br. J. Dermatol.*, **86**, 150–154.

Holmstedt, B. (1963). Structure activity relationships of the organophosphorus anticholinesterase agents. In Koelle, G. B. (Ed.), *Cholinesterases and Anticholinesterase Agents. Handbuch der Exp. Pharm.*, Vol. 15. Springer, Berlin, pp. 428–485.

Hunter, D. (1978). *The Diseases of Occupations*, 6th edn. Hodder and Stoughton, London.

Hyams, K. C., Wignall, F. S. and Roswell, R. (1996). War syndromes and their evaluation: from the US Civil War to the Persian Gulf War. *Ann. Intern. Med.*, **125**, 398–405.

Inns, R. H. and Leadbeater, L. (1983). The efficacy of bispyridinium derivatives in the treatment of organophosphate poisoning in the guinea pig. *J. Pharm. Pharmacol.*, **35**, 427–433.

Inns, R. H. and Rice, P. (1993). Efficacy of dimercapto chelating agents for the treatment of poisoning by percutaneously applied dichloro(2-chlorovinyl)arsine in rabbits. *Hum. Exp. Toxicol.*, **12**, 241–246.

Iowa Persian Gulf Study Group. (1997). Self-reported illness and health status among Gulf War veterans. *J. Am. Med. Assoc.*, **277**, 238–245.

Ireland, M. M. (1926). *Medical Aspects of Gas Warfare*, vol. XIV of *The Medical Department of the United States in the World War*. Government Printing Office, Washington, DC.

Ivanhoe, F. and Meyers, F. H. (1964). Phosgene poisoning as an example of neuroparalytic acute pulmonary edema: the sympathetic vasomotor reflex involved. *Dis. Chest*, **46**, 211–218.

Jovanović, D. (1983). The effect of bis-pyridinium oximes on neuromuscular blockade induced by highly toxic organophosphates in rat. *Arch. Int. Pharmacodyn. Ther.*, **262**, 231–241.

Juarez-Salinas, H., Sims, J. L. and Jacobson, M. K. (1979). Poly(ADP-ribose) levels in carcinogen treated cells. *Nature*, **282**, 740–741.

Kassa, J. (1998). A comparison of the efficacy of new asymmetric bispyridinium oxime BI-6 with other oximes (obidoxime, HI-6), against soman in rats. *Hum. Exp. Toxicol.*, **17**, 331–335.

Kassa, J. and Bajgar, J. (1995). Comparison of the efficacy of HI-6 and obidoxime against cyclohexyl methylphosphonofluoridate (GF) in rats. *Hum. Exp. Toxicol.*, **14**, 923–928.

Keeler, J. R., Hurst, C. G. and Dunn, M. A. (1991). Pyridostigmine used as a nerve agent pretreatment under wartime conditions. *J. Am. Med. Assoc.*, **266**, 693–695.

Khordagui, H. (1996). Potential fate of G-nerve chemical warfare agents in the coastal waters of the Arabian Gulf. *Mar. Environ. Res.*, **41**, 133–143.

Kleinberger, G., Pichler, M. and Weiser, M. (1981). 2, 3-Dimercaptosuccinic acid in human arsenic poisoning. *Arch Toxicol.*, **47**, 241–243.

Koelle, G. B. (1963). Cholinesterases and anticholinesterase agents. In Koelle, G. B. (Ed.), *Cholinesterases and Anticholinesterase Agents. Handbuch der Exp. Pharm.*, Vol. **115**, Springer, Berlin, pp. 428–485.

Koelle, G. B. (1975). Neurohumoral transmission and the autonomic nervous system. In Goodman, L. S. and Gilman, A. (Eds), *The Pharmacological Basis of Therapeutics*, 5th edn. Macmillan, London, pp. 404–444.

Leblic, C., Coq, H. M. and Le-Moan, G. (1984). Etude de la toxicité de l'eserine, VX et le paraoxon pour établir un modèle mathematique de l'extrapolation à être humain. *Arch. Belg.*, Suppl., 226–242.

Lefebure, V. (1921). *The Riddle of the Rhine*. Collins, London.

Lenz, K., Hruby, K., Druml, W., Eder, A., Gaszner, A., Kleinberger, G., Picher, M. and Weiser, M. (1981). 2, 3-Dimercaptosuccinic acid in human arsenic poisoning. *Arch. Toxicol.*, **47**, 241–243.

Ligtenstein, D. A. (1984). On the synergism of the cholinesterase reactivating bispyridinium-aldoxime HI6 and atropine in the treatment of organophosphate intoxications in the rat. PhD Thesis, University of Leiden, Netherlands.

Lindsay, C. D. and Rice, P. (1995). Changes in connective tissue macromolecular components of Yucatan mini-pig skin following application of sulphur mustard vapour. *Hum. Exp. Toxicol.*, **14**, 341–348.

Lindsay, C. D. and Rice, P. (1996). Assessment of the biochemical effects of percutaneous exposure of sulphur mustard in an *in vitro* human skin system. *Hum. Exp. Toxicol.*, **15**, 237–244.

Lipp, J. A. (1972). Effect of diazepam upon soman-induced seizure activity and convulsions. *Electroencephalogr. Clin. Neurophysiol.*, **32**, 557–560.

Lipp, J. A. (1973). Effect of benzodiazepine derivatives on soman-induced seizure activity and convulsions in the monkey. *Arch. Int. Pharmacodyn.*, **202**, 244–251.

Liu, D. D., Ueno, E., Hoi, K. and Hoskins, B. (1988). Evidence that changes in levels of cyclic nucleotides are not related to soman induced convulsions. *Neurotoxicology*, **9**, 23–28.

Lohs, von K. (1960). Zur Toxicologie und Pharmakologie organischer Phosphorsäurester. *Dtsch. Gesundheitswesen*, **15**, 2179–2133.

Lundy, P. M. and Magor, G. F. (1978). Cyclic GMP concentrations in cerebellum following organophosphate administration. *J. Pharm. Pharmacol.*, **30**, 251–252.

Lundy, P. M., Hansen, A. S., Hand, B. T. and Boulet, C. A. (1992). Comparison of several oximes against poisoning by soman, tabun and GF. *Toxicology*, **72**, 99–105.

Maksimović, M., Bosković, B., Radović, L., Tadić, V., Deljac, V. and Binenfeld, Z. (1980). Antidotal effects of bis-pyridinium-2-mono-oxime carbonyl derivatives in intoxication with highly toxic organophosphorous compounds. *Acta Pharm. Jugosl.*, **30**, 151–160.

Mann, I. (1948). An experimental and clinical study of the reaction of the anterior segment of the eye to chemical injury, with special reference to chemical warfare agents. *Br. J. Ophthalmol.*, Monogr. Suppl. XIII.

Marasas, W. F. O., Bamburg, J. R., Smalley, E. B., Strong, F. M., Ragland, W. L. and Degurse, P. E. (1969). Toxic effects on trout, rats and mice of T-2 toxin produced by the fungus *Fusarium tricinctum*. *Toxicol. Appl. Pharmacol.*, **15**, 471–482.

Marata, K., Araki, S., Yokoyama, K., Okumura, T., Ishimatsu, S., Takasu, N. and White, R. F. (1997). Asymptamatic sequelae to acute Sarin poisoning in the central and autonomic nervous system 6 months after the Tokyo subway attack. *J. Neurol.*, **244**, 601–606.

Marrs, T. C., Maynard, R. L. and Sidell, F. R. (1996). *Chemical Warfare Agents: Toxicology and Treatment*. Wiley, Chichester.

Masuda, N., Takatsu, M. and Morinari, H. (1995). Sarin poisoning in Tokyo subway [Letter]. *Lancet*, **345**, 1446.

Mattix, M. E., Hunt, R. E., Wilhelmsen, C. L., Johnson, A. J. and Baze, W. B. (1995). Aerosolized staphylococcal enterotoxin B-induced pulmonary lesions in Rhesus monkeys (*Macaca mulatta*). *Toxicol. Pathol.*, **23**, 262–268.

Maynard, R. L. (1988). *The Ethics of Chemical Warfare: an Historical Perspective*. Royal College of Defence Studies, London.

Maynard, R. L. and Beswick, F. W. (1992). Organophosphorus compounds as chemical warfare agents. In Ballantyne, B. and Marrs, T. M. (Eds), *Clinical and Experimental Toxicology of Organophosphates and Carbamates*. Butterworth–Heinemann, Oxford, pp. 373–385.

Merck Index (1989a). 11th edn. Merck, Rahway, NJ, Ref. No. 9711.

Merck Index (1989b). 11th edn. Merck, Rahway, NJ, Ref. No. 6581.

Meredith, T. J., Jacobsen, D., Haines, J. A., Berger, J.-C. and van Heijst, A. N. P. (1993). *Antidotes for Poisoning by Cyande. IPCS/CEC Evaluation of Antidotes Series*, vol 2. Cambridge University Press, Cambridge.

Meselson, M. and Perry Robinson, J. (1980). Chemical warfare and chemical disarmament. *Sci. Amer.*, **242**, 34–43.

Miskin, R. and Reich, E. (1980). Plasminogen activator: induction of synthesis by DNA damage. *Cell*, **19**, 217–224.

Monteiro-Riviere, N. A. and Inman, A. O. (1995). Indirect immunohistochemistry and immunoelectron microscopy distribution of eight epidermal–dermal junction epitopes in the pig and in isolated perfused skin treated with bis(2-chloroethyl) sulfide. *Toxicol. Pathol.*, **23**, 313–325.

Murphy, S. D. (1986). Toxic effects of pesticides. In Klaassen, C. D., Amdur, M. O. and Doull, J. (Eds), *Casarett and Doull's Toxicology: the Basic Science of Poisons*, 3rd edn. Macmillan, New York, pp. 519–581.

Nash, T. and Pattle, R. E. (1971). The absorption of phosgene by aqueous solution and its relation to toxicity. *Ann. Occup. Hyg.*, **14**, 227–233.

Nozaki, H., Aikawa, N., Fujishima, S., Suzuki, M., Shinozawa, Y., Hori, S. and Nogawa, S. (1995). A case of VX poisoning and the difference from sarin [Letter]. *Lancet*, **346**, 698–699.

Oldiges, H. and Schoene, K. (1970). Pyridinium und Imidazolinium-Salze als Antidote genüber Soman und Paraoxonvergiftungen bei Mäuse. *Arch. Toxicol.*, **26**, 293–305.

Papirmeister, B., Gross, C. L., Patrali, J. P. and Hixson, C. J. (1984a). Pathology produced by sulfur mustard in human skin grafts on athymic nude mice: I. Gross and light microscopical changes. *J. Toxicol. Cutaneous Ocul. Toxicol.*, **3**, 371–392.

Papirmeister, B., Gross, C. L., Petrali, J. P. and Meier, H. L. (1984b). Pathology produced by sulfur mustard in human skin grafts on athymic nude mice: II. Ultrastructural changes. *J. Toxicol. Cutaneous Ocul. Toxicol.*, **3**, 393–408.

Pattle, R. E. (1965). Surface lining of lung alveoli. *Physiol. Rev.*, **45**, 28–79.

Pawlowski, R. and Frosolono, M. F. (1977). Effect of phosgene on rat lungs after single high level exposure II. Ultrastructural alterations. *Arch. Environ. Health*, **32**, 278–283.

Pazdernik, T. L., Cross, R., Nelson, S., Samson, F. and McDonough, J. (1983). Soman-induced depression of brain activity in TAB treated rats: 2-deoxyglucose study. *Neurotoxicity*, **4**, 27–34.

Pearson, G. S. (1988). Chemical Defence. *Chem. Br.*, **24**, 657–658.

Peters, R. (1948). Development and theoretical significance of British Anti Lewisite BAL. *Br. Med. Bull.*, **5**, 313–318.

Peters, R. (1953). Significance of lesions in the pyruvate oxidase system. *Br. Med. Bull.*, **9**, 116–121.

Peters, R., Stocken, L. A. and Thompson, R. H. S. (1945). British Anti Lewisite [BAL]. *Nature*, **156**, 616–619.

Potts, A. M., Simon, F. P. and Gerard, R. W. (1949). The mechanism of action of phosgene. *Arch. Biochem.*, **24**, 329–337.

Prentiss, A. M. (1937). *Chemicals in War*. McGraw-Hill, New York.

Prichard, J. S. (1996). Pulmonary oedema. In Weatherall, D. J., Ledingham, J. G. G. and Warrell, D. A., II (Eds), *Oxford Textbook of Medicine*. Oxford University Press, Oxford, pp. 2495–2505.

Rengstorff, R. H. (1985). Accidental exposure to sarin: vision effects. *Arch. Toxicol.*, **56**, 201–203.

Renshaw, B. (1946). Mechanisms in production of cutaneous injuries by sulfur and nitrogen mustards. In *Chemical Warfare Agents and Related Chemical Problems*, Vol. I. US Office of Science Research and Development, National Defense Research Committee, Washington, DC, Chap. 23, pp. 79–518.

Reprint Society (1938). *The Notebooks of Leonardo da Vinci*. Reprint Society, London.

Reynolds, J. E. F. (Ed.) (1989). *Martindale: The Extra Pharmacopoeia*, 29th edn. Pharmaceutical Press, London.

Rink, S. M. and Hopkins, P. B. (1995). Direct evidence for DNA intrastrand cross-linking by the nitrogen mustard mechlorethamine in synthetic oligonucleotides. *Bioorg. Medi. Chem. Lett.*, **9**, 2845–2850.

Robin, E. D. (1979). Permeability pulmonary edema. In Fishman, A. P. and Renkin, E. M. (Eds), *Pulmonary Edema*. American Physiological Society, Bethesda, MD.

Rosen, R. T. and Rosen, J. D. (1982). Presence of four *Fusarium* mycotoxins and synthetic material in 'yellow rain'. Evidence for the use of chemical weapons in Laos. *Biomed. Mass Spectrom.*, **9**, 443–450.

Rothberg, S. (1970). Skin sensitization potential of the riot control agents BBC, DM, CN and CS in guinea pigs. *Milit. Med.*, **135**, 552–556.

Sartori, M. (1939). *The War Gases—Chemistry and Analysis*. J. and A. Churchill, London.

Scaife, J. F. (1959). Oxime reactivation studies of inhibited true and pseudocholinesterase. *Can. J. Biochem. Physiol.*, **37**, 1301–1311.

Schneeberger, E. E. (1979). Barrier function of intercellular junctions in adult and fetal lungs. In Fishman, A. P. and Renkin, E. M. (Eds), *Pulmonary Edema*. American Physiological Society, Bethesda, MD.

Schoene, K. and Oldiges, H. (1973). Efficacy of pyridinium salts against tabun and sarin poisoning *in vivo* and *in vitro*. *Arch. Int. Pharmacodyn. Ther.*, **204**, 110–123.

Sciuto, A. M., Strickland, P. T., Kennedy, T. P. and Gurtner, G. H. (1995). Protective effects of *N*-acetylcysteine treatment after phosgene exposure in rabbits. *Am. J. Respir. Crit. Care Med.*, **151**, 768–772.

Sciuto, A. M., Strickland, P. T., Kennedy, T. P., Guo, Y.-L. and Gurtner, G. H. (1996). Intratracheal administration of DBcAMP attenuates edema formation in phosgene-induced acute lung injury. *J. Appl. Physiol.*, **80**, 149–157.

Seagrave, S. (1981). *Yellow Rain: a Journey Through the Terror of Chemical Warfare*. Evans, New York.

Seidelim, R. (1961). The inhalation of phosgene in a fire extinguisher accident. *Thorax*, **16**, 91–93.

Sekijima, Y., Morita, H. and Yanagisawa, N. (1997). Follow-up of sarin poisoning in Matsumoto. *Ann. Intern. Mod.*, **127**, 1042.

Selgrade, M. K., Gilmour, M. I., Yang, Y. G., Burleson, G. R. and Hatch, G. E. (1995). Pulmonary host defenses and resistance to infection following subchronic exposure to phosgene. *Inhalation Toxicol.*, **7**, 1257–1268.

Sharabi, Y., Danon, Y. L., Berkenstadt, H., Almog, S., Mimouni-Bloch, A., Zisman, A., Dani, S. and Atsmon, J. (1991). Survey of symptoms following intake of pyridostigmine during the Persian Gulf War. *Isr. J. Med. Sci.*, **27**, 656–658.

SIPRI (1971). *The Problem of Chemical and Biological Warfare. Vol. 1. The Rise of Chemical Weapons*. Stockholm International Peace Research Institute, Stockholm.

Smith, R. P. (1986). Toxic responses of the blood. In Klaassen, C. D., Amdur, M. O. and Doull, J. (Eds), *Casarett and Doull's Toxicology: the Basic Science of Poisons*. Macmillan, New York, pp. 223–244.

Staub, N. C. (1974). Pathogenesis of pulmonary oedema. *Am. Rev. Respir. Dis.*, **109**, 356–372.

Stavrakis, P. (1971). The use of hexamethylenetetramine (HMT) in the treatment of acute phosgene poisoning. *Ind. Med. Surg.*, **40**, 30–31.

Stein, A. A. and Kirwan, W. E. (1964). Chloracetophenone (tear gas) poisoning: a clinicopathological report. *J. Forensic Sci.*, **9**, 374–382.

Sulzberger, M. B. (1943). The absence of skin irritants in the contents of vesicles. *US Navy Med. Bull.*, **41**, 1258–1262.

Szinicz, L. (1996). Non-reactivation effects of oximes. In Szinicz, L., Eyer, P. and Klimmek, R. (Eds), *Role of Oximes in the Treatment of Anticholinesterase Poisoning*. Spektrum Heidelberg, pp. 53–68.

Tammelin, L. E. (1957). Dialkoxy-phosphorylcholines, alkoxy-methyl-phosphorylthiocholines and analogous choline esters. *Acta Chem. Scand.*, **11**, 1340–1349.

Tatsuno, T. (1968). Toxicologic research on substances from *Fusarium nivale*. *Cancer Res.*, **28**, 2393–2396.

Tattersall, J. E. H. (1993). Ion channel blockade by oximes and recovery of diaphragm muscle from soman poisoning *in vitro*. *Br. J. Pharmacol.*, **108**, 1006–1015.

Taylor, P. (1980). Anticholinesterase agents. In Goodman, L. S. and Gilman, A. (Eds), *The Pharmacological Basis of Therapeutics*, 6th edn. Pergamon Press, New York, Chap. 6.

Teplitz, C. (1979). Pulmonary cellular and interstitial edema. In Fishman, A. P. and Renkin, E. M. (Eds), *Pulmonary Edema*. American Physiological Society, Bethesda, MD, pp. 97–111.

United Nations Reports: S/16433 (1984), S/17911 (1986), S/18852 (1987). United Nations Organization, New York.

US Public Health Service (1996). *Proceeding of a Seminar on Responding to the Consequences of Chemical and Biological Terrorism, July 11–14th, 1995, Bethesda, Maryland*. US Government Printing Office, Washington, DC.

van Helden, P. M., de Lange, J., Busker, R. W. and Melchers, B. P. C. (1991). Therapy of organophosphate poisoning in the rat by direct effects of oximes unrelated to ChE reactivation. *Arch. Toxicol.*, **65**, 586–593.

Vedder, E. B. (1925). *The Medical Aspects of Chemical Warfare*. Williams and Wilkins, Baltimore, MD.

Vogt, R. F., Dannenberg, A. M., Schofield, B. H., Haynes, N. A., and Papirmeister, B. (1984). Pathogenesis of skin lesions caused by sulfur mustard. *Fundam. Appl. Toxicol.*, **4**, S71–S83.

Wade, N. (1981). Toxin warfare charges may be premature [Editorial]. *Science*, **214**, 34.

Wagner-Jauregg, T. (1956). Experimentelle Chemotherapie von durch phosphorhaltige Anti-Esterasen hervorgerufenen Vergiftungen. *Arzneim.-Forsch.*, **6**, 194–196.

Warthin, A. S. and Weller, C. V. (1919). *The Medical Aspects of Mustard Gas Poisoning*. Henry Kimpton, London.

Watson, A. P., Jones, T. D. and Adams, J. D. (1992). Relative potency estimates of acceptable residues and reentry intervals after nerve agent release. *Ecotoxicol. Environ. Saf.*, **23**, 328–342.

Willems, J. L. (1989). Clinical management of mustard gas casualties. *Ann. Med. Milit. Belg.*, **3**, S1–S61.

Wilson, I. B. and Ginsburg, S. (1955). A powerful reactivator of alkyl phosphate inhibited acetylcholinesterase. *Biochim. Biophys. Acta*, **18**, 168–170.

Winternitz, M. C. (1920). *Pathology of War Gas Poisoning*. Yale University Press, Newhaven, CT.

Wolthuis, O. L. and Kepner, L. A. (1978). Successful oxime therapy one hour after soman intoxication in the rat. *Eur. J. Pharmacol.*, **49**, 415–425.

Wolthuis, O. L., Berends, F. and Meeter, E. (1981). Problems in the therapy of soman poisoning. *Fundam. Appl. Toxicol.*, **1**, 183–192.

Yamada, A. (1963). On the late injuries following occupational inhalation of mustard gas with special reference to carcinoma of the respiratory tract. *Acta Pathol. Jpn.*, **13**, 131–155.

Young, A. L., Calcagni, J. A., Thalken, C. E., Tromblay, J. W. (1978). The toxicology, environmental fate and human risk of herbicide agent orange and its dioxin. *USAF OEHL Technical Report 78–92*. National Technical Information Centre (AD-A062-143), US Department of Commerce, Springfield, VA.

Chapter 99

Nitrate, Nitrite and *N*-Nitroso Compounds

Sharat D. Gangolli

CONTENTS

- Introduction
- Dietary Levels and Estimated Human Intakes
- Endogenous Synthesis
- Toxicokineties and Metabolism
- Toxicology in Animals and Experimental Systems
- Human Effects and Epidemiological Studies
- Summary, Risk Analysis and Conclusions
- References

INTRODUCTION

This contribution is an overview of nitrate, nitrite and *N*-nitroso components with respect to their occurrence in human diet and the environment, and an estimate of human exposure from these sources. Also discussed are their endogenous formation, metabolic disposition and toxicology in experimental animals and in man.

Nitrate is an important component of man's chemical environment and the major source of human exposure is from food and drinking water. Nitrates in food may be present naturally or as an additive introduced for various technological reasons, the latter being strictly limited by regulatory control in most countries. Vegetables are the principal source of dietary nitrate but wide variations in nitrate levels have been found depending on the type of vegetable, its source, conditions of cultivation and storage. In the case of water supplies, a WHO report in 1985 on the health hazards from nitrates in drinking water noted that nitrate concentrations in surface waters in many countries had increased substantially over the previous 30–40 years and that the main reasons for this trend were the increased use of artificial fertilizers, changes in land use and disposal of waste from intensive farming (WHO, 1985).

Nitrate is readily converted in mammalian systems (mediated by bacterial and mammalian enzyme action) to nitrite, which can then react with amines, amides and amino acids to form *N*-nitroso compounds. Whereas nitrate *per se* is generally considered to be of relatively low toxicity, nitrite and *N*-nitroso compounds are known to be biologically active in mammalian systems. Hence, in assessing the health risk of nitrate to man, account must be taken of the toxicology of nitrite and *N*-nitroso compounds.

The toxicology of nitrate, nitrite and *N*-nitroso compounds has been extensively reviewed and continually updated in the light of new data emerging from ongoing research on these important chemicals. Many of the data contained in this chapter have been obtained from recent reviews (e.g. ECETOC, 1988; Speijers *et al.*, 1989; Walker, 1990; Gangolli *et al.*, 1994) which, in a number of instances, served as primary sources of information. Additionally, literature search carried out until early 1998 revealed a number of relevant research publications of interest and these have been included. However, it must be stated that this review cannot be considered to be a comprehensive survey of the subject, its main purpose rather being to focus on information which may be considered of relevance in the human risk assessment of nitrate, nitrite and *N*-nitroso compounds derived from dietary sources. Brief mention is made of human exposure to *N*-nitroso compounds from other sources, for example, by the inhalation of tobacco smoke and from cosmetic products and cutting oils.

In the literature, the dose levels of nitrate or nitrite are expressed in various ways (e.g. weight of salt, weight of ion, weight of nitrate or nitrite-N). To facilitate comparison, all dose levels are expressed as the nitrate or nitrite ion e.g., mg nitrate ion (kg body weight)$^{-1}$ day^{-1}.

This chapter consists of the following sections:

- Levels in food and drinking water and estimates of human dietary intakes; levels from other sources;
- Endogenous synthesis;
- Toxicokinetics and metabolism;
- Toxicology in animals and experimental systems
- Human effects and epidemiological studies;
- Summary, risk analysis and conclusions.

DIETARY LEVELS AND ESTIMATED HUMAN INTAKES

Nitrate and Nitrite Levels in Food and Beverages

General

Diet constitutes an important source of human exposure to nitrate and nitrite present in food either as natural components or as intentional additives. Systematic analyses for nitrate and nitrite levels in various food items, including beverages and drinking water, have been carried out and the results of some of the surveys are given in the tables. Vegetables and cured meat products are the main source of nitrate and nitrite in food but small amounts may also be present in fish and dairy products.

Vegetables

A survey of nitrate levels in a range of retail vegetables grown both within and outside the UK was carried out by the UK Ministry of Agriculture, Fisheries and Food (MAFF) and this showed considerable variations in nitrate contents (MAFF, 1992). Vegetables were grouped on the basis of average nitrate concentrations: thus, lettuce, spinach, celery and beetroot had relatively high nitrate concentrations (> 1000 mg kg^{-1}); potatoes, cabbage, spring greens had less ($100-1000$ mg kg^{-1}); and tomatoes had the lowest concentrations (< 100 mg kg^{-1}). The variation in nitrate content in fresh produce is considerable and often unpredictable even under good agricultural practice conditions. Thus, for example, nitrate levels in lettuce of Dutch, UK, Danish, German and Belgian origin were similar but significantly higher than those in lettuce of Italian and Spanish origin. These findings were mostly unrelated to the available nitrate in the soil. The results confirm other studies showing a negative correlation between nitrate levels in vegetables and daily light intensity and temperature (US Assembly of Life Sciences, 1981a).

The nitrate contents of leafy, stem and root vegetables grown under protected conditions are usually considerably higher than those in outdoor vegetables grown in the same season. This is due to the lower light intensity and higher nitrate availability under greenhouse conditions of cultivation. The higher nitrate availability is due to the mineralization of organic matter in the soil at elevated temperatures. In the above-mentioned northern European countries these vegetables can only be produced in heated greenhouses during the winter months. This results in higher nitrate contents in vegetables due to the effects of low light influx and high nitrogen mineralization. Furthermore, large differences in the nitrate content between individual plants may arise due to local differences in nitrate availability in the soil. The results of a number of other surveys are given in **Tables 1–3**. Several European countries have imposed maximum levels for nitrate in a number of vegetables. The European Union intends to set maximum levels for nitrate in vegetables shortly.

Nitrite occurs in plants at low concentrations; the concentration in fresh vegetables is generally $1-2$ mg kg^{-1} and rarely exceeds 10 mg kg^{-1} (Corre and Breimer, 1979). However, in a UK survey, potatoes have been reported to contain $2-60$ mg kg^{-1} (mean 19 mg kg^{-1}) of nitrite (MAFF, 1992).

Table 1 Average contents of nitrate and nitrite in vegetables[a]

Vegetable	Content [mg (kg fresh wt)$^{-1}$]	
	Nitrate	Nitrite
Artichoke	16	0.6
Asparagus	60	0.9
Aubergine (egg plant)	370	0.8
Beans:		
Green	466	0.9
Lima	74	1.7
Dry (navy)	18	–
Beet	3288	6.0
Broccoli	1014	1.5
Brussels sprout	164	1.5
Cabbage	712	0.8
Carrot	274	1.2
Cauliflower	658	1.7
Celery	3151	0.8
Corn	62	3.0
Cucumber	151	0.8
Endive	1780	0.8
Kale	1096	1.5
Leek	700	–
Lettuce	2330	0.6
Melon	4932	–
Mushroom	219	0.8
Okra	52	1.1
Onion	235	1.1
Parsley	1380	–
Peas	40	0.9
Pepper: sweet	165	0.6
Potato:		
White	150	0.9
Sweet	65	1.1
Pumpkin, squash	550	0.8
Radish	2600	0.3
Rhubarb	2900	–
Spinach	2470	3.8
Tomato	80	–
Turnip:		
Root	535	–
Greens	9040	3.5

[a] Data taken from Walker (1990).

Table 2 Average nitrate and nitrite levels in vegetables[a]

		Mean content [mg (kg fresh wt)$^{-1}$]	
Item	No. analysed	Nitrate	Nitrite
Lettuce:			
English	69	3900	3.0
Dutch	25	3900	ND
Spanish	15	600	11
Tomatoes:			
English	15	53	ND
Canary Islands	15	7	ND
Celery	15	3700	8.0
Potatoes	15	140	19
Cabbage	10	120	ND
Spring greens	5	280	ND
Spinach	6	390	ND
Beetroot, cooked	17	1200	< 3.0

All samples, unless stated otherwise, were of British origin purchased from retail outlets between April and May 1985.
[a] Data taken from MAFF (1992).

Table 3 Nitrate levels in crops[a]

Crop	Median range (mg kg^{-1})	Crop	Median range (mg kg^{-1})
Turnip tops	4800	Kale	30–530
Purslane[b]	1600–7200	French beans	300–530
Spinach	900–5400	Celeriac	330–490
Lettuce	750–5500	Red Cabbage	160–240
Lamb's lettuce	3000–3600	Soup greens	310–320
Chinese cabbage	3100	Cucumber	60–400
Parsley	1700–3500	White cabbage	100–270
Celery	1300–3700	Melon	150
Endive	730–4000	Potato	46–130
Beetroot	1400–3000	Paprika	16–160
Kohlrabi	2200	Tomato	6–160
Blanched celery	1800	Strawberry	72–160
Chervil	1600	Redcurrant	3–56
Oxheart cabbage	590–2600	Brussels sprout	9–40
Radish	400–1600	Chicory	30
Leek	270–2200	Apple	30
Rhubarb	400–1600	Pear	30
Cauliflower	24–960	Asparagus	28
Carrot	60–900	Savoy cabbage	110–840

[a] Data from van Duijvenbooden and Matthijsen (1989).
[b] For biodynamically grown product, 1600; for others, 4500–7200.

Cured Meats

Nitrate and nitrite levels in cured meat and meat products depend on the amounts added as a preservative and on the curing process used. In the UK, the nitrate and nitrite contents of bacon range from < 0.8 to 310 mg kg^{-1} (mean 43 mg kg^{-1}) and from < 0.5 to 76 mg kg^{-1} (mean 76 mg kg^{-1}), respectively; for ham the figures are 3–410 mg kg^{-1} (mean 22 mg kg^{-1}) and < 0.5–110 mg kg^{-1} (mean 26 mg kg^{-1}), respectively. The nitrate and nitrite levels in cured meats have shown a steady decline over

the years with improved manufacturing practice (MAFF, 1978). The results of a number of surveys of nitrate and nitrite levels in cured meats are shown in **Tables 4 and 5**.

Table 4 Nitrate and nitrite levels in cured meats[a]

		Mean (range) [mg (kg fresh wt)$^{-1}$]	
Item	No. analysed	Nitrate	Nitrite
Bacon	51	43 (ND–310)	24 (ND–76)
Ham	59	22 (3–410)	26 (ND–110)
Chopped ham/pork	22	13 (5–20)	4 (ND–15)
Tongue	18	23 (ND–82)	17 (1–71)
Corned beef	21	10 (4–17)	5 (2–8)
Luncheon meat	21	21 (6–59)	24 (1–130)
Cured pork shoulder	6	9 (ND–19)	5 (1–13)
Chicken pâté	3	12 (6–22)	4 (ND–11)
Liver sausage	3	12 (7–22)	4 (ND–11)
Liver pâté	3	23 (18–26)	7 (3–10)
Cured beef	2	29 (28–30)	11 (7–15)
Cured turkey	4	19 (13–21)	54 (1–84)

ND, not detected. Limit of detection for nitrate and nitrite, 0.8 and 0.5 mg kg^{-1}, respectively.
[a] based on data from MAFF (1992).

Table 5 Range of mean nitrate and nitrite levels in cured meat products[a]

Product	Concentration range [mg (kg fresh wt)$^{-1}$]	
	Nitrate (as $NaNO_3$)	Nitrite (as $NaNO_2$)
Preserved meat	19–49	5–39
Corned beef (canned)	60–70	15–23
Pork luncheon meat	107–205	9–23
Raw ham	204–470	21–31
Cooked ham	1295	22
Chopped ham and pork	275	22
Bacon	77–235	40–90
Sausage/sausage meat	70	50

[a] Based on data from Walker (1990).

Milk and Dairy Products

The concentration of nitrate in liquid cow's milk is low, rarely exceeding 5 mg kg^{-1}, and is not considered to be affected by the diet of the animals (US Assembly of Life Sciences, 1981a). Cheeses without added nitrate contain 1–8 mg kg^{-1} of naturally derived nitrate; a survey of Edam cheeses in the UK showed nitrate and nitrite contents of 4–27 and <0.6–1 mg kg^{-1}, respectively (MAFF, 1987). Stephany *et al.* (1978) analysed cheeses prepared from milk with added nitrate ranging from 0 to 20 g kg^{-1} $NaNO_3 l^{-1}$; the cheeses were found to contain <1–49.5 mg kg^{-1} of nitrate ion and 0.1–0.65 mg kg^{-1} of nitrite ion.

Beers

Some 172 samples of beers from 65 breweries were analysed in the UK during 1988–89 and the nitrate concentrations were found to range from 0.2 to 140 mg kg^{-1} (mean 16 mg kg^{-1}). Some 94% of the samples contained <50 mg kg^{-1} (MAFF, 1992). An earlier survey quoted a mean of 30 mg l^{-1} and a range of <10–100 mg l^{-1} for the nitrate content of beer (MAFF, 1987).

Cereals and Cereal Products

The mean nitrate content in the cereals and cereal products group in the UK dietary survey in 1987 (MAFF, 1987) was about 12 mg kg^{-1}. In the USA, mean values of 16 and 4 mg kg^{-1} were obtained for nitrate and nitrite contents, respectively (US Assembly of Life Sciences, 1981a). The RIVM survey in The Netherlands (van Duijvenbooden and Matthijsen, 1989) quotes an average figure of 10 mg kg^{-1} for nitrate in grain products.

Drinking Water

European water supplies are derived from both surface and ground waters, their proportion varying from country to country. It is estimated that about 2% of the population derive drinking water from private wells (ECETOC, 1988). The WHO review on the health hazards of nitrate in drinking water concluded that in most European countries, nitrate levels in drinking water derived from surface waters seldom exceed 10 mg l^{-1} (WHO, 1985). However, the WHO report states that nitrate concentrations in surface waters have increased substantially, especially in the last 20 years, the main factors responsible for this trend being the increased use of artificial fertilizers, change in land use and disposal of wastes from intensive animal farming. In The Netherlands, 80% of the pumping stations supply drinking water with a nitrate concentration of <10 mg nitrate ion l^{-1}, 15% with a concentration of 10–25 mg nitrate ion l^{-1} and 5% with 25–50 mg nitrate ion l^{-1} (van Duijvenbooden and Matthijsen, 1989). Because waters from different pumping stations are mixed prior to being supplied, the nitrate concentrations of drinking water supplies are generally lower. It is estimated that 55% of the drinking water supplies in The Netherlands contain <5 mg nitrate ion l^{-1}, and 20% of the drinking water supplies contain 10–21 mg nitrate ion l^{-1}.

In the UK, information provided by the Department of the Environment in 1990 indicated that most of the drinking water supplies complied with EC Directive 80/778/EEC, limiting the nitrate concentration to 50 mg l^{-1} and the nitrite concentration to 0.1 mg l^{-1} (MAFF, 1992). However, water supplies to a total of 2.4 million people contained nitrate concentrations exceeding 50 mg l^{-1} (none above 100 mg l^{-1}) (ECETOC, 1988).

Despite the EC Directive, there still exist regions in EC countries where the nitrate levels exceed the 50 mg l^{-1} drinking water limit (Institut pour une Politique Européene de l'Environnement, 1989; Varela, 1995).

N-Nitroso Compound Levels in Food and Beverages

The principal dietary sources of *N*-nitroso (N-NO) compounds are cured meats, beer, fish and cheese. There is a vast literature on the occurrence and quantification of volatile *N*-nitroso compounds in foods and a summary of selected results is shown in **Table 6**. With new developments in analytical methodology, it is now possible to quantify levels of non-volatile *N*-nitroso compounds (Massey *et al.*, 1991; Massey and Lees, 1992). In some analytical studies, 'Apparent total nitroso compounds (ATNC)' have been determined (MAFF, 1992). However, the identity of these substances is largely unknown and their toxicological significance cannot be assessed.

Table 6 Estimates of daily nitrosodimethylamine (NDMA) intakes from national dietary surveys published in 1978–90

Country	ND (μg day^{-1})	Major source (% contributed)	Reference
UK	0.53	Cured meats (81%)	Gough *et al.* (1978)
UK	0.60	Beer (81%)	MAFF (1987)
The Netherlands	0.38	Beer (71%)	Stephany and Schuller (1980)
The Netherlands	0.10	–	Ellen *et al.* (1990)
Germany	1.10	Beer (65%); cured meats (10%)	Spiegelhalder *et al.* (1980)
Germany	0.53	Beer (40%); cured meats (18%)	Spiegelhalder (1983)
Germany	0.28	Beer (31%); cured meats (36%)	Tricker *et al.* (1991)
Japan	1.8	Dried fish (91%)	Maki *et al.* (1980)
Japan	0.5	Beer (30%); fish products (68%)	Yamamoto *et al.* (1984)
Sweden	0.12	Beer (32%); cured meats (61%)	Österdahl (1988)
Finland	0.08	Beer (75%); smoked fish (25%)	Penttila *et al.* (1990)
China	No data	Marine food	Song and Hu (1988)
Italy	No data	Cured meats	Gavinelli *et al.* (1988)
Former USSR	No data	Meat and fish products	Tutelyan *et al.* (1990)

N-Nitroso Compound Levels in Other Sources: Estimates of Human Exposure

Tobacco products constitute an important source of *N*-nitroso compounds. Tobacco smoke contain three types of *N*-nitrosamines: the volatile nitrosamines (VNAs) derived from the action of nitrogen oxides on amines and residues of agricultural chemicals to form *N*-nitrosodimethylamine, *N*-nitrosopyrrolidine and *N*-nitrosodiethanolamine. Other tobacco-specific nitrosamines (TSNAs) formed are 4-(*N*-methylnitrosoamino)-1-(3-pyridyl)butanone (NNK), *N*-nitrosonornicotine (NNN), N^1-nitrosoanabasin (NAB) and N^1-nitrosoanatabine (NAT) (Hoffmann *et al.*, 1982a; Spiegelhalder and Bartsch, 1996). Up to 23 nitroso compounds in tobacco products, preformed by nitrosation processes during storage and fermentation, have been identified.

In the mainstream smoke from commercial cigarettes, levels of *N*-nitrosodimethylamine and *N*-nitrosopyrrolidine, the two most abundant VNAs present, have been found to be 20 and 110 ng per cigarette, respectively (Spiegelhalder and Bartsch, 1996). In the case of *N*-nitrosodiethanolamine, concentrations of 115–194 ppb have been found in cigarettes and in mainstream smoke the amounts reported are 24–36 ng per cigarette (Hoffmann *et al.*, 1982b).

Human exposure per day to TSNAs in tobacco users has been estimated to be 48 μg in heavy smokers, 220 μg in tobacco chewers and up to 700 μg in snuff users (Hecht and Hoffmann, 1989). Spiegelhalder (1995) has estimated the average daily exposure levels to NNN and NNK in persons smoking 20 cigarettes per day to be 1.5–6.0 μg.

N-Nitroso compounds have also been detected in cosmetic preparations, household products and cutting fluids formulated with alkanolamines such as bis- and tris (hydroxyethyl)amine, bis(2-hydroxypropyl) amine and cocoa fatty acid diethanolamides (Eisenbrand *et al.*, 1996). Most manufacturers of these product have abandoned the use of these amines in the formulation of their products in compliance with Good Manufacturing Practice recommendations by regulatory authorities in the European Union. Thus, human exposure to *N*-nitroso compounds from these sources is unlikely to present a major health hazard.

Estimated Human Dietary Intakes of Nitrate, Nitrite and *N*-Nitroso Compounds

General

Three main approaches have been used to quantify the intakes of nitrate, nitrite and *N*-nitroso compounds as follows:

- The duplicate portion technique, where one portion is used for consumption and the second for analysis;
- Analysis of all components of the diet with use of the data to calculate the likely intake from information provided by subjects on their food consumption;
- Calculation of the intake from published data on mean values of dietary components and on food consumption.

The first approach is the most difficult and time consuming but it does provide accurate data and takes account of seasonal variations and changes occurring during food preparation and cooking. The last two approaches provide estimates of mean intakes and the contribution of each dietary component. The second approach can also accommodate seasonal variations by asking food consumption per season and using seasonal data on nitrate content. Most of the published data are derived from the last two approaches. It should be noted, however, that the different methodologies give rise to different estimates of intakes and that there are further detailed differences between countries in the way national food surveys are conducted and reported. As a consequence, it is not always possible to relate comparisons of dietary intakes from country to country.

Data Obtained in Various Countries

Some of the published data on nitrate and nitrite intakes are detailed in **Tables 7–12** and data obtained in several countries are summarized in **Table 13**.

The Netherlands
The most recent estimates of nitrate intake in The Netherlands are based on a representative sample of the Dutch population using data from the Dutch National Food Consumption Survey (van Loon and van Klaveren, 1991). Information on food intake was collected

Table 7 Distribution of daily average dietary nitrate load in food groups[a]

Food group	Consumption (g day^{-1})	Content (mg kg^{-1})	Load (mg day^{-1})
Grain products	160	10	2
Potatoes	160	60	10
Vegetables/legumes	154		120
Fruit	154	20	3
Coffee/tea/nuts	34	–	–
Sugar 'visible' fats	155	–	–
Milk products	420	1	–
Cheese	25	8	–
Meat (products)	140	50	7
Eggs (products)	28	–	–
Fisheries products	14	3	–
Beer/wine/spirits	275	5	1
Total food	1		ca. 143

[a] Based on data from van Duijvenbooden and Matthijsen (1989).

Table 8 Estimated dietary intakes of nitrate and nitrite[a]

Group	Average consumption (g day^{-1})	Estimated daily intake (mg day^{-1})	
		Nitrate[b]	Nitrite[b]
Bread/cereal	0.24	(16) 3.8	(1.4) 0.34
Carcase, meat, etc.	0.059	(8) 0.48	(1.0) 0.059
Meat products	0.048	(68) 3.3	(4.9) 0.24
Fish	0.017	(11) 0.19	(1.2) 0.02
Oils/fat/eggs, etc.	0.12	(1.2) 0.14	(1.0) 0.12
Sugars and preserves	0.09	(14) 1.3	(1.0) 0.09
Green vegetables	0.05	(210) 11	(3.4) 0.17
Potatoes	0.16	(120) 19	(11) 1.8
'Other' vegetables	0.07	(140) 9.8	(1.0) 0.07
Canned vegetables	0.042	(29) 1.2	(1.9) 0.08
Fruit/products	0.091	(25) 2.3	(1.0) 0.091
Beverages	0.66	(1.9) 1.3	(1.1) 0.73
Milk	0.34	(1.4) 0.48	(1.0) 0.34)
Estimated intake		54	4.0

[a] Based on data from MAFF (1992).
[b] Figures in parentheses are average concentrations of nitrate or nitrite expressed as mg kg^{-1}.

Table 9 Contribution of various foods to the nitrate content of total diet (%)[a]

Country	Cured meats	Vegetables	Cereals	Fruit	Water
France	9	91	NDA[b]	NDA	NDA
Germany	18.5	72.5	5.5	2.9	0
Germany	7	84	3	6	+[c]
Germany	9	83	4	4	NDA
Switzerland	6.25	70	1.6	1.05	20.9
UK	2.2	67	2.8	3.0	14.1
USA	0–9.4	83–95	0.5–2.8	1.4–6	0.7–2.8

[a] Based on data from ECETOC (1988); milk and beverages excluded.
[b] No data available.
[c] The drinking water contained 50 mg l^{-1}.

Table 10 Estimated daily dietary intakes of nitrate and nitrite by analysis of diets and calculation[a]

Country	Mean daily intake (mg day^{-1})	
	Nitrate	Nitrite
France	150.7[b]	>3
Germany	68	2.6
Italy	245	–
The Netherlands	71	0.6
Norway	43	1.8
Poland:		
Adult	178	–
Child, 1–3 yr	142	4.0
Child, 3–12 months	30	1.4
Switzerland	125	–
UK	88–407	0.3–0.9
USA	53–367	0.5–3.9

[a] Based on data from Walker (1990).
[b] Excluding intakes from drinking water.

using a two-day dietary record from 5898 subjects aged 1–74 years. The survey was distributed equally over a whole year, from April 1987 to March 1988. The daily nitrate intake was calculated using the Databank on Contaminants in Food with information on the mean nitrate levels in food products from 1986 to 1989; additional information on nitrate levels in drinking water wasobtained from the Dutch Drinking Water Association. Information on the loss of nitrate during cooking was taken into account in calculating intakes. The mean nitrate intake of the total population was estimated at 113 mg day^{-1}, of which 4% was derived from drinking water, 68% from vegetables, 9% from potatoes and 19% from other sources. Among men aged 22–49 years the median nitrate intake was 95 mg day^{-1} in the period January–March, 108 mg day^{-1} in April–June, 97 mg day^{-1} in July–September and 96 mg day^{-1} in October–December. For women the comparable estimates were 96, 120, 111 and 99 mg day^{-1}, respectively. The highest median intakes were noted for children aged 1–10 years; these varied

Table 11 Estimated per capita total daily intake of nitrite (mg day^{-1}) from diet in the UK in 1985[a,b]

Source	Average daily consumption (kg day^{-1})	Nitrite content (mg kg^{-1})	Nitrite intake[c] (mg per person)
Bread and cereals	0.24	1.4 (<1.0–3.0)	0.34
Carcase meat, offal and poutry	0.059	1.0	0.059
Meat products	0.048	4.9 (1.0–17)	0.24
Fish	0.017	1.2 (<1.0–5.0)	0.02
Fats/eggs/dairy produce	0.12	1.0 (<1.0–1.0)	0.12
Sugars and preserves	0.090	1.0 (<1.0–1.0)	0.09
Green vegetables	0.050	3.4 (<1.0–20)	0.17
Potatoes	0.16	11 (3.0–26)	1.8
'Other' vegetables	0.070	1.0	0.07
Canned vegetables	0.042	1.9 (<1.0–3.0)	0.08
Fresh fruit and fruit products	0.091	1.0	0.091
Beverages	0.66	1.1 (<1.0–3.0)	0.73
Milk	0.34	1.0	0.34
Estimated intake			4.2

[a] Based on data from MAFF (1992).
[b] The UK total diet survey was based on 17 sets of samples, each set comprising of a variety of 'average diet'.
[c] The foods were prepared for consumption using distilled water.

Table 12 Analysed (A) and calculated (C) national estimates of daily dietary intakes of nitrate and nitrite[a]

Country	Basis of estimate	Intake (mg person^{-1} day^{-1})	
		Nitrate	Nitrite
France	C	110[b]	<2
Germany	C	49.3	1.72
Germany	A	55.95	2.53–3.9
Norway	C	31.4	1.17
Poland:			
Adults[c]	A	130	No data
Children (1–3 yr)[d]	A	104	2.65
Infants (0.25–1 yr)	A	21.8	0.94
Switzerland	C	91	No data
UK	C	74.4	No data
UK	A	64–297	No data
UK	C	71	No data
USA	C	100	2.6
USA	C	39	0.34
USA	C	70	0.54
USA	C	100	0.57
USA	C	75	0.77
USA	C	78	1.7
USA	C	268	0.77
USA	C	233	0.77

[a] Based on data from ECETOC (1988).
[b] Based on nitrate-free water.
[c] From meals in a students' canteen.
[d] From meals prepared in a children's home.

from 1.54 to 3.60 mg (kg body weight)$^{-1}$. No data were available on nitrite or *N*-nitroso compounds intake from this study. In a study carried by Ellen *et al.* (1990) using the duplicate portion technique, the mean intake was 52 mg nitrate ion day^{-1} and the mean intake of nitrite was <0.1 mg nitrite ion day^{-1}. The daily dietary intake of volatile *N*-nitrosamines was about 0.1 g or less.

UK

The estimated mean dietary intake of nitrate using the Total Diet Study (TDS), when distilled water was used instead of tap water in the TDS, was 54 mg day^{-1} (52 mg from food, mainly vegetables, and 2 mg from beverages) (MAFF, 1992). There was little change in the estimated average dietary intake of nitrate obtained in this 1985

Table 13 Nitrate and nitrite intakes in different countries

Country	Nitrate (mg day^{-1})	Nitrite (mg day^{-1})	Reference
Denmark	50		Statens Levneds middelinstitut (1981)
Switzerland	72		Tremp (1980)
Germany	75	3.3	Selenka and Brand-Grimm (1976)
Poland	127	8.7	Nabrzyski and Gajewska (1989)
Norway	31	1.2	Gislason and Dahle (1980)
The Netherlands	113		van Loon and van Klaveren (1991)
Sweden	48	3	Jagerstad and Nillson (1976)
USA	106	4.1	White (1975)
UK	54	2.4–4.2	MAFF (1992)
France	121	1.88	Cornee et al. (1992)
Finland	54	1.4	Laitinen et al. (1993)

survey from an earlier one carried out in 1979. The estimated dietary intakes of nitrate in different types of vegetarians ranged from 185 to 194 mg day^{-1}.

The estimated mean dietary nitrite intake from the TDS ranged from 2.4 to 4.2 mg day^{-1} (MAFF, 1992). The average daily intake of NDMA from beer, cured meats and fish was estimated to range from <0.1 to 0.6 g person^{-1} day^{-1} (MAFF, 1987).

The largest contributor to the average dietary exposure to volatile nitrosamines was alcoholic beverages, followed by fish, cured meats and cheese.

Germany

The total nitrate intake from food and drinking water was estimated to be 75 mg day^{-1} for drinking water containing 1 mg l^{-1} NO$_3$, up to 185 mg day^{-1} for drinking water containing 50 mg l^{-1} NO$_3$. Nitrite intake from food was estimated to be 3.3 mg day^{-1} (Selenka and Brand-Grimm, 1976). In a survey carried out in 1984–90 the mean daily intake of volatile N-nitrosamines from foods and beverages was found to be 0.28 g day^{-1} (Tricker et al., 1991).

Finland

A survey of nitrate and nitrite intakes in 1212 subjects aged 9–24 years, using the 48-h recall method, showed that the mean daily intakes of nitrate ion and nitrite ion from food were 54.0 and 1.4 mg, respectively (Laitinen et al., 1993). The Finnish National Board of Health's recommendation that the nitrate concentration in drinking water should be <30 mg l^{-1} shows compliance with over 99.8% of the water authorities. Assuming an average daily intake of 2 l of water, the intake of nitrate from this source would be <60 mg day^{-1}.

France

Based on new food composition tables and on the French national average food consumption, the average nitrate intake per person per day was found to be 121 mg, 85% of which was derived from vegetables, 5% from preserved and cured meats and 5% from cereal products (Cornee et al., 1992). This figure was less than half that found in 1982 (280 mg).

The average nitrite intake per person per day was 1.88 mg (43% from vegetables, 28% from cured meats and 16% from cereal products). The estimated nitrosodimethylamine (NDMA) intake per person per day was 0.25 μg, with 0.06 μg from preserved and cured meats, 0.052 μg from preserved and smoked fish and 0.026 μg from alcoholic drinks, particularly beers (Cornee et al., 1992).

Infants

Infants constitute a special case. The nitrate intake in breast-fed infants is low. In human milk, nitrate has been detected at low levels up to 5 mg nitrate ion l^{-1} (Sukegawa and Matsumoto, 1975) and did not exceed plasma levels after a nitrate-containing meal (Green et al., 1982). For infants fed on infant formulations which require dilution with water before consumption, the principal source of nitrate would be the drinking water. Assuming a fluid intake of 165 ml (kg body weight)$^{-1}$ day^{-1} for a 3-month-old infant weighing 5.6 kg, feeds prepared with drinking water containing the maximum EC limit of nitrate in water (50 mg l^{-1}) would provide a maximum nitrate intake of 46 mg day^{-1} [8.2 mg (kg body weight)$^{-1}$ day^{-1}] (MAFF, 1992). The nitrate intake in weaned infants is likely to be lower and it has been estimated that a 9–12-month-old infant might ingest about 37 mg nitrate day^{-1} (MAFF, 1987).

ENDOGENOUS SYNTHESIS

Nitrate

Experimental Animals

Studies in experimental animals have shown that nitrate can be formed endogenously by mammalian metabolic processes. Both conventional and germ-free rats maintained on low nitrate diets (<0.06 mg nitrate ion day^{-1}) excreted nitrate in excess of the intake. When the diet was supplemented with ^{15}N-labelled NaNO$_3$, about 33–50% of ^{15}N-labelled nitrate was excreted in both conventional and germ-free rats. Although about 40% of ingested nitrate was expected to be excreted in the urine (0.06 mg day^{-1}), rats excreted much more (about 0.37 mg nitrate day^{-1}). It was estimated that nitrate was synthesized in the body at the rate of approximately 1.24 mg (kg body weight)$^{-1}$ day^{-1} (Green *et al.*, 1981a). Nitrate balance studies carried out in the ferret using a ^{15}N-labelled ammonium salt led to the appearance of ^{15}N-labelled nitrate in the urine and faeces. The net biosynthesis of nitrate was found to be 0.55–0.64 mg day^{-1} (Dull and Hotchkiss, 1984).

Factors Influencing Biosynthesis

In early experiments in which rats were continuously infused with [^{15}N]ammonium acetate, or given oral [^{15}N]ammonium chloride, about 0.007–0.008% of the ammonia was converted to nitrate, confirming that ammonia could act as a precursor of nitrate (Wagner *et al.*, 1985). It was concluded that about 50% of nitrate arose from endogenous sources. A likely route for the conversion of ammonia via hydroxylamine to nitrate was confirmed when it was demonstrated that administration of hydroxylamine to rats also led to increased nitrate synthesis (Saul and Archer, 1984).

More recent experiments have shown that the major route for endogenous nitrate synthesis probably involves conversion of arginine to nitric oxide followed by oxidation of the nitric oxide to N$_2$O$_3$ and N$_2$O$_4$ (Marletta, 1988).

The arginine $\rightarrow$ nitric oxide conversion is affected by a growing family of enzymes known as nitric oxide synthases (NOS). Some of these are constitutive and some are inducible. The constitutive NOS typically produce low levels of nitric oxide for short periods (seconds) in response to intracellular messengers such as bradykinin. Inducible NOS produce higher levels over prolonged intervals (hours) in response to immunostimulants such as *E. coli* lipopolysaccharide (LPS). This process is now known to be common to many cell types including macrophages, endothelial cells, neurons, neutrophils and hepatocytes (Ignarro, 1990; Lancaster, 1992; Snyder and Bredt, 1992; Bhagat and Vallance, 1996). However, the supplementation of arginine in the diet of germ-free rats has been shown not to increase nitrate biosynthesis as measured by the urinary excretion level of nitrate (Rowland *et al.*, 1996). The infestation of Syrian golden hamsters with the liver fluke *Opisthorchis viverrini* has been found to induce nitric oxide synthase activity (Oshima *et al.*, 1994).

Some bacterial strains produce nitric oxide via reduction of nitrite (Calmels *et al.*, 1987; Ralt *et al.*, 1988). The formation of both nitrate and nitrite can be detected when experiments are carried out *in vitro*, but in the intact animal because of the efficient oxidation of nitrite by haemoglobin, only the presence of nitrate is observed in the animal. Increased nitric oxide synthesis and the urinary excretion of nitrate has been found in rats during pregnancy (Conrad *et al.*, 1993).

Humans

The biosynthesis of nitrate has also been demonstrated in several human studies. Balance studies on six elderly male subjects on a low-nitrate diet (about 0.62 mg nitrate ion day^{-1}) showed that the urinary excretion of nitrate exceeded its intake, averaging about 60 mg day^{-1} (Tannenbaum *et al.*, 1978). Similar results were obtained in young volunteers (Green *et al.*, 1981b).

Bartholomew and Hill (1984), in studies carried out on both healthy and ileostomy patients, found a 20% excess of urinary nitrate excretion over intake, suggesting that the earlier studies may have overestimated nitrate biosynthesis. However, studies using more refined analytical methodology have shown that the average excess of urinary nitrate excretion over intake was 54 mg day^{-1} [approximately 1 mg (kg body weight)$^{-1}$ day^{-1}], i.e. the same order of magnitude as the findings in the animal studies (Lee *et al.*, 1986). In a study conducted on the whole-body synthesis of nitric oxide from [^{15}N]arginine in healthy adults, Castillo *et al.* (1996) found that although only about 1.2% of plasma arginine turnover was associated with NO formation; the plasma arginine compartment served as a significant precursor pool (54%) for the whole-body synthesis of nitric oxide.

Factors Influencing Biosynthesis

The increased biosynthesis of nitrate in animals by experimentally induced infections and inflammatory reactions has also been observed in humans. Wagner and Tannenbaum (1982) observed that in a male subject on a low nitrate diet, providing an intake of 7.4 mg day^{-1}, the development of a non-specific diarrhoea led to an increase in the urinary excretion of nitrate from 43 to 280 mg day^{-1}.

In a study on hospitalized infants placed on a low dietary nitrate intake level (2–7 mg day^{-1}), those ill with acute diarrhoea had a sevenfold increase in blood nitrate levels and a 15-fold increase in urinary nitrate levels compared with infants without any gastro-intestinal disorders. The urinary nitrate excretion in the 'control' infants and in the infants with acute diarrhoea was 8.7 and 39 mg day^{-1}, respectively (Hegesh and Shiloah, 1982). Furthermore, a number of infants with diarrhoea had methaemoglobin levels exceeding 8% and a mean blood nitrate level of 37 mg l^{-1} (Hegesh and Shiloah, 1982).

Wettig *et al.* (1987) described a pregnant woman with lambliasis and a pathogenic *E. coli* infection with diarrhoea. Her nitrate intake was less than 30 mg day^{-1} but she had nitrate concentrations in morning saliva and urine of 700–900 mg l^{-1} over 6 days. Treatment with metronidazole eliminated the *Giardia lamblia* and nitrate levels in her saliva and urine fell to <100 mg l^{-1}.

These observations are all consistent with the induction of one or more nitric oxide synthases by inflammatory agents analogous to the experiments described above with animals and macrophages. This induction in humans has been difficult to demonstrate directly, but administration of [^{15}N]arginine to two volunteers resulted in the incorporation of ^{15}N into urinary nitrate in both individuals, confirming that the arginine → nitric oxide pathway exists in humans (Leaf *et al.*, 1989a, b).

Nitrite

In vitro and *in vivo* studies have shown that nitrate can be reduced to nitrite by bacterial and mammalian metabolic pathways. The widespread occurrence of nitrate reductase activity in bacteria means that the nitrite is produced endogenously at sites populated by large numbers of bacteria, namely the mouth, stomach (if the gastric pH is >5), the distal small intestine and colon, the infected urinary bladder and vagina. The amount of nitrite formed is dependent on the nitrate reductase activity of the microbial population and the availability of nitrate.

In man, saliva is the major site for the formation of nitrite. About 25% of ingested nitrate is secreted in the saliva and of this about 20% is converted to nitrite in the mouth. Thus, about 5% of dietary nitrate is converted to nitrite (Spiegelhalder *et al.*, 1976; Eisenbrand *et al.*, 1980; Walters and Smith, 1981).

A direct correlation between gastric pH, bacterial colonization and gastric nitrite concentration has been observed in healthy populations with a range of pH values from 1 to 7 (Mueller *et al.*, 1983, 1986). In individuals with gastro-intestinal disorders and achlorhydria resulting from pernicious anaemia or hypogammaglobulinaemia, gastric nitrite levels can reach 6 mg l^{-1} (Ruddell *et al.*, 1976, 1978; Dolby *et al.*, 1984).

The situation in human neonates is not clear. It is commonly asserted that infants younger than 3 months may be highly susceptible to gastric bacterial nitrate reduction because they have very little gastric acid production (Speijers *et al.*, 1989). However, Agunod *et al.*, (1969), on examining 12 infants aged 12 h to 3 months, found only one with achlorhydria. In this context, the presence of acid-producing lactobacilli in the stomach may be important as these organisms do not reduce nitrate and may maintain a pH low enough to inhibit colonization by nitrate-reducing bacteria (Bartholomew *et al.*, 1980).

As noted above, nitrite may also be produced via the arginine → nitric oxide pathway, but would be undetectable because of the rapid oxidation to nitrate. One possible example of nitrite production by this route,

however, is the methaemoglobinaemia observed in infants suffering from diarrhoea.

N-Nitroso Compounds

The possible formation *in vivo* of *N*-nitroso compounds from precursors has been extensively investigated by the following methods: (i) *in vitro* incubation of precursors under simulated salivary and gastric conditions; (ii) examination of saliva and gastric contents following administration of precursors; (iii) determination of *N*-nitroso compounds in body fluids and excreta following precursor treatment; and (iv) evidence of carcinogenicity in experimental animals following the co-administration of nitrate or nitrite and amine or amide.

Numerous *in vitro* studies have purported to simulate conditions in the saliva and the stomach, but in many cases the concentrations of nitrite used have been unrealistically high. Consequently, findings from these studies must be considered at best to be no more than an indication of a potential for nitrosation to occur (reviewed by Walker, 1990).

Walters *et al.* (1974, 1979) found that on incubating a slurry of luncheon meat (containing 30 mg nitrite ion kg^{-1}), egg and milk with human gastric juice containing 1.2 mM thiocyanate at pH 2, measurable amounts of four volatile nitrosamines were formed.

However, in another study in which a wide range of foods were incubated under similar conditions with nitrite (5–7 mg l^{-1}), no detectable amounts of volatile nitrosamines were found (Groenen *et al.*, 1982).

There is an extensive literature on the *in vivo* evidence of the nitrosation of orally administered precursor secondary and tertiary amines and amides in various species (Walker, 1990). In the context of the formation of *N*-nitroso compounds from normal dietary components, an investigation carried out on human volunteers showed that following the ingestion of meals comprising eggs, milk and luncheon meat, analyses of stomach contents revealed the presence of detectable amounts of *N*-nitrosopiperidine (NPIP) and *N*-nitrosopyrrolidine (NPYR) (Walters *et al.*, 1979). A similar study, in which volunteers were given meals with different nitrate contents (derived from vegetables) and containing meat, eggs or fish, provided further confirmatory evidence for the *in vivo* formation of volatile *N*-nitrosamines (Groenen *et al.*, 1985).

The detection and estimation of *N*-nitrosoproline (NPRO) excreted in the urine has been widely used as a quantitative measure of *in vivo* nitrosation as it is claimed to be non-carcinogenic and excreted virtually unchanged in the urine (Oshima and Bartsch, 1981). The basal rate of the urinary excretion of NPRO in subjects on a low nitrate diet is 2–7 g day^{-1} (Oshima and Bartsch, 1981).

NPRO studies carried out in the rat using ^{15}N-labelled nitrate showed that urinary ^{15}N-labelled NPRO content represented only 10–60% of the total urinary NPRO excreted, indicating that a significant amount of the total NPRO was not derived from ingested nitrate (Wagner *et al.*, 1985). Studies in humans have confirmed the animal finding that there is no correlation between dietary nitrate intake and the urinary excretion of NPRO (Tannenbaum, 1987).

Studies using ^{14}C-labelled proline in the rat have shown that nitrosation occurred to a similar extent in the presence or absence of orally administered nitrate (Mallett *et al.*, 1985). Furthermore, studies using conventional and germ-free rats showed that the gut microflora were not involved in the nitrosation of proline (Mallett *et al.*, 1985).

Male ola:SD rats were maintained on purified low-nitrate diets containing 5 or 20% lactalbumin as the source of protein and the daily urinary excretion of nitrate and NPRO was measured. Animals fed the high-protein diet consistently excreted more nitrate and NPRO than the littermates on the low-protein ration. Furthermore, whereas administered nitrite increased NPRO excretion in both groups, nitrate administration increased NPRO excretion only in the low-protein diet animals. The results suggest that protein catabolism may lead to the formation of the nitrosating agent responsible for the formation of NPRO (Mallett *et al.*, 1988). The basal urinary excretion of non-dietary NPRO was unaffected by ascorbic acid or α-tocopherol but both of these vitamins inhibited the synthesis or [15]NPRO from orally administered proline and ^{15}N-labelled nitrate (Wagner *et al.*, 1985). Conversely, endogenous formation of NPRO was increased by thiocyanate (Oshima *et al.*, 1982).

Such observations are consistent with at least two routes for NPRO formation, i.e. intragastric nitrosation via the acidic nitrite mechanism and nitrosation at some other site(s) in the body by a non-acid-catalysed mechanism that is inaccessible to orally administered ascorbic acid (Leaf *et al.*, 1989a, b; 1990). There is evidence that this latter pathway involves nitrosation via nitrosating agents rising from nitric oxide. As noted earlier, N_2O_3 and N_2O_4 are formed by oxidation of nitric oxide which then react with water to form nitrate and nitrite. Both of these compounds, however, are good nitrosating agents at or near neutral pH (Challis and Kryptopoulous, 1978).

In experiments in which both morpholine and arginine were administered to rats, levels of both nitrate and nitrosohydroxyethylglycine (NHEG), the principal metabolite of *N*-nitrosomorpholine, were higher in animals that had been treated with LPS than in non-treated controls, demonstrating that *N*-nitrosomorpholine had been formed in the LPS stimulated animals (Leaf *et al.*, 1991a, b). Administration of nitrate at levels much higher that those produced by LPS treatment led to no increase in the levels of NHEG (Leaf *et al.*, 1991a, b).

Urinary excretion of nitrosothioproline (NTPRO) has also been used as an index of *in vivo* nitrosation, but this does not always correlate with the excretion of NPRO (Elder *et al.*, 1984). Urinary levels of NTPRO are normally very low but were reported to increase to 4 g day^{-1} (a sixfold increase) after the ingestion of 217 mg of nitrate (Wagner *et al.*, 1984).

Crespi *et al.* (1986) reported that intestinal microflora did not catalyse the nitrosation of proline *in vitro* at pH > 6. This suggests that NPRO may not be an indicator of the total extent of nitrosation reactions occurring in the body. Various researchers have reported the presence of volatile nitrosamines (NDMA and NDEA) in the blood and urine of human volunteers, but as these nitrosamines are rapidly metabolised, estimates of their rates of formation *in vivo* are not accurate. Endogenous formation of NDMA has been reported in human volunteers treated with amidopyrine (Spiegelhalder, 1990), and oral or inhalation exposure to piperizine has been shown to lead to the formation of mononitrosopiperizine (Bellander, 1990).

Nitric Oxide

Although nitric oxide does not fall strictly within the framework of this review, there are some aspects of endogenous production of nitric oxide that may be relevant to this assessment. Endogenous nitrate levels reflect the total production of nitrate + nitrite arising from the arginine → NO pathway or other contributing processes. The nitrite/nitrate ratio *in vivo*, however, is unknown. There may therefore, be, locally high nitrite levels at various sites in the body, especially under conditions of infection or inflammation.

In addition, endogenous nitrate is the stable end-point from a complex series of reactions in which active intermediates are formed that can cause deamination of DNA or oxidative DNA damage. Such intermediates are probably involved in the cytotoxicity and mutagenicity that are observed in parallel with nitrate/nitrite production when cells are treated with nitric oxide (Wink *et al.*, 1991; Nguyen *et al.*, 1992; Tannenbaum *et al.*, 1994). Nitrate production by this mechanism is clearly a normal process and there is no reason to associate it with adverse effects in normal, healthy individuals.

However, the extent to which these intermediates may contribute to adverse health effects under abnormal, i.e. 'stimulated', conditions is unknown and this may be a confounding factor in the assessment of the relative risks from endogenously formed vs ingested nitrate/nitrite.

TOXICOKINETICS AND METABOLISM

The toxicokinetics and metabolic disposition of nitrate, nitrite and *N*-nitroso compounds are closely interrelated and have a pivotal role in influencing the bioavailability and toxicity of nitrite and *N*-nitroso compounds derived from ingested nitrate. Thus, both the toxicokinetics and toxicodynamics (toxic effects) of these compounds are relevant in the safety evaluation and human health risk assessment from ingested nitrate.

Nitrate

Ingested nitrate is readily absorbed from the proximal small intestine and following absorption is rapidly distributed throughout the body in both experimental animals and man (Balish *et al.*, 1981; Bartholomew and Hill, 1984). In the rat, about 50% of an oral dose was detected in the carcass within 1 h; in humans, concentrations in body fluids (serum, saliva and urine) peaked within 1–3 h (Bartholomew and Hill, 1984; Ellen *et al.*, 1982).

In most laboratory animals (except the rat) and in man, blood nitrate is selectively transported and secreted in the saliva in a dose-dependent manner by an active transport system (Witter and Balish, 1979; Fritsch *et al.*, 1985). In man the nitrate blood/salivary carrier-mediated transport system is shared by iodide and thiocyanate and the relative affinities of the three ions in the transport system are iodide > thiocyanate > nitrate; consequently, smokers who have elevated salivary thiocyanate levels were found to have lower salivary nitrate levels than non-smokers (Forman *et al.*, 1985a, b). It has been estimated that on average in humans approximately 25% of ingested nitrate is secreted in the saliva (Spiegelhalder *et al.*, 1976; Tannenbaum *et al.*, 1976).

In the rat, circulating nitrate may be secreted in the gastric and intestinal secretions into the lower bowel. This is an active transport process in the rat but not in man (Witter and Balish, 1979).

Nitrate appears in milk apparently by passive diffusion. In humans nitrate has been detected at low levels up to 5 mg nitrate ion l^{-1} (Sukegawa and Matsumoto, 1975). Concentrations in milk were not found to exceed plasma levels after a nitrate-containing meal (Green *et al.*, 1982).

Nitrate rapidly appears in the urine after ingestion. In the rat, about 55% of orally administered ^{15}N-labelled nitrate was excreted unchanged in the urine and 11% as urea and ammonia in the urine and faeces, leaving about 35% unaccounted for (Schultz *et al.*, 1985). A similar study in humans showed that about 60% of ^{15}N appeared as nitrate and 3% as urea and ammonia in the urine (Wagner *et al.*, 1983). Other studies in humans have shown that independent of dosage, about 65–70% of orally administered nitrate was excreted in the urine; excretion was maximum at about 5 h and completed within 18 h (Bartholomew and Hill, 1984). The excretion of nitrate has been reported to follow first-order kinetics with an elimination half-life of about 5 h (Green *et al.*, 1981b).

Urinary excretion of nitrate in infants has been reported to be 80–100% of the average intake (Turek *et al.*, 1980), whereas Hegesh and Shiloah (1982) claimed that the urinary nitrate excreted by infants includes endogenously formed nitrate.

Nitrate reduction to nitrite can be affected by bacterial and mammalian nitrate reductase activity; nitrate reductase activity is possessed by a wide range of microorganisms, including many resident in the mammalian gastro-intestinal tract (Hegesh and Shiloah, 1982). Mammalian nitrate reductase activity has been detected in the intestinal mucosa and liver of rats but the reaction is much slower than that of the gut flora (Schultz *et al.*, 1985; WHO, 1985).

From comparisons between germ-free and conventional rats, Ward *et al.* (1986) concluded that of the 40–50% of the dose of nitrate reduced to nitrite in conventional animals, approximately half the metabolism was mediated by mammalian nitrate reductase activity.

The widespread ability of microorganisms to reduce nitrate leads to the formation of nitrite at sites with a high microbial count, e.g. principally the mouth and stomach of some species of animals or in individuals where the pH is > 5, and in the lower gut of those species (not man) which secrete nitrate in the distal ileum. Additionally, nitrite formation can occur in the urinary tract and vagina following infection.

The rumen of ruminants (and the enlarged caecum and colon of horses) are especially suited for nitrate reduction owing to the dense microbial population and the relatively high pH (Wright and Davison, 1969).

In view of the active transport secretion of nitrate in the saliva, the oral cavity represents the most important site for the metabolism of nitrate to nitrite in humans. It has been estimated that about 25% of ingested nitrate is secreted in the saliva in man, of which about 20% is reduced to nitrite, i.e. 4–7% of the overall dose (Spiegelhalder *et al.*, 1976; Walters and Smith, 1981). Stephany and Schuller (1980) found that salivary nitrite concentrations were proportional to the amount of nitrate ingested and confirmed that the mean conversion rate of salivary nitrate to nitrite in healthy adults was approximately 6.3 mol% (i.e. about 5% by weight) of the total dietary intake.

Marked inter-individual and diurnal differences in humans have been observed in the nitrate/nitrite levels in the saliva following the oral ingestion of nitrate. Spiegelhalder *et al.* (1976) found that the ingestion of less than 54 mg of nitrate did not affect salivary nitrate and nitrite levels.

The likelihood of the reduction of nitrate to nitrite by microflora in the stomach of achlorhydric subjects and in infants has been mentioned in the earlier section dealing with endogenous synthesis.

Microbial nitrate reductase activity can be influenced by the diet. Mallett *et al.* (1984) found that pectin and other hydrocolloid food additives (guar gum, gum acacia and locust-bean gum) added at a 5% level to rat diet led to a several-fold increase in caecal nitrite production.

Nitrite

Studies on the absorption of orally administered nitrite have been complicated by the gastric pH conditions in the stomach and by its reactivity with dietary constituents and endogenous compounds. Thus, under *in vitro* simulated gastric conditions at pH < 5, nitrite rapidly disappeared and the loss was accelerated by the presence of food (Mirvish *et al.* 1975). Furthermore, nitrite could also be utilized by gut microflora as a source of nitrogen.

Absorption of nitrite in the rat has been found to be slower than that of nitrate, but some gastric absorption has been noted (Mirvish *et al.*, 1975). In mice, intestinal absorption of nitrite appeared to be faster than in the rat (Witter and Balish, 1979).

No data are available on the absorption of nitrite in man, but there is circumstantial evidence that nitrite formed by the reduction of nitrate is absorbed, leading to elevation of methaemoglobin levels in infants (Shuval and Gruener, 1972).

Nitrite is not normally detectable in body fluids and tissues of experimental animals; following i.v. injection in mice and rabbits, rapid equilibration occurs in tissues within 5 min and within 30 min the levels of free nitrite in body fluid are low (Fritsch *et al.*, 1985). The plasma half-life of nitrite in the distribution phase was found to be 48, 12 and 5 min in dogs, sheep and ponies, respectively (Schneider and Yeary, 1975). Nitrite undergoes oxidative metabolism to nitrate in the tissues and blood; the mechanism of oxidation appears to involve reaction with oxyhaemoglobin (Fe^{2+}) resulting in the formation of a methaemoglobin (Fe^{3+}) complex and the subsequent enzymic reduction to nitrate (Smith and Beutler, 1966). The reaction rate between nitrite and haemoglobin is species-dependent; in man, the reaction rate is slower than that in ruminants but faster than that in the pig (Smith and Beutler, 1966).

N-Nitroso Compounds

There is good evidence to suggest that the known volatile *N*-nitrosamines (e.g. NDMA, NDEA, NPIP and NPYR) in the diet are absorbed rapidly from the duodenum and are subsequently carried by the portal circulation to the liver (Hashimoto *et al.*, 1976). Thus, for example, NDMA is absorbed slowly from the stomach but very rapidly from the small intestine.

Spiegelhalder *et al.* (1982) found that < 1% of a dose of NDMA (0.03–300 mg per animal) was excreted unchanged in the urine of rats. The same authors also found that in man, NDMA could only be detected in the urine when administered in combination with ethanol, which is known to inhibit the metabolism of NDMA (Swann *et al.*, 1984).

Most dialkylnitrosamine studies have been shown to be metabolized by the oxidation of the carbon alpha to the nitroso group by tissue-specific microsomal multi-component mixed-function oxidase enzymes centred on cytochrome P450. It now seems reasonably certain that the cytochrome p450 system responsible for nitrosamine metabolism belongs to the 11 E subfamily of the ethanol-inducible enzymes (see reviews by Yang *et al.*, 1985; Magee, 1989). Carlson (1990) has shown that pretreatment with ethanol (10%) in the drinking water increased NDMA metabolism several-fold in the liver and lungs of treated rats. The metabolism of dialkylnitrosamines results, via an unstable intermediate, in the formation of a diazohydroxide or an alkyl diazonium ion, both of which are strong electrophilic alkylating agents (Park *et al.*, 1977, 1980).

Nitrosoproline and nitrosothioproline are not metabolized but are excreted unchanged in the urine; the metabolic fate of other non-volatile nitroso compounds remains to be elucidated.

TOXICOLOGY IN ANIMALS AND EXPERIMENTAL SYSTEMS

Nitrate

Acute Toxicity

Oral LD_{50} values are as follows:

mouse	2480–6250 mg $NaNO_3$ (kg body weight)$^{-1}$[a]
rat	4860–9000 mg $NaNO_3$ (kg body weight)$^{-1}$[a]
rat	3750 mg KNO_3 (kg body weight)$^{-1}$[b]
	rat 2450–4820 mg $NH_4 NO_3$ (kg body weight)$^{-1}$[b]
rabbit	2680 mg $NaNO_3$ (kg body weight)$^{-1}$[b]
rabbit	1900 mg KNO_3 mg (kg body weight)$^{-1}$[b]

[a]Speijers *et al.* (1989); [b]NIOSH (1987).

The oral LD_{50} in the cow was estimated to be 450 mg $NaNO_3$ kg^{-1} as a single dose but was higher (970–1360 mg kg^{-1}) when spread over a 24-h period (Crawford, 1960).

Short-term Toxicity

Rats

F-344 rats of both sexes received 0, 1.25, 2.5, 5, 10 or 20% $NaNO_3$ in the diet for 6 weeks. There was a significant reduction in weight gain in the two top dose groups and evidence of methaemoglobinaemia at autopsy. The no adverse effect dose was found to be 5% $NaNO_3$ in the diet, equivalent to a dietary intake of 2500 mg (kg body weight)$^{-1}$ day^{-1} (Maekawa *et al.*, 1982).

Wistar rats of both sexes received two different basal diets (cereal-based or semi-purified) containing 0, 1, 2, 3, 4 or 6% KNO_3 or 5% $NaNO_3$ for 4 weeks. The general condition, behaviour and survival of the animals on the two diets were unaffected. There was a small but significant dose-related increase in methaemoglobin levels in female rats at and above 2% KNO_3 in the diet but the values were still within the reference range for the strain of rats used. There was also an increase in the relative kidney weight in male animals. The no adverse effect dose was 1% KNO_3 in the diet, equivalent to 500 mg (kg body weight)$^{-1}$ day^{-1} (Til et al., 1985).

Mice

The inclusion of $NaNO_3$ in the drinking water at 1.2% for 25 weeks [approximately 2.5 g (kg body weight)$^{-1}$ day^{-1}] did not affect survival (Greenblatt and Mirvish, 1972).

Rabbits

Male animals given KNO_3 in gelatin capsules at doses of 0, 200, 400 or 600 mg (kg body weight)$^{-1}$ for 4 weeks developed dose-related effects (weight loss, tachycardia, polyuria and weakness) in all treatment groups within 2 weeks (Nighat et al., 1981).

Dogs

Two females and one male were fed a diet containing 2% $NaNO_3$ [approximately 500 mg (kg body weight)$^{-1}$ day^{-1}] for 105 or 125 days without any adverse effects reported (Lehman, 1958).

Long-term Toxicity and Carcinogenicity

Rats

Five groups of male and female rats were given $NaNO_3$ at levels of 0, 0.1, 1, 5 or 10% in the diet for 2 years. Apart from a slight depression in growth rate at the 5% level and inanition at the highest dose level, there was no evidence of any adverse effects or increase of tumour incidence in the treated animals (Lehman, 1958).

MRC-derived rats of both sexes were given drinking water containing 0 or 0.5% $NaNO_3$ [equivalent to 500 mg (kg body weight)$^{-1}$ day^{-1}] for 84 weeks and euthanized 20 weeks later. There was no statistically significant difference in tumour incidence between the two groups (Lijinsky et al., 1973).

Sprague–Dawley rats of both sexes received drinking water containing 0 or 4000 mg $NaNO_3$ l^{-1} for 14 months. No difference was observed in the methaemoglobin levels between the two groups (Chow et al., 1980).

In a comprehensive investigation, Fischer-344 rats of both sexes were given drinking water containing 0, 2.5 or 5% $NaNO_3$ [equivalent to 0, 2500 or 5000 mg (kg body weight)$^{-1}$ day^{-1}] for 2 years. The survival rate of the treated animals was significantly higher and there was a marked reduction in the incidence of mononuclear cell leukaemias compared with controls. No significant dif-

ferences were seen in the incidence of other tumour types between the test and control groups. The no observed adverse effect level in this study was reported to be 2500 mg $NaNO_3$ (kg body weight)$^{-1}$ day^{-1} [1824 mg nitrate ion (kg body weight)$^{-1}$ day^{-1}] (Maekawa et al., 1982).

Mice

In a lifetime study, groups of ICR mice of each sex were given 0, 25 000 or 50 000 mg $NaNO_3$ (kg diet)$^{-1}$. No differences in tumour incidence were seen between treated and control animals (Sugiyama et al., 1979).

Reproductive Toxicity Studies

Guinea-pigs

Sleight and Atallah (1968) gave guinea-pigs drinking water containing 0, 300, 3500, 10 000 or 30 000 mg KNO_3 l^{-1} for 143–204 days prior to mating and during pregnancy. Conception took place at all dose levels; male fertility was unaffected. Also, no significant gross or microscopic lesions were seen in the reproductive organs. Reproductive performance was unaffected except at the top dose, where the numbers of litters and live births were greatly reduced. The no observed adverse effect level in this study was 10 000 mg KNO_3 l^{-1} [equivalent to 507 mg KNO_3 (kg body weight)$^{-1}$ day^{-1} or 310 mg nitrate ion (kg body weight)$^{-1}$ day^{-1}].

Sheep and cattle

Pregnant sheep were given drinking water containing 0.3–1.2% nitrate from days 21 to 49 of pregnancy. The doses were sufficient to cause severe methaemoglobinaemia but no changes in the abortion rates were observed (Davison et al., 1965). Pregnant heifers were given a diet containing 445 or 665 mg nitrate ion from 2 months of pregnancy until parturition. The treatments produced 20–50% methaemoglobinaemia in the animals. No treatment-related effects on the outcome of the pregnancy were seen (Winter and Hokanson, 1964).

Mutagenicity

In vitro studies

No mutagenic effects were seen in bacterial systems (Salmonella typhimurium or Escherichia coli) under aerobic conditions. Under anaerobic conditions, however, nitrate was mutagenic in E. coli, probably due to the reduction of nitrate to nitrite (Kontezka, 1974). KNO_3 and $NaNO_3$ were not mutagenic in the Ames test against several strains of S. typhimurium (Ishidate et al., 1984). Ishidate et al. (1984) also found that whereas $NaNO_3$ (140 mM) produced chromosomal aberrations in Chinese hamster fibroblast cells in culture, KNO_3 (10 mM) did not have a similar effect. As NaCl (140 mM) was also found to be clastogenic in this system, it was presumed that the positive effect was probably a non-specific response due to the high osmotic pressure of the solution.

In vivo studies

Syrian golden hamsters were given 500 mg $NaNO_2$ (kg body weight)$^{-1}$ on days 11 and 12 of pregnancy. After 24 h, the foetuses were removed and used to produce embryonic cell cultures. No gene mutations, chromosomal abnormalities, micronuclei or cell transformations were seen in the cultured cells (Inui *et al.*, 1979).

Groups of mice were given two doses of 78.5, 236, 707 or 2120 mg $NaNO_3$ (kg body weight)$^{-1}$ by gavage, separated by an interval of 24 h. A small but significant increase of micronulei was seen at the 78.5 and 236 mg kg^{-1} dose levels but not at the higher dose levels when cytotoxic effects on the bone marrow were seen. An increase in chromosomal aberrations was seen only at the 707 mg kg^{-1} dose level. Rats receiving a similar treatment did not show bone marrow effects. However, groups of rats given these doses daily for 2 weeks showed a significant increase in chromosomal abnormalities at all treatment levels. It is possible that the observed effects were due to the metabolic degradation of nitrate to nitrite and the formation of *N*-nitroso compounds (Luca *et al.*, 1985).

Administration of 600 or 1200 mg $NaNO_3$ (kg body weight)$^{-1}$ day^{-1} for 2 weeks by stomach tube to male mice resulted in sperm head abnormalities at the higher dose. When mated with untreated females, no effects on fertility or litter size were observed (Alavantic *et al.*, 1988).

Thyroid Effects

Rats were given drinking water containing 40, 200, 1200 or 4000 mg nitrate ion l^{-1} for 100 days and thyroid function was assessed by ^{131}I uptake, serum iodine level, protein-bound iodine and thyroid weight and histology. Thyroid weight and ^{131}I uptake were slightly affected at all dose levels and there were associated thyroid histological changes, but there was no dose-related response in the parameters measured (Horing *et al.*, 1985; Seffner *et al.*, 1985).

Jahreis *et al.* (1987) studied the effects of administration of 3% KNO_3 in the diet for 2 days or 6 weeks to piglets (aged 56 days) on serum levels of thyroxine (T_4), triiodothyronine (T_3), nitrate, methaemoglobin and somatomedin. Sufficient iodine intake by mothers prevented a decrease in T_4 levels after 2 days of administration of KNO_3. However, after 6 weeks of treatment a striking decrease in the T_4 level was found which could not be prevented even by the addition of 0.5 mg iodine (kg diet)$^{-1}$. No adaptation to nitrate administration was observed. After 6 weeks of administration of the nitrate-containing diet to the piglets, there was a significant decrease in serum somatomedin activity which correlated with a decrease in body weight gain in the animals.

Nitrite

Acute Toxicity

The oral LD$_{50}$ values of $NaNO_2$ in mice, rats and rabbits are 214, 180 and 180 mg (kg body weight)$^{-1}$, respectively (NIOSH, 1987). The acute toxic effects of nitrite include relaxation of smooth muscle, vasodilation, lowering of blood pressure and methaemoglobinaemia.

When two doses of 100 mg $NaNO_2$ (kg body weight)$^{-1}$ were given to rats with an interval of 2 h, a high mortality occurred, whereas when the dosing interval was 4 h, none of the animals died (Druckrey *et al.*, 1963). A similar difference in toxicity was observed when rats were given divided doses of 160 or 320 mg $NaNO_2$ (kg body weight)$^{-1}$ at intervals (3 × 15 min and 4 × 30 min); this regime was found to be less toxic than single doses of 40 or 80 mg (kg body weight)$^{-1}$. Methaemoglobinaemia was used as the index of toxicity (DeVries, 1983). A likely explanation for this difference in toxicity may be the relatively short half-life of circulating methaemoglobin, reported to be 90 min in the rat (Shuval and Gruener, 1972).

Short-term Toxicity

Rats

Animals given drinking water containing $NaNO_2$ at concentrations to provide intakes of 170 and 340 mg (kg body weight)$^{-1}$ day^{-1} for 200 days showed methaemoglobinaemia, raised haematocrit, raised spleen weight in females, raised heart weight in males and changes in liver weight in females and kidney weight in both sexes (Musil, 1966).

$NaNO_2$ was administered to groups of rats of both sexes at concentrations of 0, 0.06, 0.125, 0.25, 0.5 or 1.0% in the drinking water for 6 weeks. In the 1% dose group, body weight gain was depressed by more than 10% and 4/10 females died; deaths of one male and one female also occurred in the 0.5% dose group. Methaemoglobinaemia was marked in the two top dose groups. The maximum tolerated dose was considered to be 0.25% $NaNO_2$ in the drinking water (Maekawa *et al.*, 1982).

Sprague–Dawley rats were given drinking water containing $NaNO_2$ at a concentration of 200 mg l^{-1} for 16 weeks. Blood samples taken at intervals showed methaemoglobin levels of 0.5–3.1% in the treated group and 0–1.2% in controls (Chow *et al.*, 1980).

Til *et al.* (1988) carried out a 13-week oral study of KNO_2 at concentrations of 0, 100, 300, 1000 or 3000 mg l^{-1} in the drinking water in rats. The potassium concentrations in the nitrite solutions were equalized to that of the 3000 mg KNO_2 l^{-1} solution by the addition of KCl. Body weight, food intake and food efficiency were reduced at the 3000 mg l^{-1} level in males whilst water intake was decreased in males at 1000 and 3000 mg l^{-1} and females at 3000 mg l^{-1}. There was a significant increase in methaemoglobin concentrations in the 3000 mg l^{-1} group. No impairment in renal function was observed in any of the test groups, although the relative kidney weight and plasma alkaline phosphatase activity in the 3000 mg l^{-1} group were increased. Interestingly, hypertrophy of the adrenal zona glomerulosa was observed in all the test groups. It was concluded that the no observed adverse effect level was < 100 mg KNO_2 l^{-1} in the drinking water, which is equivalent to an intake of < 10 mg KNO_2 (kg body weight)$^{-1}$ day^{-1} [6.1 mg NO_3 ion (kg body weight)$^{-1}$ day^{-1}].

A supplementary study performed by Til *et al.* (1990) revealed a no-adverse effect level of 50 mg KNO_2 l^{-1}, equivalent to 5 mg KNO_2 (kg body weight)$^{-1}$ day^{-1} [3 mg NO_2]. This effect on the adrenals was not observed in rats given nitrate in the drinking water (G. J. A. Speijers, personal communication).

Mice

$NaNO_2$ at concentrations of 1, 100, 1000, 1500 or 2000 mg l^{-1} in the drinking water for 2 weeks decreased motor activity, seemingly at high doses (Gruener and Shuval, 1973).

Black 6J mice received drinking water containing $NaNO_2$ at concentrations of 0, 100, 1000, 1500 or 2000 mg l^{-1}. A dose-related increase in methaemoglobinaemia was observed accompanied by a significant reduction in motor activity at the highest dose level. Administration of ascorbic acid restored the methaemoglobin level in the highest dose group almost to normal but did not reverse the reduced motor activity, suggesting that the latter effect was not associated with methaemoglobinaemia (Behroozi *et al.*, 1971).

Long-term Toxicity and Carcinogenicity

Rats

Gruener and Shuval (1973) administered $NaNO_2$ in the drinking water at concentrations of 0, 100, 1000, 2000 or 3000 mg l^{-1} to male rats for 2 years. The methaemoglobin levels, measured at midnight to take account of the nocturnal feeding habit of the animals and the short half-life of circulating methaemoglobin, were increased to 5, 12 and 22% of total Hb in the 1000, 2000 and 3000 mg $NaNO_2$ l^{-1} groups, respectively. The histopathological changes observed in these groups were: congestion of liver and spleen; focal inflammatory and degenerative changes in the kidneys; general emphysema, dilated bronchi and lymphocyte infiltration in the bronchial epithelium in the lungs; pronounced degenerative foci in the heart; and thin and dilated coronary arteries. The no observed adverse effect dose level was 100 mg $NaNO_2$ l^{-1}, equivalent to 5–10 mg $NaNO_2$ (kg body weight)$^{-1}$ day^{-1} [3.3–6.7 mg NO_2 ion (kg body weight)$^{-1}$ day^{-1}].

Shank and Newberne (1976) conducted a study on pregnant Sprague–Dawley rats fed from conception on a diet containing a measured average concentration of 263 ppm of $NaNO_2$ (nominal concentration 1000 mg $NaNO_2$ kg^{-1}). Pups from the F_1 litters, maintained on the same diet, were randomly selected for carcinogenicity studies and an F_2 generation was derived from the F_1 animals. The $NaNO_2$ diet feeding study was terminated at week 125 in the F_2 generation. No difference was observed in survival or tumour incidence between the test and control groups, except for a reportedly increased incidence of lymphoreticular tumours.

In a follow-up to the above study, Newberne (1978, 1979) maintained the F_1-derived rats on $NaNO_2$ at levels of 0, 250, 500, 1000 or 2000 mg kg^{-1} in the diet or 1000 or 2000 mg $NaNO_2$ l^{-1} drinking water over the lifetime of the animals. Three types of diets were studied: an agar-based semisynthetic diet, commercial chow and a refined casein-based diet. An increase in lymphoid tumours in all nitrite-treated groups relative to controls was reported. However, a peer review of the histology from the foregoing study conducted by a US Governmental Interagency Working Group arrived at a different diagnosis and reported a smaller incidence of malignant tumours. The Working Group concluded that the incidence of lymphomas and other tumours in the $NaNO_2$-treated groups was similar to that arising spontaneously in Sprague–Dawley rats and that no evidence could be adduced from the study to suggest that the ingestion of $NaNO_2$ increased the incidence of tumours (FDA, 1980a, b). Fischer-344 rats were given drinking water containing 0, 0.125 or 0.25% $NaNO_2$ from 8 weeks of age for 2 years. In high-dose females, the mean body weight was decreased by more than 10% relative to controls and there was a significant decrease in overall tumour incidence compared with controls. In part, this reduced tumour incidence arose from a reduction in monocytic leukaemias which occurs with a high incidence in this strain of rat. There was no significant difference in tumour incidence between other test groups and the controls. Survival was significantly higher in treated males than controls (Maekawa *et al.*, 1982).

A similar finding was reported by Lijinsky *et al.* (1983), who found a decrease in monocytic leukaemias in Fischer- 344 rats treated with $NaNO_2$ in drinking water at a concentration of 2000 mg l^{-1} or in the diet at 2000 mg kg^{-1}. No treatment-related changes were observed in other tumour types.

Lijinsky and Kovatch (1989) conducted a study in rats treated with $NaNO_2$ at 0.2% in the drinking water over their lifespan. Additionally, two other treatment groups were included in this study: one group on drinking water containing 0.32% sodium thiocyanate and a second group on drinking water containing both sodium nitrite (0.2%) and sodium thiocyanate (0.32%). The results showed that there was no increase in the incidence of tumours in any of the treatment groups.

Grant and Butler (1989) conducted a long-term feeding study on rats with $NaNO_2$ which was administered as part of a protein-reduced diet at dose levels of 0.2 or 0.5% (w/w) for up to 115 weeks. A dose-related decrease was noted in both the incidence and in the time of onset of lymphomas, leukaemias and testicular interstitial cell tumours. Under the conditions described in this study, $NaNO_2$ was found not to be carcinogenic when fed in the diet for up to 115 weeks, but rather to decrease the incidence of tumours in a dose-related manner.

Mice

ICR mice were given $NaNO_2$ in the drinking water at concentrations of 0, 1000, 2500 or 5000 mg l^{-1} for 18 months. No tumours attributable to treatment were observed (Inai *et al.*, 1979).

Nitrite Plus Meat Products Feeding Studies

Wistar rats were given a diet containing 40% canned meat and 0, 0.02 or 0.5% $NaNO_2$, with or without glucono-δ lactone, for 2 years. No differences were observed in the incidence of tumours or preneoplastic lesions between the treated animals and controls (van Loghten *et al.*, 1972).

In a further study on nitrite-cured meat, Olsen *et al.* (1984) conducted two-generation study on Wistar rats. Male and female animals were maintained on a basal diet or a cured meat diet initially treated with 200, 1000 or 4000 mg $NaNO_2$ kg^{-1}. The final diets as administered to the rats showed a nitrite content in the basal diet of 2 mg kg^{-1} and in the cured-meat diets of 4, 4 and 94 mg $NaNO_2$ kg^{-1}, respectively. Additionally, the highest dose cured-meat diet contained 30 g NDMA kg^{-1}. The animals were bred and the F_1 generation rats were maintained post-weaning on the cured-meat diets. Reproduction was unaffected by treatment and at termination after 122 weeks there was no significant difference in survival or incidence of malignant tumours between the nitrite treated groups and controls. However, the overall cancer incidence (total malignant tumours at all sites) was increased in the 4000 mg $NaNO_2$ kg^{-1} group. The no observed adverse effect dose level was the diet treated with 1000 mg $NaNO_2$ kg^{-1}, equivalent to a dose of 50 mg (kg body weight)$^{-1}$ day^{-1} [33 mg NO_2 ion (kg body weight)$^{-1}$ day^{-1}].

Lin and Ho (1992) conducted a study in rats fed diets containing squid (10%) or squid (10%) plus $NaNO_2$ (0.3%). Squid contains high levels of naturally occurring amines, such as trimethylamine oxide, trimethylamine and dimethylamine. The animals were treated for 10 months. Hepatocellular carcinoma (16% incidence) was induced in rats fed the diet containing 10% squid and the incidence was increased to 33% when the diet included $NaNO_2$. Partial protection against hepatic damage was afforded when ascorbic acid (0.3%) was co-administered to the animals. The authors suggested that trimethylamine oxide rather than dimethylamine may have been responsible for the induction of hepatoxicity and hepatocarcinogenicity in the study.

Reproductive Toxicity and Teratogenicity Studies

Rats

Pregnant rats were given drinking water containing 0, 2000 or 3000 mg $NaNO_2$ l^{-1} from mating to 3 weeks after parturition. The methaemoglobin levels in the controls and treated dams were 1.1, 15.5 and 24%, respectively, and a dose-dependent anaemia developed in the nitrite-treated animals. Birth weights were similar in each group but body weight gain was impaired during suckling by 48 and 72% compared with controls in the two nitrite-treated groups, although nitrite was not transferred to any appreciable extent in the milk. There was a dose-related increase of newborn mortality from 6% in the controls to 30 and 53% in the low and high dose groups, respectively (Gruener and Shuval, 1973).

Pregnant Long–Evans rats were given throughout gestation and lactation drinking water containing 0, 0.5, 1, 2 or 3 g $NaNO_2$ l^{-1}. Treatment severely affected erythropoietic development, growth and mortality in the offspring. The dose of 0.5 g l^{-1} was at or near the observed no adverse effect level. Cross-fostering indicated that treatment during the lactational period was more instrumental in producing lesions than during the gestational period (Roth *et al.*, 1987).

A three-generation study in rats and a two-generation study in Syrian hamsters, treated with dietary levels of 0 or 1000 mg $NaNO_2$ kg^{-1}, showed no effects on fertility, litter size, post-natal survival, growth rate or lifespan (Shank and Newberne, 1976).

Mice

Pregnant ICR mice were given drinking water containing either 100 or 1000 mg $NaNO_2$ l^{-1} on days 7–18 of gestation. There were no significant differences between treated and control groups in indices of developmental toxicity (litter size, foetal weight, etc.). Also, there was no evidence of teratogenic effects in this study (Shimada, 1989).

Guinea-pigs

Pregnant guinea-pigs were given single subcutaneous doses of 50, 60 or 70 mg $NaNO_2$ (kg body weight)$^{-1}$ as a 2% solution. The control and lowest treatment group had normal pregnancies while the intermediate group aborted 1–4 days after dosing. The highest dose group showed maternal deaths within 60 min. In a subsequent study, pregnant animals were given 60 mg $NaNO_2$ (kg body weight)$^{-1}$ subcutaneously and blood was collected from dams and foetuses from 0.25 to 56 h after treatment. Nitrite treatment led to deaths of 96% of the foetuses. The data suggested that foetal deaths occurred as result of hypoxia induced by maternal methaemoglobinaemia (Sinha and Sleight, 1971).

Treated females mated to at least one treated male per group received $NaNO_2$ in the drinking water at concentrations of 0, 300, 1000, 2000, 3000, 4000, 5000 or 10 000 mg l^{-1} for 100–240 days. Male fertility was not impaired. Food and water consumption and body weight gain were normal except in the top dose group. Foetal losses were total with 5000 and 10 000 mg l^{-1}, but there were no deaths at doses below 4000 mg $NaNO_2$ l^{-1}. The no observed adverse effect level was deemed to be 300 mg $NaNO_2$ (kg body weight)$^{-1}$ day^{-1} [200 mg NO_2 ion (kg body weight)$^{-1}$ day^{-1}] (Sleight and Atallah, 1968).

Mutagenicity studies

Oshima et al. (1989) conducted a short-term genotoxicity study on a commercial hickory smoke condensate, with or without added sodium nitrite, in F-344 male rats. Hickory smoke condensate [1 ml of a 10–100% (v/v) solution per rat] was given orally, either with or without $NaNO_2$ (25–100 mol per rat) to the animals. The potential of the treatments to act as glandular stomach carcinogens was assessed by measuring ornithine decarboxylase activity, replicative DNA synthesis and DNA single strand breaks in the pyloric mucosa. The results suggested that hickory smoke condensate contained substance(s) that had the potential to induce tumour-initiating and/or tumour-promoting activities and that reaction with nitrite generated new substances that could act as tumour promoters in the rat glandular stomach.

In vitro studies

Nitrous acid (HNO_2) proved mutagenic in Salmonella typhimurium and Escherichia coli (Thomas et al., 1979) and $NaNO_2$ induced reverse mutations in S. Typhimurium and chromosomal aberrations in cultured Chinese hamster fibroblast cells (Ishidate et al., 1984).

$NaNO_2$ did not cause single strand breaks in cultured mouse cells but there was a dose-related increase in gene mutations and chromosomal aberrations at high concentrations, possibly due to the deamination of bases (Kodama et al., 1976). $NaNO_2$ (2100 and 4200 mg l^{-1}) increased chromosomal aberrations, aneuploidy and malignant cell transformation in cultured newborn hamster cells (Tsuda and Kato, 1977). An increase in 6-TG mutants was produced by $NaNO_2$ in V79 hamster cells (Budayova, 1985).

Tsuda and Hasegawa (1990) found that the addition of $NaNO_2$ (5–20 mM) for 72 h to mouse BALB/c3T3 cells resulted in the induction of transformed foci (type 111 foci) in a dose-dependent manner. The treated cells produced progressively growing tumours when inoculated into nude mice. The possibility that N-nitroso compounds were formed in culture was excluded, leading the authors to conclude that nitrite per se seemed to have cell-transforming activity.

In vivo studies

Negative results were obtained in a host-mediated assay against Salmonella typhimurium at a dose level of 150 mg $NaNO_2$ (kg body weight)$^{-1}$ (Couch and Friedman, 1975) and in a mouse micronucleus test (Hayashi et al., 1981).

$NaNO_2$ (1250 mg l^{-1}) in drinking water was administered to pregnant (on days 5–18 of gestation) and to nonpregnant rats. Chromosomal aberrations were seen in the bone marrow of pregnant and non-pregnant adults and in the liver of transplacentally exposed embryos; the magnitude of the effect was greater in the embryonic liver than in the adult bone marrow (El Nahas et al., 1984).

Other studies

To test the hypothesis that nitrite may be a causative factor in cerebral glioma, VM-strain mice (a strain susceptible to glioma formation) were exposed to 0.2% $NaNO_2$ in the drinking water, both in utero and throughout their lifespan. All animals were subjected to terminal autopsy and routine histological examination. There was no excess of nervous system tumours in the test group (Hawkes et al., 1992).

To evaluate the relationship between atmospheric nitrogen dioxide exposure and the development of allergic diseases, Fujimaki et al. (1993) studied the effects of nitrite on mast cell function. Two functionally distinct types of mast cells were used, namely peritoneal mast cells (PMC) and intestinal mucosal mast cells (IMMC) of Nippostrongylus brasiliensis-infected rats. High concentrations of nitrite alone (10, 20 and 50 mM) induced histamine release from IMMC but not from PMC. Low concentrations of nitrite (< 1 mM) had no significant effect on mast cell function.

N-Nitroso Compounds

As mentioned earlier, in view of the heterogeneity and the lack of information on the identity and composition of the N-nitroso compounds present in foods or formed endogenously, it is not possible to assess the toxicology of these compounds. The known volatile N-nitrosamines commonly encountered in the Western diet (NDMA, NDEA, NPIP and NPYR), accounting for less than 10% of the apparent total nitroso compounds, have been shown to be positive in a battery of short-term mutagenicity test systems and carcinogenic in a number of animal species. The toxicity and carcinogenicity of nitrosamines have been extensively reviewed (e.g. IARC monographs) and little useful purpose would be served in attempting a survey of the subject in this chapter.

In view of the potent carcinogenicity in animal studies of some of the commonly encountered nitrosamines and the fact that many of these compounds may be formed from dietary precursors *in vivo*, an attempt has been made by Shephard *et al.* (1987) to assess the potential formation of *N*-nitroso compounds in the stomach. A simple algorithm was used which took account of the daily intake of precursor amines (amides) and the carcinogenicity of the *N*-nitroso compounds formed. From this it was concluded that dietary ureas and aromatic amines combined with a high nitrite burden could pose as great a risk as that from preformed NDMA in the diet, whereas *in vivo* intragastric nitrosation of ingested primary and secondary amines probably poses a negligibly small risk. Licht and Deen (1988) developed a theoretical model for predicting nitrosation rates in the human stomach; calculations based on their model suggest that this source of exposure may not be of sufficient magnitude to pose a serious health risk. Consequently, other possible routes and sites of endogenous nitrosation merit closer evaluation to enable a more realistic assessment of total human nitrosamine exposure to be made.

HUMAN EFFECTS AND EPIDEMIOLOGICAL STUDIES

Nitrate

Single Exposure

Estimates of the lethal dose of KNO_3 have ranged from 4 to 30 g [about 70–500 mg (kg body weight)$^{-1}$] while 30–60 g of $NaNO_3$ have been given for 2 months as an acidifying diuretic without manifestation of adverse effects (Sollman, 1957). A realistic estimate of a lethal dose for adults is about 20 g of nitrate ion or 330 mg nitrate ion (kg body weight)$^{-1}$ (Leu *et al.*, 1986).

Ellen *et al.* (1982) administered a single dose of ammonium nitrate [0.15 g (kg body weight)$^{-1}$] to 12 volunteers with no measurable haematological effects, elevation of methaemoglobin or circulating *N*-nitroso compounds. One volunteer developed diarrhoea after 7 h and another vomited after 12 min. Twelve others administered 9.5 g of $NaNO_3$ in 750 ml of intravenously over a 1-h period showed no ill effects.

Repeated Exposure

Whereas nitrate *per se* has a relatively low toxicity, most of the reported adverse effects have resulted from the reduction of nitrate to nitrite either prior to ingestion or *in vivo*. The manifestations of nitrite intoxication (methaemoglobinaemia) then become apparent.

Infants are a special 'at risk' group since neonates are deficient in methaemoglobin reductase activity and foetal haemoglobin is more readily oxidized to methaemoglobin than the mature form (reviewed in WHO, 1985). Furthermore, low gastric acid secretion favours bacterial

colonization of the stomach and the consequent enhanced microbially mediated reduction of nitrate to nitrite (Ellen and Schuller, 1983). Based on a circulating 10% methaemoglobin level as a criterion for toxicity (Winton *et al.*, 1971) and assuming 80% reduction of ingested nitrate derived from the drinking water supply used in the preparation of infant formulation to nitrite, Corre and Breimer (1979) calculated on a 'worst case' situation basis that the toxic dose of nitrate in infants is 1.5–2.3 mg nitrate ion (kg body weight)$^{-1}$.

Numerous cases of acute intoxication following the ingestion of well waters containing high nitrate contents have been reported, 97.7% of which were associated with nitrate levels of 44.3–88.6 mg nitrate ion l^{-1} (WHO, 1985). A common complicating factor in such circumstances is either the prevalence of bacterial contamination of the water supply and/or a co-existing bacterial infection. Thus, infants suffering from acute diarrhoea were found to have elevated methaemoglobin levels on a low nitrate intake (2–7 mg day^{-1}) (Hegesh and Shiloah, 1982). In one case, a dyspeptic child was found to have 72% methaemoglobinaemia associated with a drinking water nitrate concentration as low as 50 mg l^{-1} (Thal *et al.*, 1961).

There are, however, conflicting reports in the literature on the susceptiblity of infants to ingested nitrate-induced methaemoglobinaemia and even on the suggestion that an adaptation may take place to changes in the methaemoglobin response to nitrate intake (Shuval and Gruener, 1977).

Reproductive Toxicity

The death rate from malformations in infants around the time of birth was reported to be significantly higher in an area of Australia where the drinking water supply contained more than 15 mg nitrate l^{-1} than in other areas where the nitrate concentration was less than 2 mg l^{-1} (Scragg *et al.*, 1982). In a more detailed (case-control) study within the same area, concentrations of 5–15 mg l^{-1} and in excess of 15 mg l^{-1} were associated, respectively, with about three and four times the risk of malformed children when compared with a concentration below 5 mg l^{-1}. Many of the malformations involved the central nervous system. The investigators emphasized that caution should be used in interpreting these findings as the study was limited by the small size of the groups examined and confounding factors may have played a major role.

In a Canadian study, 130 infants who had CNS malformations were matched according to county and date of birth with healthy controls. For those drinking water supplied by private wells, exposure at about 26 mg nitrate l^{-1} was associated with a moderate increase in risk compared with exposure at 0.1 mg l^{-1}. A decreased risk was observed for those who drank water from municipal supplies (up to 3.3 mg nitrate l^{-1}). However, neither finding achieved statistical significance. The study was limited by the relatively small numbers examined and the investigators suggested that other factors may have been involved in the CNS malformations (Arbuckle *et al.*, 1988).

Thyroid Effects

Höring *et al.* (1988) reported preliminary results from a case control study on 12–15-year-old girls on an iodine-deficient diet, which indicated a significant increase in the incidence of goitre in the population exposed to a drinking water nitrate concentration of 22.5 mg l^{-1} compared with the population exposed to 7.5 mg l^{-1}. Van Maanen *et al.* (1994) compared the thyroid volume in populations exposed to different nitrate levels in their drinking water in The Netherlands. No iodine deficiency was observed in any of the nitrate exposure groups. A dose-dependent difference in the volume of the thyroid was observed between low and medium vs high nitrate exposure groups, showing an enlarged thyroid volume at nitrate levels exceeding 50 mg l^{-1}.

Carcinogenic Risk

Gastric Cancer

Numerous epidemiological studies have been undertaken on the relationship between nitrate intake and gastric cancer. In general, the studies were geographical comparisons of high and low gastric cancer incidence areas or case-control studies in which nitrate exposure was compared in gastric cancer patients and control populations. In both cases the variable under consideration was an estimate of exposure to environmental nitrate or some surrogate, e.g. use of well water. Geographical studies have been undertaken in a number of countries in Latin America, Europe and China.

The WHO (1985), summarizing the available evidence, concluded that no convincing evidence had emerged of a relationship between gastric cancer and the consumption of drinking water containing nitrate ion levels up to 10 mg l^{-1}. The WHO report further stated that although no firm epidemiological evidence had been found linking gastric cancer and drinking water containing higher levels of nitrate, a link could not be ruled out owing to the inadequacy of the data available. The report commented that gastric cancer was declining in most countries and that the risk from nitrate, if any, would appear to be restricted to individuals with conditions associated with low gastric acidity, rather than the population in general.

The National Academy of Science in a report in 1981 on the health effects of nitrate, nitrite and *N*-nitroso compounds came to a similar conclusion (US Assembly of Life Sciences, 1981b).

A number of geographical correlation studies have been reported in the last decade. The incidence of gastric cancer was investigated in four regions in the UK, two with a high incidence and two with a low incidence. The low-risk population was found to have 50% higher salivary levels of nitrate and nitrite than the high-risk population; the difference was not confounded by age, sex, social class, smoking or time of the last meal before saliva samples were taken. It was concluded that nitrate exposure was not a rate limiting factor and did not explain the geographic distribution of gastric cancer in the UK (Forman *et al.*, 1985a, b).

Beresford (1985) found a negative correlation between gastric cancer mortality in 229 urban areas in the UK and drinking water nitrate levels during the period 1969–73. However, both this study and that of Forman *et al.* (1985a, b) did not take account of possible long latency periods in the development of gastric cancer. A study by Clough (1983) attempted to allow for latency by comparing water nitrate levels in 1946 in 43 local authorities in Kent with gastric cancer mortality for the period 1959–73. A significant positive relationship was claimed for males but not for females.

Jensen (1982) compared cancer incidence rates for 1943–72 between Aalborg (with an elevated nitrate concentration in drinking water of 30 mg l^{-1}) and Aarhus in Denmark. A significantly moderate elevation of stomach cancer risk was found in Aalborg in both men and women. The lack of consistency in the results of geographical correlation studies is further illustrated by the fact that whereas a positive association between nitrate exposure and gastric cancer rates in Italy was found by Gilli *et al.* (1984), an inverse association or absence of association was reported by Knight *et al.* (1990) and by Leclerc *et al.* (1991) in France.

A general problem of correlation studies is that these are usually based on populations rather than on individuals, and the results, apart from being adjusted for age and sex, have often not taken into account confounding factors. A number of case-control studies (based on individuals) on the stomach cancer incidence and nitrate intakes have been reported in the last decade in which adjustments were made for other factors. Some have considered nitrate intakes from both food and drinking water, while others have only taken account of exposure from one of these sources. Those who have used both sources often categorized subjects according to the type of drinking water supply (i.e. well water or mains water supply) without attempting to quantify the actual nitrate intake from drinking water.

In a case-control study of gastric cancer by Risch *et al.* (1985), intakes of a large number of dietary items were considered among 246 cases and 246 controls. Nitrate intake, principally from vegetables, was significantly negatively correlated with cancer risk, although the nitrite intake, mainly from cured meats, was positively associated. The apparent protective effect of nitrate was reversed to a non-significantly positive association when ascorbic acid intake was taken into account.

In an Italian case-control study (consisting of 1016 cases and 1159 controls) by Buiatti *et al.* (1990), a non-significant inverse association of gastric cancer with dietary nitrate intake was found. In the report no mention was made of factors taken into account. A subsequent analysis of these data by anatomical sites within the stomach (in particular cardia) by Palli *et al.* (1992) also revealed an absence of association between stomach cancer incidence and dietary nitrate intake.

Boeing *et al.* (1991) also reported a non-significant negative association with nitrate intake in a univariate analysis in a German case-control study (143 cases; 579 controls), but this association disappeared in multivariate analysis. However, the authors did report a significantly elevated risk for users of well waters compared with users of central water supplies, but unfortunately no information was presented on nitrate levels in these well water samples. On the other hand, Rademacher *et al.* (1992) found no association with nitrate levels in water (central or private water sources) in Wisconsin using 1268 cases and an equal number of controls.

Fontham *et al.* (1986) carried out a case-control study on subjects with chronic atrophic gastritis in Louisiana (93 gastritis cases; 78 controls) and found that the gastritis cases had lower nitrate levels in their gastric juice than in the controls.

Xu *et al.* (1992) conducted a case-control involving 92 subjects in a high-risk region in China. The investigators examined the relationship between gastric mucosal lesions (including gastric cancer) and the quality of different types of drinking water and nitrate intake via water. The nitrate content in the local drinking water was generally high with a mean of 109.6 mg l^{-1} (range 4.4–497.2 mg l^{-1}). There were significant differences in the nitrate content in drinking water from different wells in qualitatively different types of waters. The histological changes were closely related to the quality of the drinking water and its nitrate content. The investigators suggested that future aetiological studies of gastric cancer should include more information on well depth, the presence of public or private wells and the nitrate content of water. As the microbiological quality of the water samples was not adequately taken into consideration, the findings in this study are difficult to evaluate.

Other Cancers

No increased risk of developing cancer of the stomach, oesophagus, bladder and lung was seen in an epidemiological study of 1327 male workers producing nitrate-based fertilizers for at least 1 year between 1946 and 1981 and who were monitored until 1981. The major nitrate exposures would have been ammonium nitrate and nitric acid. Saliva analysis indicated that exposure to nitrate had occurred (Al-Dabbagh *et al.*, 1986). Correlation studies carried out by Forman (1991) on nitrate exposure and cancers at sites other than the stomach (in particular the oesophagus) have shown inconsistent results.

Comment Regarding Nitrate and Cancer Risk

Although case-control studies on individuals are better suited than correlation studies in terms of confounding factors from other chemical exposures, problems still arise with regard to the long latency period. Furthermore, problems are frequently encountered in the accurate recall of information on food intakes and this may bias the data be a possible explanation for the inconsistent results obtained in case-control studies.

This problem can be overcome in prospective cohort studies which take accurate account of dietary nitrate intakes and the monitoring of human health. However, no prospective studies on dietary nitrate intake and cancer risk have yet been reported. Thus, the epidemiological studies that have been conducted are comparatively weak by design and the results are inconsistent. It should be pointed out, however, that the measurement of dietary nitrate intakes presents problems because of the large variations in the nitrate levels found in foods. There are at present no biomarkers of dosimetry available for nitrate exposure that can easily be applied on a large scale in epidemiological studies (Forman, 1991).

It is also important to distinguish between nitrate intake from foods and from drinking water. Vegetables are the predominant source of nitrate in the human diet and a number of studies have shown an association between high vegetable intake (e.g. in vegetarians) and a reduced risk of a variety of cancers, notably stomach cancer (for a review, see Steinmetz and Potter, 1991). It would appear that the potential adverse effects of nitrate are counterbalanced by the protective effects of other constituents present in vegetables (e.g. carotenoids, vitamin C, folic acid, flavonoids and indoles).

Forman (1991), in reviewing nitrate exposure and human cancers, came to the conclusion that the human epidemiological evidence relating environmental nitrate exposure and the risk of cancer is methodologically weak but, on balance, it does not suggest a positive association.

Nitrite

The lethal dose has been estimated to be between 2 and 9 g of $NaNO_2$, i.e. approximately 33–250 mg (kg body weight)$^{-1}$ (IARC, 1978; Corre and Breimer, 1979), with the lower doses applying to infants who are more sensitive to methaemoglobinaemia. The development of methaemoglobinaemia is commonly used as a criterion of nitrite toxicity. The normal range of methaemoglobin levels is 0.5–2%, the uppermost level being found in infants and pregnant women. Cyanosis, as evidence of toxicity, occurs at methaemoglobin levels in excess of 10%. Using this criterion, estimates of the toxic dose range from 1 to 8.3 mg $NaNO_2$ (kg body weight)$^{-1}$ (Winton *et al.*, 1971).

Few epidemiological studies have tried to evaluate the association between nitrite intake and cancer risk. As in the case of nitrate, it must be stated that an accurate assessment of nitrite intake is difficult because of the variation in its concentration in food. In a Canadian case-control study, a positive association between gastric cancer incidence and nitrite intake was found with an odds ratio of 2.6, after due adjustment had been made for dietary confounding factors (Risch *et al.*, 1985; Choi *et al.*, 1987). Buiatti *et al.* (1990) reported an increased risk of gastric cancer associated with nitrite intake, which was partly reduced after adjustment for other dietary factors. They constructed a summary index of protein and nitrite (nitrosatable–nitrosating compounds) which was positively assocated with gastric cancer. The authors also categorized the population with regard to intakes of dietary antioxidants (e.g. vitamin C and vitamin E) and found that the effect of the aforementioned summary index was the same with each category of antioxidant intake.

Boeing *et al.* (1991) reported a positive association between gastric cancer and the intake of processed meat in a German case-control study. In a prospective cohort study carried out in The Netherlands among 120 000 subjects, a positive association between processed meat intake and colon cancer incidence was found, while no association existed with fresh meat intake (Goldbohm *et al.*, 1994). These latter studies indicate a role for nitrite but also for pre-formed N-nitroso compounds. While this positive association between the intake of processed meat and the incidence of colon cancer has also been found in some other studies (Bjelke, 1980; Young and Wolf, 1988; Willett *et al.*, 1990; Thun *et al.*, 1992), other studies have failed to find an association (Stemmermann *et al.*, 1984; Phillips and Snowdon, 1985).

N-Nitroso Compounds

Since the discovery of the carcinogenicity of N-nitroso-dimethylamine (NDMA) in the rat by Magee and Barnes in the 1950s, about 300 N-nitroso compounds have been tested for carcinogenicity in experimental animals, and 85% of the 209 nitrosamines and 92% of the 86 nitrosamides have been shown to be carcinogenic in a variety of species of fish, reptiles, birds and mammals, including five species of primates (see, for example, US Assembly of Life Sciences, 1981a; IARC, 1985). Many of these compounds are potent carcinogens, producing tumours in a variety of sites in experimental animals, (Druckrey *et al.*, 1967; Preussmann and Stewart, 1984).

There is evidence that N-nitroso compounds act as carcinogens also in humans. In cancer chemotherapy, derivatives of cytostatic 2-chloroethylnitrosoureas induced an increased incidence of secondary tumours, especially leukaemias, after relatively short latency periods (Boice *et al.*, 1983). Winn (1984) reported that there was a high probability of a causal relationship between the use of chewing tobacco ('snuff dipping'), a practice prevalent in some southern states of the USA, and an increased incidence of oral cancer.

Furthermore, humans have been found to react to nitrosamines in a manner comparable to laboratory animals in terms of acute toxicity, metabolic disposition and the formation of DNA adducts (Freund, 1937; Barnes and Magee, 1954; Fussganger and Ditschuneit, 1980; Preussmann, 1990).

Intense efforts have been directed at establishing a causal association between exposure to N-nitroso compounds (pre-formed in foods or synthesized endogenously) and the incidence of cancers in humans. The intakes of nitrate and nitrite by children and their parents from foods and drinking water were estimated in a nation-wide case-control study in Finland and a study of the epidemiology of Type 1 diabetes in Finnish children. The findings of the study give evidential support to the suggestion that pre-formed nitrosamines in the diet and endogenously formed N-nitroso compounds may be associated with the development of Type 1 diabetes in children (Virtanen *et al.*, 1994). A case-control study of maternal diet during pregnancy and the risk of astrocytoma, the most common childhood brain tumour, was conducted by the the Children's Cancer Group in the USA and Canada. The study included 155 cases aged under 6 years at diagnosis and the same number of randomly selected matched controls. A trend was observed for consumption of cured meats containing pre-formed nitrosamines and precursors, but the effect of several dietary factors differing by income levels made the interpretation of results difficult (Bunin *et al.*, 1994). The conclusions of another study on the association between the maternal consumption of cured meats and vitamins and the development of paediatric brain tumours suggested that the exposure during gestation to endogenously formed N-nitroso compounds may be linked to brain tumour occurrence (PrestonMartin *et al.*, 1996). A population-based case-control study of 416 incident gliomas in adults was carried out in Australia to examine the association between dietary intake of N-nitroso compounds and precursors and the risk of glioma. The data analysed by multiple logistic regression provided only limited support to the N-nitroso compound hypothesis of glioma carcinogenesis (Giles *et al.*, 1994). A population-based case-control study was carried out in western Washington state, USA, to investigate whether the consumption of foods and beverages containing nitrosdimethylamine, nitrate and nitrite affected the risk of laryngeal, oesopheageal and oral cancers. The authors concluded that the results indicated that nitrosation may be a factor in the aetiology of upper aerodigestive tract cancers (Rogers *et al.*, 1995). A considerable number of geographical correlation studies have been conducted, but firm incontrovertible evidence is still lacking (Moller and Forman, 1991).

Human dosimetry studies have provided clear evidence of the formation of endogenous nitrosation products. Bartsch *et al.* (1990) carried out the NPRO test on subjects at high risk of cancers of the stomach, oesophagus, oral cavity and urinary bladder. In most instances higher exposures to nitroso compounds (NOC) were found in high-risk subjects but individual exposure was greatly affected by dietary modifiers or a disease state. These researchers also investigated the urinary excretion of 3-methyladenine (3-MeAde) as a marker of NOC–DNA adduct formation. Humans were found normally to excrete 3-MeAde, the origin of which is not known. Preliminary results suggested a weak correlation between basal NPRO excretion and background 3- MeAde excretion.

Stillwell *et al.* (1991) measured the urinary excretion of nitrate, NPRO, 3-MeAd and 7-methylguanine (7-MeG) in a population at high risk from gastric cancer. They observed a good correlation between urinary nitrate and NPRO for the entire population and a stronger correlation for a subset of the population with more advanced gastric pathology, i.e. with gastric metaplasia and displasia. The authors suggest that these observations are consistent with the hypothesis that urinary NPRO excretion is indicative of the involvement of *N*-nitroso compounds in the aetiology of gastric cancer.

Moller and Forman (1991), in reviewing the data on the urinary excretion of NPRO and cancer incidence in a number of studies, came to the conclusion that the NPRO test results appeared to be highest in high-risk areas but most clearly so (and only with a statistical difference) in China and Japan. The authors struck a cautionary note by stating that correlation studies may be subject to biases which arise from the presence of other, perhaps unknown, determinants of disease risks which have different prevalences in the populations studied. In the opinion of the authors, correlation studies are not ideal for the prediction of the determinants of disease risk to individuals.

To conclude, although considerable progress has been made to show that human exposure to *N*-nitroso compounds occurs from pre-formed dietary and endogenous sources, conclusive proof of a carcinogenic effect in humans from *N*-nitroso compounds is lacking.

SUMMARY, RISK EVALUATION AND CONCLUSIONS

Nitrate: Human Body Burden

Estimated Dietary Intake

Estimates of nitrate intake per day from food range from about 31 mg in Norway to 113 mg in The Netherlands

and 127 mg in Poland, 80–85% of which is derived from vegetables. In the UK the estimated mean dietary intake is 54 mg day^{-1} and for vegetarians the intakes range from 185 to 194 mg day^{-1}.

The drinking water nitrate content in The Netherlands ranges from no detectable amount to 21.0 mg nitrate ion l^{-1}. Assuming a daily intake of 2 l of drinking water, nitrate intakes would range from no detectable amount to 42 mg nitrate ion day^{-1}. Assuming an average daily intake of 108 mg of nitrate ion from food, the estimated average total dietary intake of nitrate in The Netherlands would range from 108 to 150 mg nitrate ion day^{-1}. For 60 kg adults this would give rise to dietary intakes of 1.8–2.5 mg nitrate ion (kg body weight)$^{-1}$.

In the case of infant formulations requiring dilution with drinking water, assuming a fluid intake of 165 ml (kg body weight)$^{-1}$ for a 3-month-old infant weighing 5.6 kg, the daily nitrate intake, based on the nitrate content in drinking water in The Netherlands, could be upto 3.5 mg nitrate (kg body weight)$^{-1}$. As stated earlier, this figure could rise to 8.2 mg nitrate (kg body weight)$^{-1}$ if the nitrate content of water used for preparing the formulation complied with the EC drinking water maximum limit of 50 mg nitrate ion l^{-1}.

In the UK, the average total nitrate intake in over 80% of the population provided with drinking water containing < 30 mg nitrate ion l^{-1} is estimated at about 114 mg nitrate ion day^{-1} [1.9 mg (kg body weight)$^{-1}$]. In the case of vegetarians this figure could rise to 245–254 mg nitrate ion day^{-1} [4.1–4.2 mg nitrate ion (kg body weight)$^{-1}$].

Endogenous Synthesis

The biosynthesis of nitrate in adults and infants has been estimated to be about 60 mg day^{-1} [i.e. approximately 1 mg nitrate ion (kg body weight)$^{-1}$]. Intestinal infections and diarrhoea, a not uncommon illness in infants, have been shown to induce a 7–15-fold increase in endogenous nitrate synthesis. Infections in adults have been reported to produce a similar increase.

Total body burden

In healthy adults, the estimated average total daily nitrate body burden from dietary sources (based on The Netherlands estimates) and endogenous synthesis [i.e. 1 mg nitrate ion (kg body weight)$^{-1}$] would be about 2.8–3.5 mg nitrate ion (kg body weight)$^{-1}$ and in the case of vegetarians (based on the UK estimates) it would be 5.1–5.2 mg nitrate ion (kg body weight)$^{-1}$. The total body burden in infants fed infant formulations would be up to a maximum of 4.5 mg nitrate ion (kg body weight)$^{-1}$. In the event of infections, a 7–15-fold increase in endogenous synthesis of nitrate could increase the total body burden in adults on a mixed diet to 8.8–17.5 mg nitrate ion kg^{-1} and in infants to 10.5–18.5 mg nitrate ion (kg body weight)$^{-1}$.

Nitrate: Human Body Burden

Estimated Dietary Intake

The UK survey estimated the adult intake of nitrite from foods and beverages to be in the range 2.4–4.2 mg nitrite ion day^{-1}; assuming an intake of 2 l of drinking water complying with the EC maximum permitted limit of 0.1 mg nitrite ion l^{-1} the total intake of nitrite would be 2.6–4.4 mg nitrite ion day^{-1} [i.e. 0.04–0.07 mg nitrite ion (kg body weight)$^{-1}$]. The estimated intake of nitrite by infants on infant formulations [165 ml (kg body weight)$^{-1}$] would be < 0.02 mg nitrite ion (kg body weight)$^{-1}$.

Endogenous Synthesis

In man, nitrite is formed mainly in the mouth by micro-flora-mediated reduction of salivary nitrate. About 25% of ingested nitrate is secreted in the saliva and of this about 20% is converted to nitrite; thus, about 5% of dietary nitrate is reduced to nitrite. This represents 0.09–0.13 mg nitrite ion (kg body weight)$^{-1}$ in adults on a mixed diet and about 0.21 mg nitrite ion (kg body weight)$^{-1}$ in vegetarians. In infants on formulations the amount of nitrite formed would be up to a maximum of 0.18 mg (kg body weight)$^{-1}$. Fasting levels of salivary nitrate have been reported to be about 5–10 mg l^{-1}, presumably from the endogenous nitrate pool. Salivary concentrations of both nitrate and nitrite have been found to be proportional to the amount of nitrate ingested. However, marked inter-individual and diurnal differences have been observed in the salivary concentrations of nitrate and nitrite, making it difficult to assess the extent of nitrite formation from endogenous and dietary sources of nitrate.

Total Body Burden

The estimated total body burden of nitrite in adults based on dietary intake and endogenously synthesized nitrite derived from ingested nitrate in a mixed diet is in the range 0.13–0.20 mg nitrite ion (kg body weight)$^{-1}$, and from a vegetarian diet it would be 0.25–0.28 mg nitrite ion (kg body weight)$^{-1}$. In the case of infants it would be a maximum of about 0.20 mg nitrite ion (kg body weight)$^{-1}$. These figures do not take into account the contribution to the body burden of nitrite formed from endogenously synthesized nitrate. Furthermore, gastro-intestinal and urinary tract infections are likely to increase endogenous nitrite formation.

N-Nitroso Compounds: Human Body Burden

Estimated Dietary Intake

The estimated intake of apparent total N-nitroso compounds (ATNC) in adults consuming the relevant foods in the UK survey was 36 µg N-NO day^{-1} and for 97.5th percentile consumers the intake was estimated to be 140 µg N-NO day^{-1}. Identified nitrosamines (NDMA, NDEA, NPIP, NPYR) accounted for less than 10% of the ingested ATNC.

Endogenous Synthesis

In view of the complexities of the chemistry of nitrosation products and the influence of substrate availability, nitrite ion concentration, pH conditions and reaction kinetics on their formation, it is difficult to characterize and quantify the N-nitroso compounds formed in vivo. Further complications arise from the lability and metabolic biotransformation of the reaction products. Rowland et al. (1991) have assessed endogenous N-nitrosation in man by measuring ATNC in faeces. Subjects were placed on a diet low in nitrate and ATNC for 8 days. At the end of this period ATNC in the faeces ranged from below the 40 µg N-NO kg^{-1} detection limit up to 143 µg N-NO kg^{-1} (mean 82 µg N – NO kg^{-1}). On supplementing this diet with 300 mg nitrate day^{-1}, faecal ATNC increased markedly and on the third day on this regime values were in the range 73–714 µg N-NO kg^{-1} with a mean of 307µg N – NO kg^{-1}. The results, together with the known limited occurrence of ATNC in the majority of foodstuffs tested, suggested that the ATNC in the faeces was formed endogenously from nitrosation species derived from the ingested nitrate. The urinary excretion of NPRO has been used by many researchers as an index of in vivo nitrosation reactions and the basal rate of NPRO excretion in subjects on a low nitrate diet and not dosed with nitrite or proline has been found to be 2–7 µg day^{-1} (Oshima and Bartsch, 1981). There is uncertainty, however, as to whether NPRO excretion truly reflects the total endogenous N-nitroso compounds formed. NPRO, a stable non-carcinogenic nitrosamino acid, is only readily formed and excreted unchanged, whereas NDMA and NDEA are only slowly formed but rapidly metabolized in vivo. There is evidence showing that certain drugs, e.g. amidopyrine, are nitrosatable in vivo, leading to the formation of NDMA (Spiegelhalder, 1990).

Total Body Burden

In view of the uncertainty of the identity of N-nitroso compounds in the diet and formed endogenously, it is not possible to estimate with any certainty the total body burden. Choi (1985) constructed a mathematical model to estimate both the exogenous intake and endogenous formation of nitrate, nitrite and NDMA. However, the model does not take into account variations in the metabolism of nitrate, nitrite and *N*-nitroso compounds among individuals that are due to differences in physiology, age and general health.

Toxicological Data

Nitrate: Animal Studies

Rats

The no observed adverse effect level in a 2-year carcinogenicity study carried out by Lijinsky *et al.* (1973) on MRC-derived rats was 500 mg $NaNO_3$ (kg body weight)$^{-1}$, confirming the findings of an earlier study by Lehman (1958). Maekawa *et al.* (1982) reported a no observed adverse effect level of 2500 mg $NaNO_3$ (kg body weight)$^{-1}$ in F-344 rats. The latter study was carried out up to higher dose levels, in contrast to the earlier ones where no observed adverse effects were seen at the maximum treatment dose used.

Til *et al.* (1985), based on a 4-week study of Wistar rats treated with KNO_3, reported a no-effect dose level of 500 mg (kg body weight)$^{-1}$. Adverse effects noted were the development of a dose-related small increase in methaemoglobinaemia (not exceeding 1.5%) in female animals and a dose-related increase in the relative kidney weight in males. Maekawa *et al.* (1982) found a no-effect level of 2500 mg $NaNO_3$ (kg body weight)$^{-1}$ in a 6-week study of F-344 rats.

Mice

Survival and growth were normal when $NaNO_3$ was administered at up to 5% in the diet [approximately 7.5 g $NaNO_3$ (kg body weight)$^{-1}$] to ICR mice for life. There was no treatment-related increase in tumour incidence (Sugiyama *et al.*, 1979).

Data from the above animal studies suggest that the no-effect level of 500 mg $NaNO_3$ (kg body weight)$^{-1}$ [365 mg nitrate (kg body weight)$^{-1}$] accepted by WHO (1974) may be a conservative estimate and could be increased to 2500 mg $NaNO_3$ (kg body weight)$^{-1}$ [1824 mg nitrate ion (kg body weight)$^{-1}$].

Nitrite: Animal Studies

Rats

The no-effect level in a 2-year study in rats given KNO_2 in the drinking water was found to be 10 mg $NaNO_2$ (kg body weight)$^{-1}$ (Gruener and Shuval, 1973). The main adverse effect noted was a dose-related development of methaemoglobinaemia; other effects noted included histopathological changes in the heart, lung, liver, spleen and kidney. There was no

evidence of a treatment-related increase in tumour incidence.

Various carcinogenicity studies in the rat were negative and some even showed a reduction in tumour risk (e.g. lymphomas or leukaemias) (Lijinsky *et al.*, 1983; Grant and Butler, 1989). Studies by Shank and Newberne (1976) and Newberne (1978, 1979) reported an increase in lymphoid tumours but this was ruled out by an expert peer review group after giving due consideration to the control data.

Til *et al.* (1988) carried out a 13-week study in rats treated with KNO_2 in the drinking water. Methaemoglobinaemia was significantly increased in the top-dose group (3000 mg KNO_2 l^{-1}). Interestingly, hypertrophy of the adrenal zona glomerulosa was observed in all test groups. The no adverse effect dose level was found to be lower than 10 mg KNO_2 (kg body weight)$^{-1}$.

In a supplementary study, Til *et al.* (1990) found the no-effect level for the adrenal zona glomerulosa hypertrophy to be 5 mg KNO_2 (kg body weight)$^{-1}$ day^{-1} [3 mg NO_2 ion (kg body weight)$^{-1}$ day^{-1}]. Nitrate administration in the rat failed to produce the adrenal effect. The pathological significance of this finding in the rat and its relevance to humans await clarification.

Other Effects

Nitrite has been shown to be foetotoxic in the rat and guinea-pig, due mainly to hypoxia in the developing foetuses caused by maternal methaemoglobinaemia. Nitrite gave positive results in a battery of *in vitro* and *in vivo* mutagenicity test systems.

Animal toxicity studies show that the main adverse effects of nitrite stem from the formation of methaemoglobinaemia. The animal toxicity data suggest a no adverse effect level of 10 mg $NaNO_2$ (kg body weight)$^{-1}$ [6.67 mg nitrite ion (kg body weight)$^{-1}$].

N-Nitroso Compounds: Animal Studies

Most of the volatile *N*-nitrosamines and nitrosamides so far tested in experimental animals have been found to be potent and versatile carcinogens. However, it is difficult to evaluate the animal toxicity data in terms of the carcinogenic risk from pre-formed total *N*-nitroso compounds in the human diet. As stated earlier, dietary *N*-nitroso compounds constitute a complex and ill-defined mixture containing less than 10% of identified nitrosamines. *N*-Nitroso compounds formed endogenously by the interaction of nitrite with precursor amines and amides represent potentially a more serious carcinogenic hazard. The co-administration of nitrite and precursor amines in experimental animals has been shown to be carcinogenic in many studies, but in these studies unrealistically high doses of nitrite and amines and amides were used. The relevance of the findings are therefore questionable. As mentioned earlier, carcinogenicity studies on nitrite alone have failed to demonstrate a positive effect.

Human Data: Risk Evaluation

Human Body Burden/Animal Toxicity Data Relationship

The estimated human intakes of nitrate and nitrite (based on the UK and Dutch data) are given in **Table 14**.

The observed no-effect levels of nitrate and nitrite in animal toxicity studies, accepted by JECFA and many regulatory authorities for developing acceptable daily intake (ADI) figures, are 365 mg nitrate ion (kg body weight)$^{-1}$ and 6.7 mg nitrite ion (kg body weight)$^{-1}$, respectively. Thus, the safety factors of estimated human nitrate intake as a ratio of the animal observed no-effect level in adults range from $\times 146$ to $\times 94$ in the 'worst case' intake situation, and in infants the range is from $\times 104$ to $\times 45$.

In the case of nitrite, in addition to the ingested nitrite, about 5% of the dietary nitrate is capable of being reduced to nitrite endogenously, i.e. 0.13–0.20 mg nitrite ion (kg body weight)$^{-1}$ in adults and 0.18–0.41 mg nitrite ion (kg body weight)$^{-1}$ in infants. Thus, the total nitrite exposure from dietary sources and from endogenous formation in adults ranges from 0.17 to 0.27 mg nitrite ion (kg body weight)$^{-1}$, and for infants from < 0.20 to 0.43 mg nitrite ion (kg body weight)$^{-1}$, representing safety factors of $\times 39$ to $\times 25$ in adults and $\times 34$ to $\times 16$ in infants.

These figures do not take into account endogenously formed nitrate in humans [about 1 mg nitrate ion (kg body weight)$^{-1}$] which may be available for metabolism to nitrite, thereby contributing an additional 0.05 mg nitrite ion (kg body weight)$^{-1}$ to the body pool. In the event of bacterial infections of the gastro-intestinal tract or at other sites, a condition not uncommon in infants, endogenous nitrate synthesis may be increased by 7–15-fold. This could generate 0.35–0.75 mg nitrite ion (kg body weight)$^{-1}$.

Animal studies carried out on orally administered nitrate and nitrite have shown that neither compound is carcinogenic or teratogenic. Epidemiological studies thus far have failed to provide convincing evidence that nitrate in the diet or as a result of occupational exposure is responsible for human cancers or birth defects.

Nitrite is a reactive molecule and the main site of toxic attack is the blood due to the oxidation of haemoglobin by nitrite to form methaemoglobin. The toxicological sequelae in experimental animals and in humans stem from the resulting compromised oxygen-carrying capacity in the circulation.

Infants are a special 'at risk' group as foetal haemoglobin is more susceptible to oxidation to methaemoglobin than mature haemoglobin and neonates are also deficient in methaemoglobin reductase activity. Furthermore, low gastric acid secretion in infants favours bacterial colonization of the stomach with the possibility of enhanced reduction of nitrate to nitrite.

Viewed in the light of the above comments, the adequacy of the safety margin for ingested nitrite (derived from 'free' nitrite plus 5% of nitrate in diet), estimated to be $\times 39$ to $\times 25$ in adults and $\times 34$ to $\times 16$ in infants, may need to be re-examined.

Conclusions

In assessing the health risks to man from dietary exposure to nitrate, nitrite and *N*-nitroso compounds, it is important to recognize that apart from the case of pre-weaned neonates on formulation diets prepared with drinking water, food is the main source of dietary nitrate for the human population, vegetables providing over 85% of nitrate in the diet. Furthermore, nitrite and *N*-nitroso compounds present in the diet contribute relatively small amounts to the body burden and the major source of these biologically active compounds is derived from ingested nitrate. Nitrate is readily metabolised by buccal/gastro-intestinal bacterial and by mammalian enzyme systems to nitrite, and the subsequent reactions of the endogenously formed nitrite with amines, amides and amino acids leads to the formation of *N*-nitroso compounds in the body. Thus, vegetables constitute not only the principal human dietary source of nitrate, but also indirectly of nitrite and *N*-nitroso compounds.

Nitrate *per se* is of relatively low toxicity and chronic studies have shown that it did not increase tumour incidence in experimental animals.

Nitrite has been found to be non-carcinogenic in animal studies. The main manifestation of nitrite acute toxicity in experimental animals and in humans is the elevation of circulating methaemoglobin levels and the consequent compromised oxygen-carrying capacity of the blood. A recent sub-chronic study has shown that nitrite (administered as KNO_2 in the drinking water) produced mild hypertrophy of the adrenal zona glomerulosa in the rat; this effect was not produced when nitrate was administered. The pathogenesis of the adrenal

Table 14 Estimated human intakes of nitrate and nitrite

Intake	Nitrate ion [mg (kg bw)$^{-1}$ day^{-1}] Adults	Infants	Nitrate ion [mg (kg bw)$^{-1}$ day^{-1}] Adults	Infants
Food:				
Mixed diet	1.8	–	0.04–0.07	–
Vegetarians	3.08–3.23			
Water	0–0.7	3.5–8.2	< 0.002	< 0.02
Total	2.5–3.9	3.5–8.2	0.04–0.07	< 0.02

hypertrophic effect in the rat and its toxicological relevance in the risk assessment of nitrite to humans needs to be investigated further.

Most of the volatile *N*-nitrosamines and nitrosamides so far tested have been found to be potent and versatile carcinogens affecting a variety of target sites in experimental animals. Many of these compounds are also present in minute amounts in the human diet. Additionally, the human diet contains *N*-nitroso compounds of unknown identity. Furthermore, there is clear evidence showing that nitrosation reactions can occur *in vivo*, leading to the endogenous formation of *N*-nitroso compounds. Whereas *N*-nitrosamides are direct-acting carcinogens, *N*-nitrosamines require metabolic activation to exert their carcinogenic effects. The enzyme systems responsible for the bio-activation of *N*-nitrosamines in experimental animals have also been found in human tissues. Hence it is probable that these compounds are also potential human carcinogens.

Epidemiological studies have failed to provide evidence of a causal association between nitrate exposure and human cancer incidence. Similarly, intense efforts directed at establishing a causal link between *N*-nitroso compounds, pre-formed in the diet or endogenously synthesized, and the incidence of human cancers have thus far been unsuccessful in generating clear and unequivocal evidence. On the other hand, there is convincing evidence showing that the consumption of vegetables is associated with a reduced cancer risk in humans. Vegetables, in addition to being a major contributor of dietary nitrate, are also an important source of essential micronutrients and antioxidants such as ascorbic acid, tocopherols, carotenoids and flavonoids. These components have been found to afford protection against some of the toxic effects of nitrite (e.g. methaemoglobinaemia) and prevent the formation of *N*-nitroso compounds in the body. Hence there is no firm scientific evidence to support the conclusion that dietary nitrate, derived principally from vegetables, constitutes a serious health hazard to man. However, to avoid unnecessary high peak body burdens of nitrate, it would plainly be desirable and prudent to limit nitrate levels in vegetables in keeping with good agricultural practice.

REFERENCES

Agunod, M., *et al.* (1969). Correlative study of hydrochloric acid, pepsin and intrinsic factor secretion in newborn and infants. *Am. J. Dig. Disorders*, **14**, 400–414.

Alavantic, D., *et al.* (1988). *In vivo* genotoxicity of nitrates and nitrites in germ cells of male mice. II. Unscheduled DNA synthesis and sperm abnormality after treatment of spermatids. *Mutat. Res.*, **204**, 689.

Al-Dabbagh, S. A., *et al.* (1986). Mortality of nitrate ferilizer workers. *Br. J. Ind. Med.*, **43**, 507–515.

Arbuckle, T. E., *et al.* (1988). Water nitrates and CNS birth defects: a population-based case-control study. *Arch. Environ. Health*, **43**, 162.

Balish, E., *et al.* (1981). Distribution and metabolism of nitrate and nitrite in rats. *Banbury Rep.*, No. 7, 305–317, 337–341.

Barnes, J. M. and Magee, P. N. (1954). Some toxic properties of dimethylnitrosamine. *Br. J. Ind. Med.*, **11**, 167–174.

Bartholomew, B. A. and Hill, M. J. (1984). The pharmacology of dietary nitrate and the origin of urinary nitrate. *Food Chem. Toxicol.*, **22**, 789–795.

Bartholomew, B. A., *et al.* (1980). Gastric bacteria, nitrate, nitrite and nitrosamines in patients with pernicious anaemia and in patients treated with cimetidine. *IARC Publication No. 31*. IARC, Lyon, pp. 595–608.

Bartsch, H., *et al.* (1990). Exposure of humans to endogenous *N*-nitroso compounds: implications in cancer etiology. *Mutat. Res.*, **238**, 255–267.

Behroozi, K., *et al.* (1971). Changes in the motor activity of mice given sodium nitrite in drinking solution. In *Proceedings of a Symposium on Environmental Physiology, Beersheba* (cited by Speijers *et al.*, 1987).

Bellander, T. (1990). Nitrosation of piperazine after oral intake or inhalation exposure. *Drug Dev. Eval.*, **16**, 213–233.

Bhagat, K. and Vallance, P. (1996). Nitric oxide 9 years on. *J. R. Soc. Med.*, **88**, 667–673.

Bjelke, E. (1980). Epidemiology of colorectal cancer, with emphasis on diet. In Maltoni, C. (Ed.), *Advances in Tumour Prevention, Detection and Characterisation*. Excerpta Medica, Amsterdam, pp. 158–174.

Beresford, S. A. (1985). Is nitrate in drinking water associated with the risk of stomach cancer in the urban U. K.? *Int. J. Epidemiol.*, **14**, 57–63.

Boeing, H., *et al.* (1991). Case-control study of stomach cancers in Germany. *Int. J. Cancer*, **47**, 858–864.

Boice, J., *et al.* (1983). Leukemia and preleukemia after adjuvant treatment of gastrointestinal cancer with semimustine (methyl-CCNU). *New Engl. J. Med.*, **309**, 1079–1084.

Budayova, E. (1985). Effects of sodium nitrite and potassium sorbate on *in vitro* cultured mammalian cells. *Neoplasma*, **32**, 341–350.

Buiatti, E., *et al.* (1990). A case-control study of gastric cancer and diet in Italy. II. Association with nutrients. *Int. J. Cancer*, **45**, 896–901.

Bunin, G. R., *et al.* (1994). Maternal diet and risk of astrocytic glioma in children. A report from the Children's Cancer Group (United States and Canada). *Cancer Causes Control*, **5**, 177–187.

Calmels, S., *et al.* (1987). Biochemical studies on the catalysis of nitrosation by bacteria. *Carcinogenesis*, **8**, 1085–1088.

Carlson, G. P. (1990). Induction of *N*-nitrosodimethylamine metabolism in rat liver and lung by ethanol. *Cancer Lett.*, **54**, 153–156.

Castillo, L., *et al.* (1996). Whole body nitric oxide synthesis in healthy men determined from [^{15}N]arginine to [^{15}N]citrulline labelling. *Proc. Natl. Acad. Sci. USA*, **93**, 11460–11465.

Challis, B. C. and Kryptopoulous, S. A. (1978). The chemistry of nitroso compounds. Part 12. The mechanism of nitrosation and nitration of aqueous piperidine by gaseous dinitrogen tetraoxide and dinitrogen trioxide in aqueous alkaline solutions. Evidence for the existence of molecular isomers of dinitrogen tetraoxide and dinitrogen trioxide. *J. Chem. Soc., Perkin Trans. 2*, 1296–1302.

Choi, B. C. K. (1985). *N*-nitroso compounds and human cancer: a molecular epidemiological approach. *Am. J. Epidemiol.*, **121**, 737–743.

Choi, N. W., *et al.* (1987). Consumption of precursors of *N*-nitroso compounds and human gastric cancer. *IARC Sci. Publ.*, **84**, 492–496.

Chow, C. K., *et al.* (1980). Effect of nitrate and nitrite in drinking water on rats. *Toxicol. Lett.*, **6**, 199–206.

Clough, P. W. L. (1983). Nitrates and gastric carcinogenesis. *Miner. Environ.*, **5**, 91–95.

Conrad, K. P., *et al.* (1993). Identification of increased nitric oxide biosynthesis during pregnancy in rats. *FASEB J.*, **7**, 566–571.

Cornee, J., *et al.* (1992). An estimate of nitrate, nitrite and *N*-nitrosodimethylamine concentrations in French food products or food groups. *Sci. Aliments*, **12**, 155–197.

Corre, W. J. and Breimer, T. (1979). Nitrate and nitrite in vegetables. *PUDOC Lit. Surv.*, No.39.

Couch, D. B. and Friedman, M. A. (1975). Interactive mutagenicity of sodium nitrite, dimethlyamine, methylurea and ethylurea. *Mutat. Res.*, **31**, 109–114.

Crawford, R. F. (1960). Some effects of nitrate in forage on ruminant animals. PhD Thesis, Cornell University, Ithaca, NY.

Crespi, M., *et al.* (1986). Intragastric nitrosation and precancerous lesions of the gastro-intestinal tract: testing of a hypothesis. *Proceedings of the 9th International Meeting on N-Nitroso Compounds, Vienna, 1986*. See RIVM Report 758473007.

Davison, K. L., *et al.* (1965). Responses in pregnant ewes fed forages containing various levels of nitrate. *J. Dairy Sci.*, **48**, 968–977.

DeVries, Th. (1983). *Onderzoek naar de Toxiciteit van Nitriet*. Report U 275/83 Aig, Tox St/ah Nitriet Toxiciteit, RIVM, Bilthoven (cited in Speijers *et al.*, 1987).

Dolby, J. M., *et al.* (1984). Bacterial colonization and nitrite concentration in the achlorhydric stomachs of patients with primary hypogammaglobulinaemia or classical pernicious anaemia. *Scand. J. Gastroenterol.*, **19**, 105–110.

Druckrey, H., *et al.* (1963). Quantitative Analyse der Carcinogen Wirkung von Diethylnitrosamin. *Arzneim.-Forsch.*, **13**, 841–851.

Druckrey, H., *et al.* (1967). Organotrope carcinogene Wirkung bei 65 verschiedenen *N*-Nitrosoverbindungen. *Z. Krebsforsch.*, **69**, 103–201.

Dull, B. J. and Hotchkiss, J. H. (1984). Nitrate balance and biosynthesis in the ferret. *Toxicol. Lett.*, **23**, 79–89.

ECETOC (1988). *Nitrate in Drinking Water*. Technical Report No. 27. ECETOC, Brussels.

Eisenbrand, G., *et al.* (1980). Carcinogenicity of *N*-nitroso-3-hydroxypyrrolidine and dose–response study with *N*-nitrosopiperidine in rats. *IARC Publication No. 31*, IARC, Lyon, p. 657.

Eisenbrand, G., *et al.* (1996). *N*-Nitroso compounds in cosmetics, household commodities and cutting fluids. *Eur. J. Cancer Prev.*, **5** (Suppl. 1), 41–46.

Elder, J. B., *et al.* (1984). Effect of H2 blocker on intragastric nitrosation as measured by 24-hour urinary excretion of *N*-nitrosoproline. *IARC Publication No. 57*, IARC, Lyon, pp. 969–974.

Ellen, G. and Schuller, P. L. (1983). Nitrate, origin of continuous anxiety. In Preussman, R. (Ed.), *Das Nitrosamm Pro-* blem. Verlag Chemie, Weinheim, pp. 97–134 (cited by Speijers *et al.*, 1987).

Ellen, G., *et al.* (1982). Volatile *N*-nitrosamines, nitrate and nitrite in urine and saliva of healthy volunteers after administration of large amounts of nitrate. *IARC Publication No. 41*, IARC, Lyon, pp. 365–378.

Ellen, G., *et al.* (1990). Dietary intakes of some essential and non-essential trace elements, nitrate, nitrite and *N*-nitrosamines by Dutch adults: estimated via a 24-hour duplicate portion study. *Food Addit. Contam.*, **7**, 207–221.

El Nahas, S. M. *et al.* (1984). Chromosomal aberrations induced by sodium nitrite in bone marrow of adult rats and liver cells of transplacentally exposed embryos. *J. Toxicol. Environ. Health*, **13**, 643–647.

FDA (1980a). *Re-evaluation of the Pathology Findings of Studies on Nitrite and Cancer: Histologic Lesions in Sprague Dawley Rats*. Report of the Nitrite Task Force. Food and Drug Administration, Washington, DC.

FDA (1980b). *Evaluation of the MIT Nitrite Feeding Study to Rats*. Report of the Interagency Working Group on Nitrite Research. Food and Drug Administration, Washington, DC.

Fontham, E., *et al.* (1986). Diet and chronic atrophic gastritis: a case-control study. *J. Natl. Cancer Inst.*, **76**, 621–627.

Forman, D. (1991). Nitrate exposure and human cancer. In *Nitrate Contamination—Exposure, Consequence and Control*. NATO Conference held in Nebraska, USA. Springer-Verlag, Berlin, pp. 281–289.

Forman, D., *et al.* (1985a). Nitrates, nitrites and gastric cancer in Great Britain. *Nature*, **313**, 620–625.

Forman, D., *et al.* (1985b). Nitrate and gastric cancer risks. *Nature*, **317**, 676.

Freund, H. A. (1937). Clinical manifestations and studies in parenchymatous hepatitis. *Ann. Intern. Med.*, **10**, 1144–1155.

Fritsch, P., *et al.* (1985). Excretion of nitrates and nitrites in saliva and bile in the dog. *Food Chem. Toxicol.*, **23**, 655–659.

Fujimaki, H., *et al.* (1993). Further studies on the effect of nitrogen dioxide on mast cells: effect of the metabolite, nitrite. *Environ. Res.*, **61**, 223–231.

Fussganger, R. D. and Ditschuneit, H. (1980). Lethal exitus of a patient with *N*-nitrosodimethylamine poisoning 2.5 years following the first ingestion and signs of intoxication. *Oncology*, **37**, 273–277.

Gangolli, S. D., *et al.* (1994). Assessment: nitrate, nitrite and *N*-nitroso compounds. *Eur. J. Pharmacol.*, **292**, 1–38.

Gavinelli, M. R. *et al.* (1988). Volatile nitrosamines in foods and beverages: preliminary survey of the Italian market. *Bull. Environ. Contam. Toxicol.*, **40**, 41–46.

Gilli, G., *et al.* (1984). Concentrations of nitrate in drinking water and incidence of gastric carcinomas; first description of study in the Piedmonte region, Italy. *Sci. Total Environ.*, **34**, 35–48.

Giles, G. G., *et al.* (1994). Dietary factors and the risk of glioma in adults: results of a case-control study in Melbourne, Australia. *Int. J. Cancer*, **59**, 357–362.

Gislason, J. and Dahle, H. K. (1980). Nitrat og nitritt i vart mijo og kosthold. *Norsk Vet.-Tidsskr.*, **92**, 557–567.

Goldhohm, R. A., *et al.* (1994). A prospective cohort study on the relation between meat consumption and the risk of colon cancer. *Cancer Res.*, **54**, 718–723.

Gough, D.A., Webb, K. S. and Coleman, R. F. (1978). Estimation of the volatile nitrosamine content of UK foods. *Nature*, **272**, 161–163.

Grant, D. and Butler, W. H. (1989). Chronic toxicity of NaNO$_2$ in the male F344 rat. *Food Chem. Toxicol.*, **27**, 565–571.

Green, L. C., *et al.* (1981a). Nitrate synthesis in the germ-free and conventional rat. *Science*, **212**, 56–58.

Green, L. C., *et al.* (1981b). Nitrate biosynthesis in man. *Proc. Natl. Acad. Sci. USA*, **78**, 7764–7768.

Green, L. C., *et al.* (1982). Nitrate in human and canine milk. *New Engl. J. Med.*, **306**, 1367–1368.

Greenblatt, M. and Mirvish, S. S. (1972). Dose–response studies with concurrent administration of piperazine and sodium nitrite to strain A mice. *J. Natl. Cancer. Inst.*, **46**, 1029–1034.

Groenen, P. J., *et al.* (1982). Formation of *N*- nitrosamines from food products, especially fish, under simulated gastric conditions. *IARC Publication No. 41*. IARC, Lyon, pp. 99–112.

Groenen, P. J. *et al.* (1985). Formation of nitrosodimethylamine in human gastric juice fluid after consumption of vegetables high in nitrate. In *Proceedings of the IVth European Nutrition Conference*, 1983, p. 310.

Gruener, N. and Shuval, H. I. (1973). Study on the toxicology of nitrites. *Environ. Qual. Saf.*, **2**, 219–229.

Hashimoto, S., *et al.* (1976). Dimethylnitrosamine formation in the gastro-intestinal tract of rats. *Food Cosmet. Toxicol.*, **14**, 553–556.

Hawkes, C. H., *et al.* (1992). Chronic low-dose exposure of sodium nitrite in VM strain mice: central system changes. *Hum. Exp. Toxicol.*, **11**, 279–281.

Hayashi, M., *et al.* (1981). Micronucleus tests on food additives. Annual Report. *Mutagen. Toxicol.*, **4**, 80.

Hecht, S. S. and Hoffmann, D. (1988). Tobacco-specific nitrosamines, an important group of carcinogens in tobacco and tobacco smoke. *Carcinogenicity*, **9**, 875–884.

Hecht, S. S. and Hoffmann, D. (1989). The relevance of tobacco-specific nitrosamines to human cancer. *Cancer Surv.* **8**, 273–294.

Hegesh, E. and Shiloah, J. (1982). Blood nitrate and infantile methaemoglobinaemia. *Clin. Chim. Acta*, **125**, 107–115.

Hoffmann, D., *et al.* (1982a). Tobacco specific nitrosamines: occurence and bioassays. *IARC Sci. Publ. Series No. 41*, 309–318.

Hoffmann, D. et al. (1982b). *N*-Nitrosodiethanolamine: analysis, formation in tobacco products and carcinogenicity in Syrian golden hamsters. *IARC Sci. Publ. Series No. 41*, 299–308.

Höring, H., *et al.* (1985). Zum Einfluss subchronischer Nitratappiklation mit Trinkwasser vornehmlich auf die Schilddrusse der Ratte (Radiojodtest). *Gesund Umwelt*, **4**, 1–15 (cited in ECETOC Report No. 27).

Höring, H., *et al.* (1988). Antithyroidale Umweltchemikalien. *Z. Gesampte Hyg.*, **34**, 170–173.

IARC (1978). *Monographs on the Evaluation of the Carcinogenic Risk of Chemicals to Humans. Some N-Nitroso. Compounds.* Monograph No. 17. IARC, Lyon.

IARC (1985). *Monographs on the Evaluation of the Carcinogenic Risk of Chemicals to Humans. Tobacco Habits Other Than Smoking: Betel-quid and Areca-nut Chewing; and Some Related Nitrosamines.* Monograph No. 37. IARC, Lyon.

Ignarro, L. J. (1990). Biosynthesis and metabolism of endothelium-derived nitric oxide. *Annu. Rev. Pharmacol. Toxicol.*, **30**, 535–560.

Inai, K., *et al.* (1979). Chronic toxicity of sodium nitrite in mice, with reference to its tumorigenicity. *Gann*, **70**, 203–208.

Institut pour une Politique Européenne de l'Environnement (1989). *Les Actes du Seminaire Européen Eaux-Nitrates.* Ministére de l'Environment, DPPER.

Inui, N., *et al.* (1979). Transplacental action of sodium nitrite on embryonic cells of Syrian golden hamsters. *Mutat. Res.*, **66**, 149–158.

Ishidate, M., *et al.* (1984). Primary mutagenicity screening of food additives currently used in Japan. *Food Chem. Toxicol.*, **22**, 626–636.

Jagerstad, M. and Nilsson, R. (1976). Intake of nitrate and nitrite of some Swedish consumers as measured by the duplicate portion technique. In *Proceedings of the Second Symposium on Nitrite in Meat Products, Zeist*, pp. 283–287.

Jahreis, G., *et al.* (1987). Growth impairment caused dietary nitrite intake regulated via hypothyroidism and decreased somatomedin. *Endocrinol. Exp.*, **21**, 171–180.

Jensen, O. M. (1982). Nitrate in drinking water and cancer in Northern Jutland, Denmark, with special reference to stomach cancer. *Ecotoxicol. Environ. Saf.*, **6**, 258–267.

Knight, T. M., *et al.*, (1990). Nitrate and nitrite exposure in Italian populations with different gastric cancer rates. *Int. J. Epidemiol.*, **19**, 510–515.

Kodama, F., *et al.* (1976). Mutagenic effect of sodium nitrite on cultured mouse cells. *Mutat. Res.*, **40**, 119–124.

Kontezka, W. A. (1974). Mutagenesis by nitrate reduction in *Escherichia coli*. In *Abstracts of American Society of Microbiology Annual Meeting*, Abstract No.G.106.

Laitinen, S., *et al.* (1993). Calculated dietary intakes of nitrate and nitrite by young Finns. *Food. Addit. Contam.*, **10**, 469–477.

Lancaster, J. R., Jr. (1992). Nitric oxide in cells. *Am. Sci.*, **80**, 248–259.

Leaf, C. D., *et al.* (1989a). L-Arginine is a precursor for nitrate biosynthesis in man. *Bichem. Biophys. Res. Commun.*, **163**, 1032–1037.

Leaf, C. D., *et al.* (1989b). Mechanisms of endogenous nitrosation. *Cancer Surv.*, **8**, 323–334.

Leaf, C. D., *et al.* (1990). In Moncada, S. and Higgs, E. A. (Eds), *Nitric Oxide from L-Arginine: a Bioregulatory System.* Elsevier, Amsterdam, pp. 291–299.

Leaf, C. D., *et al.*, (1991). Endogenous incorporation of nitric oxide by L-arginine into *N*-nitrosomorpholine stimulated by *Escherichia coli* lipopolysaccharide in the rat. *Carcinogenesis*, **12**, 537–539.

Leclerc, H., *et al.* (1991). Nitrates de l'eau de boisson et cancer. *Bull. Acad. Natl. Méd.*, **175**, 651–671.

Lee, K., *et al.* (1986). Nitrate, nitrite balance and *de novo* synthesis of nitrate in humans consuming cured meats. *Am. J. Clin. Nutr.*, **44**, 188–194.

Lehman, A. J. (1958). Nitrates and nitrites in meat products. *Q. Bull. Assoc. Food Drug Officers*, **22**, 136–138.

Leu, D., *et al.* (1986). Bericht über Nitrate im Trinkwasser-Standortbestimmung 1985. *Mitt. Geb. Lebensmittelunters. Hyg.*, **77**, 227–315.

Licht, W. R. and Deen, W. M. (1988). Theoretical model for predicting rates of nitrosamine and nitrosamide formation in the human stomach. *Carcinogenesis*, **9**, 2227–2237.

Lijinsky, W. and Kovatch, R. M. (1989). Chronic toxicity of sodium thiocyanate with NaNO$_2$ in F344 rats. *Toxicol. Ind. Health*, **5**, 25–29.

Lijinsky, W., *et al.* (1973). Feeding studies of nitrilotriacetic acid and derivatives in rats. *J. Natl. Cancer Inst.*, **50**, 1061–1063.

Lijinsky, W., *et al.* (1983). Species specificity in nitrosamine carcinogenesis. *Basic Life Sci.*, **24**, 63–75.

Lin, J. K. and Ho, Y. S. (1992). Hepatotoxicity and hepatocarcinogenicity in rats fed squid treated with or without exogenous nitrite. *Food Chem. Toxicol.*, **30**, 695–702.

Luca, D., *et al.* (1985). Chromosomal aberrations and micronuclei induced in rat and mouse bone marrow cells by sodium nitrate. *Mutat. Res.*, **55**, 121–125.

Maekawa, A., *et al.* (1982). Carcinogenicity studies of sodium nitrite and sodium nitrate in F-344 rats. *Food Chem. Toxicol.*, **20**, 25–33.

MAFF (1978). *Report on the Review of Nitrites and Nitrates in Cured Meats and Cheese.* FAC/REP/27. HMSO, London.

MAFF (1987). *Nitrate, Nitrite and N-Nitroso Compounds in Food.* Food Surveillance Paper No.20. HMSO, London.

MAFF (1992). *Nitrate, Nitrite and N-Nitroso Compounds in Food. Second Report.* Food Surveillance Paper No.32. HMSO, London.

Magee, P. N. (1989). The experimental basis for the role of nitroso compounds in human cancer. *Cancer Surv.*, **8**, 207–239.

Maki, T. *et al.* (1980). Estimate of the volatile nitrosamine content of Japanese food. *Bull. Environ. Contam. Toxicol.*, **25**, 257–261.

Mallett, A. K., *et al.* (1984). Hydrocolloid food additives and rat caecal microbial enzyme activities. *Food Chem. Toxicol.*, **22**, 415–418.

Mallett, A. K., *et al.* (1985). The role of oral nitrate in the nitrosation of ^{14}C-proline by conventional and germ-free rats. *Carcinogenesis*, **6**, 1585–1588.

Mallett, A. K., *et al.* (1988). Protein-related differences in the excretion of nitrosoproline by the rat—possible modifications of *de novo* nitrate synthesis. *Food Chem. Toxicol.*, **26**, 831–836.

Marletta, M. A. (1988). Mammalian synthesis of nitric oxide, nitrite, nitrate and N-nitrosating agents. *Chem. Res. Toxicol.*, **1**, 249–257.

Massey, R. C. and Lees (1992). Surveillance of preservatives and their interactions in foodstuffs. *Food Addit. Contam.*, **9**, 435–440.

Massey, R. C., *et al.* (1991). Volatile, non-volatile and N-nitroso compounds in bacon. *Food Addit. Contam.*, **8**, 585–598.

Mirvish, S. S., *et al.* (1975). Disappearance of nitrate from the rat stomach: contribution of emptying and other factors. *J. Natl. Cancer Inst.*, **54**, 869–875.

Miwa, M., *et al.* (1986). *N*-Nitrosamine formation by macrophages. *IARC Publication No. 84*, IARC, Lyon, pp. 340–344.

Møller, H. and Forman, D. (1991). Epidemiological studies of the endogenous formation of N-nitroso compounds. In *Nitrate—Exposure, Contamination and Control.* NATO Conference, Springer Verlag, Berlin, pp. 267–279.

Mueller, R. L., *et al.* (1983). The endogenous synthesis of carcinogenic N-nitroso compounds: bacterial flora and nitrite formation in the healthy human stomach. *Zentralbl. Bakteriol. Hyg. Abt. 1, Orig. Reihe, B*, **178**, 297–315.

Mueller, R. L., *et al.* (1986). Nitrate and nitrite in normal gastric juice. *Oncology*, **43**, 50–53.

Musil, J. (1966). Der Einfluss einer chronischen Natriumnitrit-intoxikation auf Ratte. *Acta Biol. Med. Ger.*, **16**, 388–392.

Nabrzyski, M. and Gajewska, R. (1989). Contents of nitrite and nitrate in the daily diets of students of a technical school and of infants and children. *Nutri. Abstr. Rev. Ser. A*, **59**, 616.

Newberne, P. M. (1978). *Dietary Nitrite in the Rat.* Final Report. FDA Contract: 74–2181. Food and Drug Administration, Washington, DC.

Newberne, P. M. (1979). Nitrite promotes lymphoma incidence in rats. *Science*, **204**, 1079–1081.

Nguyen, T, *et al.* (1992). DNA damage and mutation in human cells exposed to nitric oxide *in vitro. Proc. Natl. Acad. Sci. USA*, **89**, 3030–3034.

Nighat, S., *et al.* (1981). Induced nitrate poisoning in rabbits. *Pak. Vet. J.*, **1**, 10–12.

NIOSH (1987). *NIOSH Registry of Toxic Effects of Chemical Substances.* NIOSH, Cincinnati, Ohio.

Olsen, P., *et al.* (1984). Animal feeding study with nitrite treated meat. *IARC Publication No.57*, IARC, Lyon, pp. 667–675.

Oshima, H. and Bartsch, H. (1981). Quantitative estimation of endogenous nitrosation in humans by monitoring *N*-nitrosoproline excreted in the urine. *Cancer Res.*, **41**, 3658–3662.

Oshima, H., *et al.* (1982). Monitoring *N*-nitrosamino acid excreted in the urine and faeces of rats as an index of endogenous nitrosation. *Carcinogenesis*, **3**, 115–120.

Oshima, H., *et al.* (1989). Evidence of potential tumor-initiating and tumor-promoting activities of hickory smoke condensate when given alone or with nitrite to rats. *Food Chem. Toxicol.*, **27**, 511–516.

Oshima, H., *et al.* (1994). Increased nitrosamine and nitrate biosynthesis mediated by nitric oxide synthase induced in hamsters infected with liver fluke (*Opisthorchis viverrini*). *Carcinogenesis*, **15**, 271–275.

Österdahl, B.-G. (1988). Volatile nitrosamines in foods on the Swedish market and estimation of their daily intake. *Food Add. Contam.*, **5**, 587–595.

Palli, D., *et al.*, (1992). A case-control study of cancers of the gastric cardia in Italy. *Br. J. Cancer*, **65**, 263–266.

Park, K. K., *et al.* (1977). Mechanism of alkylation by N-nitroso compounds: detection of rearranged alcohol in the microsomal metabolism of *N*-nitrosodi-*n*-propylamine and base-catalyzed decomposition of *N*-*n*-propyl-*N*-nitrosourea. *Chem.–Biol. Interact.*, **18**, 349–354.

Park, K. K., *et al.* (1980). Alkylation of nucleic acids by *N*-nitrosodi-*n*-propylamine: evidence that carbonium ions are not significantly involved. *Chem.–Biol. Interact.*, **29**, 139–144.

Penttila, P.-L. (1990). Nitrate, nitrite and N-nitroso compounds in Finnish foods and estimation of their daily intakes. *Z. Lebendmitt. -Untersuch. Forsch.*, **190**, 336–340.

Philips, R. L. and Snowdon, D. A. (1985). Dietary relationships with fatal colorectal cancer among seventh-day adventists. *J. Natl. Cancer Inst.*, **74**, 307–317.

PrestonMartin, S., *et al.* (1996). Maternal consumption of cured meats and vitamins in relation to pediatric brain tumors. *Cancer Epidemiol. Biomarkers Prev.*, **5**, 599–605.

Preussmann, R. (1990). Carcinogenicity and structure–activity relationships of N-nitroso compounds. A review. *Drug Dev. Eval.*, **16**, 3–18.

Preussmann, R. and Stewart, B. (1984). *N*-Nitroso carcinogens. In Searle, C. E. (Ed.), *Chemical Carcinogens*, 2nd edn. American Chemical Society Monograph No. 182. American Chemical Society, Washington, DC, pp. 634–828.

Rademacher, J. J., *et al.*, (1992). Gastric cancer mortality and nitrate levels in Wisconsin drinking water. *Arch. Environ. Health*, **47**, 292–294.

Ralt, D., *et al.* (1988). Bacterial catalysis of nitrosation: involvement of the nar operon of *Escherichia coli*. *J. Bacteriol.*, **170**, 359–364.

Risch, H. A., *et al.* (1985). Dietary factors and the incidence of cancer of the stomach. *Am. J. Epidemiol.*, **122**, 947.

Rogers, M. A. M., *et al.* (1995). Consumption of nitrate, nitrite and nitrosodimethylamine and the risk of upper aerodigestive tract cancer. *Cancer Epidemiol. Biomarkers Prev.*, **4**, 29–36.

Roth, A. C., *et al.* (1987). Evaluation of the developmental toxicity of $NaNO_2$ in Long–Evans rats. *Fundam. Appl. Toxicol.*, **9**, 668–677.

Rowland, I. R., *et al.* (1991). Endogenous *N*- nitrosation in man assessed by measurement of apparent total *N*-nitroso compounds in faeces. *Carcinogenesis*, **12**, 1395–1401.

Rowland, I. R., *et al.*, (1996). Effect of dietary arginine on urinary nitrate excretion in germ-free rats. *Food Chem. Toxicol.*, **34**, 555–558.

Ruddell, W. S. J., *et al.* (1976). Gastric juice nitrite: a risk factor for cancer in the hypochlorhydic stomach? *Lancet*, **ii**, 1037–1039.

Ruddell, W. S. J., *et al.* (1978). Pathogenesis of gastric cancer in pernicious anaemia. *Lancet*, **i**, 521–523.

Saul, R. L. and Archer, M. C. (1984). Oxidation of ammonia and hydroxlamine to nitrate in the rat *in vitro*. *Carcinogenesis*, **5**, 77–81.

Schneider, N. R. and Yeary, R. A. (1975). Nitrite and nitrate pharmacokinetics in the dog, sheep and pony. *Am. J. Vet. Res.*, **36**, 941–947.

Schultz, D. S., *et al.* (1985). Pharmacokinetics of nitrate in humans: role of gastrointestinal absorption and metabolism. *Carcinogenesis*, **6**, 847–852.

Scragg, R. K., *et al.* (1982). Birth defects and household water supply. Epidemiological studies in the Mount Gambler region of South Australia. *Med. J. Aust.*, **2**, 577–579.

Seffner, W., *et al.* (1985). Zum Einfluss von subchronischer Nitratapplikation mit Trinkwasser auf die Schilddrusse der Ratte (morphologische Untersuchungen). *Gesund Umwelt*, **4**, 16–30 (cited in ECETOC Report No.27).

Selenka, F. and Brand-Grimm, D. (1976). Nitrat und Nitrit in der Ernährung des Menschen, Kalkulation der mittleren Tagesaufnahme und Abschatzung der Schwankungsbreite. *Zentralbl. Bakteriol. Hyg. Abt. 1, Orig. Reihe B*, **162**, 449–466.

Shank, R. C. and Newberne, P. M. (1976). Dose–response study of the carcinogenicity of dietary nirite and morpholine in rats. *Food Cosmet. Toxicol.*, **14**, 1–8.

Shephard, S. E., *et al.* (1987). Assessment of the risk of formation of carcinogenic *N*-nitroso compounds from dietary precursors in the stomach. *Food Chem. Toxicol.*, **25**, 91–108.

Shimada, T. (1989). Lack of teratogenic and mutagenic effects of nitrite on mouse fetuses. *Arch. Environ. Health*, **44**, 59–63.

Shuval, H. I. and Gruener, N. (1972). Epidemiological and toxicological aspects of nitrates and nitrites in the environment. *Am. J. Publ. Health*, **62**, 1045–1052.

Shuval, H. I. and Gruener, N. (1977). Infant methaemoglobinaemia and other health effects of nitrate in drinking water. *Prog. Water Technol.*, **8**, 183–193.

Sinha, D. P. and Sleight, S. D. (1971). Pathogenesis of abortion in acute nitrite toxicosis in gunea pigs. *Toxicol. Appl. Pharmacol.*, **18**, 340–347.

Sleight, S. D. and Atallah, O. A. (1968). Reproduction in the guinea-pig as affected by chronic administration of potassium nitrate and potassium nitrite. *Toxicol. Appl. Pharmacol.*, **12**, 179–185.

Smith, J. E. and Beutler, E. (1966). Methemoglobin formation and reduction in man and various animal species. *Am. J. Physiol.*, **210**, 347–350.

Snyder, S. H. and Bredt, D. S. (1992). Biological role of nitric oxide. *Sci. Am.*, **266**, 68–77.

Sollman, T. (1957). *A Manual of Pharmacology*. Saunders, Philadelphia and London.

Song, P. J. and Hu, J. F. (1988). N-nitrosamines in Chinese foods. *Food Chem. Toxicol.*, **26**, 205–208.

Speijers, G. J. A., *et al.* (1989). *Integrated Criteria Document. Nitrate Effects*. Report No. 758473007, RIVM, Bilthoven, Netherlands.

Spiegelhalder, B. (1990). Influence of dietary nitrate on *in vivo* nitrosation of amidopyrine in humans: use of the 'ethanol effect' for biological monitoring of *N*-nitrosodimethylamine in urine. *Drug Dev. Eval.*, **16**, 199–212.

Spiegelhalder, B. (1995). Environmental exposure to tobacco related NNOC. Presented at the 13th Annual ECP Symposium, October 1995, London.

Spiegelhalder, B. and Bartsch, H. (1996). Tobacco-specific nitrosamines. *Eur. J. Cancer Prev.*, **5**, (Suppl. 1), 33–38.

Spiegelhalder, B., *et al.* (1976). Influence of dietary nitrate on nitrite content of human saliva: possible relevance to *in vivo* formation of *N*-nitroso compounds. *Food. Cosmet. Toxicol.*, **14**, 545–548.

Spiegelhalder, B., *et al.* (1982). Urinary excretion of *N*-nitrosamines in rats and humans. *IARC Publication No. 41*. IARC, Lyon.

Statens Levnedsmiddelinstitut (1981). *Nitrat og Nitrit i Dansk Frugt og Grontsager*. Publication No.57. Eloni Tryk, Copenhagen.

Steinmetz, K. A. and Potter, J. D. (1991). Vegetables, fruit and cancer. I. Epidemiology. II. Mechanisms. *Cancer Causes Control*, **2**, 325–357 and 427–442.

Stemmermann, G. N. *et al.* (1984). Dietary fat and the risk of colorectal cancer. *Cancer Res.*, **44**, 1–6.

Stephany, R. W. and Schuller, P. L. (1978). The intake of nitrate, nitrite and volatile *N*-nitrosamines and the occurrence of volatile *N*-nitrosamines in human urine and veal calves. *IARC Sci. Publ.*, **19**, 443–460.

Stephany, R. W. and Schuller, P. L. (1980). The intake of nitrate, nitrite and *N*-nitrosamines and the occurrence of volatile *N*-nitrosamines in human urine and veal calves. *Oncology*, **73**, 203–210.

Stephany, R. W., *et al.* (1978). Nitrate, nitrite and *N*-nitrosamine contents in various types of Dutch cheese. *Neth. Milk Dairy J.*, **32**, 142–148.

Stillwell, W. J., *et al.* (1991). Urinary excretion of nitrate, *N*-nitrosoproline, 3-methyladenine, and 7-methylguanine in a Colombian population with high risk for stomach cancer. *Cancer Res.*, **51**, 190–194.

Stuehr, D. J. and Marletta, M. A. (1985). Mammalian nitrate biosynthesis: mouse macrophages produce nitrite and nitrate in response to *Escherichia coli* polysaccharides. *Proc. Natl. Acad. Sci. USA*, **82**, 7738–7742.

Stuehr, D. J. and Marletta, M. A. (1986). Further studies on murine macrophage synthesis of nitrite and nitrate. In *The Relevance of N-Nitroso Compounds to Human Cancer. IARC Publication No. 84*. IARC, Lyon, pp. 335–339.

Sugiyama, K., *et al.* (1979). Carcinogenicity examination of sodium nitrate in mice. *Acta Sch. Med. Univ. Gifu*, **27**, 1–6.

Sukegawa, K. and Matsumoto, T. (1975). Nitrate and nitrite contents in cow and human milk. *Eyio To Shokuryo*, **28**, 389–393.

Swann, P. F., *et al.* (1984). Ethanol and dimethylamine and diethylamine metabolism and disposition in the rat. Possible relevance to the influence of ethanol on human cancer incidence. *Carcinogenesis*, **5**, 1337–1343.

Tannenbaum, S. R. (1987). Endogenous formation of *N*-nitroso compounds: a current perspective. *IARC Publication No.84*. IARC, Lyon, pp. 292–296.

Tannenbaum, S. R., *et al.* (1976). The effect of nitrate intake on nitrite formation in human saliva. *Food Cosmet. Toxicol.*, **14**, 549–552.

Tannenbaum, S. R., *et al.* (1978). Nitrate and nitrite are formed by endogenous synthesis in the human intestine. *Science*, **200**, 1487–1489.

Tannenbaum, S. R., *et al.* (1994). DNA damage and cytotoxicity of nitric oxide. In Loeppky, R. A. and Michejda, C. J. (Eds.), *The Chemistry and Biochemistry of Nitrosamines and Other N-Nitroso Compounds*. American Chemical Society, Washington, DC, pp. 120–135.

Thal, W. *et al.* (1961). Welche Hämiglobinkonzentrationen sind bein Brunnenwasser-methämoglobinie noch mit Leben Vereinbar? *Arch. Toxicol.*, **19**, 25–33.

Thomas, H. F., *et al.* (1979). Nitrous acid mutagenesis of duplex DNA as a three-component system. *Mutat. Res.*, **61**, 129–151.

Thun, M. J., *et al.* (1992). Risk factors of fatal colon cancer in a large prospective study. *J. Natl. Cancer Inst.*, **84**, 1491–1500.

Til, H. P., *et al.* (1985). Short-term (4 week) oral toxicity in rats with nitrate added to a cereal basal diet. *CIVO–TNO Draft Report*, No. V.85.289/250458. CIVO–TNO, Zeist, Netherlands.

Til, H. P., *et al.* (1988). Evaluation of the oral toxicology of potassium nitrite in a 13-week drinking-water study. *Food Chem. Toxicol.*, **26**, 851–859.

Til, H. P., *et al.* (1990). A supplementary semichronic toxicity study of potassium nitrite in drinking water in rats. *CIVO–TNO Report*. CIVO–TNO, Zeist, Netherlands.

Tremp, E. (1980). Die Belastung der schweizerischen Bevölkerung mit Nitraten in der Nahrung. *Mitt. Gebi. Lebensmittelunters. Hygi.*, **71**, 182–194.

Tricker, A. R. and Kubacki, S. J. (1992). Review of the occurrence and formation of non-volatile *N*-nitroso compounds in Foods. *Food Addit Contam.*, **9**, 39–69.

Tricker, A. R., *et al.* (1991). Mean daily intake of volatile *N*-nitrosamines from foods and beverages in West Germany in 1984–1990. *Food. Chem. Toxicol.*, **29**, 729–732.

Tsuda, H. and Hasegawa, M. (1990). Malignant transformation of mouse BALB/cT3T cells induced by NaNO$_2$. *Carcinogenesis*, **11**, 595–597.

Tsuda, H. and Kato, K. (1977). High rate of endoreduplication and chromosomal aberrations in hamster cells treated with sodium nitrite *in vitro*. *Mutat. Res.*, **56**, 79–84.

Turek, B., *et al.* (1980). The fate of nitrates and nitrites in the organism. *IARC Publication No. 31*. IARC, Lyon, pp. 625–632.

Tutelyan, V. A., *et al.* (1990). Assay of N-nitrosamines in foodstuffs in the USSR by gas-liquid chromatography with a thermal energy analyser. *Food Add. Contam.*, **7**, 43–49.

US Assembly of Life Sciences (1981a). *The Health Effects of Nitrate, Nitrite and N-Nitroso Compounds. Part 1*. Food and Drug Administration, Washington, DC.

US Assembly of Life Sciences (1981b). Unpublished Report of the Nitrite Task Force, Bureau of Foods, US FDA. Part 1. Food and Drug Administration, Washington, DC.

van Duijvenbooden, W. and Matthijsen, A. J. C. M. (1989). *Integrated Criteria Document No.758473012*, RIVM, Bilthoven, Netherlands.

van Loghten, M. J., *et al.* (1972). Long-term experiments with canned meat treated with sodium nitrite and glucono-deltalactone in rats. *Food Cosmet. Toxicol.*, **10**, 475–488.

Van Loon, A. J. M. and van Klaveren, J. D. (1991). Nitraatinname van de Nederlandse bevolking. *Voeding*, **52**, 96–100.

Van Maanen, J. M. S., *et al.* (1994). Consumption of drinking water with high nitrate levels causes hyperthrophy of the thyroid. *Toxicol. Lett.*, **72**, 365–374.

Vanela, M. (1995). Nitrate contamination of drinking water source. In *Health Aspects of Nitrates and its Metabolites (particularly Nitrite)*. Proceedings of Council of Europe International Workshop, Bilthoven, Netherlands, November 1994. Council of Europe Press, Strasbourg, pp. 21–39.

Virtanen, S. H., *et al.* (1994). Nitrate and nitrite intake and the risk of type 1 diabetes in Finnish children. *Diabetic Med.*, **11**, 656–662.

Wagner, D. A. and Tannenbaum, S. R. (1982). Enhancement of nitrate biosynthesis by *Escherichia coli* polysaccharide. *Banbury Rep.*, No.12, 437–443.

Wagner, D. A., *et al.* (1983). Metabolic fate of an oral dose of (^{15}N)-labelled nitrate in humans: effect of diet supplementation with ascorbic acid. *Cancer Res.*, **43**, 1921–1925.

Wagner, D. A., *et al.* (1984). Modulation of endogenous synthesis of *N*-nitrosamino acids in humans. *IARC Publication No. 57*. IARC, Lyon, pp. 223–230.

Wagner, D. A., *et al.* (1985). Effects of vitamins C and E on endogenous synthesis on *N*-nitrosamino acids in humans: precursor product studies with (^{15}N) nitrate. *Cancer Res.*, **45**, 6519–6522.

Walker, R. (1990). Nitrates, nitrites and *N*-nitroso compounds: a review of the occurrence in food and diet and the toxicological implications. *Food Addit. Contam.*, **5**, 717–768.

Walters, C. L. and Smith, P. L. R. (1981). The effect of waterborne nitrate on salivary nitrite. *Food. Chem. Toxicol.*, **19**, 297–302.

Walters, C. L., *et al.* (1974). The precursors of *N*-nitroso compounds in foods. *IARC Publication No. 9*. IARC, Lyon, p. 233.

Walters, C. L., *et al.* (1979). Nitrite sources and nitrosamine formation *in vitro* and *in vivo*. *Food Cosmet. Toxicol.* **17**, 473–479.

Ward, F. W., *et al.* (1986). Nitrate reduction, gastrointestinal pH and *N*-nitrosation in gnotobiotic and conventional rats. *Food Chem. Toxicol.*, **24**, 17–22.

Wettig, K., *et al.* (1987). Stark Erhöhte Nitratsynthese bei Lambliasis in der Schwangerschaft. *Z. Klin. Med.*, **42**, 401–403.

White, J. W. (1975). Relative significance of dietary sources of nitrate and nitrite. *J. Agric. Food Chem.*, **23**, 886–891.

WHO (1985). *Health Hazards from Nitrates in Drinking Water.* WHO, Geneva.

Willet, W. C., *et al.* (1990). Relation of meat, fat and fiber intake to the risk of colon cancer in a prospective study among women. *N. Engl. J. Med.*, **323**, 1664–1672.

Wink, D. A., *et al.* (1991). DNA deamination ability and genotoxicity of nitric oxide and its progenitors. *Science*, **254**, 1001–1003.

Winn, D. M. (1984). Tobacco chewing and snuff dipping. *IARC Sci. Publ.*, **57**, 837–850.

Winter, A. J. and Hokanson, J. F. (1964). Effects of long-term feeding of nitrate, nitrite or hydroxylamine on pregnant dairy heifers. *Am. J. Vet. Res.*, **25**, 353–361.

Winton, E. F., *et al.* (1971). Nitrate in drinking water. *J. Am. Water Works Assoc.*, **43**, 95–98.

Witter, J. P. and Balish, E. (1979). Distribution and metabolsm of ingested NO_3 ion and NO_2 ion in germfree and conventional flora rats. *Appl. Environ. Microbiol.*, **38**, 861–869.

Wright, A. J. and Davison, K. L. (1969). Nitrate accumulation in crops and nitrate poisoning in animals. *Adv. Agron.*, **16**, 197–247.

Xu, G., *et al.* (1992). The relationship between gastric mucosal changes and nitrate intake via drinking water in high-risk population for gastric cancer in Moping country, China. *Eur. J. Cancer Prev.*, **1**, 437–443.

Yamamoto, M. R., *et al.* (1984). Determination of volatile nitrosamine levels in foods and estimation of their daily intake in Japan. *Food Chem. Toxicol.*, **22**, 61–64.

Yang, C. S., *et al.* (1985). Metabolism of nitrosamines by purified liver cytochrome P-450. *Cancer Res.*, **45**, 1140–1145.

Young, T. B. and Wolf, D. A. (1988). Case-control study of proximal and distal colon cancer and diet in Wisconsin. *Int. J. Cancer*, **42**, 167–175.

Chapter 100

Mycotoxins with Special Reference to the Carcinogenic Mycotoxins: Aflatoxins, Ochratoxins and Fumonisins

Pieter S. Steyn and Maria A. Stander

C O N T E N T S

INTRODUCTION

Naturally occurring toxicants produced by microorganisms, such as bacteria and fungi (moulds), contaminate foods and feeds; these foodborne hazards pose a serious health risk to mammals, fish and poultry. This chapter is exclusively dedicated to toxins produced by fungi, viz. mycotoxins, and to diseases caused by the ingestion of mycotoxins, called mycotoxicoses; the toxin production can take place in the preharvest and/or during the postharvest stage of the crop.

The well known mycotoxicologist Forgacs referred to mycotoxicoses in the early 1960s as the most neglected diseases, although many people died in Russia during World War II owing to alimentary toxic aleukia (ATA), a mycotoxicosis caused by T-2 toxin, a sesquiterpenoid mycotoxin (Ueno et al., 1972; Yagen et al., 1977). The resurgence of interest in mycotoxin research is directly related to the discovery of the aflatoxins during the 1960s, a group of structurally related hepatocarcinogens, produced on nuts and cereals by Aspergillus flavus, Aspergillus parasiticus and Aspergillus nomius, and their role in the aetiology of primary liver cancer in humans (Van Rensburg, 1986; Bressac et al., 1991 and Groopman et al., 1992). This event led to an unabated interest in mycotoxins as evidenced by the large number of monographs (Uraguchi and Yamazaki, 1978; Steyn, 1980; Lacey, 1985; Cole, 1986; Natori et al., 1989; Steyn, 1989; Smith and Henderson, 1991; Creppy et al., 1993; Miller and Trenholm, 1994; Jackson et al., 1996), numerous reviews (e.g. Steyn and Vleggaar, 1985; Pohland et al., 1992; Steyn, 1993, 1995; Beardall and Miller, 1994;

Grove 1996; Bennet and Keller, 1997) and thousands of research papers.

Mycotoxins are a chemically heterogeneous group (see **Figure 1** for the structures of representative members of the important mycotoxins) of low molecular weight compounds which are produced by the secondary metabolism of fungal genera such as *Aspergillus, Penicillium, Fusarium, Alternaria* and *Claviceps*. The mycotoxins are mostly produced by the so-called storage fungi; however, some unique mycotoxicoses such as ergotism, lupinosis and facial eczema are caused by some parasitic and saprophytic fungi (see later). It is, therefore, not surprising that mycotoxins induce powerful and dissimilar pathological effects, as shown in **Table 1**.

The mycotoxicoses are not only clinically diverse, but also often extremely difficult to diagnose owing to the numerous pharmacological effects of the causative mycotoxins. Some of the diseases associated with mycotoxins are, for example, aflatoxin [human primary liver cancer and turkey-X disease (Van Rensburg, 1986; Bressac et al., 1991)]; citreoviridin (yellow rice disease in humans); ergotoxins [ergotism, St Anthony's Fire in humans (Van Rensburg and Altenkirk, 1974)]; fumonisins [encephalomalacia in horses, pulmonary oedema in swine (Bezuidenhout et al., 1988)]; ochratoxins [nephropathy in pigs (Danish porcine nephropathy) and poultry (Pohland et al., 1992)]; phomopsin A [lupinosis in sheep (Culvenor et al., 1989)]; sporidesmin A [facial eczema in sheep (Mortimer et al., 1978)]; T-2 toxin and other trichothecene toxins [alimentary toxic aleukia (ATA)] and zearalenone (hyperestrogenism, vulvovaginitis and abortion in swine).

Table 1 Diverse biological activity displayed by some representative mycotoxins.

Mycotoxin	Biological activity	Producing Genus	
Aflatoxin B$_1$	Carcinogenicity, teratogenicity	*Aspergillus*	Büchi *et al.* (1966); Van Rensburg (1986), Groopman *et al.* (1992)
Citrinin	Nephrotoxicity	*Penicillium, Aspergillus*	Betina (1984)
α-Cyclopiazonic acid	Neurotoxicity	*Penicillium, Aspergillus*	Holzapfel (1968)
Ergotoxins (ergotamine)	Vasoconstriction, neurotoxicity	*Claviceps*	Stoll (1952); Scott *et al.* (1992)
Fumonisin B$_1$	Carcinogenicity, neurotoxicity	*Fusarium*	Bezuidenhout *et al.* (1988); Jackson *et al.* (1996)
Ochratoxin A	Carcinogenicity, nephrotoxicity	*Aspergillus, Penicillium*	Van der Merwe *et al.* (1965); Pohland *et al.* (1992); Creppy *et al.* (1993)
Patulin	Mutagenicity, antibacterial	*Penicillium*	Engel and Teuber (1984)
Penitrem A	Neurotoxicity	*Penicillium*	De Jesus *et al.* (1983); Steyn and Vleggaar (1985)
Phomopsin A	Hepatotoxicity	*Phomopsis*	Culvenor *et al.* (1989)
Sporidesmin A	Hepatotoxicity, photosensitivity	*Pithomyces*	Mortimer *et al.* (1978)
Trichothecenes (T-2 toxin)	Dermatoxicity, haematopoietic effects	*Fusarium*	Wannemacher *et al.* (1991); Plattner *et al.*, (1989); Grove (1996)
Zearalenone	Estrogenism, reproductive irregularities	*Fusarium*	Urry *et al.* (1966)

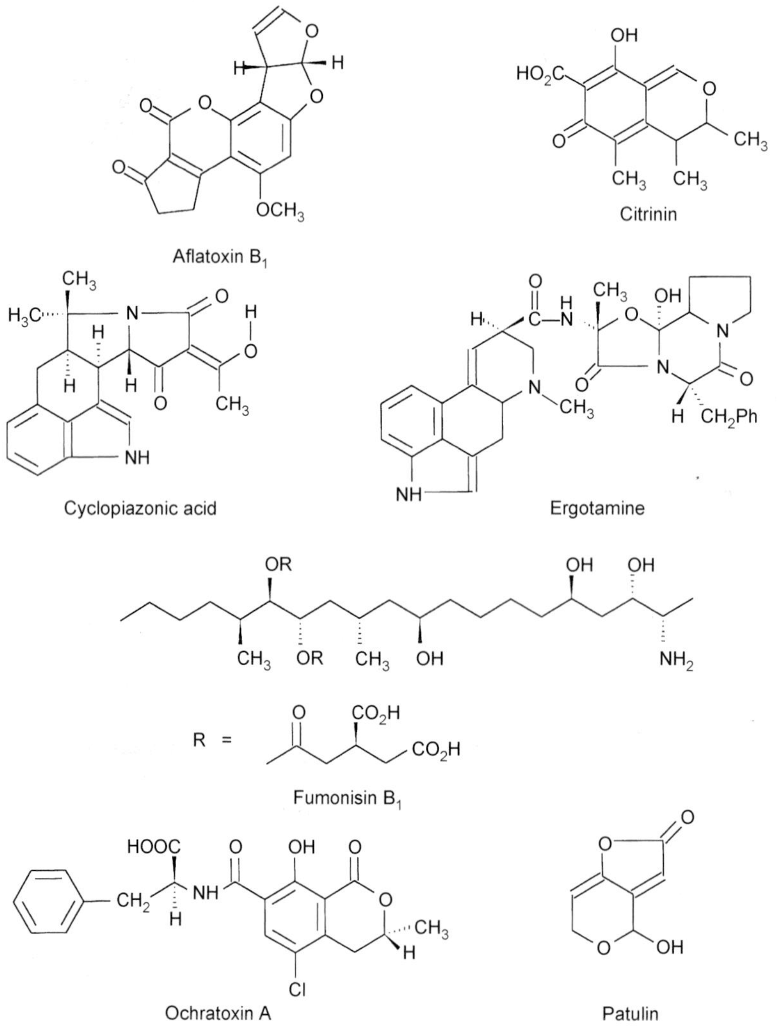

Figure 1 Structures of representative mycotoxins.

(Continued)

(Contd)

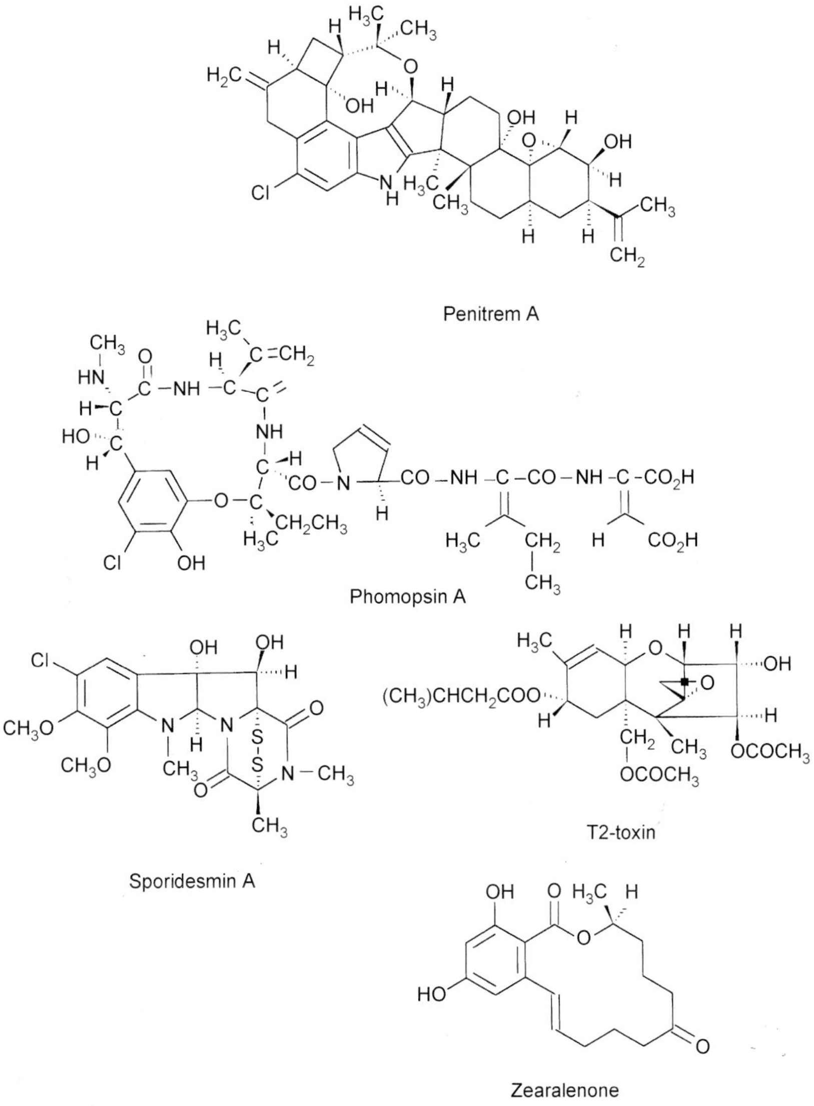

Figure 1 Structures of representative mycotoxins.

Mycotoxins are ubiquitous owing to the global distribution of toxinogenic fungi, thereby putting crops and consumers (man and animals) at risk and causing serious problems in the agricultural economies and international trade of nuts and cereals. The level of mycotoxin contamination of such commodities varies from year to year, depending on climatic conditions, commodity and location in a country. It has been estimated that one quarter of the world's food crops is at risk owing to mycotoxin contamination. Ammoniation can be effectively utilized to reduce aflatoxin levels in corn and cotton seeds by more than 99% (Lee *et al.*, 1992; Park, 1992).

Kuiper-Goodman (1989, 1995, 1996), Kuiper-Goodman and Scott (1989) and Kuiper-Goodman *et al.* (1996) have made sterling contributions to the risk assessment of mycotoxins. The human health concerns depend on the amount of the mycotoxins consumed, the toxicity of the compound (extrapolation of the test species to humans), the body weight and physical condition of the individual, the presence of the other mycotoxins as well as other dietary factors. In the case of animal mycotoxicoses, outbreaks vary according to the agricultural practice and climatic conditions in a region.

Hsieh (1990) defined the criteria of a human mycotoxicosis as follows:

- Occurrence of the mycotoxin(s) in food supplies;
- Human exposure to the mycotoxins;
- Correlation between exposure and incidence;
- Reproducibility of characteristic symptoms in experimental animals;
- Similar mode of action in humans and animal models.

The extrapolation of toxicological data from animals to humans using safety factors or other methods to arrive at an estimate of safe intake is the most challenging aspect of such assessments (Kuiper-Goodman, 1995). The extrapolation of animal toxicity data to humans is complicated by species differences in metabolic disposition, such as differences in absorption, and bonding to plasma and tissue constituents. Species differences in biotransformation as well as plasma and tissue half-life are also important.

The study of a specific mycotoxicosis requires the isolation and identification of the toxinogenic fungus involved, the chemical identification of the mycotoxin(s) and accurate and reliable laboratory methods for monitoring and regulating the mycotoxin and its metabolic products in different matrices. The toxins of most of the food-and feed-borne fungi have been characterized; the research benefited from the advent of effective and mild chromatographic techniques, high-resolution mass spectrometry (including MS–MS, GLC–MS and HPLC–MS), high-field nuclear magnetic resonance spectroscopy and single-crystal X-ray crystallography (Cole, 1986). The routine screening of food/feed samples benefited greatly from enzyme-linked immunosorbent assay (ELISA) (Morgan, 1989) and reliable analytical kits are now commercially available.

Some mycotoxins (listed in **Table 1** and **Figure 1**) are associated with specific human (Beardall and Miller, 1994) and animal mycotoxicoses (Smith and Henderson, 1991). In the following section special attention will be directed to three of the unique groups of toxins, viz. ergotoxins, sporidesmins and phomopsins.

MYCOTOXINS PRODUCED BY NON-STORAGE FUNGI

Ergotoxins

The ergotoxins (e.g. ergotamine, ergocristine, ergocryptine and ergocornine) are among the most pharmacologically active peptides and are the main alkaloids of *Claviceps purpurea*, the aetiological agent in gangrenous and convulsive ergotism. Ergotism is probably the oldest known human mycotoxicosis, known as St Anthony's Fire or the Holy Fire in the Middle Ages in Europe, and is caused by consumption of rye flour contaminated with *C. purpurea* (Stoll, 1952; Van Rensburg and Altenkirk, 1974; Lacey, 1991). As a human disease, ergotism has almost been eliminated (Scott *et al.*, 1992), but as an animal disease it can still occur widely, in the latter case also owing to contamination with *Claviceps paspali*. An isolated case of human ergotism occurred in Wollo, Ethiopia, when 150 people died due to the consumption of wild oats (*Avena abyssinica*) contaminated by a *Claviceps* species (King, 1979). The ergot alkaloids of *C. pur-*

purea are firmly associated with the plant species because the causative fungus is a specific pathogen of the rye plant.

Sporidesmins

The sporidesmins, e.g. sporidesmin A (**Table 1** and **Figure 1**), are a group of epipolythiodioxopiperazines which cause photosensitization diseases among sheep in New Zealand (facial eczema) and in South Africa [yellow thick head disease ('geeldikkop' in Afrikaans)]. In New Zealand, the saprophytic fungus *Pithomyces chartarum* infects the senescent and dead material of rye grass pastures which are consumed by sheep grazing on the new spring growth. Facial eczema frequently caused major losses, e.g. $40–100 million in 1981 (Smith, 1985). In the semi-arid Karroo region of South Africa, a similar photosensitization disease among sheep was associated with consumption of a common weed, *Tribulis terrestris*, infected with the perfect or teleomorph species *Leptosphaerulina* of which the *Pithomyces* is an anamorph (Roux, 1986). A severe outbreak of 'geeldikkop' incapacitated 250 000 sheep during a serious outbreak in 1949. Facial eczema is a secondary photosensitive expression of the toxic effects of sporidesmin on the liver (Mortimer *et al.*, 1978). In addition to its direct toxic effect on the liver parenchyma, excretion of the sporidesmin in the bile results in inflammation of the bile duct epithelium, followed by progressive necrosis of the duct wall and periductal concentric lamellar fibrosis and granulation causing the ducts to eventually become occluded (Mantle, 1991). Excretion of phylloerythrin, the product of hepatic degradation of chlorophyll, is thus impaired by the obliterative cholangitis, and the abnormally high level of phylloerythrin in the peripheral blood thus causes photosensitivity leading to oedema and inflammation of the exposed skin of sheep (Mantle, 1991).

Phomopsins

The phomopsins, a group of complex hexapeptides, containing β-dehydroamino acids, e.g. phomopsin A (**Table 1** and **Figure 1**), cause lupinosis in sheep in Australia and South Africa (Culvenor *et al.*, 1989). The phomopsins are produced by *Phomopsis leptostromiformis* (Kühn) Bubak *ex* Lind, a fungus which in nature appears to be a specific pathogen and saprophyte of *Lupinus* spp. However, it can be cultivated on cereals (maize) and liquid media and retain its toxigenicity. The liver is the major target for toxicity associated with the phomopsins; the affected liver accumulates lipids, turns yellow and becomes enlarged (Jago *et al.*, 1982). In cases of long-term exposure (low levels of the phomopsins), atrophy of the liver, fibrosis, and bile duct proliferation develop. Phomopsin A acts as a mitotic drug both *in vivo* and *in* *vitro*, and the observed symptoms of lupinosis can be related to the specific interaction of phomopsins with tubulin and microtubules (Tönsing *et al.*, 1984).

TRICHOTHECENES

This chapter is primarily dedicated to the carcinogenic mycotoxins: aflatoxins, ochratoxins and fumonisins. However, the trichothecenes are sufficiently important to warrant a brief description. The chemistry of the trichothecenes has been adequately covered by Grove (1996), who reported that a total of 182 trichothecenes, based on the trichothecane skeleton have been isolated from natural sources. They comprise 113 non-macrocyclic and 69 macrocyclic compounds.

The trichothecenes are produced by various species of *Fusarium*, *Trichoderma*, *Myrothecium*, *Verticimonisporium* and *Stachybotris* and comprise a group of closely related chemical compounds designated sesquiterpenoids. All the naturally occurring toxins contain an olefinic bond at C-9,10 and an epoxy group at C-12,13 (Grove, 1996) (see **Figure 1**). The trichothecene mycotoxins do not require metabolic activation prior to exerting their toxic effects.

The trichothecenes occur frequently in nature, and have been implicated in ATA in Russia, scabby grain intoxication (Tatsuno, 1997) and a number of animal diseases such as skin toxicity, bone marrow damage, and haemorrhagic and ill-thrift syndromes (Wannemacher *et al.*, 1991). ATA was associated with the death of more than 10% of the population in Orenburg district, close to Siberia, during the period 1942–47. The symptoms of ATA include vomiting, diarrhoea, skin inflammation, leukopenia, multiple heamorrhage and exhaustion of the bone marrow, similar to those induced by T-2 toxin. Ueno *et al.* (1972) and Yagen *et al.* (1977) concluded that T-2 toxin was the likely aetiological agent in ATA. The trichothecenes, e.g. T-2 toxin and nivalenol (NIV), induce karyorrhexis in actively dividing cells and a marked reduction in bone marrow cells and have the ability to inhibit protein and DNA synthesis and induce apoptosis in HL-60 cells (Yoshino *et al.*, 1996, 1997a, b; Sugamata *et al.*, 1997). In an *in vitro* study on T-2 toxin-induced apoptosis in human peripheral blood lymphocytes, Yoshino *et al.* (1997a) observed that the toxin affected the human peripheral blood lymphocytes, and elicited apoptic cell death, causing, in part, a marked decrease in circulating white blood cells as observed in animals which received T-2 toxin. In an ultrastructural study of apoptic cellular damage induced by acute NIV toxicoses in mice, Sugamata *et al.* (1997) observed NIV to be a potent inducer of apoptic cell death in the thymus, spleen and liver.

The trichothecenes such as T-2 toxin, diacetoxyscirpenol (DAS), vomitoxin and 4-deoxynivalenol (DON) are frequent contaminants of agricultural commodities (Tanaka *et al.*, 1988; ApSimon *et al.*, 1990; Gilbert, 1995; Scott, 1997). The trichothecenes, e.g. T-2 toxin, are optimally produced at relatively low temperatures, viz. 8–14 °C; however, Rabie *et al.* (1986) reported the production of large quantities of T-2 toxin at 25 °C by *Fusarium acuminatum*. The analytical methodology for the trichothecenes in animal feedstuffs is well established (Steyn *et al.*, 1991), e.g. by applying mass spectrometry and tandem mass spectrometry (Plattner *et al.*, 1989). Yeasts (*Kluyveromyces marxianus*) and bacteria (*Bacillus brevis*) are useful indicator organisms for the bioassay of several of the common mycotoxins. Madhyastha *et al.* (1994) evaluated the relative toxicity of 16 trichothecenes and some of their interactions by using *K. marxianus*, and found toxicity to decrease in the following order: T–2 toxin > DAS > DON > NIV.

AFLATOXINS

The deaths in 1960 in England of over 100 000 turkeys and ducklings, which consumed Brazilian peanut meal, led to the discovery of the aflatoxins, a group of hepato-carcinogenic bishydrofurano mycotoxins produced by certain strains of *A. flavus* and *A. parasiticus*. Aflatoxin B_1 (AFB$_1$) has the highest levels of occurrence and is the most carcinogenic of the known aflatoxins, while aflatoxin M_1 (AFM$_1$) is excreted in the milk of cows and has toxic properties similar to those of AFB$_1$ (Holzapfel *et al.*, 1966).

Chemistry and Metabolism

Aflatoxin B_1, B_2, G_1 and G_2 are the main metabolites of *A. flavus* and *A. parasiticus*. Büchi *et al.* (1966) elucidated the structures of the aflatoxins confirmed as by total synthesis. Aflatoxins may be classified into two broad groups according to their chemical structure: the difurocoumarocyclopentenone series (AFB$_1$, AFB$_2$, AFB$_{2a}$, AFM$_1$, AFM$_2$, AFM$_{2a}$ and aflatoxicol) and the difurocoumarolactone series (AFG$_1$, AFG$_2$, AFG$_{2a}$, AFGM$_1$, AFGM$_2$, AFGM$_{2a}$ and AFB$_3$) (Heathcote, 1984) (see **Figure 2**). Aflatoxin B_1 ($C_{17}H_{12}O_6$) is a pale-white to yellow, odourless, crystalline solid with a blue fluorescence under UV light (see **Table 2** for physical and spectroscopic data).

The aflatoxins display decreasing potency in the order $B_1 > G_1 > B_2 > G_2$, as illustrated by their LD$_{50}$ values for day-old ducklings (**Table 3**). Structurally, the dihydrofuran moiety, containing a double bond, and the substituents linked to the coumarin moiety are of importance in producing biological effects. Demethylation of AFB$_1$ leads to a toxic derivative, AFP$_1$, and hydroxylation of the bridge carbon of the furan rings to AFM$_1$, with similar toxic effects as AFB$_1$. AFM$_1$ is, however, considerably less carcinogenic than AFB$_1$.

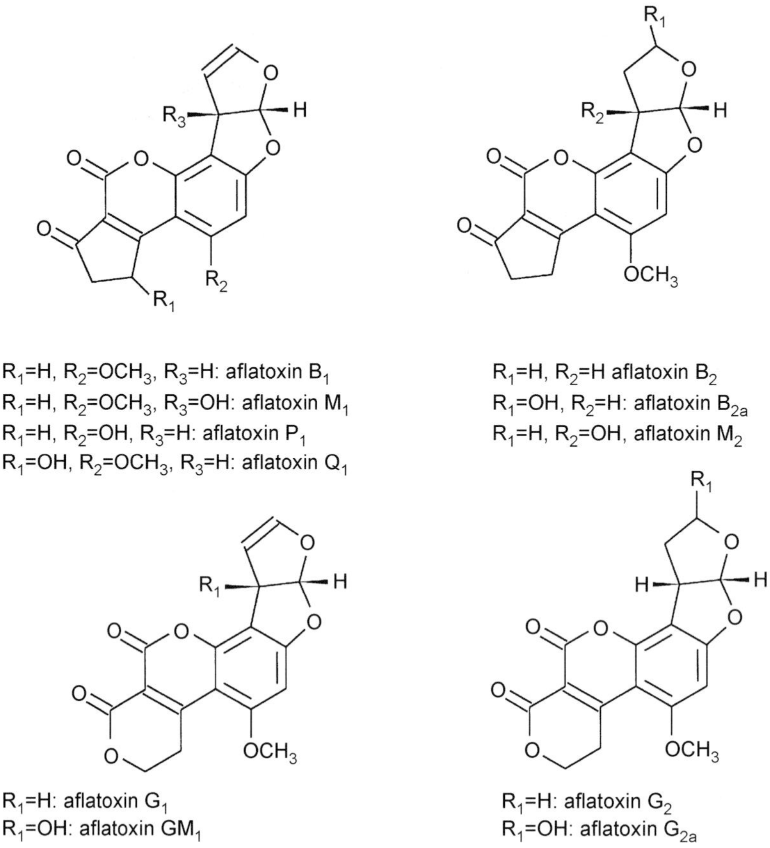

R$_1$=H, R$_2$=OCH$_3$, R$_3$=H: aflatoxin B$_1$
R$_1$=H, R$_2$=OCH$_3$, R$_3$=OH: aflatoxin M$_1$
R$_1$=H, R$_2$=OH, R$_3$=H: aflatoxin P$_1$
R$_1$=OH, R$_2$=OCH$_3$, R$_3$=H: aflatoxin Q$_1$

R$_1$=H, R$_2$=H aflatoxin B$_2$
R$_1$=OH, R$_2$=H: aflatoxin B$_{2a}$
R$_1$=H, R$_2$=OH, aflatoxin M$_2$

R$_1$=H: aflatoxin G$_1$
R$_1$=OH: aflatoxin GM$_1$

R$_1$=H: aflatoxin G$_2$
R$_1$=OH: aflatoxin G$_{2a}$

Figure 2 Structures of the important aflatoxins.

Table 2 Physical and spectroscopic data for aflatoxin B$_1$

Melting-point	269–271 °C
Optical rotation, [α]	−559 ° (concentration 625 μmol l^{-1} in chloroform)
Infrared spectrum	Strong bands at 1770, 1600, 1570, 1390 and 1310 nm
Molecular weight	312.3

Source: Pohland et al. (1982).

Table 3 Toxicities of the principal aflatoxins

Aflatoxin	LD$_{50}$ (μg per day-old duckling)
B$_1$	18
G$_1$	39
B$_2$	84
G$_2$	173
M$_1$	17
M$_2$	62

Source: Carnaghan et al. (1963); Heathcote (1984).

Biosynthesis

In an effort to control aflatoxin contamination of food and feed, scientists focused on the biosynthetic pathway of aflatoxin to understand its regulation and evolution and to eliminate the toxin from the food chain. Aflatoxin thus has one of the best studied polyketide pathways known (Trail et al., 1995). The pathway involves approximately 20 enzymes: AFB$_1$ and AFB$_2$ are produced by two parallel pathways (Bennett et al., 1994, and references cited). There are two possible initial steps: the first involves condensation of acetate and nine malonate units, whereas the alternative step involves the synthesis of a six-carbon hexanoate (Townsend, 1986) [which is then extended by a polyketide synthetase to generate a C$_{20}$ polyketide (Trail et al., 1995, and references cited; Steyn, 1980)] (see **Figure 3** for the proposed pathway). The final step in aflatoxin biosynthesis involves the oxidative cleavage and rearrangement of O-methylsterigmatocystin with loss of a C$_1$ unit (Chatterjee and Townsend, 1994).

The detection of aflatoxigenic fungi in grains, using PCR methodology, is based on three genes from the aflatoxin biosynthetic pathway (**Figure 3**) (Shapira et al., 1996). The three genes code for key enzymes involved in discrete biosynthetic steps: polyketide → norsolorinic acid (apa-2), versicolorin A → sterigmatocystin (ver-1) → O-methylsterigmatocystin (omt-1). The DNA sequences of the enzymes were established, and three primer pairs, each complementing the coding portion of one of the

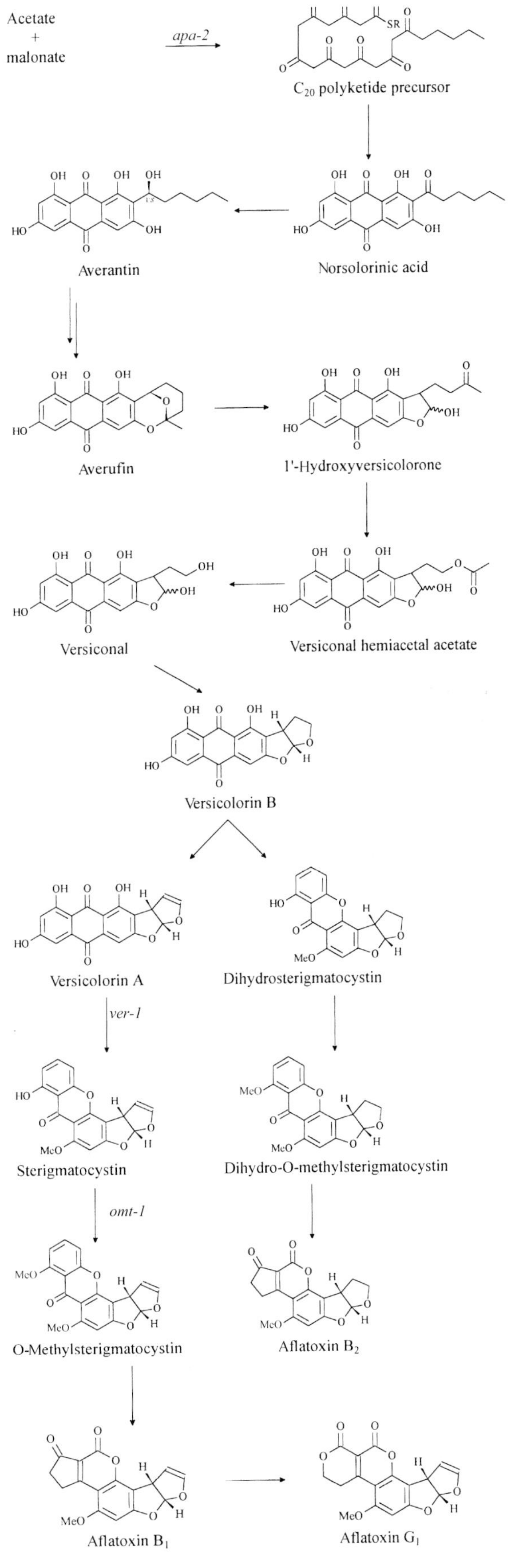

Figure 3 Biosynthesis of aflatoxin. Source: Steyn (1980); Townsend (1986).

genes were generated. The PCR technology enabled Shapira *et al.* (1996) to differentiate between the aflatoxigenic strains of *A. flavus* and *A. parasiticus* and the non-aflatoxigenic *Penicillium* and *Aspergillus* species.

Production

The aflatoxins are produced by *A. flavus*, *A. parasiticus*, *A. nomius* and *A. tamarii* (Goto *et al.*, 1996). In addition to genetic requirements for production, the yield of aflatoxin depends on the growth conditions, such as moisture, temperature (optimum conditions for *A. flavus* are 16–24% moisture at 20–38 °C), substrate, aeration (culturing moulds on a rotary shaker greatly increases yields) and other factors which affect the qualitative state of development of the mould. The yields of the different aflatoxins vary with different growth conditions, e.g. enhanced levels of AFB_1 relative to AFG_1 occur in *A. parasiticus* at elevated temperatures as a result of accelerated catabolism of AFG_1 (Detroy and Ciegler 1971, and references cited). Although 20–38 °C is the optimum temperature range for production, aflatoxin formation can also take place at temperatures as low as 7–12 °C, if an extended incubation period is utilized. Therefore, the storage of commodities at reduced temperatures cannot be used to prevent aflatoxin production. Aflatoxin production is also affected by trace metals, insecticides, herbal drugs, spices, tricarboxylic acid cycle intermediates and food preservatives, and is highly dependent on nutritional factors, e.g. sources of carbohydrates such as glycerol (Mateles and Adye, 1965) and glucose.

Determination

At first, the analysis of the aflatoxins involved the grinding of the samples, Soxhlet extraction, solvent partitioning and clean-up by SiO_2 columns followed by determination by paper chromatography, which was subsequently replaced by SiO_2 TLC (Shepherd *et al.*, 1987). A number of samples can be analysed simultaneously on one TLC plate and confirmation can be achieved by derivatization on the plate followed by a second development. The modern techniques rely on the same principles, although ready-packed clean-up columns are used which contain silica or modified silica

(especially C_{18}-bonded phase), e.g. Sep-Pak (Waters, Milford, MA, USA) and Bond-Elut (Analytichem International, Harbor City, CA, USA); however, the introduction of HPLC is replacing TLC methods in the final quantification step (Shepherd *et al.*, 1987). The problem of fluorescence quenching can be circumvented by precolumn derivatization with trifluoroacetic acid or postcolumn reaction with bromine or iodine (Shepherd and Gilbert, 1984; Kok *et al.*, 1986). The latter method has a lower detection limit of 5–30 pg of AFB_1. Cepeda *et al.* (1996) introduced cyclodextrines to increase the fluorescence of AFB_1 and AFG_1 in the postcolumn excitation of these toxins: substantial improvements (ca 30-fold) in detection limits of AFG_1 and AFG_1 were subsequently obtained by the use of heptakis-2,6-β-O-dimethyl-β-cyclodextrin. Gas chromatography–mass spectrometry (GC–MS) or liquid chromatography–electrospray ionization tandem–mass spectrometry (LC–ESI-MS–MS) can be used for confirmation of aflatoxin B_1 (Kussak *et al.*, 1995). Methods for the determination of the aflatoxins are summarized in **Table 4**.

Immunological Methods

Immunological-based screening methods for aflatoxins are rapid: the columns are commercially available and the procedures can be fully automated. Holaday–Velasco minicolumns have been widely used since 1980 in the screening of aflatoxins in corn and peanuts. A disadvantage of this method is that it relies on the characteristic fluorescence of the aflatoxins, which can be very subjective (Gilbert, 1993). There are three types of immunological based assays: batchwise quantitative methods (ELISA), semiquantitative but rapid methods for single samples, and affinity column clean-up. Agri-screen is an ELISA method and Afla-20-cup, EZ-screen and Cite-probe are all commercially available kits for aflatoxin screening, based on the principles of ELISA but using absorbed antibodies in a sandwich format. Aflatest and Oxoid are commercially available affinity columns (Gilbert, 1993). The performance of these different kits has been assessed by Dorner and Cole (1989) and Koeltzow and Tanner (1990). Radioimmunoassays (RIA) for AFB_1 had already been reported as far back as 1976 but have not been commercialized (Shepherd *et al.*, 1987).

In commercial double-antibody ELISA kits, a microtitre plate with aflatoxin–protein conjugate absorbed to

Table 4 Methods for the determination of aflatoxins

Substrate	Method	Recovery (%), detection limit	Ref.
Dust and urine	LC–MS	2 pg mg^{-1} and 50 pg ml^{-1}	Kussak *et al.* (1995)
Liquid and powered milk	Affinity column and HPLC	85.7%, 50 pg ml^{-1}	Mortimer *et al.* (1987)
Cheese	Affinity column and HPLC	75%, 5 ng kg^{-1}	Sharman *et al.* (1992)
Ground peanuts	ELISA	62–84%, 5 μg kg^{-1}	Li *et al.* (1994)

the surface of the wells is supplied. Buffer-diluted methanol extracts of the samples are pipetted separately into the wells of the titre plates, followed by a limited amount of anti-aflatoxin antibodies. There is competition between the bound aflatoxin and the aflatoxin in the sample for antibodies. The titre plate is then washed and a second antibody, with a colour-producing enzyme attached to it, is added, which binds to the anti-aflatoxin antibody bound to the well, and colour is produced with an intensity that is inversely proportional to the aflatoxin concentration in the sample, when the substrate for the colour-producing enzyme is added. In single-antibody ELISAs the colour-producing enzyme is conjugated directly to the first antibody. Although this assay is much quicker, it uses more antibodies and is therefore more expensive. Commercial ELISA kits have detection limits of about 2 μg kg^{-1} and are best suited for large batches of samples, since up to 93 samples can be assayed on one titre plate, but are not sufficiently reliable to be used as quantitative methods (Shepherd et al., 1987; Gilbert, 1993). However, recent developments have enabled this technology to be utilized with a high level of sensitivity and precision (ng kg^{-1}) (Franco, 1996).

Immunoaffinity columns consist of an anti-aflatoxin antibody bound to a gel material contained in a small plastic cartridge. In practice, the crude extract is forced through the column and the aflatoxin is left bound to the recognition site of the immunoglobulin. Extraneous material can be washed off the column with water or aqueous buffer, and the aflatoxin is obtained in a purified form by denaturing the protein gel by elution with a solvent such as methanol or acetonitrile (Gilbert, 1993). The aflatoxin in the eluate can be quantified by HPLC or with a standard UV spectrophotometer. The advantages of immunoaffinity columns are that the approach is the same for all matrices (peanuts, milk, nuts, etc.), it is much faster and cleaner than using conventional silica gel columns (there are no peak interferences when HPLC is used for quantification) and, unlike ELISA, all four aflatoxins (AFB$_1$, AFB$_2$, AFG$_1$ and AFG$_2$) can be determined individually (HPLC analysis). The disadvantage is that it is still more time-consuming than ELISA (Gilbert, 1993).

Occurrence

The aflatoxins are frequent contaminants of commodities such as corn (maize), peanuts, pecan nuts, Brazil nuts, cotton seeds, other energy-rich foodstuffs and even herbs and spices (Davis et al., 1986; MacDonald and Castle, 1996; Resnik et al., 1996). High levels of aflatoxin contamination are frequently associated with tropical climatic conditions, poor agricultural practices, drought stress and insect and mechanical damage. Internationally, due cognisance is usually given to the standards set by the US FDA (see **Table 5** for the permissible levels of aflatoxin contamination).

Table 5 Maximum levels (ppb) for aflatoxin contamination set by the US Food and Drug Administration

Substrate	Maximum Level
Food for humans and feed for some animal species	20
Milk	0.5
Feed for feedlot cattle	300
Feed for market hogs	200
Feed for breeding cattle, breeding hogs and mature poultry	100

Control and Decontamination

Ammonia has been used to destroy aflatoxins in various feedstuffs either in its gaseous form, or as an ammonium hydroxide solution (Simpson and Pemberton, 1989; Lee et al., 1992; Park, 1992). Addition to animal feeds of sequestering agents, such as activated charcoal, sodium bentonite and hydrated sodium aluminosilicate, which bind to aflatoxin and decrease its bioavailability, has been proposed as a detoxification strategy (Harvey et al., 1989; Lindemann et al., 1990; Bonna et al., 1991). Aflatoxin levels can also be reduced by the process of cooking, the dry roasting of peanuts and the popping of corn; the reduction is, however, modest (Simpson and Pemberton, 1989). Aflatoxin production can be controlled by the isolation or development of atoxigenic strains of A. flavus and A. parasiticus; these strains are able to competitively exclude toxigenic field strains from the host plant (Cole and Cotty, 1990; Cotty, 1994).

Biological Effects and Mechanism of Action

Toxicologically, the aflatoxins, particularly AFB$_1$, should be regarded as a quadruple threat, i.e. as a potent toxin, a carcinogen, a teratogen and a mutagen. AFB$_1$ induces liver cancer in all animal species tested so far and has also been linked to liver cancer in humans (Wang et al., 1996). Statistical correlations between contaminated food supplies and high frequencies of human hepatocellular carcinomas (HCC) in Africa and Asia have long implicated aflatoxins as risk factors in human liver cancer (Van Rensburg, 1986). The toxicity of AFB$_1$ toxicity varies from species to species and differences in susceptibility to aflatoxin are also found amongst individuals and between sexes (see **Table 6**). Numerous biochemical, toxicological and histological analyses have been performed to clarify the fundamental mechanisms of liver injury and hepatoma development. Molecular aetiology has substantiated the previous biostatistical studies, since AFB$_1$ causes an activation of the K1 ras proto-oncogene and modulates the p53 tumour suppressor

Table 6 Acute oral toxicities of aflatoxins

Species	LD_{50} (mg kg^{-1})						
	B$_1$	B$_2$	G$_1$	G$_2$	M$_1$	M$_2$	B$_{2a}$
Duckling	0.36	1.68	0.78	1.42	0.32	1.22	24
Rabbit	0.3						
Cat	0.55						
Pig	0.62						
Dog	0.5–1.0						
Sheep	1.0–2.0						
Guinea pig	1.04						
Monkey	2.2–7.8						
Chicken	6.3						
Rat	7.2 (M), 6 (F)						
Mouse	9.0						
Hamster	10.2						

Source: Ciegler (1975); Heathcote (1984).

gene. A molecular 'hot spot' in the *p53* gene, a G → T transversion at the third base position of codon 249, has been identified in independent studies on HCC patients from Qidong, China (Hsu *et al.*, 1991) and from sub-Saharan Africa (Bressac *et al.*, 1991). The IARC (Lyon, France) classified AFB$_1$ as a human carcinogen in 1987 and confirmed the classification in 1992.

The mutagenic and carcinogenic effects of AFB$_1$ have been well studied and are believed to arise from metabolic activation of the electron-rich dihydrobisfuran to the corresponding epoxide by the liver P450 isoenzyme CYP 2C and to a lesser extent CYP 1A2 in rats and CYP 3A4 in humans (Ishii *et al.*, 1986; Forrester *et al.*, 1990; Gopalkrishnan *et al.*, 1990). Raney *et al.* (1992) demonstrated that the AFB$_1$-epoxide occurs in *endo* and *exo* forms, each with different affinities for DNA (see **Figure 4**). The *exo*-epoxide is highly electrophilic and reacts with regions in the DNA helixes which are rich in guanine to form covalent bonds at the N-7 of guanine residues, leading to depurination and strand scission events (Essigmann *et al.*, 1982). The *Salmonella* reversion assay indicates that the *exo*-epoxide is at least 500 times more potent as a mutagen than the *endo* stereoisomer (Iyer *et al.*, 1994). AFB$_2$, on the other hand, has no double bond at this position and is practically inactive. AFB$_1$-epoxide can be metabolized further to 8,9-dihydro-8,9 dihydroxyaflatoxin B$_1$ which may bind to cellular proteins, via Schiff base formation with primary amino groups, inducing cellular injury and eventually cell death (Fink-Gremmels, 1996). In mice, virtually all the epoxidation leads to the *exo* isomer, in rats the ratio of *exo* to *endo* isomers is 32: 1 and in humans the proportion of *endo* to *exo* isomer is higher than in the rat (Neal, 1995) (see **Table 6** for toxicities). AFB$_1$-epoxide forms a conjugate with glutathione by a glutathione-*S*-transferase (GST)-mediated mechanism; glutathione is an alternative for aflatoxin to binding to other nucleophilic

centres and is apparently the most important detoxification system (Degen and Neumann, 1978; Neal, 1995). As is evident from **Figure 4**, several hydroxylations occur during the metabolism of AFB$_1$, catalysed by cytochrome P450 enzymes, leading to its secondary metabolism (AFM$_1$, AFP$_1$ and AFQ$_1$). The secondary conjugating processes involve glucuronidation, sulphation and acetylation of primary AFB$_1$ metabolites (Neal, 1995).

OCHRATOXIN A

The ochratoxins, metabolites of *Aspergillus ochraceus* Wilh. (Van der Merwe *et al.*, 1965), were the first group of mycotoxins to be discovered subsequent to the epoch-making discovery of the aflatoxins. Ochratoxin A (OTA) is a very important mycotoxin owing to its frequent occurrence in nature, its established role in Danish porcine nephropathy, and in poultry mycotoxicoses and its implicated role in Balkan endemic nephropathy and urinary system tumours in North Africa.

Chemical Characteristics and Biosynthesis of OTA

Ochratoxin A comprises a pentaketide-derived dihydro-isocoumarin moiety linked via its 12-carboxy group by a peptide bond to L-β-phenylalanine (see **Figure 5**). It forms colourless crystals when recrystallized from benzene (m.p. 90 °C with the loss of benzene) and it melts at 169–171 °C upon crystallization from xylene (Van der Merwe *et al.*, 1965).

The IR spectrum of OTA (CHCl$_3$) displays bands at 1665, 1535 and 3430 cm^{-1} (secondary amide), 1723 cm^{-1} and broad band between 2500 and 2700 cm^{-1} (carboxyl carbonyl group) and a band at 1678 cm^{-1} (lactone

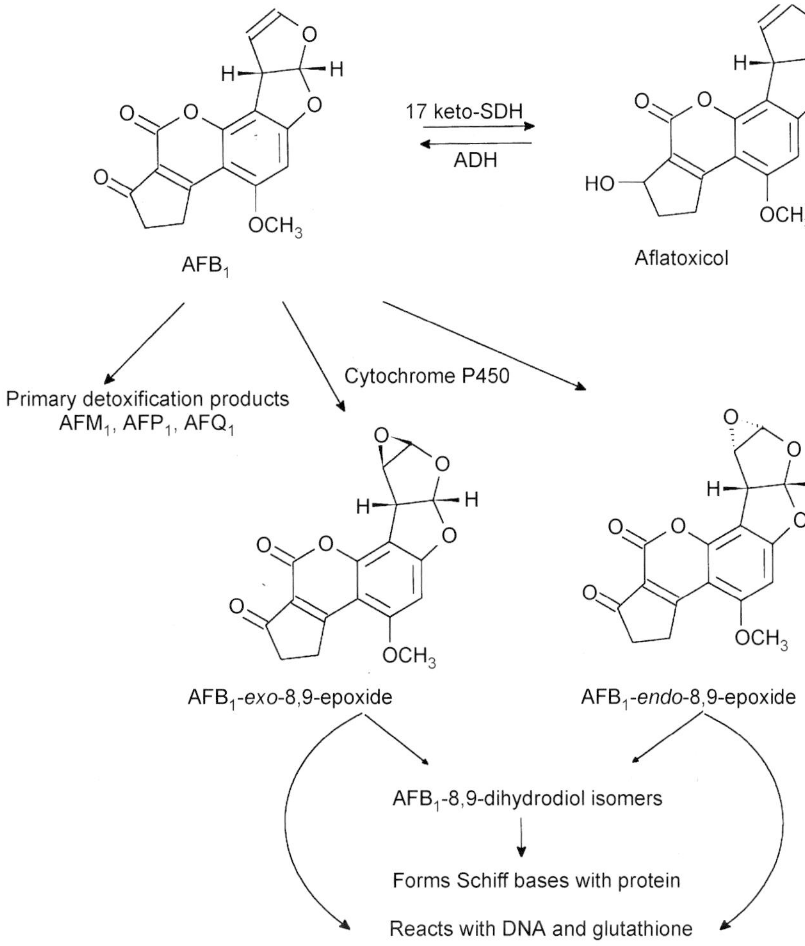

Figure 4 Metabolism of AFB$_1$. Source: Neal (1995).

carbonyl group). The UV absorption spectrum of OTA has λ_{max} 216 nm ($\varepsilon = 31\,500$) and 330 nm ($\varepsilon = 6400$) in MeOH–0.0005 M H$_2$SO$_4$. The most abundant peaks in the mass spectrum of OTA are at m/z M$^+$ 403 (13%), 359 (31%), 358 (18%), 357 (14%), 258 (52%), 257 (97%), 256 (100%), 255 (86%), 242 (49%), 241 (94%), 239 (81%) and 238 (99%).

IR spectroscopy and X-ray crystallography have demonstrated that OTA exists in solution and in the solid state in the β form, viz. the amide NH is hydrogen-bonded to the phenolic oxygen (Bredenkamp et al., 1989). ^{13}C NMR spectroscopy provided evidence for hydrogen bonding of the phenolic proton to the lactone carbonyl group (Bredenkamp et al., 1989).

The biosynthetic origin of OTA was established by employing radioactive precursors, e.g., [1-^{14}C]-and [2-^{14}C]acetate, [2-^{14}C]malonate, DL-[methyl-^{14}C]methionine and chlorine-36 (Steyn et al., 1970) and stable isotope precursors, e.g. sodium [^{13}C]formate and [1-^{13}C]- and [1,2-^{13}C]acetate (De Jesus et al., 1980). OTA is derived from combined pathways, viz. the shikimic acid pathway (phenylalanine) and the polyketide pathway

(dihydroisocoumarin); the chlorine atom is probably derived through the action of a chloroperoxidase.

Analogues of OTA

OTB, the natural dechloro analogue of OTA, is 10 times less toxic than OTA. OTA can be converted into OTB by catalytic dechlorination with palladium–charcoal and ammonium formate (Bredenkamp et al., 1989). Steyn and Holzapfel (1967) identified the methyl and ethyl esters of OTA and OTB in a culture of A. ochraceus on both sterilized cornmeal and liquid media. The toxicity of the esters of OTA is similar to that of OTA, whereas the OTB derivatives are, as to be expected, non-toxic.

OTA is hydrolysed to the non-toxic Oα (7-carboxy-5-chloro-3,4-dihydro-8-hydroxy-3-methylisocoumarin) in various organs in rats, mostly the caecum, duodenum, ileum and the pancreas, whereas the activity in the liver and kidneys is very low or non-existent in rat hepatocytes (Suzuki et al., 1977; Hansen et al., 1982; Størmer et al., 1983). OTA is chemically hydrolysed by 6 M HCl and also readily by treatment with α-chymotrypsin or

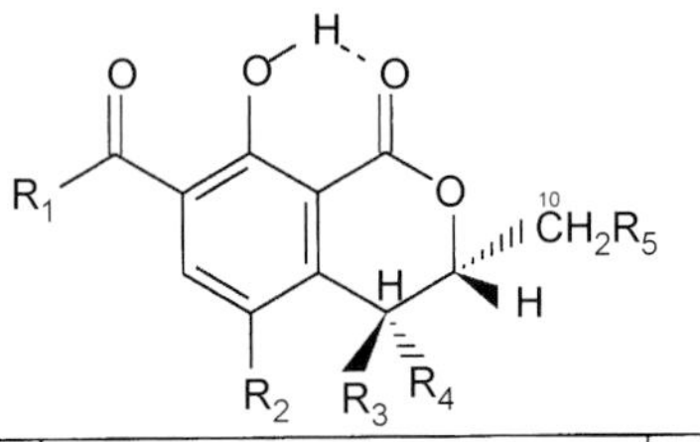

	R₁	R₂	R₃	R₄	R₅
Ochratoxin A	Phenylalanine	Cl	H	H	H
Ochratoxin B	Phenylalanine	H	H	H	H
Ochratoxin C	Phenylalanine ethyl ester	Cl	H	H	H
Ochratoxin A methyl ester	Phenylalanine methyl ester	Cl	H	H	H
Ochratoxin B methyl ester	Phenylalanine methyl ester	H	H	H	H
Ochratoxin B ethyl ester	Phenylalanine ethyl ester	H	H	H	H
Ochratoxin α	OH	Cl	H	H	H
Ochratoxin β	OH	H	H	H	H
(4S)-Hydroxyochratoxin A	Phenylalanine	Cl	OH	H	H
(4R)-Hydroxyochratoxin A	Phenylalanine	Cl	H	OH	H
10-Hydroxyochratoxin A	Phenylalanine	Cl	H	H	OH

Figure 5 Structures of the ochratoxins.

carboxypeptidase A, yielding L-β-phenylalanine and the optically active lactonic acid (OTα). OTβ, the dechloro analogue of OTα, is the hydrolysis product of OTB, and was detected in culture extracts. The less toxic ochratoxin D, 4-hydroxyochratoxin A, was isolated by Hutchison *et al.* (1971) from *P. viridicatum*. The (4R)-OH-OTA epimer is the major of the two epimers formed from OTA in human and rat liver microsomal systems under the influence of cytochrome P450s (Størmer *et al.*, 1981, 1983), while the (4S)-OH-OTA epimer is more prevalent in pig liver microsomes (Moroi *et al.*, 1985). Oster *et al.* (1991) characterized four cytochrome P450 fractions in pig liver microsomes; the two predominant forms A₂ and A₃, both with a molecular weight of 54 kDa, and the minor form Bₐ play an important role in the oxidation of OTA. These two epimers were also found in rat and rabbit liver (Størmer *et al.*, 1981) and rat kidney (Stein *et al.*, 1985). The 10-OH metabolite of OTA was formed from OTA with rabbit liver microsomal system (Størmer *et al.*, 1983). Hadidane *et al.*, (1992) discovered three natural analogues of OTA with the Phe group replaced with a serine, proline and hydroxyproline group, while Xiao *et al.*, (1996b) reported the isolation of OTα, OTβ, (4-R)-

OH-OTA, (4-R)-OH-OTB and 10-OH-OTA from a culture of *A. ochraceus*.

Five analogues of OTA, including the ethylamide of OTA (OE-OTA), the D-phenylalanine form of OTA (d-OTA), the decarboxylated OTA (DC-OTA), the *O*-methyl ether of OTA (OM-OTA) and the methyl ester of OTα (M-OTα) were synthesized using OTA or ochratoxin α by Xiao *et al.*, (1995b). The toxicities of these analogues to HeLa cells are shown in **Table 7**. Xiao and coworkers activated OTA to the N-hydroxysuccinimide ester (OTA-NHS) and OTα to acylchloride (OTα-C₁). They then used nucleophilic substitution reactions with primary amines, amino acids and alcohols to form corresponding amides and esters. OM-OTA was synthesized by the base-hydrolysis of *O*-methylochratoxin methylester. An open lactone form of OTA which is much less toxic than OTA is produced at high pH and is relatively stable at physiological pH (Xiao *et al.*, 1996a). Steyn and Payne (1998) synthesized the bromo-analog of OTA by the treatment of OTB with pyridiniumhydrobromide perbromide.

Steyn *et al.*, (1975) prepared 13 new analogues of OTA by substituting L-Phe for the L-amino acids Trp, Ala,

Table 7 The toxicity of OTA and its analogues to HeLa cells

Analogue	HeLa cell LC_{50} (mM)
OTA	0.005
OTC	0.009
OTB	0.054
d-OTA	0.163
OTα	0.56
OM-OTA	0.83
DC-OTA	7.6
OE-OTA	10.1

Source: Xiao *et al.* (1995b).

Tyr, Cys, Pro(4-OH), Glu, Met, Val, Pro, Ser, Asp, Thr and Leu. The typical lesions in cell culture which were associated with OTA toxicity were caused to various extents by all the compounds. In the group of compounds with a higher toxicity rating, four contained an aromatic ring.

Production of OTA

OTA is produced by a number of both *Aspergillus* and *Penicillium* species, as shown in **Table 8**. A number of other *Aspergillus* and *Penicillium* species were incorrectly reported to be producers of OTA owing to the difficulty associated with the correct identification of the fungi (Pitt, 1987; Samson and Frisvad, 1991).

OTA occurs extensively in many plant and animal products; the contamination is typically associated with grain stored in the temperate climate of Europe and North America. There are substantial annual variations in the OTA content of grains because the production is determined mainly by the temperature and water activity (a_w) of the substrate and the type of substrate, presence of competitive microflora, strains of fungi and the quality of the seed (Marquardt and Frohlich, 1992). The minimum a_w conditions for OTA production by, e.g., *A. ochraceus* are 0.83–0.87 and the minimum temperature is 12 °C; the optimum temperature for toxin production

Table 8 Reported OTA-producing species

Aspergillus	*Penicillium*
A. ochraceus (*A. alutaceus*)	*P. viridicatum* (*P. verrucosum*)
A. melleus (*A. quercins*)	
A. alliaceus	
A. ostianus	
A. sclerotiorum	
A. albertensis	
A. wentii	
A. auricomus	
A. niger var. niger	
A. sulphureus (*A. fresenii*)	

Source: Marquardt and Frohlich (1992); Abarca *et al.* (1994); Varga *et al.* (1996).

is 28 °C and the optimum time depends on the substrate, ranging from 7 to 14 days.

Isolation and Purification

Mouldered substrates are extracted with hot chloroform, ethyl acetate, chloroform–methanol, acidified chloroform or hexane followed by chloroform–methanol. The preliminary clean-up step is to transfer acidic components of the extract, including OTA and OTB, into a sodium bicarbonate solution, followed by acidification, extraction and column chromatography. The ochratoxins can be separated by chromatography, e.g. ion-exchange chromatography, partition chromatography on formamide-impregnated cellulose powder, column chromatography on silica gel impregnated with oxalic acid, Sephadex LH-20, Sephadex G-25, Florosil, Sephadex chromatography followed by silica gel chromatography, preparative liquid chromatography or preparative thin-layer chromatography. For final purification, OTA is crystallized from benzene, xylene or chloroform (Steyn, 1984). OTA crystallizes from xylene and chloroform without solvent of crystallization.

Analysis of OTA

Various methods for the analysis of OTA are based on TLC, HPLC and ELISA techniques.

TLC analysis is a relative inexpensive way of screening for OTA and was frequently used during the early years of mycotoxin research; it still has many applications. On TLC OTA displays an intense blue–green fluorescence under long-wavelength UV light. It is necessary to use acid modifiers (e.g. acetic acid) in TLC mobile phases (e.g. chloroform–methanol or toluene) to prevent streaking of OTA on silica gel. Problems with the rapid fading of the fluorescence intensity on the plate can be overcome by exposure of the plate to ammonia vapour, which converts the OTA into its ammonium salt, which displays a more intense blue fluorescence under UV illumination. The limits of detection for OTA on TLC are in the $\mu g\ kg^{-1}$ range. Paulsch *et al.* (1982) developed a two-dimensional TLC technique using an acidic and an alkaline developing solvent. This method, in combination with exposure of the TLC plate to methanol–ammonia, leads to a low limit of detection. Paulsch *et al.* (1982) used a simple confirmatory test for OTA based on the formation of OTA methyl ester on the TLC plate. There is an increase in the use of reversed-phase TLC (RPTLC) and high-performance TLC (HPTLC) in mycotoxin analysis. The latter has a much better efficiency of separation and uses less solvent than conventional TLC. Frohlich *et al.*, (1988) developed an RPTLC method for sample preparation in which the OTA is extracted from the spot for quantitation by direct spectrofluorimetric testing or

Table 9 Methods for the determination of OTA in different matrices

Substrate	Clean-up	Recovery (%), detection limit	Ref.
Faba beans and wheat	SPE	70%, 0.7 μg kg^{-1}	El-Banna and Scott (1986)
Wheat and barley	Acid–base solvent partition	40μg kg^{-1}	Lepom (1986)
Animal feed, grain	Two-stage SPE	90%, 5 μg kg^{-1}	Cohen and Lapointe (1986).
Wheat, barley, oats and mixed feed	1, CHCl$_3$ extraction; 2, SPE	77–96%, 0.1–0.3 μg kg^{-1}	Langseth et al. (1989).
Human blood, serum, milk and some foodstuffs	Immunoaffinity column	85%, 5–10 pg g^{-1}	Zimmerli and Dick (1995)
Human urine	Extraction, 2 $\times$ column chromatography	60–75%, 5 ng l^{-1}	Castegnaro et al. (1990)
Beer	1, SPE (C$_{18}$ silica); 2, immunoaffinity column	82–100%, 0.05–0.1 ng ml^{-1}	Scott and Kanhere (1995)

by subsequent HPLC analysis. This method has high levels of recovery (94%) and requires smaller amounts of solvents than the standard packed column methods.

HPLC separations are more efficient than those obtained by TLC and have been widely applied to the determination of OTA in various matrices (see **Table 9** for a few examples). Sample clean-up usually consists of extraction with organic solvents together with an acid to suppress the ionization of OTA, followed by further clean-up steps, e.g. with silica gel, cyano or reversed phase-solid phase extraction (RP-SPE) cartridges, immunoaffinity columns, and liquid–liquid extractions or preparative HPLC techniques. RP columns, e.g. octa-decylsilane (ODS, C$_{18}$), are usually used in quantitative HPLC separations with acidic aqueous acetonitrile or methanol as mobile phase (Van Egmond, 1991). Detection limits in the μg kg^{-1} range or lower can be obtained by using an HPLC system equipped with a fluorescence detector with excitation and emission wavelengths of 330 and 460 nm, respectively (Cohen and Lapointe, 1986).

Improved HPLC detectors such as photodiode-array detectors and improved computer search capabilities have made it possible to monitor the whole spectrum of compounds after separation, permitting further identification (Paterson and Kemmelmeier, 1990; Chu, 1992).

Jiao et al. (1991) developed a method for the identification of OTA in food samples by chemical derivatization of OTA to the O-methyl-OTA ester and GC–MS using negative ion chemical ionization. Thermospray MS has been described by Rajakyla et al. (1987) as an expensive alternative to fluorescence detection.

Radioimmunoassay (RIAs) is an analytical method that uses radioactivity for quantitative incubation of a specific antibody with a solution of unknown sample or known standard at a constant amount of labelled toxin determination of compounds. It usually involves the incubation of a specific antibody with a solution of unknown sample or known standard at a constant amount of labelled toxin followed by the separation of the free and bound toxin and the determination of the

radioactivity in the fractions (Chu, 1992). Commercial kits are available for the determination of OTA in various feeds and foodstuffs with RIA. ELISAs involve the use of antibodies generated against conjugates. These conjugates are made by linking OTA to protein (enzymes such as horseradish peroxidase) through its carboxylic acid function. Direct ELISA involves the use of a OTA–enzyme conjugate, whereas indirect ELISA uses a protein–OTA conjugate and a secondary antibody to which an enzyme has been conjugated (Morgan et al., 1986). Commercial kits like RIA are available, but the ELISA technique can be used to measure samples as small as 2.5 pg, which makes ELISA 10–100 times more sensitive than RIA (Chu, 1992).

Although substantial work is being done to improve the selectivity of the antisera used in ELISAs (Xiao et al., 1995a), the possibility of cross-reactions cannot be fully ruled out and positive findings obtained by immunoassays need to be confirmed by other techniques.

Antibody technology is used for the clean-up of cereal and animal sample extracts by utilizing immunoaffinity columns for the selective isolation of OTA (Sharman et al., 1992). Nakajima et al. (1990) prepared monoclonal antibody affinity columns for the determination of OTA in coffee by binding antibodies specific for OTA to Sepharose 4B. Immunoaffinity columns are commercially available and are used routinely in laboratories for sample clean-up followed by quantitation by HPLC or direct spectrofluorimetric measurement.

Regulations for OTA

OTA contamination is widespread in cereals, coffee, pulses, feedstuffs and other plant products. Raw agricultural products, contaminated with OTA and used as feed, can also contaminate meat and meat products of non-ruminant animals such as poultry and pigs (Van Egmond and Speijers, 1994). This problem does not occur in adult ruminants because OTA is hydrolysed by protozoan and bacterial enzymes in the fore-stomachs of these animals (IPCS, 1990). The detection of OTA in human milk indicates the carry-over of OTA from contaminated food by lactating women. Data on the occurrence of OTA in food and feed are relatively abundant for European countries but scarce for other continents. The levels of OTA contamination were found at the highest incidences in cereals (corn 10–500 μg kg^{-1}, wheat 5–135 μg kg^{-1} and barley 10–500 μg kg^{-1}) and for foodstuffs from animal products (kidneys from pigs varying from 2 to 100 μg kg^{-1}) (van Egmond and Speijers, 1994). The occurrence of OTA is related to the climate and especially the harvest and postharvest storage conditions (Pohland et al., 1992). There are 77 countries that have mycotoxin regulations and only eight have specific regulations for OTA in one or more commodities (FAO, 1996). The following factors must be taken into consideration before the limits for mycotoxins can be chosen: the availability of toxicological and analytical data, the availability of reliable analytical methods, data on the availability on the occurrence of mycotoxins in various commodities, intercountry trade and the existence of sufficient food supply (FAO, 1996). The current (proposed) limits are indicated in **Table 10**. The tolerance levels for OTA have been suggested as 1 μg kg^{-1} for infant foods and 5 μg kg^{-1} for cereals in the EU (Verardi and Rosner, 1995).

The homogeneity of OTA in products is very important; if care is not taken to ensure representative sampling, incorrect estimations of toxin concentrations will be made (FAO, 1996). Analytical quality assurance is essential to guarantee the accuracy of results and the use of reference materials (RMs) plays an important role in checking the performance of methods and proficiencies of laboratories (van Egmond, 1996). The European Commission's Standards, Measurements and Testing Programme has initiated the development of certified RMs for OTA and other mycotoxins (Wood et al., 1995).

Table 10 Limits for ochratoxin A in different commodities

Commodity	Limit (μg kg^{-1})
Children and infant foods	0.5–5
Foods	2–50
Animal feeds	5–300

Source: FAO (1996).

Ochratoxicosis

OTA is nephrotoxic to all animal species tested so far, and induces experimental liver and kidney tumours (see **Table 11**). The kidneys are the organs most susceptible to OTA, which can cause both acute and chronic kidney diseases. The renal lesions associated with the diseases include degeneration of the proximal tubules, interstitial fibrosis in the renal cortex, hyalinization of the glomeruli,

Table 11 Acute oral toxicities of the ochratoxins in different species

Species	LD$_{50}$mg (kg body weight)$^{-1}$			
	OTA	OTC	OTB	OT α
Pigs	1.0–6.0			
Chickens	3.3	4.8	41.4	22
Dogs	0.2			
Neonatal rats	3.9			
Mature rats	20–30			
Mice	46–58			

Source: Chu (1974); Krogh (1987); Kuiper-Goodman and Scott (1989).

and atrophy in the tubular epithelium (Krogh et al., 1974, 1987; Krogh et al., 1977). Pigs fed OTA showed reduced feed intake, loss of body weight, increased water consumption followed by polyurea diarrhoea, polydipsia and dehydration (Szczech et al., 1973). Residues of OTA are the greatest in the kidney, and in declining order in lean meat, liver and fat (Madsen et al., 1982). Krogh et al. (1988) reported nephropathy in pigs fed diets containing 0.2–4 mg kg^{-1} of OTA after 4-months of exposure; all lesions were confined to the kidney. Gross pathological examination of dogs administered 0.2–3 mg OTA (kg body weight)$^{-1}$ alone or in two dose combinations for 14 days indicated moderate to severe mucohaemorrhagic enteritis of the caecum, colon and rectum and enlargement of the lymph nodes, which were oedematous, hyperaemic and focally necrotic. Histopathological examination indicated that renal damage is the main feature of this toxicosis (Szczech et al., 1973). OTA inhibits cell division in these kidney cells and causes apoptic-type morphological lesions in these cells. The nuclear lesions seen in apoptosis are associated with enhanced endonuclease activity, which are responsible for DNA cleavage. OTA causes apoptosis-associated DNA degradation in human lymphocytes (Seegers et al., 1994, and references cited). OTA also causes decreased natural killer cell activity in mice (Luster et al., 1987) and the inhibition of cell division in hematopoietic stem cells (Boorman et al., 1984) and lymphocytes (Creppy et al., 1983a).

Krogh (1978) proposed that the human interstitial nephropathy diseases in the rural areas of Bulgaria, Romania and Yugoslavia might be related to a high OTA exposure. Balkan endemic nephropathy (BEN) was first identified in the 1950s and is an invariably fatal chronic kidney disease, characterized by contracted kidneys, and features changes exclusively in the renal cortex of the kidney. OTA has been found more frequently in food samples and in the serum taken from people in villages with BEN than in areas where the disease is unknown (Krogh et al., 1977; Pavlovic et al., 1979; Petkova-Bocharova and Castegnaro, 1985; Petkova-Bocharova et al., 1988). The blood of 95% of Tunisian people suffering from urinary system tumours (UST) were OTA positive, with blood concentrations higher than 90 ng ml^{-1} in several cases (Petkova-Bocharova *et al.*, 1988). OTA is also the cause of a nephropathy (Danish porcine nephropathy) affecting many pigs fed mouldy cereal feeds in Scandinavian countries. In Denmark carcasses are condemned if residue levels of OTA in the kidney exceed 25 ng g^{-1}.

Genotoxicity

OTA is a non-mutagenic carcinogen, since it has been generally negative in a number of gene mutation tests, based on both microorganisms and mammalian cells, and both with and without metabolic activation (Würgler *et al.*, 1991; Sakai *et al.*, 1992; Bendele *et al.*, 1995). However, OTA induced mutations in the modified Ames assay (Dirheimer, 1996), sister chromatid exchange in human peripheral lymphocytes *in vitro*, and SOS DNA repair in *E. coli* (Hennig *et al.*, 1991; cited by Neal, 1995). Furthermore, chromosomal aberrations could be detected after OTA exposure (Manalova *et al.*, 1990), and DNA adducts could be observed *in vivo* in the liver, kidney and spleen of rodents and humans (Pfohl-Leszkowicz *et al.*, 1993a, b) and in cytochrome P450-expressing BEAS-2B cells (Grosse *et al.*, 1994, 1995) and monkey kidney cells (Grosse *et al.*, 1995). These adducts were different for the different organs, suggesting different routes of metabolic activation. De Groene *et al.* (1996a) recently demonstrated that OTA mutagenicity requires a cytochrome P450-dependent activation step by using the *lacZ'* gene as reporter gene for mutations in cell lines expressing selected human cytochrome P450 forms. OTA-induced single-strand breaks were observed in primary rat hepatocytes (De Groene *et al.*, 1996b) and *in vivo* in rats and mice (Creppy *et al.*, 1985; Kane *et al.*, 1986).

Immunotoxicity

OTA is teratogenic to rats, mice, hamsters and chickens (Brown *et al.*, 1976; Schreeve *et al.*, 1977; Fukui *et al.*, 1987). It causes a marked increase in the number of dead and resorbed foetuses and a decrease in foetal body weight when administered to pregnant rats. Multiple gross, visceral and skeletal anomalies in pups are related to the treatment and dose of OTA administered to rats (Brown *et al.*, 1976). The subchronic exposure of Balb/c mice to OTA suppressed the antibody-production of plaque-forming cells and decreased thymocyte cell counts and the proportion of mature thymic lymphocyte (CD^{4+} or CD^{8+}) cells. The mitogenic responsiveness of thymocytes and splenocytes to concanavalin A (Con A) is also significantly decreased by OTA exposure. However, interleukin-2 production of Con A-stimulated lymphocytes, natural killer cell activity and humoral antibody titres to a viral antigen are not affected by OTA (Thuvander *et al.*, 1995). Thuvander and co-work-

ers also reported immunosuppression in Balb/c mice (Thuvander *et al.*, 1997) and Sprague–Dawley rats (Thuvander *et al.*, 1996a) after prenatal exposure to OTA. OTA exposure resulted in a decrease in proliferation and antibody, thereby indicating that subchronic, oral exposure to OTA affects certain immune functions in mice but does not suppress immune functions in the offspring (Thuvander *et al.*, 1996b).

Pharmacokinetics of OTA

About 40–65% of OTA orally administered to rats is absorbed in the small intestine, primarily in the proximal part of the jejunum. OTA has a high binding affinity for plasma constituents and binds to serum albumin and to an as yet unidentified macromolecule(s) as soon as it reaches the circulation system. This characteristic of OTA retards its elimination by limiting the transfer of OTA from the bloodstream to the hepatic and renal cells and consequently contributes to the prolonged half-life of the toxin (Chu, 1971; Stojkovic *et al.*, 1984; Kumagai, 1985; Hagelberg *et al.*, 1989). OTA also binds more specifically than plasma albumins to a smaller molecular fraction in blood (Stojkovic *et al.*, 1984). There may be a relation between the predominant nephrotoxic effect of OTA in mammals and the binding of OTA to these molecules because such molecules can easily pass through the normal glomular membrane, allowing the accumulation of OTA in the kidney (Marquardt and Frohlich, 1992). The pharmacokinetics of OTA and its metabolites in rats were recently reported by Li *et al.* (1997). The plasma half-life of OTA depends on the degree of absorption and the degree of binding to serum albumin and a number of other factors. OTA has a very high affinity for this unknown macromolecule (see above) in human serum and may therefore have a long plasma half-life (Kuiper-Goodman and Scott, 1989). The toxic activity of OTA in monkeys, with an elimination half life of 35 days and slow absorption from the gastro-intestinal tract, seems to be a good model for humans (Hagelberg *et al.*, 1989). Stein *et al.* (1985) reported an efficient reabsorption of OTA by the renal tubules of the kidney that also facilitates reabsorption of OTA into the plasma. This process in the renal proximal tubules which may be responsible for damage to the kidneys of various animal species (Szczech *et al.*, 1973; Elling, 1979; Albassam *et al.*, 1987) was reported by Jung and Endou (1989) to affect only the middle and terminal portions of the nephrons.

Rats excrete OTα, OTA and (4R)-OH-OTA mainly in the bile and urine after OTA had been administered intraperitoneally or *per os* (Støren *et al.*, 1982a, b; Xiao *et al.*, 1996b). Approximately 1–2% of the OTA was recovered as 4-OH-OTA and a total of 25–40% of the administered OTA was recovered as OTα and 6% as OTA. The relative quantity of OTA eliminated via the kidneys and the liver depends partly on the animal species, route of administration and dose, the enterohepatic recirculation, and the binding of the toxins to serum macromolecules. Data on elimination half-lifes and distribution half-lifes of other species are given in **Table 12**.

There are contradictory reports on the toxicity of OTA: some of the early reports regard OTA as the toxic agent, since its known metabolites are equally or less toxic than OTA, whereas other researchers consider the toxic effects to be due to one of its metabolites, since the simultaneous feeding of phenobarbital (phenobarbitone) increases the incidence of liver tumours seen after the feeding of OTA alone (Suzuki et al., 1986) and other more recent findings described below. Phenobarbital is known to induce the activity of various constitutive cytochrome P450 forms in the liver (Soucek and Gut, 1992). Fink-Gremmels et al. (1995) provided evidence for a number of unknown metabolites produced by metabolically competent hepatocytes, whereas Malaveille et al. (1994) discussed the formation of an OTA phenoxide radical and a thiol-derived toxic metabolite as reactive metabolites of OTA. A distinct possibility is that OTA might be metabolized, yielding both detoxified products and other metabolites responsible for the mutagenic effect described above.

Prevention of Ochratoxicoses

Superoxide dismutase (SOD) and catalase are enzymes which prevent most OTA-induced nephrotoxic effects and might be used for the prevention of such renal lesions (Baudrimont et al., 1994). Vitamin C significantly

reduces the effects of OTA on albino Swiss mice (Bose and Sinha, 1994). Other compounds that are efficient in preventing ochratoxicosis in vivo are radical scavengers, vitamins, prostaglandin synthesis inhibitors (e.g. indomethacin and aspirin), pH modifiers, and absorbent resins such as cholestyramine. (Madhyastha et al., 1992; Creppy et al., 1996). Compounds that have a high binding affinity for plasma proteins, such as piroxicam, are also promising as potential antidotes for OTA (Creppy et al., 1995). Aspartame, structurally related to OTA, prevents OTA binding to plasma proteins and is the best candidate for preventing the OTA-induced subchronic effects (Creppy et al., 1995).

A practical method to prevent ochratoxicosis is to reduce the levels of OTA contamination in foods and feedstuffs by certain cooking processes (Milanez and Leitao, 1996).

Mechanisms of Action of OTA

There appear to be a number of direct and several indirect effects of OTA. The best known effects of OTA are its effect on enzymes involved in the phenylalanine (Phe) metabolism, its effect on lipid peroxidation and its effect on mitochondrial respiration.

Inhibition of Phe-tRNA Formation

OTA inhibits protein synthesis by competition with Phe in the Phe-tRNA aminoacylation reaction catalysed by Phe-tRNA synthetase (Creppy et al., 1984). This was

Table 12 Pharmacokinetic data for OTA and some of its derivatives

Species[a]	Half-life[b]	OTA	OP-OTA	OTα	OTB	OTC	OTA-OH	Ref.
Rats (iv)	$t_{1/2\alpha}$ (min)	160 ± 17	163 ± 5	31 ± 5	14 ± 4	6 ± 1.2	19 ± 4.7	Marquardt et al. (1996)
	$t_{1/2\alpha}$ (min)	126						Galtier et al. (1979)
Rabbits	$t_{1/2\alpha}$ (min)	114						Galtier et al. (1981)
Chickens	$t_{1/2\alpha}$ (min)	30						
Cattle	$t_{1/2\alpha}$ (min)	108						Sreemannarayana et al. (1988)
Rats (iv)	$t_{1/2\beta}$ (h)	103 ± 16	50.5 ± 2.8	9.6 ± 2.3	4.2 ± 1.2	0.6 ± 0.2	6 ± 0.9	Marquardt et al. (1996)
Rats (iv)	$t_{1/2\beta}$ (h)	120						Hagelberg et al. (1989)
Rats (p)	$t_{1/2\beta}$ (h)	170						
Rats (o/iv)	$t_{1/2\beta}$ (h)	55						Galtier et al. (1979)
	$t_{1/2\beta}$ (h)	56						Ballinger et al. (1986)
Pig	$t_{1/2\beta}$ (h)	72–150						Galtier et al. (1981); Mortensen et al. (1983); Hagelberg et al. (1989).
Pre-ruminant calf	$t_{1/2\beta}$ (h)	77						Fukui et al. (1987)
Mouse	$t_{1/2\beta}$ (h)	24–48						Hagelberg et al. (1989)
Rabbits	$t_{1/2\beta}$ (h)	8.2						Galtier et al. (1981)
Chickens	$t_{1/2\beta}$ (h)	4.1						Galtier et al. (1981)
Monkeys	$t_{1/2\beta}$ (h)	840						Hagelberg et al. (1989)

[a] p = Peripherally; iv = intravenous; o = orally.
[b] $t_{1/2\alpha}$ = Distribution half-life; $t_{1/2\beta}$ = elimination half-life.

shown by Bunge *et al.* (1978), Creppy *et al.* (1979a, b) and Konrad and Röschenthaler (1977) in both bacterial and eukaryotic systems *in vitro*. This inhibition can be reversed by the administration of Phe in hepatoma cells (Creppy *et al.*, 1979a) and *in vivo* in mice (Creppy *et al.*, 1984). In addition to the inhibition of protein synthesis, the DNA and RNA synthesis may also be inhibited. Phe also provides partial prenatal protection from the teratogenic effects of OTA (Mayura *et al.*, 1984) and prevents the immunosuppressive effects of OTA in Balb/c mice (Creppy *et al.*, 1980, 1983b; Haubeck *et al.*, 1981). Creppy *et al.* (1983b) found similar inhibitory effects in the respective tRNA synthetase enzymes, when the Phe was replaced by other amino acids. Roth *et al.* (1993) reported that the inhibitory effect on Phe-tRNA synthetase alone cannot explain the inhibitory effects of OTA on growth and that other mechanisms involving OTA-activated substances must be involved. OTA also inhibits the activity of phosphoenolpyruvate carboxykinase (PEPCK) and γ-glutamyl transpeptidase and abolishes the cAMP-mediated increase in the concentration of PEPCK mRNA (Thekkumkara and Patel, 1989). Removal of the Phe moiety from OTA prevents the *in vivo* inhibition of PEPCK activity and protein synthesis (Meisner and Meisner 1981). OTA also inhibits other reactions in which Phe is involved such as those catalysed by Phe hydroxylase (Creppy *et al.*, 1990).

Lipid Peroxidation

OTA disrupts hepatic microsomal calcium homeostasis by impairment of the endoplasmic reticulum membrane, probably via lipid peroxidation (Omar *et al.*, 1991). OTA greatly enhances the rate of NADPH-or ascorbate-dependent lipid peroxidation both *in vivo* (rats) and *in vitro* (liver or kidney microsomes) as measured by malondialdehyde formation. The efficiency for lipid peroxidation enhancement is related to the presence of the phenolic hydroxyl group of the different ochratoxins and correlates well with their known toxicities (Rahimtula *et al.*, 1988, 1989). OTA stimulates lipid peroxidation primarily by chelating ferric ions (Fe^{3+}) and facilitating their reduction to ferrous ions (Fe^{2+}); the subsequent reoxidation is accompanied by O_2 consumption (Omar *et al.*, 1990). The Fe^{3+}–OTA complex produces the extremely damaging hydroxyl radical in the presence of the NADPH–cytochrome P450 reductase system and NADPH (Hasinoff *et al.*, 1990). In the presence of oxygen the OTA–Fe^{2+}–Fe^{2+}–OTA complex provides the active species which initiates lipid peroxidation. Once this process has been initiated, it can be easily propagated in the cellular environment where polyunsaturated fatty acids and oxygen are present. The oxidation of lipids by oxygen continues in a chain of radical reactions. As a consequence of this biochemical process, a wide range of degradation compounds are formed, which are chemically very reactive and produce struc-

tural injuries (Baudrimont *et al.*, 1997). There may be a connection between nephropathy caused by OTA, citrinin, iron and lipid peroxidation. Iron is presented to the tubular lumen in proteinuric states because of the glomerular leak of transferrin. Iron would be expected to be dissociated from transferrin in the tubular fluid because of its low pH and bicarbonate content, and to exist in a form that could catalyse hydroxyl radical formation. It has been suggested that if iron is available in a form capable of catalysing OH-radical formation, it could result in lipid peroxidation of tubular cell membranes (Størmer *et al.*, 1996). Lipid peroxidation caused by the free reactive oxygen species induced by OTA can be prevented in Vero cells by adding superoxide dismutase and catalase, piroxicam or aspartame to the culture medium prior to OTA addition to the medium (Baudrimont *et al.*, 1997). Pfohl-Leszkowicz *et al.* (1993a, b) linked this ability of OTA to enhance lipid peroxidation to the genotoxicity expressed by DNA adduct formation. It is also possible that the OTA-induced DNA single strand breaks in mice and rats are produced by reactive oxygen species (Creppy *et al.*, 1985; Kane *et al.*, 1986).

Inhibition of Mitochondrial ATP Production

OTA inhibits mitochondrial state 3 and 4 respiration in isolated rat liver mitochondria (Moore and Truelove, 1970) by acting as a competitive inhibitor of mitochondrial transport carrier proteins located in the inner mitochondrial membrane (Meisner and Chan, 1974; Wei *et al.*, 1985). OTA also alters the mitochondrial morphology after *in vivo* administration to rats (Suzuki *et al.*, 1975; Brown *et al.*, 1986). The mitochondrial uptake of OTA is an energy-consuming process that results in the depletion of intramitochondrial ATP and the observed ATP decrease was most pronounced in the middle (S2) and the terminal (S3) segment of the proximal tubule (Jung and Endou, 1989). Aleo *et al.* (1991) suggested that mitochondrial dysfunction is an early event during the development of OTA toxicity and that OTA toxicity to rat proximal tubules in suspension was not related to iron-mediated lipid peroxidation as measured by malondialdehyde production. The importance of the mitochondrial mechanism is not clear because OTα, which is non-toxic, was also able to inhibit mitochondrial respiration more effectively than OTA in rat liver mitochondria (Moore and Truelove, 1970).

FUMONISINS

The fumonisins are a group of mycotoxins consisting of a 2-amino-12,16-dimethylpolyhydroxyeicosane backbone esterified with propane-1,2,3-tricarboxylic acid sidechains on C-14 and C-15 (see **Figure 6**). These toxins were first discovered by a South African group led by Marasas (Bezuidenhout *et al.*, 1988; Gelderblom *et al.*,

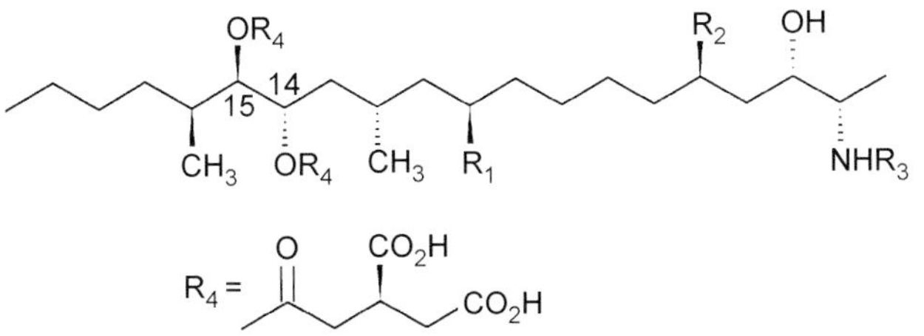

	R_1	R_2	R_3
Fumonisin A_1	OH	OH	CH_3CO
Fumonisin A_2	H	OH	CH_3CO
Fumonisin B_1	OH	OH	H
Fumonisin B_2	H	OH	H
Fumonisin B_3	OH	H	H
Fumonisin B_4	H	H	H

Figure 6 Structures of the fumonisins.

1988) after an investigation into the cause of equine leukoencephalomalacia (LEM), better known as 'hole in the head disease' in horses fed feeds contaminated with the fungus *Fusarium moniliforme*. LEM is a well known disease in many countries such as Mexico, the USA, Egypt and South Africa and causes the liquefactive necrosis of the white matter of the brain of horses and donkeys. Corn contaminated with *F. moniliforme* has also been associated with human oesophageal cancer in the Transkei area of South Africa (Rheeder *et al.*, 1992) and China (Yang, 1980; Chu and Li, 1994). Fumonisins have also been reported to cause pulmonary oedema syndrome in pigs (Harrison *et al.*, 1990) and a non-described poultry disease (ill thrift). Of the six known fumonisins, fumonisin A_1 (FA$_1$) and fumonisin A_2 (FA$_2$), the *N*-acetyl derivatives of fumonisin B_1 (FB$_1$) and fumonisin B_2 (FB$_2$), respectively, are produced in the lowest yields in cultures of *F. moniliforme* and have the lowest toxicities. These two structural analogues and FB$_4$ (**Figure 6**) do not occur under natural conditions. FB$_1$, the most abundant fumonisin in culture and naturally occurring in corn (Rheeder *et al.*, 1995), has been shown to promote tumour formation in rats and to inhibit ceramide synthetase in neuronal cells, an important enzyme in sphingolipid biosynthesis (Wang *et al.*, 1991).

Chemical Characteristics of the Fumonisins

FB$_1$ is a stable compound that persists through most normal food processing procedures (see **Table 13** for physical data for FB$_1$). Fumonisins are soluble in most polar solvents including water and are not soluble in non-

polar solvents. There is no known detoxification process for fumonisin-contaminated foods and feeds. Bezuidenhout *et al.* (1988) elucidated the structure of the fumonisins by employing NMR and mass spectrometric techniques, while the absolute configuration (see **Figure 6**) was determined by contributions from a number of workers including Blackwell *et al.* (1994a), ApSimon *et al.* (1994) and Shier *et al.* (1995) using a combination of NMR and chiral GC methods. Laurent *et al.* (1990), prepared the ammonium salt of FB$_1$, while the acetylated and methylated derivatives of FB$_1$ were prepared by Bezuidenhout *et al.* (1988) and Laurent *et al.* (1990), respectively. FB$_1$ and FB$_2$ can be hydrolysed by heating with hydrochloric acid or potassium hydroxide to yield the aminopentol of FB$_1$ and the aminotetraol of FB$_2$ (Gelderblom *et al.*, 1993).

Table 13 Physical and spectroscopic data for FB$_1$.

Melting-point	103–105 °C
Optical rotation, $[\alpha]_D$	$-28°$ (concentration 2 mg ml^{-1})
Infrared spectrum (KBr)	3450, 2934, 1729 and 1632 cm^{-1}

Production of the Fumonisins

F. moniliforme is the most important producer of the fumonisins; however, a number of other *Fusarium* species are known to be producers of these toxins, as shown in **Table 14**.

Optimum conditions for the production of fumonisins are as follows. *F. moniliforme* is grown on wet corn and incubated at 20 °C for 11–13 weeks (Alberts *et al.*, 1990; Le Bars *et al.*, 1992). The mouldy material is extracted with aqueous methanol and the fumonisin-containing extract is purified by liquid–liquid partitioning, followed by clean-up with XAD-2, silica gel and reversed-phase chromatography (Vesonder *et al.*, 1990; Cawood *et al.*, 1991). Although corn cultures are still the best way of producing large quantities of unlabelled fumonisins, liquid media are ideal for the production of unlabelled and ^{14}C-labelled fumonisins (Miller, 1994). Liquid media usually consist of a carbon source such as glucose or sucrose, a phosphate buffer (pH $\approx$ 4), and salts such as $MgSO_4$, $CaCl_2$, NaCl, NH_4Cl, Na_2SO_4 and $MnSO_4$. Alberts *et al.* (1993) developed a technique for the production of [^{14}C] FB$_1$ by *F. moniliforme* MRC 826 in 'patty' corn cultures by using L-[methyl-^{14}C]methionine as the precursor (Blackwell *et al.*, 1994b).

Table 14 Fungal producers of fumonisins

Fusarium moniliforme	*Fusarium napiforme*
Fusarium dlamini	*Fusarium proliferatum*
Fusarium nygamai	*Fusarium anthophilum*
Fusarium subglutinans	

Source: Thiel *et al.* (1991); Marasas (1996) and references cited.

Determination and Occurrence of the Fumonisins

A wide variety of extraction and clean-up methods exist for the determination of fumonisins. In general, the feeds or foods are extracted with an organic solvent mixture, followed by clean-up by liquid–liquid partitioning, solid-phase extraction, column chromatography or immuno-affinity columns. Quantitation is done by TLC (Shelby et al., 1994), HPLC (Thiel et al., 1993), post-hydrolysis GC (Sydenham et al., 1990), GC–MS (Plattner et al., 1990), liquid secondary ion mass spectrometry (LSIMS), [fast atom bombardment (FAB) MS (Korfmacher et al., 1991)] or MS–MS (Plattner et al., 1990). In many cases fumonisins are reacted with naphthalene-2,3-dicarbox-yaldehyde – potassium cyanide (Kuiper-Goodman et al., 1996), o-phthalaldehyde – mercapto–ethanol (Shephard et al., 1990), Fmoc (Holcomb et al., 1993) or 4-fluoro-7-nitrobenzofurazan (Scott and Lawrence, 1992) to yield fluorescent derivatives which can easily be detected by HPLC systems equipped with fluorescence detectors. Several immunochemical methods for the determination of FB_1 have also been developed, including ELISA with monoclonal antibodies (Azcona-Olivera et al., 1992a), polyclonal antibodies (Azcona-Olivera et al., 1992b; Usleber et al., 1994) and anti-idiotype/anti-anti-idiotype antibodies (Chu et al., 1995). Cross-reaction with FB_2 and FB_3 is very low and immunochemical methods can therefore underestimate the total concentration of fumonisins in a commodity; no cross-reaction occurs with the hydrolysed fumonisins. Schneider et al., (1995) developed a competitive direct dipstick enzyme immunoassay (EIA) and an enzyme-linked immunofil-tration assay (ELIFA) for the detection of FB_1. A nylon membrane was coated with anti-FB_1 antibodies and with anti-horseradish peroxidase (HRP) antibodies. An FB_1–HRP conjugate was used both as the labelled antigen for competitive assay of FB_1 and for non-competitive bind-ing to the anti-HRP antibodies (negative control). Immunoaffinity columns which use monoclonal antibodies are commercially available (FumoniTest, Vicam, Watertown, MA, USA) and have detection limits at ppm levels. Detection limits are reported to be 100 ppb for TLC, 50 ppb for LC–MS, and 200 ppb for ELISA (Thiel et al., 1996, and references cited).

Fumonisin contamination of corn and corn-based products has been reported on all continents. **Table 15** contains suggested safety limits for fumonisins in animal feeds (Thiel et al., 1996, and references cited), and **Table 16** contains some information regarding fumonisin contamination found in different countries. Corn (maize) is a staple food of many people living in Southern Africa; FB_1 contamination of corn may, there-fore, pose a serious threat to human health in these regions.

Table 15 Suggested safety limits for fumonisins

Species	Limit (ppb)
Cattle and poultry	50000
Pigs	10000
Horses	5000

Source: Thiel et al. (1996) and references cited.

Decontamination

The fine particulate matter (<3 mm) in corn contains the highest levels of fumonisins. By removing the 'fines' from bulk shipments of corn, the fumonisin contamination is reduced significantly (Sydenham et al., 1994). Sydenham et al. (1993b) developed a chemical method for the reduc-tion of fumonisin levels in corn by treating it with a slurry of 0.1 M calcium hydroxide for 24 h at 25 °C. The process of milling and the ammoniation treatment of contamin-ated corn also reduce the levels of fumonisins in corn products (Norred et al., 1991). All these different treat-ments suggest that the fumonisins are concentrated on the outer pericarp layer of corn kernels (Sydenham et al., 1993b).

Biological Effects and Mechanism of Action of the Fumonisins

FB_1 has been established to induce completely different toxic effects in different animal species [LEM in horses, hepatotoxic and hepatocarcinogenic to rats, and pul-monary oedema syndrome in pigs (Marasas et al., 1988; Harrison et al., 1990)]. In rats the liver is the main target for toxicity, characterized by cirrhosis and cholangiofi-brosis. FB_1 is also foetotoxic to rats, suppressing both growth and foetal bone development (Lebepe-Mazur et al., 1995). FB_1, FB_2 and FB_3 also affect the kidneys of rats after prolonged exposure, but are, according to Gel-derblom et al. (1988, 1992), not very acutely toxic to rats. Toxic response to fumonisins by rat hepatoma cell line H4TG was visible within 48 h with an IC_{50} value of $4 \mu g \, ml^{-1}$ for FB_1 and $2 \mu g \, ml^{-1}$ for FB_2 (Shier et al., 1992). IC_{50} values were not affected by the density of the cell cultures, indicating that fumonisins are not metabo-lically activated to express their toxic effects. This was confirmed by the absence of metabolites of fumonisins in the urine, bile and blood of rats fed FB_1 and FB_2 (Shep-hard et al., 1993, 1995) and in primary rat hepatocytes (Cawood et al., 1994). FA_1 and FA_2 are less cytotoxic, but PA_1 and PA_2 the hydrolysis products have similar or greater toxicity than the parent compounds (Abbas et al., 1993; Gelderblom et al., 1993). Elimination half-times of 18 and 40 min were found in toxicokinetic studies of FB_1 in blood plasma of rats and monkeys, respectively (Shephard et al., 1992, 1993). Fumonisins are non-

Table 16 References to fumonisin contamination found in different countries

Country	Commodity	Level	Ref.
Italy	Corn and corn-based foods	< 5310 ppb for FB_1, < 1480 ppb for FB_2	Doko and Visconti (1994)
Argentina	Corn	Combined fumonisin levels of 1585–9990 ppb	Sydenham et al. (1993a)
Brazil	Corn and corn-based feeds	0.2–38.5 ppm FB_1, 0.1–12.0 ppm FB_2	Sydenham et al. (1994)
USA	Corn and feeds	1.3–27.0 ppm FB_1, 0.1–12.6 ppm FB_2	Thiel et al. (1991)
India	Corn		Chatterjee and Mukherjee (1994)
Switzerland	Corn-based products		Pittet et al. (1992)
China	Corn	18–155 ppm FB_1	Chu and Li (1994)
New Zealand	Forage grass	1 and 9 ppm FB_1	Mirocha et al. (1992)

mutagenic according to the *Salmonella* test and non-genotoxic according to the DNA-repair assay with *Eschericia coli* (Gelderblom et al., 1996b) and do not induce unscheduled DNA synthesis in primary rat hepatocytes (Gelderblom et al., 1989; Norred et al., 1990). FB_1 mimics genotoxic carcinogens, in both cancer initiation and promotion (Gelderblom et al., 1992, 1994a, b) and also with respect to the induction of resistant hepatocytes in rat liver. FB_1 induces γ-glutamyl transpeptidase (GGT) and the placental form of glutathione-*S*-transferase (GSTP). These enzymes are histological markers for putative preneoplastic lesions which are initiated by genotoxic carcinogens (Gelderblom et al., 1996b). Cancer initiation is affected by the induction of 'resistant' hepatocytes, whose multiplication can be stimulated selectively by a cell proliferation stimulus in the presence of a 2-acetylaminofluorene induced mitoinhibitory effect (Gelderblom et al., 1992, 1993). When diethylnitrosamine is used as a cancer initiator, FB_1 acts as a cancer promoter, as indicated by the formation of γ-glutamyltranspeptidase and GSTP positive foci (Gelderblom et al., 1988, 1996c). Fumonisins differ from genotoxic carcinogens in the sense that their cancer initiation step requires prolonged exposure of the fumonisin while in the case of genotoxic carcinogens this step is normally completed within a few hours or days (Gelderblom et al., 1992). Gelderblom et al. (1994b), for example, found that administration of a dose of 30.8 mg of FB_1 per 100 g body weight to rats over a period of 21 days initiated cancer whereas the administration of a similar dosage over 7 days did not initiate cancer.

Of all the possible mechanisms of action of fumonisin toxicity in mammals, the one most often studied is the inhibition of sphingosine and sphinganine *N*-acyltransferase. The disruption of sphingolipid biosynthesis, by the inhibition of the conversion of sphinganine to *N*-acylsphinganines (dihydroceramides), which precedes the introduction of the double bond of sphingosine, is reported to be connected with the diseases associated with fumonisins (Wang et al., 1991). The disruption of the mechanism of sphingolipids (free long chain bases

which are important components of cell membranes) could have serious effects on cell growth, differentiation and behaviour (Merrill, 1991). This action of fumonisins has been studied in rat liver hepatocytes (Wang et al., 1991), mouse cerebellar neurons *in situ* (Merrill et al., 1993) and *in vivo* in ponies (Wang et al., 1992) and pigs (Riley et al., 1993) and leads to the accumulation of sphingoid bases, which according to Schroeder et al. (1994) is more likely to cause fumonisin mitogenicity than the inhibition of complex sphingolipid biosynthesis *per se*. Mitogens often affect cell transformations and this effect may explain the carcinogenicity of fumonisins. FB_1 and FB_2 are cytotoxic to renal epithelial (LLC-PK_1) cells and inhibit proliferation after a lag period of at least 24 h in which the cells appear to function normally. Inhibition of sphingolipid biosynthesis, with an EC_{50} of 10–15 μM for FB_1, occurred before cell proliferation and cell death, thus supporting the hypothesis that this inhibition is an early event in the toxicity of fumonisins (Yoo et al., 1992). Yoo et al. (1992), also found that the sphinganine levels increased greatly after only 6 h of exposure to 35 μM FB_1 in LLC-PK_1 cells, and that these cells are much less sensitive than primary rat hepatocytes to fumonisin inhibition of *de novo* sphingolipid biosynthesis. Riley et al. (1993) found a relationship between the lower toxicity of FB_1 to the kidneys than to the liver of Sprague–Dawley rats and the degree of disruption of the sphingolipid metabolism of these two organs. The significantly higher elevation of the levels of free sphingosine, free sphinganine, and the free sphinganine-to-sphingosine ratios found in the kidney compared with the liver were also closely reflected in the urine of the rats. Free long-chain bases and lysosphingolipids modulate intracellular signalling systems [e.g. protein kinase C, enzymes of diacylglycerol and phosphatidic acid metabolism and the tyrosine kinase activity of the epidermal growth factor (EGF) receptor], are cytotoxic to some cells and affect protein translocation, ATPases and calcium homeostasis (Riley et al. 1993, and references cited). Gelderblom et al. (1995) demonstrated that FB_1 inhibits the mitogenic response of the EGF *in vitro* in primary hepatocytes. Very little is known about mechanisms involved in the inhibition of growth-related responses in hepatocytes, although the disruption of fatty acid metabolism has been implicated as playing a role (Gelderblom et al., 1996a, 1997).

Apart from the inhibition of sphingolipid biosynthesis, FB$_1$ has also been found to effect the synthesis of cellular lipids by altering the incorporation of palmitic acid (Gelderblom et al., 1996a). Gelderblom et al. (1996a) monitored the fatty acid levels of the major phospholipids (phosphatidylethanolamine and phosphatidylcholine) and neutral lipid triacylglycerides in vitro in rat hepatocytes and in vivo in rats and found alterations in the n-6 fatty acid profiles and decreases in the free cholesterol (membrane associated) levels, which resulted in a higher phosphatidylcholine: cholesterol ratio; this suggested a more rigid membrane structure. A significant increase in the serum and the total cholesterol content of the liver was found when the highest level of 250 mg FB$_1$ kg^{-1} was administered to rats. Fumonisins may thus have important effects on membrane components, the fatty acid storage pool and the accumulation of long-chain fatty acids within the cell, which could eventually lead to the disintegration of membrane structures and eventually result in cell death (Gelderblom et al., 1996b, 1997).

Cell proliferation, an important factor in cancer initiation and promotion, is controlled by long-chain fatty acids via their control of prostaglandin levels (Cornwell and Morisaki, 1984). Prostaglandins can either inhibit or stimulate cell proliferation, depending on the cell type. In vitro studies using Balb/c 3T3 cells have shown that arachidonic acid metabolism is required for the mitogenic response of the EGF (Nolan et al., 1988; Handler et al., 1990).

Primary hepatocytes exposed to FB$_1$ showed an accumulation of polyunsaturated fatty acids. Gavino et al., (1981) demonstrated that increased levels of polyunsaturated fatty acids are associated with lipid peroxidation in normal and cancer cells, which implies that FB$_1$ can indirectly cause lipid peroxidation (see Mechanisms of Action of OTA) (Gelderblom et al., 1996b).

FB$_1$ causes lesions in the liver, kidneys, heart and lungs and subsequent death of broiler chicks (Javed et al., 1992). Qureshi and Hagler (1991) found that FB$_1$ can affect the macrophage-dependent immune system of chickens. These findings were confirmed by Chatterjee and Mukherjee (1994), who found a significant reduction in the viability and phagocytic potential of macrophages from chicken peritoneal exudate cells. Fumonisin consumption may thus result in a decreased immune response which results from FB$_1$-induced depressed macrophages and consequently leads to infections and the development of FB$_1$-induced carcinogenesis.

The short half-life of fumonisins in monkeys plasma (only trace levels are left after 4 hours) indicates that the direct measurement of fumonisins in blood is not suitable

for the determination of fumonisin exposures in animals and humans. Methods have, therefore, been developed to monitor fumonisin toxicosis in monkeys by measuring the sphingamine-to-sphingosine ratio (Shephard et al., 1993, 1996).

FB$_1$ and FB$_2$ are phytotoxic and damage weed and crop cultivars such as soybean and tomato. The primary site of fumonisin toxicity in jimson weed is the plasmalemma or tonoplast. It causes rapid, light-dependent cytoplasmic degeneration and chloroplast disruption (Abbas et al., 1992). FB$_1$ and TA-toxin produced by Alternaria alternata f. sp. lycopersici have similar structures and produce identical genotype-specific necrotic symptoms on detached leaves of resistant and susceptible tomato lines (Marasas, 1996, and references cited).

FB$_1$ and TA-toxin (see **Figure 7**) are more phytotoxic than FB$_2$ and FB$_3$ to corn and tomato seedlings and cause reductions in shoot and root length (Lamprecht et al., 1994). The mechanism of action in plants is not yet known.

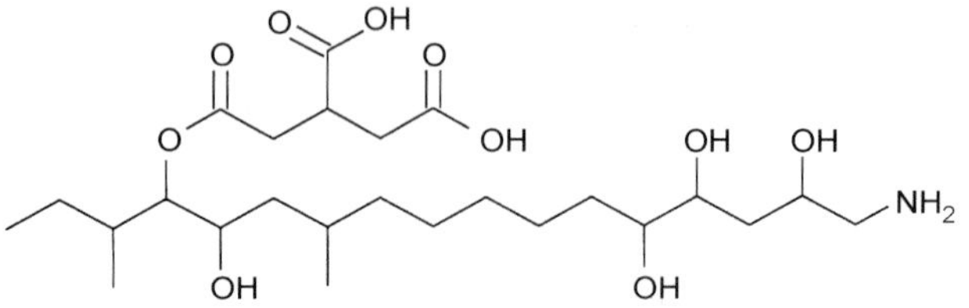

Figure 7 Structure of TA-toxin.

CONCLUSION

Sterling research is currently being done on mycotoxins. These efforts are focused on the molecular genetics of toxinogenic filamentous fungi (Bennett, 1994; O'Donnell, 1997; Bennett et al., 1994), a molecular understanding of the basic mechanism of their action, species differences in metabolism and pharmacokinetics, immunobased and physicochemical techniques for the quantification of mycotoxins, analysis of the risk involved in the exposure of man and domestic animals to mycotoxins, and the associated regulations for the control of mycotoxin contamination (Kuiper-Goodman, 1995) and applying plant molecular biotechnological techniques to breed mycotoxin-resistant cereal-and nut-producing cultivars.

ACKNOWLEDGEMENTS

Several colleagues are thanked for supplying the authors with reprints of recent papers, Mr B. E. Payne for critically reading the chapter, and Dr W. C. A. Gelderblom for valuable inputs into the fumonisin section of this review.

REFERENCES

Abarca, M. L., Bragulat, M. R., Castella, G. and Cabanes, F. J. (1994). Ochratoxin A production by strains of *Aspergillus niger* var. *niger*. *Appl. Environ. Microbiol.*, **60**, 2650–2652.

Abbas, H. K., Paul, R. N., Boyette, C. D. and Duke, S. O. (1992). Physiological and ultrastructural effects of fumonisin on jimsonweed leaves. *Can. J. Bot.*, **70**, 1824–1833.

Abbas, H. K., Gelderblom, W. C. A., Cawood, M. E. and Shier, W. T. (1993). Biological activities of fumonisins, mycotoxins from *Fusarium moniliforme*, in jimsonweed (*Datura stramonium* L.) and mammalian cell cultures. *Toxicon*, **31**, 345–353.

Albassam, M. A., Yong, S. I., Bhatnagar, R., Sharma, A. K. and Prior, M. G. (1987). Histopathologic and electron microscopic studies on the acute toxicity of ochratoxin A in rats. *Vet. Pathol.*, **24**, 427.

Alberts, J. F., Gelderblom, W. C. A., Thiel, P. G., Marasas, W. F. O., van Schalkwyk, D. J. and Behrend, Y. (1990). Effects of temperature and incubation period on the production of fumonisin B_1 by *Fusarium moniliforme*. *Appl. Environ. Microbiol.*, **56**, 1729–1733.

Alberts, J. F., Gelderblom, W. C. A., Marasas, W. F. O. and Rheeder, J. P. (1993). Evaluation of liquid media for fumonisin production by *Fusarium moniliforme* MCR 826. *Mycotoxin Res.*, **10**, 107–115.

Aleo, M. D., Wyatt, R. D. and Schnellmann, R. G. (1991). Mitochondrial dysfunction is an early event in ochratoxin A but not oosporein toxicity to rat renal proximal tubules. *Toxicol. Appl. Pharmacol.*, **107**, 73–80.

ApSimon, J. W., Blackwell, B. A., Blais, L., Fielder, D. A., Greenhalgh, R., Kasitu, G., Miller, J. D. and Savard, M. (1990). Mycotoxins from *Fusarium* species: detection, determination and variety. *Pure Appl. Chem.*, **62**, 1339–1346.

ApSimon, J. W., Blackwell, B. A., Edwards, O. E. and Fruchier, A. (1994). Relative configuration of the C-1 to C-5 fragment of fumonisin B_1 *Tetrahedron Lett.*, **35**, 7703–7706.

Azcona-Olivera, J. I., Abouzied, M. M., Plattner, R. D., and Pestka, J. J. (1992a). Production of monoclonal antibodies to mycotoxins fumonisin B_1, B_2 and B_3. *J. Agric. Food Chem.*, **40**, 531–534.

Azcona-Olivera, J. I., Abouzied, M. M., Plattner, R. D., Norred, W. P. and Pestka, J. J. (1992b). Generation of antibodies reactive with fumonisins B_1, B_2 and B_3 by using cholera toxin as the carrier-adjuvant. *Appl. Environ. Microbiol.*, **58**, 169–173.

Ballinger, M. B., Phillips, T. D. and Kubena, L. F. (1986). Assessment of the distribution and elimination of ochratoxin A in the pregnant rat. *J. Food Safety*, **8**, 1–24.

Baudrimont, I., Betbeder, A. M., Gharbi, A., Pfohl-Leszkowicz, A., Dirheimer, G. and Creppy, E. E. (1994). Effect of superoxide dismutase and catalase on the nephrotoxicity induced by subchronical administration of ochratoxin A in rats. *Toxicology*, **89**, 101–111.

Baudrimont, I., Ahouandjivo, R. and Creppy, E. E. (1997). Prevention of lipid peroxidation induced by ochratoxin A in Vero cells in culture by several agents. *Chem.–Biol. Interact.*, **104**, 29.

Beardall, J. M. and Miller, J. D. (1994). Diseases in humans with mycotoxins as possible causes. In Miller, J. D. and Trenholm, H. L. (Eds), *Mycotoxins in Grain: Compounds Other than Aflatoxin*. Eagan Press, St Paul, MN, pp. 487–539.

Bendele, A. M., Neal, S. B., Oberly, T. J., Thompson, C. Z., Bewsey, B. J., Rexroat, L. E., Carlton, W. W. and Probst, G. (1995). Evaluation of ochratoxin A for mutagenecity in a battery of bacterial and mammalian cell assays. *Food Chem. Toxicol.*, **23**, 911–918.

Bennett, J. W. (1994). From molecular genetics and secondary metabolism to molecular metabolites and secondary genetics. *Can. J. Bot.*, **73**, Suppl. 1, S917–S924.

Bennett, J. W. and Keller, N. P. (1997). Mycotoxins and their prevention. In Anke, T. (Ed.), *Fungal Biotechnology*. Chapman and Hall, Weinheim, pp. 265–273.

Bennett, J. W., Bhatnagar, D. and Chang, P. K. (1994). The molecular genetics of aflatoxin biosynthesis. In Powell, K. A. *et al.* (Eds), *The Genus Aspergillus*. Plenum Press, New York, pp. 51–58.

Betina, V. (1984). Citrinin and related substances. In Betina, V. (Ed.), *Mycotoxins: Production, Isolation, Separation and Purification*. Elsevier, Amsterdam, pp. 217–236.

Bezuidenhout, S. C., Gelderblom, W. C. A., Gorst-Allman, C. P., Horak, R. M., Marasas, W. F. O., Spiteller, G. and Vleggaar, R. (1988). Structure elucidation of the fumonisins, mycotoxins from *Fusarium moniliforme*. *J. Chem. Soc., Chem. Commun.*, 743–745.

Blackwell, B. A., Edwards, O. E., ApSimon, J. W. and Fruchier, A. (1994a). Relative configuration of the C-10 to C-16 fragment of fumonisin B_1. *Tetrahedron Lett.*, **36**, 1973–1976.

Blackwell, B. A., Miller, J. D. and Savard, M. E. (1994b). Production of carbon-14-labeled fumonisins in liquid culture. *J. AOAC Int.*, **77**, 507–511.

Bonna, R. J., Aulerich, R. J., Bursian, S. J., Poppenga, R. H., Braselton, W. E. and Watson, G. L. (1991). Efficacy of hydrated sodium calcium aluminosilicate and activated charcoal in reducing the toxicity of dietary aflatoxin to milk. *Arch. Environ. Contam. Toxicol.*, **20**, 441–447.

Boorman, G. A., Hong, H. L., Dieter, M. P., Hayes, H. T., Pohland, A. E., Stack, M. and Luster, M. I. (1984). Myelotoxicity and macrophage alteration in mice exposed to ochratoxin A. *Toxicol. Appl. Pharmacol.*, **72**, 304–312.

Bose, S. and Sinha, S. P. (1994). Modulation of ochratoxin-produced genotoxicity in mice by vitamin C. *Food Chem. Toxicol.*, **32**, 533–537.

Bredenkamp, M. W., Dillen, J. L. M., Van Rooyen, P. H. and Steyn, P. S. (1989). Crystal structures and conformational analysis of ochratoxin A and B: probing the chemical structure causing toxicity. *J. Chem. Soc., Perkin Trans.* **2**, 1835–1839.

Bressac, B., Kew, M., Wands, J. and Ozturk, M. (1991). Selective G to T mutations of p53 gene in hepatocellular carcinoma from southern Africa. *Nature*, **350**, 429–431.

Brown, M. H., Szczech, G. M. and Purmalis, B. P. (1976). Teratogenic and toxic effects of ochratoxin A in Rats. *Toxicol. Appl. Pharmacol.*, **37**, 331.

Brown, T. P., Manning, R. O. and Fletcher, O. J. (1986). The individual and combined effects of citrinin and ochratoxin A on renal ultrastructure in layer chicks. *Avian Dis.*, **30**, 191–198.

Büchi, G., Foulkes, D. M., Kurono, H. and Mitchell, G. F. (1966). Total synthesis of racemic aflatoxin B_1. *J. Am. Chem. Soc.*, **87**, 882.

Bunge, I., Dirheimer, G. and Röschenthaler, R. (1978). *In vivo* and *in vitro* inhibition of protein synthesis in *Bacillus stearothermophilus* by ochratoxin A. *Biochem. Biophys. Res. Commun.*, **83**, 398.

Carnaghan, R. B. A., Hartley, R. D. and O'Kelly, J. (1963). Toxicity and fluorescence properties of the aflatoxins. *Nature*, **200**, 1101.

Castegnaro, M., Maru, V., Maru, G. and Ruiz-Lopez, M.-D. (1990). High-performance liquid chromatographic determination of ochratoxin A and its 4R-4-hydroxy metabolite in human urine. *Analyst*, **115**, 129–131.

Cawood, M. E., Gelderblom, W. C. A., Vleggaar, R., Behrend, Y., Thiel, P. G. and Marasas, W. F. O. (1991). Isolation of the fumonisin mycotoxins: a quantitative approach. *J. Agric. Food Chem.*, **39**, 1958–1962.

Cawood, M. E., Gelderblom, W. C. A., Alberts, J. F. and Snyman, S. D. (1994). Interaction of ^{14}C-labelled fumonisin B mycotoxins with primary hepatocyte cultures. *Food Chem. Toxicol.*, **32**, 627–632.

Cepeda, A., Franco, C. M., Fente, C. A., Vazquez, B. I., Rodriquez, J. L., Prognon, P. and Mahuzier, G., (1996). Postcolumn excitation of aflatoxins using cyclodextrins in liquid chromatography for food analysis. *J. Chromatogr. A*, **721**, 59–68.

Chatterjee, D. and Mukherjee, S. K. (1994). Contamination of Indian maize with fumonisin B$_1$ and its effects on chicken macrophage. *Lett. Appl. Microbiol.*, **18**, 251–253.

Chatterjee, M. and Townsend, C. A. (1994). Evidence for the probable final steps in aflatoxin biosynthesis. *J. Org. Chem.*, **59**, 4424–4429.

Chu, F. S. (1971). Interaction of ochratoxin A with bovine serum albumin. *Arch. Biochem. Biophys.*, **147**, 359–366.

Chu, F. S. (1974). Studies in ochratoxin. *CRC Crit. Rev. Toxicol.*, **2**, 499.

Chu, F. S. (1992). Recent progress on analytical techniques for mycotoxins in feedstuffs. *J. Anim. Sci.*, **70**, 3950–3963.

Chu, F. S. and Li, G. Y. (1994). Simultaneous occurrence of fumonisin B$_1$ and other mycotoxins in moldy corn collected from the People's Republic of China in regions with high incidences of esophageal cancer. *Appl. Environ. Microbiol.*, **60**, 847–852.

Chu, F. S., Huang, X. and Maragos, C. M. (1995). Production and characterization of anti-idiotype and anti-anti-idiotype antibodies against fumonisin B$_1$. *J. AOAC Int.*, **43**, 261–267.

Ciegler, A. (1975). Mycotoxins. Occurrence, chemistry and biological activity. *Lloydia*, **38**, 21–35.

Cohen, H. and Lapointe, M. (1986). Determination of ochratoxin A in animal feed and cereal grains by liquid chromatography with fluorescence detection. *J. Assoc. Off. Anal. Chem.*, **69**, 957–959.

Cole, R. J. (1986). *Modern Methods in the Analysis and Structural Elucidation of Mycotoxins*. Academic Press, New York.

Cole, R. J. and Cotty, P. J. (1990). Biocontrol of aflatoxin production by using biocompetitive agents. In Robens, J. F. (Ed.), *A Perspective on Aflatoxin in Field Crops and Animal Food Products in the United States*. Agricultural Research Service, Beltsville, MD, pp. 62–68.

Cornwell, D. G. and Morisaki, N. (1984). FA paradoxes in the control of cell proliferation: prostaglandins, lipid peroxides and cooxidation reactions. In Proyor, W. A. (Ed.), *Free Radicals in Biology VI*. Academic Press, Orlando, FL, pp. 95–148.

Cotty, P. J. (1994). Influence of field application of an atoxigenic strain of *Aspergillus flavus* on the populations of *A. flavus* infecting cotton bolls and on the aflatoxin content of cottonseed. *Phytopathology*, **84**, 1270–1277.

Creppy, E. E., Lugnier, A. A. J., Beck, G., Röschenthaler, R. and Dirheimer, G. (1979a). Action of ochratoxin A on cultured heptoma cells – revision of inhibition by phenylalanine. *FEBS Lett.*, **104**, 287–290.

Creppy, E. E., Lugnier, A. A. J., Fasiolo, F., Heller, K., Röschenthaler, R. and Dirheimer, G. (1979b). *In vitro* inhibition of yeast phenylalanyl-tRNA synthetase by ochratoxin A. *Chem.–Biol. Interact.*, **24**, 257.

Creppy, E. E., Schlegel, M., Röschenthaler, R. and Dirheimer, G. (1980). Phenylalanine prevents acute poisoning by ochratoxin A in mice. *Toxicol. Lett.*, **6**, 77–80.

Creppy, E. E., Kern, D., Steyn, P. S., Vleggaar, R., Röschenthaler, R. and Dirheimer, G. (1983a). Comparative study of the effect of ochratoxin A analogues on yeast aminoacyl-tRNA synthesase and on the growth and protein synthesis of hepatoma calls. *Toxicol. Lett.*, **19**, 217–224.

Creppy, E. E., Størmer, F. C., Röschenthaler, R. and Dirheimer, G. (1983b). Effects of two metabolites of ochratoxin A, (4R)-hydroxyochratoxin A and ochratoxin α on the immune response in mice. *Infect. Immunol.*, **39**, 1015–1018.

Creppy, E. E., Röschenthaler, R. and Dirheimer, G. (1984). Inhibition of protein synthesis in mice by ochratoxin A and its prevention by phenylalanine. *Food Chem. Toxicol.*, **22**, 883–886.

Creppy, E. E., Kane, A., Dirheimer, G., Lafarge-Fraysinet, C., Mousset, S. and Fraysinet, C. (1985). Genotoxicity of ochratoxin A in mice: DNA single-strand break evaluation in spleen, liver and kidney. *Toxicol. Lett.*, **28**, 29–35.

Creppy, E. E., Chakor, K., Fisher, M. J. and Dirheimer, G. (1990). The mycotoxin ochratoxin A is a substrate for phenylalanine hydroxylase in isolated rat hepatocytes and *in vivo*. *Arch. Toxicol.*, **64**, 279–284.

Creppy, E. E., Castegnaro, M. and Dirheimer, G. (Eds) (1993). *Human Ochratoxicosis and its Pathologies*. John Libbey Eurotext, London, Vol. 231.

Creppy, E. E., Baudrimont, I. and Betbeder, A.-M. (1995). Prevention of nephrotoxicity of ochratoxin A, a food contaminant. *Toxicol. Lett.*, **82/83**, 869–877.

Creppy, E. E., Baudrimont, I., Belmadoni, A. and Betbeder, A.-M. (1996). Aspartame as a preventive agent of chronic toxic effects of ochratoxin A in experimental animals. *J. Toxicol.*, **15**, 207–221.

Culvenor, C. C. J., Edgar, J. A., Mackay, M. F., Gorst-Allman, C. P., Marasas, W. F. O., Steyn, P. S., Vleggaar, R. and Wessels, P. L. (1989). Structure elucidation and absolute configuration of phomopsin A, a hexapeptide mycotoxin produced by *Phomopsis leptostromiformis*. *Tetrahedron*, **45**, 2351–2372.

Davis, N. D., Currier, G. C. and Diener, U. L. (1986). Aflatoxin contamination of corn hybrids in Alabama. *Cereal Chem.*, **63**, 467–470.

Degen, G. H. and Neumann, H. G. (1978). The major metabolite of aflatoxin B$_1$ in the rat is a glutathione conjugate. *Carcinogenesis*, **11**, 823–827.

De Groene, E. M., Hassing, G. I. A., Blom, M. J., Seinen, W., Fink-Gremmels, J. and Horbach, G. J. (1996a). Development of human cytochrome P450 expressing cell lines; application in mutagenicity testing of ochratoxin A. *Cancer Res.*, **56**, 299–304.

De Groene, E. M., Jahn, A., Horbach, G. J. and Fink-Gremmels, J. (1996b). Mutagenecity and genotoxicity of the mycotoxin ochratoxin A. *Environ. Toxicol. Pharmacol.*, **1**, 21–26.

De Jesus, A. E., Steyn, P. S., Vleggaar, R. and Wessels, P. L. (1980). Carbon-13 nuclear magnetic resonance assignments and biosynthesis of the mycotoxin ochratoxin A. *J. Chem. Soc., Perkin Trans.* **1**, 52–54.

De Jesus, A. E., Steyn, P. S., Van Heerden, F. R., Vleggaar, R., Wessels, P. L. and Hull, W. E. (1983). Tremorgenic mycotoxins from *Penicillium crustosum*. Isolation of penitrems A–F and the structure elucidation and absolute configuration of penitrem A. *J. Chem. Soc., Perkin Trans.* **1**, 1847–1856.

Detroy, R. W. and Ciegler, A. (1971). Aflatoxin biosynthesis in *Aspergillus parasiticus*: effect of methionine analogs. *Can. J. Microbiol.*, **17**, 569–574.

Dirheimer, G. (1996). Personal communication.

Doko, M. B. and Visconti, A. (1994). Occurrence of fumonisins B_1 and B_2 in corn and corn-based human foodstuffs in Italy. *Food Addit. Contam.*, **11**, 433–439.

Dorner, J. W. and Cole, R. J. (1989). Comparison of two ELISA screening tests with liquid chromatography for determination of aflatoxins in raw peanuts. *J. Assoc. Off. Anal. Chem.*, **72**, 962–964.

El-Banna, A. A. and Scott, P. M. (1986). Fate of mycotoxins during processing of foodstuffs III. Ochratoxin A during cooking of faba beans (*Vicia faba*) and polished wheat. *J. Food Protect.*, **47**, 189–192.

Elling, F. (1979). Ochratoxin A-induced mycotoxic porcine nephropathy: alterations in enzyme activity in tubular cells. *Acta Pathol. Microbiol. Scand.*, **87**, 237.

Engel, G. and Teuber, M. (1984). Patulin and other small lactones. In Betina, V. (Ed.), *Mycotoxins: Production, Isolation, Separation and Purification*. Elsevier, Amsterdam, pp. 291–314.

Essigmann, J. M., Green, C. L., Croy, R. G., Fowler, K., Büchi, G. and Wogan, G. N. (1982). Interactions of aflatoxin B_1 and alkylating agents with DNA: structural and functional studies. *Cold Spring Harbor Symp. Quant. Biol.*, **47**, 327–337.

FAO (1996). *Worldwide Regulations for Mycotoxins, 1995. A Compendium*. FAO Food and Nutrition Paper. Food and Agriculture Organization, Rome.

Fink-Gremmels, J., Jahn, A. and Blom, M. J. (1995). Toxicity and metabolism of ochratoxin A. *Nat. Toxins.*, **3**, 214–220.

Fink-Gremmels, J. (1996). Personal communication.

Forrester, L. M., Neal, G. E., Judah, D. J., Glancey, M. J. and Wolf, C. R. (1990). Evidence for involvement of multiple forms of cytochrome P450 in aflatoxin B_1 metabolism in human liver. *Proc. Natl. Acad. Sci. USA*, **87**, 8306–8310.

Franco, J., (1996). Mycotoxins in nuts. In *Proceedings of the IX International IUPAC Symposium on Mycotoxins and Phycotoxins, Rome*, pp. 334–335.

Frohlich, A. A., Marquardt, R. R. and Bernatsky, A. (1988). Quantitation of ochratoxin A: use of reverse phase thin-layer chromatography for sample cleanup followed by liquid chromatography or direct fluorescence measurement. *J. Assoc. Off. Anal. Chem.*, **71**, 949–953.

Fukui, Y., Hoshino, K., Kameyama, Y., Yasui, T., Toda, C. and Nagano, H. (1987). Placental transfer of ochratoxin A and its cytotoxic effect on the mouse embryonic brain. *Food Chem. Toxicol.*, **25**, 17.

Galtier, P., Charpenteau, J. L., Alvinerie, M. and Labouche, C. (1979). The pharmacokinetic profile of ochratoxin A in the rat after oral and intravenous administration. *Drug Metab. Dispos.*, **7**, 429–434.

Galtier, P., Alvinerie, M. and Charpenteau, J. L. (1981). The pharmacokinetic profiles of ochratoxin A in pigs, rabbits and chickens. *Food Cosmet. Toxicol.*, **19**, 735–738.

Gavino, V. C., Miller, J. S., Ikharebha, S. O., Milo, G. E. and Maizewell, D. G. (1981). Effect of polyunsaturated fatty acid and antioxidants on lipid peroxidation in tissue cultures. *J. Lipid Res.*, **22**, 763–769.

Gelderblom, W. C. A., Jaskiewicz, K., Marasas, W. F. O., Thiel, P. G., Horak, R. M., Vleggaar, R. and Kriek, N. P. J. (1988). Fumonisins novel mycotoxins with cancer-promoting activity produced by *Fusarium moniliforme*. *Appl. Environ. Microbiol.*, **54**, 1806–1811.

Gelderblom, W. C. A., Marasas, W. F. O., Thiel, P. G., Semple, E. and Farber, E. (1989). Possible non-genotoxic effects of active carcinogenic components produced by *Fusarium moniliforme*. *Proc. Am. Assoc. Cancer Res.*, **30**, 144.

Gelderblom, W. C. A., Marasas, W. F. O., Vleggaar, R., Thiel, P. G. and Cawood, M. E. (1992). Fumonisins: isolation, chemical characterization and biological effects. *Mycopathologia*, **117**, 11–16.

Gelderblom, W. C. A., Cawood, M. E., Snyman, D., Vleggaar, R. and Marasas, W. F. O. (1993). Structure–activity relationships of fumonisins in short-term carcinogenesis and cytotoxicity assays. *Food Chem. Toxicol.*, **31**, 407–414.

Gelderblom, W. C. A., Cawood, M. E., Snyman, D. and Marasas, W. F. O. (1994a). Fumonisin B_1 dosimetry in relation to cancer initiation in rat liver. *Carcinogenesis*, **15**, 209–214.

Gelderblom, W. C. A., Kriek, N. P. J., Marasas, W. F. O. and Thiel, P. G. (1994b). Toxicity and carcinogenecity of the *Fusarium moniliforme* metabolite, fumonisin B_1 in rats. *Carcinogenesis*, **12**, 1247–1251.

Gelderblom, W. C. A., Snyman, S. D., Van der Westhuizen, L. and Marasas, W. F. O. (1995). Mitoinhibitory effect of fumonisin B_1 on the EGF-induced mitogenic response in primary rat hepatocytes. *Carcinogenesis*, **16**, 625–631.

Gelderblom, W. C. A., Smuts, C. M., Abel, S., Snyman, S. D., Cawood, M. E., van der Westhuizen, L. and Swanevelder, S. (1996a). Effects of fumonisin B_1 on protein and lipid synthesis in primary rat hepatocytes. *Food Chem. Toxicol.*, **34**, 361–369.

Gelderblom, W. C. A., Snyman, S. D., Abel, S., Lebepe-Mazur, S., Smuts, C. M., van der Westhuizen, L., Marasas, W. F. O., Victor, T. C., Knasmulle, R. S. and Huber, W. (1996b). Hepatotoxicity and carcinogenicity of the fumonisins in rats: a review regarding mechanistic implications for establishing risk in humans. In Jackson, L. S., De Vries, I. W. and Bullerman, L. D. (Eds), *Fumonisins in Food*. Plenum Press, New York, pp. 279–296.

Gelderblom, W. C. A., Snyman, S. D., Lebepe-Masur, S., Van der Westhuizen, L., Kriek, N. P. J. and Marasas W. F. O. (1996c). The cancer promoting potential of fumonisin B_1 in rat liver using diethyl nitrosamine as a cancer initiator. *Cancer Lett.*, **109**, 101–108.

Gelderblom, W. C. A., Smuts, C. M., Abel, S., Snyman, S. D., Van der Westhuizen, L., Huber, W. W. and Swanevelder, S. (1997). Effects of fumonisin B_1 on the levels and fatty acid composition of selected lipids in rat liver *in vivo. Food Chem. Toxicol.*, **35**, 647–656.

Gilbert, J. (1993). Recent advances in analytical methods for mycotoxins. *Food Addit. Contam.*, **10**, 37–48.

Gilbert, J. (1995). Analysis of mycotoxins in food and feed: certification of DON in wheat and maize. *Nat. Toxins*, **3**, 263–268.

Gopalakrishnan, S., Harris, T. M. and Stone, M. P. (1990). Intercalation of aflatoxin B_1 in two oligodeoxynucleotide adducts, comparative proton NMR analysis of d(ATC^{AFB}GAT).d(ATCGAT) and d(AT^{AFB}GCAT)2. *Biochemistry*, **29**, 10438–10448.

Goto, T., Wicklow, D. T. and Ito, Y. (1996). Aflatoxin and cyclopiazonic acid production by a sclerotium-producing *Aspergillus tamarii* strain. *Appl. Environ. Microbiol.*, **62**, 4036–4038.

Groopman, J. D., Hall, A. J. and Whittle, H. (1992). Molecular dosimetry of aflatoxin-N7-guanine in human urine obtained in Gambia, West Africa. *Cancer Epidemiol. Biomarkers Prev.*, **1**, 221–227.

Grosse, Y., Pfeifer, A., Mace, K., Harris, C. C., Dirheimer, G. and Pfohl-Leszkowicz, A. (1994). Biotransformation of ochratoxin A by human broncial epithelial cells (BEAS-2B) expressing human cytochrome P450s and implication of glutathione conjugation, *Toxicol. Lett.*, **74S**, 33.

Grosse, Y., Baudrimont, I., Castegnaro, M., Betbeder, A.-M., Creppy, E. E., Dirheimer, G. and Pfohl-Leszkowicz, A. (1995). Formation of ochratoxin A metabolites and DNA-adducts in monkey kidney cells. *Chem.–Biol. Interact.*, **95**, 175–187.

Grove, J. F. (1996). Non-macrocyclic trichothecenes, Part (2). *Prog. Chem. Org. Nat. Prod.*, **69**, 1–70, and references cited.

Hadidane, R., Bacha, H., Creppy, E. E., Hammami, M., Ellouze, F. and Dirheimer, G. (1992). Isolation and structure determination of natural analogues of the mycotoxin ochratoxin A produced by *Aspergillus ochraceus. Toxicology*, **76**, 233–243.

Hagelberg, S., Hult, K. and Fuchs, R. (1989). Toxicokinetics of ochratoxin A in several species and its plasma binding properties. *J. Appl. Toxicol.*, **9**, 91–96.

Handler, J. A., Danilowics, M. and Eling, T. E. (1990). Mitogenic signalling by epidermal growth factor requires arachidonic metabolism in BALB/c 3T3 cells. *J. Biol. Chem.*, **265**, 3669–3673.

Hansen, C. E., Dueland, S., Drevon, C. A. and Størmer, F. C. (1982). Metabolism of ochratoxin A by primary cultures of rat hepatocytes. *Appl. Environ. Microbiol.*, **43**, 1267–1271.

Harrison, L. R., Colvin, B. M., Greene, J. T., Newman, L. E. and Cole, J. R. (1990). Pulmonary edema and hydrothorax in swine produced by fumonisin B_1, a toxic metabolite of *Fusarium moniliforme. J. Vet. Diagn. Invest.*, **2**, 217–221.

Harvey, R. B., Kubena, L. F., Phillips, T. D., Huff, W. E. and Corrier, D. E. (1989). Prevention of aflatoxicosis by addition of hydrated sodium calcium aluminosilicate to the diets of growing barrows. *Am. J. Vet. Res.*, **50**, 416–420.

Hasinoff, B. B., Rahimtula, A. D. and Omar, R. F. (1990). NADPH–cytochrome-P-450 reductase promoted hydroxyl radical production by the iron(III)–ochratoxin A complex. *Biochim. Biophys. Acta*, **1036**, 78.

Haubeck, H.-D., Lorkowski, G., Kölsch, E. and Röschenthaler, R. (1981). Immunosuppression by ochratoxin A and its

prevention by phenylalanine. *Appl. Environ. Microbiol.*, **41**, 1040.

Heathcote, J. G. (1984). Aflatoxins and related toxins. In Betina, V. (Ed.), *Mycotoxins: Production, Isolation, Separation and Purification*, Elsevier, Amsterdam, pp. 89–130.

Hennig, A., Fink-Gremmels, J. and Leistner, L. (1991). Mutagenicity and effects of ochratoxin A on the frequency of sister chromatid exchanges after metabolic activation. In Castegnaro, M., Plestina, R., Dirheimer, G., Chernozemsky, I. N. and Bartsch, H. (Eds), *Mycotoxins, Endemic Nephropathy and Urinary Tract Tumours*. International Agency for Research in Cancer, Lyon, pp. 255–260.

Holcomb, M., Thompson, H. C., Jr., and Hankins, L. J. (1993). Analysis of fumonisin B_1 in rodent feed by gradient elution HPLC using precolumn derivatization with FMOC and fluorescence detection. *J. Agric. Food Chem.*, **41**, 764.

Holzapfel, C. W., Steyn, P. S. and Purchase, I. F. H. (1966). Isolation and structure of aflatoxins M_1 and M_2. *Tetrahedron Lett.*, **25**, 2799–2803.

Holzapfel, C. W. (1968). The isolation and structure of cyclopiazonic acid, a toxic metabolite of *Penicillium cyclopium* Westling. *Tetrahedron*, **24**, 2101–2109.

Hsieh, D. P. H. (1990). Health risks posed by mycotoxins in foods. *Korean J. Toxicol.*, **6**, 159–166.

Hsu, I. C., Metcalf, R. A., Sun, T., Welsch, J. A., Wang, N. J. and Harris, C. C. (1991). Mutational hotspot in the p53 gene in human hepatocellular carcinomas. *Nature*, **350**, 427–428.

Hutchison, R. D., Steyn, P. S. and Thompson, D. L. (1971). The isolation and structure of 4-hydroxyochratoxin A and 7-carboxy-3, 4-dihydro-3-methylisocoumarin from *Penicillium viridicatum. Tetrahedron Lett.*, **43**, 4033–4036.

IPCS, International Programme on Chemical Safety (1990). *Environmental Health Criteria, No. 105*. World Health Organization, Geneva, p. 15.

Ishii, K., Maeda, K., Kamataki, T. and Kato, R. (1986). Mutagenic activation of aflatoxin B_1 by several forms of purified cytochrome P450. *Mutat. Res.*, **174**, 85–88.

Iyer, R. S., Coles, B. F., Thier, K. D., Guengerich, F. P. and Harris, T. M. (1994). DNA adduction by the potent carcinogen aflatoxin B_1: mechanistic studies. *J. Am. Chem. Soc.*, **116**, 1603–1609.

Jackson, L. S., De Vries, J. and Bullerman, L. B. (Eds) (1996). *Fumonisins in Food*. Plenum Press, New York.

Jago, M. V., Peterson, J. E., Payne, A. L. and Campbell, D. G. (1982). Lupinosis: response of sheep to different doses of phomopsin. *Aust. J. Exp. Biol. Med. Sci.*, **60**, 239–251.

Javed, T., Bunte, R. M., Bennett, G. A., Richard, J. L., Dombrink-Kurtzman, M. A., Côté, L. M. and Buck, W. B. (1992). Comparative pathologic changes in broiler chicks on feed amended with *Fusarium proliferatum* culture material or purified fumonisin B_1 and moniliformin. In *Abstracts of 106th AOAC International Annual Meeting, August 31– September 3, 1992, Cincinatti, OH*, p. 30.

Jiao, Y., Blaas, W., Rühl, C. and Weber, R. (1991). Identification of ochratoxin A in food samples by chemical derivatization and gas chromatography–mass spectrometry. *J. Chromatogr.*, **595**, 364–367.

Jung, K. Y. and Endou, H. (1989). Nephrotoxicity assessment by measuring cellular ATP content. II. Intranephron site to ochratoxin A nephrotoxicity. *Toxicol. Appl. Pharmacol.*, **100**, 383.

Kane, A., Creppy, E. E., Roth, A., Röschenthaler, R. and Dirheimer, G. (1986). Distribution of the [³H]-label from low doses of radioactive ochratoxin A ingested by rats, and evidence for DNA single-strand breaks caused in liver and kidneys. *Arch. Toxicol.*, **58**, 219–224.

King, B. (1979). Outbreak of ergotism in Wollo, Ethiopia. *Lancet*, 1411.

Koeltzow, D. E. and Tanner, S. N. (1990). Comparative evaluation of commercially available aflatoxin test methods. *J. Assoc. Off. Anal. Chem.*, **73**, 584–589.

Kok, W. Th., Van Neer, C. H. Th., Traag, W. H. and Tuinstra, L. G. M. Th. (1986). Determination of aflatoxins in cattle feed by liquid chromatography and post-column derivatization with electrochemically generated bromide. *J. Chromatogr.*, **367**, 231–236.

Konrad, I. and Röschenthaler, R. (1977). Inhibition of phenylalanyl-tRNA synthetase of *Bacillus subtilus* by ochratoxin A. *FEBS Lett.*, **83**, 341.

Korfmacher, W. A., Chiarelli, M. P., Lay, J. O., Jr, Bloom, J., Holcomb, M. and McManus, K. T. (1991). Characterization of the mycotoxin fumonisin B₁: comparison of thermospray, fast atom bombardment, and electrospray mass spectrometry. *Rapid Commun. Mass Spectrom.*, **5**, 463–468.

Krogh, P. (1987). Ochratoxin in foods. In Krogh, P. (Ed.), *Mycotoxins in Food*. Academic Press, London, pp. 97–121.

Krogh, P., Axelson, N. H., Elling, F., Gyrd-Hansen, N., Hald, B., Hyldgard-Hensen, J., Larsen, A. E., Madsen, A., Mortenson, H. P., Moller, T., Peterson, O. K., Ravnskov, U., Rostgaard, M. and Aalund, O. (1974). Experimental porcine nephropathy. Changes in renal function and structure induced by ochratoxin A contaminated feed. *Acta Pathol. Microbiol. Scand., Sect. A.*, **246**, (Suppl), 1–21.

Krogh, P., Hald, B., Plestina, R. and Ceovic, S. (1977). Balkan (endemic) nephropathy and foodborne ochratoxin A: Preliminary results and foodstuffs. *Acta Pathol. Microbiol. Immunol. Scand., Sect. B*, **85**, 238–240.

Krogh, P., Gyrd-Hansen, N., Hald, B., Larsen, S., Nielsen, J. P., Smith, M., Ivanoff, C. and Meisner, H. (1988). Renal enzyme activities in experimental ochratoxin A-induced porcine nephropathy: Diagnostic potential of phosphoenolpyruvate carboxykinase and gamma-glutamyl transpeptidase activity. *J. Toxicol. Environ. Health.*, **23**, 1.

Kuiper-Goodman, T. (1989). Risk Assessment of Mycotoxins. In Natori, S., Hashimoto, K. and Ueno, Y. (Eds), *Mycotoxins and Phycotoxins '88*. Elsevier, Amsterdam, pp. 257–264.

Kuiper-Goodman, T. (1995). Mycotoxins: risk assessment and legislation. *Toxicol. Lett.*, **82–83**, 853–859.

Kuiper–Goodman, T. (1996). Risk assessment of ochratoxin A: an update. *Food Addit. Contam.*, **13** (Suppl), 53–57.

Kuiper-Goodman, T. and Scott, P. M. (1989). Review: risk assessment of the mycotoxin ochratoxin A. *Biomed. Environ. Sci.*, **2**, 179–248.

Kuiper-Goodman, T., Scott, P. M., McEwen, N. P., Lombaert, G. A. and Ng, W. (1996). Approaches to risk assessment of fumonisins in corn-based foods in Canada. In Jackson, L. S., De Vries, J. W. and Bullerman, L. B. (Eds), *Fumonisins in Food*. Plenum Press, New York, pp. 369–393.

Kumagai, S. (1985). Ochratoxin A: plasma concentration and excretion into bile and urine in albumin deficient rats. *Food Chem. Toxicol.*, **23**, 941–943.

Kussak, A., Nilsson, C.-A. and Andersson, B. (1995). Determination of aflatoxins in dust and urine by liquid chromatography/electrospray ionization tandem mass spectrometry. *Rapid Commun. Mass Spectrom.*, **9**, 1234–1237.

Lacey, J. (Ed.) (1985). *Trichothecenes and Other Mycotoxins*. Wiley, New York.

Lacey, J. (1991). Natural occurrence of mycotoxins in growing and conserved forage crops. In Smith, J. E. and Henderson, R. S. (Eds), *Mycotoxins and Animal Foods*. CRC Press, Boca Raton, FL, pp. 363–397.

Lamprecht, S. C., Marasas, W. F. O., Alberts, J. F., Cawood, M. E., Gelderblom, W. C. A., Shephard, G. S., Thiel, P. G. and Calitz, F. J. (1994). Phytotoxicity of fumonisins and TA-toxin to corn and tomato. *Phytopathology*, **84**, 383–391.

Langesth, W., Ellingsen, Y., Nymoen, U. and Okland, E. M. (1989). High-performance liquid chromatographic determination of zearalenone and ochratoxin A in cereals and feed. *J. Chromatogr.*, **478**, 269–274.

Laurent, D., Lanson, M., Goasdoué, N., Kohler, F., Pellegrin, F. and Platzer, N. (1990). Étude en RMN ¹H et ¹³C de la macrofusine, toxine isolée de maïs infesté par *Fusarium moniliforme* Sheld. *Analysis*, **18**, 172–179.

Le Bars, J., Le Bars, P., Dupuy, J., Baudra, H. and Cassini, R. (1992). Biotic and abiotic factors in fumonisin and accumulation. In *Abstracts of 106th AOAC International Annual Meeting August 31–September 3, Cincinatti, OH*, pp. 106.

Lebepe-Mazur, S., Bal, H., Hopmans, E., Murphy, P. and Henrich, S. (1995). Fumonisin B₁ is fetotoxic in rats. *Vet. Hum. Toxicol.*, **37**, 126–130.

Lee, L. S., Bayman, P. and Bennett, J. W. (1992). Mycotoxins. In Finkelstein, B. and Ball, C. (Eds), *Biotechnology of Filamentous Fungi. Technology and Products*. Butterworth–Heinemann, Boston, pp. 463–502.

Lepom, P. (1986). Simultaneous determination of the mycotoxins citrinin and ochratoxin A in wheat and barley by high-performance liquid chromatography. *J. Chromatogr.*, **35**, 335–559.

Li, S., Marquardt, R. R., Frohlich, A. A. and Vitti, T. G. (1997). Pharmacokinetics of ochratoxin A and its metabolites in rats. *Toxicol. Appl. Pharmacol.*, **145** (1), 82–90.

Li, S., Marquardt, R. R., Frohlich, A. A., Xiao, H. and Clarke, J. R. (1994). The development of a quantitative ELISA for aflatoxin B₁ in ground peanuts using antibodies isolated from the yolk of a laying hen. *J. Food Protect.*, **57**, 1022–1024.

Lindemann, M. D., Blodgett, D. J. and Kornegay, E. T. (1990). Further evaluation of aflatoxicosis in weaning/growing swine and its amelioration by dietary additives. *J. Anim. Sci.*, **68**, Suppl. 1, 39.

Luster, M. I., Germolec, D. R., Burleson, G. R., Jameson, C. W., Ackermann, M. F., Lamm, K. R. and Hayes, H. T. (1987). Selective immunosuppression in mice and natural killer cell activity by ochratoxin A. *Cancer Res.*, **47**, 2259–2263.

MacDonald, S. and Castle, L. (1996). A UK retail survey of aflatoxins in herbs and spices and their fate during cooking. *Food Addit. Contam.*, **13**, 121–128.

Madhyastha, M. S., Frohlich, A. A. and Marquardt, R. R. (1992). Effect of dietary cholestyramine on the elimination pattern of ochratoxin A in rats. *Food Chem. Toxicol.*, **30**, 709.

Madhyastha, M. S., Marquardt, R. R. and Abramson, D. (1994). Structure–activity relationships and interactions among trichothecene mycotoxins as assessed by yeast bioassay. *Toxicon*, **32**, 1147–1152.

Madsen, A., Hald, B. and Mortensen, H. P. (1982). Feeding experiments with ochratoxin contaminated barley for bacon pigs. 1. Influence on pig performance and residues. *Acta Agric. Scand.*, **32**, 225.

Malaveille, C., Brun, G. and Bartsch, H. (1994). Structure–activity studies in *E. coli* strains on ochratoxin A (OTA) and its analogues implicate a genotoxic free radical and acytotoxic thiol derivatives as reactive metabolites. *Mutat. Res.*, **307**, 141–147.

Manolova, Y., Manolov, G., Parvanova, L., Petkova-Bocharova, T., Castegnaro, M. and Chernozemsky, I. N. (1990). Induction of characteristic chromosomal aberrations, particularly X-trisomy, in cultured human lymphocytes treated by ochratoxin A, a mycotoxin implicated in Balkan endemic nephropathy. *Mutat. Res.*, **292**, 143–149.

Mantle, P. G. (1991). Miscellaneous toxigenic fungi. In Smith, J. E. and Henderson, R. S. (Eds), *Mycotoxins and Animal Foods*. CRC Press, Boca Raton, F.L., pp. 141–152.

Marasas, W. F. O., Kellerman, T. S., Gelderblom, W. C. A., Coetzer, J. A. W., Thiel, P. G. and Van der Lugt, J. J. (1988). Leukoencephalomalacia in a horse induced by fumonisin B₁; isolated from *Fusarium moniliforme*. *Onderstepoort J. Vet. Res.*, **55**, 197–203.

Marasas, W. F. O. (1996). Fumonisins: history, world-wide occurrence and impact. In Jackson, L. (Ed.), *Fumonisins in Food*. Plenum Press, New York, pp. 1–17.

Marquardt, R. R. and Frohlich, A. A. (1992). A review of recent advances in understanding ochratoxicosis. *J. Anim. Sci.*, **70**, 3968–3988.

Mateles, R. I. and Adye, J. C. (1965). Production of aflatoxin in submerged cultures. *Appl. Microbiol.*, **13**, 208–211.

Mayura, K., Parker, R., Berndt, W. O. and Phillips, T. D. (1984). Ochratoxin A-induced teratogenesis in rats: partial protection by phenylalanine. *Appl. Environ. Microbiol.*, **48**, 1186.

Meisner, H. (1976). Energy-dependent uptake of ochratoxin A by mitochondria. *Arch. Biochem. Biophys.*, **173**, 132–140.

Meisner, H. and Chan, S. (1974). Ochratoxin A an inhibitor of mitochondrial transport. *Biochemistry*, **13**, 2759.

Meisner, H. and Meisner, P. (1981). Ochratoxin A, an *in vivo* inhibitor of renal phosphoenolpyruvate carboxykinase. *Arch. Biochem. Biophys.*, **208**, 146.

Merrill, A. H. (1991). Cell regulation by spingosine and more complex sphingolipids. *J. Bioenerg. Biomembr.*, **23**, 83–104.

Merrill, A. H., van Echten, G., Wang, E. and Sandhoff, K. (1993). Fumonisin B₁ inhibits sphingosine (sphinganine) *N*-acyltransferase and *de novo* sphingolipid biosynthesis in cultured neurons *in situ*. *J. Biol. Chem.*, **268**, 27299–27306.

Milanez, T. V. and Leitao, M. F. (1996). The effect of cooking on ochratoxin A content of beans, variety 'Carioca'. *Food Addit. Contam.*, **13**, 89–93.

Miller, J. D. (1994). Production and purification of fumonisins from a stirred jar fermenter. *Nat. Toxins*, **2**, 354–359.

Miller, J. D. and Trenholm, H. L. (1994). *Mycotoxins in Grain: Compounds Other than Aflatoxin*. Eagan Press, St Paul, MN.

Mirocha, C. J., Gilchrist, D. G., Shier, W. T., Abbas, H. K., Wen, Y. and Vesonder, R. F. (1992). AAL toxins, fumonisins (biology and chemistry) and host specificity concepts. *Myco-pathologia*, **117**, 47–56.

Moore, J. H. and Truelove, B. (1970). Ochratoxin A, inhibition of mitochondrial respiration. *Science*, **168**, 1102.

Morgan, M. R. A. (1989). Mycotoxin immunoassays (with special reference to ELISAs). *Tetrahedron*, **45**, 2237–2249.

Morgan, M. R. A., McNerney, R., Chan, H. W.-S. and Anderson, P. H. (1986). Ochratoxin A in pig kidney determined by enzyme-linked immunosorbent assay (ELISA). *J. Sci. Food Agric.*, **37**, 475–480.

Moroi, K., Suzuki, S., Kuga, T., Yamazaki, M. and Kanisawa, M. (1985). Reduction of ochratoxin A toxicity in mice treated with phenylalanine and phenobarbital. *Toxicol. Lett.*, **25**, 1–5.

Mortensen, H. P., Hald, B. and Madsen, A. (1983). Feeding experiments with ochratoxin A contaminated barley for bacon pigs. 5. Ochratoxin A in pig blood. *Acta Agric. Scand.*, **33**, 235–239.

Mortimer, P. H., di Menna, M. E. and White, E. P. (1978). Pithomycotoxicosis 'facial eczema' in cattle. In Wylie, T. D. and Morehouse, L. G. (Eds), *Mycotoxic Fungi, Mycotoxins, Mycotoxicoses—An Encyclopedic Handbook.*, Vol. 2. Marcel Dekker, New York, pp. 63–72.

Mortimer, D. N., Gilbert, J. and Shepherd, M. J. (1987). Rapid and highly sensitive analysis of aflatoxin M₁ in liquid and powdered milks using an affinity column cleanup. *J. Chromatogr.*, **407**, 393–398.

Nakajima, M., Terada, H., Hisada, K., Tsubouchi, H., Yamamoto, K., Uda, T., Kawamura, O. and Ueno, Y. (1990). *Food Agric. Immunol.*, **2**, 189–195.

Natori, S., Hashimoto, K. and Ueno, Y. (Eds) (1989). *Mycotoxins and Phycotoxins '88*. Elsevier, Amsterdam.

Neal, G. E. (1995). Genetic implications in the metabolism and toxicity of mycotoxins. *Toxicol. Lett.*, **82/83**, 861–867.

Nolan, R. D., Danilowicz, R. M., Eling, T. E. (1988). Role of arachidonic acid metabolism in the mitogenic response of Balb/c 3T3 fibroblasts to epidermal growth factors. *Molec. Pharmacol.*, **33**, 650–656.

Norred, W. P., Plattner, R. D., Vesonder, R. F., Hayes, R. F., Bacon, C. W. and Voss, K. A. (1990). Effect of *Fusarium moniliforme* metabolites on unscheduled DNA synthesis (UDS) in rat primary hepatocytes. *Toxicologist*, **10**, 165.

Norred, W. P., Voss, K. A., Bacon, C. W. and Riley, R. T. (1991). Effectiveness of ammonia treatment on detoxification of fumonisin-contaminated corn. *Food Chem. Toxicol.*, **29**, 815–819.

O'Donnell, K. (1997). Phylogenetic evidence indicates the important mycotoxigenic strains Fn-2, Fn-3, Fn-2B and Fn-M represent a new species of *Fusarium*. *Mycotoxins*, **45**, 1–10.

Omar, R. F., Hasinoff, B. B., Mejilla, F. and Rahimtula, A. D. (1990). Mechanism of ochratoxin A stimulated lipid peroxidation. *Biochem. Pharmacol.*, **40**, 1183.

Omar, R. F., Rahimtula, A. D. and Bartsch, H. (1991). Role of cytochrome P-450 in ochratoxin A-stimulated lipid peroxidation. *J. Biochem. Toxicol.*, **6**, 203–209.

Oster, T., Jayyosi, Z., Creppy, E. E., Souhaili, A., El Amri, H. and Batt, A.-M. (1991). Characterization of pig liver purified cytochrome P-450 isoenzymes for ochratoxin A metabolism studies. *Toxicol. Lett.*, **57**, 203.

Park, D. L., (1992). Perspectives on mycotoxin decontamination procedures. *Microb. Hyg. Allerg.*, **4**(9), 21–27.

Paterson, R. R. and Kemmelmeier, C. (1990). Neutral, alkaline and difference ultraviolet spectra of secondary metabolites from *Penicillium* and other fungi, and comparisons to published maxima from gradient high performance liquid chromatograph with diode-array detection. *J. Chromatogr.*, **511**, 195.

Paulsch, W. E., Van Egmond, H. P. and Schuller, P. L. (1982). Thin layer chromatographic method for analysis and chemical confirmation of ochratoxin A in kidneys of pigs. In *Proceedings, V International IUPAC Symposium Mycotoxins and Phycotoxins. September 1–3, 1982, Vienna, Austria.* Austrian Chemical Society, Vienna, pp. 40–43.

Pavlovic, M., Plěstina, R., and Krogh, P. (1979). Ochratoxin A contamination of foodstuffs in an area with Balkan (endemic) nephropathy. *Acta Pathol. Microbiol. Scand.*, Sect B, **87**, 243–246.

Petkova-Bocharova, T. and Castegnaro, M. (1985). Ochratoxin contamination of cereals in an area of high incidence of Balkan endemic nephropathy in Bulgaria. *Food Addit. Contam.*, **2**, 267–270.

Petkova-Bocharova, T., Chernozemsky, I. N. and Castegnaro, M. (1988). Ochratoxin A in human blood in relation to Balkan endemic nephropathy and urinary system tumours in Bulgaria. *Food Addit. Contam.*, **5**, 299–301.

Pfohl-Leszkowicz, A., Grosse, Y., Kane, A., Creppy, E. E. and Dirheimer, G. (1993a). Differential DNA adduct formation and disappearance in three mouse tissues after treatment with the mycotoxin ochratoxin A. *Mutat. Res.*, **289**, 265–273.

Pfohl-Leszkowicz, A., Grosse, Y., Kane, A., Gharbi, A., Beaudrimont, I., Obtrecht, S., Creppy, E. E. and Dirheimer, G. (1993b). Is the oxidation pathway implicated in the genotoxicity of ochratoxin A. In Creppy, E. E., Castegnaro, M. and Dirheimer, G. (Eds), *Human Ochratoxicosis and its Pathologies*, Vol. 231, John Libbey Eurotext, London, pp. 177–187.

Pitt, J. I. (1987). *Penicillium viridicatum, Penicillium verrucosum* and production of ochratoxin A. *Appl. Environ. Microbiol.*, **53**, 266–269.

Pittet, A., Parisod, V. and Schellenberg, M. (1992). Occurrence of fumonisins B$_1$ and B$_2$ in corn-based products from the Swiss market. *J. Agric. Food Chem.*, **40**, 1352–1354.

Plattner, R. D., Beremand, M. N. and Powell, R. G. (1989). Analysis of trichothecene mycotoxins by mass spectrometry and tandem mass spectrometry. *Tetrahedron*, **45**, 2241–2262.

Plattner, R. D., Norred, W. P., Bacon, C. W., Voss, K. A., Peterson, R., Shackelford, D. D. and Weisleder, D. (1990). A method of detection of fumonisins in corn samples associated with field cases of equine leukoencephalomalacia. *Mycologia*, **82**, 698–702.

Pohland, A. E., Schuller, P. L., Steyn, P. S. and van Egmond, H. P. (1982). Physicochemical data for some selected mycotoxins. *Pure Appl. Chem.*, **54**, 2219–2284.

Pohland, A. E., Nesheim, S. and Friedman, L. (1992). Ochratoxin A: a review. *Pure Appl. Chem.*, **64**, 1029–1046.

Qureshi, M. A. and Hagler, W. M. (1991). Effect of fumonisin B$_1$ exposure on chicken macrophage functions *in vitro. Poult. Sci.*, **71**, 104–112.

Rabie, C. J., Sydenham, E. W., Thiel, P. G., Lübben, A. and Marasas, W. F. O. (1986). T-2 toxin production by *Fusarium acuminatum* isolated from oats and barley. *Appl. Environ. Microbiol.*, **52**, 594–596.

Rahimtula, A. D., Bereziat, J. C., Bussachini-Griot, V. and Bartsch, H. (1988). Lipid peroxidation as a possible cause of ochratoxin A toxicity. *Biochem. Pharmacol.*, **37**, 4469.

Rahimtula, A. D., Castegnaro, M., Bereziat, J. C., Bussachini-Griot, V., Broussole, L., Michelon, J. and Bartsch, H. (1989).

In Bach, P. H. and Lock, E. A. (Eds), *Nephrotoxicity*. Plenum Press, New York, p. 617.

Rajakyla, E., Laasasenabo, K. and Sakkers, P. J. (1987). Determination of mycotoxins in grain by high-performance liquid chromatography and thermospray liquid chromatography–mass spectrometry. *J. Chromatogr.*, **384**, 391–402.

Raney, K. D., Coles, B., Guengrich, F. P. and Harris, T. M. (1992). The endo-8,9-epoxide of aflatoxin B$_1$: a new metabolite. *Chem. Res. Toxicol.*, **5**, 333–335.

Resnik, S., Neira, S., Pacin, A., Martinez, E., Apro, N. and Latreite, S. (1996). A survey of the natural occurrence of aflatoxins and zearalenone in Argentine field maize: 1983–1994. *Food Addit. Contam.*, **13**, 115–120.

Rheeder, J. P., Marasas, W. F. O., Thiel, P. G., Sydenham, E. W., Shephard, G. S. and van Schalkwyk, D. J. (1992). *Fusarium moniliforme* and fumonisins in corn in relation to human esophageal cancer in Transkei. *Phytopathology*, **82**, 353–357.

Rheeder, J. P., Sydenham, E. W., Marasas, P. G., Thiel, P. G., Shepard, G. S., Schlechter, M., Stockenström, S., Cronje, D. W., Viljoen, J. H., (1995). Fungal infestation and mycotoxin contamination of South African commercial maize harvested in 1989 and 1990. *S. A. J. Sci.*, **91**, 127–132.

Riley, R. T., An, N.-H., Showker, J. L., Yoo, H.-S., Norred, W. P., Chamberlain, W. J., Wang, E., Merrill, A. H., Jr, Motelin, G., Beasley, V. R. and Haschek, W. M. (1993). Alteration of tissue and serum sphinganine to sphingosine ratio: an early biomarker of exposure to fumonisin-containing feeds in pigs. *Toxicol. Appl. Pharmacol.*, **118**, 105–112.

Roth, A., Eriani, G., Dirheimer, G. and Gangloff, J. (1993). Kinetic properties of pure overproduced *Bacillus subtilis* phenylalanyl-tRNA synthetase do not favour its *in vivo* inhibition by ochratoxin A. *FEBS Lett.*, **326**, 87.

Roux, C. (1986). *Leptosphaerulina chartarum* sp. nov., the teleomorph of *Pithomyces chartarum. Trans. Br. Mycol. Soc.*, **86**, 319.

Sakai, M., Abe, K., Okumura, H., Kawamura, O., Sugiura, Y., Horie, Y. and Ueno, Y. (1992). Genotoxicity and fungi evaluated by SOS microplate assay. *Nat. Toxins*, **1**, 27–34.

Samson, R. A. and Frisvad, J. C. (1991). Current taxonomic concepts on *Penicillium* and *Aspergillus*. In Chelkowski, J. (Ed.), *Cereal Grain Mycotoxins, Fungi and Quality in Drying and Storage*. Elsevier, Amsterdam, pp. 405–439.

Schneider, E., Usleber, E. and Märtlbauer, E. (1995). Rapid detection of fumonisin B$_1$ in corn-based food by competitive direct dipstick enzyme immunoassay/enzyme-linked immunofiltration assay with integrated negative control reaction. *J. Agric. Food Chem.*, **43**, 2548–2552.

Schreeve, B. J., Patterson, D. S. P., Pepin, G. A., Roberts, B. A. and Wrathall, A. E. (1977). Effect of feeding ochratoxin to pigs during early pregnancy. *Brit. Vet. J.*, **133**, 412–417.

Schroeder, J. J., Crane, H. M., Xia, J., Liotta, D. C. and Merrill, A. H. (1994). Disruption of sphingolipid metabolism and stimulation of DNA synthesis by fumonisin B$_1$. *J. Biol. Chem.*, **269**, 3475–3481.

Scott, P. M. (1997). Multi-year monitoring of Canadian grains and grain-based foods for trichothecenes and zearalenone. *Food Addit. Contam.*, **14**, 333–339.

Scott, P. M. and Kanhere, S. R. (1995). Determination of ochratoxin A in beer. *Food. Addit. Contam.*, **12**, 591–598.

Scott, P. M. and Lawrence, G. A. (1992). Liquid chromatographic determination of fumonisins with 4-fluoro-7-nitrobenzofuran. *J. AOAC. Int.*, **75**, 829–834.

Scott, P. M., Lombaert, G. A., Pellaers, P., Bacler, S. and Lapp, J. (1992). Ergot alkaloids in grain foods sold in Canada. *J. AOAC Int.*, **75**, 773–779.

Seegers, J. C., Lottering, M.-L. and Garlinski, P. J. (1994). The mycotoxin ochratoxin A causes apoptosis-associated DNA degradation in human lymphocytes. *Med. Sci. Res.*, **22**, 417.

Shapira, R., Paster, N., Eyal, O., Menasherov, M., Mett, A. and Salomon, R. (1996). Detection of aflatoxigenic mold in grains by PCR. *Appl. Environ. Microbiol.*, **62**, 3270–3273.

Sharman, M., MacDonald, S. and Gilbert, J. (1992). Automated liquid chromatographic determination of ochratoxin A in cereals and animal products using immunoaffinity column clean-up. *J. Chromatogr.*, **603**, 285–289.

Shelby, R. A., Rottinghaus, G. E. and Minor, H. C. (1994). Comparison of thin-layer chromatography and competitive immunoassay methods for detecting fumonisins on maize. *J. Agric. Food Chem.*, **42**, 2064–2067.

Shepherd, M. J. and Gilbert, J. (1984). An investigation of HPLC post-column iodination conditions for the enhancement of aflatoxin B_1 fluorescence. *Food Addit. Contam.*, **1**, 325–335.

Shepherd, M. J., Mortimer, D. N. and Gilbert, J. (1987). A review of approaches to the rapid analysis of aflatoxins in foods. *J. Assoc. Publ. Anal.*, **25**, 129–142.

Shephard, G. S., Thiel, P. G., Sydenham, E. W., Alberts, J. F. and Gelderblom, W. C. A. (1992). Fate of a single dose of the ^{14}C-labelled mycotoxin, fumonisin B_1 in rats. *Toxicon*, **30**, 768–770.

Shephard, G. S., Thiel, P. G., Sydenham, E. W., Alberts, J. F. and Cawood, M. E. (1993). Distribution and excretion of a single dose of the mycotoxin fumonisin B_1 in a non-human primate. *Toxicon*, **32**, 735–741.

Shephard, G. S., Thiel, P. G., Sydenham, E. W. and Snijman, P. W. (1995). Toxicokinetics of the mycotoxin fumonisin B_2 in rats. *Food Chem. Toxicol.*, **33**, 591–595.

Shephard, G. S., van der Westhuizen, L., Thiel, P. G., Gelderblom, W. C. A., Marasas, W. F. O. and van Schalkwyk, D. J. (1996). Disruption of sphingolipid metabolism in non-human primates consuming diets of fumonisin-containing *Fusarium moniliforme*. *Toxicon*, **32**, 735–741.

Shier, W. T. and Abbas, H. K. (1992). A simple procedure for the preparation of aminopentols (fumonisin hydrolysis products AP_1 and AP_2) from *Fusarium moniliforme* on solid media. In *Abstracts of 106th AOAC International Annual Meeting, August 31–September 3, 1992, Cincinatti, OH*, p. 237.

Shier, W. T., Abbas, H. K. and Badria, F. A. (1995). Complete structures of the sphingosine analog mycotoxins fumonisin B_1 and AAL toxin: absolute configuration of the side chains. *Tetrahedron Lett.*, **36**, 1571–1574.

Simpson, T. J. and Pemberton, A. D. (1989). High field ^{1}H NMR studies on the ammoniation of aflatoxin B_1. *Tetrahedron*, **45**, 2451–2464.

Smith, B. L. (1985). Recent advances in facial eczema (pithomycotoxicosis) research. In Lacey, J. (Ed.). *Trichothecenes and Other Mycotoxins*. Wiley, Chicester, pp. 325–329.

Smith, J. E. and Henderson, R. S. (Eds) (1991). *Mycotoxins and Animal Foods*. CRC Press, Boca Raton, FL.

Soucek, S. and Gut, I. (1992), Cytochrome P450 in rats: structures, functions, properties and relevant human forms. *Xenobiotica*, **22**, 83–103.

Sreemannarayana, O. A., Frohlich, A. A., Vitti, T. G., Marquardt, R. R. and Abramson, D. (1988). Studies of the tolerance and disposition of ochratoxin A in young calves. *J. Anim. Sci.*, **66**, 1703.

Stein, A. F., Phillips, T. D., Kubena, L. F. and Harvey, R. B. (1985). Renal tubular secretion and readsorption as factors in ochratoxicosis: Effects of probenecid on nephrotoxicity. *J. Toxicol. Environ. Health*, **16**, 593.

Steyn, P. S. (1980). *The Biosynthesis of Mycotoxins: a Study in Secondary Metabolism*. Academic Press, New York.

Steyn, P. S. (1984). Ochratoxin and related dihydroisocoumarins. In Betina, V. (Ed.), *Mycotoxins—Production, Separation and Purification*. Elsevier, Amsterdam, pp. 183–215.

Steyn, P. S. (Ed.) (1989). Mycotoxins. Tetrahedron Symposia in Print, No. 37. *Tetrahedron*, **45**(8).

Steyn, P. S. (1993). Mycotoxins of human health concern. In Creppy, E. E., Castegnaro, M. and Dirheimer, G. (Eds), *Human Ochratoxicosis and its Pathologies*, Vol. 231. 3–31 John Libbey Eurotext, London, pp. 3–31.

Steyn, P. S. (1995). Mycotoxins, general view, chemistry and structure. *Toxicol. Lett.*, **82/83**, 843–851.

Steyn, P. S. and Holzapfel, C. W. (1967). The isolation of the methyl and ethyl esters of ochratoxins A and B, metabolites of *Aspergillus ochraceus* Wilh. *J. S. Afr. Chem. Inst.*, **20**, 186–189.

Steyn, P. S. and Vleggaar, R. (1985). Tremorgenic mycotoxins. *Fortschr. Chem. Org. Naturst.*, **48**, 1–80, and references cited.

Steyn, P. S., Holzapfel, C. W. and Ferreira, N. P. (1970). The biosynthesis of the ochratoxins, metabolites of *Aspergillus ochraceus*. *Phytochemistry*, **9** 1977–1983.

Steyn, P. S., Vleggaar, R., Du Preez, N. P., Blyth, A. A. and Seegers, J. J. (1975). The *in vitro* toxicity of ochratoxin A in monkey kidney epithelial cells. *Toxicol. Appl. Pharmacol.*, **32**, 198–203.

Steyn, P. S., Thiel, P. G. and Trinder, D. W. (1991). Detection and quantification of mycotoxins by chemical analysis. In Smith, J. E. and Henderson, R. S. (Eds). *Mycotoxins and Animal Foods*. CRC Press, Boca Raton, FL, pp. 165–221.

Steyn, P. S. and Payne, B. E. (1998). Unpublished results.

Stojkovic, R., Hult, K., Gamulin, S. and Plestina, R. (1984). High affinity binding of ochratoxin A to plasma constituents. *Biochem. Int.*, **9**, 33–38.

Stoll, A. (1952). Recent investigations on ergot alkaloids. *Fortsch. Chem. Org. Naturst.*, **9**, 114–174.

Støren, O., Helgerud, P., Holm, H. and Størmer, F. C. (1982a). Formation of (4R)-4-hydroxyochratoxin A and ochratoxin α from ochratoxin A by rats. In *Proceedings, V International IUPAC Symposium Mycotoxins and Phycotoxins. September 1–3, 1982, Vienna, Austria*. Austrian Chemical Society, Vienna, pp. 321–324.

Støren, O., Holm, H. and Størmer, F. C. (1982b). Metabolism of ochratoxin A by rats. *Appl. Environ. Microbiol.*, **44**, 785–789.

Størmer, F. C., Hansen, C. E., Pederson, J. I., Hvistendahl, G. and Aasen, A. J. (1981). Formation of (4R)-and (4S)-4-hydroxyochratoxin A by liver microsomes from various species. *Appl. Environ. Microbiol.*, **42**, 1051–1056.

Størmer, F. C., Støren, O., Hansen, C. E., Pederson, J. I. and Aasen, A. J. (1983). Formation of (4R)- and (4S)-4-hydroxyochratoxin A and 10-hydroxyochratoxin A by rabbit liver microsomes. *Appl. Environ. Microbiol.*, **45**, 1183–1187.

Størmer, F. C., Myhre, C. and Wiger, R. (1996). Ochratoxin A induced apoptosis in HL 60 cells is enhanced by antioxidants. In Miraglia, M., Brera, C. and Onori, R. (Eds), *Proceedings of the IX International IUPAC Symposium on Mycotoxins and Phycotoxins*. Istituto Superiore di Sanità, Rome, p. 226.

Sugamata, M., Ihara, T., Todate, A., Okumura, H., Yoshino, N., Hamaguchi, M., Nakamura, K. and Ueno, Y. (1997). Apoptic cellular damages in thymus, spleen and liver after nivalenol-induced acute toxicosis in mice: a ultrastructural study. *Mycotoxins*, **45**, 39–43, and reference cited.

Suzuki, S., Kozuka, Y., Satoh, T. and Yamazaki, M. (1975). Studies on the nephrotoxicity of ochratoxin A in rats. *Bull. Environ. Contam. Toxicol.*, **43**, 180.

Suzuki, S., Satoh, T. and Yamazaki, M. (1977). The pharmacokinetics of ochratoxin A in rats. *Jpn. J. Pharmacol.*, **27**, 735–744.

Suzuki, S., Moroi, K., Kanisawa, M. and Satoh, T. (1986). Effects of drug metabolizing enzyme inducers on carcinogenesis and toxicity of ochratoxin A in mice (abstract). *Toxicol. Lett.*, **31**, Suppl., 206.

Sydenham, E. W., Thiel, P. G., Marasas, W. F. O., Shephard, G. S., van Schalkwyk, D. J. and Koch, K. R. (1990). Evidence for the natural occurrence of fumonisin B₁, a mycotoxin produced by *Fusarium moniliforme. J. Agric. Food Chem.*, **38**, 1900–1903.

Sydenham, E. W., Shephard, G. S., Thiel, P. G., Marasas, W. F. O., Rheeder, J. P., Peralta Sanhueza, C. E. P., González, H. H. L. and Resnik, S. L. (1993a). Fumonisins in Argentinian field-trial corn. *J. Agric. Food Chem.*, **41**, 891–895.

Syndenham, E. W., Thiel, P. G., Marasas, W. F. O., Stockenström, S., van der Westhuizen, L. and Shephard, G. S. (1993b). Physical and chemical procedures for the removal of fumonisins from maize. In *Proceedings of the UK Workshop on Mycotoxins, 21–23 April 1993*.

Syndenham, E. W., van der Westhuizen, L., Stockenström, S., Shephard, G. S. and Thiel, P. G. (1994). Fumonisin-contaminated maize: physical treatment for the partial decontamination of bulk shipments. *Food Addit. Contam.*, **11**, 25–32.

Szczech, G. M., Carlton, W. W., Tuite, J. and Caldwell, R. (1973). Ochratoxin A toxicosis in Swine. *Vet. Pathol.*, **10**, 347.

Tanaka, T., Hasegawa, A., Yamamoto, S., Lee, U.-S., Sugiura, Y. and Ueno, Y. (1988). Worldwide contamination of cereals by the *Fusarium* mycotoxins nivalenol, deoxynivalenol, and zearalenone. 1. Survey of 19 countries. *J. Agric. Food Chem.*, **36**, 979–983.

Tatsuno, T. (1997). Scabby wheat intoxication and the discovery of nivalenol (a review). *Mycotoxins*, **45**, 11–12.

Thekkumkara, T. J. and Patel, M. S. (1989). Ochratoxin A decreases the activity of phosphoenolpyruvate carboxykinase and its mRNA content in primary cultures of rat kidney proximal convoluted tubular cells. *Biochem. Biophys. Res. Commun.*, **162**, 916–920.

Thiel, P. G., Marasas, W. F. O., Sydenham, E. W., Shephard, G. S., Gelderblom, W. C. A. and Nieuwenhuis, J. J. (1991). Survey of fumonisin production by *Fusarium* species. *Appl. Environ. Microbiol.*, **57**, 1089–1093.

Thiel, P. G., Sydenham, E. W., Shephard, G. S. and van Schalkwyk, D. J. (1993). Study of the reproducibility characteristics of a liquid chromatographic method for the deter-

mination of fumonisins B₁ and B₂ in corn: IUPAC collaborative study. *J. AOAC Int.*, **76**, 361–366.

Thiel, P. G., Sydenham, E. W. and Shephard, G. S. (1996). The reliability and significance of analytical data on the natural occurrence of fumonisins in food. In Jackson, L., De Vries, J. W. and Bullerman, L. B. (Eds), *Fumonisins in Food*, Plenum Press, New York, pp. 145–151.

Thuvander, A., Breitholtz-Emanuelson, A. and Olsen, M. (1995). Effects of ochratoxin A on the mouse immune system after subchronic exposure. *Food Chem. Toxicol.*, **33**, 1005–1011.

Thuvander, A., Breitholtz-Emanuelson, A., Brabencova, D. and Gadhasson, I. (1996a). Influence of perinatal ochratoxin A exposure on the immune system in mice. *Food Chem. Toxicol.*, **34**, 547–554.

Thuvander, A., Funseth, E., Breitholtz-Emanuelson, A., Hallen, I. P. and Oskarsson, A. (1996b). Effects of ochratoxin A on the rat immune system after perinatal exposure. *Nat. Toxins*, **4**, 141–147.

Thuvander, A., Dahl, P. and Breitholtz-Emanuelson, A. (1997). Prenatal exposure of Balb/c mice to ochratoxin A: effects on the immune system in the offspring. *Nat. Toxins*, **4**, 174–180.

Tönsing, E. M., Steyn, P. S., Osborn, M. and Weber, K. (1984). Phomopsin A, the causative agent of lupinosis, interacts with microtubules *in vivo* and *in vitro. Eur. J. Cell. Biol.*, **35**, 156–164.

Townsend, C. A. (1986). Progress towards a biosynthetic rationale of the aflatoxin pathway. *Pure Appl. Chem.*, **58**, 227–238.

Trail, F., Mahanti, N. and Linz, J. (1995). Molecular biology of aflatoxin biosynthesis. *Microbiology*, **141**, 755–765.

Ueno, Y., Sato, N., Ishii, K., Saiha, K. and Enomoto, M. (1972). Toxicological approaches to the metabolites of the *Fusaria*. V. Neosolaniol, T-2 toxin and butenolide, toxic metabolites of *Fusarium sporotrichioides* NRRL 3510 and *Fusarium poae* 3287. *Jpn. J. Exp. Med.*, **42**, 461–472.

Uraguchi, K. and Yamazaki, M. (Eds) (1978). *Toxicology, Biochemistry and Pathology of Mycotoxins*. Halsted Press, New York.

Urry, W. H., Wehrmeister, H. L., Hodge, E. B. and Hidy, P. H. (1966). The structure of zearalenone. *Tetrahedron Lett.*, **27**, 3109–3114.

Usleber, E., Straka, M. and Terplan, G. (1994). Enzyme immunoassay for fumonisin B₁ applied to corn-based food. *J. Agric. Food Chem.*, **42**, 1392–1396.

van der Merwe, K. J., Steyn, P. S. and Fourie, L. (1965). Mycotoxins. Part II. The constitution of ochratoxins A, B and C, metabolites of *Aspergillus ochraceus* Wilh. *J. Chem. Soc.*, 7083–7088.

van Egmond, H. P. (1991). Methods for determining ochratoxin A and other nephrotoxic mycotoxins. In Castegnaro, M., Plestina, R., Dirheimer, G., Chernozemsky, I. N., and Bartsch, H. (Eds), *Endemic Nephropathy and Urinary Tract Tumours*, International Agency for Research on Cancer, Lyon, pp. 55–70.

van Egmond, H. P. (1996). Analytical methodology and regulations for ochratoxin A. *Food Addit. Contam.*, **13**, 11–13.

van Egmond, H. P. and Speijers, G. J. A. (1994). Survey of data on the incidence and levels of ochratoxin A in food and animal feed worldwide. *Nat. Toxins*, **3**, 125–143.

Van Rensburg, S. J. (1986). Role of mycotoxins in endemic liver cancer and oesophageal cancer. In Steyn, P. S. and Vleggaar,

R. (Eds), *Mycotoxins and Phycotoxins* Elsevier, Amsterdam, pp. 483–494.

Van Rensburg, S. J. and Altenkirk, B. (1974). *Claviceps purpurea*—ergotism. In Purchase, I. F. H. (Ed.), *Mycotoxins*. Elsevier, Amsterdam, p. 69.

Varga, J., Kevei, E., Rinyu, E., Teren, J. and Kozakiewicz, Z. (1996). Ochratoxin production by *Aspergillus* species. *Appl. Environ. Microbiol.*, **62**, 4461–4464.

Verardi, G. and Rosner, H. (1995). Some reflections on establishing United Community legislation on mycotoxins. *Nat. Toxins*, **3**, 337–340.

Vesonder, R., Peterson, R., Plattner, R. and Weisleder, D. (1990). Fumonisin B_1: isolation from corn culture and purification by high performance liquid chromatography. *Mycotoxin Res.*, **6**, 85–88.

Wang, E., Norred, W. P., Bacon, C. W., Riley, R. T. and Merrill, A. H. (1991). Inhibition of sphingolipid biosynthesis by fumonisins: implications for diseases associated with *Fusarium moniliforme*. *J. Biol. Chem.*, **266**, 14486–14490.

Wang, E., Ross, F., Wilson, T. M., Riley, R. T. and Merrill, A. H. (1992). Increases in serum sphingosine and sphinganine and decreases in complex sphingolipids in ponies given feed containing fumonisins, mycotoxins produced by *Fusarium moniliforme*. *J. Nutr.*, **122**, 1706–1715.

Wang, L.-Y., Hatch, M., Chen, C.-J., Levin, B., You, S.-L., Lu, S.-N., Wu, M.-H., Wu, W.-P., Wang, L.-W., Wang, Q., Huang, G.-Y., Yang, P.-M., Lee, H.-S. and Santella, R. M. (1996). Aflatoxin exposure and risk of hepatocellular carcinoma in Taiwan. *Int. J. Cancer.*, **67**, 620–625.

Wannemacher, R. W., Bunner, D. L. and Neufeld, H. A. (1991). Toxicity of trichothecenes and other related mycotoxins in laboratory animals. In Smith, J. E. and Henderson, R. S. (Eds). *Mycotoxins and Animal Foods*. CRC Press, Boca Raton, FL, pp. 499–552.

Wei, Y.-H., Lu, C.-Y., Lin, T.-N. and Wei, R.-D. (1985). Effect of ochratoxin A on rat liver mitochondrial respiration and oxidative phosphorylation. *Toxicology*, **36**, 119.

Wood, G. M., Entwistle, A. C., Farnell, P. J., Patel, S. and Boenke, A. (1995). *The Certification of the Ochratoxin A Mass Fraction of Two Wheat Reference Materials (CRMs 471 and 472)*, Document BCR/25/95. Commission of the European Communities, Brussels.

Würgler, F. E., Friedrich, U. and Schlatter, J. (1991). Lack of mutagenecity of ochratoxin A and B, citrinin, patulin and cnestine in *Salmonella typhimurium* TA 102. *Mutat. Res.*, **261**, 209–216.

Xiao, H., Clarke, J. R., Marquardt, R. R. and Frohlich, A. A. (1995a). Improved methods for conjugating selected mycotoxins to carrier proteins and dextran for immunoassays. *J. Agric. Food Chem.*, **43**, 2092–2097.

Xiao, H., Marquard, R. R., Frohlich, A. A. and Ling, Y. Z. (1995b). Synthesis and structure elucidation of analogs of ochratoxin A. *J. Agric. Food Chem.*, **43**, 524–530.

Xiao, H., Madhyastha, S., Marquardt, R. R., Li, S., Vodela, J. K., Frohlich, A. A. and Kemppainen, B. W. (1996a). Toxicity of ochratoxin A, its opened lactone form and several analogs: structure–activity relationships. *Toxicol. Appl. Pharmacol.*, **137**, 182.

Xiao, H., Marquardt, R. R., Abramson, D. and Frohlich, A. A. (1996b). Metabolites of ochratoxins in rat urine and in a culture of *Aspergillus ochraceus*. *Appl. Environ. Microbiol.*, **62**, 648.

Yagen, B., Joffe, A. Z., Horn, P., Mor, N. and Lutsky, I.I. (1977). Toxins from a strain involved in ATA. In Rodricks, J., Hesseltine, C. W. and Mehlman, M. A. (Eds), *Mycotoxins in Human and Animal Health*, Pathotox Publishers, Park Forest South, IL., pp. 327–336.

Yang, C. S. (1980). Research on esophageal cancer in China: A review. *Cancer Res.*, **40**, 2633–2644.

Yoo, H.-S., Norred, W. P., Wang, E., Merrill, A. H., Jr, and Riley, R. T. (1992). Fumonisin inhibition of de novo sphingolipid biosynthesis and cytotoxicity are correlated in LLC-PK1 cells. *Toxicol. Appl. Pharmacol.*, **114**, 9–15.

Yoshino, N., Takizawa, M., Akiba, H., Okumura, H., Tashiro, F., Honda, M. and Ueno, Y. (1996). Transient elevation of intracellular calcium ion levels as an early event in T-2 toxin-induced apoptosis in human promyelotic cell line HL-60. *Nat. Toxins.*, **4**, 234–241.

Yoshino, N., Takizawa, M., Okumura, H., Ihara, T., Sugamata, M., Tashiro, F., Honda, M., Nakamura, K. and Ueno, Y. (1997a). Nivalenol induced apoptosis in human peripheral blood lymphocytes *in vitro* and mouse peripheral blood lymphocytes *in vivo*. *Mycotoxins*, **45**, 33–37.

Yoshino, N., Takizawa, M., Tashiro, F., Honda, M. and Ueno, Y. (1997b). T-2 Toxin induced apoptosis in human peripheral blood lymphocytes *in vitro*. *Res. Commun. Biochem. Cell. Biol.*, **1**, 218–228.

Zimmerli, B. and Dick, R. (1995). Determination of ochratoxin A at the ppt level in human blood, serum, milk and some foodstuffs by high-performance liquid chromatography with enhanced fluorescence detection and immunoaffinity column cleanup: methodology and Swiss data. *J. Chromatogr.*, **666**, 85–99.

Chapter 101
Poisons of Animal Origin

Gregory P. Wedin

CONTENTS

INTRODUCTION

Poisons of animal origin is a broad topic that covers a great variety of toxic substances found in thousands of animal species. The scope of the problem that these animals pose throughout the world is presented here through a discussion of representative species whose poisons are significant hazards to humans.

It is important first to distinguish between animals that are poisonous and those that are venomous. Venomous animals, as the name implies, produce venom in specialized glands or cells that can be administered in some way to their enemy or prey. Poisonous animals, on the other hand, possess a toxin(s) within their tissue that can have deleterious effects on those who eat them.

The venom apparatus, mode of envenomation and constituents of venom vary considerably throughout the animal kingdom. Venomous animals can either bite or sting their victims and some are capable of squirting or spitting venom. The venom of most species is a unique but complex proteinaceous mixture. The biochemical and pharmacological properties of most venoms are incompletely understood owing to their complexity. Interspecies differences and difficulties in obtaining sufficient venom and in extracting individual components further complicate this issue.

An animal may use its venom offensively or defensively. For example, it may be used to subdue or kill its prey and aid in digestion. It also may be used to ward off predators. Most venoms are multi-purpose and cannot be narrowly classified. Obviously, the toxic effects that result from envenomation are greatly influenced by these functional properties and the corresponding venom constituents.

Most poisonous animals accumulate toxin through the marine food chain. The most common initial source are unicellular sea algae (dinoflagellates). A number of these dinoflagellates are responsible for the often publicized 'red tides' which are linked to poisonous shellfish.

Although people who live in regions inhabited by venomous or poisonous animals are at greatest risk of toxic exposure, such encounters can occur virtually anywhere. Venomous animals, for example, are imported by hobbyists and have been shipped inadvertently in produce or other goods. Likewise, poisonous seafood may be shipped to distant markets. This may present a therapeutic dilemma to a practitioner unfamiliar with such exposures. US Poison Information Centers are staffed with specially trained professionals who can provide expert information and advice on the management of such cases. These centres also have access to the Antivenom Index, which was developed to assist with locating the appropriate antivenin for exotic bites and stings. The Index is a joint effort of the American Association of Zoological Parks and Aquariums and the American Association of Poison Control Centers.

SNAKES

Snakes are probably the best recognized of all venomous animals. Their mystical reputation is established in ancient history, myth, magic and religion. While some people adore these creatures, others are inordinately fearful. Snakes and snakebites have been extensively studied, but much is still unknown because of the vast number and complexity of these species and their venoms.

It is estimated that up to 1 million snakebites occur annually worldwide resulting in up to 40 000 deaths. Approximately 45 000 snakebites occur in the USA each year, of which 8000 are inflicted by venomous species (Russell *et al.*, 1975). In the USA only about 9–14 deaths occur annually from venomous snakebites (Russell, 1980). Venomous snakebite is a much more significant problem in other parts of the world. In India, for example, available data suggest that up to 200 000 snakebites occur annually with approximately 15 000 deaths (George *et al.*, 1987).

Most people are bitten on the foot or leg. Accidental snakebites occur most often in children during daylight hours of warm summer months (Parrish, 1966; McNally and Reitz, 1987). On the other hand, adult men are often victims of snakebites that could be easily avoided. Careless handling of snakes has even resulted in bites to the face and tongue (Lewis and Portera, 1994).

Snakes are members of the class Reptilia. There are five families of venomous snakes, the Colubridae, Crotalidae, Elapidae, Hydrophidae and Viperidae. Over 3000 species of snakes are distributed throughout the world, primarily in temperate climates (Russell *et al.*, 1975). Approximately 300 of these snakes are significantly hazardous to man.

Only two snakes in the family Colubridae are significant hazards to man, namely the boomslang (*Dispholidus typus*) and vine snake (*Thelotornis capensis*), which are found in southern Africa (Aitchison, 1990). Their venomous bite results primarily in a consumptive coagulopathy, delayed haemorrhage and related complications. Crotalidae species are distributed throughout the world and include the pit vipers such as rattlesnakes, copperheads and cottonmouths (Kunkel *et al.*, 1983–84; Nelson, 1989). These snakes most notably produce local tissue necrosis and coagulopathies. Elapids, which are found in Asia, Australia, Africa and the Americas, include such notorious creatures as the cobras, mambas and coral snakes (Russell, 1983; Nelson, 1989). Predominantly neurotoxic effects result from the venomous bites of these snakes. The Viperidae family includes the true vipers, native to Africa, Europe and the Middle East (Nelson, 1989). The toxic effects of their bites are comparable to those of the Crotalidae. The Hydrophids include the sea snakes, which are found in the warm, shallow waters of the Indian and Pacific Oceans (Tu and Fulde, 1987). Although these snakes possess very potent neurotoxins, their short fangs and low venom output result in relatively few serious envenomations.

Toxic Manifestations

Snakes are often categorized by the primary toxic effects of their venom, but this oversimplifies the problem. For example, several species of cobra, whose venoms are considered neurotoxic, may also produce significant local necrotic and potentially lethal cardiotoxic events (Blaylock, 1982; Kunkel *et al.*, 1983–84; Minton, 1990). Likewise, rattlesnakes generally produce local tissue damage and coagulopathies but minimal neurotoxicity. The bite of the Mojave rattlesnake (*Crotalus scutulatus*), on the other hand, produces less local swelling and pain, but neurotoxic effects can predominate (Russell *et al.*, 1975; Kunkel *et al.*, 1983–84; Jansen *et al.*, 1992).

Snake venom is a complex mixture of proteins, enzymes, metals and other inorganic substances (Russell, 1983; Iyaniwura, 1991). The venom of some species, in fact, may contain up to 20 different components (Russell, 1983). In general, relatively little is known about the composition of most venoms. The complex nature of snake venom and intra-and interspecies differences contribute to the variability and perplexity of snake venom poisoning.

The potential severity of envenomation depends on a number of factors, including the species of snake, its age and size, the location, number and depth of bites and the total quantity of venom injected. Other important factors include the age and size of the victim and their general state of health. Not all strikes by snakes result in envenomation. So-called 'dry bites' may occur in up to 30% of crotalid bites, 50% of elapid bites and 75% of sea snake bites (Kunkel *et al.*, 1983–84).

Local Toxic Effects

Envenomation by Crotalids and Viperids typically results in significant local toxic effects (Russell, 1980). Pain, swelling and oedema occur soon after the bite. In severe cases, the oedema progresses rapidly. Within several hours the site may become ecchymotic and discoloured. Eccymosis may spread following the path of lymphatic drainage (Roberts and Greenberg, 1997). Vesicles may also appear, which are usually filled with clear fluid but may become filled with blood in severe cases. Local tissue necrosis also may occur, which is probably due to the direct action of venom enzymes. Pain and swelling are generally most severe following bites by eastern and western diamondback rattlesnakes and least severe following bites by copperheads and *Sistrurus* rattlesnake species (Russell *et al.*, 1975).

Coagulopathies

Snake envenomation may result in a variety of systemic manifestations. Probably the most significant but unpredictable are coagulopathies. Snakes within all families have been implicated with such disorders (Blaylock, 1982; Russell, 1983; Cable *et al.*, 1984). Both anticoagulant and procoagulant properties have been described but bleeding disorders occur most commonly. Some venoms display both properties, depending on the degree of envenomation and time course (Marsh, 1994).

Anticoagulation results from constituents of snake venom that (1) activate protein C, which initiates proteolytic inactivation of cofactors Va and VIIIa; (2) interfere with prothrombinase complex formation by direct action on phospholipids or by inhibiting the interaction between prothrombin and the activation complex; (3) digest fibrinogen enzymatically; (4) inhibit thrombin; or (5) activate plasminogen (Marsh, 1994).

Haemorrhagic toxins (haemorrhagins) that rupture the capillary endothelium have recently been identified. Snake venom usually contains multiple forms of these toxins, which are mostly zinc proteases (Marsh, 1994). This direct effect on the endothelium is complicated by other venom components or other actions of these haemorrhagins that cause fibrinolysis, inhibition of platelet aggregation, and thrombocytopenia (Hutton and Warrell, 1993).

Thrombocytopenia with or without other coagulopathies may result from intravascular clotting and consumption of platelets, sequestration of platelets at the site of envenomation or destruction of platelets by the venom (Riffer *et al.*, 1987). The degree of thrombocytopenia may directly correlate with the severity of envenomation (La Grange and Russell, 1970).

Snake venom constituents may interact at various points of the coagulation cascade to activate clotting factors V and X or even prothrombin directly (Marsh, 1994). Thrombin-like enzymes have also been identified in the venom of more than 40 crotalids and viperids (Marsh, 1994). Disseminated intravascular coagulation may complicate severe cases.

Haemodynamic and Cardiotoxic Effects

Cardiovascular shock leads to systemic complications and is a common cause of death due to crotalid envenomation (Hardy, 1986). Shock results from increased capillary permeability, which leads to third-spacing of fluids and intravascular volume depletion (Schaeffer *et al.*, 1979). Reduced cardiac output secondary to venom-induced cardiac changes and also the release of mediators such as bradykinins, histamine and serotonin may also contribute to haemodynamic compromise (Curry and Kunkel, 1985; Christopher and Rodning, 1986). Electrocardiographic abnormalities including T wave inversion and heart block have also occurred following envenomation by a number of snake species (Lalloo *et al.*, 1997).

Neurotoxicity

Neurotoxicity results from envenomation by elapids and hydrophids. The venom of these snakes are comparable but the venoms of sea snakes are more potent (Tu and Fulde, 1987). The neurotoxin of sea snakes binds to postsynaptic acetylcholine receptors, resulting in paralysis (Tu and Fulde, 1987). Respiratory paralysis is the primary cause of immediate death (Kitchens and Van Mierop, 1987). The venom of elapids such as that of the banded krait contain presynaptic neurotoxins which inhibit the release of acetylcholine at the myoneural junction (Minton, 1990). Neurotoxic signs and symptoms include diplopia, slurred speech, deafness, paraesthesiae, hyperaesthesia, muscle fasciculations, weakness, incoordination, trismus, pain, stiffness, drowsiness, apprehension, increased salivation, diaphoresis and convulsions (Russell, 1980; Blaylock, 1982; Kitchens and Van Mierop, 1987; Tu and Fulde, 1987; Nelson, 1989). Crotalid envenomation can also cause perioral paraesthesiae, muscle fasciculations, myokymia and weakness (Russell, 1980; Brick *et al.*, 1987). The Mojave rattlesnake (*Crotalus scutulatus*) is a unique crotalid in that neurotoxic manifestations predominate the clinical course.

Ocular Effects of Spitting Cobra Venom

Two species of cobra, *Naja nigricollis* and *Hemachatus haemachatus*, are capable of spraying or 'spitting' venom defensively into the eyes of a predator. The venom of these snakes produces comparable ocular effects, including intense conjunctivitis, pain, tearing, corneal oedema, de-epithelialization and opacification (Ismail *et al.*, 1993a). This corneal opacification syndrome has been attributed to the cardiotoxins in their venom (Ismail *et al.*, 1993b). Venoms from other major species of cobra that do not spit or spray venom are devoid of such activity.

Other Toxic Manifestations

Numerous other systemic toxic effects have been associated with snakebites. These may result from either direct actions of the venom or as complications of cardiovascular, neuromuscular or coagulation disorders. Renal failure may complicate crotalidae, hydrophidae and viperidae envenomation, which may result from disseminated intravascular coagulation, cardiovascular shock or haemolysis (George *et al.*, 1987; Nelson, 1989). A direct nephrotoxic effect of the venom may be the primary cause of renal dysfunction in certain cases of viperine bites (Vijeth *et al.*, 1997). Adult respiratory distress syndrome may develop in severe cases. The aetiology is unclear but shock, disseminated intravascular coagulation, multiple blood component transfusions and the venom itself have all been postulated (Curry and Kunkel, 1985). Pancreatitis and hepatocellular necrosis have also been reported following snakebite, the aetiology of which is unclear (Kjellstrom, 1989; de Silva *et al.*, 1992).

Management

Although snakebites commonly occur, treatment still remains controversial. Rather than explore fully all treatment issues and modalities, an overview of the generally accepted approach to management is presented here.

The most important first aid measures are to keep the patient calm, immobilize the bitten extremity, and transport to the nearest appropriate health care facility. Incision and suction at the bite site are generally impractical and potentially dangerous. It may be beneficial in a few select cases when it can be performed within a few minutes by a qualified individual using appropriate equipment. Likewise the use of a lymphatic tourniquet to impede venom distribution is of questionable value and hazardous if done improperly. The use of a firm bandage wrapped around the affected extremity in conjunction with immobilization has been shown to delay elapid venom distribution (Sutherland *et al.*, 1979). Such an approach may have utility in the management of elapid or hydrophid bites. The bandage is contraindicated following bites by snakes that cause tissue necrosis such as the crotalids and viperids. Cryotherapy is absolutely contraindicated.

Correct identification of the offending snake is important. Unfortunately, the victim often cannot give a sufficiently detailed description of the snake and it is usually not available for examination. The use of immunological tests to identify snake venom in serum or other materials is currently used in some countries. In Australia, for example, venom detection kits which use the enzyme-linked immunosorbent assay (ELISA) technique are an integral part of snakebite management (Minton, 1987).

Antivenin therapy is the cornerstone of snakebite management worldwide. The choice of antivenin depends on the species of snake involved and available forms of antivenin. Antivenin may be monovalent (activity against only one species of snake) or polyvalent (activity against two or more species of snake). If available, monovalent antivenin is preferable when the offending species of snake is known with certainty. However, owing to significant geographic variations of snake venom, even within the same species, monovalent antivenins are often inadequate (Gillissen *et al.*, 1994). Pooling venoms for the production of antivenin from snakes throughout the region in which the antivenin is to be used will greatly increase its clinical utility and effectiveness. In the USA, for example, Antivenin (Crotalidae) Polyvalent (Wyeth Laboratories, Philadelphia, PA) is active against all pit vipers in the Western Hemisphere and even some Asian species (Otten, 1983).

The clinical status of the patient and the offending snake species should guide antivenin therapy, but it first must be determined if the patient was envenomated. The patient should be closely monitored for the development of local or systemic signs or symptoms and laboratory changes. Approximately 4–6h of observation is generally necessary to rule out significant envenomation. There are, however, notable exceptions. Bites by the eastern coral snake (*Micrurus fulvius*), for example, may produce minimal local toxic effects but profound neurotoxicity may develop hours later. Likewise, the Mojave rattlesnake (*Crotalus scutulatus*) may produce minimal local effects but neurotoxic manifestations can be delayed (Jansen *et al.*, 1992). Accordingly, prophylactic antivenin therapy is indicated for all definite bites by the eastern coral snake and other neurotoxic snakes (Otten, 1983).

Antivenin should be administered as soon as possible following the bite. Continued absorption of venom from a depot at the bite site may prolong the clinical course. As a result, antivenin may need to be administered over a period of days. Also, antivenin therapy should not be ruled out even if the patient presents for treatment despite a significant delay if toxic effects of venom are evident (Gillissen *et al.*, 1994; Bentur *et al.*, 1997).

The dose of antivenin is dependent on the species of snake, the particular antivenin and the severity of the envenomation. It is important to note that children should receive the same dose of antivenin as adults and possibly even more (Otten, 1983).

The initial dose of Antivenin (Crotalidae) Polyvalent for crotalid bites depends on the initial severity of the bite. Russell (1983) recommends grading the severity as minimal, moderate or severe. Minimal envenomations involve only local manifestations confined to the area of the bite and should be treated with three to five vials of antivenin. Moderate envenomations that involve progressive local effects, significant systemic manifestations and laboratory changes should be treated with six to ten vials. Severe envenomation, which should be treated initially with at least ten vials of antivenin, involves the entire extremity or part and there is serious systemic toxicity and laboratory changes. Additional doses of antivenin may needed if toxic effects persist following the initial dose (Russell, 1980). In severe cases, 30 or more vials may be required. The importance for all treatment facilities to maintain adequate supplies of antivenins for indigenous snake species cannot be overstated.

Commercially available snake antivenins are derived from hyperimmunized horse serum. As a result, some patients will develop an immediate type I hypersensitivity reaction, which is IgE mediated (Otten and McKimm, 1983). To reduce the risk of unexpected hypersensitivity reactions, all patients should be skin tested prior to administering antivenin. In the event of an allergic response, the potential risks and benefits of therapy must be weighed carefully. Generally, if life or limb is at stake, antivenin therapy should commence after taking appropriate precautions. Patients who are treated with antivenin also are likely to develop a delayed immune complex reaction commonly known as serum sickness. This is an IgG-and IgM-mediated process which results in the formation of antigen–antibody complexes and the subsequent activation of the complement system (Otten and McKimm, 1983).

Acute IgE-mediated allergic reactions to antigens in the snake venom itself have also been reported (Hogan and Dire, 1990). Repeat bites or other exposure to venom or antivenin put individuals at increased risk of hypersensitivity reactions (Keyler, 1991; Kopp et al., 1993; Pearn et al., 1994). It is important to recognize that individuals who have routine contact with snakes and persons who have repeat bites can present with complex clinical findings of both allergic and toxic manifestations.

The allergenic nature of currently available antivenins is one of several barriers that limit the practical usefulness of antivenin therapy in some cases. It can lead to indecision as to whether to start therapy and restricts the dose of antivenin that can be safely administered. This is further complicated by the fact that in some cases many vials of currently available antivenins are needed to neutralize the venom adequately. Finally, antivenins are often in scarce supply owing to cost, production problems, or even political reasons in some parts of the world.

There is an urgent need for less allergenic antivenins with greater neutralizing properties at less cost. A promising approach involves the use of polyacrylamide gel affinity chromatography to produce purified antibodies (Russell et al., 1985). The superior efficacy and safety of this product have been demonstrated in both in vivo and in vitro studies (Russell et al., 1985).

Purer antivenins containing equine-derived $F(ab')_2$ have been successfully used to treat European viper bites (Karlson-Stiber and Persson, 1994). Allergic side-effects and serum sickness occurred in about 10% of treated patients.

Ovine-derived F(ab) fragments have recently been developed for a variety of snakes, including Vipera berus (common adder), Echis ocellatus (saw-scaled or carpet viper) and Micrurus fulvius fulvius (eastern coral snake). Theoretical advantages of these products include more rapid tissue penetration, larger volume of distribution and decreased risk of immune complex formation and complement-mediated anaphylactic reactions (Meyer et al., 1997). In vivo and in vitro studies have revealed increased potency and a low incidence of side-effects (Rawat et al., 1994). Early results from at least one clinical trial have been promising (Karlson-Stiber et al., 1997). Clinical efficacy was comparable to that obtained with a conventional equine $F(ab')_2$ product without the

appearance of acute anaphylactic reactions or serum sickness. One possible disadvantage of F(ab) is its rapid clearance from the bloodstream (Meyer et al., 1997). As a result, a single dose of antivenin may not persist long enough in the bloodstream to cover continued absorption of venom from the bite site. Alternative dosing regimens for F(ab) antivenins may need to be evaluated.

The application of monoclonal antibody technology may be useful for those species whose venom contains one main toxin such as the elapids (Theakston, 1989). The use of monoclonal antibodies for crotalids or viperids, on the other hand, may prove to be impractical owing to the complexity of their venoms (Sullivan, 1987; Theakston, 1989).

Local wound care should be provided as needed and tetanus immunization should be updated if necessary. Despite significant bacterial flora of the snake oral cavity, infectious complications are infrequent following snakebite. This may be due to the antibacterial activity of snake venom (Talan et al., 1991). Other factors that limit the inoculation of organisms also may reduce infectious complications. Routine prophylactic antibiotic therapy following snakebite, therefore, is generally not recommended (Talan et al., 1991; Clark et al., 1993; Kerrigan et al., 1997).

Prompt irrigation of affected eyes is important for patients exposed to spitting cobra venom. Irrigation with an aqueous heparin solution (2500 U/ml in saline) or tetracycline (1% solution) were effective in limiting the corneal opacification syndrome (Ismail et al., 1993a).

The systemic manifestations of poisonous snakebite are managed with traditional supportive measures. Since intravascular volume depletion is a primary cause of cardiovascular shock, adequate fluid replenishment is essential. Central venous pressure (CVP) and pulmonary artery wedge pressure (PAWP) should be used to guide therapy. Oxygen should be administered and appropriate respiratory support provided as needed. Whole blood or blood products may be needed to treat acute blood loss and specific coagulopathies. Anticholinesterase agents such as neostigmine bromide have been used successfully as a means to treat the paralysis of elapid bites (Blaylock, 1982; Gold, 1996, Lalloo et al., 1996). Antivenin and appropriate supportive measures, however, should be sufficient in most cases.

GILA MONSTER

The Gila monster, Heloderma suspectum, is one of only a few known venomous lizards. There are five subspecies of Heloderma: Heloderma suspectum suspectum and H. suspectum cinctum (banded Gila monster), which are found in the southwestern USA, and H. horridum horridum (beaded lizard), H. horridum exasperatum and H. horridum alvarez, which along with H. suspectum suspectum are found in Mexico (Russell and Bogert,

1981). *H. horridum alvarez* and *H. horridum horridum* are also located further south in Guatemala.

The Gila monster is known to be kept as an exotic pet, and humans may therefore be bitten and require treatment at sites far from their natural habitat. In fact, most bites by this venomous lizard result from careless handling rather than unsuspecting attacks in nature.

The Gila monster is a rather large, slow-moving, nocturnal reptile. Adults may reach 55 cm in length (Russell and Bogert, 1981). They feed mostly on small animals and have few predators other than man.

The Helodermatids have a much less sophisticated venom apparatus than snakes. It consists of two venom glands located in the lower jaw. A pair of venom ducts lead to venom-conducting grooved teeth. When the Gila monster bites it passively injects venom, which is drawn up its teeth by capillary action.

The venom apparatus is used primarily in defence. When the Gila monster bites it often holds on to crush its prey and to allow sufficient venom to be injected. The venom contains proteins and a number of enzymes. Serotonin, amine oxidase, phospholipase A, protease, lipase and hyaluronidase have all been identified (Russell and Bogert, 1981). The venom may also have bradykinin releasing activity.

Toxic Manifestations

There have been only sporadic reports of humans bitten by the Gila monster. The bite generally results in relatively minor local and systemic toxic effects. On the other hand, life-threatening reactions have been reported. Bites should be treated, therefore, as medical emergencies with appropriate evaluation and care.

The Gila monster has strong jaws which can inflict significant local pain due to mechanical trauma. Several small puncture wounds may result. Occasionally, teeth may become lodged in the tissue. Bluish discoloration around the bite may be noted but tissue necrosis is unlikely. Injected venom causes pain that can be intense and may radiate throughout the extremity.

Oedema generally develops more slowly and is less severe than that which occurs with snakebite, but in some cases it can become marked and tense (Roller, 1976; Russell and Bogert, 1981; Hooker and Caravati, 1994). This may contribute to the pain of envenomation. Lymphadenopathy and lymphadenitis have also been reported (Russell and Bogert, 1981; Bou-Abboud and Kardassakis, 1988).

Other common manifestations include generalized weakness, faintness or dizziness, diaphoresis, nausea, vomiting, hypotension and tachycardia (Hooker and Caravati, 1994). Profound hypotension has been reported in several cases (Heitschel, 1986; Piacentine *et al.*, 1986; Streiffer, 1986; Bou-Abboud and Kardassakis, 1988; Preston, 1989).

Other cardiovascular effects have been described, including non-specific electrocardiographic changes, ventricular arrhythmias and myocardial infarction (Roller, 1976; Streiffer, 1986; Bou-Abboud and Kardassakis, 1988; Preston, 1989). Impaired renal function has also been reported, which is probably a result of prolonged hypotension (Preston, 1989).

Laboratory abnormalities may include hypokalaemia and leukocytosis. Thrombocytopenia has rarely been reported (Russell and Bogert, 1981; Bou-Abboud and Kardassakis, 1988; Preston, 1989). Thrombocytopenia associated with reduced fibrinogen and increased prothrombin time, partial thromboplastin time and fibrin split products indicated a consumptive coagulopathy in two cases (Bou-Abboud and Kardassakis, 1988; Preston, 1989).

Management

Limited first aid can be provided. The first step often must be to remove the lizard, which can be difficult. Several reasonable approaches include (1) using a stick or similar device inserted in the back of the jaw to pry it off, (2) putting the affected extremity under water, thereby causing the animal to release itself, or (3) lighting and holding a match under the Gila monster's jaw. Keep the patient warm, immobilize the extremity and transport the patient to an appropriate health care facility.

The site of the bite should be thoroughly cleansed and examined for remaining teeth. An X-ray of the site may be helpful.

There is no commercially available Gila monster antivenin. Vital signs and laboratory values should be monitored closely. An electrocardiogram should also be obtained. Treatment is primarily symptomatic and supportive care.

HYMENOPTERA

Flying insects of the order Hymenoptera can be found throughout the world. Only a few of the thousands of known species are significantly hazardous to man. These include honeybees, bumblebees, wasps, hornets and yellow jackets. Honeybees and bumblebees belong to the family Apidae and the others to the family Vespidae.

Honeybees account for most apidae stings. People are most likely to be stung by honeybees when around flowering plants or if they disturb the bee's colony. The vespids are generally more aggressive and attack vigorously if disturbed. Yellow jackets tend to nest on the ground or in decaying wood. They will scavenge for food and may be pests at picnics or around garbage cans. Hornets build nests in trees or shrubs whereas wasps often nest under eaves of buildings. Venom-sensitive patients may be more likely to be stung than nonsensitive individuals. It is postulated that intrinsic attractants may account for this phenomenon (Stone et al., 1992).

Their stinging apparatus consists of a modified ovipositor that is connected to a venom sac. They grasp the victim's skin with their claws and then jab their stinger into the skin. The stinger of honeybees is barbed so it and the venom sack remain attached to the victim's skin when the bee flies away. This results in the honeybee's demise. Vespids and the bumblebee are generally able to withdraw their stingers and are capable of stinging again. Some yellow jackets, however, also may lose their stinger.

Stings from these insects may result in manifestations ranging from minor local pain and swelling to life-threatening respiratory and cardiovascular compromise. These toxic effects may result from direct local and systemic effects of the venom and also allergic reactions to venom proteins.

Toxic Manifestations

Up to 50 μl of venom may be injected with each sting. This dose is insufficient to produce systemic toxicity; however, venom constituents will produce local irritation and pain. If a person is stung many times at once then sufficient venom may be injected to produce toxicity. Systemic toxicity due to bee stings resembles an allergic reaction. Acute tubular necrosis resulting from multiple bee stings has been reported (Beccari et al., 1992). Toxicity due to vespid stings may include an acute allergic-like response followed by delayed effects such as haemolysis, rhabdomyolysis and renal failure (Bousquet et al., 1984).

The normal physiological response to a hymenoptera sting consists of a small, painful, urticarial lesion that lasts only a few hours. Approximately 10–17% of people may develop a large local reaction that includes swelling and erythema greater than 5 cm in diameter which may last more than 24 h (Maguire and Geha, 1986; Reisman, 1989). This large local reaction may have an immunological origin.

Allergic Manifestations

The allergic reactions to hymenoptera stings deserve detailed discussion. The allergic response may range from exaggerated local effects to anaphylaxis and death. It is estimated that hymenoptera stings account for at least 40–50 deaths annually in the USA, more deaths than result from all other venomous animals (Golden, 1989). The systemic allergic response to hymenoptera stings is IgE mediated. Indirect complement activation may also play a role in insect sting anaphylaxis (Van der Linden et al., 1990). There is considerable cross-reactivity among the various vespids but cross-reactivity

between vespid and bee venoms is relatively uncommon (Wright and Lockey, 1990).

The incidence of systemic allergic reactions may be as low as 0.4–0.8% in children but as high as 4.0% in adults (Settipane et al., 1972; Golden et al., 1982). Up to 10–15% of the population may be sensitized to hymenoptera venom but have not had an allergic response (Golden et al., 1982).

Systemic allergic reactions can range from mild, primarily dermatological manifestations to life-threatening anaphylaxis. Mild systemic reactions consist of generalized urticaria, angioedema, erythema and pruritus (Maguire and Geha, 1986). Gastro-intestinal symptoms may also be present. Laryngeal oedema, bronchospasm and hypotension can be life-threatening in severe cases (Maguire and Geha, 1986).

There are limited data to characterize which patients may develop none, some or all of these manifestations. Important factors include the age of the patient, history of prior stings, sensitization as documented by skin test or RAST (radioallergosorbent tests) and previous response to hymenoptera stings. Approximately 75% of the population is not sensitized to hymenoptera venom and will develop a normal local response and less than 1% will develop a systemic allergic reaction (Golden, 1989). Those who have previously had normal or large local reactions but have a positive skin test or RAST have a 10–20% risk of developing a systemic reaction (Golden, 1989). Patients with a previous history of a systemic reaction who have a positive skin test or RAST have a 50% chance of developing another systemic reaction (Golden, 1989).

It is commonly thought that patients develop more severe reactions with subsequent stings. While it is true that patients who receive repeat stings within a relatively short period (weeks to months) are more likely to develop a systemic reaction, most patients develop more mild or similar reactions with subsequent stings (Golden, 1989; Valentine et al., 1990). Insect sting allergy, in fact, is a self-limited disease for most people (Reisman, 1989). In other words, the more time between stings, the less likely a person is to have a serious systemic reaction.

The typical allergic response in children is very different to that in adults. Children are more likely to have cutaneous manifestations but less likely to develop hypotension (Golden, 1989). Also, children much less frequently develop recurrent systemic manifestations. In fact, children who have previously had non-life-threatening allergic reactions are unlikely subsequently to develop a life-threatening reaction (Schuberth et al., 1983; Valentine et al., 1990).

Management

First aid treatment for hymenoptera stings includes removing the stinger (if left behind) by scraping across

2184   General and Applied Toxicology

the site with a blunt edged object such as a dull knife or credit card. Do not grab the stinger to pull it out as squeezing the venom sack will inject more venom. The area should be washed well with soap and water. Normal local reactions can be managed by applying ice to reduce swelling, oedema and pruritus. An antihistamine such as diphenhydramine may also help relieve pruritus. Large local reactions may be helped by elevating the extremity and administering an analgesic and also a glucocorticoid such as prednisone. The combined use of H_1- and H_2-antagonists has been suggested as a means to decrease the severity of late phase cutaneous reactions (deShazo et al., 1984).

Epinephrine is the drug of choice for systemic sting reactions. Subcutaneous administration is adequate in mild to moderate cases. In the event of hypotension, epinephrine should be administered intravenously. Intravenous fluids and aggressive cardiopulmonary resuscitation should be provided if epinephrine therapy alone is not adequate. Oral or intravenous antihistamines should only be used for cutaneous manifestations of hymenoptera allergy.

Patients who are at risk of developing systemic allergic reactions should be prescribed an emergency kit that contains epinephrine for subcutaneous injection. This includes those patients with a previous history of systemic allergic effects and those who have had large local reactions and have a positive skin test or RAST.

Venom immune therapy (VIT) may be useful in selected cases. It is currently indicated for those patients who have previously had life-threatening systemic reactions and have a positive skin test or RAST (Maguire and Geha, 1986). Adults are more likely candidates than children since adults are at greater risk for developing a repeat systemic reaction. Immunotherapy, in fact, is unnecessary in most children (Valentine et al., 1990). Other patients with less severe systemic reactions who have positive skin tests or RAST may benefit from VIT, but the cost of therapy and other factors such as their age, medical history, occupation, outdoor activities or hobbies must be considered.

Conventional VIT consists of administering a gradually increasing dose of venom over 4–12 weeks to a maintenance dose of 50–100 μg. Rush protocols, in which venom doses are administered while the patient is hospitalized, achieve maintenance doses within only 4–5 days. The incidence of adverse reactions varies greatly among studies, but it seems that 50% or more of patients develop at least mild systemic effects. The variability reported may result from differences in patient populations, dosing regimens and the species of venom used for VIT. Bee venom, for example, is not as well tolerated as vespid venoms (Muller et al., 1992; Youlten et al., 1995).

Both conventional and rush VIT protocols have produced protection rates up to 97% (Golden and Valentine, 1984; Reisman and Livingston, 1992). The protection rate for honeybee venoms, however, is only about 80%.

The issue of when to discontinue VIT is still controversial. Recent evidence, however, suggests that VIT can be safely discontinued after 5 years (Graft and Schoenwetter, 1994; Golden et al., 1996).

ANTS

Ants belong to the family Formicidae and comprise the third group of venomous hymenoptera. Thousands of ant species are found throughout the world, some of which can inflict painful venomous stings. Local or systemic allergic reactions can also occur. Not all venomous ants sting. Some, such as the carpenter and weaver ants of the subfamily Formacinae, bite their prey and then spray venom into the wound. Formic acid, which is a potent cytotoxin, is the primary constituent of their venom (Rhoades et al., 1977).

Fire ants (*Solenopsis* sp.) are native to both North and South America. Fire ant envenomation is a significant health hazard in the southern USA (Blum, 1984; Stafford et al., 1989a). In fact, up to 60% of the population in an infested area are stung each year (deShazo et al., 1990). The red imported fire ant (*Solenopsis invicta*) has rapidly spread throughout the southern USA and has overtaken the less aggressive native species (*S. xyloni*), as well as the black imported fire ant (*S. richteri*). The imported fire ants of the USA are so named because they are thought to have been introduced via produce shipped from Brazil to Mobile, Alabama, in 1939.

Ants sting to subdue their prey and as a means of defence. A fire ant grasps its victim with its mandibles then, using its head as a pivot, it swings its abdominal stinger to inflict multiple stings (Diaz et al., 1989). Unlike other hymenoptera, fire ants sting slowly and may inject venom for seconds to minutes (Stafford et al., 1989b). With each sting the ant injects 0.04–0.11 μl of venom (deShazo et al., 1990).

The venom of most ants and other hymenoptera consists primarily of protein (Blum, 1984). Imported fire ant venom, on the other hand, is 90–95% piperidine alkaloids and contains only 0.1% protein (Hoffman et al., 1988a). Four proteins have been identified, namely *Sol i I, Sol i II, Sol i III* and *Sol i IV* (Hoffman et al., 1988a). All these proteins are significant allergens.

Toxic Manifestations

Toxicity associated with fire ant envenomation is normally limited to the site of the sting. *In vitro* studies indicate that the venom has haemolytic, cytotoxic, bactericidal and insecticidal properties (Adrouny et al., 1959; Rhoades et al., 1977). Multiple stings (approximately 10 000), however, have not resulted in systemic toxicity (Diaz et al., 1989).

The local response to envenomation includes an initial weal and flare reaction. Superficial vesicles with clear fluid develop at the site of the sting within 4h. This fluid is lost and replaced within 8–10h by cloudy fluid which becomes purulent. A pustule develops within 24 h, which may be surrounded by a red halo (Car *et al.*, 1957). This lesion is pathognomonic in the USA for fire ant stings (Lockey, 1990). An important complication of fire ant stings is secondary infection (Parrin *et al.*, 1981).

Large local reactions may also occur, which may be immunologically mediated (Diaz *et al.*, 1989). These reactions are characteristic of 'late-phase reactions' that occur secondary to ragweed (deShazo *et al.*, 1984). Systemic allergic reactions characteristic of those caused by other hymenoptera also may occur. The natural history of such responses has not been well studied but is probably comparable to that for other hymenoptera. Anaphylaxis may result in up to 1% of stings (deShazo *et al.*, 1990).

The prevalence of asymptomatic sensitized people to fire ant venom is comparable to that which exists for other hymenoptera, approximately 16% (Hoffman *et al.*, 1988b). Cross-reactivity may exist between bee or wasp venom and fire ant venom. *Sol i II* has been identified as the cross-reactive protein (Hoffman *et al.*, 1988b).

Neurological sequelae including seizures and mononeuropathy have also been reported (Fox *et al.*, 1982; Candiotti and Lamas, 1993). The aetiology of such reactions is not known.

Management

First aid for fire ant envenomation consists primarily of thorough washing with soap and water. Although a number of therapeutic measures have been evaluated as a means to alter the development of pustules, neither topical nor parenteral therapies had any effect on developing lesions (Parrin *et al.*, 1981). A cold compress may help relieve some swelling and discomfort. The pustules should be bandaged to prevent excoriation. Large local reactions and systemic allergic reactions should be managed as previously described for other hymenoptera.

As with other hymenoptera, the indications for immunotherapy are not clear. The relatively high risk of stings in sensitized people, however, causes many to undergo such therapy (Stafford *et al.*, 1989c). To confound the issue further, only whole body extracts are available for therapy, which contain variable quantities of venom. Some evidence of its effectiveness, however, has been presented (Hylander *et al.*, 1989).

SPIDERS

Spiders are arthropods of the order Arachnidae. Most spiders are venomous; in fact, all but two families of spiders have venom glands. Thousands of venomous spiders exist throughout the world, but only a few are of significant medical importance. Most notable are spiders of the genus *Latrodectus* and *Loxosceles*.

Black Widow Spider

The true black widow spider (*Latrodectus mactans*) is found in temperate zones of North America including all of the USA except Alaska. Other *Latrodectus* species are found throughout the world (Rauber, 1983–84). The major differences between these species are in their body markings and habitats. *L. mactans* has a characteristic shiny black coloration with a red hourglass-shaped marking on its abdomen. Generally these spiders are non-aggressive and bite defensively when threatened or disturbed. They are typically found in undisturbed, protected areas such as storage buildings, wood piles and trash heaps. Female spiders make irregular funnel-shaped webs in which to trap prey and suspend their egg sacs.

Only the females of this species are hazardous to man. The male is too small to cause significant envenomation. The black widow has claw-like hollow fangs which are connected to two venom glands in its cephalothorax. The venom glands have striated musculature which controls the injection of venom. While there are some interspecies differences in venom constituents, the toxic fraction appears to be the same (Rauber, 1983–84).

The venom of the black widow spider, which is one of the most potent of all animal venoms, is primarily neurotoxic. The venom gland contains just less than 0.2 mg of venom (Binder, 1989). The mean lethal dose ranges from 0.005 to 1.0 mg kg^{-1} in various animal species (Edlich *et al.*, 1985). The venom acts at the neuromuscular synaptic junction causing the release of acetylcholine and norepinephrine from presynaptic vesicles (Rauber, 1983–84; Binder, 1989). This results in excessive neuromuscular stimulation and, as expected, other cholinergic and adrenergic signs and symptoms. The venom causes local muscle pain initially, which then generalizes to involve primarily large muscle groups (Kobernick, 1984).

Toxic Manifestations

Most bites in humans occur above the waist on the forearm or torso (Moss and Binder, 1987). Bites are more prevalent during late summer and early autumn, when there are increased numbers of both young and mature spiders (Moss and Binder, 1987). Although the bite itself is often not initially painful and may go unnoticed, pain at the site is the most common early symptom of envenomation (Moss and Binder, 1987). Other common symptoms include abdominal pain and cramping as well as lower extremity pain and weakness. Hypertension, tachycardia, fever, leukocytosis, vomiting, restlessness, mental status changes, headache, rash, paraesthesiae, albuminuria, ptosis and periorbital oedema have also been reported. In severe cases shock, coma, respiratory failure and pulmonary oedema may occur (Binder, 1989; LaGrange, 1990). The mortality rate from black widow envenomation is probably less than 1% (Binder, 1989).

Management

There are no specific first aid measures for black widow envenomation. The bite site should be thoroughly cleansed and tetanus immunization should be updated if necessary. Medical management is primarily directed at relieving muscle spasms and pain. Calcium gluconate, administered intravenously, has been shown to be both safe and effective (Binder, 1989). Centrally acting muscle relaxants such as methocarbamol and diazepam may also provide relief. Dantrolene sodium, a direct acting muscle relaxant, has been used successfully and is reported to provide more pronounced and protracted relief (Ryan, 1983–84). Narcotic analgesics and sedatives can also be employed to help relieve pain and restlessness. Combined use of the aforementioned medications has been recommended over single drug therapy as first line treatment (Reeves et al., 1996).

An equine-derived antivenin is available but is not used routinely in the USA because of the risks associated with horse serum-based products. In one study of a small number of patients there was no demonstrable difference between those who received antivenin and those who did not in terms of length of hospitalization, ancillary drug use for pain control or clinical outcome (Moss and Binder, 1987). It is generally recommended that antivenin be reserved for cases of severe envenomation in which standard measures are inadequate. It also can be used in life-threatening situations and in those patients at high risk for severe morbidity such as the very young or old, and in those with underlying hypertension, cardiac or cerebrovascular disease. As with any equine-derived antivenin, the risk of hypersensitivity reactions must be considered and appropriate skin testing and other precautions must be taken.

Necrotic Arachnidism

Bites of some spiders result primarily in local tissue destruction. This condition has been referred to as necrotic arachnidism. The most notorious of these spiders are those of the genus *Loxosceles*. Spiders of this genus are found throughout North and South America, Africa, Australia, southern Russia, the Mediterranean and the Orient (Gendron, 1990). *Loxosceles* spiders are fawn to dark brown in colour with relatively long skinny legs and have a characteristic violin-shaped marking on its dorsal carapace (Binder, 1989). The terms brown, violin or fiddleback spider are used to describe these species. The brown recluse spider, *Loxosceles reclusa*, is the most important species in the USA. It has been extensively studied and exemplifies the toxicity associated with these spiders.

The diagnosis of brown recluse envenomation and its actual incidence are difficult to establish because of other potential causes of necrotic wounds, including bites of other spiders and confusing medical conditions such as infections or toxic epidermal necrolysis (Russell and Gertsch, 1983). Diagnostic difficulties also have hampered attempts to study various treatment modalities. For example, in one series of 95 cases of presumed brown recluse spider bite, only 17 cases could be confirmed and ultimately studied (Rees et al., 1987). A highly specific passive haemagglutin inhibition test has been described, which can serve as a useful test for determining entry into controlled treatment trials for brown recluse spider bites (Barrett et al., 1993).

The brown recluse spider is found primarily in the south-central USA (Majeski and Durst, 1976). Most reported bites have occurred in Arkansas, Kansas, Missouri and Oklahoma. These spiders inhabit primarily warm, dry, secluded places and can be found both indoors and outdoors. The household closet is the most frequently reported site of discovery (Rees and Campbell, 1989). Other potential sites include wood piles, storage buildings, stored clothing, attics, basements and other quiet locations. The brown recluse is nocturnal and, as a result, most bites occur during the night (Rees and Campbell, 1989). These spiders are most active in summer months and hibernate during the winter.

Toxic Manifestations

The venom of the brown recluse is both cytotoxic and haemolytic. At least nine proteins have been identified, most notably a hyaluronidase, which accounts for the spreading of injected venom, and sphingomyelinase D, which probably contributes to its haemolytic and cytotoxic properties (Wasserman, 1988; Hobbs and Harrell, 1989; Rees and Campbell, 1989). The quantity of venom injected is relatively small and by itself is unlikely to cause significant injury. The destructive nature of the venom is apparently faciliated by complement activation and subsequent inflammatory response (Rees et al., 1983; Hobbs and Harrell, 1989). This results in endothelial cell damage, haemorrhage, infiltration of polymorphonuclear leukocytes and thrombosis of venules and arterioles, causing necrosis (Berger et al., 1973).

The bite of a brown recluse spider results in little more than a stinging or prick sensation and may go unnoticed by the victim. The clinical manifestations following envenomation depend on the amount of venom injected, the site of envenomation and the age, underlying health and immune status of the victim (Majeski and Durst, 1976;

Wasserman and Anderson, 1983–84). Not all patients develop the characteristic necrotic lesion or potentially severe systemic effects. It may be that many bites go unrecognized because only minimal envenomation occurs and victims experience only mild discomfort that resolves uneventfully within a few days (Berger, 1973).

Most patients, even following significant envenomation, do not present for treatment until many hours after the bite, once the initial signs of a necrotic lesion become evident (Gendron, 1990). The most common presenting signs and symptoms include erythema, cellulitis, generalized rash, blister, pain, pruritus, malaise, chills and sweats (Rees *et al.*, 1987). The characteristic lesion begins as a blister with surrounding ischemic discoloration (Wasserman and Anderson, 1983–84; Hobbs and Harrell, 1989). An erythematous ring may surround this area giving a characteristic 'bulls eye' or 'halo' appearance (Wasserman and Anderson, 1983–84). The blister subsequently becomes a bluish macule, the centre of which generally sinks below surrounding tissue (Hobbs and Harrell, 1989). Over several days the necrotic lesion may progress resulting in an area of eschar which sloughs off after 7–14 days. This leaves an area of ulceration 1–30 cm in diameter (Wasserman and Anderson, 1983–84; Hobbs and Harrell, 1989). Bites in fatty areas of the body tend to become more extensive (Wasserman and Anderson, 1983–84). It may take weeks to months for this area to heal by second intention. A small percentage of patients may develop persistent lesions which could subsequently progress to the development of pyoderma gangrenosum and pseudoepitheliomatus hyperplasia (Rees *et al.*, 1987; Hoover *et al.*, 1990).

Systemic toxicity occurs less commonly and may not develop for 24–72 h after the bite. Systemic toxic effects may include fever, malaise, arthralgias, myalgias, rash, convulsions, haemolysis, thrombocytopenia, anaemia and disseminated intravascular coagulation (Wasserman and Anderson, 1983–84; Williams *et al.*, 1995). Nephrotoxicity may result as a complication of haemolysis and subsequent haemoglobinuria.

Management

The treatment of necrotic arachnidism, regardless of the spider involved, should consist of sound local wound management. This should include thorough cleansing, tetanus prophylaxis as necessary, immobilization, elevation and rest (Wasserman, 1988). Cool compresses may help relieve inflammation and pain (Gendron, 1990). A nitroglycerin patch applied to the bite site is reported to abort ischaemic damage; however, controlled clinical data are not available (Burton, 1995). Prophylactic antibiotics generally are not indicated and steroid therapy has not been found to be effective (Wasserman, 1988; Cole *et al.*, 1995). Symptomatic relief can be provided with the use of antipruritic, analgesic and antianxiety agents.

In definite cases of brown recluse spider bite, in which there is progressive local involvement, dapsone therapy may help to limit the necrotic lesion and speed healing (Berger, 1984; Cole *et al.*, 1995). It is postulated that dapsone may be effective by reducing polymorphonuclear leukocyte infiltration (King and Rees, 1983). This therapeutic modality, however, remains controversial (Phillips *et al.*, 1995). Also, dapsone itself may produce dose-dependent haemolytic anaemia, which is likely to be more severe in those with glucose-6-phosphate dehydrogenase deficiency. Dapsone should be used cautiously, therefore, and only when the diagnosis of *Loxosceles reclusa* envenomation is certain. Early excisional therapy should be avoided as it has been shown to be ineffective and potentially disfiguring or disabling (Wasserman and Anderson, 1983–84).

In cases of systemic involvement, therapy should be directed at specific complications. Systemic corticosteroids may help reduce venom induced destruction of red blood cells. Platelets and packed red blood cells may be indicated in the presence of thrombocytopenia or anaemia, respectively. Good hydration should be maintained and renal function monitored. Alkalinization of the urine is indicated in the presence of haemoglobinuria or haematuria.

A brown recluse spider antivenin has been prepared and has been shown *in vitro* to abolish the dermonecrotic activity of brown recluse venom (Rees *et al.*, 1984). In a clinical trial involving 17 patients, antivenin was comparable in effectiveness to dapsone therapy alone or dapsone in combination with antivenin (Rees *et al.*, 1987). In a rabbit model, combined dapsone and brown recluse antivenin were synergistic at improving lesion development and hastening resolution time (Cole *et al.*, 1995). Further evaluation of these therapeutic approaches is warranted. The general availability of a highly refined antivenin would be tremendous therapeutic advance for brown recluse spider bites.

SCORPIONS

True scorpions are arachnids of the order Scorpionida. There are approximately 650 species distributed worldwide, only a few of which are of significant medical importance (Curry *et al.*, 1983–84). All of these are in the Buthidae family. Scorpions primarily inhabit deserts and semiarid regions. While scorpions are native to certain locales, it is important to recognize that they may be inadvertently transported in luggage or other goods to distant areas (Trestrail, 1981).

In the USA, the most significant of all the scorpions is *Centruroides exilicauda* (bark scorpion), which is found primarily in Arizona, but also inhabits areas within New Mexico, California and Texas and also Mexico (Likes *et al.*, 1984). A number of other scorpions which can produce significant envenomation may be found in South

America, Africa, India and the Middle East (Banner, 1989).

Scorpions are nocturnal and take shelter during the day under rocks or piles of debris or may hide inside houses in clothing or shoes. The bark scorpion notoriously shelters under the loose bark of trees and in crevices of dead trees or logs (Likes *et al.*, 1984). Scorpions feed primarily on insects, spiders and occasionally other scorpions (Banner, 1989).

Scorpions have a hard exoskeleton and three primary body parts: the cephalothorax, to which are attached a pair of pincers; an abdomen, which has four pairs of legs; and a tail, which is segmented and ends in a telson which contains the stinging apparatus. The telson contains two venom glands which lead via independent ducts to the stinger. The scorpion uses its pincers to grab its prey and then arches its tail over its body and head to inject venom. Likewise, the scorpion may grab the skin of humans and sting, sometimes repeatedly, in self-defence.

Toxic Manifestations

The venom of scorpions is primarily neurotoxic. This property appears to result from its effects on the activation and inactivation of sodium channels, which ultimately results in the release of catecholamines and acetylcholine (Wang and Strichartz, 1983; Banner, 1989). Other venom fractions exhibit enzymatic, anticholinesterase, coagulopathic, haemolytic, cardiotoxic and pancreatotoxic properties (Banner, 1989).

Most envenomations occur on the extremities. Adults are most commonly stung, but children are more likely to develop serious toxicity (Curry *et al.*, 1983–84; Likes *et al.*, 1984, Berg and Tarantino, 1991). The sting of *Centruroides exilicauda* causes local pain, numbness, hyperaesthesia, salivation, agitation, wheezing, tachycardia, hypertension and muscle spasms (Likes *et al.*, 1984). In severe cases, cranial nerve and somatic motor abnormalities such as eye movement disorders, blurred vision, tongue fasciculations, difficulty in swallowing and jerking of the extremities may develop (Curry *et al.*, 1983–84). Respiratory failure, pulmonary oedema, multiorgan failure and rhabdomyolysis have been described in severely envenomated children (Berg and Tarantino, 1991).

Centruroides and *Tityus* scorpions are of significant importance in South America. Clinical manifestations are similar to those produced by other scorpions and result from excess neurotransmitter release from the sympathetic and parasympathetic nerve endings and adrenal medulla. Severe envenomation may result in cardiocirculatory failure and pulmonary oedema (Hering *et al.*, 1993) *Tityus* scorpion envenomation may also produce significant local pain and erythema. This species has also been reported to produce pancreatitis (Bartholomew, 1970).

In South Africa, the most important genera of scorpions include *Parabuthus* and *Bothotus*. These scorpions

most commonly sting their victims; however, certain species of *Parabuthus* are also capable of squirting venom up to 1 m (Newlands, 1978). If the venom enters the eye or open wound it can cause toxicity comparable to that of the spitting cobra. Local effects following envenomation by these South African scorpions includes local burning and possibly swelling. Systemic toxicity may include muscle contractions, convulsions, perspiration, salivation, tachycardia, arrhythmias and irregular respirations (Newlands, 1978). Death may result from respiratory or cardiac failure.

Red scorpion (*Mesobuthus tamulus*) envenomation in India can cause severe toxicity and death. Excessive release of catecholamines can result in myocardial damage, arrhythmias, cardiac failure and pulmonary oedema (Alagesan *et al.*, 1977; Rajarajeswari *et al.*, 1979; Bawaskar, 1982). Other reported manifestations in both fatal and non-fatal cases include profuse sweating, mydriasis, vomiting and priapism (Bawaskar, 1982).

The Middle East and northern Africa are inhabited by the yellow scorpion (*Leiurus quinquestriatus*) and also *Androctonus* and *Buthus* species. The yellow scorpion also causes excessive release of catecholamines, which can result in myocardial damage and congestive heart failure (Barzilay *et al.*, 1982). Arrhythmias and pulmonary oedema have also been reported (Alagesan *et al.*, 1977; Rahav and and Weiss, 1990). Pancreatitis is a common complication of envenomation by the yellow scorpion and may explain the abdominal pain and vomiting commonly seen following envenomation (Sofer *et al.*, 1991).

Management

First aid for scorpion envenomation consists of good local wound care, including thorough cleansing and tetanus prophylaxis if necessary. Cold compresses can be applied to help relieve pain and inflammation if present. Systemic manifestations of envenomation can generally be managed conservatively with traditional supportive measures. Atropine sulphate may be indicated to control excessive parasympathetic manifestations; however, often this is not necessary (Banner, 1989). Clinical reports describe the successful management of the cardiovascular manifestations of scorpion envenomation with beta blockers, calcium channel blockers, vasodilators such as hydralazine and angiotensin converting enzyme inhibitors (Gueron *et al.*, 1992). The selection of specific therapy should be based on the clinical findings and manifestations of the patient. Prazocin is first-line treatment in India for hypertension and pulmonary oedema caused by the red scorpion, *Mesobuthus tamulus* (Bawaskar and Bawaskar, 1997). Sodium nitroprusside is used for severe cases of pulmonary oedema.

Antivenin therapy has an important role in therapy for scorpion envenomations in some parts of the world.

Antivenin is available in India, Israel, South Africa, North Africa and Mexico (Banner, 1989). In the USA, an antivenin for *C. exilicauda* has been derived from goat serum, but it is not approved by the Food and Drug Administration (Rachesky *et al.*, 1984). It has been used safely and successfully to relieve severe signs and symptoms of envenomation (Gateau *et al.*, 1994). Experience with antivenin in other parts of the world is also limited and issues relative to safety, efficacy and specificity remain to be resolved (Banner, 1989).

JELLYFISH

The phylum Cnidaria (formerly Coelenterata) includes the subphylum Scyphoza, the true jellyfish. The Portuguese man-o'-war, although generally considered a jellyfish, is actually a Cnidarian of the subphylum Hydrozoa. Because of marked similarities, however, the Portuguese man-o'-war will be discussed here with the true jellyfish.

The most notable of these species are the box jellyfish (*Chironex fleckeri*), which inhabits the coastal waters of Australia and the Indo-Pacific region, the Portuguese man-o'-war (*Physalia physalis*), located in the more tropical waters of the Atlantic, the sea nettle (*Chrysaora quinquecirrha*), which is endemic to the Chesapeake Bay and the mid-Atlantic costal waters of the USA, and the Pacific Portuguese man-o'-war (*Physalia utriculus*), which is often responsible for stings in Hawaiian waters. Other species of jellyfish also may be found in these and other waters throughout the world.

The hanging tentacles of jellyfish contain thousands of stinging organelles known as nematocysts. Within the nematocyst is a coiled thread-like structure coated with venom. In response to pressure or changes in osmolarity, the nematocyst fires its thread, which can penetrate the skin to cause envenomation.

The venom of jellyfish contains various polypeptides and enzymes. It is both toxic and allergenic. In animal studies the venom has been shown to produce dermonecrosis, vasopermeability, haemolysis, cardiotoxicity, neurotoxicity, musculotoxicity and cytotoxicity (Burnett and Calton, 1987a). A kinin-like fraction has also been identified which is believed to account for pain (Burnett and Calton, 1987a).

Toxic Manifestations

The most common manifestations from Cnidaria envenomation are local toxic effects. Severe systemic and allergic reactions may also occur. The severity of envenomation is dependent on a number of factors, including the species of jellyfish, the extent and duration of contact with tentacles and the resultant number of fired nematocysts, the amount of venom available in the nematocyst

at the time of firing, the thickness of the skin and the size, age and underlying health of the victim (Burnett *et al.*, 1987a; Lumley *et al.*, 1988).

Skin contact with jellyfish tentacles typically results in linear, urticarial and painful eruptions which result from the direct toxic effects of the venom (Burnett and Calton, 1987a). The sting of the Portuguese man-o'-war is generally considered more painful than that of the sea nettle and the local pain from envenomation by the box jellyfish can be excruciating (Burnett *et al.*, 1987a). The resultant lesions may be vesicular, haemorrhagic, necrotizing or ulcerative (Burnett *et al.*, 1987a). Subacute or chronic reactions may include localized hyperhidrosis, desquamation, lymphadenopathy, angioedema, urticaria, keloid formation, hyper- or hypo-pigmentation, local fat atrophy, contractions, vasospasm, gangrene and nerve damage (Burnett *et al.*, 1987a; Burnett and Calton, 1987b).

An allergic response may contribute to the local effects (Burnett *et al.*, 1983). In fact, a large local reaction comparable to that seen with hymenoptera stings has been described (Burnett and Calton, 1987a). Delayed, persistent or recurrent eruptions at the site of the initial sting and at distant sites have also been reported (Burnett *et al.*, 1983, 1987b; O'Donnell and Tan, 1993). It has been postulated that an antigen depot must exist for this to occur. There is also evidence that individuals may cross-react with different animals of this phylum (Burnett *et al.*, 1987b). The potential for an anaphylactic reaction must be considered.

Jellyfish stings to the cornea cause intense pain, tearing and photophobia. The injuries are typically self-limited without long-term sequelea. Unusually severe reactions consisting of iritis, mydriasis, loss of accommodation and increased intraocular pressure have been reported (Glasser *et al.*, 1992).

Jellyfish envenomation may result in severe systemic toxic reactions and even death. The most common systemic toxic effects include headache, nausea, vomiting, malaise, weakness, perspiration and lacrimation (Burnett *et al.*, 1987a). More severe manifestations include hypotension, cardiac conduction disturbances, arrhythmias, respiratory depression, pulmonary oedema and cardiovascular collapse.

Death from jellyfish envenomation may result from either allergic or toxic mechanisms. The box jellyfish is the most toxic of all marine animals and has been implicated in most jellyfish-related fatalities. It is not clear whether death results due to cardiotoxicity or respiratory failure (Lumley *et al.*, 1988; Stein *et al.*, 1989). The precise aetiology, in fact, may be dose dependent (Lumley *et al.*, 1988).

Management

Victims of jellyfish envenomation should be kept quiet and the affected limb should be immobilized because muscle activity may increase the firing of nematocysts. The exposed area should be rinsed with sea water. Fresh water is contraindicated as this too will increase nematocyst firing due to the osmotic change.

The next step is to inactivate the nematocysts, which is a species specific process. For most species this can be accomplished by flooding the area with household vinegar (5% acetic acid). In the event of sea nettle or lion's mane jellyfish envenomation, a baking soda slurry is more appropriate (Burnett and Calton, 1987b). Nematocysts can then be removed from the skin by scraping with a blunt-edged object such as a sea shell or credit card or by shaving with a razor. Application of a cold pack may help relieve mild to moderate pain (Exton et al., 1989). Topical anaesthetics or steroid creams and oral analgesics may benefit some patients. Hyperpigmentation can be treated with a bleaching agent such as topical hydroquinone (Kokolu and Burnett, 1990).

Topical corticosteroids and cycloplegics are recommended as initial treatment for corneal jellyfish stings (Glasser et al., 1992). Topical or systemic therapy for increased intraocular pressure should be administered as needed.

Systemic manifestations are managed with traditional supportive measures. The definitive treatment of box jellyfish envenomation is a specific antivenin from the Commonwealth Serum Laboratory in Australia (Holmes, 1996). The calcium-channel antagonist verapamil hydrochloride has been shown to inhibit the action of box jellyfish cardiotoxin and prolong survival in mice (Burnett and Calton, 1983). This finding has been extended to other jellyfish species (Burnett et al., 1985).

Antihistamines may be useful if there is evidence of an allergic response to the venom. Anaphylactic reactions should be managed accordingly. In the event of recurrent dermal eruptions, a tapering dose of a corticosteroid may be employed.

In addition to the Portuguese man-o'-war, another important Hydrozoan is fire coral. The fire coral, while not a true coral, is so named because of its marked resemblance to these species. Polyps which contain nematocysts protrude through pores of its calcareous skeleton. It typically produces only mild dermatitis and burning discomfort (Kizer, 1983–84). The subphylum Anthosa includes the sea anemones, which also contain modified nematocysts capable of inflicting stings and local effects as described for other cnidarians.

STINGRAYS

Another important costal hazard is the stingray. Approximately 20 species have been described (Fenner et al., 1989). These creatures are often found partially buried in the sand and are a significant hazard to beachcombers and to those who swim or play in shallow water. Although normally very docile, if they are stepped on or otherwise abruptly disturbed, stingrays will lash their tails forward and sting with a spine located near the base of the tail. Some species of stingray contain more than one spine and are capable of inflicting multiple simultaneous stings (Grainger, 1987).

The stinging spine(s) of stingrays is (are) covered by a venom-containing integumentary sheath. As the spine enters the victim, this sheath may rupture, resulting in the release of venom into the wound. The spines of stingrays vary by species and may range from 2.5 to 12 cm in length (Grainger, 1985). The spine is curved and serrated, enabling it to inflict significant trauma in addition to envenoming the victim. A large stingray, in fact, is capable of inflicting fatal traumatic injury (Russell et al., 1958).

Toxic Manifestations

Most stings are to the lower extremities (Russell et al., 1958). The upper extremities, abdomen or thorax may be involved due to careless handling or under extraordinary circumstances. The stingray's venom consists of a heat-labile protein that causes intense pain at the site of the sting which is out of proportion to the physical trauma. In the event that the wound is not characteristically painful and other toxic manifestations do not occur, it is likely that the integumentary sheath had already been lost or it was not disrupted during the sting.

The venom can produce local tissue necrosis which complicates the healing process (Fenner et al., 1989). It has also been shown in animal models to possess both cardiotoxic and neurotoxic properties (Russell et al., 1958). Systemic manifestations from envenomation may include nausea, vomiting, diarrhoea, salivation, generalized oedema, headache, vertigo, syncope, respiratory depression and distress, cardiac conduction disturbances and arrhythmias, hypotension, muscle cramps, fasciculations, tremor and seizures and death (Russell et al., 1958; Grainger, 1985; Ikeda, 1989). Secondary infection is also possible.

Management

First aid for stingray envenomation consists of washing the wound with sea water and as soon as possible soaking the site in water which is as hot as the patient can tolerate for 30–90 min. This is done to denature the thermolabile venom (Russell et al., 1958; Fenner et al., 1989). The wound should then be surgically explored to remove any remaining fragments of the sheath or spine. Necrotic tissue should be debrided and an antiseptic should be used to cleanse the wound, which should be left open to heal by natural intention. Tetanus immunization should be updated if necessary and prophylactic antibiotics should be administered in serious cases (Fenner et al.,

1989). Narcotic analgesics may be necessary to control pain. No antivenin is available and systemic manifestations should be managed with traditional symptomatic and supportive care.

STINGING FISHES

Other venomous underwater creatures include fresh and salt water fishes. Common examples include the lionfish, scorpion fish, stonefish, catfish and weever fish. All these fish sting with venomous spines on their fins. The sting of these fish is much less traumatic than that associated with the stingray, but in other respects their stings are very similar.

Fish stings may be inflicted in those who swim or recreate in the oceans, seas or lakes, in those who fish for recreation or commercially, and in hobbyists who may keep a venomous species in an aquarium. The lionfish is popular with salt water aquarists and has been responsible for many stings to the hand and fingers (Kizer et al., 1985; Trestrail and Al-Mahasneh, 1989).

Toxic Manifestations

Fish stings result in an initial sharp, stabbing pain when the spine penetrates the skin. In some cases the spine may break free and remain lodged in the wound. Severe pain may ensue which can radiate to involve the entire extremity. The pain may become excruciating and incapacitating in some cases. Pronounced local swelling occurs commonly and vesicles may form at the puncture sites (Auerbach et al., 1987). The vesicular fluid can itself be harmful and prompt drainage of the fluid is recommended. Delayed onset of Raynaud's phenomenon following a weever fish sting to the finger has been reported (Carducci et al., 1996).

Systemic manifestations may occur with significant envenomation resulting from multiple stings or single stings from certain species such as the stonefish. These toxic effects may include nausea, vomiting, diaphoresis, bradycardia or tachycardia, conduction disturbances, hypotension, myocardial ischaemia, respiratory distress, pulmonary oedema, muscle tremor, weakness, delirium, convulsions and death (Kizer et al., 1985; Ell and Yates, 1989; Lehmann and Hardy, 1993). Systemic manifestations may be delayed (Bangh, 1997).

Management

As with the stingray, the venom of these fish consists primarily of heat labile proteins. Accordingly, first aid treatment should include immersion of the affected site in water as hot as the patient can tolerate for 30–90 min. Afterwards the site should be thoroughly cleaned and in

some cases the wound may need to be surgically explored to remove any remaining spine. Tetanus immunization should be updated as necessary. Prophylactic administration of antibiotics is not routinely necessary. Catfish stings may pose a greater risk of infection and should be managed accordingly (Baack et al., 1991).

Failure to treat these inflictions promptly may result in significant tissue necrosis, permanent scaring and physical impairment (Kasdan et al., 1987; Mann and Werntz, 1991). Systemic manifestations should be managed with traditional supportive and symptomatic measures. An antivenin is available for the management of stonefish envenomation.

POISONOUS FISH AND SHELLFISH

In addition to those animals which can cause human poisoning by envenomation, several toxic syndromes may result from ingestion of various fish and shellfish. In some cases these animals excrete the toxin, but most concentrate toxins that are produced by dinoflagellates or bacteria. Fish can be categorized based on the tissue which contains the toxin (Halstead, 1964).

Ichthyosarcotoxic fish, which cause most poisonings, have toxin in muscle, viscera, skin or mucus. Ichthyootoxic fish produce toxin which is concentrated in the gonads. Ichthyohaemotoxic fish, which rarely produce poisoning, have toxin in their blood. Toxic syndromes resulting from ingestion of poisonous aquatic life are unlike traditional food poisoning, which is associated with ingestion of microbial-contaminated foods.

Ciguatera Fish Poisoning

Ciguatera intoxication is the most common type of ichthyosarcotoxic fish poisoning. The primary responsible toxin, ciguatoxin, is produced by the dinoflagellate *Gambierdiscus toxicus* (Eastaugh and Shepherd, 1989). Although it has anticholinesterase activity, its primary mechanism of action is thought to be from competitive inhibition of calcium-regulated sodium channels (Eastaugh and Shepherd, 1989). Ciguatoxin is a heat-stable, lipid-soluble compound that is resistant to gastric acid (Eastaugh and Shepherd, 1989). It can be excreted in breast milk, which can cause toxicity in nursing infants (Blythe and deSylva, 1990). Maitotoxin, scaritoxin, lysophosphatidylcholine, ATPase inhibitor and possibly an indole-positive toxin may also contribute to toxicity (Sims, 1987). Toxins are concentrated up the food chain and, as a result, large fish are most likely to cause human poisoning. Hundreds of fish species have been reported to harbour ciguatoxin; common examples include the barracuda, grouper, snapper, amberjack and sea bass (Halstead, 1964).

Most outbreaks of ciguatera intoxication occur in the Caribbean and South Pacific. In the USA, most cases have been reported in Hawaii and Florida (Hughes and Merson, 1976). Ciguatera poisoning, however, has also been associated with ingestion of fish caught from the southeastern US coastal waters as far north as North Carolina (Morris et al., 1990). The ability readily to transport fish great distances may result in ciguatera poisoning in virtually any geographic region. People of Chinese or Philippine descent are likely to be more severely affected and Hawaiians least affected (Sims, 1987). This ethnic variation is not well understood.

Toxic Manifestations

Ciguatera poisoning affects primarily the gastro-intestinal and nervous systems. Signs and symptoms usually develop within 6 h; however, there is considerable variability. Common gastro-intestinal effects include diarrhoea, vomiting and abdominal pain (Morris et al., 1982). These symptoms generally occur early and resolve within 24 h. Other initial symptoms may include malaise, pain and weakness in the lower extremities, dysesthesias including reversal of hot and cold sensation, pruritus and paraesthesiaes around the mouth and of the extremities (Hughes and Merson, 1976; Morris et al., 1982). These effects may persist for weeks or months. Other common findings include rash, dry mouth, metallic taste, myalgias, arthralgia, visual disturbances, and a sensation of loose teeth. Bradycardia, hypotension and respiratory paralysis may occur in severe cases (Hughes and Merson, 1976).

Management

Gastro-intestinal decontamination may be helpful if the toxic nature of the fish is recognized soon after ingestion. Treatment is primarily symptomatic and supportive care. Fluid and electrolyte balance should be monitored as well as the electrocardiogram. Atropine and intravenous fluids have been effective in the treatment of bradycardia and hypotension. Mannitol was found to improve dramatically the neurological and gastro-intestinal toxicity in a group of 24 patients (Palafox et al., 1988). Mannitol has also been shown to benefit patients with chronic symptoms even with delayed administration (Blythe et al., 1992; Eastaugh, 1996). It is postulated that mannitol may have inactivated the toxin or competitively inhibited its action on the sodium channel (Palafox et al., 1988). The possibility that ciguatera may cause oedema in the nervous tissue, which mannitol could reverse, has also been hypothesized (Palafox, 1992).

Paralytic Shellfish Poisoning

Paralytic shellfish poisoning results from ingestion of contaminated bivalve molluscs such as clams and oysters. These molluscs concentrate neurotoxins known as saxitoxins, which are produced by a number of dinoflagellates including those of the *Gonyaulax* and *Pyridinium* species (Eastaugh and Shepherd, 1989; Rodrigue et al., 1990). The toxin is a water-soluble, heat-and acid-stable compound which cannot be destroyed by ordinary cooking (Auerbach and Halstead, 1989). The toxin acts by interfering with sodium conductance, thereby inhibiting neuromuscular transmission.

Toxic Manifestations

As the name implies, paralytic shellfish poisoning affects primarily the nervous system. Prominent toxic effects include paraesthesiae of the lips, face and extremities, headache, weakness, dizziness, vertigo and difficulty in walking (Hughes and Merson, 1976; Eastaugh and Shephard, 1989). A sensation of floating has also been described (McCollum et al., 1968). In severe cases, muscle paralysis may occur. Death may result due to respiratory arrest if adequate life support cannot be provided. Some neurological symptoms such as headaches, memory loss and fatigue may persist for up to 2 weeks (Rodrigue et al., 1990).

Management

Gastro-intestinal decontamination should be performed if the toxic nature of the mollusc is recognized soon after consumption. The remainder of therapy is basically symptomatic and supportive care. Respiratory function should be monitored closely with ventilatory assistance provided as needed.

Neurotoxic Shellfish Poisoning

A milder intoxication, known as neurotoxic shellfish poisoning, results from ingestion of shellfish contaminated with brevitoxins, produced by the dinoflagellate *Ptychodiscus brevis* (Sakamoto et al., 1987). These toxins stimulate post-ganglionic cholinergic nerve fibres (Grunfeld and Spiegelstein, 1974; Asai et al., 1982). The coastal waters of western Florida, Texas and North Carolina have been affected by *P. brevis* (Sakamoto et al., 1987; Morris et al., 1991). Toxic manifestations include nausea, vomiting, diarrhoea and paraesthesiae. As with ciguatera poisoning, patients may experience the hot–cold reversal phenomenon (Hughes and Merson, 1976; Sims, 1987).

Domoic Acid Intoxication

A unique toxic syndrome has been described that resulted from ingestion of contaminated mussels from Prince Edward Island in Canada (Perl et al., 1990).

Domoic acid was implicated as the responsible toxin, which was apparently produced by the marine algae *Nitzschia pungens*. Domoic acid is an excitatory neurotransmitter structurally similar to glutamic acid and kainic acid (Teitelbaum *et al.*, 1990).

The most common acute symptoms of intoxication included nausea, vomiting, abdominal cramps, diarrhoea, headache and memory loss (Perl *et al.*, 1990). In severe cases altered mental status, seizures, myoclonus and cardiovascular instability resulted. Death was reported in four cases. The initial widespread neurotoxicity and subsequent chronic residual memory impairment differentiates this syndrome from either paralytic or neurotoxic shellfish poisoning.

Tetrodotoxic Fish Poisoning

Tetrodotoxication is primarily associated with ingestion of the puffer fish and related fish of the order Tetraodontiformes. Other animals also may contain this neurotoxin, for example the Californian newt (*Taricha torosa*), Pacific goby (*Gobius criniger*) and Costa Rican frog (Tibballs, 1988). Two species of gastropod molluscs collected off the southern coast of Taiwan have also been implicated in an outbreak of tetrodotoxin poisoning (Yang *et al.*, 1995).

Tetrodotoxin acts similarly to saxitoxin in that it blocks neurotransmission by action on sodium channels (Narahashi, 1972). This results in motor, autonomic and sensory nerve impairment (Tibballs, 1988). It also has direct action on the medulla, stimulating the chemoreceptor trigger zone and depressing the respiratory centre (Eastaugh and Shepherd, 1989).

Toxic Manifestations

Prominent signs and symptoms of intoxication include persistent vomiting, paraesthesiae, weakness, respiratory impairment, hypotension and bradycardia (Sims and Ostman, 1986; Tibballs, 1988). Hypertension has been reported in patients with pre-existing hypertensive disease (Deng *et al.*, 1991; Yang *et al.*, 1995). The precise mechanism of the hypertensive response is not understood. Other manifestations may include headache, dilated pupils, salivation, diaphoresis, myalgias, dysarthria, ataxia, muscle fasciculations and seizures (Sims and Ostman, 1986). Death may result in severe cases due to respiratory failure or cardiovascular collapse.

Management

Treatment is primarily symptomatic and supportive care. Gastric lavage should be performed if it can be done soon after ingestion. Activated charcoal is also recommended. Ventilatory assistance may be required in severe cases. Hypotension and bradycardia should be managed with atropine and fluid therapy. Vasopressors, such as dopamine hydrochloride, may be required.

Scombroid Fish Poisoning

Scombroid fish poisoning is a toxic syndrome that resembles an acute allergic reaction. It results from ingestion of spoiled fish that is contaminated with histamine and possibly other toxins. These scombrotoxins are heat stable and, therefore, not destroyed by cooking. Histamine is formed as a result of bacteria that cause enzymatic decarboxylation of histidine, which is normally present in the flesh of certain fish species (Lerke *et al.*, 1978). Fish most commonly involved are those of the suborder Scombroidei such as the tuna, mackerel, bonito, skipjack and saury. Other marine fish such as the mahimahi have also been implicated in outbreaks of scombroid intoxication (Eastaugh and Shepherd, 1989).

Although histamine is an important factor in the pathogenesis of scombroid poisoning, the exact mechanism is still unclear. Histamine has limited activity when administered orally due to rapid metabolism and elimination in the urine (Garrison, 1990). However, markedly elevated urinary histamine concentrations have been measured in symptomatic patients after ingestion of scombrotoxic fish (Morrow *et al.*, 1991). This evidence and the effectiveness of antihistamines to relieve symptoms of scombroid intoxication implicate histamine as the causative toxin. Other substances in spoiled fish such as cadaverine or putrescine might inhibit histamine-metabolizing enzymes, thereby allowing the absorption of histamine (Auerbach, 1990). This is an area that warrants further investigation.

Toxic Manifestations

Scombroid intoxication usually results in a relatively mild, self-limited syndrome, which typically begins within 1 of ingestion and lasts for 8 h or less (Merson *et al.*, 1974; Hughes and Merson, 1976). Typical manifestations include nausea, diarrhoea, abdominal cramps, vomiting, throbbing headache, oral blistering or burning sensation, flushing, burning sensation of the skin and urticaria. Tachycardia, palpitations, bronchospasm and respiratory distress may also occur (Merson *et al.*, 1974; Hughes and Merson, 1976; Blakesley, 1983).

Management

Treatment is primarily symptomatic and supportive care. If the fish is recognized as poisonous soon after ingestion, the gastro-intestinal tract should be decontaminated. Antihistamines such as diphenhydramine are the mainstay of therapy. The use of cimetidine in a few cases has been shown to relieve dramatically the signs and symptoms of scombroid intoxication (Blakesley,

1983; Auerbach, 1990). Bronchodilators may be needed in the event of bronchospasm.

It is important to differentiate between scombroid poisoning and fish allergy. An incorrect diagnosis of fish allergy will unnecessarily limit the diet of the patient. Considerations include the patient's prior response to ingestion of the implicated fish species and the response in others who consumed the same meal (Taylor *et al.*, 1989). The food can be analysed for the presence of histamine, but at this time there are no diagnostic tests that can be performed on the patient (Lerke *et al.*, 1978; Taylor *et al.*, 1989).

Diarrhoeic Shellfish Poisoning

Several species of the dinoflagellate *Dinophysis* produce okadaic acid, the causative agent in diarrhoeic shellfish poisoning (DSP). As the name implies, consumption of contaminated shellfish produces gastroenteritis within 30 min up to 2 h. DSP is a worldwide public health problem with documented outbreaks in Japan, Europe, Chile, Thailand, Nova Scotia and New Zealand (Tester, 1994).

REFERENCES

Adrouny, G. A., Derbes, V. J. and Jung, R. C. (1959). Isolation of a hemolytic component of fire ant venom. *Science*, **130**, 449.

Alagesan, R., Srinivasarnghavan, J., Balambal, R., Haranath, K., Subramanyam, N. and Thiruvengadam, K. V. (1977). Transient complete right bundle branch block following scorpion sting. *J. Indian Med. Assoc.*, **69**, 113–114.

Aitchison, J. M. (1990). Boomslang bite—diagnosis and management: a report of 2 cases. *S. Afr. Med. J.*, **78**, 39–42.

Asai, S., Krzanowski, J., Anderson, W. H., Martin, D. F., Polson, J. B., Lockey, R. F., Bukantz, S. C. and Szentivanyi, A. (1982). Effects of the toxin of red tide, *Ptychodiscus brevis*, on canine tracheal smooth muscle: a possible new asthma-triggering mechanism. *J. Allergy Clin. Immunol.*, **69**, 418–428.

Auerbach, P. S., McKinney, H. E., Rees, R. S. and Heggers, J. P. (1987). Analysis of vesicle fluid following the sting of the lionfish *Pterois volintans*. *Toxicon*, **25**, 1350–1353.

Auerbach, P. S. and Halstead, B. W. (1989). Hazardous aquatic life. In Auerbach, P. S. and Geehr, E. C. (Eds), *Management of Wilderness and Environmental Emergencies*, 2nd edn. C. V. St Louis, MO, pp. 931–1028.

Auerbach, P. S. (1990). Persistent headache associated with scombroid poisoning: resolution with oral cimetidine. *J. Wild. Med.*, **1**, 279–283.

Baack, B. R., Kucan, J. O., Zook, E. G. and Russell, R. C. (1991). Hand infections secondary to catfish spines: Case reports and literature review. *J. Trauma*, **31**, 1432–1436.

Bangh, S. A. (1997) Lionfish envenomation with delayed onset of systemic symptoms (Abstract). *J. Toxicol. Clin. Toxicol.*, **35**, 530.

Banner, W. (1989). Scorpion envenomation. In Auerbach, P. S. and Geehr, E. C. (Eds), *Management of Wilderness and Environmental Emergencies*, 2nd edn. C. V. Mosby, St Louis, pp. 603–616.

Barrett, S. M., Romine-Jenkins, M. and Blick, K. E. (1993). Passive hemagglutination test for diagnosis of brown recluse spider bite envenomation. *Clin. Chem.*, **39**, 2104–2107.

Bartholomew, C. (1970). Acute scorpion pancreatitis in Trinidad. *Br. Med. J.*, **1**, 666–668.

Barzilay, Z., Shaher, E., Motro, M., Shem-Tov, A. and Neufeld, H. N. (1982). Myocardial damage with life-threatening arrhythmia due to a scorpion sting. *Eur. Heart J.*, **3**, 191–193.

Bawaskar, H. S. (1982). Diagnostic cardiac premonitory signs and symptoms of red scorpion sting. *Lancet*, **1**, 552–554.

Bawaskar, H. S. and Bawaskar, P. H. (1997). Scorpion envenoming and the cardiovascular system. *Trop. Doct.*, **27**, 6–9.

Beccari, M., Castiglione, A., Cavaliere, G., d'Aloya, G., Fabbri, C., Losi, B., Ranzini, C., Ramagnoni, G. and Sorgato, G. (1992). Unusual case of anuria due to African bee stings. *Int. J. Artif. Organs*, **15**, 281–283.

Bentur, Y., Zveibel, F., Adler, M. and Raikhlin, B. (1997). Delayed administration of *Vipera xanthina palaestinae* antivenin. *J. Toxicol. Clin. Toxicol.*, **35**, 257–261.

Berg, R. A. and Tarantino, M. D. (1991). Envenomation by the scorpion *Centruroides exilicauda* (*C. Sculpturatus*): severe and unusual manifestations. *Pediatrics*, **87**, 930–933.

Berger, R. S. (1973). The unremarkable brown recluse spider bite. *J. Am. Med. Assoc.*, **225**, 1109–1111.

Berger, R. S., Adelstein, E. H. and Anderson, P. C. (1973). Intravascular coagulation: the cause of necrotic arachnidism. *J. Invest. Dermatol.*, **61**, 142–150.

Berger, R. S. (1984). Management of brown recluse spider bite. *J. Am. Med. Assoc.*, **251**, 889.

Binder, L. S. (1989). Acute arthropod envenomation. *Med. Toxicol. Adverse Drug. Exp.*, **4**, 163–173.

Blakesley, M. L. (1983). Scombroid poisoning: prompt resolution of symptoms with cimetidine. *Ann. Emerg. Med.*, **12**, 104–106.

Blaylock, R. S. M. (1982). The treatment of snakebite in Zimbabwe. *Cent. Afr. J. Med.*, **28**, 237–246.

Blum, M. S. (1984). Poisonous ants and their venoms. In Tu, A. T. (Ed.), *Insect Poisons, Allergens and Other Invertebrate Venoms*. Marcel Dekker, New York, pp. 225–242.

Blythe, D. G. and deSylva, D. P. (1990). Mother's milk turns toxic following fish feast. *J. Am. Med. Assoc.*, **264**, 2074.

Blythe, D. G., deSylva, D. P., Fleming, L. E., Ayyar, R. A., Baden, D. G. and Shrank, K. (1992). Clinical experience with iv mannitol in the treatment of ciguatera. *Bull. Soc. Pathol. Exp.*, **85**, 425–426.

Bou-Abboud, C. F. and Kardassakis, D. G. (1988). Acute myocardial infarction following a Gila monster (*Heloderma suspectum cinctum*) bite. *West. J. Med.*, **148**, 577–579.

Bousquet, J., Huchard, G. and Francois-Bernard, M. (1984). Toxic reactions induced by hymenoptera venom. *Ann. Allergy*, **52**, 371–374.

Brick, J. F., Gutmann, L., Brick, J., Apelgren, K. N. and Riggs, J. E. (1987). Timber rattlesnake venom-induced myokymia: evidence for peripheral nerve origin. *Neurology*, **37**, 1545–1546.

Burnett, J. W. and Calton, G. J. (1983). Response of the box-jellyfish (*Chironex fleckeri*) cardiotoxin to intravenous administration of verapamil. *Med. J. Aust.*, **2**, 192–194.

Burnett, J. W., Cobbs, C. S., Kelman, S. N. and Calton, G. J. (1983). Studies on the serologic response to jellyfish envenomation. *J. Am. Acad. Dermatol.*, **9**, 229–231.

Burnett, J. W., Gean, C. J. and Calton, G. J. (1985). The effect of verapamil on the cardiotoxic activity of Portugese man-o'-war (*Phisalia physalis*) and sea nettle (*Chrysaora quinquecirrha*) venoms. *Toxicon*, **23**, 681–689.

Burnett, J. W. and Calton, G. J. (1987a). Jellyfish envenomation syndromes updated. *Ann. Emerg. Med.*, **16**, 1000–1005.

Burnett, J. W. and Calton, G. J. (1987b). Venomous pelagic coelenterates: chemistry, toxicology, immunology and treatment of their stings. *Toxicon*, **25**, 581–602.

Burnett, J. W., Calton, G. J., Burnett, H. W. and Mandojana, R. M. (1987a). Local and systemic reactions from jellyfish stings. *Clin. Dermatol.*, **5**, 14–28.

Burnett, J. W., Hepper, K. P., Aurelian, L., Calton, G. J. and Gardepe, S. F. (1987b). Recurrent eruptions following unusual solitary coelenterate envenomations. *J. Am. Acad. Dermatol.*, **17**, 86–92.

Burton, K. G. (1995). Nitroglycerine patches for brown recluse spider bites. *Am. Fam. Physician*, **51**, 1401.

Cable, D., McGehee, W., Wingert, W. A. and Russell, F. E. (1984). Prolonged defibrination after a bite from a 'nonvenomous snake'. *J. Am. Med. Assoc.*, **251**, 925–926.

Candiotti, K. A. and Lamas, A. M. (1993). Adverse neurologic reactions to the sting of the imported fire ant. *Int. Arch. Allergy Immunol.*, **102**, 417–420.

Car, M. R., Derbes, V. J. and Jung, R. (1957). Skin responses to the sting of the imported fire ant (*Solenopsis saevissima*). *Arch. Dermatol.*, **75**, 475–488.

Carducci, M., Mussi, A., Leone, G. and Catricala, C. (1996). Raynaud's phenomenon secondary to weever fish stings. *Arch. Dermatol.*, **132**, 838–839.

Christopher, D. G. and Rodning, C. B. (1986). Crotalidae envenomation. *South. Med. J.*, **79**, 159–162.

Clark, R. F., Selden, B. S. and Furbee, B. (1993). The incidence of wound infection following crotalid envenomation. *J. Emerg. Med.*, **11**, 583–586.

Cole, H. P., Wesley, R. E. and King, L. E. (1995). Brown recluse spider envenomation of the eyelid: an animal model. *Ophthal. Plast. Reconstr. Surg.*, **3**, 153–164.

Curry, S. C., Vance, M. V., Ryan, P. J., Kunkle, D. B. and Northey, W. T. (1983–84). Envenomation by the scorpion *Centruroides sculpturatus*. *J. Toxicol. Clin. Toxicol.*, **21**, 417–449.

Curry, S. C. and Kunkel, D. B. (1985). Death from a rattlesnake bite. *Am. J. Emerg. Med.*, **3**, 227–235.

Deng, J. F., Tominack, R. L., Chung, H. M. and Tsai, W. J. (1991). Hypertension as an unusual feature in an outbreak of tetrodotoxin poisoning. *J. Toxicol. Clin. Toxicol.*, **29**, 71–79.

deShazo, R. D., Griffing, C., Kwan, T. H., Banks, W. A. and Dvorak, H. F. (1984). Dermal hypersensitivity reactions to imported fire ants. *J. Allergy Clin. Immunol.*, **74**, 841–847.

deShazo, R. D., Butcher, B. T. and Banks, W. A. (1990). Reactions to the stings of the imported fire ant. *N. Engl. J. Med.*, **323**, 462–466.

de Silva, H. J., Ratnatunga, N., de Silva, U., Kularatne, W. N. S. and Wijewickrema, R. (1992). Severe fatty change with hepatocellular necrosis following bite by a Russell's viper. *Trans. R. Soc. Trop. Med. Hyg.*, **86**, 565.

Diaz, J. D., Lockey, R. F., Stablein, J. J. and Mines, H. K. (1989). Multiple stings by imported fire ants (*Solenopsis*

invicta), without systemic effects. *South. Med. J.*, **82**, 775–777.

Eastaugh, J. and Shepherd, S. (1989). Infectious and toxic syndromes from fish and shellfish consumption. *Arch. Intern. Med.*, **149**, 1735–1740.

Eastaugh, J. (1996) Delayed use of intravenous mannitol in ciguatera (fish poisoning). *Ann. Emerg. Med.*, **28**, 105–106.

Edlich, R. F., Rodeheaver, G. T., Feldman, P. S. and Morgan, R. F. (1985). Management of venomous spider bites. *Curr. Concepts Trauma Care*, **7**, 17–20.

Ell, S. R. and Yates, D. (1989). Marinefish stings. *Arch. Emerg. Med.*, **6**, 59–62.

Exton, D. R., Fenner, P. J. and Williamson, J. A. (1989). Cold packs: effective topical analgesia in the treatment of painful stings by *Physalia* and other jellyfish. *Med. J. Aust.*, **151**, 625–626.

Fenner, P. J., Williamson, J. A. and Skinner, R. A. (1989). Fatal and non-fatal stingray envenomation. *Med. J. Aust.*, **151**, 621–625.

Fox, R. W., Lockey, R. F. and Bukantz, S. C. (1982). Neurologic sequelae following the imported fire ant sting. *J. Allergy Clin. Immunol.*, **70**, 120–124.

Garrison, J. C. (1990). Histamine, bradykinin, 5-hydroxytryptamine, and their antagonists. In Gilman, A. G., Rall, T. W., Nies, A. S. and Taylor, P. (Eds), *Goodman and Gilman's The Pharmacological Basis of Therapeutics*, 8th edn. Pergamon Press, New York, pp. 575–599.

Gateau, T., Bloom, M. and Clark, R. (1994). Response to specific *Centruroides sculpturatus* antivenom in 151 cases of scorpion stings. *J. Toxicol. Clin. Toxicol.*, **32**, 165–171.

Gendron, B. P. (1990). *Loxosceles reclusa* envenomation. *Am. J. Emerg. Med.*, **8**, 51–54.

George, A., Tharakan, V. T. and Solez, K. (1987). Viper bite poisoning in India: a review with special reference to renal complications. *Renal Failure*, **10**, 91–99.

Gillissen, A., Theakston, R. D. G., Barth, J., May, B., Krieg, M. and Warrell, D. A. (1994). Neurotoxicity, haemostatic disturbances and haemolytic anaemia after a bite by a Tunisian saw-scaled or carpet viper (*Echis 'pyramidum'-complex*): failure of antivenom treatment. *Toxicon*, **32**, 937–944.

Glasser, D. B., Noell, M. J., Burnett, J. W., Kathuria, S. S. and Rodrigues, M. M. (1992). Ocular jellyfish stings. *Ophthalmology*, **99**, 1414–1418.

Gold, B. S. (1996). Neostigmine for the treatment of neurotoxicity following envenomation by the Asiatic cobra. *Ann. Emerg. Med.*, **28**, 87–89.

Golden, D. B. K., Valentine, M. D., Kagey-Sobotka, A. and Lichtenstein, L. M. (1982). Prevalence of hymenoptera venom allergy. *J. Allergy Clin. Immunol.*, **69**, 124.

Golden, D. B. K. and Valentine, M. D. (1984). Insect sting allergy. *Ann. Allergy*, **53**, 444–449.

Golden, D. B. K. (1989). Epidemiology of allergy to insect venoms and stings. *Allergy Proc.*, **10**, 103–107.

Golden, D. B. K., Kwiterovich, K. A., Kagey-Sobotka, A., Valentine, M. D. and Lichtenstine, L. M. (1996). Discontinuing venom immunotherapy: outcome after five years. *J. Allergy Clin. Immunol.*, **97**, 579–587.

Graft, D. F. and Schoenwetter, W. F. (1994). Insect sting allergy: analysis of a cohort of patients who initiated venom immunotherapy from 1978 to 1986. *Ann. Allergy*, **73**, 481–485.

Grainger, C. R. (1985). Stingray injuries. *Trans. R. Soc. Trop. Med. Hyg.*, **79**, 443–444.

Grainger, C. R. (1987). Multiple injuries due to stingrays. *J. R. Soc. Health*, **107**, 100.

Grunfeld, Y. and Spiegelstein, M. Y. (1974). Effects of *Gymnodinium breve* toxin on the smooth muscle preparation of guinea-pig ilium. *Br. J. Pharmacol.*, **51**, 67–72.

Gueron, M., Ilia, R. and Sofer, S. (1992). The cardiovascular system after scorpion envenomation. A review. *J. Toxicol. Clin. Toxicol.*, **30**, 245–258.

Halstead, B. W. (1964). Fish poisonings—their diagnosis, pharmacology and treatment. *Clin. Pharmacol. Ther.*, **5**, 615–627.

Hardy, D. L. (1986). Fatal rattlesnake envenomation in Arizona: 1969–1984. *J. Toxicol. Clin. Toxicol.*, **24**, 1–10.

Heitschel, S. (1986). Near death from a Gila monster bite. *J. Emerg. Nurs.*, **12**, 259–262.

Hering, S. E., Jurca, M., Vichi, F. L., Azevedo-Marques, M. M. and Cupo, P. (1993) 'Reversible cardiomyopathy' in patients with severe scorpion envenoming by *Tityus serrulatus*: evolution of enzymatic, electrocardiographic and echocardiographic alterations. *Ann. Trop. Paediatr.*, **13**, 173–182.

Hobbs, G. D. and Harrell, R. E. (1989). Brown recluse spider bites: a common cause of necrotic arachnidism. *Am. J. Emerg. Med.*, **7**, 309–312.

Hoffman, D. R., Dove, D. E. and Jacobson, R. S. (1988a). Allergens in *Hymenoptera* venom. *J. Allergy Clin. Immunol.*, **82**, 818–827.

Hoffman, D. R., Dover, D. E., Moffitt, J. E. and Stafford, C. T. (1988b). Allergens in *Hymenoptera* venom. *J. Allergy Clin. Immunol.*, **82**, 828–834.

Hogan, D. E. and Dire, D. J. (1990). Anaphylactic shock secondary to rattlesnake bite. *Ann. Emerg. Med.*, **19**, 814–816.

Holmes, J. L. (1996). Marine stingers in far north Queensland. *Aust. J. Dermatol.*, **37**, S23–S26.

Hooker, K. R. and Caravati, E. M. (1994). Gila monster envenomation. *Ann. Emerg. Med.*, **24**, 731–735.

Hoover, E. L., Williams, W., Koger, L., Murthy, R., Parsh, S. and Weaver, W. L. (1990). Pseudoepitheliomatous hyperplasia and pyoderma gangrenosum after a brown recluse spider bite. *South. Med. J.*, **83**, 243–246.

Hughes, J. M. and Merson, M. H. (1976). Fish and shellfish poisoning. *N. Engl. J. Med.*, **295**, 1117–1120.

Hutton, R. A. and Warrell, D. A. (1993). Action of snake venom components on the haemostatic system. *Blood Rev.*, **7**, 176–189.

Hylander, R. D., Ortiz, A. A., Freeman, T. M. and Martin, M. E. (1989). Imported fire ant immunotherapy: effectiveness of whole body extracts. *J. Allergy Clin. Immunol.*, **83**, 232.

Ikeda, T. (1989). Supraventricular bigeminy following a stingray envenomation: a case report. *Hawaii Med. J.*, **48**, 162–163.

Ismail, M., Al-Bekairi, A. M., El-Bedaiwy, A. M. and Abd-El Salam, M. A. (1993a). The ocular effects of spitting cobras: I. The ringhals cobra (*Hemachatus haemachatus*) venom-induced corneal opacification syndrome. *J. Toxicol. Clin. Toxicol.*, **31**, 31–41.

Ismail, M., Al-Bekairi, A. M., El-Bedaiwy, A. M. and Abd-El Salam, M. A. (1993b). The ocular effects of spitting cobras: II. Evidence that cardiotoxins are responsible for the corneal opacification syndrome. *J. Toxicol. Clin. Toxicol.*, **31**, 45–62.

Iyaniwura, T. T. (1991). Snake venom constituents: Biochemistry and toxicology (Part 1). *Vet. Hum. Toxicol.*, **33**, 468–474.

Jansen, P. W., Perkin, R. M. and Van Stralen, D. (1992). Mojave rattlesnake envenomation: prolonged neurotoxicity and rhabdomyolysis. *Ann. Emerg. Med.*, **21**, 322–325.

Karlson-Stiber, C. and Persson, H. (1994). Antivenom treatment in *Vipera berus* envenoming—report of 30 cases. *J. Intern. Med.*, **235**, 57–61.

Karlson-Stiber, C., Persson, H., Heath, A., Smith, D., Al-Abdulla, I. H. and Sjostrom, L. (1997). First clinical experiences with specific sheep Fab fragments in snake bite. Report of a multicentre study of *Vipera berus* envenoming. *J. Intern. Med.*, **241**, 53–58.

Kasdan, M. L., Dasdan, A. S. and Hamilton, D. L. (1987). Lionfish envenomation. *Plast. Reconstr. Surg.*, **80**, 613–614.

Kerrigan, K. R., Mertz, B. L., Nelson, S. J. and Dye, J. D. (1997) Antibiotic prophylaxis for pit viper envenomations: prospective, controlled trial. *World J. Surg.*, **21**, 369–373.

Keyler, D. E. (1991). Snake venom or antivenom induced urticaria. *Vet. Hum. Toxicol.*, **33**, 283–284.

King, L. E. and Rees, R. S. (1983). Dapsone treatment of a brown recluse bite. *J. Am. Med. Assoc.*, **250**, 648.

Kitchens, C. S. and Van Mierop, L. H. S. (1987). Envenomation by the eastern coral snake (*Micrurus fulvius fulvius*). A study of 39 victims. *J. Am. Med. Assoc.* **258**, 1615–1618.

Kizer, K. W. (1983–84). Marine envenomations. *J. Toxicol. Clin. Toxicol.*, **21**, 527–555.

Kizer, K. W., McKinney, H. E. and Auerbach, P. S. (1985). Scorpaenidae envenomation. A five-year poison center experience. *J. Am. Med. Assoc.*, **253**, 6, 807–810.

Kjellstrom, B. T. (1989). Acute pancreatitis after snake bite. *Acta Chir. Scand.*, **155**, 291–292.

Kobernick, M. (1984). Black widow spider bite. *Am. Fam. Physician*, **29**, 241–245.

Kokolu, F. and Burnett, J. W. (1990). Treatment of a pigmented lesion induced by a *Pelagia noctiluca* sting. *Cutis*, **46**, 62–64.

Kopp, P., Dahinden, C. A. and Mullner, G. (1993) Allergic reaction to snake venom after repeated bites of *Vipera aspis*. *Clin. Exp. Toxicol.*, **23**, 231–233.

Kunkel, D. B., Curry, S. C., Vance, M. V. and Ryan, P. J. (1983–84). Reptile envenomations. *J. Toxicol. Clin. Toxicol.*, **21**, 503–526.

La Grange, R. G. and Russell, F. E. (1970). Blood platelet studies in man and rabbits following crotalus envenomation. *Proc. West. Pharmacol. Soc.*, **13**, 99–105.

LaGrange, M. A. C. (1990). Pulmonary oedema from a widow spider bite. *S. Afr. Med. J.*, **77**, 110.

Lalloo, D. G., Trevett, A. J., Black, J., Mapao, J., Saweri, A., Naraqi, S., Owens, D., Kamiguti, A. S., Hutton, R. A., Theakston, R. D. G. and Warrell, D. A. (1996). Neurotoxicity, anticoagulant activity and evidence of rhabdomyolysis in patients bitten by death adders (*Acanthophis* sp.) in southern Papua New Guinea. *Q. J. Med.*, **89**, 25–35.

Lalloo, D. G., Trevett, A. J., Nwokolo, N., Laurenson, I. F., Naraqi, S., Kevau, I., Kemp, M. W., Hooper, R. J. L., Theakston, R. D. G. and Warrell, D. (1997). Electrocardiographic abnormalities in patients bitten by taipans (*Oxyuranus scutellatus canni*) and other elapid snakes in Paupua New Guinea. *Tran. R. Soc. Trop. Med. Hyg.*, **91**, 53–56.

Lehmann, D. F. and Hardy, J. C. (1993). Stonefish envenomation. *N. Engl. J. Med.*, **329**, 510–511.

Lerke, P. A., Werner, S. B., Taylor, S. L. and Guthertz, L. S. (1978). Scombroid poisoning: report of an outbreak. *West. J. Med.*, **129**, 381–386.

Lewis, J. V. and Portera, C. A. (1994) Rattlesnake bite of the face: case report and review of the literature. *Am. Surg.*, **60**, 681–682.

Likes, K., Banner, W. and Chavez, M. (1984). *Centruroides exilicauda* envenomation in Arizona. *West. J. Med.*, **141**, 634–637.

Lockey, R. F. (1990). The imported fire ant: immunopathologic significance. *Hosp. Pract.*, **25**, 109–112, 115–124.

Lumley, J., Williamson, J. A. Fenner, P. J., Burnett, J. W. and Colquhoun, D. M. (1988). Fatal envenomation by *Chironex fleckeri*, the north Australian box jellyfish: the continuing search for lethal mechanisms. *Med. J. Aust.*, **148**, 527–534.

McCollum, J. P. K., Pearson, R. C. M., Ingham, H. R., Wood, P. C. and Dewar, H. A. (1968). An epidemic of mussel poisoning in north-east England. *Lancet*, **2**, 767–770.

McNally, S. L. and Reitz, C. J. (1987). Victims of snakebite: a 5-year study at Shongwe Hospital, Kangwane, 1978–1982. *S. Afr. Med. J.*, **72**, 855–860.

Maguire, J. F. and Geha, R. S. (1986). Bee, wasp and hornet stings. *Pediatr. Rev.*, **8**, 6–11.

Majeski, J. A. and Durst, G. G. (1976). Necrotic arachnidism. *South. Med. J.*, **69**, 887–891.

Mann, J. W. and Werntz, J. R. (1991). Catfish stings to the hand. *J. Hand Surg.*, **16A**, 318–321.

Marsh, N. A. (1994). Snake venoms affecting the haemostatic mechanism—a consideration of their mechanisms, practical applications and biological significance. *Blood Coag. Fibrinol.*, **5**, 399–410.

Merson, M. H., Baine, W. B., Gangarosa, E. J. and Swanson, R. C. (1974). Scombroid fish poisoning: outbreak traced to commercially canned tuna fish. *J. Am. Med. Assoc.*, **228**, 1268–1269.

Meyer, W. P., Habib, A. G., Onayade, A. A., Yakubu, A., Smith, D. C., Nasidi, A., Daudu, I. J., Warrell, D. A. and Theakston, R. D. G. (1997). First clinical experiences with a new ovine Fab *Echis ocellatus* snake bite antivenom in Nigeria: randomized comparative trial with Institute Pasteur Serum (Ipser) Africa antivenom. *Am. J. Trop. Med. Hyg.*, **56**, 291–300.

Minton, S. A. (1987). Present tests for detection of snake venom: clinical applications. *Ann. Emerg. Med.*, **16**, 932–937.

Minton, S. A. (1990). Neurotoxic snake envenoming. *Semin. Neurol.*, **10**, 52–61.

Morris, J. G., Lewin, P., Hargrett, N. T., Smith, C. W., Blake, P. A. and Schneider, R. (1982). Clinical features of ciguatera fish poisoning: a study of the disease in the US Virgin Islands. *Arch. Intern. Med.*, **142**, 1090–1092.

Morris, P. D., Campbell, D. S. and Freeman, J. I. (1990). Ciguatera fish poisoning: an outbreak associated with fish caught from North Carolina coastal waters. *South. Med. J.*, **83**, 379–382.

Morris, P. D., Campbell, D. S., Taylor, T. J. and Freeman, J. I. (1991). Clinical and epidemiological features of neurotoxic shellfish poisoning in North Carolina. *Am. J. Publ. Health*, **81**, 471–474.

Morrow, J. D., Margolies, G. R., Rowland, J. and Roberts, L. J. (1991). Evidence that histamine is the causative toxin of scombroid-fish poisoning. *N. Engl. J. Med.*, **324**, 716–720.

Moss, H. S. and Binder, L. S. (1987). A retrospective review of black widow spider envenomation. *Ann. Emerg. Med.*, **16**, 188–192.

Muller, U., Helbling, A. and Berchtold, E. (1992). Immunotherapy with honeybee venom and yellow jacket venom is different regarding efficacy and safety. *J. Allergy Clin. Immunol.*, **89**, 529–535.

Narahashi, T. (1972). Mechanism of action of tetrodotoxin and saxitoxin on excitable membranes. *Fed. Proc.*, **31**, 1124–1132.

Nelson, B. K. (1989). Snake envenomation: incidence, clinical presentation and management. *Med. Toxicol. Adverse Drug. Exp.*, **4**, 17–31.

Newlands, G. (1978). Review of Southern African scorpions and scorpionism. *S. Afr. Med. J.*, **54**, 613–615.

O'Donnell, B. F. and Tan, C. Y. (1993). Persistent contact dermatitis from jellyfish sting. *Contact Dermatitis*, **28**, 112–113.

Otten, E. J. (1983). Antivenin therapy in the emergency department. *Am. J. Emerg. Med.*, **1**, 83–93.

Otten, E. J. and McKimm, D. (1983). Venomous snakebite in a patient allergic to horse serum. *Ann. Emerg. Med.*, **12**, 624–627.

Palafox, N. A., Jain, L. G., Pinano, A. Z., Gulick, T. M., Williams, R. K. and Schatz, I. J. (1988). Successful treatment of ciguatera fish poisoning with intravenous mannitol. *J. Am. Med. Assoc.* **259**, 2740–2742.

Palafox, N. A. (1992). Review of the clinical use of intravenous mannitol with ciguatera fish poisoning from 1988 to 1992. *Bull. Soc. Pathol. Exp.*, **85**, 423–424.

Parrin, J., Kandawalla, N. M. and Lockey, R. F. (1981). Treatment of local skin response to imported fire ant sting. *South. Med. J.*, **74**, 1361–1364.

Parrish, H. M. (1966). Incidence of treated snakebites in the United States. *Publ. Health Rep.*, **81**, 269–276.

Pearn, J. H., Covacevich, J., Charles, N. and Richardson, P. (1994). Snakebite in herpetologists. *Med. J. Aust.*, **161**, 706–708.

Perl, T. M., Bedard, L., Kosatsky, T., Hockin, J. C., Todd, E. C. D. and Remis, R. S. (1990). An outbreak of toxic encephalopathy caused by eating mussels contaminated with domoic acid. *N. Engl. J. Med.*, **322**, 1775–1780.

Phillips, S., Kohn, M., Baker, D., Vander Leest, R., Gomez, H., McKenney, P., McGoldrick, J. and Brent, J. (1995). Therapy of brown spider envenomation: a controlled trial of hyperbaric oxygen, dapsone, and cyproheptadine. *Ann. Emerg. Med.*, **25**, 363–368.

Piacentine, J., Curry, S. C. and Ryan, P. J. (1986). Life-threatening anaphylaxis following Gila monster bite. *Ann. Emerg. Med.*, **15**, 959–961.

Preston, C. A. (1989). Hypotension, myocardial infarction, and coagulopathy following Gila Monster bite. *J. Emerg. Med.*, **7**, 37–40.

Rachesky, I. J., Banner, W., Dansky, J. and Tong, T. (1984). Treatments for *Centruroides exilicauda* envenomation. *Am. J. Dis. Child.*, **138**, 1136–1139.

Rahav, G. and Weiss, A. T. (1990). Scorpion sting-induced pulmonary edema: scintigraphic evidence of cardiac dysfunction. *Chest*, **97**, 1478–1480.

Rajarajeswari, G., Sivaprakasam, S. and Viswanathan, J. (1979). Morbidity and mortality pattern in scorpion stings. *J. Indian Med. Assoc.*, **73**, 123–126.

Rauber, A. (1983–84). Black widow spider bites. *J. Toxicol. Clin. Toxicol.*, **21**, 473–485.

Rawat, S., Laing, G., Smith, D. C., Theakston, D. and Landon, J. (1994). A new antivenom to treat eastern coral snake (*Micrurus fulvius fulvius*) envenoming. *Toxicon*, **32**, 185–190.

Rees, R. S., O'Leary, J. P. and King, L. L. (1983). The pathogenesis of systemic loxoscelism following brown recluse spider bites. *J. Surg. Res.*, **35**, 1–10.

Rees, R. S., Nanney, L. B., Yates, R. A. and King, L. E. (1984). Interaction of brown recluse spider venom on cell membranes: the inciting mechanism? *J. Invest. Dermatol.*, **83**, 270–275.

Rees, R., Campbell, D., Rieger, E. and King, L. E. (1987). The diagnosis and treatment of brown recluse spider bites. *Ann. Emerg. Med.*, **16**, 945–949.

Rees, R. S. and Campbell, D. S. (1989). Spider bites. In Auerbach, P. S. and Geehr, E. C. (Eds), *Management of Wilderness and Environmental Emergencies*, 2nd edn. C. V. Mosby, St Louis, pp. 543–561.

Reeves, J. A., Allison, E. J. and Goodman, P. E. (1996). Black widow spider bite in a child. *Am. J. Emerg. Med.*, **14**, 469–471.

Reisman, R. E. (1989). Studies of the natural history of insect sting allergy. *Allergy Proc.*, **10**, 97–101.

Reisman, R. E. and Livingston, A. (1992). Venom immunotherapy: 10 years of experience with administration of single venoms and 50 μg maintenance doses. *J. Allergy. Clin. Immunol.*, **89**, 1189–1195.

Rhoades, R. B., Schafer, W. L., Newman, M., Lockey, R., Dozler, R.M., Wubbens, P. F., Townes, A. W., Schmid, W. H., Neder, G., Brill, T. and Wittig, H. J. (1977). Hypersensitivity to the imported fire ant in Florida. Report of 104 cases. *J. Fla. Med. Assoc.*, **64**, 247–254.

Riffer, E., Curry, S. C. and Gerkin, R. (1987). Successful treatment with antivenin of marked thrombocytopenia without significant coagulopathy following rattlesnake bite. *Ann. Emerg. Med.*, **16**, 1297–1299.

Roberts, J. R. and Greenberg, M. I. (1997). Ascending hemorrhagic signs after a bite from a copper head. *N. Engl. J. Med.* **336**, 1262–1263.

Rodrigue, D. C., Etzel, R. A., Hall, S., DePorras, E., Velasquez, O. H., Tauxe, R. V., Kilbourne, E. M. and Blake, P. A. (1990). Lethal paralytic shellfish poisoning in Guatemala. *Am. J. Trop. Med. Hyg.*, **42**, 267–271.

Roller, J. A. (1976). Gila monster bite (Letter). *J. Am. Med. Assoc.*, **235**, 249–250.

Russell, F. E., Panos, T. C., Kang, L. W., Warner, A. M. and Colket, T. C. (1958). Studies on the mechanism of death from stingray venom a report of two fatal cases. *Am. J. Med. Sci.*, **235**, 566–584.

Russell, F. E., Carlson, R. W., Wainschel, J. and Osborne, A. H. (1975). Snake venom poisoning in the United States: experiences with 550 cases. *J. Am. Med. Assoc.*, **233**, 341–344.

Russell, F. E. (1980). Snake venom poisoning in the United States. *Annu. Rev. Med.*, **31**, 247–259.

Russell, F. E. and Bogert, C. M. (1981). Gila monster: its biology, venom and bite—a review. *Toxicon*, **19**, 341–359.

Russell, F. E. (1983). *Snake Venom Poisoning*. Scholium International, Great Neck.

Russell, F. E. and Gertsch, W. J. (1983). For those who treat spider or suspected spider bite (Letter to the Editor). *Toxicon*, **21**, 337–339.

Russell, F. E., Sullivan, J. B., Egen, N. B., Jeter, W. S., Markland, F.S., Wingert, W. A. and Bar-Or, D. (1985). Preparation of a new antivenin by affinity chromatography. *Am. J. Trop. Med. Hyg.*, **34**, 141–150.

Ryan, P. J. (1983–84). Preliminary report: experience with the use of dantrolene sodium in the treatment of bites by the black widow spider *Latrodectus hesperus*. *J. Toxicol. Clin. Toxicol.*, **21**, 487–489.

Sakamoto, Y., Lockey, R. and Krzanowski, J. (1987). Shellfish and fish poisoning related to the ingestion of toxic dinoflagellates. *South. Med. J.*, **80**, 866–870.

Schaeffer, R. C., Pattabhiraman, T. R., Carlson, R. W., Russell, F. E. and Weil, M. H. (1979). Cardiovascular failure produced by a peptide from the venom of the southern pacific rattlesnake *Crotalus viridis heller*. *Toxicon*, **17**, 447–453.

Schuberth, K. C., Graft, D. F. and Kagey-Sobotka, A. (1983). Do all children with insect allergy need venom therapy? (Abstract). *J. Allergy Clin. Immunol.*, **71**, 140.

Settipane, G. A., Newtead, G. J. and Boyd, G. R. (1972). Frequency of hymenoptera allergy in an atopic and normal population. *J. Allergy Clin. Immunol.*, **50**, 146–150.

Sims, J. K. and Ostman, D. C. (1986). Pufferfish poisoning: emergency diagnosis and management of mild human tetrodotoxication. *Ann. Emerg. Med.*, **15**, 1094–1098.

Sims, J. K. (1987). A theoretical discourse on the pharmacology of toxic marine ingestions. *Ann. Emerg. Med.*, **16**, 1006–1015.

Sofer, S., Shalev, H., Weizman, Z., Shahak, E. and Gueron, M. (1991). Acute pancreatitis in children following envenomation by the yellow scorpion *Leiurus quinquestriatus*. *Toxicon*, **29**, 125–128.

Stafford, C. T., Hutto, L. S., Rhodes, R. B., Thompson, W. O. and Impson, L. K. (1989a). Imported fire ant as a health hazard. *South. Med. J.*, **82**, 1515–1519.

Stafford, C. T., Hoffman, D. R. and Rhoades, R. B. (1989b). Allergy to imported fire ants. *South. Med. J.*, **82**, 1520–1527.

Stafford, C. T., Rhoades, R. B., Bunker-Soler, A. L., Thompson, W. O. and Impson, L. K. (1989c). Survey of whole body-extract immunotherapy for imported fire ant- and other hymenoptera-sting allergy. *J. Allergy Clin. Immunol.*, **83**, 1107–1111.

Stein, M. R., Marraccini, J. V., Rothschild, N. E. and Burnett, J. W. (1989). Fatal Portuguese man-o'-war (*Physalia physalis*) envenomation. *Ann. Emerg. Med.*, **18**, 312–315.

Stone, B. D., Hutcheson, P. S., Evans, R. G. and Slavin, R. G. (1992). Increased incidence of stings in venom-sensitive patients. *Ann. Allergy*, **69**, 445–446.

Streiffer, R. H. (1986). Bite of the venomous lizard, the Gila monster. *Postgrad. Med.*, **79**, 297–299, 302.

Sutherland, S. K., Coulter, A. R. and Harris, R. D. (1979). Rationalization of first-aid measures for elapid snakebite. *Lancet*, **1**, 183–186.

Sullivan, J. B. (1987). Past, present, and future immunotherapy of snake venom poisoning. *Am. Emerg. Med.*, **16**, 938–942.

Talan, D. A., Citron, D. M., Overturf, G. D., Singer, B., Froman, P. and Goldstein, E. J. C. (1991). Antibacterial activity of crotalid venoms against oral snake flora and other clinical bacteria. *J. Infect. Dis.*, **164**, 195–198.

Taylor, S. L., Stratton, J. E. and Nordlee, J. A. (1989). Histamine poisoning (scombroid fish poisoning): an allergy-like intoxication. *J. Toxicol. Clin. Toxicol.*, **27**, 225–240.

Teitelbaum, J. S., Zatorre, R. J., Carpenter, S., Gendron, D., Evans, A. C., Gjedde, A. and Cashman, N. R. (1990).

Neurologic sequelae of domoic acid intoxication due to the ingestion of contaminated mussels. *N. Engl. J. Med.*, **322**, 1781–1787.

Tester, P. A. (1994). Harmful marine phytoplankton and shellfish toxicity: potential consequences of climate change. *Ann. N. Y. Acad. Sci.*, **740**, 69–76.

Theakston, R. D. G. (1989). New techniques in antivenom production and active immunization against snake venoms. *Trans. R. Soc. Trop. Med. Hyg.*, **83**, 433–435.

Tibballs, J. (1988). Severe tetrodotoxic fish poisoning. *Anaesth. Intensive Care*, **16**, 215–217.

Trestrail, J. H. (1981). Scorpion envenomation in Michigan: three cases of toxic encounters with poisonous stow-aways. *Vet. Hum. Toxicol.*, **23**, 8–11.

Trestrail, J. H. and Al-Mahasneh, Q. M. (1989). Lionfish string experiences of an inland poison center: a retrospective study of 23 cases. *Vet. Hum. Toxicol.*, **31**, 173–175.

Tu, A. T. and Fulde, G. (1987). Sea snake bites. *Clin. Dermatol.*, **5**, 118–126.

Valentine, M. D., Schuberth, K. C., Kagey-Sobotka, A., Graft, D. F., Kwiterovich, K. A., Szklo, M. and Lichtenstein, L. M. (1990). The value of immunotherapy with venom in children with allergy to insect stings. *N. Engl. J. Med.*, **323**, 1601–1603.

Van der Linden, P. W. G., Hack, C. E., Kerckhaert, J. A. M., Struyvenberg, A. and Van der Zwan, J. C. (1990). Preliminary report: compliment activation in wasp-sting anaphylaxis. *Lancet*, **336**, 904–906.

Vijeth, S. R., Dutta, T. K. and Shahapurkar, J. (1997). Correlation of renal status with hematologic profile in viperine bite. *Am. J. Trop. Med. Hyg.*, **56**, 168–170.

Wang, G. K. and Strichartz, G. R. (1983). Purification and physiological characterization or neurotoxins from the venoms of scorpions *Centruroides sculpturatus* and *Leiurus quinquestraitus*. *Mol. Pharmacol.*, **23**, 519–533.

Wasserman, G. S. and Anderson, P. C. (1983–84). Loxoscelism and necrotic arachnidism. *J. Toxicol. Clin. Toxicol.*, **21**, 451–472.

Wasserman, G. S. (1988). Wound care of spider and snake envenomations. *Ann. Emerg. Med.*, **17**, 331–1335.

Williams, S. T., Khare, V. K., Johnston, G. A. and Blackall, D. P. (1995). Severe intravascular hemolysis associated with brown recluse spider envenomation: a report of two cases and review of the literature. *Am. J. Clin. Pathol.*, **104**, 463–467.

Wright, D. N. and Lockey, R. F. (1990). Local reactions to stinging insects (*Hymenoptera*). *Allergy Proc.*, **11**, 23–28.

Yang, C. C., Han, K. C., Lin, T. J., Tsai, W. J. and Deng, J. F. (1995). An outbreak of tetrodotoxin poisoning following gastropod mollusc consumption. *Hum. Exp. Toxicol.*, **14**, 446–450.

Youlten, L. J. F., Atkinson, B. A. and Lee, T. H. (1995). The incidence and nature of adverse reactions to injection immunotherapy in bee and wasp venom allergy. *Clin. Exp. Allergy*, **25**, 159–165.

FURTHER READING

Auerbach, P. S. (1990). Marine envenomations. *N. Engl. J. Med.*, **325**, 486–493.

Golden, D. B. K., Kwiterovich, K. A., Kagey-Sobotka, A., Valentine, M. D. and Lichtenstein, L. M. (1996). Discontinuing venom immunotherapy: outcome after five years. *J. Allergy Clin. Immunol.*, **97**, 579–587.

Karlson-Stiber, C., Persson, H., Heath, A., Smith, D., Al-Abdulla, I. H. and Sjostrom, L. (1997). First clinical experiences with specific sheep Fab fragments in snake bite. Report of a multicentre study of *Vipera berus* envenoming. *J. Intern. Med.*, **241**, 53–58.

Marsh, N. A. (1994). Snake venoms affecting the haemostatic mechanism—a consideration of their mechanisms, practical applications and biological significance. *Blood Coag. Fibrinol.*, **5**, 399–410.

Russell, F. E. (1983). *Snake Venom Poisoning*. Scholium International, Great Neck.

Watters, M. R. (1995). Organic neurotoxins in seafoods. *Clin. Neurol. Neurosurg.*, **97**, 119–124.

Valentine, M. D., Schuberth, K. C., Kagey-Sobotka, A., Graft, D. F., Kwiterovich, K. A., Szklo, M. and Lichtenstein, L. M. (1990). The value of immunotherapy with venom in children with allergy to insect stings. *N. Engl. J. Med.*, **323**, 1601–1603.

INDICES

SUBJECT INDEX

This Index contains topics, biological terms and normal endogenous biological materials.

actin-binding proteins, as calpain substrate 189–90
actinic elastosis 836
α-actinin 894
actinomyces 562
actinomyosin 939
actinomyosin adenosinetri-phosphatase 818, 950
activated partial thromboplastin time 361, 389
activation *see* enzymes
activators, rubber industry 2014, 2016
active energy dependent transport 547
'active metabolites' 870–2
active oxygen species 240
active transport 548
actual received dose 149
actuarial tables 1749
acute dermal toxicity *see* skin
acute dietary testing, LC$_{50}$ 1344–5
acute exposure *see* acute toxicity studies
acute lethality testing 35
acute myeloid leukaemia, oncogene activation 1457
acute overdose, commonly encoutered substances 1496
acute phase proteins 367
acute reference dose (ARfD) 1603, 1609, 1993
acute renal failure 685
acute toxicity studies
  advantages 55–6
  animal species choice 325
  animal welfare 493
  classification 5
  data interpretation 327–8, 331–2
  definitions 34–5, 1446, 1772
  dermal *see* skin
  development of assessment 35–8
  dose level selection 325–6
  factors affecting 45
  factors affecting metabolism and toxicity *326*
  Good Laboratory Practice (GLP) 440
  inhalation 46, 327
  intepretation 1337–8
  interspecies extrapolation 1447
  LD$_{50}$ values 13, 16, 39, 326, 425, 1593
  lethal injury to heart 821
  long-term effects 55

  metabolic consequences *325*
  new substances 1591, 1622
  non-rodent 44–5
  oral tests *324*, 326–7, 1329, 1343–4
  parameters studies 39–40
  parenteral 47
  pesticides 1609
  pharmaceuticals 1616
  principles and procedures 38–50
  protocol design 40–2, 325–8
  rationale, design and use 1331–4
  refinement 495–9
  replacement 499
  screening 35
  statistical design 495
  testing for effects 33–54
  wildlife toxicology 1329–34
acyl-CoA:amino acid *N*-acyltransferases *216*
adaptation, rate 651
adaptive DNA repair pathway 1023–4
adaptive enzyme induction 6
adder, common (*Vipera berus*) 2181
addictive behaviours, management 1444
addictive substances 1151, 1443
addition reactions 613
additive effects 20, 50, 1416, 1787
  see also mixtures of chemicals
additives *see under* food; plastics; rubber
adducts 161–2, 1026–7, 1636
  see also macromolecular adducts
adenohypophysis 372, 980–1
adenoma, biomarker 1856
adenosine 806
adenosine diphosphate (ADP), and apoptosis 191, 192
adenosine monophosphate *see* cyclic adenosine monophosphate
adenosine triphosphatase (ATPase) 341, 343, 366, 631, 642
  actinomyosin 818
  Ca^{2+} 156, 806, 809
  Mg^{2+} 341
  Na$^+$/K$^+$ *see* sodium/potassium
  ouabain-sensitive 812
adenosine triphosphate (ATP)
  and apoptosis 185
  cardiac toxicology 806–7
  clinical chemistry 366
  depletion 190

  hepatotoxicity 868
  levels, as biomarker 1848
  neurotoxicity 631, 642
  pathology 341, 343
  pulmonary toxicology 185, 722
  reduced synthesis 681
  skeletal muscle toxicity 938
  sulphation 105
  synthesis 127
  weigh-master role 166
S-adenosylmethionine 109
adenovirus, and apoptosis 194
adenylate cyclase 779, 785, 819, 820, 982
adenylate kinase 357
adhesion molecules 168, 189–90
adhesions 532
adhesives 1295
ADI *see* acceptable daily intake
adipose tissue 810–11
  accumulates pesticide residues 1343
  adrenal hormone action 370
  biomarker 1589, 1858
  biomonitoring 1844, 1905, 1906
  dioxin levels 88
  distribution in 70, 71
  interspecies 88
  nitrate and nitrite levels 2116, 2117
  organic solvents 2038
  PBPK studies 89–90, 144
  PCBs 810–11
  PCBs in 642
  pharmacokinetic analysis 284
  as protective against dioxin 283–4
  as storage site 17
  styrene levels 2020
ADME (absorption/distribution/metabolism/excretion) studies 67–8
Administration of Radioactive Substances Advisory Committee 466
administration route
  see also exposure route
  drug(s) 21
  synthetic materials 1739
  toxicants 1504
  in toxicity testing 1616, 1622
ADP *see* acoustic distortion product; adenosine diphosphate
adrenal cortex 179, 346, 984–6

adrenal gland
   clinical chemistry 370
   drug toxicity *369*
   hypertrophy, nitrites 2135,
      2136–7
   in vitro test *418*
   radiation-induced changes 1691
   susceptibility to drug-induced
      lesions 369
   tumours in plastics industry 2022
   weight 346
adrenal medulla *986*
adrenaline (epinephrine) 262, 547,
   808, 2184
α-adrenergic receptors 808, 813
β-adrenergic receptors 808, 813,
   896
adrenocorticotrophic hormone
   (ACTH) 369–70, 980
adsorption on storage 1909
adult respiratory distress syndrome
   (ARDS) 732, 2179–80
adult/developmental toxicity (A/D)
   ratio 1187–8
adverse effects 21–2, 34
   acute toxicity studies 38
   biomarker 1842
   definition 4, 34, 1394
   distasters 1427, 1437, 1450
   factors affecting 21–2
   from fires 1924–5
   human studies 456
   predictability 1438
   risk assessment 1754
   and safety of medicine 1426,
      1429
   synthetic materials 1738, 1739,
      1740
   types 21
advisory committees (UK) 1578,
   1594, 1595, 1637
aerial spraying 1339, 1341, 1355,
   1727
aerodynamic diameter formula 590
aerosols
   aerodynamic size distribution
      598
   chemical 315
   concentration 598
   deposition mechanisms 588, 590
   dose–response assessment 1762
   electrostatic charge 592
   environmental 599
   exposure 603
   eye irritation tests 740

generation from liquids 594–5
generation from solids 596–7
generator diagrams *596*
inhalational toxicity 590–2
mixtures 315–16
particle size 16, 595
particulate sampler *598*
physics 588
repeated exposure studies 60
respiratory tract potency *625*
skin deposition 605
spectrometry 599
toxicity 46
toxicity testing 316
water inhalation study 604
aerospace workers and idiopathic
   environmental illness 1705,
   1708–9, 1710
affinity chromatography 372, 2152,
   2153
affinity constant 84
Afghanistan, chemical warfare
   2080
aflatoxicosis 1994
African scorpions 640
African swine fever virus, and
   apoptosis 194
agarose gel electrophoresis 187,
   188
agave (*Agave lecheguilla*) 1519,
   1523
Agave lechaguilla see agave
age effects
   and clearance 84
   drug safety 1439
   on metabolism 115, 1417
   on microbial metabolism 572
   PBPK modelling 89
   on radiation toxicology 1683,
      1692, 1693
   and response to toxic agents 15,
      21, 1416, 1417
   steady state concentration and 83
ageing, role of genetic mutations in
   1037
Agelaius phoeniceus see blackbird,
   red-winged
Agelenopsis see spiders
Agency for Toxic Substances and
   Disease Registry (USA) 669,
   1749
agonal signs 41
agonosis 43
agoraphobia, toxic 1709

agranulocytosis 394–5, 1426, 1427
Agreement on Sanitary and
   Phytosanitary Measures (WTO)
   1569, 1649
Agreement on Technical Barriers to
   Trade (WTO) 1569
Agricola, Georgius 1474
agricultural biotechnology 1454,
   1459
agricultural chemicals
   see also herbicides; insecticides;
      pesticides *and Chemical Index*
   cartilage and bone toxicity 965
   combustion products 1919
   human studies 453
   industry 438
   pharmacogenetics 215
   plant-protection products 1548
   regulatory aspects 1548, 1960
   reproductive toxicity 1143
   and wildlife toxicology 1328,
      1343, 1347
Agricultural Chemicals Regulation
   Law (Japan) 37
Agricultural Compound Unit (New
   Zealand) 1611
agricultural effluents 1340, 1343,
   1351, 1354–5, 1514
Agricultural Pests Control Act 1927
   (Canada) 1600
agricultural soils 1377, 1383
agricultural waste, disposal 2114
agricultural workers
   pesticide exposure 605, 1548,
      1993
   reproductive risks 463
   risks of death 1825, 1830
agrochemicals *see* agricultural
   chemicals; pesticides
Agrostemma gigatho see corn cockle
AHH *see* arylhydrocarbon
   hydroxylase
AhR *see* aromatic hydrocarbon
   receptor
α-AIB *see* α-aminoisobutyric acid
AIDS 229, 1003–4
air
   see also indoor air
   expired *see* breath
   filtration 488, 512, 514
   patterns of exposure to 603
air conditioning systems *see* heating,
   ventilation and air conditioning
   systems
air jet mills 597

air pollution 8, 315, 316, 1265–7
see also air pollution; indoor air
contaminants; summer smog;
winter smog
adduct immunoassays 1886
cadmium 2052
definition of adverse health
effects 1283–4
from disasters 1828, 1832, 1833
IEI and 1706
mercury 2057–8
modelling 1772
monitoring 149, 1778, 1904
neonatal toxicity 1227
patterns of exposure to 1267–8
RfC 1760
toxicological aspects 1274–83
variety 1446
in workplace 1909
air–water partition coefficient 582
airborne industrial chemicals 1487
airborne occupational exposure
limits 1481
airborne particulates 565
aircraft fires 1921, 1923
airflow patterns 590–1
airway *see* respiratory system
ALA *see* aminolaevulinic acid
ALAD *see* δ-aminolaevulinic acid
dehydrogenase
alanine aminopeptidase (AAP) *356,
363*
alanine aminotransferase (ALT)
assays 1462
biomarkers 1857, 1858, 1859,
1860, 1861, 1862
clinical chemistry 355–6, 359,
363, 366
hepatotoxicity 43, 868
alanine–valine substitution 283
ALARA *see* as low as reasonably
available
albinos, chemical distribution in
tissues 129
albumin
adducts 1893
in BALF, dose-response
assessment 1762
binding 368, 371
as biomarker *678*, 1845, 1858,
1860, 1861, 1880, 1910
circadian toxicology 253
clinical chemistry 355, 358, 361,
363, 364, 366, 367
electrophoretic techniques 368

excretion 682
[125]I-labelled 722
as mouse allergen 511
pancreatic toxicology 897
alcohol dehydrogenase 103, 104,
216, 235–40, 429, 2040
alcoholic disease
acute rhabdomyolysis 940–1
chronic myopathy 941–2
flushing 238
liver 237
pancreatitis 237
alcoholism 236, 237, 757
aldehyde dehydrogenase (ALDH)
103, *216*, 236–40, 2016
aldehyde oxidase 103, *216*, 238,
239
aldo-keto reductases *216*, 241–3,
242
aldolase 941
aldose reductases 241, *242*, 762–3
aldosterone 985, 1859
Alfred P. Murrah Federal Building
bombing 1721
algae 1548, 2193
see also microalgae
alicyclic hydroxylations 101
Aliens of America 1725
alimentary toxic aleukia (ATA) 394
alimentary tract 19, 1689, 2145,
2149
see also specific areas
aliphatic hydroxylations 100–1
aliphatic sulphation *106*
alkaline phosphatase (AP) 337,
344–5, *355–6*, 385, 873, 1462,
1849, 1859, 1860, 1862
alkaline unwinding assay 1845
alkylation 8, 159
O⁶-alkyldeoxyguanine-DNA
alkyltransferase 1892
alleles *see* genes; genetic
allergens
see also Chemical Index
contact 708, 710
pyrethroids 1999
allergic challenge testing 1780
allergic contact dermatitis 7, 23,
510, 511, 711, 830, 834–6,
838–40, 1779, 2062–3
allergic reaction
to animal stings 2181, 2183,
2189
as biomarker 1847
to drugs 21, 1427, 1438

to laboratory animals 511–14,
1530
to latex 510–11, 1667
to meat wrapper 1915
to nitrites 2128
ozone and nitrogen dioxide
effects 1279–80
pathogenesis 703–4
and peripheral sensory irritation
615
respiratory 701
allergic rhinitis 1703, 1715, 1716
allergic sinusitis 1703, 1711
allergy
compound 840
concept 524, 1416, 1704
alligators, environmental endocrine
effects 1407
allometry 51, 52, 88–9, 91, 92,
1834
alloys, medical devices 1734
alopecia 40, 41, 235, 1696, 2015
alphabet bomber 1725, 1728
alphafetoprotein, biomarker 1849
alprazolem 4-hydroxylase *217*
ALS *see* amyotrophic lateral
sclerosis
ALT *see* alanine aminotransferase
Alternaria spp. 2145
'alternative' remedies 1550
alternative testing methods 36,
52–3
alveolar air
–blood interface 590
biomonitoring 607
alveolar buds 340
alveolar cells 128, 722, 723, 725,
728, 731, 1690
alveolar deposition 46, 316, 591,
592
alveolar haemorrhage 728
alveolar macrophages 315, *417*
alveolar oedema 722
alveolar proteinaceous material 728
alveolar surface area 590
alveolitis 729
Alzet osmotic minipump 528
Alzheimer's disease 166, 634, 635,
1379–80, 2060
Amanita spp. *see* mushrooms
Amaranthus spp. *see* pigweed,
rough
amberjack 2191
ambient monitoring 461, 1602
amenorrhoea 1156

American Academy of Forensic Sciences 1491

American Antivivisection Society 486

American Association for the Accreditation of Laboratory Animal Care 487

American Association of Clinical Chemists 1491

American Association for Laboratory Animal Science 492

American Association of Poison Control Centers 459

American Association of Poisons Control Centers, National Data Collection System 38

American Board of Forensic Toxicology (ABFT) 1489, 1491

American College of Toxicology 493

American Conference of Governmental Industrial Hygienists (ACGIH)
  behavioural toxicity studies 668
  biological monitoring 1485, 1910
  mixed route of exposure 603, 606
  occupational toxicity studies 1458, 1475, 1477
  origins 1482
  peripheral sensory iritation studies 625
  threshold limit values 1483, 1594

American Crop Protection Association (ACPA) 1602

American Medical Association (AMA) *402*, 486

American National Standards Institute (ANSI) 1458, 1662

American Society for Testing and Materials (ASTM), and wildlife toxicology 1328

American Veterinary Medical Association 487, 497

Ames test 279, *403*, 499, 565, 567, 1045–6, 1383, 1434, 1448, 1479, 1756
  see also mutation tests; *Salmonella triphimurium*

amidases, hydrolysis 105

amide hydrolysis 105

amine group oxidation 102

amine oxidase (AO) 238–9

amino acid transferase 372

amino acids
  as biomarker 1849, 1861
  conjugation 98, 109
  metabolism 105, 568
  modification 159
  necessary for bone growth 971–2
  substitution 231
  transport system *681*

aminoaciduria 679, 1862

γ-aminobutyric (GABA) receptors 632, 634, *641*, 651, 1244

γ-aminobutyric (GABA) synapse 640

aminoglycoside nephrotoxicity cascade *687*

α-aminoisobutyric acid (α-AIB) 1255, 1256

δ-aminolaevulinic acid (ALA) 392, 1343, 1461

δ-aminolaevulinic acid dehydrase (ALAD)
  as biomarker 1848, 1864, 1867
  biomonitoring 1906
  haematotoxicity 392
  lead inhibition 1345, 2056
  nephrotoxicity 683
  wildlife toxicity 1344

δ-aminolaevulinic acid synthetase, as biomarker 1863–4

aminophospholipid translocase, and apoptosis 183

ammoniation of cereals 2147, 2153

amnesia, predictability in animal tests 1438

amphibians 111, 178, 1327, 1330, 1353

amphiphilic agents 730, 945

Amsinkia intermedia see fiddleneck

amylase *356*, 365, 547, 572, 897

amyloid 296, 367

amyloidosis 943

amyotrophic lateral sclerosis (ALS) 239, 636

Anabaena, blue–green algae toxicity 1516

anaemia
  and arsenic 2051
  and benzene 100
  clinical chemistry 366
  erythropoietin therapy 1971
  and fungicides 2003
  haematotoxicity studies 389, 390
  and lead 2056
  megaloblastic 389–90, 391

microcytic 389–90, 391
  and organic solvents 2037
  parenteral toxicity studies 535
  pernicious 562, 1125

anaemic hypoxia, from fires 1920, 1921

anaerobic bacteria, in large intestine 562–3

anaerobic cabinets 563

anaerobic pyrolysis 1916

anaesthesia/anaesthetic agents
  for blood sampling 386–7
  cardiac toxicity 817–18
  clinical chemistry 357, 362
  forensic analysis 1491, 1495
  inhalation *498*, 2030
  for injections 527
  local 522, 741, 816, 817, 946–7, 955–6
  neurotoxicity 641
  occupational exposures 1463
  pancreatic toxicity 898
  potency 2030
  regulatory aspects 1548
  reproductive toxicity 1145, 1156, 1465
  as sign of toxicity 40, 41
  and spontaneous abortion 1464

analgesia/analgesics 40, 41, 219, 386, 460, 536

analysis of variance (ANOVA) 1177
  see also statistical analysis

analytical chemistry 1941–2

analytical measures of exposure 1461

analytical methods 358, 1446–7, 1646–7

anaphylactoid reactions
  adverse drug reaction 1427, 1438
  food additives and 1986–7
  insect stings and 2183
  laboratory occupational hazard 511
  parenteral toxicity 522, 535
  regulations 1549

Anas americana see wigeon, American

Anas platyrhynchos see mallard

Anas rubripes see black duck

anatomical site concentration differences 1495

Androctonus see scorpion

androgen 984, 1394–5, 1400, 1403

androgen receptor (AR) 689, 983–4
androgen receptor antagonists 1328
androgenic binding protein 372
androgenic hormone-related
  processes 1401
anemone, Bermuda 820
Anemonia sulcata 820
aneuploidy 1081, 1141
angina 394, 460, 527, 805, 822
angio-oedema, LAA 512
angiogenesis 282
angiography 756
angiosarcoma, and vinyl chloride
  1771
angiotensin 675, 684
aniline 4-hydroxylase 217
animal carcinogenesis, and human
  risk 1536–9
animal care *see* animal welfare
Animal Cruelty Act 1876 (UK) 486
animal feeds 444, 1514, 1515,
  1518, 1648, 2158–9
  see also cattle, *etc.*
animal grooming, exposure 603,
  604
animal hair, LAA 511
animal housing 489–90, 740
animal husbandry 323–4, 490–1
animal– plant warfare 215
Animal Remedies Act 1956
  (Ireland) 1558
animal rights 36, 485, 493
Animal (Scientific Procedures) Act
  (UK) 36, 1960
animal stings and bites
  cardiotoxicity 2179, 2189, 2190
  neurotoxicity 2179, 2188, 2190
  pancreatic toxicity 2180, 2188
  respiratory toxicity 2179–80,
    2189
  skin damage 2178, 2182, 2183,
    2185, 2187, 2189
animal studies
  see also inter/intraspecies *and*
    also specific types of animals,
    e.g. rat; species; strains
  acute toxicity 38–50, 1741
  antidotal assessment *431–2*
  behaviour, ethological analyses
    653–4
  cardiotoxicity 815
  combustion 1925–6
  comparability of groups 57
  cytogenetic assays 1083, 1086–7

dietary restriction 323
drugs 527, 1430–1
endangered species, biomarker
  1845
endogenous synthesis of nitrates
  2118–19
ethics 1957, 1958, 1959
factors influencing toxicity
  15–16
gastro-intestinal flora 561–4
harmonization 37–8
hazard bioassays 28, 1754–5,
  1763
health status 57
immunotoxicology 1005, 1006–9
intraocular pressure (IOP) values
  749
legal limitations 1591, 1664
long-term 1618–20
methodology 1536
mixed exposure to toxins 604–5
MRLs 1643
multi-generation 604
nitrate/nitrite/*N*-nitroso toxicity
  2123–5, 2135–6
number of animals needed 25
pancreatic cancer 922–6
particulates ingestion 1772
of pharmaceuticals 1616
placental toxicity 1243, 1247–8,
  1250–4
protocol design 22–5, 40–2,
  1964
Redbook protocols 1635, 1659
reduction/replacement 52, 53,
  148, 402, 499–500, 1622
repeated exposure protocols 57
reproductive toxicity 1137–40,
  1142–3
research programmes 1940, 1941
safe dose 91
skin irritation tests 832, 843–4
skin sensitization tests 841–3
species choice 1039, 1314
synthetic materials 1739, 1741,
  1742
teratogenicity 1169–79, 1181–8,
  1189, 1222, 1245–6
tightly specified 1535
toxicity testing 2
use of laboratory animals 402
variables 431
weight gain 323
animal technician, antineoplastic
  drugs exposure 515

animal toxins 820–1, 1444,
  2177–99
animal welfare 485–507
  humane treatment 401
  humane treatment diagram *502*
  information resources 471
  legislation/policy 36, 486–7
  quality assurance 444
  regulations 61, 64, 1734, 1740
  responsibility 500–1
  severe pain or distress signs *497*
Animal Welfare Act 1970 (US) 486
Animal Welfare Act 1995 (US) 487,
  501
Animal Welfare Act (USA) 36, 486,
  1664
anisocytosis 391
ankylosing spondylitis, radiation-
  induced 1692
annular furnace 1926
anogenital distance 1406
Anolis carolinenis see lizard, green
  anole
Anopheles albimanus see mosquito
anophthalmia 758
anorexia 283, 814, 815–16, 1351–2,
  1724
  see also feeding behaviour;
    starvation
anosmia 21
ANOVA *see* analysis of variance;
  statistics
anoxia 785, 1510–11, 1848, 1869
Anser anser see goose, greylag
ANSI *see* American National
  Standards Insitute
antagonistic interactions 20, 50,
  305, 306, *313*, *426*, 1395, 1416
antagonists 33, 35, 126
Antarctica *see* polar regions
anthelmintics 527, 634, 641, 1999
Anthosa 2190
anthrax disease 1726
anthropogenic origins, chemical
  hazard 1328, 1330
anthropogenic pollution 1329, 1370
  see also pollution
anthroposophic medicines 1550
antiabortefacient 1392
antiallergy drugs 262–3
antianginal drugs *220*
antiarrhythmics *219*, 817–18
antibiotic resistance genes 1024–5

antibiotics *522*, 532, 819–20, 1146
  see also specific antibiotics, e.g.
    penicillin (*in Chemical Index*)
  anaphylactic reactions 1549
anticancer drugs 261–2
  and female reproductive disorders
    1465
  and gut microflora 572
  molecular interactions 163
  for phosgene toxicity 2099
  supplies in CB attack 1729
antibodies
  for adduct analysis 1885
  antiCD₃, and apoptosis 188
  antiheroin 942
  anti-latex IgE 510
  antinuclear 682
  as biomarker 1848
  biotinated 338
  for ochratoxin analysis 2158
anticaking agents 1985
anticarcinogens 157
anticholinesterase properties 29,
  429, 636, 1475, 1554, 1996
anticholinesterases
  behavioural effects 1348–9,
    1351, 1352
  and brain cholinesterase levels
    1344
  clinical chemistry 368
  design of studies 328
  differential toxicity 1335
  intermittent exposure 1351
  natural exposure 1351
  as pesticides 1994, 1995–8
  and predation behaviour 1348
  reproductive effects 1352
  safety studies 1444
  secondary toxicity 1341–2
  for snakebites 2181
  sporadic lethality 1328
  wildlife toxicology 1329, 1343
Anticipated Residue Contribution
  1602
anticoagulants 229, 230, 357, 387,
  756, 989, 1345, 1455, 1510–11
antidegradants 2014
antidiuretic hormone *see* arginine
  vasopressin
antidotes 425–51
  additive 433
  antagonism 430
  comparison 432–3
  detoxifying *426*
  direct *426*

dose assessment 432
efficacy 430–3
enzyme-catalysed reaction 428–9
enzyme-poison complex reaction
  429–30
evaluation 1452
experimental assessment 431–2,
  431
forming detoxifying substance
  429
mechanism of action *426*–30
new 426
pharmacological *426*, 430
phenobarbital index 460
prophylactic administration 432
related mechanisms 430
studies 25
synergistic 433
in toxicology laboratory 516
antifertility 523
antifreeze 1510
  see also ethylene glycol *in
    Chemical Index*
antigen-presenting cells (APCs)
  1000
antigenic determinants 338, 997
antigens 549
antimetabolites 261
antimicrobials
  see also antibiotics
  microbiological endpoints 1645
antioxidant(s)
  and apoptosis 191
  biochemistry 127
  as biomarkers 1847, 1867, *1868*
  defence systems 158, 168,
    1867–9
  dietary role 1978–9, 1982–3,
    1984, 1985–6
  function of cells 160
  in IEI 1705
  neurotoxicity 634
  nitrite intake and 2132, 2137
  regulations 1552, 1653
  response element 277
  in rubber industry 2017
antiozonants 2017
antisense oligonucleotides 196
antisera 428
antistatics 2023
antitack agents 2014, 2017
antitoxins, in CB attack 1729
α₁-antitrypsin deficiency 29
Antivenom Index 2177

antivivisection *see* animal rights
ants 2184–5
anuria 40, 41
anus
  mucosal radiation-induced
    changes 1689
  and peroral toxicity 545
anutrient chemicals 216–17
anxiety, in idiopathic environmental
  illness 1708, 1709, 1710,
  1714
AOELs *see* acceptable operator
  exposure levels
aortic anatomy 805
aortic aneurysm, in firefighters
  1928, 1929
AP *see* alkaline phosphatase
AP-1 transcription factor 168
Apaf *see* apoptotic protease
  activating factors
APCs *see* antigen-presenting cells
apical junctions 548
Apidae 2182
aplastic anaemia *389–90*, 1438,
  1634
apnoea 40, 41, 615
APO1, and apoptosis 193
Apocynum spp. *see* dogbane
apolipoproteins 367
apoptogens 197
apoptosis 175–202
  biochemistry 126, 187–90
  definition 175
  distinguishing features 177
  drug- and chemical-induced
    197–200
  from radiation 1690
  genetic regulation 192–7
  induction phase 192
  inhibition 1127–8
  initiation 192
  liver remodelling by 880–1
  molecular and cellular concepts
    157, 163–9
  morphological features 176,
    183–7
  mycotoxins and 2149
  occurrence 178–9
  ototoxicity 792
  and p53 1031
  pathology 338, 340, 344
  pathophysiology 178
  response levels 177–8
apoptotic bodies, formation 183

apoptotic protease activating factors
Apaf 164–5
APAF-1 195
apparent safety margin overestimation 87
apparent volume of distribution 70,
75, 78, 79, 87, 89
applanation tonometry 749
apples, nitrate levels 2113
applied toxicology 1941–2
approvals 1543
approximate lowest lethal
concentration 46
approximate methods, cost-
effectiveness 1331
aquaculture 636, 1548
aquatic environments 317
aquatic toxicology 3, 1309–25
acute and chronic toxicity 49,
1315–16
biochemical techniques 1317
biomarkers 1319
chemical assessment 1312–13
choice of species 1314
comparative species sensitivity
1319–20
concepts and principles 1311–15
definition of terms 1311–12
environmental and ecological
contributions 1314–15
exposure, bioavailability and
toxicity estimates 1313
hazard evaluation and risk
assessment 1318–19
history of 1309–10
and law 1311
links to human health 1310
microcosm and mesocosm
techniques 1318, 1319
microscale testing 1320
minimum time to toxic effect and
toxicity curve 1314
modelling techniques 1316–17
objectives and scope 1310
practice of 1310–11
predictive techniques 1315
quantitative structure–activity
relationships 1317
sediment toxicity 1319
test principles 1314
aqueous humour, prostaglandins
741
aqueous solutions 1683, 1777–8
AR see androgen receptors

arachidonic acid 185, 191, 792,
981, 1867, 1981
arachidonic acid epoxygenase *217*
Arachnidae 2185
arbitration, EU procedures 1625–6,
1641
arc welders, biomonitoring 1904
Arctic *see* polar regions
Ardea herodias see heron, great blue
area under curve (AUC)
age-related changes 84
bioavailability calculation 75
calculation 79, 80
chronic intake 82, 83
clearance 79, 80
dioxin 88
drug interactions 22
extent of distributions 78
parenteral toxicity 523
PBPK modelling 148, 149
percutaneous absorption 19
pharmacogenetics 236
regulations 1620
scaling factors 1769
steady state 81
area under first moment of
concentration–time curve
(AUMC) 84–5
arene oxide 100
ARfD *see* acute reference dose
Argentina, fumonisin contamination
of cereals 2165
arginine, species differences in
conjugation 111
arginine vasopressin, as biomarker
1859
Argiope spp. *see* spiders
argyrophil staining 343–4
arid regions, water quality 1340
Aristolochia spp., MRLs 1642
Aristotle 35
arithmetic mean 1782
Armageddon 1728
arms, male adult skin surface area
583
aromatase inhibition, assay 1403
aromatic hydrocarbon receptor
(AhR) 564, 1395, 1756, 1892
aromatic hydroxyl groups,
sulphation *106*
aromatic hydroxylations 100, 110
arrhythmias *see* cardiac arrhythmias;
ventricular arrhythmias
arrow worms *see Chaetognaths*

arsenite methyltransferase activity
2050
Artemia spp. *see* brine shrimp
arteritis, statistical analysis 296
artery, clearance 74
arthritis 263, 266
arthropods 1341, 1999
artichokes, nitrate and nitrite levels
2112
artifact-free techniques 19, 60
artificial flavours 1654
artificial respiration, in nerve agent
toxicity 2092
artificial sweeteners 1431, 1552,
1653
Aryan Nations 1727
aryl hydrocarbon hydroxylase
(AHH) 29, 1865
aryl hydrocarbon nuclear
translocator (ARNT) 282
aryl hydrocarbon receptor *281*, 283
as low as reasonably available
(ALARA) 1752
Asahara, Shoko 1728
asbestos-related disease 1445
Asclepia spp. *see* milk weed
ASFV-HMWF-5-HL, and apoptosis
193
ash from volcanoes 1815, 1816,
1817
asialo GM1 341
Asian women, lower incidence of
breast cancer 1398
L-asparaginase 993
asparagus, nitrate and nitrite levels
2112, 2113
aspartate aminotransferase (AST)
366
acute toxicity 43
as biomarker 1848, 1857, 1858,
1859, 1860, 1861
clinical chemistry 355–6, 358,
366
hepatotoxicity 868
levels following CO_2 in rats 61
wildlife toxicity 1345
aspartic acid *1878*
aspase activity 164
Aspergillus spp. 1301
A. albertensis 2157
A. alliaceus 2157
A. auricomus 2157
biological activity 2146
as carcinogen 1982

azo reductase enzymes 564
azo reduction 104
azo structures 1041, 1079, 1090

B

B lymphocytes 341, 998
baboon, sequenced CYP genes *216*
Bacillus anthracis 1726, 1727
Bacillus brevis 2149
background levels of toxins 1781,
    1792, 1893–4
background pathology 295
bacon, nitrate and nitrite levels
    2113
bacteria
    as CB weapon 1726
    as chemical warfare agents *2082*
    foodborne hazard 2145
    for *in vitro* testing 52
    metabolism 72
    Microtox 1319, 1320
    mutagenic 128
    Mutatox 1320
    nitric oxide production 2119
bacterial mutation tests 1041–50,
    1756
bacterial reductases 565
bactericides 34
Bacteroides 562, 563
baculovirus, and apoptosis 195
bad, and apoptosis 193, 194
bak, and apoptosis 193
BAL *see* biomonitoring action levels
balance disorders 787–95
Balb/c 3T3 cells *410*
BALF *see* broncheoalveolar lavage
    fluid
Balkan endemic nephropathy 2154,
    2159
banana 222
bandaging for snakebite area 2180
banded krait 2179
Banisteriopsis caapi 222
banned and restricted substances,
    OECD inititatives 1571
barbiturate-type inducer 113
bark scorpion *see* scorprion
barracuda 2191
barrier cream 511
Bartlett test 300
basal cell carcinomas 837
basal cells 779
basal lamina 340
base-pair transformation 7–8

base-set data requirements 1479,
    1480, 1590–1
basement membrane 383
basic drug screen (BDS) 1500,
    1502, 1504
basic fucsin-picric acid method 343
basilar membrane 776, 778, 780,
    781, 786
basilar papilla 791
basophilic granules 175
basophils 263, 384
Basque separatists 1727
BAT *see* best available technology;
    Biologische Arbeitsstoff-Toleranz-
    Wert
bathmotropic effects 43
bats, susceptibility to pesticides
    1339
battery manufacture workers 668
BAX 168, 191, 194, 197
BAX protein up-regulation, NSAIDs
    and 132
BCF *see* bioconcentration factor
BCL_2 168, 189, 200
bcl-2, and apoptosis 192, 193, 194,
    195, 197, 199
bcl-w, and apoptosis 194
bcl-XL, and apoptosis 191, 193
bcl-Xs, and apoptosis 193
BCL/D1 cells *410*
BEAM *see* brain electrical activity
    mapping
beans
    nitrate and nitrite levels
        2112–13, 2115
    ochratoxin analysis 2158
    toxicity 1983
bedding 58, 356, 512, 514
beef
    ingestion, standard assumptions
        1773, 1775
    nitrate and nitrite levels 2113
beer
    and degreasers' flush 1415
    nitrate, nitrite and NDMA levels
        2113–14, 2115, 2118
    ochratoxin analysis 2158
bees 1646, 1647, 2181
beet (*Beta vulgaris*)
    nephrotoxicity 1522
    nitrate and nitrite levels 2112–13
beetle, grandis 259
behavioural aberrations
    adverse drug reaction 1430
    as biomarker 1846, 1855–61

field studies 1354
from fires 1920, 1921
quantification 1353
wildlife species 1327, 1328,
    1345–7
behavioural approaches, in IEI
    treatment 1714, 1716
behavioural assessments 39, 45,
    657–8
behavioural conditioning, in IEI
    1707–8
behavioural response audiometry
    780
behavioural thermoregulation
    664–5
behavioural toxicity 23
    aggression induction 653
    assessment 650–73
    athletic performance 652
    cognitive tests 656–7
    complex schedules 660–1
    discrimination performance
        661–2
    endocrine disruption 653
    EPA guidelines 665
    EU guidelines 665
    functional observation batteries
        (FOB) *651*
    habituation phenomenon 651
    human testing 666–9
    lead 2056
    motor function 651–3, 654,
        662–4
    naturalistic behaviour 653
    neonatal testing 665–9
    organic solvents 2036, 2041–2
    organophosphates 1997
    reinforcer types 664–5
    risk assessment 670
    safety studies 1443
    schedule-controlled operant
        behaviour *658–9*
    schizophrenia 665
    sensory function 654–6
    sensory testing 661–2
    sexual behaviour 653
    simple schedules 659–60
    tests for children 669
BEI *see* biological exposure indices
Beirut bombing 1721
Belgium, nitrate levels 2112
bench mechanics biomonitoring
    1904
bench-scale extraction experiments
    1777–8

benchmark dose models (BMD) 1180–1, 1761–2, 1781, 1786, 1787

benchmark value (UK) 1486

benefits of drugs 35

Benirschke bodies 175

benzene hydroxylase 257

benzodiazepine receptor binding, effects on toxicity 16

benzoxazinorifampicin 30-hydroxylase *217*

Bernard, Claud 36, 1935

best available technology (BAT) 1752

best guesses 28

best-fit predictions 1763, 1766

Beta vulgaris see beet

beverages *see* drinks

BHK cells *410*, 412

Bhopal disaster 2, 38, 1724, 1819, *1820*

BHRF1, and apoptosis 193, 194

bias 1450, 1958

bicarbonate secretion, ductal cells 897

bifidobacteria 563, 572

bik 1, and apoptosis 193

bile
autopsy samples 1495
circadian toxicology 255
clinical chemistry 371
drainage *854*
excretion 18, 72, 79, 255, 523, 525, 555
flow, as biomarker 1843, 1849, 1859, 1864
and gastro-intestinal microflora 562
glucuronides 272
half-life extension 556
NSAIDs and 132
substance transport 564

bile acids 43, 255, 355, 360, 567–8, 864, 1843, 1858, 1879

bile canaliculi 338, 360, 854, *856, 857*, 860, *861*, 865

bile duct 274, 866, 881–3

bile pigments, as biomarker 1858

bile salts 860, 864

biliary system 359

bilirubin
as biomarker 1843, 1848, 1849, 1858, 1860, 1861
clinical chemistry 355, 358, 360, 362

haematology 391

bilirubin–glucuronyl transferase 867

bilirubinuria 360

binary interactions 313

binary weapon system 2080

binding 17

binding values, EU 1595

binomial theorem 1353

bioabsorbable sutures 1744–5

bioaccumulation 460, 1311, 1315, 1318, 1565

bioactivation 157

bioamplification, methylmercury 1378

bioassays 336, 1331–2

bioavailability
and absorption rate 75, 76
acute toxicity 39
age and 84
cutaneous 581
definition 69
in drinking water 1381
effects on 45
estimation 76, 146, 581
exposure assessment process 1777–9
and pH 1376–81
and plasma clearance calculation 79
repeated exposure studies via nutrition 59

biochemical basis of toxicity 125–36

biochemical biomarkers 1338, 1848

biochemical differences, intra-specific 1509

biochemical end-points 432

biochemical function reserves 10

biochemical processes, disturbance 127

biochemical uncoupling agents 6

biochemistry, in repeated exposure studies 61, 63

Biocidal Products Directive, EU Directive 98/8/EC 1611

biocides 39

biocompatibility
medical devices 1666, 1670, 1672
of synthetic materials 1731–2, 1733, 1738
testing 1038–42, 1679, 1743, *1745*

bioconcentration 1311, 1315

bioconcentration factor (BCF) 1311–12, 1318

biodegradation
medical devices 1735, 1742–3, 1744–5
testing 1565

biodistribution 17

biogenic amines, concentration in lung 128

biogeochemical cycles 1365, 1370

biohandling 17–18

biological approach to toxicology 1447–8

biological effect monitoring, in the workplace 1485–6

biological effectiveness of radiation 1689

Biological Effects of Ionizing Radiation III, Committee of the US National Academy of Science 1694

biological exposure index (BEI) 149, 603, 606, 1447, 1485, 1910–11

biological functions, and toxicology 1940

biological markers *see* biomarkers

biological monitoring *see* biomonitoring

biological product, definition 1973

biological protection, PSI 615

biological rhythms *see* biorhythms

biological risk assessment 28

biological terrorism *see* terrorism

biological testing, medical devices 1668

biological tolerance values for working materials (BAT values) 1485

biological toxins 816, 1143, 1146

biological variation 356, 358

biological warning, PSI 615

biologically active principles (BAPs), as flavourings 1655

biologically based modelling 1770

biologically effective dose 1877

Biologische Arbeitsstoff-Toleranz-Wert (BAT) 1485, 1911

Biologische Bundesanstalt für Land- und Forstwirtschaft (BBA) 1607

bioluminescence 370

biomagnification 1312

biomarkers 1849–54
acetylcholinesterase activity 1462

biomarkers (*Contd.*)

affected by drugs 1417

aquatic toxicity 1319

aselective 1845

assay utility 1461

behavioural and clinical 1846, 1855–61

bridging 1464

in cancer epidemiology 1538

changes in response to health status *1850*, 1851

clinical 364, 1848, 1855–61

definition 1538, 1841, 1842–3

in developmental and reproductive system 1464–5

of disease 461

effect and response 1843, 1847, 1855–73

effective dose 1842, 1843, 1844–5, 1848

in endocrine assays 1403–4

environmental 1531, 1870

enzyme levels 1848, 1865–9

in epidemiology 1457, 1534, 1538

ethics 1893–4

exposure 606–7, 1461, 1538, 1842, 1843–5, 1847, 1856, 1875–90, 1893

foetal development 1465

in hazard and risk assessment 1344, 1408, 1460, 1461–2

identification 1841–2

for IEI 1715

integrated approach 1850–3

internal dose 1844, 1876–7

invasive 1846–8

multi-biomarker approach 1850, 1851

National Research Council 1464

non-destructive 1842

non-invasive 1842, 1845

paradigm *1875*, 1876

pathology 1846–8

pharmacogenetics 225

present status 1841–2

protein synthesis 1848–9, 1869

quantal relevance 1893

selective 1845

susceptibility 461, 1843, 1847, 1850, 1875, 1890–2

toxicokinetics 72

types 1842, 1876

urinary 1861–5

validation 1892–4

for wildlife species 1345, 1407–8

biomaterials 340, 1732

see mainly medical devices

Biometric Testing Inc. 437

biomonitoring 461, 464, 1460, 1602, 1876

action levels (BAL) 1910–11

case study 1778–9

concentration units 1907–8

effects 1906–7

environmental health risk assessment 1876

ethical aspects 1911–12

genotoxic end-points 1906–7

human testing 461, 464, 1780

in IEI 1712

intepretation of data 1909–11

multiple route toxin estimation 606

occupational exposures 149, 1460, 1485–6, 1899–914

reference limits 1909–10

regulations 1602

selectivity 1904

sources of error 1908–9

specimens used 1907

standards 1485

toxicological end-points 1906

biopharmaceutics 1963, 1964–74

bioprotective mechanisms 6

bioremediation 1372–3

BioResearch Monitoring Program 438

biorhythms 251–2, 356

biostatistical uncertainty 1956

biotechnology 335, 428, 1454–5, 1459, 1460, 1462, 1463, 1963–75

biotechnology products 1454, 1455, 1548, 1553, 1558, 1584, 1623, 1628–9, 1638, 1640

biotherapeutics 1964

biotransformation 17–18, 51–2, 53, 97–124, 216, 306, 465

see mainly metabolism

birch pollen 623

bird repellents 1347

birds

see also chicken; poultry; wildlife species

acute oral toxicity tests 1329

and apoptosis 178

aquatic toxicity 1316

chronic reproduction tests 1350–1

comparative toxicology 1334–5

dermal tests 1331

dietary toxicity tests 1329

eggs *see* eggs

environmental contaminants sensitivity 1334

food contamination 1825

inhalation and oral toxicity studies 1331

as model species 1327, 1349

N-nitroso compounds toxicity 2132

organophosphorus toxicity 1328, 1523

pesticide sensitivity 1329, 1335, 1338

phenol metabolism 111

secondary toxicity 1524

sodium monofluorate toxicity 1524

strychine toxicity 1524

studies 45

subacute dietary toxicity test 1333–4

toxic vapours sensitivity 1509

toxicokinetic studies 1347

birdsfoot trefoil (*Lotus corniculatus*) 1519

Birkbeck granules 340

birth defects 281, 1818, 1929, 1948–9, 1952

see also cleft lip and palate; teratogenicity

bite, infection transmission 514

bitterweed (*Hymenoxys*), hepatoxicity 1519

black body agents 2080

black duck (*Anas rubripes*), eggshell thinning 1350

black grease-wood (*Sarobatus vermiculatus*), nephrotoxicity 1522

black locust (*Robinia pseudoacacia*), toxicity 1518, 1519

black smoke 1266, 1268, 1271

black widow spider 640, 2185–6

blackbird, red-winged (*Agelaius phoeniceus*) 1335, 1352

blackfoot disease 1382, 2051

bladder *see* urinary bladder

bleomycin hydrolase 729

blepharitis, grading system 742–*3*

blepharoconjunctivitis 738

blepharospasm 8, 41, 614, 620, *621*, 622, 755
blind slide reading 337
blindness 130, 425, 643, 765, 1430
blink reflex 620, 741
Bliss independence 305
blister base technique 623
blister beetles 1518
blistering agents 1724
blood
    acetylcholinesterase activity in nerve gas toxicity 2091–2
    affinity for substance 77
    alcohol concentration (BAC) 939, 1491, 1916
        see also alcohol; ethanol (*in Chemical Index*)
    arsenic levels 2052
    BALs 1910
    biomarkers 1847, 1876–7, *1879*
    biomonitoring 606, 1899, 1905, 1906, 1907
    bismuth levels 2061
    cadmium levels 2053, 2054
    CB agents 1724
    cholesterol levels, diet and 1978
    clotting *see* blood coagulation
    composition, interspecies 88
    concentration, peak circulating, scaling factors 1769
    contamination 1909
    copper levels 2064
    distribution 70
    interaction with medical devices 1734, 1735, 1736, 1741
    lead levels 606, 2055, 2056, 2057
    mercury levels 2058, 2060
    occult 364–5
    ochratoxin analysis 2158
    in PBPK 145
    reaction to implantation 539
    sampling 45, 67, 75, 385–8
    see also biochemistry; haematology
    toxicant concentration 1504
    toxicity *see* haematotoxicity
blood cells, radiation-induced changes 1685
blood coagulation 229, 264, 361, 367, 388–9, 821, 861, 1964, 1970, 2006
blood coagulopathy from snakebite 2178–9

blood components, storage bags 1737
blood dyscrasias 1427, 1520, 1634
blood flow 74, 254, 256, 1713
    see also circulation
blood gases, in IEI 1709, 1713
blood plasma cholinesterase 1354, 1355
blood pressure 264, 460, 614, 615, 1979
    see also hypertension; hypotension
blood products, medicinal use 1548
blood proteins, mutations radiation-induced 1694
blood tests *355*, 1713
blood transfusions, in treatment of rodenticide toxicity 1511
blood urea nitrogen (BUN) 1462, 1858, 1859, 1860, 1861
blood vessels 336, 1691, 1908
blood–brain barrier 17, 254, 569, 632–3, 2030, 2055, 2059–60
blood–gas partition coefficients of organic solvents 2029
blood–organ barrier 71
blood–perilymph barrier 779, 786
blood–placenta barrier 2055, 2059
blood–testes barrier (BTB) 372, 1141, 1463
blood–tissue equilibrium 71
Bloodborne Pathogen Standard 1459
Bloom's Syndrome (BS) 1034
blowing agents 2014, 2017, 2021–2, 2023
blue baby syndrome
    see methaemoglobinaemia
Blue Book 1657
blue–green algae toxicity 1516
BMD *see* benchmark dose
body, as two compartment system 77
body burden
    assessment 1905
    cadmium 2054
    nitrate, nitrite and *N*-nitroso compounds 2133–5, 2136
    and occupational exposure 88, 1905
    parent compound 86
    PCBs 1780
    rate of change 79
    safety margin calculations 91
    total 88, 149

body fluids 1848, 1877, 1941–2
body posture, as source of error in biomonitoring 1908
body weight 538
    in acute toxicity testing 39
    allometric scaling 51
    appropriate distribution 1782
    changes, as biomarker 1846, 1855, 1859
    decrease 283
    determination 42
    energy consumption and 1980
    measurement 61, 64, 89
    related to LD_{50} 51
    related to surface area 92
    in repeated exposure tests 63
    rule 51
    scaling factors 1769
    standard assumptions 1773
bolus 19, 55
bonding agents, in rubber industry 2014
bone
    autopsy samples 1495
    biomarkers 1844, 1859
    biomonitoring 1905
    calcified 341
    cancer radiation-induced 1693
    embryology 966, 968–70
    examination 343
    formation 2068
    fractures, cadmium levels and 2053
    lead uptake 2055, 2056
    and medical devices 539, 1735, 1736, 1741
    mineralization 342
    physiological aspects 968
    radiation-induced changes 1691–2
    resorption 675, 2068
    as storage site 17
    structure and function 966–7
    toxic damage 968–75
bone marrow
    benzene toxicity 16, 56, 100
    biopsies 341
    chromosomal aberrations 24, 276
    circadian toxicology 256, 260
    haematology 383, 385
    Lewisite toxicity 2089
    management 2087
    mustard gas toxicity 2086
    myeloperoxidase 240

bone marrow (*Contd.*)
   nephrotoxicity 675
   nitrate toxicity 2125
   organic solvent toxicity 2037
   peroxidases 103
   radiation-induced changes 1685,
     1686, 1690
   sampling 388
   suppression, cytokines for 1971
Bonferroni *t* test 1332
bonito 2193
Boolean operators 479
boomslang (*Dispholidus typus*)
   2178
borderline products, regulatory
   aspects 1553
Borgias 35
Bothotus see under scorpion
Bothrops spp. *see* snakes, crotaline
botulism 428, 549, 633, 640, 1340,
   1513, 1726, 1989, 2104
Bouin's stain 336, 345
bound residues, guidelines 1636
bounding information 1766–7, 1786
bowel *see* large intestine
Bowman's membrane *410*
box jellyfish (*Chironex fleckeri*)
   2189
Box–Behnken designs 314
bracken fern, toxicity to horses
   1519
bradycardia 40, 41, 43, 614, 615,
   811, 823, 824
bradykinin, NOS and 2119
bradypnoea 40
Braer disaster 1826–7
brain
   biomarkers 1866
   cholinesterase 1338, 1343, 1344,
     1351, 1354, 1523, 1996
   drug damage 103
   electrical activity mapping
     (BEAM) 1713, 1716
   enzyme distribution 1857
   fog 1709
   free radical damage 634
   haemorrhage 1217
   hypoglycaemia 636
   imaging 1707
   immersion fixation 347
   iron levels 634
   ischaemia 636
   lead damage 2055–6
   mercury concentration 570
   morphometry 339

MPTP oxidized 132
NQO2 in 240
organic solvent damage 2029,
   2030, 2035, 2036, 2040
perfusion fixation 347
pesticide residues 1343
pharmacogenetics 232
radiation damage 1690–1
tumours 1928, 1929, 2015, 2019,
   2132
weight 64, 1856
brainstem, in ALS 239
Branta canadensis see goose,
   Canada
Brassica spp. *see* broccoli; brussels
   sprouts; cabbage; kale
Brazil, fumonisin contamination of
   cereals 2165
BRCA1, as biomarker 1850
bread, contamination 1824, 1825,
   2116, 2117
breakfast cereals
   see also cereals
   fortification 1552
breast
   cloned enzymes 242
   irradiation 1691, 1693
breast cancer
   cyclic induction 266
   and dietary fat 1980, 1981
   endocrine related 1399
   environmental effects 1392,
     1399–400
   hormone treatment 1392
   interspecies variation 278, 279
   MCF-7 cells 1402
   and organochlorine compounds
     1400, 1995
   and PCBs 163
   in plastics industry 2020, 2021
   rarer in Asian women 1398
   risk 572
   in rubber industry 2015
   and selenium 1983
   surgery, and fertility cycle 266
   tamoxifen treatment 284
breast–ovary cancer genes,
   biomarker 1850
breast-feeding 1224–7
breath
   apparatus in PBPK *146*
   biomarker 1845, 1848, 1855,
     1867
   biomonitoring 1907
   elimination in 72

source of cP450-generated
   metabolism 1865
tests 365
breathing
   laboured 497
   patterns 262, 1713, 1920
   rate *see* respiratory rate
   zone 607
breathing apparatus, for firefighters
   1938
breeding colonies 357
BRI *see* building-related illness
brine shrimp 414
brine shrimp (*Artemia* spp.) 1187
Brinvilliers, Marquise de 35
British Library 477
British Pharmacopeia 536, 537
British Toxicology Society 326,
   425
broccoli
   see also kale
   nitrate and nitrite levels 2112
broncheoalveolar lavage 704, 722,
   729
broncheoalveolar lavage fluid
   (BALF) 1762
bronchi 20, 46, 262, 343, 510
bronchiolar cells 722, 726, 732
bronchioles, inhalation effects 20
bronchitis 1269–70, 1961
bronchodilators *220*, 262–3, 810
bronchospasm 252
Bronsted acidity 614
broom, toxic ingredients 1552
broomweed (*Gutierrezia
   microcephala*), reproductive
   toxicity 1521
Brownian diffusion 591
Brunner's glands 545
brush borders 345, 363, 678, 680,
   681, 683, 688, 690
brussels sprouts, nitrate and nitrite
   levels 2112–13
BS *see* Bloom's Syndrome
BTB *see* blood–testes barrier
bubblers 594
bubonic plague bacteria 1727
buccal
   see also oral
   absorption 545
   cavity 545
   microflora 561–2
   mucosa, radiation-induced
     changes 1689

buckwheat (*Fagopyrum esculantum*), photosensitization effects 1523

Buehler technique 841, 1005

Buenos Aires, car bombing 1722

buffers, biomonitoring 1904

bufuralol 1′-hydroxylase 217

building materials 1295, *1296*, 1298, 1304

building-related illness (BRI) 1292

Bulgarian agents and CB weapons 1727

bulking agents 1552, 1653, 1985

bullfrog (*Rana catesbeiana*) 1330–1, 1353

bumblebee 2182

bundle of His 805

Bureau of Biologists (USA) 1973

Bureau of Chemistry (USA) 1534

Bureau of Medical Devices and Diagnostic Products (USA) 1662

burns 833, 1724, 1818, 1916, 1917, 1927, 2087

Bursa of Fabricius 385

Buteo jamaicensis see hawk, red-tailed

Buthidae 2189

Buthus see scorpion

buttercup (*Ranunculus* spp.), toxicity 1518, 1520

butyrylcholinesterase 368, 429, 824, 1730, 1866

butylhydroperoxide, as biomarker 1868

by-products in rubber manufacture 2014

bystander risk *see* occupational risk

C

c-fibres 612, 1705

c-fos 16, 168, 190, 193, 195

c-jun 168, 190, 193, 195

c-myc 167, 189, 193, 196

C-reactive protein (CRP) 366–7

C-S lyase 568

cabbage, nitrate and nitrite levels 2112–13

CAC *see* Codex Alimentarius Commission

cacosmia 1708

CADDY project 1609

cadherin, as calpain substrate 189–90

caecum 521, 545, 556, 605, 1985, 1986, 1987, 1990

Caenorhabditis elegans 177, 190, 194, 1092, 1189

caeruloplasmin binding to copper 2064

caffeine *N*-3 demethylase *217*

caged field trials 1349–50

caging 58, 356, 512, 514

calcineurin, as calpain substrate 190

calcitonin 968

calcium
- –calmodulin–calcineurin signalling 684
- –phosphate balance 1987
- -dependent and papain-like proteases *see* calpains
- adenosine triphosphatase *see* adenenosine triphosphatase, Ca^{2+}
- and apoptosis 187, 188, 189, 192
- as calpain substrate 190
- cardiac toxicology 809, 811, 812
- CO$_2$ effects 61
- compartmentation changes 167
- dysregulation 198
- extra-skeletal binding 973
- homeostasis 127, 156, 163–4, 1859, 2036, 2059, 2162
- intracellular *164*, 168, 194, 807–8, 813, 982
- and lead uptake 2055
- in outer hair cells, organ of Corti 787
- in pancreatic juice 897
- skeletal muscle toxicology 939

calcium channel(s) 639, 806, 817, 818, 2066

calcium channels blockers 956

calcium phosphate, in tooth enamel 967

calcium pumps 156, 938

calmodulin, interaction with lead 2055

calmodulin-dependent kinase 190

calpain 164, 189, 191, 193

calreticullin induction 168

Calycanthus spp. *see* sweet shrub

CAM *see* chorioallantoic membrane assay

camel, lens 242

Cameroons lake disaster 38, 1817

cAMP *see* cyclic adenosine monophosphate

Canada
- classification and labelling requirements 1477, 1603–4
- food additives regulation 1659
- food contact materials regulation 1659
- nitrite levels 2132
- pesticide regulation 1600, 1601
- risk assessment 1602–3

Canadian Council on Animal Care 486

cancer
- *see also* carcinogenesis *and individually named organs*
- and acetylation status 112
- and apoptosis 163
- bioassays, dose selection 148
- chemotherapy *see* chemotherapy
- chronotherapy 266
- circadian radiosensitivity 260
- determination of cause 1952
- development stages 1875
- diet and 1980–3
- DNA degradation pattern 187
- endocrine-related 1391
- following Seveso disaster 1818
- genetic aspects 1538, 1847, 1891
- incidence, USA 1787
- potency factors (CPF) 1751, 1764–6, 1771, 1782, 1786
- prevention programmes 1940, 1942
- radiation-induced 1695, 1821
- registration records 1532, 1533
- research history 1944
- risk assessment 148, 1782, 1784, 1790, 1830, 2050

Cancerline 1947

Candida albicans 413

cannibalism in animals 58

CAP *see* compound action potential

capillaries, dermis 829

capsules, dosing procedures 60

car
- *see also* automobile(s)
- accidents *see* road traffic accidents
- bombs 1722

carbohydrate 115, 1966

carbonating agents 1985

carbonic anhydrase 159, 160

carbonyl reductase 104, *216*, 241, *242*, 243

carboxyhaemoglobin (COHb) 150, 1843, 1920, 1921, 1924, 1927

carboxyhaemoglobinaemia *392*
carboxylators 238
carboxylesterases 105, 1866
carboxylic acid ionophores 821
carcass searches 1354
carcinoembryonic antigen (CEA), as
    biomarker 1849
carcinogen(s)
    see also specific types, e.g.
        aflatoxin (*in Chemical Index*)
    –protein adducts 225
    acceptable risk level 1787, 1788
    added risk 1786
    antagonistic interactions 314
    apoptosis 198
    binding 571
    classification 1537, 1593, 1766
    determining safe exposures 1484
    dose-response assessments 1759,
        1763–5, 1766
    epigenetic 7, 128, 314
    exposure to 225
    in fires 1821
    in food 1981–2
    genotoxic 8
    mixtures 314–15
    naturally occurring 1981
    PBPK modelling 1770
    primary 7
    promoters 314
    risk assessment 1751, 1753,
        1754, 1755
    scaling factors 1769
    synergism 314–15
    synthesis 566–7
    toxicokinetics 85
    trace quantities 1574–6
    ultimate 7
Carcinogen Assessment Group
    (USA) 147
Carcinogen guidelines (EPA) 1766
Carcinogen Potency Database
    (CPDB) 1105, 1111
carcinogenesis/carcinogenicity
    see also genetic carcinogens;
        genetic toxicology; *individually
        named organs*
    acetylaminofluoroene 110
    acrylamide 1455
    as adverse drug reaction 1427
    aflatoxins 1537, 2154
    4-aminobiphenyl 1537
    anabolic steroids 1549
    animal studies 1536–8
    aromatic amines 120

arsenic 1382, 2051
asbestos 1537
benzene 1455, 1537
benzidine 1537, 1587
beryllium 2061
bioassays 2, 336
biochemistry 126
biomarker 1845, 1849–50, 1856,
    1866, 1867, 1875, 1886
biomonitoring 1904–5, 1906–7,
    1911
bis(chloromethyl) ether 1537
cadmium 2053–4
chlorambucil 1537
chlorination byproducts 1383–4
chloroform 1455
chromium 1539, 2062
coal tars 1537
cutaneous 836, 837
cyclophosphamide 1537
definition 7
dichloromethane 1537
dietary factors 58, 1980–1
diethylstilbeostrol 1537
dioxins 87
epidemiology 1537
erionite 1537
erythrosine (FD&C Red 3, E127)
    1553
ethylene oxide 1455
in firefighters 1929
food products 1563
formaldehyde 1455, 1456, 1537
fumonisins 2165
and gastro-intestinal microflora
    561
genetic factors 1027–35,
    1099–101
herbicides 2005
heterocyclic amines 274
hydrazine 1455
initiation 314
interspecies extrapolation 1536
liver enlargement and
    remodelling by 880–1
medical devices 1734, 1735,
    1742
melphalan 1537
methotrexate 1455
methoxsalen + UV-A 1537
mineral oil 1537
multistage model 314
2-naphthylamine 1537
nickel 1537, 1539, 2063

nitrates 1382, 2124, 2130–1,
    2137
nitrites 1383, 2128
nitrobenzene 104
N-nitroso compounds 1383,
    2132
non-genotoxic 1034–5, 1101–2,
    1119–20, 1121
organic solvents 2036, 2037,
    2039
organophosphates 1998
and parenteral toxicity 525–6
phenol 1455
piperidine 1455
plastics industry 2019–23
promotion 314
radiation-induced 1692–3, 1697
radon 1538
rubber industry 2014–19
saccharin 1537, 1553
selenium 2065
shale oils 1537
species differences 59
testing
    alternative tests 64, 401
    guidelines 1434–5
    long-term 356, 1618–19
    new substances 1591,
        1618–19, 1628
    and parenteral toxicity 64,
        401, 521
    repeated-dose 64, 330
    replacement tests 499
    veterinary drugs 1643
tobacco smoke 1537, 1538
transplacental 1207–9
TSG and 1892
urea 1455
vinyl chloride 1417, 1537, 1551
wastes 1827–8
wood dust 1475
carcinoma *see* cancer
Carcinus aestuarii, biomarker 1852
cardiac, *see also* heart
cardiac action potential 805
cardiac anomalies 1465
cardiac arrest 50
cardiac arrhythmias 806, 807, 808,
    810, 814, 816, 823
    acute toxicity 40, 41, 43, 50
    and adverse drug reactions 1427,
        1429, 1430
    and barium 1757
    clinical chemistry 366
    ECG 806

cardiac arrhythmias (*Contd.*)
  and fires 1921, 1923
  and halogenated hydrocarbons
    461, 1505
  and organic solvents 2036, 2037
  and organophosphates 1997
  and terfenadine 125–6
  'torsade de pointes' 824
cardiac chrono-pathology 264
cardiac conduction pathway 343,
  805
cardiac contraction 805–6
cardiac myocytes 807
cardiac myopathy 43, 2064
cardiac output 83, 92, 364, 366
cardiac puncture 357
cardiac stimulants 220
cardiac toxicity *see* cardiotoxicity
cardiac toxicology 803–26
cardiac tumours, in rubber industry
  2015
cardiac weight 343
cardinal, northern (*Cardinalis
  cardinalis*), subacute feeding trials
  1338
Cardinalis cardinalis see cardinal,
  northern
cardiomyopathy 807, 813, 942,
  1430
cardiopathy, selenium deficiency
  2065
cardiotoxic agents 807–16
cardiotoxicity
  adverse drug reactions 1427,
    1438
  animal stings 2179, 2189, 2190
  biochemical basis 806–7
  clinical chemistry 366
  fluoroacetate 6
  mechanisms 816–24
  nitrites 2126
  organophosphates 1998
  pathological basis 807
  pharmacogenetics 240
  signs 40, 43
  terfenadine 38
cardiovascular agents 25, 1439
cardiovascular effects
  collapse 15, 1984
  and drinking water hardness
    1381
  in firefighters 1928–9
  of Gila monster bite 2182
  in vitro test systems *417*

organic solvents 2041
plant toxins 1522
radiation-induced 1691
Seveso disaster 1818–19
cardiovascular system 343
carnitine acyltransferase 1866, 1868
Carolina jessamine (*Gelsemium*
  spp.), neurotoxicity 1520, 1521
carpenter ant 2184
carpet, IEI and 1708
carrier proteins 371
carrion-eating species *see* predatory
  species
carrot, nitrate and nitrite levels
  2112–13
Carson, Rachel 1599
cartilage
  articular 342
  embryology 966
  physiological aspects 968
  radiation-induced changes
    1691–2
  structure and function 966–7
  toxic damage 968–75
cartridge respirators 516
CAS *see* Chemical Abstracts
  Service
cascade impactor 598, *599*
CASE *see* computer-automated
  structure evaluation
case-control studies 1456, 1466,
  1529, 1532–3, 1539, 1755
case-referent studies *see* case-
  control studies
caspases 164–5, 191, 194–5
cassava 900, 918, 920, 1553, 1984
cassia, toxic to domestic animals
  1513
castor oil plant (*Ricinus communis*),
  toxicity 345, 1518, 1519, 1727
cat
  see also domestic animals
  acetaminophen (paracetamol)
    susceptibility 1509
  aflatoxin LD$_{50}$ 2154
  allergenic sebaceous glands 512
  allergens 511–12
  aminophenol hydroxylation 11
  benzoic acid lethality 535
  blood pressure response to
    depressors 535
  chlorate herbicides susceptibility
    1512
  common toxicoses 1510–13

ethylene glycol toxicity 110
food contamination 1825
garbage toxicity 1512
human contact 490
LAA 511
phenol metabolism 111
pyrethrin/pyrethroid toxicity
  1510
stratum corneum skin
  permeability *579*
vomiting reflex 546
cat scratch disease 514
catalase 158, 344, 809, 1866, 1868,
  2161
catalepsy 40, 41
cataract 20, 160, 758, 762–4, 1430,
  1687–8, 2003, 2004
catechol *O*-methyltransferase *216*,
  813
catecholaminergic systems 641, 808
catecholamines 346, 806, 813
catfish 2191
cations
  complexing 1368, 1369
  soil storage 1369
cattle
  see also ruminants
  blue–green algae toxicity 1516
  cornea *410*
  CYP 216
  CYP genes 216
  ginger neuropathy 1824
  lead toxicity 1515
  methionine salt 532
  molybdenum toxicity 1515
  nitrate toxicity 1509, 2123, 2124
  ochratoxin toxicity 2161, 2164
  salt toxicity 1517
  selenium toxicity 1515
  T_3 and T_4 concentration 371
cattle feed, contamination 1554,
  2153
caudal vein lesions 529
cauliflower, nitrate and nitrite levels
  2112–13
causal factors in legal matters 1952
cause of death, inaccuracies on
  death certficates 1529
cause–effect relationship 1354
CB *see* terrorism, chemical and
  biological
CBN *see* contraction band necrosis
CC10 *see* Clara cell protein
CCK *see* cholecystokinin;
  cholecystokinin-pancreozymin

CD surface membrane antigen
see cell-surface differentiation
antigens
CD4+ T lymphocytes 703
CD-ROM 481–2
CDC *see* Centres for Disease
Control
cdk, and apoptosis 193
CEA *see* carcinoembryonic antigen
Ced 187, 190, 193, 194, 195
CEDA *see* cloned enzyme donor
immunoassay
ceiling value, definition 1484
celeriac 1005, 2113
celery, nitrate and nitrite levels
2112–13
Cell Products Safety Commission
(WHO) 1463
cell-free versus cell-based metabolic
activation systems 1040
cell-mediated (type IV) immunity
126, 834
cell-surface differentiation (CD)
antigens 187, 193, 998, 999–1000
cell(s)
adaptive responses 157
antioxidant function 160
apoptosis *see* apoptosis
chemical exposure 126
concepts in toxicology 155–7,
163–6
culture additions, toxic hazard
1454
culture methodology 847
culture techniques, synthetic
materials 1740
cycle 258, 1030–1
for cytotoxicity testing 52–3
membrane damage 52
morphology 52
proliferation 52
viability 52
damage, biomarker 1848, 1850,
1856
death *see* mainly apoptosis;
necrosis
death
radiation-induced 1684, 1685
rates, PBPD model 1770
defence mechanism 10
differentiation, and p53 1031
function maintenance 127
homeostasis 158
hyperplasia 556
injury 53, 178

karyorrhexis, mycotoxins and
2149
life-span 1685
line, enzyme expression 135
membrane absorption 69
necrosis *see* necrosis
proliferation 160, 314, 340, 344,
604, 1856
radiation-induced changes 1684,
1695
replication, increased 126
self-deletion 157
shape, calpains and 190
shrinkage 183
stimulating factors, toxic hazards
1455
stress responses 166–9
transformation 413
turnover increase consequences
1750, 1766
water balance, biomarker 1843
celluria 362
cement 577
Center, *see also* Centre
Center for Biologic Evaluation and
Research (US) 1665
Center for Devices and Radiological
Health (CDRH) (US) 1664, *1665*
Center for Drug Evaluation and
Research (USA) 1615, 1665
Center for Veterinary Medicine (US)
1633–8
Centers for Disease Control (CDC)
(US) 1459
Central Bank (Colombo) bomb
1722
central compartment 77, 78
Central Composite designs 314
central nervous system (CNS)
see also nervous system
acetylcholinesterase 368
age effects of drugs 1439
anticholinesterase effects 1995–6
axons 631
cardiotoxicity 805
chlorinated hydrocarbons 1510,
1518
defects 1465
depression
organic solvents 2030, 2033,
2035, 2036, 2037, 2038,
2039, 2040, 2041
plastics industry 2020, 2021
potatoes 1984
rubber industry 2015

development 1696
dichloromethane toxicity 1475
distribution in 71
dogs 1513
ethanol toxicity 1455
function, fire effect 1920, 1923
hexane 1455
horses 1519
and IEI 1704, 1706–7, 1713,
1716
injury 8
insecticide effects 2000
lead toxicity 1513, 1515, 1523
lindane effects 1995
medical devices toxicity testing
1741
mercury toxicity 1475, 2059
naphthalene 1455
neurotoxins 126–7
nitrate toxicity 2129
nitrogen toxicity 1514
organophosphate toxicity 1997
plant toxicity 1520
radiation injury 1685
toluene toxicity 1455
trichloroethylene toxicity 1475
trophic disease, growth factors
therapy 1972
tumours in plastics industry 2021
xylene toxicity 1475
Central Pharmaceutical Affairs
Council (Japan) 1566
central respiratory depression 811
Centre, *see also* Center
Centre for Medicines Research
(UK) 1431, 1435
centrilobular necrosis 872
Centrocercus urophasianus
see grouse, sage
Centruriodes spp. *see* scorpions
CEPEX *see* Controlled Ecosystem
Pollution Experiment
ceramics 1734, 1738
ceramides 191, 195, 828
cereals
aflatoxin 2150, 2153
ammoniation 2147, 2153
contamination 1823, 1825, 1982
dust, respiratory effects 1475
ergotoxin 2148
flour treatment agents 1552,
1985
fumonisin 2163, 2165
mercury contamination 1249

cereals (*Contd.*)
  nitrate and nitrite levels 2114, 2115, 2116, 2117, 2118
  ochratoxin 2158–9
  phomopsin 2148
  sporidesmin 2148
cerebellar ataxia 235
cerebellar cortex, methylmercury damage 643
cerebellar granular cells 166, 636
cerebral blood flow, CO and HCN toxicity studies 1924
cerebral cortex 239, 637
cerebral glioma, nitrites 2128
cerebral nuclei 347
cerebral palsy, from mercury toxicity 2059
cerebral pressure, high 636
cerebral syndrome, from radiation 1685
cerebrospinal fluid (CSF) 254, 537, 1848
cerebrovascular radiation damage 1687
cerebrum 347
certain effective dose *see* ED_{100}
certain lethal dose *see* LD_{100}
certification 1491, 1543, 1546
cervical cancer 1693, 1982
cervical dislocation *498–9*
cervical intra-epithelial neoplasia, biomarker 1856
Chaetognaths 1314
chain of evidence 1491, 1494
challenge procedures, in IEI 1713
chaperone molecules 167
chaperonin, as biomarker 1848, 1869
CHD *see* coronary heart disease
Chediak–Higashi syndrome 1034
cheese
  aflatoxin determination 2152
  nitrate, nitrite and NDMA levels 2113, 2115, 2118
  starter cultures 1645
chelation therapy 2, 3, 367, 426, 427–8, 552, 1513, 1515, 2068–9
chemical(s) 1347
  see also Chemical Index for specific chemicals
  –chemical interactions *see* drug interactions; mixtures
  –receptor interactions 34
  activation 564–6

avoidance, absent in wildlife species 1347
bioavailability estimation 581
burns 833
carcinogenic 7
catastrophes *see* disasters
causing respiratory allergy 702
concentration, and surface contact area 578
deterioration on storage 1909
effects 215–50
exposure assessment 461–2
factory biomonitoring 1904
hazards 1328, 1330, 1338–44, 1418–19, 1675
health surveys 461–4
industry 2, 1347, 1463
labelling 448
metabolism 216–18
mixtures *see* mixtures of chemicals
nomenclature 480
occupational exposure 461–4
percutaneous absorption 583, *583*
pollutants 215
preparations 1557, 1606
renal effects 678–92
respiratory sensitization 701–19
screening, in wildlife toxicology 1327, 1329
in soil 582
spillages 1339–440, 1545
  see also disasters
substances
  databases 1456
  definition 1557
  human toxicity 1547
  misuse 1339–440, 1524
  multiple uses 1544, 1547
  new 1443, 1448, 1452, 1544
  notification 1545
  toxicological studies 1606
terrorism *see* terrorism
as therapeutic agents 460–1
treatment, field study evaluation 1352
vapours, percutaneous absorption 584
warfare 1035
  agents 1444, 1547, 2079–109
  see also acetylcholin-esterase; *specific agents (in Chemical Index)*;

mechanisms of toxicity 938; studies 25, 38
  alleged 2104–5
  antidotes 2068
  casualties 2080, 2082–3
Chemical Abstracts Service 480
Chemical Agents Directive, EU 1481
Chemical Carcinogenesis Research Information System (CCRIS) 1677
Chemical Hazard Data Availability Study 1587
Chemical Industries Association (UK) 1486
Chemical Industry Institute of Toxicology (US) 341, 1942
Chemical Manufacturers Association (US) 1676
Chemical Mutagens, Principles and Methods for Their Detection 1038
Chemical Substances Control Law (Law 44) (Japan) 37, 1565
Chemicals (Hazard Identification and Packaging) Regulations (CHIP) 1476–7
chemoreceptors 546, 1920
chemosis 40, 41, *741–2, 742–3*, 745
chemotherapy
  and apoptosis 197
  biomarkers 1862
  DNA modification 1878–9, 1886
  infusion 530
  molecular interactions 163
  ovarian dysfunction 1152–3
  and parenteral toxicity 532
  pharmacogenetics 238
  poultry toxicity 1520–2
  reproductive toxicity 1146
  safety 1971–2
  skeletal muscle toxicity 943, 945
  toxicokinetics 92
Chenopodium spp. *see* lambs-quarters
Chernobyl disaster 1443, 1724, 1820–1
Chernoff–Kavlock assay 1186
chervil, nitrate levels 2113
Cheyne–Stokes sign 40, 41
chicken (*Gallus domesticus*) 234
  see also poultry
  aflatoxin LD_{50} 2154
  aminophenol hydroxylation 110

chicken (*Gallus domesticus*)
  (*Contd.*)
  and apoptosis 178
  arsenic in feed 1951–2
  biliary excretion 555
  contaminated drinking water
    1340
  eggs 233
  eye tests 751
  fumonisin toxicity 2165
  heterocyclic amines 271
  intravenous injection site 526
  liver 234
  malathion sensitivity 1342
  neurological tests 23
  neurotoxicity 638, 1824
  nitrate and nitrite levels 2113
  ochratoxin toxicity 2160, 2161
  organophosphate studies 1997
  studies 792
chicory, nitrate levels 2113
chief cells 545
child-resistant packaging 1603,
  1604
childhood syndromes, associated
  with tumour suppressor genes
  1032
children
  see also neonates
  air pollution studies 1270–1,
    1273–4
  allergic reaction to insect stings
    2183
  cancer 1464, 1465, 1820
  in clinical trials 1618
  CNS defects from plastics
    industry 2020
  copper toxicity 2064
  drug therapy 1227–9
  exposure assessment 1776, 1782,
    1783
  eye injuries 737
  informed consent 455
  iron levels 2065
  lead toxicity 639, 973, 1205,
    1227, 1769, 2055, 2056, 2057
  mass poisoning 460
  mercuric toxicity 2058, 2059,
    2060
  nitrate levels 2116–17, 2118,
    2122, 2129, 2132, 2133, 2136
  nitrite intakes 2134, 2136
  ochratoxin regulations 2158–9
  over-the-counter (OTC) drugs
    1228–9

passive smoking 1267, 1273
poisoning statistics 38
radiation injury 1691, 1694,
  1695, 1697
risk assessment 1754
screening, biomarkers 1845
selenium deficiency 2065
skin reactivity of 831
snakebites 2178
testing initiative 1587
thyroid cancer 1820
Chile, deliberate food poisoning
  1724
chimeric animals 1964
chimney sweeps, scrotal cancer 2,
  1474
chimpanzee *579*, 1971, 2050
China
  fumonisin contamination of
    cereals 2165
  nitrate levels 2114, 2131
  N-nitroso compounds levels
    2133
Chinese cabbage, nitrate levels
  2113
Chinese hamster ovary (CHO) cells
  24, 752, 753
  and apoptosis 196, 198
  cytogenetic assays 1081, 1082,
    1083, 1084, 1434
  β-hexosaminidase *412*
  Hgprt gene 1051, 1053
  mutant UV-1 1023
  and nitrates/nitrites 2124–5,
    2128
  recombinant human
    erythropoietin cloning 1971
  V79 system 1051–3, 1083
Chinese restaurant syndrome 1988
CHIP *see* Chemicals (Hazard
  Identification and Packaging)
  Regulations
chiral factors in metabolism 115
Chironex fleckeri see box jellyfish
chitin synthesis inhibitors 2000
chlor-alkali workers 663
chloracne 284, 838, 1444, 1554,
  1818
chloride channels 641, 764, 897
chloride ion 104
chlorination 1381, 1383–4
chlorine-containing wastes 281
chlorofluorocarbons, natural 1366
chloroquine myopathy 944

chlorzoxazone 6-hydroxylase *217*
choking agents 1724
cholecystokinin (CCK) 880, 897,
  992
cholecystokinin-pancreozymin 895
cholelithiasis 883
cholera 820, 1310
cholestasis 132, 356, 359, 361,
  883–4, 1843, 1849, 1858, 1859,
  1860
cholesterol 370, 823, 860, 862, 938,
  1978
cholesterol ester hydrolase 897
cholesterol lowering agents 946
cholesterol stones 898
cholostrum 549
cholic acid, as biomarker 1858
cholinergic agonists 897
cholinergic cells, damage 642
cholinergic fibres 615
cholinergic muscarinic system,
  radiation-induced changes 1689
cholinergic reflex mechanisms 256
cholinergic symptoms from
  anticholinesterases 1995
cholinergic synapses 6
cholinergics 808
cholinesterase *216*, *356*, 359,
  368–9, 466, 760, 1342, 1485,
  1906
cholinesterase inhibitors 369, 823,
  1337, 1345, 1906, 1996, 2006
Chondodendron toxicity 34
chondritis, radiation 1691
chondrocytes 342
chondrodystrophies 965, 969
chondrogenesis 966, 968
choreiform movements 638
choreoathetosis/salivation (CS)
  syndrome 1244
chorioallantoic membrane *411*, 499,
  752
chorionic gonadotrophin 538
Christison, Robert 1490
chromaffin reaction 346
chromatid damage, biomarker 1848
chromatin 161, 164, 183, 187, 189,
  2054
chromatographic methods
  see also specific methods
  in forensic testing 1497–500
chromodacryorrhoea 40, 41
chromophores 337, 836–7

chromosomal aberrations
  bioassay 1460, 1479
  biomarkers 1841, 1848, 1877
  biomonitoring 1906
  centric fusions 1080
  clastogenic potential 24
  deletions and deficiencies 1080
  in firefighters 1929
  fungicides 2002
  and gastro-intestinal microflora
    567
  individual 1078–81
  inversions 1080
  in leukaemia 395
  medical devices and 1742
  nitrates and 2124
  nitrites and 2128
  organic solvents and 2037, 2039
  in plastics industry 2020
  radiation-induced 1684, 1693,
    1694, 1695–6
  reciprocal translocations 1080
  reproductive toxicity 1144
  in rubber industry 2015
  set 1081
  following Seveso disaster 1818
chromosome 2q33 239
chronic carcinogenesis assay 499
chronic exposure toxicity studies
  animal welfare 499
  assessment 1772
  biomarkers 1893
  classifcation 5
  definitions 1446
  design 323
  education 1940
  food toxicology 1977
  medical devices 1735, 1742
  peroral toxicity 550
  repeated exposure 57, 64–5
  toxicokinetics 80–90
chronic fatigue syndrome 1703,
  1710, 1714, 1715
chronic neurological disease 566
chronic obstructive pulmonary
  disease (COPD) 224
chronic ocular hypertensive rabbit
  model 749
chronic papillary injury 688
chronic postviral syndrome 1710
chronic reproduction tests 1350–1
chronic toxicity test studies, oral
  324
chronicity trials 1350–2

chronobiology, hypertension 264
chronophysiology, blood clotting
  264
chronotherapy 252
chronotropic effects 43, 805, 816
Chrysanthemum 639
Chrysaora quinquecirrha *see* sea
  nettle
chylomicrons 367, 548, 557
chyme 546, 548
chymotrypsin 365
chymotrypsinogen 897
cicatricial ectropion 756
Cicuta spp. *see* water hemlock
cigarette smoke *see* smoking;
  tobacco smoke
ciguatera fish 2191–2
Cillus cereus 823
cinchona tree 817
circadian toxicology 251–70
  absorption variation 253
  effects on toxicity 16
  pharmacodynamics 252
  pharmacokinetics 252–6
  radiosensitivity 260
  repeated exposure studies 58
  rhythms 251, 252–6, 259, 370,
    749, 1419
  time 252
  and variability of results 265
circulation 545, 547, 548
cirrhosis 236, 867, 873–4, 942, 943
  see also hepatotoxicity; liver
civatte bodies 175
CK *see* creatine kinase
claims, in labelling and advertising
  1674
clam toxicity 2192
Clara cells 128, 132, 590, 722, 731,
  2004
Clara cell protein 1276, 1859
clarifying agents 1985
classification and labelling
  see also EU Directive
    88/379/EEC
  Canadian requirements 1603–4
  chemical hazards 1675
  claims 1674
  commercial products 1603–4
  dangerous substances and
    preparations 1590, 1593–4
  dosing procedures 44
  EU requirements 1479, 1486,
    1557, 1609–10, 1627, 1628

  harmonization 1478
  in hazard identification 1476–8
  household products 1589,
    1603–4
  industrial chemicals 1545, 1551
  plant protection products 1610
  risk and safety phrases 1477,
    1487, 1557, 1594, 1603
  of substances 44
  symbols used 1477, 1557, 1594,
    1603
  US requirements 1603–4
  veterinary drugs 1637
*Classification of pesticides by
  hazard* 37
clastogenesis 7, 24
  see chromosomal aberrations
Claviceps spp. 2145, 2146
  C. paspali 2148
  C. purpurea 1516, 2148
clay soils 1367, 1369
Clean Air Act (1956) (USA) 1270,
  1272
Clean Air Act (USA) 1750, 1752
clearance 45, 74, 78–80, 1544,
  1546
  see also excretion; metabolism
cleft lip and palate 258, 965, 969,
  972, 1188–9, 1217, 1465
clinical biomarkers 1855–61
clinical chemistry 62, 332, 355–99
clinical ecology 1450
clinical laboratories, source of
  biological hazards 1459
clinical observations, toxicity signs
  61
clinical research, and drug
  regulation 1439
clinical signs (*general only*) 39,
  40–4, 45, 63
clinical toxicology (*general only*) 3,
  1877, 1941–2
clinical trials 457
  and adverse drug reactions 1435
  anticarcinogen 278
  certificates 1425, 1622
  ethics 1955, 1958
  EU requirements 1622–3
  exemption 2, 1439, 1543, 1622
  new pharmaceuticals 1622–3
  non-clinical safety studies 1616
  patient selection criteria 1435,
    1439
  phases I–III 1616
  randomized 425

clinical trials (*Contd.*)
  recruitment of subjects 1617–18, 1622
  statistical factors 1439
clinicians, responsibilities 1426, 1438
clofibrate-type inducer 113
cloned enzyme donor immunoassay (CEDA) 1502
cloning 218, 229, 230, 236, 239, 240
clonogenic cells, radiation-induced changes 1684
closed patch method, synthetic materials testing 1740
Clostridium spp. 563, 568
  C. basili 640
  C. botulinum 1512, 1513, 1726, 1727, 1989
clot busters, safety evaluation 1970
clothing, and reduction of percutaneous uptake 584
clotting *see* blood, coagulation
clover, alsike (Trifolium hybridum) 1519, 1523
clusterin mRNA, and apoptosis 1690
clustering, in occupational or geographical areas 1533
CM *see* cochlear microphonic potential
Cnidera 2189
CNS *see* central nervous system
coagulation *see* blood, coagulation
coagulative myocytosis
  see contraction band necrosis (CBN)
coalitive effects of substances 50
coalminers, risk of death 1830
cobra *see* snakes
cocarcinogens 7
coccidiostats 1520–1
cochlea 347, 776–81, 784, 786, 789–91, 793–5
cochlear microphonic potential (CM) 781, 783, 785, 787
Cochran–Armitage trend test 300
Cockayne's syndrome 1034
cocklebur (*Xanthium* spp.), toxicity 1518, 1520
cockroach, Madeira 259
cocoa, fatty acids 2115
Code of Federal Regulations 1658, 1662–4
Codex Alimentarius 1648, 1649

Codex Alimentarius Commission (CAC) 2, 3, 1570, 1659
Codex Alimentarius Commission on Pesticide Residues (CCPR) 1611
Codex committees 1570, 1648, 1649
coefficient of variation 358
coefficients of regression 51
coffee 2115, 2158
cognitive impairment 642, 2056, 2059
cognitive-behavioural therapy 1714
COHb *see* carboxyhaemoglobin
cohort studies 1466, 1529, 1531–2
  see also case-control studies
coke emissions 306, 1886
cold medications 814
colic, horses 1518
coliform bacteria, in garbage toxicity 1512
Colinus virginianus see northern bobwhite
colipase 897
collagen
  as biomarker 1859, 1880
  and cartilage and bone toxicity 967
  clinical chemistry 364
  and cutaneous toxicity 829
  fibres 343
  orientation 342
  pathology 342, 343
  synthesis 315, 970
  Type I 864, 1859
  Type IV 894
collagenase 159, 271, 278
colliculi 232
colloidal osmotic effect 367
coloboma 758
Colombo bombing 1722
colon
  cancer
    see also colorectal cancer
    bile acids in 568
    and diet 58, 1981
    in firefighters 1928, 1929
    and gastro-intestinal microflora 566, 567
    in germ-free rat 569
    and lignans 571
    and nitrites 2132
    pharmacogenetics 240
    phenotypes 1891
    in rubber industry 2015
    and selenium 1983

contents sampling 563
crypt cells 567
epithelium 561
modelling 556
radiation-induced mucosal changes 1689
substance transport 564
colony-forming unit-spleen assay 383
colony-stimulating factors, transgene models 1964
Color Additive Amendments *see* Delaney Clause
colorectal cancer 274, 567
  see also colon cancer; rectal cancer
  and diet 1981, 1982
  phenotypes 1891
colorimetric methods, in forensic testing 1490, 1497–500
colostomic stomatitis 524
colour discrimination 738, 756
colour vision 756, 757
Colubridae 2178
Columba livia see pigeon, domestic
columnar cells 545, 828
coma 39, 235, 1758
COMARE *see* Committee on Medical Aspects of Radiation in Environment
combination index 312
combination therapeutic devices 1746
combustion, incomplete 315
combustion toxicology 24–5, 593, 616, 1915–33
  see also fire
comedones 838
comfrey 1552, 1554, 1981
Commander Nero of Force Majerius 1724–5, 1728
commercial products, classification and labelling 1603–4
Committee on Medical Aspects of Radiation in Environment (COMARE) 1695
Committee for Proprietary Medicinal Products (CPMP) (EU) 1426, 1429, 1436, 1438, 1557, 1558, 1621, 1623, 1627, 1639
Committee on Safety of Drugs (UK) 1425, 1546, 1637
Committee on Safety of Medicines (UK) 1425, 1428, 1435, 1559, 1627, 1637

Committee on Scientific Dishonesty (Denmark) 1958
Committee on Toxicology (USA) 1935
Committee for Veterinary Medicinal Products (CVMP) (EU) 1638, 1639, 1641
common chemical sense 612
Common Sense Initiative, US EPA 1587–8
communication
    amongst peers 1940
    by expert witness 1948
    for risk management 1814, 1829, 1911
communications industries, radiofrequency radiation 1418–19
companion animals *see* domestic animals
comparative toxicology of birds and mammmals 1334–5
    see also extrapolation, inter-species
comparison subjects 1531–2, 1533
compartment syndromes 940
compartment system for distribution 77, 78, 79, 1768
compartmentalization 141
compensation 1716, 1959
Competent Authorities 1557, 1578, 1590, 1591
competitive agonism 305, 626
competitive binding assays 1402
competitive inhibition 305
complete negative correlation 304–5
complete positive correlation 304
complexation reactions 1366
component interaction analysis 305
compound action potential (CAP) 781, 783, 785, 786, 787
compound effect summation 303
Comprehensive Environmental Response, Compensation and Liability Act (USA) 1750
computers and computer-aided systems 39
    programs for fraud 1958
    quantitative structure-activity response (QSAR) models 52, 53
    standard operating procedure (SOP) 448

structure evaluation (CASE) 713, 1103
    in tests 667, 668, 754
concentration–dose addition 304
concentration–effect curve 748
concentration–time curve 1834, 1835
    see also plasma
Concise International Chemical Assessment Documents (CICADs) 1592, 1612
concussion 636
condensation generators 594
Condylactis gigantea see anemone, Bermuda
confidence limits, in PBPK modelling 150
confidentiality of data 1894, 1911, 1957
confocal microscopy 339, 347
    through focusing (CMTF) 748
confounders, multiple 1447
confoundings 1531, 1535
confusion 1758
congenital malformations 510, 1219–22, 1419, 1697, 2041
Conium maculatum see hemlock
conjugation reactions 17, 18, 105–9, 216, 359, 1334
conjunctival chemoreceptors 755
conjunctival damage 605, *741*
conjunctival fibroblasts 757
conjunctival haemorrhage 742
conjunctival hyperaemia 614, 738, *741–2, 742–3*
conjunctival redness 622
conjunctivitis 40, 41, 510, 512, 738, 756
connective tissue 343, 530
consent for testing 1957
conservatisms, compounding 1782
constant relative density 1908
constants 1834–5
constipation 40, 2061
construction industry, risk of death 1830
consultations by IEI patients 1712, 1716
Consumer Labelling Initiative (CLI) (US) 1589, 1603
Consumer Product Safety Act (USA) 37, 1589
Consumer Product Safety Commission (CPSC) (USA) 37, *413*, 1589, 1750

consumer products 303, 1550, 1595
Consumer Protection Act (UK) 1550
consumer safety 471
contact dermatitis *see* dermatitis
contact lenses 1667
container closure systems 1603, 1604, 1737
contraceptive steroids, environmental oestrogen effects 1565
contraceptives, regulatory aspects 1548, 1549
contraction band necrosis (CBN) 813–14, 819, 820
contrived field tests 1352
control animals 59, 61, 64–5
Control Limits, Health and Safety Executive (UK) 1594
Control of Pesticides Regulations (UK) 1546
control substances, for validation of endocrine activity screens 1403
Control of Substances Hazardous to Health (COSHH) (UK) 37, 463, 1481, 1594, 1596
Controlled Ecosystem Pollution Experiment (CEPEX) 1318
controlled field studies 1327, 1328
    aquatic toxicology 1318, 1319
controls, in IEI 1705
Convalaria spp. *see* lily-of-the-valley
convulsants 640–1
convulsion *see* seizure
Conway microdiffusion dish *1497*
cooking methods *see* food
Coombs test 391
Cooper Committee, Study Group in Medical Devices 1662
coordination tests 654
copper smelting industry 1246
copperhead 2178
coprophagy prevention 604
coproporphyria 1705, 1864
coproporphyrinogen as biomarker 1864
coral (*Goniopora* spp.) 819, 820
cormorant, double-crested (*Phalacrocorax auritus*) 1329, 1355
corn
    see also cereals
    nitrate and nitrite levels 2112

corn cockle (*Agrostemma gigatho*), toxicity to food-producing animals 1518

cornea
ALDH3 activity 237
changes 40, 41, 44
chemoreceptors 755
ciliary nerve PSI stimulation 619
dehydration 747
deposits 757
epithelium 741, 746, 751
injury 738, *741*, *745*, 746, 747, 748, 750
isolated tissue tests 751–2
neovascularization 742
oedema 738, 747
opacity 741–2, 745, 748, 751
pathology 347
permeability 741, 746, 753
protein *410*, 752
re-epithelialization 746
revascularization, grading system 742–3
swelling 748
thickness 496, 738, 746, 747–8, *748*
transplants, growth factor therapy 1972
ulceration, FDA grading 745

corned beef, nitrate and nitrite levels 2113
coronary arteries 264, 343, 523, 805, 812, 1929, 2126
coronary heart disease (CHD) 1978, 1979–80
coronary thrombosis, diet and 1978
corpus luteum 372
correlation coefficients 89
correlation spectroscopy, biomarkers 1862
corrosion, local effect 19
corrosive effects 1455
corticotrophic releasing hormone (CRH) *369*
Corydalis spp. *see* fitweed
Corynebacterium diphtheriae 639
COSHH *see* Control of Substances Hazardous to Health; Control of Substances Hazardous to Health Regulations
Cosmetic Products (Safety) Regulations 1989 (UK) 1550
Cosmetic, Toiletry and Fragrance Association 503

cosmetics
air pollution 1298
cutaneous toxicity 828, 835
definition 1550
EU regulations 1559–60
and gastro-intestinal microflora 564
human testing 464
hypersensivity reactions 1550
mixtures 606
N-nitroso compounds 2115
neonatal toxicity 1226
permitted/prohibited lists 1557, 1559–60
phamacogenetics 215, 230
regulatory aspects 1544, 1550
cost-benefit analyses 28, 1789, 1792
cost-effectiveness, approximate methods 1331
co-substrates 429
cottonmouth 2178
Coturnix japonica see quail, Japanese
cough 512, 614
coumarin 7-hydroxylase *217*
Council for the Defense of Medical Research 486
Council of Europe 37, 1571
Committee of Experts on Flavouring Substances 1657
Committee of Experts on Materials and Articles Coming into Contact with Food 1657
Council of the European Communities 486
Council for International Organizations of Medical Science 454, 486
councilman bodies 175
counselling for test results 1957
counterterrorism forces 1721
courtroom, expert witness in 1950–1
covalent binding 6, 127–8, 230
coverings or coating, for foods 1654
cow *see* cattle
cowbird, brown-headed (*Molothus ather*) 1347
cowpox virus, and apoptosis 195
CPDB *see* Carcinogen Potency Database
CPF *see* cancer potency factors
CPK *see* creatine phosphokinase

CPSC *see* Consumer Product Safety Commission
crab
biomarker 1852
horseshoe 402, 537
cranial nerve paresis 757
craniorachischisis 969
crayfish 820
CRC Critical Reviews in Toxicology 1676
creatine, as biomarker 1859, 1861, 1862
creatine kinase (CK)
as biomarker 1848, 1857, 1858, 1861, 2031
clinical chemistry 355–6, 357, 366
half-life 1858
levels following CO_2 in rats 61
pathology 343
and skeletal muscle toxicity 939, 940, 941, 943, 944, 951
as substrate 160
creatine phosphate 807
creatine phosphokinase (CPK) 531, 534, 1860
creatinine 43, 1859, 1860, 1861
creatinine-corrected units 1908
credibility 25, 1557, 1579
Creutzfeld–Jacob disease 1964
criminal poisoning *see* poisoning
cristate 778
criterion of judgment in legal matters 1952
critical illness myopathy 947
Critical Incident Stress management 1729
CrmA, and apoptosis 193, 195
cross-sectional studies 1456, 1534
cross-tachyphylaxis 612
Crotolaria spp. *see* rattlebox
Cruelty to Animals Act (UK) 36
crustaceans 1311, 1314, 1318, 1319–20, 2052
see also individual species
cryomicrotome 751
cryopreservation techniques 271
crypt assay reports on radiation 1689, 1690
cryptorchidism 1248
Crystal Ball software 1782
p-crystallin *242*
crystalluria 363
crystal violet staining 753
CS-syndrome 1998

CSF *see* cerebro spinal fluid
CTL *see* cytotoxic T lymphocyte assay
cubital vein sampling 1909
cucumber, nitrate and nitrite levels 2112–13
cultural factors, in medical practice 1567
cumulative dermatitis *see* dermatitis
cumulative frequency distribution curve *see* dose–response curve
cumulative toxicity 5, 6, 555
Cupressus macrocarpa see cypress, Monterey
curare 34
curing agents, rubber industry 2014, 2017
curlydock (*Rumex* spp.), nephro-toxicity 1522
Current Contents 475, 1677
cutaneous *see* dermal; skin
cuticular plate 776, 782
cutting fluids, *N*-nitroso compounds 2115
Cyanocitta cristata see jay, blue
cyanogenic plants 1522
cyanosis 40, 728
cycad nut, as carcinogen 1981
cyclic adenosine monophosphate (AMP) 191, 808, 817, 820, 895, 896, 897, 985
cyclin D, and apoptosis 193
cyclin gene, biomarker 1850
cycloplegia 738, 759
Cymopterus watsonii see spring parsley
cynomolgus monkeys, microsomes 272–3
Cynomys spp. *see* prairie dog
CYP
    see also cytochrome P450
    CYP1A1 114, 867, 1891, 1892
    CYP1A2 114, 867, 871, 1891
    CYP1A4 114
    CYP2A6 230–2, *232*
    CYP2B 867
    CYP2C9 228–30, 228
    CYP2C18 871
    CYP2C19 225–8, 226–7
    CYP2D6 112, 1891
    CYP2D
        clinical toxicities 222
        genotype detection *219*
        and hepatotoxicity 871
        and lung cancer 224–5

polymorphism 218, *219–21*, 222–5
substrates 218, *219–21*, 222
toxicological significance 222–5
CYP2E1 867, 872, 2032
CYP3 867
CYP3A5 871
dog 216
pharmacogenetics 216
polymorphisms 218–32, 1891
cypress, Monterey (*Cupressus macrocarpa*), reproductive system toxicity 1521
Cyprus, CB agent threat 1724–5
cysteine 108, 131, 1862, *1878*, 1883
cysteine conjugate β-lyase 108, 691–2
cysteine sulphydryl group 607
cysteinyl glycinase 107
cystic fibrosis 897, *898*, *901*, 902
cystitis radiation-induced 1691
cytochemistry 337–8
cytochrome 862–3
cytochrome *a* 807
cytochrome *a₃* 807, 1921
cytochrome *b* 807
cytochrome *b₅*, induction 1866
cytochrome *c* 164, 192, 807
cytochrome *c₁* 807
cytochrome *c* reductase 254
cytochrome oxidase 34, 765, 821, 939, 1920, 1923, 1924, 2040
cytochrome P450 6
    see also CYP
    and acetaminophen toxicity 116, 132
    activation reactions catalysis 18
    activity 1402
    aflatoxin metabolism 2154
    as biomarker 1842, 1843, 1848, 1865, 1870, 1886, 1891
    and bromobenzene toxicity 118
    and carbon tetrachloride toxicity 117, 118
    development 115
    and drug interactions 21–2
    and electrophiles 161
    and environmental oestrogen toxicity 1403
    and eye toxicity 763
    and gastro-intestinal microflora 568
    and halothane toxicity 132

and hepatotoxicity 862–3, 866, 867, 871, 872–3
inducers 114
inhibitors 50
interactions 1437
interspecies variation 273, 279
in liver microsomes 280
and metabolism 72, 98–100, 101, 102, 104, 105, 112, 113, 272
and nephrotoxicity 688, 689, 693
and nitrosamine metabolism 2123
nutritional effects 115
occupational toxicity 1429
oxidases 571
pathology 347
role elucidation 135
species differences 110
and systemic pulmonary toxicity 726, 729, 730, 731, 732
cytochrome P450 mono-oxygenases 216, *217–18*, 589
cytochrome P450 reductase 240
cytocochleagrams 782–3
cytogenetic damage, consequences of 1079
cytogenetic studies
    see also in vitro and *in vivo* studies
    in vitro 403, 1081–5
    in vivo 403, 1085–8
cytokines
    as biomarkers 1869
    cardiac myocyte exposure to 812
    cellular concepts 168
    effects, gene transfer studies 1964
    fingerprinting 710–12
    functional subpopulations 703–4
    IEI and 1705
    immunotoxicity 999, 1001–3, 1011, 1012
    mediators in irritant dermatitis 834
    ozone exposure 1276
    production from synthetic materials 1732
    profiles 707
    secreted by Kupffer cells 864
cytology, urine 362–3
cytoplasmic membrane distribution 71
cytoplasmic receptor genes, polymorphism 1892

cytoplasmic vacuolization 551
cytoskeletal active compounds 638
cytoskeletal effects of metal toxins 2067–8
cytoskeletal proteins 631
cytosolic binding proteins 126
cytosolic enzymes 98, 105, 108, 109
cytosolic glutathione transferase 118
cytosolic receptors 126
cytosolic reductase 104
cytosolic SOD activity biomarker 1868
cytostatic drugs 515
cytotoxic agents 258, 522, 536, 1463, 1766
cytotoxic hypoxia from fires 1920
cytotoxic T lymphocyte assay (CTL) 1007
cytotoxic/suppressor T cells 341
cytotoxicity 126
  assays 752–5
  index 52
  mechanism 136
  medical devices 1734, 1735, 1740, 1743

D

D$_{50}$ *see* mean aerodynamic diameter
dab, North Sea (*Limanda limanda*) 1870
Dad-1, and apoptosis 193
DADs *see* delayed after-polarizations
dairy foods 1773, 2113, 2115, 2117
damage *see* DNA, damage
damage inducible (*din*) genes 1022
dander 511, 1300
  see also hair
danger symbols 1477, 1603
Dangerous Chemical Substances and Proposals Concerning Their Labeling (USA) 37
dangerous dose 1831
Dangerous Properties of Industrial Materials 1476
Dangerous Substances Directive
  see EU, Directive 67/548/EEC; EU, Directive 79/831/EEC
dangerous substances and preparations, EU regulations 1590, 1593–4, 1609–10
Danish, *see also* Denmark

Danish painters' disease *see* organic solvent syndrome
Danish porcine nephropathy 2145, 2154, 2160
Daphnia spp. 1318, 1320
  D. magnus 408
data
  interpretation 1941
  monitoring 1958
  requirement, regulatory procedures 1572–3, 1601
  transformation, in exposure reconstruction 1458
databanks 481
databases 477–81
  chemical substances 1456
  chromium exposures 1457–8
  clinical chemistry 358
  control 59
  for expert witness 1947
  indexing 480
  limitations 1461
  pesticides 1603
  toxicity criteria 1759, 1766
  in toxicology 39, 53, 1676, 1939, 1943
Datura stramonium see jimsonweed
Daubert decisions 1947, 1948–50
Davidson's fixative 336, 347
DBA *see Dolichos biflorus* agglutinin
De Materia Medica 35
De Venenis 35
deacetylation, acetaminophen 117
deafness *see* hearing loss
dealkylation 101–2
deamination 101–2
death
  causes 1502, 1529
  certificates 1529, 1535
  following testing in animals 8–9
  from poisoning 38, 1353, 1444, 1489–90
  from whole-body irradiation 1686
  genes 194
  medicolegal investigation 1489
  as quantal response 13
  receptors 196
  records, use in epidemiology 1532
  risk of 1830
  see also lethality
death camas, *Zygadenus* spp., cardiovascular effects 1522

debrisoquine 4-hydroxylase *217*
debrisoquine hydroxylation defect 218
decalcification 342, 782
decapitation 497, *498*–9
dechlorination 104, 566
decision-making tools 1787, 1791, 1829
Declaration of Helsinki 454
decomposed remains 1495, 1496, 1503
decontamination procedures 1511, 1729
deconvolution 655
Dedrick plots 89
default assumptions 603, 1784–5, 1787
definitive tests, field studies 1353–4
degeneration 340
degradation 1734, 1779–80
degreasers' flush 1415
dehalogenation 98, 104
dehydration 367, 1687
dehydration constant 613
7-α-dehydroxylation 567
Delaney Clause, Food, Drug and Cosmetics Act 1938 (USA) 1552–3, 1561, 1563, 1658, 1749
delayed after-polarizations (DADs) 812
delayed hypersensitivity response (DHR) 1007
delayed polyneuropathy 329
demethylation 115, 222, 225–6, 569–70, 572
demographic expansion 1443
demyelination 347, 638, 639, 822, 944
dendrites 631, 703
Denmark
  Committee on Scientific Dishonesty 1958
  nitrate and nitrite levels 2112, 2118, 2130
dental amalgam 1204, 1227, 1249
dental caries 1381
dental exposure, mercury 643
dental workers, latex allergy 510
dentifice 967
dentine 967, 1735, 1736, 2057
dentists, female 1204
dentition 343
  see also teeth
deoxyadenosine *1878*
deoxycytosine *1878*

deoxyguanosine 1878, *1881*
deoxynucleotidyl transferase 340
deoxypyridinoline, as biomarker 1859
deoxyribonucleic acid *see* DNA
Department of Agriculture (USA)
    acute toxicity studies 36
    and agricultural biotechnology 1459
    animal test reduction 494
    animal welfare 486, 496
    Food Safety Inspection Service 1563
    National Food Consumption Survey 1602
    obligations 1599
    regulatory efforts 1561
    veterinary drug regulation 1633–8
    wildlife protection 1347
Department of Defense (USA) 824
Department of the Environment (USA) 1090
Department of Health (UK) 439, 450, 454
Department of Trade and Industry (UK) 459
Department of Transportation (USA) 496, 1588–9
dephosphorylation 429
depolarization 639, 640, 938
depolarizing after-potentials 824
depression
    chronotherapy 266
    in IEI 1707, 1708, 1709, 1710, 1714, 1715
    organic solvents 2030, 2033, 2035, 2036, 2037, 2038, 2039, 2040, 2041
    pharmacogenetics 234
    plastics industry 2020, 2021
    potatoes 1984
    rubber industry 2015
dermal/dermis *see mainly* skin
dermal bioavailability 581, 584
dermal exposures 604, 1339
dermal to inhalation extrapolation 148
dermal toxicity test, in hairless mice 605
dermatitis
    contact 7, 23, 510, 511, 711, 830, 834–6, 838–40, 1779, 1985, 2062–3

    see also allergic contact dermatitis
    cumulative 833
    from rotenone 1999
    in IEI 1715
    occupational 1415
dermatological effects, predictability in animal tests 1438
Derris spp.
    D. eliptica 1999
    D. mallaccensis 1999
Descartes, R,n, 36
descriptive studies, methodology 1533
desensitization 626, 1714
desiccants 2006
design of studies 22–5, 148, 1964
    see also individual study types
designer drugs 1392, 1491
designer species 135
detection methods, specific and non-specific 67
deterministic effects of radiation 1684, 1685–92
dethiolase enzyme 160
detoxification 17, 18, 19, 56, 228, 357, 427, 545
    antidotal studies 427
    and biohandling 17, 18
    by enzymes *224*
    clinical chemistry 357
    endogenous 431
    in liver 19, 1329
    ovarian, impaired 1150
    and pancreatic disease 911–12
    pathways 272
    peroral toxicity 545
    pharmacogenetics 228
    repeated-dose toxicity studies 56, 328
    treatment for IEI 1715
    vs toxication 116–21
Deutsche Forschungsgemeinschaft 1910
developing countries
    chlorinated hydrocarbon toxicity 1510
    mycotoxin toxicity 1524
    paraquat 1512
    pesticide morbidity and mortality 1548
    pollutant emissions 1371
    regulation less stringent 1544
    WTO membership 1570
developmental delay 239

developmental toxicity 8, 1167–201
    see also congenital mal-formations; embryo toxicity; foetal toxicity; reproductive toxicity
    alternative testing 415
    development stage and type of effects 1218–22, 1234–6
    endocrine-related 1399
    and environmental endocrines 1406–7
    interspecies variation 283
    lead 2056
    male-mediated 1185
    mechanisms 1188–91
    neurotoxicity 642, 655, 669, 1467
    organic solvents 2041
    postnatal evaluations 1181–5
    radiofrequency radiation 1419
    regulatory health assessment 1179–81
    screening protocols 1185–8
    Segment II study 1169, 1176–9
developmentally relevant genes 1190–1
device master file 1679
dextran-coated activity charcoal technique 982
dextromethorphan *O*-demethylase *217*
DHEA *see* dihydroepiandrosterone
DHR *see* delayed hypersensitivity response
diabetes 132, 263, 1427, 1969, 2132
diabetes mellitus 1037, 1216
diabetic cataract 160, 764
diabetogenic substances 991–3
diacylglycerol, and apoptosis 190, 191
diagnostic equipment 1661
diagnostic pharmaceuticals, regulatory aspects 1548
diagnostic recombinant products 1966
diagnostic tests, biotechnological 1454
diagonal radioactive zone 1890
dialkylphosphoryl-enzyme complexes 429, 1996
Dialog 1947
dialysis 363, 425, 523, 535, 724, 1379, 2060
diamine oxidase, oxidation 103

diaphoresis 41
diarrhoea
    and acute toxicity 40, 41
    bismuth for 2061
    clinical chemistry 364
    from shellfish toxicity 2194
    from sweeteners 1990
    nitrate excretion 2119, 2129,
        2133
    phamacogenetics 235
    radiation-induced 1689
DIC microscopy see differential
    interference contrast microscopy
Dicentra cucullaria see Dutchman's
    breeches
Dichapetalum cymosum 34
1,1-dichloroethylene 2-hydroxylase
    217
Dicks, The 2102
Dictyostelium discoides 414
diet see food; nutrition
Dietary Risk Evaluation System
    1602–3
diethylstilboestrol 988
differential interference contrast
    (DIC) microscopy 781
diffusion 46, 73, 97, 143, 547, 579,
    582, 1739
diffusion constant 578, 579
digestive proenzymes 545
digestive secretions 252
digestive system 40, 343–4, 1689
Digitalis purpurea see foxglove
digoxin toxicity 427
dihydroepiandrosterone (DHEA)
    984–5
dihydrofolate reductase 256
13,14-dihydro-15-ketoprostaglandin
    FU2αu 243
dihydropyrimidine dehydrogenase
    216, 235, 261
dilution 25, 26
dimethylamine, as biomarker 1862
7,12-dimethylbenz[a]anthracene
    hydroxylase 217
N,N-dimethylglycine, as biomarker
    1862
DIN 53-438 1926
din genes see damage inducible
    genes
dinoflagellates 2192
Dinophysis spp. 2194
Dioscorides 35, 472
dioxin-contaminated soil study 606
diphosphate kinase 261

diphtheria 36
diplopia 757
Dipodomys spp. see kangaroo rat
Director for Graduate Education
    1936–7
disasters 1811–39
    see also specific events e.g.
        Chernobyl, Seveso
    accepted 1814
    accetable 1814
    chemical 1443, 1452
    dilute 1828
    disseminated 1814, 1832
    environmental 1443
    involuntary 1814
    man-made 1815, 1818–26
    natural 1813, 1814–17
    objective 1814
    overt 1828, 1829–32
    perceived 1814
    prevention 1828–37
    risk and benefit 1814
    safety regulations 1443–4
    spillages 606, 1339–440, 1545,
        1551
    theory 1811–14
    tolerable 1814
    types 1814–28
    voluntary 1814
discharge 41
Discourse: the principles of
    philosophy 36
disease
    co-existing, risk assessment 28
    definition 1527
    processes, spontaneous, in
        studies 65
    states, effect on metabolism
        114–15
dishonesty in testing and publication
    1958
disinfectants 1464, 1611
Dispholidus typus see boomslang
disposable syringes 1672–3
disruptive behaviour 664
dissertation in toxicology 1939
dissolution, incomplete 70
dissolution–precipitation reactions
    1366
distal convoluted tubule 363
distribution
    of distributions 1782, 1783
    and dose-dependent kinetics 83
    extent 70–2, 78
    interspecies 88

    multiple route exposure 606, 607
    of organic solvents 2029
    phase 75, 76–7
    rate 70, 76–8
    repeated exposure 67, 70–2,
        76–8
diuresis 40, 41, 523, 681
diuretic response 362
diurnal variations 81–2, 252, 365,
    373, 1908
dizziness 236, 785, 788
DNA
    adducts 161–2, 224, 271, 272
        analysis 1317, 1887–90
        biomarkers 1841, 1842, 1844,
            1845, 1847, 1878, 1880–2,
            1885–90
        in firefighters 1929
        formation 285
        in hepatocytes 284
        as indicators of exposure 1457
        in occupational epidemiology
            1457
        in oral toxicity test 604
        and spontaneous abortion
            1465
        in test animal livers 275
    antibodies 1885
    and apoptosis 187
    breakdown 177
    cloning 218
    colonic mucosa and FP 567
    covalent binding 272
    crosslinks 730
    damage
        analysis 1845, 1849, 1867
        biochemistry 126
        ceramide 191
        and genotoxicity 126
        mechanism 128
        nitric oxide 2121
        nitrites 2128
        ochratoxins 2159
        radiation 1684, 1695
        tumour risk assessment 1763
    fingerprinting 215
    fragmentation 132, 163, 189,
        1847, 1848
    gene regulation 1019
    hepatocytes 275
    hydroxylation 285, 633, 1867
    injury see DNA, damage
    interactions 128, 162, 163
    ladder development 187, 188,
        189

DNA (*Contd.*)
 lung 723
 mapping and sequencing
  see human genome project
 metabolism 391
 microinjections into pronucleus
  1964
 as molecular target 160–2
 mustard gas binding 2084
 mutation and cancer 1027–35,
  1099–101
 PCR amplification 218
 plasmids 1024–5
 point mutations 1025–7
 probes 239, 563
 proteins 1966–8
 recombinant technology 1723,
  1963, 1964, 1965, 1966
 repair
  adaptive pathway 1023–4
  and apoptosis 195
  arsenic 2052
  cadmium 2054
  carcinogen effect 314
  chromium 2062
  enzymes 8, 1892
  error-prone and post-
   replication 1022–3
  excision 1020–2
  inhibition 261
  mechanism 6, 164, 1882
  mismatch 1023
  and mutagenicity 1019–24
  ootocytes 1150–1
  and plasmids 1025
 replication 195
 response elements 722
 sequencing 218, 229
 size and stereochemical
  properties of interacting
  molecule 162
 strand breakage 390, 567, 634
 structure 1017–19
 synthesis
  and apoptosis 198
  cardiac toxicity 808–9
  circadian 256, 258
  fertility cycle variation 266
  inhibition 261
  reproductive toxicity 1142,
   1145
  skin 258, 833
  unscheduled (UDS) 271, 567,
   1104
 thymus 284

transcription 1019
translation 1019
DNA acetyltransferase 273
DNA polymerase 340
DNA sulphotransferase 273
DNA-derived therapeutic products
 1966
DNAse 189, 897
Doctor of Philosophy requirements
 1938, 1939
dog
 acute toxicity studies 45
 aflatoxin LD$_{50}$ 2154
 allergens 512
 ALP isoenzyme 359
 alternative tests to 402
 aminophenol hydroxylation 110
 anaesthesia 387
 atrioventricular node 343
 biceps femoris absorption 531
 biliary excretion 555
 bilirubin 360
 blood collection and sampling
  357, 386, *386*
 body weight/surface area
  difference 92
 breathing rate 46
 cancer studies in plastics industry
  2021
 carbamate herbicide toxicity
  1512
 ceftizoxime clearance 89
 chlorphenoxy herbicide toxicity
  1512
 cholecalciferol toxicity 1511
 cholinesterase inhibition 369
 combustion toxicity studies 1924
 common toxicoses 1510–13
 CYP genes 216, *216*
 dander allergen 512
 developmental period 1696
 exercise pens 490
 fungicide toxicity 2002, 2003
 garbage toxicity 1512
 hair allergen 512
 HDL fraction 367
 herbicide toxicity 2005
 hexobarbitone toxicity 111
 hydrogen cyanide toxicity 2102
 intravenous injections 526, 529
 intubation 544, 549
 ischaemic damage 336
 islet cell 346
 left ventricle papillary muscles
  damage 336

liver amine oxidase (AO) 238
long bone haematopoiesis 383
longissimus dorsi absorption 531
mab markers 338
methaemoglobin model 393
neurotrophic factor
 pharmacokinetics 1972
nitrite toxicity studies 2123
ochratoxin toxicity 2159
osmotic minipump 528
phosgene 2097
pulmonary oil microembolism
 534
repeated exposure studies 59
reproductive cycle 372
saliva allergen 512
secondary toxicity 1510
sinuatrial node 343
stratum corneum skin
 permeability *579*
tPA safety evaluation 1970
treatment groups 358
troponin measurement 366
tumorigenicity of medical devices
 1742
vomiting reflex 546
zinc intoxication 1513
dogbane (*Apocynum* spp.),
 cardiovascular effects 1522
Dolichos biflorus agglutinin (DBA)
 1061
Doll, Richard 1529, 1536, 1539
Domagk, Gerhard 34
domestic animal toxicity 1510–13
Domestic Preparedness Program
 (USA) 1729
dominant lethal mutation 523,
 1038, 1060–1, 1143, 1144
dominant oncogenes
 see proto-oncogenes
doomsday cults 1728
dopamine 16, 642–3, 1348, 2039
dopamine agonists and antagonists
 1328
dopamine oxidase, inhibition by
 disulfiram 2016
dorsal root ganglia 347
dose
 -dependent kinetics 21, 83–5
 additivity 303, 309, *313*
 administered 79
 in animal bioassay 1750
 calculation 1774–5
 definition 9

dose (*Contd.*)

environmental endocrines 1396–7

escalation study 1616

level, grouping 303

limit 42

loading 88

mode in chronic studies 65

and plasma clearance calculation 79

range 39, 44

selection 65, 92, 148, 1619–20

dose–effect *see* dose–response

dose–mortality data 13

dose–response curve

see also area under curve (AUC)

acute toxicity 13–15, 47

comparison 312

cumulative 47–8

estimation 1330

mixtures 304, 311, 312

nature of 9–12

non-monotonic 1397

non-threshold 1397

normal distribution *47*

population studied and 1835, *1836*

safety margins 91

shape 1337, 1397, 1416, 1451, 1452, 1575

sigmoidal 49, 128

skewed *48*

slope 1331–2

statistical reliability 1331

subchronic toxicity tests 1344

dose–response functions 659

dose–response relationship 4, 8–15

see also exposure–response relationship

acute lethal toxicity 13–15

acute toxicity testing 35–6, 47

animal studies protocol design 42, 60

assessment 1460

chronic toxicity studies 64

comparison 1333

controlled experiments 1447

design of studies 22

developmental toxicity 1178, 1180–1

in epidemiology and toxicology 1530

evaluation 433, 1461

explaining in court 1951

eye toxicity 739

hazard and risk assessment 38

human studies 453, 456, 1534, 1574

immunotoxicity 1003

modelling 1834

nature of relationship 9–12

ozone concentrations 1274, 1276, *1277*

of pollutants 1870

prediction 1574

peripheral sensory irritation (PSI) 625

quantifiable 1448

radiation 1693

risk assessment and 1750, 1752, 1758–71, 1792

alternative models 1766

biologically based models 1770

carcinogens 1763–5

case studies 1761–2, 1770–1

epidemiology in context 1770

issues 1766

non-carcinogens 1759–62

PBPK models 1767–9, 1770–1

presentation of risk ranges 1766–7

route-specific toxicity criteria 1765–6

scaling factors 1769

statistical considerations 47–8

surface analysis 306

dosimetric scaling in humans 147

dosimetry 1457, 1460–1

dosing

characteristics 16, 56

continuous vs bolus 555

procedures 44, 59–60

timing effects 16

vehicle 446, 551–2, 557

dossier of toxicity 1447, 1448, 1601, 1605, 1606, 1608, 1609

double data entry 1958

dove, ringed turtle-, (*Streptopelia risoria*), behavioural studies 1347–8

Dow Corning Corporation, Memorandum of Understanding 1585

Down's syndrome 1081, 1144

Draize test *see* eye irritation test

drinking water

see also water

and air pollution 1293

aluminium content 1379

arsenic content 1382, 2050, 2051, 2052

cadmium content 2052

carcinogenicity 554, 1383

cardiotoxicity 822

chemical composition 1381

chlorination 1295, 1381, 1383–4

chronic study 550

contamination *see* pollution

copper content 1380

dosing procedures 59–60

environmental exposure 603

exposure length 604

as exposure route 1381

fluoride content 1381

hardness, and cardiovascular disease 1381

human health aspects 1381–6

ingestion, standard assumptions 1773, 1776

lead content 1378, 2055

level of concern (DWLOC) 1603

MCLs 1790

mercury content 2057

mixed routes of exposure 607

mixtures of chemicals 314

neonatal toxicity 1227

nitrate contamination 566, 1382–3, 1514, 2111, 2114, 2116, 2117, 2118, 2129, 2130, 2131, 2133

nitrites 2134

peroral toxicty 543

pesticide exposures 1603

pH 1376–7, 1378

placental toxicity 1248

pollution 1376, 1824–5, 1832

in pyrogen test 536

regulatory standards 1381, 1383, 1448, 1609, 1673

RfD 1760

sensitivity analysis 1786

standards 1784

test material in 549

toxicity assessment 306

drinks 303

adulteration 1823–4

interaction with drugs 21

mass poisoning 1823–4

nitrate and nitrite levels 2112–14, 2115, 2116, 2117

driving under the influence of
alcohol (DUI) 1491
see also alcohol (*in Chemical
Index*)
driving under the influence of drugs
other than alcohol (DUID) 1491
dromotropic effects 43
Drosophila melanogaster 216, 414,
1050, 1056–8, 1092, 1189, 1190,
1869
drowning 814
drowsiness 43, 460
drug(s)
absorption categories 552
abuse/misuse
behavioural toxicity 664
cardiotoxicity 813–15
cross-reactivity 1501
eye toxicity 757
forensic analysis 1491, 1495
immunotoxicity 1003
medicinal use 1550
occupational toxicity 1416
regulatory aspects 1550
reproductive toxicity 1143,
1146, 1151, 1154, 1224,
1254–7
safety aspects 1444
screening (DAS) 1502, 1503
administration route 21
adverse effects *see* adverse drug
reactions
anti-inflammatory 263
anticancer 261–2
biomaterials and 1745–6
carcinogenicity testing 1618–19
and chemical toxicity 460–1,
1417
circadian toxicology 252–4
clinical trials 457
combinations 1504
controlled and scheduled (UK)
1545
delivery system development
1966
dependence, adverse drug
reaction 1430
development and toxicity testing
265–6, 1436–7, 1974
dietary inclusion 523
disasters 1426–9, 1439–40, 1634
efficacy 1425, 1426, 1429, 1562
evaluation and approval 1425
forensic analysis 1495, 1501
gastro-intestinal absorption 521

gut microflora metabolism 572
human testing 453
interactions 21
acute toxicity 38, 50
drug–chemical interaction,
pregnant women 1216,
1217
drug–drug interactions 125–6
drug–food interactions 125–6
FDA guidance 1438–9
and metabolism 113
occupational toxicity 1415–16
prediction 1437–9
regulation 1426
studies 1565
liver detoxification 344
manufacturers *see* pharmaceutical
companies
metabolic effects 109–10
metabolism 216–18, 863, 866,
910
and myopathies 942–7
neuroleptic 264–5
over-the-counter *see* over-the-
counter drug(s)
oxidation consequences 215–18
and pancreatitis 915–20, 991–3
processing 1968
prohibited list 1550
pulmonary excretion 256
receptor theory of drug action 34
reduction 215–18
regulatory aspects
and clinical research 1439
EU 1557–9, 1621–30
history 1634
Japan 1544, 1565–7
Norway 1544, 1568–9
patterns 1543
processing 1972–3
USA 1544, 1615–20, 1662,
1665
safety
and efficacy 1549
margin calculations 91
regulatory aspects 1425,
1429–34, 1622, 1634
requirements, UK 1425
seasonal exposure 267
side-effects *see* adverse effects
specialized uses 1548
substrates for CYP2D6
polymorphism *219–21*
surveillance schemes 457–8
targeting 1966

testing
forensic 1495, 1501
guidelines 2, 40
on healthy human volunteers
1546
and thrombocytopenia 395
toxic-therapeutic ratio 260
toxicity 21–2, 1425–41, 1549
Type A and B action 21
veterinary *see* veterinary drug(s)
Drug Safety Research Trust 458
Drugs, Cosmetics and Medical
Instruments Law (Japan) 37
dry cleaning industry *678, 2037*
see also service industries
dry eye syndrome 755
DT diaphorase *see* quinone
reductase
dually perfused human placental
cotyledon 1236–7
Duboscq colorimeter 1490
ducks *see* poultry
duct of Santorini 894
duct of Wirsung 894
ductal cells, pancreas 897
Dunlop Committee *see* Committee
on Safety of Drugs
duodenal absorption 69
duodenal chyme 545
duodenal mucosa 545
duodenal ulcer 227, 236
duodenum 545, 546, 556
Durham–Humphrey amendment,
Food, Drug and Cosmetics Act
1938 (USA) 1562
dust
acute toxicity 46
aflatoxin determination 2152
cereals, respiratory effects 1475
chemical contaminants absorbed
on 1299
effects 20
emissions 1815, 2015
exposure 603
generation systems 596–7
inhalation dose calculation 1774,
1775
organic and inorganic 1299
resuspension 1300
as source of contamination of
samples 1909
Dutchman's breeches (*Dicentra
cucullaria*), neuroxicity 1520
dyaphyseal dysgenesis 972
dyes 39, 163, 918, 2014

dyschromatopsia 756
dyskinesia, predictability in animal tests 1438
dysphasia from peroral exposure 19
dyspnoea 40, 41, 512, 728, 731
dystrophic calcification 727

E

E1B19K, and apoptosis 194
E_{50} values 752, 753
E-numbers 1655
eagle, bald (*Haliaeetus leucocephalus*) 1329, 1341
Eagle River Flats, Alsaka 1341
ear
  canal, parathion percutaneous absorption 578
  inner 347, 775–83, 784–96
  melanin in 129
early warning systems 457, 1729–30
Earth Summit *see* United Nations Conference on Environment and Development
earthworms
  as biomarkers 1866
  contact lethality test *408*
  Eisenia foetida 408, 409
  Lumbricus rubellus 408, 409
  toxicity rating 408, *409*
Ebers papyrus 35, 472, 1527
Ebstein's anomaly of tricuspid valve 1205
EC_{50} (median effective concentration) 1312, 1313, 1315
  for blepharospasm 620
  choosing 48
  data for modelling 1834
  sensory irritants *624*
  subchonic toxicity testing 1345
ecdysone agonists 2000
ECG *see* electrocardiogram
Echinaceae purpurea, MRLs 1642
Echis ocellatus see viper, saw-scaled/carpet
Echium plantagineum see viper's bugloss
echothiophate, eye absorption systemic toxicity 762
ecoepidemiology 1407
ECOFRAM *see* Ecological Committee on FIFRA Risk Assessment Methods

Ecological Committee on FIFRA Risk Assessment Methods (ECOFRAM) 1328, 1352
ecological fallacy 1755
ecological health and integrity 1314–15
ecological toxicology, definition 1328
ecotoxicology *see* environmental toxicology
ectoderm 828
ectoparasiticides 1633, 1636–7, 1649, 1993, 1995
eczema 510, 1430, 2145, 2148
ED_{50} (median effective dose) 301
ED (exposure dose) 4, 9, 13, 18
  ED_{01} 48
  ED_{50} 9–10, 11, 36, 39, 48, 2030
  ED_{99} 11
  ED_{100} 48
edge associations, critical 1353
editorial review 457
Edman degradation 1883–4
EDSTAC *see* Endocrine Disrupter Screening and Testing Advisory Committee
Edward syndrome 1081
EEG *see* electroencephalogram
effect addition 304
effective dose 323, 1842, 1843, 1844–5, 1848
efficacy
  antidotes 430–3
  and drug safety 1549
  pesticides 1601
  testing 1573
  veterinary drugs 1634
EGF *see* epidermal growth factor
eggs
  bioassay 1334
  nitrate, nitrite and *N*-nitroso levels 2115, 2116, 2117, 2120
  single-dose acute tests 1330
  suceptibility to xenobiotics 1330
  tainted 234
eggshell thinning
  brown pelican 1351
  and chlorinated hydrocarbons 1329, 1343, 1345, 1548
  poultry 1520
  raptorial birds 1351, 1354
  waterfowl 1354
egr-1, and apoptosis 193

Egypt
  ancient writings 1489, 1527
  chemical warfare 2080
EINECS *see* European Inventory of Existing Commercial Chemical Substances
ejaculatory function 1142
EKA *see* exposure equivalents for carcinogenic chemicals
EKG *see* electrocardiogram
elastic fibres 829
elastic stain 336
elastomers 2013
elderly people
  adverse drug reactions 1427, 1428, 1439
  skin reactivity 831
  statistical artefacts 1529
electric shock, aggression 653
electricity, sensitivity 1714
electrocardiogram (ECG/EKG) 39, 805–6
  abnormalities *see* cardiac arrhythmias
  changes 809, 811, 817, *818*, 819, 822, 823
  P wave 805, 806, 807
  P–R interval 822
  Q–T interval *806*, 817, 819, 823
  QRS complex 805, 817
  recording 45
  S–T segment 805, *806*, 809, 811, 819, 823
  T-wave 805, 806, 809, 823
  U-wave 823
electrochemical conductance, for DNA adduct analysis 1889
electrode paste production workers, exposure risks 1886
electroencephalogram (EEG)
  activity 251
  following organic solvents 2032
  in IEI 1707, 1713
  radiation-induced changes 1691
electrolyte(s)
  balance 363–4, 366–7
  disturbances, ethanol myopathy 938, 940
  forensic analysis 1495, 1498
  imbalance 1757
  transport, radiation-induced changes 1689, 1690
electromagnetic flowmeter 679
electromagnetic radiation 1418–19

electromyocardiogram (EMG) 943, 944
electron(s)
 -withdrawing group 221–2
 donor 238
 ejection 1683
 impact (EI) 1499
 secondary 1683
 transfer 1985
 transport chain 635
electron microscopy 338–9, 764, 781, 782, 787, 790, 867–8
 ethanol myopathy 938
 soft tissue tumours 340
electron spin resonance 619
electronic bibliographic databases 474
electronic literature sources 477–81
electronics industries, radiofrequncy radiation 1418–19
electro-oculography 756
electrophiles 100, 130, 156, 161, 162, 167–8
electrophoresis 187, 188, 366, 367
electroplaters, biomonitoring 1904
electroretinography 756, 764
Elementa Medicinae et Chirurgiae Forensis 36
elements, speciation 1365
elephant, weight 51
elimination *see* excretion
ELISA *see* enzyme-linked immunosorbent assay
elixirs, toxic 1426–8
E_m *see* resting membrane potential
emaciation 41
embolization, arterial 814
embryo, parenteral toxicology 528
embryogenesis 178, 1464, 1684
embryolethality 528, 1243
embryonic stem cells, gene transfer 1964
embryotoxicity
 see also congential malformations; developmental toxicity; placenta; skeletal abnormalities
 cadmium 2053
 circadian toxicology 258
 dioxin 284
 disulphide formation and 159–60
 fungicides 2002
 organic solvents 2040, 2041
 placental toxicity 1243

in pregnant rat 534
 radiation 1696, 1697
emergency planning 1728, 1729, 1814, 1832, 1836–7
Emergency Planning and Community Right-to-know Act 1589–90
emesis *see* vomiting
EMG *see* electromyocardiogram
EMIT *see* enzyme-multiplied immunoassay technique (EMIT)
emphysema 29, 722, 732, 1928
employees, education and training 1463
employers, responsibilities 1481
emulsifiers 1552, 1653, 1985, 1987–8
enantioselective metabolism 226
encapsulation dosing procedures 60
encephalomalacia, horses 2145, 2163
encephalopathy 235, 1430, 2031
endive, nitrate and nitrite levels 2112–13
endocarditis 814
endocardium, pathology 343
endocochlear potential (EP) 777, 781, 785, 787
endocrine
 -active compounds, definition 1394
 disruption 664, 980–1, 1316, 1392–3, 1394, 1400, 1534
 feedback axis 369
 function 369–73, 1395–6, 1400–1
 glands, definition 1395
 homeostasis 1391
 hormone assays 981–3
 hyperplasia 346
 mimic, definition 1394
 modulation *see* endocrine, disruption
 myopathies 947–50
 receptors 983–4, 1402
 system 979–95
  male, toxins affecting 1146–7
  pathology 346
  radiation-induced changes 1691
  signs of toxicity 40, 1391–414
  target organ toxicity 984–93
  tissues 1395

Endocrine Disrupter Screening and Testing Advisory Committee 1393–5, 1400, 1401, 1402, 1403, 1408
endocytosis 680, 682, 685, 693
endocytotic vesicles 791
endolymph, cochlea 775, 776, 777, 779, 780, 784, 789, 795
endometrial cancer 135, 458, 1392, 1399, 1400
endometrial glands, premenstrual, basophilic bodies in 175
endometrial ischaemic death 177
endometrium, pathology 346
endoneural capillary system 633
endonucleases 127, 187, 1963
endoperoxides in diet 1980
endoplasmic reticulum
 see also rough or smooth endoplasmic reticulum
 circadian toxicology 254
 cytochrome P450 in 99
 distribution 71
 enzymes 98, 156
 hepatotoxicity 861, 868
 outer hair cells 786
 pathology 338, 344
 peroral toxicity 548
 pharmacogenetics 232
 stress components 168
endorphins, in human placenta 1256
endothelial bone 966
endothelial cells 632, 633, 2119
endothelium 383
endotoxins
 in animal husbandry 1516–17
 cardiotoxicity 819–20
 concentration 537
 parenteral toxicity 536
 and TNF, toxicology 259
endotracheal route of exposure 59
energy
 deposition 1683
 in experimental carcinogenesis 1980–1
 intake 92
 requirements of body 127
 stressors 1329
Enforcable Consent Agreements (ECAs) 1585
engineering controls 461, 514
enhancement of toxicity 21
enkephalins, in human placenta 1256

enterochromaffin cells 343–4
enterococci 562
enterohepatic circulation 18, 555–6, 557, 568–9, 570, 689
enterooxyntin 546
enterotoxaemia, domestic animals 1512
enterotoxicosis, domestic animals 1512
environmental carcinogens, biomarker 1849
Environmental Chemicals Data and Information Network 481
environmental conditions
   and chemical toxicity 1419
   improvements in quality 1370–1
   PBPK modelling 147–8
   repeated exposure studies 57–8
environmental contaminants
   see environmental pollutants
environmental costs 1752–3
environmental disasters 1443
   see also disasters
environmental endocrines
   see also environmental oestrogens
   debate 1400, 1404
   developmental effects 1406–7
   dosage 1396–7
   effects on wildlife populations 1407
   and human disease 1399–400
   low-level exposure 1395
   regulatory issues 1393–4
   screening and testing 1401–4, 1407–8
   toxicology 1391–414
environmental epidemiology 1529
environmental exposure 19, 606
   regulatory aspects 1415
   renal dysfunction markers 678
   safety margins 91
   to dioxin 87
   to organic solvents 2037
environmental factors
   affecting metabolism 109–10, 112–14
   interactions 1415–24
   pesticide residue effects 1548
   and toxicity 16, 21, 45
environmental field sampling 1781
environmental groups 1945
environmental guidelines
   see guidelines

Environmental Health Criteria (IPCS publications) 476, 1571, 1592, 1612, 1759
environmental health effects 1534
environmental illness *see* idiopathic environmental illness
environmental influences, on response to toxic agents 1418–19
environmental monitoring 1460
Environmental Mutagen Information Center 478
Environmental Mutagen Society 1038
environmental neurotoxins, abnormal tremor 663
environmental oestrogens
   see also environmental endocrines
   breast cancer 1392
   effects on fish 1565
   EPA (USA) investigations 1393–4
   epidemiological and toxicological co-operation 1534
   exposure 1398
   human health effects 1392
   hypothesis 1399
   regulatory focus 1529
   reproductive effects 1565
   unreproducible experiments 1404–5
environmental pollutants 524, 1464, 1564
   persistent 1553–4
environmental pollution
   biomarkers 1531, 1841, 1842, 1866, 1870
   by industrial chemicals, in Japan 1547
   human health effects 1530–1
   IEI and 1711
   mercury 1826, 2057
Environmental Protection Agency (EPA) (USA)
   acute toxicity studies 37, 45
   and agricultural biotechnology 1459
   air pollution studies 1269, 1292
   attitude to epidemiology 1528
   ban on chorinated hydrocarbons 1329
   biopharmaceutics regulations 1973
   Carcinogen Assessment Group 147, 1763–4, 1770

   Common Sense Initiative 1587–8
   developmental neurotoxicity guidelines 1467
   education 1936
   environmental oestrogen investigation 1393–4
   Existing Chemicals Program 1586–90
   exposure calculations 1775
   field studies requirements 1327, 1328, 1353
   formation 1599
   guidelines 1637
   industrial chemicals regulation 1545, 1581–6
   master testing List (MTA) 1585
   multigeneration testing protocol 1406
   Office of Pollution Prevention and Toxics (US) 1581
   pathology 347
   PBPK modelling 1769
   'pen-in-field' protocol 1349
   peroral toxicity 550
   pesticide MRLs 1563
   Pollution Prevention Recognition Program 1583
   powers 1459, 1480–1
   pre-manufacturing notice 1557
   quality assurance 437
   reference guidelines 1352
   registration of end-use product 1350, 1352, 1353
   regulatory function 1328
   reproductive risk assessment guidelines 1467
   risk assessment 1749, 1751, 1752, 1756, 1784, 1788–9
   subchronic toxicity test 1344
   surface area scaling factors 1769
   threshold margin of safety for wildlife 1331
   veterinary drug regulation 1633–8
   Worker Protection Standard 1603
environmental regulations
   see regulatory aspects
environmental risk assessment
   see under risk assessment
environmental somatization 1709, 1715
environmental sources of toxic exposure 1444

environmental stressors 1353, 1407, 1848
Environmental Teratology Information Center 478
environmental toxicology 2, 3, 27, 642–3, 1319–20, 1328, 1450–1
enzymatic detoxicants *426*
enzymatic testing, in field studies 1354
enzyme(s)
  abbreviations *356*
  and absorption 70
  activation 121, 224, 564–6
  activities, PBPK modelling 89
  and acute toxicity 35
  aflatoxin metabolism 2150
  assays 45
  biomonitoring 1906
  catalysis 98
  cDNA cloning 135
  changes, as biomarker 1848, 1856–8, 1860, 1867
  detoxification activities, cellular sensing 157
  dialkyl phosphorylated 429
  digestive 88
  distribution in tissues 1857
  EC numbers 356
  engineering 1454
    see also biotechnology industries
  exogenous 429
  as food additives 1552
  gastrointestinal function 365
  half-life 1857, 1858
  hydrolysis 18, 1883
  inactivation 127, 130
  inducibility 100
  induction 113
    adaptive 6
    as biomarker 1847, 1848, 1856, 1865–6
    in chronic intake 83, 90
    consequences 114
    as double-edged tool 911
    extrahepatic 911
    from organic solvents 2032–3
    hepatic 866–7, 910–12
    non-cP450 1866
    pancreatic 911–12
  inhibition 6, 8, 114, 159, 1847, 1848, 1866–7
  inhibitors 1455
  localization 1857
  metabolic 73

in nucleic acid manipulation 1965
  oxidative 102–3
  Phase I and II 216
  plasma 359–60
  polymorphisms, biomarker 1850
  preparations 1985
  restriction, history of 1963
  stabilization 113
  synthesis, pancreatic 895
  urinary 363, 367
  xenobiotic metabolism 1890–2
enzyme immunoassay (EIA) 370, 1501–2, 1503
enzyme–substrate theory 34
enzyme-linked immunosorbent assay (ELISA)
  adducts 1885, 1887, 1889
  aflatoxin 2152–3
  biotechnology products 1972
  in clinical chemistry 360
  in endocrine toxicology 983
  in forensic testing 1502
  laboratory ocupational hazard 510
  ochratoxin 2158
  in respiratory toxicology 706, 710
  snake venom 2180
enzyme-multiplied immunoassay technique (EMIT) 983, 1501
enzymuria 685, 687
eosin staining 345
eosinophilia 384, 389, 728
eosinophilia–myalgia syndrome (EMS) 395, 946, 1463, 1553, 1568
eosinophilic pneumonitis *727*
eosinophils 702, 729
EP *see* endocochlear potential
EPA *see* Environmental Protection Agency
epicardium 804
epichlorohydrin 1035
epicutaneous techniques, sensitization studies in animals 841–2
epidemic, definition 1527
epidemiological studies 454, 457
  biomarkers 1538
  breast cancer 571
  definition 1527
  end-points 1529–30
  environmental 1529, 1534

health and chemical exposure 461
  hepatocellular cancer 274
  historical aspects 1527–9
  and idiopathic environmental intolerance 1716
  laboratory workers 515
  methodology 1529, 1535
  nitrates, nitrites and *N*-nitroso compounds 2129–33
  observational 1456
  organic solvent toxicity 2041–2
  prognostic criteria 1450
  protein and colonic cancer 568
  reproductive outcomes 1463
  risk assessment 1755–6, 1770
  study designs 1531–4
  techniques 22, 25
  teratogenic eye toxicity 758–9
  and toxicology 1449, 1455–7, 1527–42
  workforce health status 464
epidermal growth factor (EGF) 729, 1972
epidermal growth factor (EGF) receptor 189–90
epidermis 828
  back-diffusion 582
  circadian toxicology 258
  diffusion 46
  keratinocytes 411–*12*, 413
  lichenification 835
  pathology 340
  thickness 583
epididymides 371
epigenetic *see* non-genotoxic
epiglottis 544
epilation radiation-induced 1688
epilepsy 166, 2030
epinephrine *see* adrenaline
epineurum 633
epithelial cells
  and apoptosis 199
  lining 548
  proliferation 126
  radiation-induced damage 1690
epithelium, passage across 70
epoxide hydrolase
  as biomarker 1866
  biotransformation 115
  bromobenzene toxicity and 118
  catalysis 130–1
  induction 1866
  interspecies extrapolation 279

European Union (EU) Regulations
258/97 (Novel Foods) 1560
541/95 1629
542/95 1629, 1640
1069/98 1629
1146/95 1629
2232/96 1655
2309/93 1621, 1623, 1625, 1629, 1639
2377/90 1638, 1643, 1644
euthanasia 61, 496–7, 497–8, *498*
evaporation on storage 1909
evaporimeter 845
evoked potentials 661, 1713
evolution 215
ex vivo studies 52
examination for toxicology 1938–9
Excerpta Medica 473
excipient solvents 533–4
excision repair of DNA 1020–2
excitable membrane function 126–7
excitotoxicity 166, 631, 634, *635*, 644
excitotoxins *634–6*
excretion 18, 67, 72–3, 74–5, 78–80
   see also metabolism
   dose-dependent kinetics and 83
   extent 73
   first-order 73
   half-life, concentration 86
   interspecies 88
   rate 72–3, 79
   rate constant 77, 80, 86
   saturation 83, 84
   sigma minus method 85
excretory products, as biomarkers 1849
exemption, from routine testing 1601
exencephaly 528
exercise
   avoidance 665
   variables 356
exhaled air 552, 581
EXICHEM database 1571
Existing Chemicals Program, EPA (USA) 1586–90
existing drugs, MRLs 1647
existing industrial chemicals, EU regulation 1592–6
existing plant protection products 1608–9
existing products, dossiers 1608

Existing Substances Regulation, EU 1480, 1590, 1608
exocrine cells 545
exogenous dyes 360–1
exogenous enzymes 429
exophthalmos 40, 41
experimental design 293–5, 299–300, 455
   see also study design
experimental errors 294
experimental hypo-responders 294
experimental myopathies 950–5
Experimental Use permits (EUPs) 1600
expert advice 1449, 1639
expert report, EU requirements 1627
expert systems 1449
Expert in Toxicology, DGPT 1943
expert witness 1946–51
export and import of chemicals, US 1588
exposure
   acute toxicity 34–5
   assessment 1460, 1752, 1772–86
      biomarkers 1461, 1538
      in occupational setting 1456
      retrospective 1770
      temporal relevance 1893
   -based finding 1583
   biomonitoring 1899–906
   chamber 593
   characteristics, effects on toxicity 16
   chemical 1328, 1474
   control, in IEI 1716
   data 1530
   definition 1750
   dose *see* ED
   –effect relationship 1313, 1315
   environmental 606
   equivalents for carcinogenic chemicals (EKA) 1911
   estimates, statistical and analytical issues 1781–2
   expression 147
   groups, choosing 60–1
   history in IEI 1711
   index 128
   intermittent 1351
   limits, occupational, PBPK modelling 149
   measurement 1530–1
   misclassification risk 1755
   nose-only 604

parameters 45
pathways 1772, 1787
patterns 1474, 1535–6
potency index 91
reconstruction, data transformation 1458
repeated *see* repeated exposure toxicity
retrospective measurement 1530
route 5, 17, 18–20
   effects 45
   mixed/multiple 603–9, 1904–5
   and nephrotoxicity 704–5
   occupational toxicity 1464, 1485
   of organic solvents 2029
   PBPK modelling 147–8
   pesiticides 1993
   in protocols 40
   regulatory aspects 1548, 1619
   in repeated exposure studies 59
   risk assessment 1754
   -to-route extrapolation 1766, 1769
   secondary 60
   soil and groundwater 1366
   -specific toxicity criteria 1765–6
   and total body burden 149
scenario construction 1772–3
single (acute) 55
sources, wildlife toxicology 1339–42
studies 23
systems 592–3
time (duration) 13, 20, 1739, 1745, 1772, 1786
whole body 604, 623
withdrawal 1715
Exposure factors handbook 1775
exsanguination *498–9*
extenders in rubber 2017
external chain of custody 1491
external dose *see* exposure dose
extracellular fluid 549, 675
extraction
   procedure 1369, 1739
   ratio 74
extrahepatic enzyme induction 911
extrahepatic toxins 133
extramedullary haemopoiesis, spleen 341
extraocular muscles 614, 757

extrapolation

see also interspecies extrapolation

disaster studies 1833, 1834

exudates 41, 342

exudation 539

eye

see also ophth- and parts and diseases of the eye

acute inflammatory reaction 755

adverse drug reactions 1427

allergic response 512

arsenic retention 2051

blinking 739

chemical injuries 737–8

concentration-response for threshold sensation 616

contact of substance with 19, 20

cosmetics 759

cytotoxicity assays 752–5

enucleated methods 751–2

episceral venous complex 614

exposure to toxins 605

fixation 336, 347

hypertension 614, 757

hypoplasia 758

inferior conjunctival sac for material testing 739, 740

inflammation signs 738

injury 8

disasters 1814, 1819

fires 1920, 1925, 1928

fungicides 2003

jellyfish venom 2189

Lewisite 2089

methanol 2040

mustard gas 2084, 2087

nerve agents 2091

phosgene 2098

radiation 1684, 1687–8, 1696

riot control agents 2104

scoring system 741

scorpion venom 2188

snake venom 2179

volcanoes 1816

intraocular pressure (IOP) measurements 748–50

irrigation 741, 2013, 2016, 2020, 2021, 2032, 2181

irritation 622–3, 737–55

see also eye irritation tests

itching as allergic response 512

local anaesthesia effects 747

malformations 757

metabolism 756

peripheral sensory irritation 614, 755

signs of toxicity 44

slit-lamp biomicroscopy 746

and systemic toxicity 755–9, 759–64

tests in repeated exposure 63

toxicology 737–74

toxin absorption sites 759–60

triparanol toxicity 1634

eye drops, vasoconstrictor effects 1550

eye irritation tests 23, 25, 738–46

alternative methods 410, 747–55

animal welfare 494, 499

computer-based modelling 754

Draize scoring 496, 740–1, 744–6, 752

human studies 466

immunotoxicology 1005

in vitro 739

modification 466

rabbit studies 745, 841, 843–4

results 742, 744–6

F

FA see Fanconi's anaemia

fabrics, biocompatibility testing 1738

facial parasthesia 524

facial warming 236

FACScan flow cytometer 680

factor IX 1965

factor VIII 1965, 1966, 1970

factor VII

and diet 1980

factorial designs 313

Factories Inspectorate (UK) 1960

factory

see also occupational toxicology; workplace

biomonitoring 1904

emissions, inhalation exposure 606

facts, real vs junk science 1946–7

factsheets 1448–9

FAD see flavin

faecal excretion 18

dioxin 90

elimination rate constant calculation 86

mecury 2059

sigma minus method 85

toxicokinetics 69, 70, 72

faeces

absence 40

bacterial flora 563

bolus weight 1645

chemical excretion 581

clinical chemistry 362

mutagenic activity 566

N-nitroso compounds 567

stained 40

FAEES see fatty acid ethyl esters

Fagopyrum esculentum see buckwheat

FAK see focal adhesion kinase

Falco peregrinus see peregrine falcon

fallopian tubes see oviducts

false positives 404, 1501

familial motor neuron disease 239

family environment see home environment

Fanconi's anaemia (FA) 1033–4

FAO see Food and Agriculture Organization

farm animal studies 45

farm animals, see also food-producing animals and specific animals

farmers see agricultural workers

Farr, William 1527, 1528, 1529

Fas 190, 191, 193, 195–6, 199

fasciculations 40, 41, 430, 950, 951

Fasciola hepatica see liver fluke

fasciotomies 941

fast twitch fibres 342

fasting see feeding behaviour

fat

see also adipose tissue

dietary 58, 1980

heated, as source of oxygen free radicals 1979

partition coefficients of organic solvents 2029

in tissues, interspecies 88

fat cells 829

fat storage cells see Ito cells

fatigue 1686, 1687, 1703, 1706, 1724

fatty acids

composition changes with organic solvents 2036, 2037

essential 1979–81

metabolism 99, 1868

monounsaturated 1978

non-esterified 367

oxidation 869

fatty acids (*Contd.*)
  pharmacogenetics 216
  polyunsaturated 1980
  saturated, blood cholesterol and 1978
  storage pool, fumonisins and 2165
fatty liver-haemorrhagic syndrome (FLHS) 233–4
fault indemnity 1959
fault tree analysis 1832
FBI forensic laboratories 1942
FCA test *see* Freund's Complete Adjuvant test
FDA *see* Food and Drug Administration (FDA) (USA)
FDCs *see* follicular dendritic cells
fecundity 1465, 1846
Federal Insecticide, Fungicide and Rodenticide Act (FIFRA) (USA) 37, 487, 1328, 1350, 1459, 1467, 1563, 1599, 1600, 1636, 1750
feedback mechanisms 546, 980–1, 986–7
feeding behaviour 1328, 1347, 1351
feeding studies, chemical effect on renal function 678
feedstock chemicals, occupational exposures 1463
feedstuffs *see* animal feeds
feet *see* foot
female reproductive system 1147–56
  see also pregnancy
  drug and chemical effects 1155–6
  exercise effects 1156
  health evaluation 1465–6
  occupational hazards 1465–6
  physiology 1147–9
  toxic mechanisms 1149–55
feminization 654, 862, 1226–7
femoral blood concentrations 1495, 1504
femur 341
Fenton reaction 633, 641
feral animals *see* wildlife species
fermentation
  peroral toxicity 545
  plants, source of biological hazards 1459
  process, biopharmaceutics regulations 1973

ferret
  black-footed ferret (*Mustela nigripes*) 1347
  Siberian (*Mustela evermanni*) 1346
  studies 45, 110, 2199
ferritin 2065
ferrochelatase 392, 1864, 1906, 2056
fertility 465
  see also reproductive system
  cycle, toxicology 266
  female 1465
  and fungicides 2002
  male 62, 1464
    see also sperm quality
  and organic solvents 2041
  and radiation 1688, 1696
  reduced 1463
  study, Japanese requirements 1567
  toxic effects on 23–4
fertilization, regulation 1464
fertilizers 1371–2, 1383, 1514, 2114
fescue, tall (*Festuca arundinaceae*), reproductive system toxicity 1521
Festuca arundinacea see tall fescue
FETAX system *see* frog embryo teratogenesis assay: *Xenopus*
FEV *see* forced expiratory volume
fever 169, 235, 265
fibre inhalation 20
fibrinogen 264, 366, 2179
fibrinolysis 264, 385
fibroblasts 196, 315, *412*, 530, 567, 728, 810, 829
fibromyalgia 1703, 1710, 1714
fibronectin 342
fibrosis 6, 19, 807, 873–4
Fick's law 46, 143, 578, 582
fiddleback spider 2186
fiddleneck (*Amsinkia intermedia*), hepatoxicity 1519
field studies
  animal behaviour 1346
  definitive tests 1353–4
  ecology 1327
  EPA guidelines 1353
  granular formulations 1350
  non-destructive sampling 1345
  population estimation 1353
  screening tests 1353–4
  statistical analysis 1353
  test design 1354

FIFRA *see* Federal Insecticide, Fungicide and Rodenticide Act
figure-of-eight mazes 651
filamin, as calpain substrate 189–90
fillers 2014, 2022
filter cages 514
fine needle aspiration 344
finger-prick blood samples 19
fingernails *see* nails
Finland
  BALs 1910, 1911
  nitrate, nitrite and *N*-nitroso levels 2114, 2118, 2132
Finnish Institute of Occupational Health 666
fire ants (*Solenopsis* spp.) 2184
fire coral jellyfish 2190
fire extinguishers 460
firefighters
  risks 1821, 2033
  toxicity studies 1916, 1920, 1926–9
fires
  see also combustion
  airport 1821–2
  atmosphere in 1916–17, 1920–4
  combustion products 1915–16, 1924
  deaths in 1494–5, 1917
  disasters 1821–3
  exposure tests 24–5
  hazard investigation 1924–7
  incapacitating factors 1920
  nature and toxicity of atmospheres 1917–19
fireworks 1524
first-aid management 22
first-order reactions 69, 73, 74, 75, 79–80, 84
first-pass metabolism 22, 56, 69–70, 545, 548, 552
fish
  acute toxicity studies 38
  alternative testing 407
  aluminium toxicity 1379
  and apoptosis 178
  arsenic levels 2052
  biomarker 1852, 1866, 1867, 1869
  CHD and 1980
  dioxin 281
  environmental endocrine effects 1407
  environmental oestrogen effects 1565

fish (*Contd.*)
  farming 1548, 1648
  gonadal recrudescence assay
    1403, 1408
  heterocyclic amines 271
  ingestion, risk assessments 1780,
    1785
  liver oils 1552
  mercury toxicity 1249, 1310,
    1826, 2057–8
  MRLS 1646, 1647
  nitrate, nitrite and *N*-nitroso
    levels 2114, 2115, 2116, 2117,
    2118, 2120, 2132
  oil spillage and 1826–7
  phenol metabolism 111
  poisonous 2191–4
  pollutants in 1870
  predatory 1378, 1379
  scombrotoxic 1554
  stinging 2191–2
  toxicology studies 45, 790, 1311,
    1314, 1316, 1318, 1319–20
  vitellogenin 1407, 1408
Fish and Wildlife Service (USA)
  1331, 1332
fish-eating human populations,
  methylmercury exposure 1379
fish-eating wildlife species 1329,
  1339–440
fish-odour syndrome 233–4
Fisheries Act (Canada, 1971) 1311
fishermen, risk assessment 1775,
  1780, 1826, 1830
Fisher's exact test 300, 301
fit *see* seizure
fitweed (*Corydalis* spp.),
  neurotoxicity 1520
five-day dietary tests 1335–6
fixation 336, 338, 339
fixed dose procedures 44, 326
flame, trauma from 1916
flame photometry 367
flame retardants 2014, 2022
flaming, combustion 1916
flashover 1822
flatulence 40
flavin (FAD), reduction 104
flavin monooxygenase (FMO) 102,
  216, 232–3, 725
flavoprotein cofactors 103
Flavor and Extract Manufacturers'
  Association 1658
flavours and flavour enhancers
  1985, 1988

regulatory aspects 1552, 1653,
  1654, 1655, 1656–7
flea and tick control products,
  toxicity 1510
flip-flop kinetics 75
floating necrosis 872
floor and furniture waxes 1295
flounder, European (*Platichthys
  flesus*) 1870
flour *see* cereals
fluctuation tests 1048
fluidized beds 597
fluorescein
  flare 746
  fundus angiography 764
  permeability 751
  retention 752
  staining 746, 751, 752
fluorescence microscopy 346,
  781–2
fluorescence spectrometry *680*,
  1882, 1889
fluorescent polarization
  immunoassay (FPIA) 1502
fluoridation, water 1534
fluoroacetyl coenzyme A 6
fluorochromes 1848
fluorometer 750
fluorophotometry 746
flushing 114, 460
flux 578, 582
fly
  see also Drosophila
  house 259
FMO polymorphisms 233–5
foaming agents 1985
FOB *see* functional observational
  battery
focal adhesion kinase (FAK2), and
  apoptosis 195
focal granulomatous plaques 532
focal hyperplasia, incidence 296
focal myopathies 946–7
focal necrosis 539
fodrin 189–90, 195
foetal alcohol syndrome 660, 757,
  758, 2040
foetal development 1465
  biomarkers 1465
  and lead 1487
  PCBs damage 642
  regulation 1464
  stages and types of effects
    1218–22
foetal distress syndrome 1427

foetal exposure and eye toxicity
  758–9
foetal heart rate 1216
foetal loss 1465, 1466, 1530
  see also abortion, spontaneous
foetal malformation, in mouse
  inhalational study 604
foetal metabolism 1240
foetal metallothionein gene
  expression 2067
foetal Minamata disease 1249
foetal toxicity *see* foetotoxicity
foetotoxicity
  arsenic 2051
  CO 1921–2
  dioxin 282, 1818
  firefighters 1929
  food contamination 1825
  fumonisins 2164
  fungicides 2002, 2003
  interspecies variation 281
  lead 1205, 2055, 2057
  lithium 1205–6
  mercury 2057, 2058, 2059
  methylmercury 1204
  nitrites 2128, 2135
  non-lethal 8
  organic solvents 2041
  placental toxicity 1243
  radiation 1696, 1697
  reproductive studies 23
foliage, herbicide/pesticide residues
  1341, 1349, 1518
follicle stimulating hormone (FSH)
  986–7
  as biomarker 1858
  breast cancer surgery 266
  dioxin effects 163
  female 1147, 1148, 1151, 1155
  male 1141, 1143
follicular cell tumours in plastics
  industry 2022
follicular dendritic cells (FDC)
  1000
follow-up period, cohort studies
  1531
food 316–17
  see also nutrition
  allergies 1706, 1986
  cardiotoxic materials in 823
  consumption 39, 61, 63, 83, 84,
    1846, 1855, 1859
  contamination
    accidental 1824–5
    adulteration 1823–4

food

contamination (*Contd.*)
aluminium 2060
amines 103
BaP 569
cadmium 1377, 2052–3
carbamates 1998
carcinogens 1763
CB agents in 1724
chemical 1551, 1554, 1563, 1780
dioxin 88
disasters 1823–4
and gastro-intestinal microflora 571
heterocyclic amines 272
lead 2055
microbiological 1551
myocotoxins 2145, 2147, 2153
nitrate, nitrite and *N*-nitroso compounds 566, 2112–18, 2120, 2121, 2134–5, 2136
ochratoxin 2158–9
PAH 1791
pesticides 1563, 1994
prevention 1832
regulatory aspects 1553–4
storage-related 1825
cooking methods 1780, 1886, 1982, 2161
DEHA migration into 466
–drug interactions 21, 125–6
factors, European 1646
flavourings *see* flavours and flavour enhancers
functional (FOSHU) 1551–2, 1567–8
intake 252
intolerances 1986
labelling 1560
MRL 1610
novel 1546, 1551, 1553
phyto-oestrogens 570–1, 1392, 1398
poisoning *see* food, contamination
processing 1982
plants, source of biological hazards 1459
production, Japanese regulation 1567–8
products 1551–4, 1563
regulatory aspects 1546, 1551–2, 1567–8

safety assessment, veterinary drugs 1634–5
simulants 1657
sources, contaminated 1339, 1355, 1444
for specific health uses (FOSHU) *see* food, functional
toxicology 1977–84
Food Additive Amendment, Food, Drug and Cosmetics Act 1562
food additives
ADI 1656
authorization 1655–7
carcinogenicity 1125
classification 1984
cutaneous toxicity 835
generally recognized as safe (GRAS) 1563, 1658
immunotoxicity 1004
margin of safety 316
molecular targets 163
MRLs 3
not approved 1656
permitted list systems 1552
pharmacogenetics 215
recommended daily allowance 316
regulatory aspects 1544, 1552–3, 1653–60
Canada 1659
EU 1653, 1655–7
USA 1562–156, 1658–9
reproductive toxicity 1139
safety margin calculations 91
toxicology 1656, 1659, 1977, 1984–90
toxokinetics 67, 70
Food and Agriculture Association, Codex Alimentarius Commission 1570
Food, Agriculture, Conservation, and Trade Act 486
Food and Agriculture Organization (FAO) 462, 1960
food chain
human, contamination 1373, 1375, 1376
mercury 1825–6
oil spillages 1826–7
PCBs in 642
pharmacogenetics 215
radioactivity 1821
toxin accumulation by animals 2177

food chemicals, regulatory aspects, EU 1560
food contact materials 1653–60
Food and Drug Administration (FDA) (USA)
acute toxicity 36, 37, 40
aflatoxin levels 2153
and agricultural biotechnology 1459
biopharmaceutics regulations 1973
cardiotoxicity 815
congressional committees 1664
drugs 2, 1438–9
education and 1935
and environmental oestrogen toxicity 1394
eye lesions grading system *742*
food additives regulation 1562–3
and gastro-intestinal microflora 565
guidelines 1426, 1636
history 1534
human studies 460
medical device monitoring 1662, 1733, 1734, 1735, 1743, 1744
mutagenicity 1038
pre-marketing approval of food additives 1658
quality assurance 437
Red Apple Conference Center, Arkansas 450
regulatory procedures 1561–4, 1615
reproduction and teratogenicity study 137–8, 1168
risk assessment 1750, 1769
toxicology testing guidelines 1635
veterinary drug regulation 1633–8
Food and Drugs Act 1906 (USA) 1534, 1544, 1561, 1599
Food and Drugs Act 1920 (Canada) 1600, 1659
Food and Drugs Act 1925 (UK) 1637
Food, Drugs and Cosmetics Act 1938 (USA) 36, 37, 1426, 1544, 1562, 1599, 1634, 1658, 1750, 1935
Delaney Clause 1552–3, 1561, 1563, 1658, 1749
Durham–Humphrey amendment 1562

Food, Drugs and Cosmetics Act
1938 (USA) (*Contd.*)
  Food Additive Amendment 1562
  Kefaufer–Harris amendment
   1562
  Miller amendment 1599
  Pesticide Chemical Amendment
   1563
Food, Drugs and Insecticide
  Administration (US) 1561
Food and Environmental Protection
  Act 1985 (UK) 1546
Food Quality Protection Act 1996
  (USA) 1393, 1599, 1602, 1603,
  1604
Food Safety Inspection Service
  (USA) 1563, 1637
food supplements, regulatory
  aspects 1551–2
food-producing animals
  common toxicoses 1513–17
  neurotoxicity 1520
  pharmaceutical treatment 1549
food-producing plants 1548, 1554
foods, functional (FOSHU),
  regulatory aspects 1546, 1551–2
foot
  male adult skin surface area 583
  parathion percutaneous
   absorption *578*
  splay measurement for delayed
   neuropathy 654
forage 1515, 1518
forced expiratory volume (FEV)
  510, 512, 1270–1, 1273, 1274,
  1277, 1279
forced vital capacity (FVC) 512,
  1270–1, 1273, *1277*
forearm, absorption *577*, *578*, 580
forebrain 347
forehead *577*, *578*
foreign body response 532, 1130–1,
  1679–80, 1732
foreign manufacturing approvals,
  Japan 1566
forensic toxicology 3, 1489–507,
  1941–2
  certification 1491
  definition 1489
  exposure biomarkers 1877
  instrumentation 1491
  interpretation of results 1504–5
  laboratory protocols *1503*
  professional organizations 1491
  responsibilities 1491, 1494

specimens
  collection 1495–6
  identification and storage
   1491–4
forensic urine drug testing (FUDT)
  1491
fore*seeable* events 1832–3
forestomach 551, 554, 556, 557,
  1986, 2020, 2021
forestry products industry, source of
  biological hazards 1459
Forgacs 2145
Formicidae 2184
formulation 16, 37, 70
fortified foods 1552
forward mutation tests 1049–50
FOSHU *see* foods, functional
fossa cubitalis, parathion
  percutaneous absorption *578*
fossil fuels 1265, 1267, 1274
foundry workers, exposure risks
  1886, 1887
fox, kit (*Vulpes macrotis*) 1347
foxglove (*Digitalis purpurea*) 34,
  1522
FPIA *see* fluorescent polarization
  immunoassay
Fragrance Industry Manufacturers
  Association 1676
FRAME *see* Fund for the
  Replacement of Animals in
  Medical Experiments
frameshift mutation 8
Framingham Heart Study 1529
France
  BALs 1910
  legal restrictions 1547
  nitrate and nitrite levels 2116,
   2117, 2118
fraud 1958
fraudulent medical devices 1662
fraudulent practice 293
fraudulent toxicological data 1561,
  1563–4
fraudulent treatments 1561–2
free radical oxidation products
  (FROPS) 896
free radicals 161, 240, 633–4, 1683,
  1705, 1867
  see also oxygen free radicals
Free–Wilson system 1103
Freedom of Information Act (USA)
  1561, 1562, 1578
Freedom of Information Summary
  1634

freezants 1985
Freund's Complete Adjuvant (FCA)
  test 841, 842, 1005
frictional trauma 830
fried meat *see* meat, fried
frog
  African clawed (*Xenopus laevis*)
   414, 1187, 1209, 1403
   embryo teratogenesis assay
    1187, 1209
  Columbian (*Phyllobates
   aurotaenia*) 816, 818
  Costa Rican 2193
  flexor reflex *620*, *623–4*
  metamorphosis assay 1403
FROPS *see* free radical oxidation
  products
frostbite 837
fruit
  ingestion, standard assumptions
   1773
  nitrate and nitrite levels 2113,
   2115, 2116, 2117
  toxicity and 1983–4
fruit fly *see Drosophila
  melanogaster*
Fry–Lee test 300
Frye rule 1948, 1949
FSH *see* follicle stimulating
  hormone
fugacity, models incorporating 1778
full-face air-supplied devices 516
fumes, in rubber industry 2014,
  2015
fumigants for rodents 2006
function foods *see* foods, functional
functional disorders, covert 657
functional observational battery
  (FOB) 63
functional toxicity detection 23
Fund for the Replacement of
  Animals in Medical Experiments
  (FRAME) (UK) 504
fungi 462, 1301–2, 1369
  see also mycotoxins
fungicides 990, 1151, 1226, 1249,
  1998
furnaces for combustion studies
  1926
Fusarium spp. 2145, 2146, 2149
  F. acuminatum 2149
  F. dlamini 2163
  food toxicology 1982
  fungi-infected grain 823, 1252–3
  F. moniliforme 1516, 1520, 2163

Fusarium spp. (*Contd.*)
  mycotoxins 1516
  F. nygamai 2163
  F. solani 726
  F. subglutinans 2163
Fusobacterium 563
FVC *see* forced vital capacity

G

G1-S phase 260
G2-M phase 260
GABA *see* γ-aminobutyric acid
GADD 153, 167, 168
gait abnormality 40, 41, 1997
galactorrhoea, adverse drug reaction
  1430
galactose, and apoptosis 183
galactosidase, as biomarker 1862
galactosylhydroxylysine, as
  biomarker 1859
Galen 35, 460
gallbladder
  passage of drugs and chemicals
    557
  tumours 2018
gallstones 898, 899, 1843
Gallus domesticus see chicken
Gambierdiscus toxicus 819, 2191
game species
  cadmium levels 1375, 1378
  feeding trials 1330
  mercury concentration 1355
  xenobiotic tolerance 1337–8
gametogenesis, regulation 1464
gangrene 1382, 1516
  see also necrosis
gap junctions 779, 806, 810, 854
garbage toxicity, domestic animals
  1512–13
Gardener's syndrome 1034
gardening, biomonitoring 1780
Gardner hypothesis 1695
garlic as antioxidant 1984
gas chromatography 597, 1491
gas chromatography–mass
  spectrometry (GC–MS) 597,
  1499–500, 1503, 1504
gas masks for CB attack 1729
gas stoves 1278, 1279, 1296
gas–liquid chromatography (GLC)
  367, 1499, 1500, 1502–3
gases
  see also war gases
  absorption 589–90

aliphatic 2034
atmosphere analysis 597
atmosphere generation 594
biomonitoring 1907
exposure 20
incidents, risk of death 1830
indoor air pollutants 1296–8,
  1303
inorganic 1296
lake emissions 181
mixtures 315–16
mortality data 1834–5, 1917
in repeated exposure studies 60
rubber industry emissions 2015
sampling 597
toxicity 46
uptake, PBPK modelling *146*,
  148–9
volcanic 1815
gasping 41
Gasserian ganglia 347
gastric, *see also* gastro-intestinal
gastric acid secretion 227
gastric cancer *see* stomach cancer
gastric contents 1495, 1504
gastric fluids, bench-scale extraction
  experiments 1777–8
gastric mucosa 108, 547
gastric parietal cells 365
gastric secretion 546
gastric ulcer 227, 236, 2061
gastrin 365, 546, 547
gastro-enteric target 524–6
gastro-intestinal tract
  see also specific areas, e.g.
    stomach
  absorption 19
    aluminium 2060
    cadmium 2052–3
    lead 2055
    mercury 2058
    parenteral toxicity 521, 523
    peroral toxicity 552
    tin 523
    toxicokinetics 67, 69, 75
    zinc 2066
  atresia 1348
  cancer 235, 2002
  clinical chemistry 364–7
  epithelium 338, 343
  flora 561–76
    detoxification 569–71
    factors affecting metabolism
      and toxicity 571–3
    human 1645

    and parenteral toxicity 521,
      522
    and peroral toxicity 555, 556
    protective effects 569–71
    species differences and
      metabolism 572
  haemorrhage 132, 282, 458
  and idiopathic environmental
    intolerance 1704
  and metabolism 98
  mucosa 105, 339, 551
  nitrobenzene reduction 104
  and parenteral toxicity 522, 530,
    532
  pathology 343
  PBPK studies 89–90
  pH 252
  toxicity
    adverse drug reactions 1427,
      1438
    arsenic 1515, 2051
    copper 1380
    domoic acid 2193
    fish poisoning 2192
    food additives 1986
    food contamination 1825
    garbage poisoning 1512–13
    herbicides 2004, 2006
    horses 1519
    houshold product ingestion
      1512
    iron 2065
    lead 1475
    mushrooms 1513
    mycotoxins 1516
    nitrates 2119
    nitrites 2120
    nitrogen 1514
    potatoes 1984
    radiation 1684, 1685, 1686,
      1687, 1689
  trace element uptake deficiency
    2049
  ulceration 363, 365, 524, 525,
    1430
gastro-oesophageal junction, in
  peroral toxicity test 553
gatekeepers, trial judges 1949
gaussian distribution 11, 12, 322,
  1785
gavage 55, 59, 549, 550, 551
  acute toxic response 555
  dosing 67, 75, 554, 604
  oesophageal injury to treated rats
    553–*4*

geeldikkop 2148
GEES *see* generalized estimating equations
gel electrophoresis *219*, 1845
gel filtration 363
gelatin capsules 549
gelling agents 1985
Gelsemium spp. *see* Carolina jessamine
gelsolin, and apoptosis 195
gender differences
   AITC 134
   and behaviour 664
   cadmium toxicity 1374, 2053
   enzyme induction 2033
   in idiopathic environmental intolerance 1707
   metabolism 111
   nephropathy 129
   nitrate intakes 2116
   nucleus of the preoptic area 1406
   pesticide sensitivity 1338
   radiation toxicology 1683, 1692
   and response to toxic agents 1343, 1416
gene–environment interactions 215
General Agreement on Tariffs and Trade (GATT) 1569, 1611, 1649
general drug screen (GDS) 1502, 1503
general population *see* population
generalized estimating equations (GEES) 1178
generally recognized as safe (GRAS) 725, 1563, 1658
genes
   see also specific genes
   amplification 339, 1967
   developmentally relevant 1190–1
   dosage 162
   expression 53, 169
   families 99
   loci 236
   mapping 1091
   mutation *see* mutagenicity
   new variants 215
   phenotypes and genotypes 218
   rearrangements 340
   and regulation of apoptosis 193
   sequencing 1548
   stress-related 167
   superfamily 216–18
   transcription activation 126, 2067

genetic abnormalities
   biochemistry 126, 128
   as biomarker 1848, 1849
   from radiation 1683, 1693, 1695
   molecular concepts 157, 162, 163, 168
genetic code 1017, *1018*
genetic engineering 1963
genetic factors
   in acetylation 108
   affecting drug effects 110
   and metabolism 111–12
   and response to toxic agents 1338, 1416
genetic manipulation 135
genetic modification 1454, 1553
   see also genetic enginering
genetic polymorphisms
   see polymorphisms
genetic predisposition 461
genetic risks, in radiation studies 1694
genetic screening 235
genetic toxicology
   guidelines 1038–9, 1061
   in vitro test systems 1039–58
   interpretation of data 1064–5
   mammalian mutation tests 1051–6, 1058–61
   restriction site mutation analysis 1062
   tissue-specific genetic polymorphisms 1061–2
   transgenic models 1062–4, 1111–14
genetic variants 238
genetically engineered products, testing 1463
genetically modified organisms (GMOs) 1459, 1548, 1560, 1584, 1628, 1629
genetically susceptible subpopulations 28–9
genetics, applied 1963
Geneva Protocol 2080
genito-urinary cancer in firefighters 1928, 1929
genomic instability radiation-induced 1695–6
genotoxic carcinogens 8, 874, 1101–6, 1114, 1434
   see also rodent carcinogenicity tests
genotoxic chemicals 7, 1484

genotoxic initiators 7
genotoxicity 8
   2-naphthylamine 134
   arsenic 2051
   bioassays 1460
   biochemistry 128
   biomarker 1845
   biomonitoring 1906–7
   dose extrapolation 1766
   firefighters 1929
   fumonisins 2165
   human studies 465
   Japanese test battery 1567
   medical devices 1734, 1735, 1742
   nitrites 2128
   ochratoxins 2160
   organic solvents 2040
   PBPK modelling 1770
   plastics industry 2020
   risk assessment 1750
   rubber industry 2015
   testing 24, 1435, 1448
      EU requirements 1622
      extrapolation 1435, 1448
      harmonization 1573
      new pharmaceuticals 1617, 1618–19
      new substances 1591
      replacement tests 499
   toluene exposure 1456
genotype 218, 1850
GENSTAT statistical program 301
geographic distribution 1527
geographical location 1910
geometric mean 1781, 1782
George III, King 1849
gerbil, aminophenol hydroxylation 110
Gerbillinae, interspecies differences 283
germ cells
   acrosome 345
   assays 1086, 1088
   chromosomes 1145
   damage from radiation 1684, 1688, 1692
   pathology 336
germ layer differentiation 8
German Society of Experimental and Clinical Pharmacology and Toxicology 1943
germander (*Teucrium* spp.), adverse effects 1427

Germany
BALs 1910, 1911
Biologische Bundesanstalt für
Land- und Forstwirtschaft
(BBA) 1607
CB agent threat 1724
chemical warfare 2079, 2080,
2100
classification and labelling 1477
MAK values 1483–4, 1594
nitrate and nitrite levels 2112,
2114, 2116, 2117, 2118, 2131,
2132
Technische Richtkonzentrationen
(TRK) values 1484, 1594
toxicology education 1943
germinal follicles 341
GESAMP (Working Group on the
Evaluation of Harmful Substances
Carried by Ships) 1310–11
gestation 23, 758–9, 1696
Gettler, Alexander O. 1490–1
GFR *see* glomerular filtration rate
GGTP *see* γ-glutamyl transpetidase
GH *see* growth hormone
Giemsa stain 341
Gila monster (*Heloderma horridum*;
H. suspectum) 2181–2
ginger paralysis 1824
glabrous skin 829, 830
glandular stomach 546, 556
glass fibre emissions 1293
glass for samples, contamination
from 1909
glaucoma 20, 757
glaucopsia 738
glazing agents 1653, 1985
glial cells 347, 631, 632, 634, 643
glial fibrillary acid protein 347
GLIM statistical program 301
glioma, *N*-nitroso compounds 2132
gliosis 631
GLOBAL dose–response computer
programs 1764, 1771
global revolutionary group 1728
globulins 253, 367, 368, 897
see also microglobulins
glomerular basement membrane
336
glomerular filtration 255–6, 257,
362, 428, 684, 686, 1462
glomerular function 72, 362
glomerular mesangial cells 183
glomerular permeability 363

glomerulonephritis, mercury-
induced 682
glomerulus 345, 363
*Glossary for Chemists of Terms used
in Toxicology* 1811–12
glove powder 510
gloves 510, 583
GLP *see* good laboratory practice
D-glucaric acid as biomarker 1865
glucocorticoid receptor-binding
protein 2066
glucocorticoids 187, 188, 1869
glucogenesis 283, 939
glucose
as biomarker 1861
conjugation 107
homeostasis 283
levels following CO_2 in rats 61
necrosis prevention 166
plasma measurements 365
uptake, organ of Corti 790
urine levels *see* glycosuria
glucose transporters 779
glucose-1-phosphate,
glucuronidation 106
glucose-6-phosphatase 383, 391,
868, 872
glucose-6-phosphate dehydrogenase
28, 159, 337, 344, 384, 2187
β-glucosidase 566, 571–2
glucosuria 683
see also glycosuria
glucuronic acid 18, 106, *107*, 111,
116, 132, 236, 371, 862, 1866
β-glucuronidase 272, 556, 568–9,
572, 1228
glucuronidation 98, 106–7, 114,
115, 255, 568
glucuronosyl-*S*-transferases (GST)
markers 135, 1866, 1891
glues 1961, 2029, 2036
glutamate 166, *1878*
glutamate dehydrogenase 356, 359,
1857
glutamate receptors 634
glutamine 106, *107*, 109
γ-glutamyl transferase (GGT) 107,
363, 1849, 1862, 2059
γ-glutamyl transpeptidase (GGTP)
43, 337, 344, 1255–6
γ-glutamylcysteinylglycine 107,
130
glutaredoxin (GRX) 160

glutathione
activities 255
and apoptosis 191
as biomarker 1842, 1848,
1862–3
biomarker 1842, 1843, 1891
circadian toxicology 257
conjugation 18, 98, 107, 116–17,
121, 130, 131, *134*, 1865
depletion 28, 158
metabolism and 104, 105
oxidative stress and 158
glutathione peroxidase 127, 158,
793, 1276, 1870
glutathione reductase 104, 729,
793, 1857, 1868–9, 1870
glutathione *S*-transferase
biomarker 1850, 1865, 1868,
1870
biotransformation 107, 115, 118
catalysis 130
clinical chemistry 359, 363
in epidemiology 1537–8
hepatotoxicity 871
interspecies extrapolation 279
pathology 344
pharmacogenetics 281
glutathione-protein mixed
disulphides 159
glutathione/GSSG ratio 191, 255,
1868–9
S-glutathionylation reactions 160
gluten-free products 1553
glyceraldehyde-3-phosphate
dehydrogenase 160, 1843
glycine 18, 109, 111
glycocholic acid, as biomarker
1858
glycogen 862, 1861
glycogen phosphorylase b 160
glycolysis 357, 939
glycoproteins, as biomarker 1856
glycosaminoglycan metabolism 758
glycosuria 332, 362, 679, 686, 689,
690, 1862
GM-CSF *see* granulocyte–
macrophage colony-stimulating
factor
GMOs *see* geneticaly modified
organisms
gnotobiotic animal studies 1645
goat *216*, 371, 579, 1515
Gobius criniger see goby, Pacific
goblet cells 545, 755, 1690

guidelines
  endocrine disrupting effects
    1400
  environmental 1763–4, 1770,
    1775
  harmonization 1636
  in vitro cytogenetic assays (UK)
    1081, 1083, 1084
  for testing 31, 1434–6
Guidelines for Testing of Chemicals
  37
guinea pig
  aflatoxin LD$_{50}$ 2154
  allergens 511
  aminophenol hydroxylation 110
  anaphylaxis 535
  arsenic metabolism 2050
  β-glucuronidase and β-
    glucosidase 572
  biliary excretion 555
  blepharospasm test *612, 613,*
    619, 620, 621, 623–4
  brain FMO 232
  breathing rate 46
  cancer studies in rubber industry
    2018
  chemical respiratory sensitization
    assessment 705–6
  cortisol as plasma maker 356
  CYP genes 216
  dermal studies 46
  developmental period 1696
  dioxin toxicity 85, 87, 282
  famciclovir conversion 239
  gastro-intestinal tract 544
  HDL fraction 367
  hepatocyte LD$_{50}$ for dioxin 284
  hepatotoxicity marker 359
  hypersensitivity reactions 340
  interspecies differences 274–5,
    283
  intravenous injection site 526
  LAA 511
  LD$_{50}$ intravenous dosing 525
  lens 242
  liver 872
  model for interferon testing 1971
  nerve agents 2091, 2093
  nitrate toxicity 2124
  nitrite toxicity 2127–8, 2135
  organic solvents 2041
  ototoxicity studies 776, *778,*
    783, 789, 792, 794
  pseudoeosinophils 385

repeated-dose studies 329
respiratory effects of sulphuric
  acid 1281
respiratory hypersensitivity 705
safety of biologicals 535
skin sensitization tests *841,* 842,
  1005
stratum corneum skin
  permeability *579*
T$_3$ and T$_4$ concentration 371
Gulf War 2081
Gulf War syndrome 28, 2096
Gulf War Veteran's Illness,
  Presidential Advisory Committee
  1729
gulls
  environmental endocrine effects
    1407
  herring 654
  laughing (*Latrus atricilla*),
    aberrational behaviour 1348
  PCBs in 642
gut *see* gastro-intestinal tract
Gutierrezia microcephala
  see broomweed

H

h-gate 639, 640
Ha-ras, and apoptosis 189
Haber rule 327, 1834–5
Haber–Weiss reaction 633
habitat 1328, 1407
habituation, in motor activity *652*
haem
  iron absorption 2065
  metabolism 2068
  synthesis 1863–4, 2056
haem oxygenase isozyme-1 2066
haemabsorbents 1734–5
haemagglutination 338
haemangiomas 1248
haemangiosarcoma 1533, 2015
haemapoietic system tumours 2019
haematochromatosis 869
haematocrit 364, 387
haematology 39, 62
  acute toxicity 39
  insecticide studies 2000
  in long-term toxicity studies
    331–2
  in repeated exposure studies 61,
    62, 63
  test abnormalities 389–96

haematopoiesis
  and apotosis 179, 191
  haematology 383–4, 391
  and hepatotoxicity 865
  pathology 336, 341
  pharmacogenetics 240
  radiation-induced changes 1684,
    1685, 1686, 1696
  signs of toxicity 43–4
haematopoietic stimulating factors
  1971
haematotoxicity
  adverse drug reactions 1427,
    1438
  benzene 1475
  lead 1475, 1513
  nitrobenezene 104
  organic solvents 2033, 2041
  pharmacogenetics 241
  rodenticide toxicity 1511
  snake venom 2179
haematoxylin staining 345
haematuria 43
haemochromatosis 902, 2065
haemocompatibility of medical
  devices 1735, 1741
haemoconcentration 357
haemodyalysis 941
haemoglobin (Hb)
  abnormal 384
  adducts, as indicators of exposure
    1457
  in antidotal studies 429
  biomarker 1845, 1879–80,
    1883–4, 1890, 1892–3
  carbon monoxide binding 430,
    1282, 1921
  and cardiotoxicity 821
  clinical chenistry 358, 364
  foetal 394
  genotyping 1890–1
  glycosylated 365
  in haematology 384, 387
  physiology 392
  Soret band 368
  synthesis, biomonitoring 1906
haemoglobinuria 367
haemolysis
  and alternative testing 410, 413
  clinical chemistry 357
  in haematology 383
  nitrobenzene effects 104
  oxidant effects 28
  test for synthetic materials 1741
haemolytic anaemia 384, *390,* 391

haemolytic jaundice 360
haemoperfusion 425, 724
haemorrhage
    alveolar 728
    brain 1217
    clinical chemistry 367
    conjunctival 742
    gastro-intestinal tract 132, 282,
        458
    kidney 344
    pericardial 807
    radiation-induced 1686, 1688
    subendocardial 814
    traumatic 539
haemorrhagic cystitis 1430
haemorrhagic pancreatic necrosis
    899
haemosiderosis 535
haemostasis 385
Hague Convention 2079
Hahnemann, Samuel 2
hair
    analysis 1496
    autopsy samples 1495
    biomonitoring 606, 1907
    contaminated 1355
    depigmented 1515
    elimination via 18, 72
    follicles 46, 256, 577, 830, 847
    and indoor air pollution 1300
    LAA 511
    loss 1511, 1515, 1519
    mercury levels 2059, 2060
    removal 46
hair cells, organ of Corti (HCs)
    776–8, 780, 782–7, 788–95
hair dyes and products 230, 1550
hair/beauty establishements
    see service industries
Halabja chemical war effects 2080
Haldane coefficient 393
half-life
    absorption 69
    as biomarker 1879
    biomonitoring 1905–6
    data in risk assessment 1780,
        1792
    elimination, calculation 86
    human studies 462
    interspecies 51
    reducing 97
    relationship to clearance 79–80
    scaling factors 1769
    short-range toxins 131
    terminal 77, 84

toxicokinetics 73–4
    using MRT 85
Haliaeetus leucocephalus see eagle,
    bald
Halichondria spp. *see* sponges,
    marine
Halley, Edward 1528
hallucinations from solvent abuse
    2029, 2036
halogen atoms, oxidation 101
Halotegon spp., nephrotoxicity
    1522
ham, nitrate and nitrite levels 2113
hamster
    see also Chinese hamster ovary
        (CHO) cells
    acetaminophen toxicity 110
    aflatoxin toxicity 2154
    aminophenol hydroxylation 110
    arsenic toxicity 2050, 2051
    brain FMO 232
    cadmium toxicity 2054
    cancer studies in plastics industry
        2019
    CYP genes 216
    developmental period 1696
    dioxin toxicity 85, 282
    gallium toxicity 2063
    gene mutation assay 24
    β-glucuronidase and β-
        glucosidase 572
    hepatotoxicity testing *417*
    indium toxicity 2063
    interspecies differences 274–5,
        283
    LAA 511
    laryngeal tumours 525
    lung culture *417*
    NAT enzymes 108
    nitrate toxicity 2126
    nitrite toxicity 2127
    NOS 2119
    ochratoxin toxicity 2160
    oestrogen effect on liver 284
    tamoxifen protection against
        hepatocarcinogenesis 284
hand
    percutaneous 577, 578, 583
    washing, and response to toxic
        agents 1417
Haplopappus heterophylus
    see goldenrod, rayless
haptens 705, 835–6
haptoglobin 254
hard metal 1904, 2063, 2064

hardeners, in plastics industry 2022
harm criterion 1812, 1829, 1830,
    1831
harmonization
    see also International Conference
        on Harmonization
    of classification systems 1478
    Council of Europe 1571
    of drug safety regulations 1426,
        1430, 1431–4, 1622
    European 1572, 1590, 1654
    guidelines 1636
    international 37–8, 55, 1611,
        1662
    Nordic Community 1572
    OECD 1572, 1612
    of pesticide regulations 1605,
        1611
    of regulatory issues 1546–7,
        1604, 1648–9
    of toxicological testing
        requirements 1567
Harmonized Electronic Dataset
    1480
harrassment, peripheral sensory
    irritant effects 615
hawk, red-tailed (*Buteo jamaicensis*)
    1342, 1355
HAZARD 1 Fire Hazard
    Assessment Method 1927
Hazard Communication Standard
    37, 1477
hazard index 312–13, *313*, 1787
hazard quotient 312, 1786–7
hazardous exposures, routes and
    nature 509–10
Hazardous Materials Transportation
    Act (USA) 37
Hazardous Substances Act (USA)
    37
Hazardous Substances Data Bank
    481, 1677
hazardous wastes, sites 669
hazards 1811–12
    acute 1338–44
    affected by physical agents
        1418–19
    analysis 27–9, 38, 1927
    anthropogenic 1328–30
    assessment 475
    classification and labelling 36–7,
        1476–8, 1610, 1675
    definition 34, 1449, 1811
    EU criteria 1486, 1557

hazards (*Contd.*)
  evaluation 554–7, 1318, 1332, 1415–24, 1449–50
  identification 314, 456, 1460, 1461, 1476–8, 1536–8, 1753–8
  impact severity 1960
  prediction, probabilistic methods 1328
  relationship to risk 1812
  risk assessment *1829*
Hb *see* haemoglobin
HBV *see* hepatitis B virus
HCs *see* hair cells, organ of Corti
HDL *see* high-density lipoprotein cholesterol
head
  male adult skin surface area *583*
  trauma 636
head-only exposure 46
headache 43, 454, 460, 515
headlice 460, 1995
headspace generation 594
health, vs survival 1961
health care workers
  biological hazards 1459
  cytotoxic material studies 515
  exposure to medical devices 1679
  laboratory hazards 510
  reproductive risks 463
health effects, planning 1832
Health Effects Assessment Summary Tables 1759
health guidance values, UK 1486
Health Industry Manufacturers Association (HIMA) 1743
health information systems 1661–2
health insurance, permitted/proscribed lists 1544–5
health products, toxicological effects 1552
Health Protection Branch, Health Canada 1659
Health Research Extension Act 487
health risk
  assessment 147–8, 1461–2
  assessment *see mainly* risk assessment
Health and Safety at Work Etc. Act 1974 (UK) 1481, 1545, 1547, 1595–6
Health and Safety Commission (UK) 1481, 1594, 1595

Health and Safety Executive (UK) 459, 1486, 1545, 1590, 1594, 1595, 1695, 1812
Health and Safety Guides (IPCS publications) 1571
Health and Safety Laboratory (UK) 1910
health and safety regulations 36–7
health status 1416, 1504–5, 1509–10, 1531
health supplements 1550, 1551, 1552, 1567
health surveillance 467, 1485–6
health surveys 461–4
healthy human volunteers 1546, 1547
healthy worker effect 1532, 1535
hearing loss 643, 655, 784, 785, 786, 787–95
hearing problems 130
heart 343
  see also cardiac; cardio-; coronary heart disease; myocardial; myocardium
  anatomy *804*, 805
  block 43
  blood, forensic sampling 1495, 1496, 1504
  clinical chemistry 365–7
  disease 1427, 1456, 1928
  embryology 803–4
  enzyme distribution 1857–8
  failure, congestive 285, 366, 808, 812
  left atrium 805
  left ventricle 343, 805
  muscle, biomarker 1848
  normal contraction 805–6
  NQO2 in 240
  oxidation in 103
  radiation-induced changes 1691
  rate, as biomarker 1855
  right atrium 805
  right ventricle 805, 814
  and taurine 361
  weights 336, 343
heat 1343, 1418–19
heat inducible genes 2066
heat shock 169, 196
  cognate protein 2066
  elements 2066–7
  factors (HSFs) 167, 2066
  proteins (hsp)
    and apoptosis 193

  as biomarkers 1842, 1848, 1869
  environmental enzyme toxicity 1395
  interspecies variation 281
  metal toxicity 2066–7
  molecular concepts 163, 167, 168, 169
heating appliances 1278, 1300
heating, ventilation and air conditioning (HVAC) systems 515, 1293–5, 1300
heavy metals 3, 58, 1712, 1848, 1868
  see also metals
HEDSET *see* Harmonized Electronic Dataset
Heinz bodies 384, 391, 393
HeLa cells 410, 2157
Helenium spp. *see* sneezeweeds
Helicobacter pylori infection 562
heliotrope (*Heliotropum* spp.) 133, 1519
hellebore
  false (*Veratrum*) 818
  false (*Veratrum californicum*), reproductive system toxicity 1521
Helly's fluid 345
Heloderma see Gila monster
helper T cells 341, 1704
Helsinki declaration on human experiment 1958
HEMASTIX reagent strip 495, 496
hemlock (*Conium maculatum*) 34, 1521
hen *see* chicken
henbane (*Hyoscyamus niger*), neurotoxicity 1521
Hep-G$_2$ cells, and apoptosis 191
hepatectomy, partial 284
hepatic, *see also* liver
hepatic angiosarcoma, adverse drug reaction 1430
hepatic circulation *see* liver, circulatory system
hepatic cytochrome P450 255, 272
hepatic injury *see* hepatotoxicity
hepatic microsomal oxidase 255
hepatic mixed function oxidase activity 58
hepatic monoesterase 1337, 1339, 1342, 1345
hepatic monooxygenase 1329, 1334
hepatitis 132, 236, 1427, 2064

hepatitis B (HBV) 274, 1100
hepatocarcinogenesis
  see also specific carcinogens, e.g.
    aflatoxins *in the Chemicals*
    Index
  aflatoxin B1 278
  biomarkers 1869
  circadian toxicology 259
  interspecies variation 271, 275
  oestrogen induced 284
  and parenteral toxicity 526
  protective clinical trials 278
hepatocarcinoma
  and aflatoxins 1538, 1982, 2145,
    2153–4
  aromatic amines 120
  benzopyrene 130
  diet effects 58
  epidemiological studies 274
  and mycotoxins 1883
  nitrites 2127
  and peroral toxicity 551
  pharmacogenetics 235, 240
  in plastics industry 2022
  rat and mouse 1127–9
  in rubber industry 2018
  in Thailand 278
  and vinyl chloride 1456, 1475,
    1538
hepatocellular hypertrophy 338
hepatocellular necrosis from snake
  venom 2180
hepatocytes
  in alternative testing 416, 418
  apoptosis *179, 180, 181–2,* 198
  biliary dysfunction *417*
  biomarkers 1843, 1862, 1880
  cadmium binding 2053
  calcium homeostasis and 156
  carbonic anhydrase III 160
  clinical chemistry 359
  damage marker 359
  DNA 275
  embryonic 865
  enzyme induction and 113
  functions 860–5
  gap junctions 854
  GST A1 induction 274
  hypertrophy 344
  incubation with tamoxifen 285
  and laboratory occupational
    toxicity 551
  modelling 306
  NOS and 2119
  organocytosis 183

peroxisome proliferation *417*
relationship to sinusoid and
  Kupffer cells *857*
structure 860, *861*
test system 407
in toxicological tests 271
hepatosomatic index 1870
hepatotoxicity
  see also liver
  acetaminophen (paracetamol)
    110, 113, 116–17, 1427
  activation of toxins 868–73
  acute 868
  adverse drug reactions 1427
  aflatoxins 274, 1516
  alkaloids 133
  biomarker 1842, 1843, 1845,
    1849, 1858, 1859, 1860, 1862,
    1887
  blue–green algae toxicity 1516
  bromobenzene 100, 118, 133
  carbon tetrachloride 16, 117–18
  and cardiotoxicity 810
  chloroform 111
  chronic, agents causing 877
  circadian toxicology 257
  clinical chemistry 358
  copper 2064
  death from 15
  dioxin 1818
  dose–response relationship 56
  ethanol 28, 199
  evaluation 1462
  food contamination 1825
  fumonisins 2164–6
  fungicides 2002
  haloalkanes 121
  hepatic enzyme inducers 135
  herbicides 2005
  in horses 1519
  in vitro test systems *417*
  isoniazid 119
  marker 359
  metabolism 133
  methanol 119
  neomycin 1455
  and nephrotoxicity 691
  nitrites 2126
  NSAIDs 132, 136
  nutrition effects on metabolism
    115
  OCs 1995
  oestrogen-induced 284
  organic solvents 2029, 2033,
    2035–6, 2037, 2039, 2041

PCBs 1554
and peroral toxicity 551, 552
pharmacogenetics 230–1, 239
phenacetin 103
phomopsins 2148
plasma enzyme assessment 355,
  361
predictability in animal tests
  1438
protection from *201*
radiation 1684, 1685, 1690, 1696
repeated exposure studies 56
signs 43
solvents 133–4
sporidesmins 2148
and time of dosing 16
toluene 1456
toxic changes 867–84
toxic plants 1519
white phosphorus 1511
herbicides
  aquatic toxicity 1313
  circadian toxicity 259
  domestic animal toxicity 1510,
    1511–12
  endocrine toxicity 990
  groups 1998, 2003, 2004–6
  and habitat quality 1328
  interspecies variation 281
  nestling studies 1349
  neurotoxicity 638
  pancreatic toxicity 927
  pulmonary toxicity 43
  in warfare 2105
hereditary effects from radiation
  1684, 1692, 1693–6
hereditary thymine-uraciluria 235
heritable chromosome assays 1086
heritable defects and genetic
  damage 1035–8, 1101
heritable translocation tests 1143
heron
  black-crowned night-herons
    (*Nycticorax nycricorax*) 1340
  great blue (*Ardea herodias*) 1329
Herpes simplex 836
herring gull 654
Hershberger assay 1403
heterochomatin 160
heterophils 385, 539
heterozygosity 234
HGMP *see* Human Genome
  Mapping Project (HGMP)
high-density lipoproteins (HDL)
  367, 1978

high-dose effects *see* maximum tolerated dose (MTD), evaluation of
high-dose testing 1434
high-explosive (HE) shells 2102
high-molecular-weight substances, characteristics 1966
high-pressure liquid chromatography (HPLC) 597, 712, 1455, 1491, 1500, 1862, 1882, 2158
high-production-volume (HPV) chemicals 1480, 1585, 1587, 1592
high-throughput screens 1401, 1402
high-toxicity laboratory 515
Hill criteria 1755–6
HIMA *see* Health Industry Manufacturers Association
hippocampal granule cells 638
hippocampal responses to ischaemia 168
Hippocrates 35, 460, 472, 1841, 1849
Hiroshima 1692, 1693, 1697
his genes 1042
histamine decarboxylase 344
histamine-like substances, release radiation-induced 1688
histidine 24, 764, *1878*, 1882, 1883
histidine genes *see his* genes
histiocytes 532
histochemistry 337–8
histology 39, 61, 64
histology technicians, exposure to chemicals 515
histones 160–1, 190, 1880
histopathology 331, 335–7, 531, 539, 1846, 1847, 1856
    eye irritation tests 746
historical aspects
    biotechnology 1963–4
    chemical exposures 1474
    occupational exposure limits 1482
    toxicology 1–4, 35–6, 1489–91, 1731–2, 1935–6, 1944
    warfare agents 2079–81
history (patient), risk assessment development 1750
HIV *see* human immunodeficiency virus
hives 510
HL-60 cells, and apoptosis 199
HLA *see* human leukocyte antigen

HLA-DPB1 as biomarker 2061
Hodgkin's disease 395, 1692
Hohenheim, P.A.T.B. von 36
holding rooms for animals 58
hole in the head disease 2163
holocytochrome *c* 165
Holy Fire 2148
home environment, effect on toxicity 1415, 1416, 1417–18
Home Office (UK) animal studies statistics 38, 53
homeopathy 2, 1451, 1550
homeostasis 34, 159, 192, 370, 1397–8
homicide 543
    see also poisoning, homicidal
homocysteine, CHD and 1979
homogeneity tests, standard operating procedure (SOP) 446
honey 1646, 1647, 1984
honeybee 2182
hoof abnormalities, selenium toxicity 1519
hormesis 1397, 1445, 1451–2, 1951–2
hormone assays 981–3
hormone replacement therapy 458, 1398
hormones 879, *981*, 1395
    see also individual hormones
hornet 2182
horse
    arsenic toxicity 1518
    common toxicoses 1517–20
    CYP genes 216
    encephalomalacia 2145
    fumonisin toxicity 2164
    gastro-intestinal problems 1519
    lead toxicity 1518
    leukoencephalomalacia 1520, 2163
    liver failure 1519
    mycotoxin toxicity 1516, 1520
    nervous system disorders 1519
    nitrate/nitrites 1519, 2122, 2123
    plant toxicity 1518–19
    snake bites 1517
    stratum corneum skin permeability *579*
    sudden death 1519
    T_3 and T_4 concentration 371
horseradish 134
horseradish peroxidases 103
horsetail, neurotoxic to horses 1519

hospital
    admissions due to toxic exposures 1444
    needs in CB attack 1729
host-cell derived proteins, as impurities 1968
house dust mites 1302
household products
    see also cleaning products *in Chemical Index*
    adverse effects 1450
    allergy 1704
    classification and labelling 1589, 1603–4
    domestic animal toxicity 1510, 1512
    human studies 464
    N-nitroso compounds 2115
    potentially hazardous 1443
    regulatory aspects 37
    risk assessment 1444
housing
    conditions 58
    as exposure factor 604
Howell–Jolly bodies 391
HPLC *see* high-pressure liquid chromatography (HPLC)
HPV *see* human papilloma virus
HSF *see* heat shock factors
hsp *see* heatshock proteins
human activity, and soil composition 1329
human chorionic gonadotophin assays 1465
Human Fertilisation and Embryology Act 1990 454
Human Genome Mapping Project (HGMP) 1090–2
human immunodeficiency virus (HIV) 159, 636, 814, 1957
human leukocyte antigen (HLA) 1037
human papilloma virus (HPV) 1100
human populations, immunotoxicity 1005–6
human studies 25, 453–70
    see also interspecies extrapolation
    acute toxicity testing 33, 38, 55
    aluminium toxicity 1379, 2060
    anaesthesia 104
    antidotal assessment 433
    and apoptosis 178
    aquatic toxicology 1310
    barbiturate metabolism 111

human studies (*Contd.*)
  behavioural toxicity testing 666–9
  breathing rate 46
  bufarolol toxicity 115
  cadmium toxicity 2053–4
  carcinogenicity, prediction from animal testing 1536–8
  case surveillance 458
  case–control studies 455, 458
  ceftizoxime clearance 89
  cohort studies 455
  combustion studies 1926–7
  cyanide toxicity 1923
  cytochrome P450 enzymes 99
  data evaluation 455–6
  data sources 456–7
  developmental period 1696
  dioxin toxicity 87, 88, 90
  DNA repair deficiency syndromes 1033–4, 1101
  dose–response relationship 1534
  dosimetric scaling in 147
  effect studies 465–7
  environmental endocrine toxicity 1399–400
  environmental toxicity 1328, 1376–81, 1530–1, 1534
  epidemiological studies 455
  epithelial cells, apoptosis 199
  ethics 1535
  ethylene glycol toxicity 55
  exposure assessment case study 1778
  exposure to toxicity test 605–7
  eye toxicity 759
  factors affecting metabolism 109–10
  food chain contamination 1373, 1375, 1376
  furan toxicity 90
  genetic factors 110, 111–12
  genome mapping 216–17, 1090–2
  harmonization problems 1567
  hazard evaluation 28–9
  hepatic enzyme inducers 135
  hydrogen cyanide toxicity 2101
  hypothesis testing 455
  indoor air contaminants 1292–3, 1294
  irritant or allergic dermatitis 838–40
  isoniazid toxicity 119–20
  justification 464–5
  kinetic behaviour prediction 147
  latency period 456
  Lewsite effect 2088–9
  male adult skin surface area 583
  mercury levels 2058
  metabolism 146, 466–7
  methanol toxicity 119
  methodology 1536
  monitoring of environmental mutagens 1090
  MPTP toxicity 132
  NAT enzymes 108
  nephropathy 2154, 2159
  nerve agents toxicity values 2091
  nitrate, nitrite and *N*-nitroso compounds 2115–18, 2121, 2122, 2123, 2129–31, 2133–5, 2136
  nitrates, endogenous synthesis 2119–20
  nitrogen dioxide exposure 51
  organic solvents toxicity 2033–4, 2037
  organophosphate toxicity 955
  organophosphates 955
  percutaneous absorption 580
  pharmacokinetic studies 466–7
  pharmacology clinical trials 1616
  protein content 1869
  PSI studies 622–3
  quantitative evaluation 456
  radiation toxicity 1686, 1693, 1696
  relevant data 572
  riot control agents 2013
  risk assessment 1449–50, 1755
  safety margin calculations 91
  stratum corneum skin permeability 579
  sulphur mustard vapour effects 2084
  surveillance schemes 456–7
  synthetic materials sensitization tests 1740
  tissue preparations for safety evaluations 135
  toxicity data 453–70
  weight 51
humane animal research 493–501
humectants 1985
humidity 16, 58, 1419
humus 1367, 1368
Huntington's disease 166, 634, 636
Huskvarna, chronic renal disease 1428
Hussein, Sadam 1723, 1726
HVAC systems *see* heating, ventilation and air conditioning systems
hyaline droplets 63, 64, 691
hyberbaric oxygen therapy 1921
hybrid site-specific proteins 1966
hybridoma technology 1454, 1966
  see also biotechnology industries
Hydra attenuata 414, 1187
hydration 98, 105
hydrocarbon nuclear translocator protein 163
hydrocephalus 1217
hydrocortisone *see* cortisol
hydrogen bonds 613–14, 1369
hydrogen peroxidase 633
hydrogen peroxide 127, 1867, 1868
hydrological cycle 1370
hydrolysis 17, 98, 105, 110, 216, 254, 255, 523, 550
hydrophilic and hydrophobic species 547
hydroxybutyrate dehydrogenase, as biomarker 1860
17-hydroxycorticosteroid, as biomarker 1865
6β-hydroxycortisol, as biomarker 1865, 1867
hydroxyl radical 127
hydroxylation 100–2, 110, 112, 115, 221, 225, 226, 229, 230, 231, 240, 272, 273, 277
hydroxyproline, as biomarker 1859
20β-hydroxysteroid dehydrogenase 241
5-hydroxytryptamine 222, 236, 547, 632, 641, 706, 730, 815, 834, 956-7, 1960, 2039
Hydrozoa 2190
hygienic research 2013
hymenoptera 2182–5
Hymenoxys spp. *see* bitterweed
Hyoscamus niger see henbane
hyothalamic–pituitary–gonadal axis, assay 1403
hyper-responders 294
hyperactivity 41, 1986
  see also attention disorders
hyperaemia, in human subject PSI 623
hypercalcaemia, ECG/EKG profile *806*

hypercarbia 765
hypercholesterolaemia 823, 1978
hyperestrogeneism 2145
hypergastrinaemia 1125, 1126
hyperglycaemia, and adverse drug reactions 142
Hypericum perforatum see St John's wort
hyperinsulinaemia 815
hyperkalaemia 532
hyperlipidaemia 358, 364, 815, 1427
hypernatraemia 364
hyperosmia in IEI 1708
hyperoxia 724, 728, 764, 765
hyperparathyroidism 900, 949–50
hyperplasia 556
hyperpnoea 41
hyperproteinaemia 367
hypersensitivity reactions
    acute toxicity 41
    in eye 20
    immunotoxicity 1004–5
    myocarditis 807
    systemic pulmonary toxicity 726, 729
    to cosmetics 1550
    to drugs 21
    to snake venom 2180–1
    type I 510
    type IV 510
hypersusceptible (hyperreactive) groups 9, 12, 14, 1831, 1833, 1835
hypertension 21, 264, 822, 823, 1216
hyperthermia 6, 40, *522*
    see also heat
hyperthyroidism 948–9
hypertonia 40, 41
hypertrophy 685
hyperventilation 1709, 1713, 1714
hypervitaminosis A 969, 972
hypnotics *536*, 1491, 1495
hypoactivity 41
hypocalcaemia 365, 530
hypocarbia 1709
hypochlorhydria 562
hypochondria 1709, 1711
hypogammaglobulinaemia 562
hypoglossus nucleus 642
hypoglycaemia 283, 365, 458, *806*, 982
hypoglycaemic drugs *220*, 228, 365
hypokalaemia 1430

hypokalaemic myopathy 940, 941, 945
hypolipidaemic agents 367, 368, 920, 922, 1978
hypomagnesaemia 683, 940
hyponatraemia 364
hypophosphataemia 940
hypopnoea 40
hypoproteinaemias 367
hyposusceptible (hyporeactive) groups 9
hypotension 944
hypothalamic–pituitary–endocrine axis *369*, 1400
hypothalamic–pituitary–ovarian axis 372, 1147–8, 1151
hypothalamic–pituitary–testicular axis 371, 1140–1
hypothalamic-releasing hormones 981
hypothalamus 251, 346, 347, *369*
hypothermia 40, *522*
    see also heat
hypotheses in toxicology 1939
hypothyroidism 949, 950
hypotonia 40, 41
hypovolaemic shock 822
hypoxaemia 26, 56, 1920
hypoxanthine-guanine phosphoribosyl transferase (HGPRT) 24
hypoxia 6, 168, 808, 969, 1216, 1920

I

I-bands 938
Ia antigen 340
IAP, and apoptosis 195
IARC *see* International Agency for Research on Cancer
IATA *see* International Air Transport Association
iatrogenic disease 938, 1446
ICAD, and apoptosis 195
ICAO *see* International Civil Aviation Organization
ICE *see* interleukin-1-converting enzyme
ICH *see* International Conference on Harmonization
ichthyootoxic fish 2191
ichthypsarcotoxic fish 2191
ICRP *see* International Commission on Radiological Protection

ICSH *see* interstital cell stimulating hormone
icterus 360
ID$_{50}$ 34–5, 52, 1876–7
idiopathic environmental illness (IEI) 1703–20
    aetiological theories 1704–7
    as behavioural phenomenon 1707–9
    evaluation and diagnosis 1711–13
    as illness belief system 1710–11
    as misdiagnosed illness 1709–10
    prevalence 1704
    research recommendations 1715–16
    social and political implications 1716–17
    treatment 1713–15
idiosyncratic reactions 4, 21, 1416, 1549
IEI *see* idiopathic environmental illness
IFN *see* interferon
Ig *see* immunoglobulin
IH *see* inhibition concentration
Iito (fat storing/stellate) cells 864–5
IL *see* interleukin
IL-2 gene expression 191
ileum 562
illness belief system, IEI as 1710–11
ILO *see* International Labour Organization
ILSI *see* International Life Sciences Institute
imaging systems 1661
imidazole *N*-methyltransferase *216*
immediate-type allergic reactions 704
immersion fixation 339
immune haemolytic anaemia 1438
immune sensitization test for synthetic materials 1740
immune system 997, *998*
    cell mechanisms 998–1001
    cell-mediated responses 126
    compromised 1416
    cytokines 1001–3
    detecting changes 1969
    disorders, 5-HT inhibitors 1960
    functions, biomarker 1849
    immature 1337
    long-term effects 1446
    modulation 409

immune system (*Contd.*)
  related parameters 1008, 1009
  type 2 responses 710
immune-complex-type
  glomerulonephritis 682
immune-mediated reactions 6–7,
  19, 23, 178
immuno-allergic reactions 1444
immunoassays 367, 371, 514, 1491,
  1500–2
  see also enzyme-linked
    immunosorbent assay; enzyme-
    multiplied immunoassay
    technique
immunobiology, respiratory
  sensitization to chemicals 702–13
immunochemical analysis,
  macromolecular adduct 1885–7
immunocytochemistry 336, 338,
  339, 340, 342
immunoelectrophoresis 368
immunoenzymometric methods 365
immunogenicity 1964, 1967
immunogens 1302
immunoglobulins
  biomarker 1848
  Ig 999
  IgA 868
  IgE 510, 512, 682, 702–4, 705,
    999, 1004
  IgG 682, 1004
  IgM 1004
  and neonatal immunity 549
immunohistochemistry 237, 239,
  342
immunoinhibition methods 366
immunological testing, in IEI 1713
immunological theories, of
  idiopathic environmental
    intolerance
    aetiology 1704–5
immunoradiometric assays (IRMAs)
  983
immunosuppression 7, 85, 389,
  1003–4
  biomarkers 1862
  and carcinogenesis 1130, 1131
  fumonisins 2165
  haematotoxicity 389
  mycotoxins 1516
  myopathies 946, 948
  nephrotoxicity 684–5
  repercussions 7
  toxicokinetics 85
immunosurveillance 8

immunotherapy 428, 1967–8, 2184
immunotoxicology 997–1016
  animal studies 1005, 1006–9
  biomarkers 1875
  dioxin 87
  in human populations 1005–6
  hypersensitivity 1004–5
  immunosuppression 1003–4
  in vitro studies 1009–10, 1012
  molecular 1011–12
  ochratoxins 2160
  organometallic compounds 2001
  procedures 1967–8, 1974
  risk assessment 1756
  testing 1448
  wastes 1827–8
implant 60, 530, 1731, 1741
  see also medical device
implantation 539, 1464
imposex, molluscs 1407
impurities, importance in toxicology
  1445–6
in situ hybridization 239, 345
in vitro diagnostic devices 1661,
  1667
in vitro fertilization, legal
  restrictions 1547
in vitro studies 52–3, 401–24, 453,
  1449
  acute toxicity 52–3
  developmental toxicity 1184,
    1186–7, 1188, 1247
  genetic toxicology 1039–58
  haemolysis test for synthetic
    materials 1741
  human studies 453
  immunotoxicology 1009–10,
    1012
  in vivo correlations 1438
  metabolic activation 1039–41
  ototoxic effect of salicylates 786
  percutaneous absorption 580
  skin irritation and sensitization
    845–7
  toxokinetics 67
  UK guidelines 1081, 1083, 1084
in vivo studies
  design 44–5
  in vitro correlations 1438
  limitations *404*
  percutaneous absorption 579–80
  rationale *404*
inborn errors 234, 2049
incinerator emissions 606, 1776,
  1780

increased capillary fragility 385
indentation tonometry 749
independent effects of mixed
  chemicals 20
independent expert advice 1544,
  1562, 1578, 1638, 1658
independent joint action 304
index of exposure 128
Index Medicus 473, 478
indexing 474
India
  ancient writings 1489
  childhood cirrhosis 2064
  fumonisin contamination of
    cereals 2165
Indian cobra venom 820
indicative limits, EU 1595
indigenous compounds 1890
indigestion, in laboratory workers
  515
individual response 8, 135–6, 1708
indoor air, pollution 626
indoor air contaminants 1291–307
  building improvement plans
    1304
  gases 1296–8, 1303
  human health 1292–3, *1294*
  microbial 1303
  and outdoor (I/O) concentrations
    1291–2, 1295
  outdoor sources 1293
  particulates 1298–302, 1303
  sampling and characterization
    1302–3
  sick building syndrome (SBS)
    1292, 1299
  sources 1293–6
induction pathway 189
induction pathway *see mainly*
  enzyme induction
inductive period, skin sensitivity
  835
industrial accidents 737, 1547,
  1818–21, 1830
Industrial Bio-Test 437
industrial chemicals
  classification and labelling 1545,
    1551
  notification 1545
  occupational hazards 1550
  OECD inititatives 1571
  product information 1456
  as raw materials 1549, 1550
  regulatory aspects 1550–1,
    1581–90

industrial chemicals (*Contd.*)
  EU 1556–7, 1590–6
  Japan 1545, 1564
  UK 1595–6
  USA 1545
  reproductive toxicity 1111,
    1139–40, 1146, 1156, 1465
  risk assessment and management
    1460–1
  safe working practices 1545,
    1551
  sperm evaluation studies 1467
  spillages 1551
  toxicological testing 1545, 1551
  workplace exposure limits 1545,
    1551
industrial effluents/emissions
  environmental oestrogen effects
    1565
  field study evaluation 1352
  and habitat quality 1328
  Japanese experience 1564
  treatment processes 1565
  wildlife toxicity 1339, 1343
industrial hygiene data, IEI 1712
industrial hygienist 1458, 1530
industrial products, risk assessment
  1444
industrial safety regulations 1960
industrial site evaluation 1772,
  1792
industrial toxicology
  see occupational toxicology
industrialized areas, pollution 316
industry, environmental effects
  1328, 1373–4
Industry Health and Safety Law
  1972 (Japan) 1565
infared thermography 844
infections 814, 2133
inferior olive nucleus 642
infinite dose situation 582
inflammatory agents, NOS induction
  2120
inflammatory bowel disease 900
inflammatory mediators 1705,
  1715–16
inflammatory response
  and apoptosis 196
  avoidance 176
  as biomarker 1843, 1855
  cellular effects 126
  chronopathology 263
  circadian toxicology 263
  definition 6

dose–response relationship 9
eye 20
  and idiopathic environmental
    intolerance 1705–6
  local effect 19
  molecular concepts 169
  and necrosis 164, 177
  pathology 340, 343
  peripheral sensory irritation 611
  skin 837
  to Lewisite 2089
  to sulphur mustard 2085
influenza virus, biomarker 1849
influenza-like syndrome from PTFE
  1915
information resources 471–83
  see also databases
information sharing 1959
information sources, safety
  assessment 1675–7
infradian frequency 251
infrared spectroscopy 597, 712
infusion techniques 522, 527–8
ingestion
  see also peroral
  of contaminated food and water
    1339
  standard assumptions 1773
  workplace exposures 1474
inhalable fraction 461, 592
inhalant abuse 2029, 2038
inhalation 20
  acute toxicity 46
  aerosol container closure systems
    1737
  cadmium 2052, 2053
  CB agents 1724
  chamber 46
  dosing 432, 523
  exposure route 59, 60, 604,
    1474, 1504
  extrapolation from oral data 148,
    1832
  gases, mortality data 1834–5
  hydrogen cyanide *2101*
  lead 2055
  mercury 2058
  metabolites formed during
    exposure 148
  of mixtures 21
  nickel 2063
  nitrogen dioxide 51
  organic solvents 2029
  PBPK modelling 145, 1768

and peripheral sensory irritation
  623
risk assessment 461
risks 1773, 1780
testing
  determination of LC_{50} 49
  interpretation of results 26
toxicology 20, 46, 588–601
vs percutaneous route 19
xenobiotics 1339
inherited cancer genes 1101
inherited somatic mutations 1538
inhibin B, as biomarker 1858
inhibition 305
  concentration (IH) 1312
  factor 584
initiator(s) 566, 2023
initiator, -promoter scheme 7
injection
  fever 537
  site, carcinogenesis 1130–1
  subcutaneous 523
  technique 526–7
injury without warning, peripheral
  sensory irritation 615–16
innervation 545–6
innovatory products, definition
  1623
inotropic effects 805, 808, 816, 818
Insecticide Act 1910 (USA) 1599
insecticides 2, 259, 460, 524, 641,
  824, 1994–2000
  *see also individual compounds in
    Chemical Index*
  biological origin 1999–2000
  biomonitoring 1902
  cardiotoxicity 824
  circadian toxicology 259
  domestic animal toxicity 1510
  effects 651
  and environmental toxicology 2
  in food chain 1826
  forensic analysis 1491
  human studies 460
  and invertebrate food base 1328
  mammalian selectivity ratio
    (MSR) 1547
  metabolism 101
  molecular interactions 163
  neurotoxicity 43, 641
  parenteral toxicity 524
  placental toxicity 1242–5
  poultry toxicity 1523

insecticides (*Contd.*)
  species sensitivity differences
    110
  time course of effects 1956
  wildlife toxicity 1341
insects 38, 111, 178, 462, 1994,
  1999–2000, 2182–4
insertion sequences 1027
Institute of Occupational Health
  (Finland) 1910
Institution of Chemical Engineers,
  hazard definition 1811
institutional animal care and use
  committee 487, 501–3
institutional review board 454
instrumentation, forensic toxicology
  1491
insulin 346, 458, 522, 527, 530,
  982, 991, 1455, 1965, 1966,
  1969-70
  see also diabetogenic substances
insurance risk tables 1749
integrated field and laboratory
  studies 1354–5
Integrated Risk Information System
  (IRIS) 1759
Integrated Uptake and Exposure
  Biokinetic Model 1769
integrin, as calpain substrate
  189–90
integumentary signs of toxicity 40
intellectual property rights 1569
interaction factor 313
interactive effects
  chemicals within cells 158
  drugs *see* under drugs
  mixed chemicals 20, 305,
    306–13
  PBPK modelling 148–9
  toxic 1342–3
  zero response surfaces *310*
Interagency Coordinating
  Committee on the Validation of
  Alternative Methods 411
intercalcated discs 804, 813
interferons (IFN) 115, 703, 710–*11*,
  999, 1002, 1455
intergeneric microorganisms 1584
Intergovernmental Forum on
  Chemical Safety 1592
interindividual *see* intraspecies
interlaboratory testing 16, 49, 626
interleukin-1 converting enzyme
  (ICE), and apoptosis 194, 195

interleukins 185, 1972
  after exposure to TMA *711*
  as biomarkers 1869
  in IEI 1704, 1706
  IL-1 265, 533, 722, 729, 864,
    1000, 1001, 1002, 1012
  IL-2 265, 266, 341, 999, 1002,
    1012
  IL-3 999, *1002*
  IL-4 682, 703, 999, 1000, 1002
  IL-5 703, 999, 1002, 1012
  IL-6 703, 864, 999, 1002, 1276
  IL-7 1002
  IL-8 1002
  IL-10 703, 999
  IL-12 999
  IL-13 703, 999
intermediate cells, cochlea 779
intermediate syndrome 426, 1996,
  1997
internal dose *see* ID$_{50}$
Internation Chemical Safety Cards
  1571
International Agency for Research
  on Cancer (IARC) 1104–6, 1383,
  1434, 1537, 1571
International Air Transport
  Association (IATA) Restricted
  Articles Regulations 37
International Association of
  Forensic Toxicologists 1491
International Civil Aviation
  Organization (ICAO) 37
International Commission on
  Radiological Protection (ICRP)
  1684
International Conference on
  Harmonization (ICH)
  data collection 1436
  genotoxicity testing 1039
  guidelines 1138, 1169, 1430,
    1434–5, 1436, 1439, 1627,
    1630
  medical devices 1662, 1667
  pharmaceutical safety testing 2,
    1426, 1430, 1622
  registration 1546–7
  Safety Working Group Consensus
    Regarding New Drug
    Applications 40
international copyright law 475
International Council for Laboratory
  Animal Science 486

International Court of Justice 1572
International Covenant on Civil and
  Political Rights 453–4
International Environmental
  Information System
  (INFOTERRA) 1571–2
international estimated daily intake
  for the European diet (IEDI) 1609
International Federation of
  Pharmaceutical Manufacturers
  Associations (IFPMA) 1431
International Labour Organization
  (ILO) 476, 482
International Life Sciences Institute
  (ILSI) 1106
international normalized ratio (INR)
  229
International Organization for
  Standardization (ISO) 461, 536,
  538, 592
  exposure assessment 461
  extracts of solids 538
  inhalable fraction 592
  ISO 10993 testing standards
    1670
  medical device testing 1668–71
  medical devices guidelines 536,
    1662, 1733–7, 1738, 1742,
    1743, 1744
international organizations,
  regulatory powers 1569–72
international periodicals directories
  475
International Programme on
  Chemical Safety (IPCS) 459,
  1452, 1570, 1571, 1592, 1612,
  1659, 1703, 1759
  see also Environmental Health
    Criteria
International Register of Potentially
  Toxic Chemicals (IRPTC) 1571
international regulation 1648–9
International System for Human
  Cytogenetic Nomenclature (ISCN)
  1083
International Uniform Chemicals
  Information Database 481
International Workshop on
  Immunotoxicology and
  Immunotoxicity of Metals 1009
Internet 53, 477, 482, 1723, 1759,
  1947
internodal pathways 850

interspecies extrapolation 147,
271–90, 1435–7, 1447–8, 1449,
1461, 1754–5, 1763, 1769
see also interspecies variability
acute toxicity 28, 51, 55
agrochemical toxicity 25
allometric scaling 51
appropriateness 1754–5
arsenic toxicity 2052
carcinogenicity 1536
chronic high dose studies 80–90
dioxin body burden 88
dose–response assessments
1758–9, 1760, 1763
dosimetric scaling 147
environmental endocrine toxicity
1391, 1392–3
in vitro tests 53
inter-route 147–8, 1766
legal matters 1952
low-dose risk 90–1
mathematical modelling 1941
mycotoxin data 2148
nitrate/nitrite toxicity data 2136
occupational toxicity 1461
organic solvents 2041–2
PBPK modelling 51–2, 607,
1767–9, 1771
and prediction 1534
problems 430
radiation data 1694, 1695
regulatory aspects 1430–1, 1574,
1575
repeated exposure studies 59
risk assessment 1447–8, 1449
role of toxicokinetics 67
safety evaluations and 135
therapeutic protein testing 1967
interspecies variability
see also interspecies
extrapolation
acute toxicity 45, 50–2
adducts *275*
AITC 134
cadmium toxicity 2054
clinical chemistry 371
dioxin toxicity 282
disaster studies 1834
domestic animals 1509
dose adjustment 147, 1758
erythrocyte fragility test 1741
haematology 385
immunogenicity 1964
metabolism and 110–11
in metabolism of tamoxifen 285

MPTP susceptibility 132
negligible risk and 90
prenatal toxicity 282
peripheral sensory irritation 626
safety margin calculations 91, 92
study design 135, 322
testicular atrophy 82–3
uncertainty factors 1760
interstital cell stimulating hormone
(ICSH) 987
interstitial fibrosis *727*, 807
interstitial oedema 722
interstitial pneumonitis *727*
interstitial pulmonary fibrosis 315
intertest comparability 1352
intervention studies, methodology
1534
intestine
see also gastro-intestinal
absorption 69, 88
bacterial metabolism, dietary
modification *573*
biomarkers *1879*
blood flow 252
crypt cells, apoptosis 179
epithelium 197, 337, 524, 548,
1684
half-life extension 556
hydrolysis 523
mouse dermal toxicity test 605
mucins 561
mucosa 368, 547, 568
peroxidases 103
segments, interspecies
extrapolation 555
toxicity 556
villi 545, 554, 1687, 1689, 1690
intolerance 4, 21
INTOX system 459
intoxication, definition 1445–6
Intra-agency Regulatory
Alternatives Group 411
intra-alveolar oedema 732
intra-arterial route 527
intracellular fluid 70
intracerebral route 47, 524, 527,
641, 644
intracerebroventricular route 527,
528
intracranial pressure, raised 1427
intracutaneous route, local reaction
538–9
intracutaneous testing, synthetic
materials 1741
intradermal techniques 841, 842

intragastric route, varying LD_{50} 525
intraluminal instillation 525
intramembranal bone 966
intramuscular myodegeneration 522
intramuscular route 523, 526–7,
531–2
intramuscular route of exposure 19,
47, 55
intramuscular toxicity 412
intramyelinic oedema *638*, 639
intraocular pressure 496, 614,
748–9, *749*, *750*
intraocular tissue, medical devices
toxicity testing 1741
intraperitoneal route
activity promotion 532
acute toxicity 47
animal dechlorination reactions
566
bioavailability 533
in carcinogenicity studies 525
LD_{50} 525, 534
liver change 533
neonatal mouse 525–6
neurotoxicity 642
parenteral toxicity 523, 526,
532–3
synthetic materials 1739–40
visceral penetration risk 526
intrapleural route 525, 527
intrapulmonary injection, lung
squamous cell carcinoma 525
intraspecies variability
acute toxicity 45
AhR differences 1892
biochemical 1509
disaster studies 1834
DNA repair 1892
dose–response assessments 1760
extrapolation by *in vitro* testing
53
genetic polymorphism 1890
similarities and differences in
acute testing 50–2
tools to examine 135
intrathecal route 527
intratracheal route 432
intrauterine contraceptive devices
1674
intrauterine development 8
intrauterine growth retardation
(IUGR) 1219, 1254–7, 1696
intrauterine position effects 1406
intravascular injection, distribution
and 70

intravenous route
    acute toxicity 47
    alternative testing 412
    artefacts and alterations 529–30
    by injection 526
    by osmotic minipump 528
    in carcinogenicity studies 525
    comparison with oral data 75
    distribution and 70, 78
    guidelines 523
    nausea and vomiting 524
    and plasma clearance calculation 79
    repeated exposure 55, 59
    solution bags 1737
    statistical moment analysis 85
intravitreal route 644
intrinsic toxicity 523–4
inulin as marker 1972
invertebrates 38, 1327, 1328, 1349, 1355
    see also specific invertebrates
investigation brochure (IB) 1623
investigational device exemption (IDE) 1662, 1663
Investigational New Animal Drugs Application (INAD) (USA) 1634
Investigational New Drug Application (IND) 1546, 1615
iodotyrosine 1868
ions
    exchange–adsorption reactions 1366
    transport 754, 779, 784–7, 790, 807, 938–9, 1843
    transporters 189–90
ion channels 777
    neurotoxins 639–40
ionization 1683
ionized molecules, absorption 69
ionizing radiation 464, 1154, 1464, 1465
ionotropic effects 43
IORT treatment for radiation injury 1689
IPCS see International Programme on Chemical Safety
IQ 566
Iran–Iraq chemical warfare 2080
Iraq 1249, 1726–7, 1825–6, 2080
iris, injury 741, 745
Irish Republican Army 1727, 1730
iritis 40, 41, 742–3
IRMAs see immunoradiometric assays

irradiation see radiation
irrigation, and soil salinization 1371
irritant dermatitis 832–4, 838–40
irritants 40, 1455, 1475
    see also eye; lung; mucous membrane; peripheral sensory; respiratory tract; skin
    acute toxicity 40
    airborne toxicants 1487, 1828
    chemical warfare 2080
    effects 56
    fires 1821
    medical devices 1734, 1735, 1740–1
    occupational toxicity 1455, 1475
    testing 839
      see also eye irritation testing
    vapours 589–90
irritation
    see also eye; lung; mucous membrane; peripheral sensory; respiratory tract; skin
    cumulative 60
    definition 611
    lung or skin 1474
    peripheral sensory (PSI) 23, 611–30
    primary 23
    testing 25
irritative/corrosive effects 1475
ischaemia
    clinical chemistry 364
    hippocampal responses 168
    myocardial 805, 815
    nephrotoxicity 681, 684
    NMDA 166
    pathology 343
    reperfusion 158
    stria vascularis 785, 786
ISCN see International System for Human Cytogenetic Nomenclature
Islamic extremists 1722
ISO see International Organization for Standardization
isoboles 307–11, *309*
isobolograms 311, 312
isocitrate dehydrogenase *356*, 939
isoelectric focusing 752
isoenzymes 355, 363
isoleukotrienes 896
isomers 115
isoniazid-type inducer 113
isopleths 1833, *1835*, 1836

isoprostanes 896
Israel, deliberate food poisoning 1724
itai-itai disease 1373, 1564, 2053
Italy
    fumonisin contamination of cereals 2165
    nitrate and nitrite levels 2112, 2114, 2116, 2130, 2131
Iva augatifolia see sumpweed

J

J-receptor 615
Japan
    see also Matsumoto; Minamata; Tokyo
    cosmetics regulation 1550
    deliberate food poisoning 1724
    drug regulation 1428, 1430, 1544, 1565–7
    environmental pollution by industrial chemicals 1547
    food production regulation 1567–8
    foreign manufacturing approvals 1566
    functional foods regulation 1552, 1567–8
    government ministries 438
    industrial chemicals regulation 1545, 1564
    marketing authorization 1566
    mercury-exposed pregnant women 1249
    nitrate levels 2114
    N-nitroso compounds levels 2133
    post-war radiation exposure 1035
    pre-manufacturing notification 1565
    regulatory processes 1554–5, 1564–8, 1649
    reproductive toxicological testing 1567
    sarin gas attack see under sarin
    Tokyo subway sarin gas attack 955
jaundice
    acute toxicity 41
    from food contamination 1825
    from NSAIDs 132
    and hepatic necrosis 1426, 1427

jaundice (*Contd.*)
   human studies 460
   predictability in anaimal tests
      1438
jaw 577, *578*
jawbone necrosis, white phosphorus
   1475
jay, blue (*Cyanocitta cristata*) 1338
JECFA *see* Joint Expert Committee
   on Food Additives
jejunal absorption 69
jellyfish 2189–90
   lion's mane 2190
jet lag 252
jimsonweed (*Datura stramonium*)
   1521, 2165
Jinzu River, cadmium toxicity 2053
JMPR *see* Joint Meeting on
   Pesticide Residues
jogger's dilemma 665
Johns Hopkins Center for
   Alternatives to Animal Testing
   504
Joiner vs General Electric 1949
Joint Expert Committee on Food
   Additives (JECFA) 3, 1570, 1636,
   1643, 1648–9, 1657, 1659, 1984
Joint Meeting on Pesticide Residues
   (JMPR) 3, 462, 1570, 1611–12,
   1649
judges in toxicological cases 1949,
   1950–1
jugular vein 357, 386, 545
Jun protein 240
jun-kinase 195
junk science 1946–7, 1949
juries 1946, 1950–1
juvenile hormone analogues
   1999–2000
juxtaglomerular apparatus 345
juxtamedullary nephrons 676

K

kainate receptor 636
kale (*Brassica* spp.)
   as antioxidants 1984
   cardiovascular effects 1522
   nitrate and nitrite levels 2112–13
   pharmacogenetics 234
Kamikuishiki sarin production 1726
kangaroo rat (*Dipodomys* sp.) 1347
Kaposi's sarcoma 814
karyolysis 821
karyorrhexis 821

Kefaufer–Harris amendment, Food,
   Drug and Cosmetics Act 1938
   (USA) 1562
keratin, arsenic in 2050–1, 2052
keratinization 828
keratinized stratified squamous
   epithelium 544
keratinocytes
   and cutaneous toxicity 828, 830,
      831, 847
   life cycle 179
   necrosis 748
   UV radiation and 167
keratitis 742–3, 744
keratohyalin 828
keratonus 742
keratopathy 756, 757
Keshan disease 823, 2065
kestrel, American 1345, 1348,
   1349, 1350
keto group, reduction 104
ketone reductase 242
6-ketoprostaglandin F$_1$,
   biomonitoring 1910
kidney
   see also nephrotoxicity; renal
   aminoglycoside elimination 789
   autopsy samples 1495
   biomonitoring 1905, 1906, 1910
   cancer 135, 241, 1032, 2018
      see also kidney, tumours
   clinical chemistry 361–4
   column of Bertin 675
   concentration ability 362
   congestion 344
   damage *see* nephrotoxicity
   DCVC 167
   diuretic action site 785
   dysfunction, as biomarker 1849,
      1859, 1860, 1861–2
   electrolyte balance 366
   enlargement, and food additives
      1985
   enzymes
      biomarkers 1861–2
      microsomal 107
      peroxidases 103
      sulphation 105
   erythropoietin 384
   excretion 18, 255–6
      biochemistry 129
      blood flow in neonates 83
      clearance calculation 80
      plasma clearance and 79
      sulphonamide 129

   and toxicity 21
   toxicokinetics 72
   failure 900, 940, 941
   FMO expression 232
   function 678–80
      assessment 1861
   GGT marker 359
   haemorrhage 344
   hyaline droplet 64
   injury 680–92, 1462
   in metabolism 254
   metal binding 128
   metanephric 414
   neonatal glomerular filtration rate
      1228
   optimal drug timing 261
   pathology 344
   PBPK studies 89, *90*, 144
   and reductive stress 168
   renin cells 340
   structure and function 675–8
   as target organ 43
   taurine 361, 1862
   transplantation 900
   transplants, HPLC 1862
   tubular cells 56, 183
   tumours
      in firefighters 1928
      fungicides 2002
      ochratoxins 2159
      in plastics industry 2022
   weight 336, 344, 1861
KIMS *see* kinetic interaction
   microparticles in solution
kinases 190, *216*
kindling, limbic, in IEI 1706
kinetic interaction microparticles in
   solution (KIMS) assay 1502
kinetics
   see also pharmacokinetics;
      toxicokinetics
   biomonitoring 1905–6
   dose-dependent 83–5
   flip-flop 75
   Michaelis–Menten 84
   transition 1890
   variation in biomonitoring
      1908–9
Kings Cross fire 1822–3
kinins 361, 675, 834
Klebsiella pneumoniae 1278
Kluyveromyces marxianus 2149
knock-down agents 2080

knowledge-based system,
Estimation and Assessment of
Substance Exposure (EASE)
1479
Kochia scoporia, hepatoxicity 1519
Koch's postulates 1952
kohlrabi, nitrate levels 2113
Kosteve, Vladimir 1727
Koupparis, Panos 1724–5
Krebs cycle *see* tricarboxylic acid
cycle
krill *see Euphausiids*
Kruskal–Wallis one-way ANOVA
300
Kupffer cells 200, 274, 385, *857*,
858, 862, 864, 873, 881
Kurbegovic, Muharem 1725
Kussmaul sign 40
kwashiorkor 823, 897, 903, 910
see also protein deficiency
kyphosis 41

L

L929 cells *410*
L5178Y mutation test 1434
LAA *see* laboratory animal allergy
labelling *see* classification and
labelling
laboratory
accreditation 492–3
animals *see* animal welfare and
animal studies
animals, allergy to 511–14, 516
practice
see also interlaboratory
ethical aspects 1958
reproducibility of results 1893
samples, sources of error 1911
toxicology 3
studies
animal behavioour 1346
forensic 1489
reproductive behaviour
1347–8
workers
and congenital malformation
510
latex allergy 510
Laboratory Animal Technician
certification (US) 492
Laboratory Animal Welfare Act
(US) 1966 486
lachrymation
and accidents 8

acute toxicity 40, 41
as allergic response 512
from nerve gas 605
grading 742–3
peripheral sensory irritation 614
reflexes 755
lactate dehydrogenase (LDH)
acute toxicity 43
assays 1462
in BALF, dose–response
assessment 1762
biomarker 1848, 1858, 1859,
1860, 1861, 1862
cardiotoxicity 806
clinical chemistry 355–6, 359,
366
isoenzymes 366, 372
pathology 343
and wildlife toxicity 1345
lactation 23, 340, 1548, 1549
lactic acid producing bacteria (LAB)
571–2
lactic acidosis 126, 1430, 1438
lactic aciduria 679, 1862
Lactobacillus 562
lactoferrin 897
lactoperoxidase 103
lactotrophic hormone (prolactin)
980
Lactrodectus mactans see black
widow spider
lag phase prior to absorption 69, 75
Lake Nyos disaster 1817
LAL test 537
lamb's lettuce, nitrate levels 2113
lambsquarters (*Chenopodium* spp.),
nephrotoxicity 1522
laminar flow cabinets 515
laminin, mustard gas and 2085
lamins, and apoptosis 190, 195
land-use planning 1831, 1832, 1836
Langerhans cells 340, 828, 830,
835, 991
lanolin 835, 836
Lantata camara, hepatotoxicity
1519
lapilli 1815, 1816
large intestine
microflora 562–4, *564*
modelling 556
mucosal oxidases 571
predominant organism
identification 563
rate of transfer 69

Larus argentatus 654
laryngeal nerve, peripheral sensory
iritation stimulation 619
larynx
cancer 1456, 1982, 2132
granulomas 27
mouse dermal toxicity test 605
laser Doppler flowmetry 845
last measured concentration 79
late asthmatic response 510
latency period 1531
latency to toxicity 5, 6
before tumour appearance 64
and LD_{50} 15
phosgene-induced 2098
radiation-induced 1692
repeated exposures 56, 63
risk assessment and 1755
skin absorption 1778
lateral cisternae system, outer hair
cells 786, 787
lateral plasma menbrane, outer hair
cells 786
lateralization technique, in human
subject PSI 623
latex industry 2018
lathyrism 634
Lathyrus sativas 634
Latrus atricilla see gull, laughing
laundromats 1216, 1226
lauric acid 12-hydroxylase *217*
lava 1815, 1816
Law 44, Chemical Substances
Control Law, (Japan) 1565
law, *see also* legal aspects of
toxicology
law enforcement, use of toxic
chemicals 1547
LC *see* Langerhans cells
LC_{50} (median lethal concentration)
13
acute toxicity 36
age effects 1337
alternative testing 407
aquatic toxicity 1312, 1313,
1315
caution/reproducibilty 1337
choosing 48
combustion studies 1926, 1927
data for modelling 1834
defining 46, 49
determination 49
mixtures 317
nitrogen dioxide 51
repeated exposure toxicity 55

leukaemia (*Contd.*)
  nitrates 2124
  organic solvents 2037
  and parental occupational
    exposure 1465
  plastics industry 2020
  radiation 1464, 1692, 1693,
    1695, 1697
  rubber industry 2015, 2018
  toxicology 395
leukaemogenesis 395
leukocytes 384–5, 833
  acetylation enzymes 108
  biomarkers 1845, 1880, 1892
  clinical chemistry 362–3
  count 61, 387, 388
  and cutaneous toxicity 833
  DNA 1882, 1885, 1886, 1891
  parameters 388
  and parenteral toxicity 533
  pathology 341
leukocytosis 389
leukoencephalopathy, radiation-
  induced 1691
leukopenia 235, 389, 394, 2089
leukotrienes 702, 845, 1981
  role in respiratory damage from
    fires 1917
Leydig cells 371, 987–8, 1464,
  1859
LH *see* luteinizing hormone
Li–Fraumeni syndrome 1031–2
liability 1948, 1959
libido 1142, 1146, 1154–5
Libya, chemical warfare 2080–1
licences 1543
licensing, UK 1546
Licensing Authority (UK) 1559,
  1627
lichen planus, civatte bodies 175
lichenification of epidermis 835
life span 1769, 1773
ligand exchange 1369
ligand-protein theory 34
light microscopy 781, 782, 951,
  952
light-induced cutaneous toxicity
  836–7
lightning, risk of death 1830
lily-of-the-valley (*Convalaria* spp.),
  cardiovascular effects 1522
lima beans, toxicity 1984
Limanda limanda see dab, North
  Sea
limb explants 967

limbic kindling in IEI 1706
limit of detection (LOD) 1781–2
limit tests 44, 45
Limited Announcements, New
  Substances Notification Scheme
  1590
limits of detection 1563
Limulus spp.
  amoebocyte lysate test 53, 413,
    537
  L. polyphemus 537
line transect sampling 1353
linoleic acid deficiency, effect on
  metabolism 115
lionfish 2191
lipaemia 357
lipases 156, 347, 356, 365, 897
lipid(s)
  barrier 69
  clinical chemistry 361, 365, 367,
    370
  damage 104, 128
  deficiency, effect on metabolism
    115
  lowering drugs 1124
  metabolism 868–9, 939
  pathology 355
  peroxidation 6
    biochemistry 127, 136
    as biomarker 1848, 1867
    and carbon tetrachloride
      toxicity 118
    in cardiotoxicity 807, 808,
      809
    in cartilage and bone toxicity
      872
    in cutaneous toxicity 837
    in eye toxicity 757
    and gastro-intestinal
      microflora 570
    human placenta 1246
    induction 167
    in nephrotoxicity 687
    ochratoxin and 2162
    pharmacogenetics 158, 237,
      240
  solubility 69, 71, 143
  as targets 34
  tests 359
  theory of inhalation anaesthetics
    2030
lipid hydroperoxides 6, 158, 1866
lipid peroxidase 764
lipofuscin 867
lipophilic pathway 581

lipophilicity 131, 581
lipoproteins 815, 868–9
liposomes 570
lipoxygenases 158, 159
lipstick 606
liquid chromatography 1500
liquid formulations, toxicity 1338
liquid scintillation counting 534
liquids, assessing chemicals in
  1777–8
Lisa ramada 1870
Listeria monocytogenes 1007
literature for expert witness 1947
literature review, tier testing *403*
litter, non-contact absorbent 514
liver
  see also hepatic, hepato-
  acetylation enzymes 108
  adrenal hormone action 370
  alcohol dehydrogenase 242
  alcoholic disease 236
  amine oxidase (AO) 238
  anatomy and physiology 853–9,
    860–5
  apoptosis 132, 198
  autopsy specimens 1495, 1496
  azoreduction 564
  bile acids 567
  bioavailability alteration 555
  biomarkers *1879*
  biomonitoring 1905
  blood flow 254, 2033
  cancer *see* hepatocarcinoma
  carbonyl reductase 242
  cell, *see also* hepatocyte
  cell nuclei
    accumulation of Ca^{2+} 187–8
    peroxisome proliferator 2022
    regeneration 126
  cholinesterase 368
  circadian blood flow 254
  circulatory system 545, 548,
    552, 556, 853–4, *855*, 856, *858*,
    859
  cirrhosis *see* cirrhosis
  clearance/excretion assays 1462
  clinical chemistry 358–61
  cytochrome P450 99, 218, 274,
    277
  cytosol enzyme reduction 104
  damage *see* hepatoxicity
  dechlorination reactions 566
  detoxification 19, 344
  development 865–6
  dioxin accumulation 88

liver (*Contd.*)
  disease
    apoptosis in 175
    effect on metabolism 114–15
    and forensic testing 1504–5
    porphyria 29
  ducts 545
  dysfunction and injury 1462
  enlargement 880–1, 1986
  enzyme induction 135, 910–11
  enzymes 98
    biomarker 1843
    biotransformation 98
    distribution 1857
    excereration 21, 1462
    following carbon tetrachloride 1857, *1858*
    hydration 105
    induction 135, 910–11
    reduction 104
    sulphation 105
    systems 550
  erythropoietin 384
  failure 943
  fatty 1862, 1863
  FMO expression 232
  forensic toxicology 1504
  function tests 359
  gene product excretion 217–18
  glucuronide conjugate formation 556
  glutathione conjugation 107
  haemopoiesis 383
  half-life extension 556
  innervation 854
  Kupffer cells 103, 385
  mercury uptake 2058
  metabolic function 70, 148, 254, 272
  microsomes 107, 111, 274, 285
  mitochondrial enzymes 103
  mitoinhibitory pathways 126
  morphometry 339
  necrosis 6, 102, 281, 360, 361, 1430
  nodules 565
  normal adaptive changes 866–7
  NQO 240
  oxidative stress 912
  parenchymaal organization 855–9
  PBPK studies 89–90
  perfusion, furan 90
  pesticide residue accumulation 1343
  pharmacokinetic analysis 284
  portal exposure 603
  remodelling 880–1
  substance activation in 19
  as target organ 43, 131
  taurine 1862
  as tissue compartment in PBPK 144
  tissue in mutagenicity tests 1039–41
  toxicity *see* hepatotoxicity
  for toxicokinetic modelling 307
  transplant 884
  tumours
    see also hepatocarcinoma
    diet effects 58
    dioxin 88
    food additives and 1986
    fungicides 2002
    ochratoxins 2159
    and peroxisome proliferators 7
    plastics industry 2019, 2020–1, 2022, 2023
    rubber industry 2015, 2016, 2018
    vinyl chloride 1771
  vulnerable to xenobiotics 1462
  weight 336, 344, 1859
  xenobiotic metabolism 1339
liver fluke (*Fasciola hepatica*) 882, 2119
liver pate, nitrate and nitrite levels 2113
liver sausage, nitrate and nitrite levels 2113
lizards
  acute testing 1353
  green anole (*Anolis carolinenis*) 1330–1
  venomous 2181–2
LLNA *see* local lymph node assay
LMS *see* multistage model, linearized version
LMW5-HL, and apoptosis 194
Loa loa control 1999
loading dose 88
LOAEL *see* lowest observed adverse effect level
lobbies for anti-vivisection 36
Lobelia spp. *see* wild tobacco
lobster studies 820

local anaesthetics *see* anaesthesia/ anaesthesia/anaesthetic agents, local
local effects 5
local lymph node assay (LLNA) 708, 842–3, 1005, 1009, 1010
local tolerance studies 1616–17, 1628
lock and key receptor–ligand model 1397
locoweed, neurotoxic to horses 1519
LOD *see* limit of detection
Loewe additivity 304
log-normal distribution 47
log-probit plot 10, 12, 13, 48, 431
logistic function 49
logit analysis 49, 1331–2
Lonchocarpus utilis 1999
London principles report 1756
London smog 1265, 1268–9
long-term carcinogenicity studies 1618–19
long-term effects 1446, 1451
long-term toxicity studies, Good Laboratory Practice (GLP) 440
loop of Henle 345, 363, 675, 785
Los Angeles
  CB agent threat 1724, 1725
  smog 1265–6, 1275, 1278
Lotus corniculatus see birdsfoot trefoil
Lotus tetragonolobus 345
Louis-Bar syndrome *see* ataxia telangiectasia
Love Canal (USA) disaster 1372, 1827–8
low birth weight 1464, 1465
low linear energy transfer 1683
low volume eye test (LVET) 739
low-density lipoproteins (LDL) 367, 1978
low-dose effects 1397, 1404, 1451–2, 1460, 1563
  see also hormesis
lowest observed adverse effect level (LOAEL) 57, 60, 1180, 1181, 1483, 1759–60, 1787
Loxosceles spiders 2186–7
LS cells *410*
LT_{50} 13, 1314
luncheon meat, nitrate, nitrite and *N*-nitroso levels 2113, 2120

lung

see also pulmonary

ADLH in 237

cancer

β-carotene and 1983

biomarkers 1880, 1892

deaths, estimates 1751

in firefighters 1928, 1929

and formaldehyde 1456

from dioxin 88

interspecies variation 278

mechanistic data 224–5

miners 1538

nickel 2063

nitrates 2131

occupational toxicology 1474

organic solvents 2042

and organohalides 1457

pharmacogenetics 223–5, 241

phenotypes and 1891

phenotyping studies 224

radiation-induced 260

radon exposure 1293

and silicosis 1457

in smokers, polymorphisms
and 135

and smoking 1529, 1538

carbonyl reductase 242

cells, regeneration 126

chromium absorption 2062

circadian blood flow 254

congestion 342

culture *417*

cytokines 728

damage *see* lung, toxicity

embolism 731

enzyme hydration 105

fibrosis 722

function studies *see* ventilatory
capacity

immersion fixation 342

lead absorption 2058

lipid peroxidation 315

metabolism 254

mouse dermal toxicity test 605

necrosis and vasculitis 281

NQO2 in 240

oedema 342, 726

oxidative injury 722

pathology, LDH in BALF and
1762

PBPK studies 89–90

perfusion fixation 342

peroxidases 103

pleural effusions 342

tissue, biomarkers 1880, 1885

toxicity

acute 56

adverse drug reaction 1430

alkaloids 133

arsenic 2051

asbestos 1475

assessment 722–3

biochemistry 132

biomarkers 1858

cadmium 1475

herbicides 2004

inhalation 20, 46, 1814, 1819,
1828

injury sites 722

lead 1474

miners 1827

mustard gas 2086

nerve agents 2091, 2096–100

nitrites 2126

organ selectivity mechanisms
721

organic solvents 2032

PCBs 131

phosgene 2098

primary 26

radiation 1684, 1685, 1690,
1695

signs 43

sites 722

smoke 1821

systemic 721–36

warfare agents 2082

weight, dose–response
assessment 1762

lupin (*Lupinus* spp.) 1519, 1521,
2148

lupinosis 2145, 2148–9

Lupinus spp. *see* lupin

lupus syndrome, acetylation status
and 112

luteinizing hormone (LH) 163, 266,
369, 371, 986–7, 1141, 1147,
1151, 1155, 1351

luteinizing releasing hormone
(LRH) *369*

Lycium spp. *see* matrimony vine

lymph 549, 552

lymph nodes 341, 710, *711*

assay, synthetic materials testing
1740

lymphadenitis 514

lymphadenopathy 534

lymphangiomas 1248

lymphatic drainage, liver *854*

lymphatic system 40, 341, 547,
548–9, 1694

lympho-haematopoietic cancers in
firefighters 1928, 1929

lymphocytes 998–1000

and apoptosis 196

counts following CO_2 in rats 61

cytogenetics 515, 1082

haemtology 385

pharmacogenetics 235

radiation-induced changes 1685,
1686, *1687*

lymphocytolysis 525

lymphocytopaenia, and food
additives 1987

lymphoedema 230

lymphoid cells, apoptosis 179

lymphoid follicle aggregates 549

lymphoid germinal centres, tingible
bodies in 175

lymphoid sheaths, morphometric
analysis 341

lymphoid tissue 341

lymphoid tumours, nitrites 2126,
2135

lymphokine-activated killer cells
343

lymphoma

mouse dermal toxicity test 605

murine B-cell, and apoptosis 198

in plastics industry 2019, 2022

in rubber industry 2015

statistical analysis 296

lymphopenia 389–90

lymphosarcoma, in rubber industry
2015

lysine *1878*

lysophospholipid (PAF) 896

lysosomes

in cutaneous toxicity 833

enzyme release 177

in eye toxicity 757

liver 860, *861*, 862, 864, 869–70

membrane stability 1317

in nephrotoxicity 685

in pancreatic juice 894, 897

pathology 340

lysozyme 340, 2053

M

M cells 344, 549

m-gate 639

MAb techniques *see* monoclonal
antibody techniques

mackerel 2193
macrocytosis 391
α2μ-macroglobulin 367
macromolecular adducts 128, 1460, 1877–82
  biochemistry 128
  as biomarkers 1461, 1877–82
  biomonitoring 1904
  formation 1457, 1460
  immunochemical methods of analysis 1885–7
  occupational toxicity 1460
  physical methods of analysis 1882–5
macromolecular reaction products 1877
macromolecular synthesis 1964, 1965–6
macromolecules 127–8, 549
macrophage inflammatory protein-1α 729
macrophages
  and apoptosis 199, 200
  biomarker 1843, 1855
  in cutaneous toxicity 829
  foamy 1978
  haematology 385
  in immunotoxicology 997, 998, 999, 1000–1
  in inflammation 126
  in neurotoxicology 632
  NOS and 2119
  pathology 343
  phagocytosis by 183
  in systemic pulmonary toxicity 731
macular oedema 756
Magendie 36, 1935
maggots 1495, 1496
magma 1815
magnesium 635
magnetic resonance imaging (MRI) 496, 756, 941
magnocellular reticular nuclei 232
Magnusson–Kligman maximization test 1591
magpie, black-billed magpie (*Pica pica*) 1342, 1355
Maimonides, Moses 35, 472
major histocompatibility complex (MHC)
  class II 999, 1000, 1001
  genotype 215
  in immunotoxicology 997, 998
  in neurotoxicology 632

MAK *see* Maximale Arbeitskonzentrationen Commisssion
malaria 460, 944, 1994, 2000
male-mediated teratogenicity 1185
malformations
  see also congenital malfromations; mutagenicity; teratogenicity
  adverse drug reaction 1465
  cogenital 510, 1219–22, 1419, 1697, 2041
  in laboratory workers 510
  and nitrates 2129
  and occupational exposures 1465
  radiation-induced 1696
  and selenium 1351
  selenomethione 1354
malignant carcinoid syndrome 815
malignant melanoma, treatment 1964
malingering 1911
mallard (*Anas platyrhynchos*)
  avian embryo bioassay 1334
  behavioural studies 1346, 1348
  dermal exposure to pesticides 1331, 1339
  dose–response anomalies 1330
  as model species 1329
  organophosphorus toxicity 1337
  pesticide toxicity 1335–6, 1339
  reproduction tests 1350, 1351
  secondary toxicity 1342
  sodium cyanide toxicity 1331
  subacute toxicity testing 1332, 1333–4
Mallory bodies 867
Mallory Heidenhaim stain 64
malnutrition 562
mamba 2178
mammalian cells 196, 1684
mammalian mutation tests 1051–6, 1058–61
mammalian selectivity ratio (MSR), insecticides 1547
mammals
  see also specific mammals
  acute toxicity studies 38, 1329
  adenocarcinomas, diet effects 58
  and apoptosis 178
  biomarkers 1858, 1866, 1867, 1869
  biotechnology 1965–6
  comparative toxicology 1334–5

endogenous synthesis of nitrates 2118–19
genotoxicity 128
GI system, radiation-induced changes 1687
glands peroxidases 103
herbicide toxicity 2006
N-nitroso compounds toxicity 2132
palate development 179
phenol metabolism 111
reproductive system radiation-induced changes 1684, 1688
reproductive toxicity studies 1185
weight 51
mammary ducts 340
mammary epithelial cells 278
mammary gland 340–1
mammoplasty 279
Man with 21 Faces, The 1724
man *see* humans
Manchester Airport crash 1821–2
mania 263
manic-depressive patients 523
Mann–Whitney U test 300
mannosamine, and apoptosis 183
Mantel–Haentzel procedure 1960–1
manufacturers, responsibilities 1480
manufacturing industries
  see also industrial/y radiofrequency radiation 1418–19
manufacturing procedures, for biopharmaceutics 1972–3
manufacturing workers, exposure to medical devices 1679
manure, decomposition 1455
MAO *see* monoamine oxidase
MAPP kinase pathway 163
Marascuilo and McSweeney test 300
Margin of Exposure (MOE) 1602
margin of safety 11
marginal cells, cochlea 779
Marine Environment Research Laboratory (MERL) 1318
marine sponges (*Halichondria* spp.) 817
mark–recapture methods 1353, 1354
marker residue, residue depletion studies 1646
market basket approach 1646

marketing authorization
EU procedures 1544, 1622,
1623–7
Japan 1566
'need' clause 1568–9
renewals and variations 1629–30
responsibilities of holder 1625,
1629
UK procedures 1627
marketing of toxicologist 1947
Markov, Georgi 1727
marmoset monkey
see under monkey
Marsh test, arsenic 1490
masculinization in women 862
mass intoxication 1445
mass median aerodynamic diameter
(MMAD) 20, 1762
mass median diameter (MMD)
1281
mass spectrometry 1500, 1501
in forensic toxicology 1491
of macromolecular adducts
1882, 1883, 1885, 1889
mass transfer 582
mass-transfer coefficients 582
mast cells
in alternative testing 412
in cutaneous toxicity 829, 830,
833
function, nitrites and 2128
hyperplasia radiation-induced
1690
in immunotoxicity 997, 1000
in nephrotoxicity 702, 706
in respiratory sensitization 707
Master of Science requirements
1938, 1939
Master testing List (MTA), US EPA
1585
MAT *see* mean absorption time
matching, comparison group 1533
MATCs *see* maximum acceptable
toxicant concentrations
Material Safety Data Sheet (MSDS)
37, 516, 833, 1448–9, 1459, 1478,
1712
maternal acidosis 1189
maternal toxicity
and childhood tumours 1465
developmental effects 758–9
drug levels in breast milk
1225–6
factors influencing transplacental
transfer 1241–2

in mouse inhalation study 604
risk assessment 1754
mathematical modelling 581, 1451,
1461, 1563, 1575
matrimony vine (*Lycium* spp.),
neurotoxicity 1521
matrix attachment regions 189
Matsumoto, sarin incident 1721,
1723, 1726, 1729
Maximale Arbeitskonzentrationen
Commission (MAK) 1477, 1482,
1483–4, 1485, 1594
maximally exposed individual
(MEI) 1775
maximally tolerated does (MTD)
1619
maximization patch method,
synthetic materials testing 1740
maximum acceptable toxicant
oncentrations (MATCs) 1316
maximum allowable concentrations
(MAC) 1482
maximum contamination limits
(MCL) 1784, 1790
maximum exposure limit (MEL)
(UK) 1484, 1594
maximum feasible dose, in dose
selection 1620
maximum lifespan potential (MLP)
89
maximum likelihood method 44
maximum residue level (MRL) 3,
1563, 1570, 1574, 1603, 1609,
1610, 1611, 1639–40
animal testing 1643
establishing 1647–8
EU regulation 1641–3
existing drugs 164
fish 1646, 1647
pesticides 1993
pollutants 3
practicability 1646
regulatory aspects 1563, 1570,
1574, 1603, 1609, 1610, 1611,
1639–40
toxicity testing 1643, 1644
maximum safe concentration,
residues 1635
maximum tolerated dose (MTD)
carcinogenicity 1106–7
chronic studies 65
definition 1755
epidemiology 1535
evaluation of 1110–11
PBPK modelling 148

repeated exposure 60
subchronic studies 62
Mayo Clinic 815
maze techniques 657
MCF-7 breast cancer cell assay
1402
McKone's model 582
MCL *see* maximum contamination
limits
mcl-1, and apoptosis 193
McNemar's test 301
MCV *see* mean corpuscular volume
McVeigh, Timothy 1722
MDCK cells *410*
mean absorption time (MAT) 75
mean cell volume 387
mean corpuscular haemoglobin
content (MCHC) 387
mean corpuscular volume (MCV)
389
mean residence time (MRT) 75,
84–5
meat
and cancer 1981, 1982
cooked 274
cured/processed 2113, 2114,
2116, 2118, 2132
dioxin 281
fried 566
ingestion, risk from 1772
nitrate and nitrite levels 2113,
2114, 2115, 2116, 2117, 2118,
2127, 2132
PAHs 1791
radioactivity 1821
raw, inspection 1637
red, drug residues 1647
Meat Inspection Act (USA) 1563
meat wrapper allergy 1915
mechanoreceptors 661
mechanotransduction 776
media involvement 1576
median effective concentration
see EC_{50}
median effective dose *see* ED_{50}
median effective time *see* ET_{50}
median eminence 347
median lethal concentration
see LC_{50}
median lethal dose *see* LD_{50}
median lethal molar concentration
49
median lethal time *see* LT_{50}
median response 12

mediastinitis from peroral exposure 19
Medicaid 458
Medical and Biologic Effects of Environmental Pollutants 1676
Medical Device Amendment 1976 (USA) 1662, 1663, 1733
medical devices
  American National Standards Insitute (ANSI) 1662
  biocompatibility 1666, 1670, 1672, 1738–42
  biological testing 1668
  chemical characterization 1742–3
  classification 1666, 1667–8, 1671–2, 1734–7
  combination product 1733
  definition 1661, 1732–3
  direct contact 1732–3
  duration of contact 1734
  external 1735
  finished product 1733
  fraudulent 1662
  Good Laboratory Practice 1664
  guidelines 1733–7
  historical aspects 1662, 1733–4
  implantable 1732, 1735
  implantation tests 539
  indirect contact 1733
  International Commission on Harmonization 1662, 1667
  materials and components 1672–3, 1731
  non-implantable 1732
  parenteral toxicity 523, 538
  potential toxicity 1643
  premarketing procedures 1663–4, 1737–8
  public perception 1674
  raw materials 1672–3
  regulatory aspects 1548–9, 1562, 1661–81
    EU 1671–2
    US 1662–5
  risk assessment 1743–6
  sterilization 1667, 1668, 1679–80, 1740
  surface 1735
  target organ toxicity 1734
  testing 1672–80
    International Standards Organizations (ISO) 1662
    ISO 1668–71
    needs 1734–8

United States Pharmacopeia 1668, 1669
  toxicity testing 1665–72
  toxicology 1731–47
  uses and abuses 1672
  vs drug 1733
medical ethics *see* ethical issues
medical evaluation, postplacement periodic 513–14
medical examinations 462
Medical Examiner's Office, New York 1490
medical industries, radiofrequency radiation 1418–19
Medical Literature Analysis and Retrieval System (MEDLARS) 478
medical planning 1837
medical practice, cultural factors 1558, 1567
medical products 522
Medical Research Council (UK) 454
Medical Research Council Ethics Series 1958
medical screening, in the workplace 1460
medical and surgical supplies 1661, 1667
medical surveillance 462, 1460
medical toxicology 1443, 1444–5, 1447, 1452
Medicines Act 1968 (UK) 1425, 1546, 1627, 1637, 1638
Medicines Act Leaflet, MAL 4 1622
Medicines Commission (UK) 1425
Medicines Control Agency (UK) 458, 1425, 1436, 1578, 1627, 1638
MediConf 473
MEDLARS *see* Medical Literature Analysis and Retrieval System
Medline 1676–7, 1943, 1947
medulla 546
medulla oblongata 347
megakaryocytes 385, 395
'megalin' receptor 791
mehrotoxicity, lead 2056
MEI *see* maximally exposed individual
meiosis 40, 41, 605
MEL *see* maximum exposure limit
melanin 129
melanocytes 779, 830
melanogenesis 779

melanomas 837
melanosome 830
melatonin 163
melon, nitrate and nitrite levels 2112–13
membrane
  ion pumps 126–7
  permeability 252
  phospholipids, methylation 896
  receptors 163
membranous labyrinth 775
Memorandum of Understanding, Dow Corning Corporation 1585
memory disturbances in IEI 1707
memory search 667
Menière's disease 787
meningitis, and adverse drug reactions 1427
Menkes disease 2064
menstrual function 234, 251, 340, 830, 1148–9, 1463, 1464, 1465
mental health needs in CB attack 1729
mental retardation radiation-induced 1696, 1697
mentors in toxicology 1937, 1939, 1942
mephenytoin 4′-hydroxylase *217*
mephenytoin, metabolic pathways *225–6*
β-mercaptopyruvate sulphur transferase 428
Merck Index 222, 1677
MERL *see* Marine Environment Research Laboratory
Merrell Dow Pharmaceuticals 1948–9
mescal beans (*Sophora* spp.), neurotoxicity 1520, 1521
mesenchymal cells 340, 804
mesenchymal induction 968–9
MeSH (Medical Subject Heading) 480
Mesobuthus tamulus see scorpion, red
mesocosm *see* controlled field study
mesoscale models 1781
mesothelioma 1131, 2017
MEST *see* mouse ear swelling test
meta-analysis 1456–7
metabolic acidosis 2040
metabolic activation 17, 18, 52, 56, 130–5, 545, 1039–41, 1056
metabolic clearance calculation 80
metabolic constants 145–6

metabolic inhibitors 870
metabolic phenotyping 112, 265
metabolic poisons 604, 807
metabolic polymorphisms, and
  cancer 1538
metabolic rates 72–3, 357
metabolic retroversion 234
metabolic theory of idiopathic
  environmental intolerance
  aetiology 1705
metabolism 67, 74–5
  see also biotransformation;
    inborn errors of metabolism;
    kinetics; toxicokinetics
  affecting biological activity 97
  bacterial 72
  biomarkers of susceptibility
    1850, 1877
  in biomonitoring 461
  BPK modelling and 148
  definition 72
  dose-dependent kinetics and 83
  of drugs 21, 22
  effects 21, 65
  enzyme-catalysed 73
  extent 73
  factors affecting 109–15
  first-pass 22, 69–70, 73, 523
  incomplete absorption and 70
  inhibition 114
  intermediary 92, 98, 159
  interspecies differences 85
  major reactions 98
  mixed routes of exposure 606,
    607
  molecular concepts 157–8
  in multiple route exposure 606
  pharmacogenetics 215
  phase 1 reactions 98–105, 110,
    115
  phase 2 reaction 105–9, 110–11,
    115
  and plasma clearance 79
  products 97
  reducing excretion 98
  in repeated exposure studies 56
  saturation 85
  scaling factors 1769
  studies 24
metabolites
  as biomarkers 607
  biomonitoring 1906, 1907
  relationship with macromolecular
    adducts 1878, 1879
  sigma minus method and 86

toxic 429, 1329
  ethical issues 1956–7
  toxicokinetics 72
metal smelters, and plant metal
  concentrations 1373
metal storage diseases 902
metal workers, risks 1463, 1474
metal-based compounds, toxic-
  therapeutic ratio 260–1
metallothionein 1848, 1869, 1870,
  2053, 2054, 2059, 2067
metals
  see also heavy metals
  biocompatibility testing 1738
  cardiotoxicity 822
  chelation 1985
  fume fever 2066
  fungal extraction from soil 1369
  hepatotoxicity 822, 870
  immunotoxicity 1004
  indestructibility 1366
  medical devices 1734
  occupational exposures 1463
  placental toxicity 1245–6
  teratogenicity and embryotoxicity
    1203–9
metamorphosis, and apoptosis 178
metaphase analysis 1085, 1088
metaphysis 342, 966
metastatic mineralization 969
methaemoglobin 15, 384, 392-3,
  428, 432, 565, 572, 2120, 2123,
  2125–6, 2129, 2131, 2135, 2136
methaemoglobin reductase 392
methaemoglobinaemia
  in acute toxicity 28
  adverse drug reaction 1430
  antidotal studies 429
  biochemistry 127
  compounds producing 393
  drinking water toxicity 1383
  effect 392
  and fire intoxication 1920
  and gastro-intestinal microflora
    565, 572
  haematotoxicity 391, 392
  herbicide toxicity 2005
  hydrogen cyanide toxicity 2102
  insecticide toxicity 2000
  in neonates, food additives and
    1989
  and nitrate-accumulating plants
    1522
  nitrobenzene toxicity 104
  spectrophotometry 393

methaemoglobinuria 384
5-methyl hydroxylation 227
methylation 18, 98, 109, 896, 2050
methyltransferases 109
MFO system see mixed function
  oxidase system
Mg^{2+}-ATPase 341
MHC see major histocompatibility
  complex
MIC_{50} 1645
mic, biomarker 1849
Michaelis constant 146
Michaelis–Menten kinetics 84, 90,
  145, 305
micro-organisms, pathogenic, in
  sewage sludge 1372
microalgae 1310, 1314, 1318,
  1319–20
  see also micro-organisms
microbial, see also micro-organisms
Microbial Commercial Activity
  Notice (MCAN) 1584
microcapsule, liver kidney and
  spleen weight decrease 551
microcephaly, radiation-induced
  1696, 1697
micrococci 562
microcosms, aquatic toxicology
  1318, 1319
microdensitometry, integrating 338
microdialysis 644
microdiffusion 1497
microencapsulation 60, 550
micro-exposure techniques 1775
microglia 338, 632, 633
microglobulins
  biomonitoring 1906, 1910
  and cadmium toxicity 2053
  clinical chemistry 363
  labioratory occupationa risks 511
  measurement 63
  nephropathy marker 129, 271,
    678, 692, 1374
micrognathia 972
micronuclei 1848
  assays 1085, 1087–8, 1460
micronutrient deficiencies 913–14,
  1551–2
micro-organisms
  and building/interiors materials
    1295
  catalytic propeties 1368
  as CB weapon 1723, 1726
  emitted volative organic
    compounds 1298

micro-organisms (*Contd.*)
  food contamination 1551
  HVAC-treated air 1295
  indoor pollution 1293, 1301–2
  metabolism, age effect 572
  methylation 109
  nitrate reduction 2122
  regulatory aspects 1605
  sampling strategies 1303
  toxicological testing 1607
microphthalmia 758, 2002
microprocessor-controlled pump
  527
microscale models 1320, 1781
microscopy
  see also specific methods, e.g.
    confocal microscopy
  examinations of inner ear 781–3
microsomes
  aflatoxin B_1 production 276
  conjugation 360
  enzymes 104, 105, 111, 115,
    1995
    methyltransferases 109
    monooxygenases 113, 114
    oxidases 878–9, 1986
    reductase 104
  fractions
    cytochrome P450 in 99
    modelling 306
  interspecies differences 272
  modelling 307
  N-hydroxylation 273
microtox test 753
microtubule associated proteins
  189–90
microtubules 631, 638, 942–3
Microtus spp. *see* voles
microvilli 88, 545, 776
microvillus plasma membrane,
  human placenta 1238
microwave cooking 274
microwave irradiation 497, *498–9*
Micrurus fulvius see coral snake,
  eastern
midazolam hydroxylases *217*
midbrain 347
middle ear 347, 787
migration, chemical 1654, 1655,
  1657
migration inhibition factor 413
migratory behaviour, white-throated
  sparrow (*Zonotrichia albicollis*)
  1348
mild secretion 372

military training facilities,
  contamination 1341
milk
  aflatoxin determination 2152,
    2153
  allergen studies 1005
  elimination via 18, 72
  exposure to dioxin 88
  ingestion, risk from 1772
  mercury levels 2059
  nitrate, nitrite and *N*-nitroso
    levels 2113, 2115, 2116, 2117,
    2118, 2120, 2122
  OC expression in 1995
  ochratoxin levels 2158–9
milkweed (*Asclepsia* spp.),
  neurotoxicity 1519, 1520
millennarian cults 1728
Miller amendment, Food, Drug and
  Cosmetic Act 1599
Minamata disaster 643, 665,
  1564–5, 1826, 1828, 2057
mine(s)
  see also mining
  ponds, contaminated 1340
  tailings 1331, 1355, 1373
Mine Safety and Health Act 1977
  (USA) 1589
Mine Safety and Health
  Administration (USA) 1588–9
mineralocorticoids 984, 985
minerals 548, 972–4
  see also food supplements
miners, risks 1474, 1538, 2051,
  2057
miniature diffusion cells 528
minimal inhibitory concentration
  see MIC
minimal risk 454, 465
minimum body burden 86
minimum effective dose *see* ED_{01}
minimum irritation concentration
  619
minimum lethal dose (MLD)
  see LD_{01}
minimum pre-marketing data set,
  EU 1583, 1584
mining
  see also mine(s)
  disasters 1827
  and soil and water toxicity
    1373–4, 1382
Ministry of Agriculture, Fisheries
  and Food (UK) 1637

Ministry of Health and Welfare
  (Japan) 330, 1565, 1566
Ministry of International Trade and
  Industry (Japan) 1565
Ministry of Labour (Japan) 1565
MINITAB statistical program 301
mink (*Mustela vison*), routine
  testing 1350
miscarriage *see* abortion,
  spontaneous
misconduct and publication 1958
misdiagnosis, IEI and 1709–10
mistletoe (*Phoradendron* spp.),
  toxicity 1518, 1552
mists *see* aerosols
Misuse of Drugs Act 1971 (UK)
  1545
Mithridates VI 35
mitochondria
  activity 359
  acyltransferase enzyme 109
  in antidotal studies 428
  ATP production inhibition by
    ochratoxin 2162
  beta-oxidation by 939
  Ca^{2+} ATPases 156
  calcification 821
  and cardiotoxicity 808, 809, 811,
    813, 820
  complexes 634
  cytochrome P450 99
  cytotoxic response 752
  dehydrogenases 413
  electron transport 633, 1999
  enzymes 98, 103, 337
  in excitatotoxicity 635
  function 163, 166, 192
  genome 161
  liver 860, *861*, 868
  membrane potential 192
  and nephrotoxicity 684, 691
  and neurotoxicity 631
  oxidative stress and 160
  permeability transition, and
    apoptosis 192
  and pharmacogenetics 237
  rat studies 810
  respiration 685, 687
  SOD activity biomarker 1868
  structural changes 683
  swelling 192, 815, 818, 819, 821
mitogen-activated protein kinase/
  extracellular signal regulated
  kinase 195
mitoinhibitory pathways 126

mitosis 340, 544

mitotic index, fertility cycle variation 266

mitotic rate 256

mixed function oxidase 725, 732, 1317

mixed leukocyte reaction (MLR) 1000, 1007

mixed routes of exposure 603–9

mixtures
  acute effects assessment 49–50
  additivity 50, 312
  analysis 305
  antagonism 50, 309, 312
  binary 312
  biomarkers 1841
  chemical 303–19
  complex 314
  effects 20–1, *308*
  factorial designs 313
  interaction 148–9, 309, 313–14
  occupational toxicity hazard 1418
  organic solvents 2033, 2042
  risk assessment 1751
  simple 314
  study methods 305–14
  synergy 309, 312
  toxicity studies 303
  whole 306

mixtures of chemicals, occupational toxic hazard 1418

MKV *see* Moolgavkar–Knudson–Venzon

MLD *see* LD$_1$

MLP *see* maximum lifespan potential

MLR *see* mixed leukocyte reaction

MMAD *see* mass median aerodynamic diameter

MMD *see* mass median diameter

mode of action, risk assessment 1754

model species
  see also species
  for drug testing 1431
  human genome project 1092
  reproductive studies 1328
  wildlife 1327

modelling
  see also mathematical modelling
  chronic ocular hypertensive rabbit 749
  computer-based eye irritation tests 754

gastro-intestinal parameters 556–7
  mathematical for percutaneous toxicity 581
  physicochemical properties based 581–2
  physiologically based pharmacokinetic 607
  risk assessment 1575
  skin absorption 578
  two-compartment for biomonitoring 606

modified reproduction tests 1351–2

modified starches 1552, 1653

modifying factor 1759–60

modulus 776

molar units in biomonitoring 1907

molarity, definition 1446–7

molecular biology
  definition 1965
  technology 336, 339–40
  and toxicology 136
  use 1966

molecular epidemiology 1457, 1534, 1538

molecular immunotoxicology 1010–12

molecular orbital energies 713

molecular probes 339

molecular targets 158–63

molecular toxicology 155–74

molecular volume, definition 597

molecular weight (MW) of toxic agent 1217

molluscicides 1998, 2006

molluscs 1407, 1866, 2192

Molothus ather see cowbird, brown-headed

molybdenum cofactor deficiency 239

molybdenum hydroxylase 239

Mon Voisin, Madame 35

monitored release schemes 1960

monitoring
  see also screening
  ambient 461
  ambient and biological 1602
  biological 461, 464
  personal 461
  pollutants 1460
  to prevent CB incidents 1728
  for toxicity 61–2

monkey studies
  acute toxicity 45
  aflatoxin LD$_{50}$ 2154

ceftizoxime clearance 89

circadian variation 254

CYP genes 216

delayed spatial alternation 660–1

dioxin exposure 87

fumonisin toxicity 2165

hepatic microsomes 273

interferon testing model 1971

intubation 544, 549

IQ 272

LDL fraction 367

liver 274, 872

marmoset
  arsenic metabolism 2050
  β-glucuronidase and β-glucosidase 572
  intravenous injection site 526

mercury toxicity 2058, 2059

MPTP toxicity 132

nerve agent toxicity 2095

ochratoxin pharmacokinetics 2161

ototoxicity 787

patas monkey 787

pharmacodynamic and pharmacokinetic toxicity 329

phosgene 2097

progesterone level 372

reproductive cycle 372

rhesus monkey
  biliary excretion 555
  dioxin susceptibility 282
  experimental toxicity 429
  internal carotid artery infusion 530

spatial contrast ssensitivity 661

squirrel monkey 663

stratum corneum skin permeability *579*

vomiting reflex 546

monkey virus B, infection transmission 514

monkshood (*Aconitum napellus*) 34, 818

monoamine oxidases (MAO) 103, 114, 222, 814, 939

Monoclonal Amphetamine/Metamphetamine Assay (EM) EMIT immunoassay 1501

monoclonal antibodies
  see also biotechnology products
  in antidotal studies 426
  development 1964, 1965, 1967, 1973–4
  endocrine toxicology 983

monoclonal antibodies (*Contd.*)
 IgE 707
  measurement 366
  in occupational toxicology 1454
  in pathology 341, 344
  pharmacogenetics 230
  poisoning antidotes 428
monocytes 385
monodealkylation 429
monogastric species 1509, 1513
*Monographs on the Evaluation of
 the Carcinogenic Risk (of
 Chemicals) to Humans* 476
mononuclear blood cells 277
mononuclear phagocytes 533
monooxygenases 115, 343
Monte Carlo analysis 1758,
 1782–5, 1789–90, 1791
mood 222, 1714
Moolgavkar–Knudson–Venzon
 (MKV) model 1770
morbidity
  in acute toxicity testing 39
  statistics, interpretation 1533
Morinaga incident 2051
morphine placental opioid system
 1256–7
morphological teratogenic effects 8
morphometric analysis 339, 342,
 722
Morris water maze 657
MORT-1, and apoptosis 193
mortality
  see also death; lethality
  rates, regional 1531–2
  statistics, availability 1533
  and survival, field testing 1354
mosquito
  Anopheles albimanus 216
  control 1998
  larva 259
most likely estimate scenarios 1775
motion sickness 527
motor activity changes 41
motor end plates,
 acetylcholinesterase 368
motor neurone disease (ALS) 239,
 635
motor system impairment 655
mould-release agents, rubber
 industry 2014, 2017
Mount St Helens 1816–17
mouse
  activity promotion 532
  acute lethality studies 428

adrenal medulla 346
aflatoxin LD$_{50}$ 2154
age effects on metabolism 115
aggressive behaviour 653
AITC toxicity 134
allergens 511
amine oxidase (AO) 239
apoptosis 178, 193, 197
arsenic metabolism 2050
aryl hydrocarbon receptor-
 deficient 281
barbiturate metabolism 111
bite infection transmission 514
blood sampling site *386*
body weight
  and LD$_{50}$ 51
  /surface area difference 92
bone marrow 385
brain FMO 232
breast cancer surgery timing 266
breathing rate 46
bromobenzene toxicity 118
cadmium toxicity 2054
cancer studies 262, 278, 291
  non-genotoxic 1120, 1131–2
  in plastics industry 2019,
   2021, 2022, 2023
  in rubber industry 2015, 2016,
   2018
  skin 315
cardiac puncture 387
ceftizoxime clearance 89
circadian variations 252–3, 255,
 256
cleft palate effect of dioxin 282
combustion toxicity studies
 1924, 1926
cornea, permeability procedure
 750
CYP genes 216
dechlorination reactions 566
deer (*Peromyscus maniculatus*)
 1335
dermal studies 46, 554, 1944
designer 1964
developmental period 1696
dietary studies 58, 1982, 1985,
 1986
dioxin toxicity 85, 282
dominant lethal test 1060–1
ear, model for skin 340
ear swelling test (MEST) 842
embryo limb bud testing 414
eye/permeability test *410*
FMO expression 232

fungicide toxicity studies 2004
furan toxicity 90
gastro-intestinal microflora 563
germ cell cytogenetic assays
 1088
β-glucuronidase and β-
 glucosidase 572
hair follicle allergen 511
hairless, in dermal contact test
 605
HDL fraction 367
hepatic enzyme inducers 135
hepatocarcinogenesis 271
hepatocytes, apoptosis from
 acetaminophen *179*
herbicide toxicity studies 2004,
 2005, 2006
heterocyclic amines 272
hexobarbitone toxicity 111
hydration and renal clearance
 533
hypersensitivity reactions 1005,
 1007
IgE test 704, 707–10
interleukin-2 343
interspecies difference 274–5,
 283
intestinal studies 260
intravenous injection sites 526
irradiation toxicity 1951
isotonic saline LD$_{50}$ 533
killer cells 341
L929 fibroblasts *410*
LAA see Laboratory animal
 allergy
LD$_{50}$ 407–8, 525
[14]C-leucine label *412*
liver
  apoptosis 199
  electrophoretic variants 239
  microsomes 279
  tamoxifen metabolites 285
  toxicity 257, 551, 853, 866,
   872, 1825
  tumours 526, 1127–9
lymphoma
  cell cultures 407–8
  L5178Y TKS+/-s assay
   1053–4
macrophage, and apoptosis 199
medullary space 383
mercury toxicity 2059
metallothionein role studies 2067
methaemoglobinaemia,
 insecticide 2000

mouse (*Contd.*)

methylmercury 570

microcapsule dosage 551

motor activity 651

nasal passages 342

nerve agents toxicity 2091

neurotoxicity test *417*

NIH 3T3 fibroblasts 1099–100

nitrate toxicity 2123, 2124, 2125, 2135

nitrite toxicity 2123, 2125, 2126, 2127, 2128

nitroreduction and liver and lung tumours 565

ochratoxin toxicity 2160, 2161, 2162

orbital sinus blood sample 387

organic solvents toxicity 2041

organophosphate toxicity 638, 1997

osmotic minipump 528

otötoxicity 791, 795

parathion toxicity 1342

PCB toxicity 131

percutaneous absorption 577, 579

phosgene toxicity 2097

plethysmography 623–4, 625

pregnant, subcutaneous dosing 528

PSI plethysmography *621*

PSI respiratory rate depression *620*

radiation studies 260, 1694, 1695, 1696

repeated exposure studies 59

reproductive cycle 372

respiratory rate depression *613*

respiratory sensitization assessment 706–7

skin *see* mouse, dermal studies

somatic spot test 1058–9

specific locus test 1059–60

sperm analysis 1142

spinal cord amine oxidase (AO) 239

stratum corneum skin permeability *579*

sulphur mustard toxicity 2084

teratogenicity study 258

testicular atrophy 82–3

³H-thymidine label *412*

toxicity rating scheme 408

transgenic 1062–4

tumorigenicity

of high-fat diet 1980

of medical devices 1742

of radiation 260

upper GI tract 544

urinary allergens 511, 514

white-footed (*Peromyscus leucopus*) 1345

wood, biomarkers 1866

mouth *see* buccal; oral; peroral

moving average method 49

MRI *see* magnetic resonance imaging

MRL *see* maximum residue level

mRNA *see* RNA, messenger

mrp *see* multidrug resistance-associated proteins

MRT *see* mean residence time

MSDS *see* Material Safety Data Sheet

Msp1, lung cancer and 1891

MTD *see* maximum tolerated dose

MTT assay 752

mucin 338, 343

mucociliary escalator 604, 605

mucofilaments 340

mucopolysaccharides 829, 966, 967, 969

mucoprotein 897

mucosal epithelium 549

mucous membranes

contact with medical devices 1735, 1736

irritation 2006, 2032

radiation-induced changes 1689, 1690

mucus

ductal cells 897

in oral exposure 604

muffle furnace 1926

Muller cells 644

Mullerian duct regression 179

mullet, grey *see Lisa ramada; Oedalechilus labeo*

multidrug resistance-associated proteins (mrp) 864

multigeneration tests 1143, 1185, 1406

multimedia applications 475

multinuclear giant cell 539

multiple chemical sensitivity syndrome 1416, 1450

see also idiopathic environmental illness

multiple dosing combinations 433

multiple myeloma from organic solvents 2037

multiple route exposure 606, *608*

multi-species toxicity studies 1430–1

multistage models 1537, 1764, 1766, 1771

Musca domestica 216

muscarinic cholinergic receptors 430

muscarinic receptor-associated effects 1242

muscarinic receptors, stimulation by airborne agents 605

muscle

adrenal hormone action 370

cell damage, biomarker 1848, 1860

damage 342

distribution in 70

enzyme distribution 1857

fibres 539, 938, 939, 941, 942, 944

function 126–7

ginger toxicity 1824

implant testing 1741

injury

biomarkers 1861

signs 40

irritancy 413

iso-enzymes, as biomarker 1861

metabolism radiation-induced changes 1689

necrosis 951–5

PBPK studies *90*, 144

musculoskeletal system 341–2, 1691–2

mushrooms

Amanita spp.

acute toxicity 34

neurotoxicity 634

A. phalloides 34

as carcinogens 1981

nitrate and nitrite levels 2112

toxic metal concentrations 1369

veterinary toxicology 1513

mussels

biomarkers in 1866

Mytilus edulis 1870

toxicity 634, 2192–3

mustard, AITC in 134

Mustela spp.
  M. evermanni see ferret, Siberian
  M. nigripes see ferret, black-
    footed
  M. vison see mink
mutagenic, *see also* carcinogenesis;
  genetic damage; genetic
  toxicology
mutagenic carcinogens 873
mutagenic hepatocarcinogens
  874–6
mutagenicity 7–8, 24, 523, 567,
  571
  aflatoxin 2154
  arsenic 2052
  biomarker 1867
  definition 7–8
  ethidium bromide 1455
  fungicides 2002
  and gastro-intestinal microflora
    571
  herbicides 2005
  nitrates 2124–5
  nitrites 2128
  OCs 1995
  organophosphates 1997–8
  and parenteral toxicity 523
  and peroral toxicity 567
  in plastics industry 2019, 2020,
    2021
  in rubber industry 2015
  site-directed 1966
  testing 2, 24, 401, 1434–5, 1567,
    1573, 1628
mutagens *see mainly specific types,*
  e.g. benzo[a]pyrene in Chemical
  Index
mutagens
  determining 'safe' exposures
    1484
  literature on 1038
  risk assessment 1751, 1756
'MutaMouse' *see* transgenic models
mutation
  assay 24
  biochemistry 126, 128
  lung or skin 1474
  from medical devices 1742
  PBPD model 1770
  pharmacogenetics 226
  from radiation 1684, 1688, 1692,
    1693, 1694, 1695
mutual acceptance of data (MAD)
  (OECD) 1564, 1570, 1591

Mutual Recognition (decentralized)
  Procedure, EU 1625–6, 1640–1
Mutual Recognition Facilitation
  Group (MRFG) 1625
myasthenia gravis, treatment 1995
Mycobacterium tuberculosis 841
mycotoxicoses 2145, 2147, 2154
mycotoxins 2145–76
    see also specific mycotoxins,
      e.g. aflatoxin
    as CB weapon 1726
    food contamination 1994
    human studies 462
    indoor air pollution 1301–2
    metal extraction from soil 1369
mydriasis 40, 41, 759
myelin 64, 347, 2037
myelin cells 631
myelinopathies 638–9
myeloid cell types 383
myeloid inclusion bodies 818
myeloperoxidase 103, 112, 240
myelotoxicity 241, 265, 2037
myocardial damage 366
myocardial fibrosis 814–15
myocardial hypertrophy 815
myocardial infarction 229, 264,
  367, 814, 823
myocardial ischaemic necrosis, diet
  and 1978
myocardial necrosis 808, 814, 818,
  821
myocardial scar tissue 343
myocardium 336, 343, 804, 805,
  821
myocytes 804
myocytolysis 807
myoepithelial cells 340, 341
myofibrillar alteration 807
myofibrillar degeneration *see*
  contraction band necrosis (CBN)
myofibrillar lysis 807
myoglobin 340, 342, 360, 384, 941
myoglobinaemia 941
myoglobinuria 942, 1861
myopathies 366, 1997
  drug(s)-induced 942–7
myosin 341, 343, 894
myosin ATPase 342
myotactic reflex 42
Myrothecium spp. 2149
Mytilus edulis see mussels
myxoedema, radiation-induced
  1691

N

Na+/K+ *see* sodium/potassium
NAD 190, 191, 237–8, 240
NADH2 diaphorase 344
NADH 103, 104, 753
NADH dehydrogenase flavin 809
NAD(P)H: quinone oxidoreductase
  216, 240
NADP/NADPH ratio 191
NADPH
  cP450 reductase induction 1866
  generation 28
  in haematology 384
  oxidation 99, 102–3
  pharmacogenetics 232, 240–1
  redox cycling and 127
  reduction 104
  in systemic pulmonary toxicity
    724, 730
NAFTA *see* North Atlantic Free
  Trade Areas
Nagasaki bombing 1692, 1693,
  1697
nails 18, 606, 1495, 1907
Naja nigricollis see cobra
narcosis 8, 25, 2034
narcotics 2030
nasal congestion, as allergic
  response 512
nasal discharge 40
nasal epithelium, histopathology
  315
nasal mucosa
  cytotoxicity from formaldehyde
    16
  epithelium, glutaraldehyde effects
    62
  eye effects and 20
  irritation 315
  nerve PSI stimulation 619
  site of eye drug absorption
    759–60
  toxicity 56
nasal particle disposition 46
nasal PSI 614
nasal resistance, IEI and 1705
nasal sinuses 342
nasal tumours 16, 2018, 2020, 2063
nasal turbinates 704
nasal washings in IEI 1715–16
nasolacrimal ductules 755
nasolacrimal occlusion 760
nasopharyngeal region inhalation
  toxicity 46

NAT *see N*-acetyltransferase

national approaches, regulatory aspects 1547

National Cancer Institute (USA) 551, 765, 1434

National Estimated Daily Intake (NEDI) 1602

National Fire Protection Assocation (NFPA) (US) 1458

National Food Consumption Survey (USA) 1602

National Health Services Central Register (UK) 1531

National Institute of Building Sciences (USA) 1927

National Institute of Environmental Health Sciences (USA) 1935, 1936, 1942

National Institute for Occupational Safety and Health (NIOSH) (USA) 481, 650, 1458, 1588–9, 1677, 1936

National Institutes of Health (NIH) (USA), guidelines 1459

National Library of Medicine (USA) 478, 1676–7

National Pollutant Discharge Elimination System (NPDES) 1311

national population
see also population
as comparison subjects 1531

National Research Council (USA) 1752
biomarker paradigm 1464, 1875

National Residue Program, Food Safety and Inspection Service 1637

National Theoretical Maximum Daily Intake (NTMDI) 1602

National Toxicology Program (NTP) (USA)
carcinogenicity 1102, 1106, 1108, 1434
cutaneous toxicity 835
education 1940
immunotoxicity 1006–7
pathology 341, 344, 346
reproductive toxicity test protocol 1140
safety aspects 1968

natriuretic hormone 364

natural disasters, toxic effects 1444

natural flavours 1654

natural killer (NK) cells 188, 343, 865, 999, 1001

natural selection 215

natural toxicants 1366, 1371, 1534, 1554, 1977

naturally occurring toxicity 1366, 1371, 1534, 1554, 1977

nature-identical flavours 1654

nausea 43, 524, 811

Nazi physicians 453

nbk, and apoptosis 193

NCEs *see* normochromatic erythrocytes

NDMA, false conclusion 298

near-maximum lethal toxicity 13

near-threshold lethal toxicity 13

nebulization 595

neck
male adult skin surface area *583*
radiation-induced tumours 1691

necrogens 197

necropsy
see also autopsy; post-mortem
acute toxicity 39
dermal toxicity test 605
gross 42, 45
procedures 62
in repeated exposure studies 61, 64

necrosis
and acute toxicity 40, 42
arachnidism 2186–7
biochemical changes 126, 187, 188
cause 6, 126
characterization 176
and circadian toxicology 255
definition 6, 175
distinguishing features 177
ergot toxicity 1516
molecular concepts 163–9
morphology 183
nitric oxide 199
secondary 187
zonal 6

necrotizing myopathies 942
see also muscle necrosis

necrotizing vasculitis 822

'need' clause, marketing authorizations 1568–9

needles, stainless steel, for sampling 1909

negative control substances 340

negative effects 1450–1

negligence 1450

Neisseria spp. 562

nematocysts 787
on jellyfish 2189, 2190

nematodes 177, 178, 1999

neo-Nazis 1728

neon ions, radiation-induced changes 1690

neonatal mouse test 525

neonates
blood flow 83
development 8
dioxin exposure 88
exposure via milk 72
food additives consumption 83–4, 1985, 1989
hGH safety 1970
metabolism 115
mortality 1203
neoplasia 7
nitrite levels 2120
peroral toxicity 549
prenatal treatment effects 651
toxicology 1224–9

neoplasia *see* mainly cancer; tumours

neoplasia
aberrant crypt foci 571
and peroxisome proliferation 1124

NEP *see* neutral endopeptidase

nephritis-like reaction, radiation-induced 1691

nephro-, *see also* kidney; renal

nephrocalcinosis 357, 1430

nephron 345, 676

nephropathy *522*, 685
adverse drug reaction 1430
analgesic 679, 688
humans 2154, 2159
and parenteral toxicity 522
pigs 2145, 2154, 2159
poultry 2145
predictability in animal tests 1438
urinary markers *678*

nephrosclerosis, food additives and 1986

nephrotic syndrome 682

nephrotoxicity
adverse drug reactions 1427, 1430
bismuth 2061
bromobenzene 118
cadmium 1373–4, 1475, 2053, 2054

nephrotoxicity (*Contd.*)
  cholecalciferol 1511
  and circadian toxicity 256
  clinical chemistry 355, 361, 362, 367
  copper 1514–15
  ethylene glycol 1426, 1428, 1512
  evaluation 1462
  furosemide 198
  gallium 2063
  haloalkanes 121
  herbicides 2004, 2005, 2006
  indium 2063
  lead 1475, 1515
  metal-based compounds 260–1
  mycotoxin 1516
  nitrite 2126
  organic solvents 2029, 2035, 2036, 2038, 2041
  organophosphates 1998
  and parenteral toxicity 523
  PCBs 131
  pesticide residues 1343
  phenacetin 1428
  plants 1522
  radiation 1685, 1691, 1696
  reactive intermediates 131
  responses 675–700
  signs 43
  snake venom 2179
  sulphonamides 98
  test systems *417*
  uranium 1475
  white phosphorus 1511
nephrotoxins 305, *417*, 680, 1862
Nerium oleander *see* oleander
Nero 35
nerve agents 1721–30, 1996–7, 2089–96
  absorption 2090–1
  clinical effects 2091
  clinical investigations 2091–2
  half-lives 2091
  history 2080, 2081
  long-term effects 2095–6
  mechanism of action 2091
  military use 2090
  pesticides 1996–7
  physicochemical agents 2090
  prognosis for casualties 2095
  terrorist use 1721–30, 2090
  toxicity 2090
    management 2092–5
  types 2082

nerve cells 179, 195, 631–2, 643
  see also neurons
nerve growth factors 178
nervous system
  see also neural, neuro-
  and apoptosis 178
  cells *see* nerve cells; neurons
  demyelination, organophosphorus pesticides 1333
  development, in tadpoles 1956
  function 126–7
  immature 1337
  nerve terminals 631, 640–1
  OC effects 1995
  organophosphate toxicity 1997
  pathology 346–7
  radiation-induced changes 1690–1
  sprouting 631
  toxicity *see* neurotoxicity
nesting behaviour 1352, 1353
'net acid gas' 1266
net affinity 427
Netherlands
  nitrate and nitrite levels 2112, 2114, 2115, 2116, 2118, 2132, 2133
  novel food controls 1546
  occupational exposure levels 1594
Netherlands Animal Welfare Society 486
network theory of molecular mechanisms *157*
neural crest, test system 414
neural membranes, and organic solvents 2030, 2038
neural pathway methods for PSI recording 619–21
neural tube defects *see* spina bifida
neurasthenia 1710
neurobehavioural effects
  fires 1920
  lead 2055, 2056
  malformations 8
  organic solvent syndrome 1529
  organic solvents 2032
  protein deficiency and 16
  screening 495
neuroblast cell, radiation-induced changes 1697
neurocognitive function in idiopathic environmental intolerance 1707

neurodegenerative disorders, mechanisms 636
neuroendocrine activity
  assay 1328
  radiation-induced changes 1690
neurofibrillary degeneration, aluminium 1379
neurofilaments 631, 637, 638
neurogenic inflammation in IEI 1715–16
neuroleptanalgesic 539
neuroleptic drugs 264–5, 1430
neurological disease, and apoptosis 178
neuromuscular junctions 6, 790
neuromuscular symptoms, radiation-induced 1686
neuromuscular transmission 950–1
neuron(s) 631
  chemical lesions 641–2
  cholinergic 638
  degeneration 631
  inability to regenerate 126
  NOS and 2119
  radiation-induced changes 1690
  -specific enolase 344, 2031
neuropathy
  delayed-onset peripheral 55
  from ginger 1824
  from honey 1984
  skeletal muscle toxicity 944
  from solvents 131
  target esterase (NTE) 638, 2095
  from toxic oil syndrome 1824
neurophysiological effects in idiopathic environmental intolerance 1716
neuropsychological testing in idiopathic environmental intolerance 1713
neuroretina 756
neurosensory epithelia *see* organ of Corti
neurotoxic esterase, biomarker 1345
neurotoxic theories of idiopathic environmental intolerance aetiology 1706–7
neurotoxicity 631–47
  adverse drug reactions 1427, 1430
  aluminium 1380, 2060
  animal stings and bites 2179, 2188, 2190
  avermectins 1999

neurotoxicity (*Contd.*)
   and behavioural toxicity 651
   biochemistry 126–7
   biomarkers 1875
   bismuth 2061
   blue–green algae toxicity 1516
   dose–response assessment 1758
   ethylene oxide 1455
   fires 1920, 1921
   FOB screen 63
   food contamination 1825
   horses 1519
   in vitro test systems *417*
   lead 1518, 2055
   and lethal synthesis 6
   mercury 1564–5, 2058
   methylmercury 569–70
   MPTP 132
   NMDA 166
   organic solvents 2030–2, 2034
   placental toxicity 1244, 1246
   predictability in animal tests
      1438
   pyrethroids 1998
   radiation 1686, 1687
   risk assessment 1756
   shellfish 2192
   signs 40, 43
   sodium chloride 1517
   tests 23
   transport mechanism 632
   vincristine 1455
   vitamin B_6 1552
neurotransmitters 632, 640, 642,
   643
neurotrophic factors 788
neutral endopeptidase (NEP), IEI
   and 1705
Neutral Red uptake assay 753–4
neutrons 1683
   activation measurement
      biomonitoring of cadmium
      1905
   radiation-induced changes 1690,
      1693
neutropenia 394–5, 1549
neutrophil leukocytosis 535
neutrophils 103, 200, 384, 1686,
   1843, 2119
New Animal Drugs Application
   (NADA) (USA) 1634
new chemical substances
   see also novel foods and food
      ingredients
   dossier 1601, 1605, 1606

regulatory aspects
   EU 1478–9, 1627–9
   USA 1582–6
   toxicological studies 1557, 1565,
      1581, 1606
New Chemicals Program (USA)
   1583
New Drug Application (NDA)
   (USA) 1562, 1615, 1974
New Drug Approval (USA) 1544
New Zealand
   Agricultural Compound Unit
      1611
   fumonisin contamination of
      cereals 2165
newborn *see* neonate
newt, Californian (*Taricha torosa*)
   818, 2193
NF_{kb}-dependent genes 168
NFPA *see* National Fire Protection
   Association
nicotine adenosine dinucleotide
   phosphate *see* NADHP
nicotinic receptor-associated effects
   1242
nictitating membrane changes 42
nifedipine dehydrogenase *217*
nigericin, and apoptosis 192
Nightingale, Florence 1529
nightshades (*Solanum* spp.),
   neurotoxicity 1521
NIH *see* National Institutes of
   Health
Niigata disaster 1826, 1828, 2057
NIOSH *see* National Institute for
   Occupational Safety and Health
nitrate reductase 562, 567, 572,
   2122
nitrate-accumulating plants, and
   methaemoglobinaemia 1522
nitric oxide synthases (NOS) 812,
   2119–20
nitrite reductase 567
nitro reduction 104
nitroreductase *216*
nitrosation reactions 567
Nitzschia pungens 634, 2193
NK cells *see* natural killer cells
NMR *see* nuclear magnetic
   resonance
no correlation 304–5
no observed adverse effect level
   (NOAEL)
   behavioural toxicity 657

developmental toxicity 1172,
   1179, 1180
disadvantages 1761
human studies 462
mixtures 314
occupational toxicity 1483
regulations 1574, 1612
repeated exposure studies 56, 57,
   60
in risk assessment 1757,
   1759–61, 1787
as safe dose in animals 91
study design 322
no observed effect concentration
   (NOEC) 1312, 1316, 1318
no observed effect level (NOEL) 12
   air pollutants 316
   antidotal studies 433
   regulations 1448, 1449, 1451,
      1602, 1635, 1643
   repeated exposure studies 56, 60,
      64
NOAEL *see* no observed adverse
   effect level
Nobel, Alfred 460
nodes of Ranvier 631, 637
NOEC *see* no observed effect
   concentration
NOEL *see* no observed effect level
noise *see* ototoxic interactions
non-bacterial thrombotic
   endocarditis 814
non-carcinogens
   dose–response assessments
      1759–62
   risk expression 1786–7
non-clinical safety studies 1616–18
non-competitive inhibition 305
non-genotoxic (epigenetic)
   carcinogens 7, 126, 1119–20,
      1131–2
non-Hodgkin's lymphoma 1995,
   2005
non-invasive procedures 62
non-linear kinetics *see* dose-
   dependent kinetics
non-mutagenic hepatocarcinogens
   876–81
non-necrotizing arteritis 1551
non-protein nitrogen compounds,
   toxicity 1514
non-reproducible results 1445
non-sensory epithelia 778–9
non-specific cholinesterase 368
non-specific effects 35

non-threshold effects 1758
noradrenaline 808, 812, 813, 2039
Nordic countries, regulatory procedures 1568–9, 1572
Nordic Working Group on Food Toxicology 1568
norepinephrine *see* noradrenaline
normal equivalent deviant ranges 48
normit chi-squared-squared method 49
normoblasts 384
normochromatic erythrocytes (NCEs) 1087
Norsk Medisinaldepot 1568
North American Free Trade Agreement (NAFTA) 2, 1604, 1649
northern bobwhite (*Colinus virginianus*)
  anticholinesterase exposure 1351
  avian embryo bioassay 1334
  behaviour 1346, 1348, 1352
  chronic testing 1350
  dose–response anomalies 1330
  fenthion toxicity 1338
  inhalation and oral toxicity studies 1331
  as model species 1329
  parathion toxicity 1351
  reproduction tests 1350, 1351
  subacute testing 1332, 1333–4, 1338
  subchronic toxicity testing 1344
Norway
  nitrate and nitrite levels 2116, 2117, 2118, 2133
  pharmaceuticals regulation 1544, 1568–9
NOS *see* nitric oxide synthases
nose
  -only exposure 60
  see mainly nasal
Notice of Commencement of Manufacture 1583
Notice to Applicants 1621
notification, meaning 1546
Notification of New Substances (NONS) Regulations (EU) 1478
Notification of New Substances Regulations (UK) 37, 1590
notification schemes 1543, 1545
novel foods and food ingredients 1551, 1553, 1560

NPDES *see* National Pollutant Discharge Elimination System
nQUERY ADVISOR statistical program 301
NTP *see* National Toxicology Program
NUC, and apoptosis 189
nuclear, fear of word 1959
nuclear aberrations 571
nuclear chromatin 681
nuclear condensation 183
nuclear disaster 1443, 1820–1
nuclear industry, and radiation damage 1692
nuclear magnetic resonance (NMR) spectroscopy 234, 364, 678–9, 1849, 1850–1, 1862
nuclear proteins, ribosylation 190
nuclear receptor genes, polymorphism 1892
nuclear scaffold structures 163
nuclear transport, *bcl-2* gene and 194
nuclear waste 1313
nuclear weapons 1444, 1723
37 kDa nuclease, and apoptosis 189
nuclease P_1 treatment method 1887, 1888–90
nucleic acid
  damage by free radicals 1683
  interactions with toxins 163
  modification, endogenous 1878–9
  replication interference 8
  study 1965
  as targets 34, 160–2
nucleophiles 684, 689, 835
nucleophilic sites in genome 161
5-nucleotidase 337, 344–5, *356*, 359
nucleotide monophosphate 261
nu,e ardente 1815
null genotype 1891
Nuremberg Code 453
nutrition
  see also food
  antioxidants 158
  balanced 317
  as biomarker 1845
  biomonitoring 1780, 1907
  bone and cartilage growth needs 969–70
  deficiencies 8, 317, 792, 823, 969–74, 1977, 2064–5
  and diet 1551, 1980–3

dosing procedures 59–60
drug inclusion 523
and drug metabolism 113
exposure 19
  risk assessment 1602–3
fibre 561, 572
gut microflora metabolism 572–3
habits
  inter-ethnic variations 1646
  poor 1552
hazard evaluation 28
imbalance 316–17
and indoor air contaminant effects 1292
ingestion, standard assumptions 1773
maternal diet and foetal growth 1217
and metabolism 109–10, 115
and radiation effects 1690
repeated exposure studies 58
restriction 323
science development 1977
selenium requirements 2065
in standard operating procedure (SOP) 446
status 15–16, 366, 938, 939, 1690
and toxicity 15–16, 21, 1415, 1416, 1417, 1977–83
toxicokinetics studies via 75
tumour-promoting activity 568
variables 356
vascular disease and 1978–80
Nutrition Canada Survey 1602
nuts
  aflatoxin contamination 2153
  nitrate levels 2115
  toxicity and 1983–4
Nycticorax nycricorax see heron, black-crowned night-
nystagmus 40, 42, 757, 788

O

OAEs *see* otoacoustic emissions
oak (*Quercus* spp.), toxicity 1513, 1518, 1522
obesity *see* size factors
obsessive-compulsive disorder, IEI and 1709
obstructive nephropathy, adverse drug reaction 1430
Occam's razor, ethics 1957

occult blood 364–5
occupational disease 701
occupational epidemiology, definition 1456
occupational exposure
see also idiopathic environmental illness; occupational hazards
  acute toxicity 46
  aluminium 2060
  arsenic 1246
  asbestos 1006
  beryllium 2061
  biomarkers 1877, 1886
  biomonitoring 1899–914
  cadmium 2053–4
  carbon monoxide *1283*
  chromium 2062
  dioxin 88
  guidelines 57, 618
  human studies 466
  lead 2055, 2056
  mercury 643
  metals, during pregnancy 1203, 1204, 1205, 1206
  nickel 2063
  nitrogen oxide 1278
  organic solvents 2031, 2033, 2037, 2039
  paternal 1464
  PBPK modelling 148, 149
  PEL 606
  pesticides 1548, 1993
  peripheral sensory irritation effects 616
  regulatory aspects 1415, 1752
  reproductive system toxins 1138, 1150, 1156
  rubber industry 2015
  safety margins 91
  tetrachloroethelene, perinatal exposure 1216–17, 1226
  TLV 606
  to toxins 266, 605, 1444
  veterinary drugs 1637
occupational exposure limit (OEL) 1481–5
  airborne 1481
  biological monitoring 1910
  definition 1481–2
  EU 1483, 1594–5
  health-based 1483–4
  historical aspects 1482
  in-house 1486
  lists 1482–3, 1484–5, 1486

Maximale Arbeitskonzentrationen Commission 1482
  PBPK modelling 149
  percutaneous toxicity 584
  peripheral sensory irritation 625–6
  regulations 1459, 1594
  toxicological background 1483–5
  USSR (former) 1482
occupational exposure standard (OES), UK 1483–4
occupational factors 1415–24
occupational hazards 509–20, 828
  see also occupational exposure
  allergic reactions 509
  cancer risk prediction 1770
  disturbance of mood and sleep 515
  evaluation 27
  exhaust hoods 510
  gloves 510
  industrial chemicals 1550
  infection 509
  lymphocyte cytogenetics 515
  mixing operations 510
  physical injury 509
  protective clothing 510
  reproductive effects 510, 1465–7
  sister chromatic exchanges 515
  socially acceptable 1474
  target tissues 1753
  test diets 510
  urine mutagenicity 515
  zoonoses 514–15
occupational history 1531
occupational hygiene 584, 1473, 1487
occupational industrial exposures, and metabolism 112–13
occupational legislation 1458–9
occupational medicine 456, 1458
occupational mortality 1529
occupational risks 1476, 1602, 1830
Occupational Safety and Health Act 1970 (USA) 37, 1453, 1458, 1467, 1481, 1482, 1588
Occupational Safety and Health Administration (OSHA) (USA)
  acute toxicity 37
  laboratory occupational toxicity 515
  mixed routes of exposure 603
  multistage risk models 1537

permissible exposure limits (PELs) 660, 1482
  regulations 1435, 1453, 1477, 1481, 1588
  risk assessment 1749
occupational safety recommendations 1648
occupational sensitization, chemical route 705
occupational surveillance programme 464
occupational toxicology 1453–71, 1473–88
  definition 3
  history 2
ochratoxicosis 2159–60, 2161
octanol–water partition coefficient 145, 581–2, 613, 810, 1312, 1315, 1317, 1318, 2030
ocular *see* eye
oculomucocutaneous syndrome 1427, 1438, 1549
odds ratio (OR) 1533
odour intolerance in idiopathic environmental intolerance 1704, 1705, 1706, 1707–9, 1714, 1716
OECD *see* Organization for Economic Cooperation and Developemt
Oedalechilus labeo 1870
oedema
  acute alcoholic rhabdomyolysis 940
  acute toxicity 40, 42
  cellular 815, 822
  dermatitis 832, 835
  dioxin toxicity 282
  pathology 342
  stria vascularis 785
  synthetic materials testing 1741
oedematous pancreatitis 898, 906–7
OEL *see* occupational exposure limit
oesophagus
  blood supply 545
  cancer
    in firefighters 1929
    from fumonisins 2163
    and mycotoxin toxicity 1516
    from nitrates 2131
    from *N*-nitroso compounds 2132, 2133
    in rubber industry 2015
  drug transport 555
  epithelium 544, 554

organ(s) (*Contd.*)
    transplantation 684
    weight
        analysis, PBPK modelling
            145
        as biomarker 1846, 1855–6
        checks 45
        in long-term toxicity studies
            331
        pathology 336
        in repeated exposure studies
            61, 64
organ of Corti 347, 776–8, 780,
    781–3, 787, 790
organic matter, in soil 1368, 1369
organic solvent syndrome (Danish
    painters' disease) 1527, 1529,
    1539
Organization for Economic
    Cooperation and Development
    (OECD) 2
    acute toxicity studies 36, 37
    animal testing harmonization
        501
    aquatic toxicology initiatives
        1311, 1314
    banned and restricted substances
        1571
    existing substances, risk
        assessment programme 1480
    guidelines 326, 439, 465, 1139,
        1400, 1404, 1436, 1612
    harmonization 1478, 1572, 1612
    high production volume (HPV)
        chemicals program 1480, 1585
    industrial chemicals 1571
    information resources 482, 487
    mutual acceptance of data
        (MAD) 1564, 1591
    *Principles of Good Laboratory
        Practice* 439, 442, 445, 1591
    regulatory procedures 1570–1
    and wildlife toxicology 1328
    Working Group on Endocrine
        Disrupters 1393, 1401
organizational information resources
    482
organogenesis 23
organophosphate anticholinesterases
    6, 12, 25, 329
ornithine carbamyltransferase 356,
    359, 1345
ornithine conjugation 109, 111
ornithine decarboxylase gene 167
orosomucoid 254

orotate phosphoribosyltransferase
    261
Orphan Drug Act 1984 (USA) 1662
orphan drug procedure 2
Osaka, CB incident 1726
OSHA *see* Occupational Safety and
    Health
osmolality 332, 362, 364, 365, 366
osmotic load, high 521
osmotic minipump 60, 528–9
osprey (*Pandion haliatus*) 1329,
    1341
osteitis, radiation 1691
osteoblasts 968, 1858
osteocalcin 1859
osteoclasts 1858
osteogenesis 968
osteomalacia 1427
osteopathy, adverse drug reaction
    1430
osteoporosis 973, 1859
osteosarcommas 1081
OTC *see* 'over-the-counter' drugs
otoacoustic emissions (OAEs) 781,
    783, 786
ototoxic interactions 795–6,
    1418–19, 1430
outer root sheath, hair follicles 830
ovarian cancer 278, 1400
ovarian cells, apoptosis 179, 196,
    198
ovarian receptors 372
ovary
    clinical chemistry 372–3
    cloned enzymes 242
    cycles 1148–9
    development 1148
    drug toxicity 369, *369*, 987,
        1152–3
    hypothalamic–pituitary pathway
        1148
    pathology 346
    physiological considerations
        986–7
    radiation-induced injury 1685,
        1688
    weight 336
over-the-counter (OTC) drugs 1562
    availability 1550
    children 1228–9
    cross-reactivity in testing 1501
    demand for 1549–50
    in pregnancy 1215, 1222–4,
        1226
overdosage 4, 21, 116

overexposure 22
oviducts 1149
ovulation 372, 1148–9
owl, barn (*Tyto alba*) 1355
Oxford Childhood Cancer Study
    1697
oxidants 28, 158, 192
oxidase, mixed function 373
oxidation 17, 98–103
    β-oxidation 109, 939
    circadian toxicology 254
    cytochrome P450-dependent
        221, *227*, 228, 232
    drugs 114–15
    FMO substrates *233*
    genetic polymorphisms 218–43
    non-cytochrome P450-dependent
        102–3
    N-oxidation 102–3, 233, 234,
        272
    pharmacogenetics 216, 226, 232
    S-oxidation 101–2, 233
    species differences 110
oxidation state 1365
    see also speciation
oxidation–reduction P450 systems
    254–5
oxidation–reduction reactions 1366
oxidative haemolysis 391
oxidative metabolism 218, 280,
    315, 785
    see also oxidation
oxidative phosphorylation 127, 794,
    806, 811, 813, 821, 822, 939, 969
oxidative pyrolysis 1916
oxidative reactions 564
oxidative stress
    and apoptosis 191–2, 199
    as biomarker 1845, 1848, 1866,
        1867, 1869
    cell killing 166
    DNA adducts from 1881
    in eye toxicity 762–3
    in haematology 391
    in liver 912
    molecular concepts 158, 159–60,
        168–9
    and nephrotoxicity 681
    in other pancreatic diseases
        909–10
    in pancreatic disease 904–14
    pharmacogenetics 240
    role 163
oxirane ring 100
oxireductase 238

oxygen
availability 127, 1919
blood gas level, in fires 1920
depletion from fire 1916
free radicals, sources 1979
metabolites 158
oxidation reactions and 99
reduction 104
as target 34
oxyhaemoglobin dissociation curve 384, 393, 1921, 1922
oxyradicals, as biomarker 1867
oyster, toxicity 2192

P

P13 kinase, and apoptosis 191
p53
and apoptosis 189, 193, 195, 196
as biomarker 1849
expression, nitric oxide synthesis and 200
induction, radiation-induced 1690
molecular concepts 168
mutations 1427, 1429, 1457, 1538
suppressor gene 1030–1, 1101
in testing 1448
transcription factor 168
and tumorigenesis 1892
P450 *see under* cytochromes
pachymetry 738
packaging
see also classification and labelling; food contact materials
CB agents threats 1724
requirements 36–7
synthetic materials 1736–7
packed cell volume (PCV) 387
paclitaxel 6-hydrogenase *217*
paedatric *see* child/ren
paints and varnishes 1417, 1418, 1419, 1704, 1708, 2055
palate 179, 191
see also cleft lip and palate
Palestinians, deliberate food poisoning 1724
palm, permeability 577, *578*
palpation 45
palpitation 236
Palythoa 820

pancreas
acinar cells 895–7
anatomy and physiology 894–5, 991
cancer 132–3, 235, 898, 901–2, 920–6, 2015
diseases and definitions 897–8
drug and chemical toxicity 369, 910–27
ducts 545, 897
evolution 893, 894
in vitro test system *418*
in miscellaneous systemic diseases 902–3
peroral toxicity 547
secretion 364, 546, 894, 897
toxicity, oxygen free radical 903–10, 912–14
pancreastasis 908–9
pancreatitis
acute 897, 898–900, 906–10, 915–17, 991–3
chronic 900–1, *902*, 917–20
drug(s)-induced pancreatitis 915–20, 991–3
from animal stings and bites 2180, 2188
recurrent (non-gallstone) 909
tests 365
pancytopenia 389–90, 394
Pandion haliatus see osprey
panic attacks in IEI 1708, 1709, 1710, 1714
pannus 742
Paoli Railroad Yard PCB litigation 1949
Papanicolaou stain 344
papillary muscles 343
papillotoxic agents 363
paprika, nitrate levels 2113
PAPS *see* 3′-phosphoadenosine-5′-phosphosulphate
papules 835
para-acute dosing 39
Parabuthus see scorpion
Paracelsus 36, 47, 472, 1474, 1547, 1937
paracrine effects 981
paradigm shift, in environmental toxicology 1749–50
paraesthesia 465, 1999
paraffin wax embedding 338
paralysis 42, 1824, 1997, 2192
paraparesis 634
parasitic infections 365, 367

parasthesia, facial 524
parathyroid gland 369, 1691
parathyroid hormone (PTH) 949–50, 968
paravertebral muscles, implantation into 539
parenchymal cells of liver, radiation-induced changes 1684, 1685
parenteral infusions 522, 533–5
parenteral routes 60, 526–9
see also specific route, e.g. intravenous
parenteral toxicity 521–42
acute 46
alternative testing 412–13
indications 522–6
long-term studies 521
parietal cells 545, 546
parkinsonism
adverse drug reaction 1430
free radicals 634
genetic suscepibility 29
MPTP and 132
neurotoxicity 635, 636, 641
pharmacogenetics 29, 223, 225, 232
Parkinson's disease
see parkinsonism
paroxysmal atrial tachycardia (PAT) 811
parsley, nitrate and nitrite levels 2112–13
partial addition, mixture effect *313*
partial hepatectomy as promoter 566
particle accelerators 1683
α-particles 1683
particles *see* particulates
particulates
see also winter smog/particulates complex
atmosphere analysis 597–9
atmosphere generation 594
breathing zone samples 598
characterization and sources 1299
deposition 46, 592
dispersion system 596
dose–response assessment 1762
effects on human populations 1281–2
from volcanoes 1815
gravitational sedimentation 591
high-energy 1683
'higher risk' 592

particulates (*Contd.*)
  impaction 591
  ingestion 1772
  inhalation 20, 21
  interception 591
  light scattering properties 599
  mixtures 315–16
  processes causing changes to 1300
  pulmonary deposition 316
  sampling 1303
  sink effect 1299–300
  size and shape 391, 590, 598, 605, 618, 1298–9, 1814
  sulphates 1281
  suspended (SPM) 1266, 1299
partition coefficients 89, 143, 145, 578, 579, 582, 2030
parvalbumin 808
PAS *see* periodic acid–Schiff reaction
passerine birds
  acute toxicity testing 1330, 1331
  dermal exposure to pesticides 1339
  reproductive success 1352
  xenobiotic tolerance 1337–8
passive diffusion 547
passive smoking 1416, 1417, 1905
passive smoking *see* smoking
PAT *see* paroxysmal atrial tachycardia
Patau syndrome 1081
patch tests 838–40
pate, nitrate and nitrite levels 2113
patent protection 1569
paternal workplace exposures 1464
pathological effects
  as biomarker 1846, 1855–7
  in legal matters 1952
  on metabolism 114–15
  repeated exposure 62
pathological techniques 335–53
patient compliance and drug toxicity 21
Patient Information Leaflet 1627
Patriot's Council 1727
pattern recognition 1849
Patty's Industrial Hygiene and Toxicology 1476
Pavlovian conditioning in IEI 1708
PBPD *see* physiologically based pharmacodynamic
PBPK 1416

PBPK *see* physiologically based pharmacokinetic (PBPK) modelling
PCEs *see* polychromatic erythrocytes
PCR *see* polymerase chain reaction
PDP *see* postdrug potentiation
PDR *see* postdrug repetition
peak expiratory flow rate 510
peanuts 1982, 2152
pear, nitrate levels 2113
peas, nitrate and nitrite levels 2112, 2115
pectin increase in nitrite production 2122
pedosphere, definition 1365
peer review 474, 1941
Peganum harmala 222
PEL *see* permissible exposure limit
Pelecanus occidentalis see pelican, brown
pelican, brown (*Pelecanus occidentalis*) 1329, 1351
pembe yara 1226
'pen-in-field' protocol 1349
penetration phase, chemical 578
Penicillium spp. 1253, 1301, 1516, 1982, 2145, 2146
pentose phosphate metabolism 166
peppers, nitrate and nitrite levels 2112
pepsin 547
pepsinogen 365, 545
peptic ulceration 365
peptide bond cleavage in adduct analysis 1883
peptides, as impurities 1969
peptidyl-prolyl *cis-trans* isomerase 684
Peptococcus 568
Peptostreptococcus 568
percentile cumulative response 48
perception 222
perception-altering 222
percutaneous absorption
  calculations 583–4
  chemical liquids *579*
  chemical vapours *584*
  determination 578–83
  factors affecting 577–8
  mixtures 21
  pharmacokinetic models 582–3
  rate 585
  repeated exposure 55, 59
  studies 579–80

percutaneous hazard *see* dermal exposure
percutaneous permeability coefficients 580
percutaneous toxicity 432, 577–86
peregrine falcon (*Falco peregrinus*) 1329, 1341
perfume allergy 1704, 1708
perfused organs 416
perfusion fixation 339
periarteritis, statistical analysis 296
peribiliary plexus 854, *855*
pericardial effusion 814
pericarditis 807
pericardium 343, 804, 807
perichondrial ossification, rat foetus *967*, *970*
perilymph 775, 776, 779–80, 786, 789, 794, 795
perineum, male adult skin surface area *583*
perineurium 633
periocular blood vessels 20
periodic acid–Schiff reaction (PAS) 336, 345, 867
periodic audit testing 1679
periodic safety update reports (PSUR) 457, 1629
peri-orbital oedema 510
peripheral blood smears 341
peripheral blood specimens, post-mortem 1495
peripheral circulation *369*
peripheral compartment 77, 78, 141
peripheral nervous system (PNS) 178, 631
  see also nervous system
peripheral neuropathy 638
  acetylcholinesterase inhibition 12
  acrylamide 1455
  adverse drug reaction 1430
  arsenic compounds 1515
  n-hexane 1475
  induction 662
  lead 1475
  mercury 1475
  mushroom toxicity 1513
  organic solvents 2030, 2035, 2040
  pyrethroids 1998–9
  and skeletal muscle toxicity 941–2
peripheral sensory irritation (PSI) 8, 23, 611–29

periphlebitis 529
peri-postnatal period 1138
peristalsis 545, 562
peritoneal fluid 533
peritoneal sensitivity 526
peritonitis from peroral exposure 19
permeability
  barrier 71
  coefficient 579, 584
  constant 46, 1777–8
permeation enhancers 759
permissible exposure limits (PELs)
  603, 606, 1458, 1482, 1588
permits 1543
permitted/proscribed list systems
  1543, 1544–5, 1552, 1557,
  1559–60
Peromyscus spp.
  P. leucopus see mouse, white-
    footed
  P. maniculatus see mouse, deer
peroral route 19, 59
  absorption 67
  comparison with intravenous data
    75
  dose calculation 1774–5
  interspecies differences 15
  procedures 59, 549–54
peroral toxicity 543–59
  anatomical and physiological
    considerations 554–5
  carcinogenicity 554
  chronic irritation 554
  direct contact effects 553–4
  first-pass effect considerations
    555
  gastro-intestinal parameters in
    modelling 556–7
  gavage dosing toxicity 554
  hazard evaluation 554–7
  irritant reponse and forestomach
    tumours 554
  localized effect considerations
    556
  oesophageal perforation 553
  strictures 553
  ulcerations 553
peroxidases 103, 337–8, 364, 370,
  1868
peroxisomes
  proliferation 271, 860, *861*, 867,
    869, 1124, 1403, 2005
  proliferators 7, 126, 135, 878
peroxy radicals 6
persistent (permanent) toxicity 5, 6

person-years, definition 1532
personal habits 28, 1474
personal and lifestyle influences,
  and response to toxic agents
  1416–17
personal protective equipment
  149–50, 463, 514, 515, 1485,
  1551, 1648, 2081, 2092, 2103
personal sampling 461, 1530
personality disorder, idiopathic
  environmental intolerance and
  1709
personnel records 1458, 1528, 1531
Pest Control Products Act 1939
  (Canada) 1600
Pest Management Regulatory
  Authority (Canada) 1600
pest resistance, genetically modified
  1553
pesticide(s)
  see also insectides;
    organophosphates (*in Chemical
    Index*; rodenticides
  acute toxicity studies 39
  additive effects 50
  aerial application 1339, 1341,
    1355
  aquatic toxicity 1313, 1315–16
  authorization, EU 1604–10
  avian embryo bioassay 1334
  behavioural effects 1348
  biomonitoring 1906
  carcinogenicity 1111, 1123, 1127
  cartilage and bone toxicity 965
  chemical variety 1445
  classification 1993, 1994
  databases 1603
  definition 1600, 1993
  deregistration 1601
  in diet 58
  differential sensitivity 1336
  differential toxicology 1547
  domestic animal toxicity 1510
  in drinking water 1603
  efficacy data 1601
  exposure data quality 1530
  exposure routes 59, 1548
  forensic testing 1504
  formulations 1338–9, 1340, 1341
  gender differences in
    susceptibility 1338
  human studies 25
  IEI and 1708
  indoor air pollution 1299
  and menstrual disorders 1465

metabolism 101, *102*
misunderstanding and misuse
  1339
mixtures 305, 314, 2007
MRLs 3, 1563
natural toxicants in foods and
  1983
new 1601, 1602, 1605–8
nomenclature 1547
occupational exposures 1463,
  1530, 1535
organophosphate 259
and parenteral toxicity 523
pharmacogenetics 232
plant protection 1548
pre-marketing authorization
  1543, 1557
probabilistic methods of hazard
  prediction 1328
production industries,
  reproductive risks 1463
regulations 37, 1544, 1547–8,
  1557, 1600, 1605–8, 1960
  Canada 1600
  harmonization 1605, 1611
  US 1599, 1600
reproductive toxicity 1138–9,
  1145–6
residues
  environmental effects 1548,
    1565
  food contamination 1563
risk assessment 462–3, 1444
safety margin calculations 91
skeletal muscle toxicity 955
in soil–water systems 1371
species sensitivity differences
  110
spillage and misuse 1339–440
stability 1548
storage stites in body 17
toxicology 259, 1993–2011
toxokinetics 67
Pesticide Chemical Amendment,
  Food, Drugs and Cosmetics Act
  1563
Pesticide Fact File 1947
Pesticide Forum, OECD 1612
Pesticide Handlers Exposure
  Database (PHED) 1602
Pesticide Safety Precaution Scheme,
  UK 1546
Pesticides Safety Directorate (PSD)
  (UK) 1607

PET scan in idiopathic
  environmental intolerance 1707,
  1713, 1716
Peter of Albanos 35
petrous bone, decalcification 347
pets *see* domestic animal
Peyer's patches 344, 549, 557
PGF synthase, ox lung cloned *242*
pH
  effects on absorption 547
  factors affecting 546–7
  of formulation 46
  modifiers, prevention of
    ochratoxicosis 2161
  urine in long-term toxicity studies
    332
phagocytes 200, 731, 908–9
phagocytosis 6, 176, 183, 384, 534,
  997
Phalacrocorax auritus
  see cormorant, double-crested
Phalaris 222
Pharmaceutical Affairs Bureau
  (Japan) 1566
Pharmaceutical Affairs Law (Japan)
  1544, 1566
pharmaceutical industry
  development 2
  responsibilities 1426, 1438
  restrospective data 1435
  safety standards 1439
pharmaceutical use, biotechnology
  products 1548, 1558
pharmaceuticals *see* drugs
pharmacodynamics
  in acute toxicity testing 34, 39
  differences, uncertainty factors
    and 1762
  in dose selection 1620
  extrapolation studies 1438
  interactions 1416
  peroral 543
  testing, in marketing
    authorization applications
    1628
pharmacogenetics 215–18
pharmacogenotyping 222
pharmacokinetics
  aberrant 125–6
  acute toxicity testing 39
  basic concepts 73–5
  biomonitoring 461, 607
  chronic studies 65
  circadian 252–6
  definition 67

derivation 73–80
differences, RDDRs and 1762
dose–response assessments 1758
end-points, in carcinogenicity
  testing 1620
of ethanol 552
interactions 1416
models 19–20, 582–3
order of reaction 73
parameters and constants 68–73
peroral toxicity 543
regulations 1436, 1438, 1443
in repeated exposure studies 56
scaling, physiologically based
  51–2
studies 24, 1616, 1646
testing, in marketing
  authorization applications
  1628
'worst-case' scenario 19–20
pharmacological effects 8
pharmacological toxicology 3
pharmacology 125, 1547
pharmacovigilance 1629, 1640
pharyngeal cancer in firefighters
  1929
pharyngeal mucosa,
  radiation-induced changes 1689
pharyngeal particle deposition 46
pharynx 544
Phase I and II enzymes and
  reactions 17–18, 216, 254, 273,
  568
phase-contrast microscopy 781
Phaseolus vulgaris 345
Phasianus colchius see pheasant,
  ring-necked
pheasant, ring-necked (*Phasianus
  colchius*) 1332, 1333–4, 1340,
  1341
phenotypes
  ADH 236
  ALDH 237
  as biomarker 1847, 1890–1
  and biotransformation 112
  debrisoquine 223
  ethnic differences 236
  functional 218
  metabolic 265
  pharmacogenetics 231
  studies 224
  tests 222
phenyalanine-free amino acid
  mixtures 1553

phenylalanine-tRNA formation
  inhibition 2161–2
S-phenylcysteine adduct analysis
  1882
phenylketonuria, food additives and
  1990
Philadelphia chromosome 1080,
  1099
PhIP$_2$ *see* phosphatidylinositol
  4′,5′-bisphosphate; phospholipid
phlebitis 529
phobic disturbance in IEI 1709
phocomelia 1430, 1956
  see also thalidomide *in Chemical
    Index*
Phomopsis spp. 2146
  P. leptostromiformis 2148
Phoradendron spp. *see* mistletoe
phosphatases, as calpain substrate
  190
phosphate molecule synthesis
  interference 6
phosphatidylchlorine 896
phosphatidylserine 187
phosphatidylserine receptors 183
3′-phosphoadenosine-5′-
  phosphosulphate (PAPS) 105, *106*
phosphodiester alkylation 162
phosphodiesterase, inhibition 817
phosphoenolpyruvate carboxykinase
  283
phosphoglycerate kinase 372
phospholipases 127, 129, 190
  A 195
  A$_2$ 897, 899, 938
  C (PLC) 896
phospholipidosis 338, 344, *730–1*,
  756, 1430
phospholipids 191, 254, 255, 367,
  548, 685, 807, 809, 860, 938
phospholipids, attack 1867
phosphorus-32 postlabelling 279,
  280, 284, 1845, 1846, 1849,
  1888–90
photoallergy 837
Photobacterium phosphoreum 753
photocell arrays 651
photochemical air pollution
  see summer smog/photochemical
    complex
photoimmunotoxicity 836
photoperiod effects on toxicity 16,
  58
photophobia 756, 757
photoreceptors 757

photosensitivity 1427, 1428, 1430, 1438

photosensitization 413, 415, 836–7, 1523, 2148

phototoxic retinopathy 490

phototoxicity 340, 413, 415, 837

Phyllobates aurotaenia see frog, Columbian

Physalia physalis see Portuguese man-o'-war

Physalis spp. *see* groundcherry

physical abuse, IEI and 1710

physical agents, effect on chemical hazards 1418–19

physical examination
  in acute toxicity 45
  in idiopathic environmental intolerance 1711, 1712

physical mechanisms of IEI aetiology 1704–7

physical and mental development, and environmental endocrines 1392

physical stress effects 167

physical trauma from fire 1916

physician, approach to toxicology 1447–8

physiological function in acute toxicity testing 39

physiological indicators of health, wildlife species 1327, 1328

physiological parameters, allometric scaling 51

physiological variation in biomonitoring 1908

physiologically based pharmaco-dynamic (PBPD) model 1770

physiologically based pharmacokinetic (PBPK)
  modelling 141–50
   acute toxicity studies 51–2, 53
   applications in toxicology 147–9
   case study 1770–1
   chronic high-dose studies 88, 89–90
   classical vs 141–2
   clearance studies 74
   definition 141
   determining parameter values 145–7
   development 143–7
   dose–response assessment 1767–9
   environmental health risk assessment 1792

establishing an adjusting occupational exposure limit (OEL) 149

formulation of mathematical relationship 144–5

inhalation model *1768*

metabolic interactions in chemical mixtures 148–9

mixed routes 607, 608

occupational toxicity 1416, 1460

parameters 1768

peroral toxicity 543, 556

personal protective equipment evaluation 149

refining experimental design in toxicity testing 148

and reformulation 147

route-to-route extrapolation 1766

safety margins 91

scaling 51–2

theory and principle 143

tissue compartments selection 144

uncertainties and limitations 149–50

validation 1780

phyto-oestrogens 570–1, 1392, 1398, 1403, 1404, 1407

Phytolacca dodecandra see pokeweed

phytometabolism, organophos-phorus insecticides 1341

phytoplankton 1310

phytoremediation 1373

Pica pica see magpie, black-billed

piezobalances 599

pig
  aflatoxin toxicity 2145, 2153, 2163, 2164
  arsenic toxicity 1515
  CYP genes 216
  fetal eye *in vitro* cornea, preparation 752
  FMO expression 232
  intraperitoneal dosing necrosis 534
  monogastric 1513
  mustard gas 2085
  mycotoxin toxicity 1516
  nerve agents 2094
  nitrite levels 2123
  ochratoxin toxicity 2158, 2159, 2161, 2164
  phenol metabolism 111
  salt toxicity 1517

sciatic nerve injection damage 531

selenium toxicity 1515

stratum corneum skin permeability *579*

sulphonilamide residues 1637

T_3 and T_4 concentration 371

testicular cloned aldo-keto reductase *242*

trichlorfon toxicity 636

pig farming, toxic gases 1516–17

pigeon
  arsenic metabolism 2050
  domestic (*Columba livia*), behavioural testing 1346
  performance after carbon disulphide exposure *660*

pigmentation 830, 836, 837, 2190

pigweed, rough (*Amaranthus* spp.), nephrotoxicity 1522

pike *see* fish, predatory

piloerection 40, 42

pineapple 222

pink disease 2058

pinna 780
  reflex 42

pinocytosis 547, 549

pinprick tests, in LAA 512

Pinus ponderosa see ponderosa

pit cells 865

Pithomyces 2146
  P. chartarum 2148

pituitary gland 298, 346, 369, 1691

pituitary hormones 369, 371, 950

pituitary–target organ feedback systems 980–1

pituitary–thyroid axis 371

pK of formulation 46

pK_a 546

PKC *see* protein kinase C

placebo 425, 1715

placenta
  as barrier 17
  blood vessels 1237–8
  chemical toxicity 1241–2
  clinical chemistry 372
  cloned enzymes 242
  and drugs of abuse 1254–7
  metabolism 1240
  pathology 344
  structure and function 1233–9
  tissue evaluation 1236–9
  trophoblasts 1255–6
  villus tissue and cells 1238–9

placental transfer 1239–40, 1242
   amino acids 1255–7
   dioxins and PCBs 1250–1
   insecticides 1242–5
   metals 1245–50
   myotoxins 1251–4
   neonatal toxicity 1217
plagiarism 1958
plague, epidemiology 1528
Planaria 414
planimetry 746
plant (industrial) *see* industrial site
plantar nerve 637
plant(s)
   and apoptosis 178
   biotechnology 1965–6
   cadmium levels 1375
   cardiovascular toxicity 1522
   edible 566
      see also specific food plants
   gastro-intestinal toxicity 1518
   genetic modification 1454
   metal concentrations 1373
   mutagenicity tests 1039
   nephrotoxicity 1522
   neurotoxic 1520, 1521
   photosensitization 1523
   protection products 1557,
      1608–9, 1610
   psychedelic properties 222
   reproductive toxicity 1521
   soil partition factor 1786
   toxicity
      to domestic animals 1513
      to food-producing animals
        1517, 1518
      to horses 1518–19
   uptake from soil 1369
Plant Pest Act (USA) 1459
Plant Protection Products Directive
   91/414/EEC 1557, 1605
plasma cholinesterase inhibition
   1996
plasma clearance 76, 79, 89
plasma concentration 84, 86
plasma concentration–time curve
   581
   see also area under curve
   chronic intake 80, 81, 82
   determination 75
   and distribution 76, 77, 78
   first-order 74
   interspecies 89
   intravenous dose 70, 76

   oral doses 75
   zero-order 74
plasma distribution 70
plasma enzymes 105, 355, 359–60
plasma half-life 255
plasma membrane 156, 163, 860,
   1684
plasma proteins 254, 367–8, *522*,
   861, 862
   binding 71, 1226, 1228
plasmapheresis 941
plasmids 1024–5, 1043–4
plasminogen activation by snake
   venom 2179
plasminogen activation tests, eye
   753
plastic embedding procedures 339,
   347
plasticizers 2023
plastics
   additives 2021–3
   biocompatibility testing 1738
   classification 1733
   industry 2018–23
   for samples, contamination from
      1909
plate incorporation methods 1045–6
platelets 264, 385, 387–8, 815,
   1686, *1687*
Platichthys flesus see flounder,
   European
plausible risks 1766, *1767*, 1787,
   1788
PLC *see* phospholipidase C
Plenck, Joseph 36, 1490
pleural cells 533
pleural effusion 724
plumbing *see* water distribution
   systems
pluripotent stem cells 383
Plutarch 2079
PM$_{2.5}$ 314, 592, 599
PM$_{10}$ 592, 599
PM *see* particulates
PMN *see* premanufacture notice
PMS *see* post-marketing
   surveillance
pneumoconiosis 1827, 2064
pneumonitis *727*, 1690, 2004, 2061
poikilocytosis 391
point estimate approach 1782,
   1784, 1786
point mutations 7–8, 1025–7,
   1028–30

poison control centers (PCCs) 459,
   471, 737
Poison and Drug Act 1964
   (Norway) 1568
poison hemlock *see* hemlock
poison ivy 835, 836
'poison squad' 1534
poisoning (general only)
   common cause of death 1444
   criminal 1444
   of domestic animals 1509
   fatal, quantification 1353
   homicidal, historical 1489–90
   management 1447
poisonous animals 2177, 2191–4
poisons
   see also animal toxins
   analytical detection 1502–3
   antidotal efficacy assessment
      432
   toxicology 425–6
Poisons and antidotes 35
Poisons Information Centers (USA)
   2177
poisons information services 3
pokeweed (*Phytolacca dodecandra*),
   toxicity 1518
Poland
   BALs 1910
   nitrate and nitrite levels 2116,
      2117, 2118, 2133
polar bears, PCBs in 642
polar moiety in phase II reaction
   105
polar pathway 581
polar regions 1370, 1374
polarized light microscopy 342, 343
polishers, biomonitoring 1904
political controversies 1448, 1563,
   1575, 1649–50
pollen 623, 1301
Pollutant Responses in Marine
   Animals (PRIMA) 1316
pollution (general only)
   see also air; environmental;
      water
   hotspots 1449
   not necesarily increasing 1370–1
   prevention, New Chemicals
      Program 1583
Pollution Prevention Recognition
   Program (USA) 1583
poly(ADP-ribose) polymerase, and
   apoptosis 190, 195

polyamine transport mechanism 128

polychotomous response 47

polychromatic erythrocytes (PCEs) 1087

polyclonal antibodies 982

polyclonal antisera 338

polycythaemia 389, 391–2

polyethylene tubing 526

polyfume fever 1915

polygenic mutations in multifactorial conditions 1037

polygraph tests 1948

polyhydramnios 1206

polymer industry 1734, 1915, 1917, 2013–28

polymerase chain reaction (PCR)
    ADH 236, 237
    CYP2D6 218, 219
    in pharmacogenetics 218, 229, 234, 235
    safety technology 1966

polymeric matrix testing 1742

polymodal nociceptor 612

polymorphisms 21, 38, 112, 135, 217–43, 274, 1549, 1890

polymorphonuclear leukocytes 384, 533

polymorphs 384

polymyositis 943

polyneuropathy, organophosphate-induced delayed 1996, 1997

polyuria 40, 42, 43, 362, 682

ponderosa (*Pinus ponderosa*), reproductive toxicity 1521

pons 347

pony *see* horse

POPs *see* progesterone-only oral contraception

population
    -based studies, male reproductive health 1466
    composition ratios 1353
    dynamics 1327
    estimation, in field testing 1353
    exposures 1535
    risk 1813
    size, as biomarker 1846, 1847

porcelain factory biomonitoring 1904

pork
    heterocyclic amines 271
    nitrate and nitrite levels 2113

porphobilinogen, as biomarker 1864

porphyria 383, 392, 1705, 1713

porphyria cutanea tarda 29, 1226

porphyrin
    biomarker 1849, 1863–5
    as biomarker 1461
    clinical chemistry 362
    complex 99
    dioxin-induced 1818
    excretion, arsenic and 2051
    hepatic 29
    metabolism 2068
    synthesis 1863–4

porphyrinuria 2063

portal vein 545, 555, 556

Portuguese man-o'-war (*Physalia physalis*) 2189

positive control substances 340

positive/negative lists *see* permitted/proscribed lists

post-drug potentiation (PDP) 950–1

post-drug repetition (PDR) 950

poster presentations 1941

post-marketing authorization procedures, EU 1629–30

post-marketing surveillance (PMS) 22, 457, 1960

post-mortem drug testing 1501

post-mortem interval 1495

post-natal evaluations, teratogenicity 1181–5

post-natal growth 969–70

post-registration observations 1435

post-traumatic stress disorder 1707

post-traumatic syndrome 1825, 1828

posture 252

potassium changes, as biomarker 1861

potassium channels 639, 805, 806, 822, 897

potato
    see also Solanum spp.
    nitrate and nitrite levels 2112–13, 2115, 2116
    toxicity 1984

potency 39

Potential Daily Intake (PDI) 1602

potentiation 20, 50, 305, 306, *313*

Pott, Percival 472, 1474

potters 456

poultry
    see also specific types, e.g. chicken
    aflatoxin toxicity 2145, 2149, 2154

cardiotoxicity 819

common toxicoses 1520–4

fumonisin toxicity 2163

mycotoxin toxicity 1524

ochratoxin regulations 2158

salt toxicity 1522–3

Poultry Products Inspection Act (USA) 1563

PPARα *see* peroxisome proliferation associated receptor

prairie dog (*Cynomys* spp.), poisoned 1347

prandial state 552–3, 557

prealbumin 254, 371, 511

precipitation on storage 1909

preconceptual irradiation 1695

precursors for *in vitro* testing 52

predation
    see also feeding patterns; secondary toxicity
    pesticide effects 1348

predator species
    eggshell thinning 1351, 1354, 1548
    secondary/tertiary toxicity 1341, 1346–7

pre-derived cancer values 1758

pre-derived non-cancer values 1758

pre-employment medical screens 513

pre-existing disease 461

pregnancy
    chemical and drug exposure 1216–24
    detection 1465
    diethylstilboestrol effects 1406
    and drug toxicity 21
    exposure to metal compounds 1203–6
    and increased susceptibility to toxicants 1464
    17β-oestradiol levels 1398
    outcome abormalities radiation-induced 1694
    pathology 340
    studies of chemicals and 23
    viral infections and neurotoxicity 665

Pregnancy Discrimination Act 1467

pregnant women, in clinical trials 1618

pre-historic toxicology 1527

pre-incubation tests 1047–8

pre-keratins 828

pre-leptone spermatocyte radiation-induced changes 1688
preliminary safety data 464–6
pre-manufacture notice (PMN) 1459, 1545, 1581
exemption 1581
Japan 1565
USA 1557
pre-marketing approval, medical devices 1663–4
pre-marketing authorization
drugs 1543, 1544
EU 1551, 1552, 1557
food additives, USA 1658
novel foods, EU 1551, 1553
pesticides 1543, 1557
terminology 1543
veterinary medicines 1558
pre-marketing notification 37, 1545, 1557
pre-Marketing Notification of New Chemicals Act (USA), amendment 37
premature ventricular contraction (PVC) 811, 818
prematurity 1464, 1465
prenatal irradiation effects 1696–7
pre-neoplastic foci 692
preputial separation, in juvenile male rats 1406
prescribers *see* clinicians
prescription medications, cross-reactivity in drug testing 1501
presentation, effects on toxicity 16
preservatives 1552, 1560, 1611, 1653, 1985, 1988–9
pre-synaptic terminal 813, 814
prey base, removal by anticholinesterase 1352
Preyer's reflex 42, 780
PRIMA *see* Pollutant Responses in Marine Animals
primary effects 26
'primary irritation' *see* chemical burns; irritation
primary literature 475
primates
see also humans
combustion toxicity studies 1923
human contact 490
metanol toxicity 119
model for interferon testing 1971
prime toxicant 307

printing industry
noise and chemical hazards 1418
reproductive risks 1463
prions, as impurities 1968
probabilistic analysis 1328, 1449, 1782–4, 1785, 1792
probability
density functions 1784
distribution 1782
quantifying 1573, 1574
of response 48
probe, labelled DNA 239
probit analysis 48, 49, 493, 1331–2, 1334, 1344–5, 1763
procarboxypeptidase 897
procarcinogens 7
procaspases 164, 191
process flavourings 1654
proctitis 524
prodromal syndrome, radiation-induced 1686
product(s)
databases 1448–9
factsheets 1448–9
formulation, differential hazard 1338–9
licence 1425
and process validation 1678
safety 402, 403, 738, 755
toxicology 3
Product Licence (UK) 1544, 1627
Product License Application (USA) 1974
Product Stewardship agreements 1585
proelastase 897
professional organizations, forensic toxicology 1491
Professors in Toxicology 1937
progesterone 266, 372, 534–5, 1149, 1155–6, 1403
prognostic criteria and factors 1450
programmed cell death
see apoptosis
'prohaptens' 836
prokaryotes 216, 1019, 1966, 1969
prolactin 372
prolactin effects, assay 1328
prolapsus 42
proliferating cell nuclear antigen 338
proline nitrosation 2121
promoters 7, 88, 126, 566
pronase in adduct analysis 1883
pro-oxidants 168

Propionibacterium 563
proportional mortality ratio (PMR) 1532
prospective cohort studies 1456, 1532
prospective studies, ethical issues 1435
prostaglandin synthases 103, 241, 678, 729, 732
prostanoids, concentration in lung 128
prostate
cancer 1983, 2015, 2054
cells, apoptosis 179, 196
-specific antigen (PSA), biomarker 1849
prostatic acid phosphatase DNA adduct analysis 1890
prostheses 523
see also medical devices
prostration 40, 42
protease inhibitors, adverse effects 1427
proteases 127, 156, 194, 1883
proteasomes 164
protection ratio 433
protective clothing *see* personal protective equipment
protective proteins, as biomarker 1847
protein(s)
see also specific types, e.g. heat-shock proteins
adducts 1843, 1844, 1845, 1847, 1877–80, 1887
antibodies 1885
attack 1867
binding 51, 71, 73, 126, 128
C, activation by snake venom 2179
catabolism 159
cell cycle involvement 168
changes, as biomarker 1858–9
damage, metal toxicology 2066
deficiency 16, 115, 970–1
see also kwashiorkor
degradation 1883–4
dietary 58, 2120
engineering 1454
see also biotechnology industries
as impurities 1969
inhibition 189
interactions with chemicals 85
interactions with toxins 163

protein(s) (*Contd.*)

  levels in BALF, in dose–response assessment 1762

  modification, endogenous 1878

  phosphatase inhibitor 199

  post-translation modification 1878

  synthesis 113, 114, 188, 1843, 1848–9, 1862–3, 1869

  as targets 34, 159–60

  therapeutic 1964–74

  thiols 128

  tissue content, interspecies 88

  visualization, as biomarker 1856

protein kinases 190

  C (PKC) 190, 195, 808, 896, 2055

proteinase-K, in adduct analysis 1883

proteinuria 43, 363, 367, 678, 682, 685, 687, 689, 690

proteolysis 819

proteolytic enzymes 701

proteomics 169

prothrombin 361, 389, 2179

prothrombinase 2179

protista for *in vitro* testing 52

proto-oncogenes 364, 395, 1028–30, 1099–100

protocol design 40–2, 64–5

protoporphyrin 1864, 1906

provisional tolerable weekly intake (PTWI) 91

provocation-neutralization in IEI 1713, 1714

proximal tubule 345, 362, 363, 676

pruritis 510

PSA *see* prostate-specific antigen

pseudoallergic reactions 1986–7

pseudocholinesterase 29, 1906

  see also butyrylcholinesterase

pseudoeosinophils 385

pseudogene *216*, 230, 237

pseudohypoparathyroidism 950

pseudomembranatous colitis 1438

Pseudomonas 536, 1301

pseudoperoxidase activity 364

psychedelic drugs *220*

psychedelic effects 222

psychiatric disorders in IEI 1707, 1709, 1710, 1714, 1716

psychiatric evaluation in IEI 1712, 1715

psychoactive drugs, forensic analysis 1491

psychogenic asthma attacks 1708

psychological disturbance, adverse drug reactions 1427

psychological stress 1708, 1710, 1729, 1927

psychomotor retardation 235

psychosomatic symptoms, idiopathic environmental intolerance and 1711

psychotomimetic agents 2082

psychotropic drugs 264–5, 1443

psychotropic effects 223

PTH *see* parathyroid hormone

ptosis 40, 42, 757

PTWI *see* provisional tolerable weekly intake

Ptychodiscus brevis 2192

public health

  pests, pesticide efficacy 1601

  protection 1426

Public Health Service 487

public hygiene insecticides, EU regulation 1611

public perception

  of medical devices 1674

  of risk 1576–8, 1959

  of science 1959

public relations 1576

public risk 1812–13

public safety, regulatory aspects 1439

PUFA *see* polyunsaturated fatty acids

puffer fish 34, 639, 816, 2193

pugilist brain 636

pulmonary, *see also* lung

pulmonary alveolar proteinoses *727*

pulmonary arterial hypertension 730

pulmonary cadmium absorption 2052

pulmonary capillaries 724, 728

pulmonary damage, from riot control compounds 2013

pulmonary drug excretion 256

pulmonary endothelial cells 730

pulmonary epithelium, target tissue 128

pulmonary exposure to chemicals 603

pulmonary fibrosis 725, 728, 731, 1430, 2060

pulmonary function tests in idiopathic environmental intolerance 1709

pulmonary hyperplasia 728

pulmonary hypersensitivity 702

pulmonary hypertension 730, 815

pulmonary lipid embolism *727*

pulmonary lipidosis 730–1

pulmonary oedema 724, *727*, 732

  acute 809

  from fires 1917

  from organic solvents 2036–7

  from phosgene toxicity 2099

  interstititial 728

  in pigs 2145, 2163, 2164

pulmonary ossification *727*

pulmonary phospholipidosis *730–1*

pulmonary pneumocytic dysplasia 728

pulmonary surfactant 731

pulmonary system 342

pulmonary toxicity, systemic 721–36

pulmonary uptake of organic solvents 2029

pulmonary vascular leak syndrome 343

pulmonary vasculitis *727*

pulse exposures 1535, 1536

pulse rate 264

pulsed field gel electrophoresis 563

pumpkin, nitrate and nitrite levels 2112

pupillary reflex 42, 45, 764

Pure Food and Drug Act (USA) 36

Purkinje cells 637, 643

Purkinje fibres 805, 816, 818

  see also ventricular ectopic pacemaker activity

purslane, nitrate levels 2113

purulent exudate 530

PVC *see* premature ventricular contraction

pyknosis 821

pyloric sphincter 545

Pyrethrum cinariaefolium 34

pyrexia 127

Pyridinium spp. 2192

pyridinoline, as biomarker 1859

pyroclastic debris 1815

pyrogen test 535–6

pyrogenicity 522, 535

pyrogens, as impurities 1968

pyrolysis 315, 1916, 1919–20

Q

Q fever, infection transmission 514
QA *see* quality assurance
QEEG *see under* electro-encephalogram
QRA *see* risk assessment, quantitative
QSAR *see* quantitative structure-activity relationship
quadriceps, risk in intramuscular dosing 527
quail *see* northern bobwhite
quail
    Japanese (*Coturnix japonica*)
        age effect on LC_{50} 1337
        carbofuran sensitivity 1342
        dose–response anomalies 1330
        as model species 1344
        parathion sensitivity 1342
        subacute toxicity testing 1332, 1333–4
quality assurance 293, 437–51, 1563–4, 1664
quality control 45, 535–9, 1628, 1973
quantal response 9, 10–11, 13
quantified risk analysis 1829
quantitative structure–activity relationship (QSAR) 317, 613, 1449
    see also strcture–activity relationship
quantity of absorbed dose per unit mass 1684
quarrying, risk of death 1830
quasi-folded proteins 167
Quercus spp. *see* oak
questionnaires 1450, 1529–30
quinone oxidoreductase 104, 240–1
quinone reductase, DT diaphorase 104

R

R-*ras*, and apoptosis 193
rabbit
    acute toxicity 45
    adrenaline 529
    aflatoxin LD_{50} 2154
    aluminium toxicity 427
    amphetamine metabolism 102
    arsenic metabolism 2050
    baseline temperature 536

biliary excretion 555
blood sampling 386
cardiotoxicology 811, 813, 818
cornea, epithelial cells and plasminogen activator 753
coronary artery test systems *417*
cyanide toxicity *760*
cyotchrome P450 antibodies 218
CYP genes 216
dermal and oral 46
developmental period 1696
dioxin susceptibility 282
endotoxin sensitivity 536
ethylene glycol toxicity 110
eye irritation tests 739
eye toxicity 409, 410
FMO expression 232, 233
gastric pH 555
β-glucuronidase and β-glucosidase 572
HDL fraction 367
hepatotoxicity marker 359
hexobarbitone toxicity 110, 111
immature 536
in vitro lung tests *417*
interferon testing model 1971
intra-arterial dosing 527
intravenous injection site 526
kidney ketone reductase 242
LAA 511
long bone haematopoiesis 383
muscle implantation 535
NAT enzymes 108
neuropathy from ginger 1824
nitrate toxicity 2123, 2124
nitrite toxicity 2123, 2125
ochratoxin pharmacokinetics 2161
oral drug administration 522
N-oxidation inhibition 232
parenteral techniques 526
phosgene 2097
pulmonary oil microembolism 534
pyrogen test 522, 526, 535, 536
replacement 402
sacrospinal muscle 342
skin irritation studies 843
sperm analysis 1142
stomach pH 555
stratum corneum skin permeability *579*
synthetic materials testing 1741
tPA safety evaluation 1970
upper GI tract 544

water injections 533
weight 51
wild 1350
race *see* ethnic factors
rad (unit) 1684
radial arm maze 657
radiant furnace 1926
radiation
    see also ultraviolet light
    absorption 1683
    and apoptosis 188, 1690
    β-radiation 599
    biomarker 1849
    dose–response model 1766
    exposure 1035
    γ-radiation 1683, 1693
    hormesis and 1951
    -induced lethality 260
    ionizing
        and apoptosis 177, 191, 199
        carcinogenesis 1692–3
        cellular stage 1684
        densely ionizing 1683
        deterministic effects 1685–92
        hereditary effects 1693–6
        nature of action 1683–4
        partial body 1685, 1687–92
        physical and chemical stages 1683
        prenatal 1696–7
        reproductive toxicity 1154
        stochastic effects 1692–7
        tissue 1684
        toxicology 1683–701
        whole-body 1685, 1686–7
    lung toxicity 728
    and menstrual disorders 1465
    occupational exposures 1463
    radiofrequency, toxicity 1418–19
    sickness, acute 1820
    toxicology 260
radicals, reactions 161
radioactive zone, diagonal 1890
radioactivity
    accidental release 1820, 1828, 1833
    bioavailability 581
radioallergosorbent test (RAST) 510, 513, 514
radiofrequency radiation
    see radiation, radiofrequency
radioimmunoassay (RIA) 371, 982–3, 1502, 1885, 1889, 1967, 2158

radioimmunometric measurement 365

radiolabelling studies 67, 70, 72, 982

radiological contrast media, regulatory aspects 1548

radionuclides 11683

radioprotectants 1690

radiosensitivy, circadian 260

radiotelemetry 1353, 1354

radish, nitrate and nitrite levels 2112–13

rainbow trout *see* trout, rainbow

raising agents 1985

Ramazzini, Bernadino 1474, 1528

Rana catesbeiana see bullfrog

random audit programme 516

random sampling programmes 1781

randomization 294, 1353, 1535

Ranunculus spp. *see* buttercup

rape (plant) *see* kale

rape*seed* 234

rape*seed* oil, adulterated 1551

rapid acetylator phenotype 274

rapid eye movements 251

raptorial birds *see* predatory species

ras
    and apoptosis 195
    biomarker 1849, 1892
    carcinogenicity 1100–1, 1113–14
    mutagenicity 1029–30
    oncogene activation, and solvent exposure 1457

RAST *see* radioallergosorbent test

rat
    acetaminophen toxicity 110, 117
    acetylaminofluorene toxicity 110
    acrylamide neurotoxicity 637
    acute myelogenous anaemia model 527
    acute toxicity studies 38, 257
    adenocarcinoma by pancreas implantation 525
    adipose tissue dioxin level 282
    adrenal glucocorticosteroid 356
    aflatoxin LD_{50} 2154
    age effects on metabolism 115
    aggressive behaviour 653
    AITC toxicity 134
    ALP activity 355
    amine oxidase (AO) 238, 239
    aminophenol hydroxylation 110
    arsenic metabolism 2050
    aryl hydrocarbon hydroxylase 524

aspirin hydrolysis 525

behavioural testing 1346

benzo[*a*]pyrene 278, 279

bile 569

biliary excretion 555

bilirubin 360

bladder carcinogenesis 1129–30

blood sampling site *386*

body weight/surface area difference 92

bone marrrow 385

brain
    atrophy by MAM 636
    FMO 232

breast tumour induction 266

breathing rate 46

cadmium 2054

carbaryl 1342

carbon tetrachloride hepatotoxicity 1857, *1858*

carcinogenicity studies 291, 336, 1127–9, 2015, 2016, 2018, 2019, 2020, 2021, 2022

carcinoid gastic tumours 1124–7

cardiac puncture 387

cardiotoxicity 527, 813

ceftizoxime clearance 89

ChE inhibition 369

chemical $LD_{50}s$ 408

chlorine irritant effects 613

circadian variations 253, 254, 255

clotting function tests 388

CO_2 studies 61

cocaine toxicity 528

colon
    carcinomas 568
    FC-12 567
    nitrosation reactions 567

combustion toxicity 1923, 1924, 1926

contaminated arthopods 1341

coronary artery test systems *417*

coumarin hydroxylation *231*

creatine kinase 412

CYP genes 216

cytochrome P450 3A 285

dechlorination reactions 566

dermal toxicity 46

developmental period 1696

dietary studies 1982, 1985, 1986, 1987, 1990

dimethoate toxicity 1335

dioxin toxicity 85, 87, 88, 90, 282, 284

dose–response assessments 1760–1, 1762

drug dosage by gavage 553

ejaculation latency 653

embryo toxicity and oxidative stress 159–60

epididymis ABP 372

epoxide hydrolase 279

ethylene glycol toxicity 55, 110

exhaled air 552

extrapolation of results 53

famciclovir conversion 239

female reproductive system 1244, 1245

foreign body carcinogenesis 1130–1

forestomach 551, 555

fumonisin toxicity 2164, 2165

fungicide toxicity 2002, 2004

gastric ulceration 524

gender differences 129, 272–3, 1338

germ-free 566

GGT 359

giant cell granuloma 529

glomerular filtration rates 356

glucocorticosteroid as plasma marker 356

β-glucuronidase and β-glucosidase 572

gnotobiotic 564

haematotoxicity 104

halothane toxicity 104

Hb 1883

HDL fraction 367

hepatocyte DNA repair test 1434

herbicide toxicity 2004, 2005, 2006

heterocyclic amines 272

hexobarbitone toxicity 110, 111

$HgCl_2$ autoimmune response 682

hGH safety evaluation 1970

IgE antibody response 704

ileum length 554–5

in vitro lung tests *417*

inability to vomit 524

infusion systems 527

interspecies differences 274–5, 279, 283

intestinal absorption 546

intravenous dosing
    and hypotensive bradycardia 533
    injection sites 526

rat (*Contd.*)

   intromission latency 653

   islet cell 346

   jejunum length 554–5

   LAA 511

   LDH activity 355

   liver

     apoptosis 199

     carcinogenesis 259, 271

     enzyme inducers 135

     hepatotoxicity 230–1, 359, 417, 853, 866, 872

     interspecies differences 279

     necrosis 361

     pathology 344

     thyroxine excretion 1123

   male, testosterone 511

   mammary gland 278, 571

   medullary space 383

   MeHg in faeces 570

   mercury 2058

   metallothionein gene expression 2067

   methionine salt, intramuscular dosing 532

   methotrexate, circadian response 261

   microflora 563, 565

   microsomes 279

   milk allergen studies 1005

   mitochondria 810

   as model species 1335

   motor activity 651

   muscle necrosis 951–5

   myelosuppression 527

   nasal passages 342

   nasal turbinate structure 592

   nephritis 511

   nerve agents 2091

   nitrate, nitrite and *N*-nitroso toxicity 2120, 2122, 2123–4, 2125–8, 2135, 2199

   NMR of urine *679*

   nutrient requirements for trace elements and vitamins 604

   nutrition effects on metabolism 115

   ochratoxin pharmacokinetics 2161, 2162

   ocular teratogenesis 758

   olfactory bulb of brain 232

   orbital sinus blood sample 387

   organic solvents 2041

   organophosphate studies 1997

   oropharynx bacterial infection 514

   ototoxicity 794

   ozone toxicity studies 1275, 1276

   parenteral techniques 526

   PCB toxicity 131

   peritoneal cells *411*

   peritonitis 532

   pesticide sensitivity 1338

   phosgene 2097

   phrenic nerve test *417*

   plasma ALP 359

   poisons 2006

   prandial state bioavailability 552

   preferred intraperitoneal dosing 526

   pregnant, osmotic minipump use 528

   proteinuria 511

   proximal tubule 345, 417

   pulmonary fibrinogenesis 527

   pulmonary oil microembolism 534

   renal tubule 680, 1862

   repeated acquisition task 661

   repeated exposure studies 59

   reproductive cycle 372

   reproductive system *see* rat, female/male

   respiratory tract deposition pattern of particles *589*

   riot control agents 2013

   running wheel 652, 664

   skin permeability 584

   splanchnic artery necrosis 527

   stomach

     absorption 546

     section 544

   strain, survival 323

   strain differences 239

   subcutaneous sarcoma 530

   sulphur mustard 2084, 2086

   T_3 and T_4 concentration 371

   tamoxifen 285

   target tissues for non-mutagenic carcinogens *1120*

   testis

     ABP 372

     atrophy 82–3

     toxicity 372

   thromboarteritis 529

   troponin measurement 366

   tumorigenicity of medical devices 1742

   upper GI tract 544

   urinary aeroallergens 514

   urinary biomarkers *1864*, 1885

rat bite fever 514

rate constant 70, 73, 77, 79, 86

rattlebox

   (*Crotolaria* spp.) 133, 730, 1519

   (*Sesbiana* spp.) 1518

rattlesnake 2178

   Mojave (*Crotalus scutulatus*) 2178, 2179, 2180

   Sistrurus 2178

   western diamondback 2178

raw materials, medical devices 1672–3

ray designs 306

Raynaud's phenomenon 2019

Rb see retinoblastoma gene

RD_{50} (respiratory depression) 612–13, 620, 621–2

RDA *see* recommended daily allowance

RDDR *see* regional deposited dose ratios

reactions

   see also first-order reactions

   order 73–5

reactivation 429, 430

reactive airways dysfunction syndrome 1915

reactive effects 35

reactive intermediates 130–2, 133–5, 157–63

reactive metabolite 223

reactive oxygen species (ROS) 34, 127, 128, 192, 199, 635, 643, 684, 691

reactive radical metabolites 104

reality checks on model results 1781

reanl cells, regeneration 126

Reaper, and apoptosis 193, 195

reasonable man, legal concept 1677–8

reasonably maximal exposure scenarios 1775

receptor

   agonists 631

   antagonism 430

   binding assays 1402–3

   definition 1395

   interaction 6

   ligand binding, transcriptional activity 1402

   -mediated events 126

regulatory procedures (*Contd.*)
Nordic Council 1568–9
patterns 1543–7
reinforcing agents in rubber industry 2017, 20114
Reissner's membrane 776, 780, 782
relative potency factor 311
relative risk (RR) 1533
release pathways 189
release testing 1678
relevance of expert witness report 1949
reliability of expert witness report 1949
religious conflicts 1723
religious cults 1728
REM *see* rapid eye movements
Remote Access to Marketing Authorizations (RAMA) 1436
renal, *see also* kidney; nephro-
renal blood flow 254, 255
renal cells
apoptosis 179
damage, extrapolation studies 1754
epithelial 362
renal clearance assessment 1861
renal insufficiency 943
renal papilla 345
renal tubules 256, 257, 337, 338, 345, 685
renal vascular resistance 678, 684
renin 345, 364
–angiotensin system 370, 684
repeated application irritation testing 844
repeated dose toxicity studies 328–31, 1591, 1616, 1618, 1622
repeated exposure toxicity 22, 55–66
repeated insult patch testing (RIPT) 839–40
replication factor C, and apoptosis 195
reporter gene assays 1402
reports from students 1940–1
Reports of the Scientific Committee for Food, EU 1656
reproducibility of results 45
reproductive efficiency, epidemiological measurement 1529–30

reproductive system
see also female reproductive system; male reproductive system
cell changes 179
clinical chemistry 372
genetic mutations 1038
male 1140–7
environmental effect *see* sperm count
environmental endocrine effects 1391, 1399, 1400
occupational hazards 1466–7
physiology 1140–2
toxic agents 1142–7
workplace semen samples 1529
pathology 345–6
plant toxicity 1521
screening tests in animals 1137–40, 1142–3
weight 1395, 1400, 1402–3, 1407
reproductive toxicity
biomarkers 1858–9
carbamate pesticides 1351
classification 1593
diethylstilboestrol 1392
dioxin 87
environmental oestrogens 1565
fungicides 2002, 2003
laboratory studies 1347–8
mechanisms 1464
medical devices 1734, 1735
model species 1328
mycotoxin 1516
new drugs 1617–18
nitrates 2124, 2129–30
nitrites 2127
occupational hazards 1463–7, 1929
organic solvents 2041
organophosphorus pesticides 1351
prednisone 1455
radiation 1684, 1688–9
rifampin 1455
risk assessment 1467, 1751, 1756
streptomycin 1455
studies 8, 23–4, 1137–8, 1168–9
testing 499, 1329, 1567, 1628
toxicology laboratory 510

wildlife species 1327, 1328, 1339–440
xenobiotic effects 1347–8
reptiles
phenol metabolism 111
studies 790
wildlife toxicology 1327, 1330, 1353
RER *see* rough endoplasmic reticulum (RER)
research
ethics committees 1960
experience for toxicology 1939–40
laboratories, source of biological hazards 1459
and risk assessment 1753
reservoir effect 577, 579
residence time, standard assumptions 1773
residual capacity, inhalation toxicity 46
residuals 75, 77
residue file, EU Regulation 2377/90 1643, 1644
residues
analysis 1354
cut-off assessment 1635
depletion studies 1646
maximum safe concentration 1635
monitoring 1637
surveillance, UK 1647–8
wildlife species 1327
resin
embedded sections 339
manufacture, formaldehyde exposure 1456
resistant starch 561
resorption phase, chemical 578
Resource Conservation and Recovery Act (USA) 1749–50
resources 1957, 1961
respirable fraction 461, 512, 592
respirators 149–50, 584, 1714
respiratory allergens 702, 706, 712
respiratory allergy 701
respiratory depression *see* RD_{50}
respiratory homeostasis maintenance drugs 25
respiratory irregularities 42
respiratory protective equipment 514, 516

respiratory rate 45, 46, 307, 612–13, 620, 621–2, 1776
respiratory sensitization 701–19, 1484
respiratory symptoms in IEI 1712
respiratory system
    aerosol PSI *625*
    airflow patterns *591*
    allergic response 512
    anatomical structure 590
    biopsies in IEI 1706
    function tests 513
    in vitro test systems *417*
    irritation 23, 56, 614–15
    muscle paralysis, anoxia 1510–11
    particle deposition 590–2
    resistance 466
    response to reactive chemicals 1474
    route of exposure 59
    wood workers 1456
respiratory toxicity
    see also inhalation toxicity; summer smog; winter smog
    animal stings and bites 2179–80, 2189
    anticholinesterases 1996
    arsenic 2051
    bleomycin 1455
    chromium 2062
    etheylenediamine 1475
    firefighters 1928
    fires 1916, 1917, 1921, 1923, 1925
    formaldehyde 16
    glutaraldehyde 62
    grain dust 1475
    herbicides 2006
    idiopathic environmental intolerance and 1704, 1705–6, 1712, 1716
    diisocyanates 1475
    kaolin 1475
    meat wrapper films 1915
    mercury 2058
    mustard gas 2086, 2087
    mycotoxins 1516
    nerve agents 2092
    nickel 2063
    nitrate 1514
    nitrogen dioxide 1279
    organophosphates 1997
    ozone 1276
    paraquat 1512

particle size of substance effects 16
phosgene 2098
plastics industry 2020, 2021, 2022
radiation 1687, 1690
rodenticides 1511
rotenone 1999
rubber industry 2014, 2015
signs 40
solder flux 1475
toluene diisocyanate 1456
toxic gases 1517
toxic oil syndrome 1824
volcanoes 1815, 1816
wood dust 1475
response
    addition 304
    –duration histograms 744, 745
    50 response point 9–10
    surface analysis 311
responsibility
    for drug interactions 1438
    for occupational risk management 1476
resting membrane potential (E_m) 816
restricted products, classification and labelling 1603–4
restriction site mutation analysis 1062
reticulin 341
reticulocyte 384
reticulocytosis 385, 388, 391
reticuloendothelial system 183, 360
reticulosarcoma 296, 2015
retina
    dysgenesis 758
    gliosis 758
    infarction 756
    ischaemia 765
    melanin in 129
    pathology 347
    periarteritis 756
    pigment epithelium 765
    toxicity 530, 764–5
retinoblastoma(s) 1032, 1081
retinoblastoma(s), (*Rb*) gene 193, 1849, 1850
retinol binding protein 678, 1906, 1910, 2053
retinopathy 129, 756, 1430
retinoscopy 764
retro-orbital plexus 357
retroperitoneal fibrosis 1438

retrospective (historical) studies 1435, 1531
retroviral infection, gene transfer 1964
reverse pharmacogenetics 228
reversibility of toxicity 63
R_f values *see* chromatographic methods
RfC *see* reference concentration
RfD *see* reference dose
rhabdomyolysis 940, 941, 942, 943, 946
rhabdomyosarcoma 262, 531
rhesus monkey *see* under monkey
Rheum rhaponticum see rhubarb
rheumatoid arthritis 263, 265, 764, 944
Rhine (river) 1370
rhinitis 510, 512, 513, 701, 758, 1703, 1715, 1716
rhinoconjunctivitis 512
rhinorrhoea 40, 512
Rhododendron spp.
    R. aricacea 818
    toxic to domestic animals 1513
rhubarb (*Rheum rhaponticum*) 1522, 2112–13
RIA *see* radioimmunoassay
ribonucleic acid *see* RNA
ribonucleic reductase 261
ribose, conjugation 107
ribosomes 681, 860
Ricinus communis see castor oil plant
rickets 1427
rickettsia as CB weapon 1726
RIDIT analysis 49
right-wing anti-government groups 1728
righting reflex 40, 42
rights of individuals, ethics and biomonitoring 1911
ring sideroblasts 391
ringworm, irradiation 1693
riot control compounds 2102–4
RIP, and apoptosis 196
RIPT *see* repeated insult patch testing
rising dose procedures 44
risk(s)
    assessment 27–8
        acceptable risk level 1787, 1788, 1829
        added risk calculation 1786
        behavioural toxicity 670

risk(s)
assessment (*Contd.*)
biomarkers 1408
confidence in figures 1790
contaminated soil 582
contribution of human health
toxicology 1833–6
development 1749
dietary exposure 1602–3
disasters 1813–14, 1929–32
dose–response assessment
1758–71
ecological 1318–19
environmental 657, 1749–809
ethical issues 1960–1
existing substances
programme, EU/OECD
1480
genetically modified
organisms 1628, 1629
guidelines 1751, 1763
and hazard 1536–8, 1811
health surveys 462–3
how it works 1749–52
human studies 38, 461,
1449–50
industrial chemicals 1460–1
information resources 475
intolerable 1829
justifiable 1829
language 1557, 1579
medical approach 1449
medical devices 1674, 1743–6
medical impact 1444
mixed routes of exposure 607,
608
mycotoxins 2147
nitrates and nitrites 2136
occupational and
environmental factors
1415–24
overestimations 1751, 1756,
1771, 1781, 1787, 1835
paradigm 1473, 1753
PBPK modelling 147–8
in peroral toxicity 554–7
potential 1752–3
process 1752, 1753–91, 1941
quantitative 1537, 1752, 1792
radiation 1693, 1694
regulatory aspects 1479,
1480, 1573–4, 1750
reliability 1456
standardization 1751

statistical and analytical issues
1781–2
study design 25
toxicity tests 275
toxokinetics for 90–2
underestimation 1756, 1781,
1835
avoidance 1955
-based sampling plan 1792
characterization 456, 1460,
1461, 1753, 1786–91
communication and perception
1576–8, 1911, 1959
definition 1449, 1812
factors 1576–8, 1978
index 149
individual 1812–13
management
biotechnology industry 1462
environmental exposure 603
environmental health 1750
health
and chemical exposure
461; surveys 463–4
industrial chemicals 1460–1
mixed routes of exposure 607,
608
PCBs 1588
regulatory aspects 1574
strategies 1586
negligible 90
phrases (R-phrases) 1477, 1487,
1557, 1594, 1603
potential 1960
reduction 1813–14
regulatory aspects 1573–8
relationship to hazard .1812
societal 1812–13, 1833
Risk Assessment Directive, EU
1479
*Risk assessment in the Federal
Government: managing the
process* 1750
Risk Assessment Regulation, EU
1480
@RISK software 1782, 1784
rivers
improved quality 1370
pollution 1866
RME (EPA-type default point
values) risks 1784–5, 1788
RNA
messenger (mRNA) 113, 195,
346, 712, 785, 788, 808–9,
1011–12, 1019, 1080, 1865

and mutagenicity 1019
and reproductive toxicity 1145
ribosomal (rRNA) 1019
synthesis inhibition 188, 189
transfer (tRNA) 1019, 1026
RNAse 897
road traffic accidents 1830, 1921
robin, American (*Turdus
migratorius*) 1341
Robinia pseudoacacia see black
locust
rodent(s)
see also specific rodents, e.g. rat
bone marrow metaphase analysis
1088
forestomach 544
fungicide toxicity 2002
glandular stomach 544
herbicide toxicity 2005
lindane toxicity 1995
liver
cellular alteration 344
glutathione activity 338
glycogen activity 338
oncogene expression 344
long-term feeding studies 323
mammary tumour induction 278
metal teratogenicity 1206–9
mouth lining 544
nitrogen oxide studies 1278–9
oesophagus 544, 553
tail vein blood sampling 386
tests
20-day pubertal female assay
with thyroid 1403
bioassays 1535, 1537, 1763,
1767
carcinogenogenicity 1106–14
DNA damage 126
long-term 1753
micronucleus 1087–8
neurological 23
species requirements 1573
teratogenicity bioassays
1207–9
weight 51
vinyl chloride toxicity 1771
vomiting response 553
wild 1335, 1350
rodenticides 523, 1345, 2006–7
decontamination procedures
1511
domestic animal toxicity
1510–11
EU regulation 1611

rodenticides (*Contd.*)
  and parenteral toxicity 523
  poultry toxicity 1524
  testing 45
  wildlife toxicity 1345
  yellow phosphorus 1523–4
ROELEE 84 statistical program
  301
Romanowsky stain 336, 341, 385,
  1087
roofing workers, exposure risks
  1886, 1887
rooting powders 2005
rope of death 222
ROS *see* reactive oxygen species
rose allergy 1708
rotarod techniques 654
rotating brush generators 596
Rotating Table Dust Generator *596*
rough endoplasmic reticulum (RER)
  860, *861*, 864, 894, 895
route of administration
  see administration route
route of exposure *see* exposure route
Royal College of Physicians of
  London 433, 454
Royal Society (UK), Study Group of
  Risk Assessment 1811
Rp-2/Rp-8, and apoptosis 193
RTECS *see* Registry of Toxic
  Effects of Chemical Substances
rubber industry 564, 1667, 1738,
  2013–18
*Rules governing medicinal products
  in the European Union* 1621,
  1627
rumen
  see also forestomach
  microflora, in nitrogen toxicity
   1514
Rumex spp. *see* curlydock
ruminants 527, 544, 1509, 2122
  see also cattle; forestomach
  wild 1375, 1378
running memory 667
running wheels 651
Russia *see* USSR (former)
rye *see* cereals

S

S9 fraction preparation 1040–1
β-S100 biomarker 2031
S phase 256
S-PLUS statistical program 301

SA node *see* sinoatrial node
Saccharomyces cerevisiae see yeast
saccule 778
sacrifice animals 61, 65
safe dose 91
Safe Drinking Water Act (USA)
  1393, 1750
Safe Medical Devices Act 1990
  (USA) 1662
safe working practices, industrial
  chemicals 1545
safety
  see also apparent safety margin
  assessment 35, 36, 135, 1941
   acute toxicity 35, 36
   biochemistry 135
   biodrugs 1967–9
   biomaterials 1738–9, 1746
   education 1941
   information sources 1675–7
   medical devices 1675–7
   packaging materials 1737
   pre-clinical 1968
   reference sources 1676–7
   transgene models 1964
  assurance procedures 91–2
  definition 34
  demonstration in acute toxicity
   studies 38–9
  factors (coefficients)
   factsheets 1448
   food 316
   Food and Drug Administration
    (FDA) (USA) 1635
   indoor air pollution 316
   new chemicals 1448
   occupational toxicity 1461
   regulations 1575, 1643
   study design 322
  file, EU Regulation 2377/90
   1643, 1644
  margin in risk assessment 91
  needs in CB attack 1728
  parameters, medical devices
   1737–8
  pharmacology 125, 1616
  phrases (S-phrases) 1477
  ratios *11*
  regulations 1960
  symbols 1594
  testing 1621, 1628–9
Safety Association of Marketed
  Medicine 458
sago palm *seeds* 635
Saimiri sciureus 663

St Anthony's Fire 2145, 2148
St Johns wort (*Hypericum
  perforatum*), photosensitization
  effects 1523
saline, percutaneous absorption *in
  vitro* studies 580
salinity changes as biomarker 1842,
  1848, 1869
saliva 18, 72, 562, 1845, 2120,
  2122, 2134
salivary glands 237, 343, 1689
salivation 42, 497
salmon lice control 636
Salmonella spp.
  in garbage toxicity 1512
  and gastro-intestinal microflora
   561, 565, 572
  /microsome assay 566
  S. typhimurium 272, 279, 499,
   566
   mutagenic DNA repair 1022,
    1025
   mutation tests 1042, 1043–6,
    1049, 1050, 1102, 1103–4,
    1185–6
   toxicity studies 24, 2124,
    2128
  S. typhosa 536
salmonids (fish) 1311, 1314
SALT *see* skin-associated lymphoid
  tissue
sampling
  contamination 1909
  misuse 1911
  pollutants, in samples 1909
  procedures, validation 1893
  sources of error 1908–9
  standardization 1908
  strategies 1530, 1905
San Francisco Bay Area Region
  Poison Control Center 737
sandwich enzyme immunoassay
  514, 983
sanitary and phytosanitary measures
  3
SAR *see* structure–activity
  relationships
sarcolemma 539, 808
sarcomas 837
  herbicides 2005
  induction 530–1
  spleen 565
  subcutaneous 522, 529, 530
sarcoplasmic calcium 938

sarcoplasmic reticulum 808, 809, 812, 813, 816, 820, 821, 938, 939

Sarobatus vermiculatus see black grease-wood

SAS statistical program 301

sassafras 1552, 1981

saury 2193

sausage, nitrate and nitrite levels 2113

SBS *see* sick building syndrome

scabby grain intoxication 2149

scabies 460

scala media 776, 779, 789

scala tympani 776, 779

scala vestibuli 776, 779

scalds, deaths from 1917

scale containment 1960

scaling factors in risk assessment 1769

scalp 577, 578

scanning calorimetry 619

scanning electron microscopy (SEM) 339, 347, 756, 782

scanning lens monitoring 756

scanning synchronous fluorescence spectrophotometry 1882, 1889

scar formation 177

scatter diagrams 1836

scavenger systems 515

SCE *see* sister chromatid exchange

Schiff's reaction 344

Schistosomas haematobium 636

schistosomiasis treatment 1995

schizophrenia as neurotoxic process 665

Schlick atomiser 595

Schmiedeberg 1935

Schmorl's stain 867

Schwann cells 631, 639

sciatic nerve 527, 531

Science and judgments in risk assessment 1752

Scientific Committee on Animal Nutrition (EU) 1648

Scientific Committee on Cosmetology (EU) 1560

Scientific Committee on Food (EU) 91, 1560, 1655–6, 1657

Scientific Committee for Occupational Exposure Limits to Chemical Agents (SCOEL) 1595

scleroderma 944, 2019

scombroid fish 2193–4

scorpion fish 2191

scorpions 2187–8
  Androctonus 820, 2188
  Bothotus 2188
  Buthus 2188
  Centruroides 820, 2187–8, 2189
  Mesobuthus tamulus 2188
  Parabuthus 2188
  Tityus 820, 2188

scramblase 187

screening
  see also monitoring; testing
  definition 1394
  information data set (SIDS) 1480, 1585, 1587
  level assessments 1586
  objectives 1400
  protocols, developmental toxicity 1185–8
  tests
    environmental endocrines 1407–8
    field studies 1353–4
    forensic toxicology 1497
    standardized 1328

scrotum 577, 578
  cancer 2, 456, 1474

sea anemones 640, 2190

sea bass 2191

sea nettle (*Chrysaora quinquecirrha*) 2189

sea snake 2178, 2179

sea urchin *414*
  aquatic toxicology 1319, 1320

seafood
  see also shellfish *and individual foods, e.g.* mussels
  arsenic 1382
  histamine 823
  methylmercury 1564–5

seagulls, PCBs in 642

seals, PCBs in 642

seasonality, and xenobiotic toxicity 1342–3, 1419

sebaceous glands 46, 829–30

sebum 830

Second World War *see* Word War II

second-hand smoke *see* passive smoking

secondary effects 4, 21, 26, 125

secondary/tertiary toxicity
  anticholinesterases 1341–2
  birds 1524
  carrion-eating species 1341
  dogs 1510
  famphur 1342

laboratory testing 1353
  predator species 1341, 1346–7

secrecy 1961

Secretary of Agriculture (US) 486

secretin 895

security against terrorism 1721

sediments
  field sampling 1781
  toxicant dispersal 1832
  toxicity, aquatic toxicology 1319

*see*d dressings, toxicity 1825–6

*see*ds
  chemically treated 1341, 1343
  contaminated 1339
  mercury toxicity 2057

segmental necrosis 944

seizure-related deaths 1494, 1504

seizures
  in acute toxicity 40, 41
  in animals 497, 644
  diazepam for 430
  herbicide toxicity 2006
  neurotoxicology 641
  pharmacogenetics 235, 239
  solvent abuse 2029
  strychine toxicity 1510

selective ion monitoring (SIM) 1500

selective ion monitoring (SIM), GC mass spectrometry (SIM-GCMS) 231

seleniferous plants 1519

self-medication 1549

self-poisoning (acute overdose), commonly encoutered substances 1496

Sellafield 1695

SEM *see* scanning electron microscopy

semen
  see also sperm
  analysis 1467
  quality 1145–6, 1463, 1466
  samples 1529

semi-automated digital image analysis 339

semi-quantitative prognostic criteria 1450

seminal fluid 372

seminiferous epithelium 345

seminiferous tubules 346, 371–2

Senecio spp. *see* groundsel

sensation changes 40

sensitive population, response to toxic agents 1416

sensitivity 47, 150, 1785–6, 1833–4
sensitization
    contact 340
    effects, OEL notation 1485
    lung or skin 1474
    medical devices 1734, 1740
    patch testing 838–9
sensory irritation 21
    see also peripheral sensory
        irritation
    biological models 619–22
    chemical models 618–19
    concentration-response data 616
    cutaneous toxicity 832–3
    determination methods 618–23
    effective concentration (EC) 616
    exposure dosage *617*
    incapacitating concentration (IC)
        617
    mixtures 307
    peripheral 611–29
    response 616–18
    significance 615–16
    in warfare 2082
sensory nerve fibres, IEI and 1706
sensory nerve receptors 612, 623
sensory thresholds 655
sentinel animals 58, 1870
sepiapterin reductase *242*
sequential dosing procedures 44
serine *1878*
serotinergic system 222, 223
serotonin *see* 5-hydroxytryptamine
    (5HT)
Sertoli cells 346, 371–2, 418, 1141,
    1142, 1404, 1464
serum
    biochemistry as biomarker
        1858–9, 1929
    horse butyrylcholinesterase 429
    lipid, dioxin levels 282
    parameters 43
    sickness 1549, 2181
    tests 355
service industries, toxic exposures
    1453
Sesbania spp. *see* rattlebox
set dose procedures 44
SETAC *see* Society of
    Environmental Toxicology and
    Chemistry
seventh amendment, EU 1590
Seveso disaster 2, 38, 1443, 1444,
    1724, 1818–19

sewage
    aquatic toxicity 1310
    environmental oestrogen efffects
        1565
    sludge 1371–2
    treatment plants, hormone levels
        1407
sex
    see also gender differences
    chromosome, abnormalities
        1081, 1694
    hormone binding globulin
        (SHBG) 372, 1398
    hormones and agonists 1129
    -linked conditions 1036, 1056–7
    ratios, altered 1392
sexual abuse, idiopathic
    environmental intolerance and
    1710
sexual assault, and acid phosphatase
    1495
sexual behaviour 664
    see also libido
sexual changes, as biomarker 1855
sexual differentiation 179
Sgp-2, and apoptosis 193
sheep
    aflatoxin toxicity 2154
    copper toxicity 1514
    CYP genes 216
    facial eczema 2145, 2148
    herbicide toxicity 2006
    lupinosis 2145, 2148
    methionine salt 532
    nitrate toxicity 2124
    nitrite levels 2123
    pharmacogenetics 223
    selenium toxicity 1515
    T_3 and T_4 concentration 371
Sheffield (Brightside) disaster 1821
shellfish
    see also seafood
    biomarkers 1852
    cadmium concentrations 822
    contamination 1825
    diarrhoeic 2194
    neurotoxicity 639, 2192
    oil contamination 1826–7
    paralytic 2192
    poisonous 2177, 2191
    saxitonin toxicity 1554
    toxin 816
shift work 1419
Shigella spp. 561

shipping
    and aquatic toxicity 1310–11
    disasters 1826–7
ships, anti-fouling 1548
shock-associated odour 666
shop workers, risk of death 1830
short-chain fatty acids 561
short-range toxins 131
short-term exposure limit 625
short-term mutagenicity tests 1434
short-term repeated dose studies 5,
    39, 57
showering exposure 1773, 1780,
    1786
shrew 51, 1866
shrimp *see* brine shrimp
sialic acid biomonitoring 1910
sick building syndrome (SBS)
    1292, 1299, 1530, 1703
sickle cell anaemia 384
side-effects 4, 21, 1435
sideroblastic anaemia 389, 391
siderophagocytosis 532
Sidman avoidance 657
SIDS *see* screening information data
    set
sigma minus method 80, 85
signal transduction 159, 163–4,
    169, 190, 194
signalling 190, 202
significant new use notice (SNUN)
    1583
significant new use rule (SNUR)
    1581, 1583, 1587
Silent Spring 2
silicon microphysiometer 753, 847
silicone biocompatibility testing
    1738
silicosis 1475
silk combustion products 1923
silo filler's disease, nitrogen dioxide
    1517
simian virus 40 415
simple dissimilar action 304–5
simple independent action 304
simple joint action 304
simulated field trials *see* caged field
    trials
single application irritation testing
    see Draize test
Single European Act 1987 1555
single-dose toxicity studies
    see also acute toxicity testing
    embryotoxicity 1334
    LD_{50} test 1328

single-dose toxicity studies (*Contd.*)
  oral 1330, 1332–3, 1335–6
  regulations 1616
single-generation reproduction
  studies 1328
singlet oxygen $^1O_2$ 127
sink effects
  indoor air particles 1299–300
  ozone and nitric oxide 1274–5
sinoatrial (SA) node 805, 808, 811,
  817
sinus arrest 811
sinus tachycardia 819
sinusitis 1703, 1711
sinusoid epithelial cells 855, 856,
  857, 858, 864, 881
sinusoids 545
SIRC cells 410
sister chromatid exchange assays
  (SCE) 276, 515, 567, 1088–90,
  1460
Sistrurus see rattlesnake
site-of-contact effects 1474
sixth amendment *see* EU Directives,
  79/831/EEC
size factors
  obesity 366, 1981
  and response to toxic agents
  1416
SK *see* ethyl bromoacetate
skeletal, *see also* bone; cartilage
skeletal abnormalities 40, 951, *952,
  966*, 968–70, 972, 1217, 1245–6
skeletal fluorosis 1381
skeletal muscle
  autopsy samples 1495
  biomarker 1848
  enzyme distribution 1858
  fibre simplification 342
  necrosis 366
  NQO2 in 240
  nuclei ATPase activity 187
  toxicity 938–64, 1512
skeletal remains, forensic
  examination 1495, 1496
skin
  see also cutaneous; dermal;
    percutaneous; subcutaneous
  abrasions 46, 363
  absorption
    human studies 463, 465
    of lead 2055
    modelling 578
    of organic solvents 2029–30

as source of error in
  biomonitoring 1908
time factors 1778
toxicokinetics 69, 70, 75
adipose layers reached by soil
  chemical 582
allergic response 512
animal and human 584
and apoptosis 197
assessment 340
barrier function 577
cancer 836, 837
  arsenic 1382, 2051
  biomarkers 1892
  and dietary fat 1980
  interspecies variation 278
  mixtures 315
  occupational toxicity 1474
  in plastics industry 2019,
    2020
  in rubber industry 2015
  and ultraviolet light 1538
cells *see* keratinocytes
condition, as biomarker 1855
contact studies 60, 1735, 1736,
  1740–1, 1765
damage
  animal stings and bites 2178,
    2182, 2183, 2185, 2187,
    2189
  in disasters 1814
  fungicides 2002
  lake gas 1817
  Lewisite 2088, 2089
  radiation 1684, 1685, 1688
  rubber chemicals 2014, 2016
  sulphur mustard 2084, 2085,
    2087
  toxic oil syndrome 1824
disorders
  adverse drug reactions 1427
  predictability in animal tests
    1438
dosing 523
exposure 19–20
  see also percutaneous;
    subcutaneous
  assessing 1777–8, 1780
  dose calculation 1774, 1775
  sensitivity analysis 1786
  soil 1776–7, 1778
  standard assumptions 1773
  to chemicals 605
functions 830–1
in humans 623

hydration 46
irritation
  alternative tests 411–12
  analogy 754
  characterization of 834
  cumulative 60
  nickel 2062–3
  organic solvents 2032
  primary 23
  repeated exposure 56
  results evaluation 844–5
  selected microscopic changes
    833
  tests 494
lotions 605
mouse dermal toxicity test 605
notation 603
oncogenicity bioassay 58
painting study 554
penetration studies 499, 578, 580
permeability 579
pigmentation, arsenic 2051
prick tests 510, 513
sensitization 413
structure 577–8, 828–30
surface areas, 'rule of nines'
  estimation 583
tags and papillae 1248
as tissue compartment in PBPK
  144
toxicity
  acute 46
  diisocyanates 1475
  effects 829, 831–8
  in vitro assays 845–7
  in vivo results 844–5
  OEL notation 1484–5
  signs 44
  testing 327, 838–44
  xylenes 1475
skin-associated lymphoid tissue
  (SALT) 830–1
skipjack 2193
SLE *see* systemic lupus
  erythmatosus
sleeping
  problems in IEI 1714
  sickness 1994
  time, as biomarker 1855
slimming aids 1551
slit-lamp biomicroscopy 496, 738,
  746, 747, 751, 756
slow acetylators 273
slow twitch fibres 342

small business sector 1453, 1481, 1487

small intestine 552, 562

small mammals
feeding trials 1330
subacute dietary toxicity test 1333–4

SMART *see* somatic mutation and recombination test

smelter factory 1904, 2051

smog, *see also* London smog

smoke from fires 46, 1821–3, 1916, 1917, 2128
see also tobacco smoke

smoked foods 1982

smokers/ing
adducts in 1883, 1885, 1890
biomarkers 1845
biomonitoring 1904, 1905
cadmium 2052
and cancer 1538, 1981
carbon monoxide levels 607
β-carotene and 1983
CHD and 1978
contamination 1915
drug metabolism 113
effect on COHb levels 1921
ethylene oxide 1784
hazards 28, 1439
Hb adducts 1883
idiopathic environmental intolerance and 1705
interaction
with asbestos exposure 1417
with chemicals, in firefighters 1929
with lead exposure 1417
laboratory ban 516
and lung function tests in firefighters 1928
nitrate metabolism 2122
nitrosamine adducts 1885
N-nitroso compounds 2115
PAHs 1886
passive *see* passive smoking
and phenotypes 1891
polycythaemia 391
and reference limits 1910
risks 223, 274, 279, 513, 1529, 1751
as source of error 1908
vitamin E and 1983

smokestacks 1376

smooth endoplasmic reticulum 105, 113

smooth muscle 460

snails, aquatic toxicity 1316

snakebites
acute toxicity 38
horses 1517
management 2180–1
phosphodiesterase DNA adduct analysis 1890
statistics 2178
toxic manifestations 2178–80

snakeroot, white (*Eupatropium rugosum*), neurotoxicity 1519, 1520

snakes 2177–81
cobra (*Hemachatus haemachatus*; *Naja nigricollis*) 820, 2178, 2179, 2180
coral snake (*Micrurus fulvius*) 2178, 2180, 2181
crotaline
(*Bothrops* spp.) 957
rattlesnake (*Crotalus scutulatus*) 2178, 2179, 2180
pit viper 2180
saw-scaled/carpet viper (*Echis ocellatus*) 2181
sea snake 2178, 2179
viper 2178

snapper 2191

sneezeweeds (*Helenium* spp.), hepatoxicity 1519

sneezing 512, 614, 2102

Snow, John 1528

snuff 2115, 2132

Soap and Detergent Association 503

soaps, allergy 1704

social and regulatory toxicology 1447

Social Security Act 1975 511

societal differences and risk acceptance 1961

Society of Environmental Toxicology and Chemistry (SETAC) 1316, 1328

Society of Forensic Toxicologists 1491

Society of Toxicology (SOT) (USA) 39, 326, 402, 425, 472, 493, 1770, 1935–6

socioeconomic factors in air pollution studies 1272, 1274

Socrates 1489

SOD *see* superoxide dismutase–catalase system

sodium changes, as biomarker 1861

sodium channel blockers 1510

sodium channels 639, 640

sodium/potassium (Na+/K+)
ATPase
and cardiotoxicity 807, 808, 809, 811, 812, 816, 818, 821, 823
and ototoxicity 779, 785
pathology 341
species differences 286
pump 812, 818, 822

soil(s) 577
absorption, in disasters 1828
agricultural 1376
buffering capacity 1376
cation storage 1369
chemical bioavailability 1777, 1778
chromium contamination 1778–9, 1780
composition 1329, 1367
definition 1366
dioxin contamination 281, 606, 1818
field sampling 1781
forming factors 1367
horizons 1367
ingestion 1773, 1774, 1775–7, 1782–3, 1788
lead contamination 1780
loading 582
material binding, cycling and transformation 1368–70
matrix, movement to skin 582
mineralogical and chemical composition 1367–8
mining activities contamination 1373
natural 1375–6
nature and properties 1366–8
near waste disposal sites 1372
nitrate contamination 2112
organic contaminants 1369
organic matter 1368, 1369
PAH contamination 1791
parent material 1367
particles, surface area 1367
pH 1368
profiles 1367
reference values for metal contamination 1373
salinization 1371

soil(s) (*Contd.*)
  self-purification 1370
  solution 1367, 1368
  texture 1367
  toxicant dispersal 1832
  wildlife hazard 1340–1
soil(s)–water systems
  acidification 1376
  interrelated 1365
  pollution 1370–81
  selenium 1380
Solanum spp. *see* nightshades
solder flux, respiratory effects 1475
soldering, lead neurotoxicity 639
Solenopsis spp. *see* fire ants
solid–water interface 1365, 1368
solvent(s)
  see also organic solvents (*in Chemical Index*)
  abuse 2029
  extraction 367
  in food 1985
  idiopathic environmental intolerance and 1708
  intoxication 1715
  in plastics industry 2023
  in rubber industry 2014, 2017–18
somatic cell assays 1085–6
somatic effects of radiation 1684, 1692
somatic mutation and recombination test (SMART) 1057
somatization, IEI and 1709, 1715
somatosensory discrimination 661
somatotrophs *see* growth hormone (GH)
somnolence 42
Sophora spp. *see* mescal beans
SOPs *see* standard operating procedures
sorbitol dehydrogenase 356, 359, 1462
sorghum, cyanide-containing plant 1519
SOT *see* Society of Toxicology
soybean fumonisins 2165
SP-1 transcription factor 168
space of Disse 855, *858*, 864
Spain
  nitrate levels 2112
  toxic oil syndrome 38, 1444, 1551, 1554, 1568, 1824

sparrow
  house, subacute feeding trials 1338
  white-throated (*Zonotrichia albicollis*), migratory behaviour 1348
spasticity 42, 1983
spatial processing 667
special sense organs 346–7
speciality medical devices 1661, 1667–8
speciation
  arsenic 1382, 1515
  chromium 1458
  elements 1365
  mercury 1378
  terminology 1445
species
  see also model species
  affecting toxicity 2, 15
  differences *see* interspecies variability
  diversity 1327
  overcrowding 1842
  selection 59, 293, 739, 1967
  sensitivity in repeated exposure studies 59
specific effects 35
specific gravity 362
specific ion electrodes 367
specific locus test 24, 1143
specimen sampling *see* sampling
SPECT in idiopathic environmental intolerance 1707, 1713, 1716
spectrofluorimetry 1498
spectrometry *see* specific techniques
spectrophotometry 597, 982, 1491, 1498, 1882, 1889
  see also specific techniques
spectroscopic methods
  see also specific techniques
  in forensic testing 1497
speech problems, and PCBs 642
sperm
  see also semen
  analysis 1142, 1143
  clinical chemistry 362
  count
    as biomarker 1858
    environmental encrocrine effects 1391, 1392
    reduced 1392, 1399, 1404, 1464
  variability 1399

morphology, glutaraldehyde effects 62
  quality 1464, 1466–7
spermatids 346
spermatocyte 372
spermatogenesis 371, 1141–2
  clinical chemistry 371
  dibromochloropropane (DBCP) effects 1466
  nitrate effects 2125
  organic solvent effects 2041
  radiation effects 1688–9
  semen analysis 1467
  toxins affecting 1145–6
sphincter of Oddi 894
sphinganine inhibition, fumonisins 2165
sphingomyelin pathway, and apoptosis 191
sphingomyelinase D, in spider venom 2186
sphingosine inhibition, fumonisins 2165
spiders 2185–7
  Agelenopsis 820
  Argiope spp. 820
  black widow spider 640, 2185–6
  brown spider 2186
  necrotic effects 2186–7
spillages, chemical 606, 1339–440, 1545, 1551
spina bifida 969, 1216, 1696
spinach, nitrate and nitrite levels 2112–13
spinal cord
  amyotrophic lateral scoliosis (ALS) 239, 1983
  glycine receptor antagonist 641
  neurotoxic action 640
  organic solvent toxicity 2031
  pathology 347
  peroral toxicity 546
  radiation-induced damage 1690
spinal reflex check 45
spiral ligaments 779, 785, 795
spirits, nitrate levels 2115
spleen 103, 341, 383, 565, 1762, 2126
spleen colony formation (CFU-S) 260
splenomegaly 391
SPM *see* particulates, suspended
spongiform encephalopathy, adverse drug reaction 1430
spongiotrophoblast 282

spontaneous abortion *see* abortion

spraying, metabolic excretion 460

spring greens, nitrate and nitrite levels 2113

spring parsley (*Cymopterus watsonii*), photosensitization effects 1523

SPSS statistical program 301

spurge (*Euphorbia* spp.), toxicity 1518

squamous cell carcinomas 837, 1692

squamous epithelium, mitosis 340

squamous metaplasia from formaldehyde 16

squirrel monkey 663

Sri Lanka, deliberate food poisoning 1724

Stabe, Casina 1528

stability data, in marketing authorization application 1628

stability tests, standard operating procedure (SOP) 446

stabilizers 1552, 1653, 1985, 2022

Stachybotris spp. 2149

stacks *see* incinerators

staggers 223

staining techniques 64, 342

stakeholders in risk assessment 1829

Standard Operating Procedures (SOPs) 293, 444, 445, 446, 447–8

standard texts 475–6

standardized mortality ratio (SMR) 1532

Standing Committee on Plant Health (EU) 1605, 1607–8, 1610

Stanford–Binet intelligence test 669

stapes 776

Staphylococcus spp.
  enterotoxin B 1690
  in garbage toxicity 1512
  in intestine 562

starling, European (*Sturnus vulgaris*) 1348, 1349, 1352

startle reflex 42

starvation
  see also anorexia; feeding behaviour
  effect on metabolism 115

Stas–Otto method 1490

static monitoring, exposure data 1530

statistics 291–302
  acute toxicity testing 45, 47–50, 1331–2
  age adjustment 298
  analysis of variance (ANOVA) 1177
  bias 291
  bioassay 1331–2
  chance 291
  clinical trials 1439
  combination 296, 297
  comparison methods 292, 300–1
  confidence interval 292
  confounding variables 301
  continuous data 301
  control groups 297, 298
  correlation coefficients 301
  developmental toxicology 1177–8
  dose-related trend 300
  false conclusion 298
  false positive 291
  field studies 1353
  formal models 296
  heterogeneity 300
  hypothesis testing 292
  LD_{50} 301
  low-dose extrapolation 297–8
  meta-analysis 1456–7
  misuse 1533
  multivariate methods 301
  NOEL estimation 297–8
  non-parametric methods 297
  null hypothesis 300
  observation context 298
  paired data 301
  pairwise comparison 300
  pooled data 297
  probability 292
  ranked data 301
  response variable 300
  software 301
  stratification 297
  subchronic toxicity testing 1344–5
  survival differences 298
  tests 292, 300–1, 1332
  time-to-tumour models 296
  trend analysis 297
  variables 295–6, 301
  wildlife toxicology 1330, 1331

statum granulosum 828

STATXACT statistical program 301

steady state 80–2, 83, 87, 582

steam distillation 1497

stellate cells *see* Ito cells

stem cells 383, 1684, 1686, 1687

stercobilinogen 360

stereocilia 776–7, 782, 790–1

stereospecificity 614

stereotactic injections 641

sterility, radiation-induced 1688

sterilization 1454, 1455, 1667, 1668, 1679–80

sternum, bone marrow 341

sternutators 2102

steroid binding proteins 1892

steroid hormone assays 1317

steroid receptors 126, 984

steroid-type inducer 113

steroidogenesis, *in vitro* assay 1402

Stevens–Johnson syndrome 755

stillbirths 1203, 1205

stinging *see* sensory irritation

stingrays 2190–1

stochastic reinforcement of waiting 660

stochastic response to radiation 1684, 1685

stomach
  see also forestomach; gastric; gastro-
  absorption 69
  ALDH3 in 237
  cancer
    gastric carcinoma 240
    nitrates 2130–1
    nitrites 2132
    N-nitroso compounds 567, 2132
    in plastics industry 2022
    in rubber industry 2015
    vitamin C and 1982
  carcinoid tumours 1124–7
  dosing into 549
  modelling 556
  mucosal radiation-induced changes 1689
  occlusion 11
  secretions 546

stomatitis 235

stonefish 2191

storage sites 17

strain
  differences, and metabolism 111
  and sensitivity in repeated exposure studies 59
  and toxicity 15, 2054

stratum corneum
  absorption 69
  chemical crossing estimation
    model 582
  cutaneous toxicity 828, 830, 831,
    833, 843, 845, 847
  diffusion 46, 582
  fat content 583
  penetration phase 578
  percutaneous toxicity 577
  and transfer rate 578
stratum germinativum (basal layer)
  828
stratum lucidium 828
stratum spinosum 828
Straub tail 42
strawberry, nitrate levels 2113
Streptobacillus meliniformis 514
Streptococcus 562
streptokinase 366, 538
Streptomyces spp.
  S. avermitilis 1999
  S. cinnamonensis 819
  S. cuspidosporus 765
  S. sparsogenes 765
Streptopelia risoria see dove, ringed
  turtle-
stress
  -activated protein kinase, and
    apoptosis 195
  cellular responses 166–9
  and chemical toxicity 1419
  clinical chemistry 357
  and cocaine toxicity 1419
  detection with polygraph 1948
  following disasters 1828
  effect on toxicity 1417
  in firefighters 1928–9
  following food contamination
    1825
  in mouse inhalational study 604
  reduction techniques 1714, 1729
  -related autonomic reaction in IEI
    1708
  as source of error in
    biomonitoring 1908
  variables 356
  following volcanic eruption 1817
stress proteins 168, 1461, 1847,
  1869, 2066–7
stressors
  endogenous and exogenous
    1337–8
  and reproductive failure 1465

stria vascularis
  amnioglycosides effects on
    792–3
  cis-Platinum effects on 793–4
  in ototoxicity 779, 780, 782,
    784–5
  trimethylin effects on 794, 795
structure–activity relationships
  (SAR)
  and alternative testing 407, 411
  and animal welfare 499
  and aquatic toxicity 1315
  and cutaneous toxicity 846
  in environmental health 1756
  and eye toxicity 754
  genotoxic carcinogens 1102–4
  and hepatotoxicity 876
  and nephrotoxicity 701, 706
  new chemical substances 1581
  in new product testing 1635
  oestrogen agonists and
    antagonists 1401
  and parenteral toxicity 524
  regulatory aspects 1583–4, 1618,
    1635
  and repeated exposures 61
  and respiratory toxicity 712–13
  in risk assessment 1449
student presentations in toxicology
  1940–1
student–mentor relationship 1937,
  1939
Student's *t*-test 300
study design and conduct 22–5
Study Director 386, 439, 440,
  441–2, 444, 449
Study Group on Combination
  Effects 304
Study Group on Medical Devices
  (Cooper Committee) 1662
stupor 42
Sturnus vulgaris see starling,
  European
styrene, vapour and colour vision
  impairment 756
styrene epoxygenase *217*
subacute intoxication, definition
  1446
subacute myelo-opticoneuropathy
  (SMON), and clioquinol 1427,
  1428, 1566
subacute toxicity studies 39
  design 328–31, 1534
  dietary tests 1333–4
  feeding trials, in captivity 1338

LD$_{50}$ protocol 1330
repeated exposure 57
reproducibility 1332, 1448
subadditivity 305, 1416
subarachnoid space 779
subchronic toxicity studies 39
  design 328–31
  environmental health risk
    assessment 1772
  Good Laboratory Practice (GLP)
    440
  medical device testing 1742
  oral tests 324
  repeated exposures 57, 62–4
  wildlife toxicity 1344–5
subcutaneous, *see also* skin
subcutaneous exposure 19, 47,
  525–6, 530–1
subcutaneous implantation 528
subcutaneous infection 530
subcutaneous injection 525
subcutaneous sarcoma 530
subdural haematoma 636
subendocardial haemorrhage 814
sublethal toxicity 15, 1333, 1353,
  1831
sublingual neutralization for
  idiopathic environmental
  intolerance 1715
subspecialities of toxicology 3
substance P, idiopathic
  environmental intolerance and
  1705
substantia nigra 103, 223, 232, 641
substrate specificity 233, 241
succinate, as biomarker 1862
succinate dehydrogenase 342
succinyl-coenzyme A 392
sudden death, horses 1519
sugar
  and lectins 183
  nitrate and nitrite levels 2115,
    2116, 2117
suggestive responses in idiopathic
  environmental intolerance 1708
suicide 38, 234, 543, 1443, 1444
suicide substrates enzyme
  inactivators 130
suing expert witness 1948
sulphaemoglobinaemia 391
sulphatase 568
sulphate 16, 18, 105
sulphation 98, 105–6, 115, 255
sulphomucin 897
sulphonation 528

sulphones 101
sulphotransferases 105–6, 216, 272–3, 285
Summary of Product Characteristics (SmPC) 1438, 1623, 1627
summer smog/photochemical complex 1265–6, 1267, 1273–80
sumpweed (*Iva augatafolia*), reproductive system toxicity 1521
suntan, artificial 1550
superfusion chamber 751
superoxide anion radical O_2^- 127, 1867
superoxide dismutase (SOD) 127, 158, 239, 636, 809, 1867–8, 2161
superoxide dismutase (SOD)–catalase system 1276
supervised trials median residue (STMR) 1609
suppliers, responsibilities 1476, 1480, 1481
supply-side testing programs 1478–81
suppressor genes 162
suppressor mutations 1026
supra-additive interactions *see* synergistic interactions
sural nerve 637
surface area
   and body weight 51, 92
   scaling factors 1769
   sensitivity analysis 1786
   soil and groundwater toxicity 1367, 1369
   soil particles 1367
surface exposures, in the workplace 1474
surrogate data 1602
surrogate models, for human exposures 1534
surrogate species *see* model species
Surveillance of Work Related Occupational Respiratory Disease (SWORD) (UK) 701
survival
   factors, and apoptosis 193
   genes 194
   vs health 1961
Susrata 1731
sutures, bioabsorbable 1744–5
sweat
   bench-scale extraction experiments 1777–8
   chromium toxicity 1779

diffusion 46
excretion 18
radioactivity excretion 581
sweat glands 577, 829, 847
Sweden, nitrate and nitrite levels 2114, 2118
Swedish National Food Administration 1379
Swedish National Institute of Occupational Health 668
sweet potatoes 726
sweet shrub (*Calycanthus* spp.), neurotoxicity 1520
swine *see* pigs
Swiss roll techniques 343
Switzerland
   BALs 1910
   fumonisin contamination of cereals 2165
   nitrate and nitrite levels 2116, 2117, 2118
symbols, in classification and labelling 1477, 1557, 1594, 1603
sympathetic nervous system 368, 1142
sympathomimetic drugs 219, 1438
symposium format progress reports 1940–1
symptom diary 1712
symptom questionnaires 1530
synaptic clefts 640
synaptic vesicles 632
Synechocystis spp. 1092
synergistic interactions 20, 28, 50, 305, 306, 313, 1395, 1405–6, 1416
synthetic hormones 1455, 1465
synthetic materials 1731, 1739
synthetic protein membranes 754
synthetic reactions 216
Syrian golden hamster *see* hamster
SYSTAT statistical program 301
systemic absorption 523
systemic circulation 555, 603
systemic lupus erythematosus (SLE) 764, 944
systemic toxicity
   acute 35, 56
   aflatoxins 1516
   definition 5
   fires 1917
   medical devices 1735
   synthetic materials testing 1741
   testing 40

T

T_3 *see* triidothyronine, thyroid hormones
T_4 *see* tetraiodothyronine (thyroxine), thyroid hormones
T cell(s)
   and apoptosis 188
   functional subpopulations 703–4
   helper (Th cells) 703, 729, 998–9
   hybridomas, and apoptosis 190
   and immunotoxicity 998–1000, 1012
   in latex allergy 510
   lifespan 1882
   mitogen 710
   pathology 341, 343
   response 682
   skin-infiltrating 830, 835
   subset alterations in IEI 1704
   Swiss mouse fibroblast cell line 413
   thymocytes 341
   zones 341
T cell receptor (TCR) complex 998
T syndrome 1244, 1998
tables for computation 49
tachycardia 40, 42, 43, 460, 811, 824
tachyphylaxis 612, 619, 725
tachypnoea 40, 42
tacrolimus, diabetogenic effect 764
tadpole tail regression 178
talin, as calpain substrate 189–90
Tamil guerillas 1724
Tamm–Horsfall glycoprotein 362, 678
tampons 1667
tandem mass spectrometry 225
Tantramar copper swamp 1368
tapwater *see* drinking water
tardive dyskinaesia 663
target organ(s)
   accumulation testing 1967
   acute toxicity 15, 39, 43
   biochemistry 128–30
   for cell apoptosis by toxins 184–6
   dose 9, 91, 147
   identification in acute toxicity testing 39
   medical devices toxicity 1734, 1741
   regulatory aspects 1676

target organ(s) (*Contd.*)
  residue depletion studies 1646
  risk assessment 1754, 1787
  toxicity models 415–16, 418
  toxin distribution 603
  toxokinetics 67
Target of Organ Toxicity Series 1676
target population, risk assessment 1754
target receptor, chemicals acting on *307*
target species 1646, 1754
target tissue *see* target organ(s)
Taricha torosa see newt, Californian
tarragon, as carcinogen 1981
taste loss, adverse drug reaction 1430
taurine 109, 111, 1862–3
taurocholic acid, as biomarker 1858
Taxus spp. *see* yew
TC_{50} *see* threshold concentration
TCR *see* T cell receptor complex
TD_{50} values *see* tumour(s)
TDI *see* tolerable daily intake
tea 1824, 2115
teased nerve fibre preparations 347
technical dossier 1590–1
technical training 492
technical-grade material, used for testing 1338–9
technician training *404*
Technische Richtkonzentrationen (TRK) values 1484, 1594
tectorial membrane 776
teeth
  enamel 967, 972, 973
  fillings 643
  pathology 343
  toxicant levels as biomarker 1844
TEF *see* toxicity equivalence factors
teleosts, biomarkers 1869
temperature
  see also heat
  ambient 46
  and behaviour 664
  changes as biomarker 1842, 1848, 1855, 1869
  and chemical toxicity 1419
  and combustion products 1919–20
  effects on toxicity 16
  environmental, repeated exposure studies 57–8

extremes, and xenobiotic toxicity 1342–3
tephra 1815, 1816
teratogenicity 8
  see also developmental toxicity; mutagenicity
  actinomycin 1455
  in avian embryo testing 1334
  as biomarker 1848, 1869
  and circadian toxicology 258
  dioxin 1818
  fungicides 2002, 2003
  herbicides 2005
  indium 2063
  and mutagenicity 1038
  nitrites 2127
  organic solvents 2041
  and placental toxicity 1243
  in pregnant rat 534
  retinoids 1549
  risk assessment 1751
  testing 1448, 1643
  thalidomide 1427
  veterinary drugs 1643
  vitamin A 1552
  wastes 1827–8
  zinc deficiency 2066
teratogens 85
teratology studies 23, 329, 465, 1567
terminal half-life 77, 84
terminal slope 79, 85
terrestrial field studies 1352–4
territory mapping 1353
terrorist attacks with chemical and biological (CB) agents 1721–30, 1827
tertiary toxicity *see* secondary/ tertiary toxicity
test(ing)
  abnormal 537–8
  adminstration route 1622
  alternative 415, 1957
  base-set 1479, 1480
  battery 1573, 1617, 1621, 1635
  British, European and American 538
  colour additives 1659
  consent to 1957
  definition 1394
  dosimetry 588–9
  and drug development 265–6
  ethics 1957–8
  facilities 444
  food additives 1656, 1659

food contact materials 1657
forensic 1502–4
guidelines
  FDA 1635
  OECD 1612
harmonization 1567
human exposure 605–7
industrial chemicals 1545
inherent errors 1957
interpretation 1956
local reaction 538–9
in marketing authorization applications 1628
maximum residue levels (MRLs) 1643, 1644
medical devices 1665–72
methods 1591–2
micro-organisms 1607
misconduct and 1958
objectives 1400, 1958–9
paradigm 1737, 1743, *1744*
quality assurance 1563–4
repeated exposure studies 58–9
species *see* model species
study design 1539
substances 444–5, 448
systems 401–24
  characteristics 404–9
  developmental toxicity considerations *414*
  in vitro 405, 406–7, 412
  limitations *404*
  structure–activity relationships 414
  validation *406*
variability 1332
veterinary drugs 1635
testimony of expert witness 1950
testis
  atrophy 82–3, 131, 1985
  cadmium toxicity 2054
  clinical chemistry 371–2
  cloned enzymes 242
  culture assay 1402
  damage, adverse drug reaction 1430
  distribution in 71, 1858
  drug toxicity 369, *369*
  dysfunction 372
  fixation 336
  food additives toxicity 1985
  fungicide toxicity 2054
  injury, biomarkers 1858–9, 1860, 1861, 1862
  interstitial cells 371

thyroid gland (*Contd.*)
  in vitro test *418*
  pathology 346
  physiological considerations
    988–9
  toxic conjugate effect 569
  toxicological effects 369, 989–91
  weights 336
thyroid hormone(s)
  clinical chemistry 365, 369, 371
  dioxin effects 163
  and nervous system development
    642
  -related processes 1401
  thyroxine (T_4) 369–70, 984, 989,
    990, 1122
  triiodothyronine (T_3) *369–70*,
    989
thyroid receptors 984
thyroid stimulating hormone (TSH)
  980, 990–1, 1121, 1123
thyrotrophic 4-methylhydroxylase
  217
TI_{50} *see* therapeutic index
tibial nerve 637
tidal volume 46, 615
Tier I screens (TIS) 1184–5
tight junctions 777, 779
timber *see* wood
time
  above tissue concentration,
    scaling factors 1769
  of death, investigation 1495
  -dependent sensitization in IEI
    1706–7
  effects, repeated exposure studies
    58
  factors, models incorporating
    1778
  –response relationship of
    pollutants 1870
  to toxic effect 15
  -weighted average (TWA) 1459,
    1484, 1588
timing of sampling 1908, 1910
tinea capitis, irradiation 1693
tingible bodies 175
tinnitus 130, 785, 786
tissue(s)
  see also target organ(s)
  affinity for substance 77
  –air partition coefficients 145
  –blood partition coefficient 145,
    146

compartment choice in PBPK
  144
contact with medical devices
  1735, 1736
cytokinetics 256
distribution 88, 128–30
enzyme levels, as biomarkers
  1865–7
fibrosis from radiation 1686
fixation 64, 336
forensic toxicology
  measurements 1941–2
inflammation or damage, lung or
  skin 1474
levels 45, 53
pathology 62, 1855
permeability 17
protein binding 71
rejection, HPLC 1862
response to implants 1731, 1732,
  1736
sensitivity in chronic studies 65
solubility 143
-specific genetic polymorphisms
  1061–2
specificity 128–38, 178
susceptibility patterns 256
Tityus see scorpion
TLC *see* thin layer chromatography
TLV *see* threshold limit value
TNF *see* tumour necrosis factor
TNF-R-associated death domain
  (TRADD) 193, 196
TNF-related apoptosis-inducing
  ligand (TRAIL) 196
tobacco
  chewing 2132
  replacement 220
  smoking *see* smokers/ing
  wild (*Lobelia* spp.), neurotoxicity
    1521
toenails *see* nails
Toffana, Mme 1490
Tokyo sarin incident 1721, 1723,
  1726, 1728, 1729, 1730, 1827
tolerable daily intake (TDI) 91,
  1574
tolerance, repeated-dose toxicity
  studies 328
tomato
  fumonisins 2165
  nitrate and nitrite levels 2112–13
tongue 343, 545
tongue (food), nitrate and nitrite
  levels 2113

tonometry 756
tooth *see* teeth
toothpaste 230
top dose 60
topoisomerases, and apoptosis 190
torsade de pointes see cardiac
  arrhythmias
torsion 42
torso, male adult skin surface area
  583
torts, toxic 1946
torture, use of toxic chemicals 1547
total body dose, biodegradable
  biomaterials 1745
total suspended particulates (TSP)
  1269, 1270, 1271, 1272
total volatile organic compounds
  (TVOCs) 1297–8, 1302
tourniquet as source of error in
  biomonitoring 1908
TOXBACK 1947
toxic cardiopathy 821–4
Toxic and Deleterious Regulation
  Law (Japan) 37
toxic dose 323
toxic equivalency factor 304, 1416
Toxic Exposure Surveillance System
  459
toxic gases, in animal husbandry
  1516–17
toxic interactions *see* interactive
  effects, toxic
toxic metabolites *see* metabolites,
  toxic
toxic myocarditis 807
toxic oil syndrome 38, 1444, 1551,
  1554, 1568, 1824
Toxic Release Inventory 1587,
  1589–90
toxic shock syndrome 1674
toxic stress 807
Toxic Substances Control Act 1976
  (TSCA) (USA)
  acute toxicity 37
  animal welfare 487
  behavioural toxicity 650
  chemical testing program
    1584–5
  environmental health risk
    assessment 1750
  industrial chemicals 1557
  information gathering authorities
    1586
  notification schemes 1545

Toxic Substances Control Act 1976
(TSCA) (USA) (*Contd.*)
  occupational toxicity 1459,
    1467, 1480–1
  pathology 347
  peroral toxicity 550
  wildlife toxicity 1328, 1334
toxic torts 1946
toxic wastes *see* waste disposal sites
toxic–therapeutic ratio 252, 260
toxication 116–21, 1329
toxicity (*general only*)
  action 34
  administration routes 1504
  biochemical basis 125–36
  circadian 257–65
  classification and labelling 5,
    1610
  data
    New Substances Notification
      Scheme 1590
    regulatory uses 1648
  in dead animals 23
  definition 4, 34, 1750
  description and terminology 4–6
  elimination by genetic
    manipulation 1553
  end-points, in carcinogenicity
    testing 1620
  equivalence factors (TEF) 1756,
    1757
  information sources 1759
  mechanisms 125–6
  monitoring 61–2
  nature of 6–8
  overt signs 1354
  ranking 36–7
  recommended procedures 63
  seasonal exposure 267
  species-specific 405
  subchronic 465
  testing *see* test(ing)
  types 328
toxicodynamics 34, 67, 92, 305,
  1444, 1446
toxicokinetics 67–95
  see also pharmacokinetics
  and biomonitoring 1485
  bird studies 1347
  clinical trials 1616
  definition 67
  extrapolation studies 1436
  human 1446
  medical devices 1742
  parameter selection 92

  physiologically based studies
    306
  safety studies 1443, 1444
  separation from toxicodynamic
    aspects 92
  steady-state 1835
  wildlife studies 1353
toxicological disasters *see* disasters
Toxicological Excellence in Risk
  Assessment 1759
toxicological hazards *see* hazards
toxicological risk *see* risk
toxicologist
  co-operation with epidemiologists
    1538
  duties 1955–7
  education 1935–44, 1951
toxicology (*general only*)
  *see also specific subjects, e.g.
    legal aspects of toxicology, etc.*
  applied 1941–2
  chemical and analytical methods
    1447
  databases 1676
  definition 155, 1443
  education 1935–44
  endpoints 1529
  and epidemiology 1527–42
  etymology 1547
  experimental 1534
  historical aspects 1474–6,
    1489–91, 1527
  laboratory 509–20
  methodological differences from
    epidemiology 1535
  pathological techniques 335–53
  studies
    design 22–5, 322–34
    review 25–7
Toxicology Training Program
  (USA) 1935
Toxicology Data Bank 1677
toxicovigilance 458–60
toxinology 3
TOXKITS 1320
Toxline 478, 1676, 1943, 1947
Toxnet 1677, 1759
trachea 20, 46, 342, 544, 605
tracheobronchial system 591, 1814,
  1859, 1885
tracing, vital status 1531
TRADD *see* TNFR-associated death
  domain
trade barriers and disputes 1648–9

Trade-related Aspects of Intellectual
  Property Rights 1569
TRAIL *see* TNF-related apoptosis-
  inducing ligand
training programme, for respirator
  use 516
Trait, de toxicologie 36
trans-species *see* interspecies
N,O-transacetylation 108–9
transaminases 43, 868, 1462
transcriptase-polymerase chain
  reaction (PCR) 712
transcription
  activation 113
  activity 1402
  factors 190
  and hepatotoxicity 866–7
  interspecies variation 281
  mutagenicity 1019
  pharmacogenetics 232, 235, 240
  proteins 168
transdermal *see* skin
transducer radiotelemetry system
  749
transduction channel of hair cells
  790, 791
transduction pathways, and
  apoptosis 190
transfection, endocrine receptors
  1402
transferrin 1910, 2065
transforming growth factor (TGF)-β
  193, 729, 1690, 1972, 1929
transgene technologies 1964
transgenic animals 135, 682,
  1062–4, 1111–14
transglutaminases 177, 189
transient effects 5, 6, 1179
transition kinetics 1890
transition mutations 162
translation of mRNA 1019
translocator protein 281
transmission electron microscopy
  338–9, 756
Transparency Directive, EU 1545
transparency in risk estimates 1788
transplacental transport 1464, 1465
transport
  active 73
  atmospheric 1371, 1374–5
  mechanisms 1367, 1371
  requirements 37
  in soil 1367, 1370
  transplacental 1464, 1465
transulphuration 428

trapezoidal rule 79, 84–5

trauma
  see also stress
  in fires 1927
  from NMDA 166
  from parenteral injections 60
  injuries 1503
  linked to alcohol and drug use
    1444

treat and plate tests 1048–9

Treatise on Poisons 1490

treatment, toxic exposures 1444

Treaty of Maastricht 1992 1555,
  1556

Treaty of Rome 1555, 1621

tree nuts, as carcinogen 1982

tremor 40, 42, 497, 663

Treponema pallidum 1092

Trevan approach 36, 40

Tribulis terrestris 883, 2148

tricarboxylic acid cycle (Krebs
  cycle, TCA) 6, 337, 634, 643,
  822

Trichinella spiralis 1008

Trichoderma spp. 2149

Trichodesma europeum,
  hepatotoxicity 1519

trichothiodystrophy (TTD) 1034

trichrome stain 336

Trifolium hybridum see clover,
  alsike

trigeminal chemoreceptors 626

trigeminal nerve, peripheral sensory
  irritation effects 615

triglycerides, as biomarker 1848,
  1858, 1859, 1860, 1863

trimethylamine *N*-oxide, as
  biomarker 1862

trimethylaminuria 234

Tripartite Agreement 1662, 1733

TRK *see* Technische
  Richtkonzentrationen

tRNA *see* RNA, transfer

trophic factor withdrawal 178

trophoblastic tissue, human placenta
  1238

tropics 566

tropomyosin 343, 366, 894

trout
  rainbow (*Oncorhynchus mykiss*)
    409, 1311
  test system *414*

TRPM-2, and apoptosis 193

TRX *see* thioredoxin

trypsin protein catabolism 159

trypsinogen 899

tryptophan *1878*

tryptophan fluorescence
  spectroscopy 756

TSCA *see* Toxic Substances Control
  Act

TSCA Experimental Release
  Application (TERA) 1584

TSG *see* tumour suppressor genes

TSH *see* thyroid stimulating
  hormone

TSP *see* total suspended particulates

TTD *see* trichothiodystrophy

tuberculosis 514, 757

tubulin proteins 2067

tumorigenicity
  adriamycin 1455
  benzo[*a*]pyrene 115
  biomarkers 1848, 1892
  definition 7
  in environmental health risk
    assessment 1766
  fat in diet and 1980
  and gastro-intestinal microflora
    565
  medical devices 1742
  OCs 1995

tumour(s)
  see also carcino-; neoplasm *and*
    specific types of tumour, e.g.
    sarcoma
  apoptosis machinery 202
  blood flow 256
  cells 238, 1080–1
  dose reducing tumour incidence
    50% (TD$_{50}$) 274
  genes, biomarker 1849–50
  incidence
    and diet 16, 58
    latency to 64
    nitrates 2124
    nitrites 2126, 2127, 2128,
      2135
    random differences in controls
      65
  initiating activity 567
  markers 1849–50
  PBPK modelling 1770
  production, LMS 1764
  promoters, synthesis 567–9
  promoting activity, FC 567
  risk assessment 1754, 1755
  suppressor genes (TSG) 192,
    1030, 1032, 1100–1, 1849,
    1892

tumour necrosis factor(s) (TNF)
  and apoptosis 192, 193, 195, 196
  circadian toxicity 259, 265
  immunotoxicity 1001, 1002
  nephrotoxicity 703
  systemic pulmonary toxicity
    722, 729
  TNF-α 191, 199, 864, 873, 999,
    1000, 1001
  TNF-β 864
  TNF-L 195

tumour necrosis factor receptor
  (TNF-R) 163, 193, 196

tuna 2193

tunnel disasters 1827

Turdus migratorius see robin,
  American

turf farms 1329, 1348

turkey
  see also poultry
  nitrate and nitrite levels 2113
  X disease 2145

turnip, nitrate and nitrite levels
  2112–13

TVOCs *see* total volatile organic
  compounds (TVOCs)

TWA *see* time-weighted average

twins, cancer study radiation-
  induced 1697

two-generation studies 83, 1404,
  1405

Tympanuchus phasianellus
  see grouse, sharp-tailed

typhus 2

tyre
  curing fumes 2014
  workers, risks in rubber industry
    2015, 2017

tyrosine residues 370

Tyto alba see barn owl

U

U1-70 kDa, and apoptosis 190, 195

ubiquitin, as biomarker 1848, 1869

UCR *see* unit cancer risks

UDP-glucosyltransferases *216*

UDP-glucuronyltransferase 285,
  1403

UDS *see* unscheduled DNA
  synthesis

UF *see* uncertainty factor

ulceration 340, 343, 363, 365, 524,
  525, 553, 745, 1430, 1686, 1689

ulcerative colitis 565

ulcerogenic drugs 364
ultradian frequency 251
ultrafiltration 363
ultra-rapid metabolizers 224
ultrasound techniques 747, 951, 1216
ultraviolet
  filters, in cosmetics 1560
  light
    absorbers in plastics industry 2022
    and apoptosis 199
    arsenic interaction with 2052
    circadian toxicity 252
    cutaneous toxicity 836, 837
    DNA damage 1892
    in epidemiology 1538
    gene expression alterations 167
    mutagenic DNA repair 1019–20, 1023, 1025, 1034
umbilical cord, blood lead levels 2057
*umu*DC genes 1022
uncertainty factor (UF) 13, *91*, 313, 1759–60, 1787
unconditioned response to odour 1707–8
underground storage tanks 1372
uniform resource locator (URL) 482
unit cancer risks (UCR) 1764–5
United Kingdom (UK)
  BALs 1910, 1911
  benchmark value 1486
  chemical warfare 2080
  nitrate and nitrite levels 2112, 2114, 2116, 2117–18, 2130, 2133, 2134
  toxicology education 1942–3
United Nations
  Committee of Experts on the Transport of Dangerous Goods 37
  Conference on Environment and Development 1478
  Conference on Environment and Health 1592
  Environment Programme 476
    see also International Program on Chemical Safety
  human studies 453
United States of America (USA)
  Army 824
  BALs 1910

biotechnology products regulation 1584
chemical warfare 2080
chemicals export and import 1588
classification and labelling requirements 1477, 1603–4
Congress 438, 486
consumer protection 1589
cosmetics regulation 1550
dietary exposure, risk assessment 1602–3
drug regulation 1544, 1615–20
food additives regulation 1658–9
fumonisin contamination of cereals 2165
harmonization of regulation 1649
industrial chemicals regulation 1581–90
medical devices regulation 1662–5
new chemicals, regulatory program 1582–6
nitrate, nitrite and *N*-nitroso levels 2113, 2116, 2117, 2118, 2131, 2132
occupational and bystander risk assessment 1602
pesticide regulation 1599, 1600, 1601
supply-side testing and risk assessment 1480–1
toxicology education 1935–42
veterinary drug regulation 1633–8
worker protection 1588–9
United States Department of Agriculture (USDA)
see Department of Agriculture (USA)
United States Pharmacopeia
  medical device testing 1668, 1669
  parenteral toxicity studies 536
  plastics classification 1733
University of Pittsburgh combustion device 1926
University of Surrey toxicology curriculum 1942–3
unscheduled DNA synthesis (UDS) 271, 567, 1104
up-and-down procedure 326

uracil NDA glycosulase 1892
urea 43
  see also blood urea nitrogen
ureter 1691, 1928
uricase 344
uridine diphosphate glucuronic acid
  see UDP
uridine kinase 261
uridine phosphorylase 261
urinalysis 61, 62, 63, 332, 362, 1460, 1466
urinary bladder
  AITC toxicity 134
  cancer
    acetylator status and 28, 1891
    adverse drug reaction 1430
    aromatic amines 120
    circadian studies 258
    in firefighters 1928
    food additives and 1990
    isoniazid 112
    nitrates 2131
    N-nitroso compounds 2132
    and phenotypes 1457, 1891
    in plastics industry 2021
    ras genes 1029–30
    in rubber industry 2015
    and smoking 1538
  carcinogenesis 258, 566, 1129–30
  epithelium 339
  mucosa 345
  pH 135
  radiation-induced changes 1691
  stones, and food additives 1987
urinary excretion 18
  arsenic 2052
  and bioavailability calculation 76
  biomarkers 1844, 1845, 1846, 1847, 1848, 1849, 1855, 1859, 1861–5, 1876–7, *1879*, 1885
  cadmium 2054
  clearance rate calculation 80
  elimination rate constant calculation 86
  radioactivity elimination 72
  sigma minus method 85
urinary protein
  as biomarker 1861, 1906
  clincal chemistry 363
  LAA 511
urinary tract 344–5, 1691, 2154

vestibular toxicity, caloric or
rotational stimulation 788
Vesuvius 1815–16
veterinary drugs
abuse potential 1637
classification and labelling 1637
efficacy studies 1634
food safety assessment 1634–5
legal violations 1637, 1647,
1648
MRLs 1642
non-therapeutic 1549
occupational exposures 1637
pesticidal ingredients 1548
pre-marketing authorization
1558
regulations 1549, 1633–52
residues 1563, 1574
socioeconomic aspects 1649
toxicological testing 1635
variation in use 1640
withdrawal period 1636, 1647
veterinary facilities, source of
biological hazards 1459
Veterinary International Conference
on Harmonization (VICH) 2,
1649
veterinary medicine 491, 522, 531
Veterinary Medicines Directorate
(UK) 1638
Veterinary Pharmaceutical
Committee 1639
Veterinary Products Committee
(UK) 1637
veterinary toxicology 3, 1509–26
vial equilibrium technique 145
vibration 662, 1418–19
Vibrio cholera 820
VICH *see* Veterinary International
Conference on Harmonization
video tape in courtroom 1951
Vietnam, chemical warfare 2080,
2105
vimentin, and apoptosis 195
vine snake (*Thelotornis capensis*)
2178
vinyl chloride workers,
haemangiosarcoma 1533
violence, risk of death 1830
violin spider 2186
viper 2178
pit 2180
saw-scaled/carpet (*Echis
ocellatus*) 2181
Vipera berus see adder, common

Viperidae 2178
viper's bugloss (*Echium
plantagineum*), hepatoxicity 1519
viral hepatitis 868
virtually safe doses (VSD) 1764–5
Virus Act (USA) 36
viruses
carcinogenicity 1100
as CB weapon 1726
as chemical warfare agents *2082*
as impurities 1968
regulation *see* micro-organisms
viscosity of formulation 46
visual cortex, methyl mercury
damage 643
visual dysfunction/impairment 129,
614, 615, 738, 757, 765
visual evoked potentials 756
vital fluorescent labels 342
vital status, tracing 1531
vitreous humour, forensic testing
1495, 1503, 1504
vitronectin 187
vitronectin receptors 183
VLDL *see* very low density
lipoproteins (VLDL)
VOCs *see* volatile organic
compounds
volatile screen (VS) 1502
volatile toxins 1491, 1495
volcanoes 1815–17
voles (*Microtus* spp.) 1335
voltage activated channels 639
volume
effects on absorption 547
factors affecting 546–7
voluntary consent 453
voluntary regulation schemes 1543,
1545–6, 1586, 1589, 1637
volunteer testing 567, 1960
Volvariella volvacea 820
volvulus 364
vomiting
in acute toxicity 40, 41
agents in warfare 2028
cardiac toxicity 811
centre 546
clinical chemistry 364
human studies 460
induction 1511
peroral toxicity 549
protective reaction 1347
response 553
vomiting (emesis) 40, 41, 364, 549

von Kossa stain 342
VSD *see* virtually safe doses
vulcanization 2016
vulcanizers 2015
Vulpes macrotis see kit fox
vulvovaginitis 2145

W

Wallerian degeneration 347
waltzing syndrome 638
warble fly control 1342, 1355
warfare
agents *see* chemical warfare
agents; nerve agents
radiation effects in 1692, 1693
S-warfarin 7-hydroxylase *217*
wartime, development of toxicology
during 2
wasps 2182
waste disposal
disasters 1827–8
from farms 2114
regulations 1960
sites 314, 669, 1372–3
wasting syndrome 283
water
see also drinking water;
groundwater
acidification 1376
aerosol 604
aluminium levels 2060
consumption in studies 61, 63
contaminated 1339, 1340, 1828
field sampling 1781
fluoridation 1534
hardness *see* drinking water
increased consumption in
poisoning 1523, 1524
intake variables 356
mixed routes of exposure 607
natural chemical composition
1370
pH
and methylmercury 1379,
1380
and selenium 1380
pollution 1870
see also aquatic toxicology
quality 1340, 1673
self-purification 1370
solubility 71
trace metals anthropogenic inputs
1370

water distribution systems
asbestos content 1380
CB agents and 1727
copper content 1380
corrosion 1377
lead content 1378
pesticide exposure 1993
water hemlock (*Cicuta* spp.),
neurotoxicity 1519, 1520
water-soluble formulations,
availability and toxicity 1340
waterborne diseases 1383, 1384
waterfowl
eggshell thinning 1354
lead toxicity 1340–1, 1343, 1523
nest and brood abandonment
1348
nesting grounds 1355
susceptibility to diazinon 1328
watermelon, aldicarb contamination
1548
waxes 1295
weakness 460
weaver ant 2184
weavers 456
*Webster's New Collegiate
Dictionary* 425
Wechsler Intelligence Scale for
Children 669
weedkillers *see* herbicides
weeds 462
weever fish 2191
weigh-masters 164, 166
weight
see also size factors
loss 235
weight-of-evidence (WOE)
classification 313, 1757
welding fumes 314
Western blot methods 235, 273, 510
wetlands, drainage 1355
whale
blue, weight 51
mercury toxicity 2057
wheat *see* cereals
wheezing, as allergic response 512
white blood cells *see* leukocytes
white supremacist groups 1728
WHO *see* World Health
Organization
whole-body concentration,
dosimetric scaling 147
widgeon, American 1328, 1350
Wilcoxon matched-pair signed-ranks
test 301

wild tobacco (*Lobelia* spp.),
neurotoxicity 1521
wildlife species
acute toxicity 1329–34, 1338–44
and agricultural chemicals 1328,
1343, 1347
behavioural aberrations 1327,
1328, 1345–7
biomarkers 1345, 1407–8, 1866
in captivity 1338, 1343, 1345,
1349
chemical screening 1327, 1329
endocrine disruption 1392–3
energy stressors 1329
environmental endocrine effects
1407
exposure effects 1328
exposure sources 1339–42
feeding habits 1328
feeding patterns 1347
fish-eating 1329, 1355
laboratory tests 1345
lack of chemical avoidance 1347
lead toxicity 1340–1
physiological indicators of health
1327, 1328
reproductive impairment 1327,
1328
residue burders 1327
soil hazards 1340–1
species studies 45
sublethal exposures 1333,
1344–54
susceptibility to toxic chemicals
1328–9
test protocols 1330–4
toxicology 1327–64
water requirements 1440
white phosphorus toxicity
1340–1
xenobiotic tolerance 1344
Wiley, Harvey 1534
Wilms' tumour 262, 1032, 1464
Wilson's disease 427, 869, 897,
902, 910, 2064, 2068
wine, nitrate levels 2115
winter smog 1265, 1266, 1268–73,
1272, 1273
withdrawal or deficiency syndromes
1451
see also negative effects
withdrawal periods, veterinary drugs
1636, 1647
Withering, William 2
witness *see* expert witness

Wolffian duct differentiation 179
wood
burning 1917–18, 1935
dust, respiratory effects and
carcinogenicity 1475
preservation 1790, 1995, 1998,
2001, 2002, 2004
protection 1548
woodworkers, respiratory function
1456
wool, combustion products 1923
Worker Protection Standard (US)
1588–9, 1603
workers
exposure studies 467, 1755
older 46
protection 604, 1588–9
working groups, EU 1643, 1656,
1657
workplace
see also occupational toxicology
atmosphere 314
exposure guidelines 755, 1545,
1551
exposures 1474
eye safety 755
improvement, ethics and 1911
management, and LAA 513–14
monitoring 1460, 1463
reproductive hazards 1463–7
standards 1459
Workplace Hazardous Material
Information System (WHMIS)
(Canada) 1477
World Health Organization (WHO)
see also International Programme
on Chemical Safety
air pollution studies 1268, 1271,
1272, 1273, 1274, 1280, 1292
Air Quality Guidelines for
Europe 1271, 1279, 1282
Cell Products Safety Commission
1463
Codex Alimentarius Commission
1570
Expert Group of pesticide
residues 1960
–FAO Joint Expert Committee on
Food Additives 91
Food Additives Series 1659
human studies 454, 458, 462
information 476, 482
parenteral toxicity studies 531
pathology studies 341

World Health Organization (WHO)
acute toxicity studies 37
World Medical Association 454
World Trade Center bombing
1722–3
World Trade Organization (WTO)
1569–70, 1649
World War I, chemical warfare
2079–80, 2083, 2089, 2096, 2098,
2100, 2102
World War II 453, 460, 472, 2080,
2100, 2102, 2145
worst-case scenario 19–20, 1775
wound-healing properties of growth
factors 1972
Wright Dust Feed Mechanism 596
Wright nebulizer 595
Wright's stain 1087

X

X-linked conditions *see* sex-linked
conditions
X-ray diffraction 619
X-ray fluorescence spectrometry for
biomonitoring 1905
X-rays 634, 1683, 1693
xanthine dehydrogenase 238
xanthine oxidases 101, 103, 238–9
Xanthium spp. *see* cocklebur
xenobiotics
additive effects 1342
dermal exposure 1339, 1349
dietary presentation 1337
endocrine active

see environmental oestrogens
exposure routes 1339
exposure sources 1339–42
hepatic monoesterase (HMO)
metabolism 1339
ingestion 1339
inhalation 1339, 1349
interactions with natural stressors
1342–3
metabolism 215, 216, 1337
monooxygenase metabolism
1329
pharmacogenetics 215
recovery from exposure to 1346
reproductive toxicity 1347–8
secondary effects 1444
susceptibility 1338, 1343
tolerance 1337–8, 1344
toxicity determinants 1329
wildlife toxicity 1327, 1344
Xenopus laevis see frog, African
clawed
xeroderma pigmentosa 1033, 1892

Y

yeast (*Saccharomyces cerevisiae*)
52, 1019, 1022, 1092
Yellow Book 37
Yellow Card scheme 458
yellow jacket 2181
yellow rice disease 2145
yellow scorpion (*Leirus
quinquestriatus*) 820, 2188
yellow thick head disease 2148

Yersinnia pestis 1727
yew (*Taxus* spp.), cardiovascular
effects 1522
yoghurt
live 1552
starter cultures 1645
'Yokkaichi asthma' 1280
yolk sac 383
Yousef, Ramzi 1722–3
youth culture 222
Yun Chi Ch'i Ch'ien 35

Z

Z-band 813, 819
Z-discs 938
Zenker's stain 345
zero-order absorption 69
zero-order reaction 73, 84
zinc deficiency syndrome,
acrodermatitis enteropathica 1565
zinc proteases, in snake venom
2179
zinc protoporphyrin 392, 1485
zoanthids *see Palythoa*
Zollinger–Ellison syndrome 1125
Zonotrichia albicollis see white-
throated sparrow
zoonoses 514–15
Zopyrus 35
Zygadenus spp. *see* death camas
zygote 8, 1684
zymbal gland tumours 2015, 2021

CHEMICAL INDEX

This Index contains xenobiotics (industrial chemicals, drugs and foreign environmental materials) and their metabolites. Naturally occuring and biological substances are to be found in the Subject Index.

A

abamectin 1994, 1999
ABP *see* 4-aminobiphenyl
abrin 184, 2104
acephate, behavioural effects 1348
acetaldehyde 236, 237, 239, 315, 613, 813, 917, 920, 1927, 2040
acetaminophen (paracetamol)
  activation pathways 689
  acute overdose 1496
  adduct formation 159, 1887
  age effects 1417
  alternatives to 417
  antidotal studies 426, 430
  and apoptosis 179, 180, 184, 185, 198, 199, 200, 201
  biomarkers 1842–3, 1845
  circadian toxicity 252, 255, 257
  cyanide lacing 1724
  DNA effects 188
  elixir 1426–7
  eye toxicity 763
  foetal effects 1223
  forensic screening tests 1497
  gastro-intestinal microflora 569
  hepatoxicity 6, 130, 131, 688, 853, 871, 873, 877, 881
  in vivo studies 417
  kidney response 688–9
  LD_{50} 51
  metabolism 116–17
  pancreatic toxicity 911, 916
  protective system against 157
  skeletal muscle toxicity 940
  toxicity 125, 1427, 1430
    to domestic animals 1509, 1510
acetates 428, 2032
acetazolamide 807, 1417
acetic acid 752, 1514, 1918, 1919, 1989
acetohexamide 242
acetone
  biomonitoring 1900, 1907
  cytogenicity 1082

forensic toxicology 1503
from polypropylene combustion 1919
indoor air quality 1298
metabolism 2041
mixed route of exposure 605
PBPK modelling 142
peripheral sensory irritation 623
in plastics industry 2020, 2023
acetonitrile 1455, 1922
acetophenone 242
N-acetoxyaminofluorene 120
acetyhalenes 2034
acetylaminofluorenes 106, 107, 110, 111, 875, 883, 1866
acetylaminophen, hydroxylation 102
N-acetyl-*p*-aminophenol 688
N-acetyl-*p*-benzoquinonimine (NABQI) 117, 130, 132, 159, 430, 688, 763, 1842–3
acetylcholinesterase inhibitors (AChE-Is) 950–5, 1242–3
N-acetylcysteine (NAC)
  acetaminophen antidote 132
  antidotes 426, 430, 433
  apoptosis and 199
  biomarker 1865
  conjugation 107, 108
  formation 1865
  metabolism 108, 116, 118, 131, 134
  for mustard gas respiratory tract lesions 2087
  pancreatic toxicity 908
  for phosgene poisoning 2099
acetylene 2034
3-acetyl-2,5-hexanedione 637
acetylhydrazine 28, 119
acetylisoniazid 119
N-acetyl-5-methoxytryptamine *see* melatonin
N-acetylprocainamide 84
acetylpyridine 642
β-acetylpyridine 642
acetylsalicylic acid *see* aspirin

AChE-Is *see* acetylcholinesterase inhibitors
acid(s)
  irritant properties 2032
  organic 1496, 2003
acid aerosols 1280–1
α-1 acid glycoprotein 253–4
acid anhydrides 701, 2020
acid precipitation *see Subject Index*
acid saccharin (SAC) 1130
acid sulphates 1266
acifluorfen 259
aconite 2, 34, 1490
aconitidine 639
aconitine 639, 757, 818, 821
acridine 1145
acriflavine 821
acrolein
  cardiac toxicity 810
  as combustion product 1821, 1927, 1928
  death from 26
  eye toxicity 738
  hepatotoxicity 872
  metabolism 103
  mixtures 315
  pancreatic toxicity 917
  peripheral sensory irritiation 613, 626
  systemic pulmonary toxicity 729
  vapour 21
acronitrile 1880, 1884
acrylamides
  behavioural toxicity 654, 661, 662
  biomarker 1880, 1884
  neurobehavioural effects 16
  neurotoxicology 637
  occupational toxicology 1455
  in plastics industry 2021
  regulations 1430, 1587
acrylates 835, 2022
acrylonitrile 142, 985, 1900, 1922, 1929, 2015, 2021
acrylonitrile–butadiene rubber 2013
acrylonitrile–butadiene–styrene 626

actinomycin 163, 184, 188, 199, 262, 727, 974, 1145, 1455
Adamsite *see* chlorodihydro-phenarsazine
adenosylcobalamin 2064
adipates 2017, 2022
adiponitrile 1922
adrenaline/lidocaine combination 947
adrenergic agonists and antagonists 16, 430, 433
adriamycin (doxorubicin)
  and apoptosis 184, 185, 192, 1430, 1861
  biomarker 1861, 1867
  cardiac toxicity 808–9, 821
  circadian toxicology 255, 262
  hepatotoxicity 872
  mechanism of action 127
  orrupational toxicology 1455
  pancreatic toxicity 904, 926
  parenteral toxicity 524, 527
  pharmacogenetics 240
  skeletal muscle toxicity 945
  systemic pulmonary toxicity 727
  toxic reactions 1430
AF-2 *see* furylfuramide
AF64A 642
AFB1 oxides 276
aflatoxicol 2149
aflatoxins 2145, 2149–54
  A$_1$ 882
  B$_1$ 231, 271, 274–8, 569, 571, 1042, 1044, 1251–2
    adducts 1883, 1885, 1886–7
    8,9-epoxygenase 217
    hepatocarcinogenesis 278
    -2,3-oxide, hepatotoxicity 130
    phase I and II metabolism 276, 277
    stereochemical factors and 162
  B, in diet 1982
  biomarkers 1845, 1848, 1880, 1881, 1882
  G$_1$ 1251–2
  hepatotoxicity 58, 877, 1537, 1538
  N^7-guanine, DNA adducts 1885
  and *p53* mutation 1457
  toxicity to food-producing animals 1515–16, 1524
  veterinary toxicology 1516, 1520
8-AG *see* 8-azaguanine (8-AG)
agarose 368

Agent Orange *see* 2,3,7,8-tetra chlorodibenzodioxin (TCDD)
aglycone 556
β-agonists
  ban 1647–8
  testing 1554
AITC *see* allyl isothiocyanate
ajmaline 219, 222, 223
alachlor 2003, 2005
β-alanine 235
Alar 1790
alclofenac 1960
alcohol
  see also ethanol and other specific alcohols
  abuse 2040–1
  acute overdose 1496
  aggressive behaviour after 653
  consumption, hazard evaluation 28
  intoxication hindering escape from fire 1916
  metabolism 113, 114, 235
  teratogenicity 258
aldehydes 307, 315, 530, 1275, 1298, 1868
  air pollution 1298
  biomarker 1867, 1868
  chlorination byproduct 1383
  irritant properties 2032
  metabolism 103, 104
  mixtures 307, 315
  parenteral toxicity 530
  reduction 104
aldesleukin 1965
aldicarb 101, 102, 1006, 1336, 1341, 1347, 1548, 1994, 1998
aldomet *see* α-methyldopa
aldosterone 364, 369–70, 675
aldrin 641, 879, 1243–4, 1329, 1994
alfoxolone 641
alginic acid 1985
alicylic solvents 2037
aliphatic alcohols 757–8, 2023
aliphatic hydrocarbons 1504, 2034–7
aliphatic nitriles, unsaturated 551
aliphatic solvents 2034–7
alkali compounds 1987
alkali elements 1381
alkaline earth elements 1381
alkaloids
  indole 222–3
  nicotinic 1520, 1521

pyrrolizidine 133, 730, 872, 873, 881, 882, 1981
  veterinary toxicology 1519, 1520, 1521
  vinca 638, 942, 943, 992, 1152, 1153
alkanes 1868, 2034–5
alkanolamines 2115
n-alkenals 1867
alkenes 104, 161, 1879, 2034–5
N^3-alkyladenine 1885
n-alkylamines 612
alkylating agents 527, 1104, 1144, 1146, 1465, 1882, 1883
alkylbenzenes 149, 2032
alkylene epoxides 7
N^1-alkylgaunine, DNA adducts 1885
0^6-alkylguanine
  biological activity 2146, 2153–4
  biomarker 1865
  biosynthesis 2150–2, 2151
  characteristics 2035
  chemical structure 2146, 2150
  competing pathways 115–17
  control and decontamination 2153
  determination 2152
  DNA adducts 115, 1881, 1883, 1885, 1917, 1918, 1919, 2151
  enzyme induction 1866
  equine-derived 2186
  fish poisoning 2193
  from polymers 1917, 1919
  Hb adduct levels 1880
  immunological screening 2152–3
  LD$_{50}$ 2150, 2154
  metabolism 71, 105, 110, 113, 114, 1883, 2149, 2155
  occurrence 2153
  physical and spectroscopic data 2150
  production 2152
  renal clearance 97
  scorpion sting 2188–9
  spider bite 2187
alkyl-lead 2054–5
alkyloctyl phosphorofluoridates 638
alkylsulphonic esters 2022
alkynes 2034
allergens 53, 262, 511–12, 702, 1299, 1300–1, 1302
allethrin 824, 1244
alloxan 881, 991, 992
alloys 2049, 2064

allyl alcohol 103, 255, 810, 872, 873, 882, 920
allylaldehyde 103, 119
allylamine 103, 809–10
allyl formate 881, 882, 883
allylglycine 641
allylisopropylacetamide 114
allylisothiocyanate 126
allyl isothiocyanate (AITC) 134
ALO1576 763
L-alosine 634
alphaxalone 1427, 1438
alprazolam 1495
alprenolol 219, 760
alteplase 1965, 1966
alum 1824
aluminium 2060
   and acid precipitation 1377
   and Alzheimer's disease 1379–80
   in antacids 1380
   antidotes 427
   biomonitoring 1900, 1904, 1905, 1907
   biovailability 1380, 1381
   cartilage and bone toxicity 973
   in drinking water 1379, 1381
   as environmental pollutant 1379–80
   ligands 1365–6, 1369
   mobilization 1379
   neurotoxicity 1379, 1380
   placental toxicity 1245–6
   solubilization 1371
   speciation 1365–6
   toxicity 1379
aluminium hydroxide 2022
aluminium phosphide 2006
aluminium sulphate 1824
amalgams 2049
amanitines 34, 870, 1513
amantidine 1495
amethocaine hydrochloride 2087
amidarone (Cordarone X) 1427
amidephrine 15
amidopyrine 1426
amiflamine 219
amikacin 685, 787, 788
amines 305, 2014, 2023, 2032
amino acid pyrolysates 1038
amino acids 548, 1983
aminoacridines 163
D,L-aminoadaptic acid 644
aminoalkyltrialkoxydisilane 11
2-aminoanthracene 1046, 1047

p-aminoazobenzene 2023
3-aminobenzamide 190, 200, 201
aminobenzene 1146
p-aminobenzoic acid 105
aminobenzotriazole 872, 1865
4-aminobiphenyl (ABP) 225, 1537, 1845, 1880, 1891
γ-aminobutyric acid (GABA) antagonist 641
aminocyclohexanols 71–2
2-amino-3,6-dihydro-3-methyl-7*H*-imidazo[4,5-*f*]quinoline-7-one 566
4-aminodimethyaniline 565
2-amino-3,8-dimethylimidazo [4,5-*f*]quinoxaline 272, 274, 1061
3-amino-1,4-dimethyl-5H-pyrido [4, 3-b]indole(Trp-P-1) 571
aminofluorene 120
aminoglutethimide 1121
aminogluthemide 1395
aminoglycosides 129, 130, 522, 685–6, 784, 787–93, 795–6, 819
p-aminohippurate 129, 364, 679, 1462
2-amino-3-methyl-3*H*-imidazo [4,5-*f*]quinoline 272, 274, 566
2-amino-1-methyl-6-phenylimidazo [4,5-*b*]pyridine 272, 274, 1881
3-amino-1-methyl-5H-pyrido [4, 3-b]indole 571
1-amino-2-naphthol 565
6-aminonicotinamide 972
aminonitriles 1983
aminophenols 110, 113, 117, 390, 393, 680, 688–9, 1907
aminophylline 816
aminoplasts 2018
β-aminopropionitrile 974
4-aminopropiophenone 393, 429
p-aminopropiophenone, for hydrogen cyanide poisoning 2102
aminopyridines 817, 822
aminopyrine 113, 2121
aminosalicylic acid (5-ASA, PAS) *see* aspirin; salicylates
amiodarone 219, 730, 755, 757, 818, 943–4, 945, 989, 1428
amitraz 1994, 2000
amitriptyline 51, 219, 264, 807, 819, 1495
amitrole 990, 2006
amitryptyline 1495

ammonia 117, 362, 568, 589, 751, 1297, 1516–17, 2018, 2119
ammonia compounds, in food 1514, 1987
ammonium bisulphate 1281
ammonium bisulphite 1281
ammonium hexachloroplatinate 711
ammonium hydroxide 752
ammonium metabisulphate 1281
ammonium phosphate 1514
[S]15[s]N-ammonium acetate 2119
[S]15[s]N-ammonium chloride 2119
ammonium sulphate 1266, 1281
ammonium sulphite 1281, 1987
ammonium tetrachloroplatinite 711
amoscanate 764
amoxapine 945, 1495
amoxycillin 2099
amphenidone 1634
amphetamines
   cardiac toxicity 808, 814
   controlled drug 1545
   derivatives 218
   forensic analysis 1491, 1503
   immunoassays 1501
   metabolism 102
   misuse 1550
   pharmacogenetics 219
   reproductive toxicity 1146
   risk acceptance 1960
   site-dependent blood concentrations 1495
   skeletal muscle toxicity 942
   steam distillation 1497
amphiphilic drugs 385, 730–1, 945
amphotericin B 536, 819, 945
ampicillin 756, 807, 1025
amygdalin 566
amyl nitrate 1550
amyl nitrite 3, 393, 426, 429, 460
anabolic steroids 815, 948, 1146, 1549, 1554
anastrozole 1403
anatoxin A 1516
androgen 370–1
andromedol 1984
angiotensin converting enzyme inhibitors 2188
anilines
   and anaemia 390
   biomonitoring 1900, 1907
   and gastro-intestinal microflora 565
   haemoglobin toxicity 393

anilines (*Contd.*)
  herbicides 2003, 2005
  metabolism 104, 110
  in oils 1824
  toxic reactions 1430
annatto, in food 1987
Antabuse *see* disulfiram
antacids 1380, 2060–1
anthracyclines 127, 807, 808–9
anthrax 1726–7
anthrocyanins 1987
α_1-antichymotrypsin 340
anticancer drugs 240, *240*, 258,
  262, 683–4, 727–9, 756–7, 1866
anticholinergic drugs 429, 430,
  1430
anticoccicidal drugs 1648
anticonvulsants 225, 258, 2092
antidepressants 218, *219*, 232, 819,
  1146, 1491, 1496, 1504, 1714
antidiabetic drugs 241
antiemetic drugs 229
antiepileptic drugs 1494
antifoaming agents 1985
antifouling compounds 1548, 1611,
  2001
antifreeze 1512
  see also ethylene glycol
antigenic agents 536
antihaemophilic factor 1965, 1970
antihistamines *219*, 262, 1127,
  1223, 1427, 1429, 1550, 2184,
  2190
antihypertensive drugs *219*
anti-inflammatory drugs 263, 1438
  see also non-steroidal anti-
    inflammatory drugs
antimalarial drugs 227
antimony 1451, 1489, 1491, 1496,
  1907
antimony trioxide 2018, 2022
anti-oestrogens *220*, 1392, 1403
  see also tamoxifen
antiperistaltic drugs *220*
antipsychotic drugs *219*
antipyretics *536*, 688
antipyrine 114–15, 253, 395
antirheumatic agents 1439
antisecretory drugs 1124, 1125–7
α_1-antitrypsin 254
antituberculosis drugs 119, 391
antitussive drugs *220*
antiulcer drugs 16
antivenin 2180
anxiolytics 641, 819

apamin 820
aphidicolin 185
apocynamarin 1522
apomorphine 1403, 1511, 1520,
  1547
appetite suppressants *220*
aprindine 219
1-(β-D-arabinofuranosyl)cytosine
  (Ara-C) 185, 195, 199
Ara-C *see* 1-(β-D-arabinofuranosyl)
  cytosine
arene oxides 130
arginine 229, 2119
aristolochic acid 554
Arochlor 24, 1254, 1343, 1348,
  1866
  see also polychlorinated
    biphenyls
aromatase inhibitors 1395
aromatic acids 109
aromatic amines 7, 28, 456, 874–6,
  1039, 1041, 1056, 1057, 1079,
  1104
  adducts 162
  biomarkers 1880, 1882, 1885,
    1886
  biomonitoring 1904
  carcinogenesis 7, 1104, 2015
  cytogenicity 1079
  human studies 456
  metabolism 112, 120
  mutagenicity 1039, 1041, 1056,
    1057
  reaction with DNA 161
  susceptibility 28
aromatic amino acids 568
aromatic hydrocarbons 2037–40
  acute overdose 1496
  and blood–testis barrier 1463
  forensic testing 1504
  inducing GSTs 1866
  toxicity 2030
aromatic hydroxylamines 1867
arsenates 2050
arsenic 2050–2, 2066
  acute overdose 1496
  animal toxicity 1513, 1518,
    1951–2
  anthropogenic emissions 1370
  antidotes 427
  biomarker 1864
  biomonitoring 1900, 1904, 1907
  carcinogenic 1382
  cardiac toxicity 822
  in drinking water 1382

  forensic testing 1491, 1504
  gastro-intestinal toxicity 1515
  general symptoms 1513
  in groundwater 1382
  hepatotoxicity 870, 881, 882
  in humus layer 1375
  as impurity in fertilizer 1371
  marketing controls 1595
  Marsh test 1490
  in mining areas 1382
  as natural poison 34
  nephrotoxicity 6
  ototoxicity 784
  PBPK modelling 142
  poisoning 1382, 1490
  reproductive toxicity 1156
  and skin cancer 1382
  in soils 1329, 1373
  solubilization 1371
  speciation 1382, 1515
  teratogenicity 1206, 1246–7
  and vascular disease 1382
arsenic compounds
  organic *see* organoarsenicals
  peripheral neuropathy 1515
  rodenticides 1510–11
  toxicity to animals 1512, 1515
arsenic oxide 2014
arsenic sulphide 2050
arsenic trioxide 1900, 2050, 2051
arsenic trisulphide 2050
arsenilic acid 1515
arsenite 2066
arsenobetaine 2052
arsenopyrite 2050
arsine 390, 2082
artificial sweeteners 1431, 1552
arylamides 101
arylamines 28, 101, 108–9
arylesterase 216
aryl hydrocarbons 867
arylhydroxamic acid 109
arylphosphates 2022
AS *see* ascorbic acid (AS)
5-ASA *see* aminosalicylic acid
asbestos
  binding values (EU) 1595
  carcinogenicity 1131, 1537
  as combustion product 1927,
    1929
  environmental source 1380
  health hazard 1380
  human studies 456, 463
  immunotoxicity 1006
  inhalation 1446

asbestos (*Contd.*)
  lung disease 1475
  occupational exposure 1456, 1487
  parenteral toxicity 525
  in plastics industry 2022
  release in fires 1821
  and smoking 28, 1417, 1445
  in water distribution systems 1377
  workplace exposure 1475
ascorbic acid (AS) 1130, 2121, 2137
  see also vitamin C
aspartame 1653, 1989, 2161
L-aspartate 634
asphalt 922
aspirin
  see also salicylates
  acute toxicity 51
  cardiac toxicity 807
  cartilage and bone toxicity 969
  circadian toxicity 263
  endocrine toxicology 991
  and gastro-intestinal microflora 565
  haematotoxicity 390, 391
  neonatal toxicity 1223
  nephrotoxicity 688
  ototoxicity 786
  pancreatic toxicity 908
  parenteral toxicity 525
  peroral toxicity 549, 552
atrazine 607, 2003, 2006
atropine
  antidotal studies 429, 430, 1355, 1510, 1998
  for carbamate poisoning 1998
  cardiac toxicity 824
  for fish poisoning 2192
  laboratory occupational hazard 516
  for OP poisoning 1998
  peroral toxicity 548
  placental toxicity 1256
  skeletal muscle toxicity 955
  in toxic plants 1521
  toxic reactions 1430
  treatment of nerve agent poisoning 2090, 2092, 2093–4
atropine sulphate, for scorpion bite 2188
ATX-II 820
auramine 463
auritricarboxylic acid 188, 198

averantin 2151
avermectins 641, 1999
averufin 2151
AY-9944 730
8-azaguanine (8-AG) 1052
azaserine 58, 924, 925
azathioprine 915, 917, 945, 1010, 1153
azides 392
azinophos methyl 1335
5-(aziridin-1-yl)-2,4-dinitro-benzamide 241
azobisformamide 2014, 2017, 2023
azobisisobutyronitrile 2023
azo compounds 564–5, 2022, 2023
azodicarbonamide 2022
azo dyes 7, 240, 1986
azoles 2001, 2003
azothioprine 727, 764
azoxymethane 571
azoxystrobin 1608
AZT *see* zidovudine

B

bacitracin 1648
bacitracin zinc 538
baking soda 2190
BAL *see* dimercaprol
banamine hydrochloride 1518
BAPP *see* 2,2-bis(4-amino phenoxyphenyl) propane
barbital 553
barbiturates
  acute overdose 34, 1496
  behavioural toxicity 651
  clinical chemistry 357
  controlled drug 1545
  in drug combinations 1504
  drugs of abuse screen (DAS) 1503
  forensic analysis 1491
  haematology 390–1
  induction 113, 114
  injection 498
  metabolism 111, 113, 114, 115
  neurotoxicity 641
  pharmacogenetics 226
  reproductive toxicity 1151
  skeletal muscle toxicity 944
  toxicity study design 325
barium 805, 822, 1757
barium chloride 1757
barium oxide 2022
barium sulphate 1757

bases, absorption 69
batrachotoxins (BXT) 639, 816, 818, 821, 824, 2104
Baytex 4 *see* fenthion
BBN *see* N-butyl-N-(4-hydroxy-butyl)-nitrosamine
BCLE *see* butyryl cholinesterase
BCNU *see* 1,3-bis(2-chloroethyl)-1-nitrosourea
beetroot red 1987
belladonna 2
Bendictin 1948–9
benomyl 758, 2000, 2002
benoxaprofen (Opren) 132, 1427, 1428, 1438, 1439
bentazon 259
benzaldehyde 237, 239, 613, 2038
benz[*a*]anthracene 280, 1791, 2017
benzene 2037
  air pollution 1267, 1298
  and alcohol 2033
  and apoptosis 184
  biomarkers 1867, 1882, 1884
  biomonitoring 1900, 1904, 1907, 1908, 1910
  carcinogenicity 1455, 1537, 2015
  characteristics 2035
  chromosomal abnormalities 395
  circadian toxicity 257
  as combustion product 1927
  in diet 1981
  early research 1482
  epidemiology 2042
  excretion 98
  exposure routes 607
  haematology 390, 395, 1475
  human studies data 463
  immunotoxicity 1004
  impurity in toluene 1445–6
  interactions 2034
  marketing controls 1595
  metabolism 100, 103, 2032, 2038
  ototoxicity 795
  PBPK modelling 142, 150
  pharmacogenetics 240–1
  risk assessment 1770
  rubber additive 2014, 2017, 2018
  in styrene 2039–40
  with toluene, PBPK modelling 149
  toxic reactions 1430
  vapour 16, 56
benzene-*trans*-1,2-dihydrodiol 105

bufuralol 115, 116
bumetamide 785, 795
bupivacaine 529, 947, 955–6
busulphan 727, 1153
butadiene 59, 142, 1880, 1883,
    2013, 2015, 2034
butane 1867, 2034
butane-1,4-diol diglycidyl ether
    2020
butanol 199, 1888, 2018
butazone 1298
buthionine sulphoximine 185, 792
butoxyacetic acid 19
2-butoxyethanol acetate 19, 142,
    1900, 1907
Butter Yellow *see* dimethylamino-
    azobenzene
butylated hydroxyanisole (BHA)
    200, 553–4, 1125, 1131, 1985
butylated hydroxytoluenes (BHT)
    carcinogenicity 1127
    as food additives 1985
    hepatotoxicity 862, 879, 883
    metabolic activation 726
    mixtures 315
    parenteral toxicity 532
    as rubber additives 2014, 2017
    systemic pulmonary toxicity 725
butylated phenols 1866, 1900,
    1907, 1985
butylated triphenyl phosphate (BTP)
    986
butylbutyryl lactate 1988
butyl 2-chloroethyl sulphide 757
2,6-di-*tert*-butyl-*p*-cresol
    see butylated hydroxytoluenes
    (BHT)
butyl digol 751
tert-butylhydroperoxide 199
N-butyl-*N*-(4-hydroxybutyl)-
    nitrosamine (BBN) 1990
butyl peroxide 2016, 2023
N-*tert*-butyl-α-phenylnitrone 634
butylphenyl phthalate 1404–5
butyl rubber 2013
tert-butyl nitrite 15
butyraldehyde 613
butyric acid 1125
BW-755C 1917
BXT *see* batrachotoxins
BZ-9 759
BZ *see* 3-quinuclidinyl benzoate

BzAO inhibitors *see* benzylamine
    oxidase inhibitors

C

C2-ceramide 185
cadaverine 2193
cadmium 2052–4
    anthropogenic emissions 1370,
    1373
    antidotes 427
    and apoptosis 184, 200
    aquatic toxicity 1310
    associated with zinc 1374
    behavioural toxicity 659
    biomarker 1844, 1848, 1861,
    1869, 1870
    biomonitoring 1485, 1900, 1904,
    1905, 1906, 1907, 1908, 1909,
    1910
    cartilage and bone toxicity 974,
    2068
    chelation therapy 2068
    circadian toxicology 257
    as environmental pollutant 1370,
    1373–4, 1377–8
    in food 1375, 1377, 1378
    hepatotoxicity 873
    as impurity in phosphate
    fertilizers 1369, 1371, 1372
    itai-itai disease 1564
    leaching 1377
    lung disease 1475
    and metallothionein 2067
    mixtures 313
    nephrotoxicity 682–3, 1373–4,
    1475
    placental toxicity 1247–8
    in plants 1369
    in sewage sludge 1372
    in soils 1329, 1371, 1372, 1373,
    1375, 1377
    sperm evaluation studies 1467
    in tobacco smoke 1377
    toxicity 1765, 1952
    in water distribution systems
    1377, 1382
cadmium compounds
    in plastics industry 2022, 2023
    in rubber 2016, 2017
cadmium sulphide 2014, 2050
cadmium yellow 2050
caeruloplasmin 367
caesium 805, 1960
caffeine
    and apoptosis 200

    and cancer 1891
    cardiac toxicity 816, 822
    developmental effects 1416,
    1417
    distribution 71
    interaction with industrial
    chemicals 1417
    interspecies pharmacokinetics 89
    metabolism 113, 217
    pancreatic toxicity 922
    pharmacogenetics 217–18
    site-dependent blood
    concentrations 1495
calamine 2052
calcitriol 973, 2068
calcium
    apoptosis and 200
    cadmium interference 2054
    and cartilage and bone 965, 968,
    972
    in drinking water 1381, 1382
    and nephrotoxicity 675
    tests 355, 364, 366
calcium antagonist drugs 1956
calcium arsenate 2050
calcium channel blockers 1504,
    2188
calcium chloride 969, 2018
calcium disodium edetate 433, 1515
calcium gluconate 2186
calcium ionophores 956
calcium nitrate 2018
calcium nitride 2068
calcium oxide 833, 2022
calmidazolium 819
calmodulin 808
calomel *see* mercury(I) chloride
calpain 636
calphostin C 185
calycanthine 1520
campothecin 195
Can f 1 allergen 512
cannabis
    drugs of abuse screen (DAS)
    1503
    epidemiology 1545
    ethics 1960
    eye toxicity 757
    forensic analysis 1491, 1495,
    1500
    pharmacogenetics 229
    L-Δ⁹-tetrahydrocannabinol 818,
    1151–2
    α-tetrahydrocannibol 229
    THC 229

cantharidin 1518
canthoxanthin 1987
caproic acid 1989
caprolactam 1537
capsaicin 612
captan 2001, 2002
captofol 2001, 2002
caramel 1987
carbadox 1648

carbamazepine 10,11-oxide 130
carbamazine 253–4
carbapenems 686
carbaryl 24, 227–8, 1243, 1342, 1523, 1548, 1994
carbendazim 2000, 2002
carbenoloxone 945
carbimazole 1549
carbinolamine 102
carbocations, reaction with DNA 161
carbofuran 1331, 1336, 1339, 1341, 1342, 1347, 1348, 1350
carbohydrates 359, 370, 1981
carbolines 222, 223, 641
carbon, from wood burning 1917
carbonates 2014, 2017
carbon black 1282, 2014, 2017
carbon dioxide
  acute toxicity 38
  air pollution 1296
  Bhopal disaster 1819
  blood analysis 61
  with CO 1924–7
  as combustion product 1928
  fires 1821
  formate oxidation 2040

  from lake water 1817
  from volcanoes 1815
  from wood burning 1917–18
  and gastro-intestinal microfloral 563
  inhalational toxicity 590
  metabolism 2036, 2041
  in plastics industry 2021
  removal in inhalational studies 592
  tests 357
carbon disulphide
  acute toxicity 43
  behavioural toxicity 660
  biomonitoring 1900
  eye toxicity 756
  and heart disease 1456
  human studies 463
  as inhibitor 114
  neurotoxicity 637
  ototoxicity 784
  sperm evaluation studies 1467
  toxicity 637, 1430
carbon monoxide (CO)
  acute overdose 1496
  air pollution 1267, 1268
  analysis in tissues 1491
  in animal husbandry 1516–17
  antidotes 426, 430
  biomarkers 1842
  biomonitoring 1485, 1900, 1905, 1908, 1910
  with carbon dioxide 1924–7
  cardiac toxicity 821
  and cardiovascular disease 34
  in combustion products 1917–18, 1920–2, 1927, 1928, 1929
  dose–response assessment 1758
  early OEL 1482
  effects on humans 1282–3
  in fires 1821, 1822
  foetal half-life 1922
  forensic analysis 1491, 1495
  from lake water 1817
  from volcanoes 1815
  and haemotoxicity 384, 391–4
  with HCN 1924
  indoor sources 1296
  microdiffusion 1497
  mixed routes of exposure 607
  neonatal toxicity 1218
  quantitative analysis 1490
  in smoke 1446
  in tobacco smoke 28

  toxicity, elevated temperature and 1919–20
  toxicokinetics 1282
carbon steel 2064
carbon tetrachloride 2035–6
  activation 6
  alcohol and 2033
  biomarker 1857, 1858, 1859, 1861, 1862, 1867
  biomonitoring 1900, 1907
  cardiac toxicity 810, 821
  characteristics 2035
  with chlordecone 149
  circadian toxicology 257, 259
  epdemiology 2042
  genotoxicity 200
  hepatotoxicity 16, 56, 132, 869, 872, 873, 877, 881
  human studies 463
  as impurity in trichloroethylene 1445
  as inhibitor 114
  interactions 2033
  metabolism 104, 115, 117–18
  with methanol 149
  pancreatic toxicity 900, 914, 916, 920, 927
  PBPK modelling 142, 150, 1767
  percutaneous toxicity 585
  peroroal toxicity 551
  systemic pulmonary toxicity 731
  toxicity enhanced by ketones 1418
  toxic reactions 1430
carbonyl fluoride 1915, 1918
carboplatin 260–1, 784
carboxyatractyloside 1518, 1520
carboxyhaemoglobin 393–4, 1267, 1282, 1283, 1494–5, 1504, 1905
carboxylic acids 131
carboxyphosphamide 238
cardenolides 1520
cardiac glycosides 237, 285, 428, 808, 811–12, 818, 821, 1549
carisprodol 1495–6, 1503
carmustine see 1,3-bis (2-chloroethyl)-1-nitosourea
carotenes/carotenoids
  as antioxidants 158, 1978, 1982, 1983, 2137
  in foods 1653, 1987, 2131
carprofen 1642
catecholamines 256, 346, 357, 632
catechols 100, 990
Cau p 1 allergen 511

Cau p II allergen 511
ceftazidime 687
ceftizoxime 89
cellulose 1552, 1985, 2022
cellulose acetate 368
Centruroides toxin 820
cephaloglycin 686, 687
cephaloridine 686–8
cephalosporins 127, 128, 129, 390, 552, 686, 687
CFCs *see* chlorofluorocarbons
chaconines 1521, 1984
channel black 2017
charcoal 425, 2153
chenodeoxycholic acid 360, 567
chlomipramine 219
2-chloracetophenone 2102
α-chloralose 2006
chlorambucil 191, 727, 1537
1-chloramitriptyline 730
chloramphenicol
    adverse drug reactions 1438, 1439
    cardiac toxicity 807
    drops for mustard gas eye damage 2087
    eye absorption and aplastic anaemia 761
    and gastro-intestinal microflora 569
    haematotoxicity 390–1, 395, 1634
    maximum residue limits (MRLs) 1642
    parenteral toxicity 533–4
    therapy for phosgene poisoning 2099
chlorate herbicides 1512
chlordane 879, 1226, 1243–4, 1342, 1343, 1523
chlordecane 637
chlordecone (Kepone) 142, 149, 879, 1146, 1154, 1244, 1418, 1475
chlordiazepoxide 1495
chlorendic acid 2022–3
chlorfenvinphos 142
chlorhexidine 1642
chloride 355, 364, 428, 1504, 2102
chlorinated cyclodienes 1243–4
chlorinated hydrocarbons
    acute overdose 1496
    banned by US EPA 1329
    behavioural effects 1346
    brain residues 1343

cardiac toxicity 804
and CNS 1510, 1518
domestic animal poisoing 1510
and eggshell thinning 1343, 1345
equine poisoning 1518
forensic analysis 1491, 1504
and hepatic monoesterase (HMO) activity 1342, 1345
human studies 461
indoor sources 1295
and menstrual disorders 1465
microdiffusion 1497
persistence in environment 1510
poisoning, developing countries 1510
poultry poisoning 1523
reproductive effects 1339–40, 1350
secondary poisoning 1341
in soil and groundwater 1372
stability 1329, 1341
chlorinated phenols 1310, 1366, 1373, 1383
chlorinated solvents 39
chlorine
    as chemical warfare agent 2082, 2096
    dangerous dose 1831
    in fires 1821
    gas 1724
    peripheral sensory irritation 626
    risk assessment 1832–3
    in rubber 2018
    soil content 1328
chlorine dioxide 989
chloroacetaldehyde 100–1
chloroacetone 2102
chloroacetophenone (CN) 623, 744, 745, 748, 750, 751, 2103
chloroalkanes 142, 2022
chloroalkyl thio compounds 2001, 2002
chlorobenzenes 1372, 1900
2-chlorobenzylidine malononitrile (CS) 623, 745, 2080, 2082, 2103, 2104
2-chlorobuta-1,3-diene *see* chloroprene
chlorocatechols 1907
chlorocresol 535
chlorocyclizine 730
chlorodihydrophenarsazine (DM) 2081–2, 2082, 2102, 2103
2-chloroethylnitrosoureas 2132
chlorofluorocarbons 460

chloroform 2036
    anaesthesia 2, 2030
    biologically based model 1770
    bounding information 1767
    carcinogenicity 1455
    cardiac toxicity 810
    chlorination byproduct 1383
    circadian toxicity 255, 257
    cytotoxicity 126
    dose–response model 1764
    genotoxicity 200
    hepatotoxicty 877
    injection 498
    kidney response 689–90
    maximum residue limits (MRLs) 1642
    metabolism 104, 111, 2036
    Monte Carlo analysis 1784
    natural 1366
    PBPK modelling 142
    percutaneous toxicity 583
    peroral toxicity 551
    risk assessment 1757, 1766
α-chlorohydrin 1147
chloromethyl methyl ether 1537
chloropentafluorobenzene 142
chlorophacinone 2006
chlorophenols 21, 38, 1900, 1907
chlorophenoxy acids 1900
p-chlorophenylalanine 763
chlorophyll 384, 1987, 2148
chloroprene 1464, 2015
2-chloropropionate 634
chloroquine 128, 129, 393, 730, 755, 756, 942, 944, 945, 1861
3-chlorostyrene 612
chlorothalonil 2001, 2004
chlorothiazide 548
chlorotrifluoroethylene 691
chlorozotocin 727
chlorpheniramine 219, 1495
chlorphenoxy herbicides 1512
chlorphentermine 730
chlorpromazine
    apoptosis and 188, 198
    cardiac toxicity 816, 819
    hepatotoxicity 859
    maximum residue limits (MRLs) 1642
    mg/kg 264
    peroral toxicity 553
    pharmacogenetics 219, 233
    systemic pulmonary toxicity 730
    tests 366
    tissue specificity 129

chlorpropamide 755

chlorprotixen 219

chlorpyrifos 1336, 1340

chlorthalidone 807

chlorzoxazone 241

cholecalciferol *see* vitamin D$_3$

cholecystokinin 184, 547

cholesterol 255, 355, 361, 367, 548

cholesteryl hemisuccinate 200

cholestyramine 255, 895

cholic acid 360, 567

choline 1518

cholinolytics 2093–4

CHP *see* cyproheptadine

chromium 2061–2, 2066
    apoptosis and 200
    bioavailability 1778–9
    biomonitoring 1780, 1900–1,
      1904, 1907, 1909, 1910
    carcinogencity 1539
    cardiac toxicity 823
    causing apoptosis 185
    cutaneous toxicity 835
    dose–response assessment 1760
    in drinking water 1381, 1382
    genotoxicity 200
    in home environment 1418
    industrial hygiene database
      1457–8
    mixed routes of exposure 604
    nephrotoxicity 680, 683
    PBPK modelling 142
    route-specific toxicity criteria
      1765
    in sewage sludge 1372
    in soils 1329, 1373
    speciation 1458

chromium compounds 200, 1537,
    2014, 2017, 2023

chromogranin A 344, 346

chrysene 1791

cicutol 1520

cicutoxin 1520

cigarette smoke *see* tobacco smoke

ciguatoxin 819, 821, 823, 2191

cimetidine 572, 1010, 1146, 1215,
    2193

cinchona 2

cinnabar 2057

circatrigintan 251

circavigintan 251

cis-dichlorodiammineplatinum II
    (cis-DPP)
    see cisplatin

cismethrin 529, 534

cisplatin
    and apoptosis 185
    circadian toxicology 254, 256,
      260, 262
    eye toxicity 765
    nephrotoxicity 683–4
    ototoxicity 784, 793–4, 795
    parenteral toxicity 524
    regulations 1430
    respiratory sensization 711

cis-platinum *see* cisplatin

citalopram 219, 730

citral (3,7-dimethyl-2,6-octadien-
    1-al) 551, 554

citrate 644

citreoviridin 2145

citric acid 1985

citrinin 2146

clarithromycin 1429

clays 2014, 2017

cleaning agents 461

cleaning products 920, 1512, 1550,
    1603
    see also household products *in*
      Subject Index

clemastine 219

clenbuterol 1863

clindamycin 531, 1438

clioquinol 1427, 1428, 1438, 1565,
    1566

clodronate 184

clofibrate 113, 114, 867, 883, 946,
    1866

cloforex 730

cloxacillin 537

clozapine 219, 663

CN *see* 2-chloroacetophenone

CO *see* carbon monoxide

coal burning 1266, 1267–8, 1270,
    1283

coal dusts, occupational exposure
    1456

coal gas poisoning, CO Hb
    concentration 1921

coal tars 1537, 2004

cobalt 2064
    antidotes 426
    biological monitoring 1901,
      1904, 1907, 1909, 1910
    cardiac toxicity 821, 822
    cutaneous toxicity 835
    in drinking water 1381
    endocrine toxicology 992
    haematotoxicity 391
    hepatotoxicity 870

cobalt chloride 114

cobalt compounds 426

cobalt-containing cyanide activities
    428

cobalt edetate 516

cobalt histidine 428

cobalt naphthenate 2020

cobalt sulphate 1430

cocaine
    abuse 1550
    acute overdose 1496
    cardiac toxicity 813–14
    controlled drug 1545
    drugs of abuse screen (DAS)
      1503
    eye toxicity 758
    forensic analysis 1491, 1504
    hepatotoxicity 872
    and idiopathic environmental
      illness 1706, 1708
    placental toxicity 1257
    site-dependent blood
      concentrations 1495
    and stress 1419

cochineal 1653, 1987

codeine 219, 222, 1491, 1504

colchicine 16, 184, 185, 199, 391,
    637, 638, 867, 942–3, 1642

colour additives 1552, 1560, 1658,
    1659, 1985, 1986–7, 2017
    see also food colourings

compound 1080 *see* fluoroacetate

concanavalin A 338, 710

condylactis toxin (CTX) 820

conicine 34

coniine 1521

convallamarin 1522

convallarine 1522

convallatoxin 1522

cooking fats 274

cooking oil 642

cooking oils 38

copper 2064, 2066
    anthropogenic emissions 1370
    biomarker 1869
    cardiac toxicity 823
    and cartilage and bone toxicity
      973, 974, 2068
    causing apoptosis 184
    chelation therapy 2068
    in drinking water 1380
    from mining sites 1373
    gastro-intestinal symptoms 1380
    haematotoxicity 390
    hepatotoxicity 870

copper (*Contd.*)
  historical refrences 1489
  as impurity in fertilizer 1371
  metallothionein and 2067
  natural high concentrations 1366
  pancreatic toxicity 927
  in sewage sludge 1372
  in soils 1329, 1373
  toxicity to animals 1509, 1514–15
  in water distribution systems 1377
copper acetate 533
copper compounds, in rubber 2016
copper sulphate 2000, 2001
coproporphyrin III 392, 2051
corn oil 58, 75, 547, 551, 555, 556, 750, 925
corrosive sublimate *see* mercuric chloride
corticol 262
corticosteroids
  cartilage and bone toxicity 969
  deficiency 948
  excess 947–8
  eye toxicity 757–8, 762
  HSF-1 expression 167
  neonatal toxicity 1216
  over-the-counter availability 1550
  for radiation skin changes 1688
  skeletal muscle toxicity 942, 947–8
  skin toxicity 834, 1549
  teratogenicity 258
  tests 370
  therapy for phosgene poisoning 2099
corticosterone 369–70, 985
corticotropin 1642
cortisol (hydrocortisone) 263, 369–70, 985
cortisone 530, 758, 969, 985
cotinine 221, 239, 1905
cotton 259, 638
coumarins 184, 230–1, 882, 1655, 2006, 2023
coumarol 396
coumarone 231
coumoestrol 1396, 1403
CR *see* dibenz[b,f]-1,4-oxazepine
creatine 272
creatinine 355–6, 362, 685, 1462
creosote 2001, 2004
cresols 568, 1417, 1904, 1907

cristobolite 1815
crocidolite 1446
crotonaldehyde 613
croton oil 844
crystallins 242
crystal violet 745, 753
CS *see* 2-chlorobenzylidine malononitrile
cumene 626
cutting oil 27, 39
cyanate 638
cyanide 2082
  see also sodium cyanide
  acute overdose 1496
  analysis in tissues 1491
  animal euthanasia 498
  antidotes 3, 25, 426, 428, 431, 1924
  biomonitoring 1905
  cardiac toxicity 807, 821
  in cassava 1553
  and collective suicide 1443
  as combustion products 1921, 1923
  conjunctival sac LD_{50} 760
  elimination by genetic manipulation 1553
  endocrine toxicology 989
  enzyime inhibition 6, 34
  eye toxicity 760
  food poisoning 1724
  forensic testing 1504
  from *Euphorbia* spp. 1518
  from lake water 1817
  and gastro-intestinal microflora 566
  microdiffusion 1497
  in mine ponds 1340
  repeated doses 328
  risk assessment 1750, 1777
  in smoke 1446
  in sorghum 1519
  steam distillation 1497
cyanmethaemoglobin 392, 429
cyanocobalamin *see* vitamin B_{12}
cyanofenphos 1997
cyanogen bromide 1455, 2102
cyanogen chloride 1724
cyanogenic glycosides 566, 917, 918, 919
cyanogens 1919, 1922, 1983–4
1-cyano-2-hydroxy-3-butene 184, 919
cyanopyrethroids 524
cyanuric chloride 626, 711

cycad toxin 635
cycasin 566, 636, 876, 936, 991, 1981
cyclamate 82, 573, 1990
cyclodienes 1995
cyclohexane 101, 2035
cyclohexane carboxaldehyde 613
cyclohexanols 71, 101
cyclohexene oxide 279
cycloheximide 184, 188, 198, 869, 974, 1862
cyclohexylamine 71–2, 82, 1989
cyclohexyl benzoate 1915
cyclohexyl methyl phosphono-fluoridate (GFF) 1724, 2089, 2090
cyclohexylthiophthalimide 2014
cyclopamine 1521
cyclopentalate 761
cyclopentate 761
cyclophosphamide
  carcinogenicity 1537
  cardiac toxicity 809
  causing apoptosis 184
  circadian toxicity 257, 258, 262
  as inhibitor 114
  metabolic activation 729
  occupational hazards 515
  parenteral toxicity 524
  pharmacogenetics 237
  pulmonary toxicity 727–9
  reproductive toxicity 1144, 1145, 1146, 1150, 1152
  toxic reactions 1430
cyclopropane 818
cyclosporins 16, 22, 192, 684–5, 908, 915, 1010, 1430, 1862
cycloxyarylamine 109
cyfluthrin 1998
cyhalothrin 1245
α-cylcopiazonic acid 2146
cypermethrin 466, 651, 1244, 1245, 1994, 1998
cyphenothrin 1244
cyproconazole 2001
cyproheptadine (CHP) 991–2
cyproterone acetate 184, 879, 880, 1129, 1155
cyromazine 1994
cysteamine 426, 985
cysteine 71, 229, 234, 636, 690
L-cysteine sulphanate 634
3-cystein-S-yl-4′-hydroxyaniline 688
cytarabine 727

dichlorodiphenyltrichloroethane (DDT) (*Contd.*)

ethanol (*Contd.*)
    treatment for ethylene glycol
        toxicity 1512
    volatile screen 1502
ethanolamine 1455
ethchlorvynol 1496, 1497
ethene *see* ethylene
ether 357, 498
    see also diethyl ether
ethidium bromide 163, 1455
ethinyloestradiol 22, 284, 569, 879,
    1129, 1392, 1397
ethion 1335
ethionine 882, 883, 971–2, 1862
ethoprop 1336
ethoxyacetic acid 1907, 2041
6-ethoxy-1,2-dihydro-2,2,4-
    trimethylquinolone 2017
2-ethoxyethanol 1901, 2030, 2033,
    2041
2-ethoxyethyl acetate 1901
ethoxyquine 130
ethyl acetate 142, 2034
ethyl acrylate 142, 148, 547, 554
ethyl aminobenzoate 413
ethylbenzene 612, 1901, 2033,
    2035
ethyl bromoacetate (SK) 2102
ethyl chlorosulphonate 2102
ethyldeshydroxysparsomycin 765
1,1′-ethylene-2,2′bipyridylium 724
4′-ethylenebis(2-chloroaniline),
    biomonitoring 1902, 1907, 1910
ethylene-bisdithiocarbamates 1123,
    2000, 2001
ethylene bis(tetrabromo)
    isophthalimide 2022
ethylenediamine (EDA) 59, 1475
ethylenediamine tetra-acetic acid
    (EDTA) 357, 384, 388, 535, 622,
    973
ethylene dibromide 880, 1038,
    1145, 1146, 1377, 1467, 1557,
    1770
ethylene dichloride 142, 1557
ethylene (ethene) 259, 1880, 1881,
    1883, 1901, 2019
ethylene glycol
    antidotes 15, 426, 429
    dinitrate biomonitoring 1901,
        1907
    in elixirs 1634
    LD$_{50}$ 15, 55
    metabolism 97, 110, 2032
    mixtures 49

peroral toxicity 553, 555
    pharmacogenetics 237
    toxic reactions 1430
ethylene glycol monoethers 553
ethylene glycol–xylene, Seveso
    disaster 1818
ethylene oxide
    biomarkers 1845, 1865, 1879,
        1882
    biomonitoring 1901
    DNA adducts 1881, 1885, 1886
    exposure levels 1484
    Hb adducts 1880, 1883–4
    interspecies variations in toxicity
        274
    mixtures 21
    mutagenicity 1035
    PBPK modelling 142
    in plastics industry 2019
    prohibited 1557
    reroductive toxicity 1156
    and spontaneous abortion 1464
    toxic hazard 1455
ethylene–propylene rubber 2013
ethylenethiourea (ETU) 2001,
    2002, 2014, 2016
ethyleneurea 1766
ethyl glycol (EG) 1189
2-ethylhexanoic acid 466
2-ethylhexanol 550
5-ethylidene-2-norbornene (ENB)
    61–2
N-ethylmaleimide 816
ethylmaltol 1988
ethyl mercury 681
ethylmethane sulphonate 200, 1023,
    1052, 1145
ethylmethylphenyl glycidate 1988
ethylmorphine 111, 113, 219, 255
N-ethylmorpholine 738
o-ethyl-o,p-nitrophenyl phenyl-
    phosphothioate 1335, 1342, 1345,
    1997
N-ethyl-*N*-nitrosourea 1030
ethylnodiol diacetate 879
ethyl octyl phosphorofluoridates
    638
4-ethyl-1-phospha-2,6,7-
    trioabicyclol[2.2.2]octane-1-oxide
    1925
N-ethylpiperidine 738
p-ethyl phenol 570
ethylvanillin 1988
etidocaine 529
etoposide 185, 199, 200, 262, 727

etretinate 946
ETU *see* ethylenethiourea
eugenol 708
euphorbin 1518
euphoron 1518
exhaust fumes *see* diesel
    combustion products;petrol/diesel
    fumes

F

Fab fragments 426, 428, 1447,
    2181
fagopyrin 1523
famciclovir 239
famphur 1341, 1342, 1355
fatty acid ethyl esters (FAEEs) 813
FC-11 *see* trichlorofluoromethane
FC-12 *see* dichlorodifluoromethane
FC-14 *see* dichlorotetrafluoroethane
fecapentaenes 567–8
Fed d 1 allergen 512
felodipine 22
fenabutatin oxide 2001
fenbuconazole 2001, 2003
fenclofenac (Flenac) 569, 1427,
    1428
fenfluramine 220, 730, 804, 815,
    1155, 1427
fenitrothion 1335, 1994
fenofibrate 859
fenoldopam mesylate 527, 821
fenoprop 2003, 2005
fenoxycarb 2000
fenpropimorph 2001, 2004
fensulfothion 1336, 1337
fentanyl citrate 527, 539
fenthion 1338, 1340, 1341, 1346,
    1352
fentin 2000, 2001
fenvalerate 1244, 1245
feprazone (Methrazone) 1427
ferbam 2000, 2001
ferric compounds *see* iron(II)
ferritin 822
ferrocyanides 1985
ferro-manganese alloy production
    668
ferrous compounds *see* iron(II)
fertilizers 305
fexofenadine 1429
fibreglass 2019
fibroblast growth factor 1972
fibronectin 342
filgrastim 1965

finasteride 1403
fipronil 1994, 2000
flavonoids 566, 1429, 1984, 2131, 2137
flax*seed* flour 570
flecainide 220, 222
flectol H 882
fluanisone 527, 539
fluazifop 142, 259
fludarabine 727
flumazanil 426, 430, 433
flumethrin 1994, 1998
flunisolide 758
fluoran 1987
fluorescein 746, 751, 752, 753, 760
fluoride
    acute overdose 1496
    analysis in tissues 1491
    biomonitoring 1901, 1907, 1910
    bound by ligand exchange 1369
    cartilage and bone toxicity 967, 973
    in drinking water 1381
    PBPK modelling 142
    storage sites 17
fluorocarbons 1455
fluorocene 338
fluorochrome penetration 750
fluorocitrate 643
fluorodeoxyuridine 185, 261
fluoroelasomers 2013
fluoropyrimidines 261
5-fluoropyrimidin-2-one 238
fluoroscein dyes 1987
fluorotrichloromethane 1901, 1907
5-fluorouracil
    causing apoptosis 184
    circadian toxicology 261, 266
    interaction with sorivudine 1565
    neurotoxicology 643
    pancreatic toxicity 926
    parenteral toxicity 524
    peroral toxicology 548
    pharmacogenetics 235, 238
    systemic pulmonary toxicity 727
fluoxetine 220, 232, 730, 1495
flupentixol 220
fluphenazine 220
flurandrenolide 758
flutamide 1403
[tau]-fluvalinate 1642
folate 257, 391, 972, 2040, 2131
folcodine 220
follicle stimulating hormone (FSH) 369, 371, 1965

folpet 2001, 2002
food colourings 530, 564, 1123, 1653
formaldehyde
    antidotal studies 429
    carcinogenicity 1456, 1537
    chemical mixtures toxicity 315
    as combustion product 1929
    in diet 1981
    dose profiling 16, 56
    eye toxicity 765
    idiopathic environmental illness 1705, 1706, 1709, 1713
    indoor sources 1295, 1298
    inhalation toxicity 20, 589
    irritant effects 16, 1475
    lung cancer 1456
    metabolism 119
    methanol oxidation 2040
    mixtures 21
    mutagenicity 1038
    occupational hazards 510, 515
    pancreatic toxicity 902
    peripheral sensory irritation 623, 626
    pharmacogenetics 237
    from polyethylene 1918–19
    reproductive toxicity 1156
    respiratory sensitization 16, 707–11
    risk assessment 1757, 1766
    in rubber 2016, 2018
    toxic hazard 1455
    from wood burning 1918
formalin 510
formate 119, 429, 765, 1455, 1901, 1907, 2040, 2041
2-formyl-3,4-dihydro-2*H*-pyran 738
Fos protein 240
fostriecin 199
fotemustine 727
Fowler's solution 460
FPL 52757 863–4, 881, 882
frusemide *see* furosemide
FTY 720 184
5-FU *see* 5-fluorouracil
fuel oil 922
Fuller's earth, decontaminant 2083, 2087, 2092
fulvic acids 1368
fumaric acid 549, 1985
fumonisins 1252–3, 2145, 2146, 2162–6
    A_1 2163
    A_2 2163

    B_1 1515–16, 1520, 2146
    B_2 2163
    B_3 2163
    B_4 2163
furan-2-al *see* furfural
furans 90, 132, 142, 726–7, 1756, 1757
furazolidone 819, 1642
furfural 237, 1901
furnace black 2017
furoic acid 1907
furosemide (frusemide) 184, 198, 253, 785, 795, 915, 1010, 1430
furylfuramide (AF-2) 1038

G

GA *see* tabun
gadolinium chloride 873, 881
galactoflavine 972
galactosamine 6, 184, 1860, 1861
galena *see* lead sulphide
gallic acid 1518, 1522
gallic acid esters 1985
gallium 2063
gallium arsenide 2050, 2063
ganglio-*n*-tetrosylceramide *see* asialo GM1
gas, bottled 920
gasoline *see* petroleum products
GB *see* sarin
GD *see* pinacolyl methylphosphono-fluoridate
GE *see* isopropyl ethylphosphono-fluoridate
gelsemine 1520
genestein 1396
genistin 197, 570
gentamicin
    cardiotoxicity 819
    circadian toxicology 16, 265
    nephrotoxicity 685
    ototoxicity 789, 792, 795
    parenteral toxicity 531, 537
    tissue take-up 128, 129
    toxic reactions 1430
gentian violet 738
germanium 1567–8
germanium compounds 1552
gestodene 1427, 1428–9
GF *see* cyclohexyl methyl-phosphonofluoridate
gigathenin 1518
ginerol 806
ginseng 1552

gitoxin 237
glass 2022
gliotoxin 197
glucagon 346, 547, 759, 991
D-glucaric acid 1848
glucocorticoids 757, 758
    antidotal studies 428
    and apoptosis 197
    endocrine toxicology 984, 985,
      990–1
    for insect stings 2184
    manufacture, toxic hazards 1455
    for mustard gas respiratory tract
      lesions 2087
    skeletal muscle toxicity 947
    therapy for phosgene poisoning
      2099
gluconate 428
glucono-δ-lactone 2127
glucose 355–6, 358, 362, 684,
    1495, 1496, 1504
glucosinolates 1983, 1984
glucuronides 107, 537
glufosinate 2003, 2006
glutamate 115, 632, 634, 1988
glutamate antagonists 635
glutamine 236
glutaraldehyde 26, 62, 548, 701,
    711
glutathione
    circadian toxicology 257
    haematotoxicity 384, 393
    interspecies varation in toxicity
      277
    metabolism 100
    mixtures 315
    nephrotoxicity 681
    neurotoxicity 634
    pathological changes 344
    systemic pulmonary toxicity 724
    tests 361
glutathionine 262
glutethimide 1122, 1496, 1503,
    1545
glycerol 2022
glycerol formal 534
glyceryl dinitrates 1907
glyceryl triacetate 740, 750
glycidyl ethers 1884, 2023
glycine 236, 392, 632
glycoconjugates 343
glycogen 336
glycol ethers 585, 804, 1156, 1467,
    2023, 2032, 2041
glycolic acid 2032

glycols 2014, 2020
glycoproteins 338, 364
glycosaminoglycans 342
glycosides
    cardiac 237, 285, 428, 808,
      811–12, 818, 821, 1549
    cytogenicity 1090
    in toxic plants 1522
glycosides food toxicology 1983–4
glyphosate 1512, 2003, 2006
gold 390, 395, 870, 1003, 1004,
    1130, 1489
gossypol 185, 1553
grain dusts 701
gramicidin D 819
granisetron 220
grayanotoxins (GTX) 639, 818,
    821, 824
griseofulvin 552, 569, 867, 870
growth factors 1972
GTX *see* grayanotoxins
guanethidine 1427
guanoxan 220
N^7-guanyl-aflatoxin B1 1845
S-[2-(*N*-guanyl)ethyl]glutathione
    121
guanylic salts 1988
guianidine derivatives 2016

H

H1-blockers 738
H_2 antagonists *see* histamine H_2
    antagonists
H7 191, 199
H16 426
haematoporphyrin 762
haemocyanin 384
haemophilus B, conjugate vaccine
    1965
haemoprotein 254
haemorrhagins 2179
haemosiderin 2065
Hagedorn oximes 429, 2094, 2095
haloacetonitriles 1383
haloalkanes/haloalkenes 121, 161,
    690–1, 871, 2032
haloethylglutathione 121
halogenated compounds, forensic
    screening tests 1497
halogenated hydrocarbons
    abusive use 1505
    aliphatic 313
    aromatic 810–11, 872, 911, 917,
      922, 1004

    chlorination byproducts 1383
    metabolism 104
    nephrotoxicity 689–91
    protein adducts 1887
    steam distillation 1497
halogens, bioavailability in drinking
    water 1381
haloperidol 220, 243, 264, 553,
    663, 1403
halothane
    activation 132
    adverse drug reactions 1438,
      1439
    anaesthesia 2030
    animal euthanasia 498
    biomarker 1849
    biomonitoring 1901
    cardiac toxicity 810, 818
    cartilage and bone toxicity 966
    metabolism 101, 102, 104
    reproductive toxicity 1145
    tests 357
haloxyfop 2003, 2005
harmaline 222, 223
harmalol 222
harman 222
harmine 222
hashish *see* cannabis
HCH *see* hexachlorocyclohexane
heavy metals 2049
    and acid precipitation 1377
    animal toxicoses 1513, 1523
    cartilage and bone toxicity 965
    combustion products 1919
    as contaminants in food crops
      1369
    endocrine toxicity 987–8
    environmental contamination
      1564
    forensic analysis 1491, 1495,
      1497
    groundwater contamination 1369
    human studies 461
    and menstrual disorders 1465
    natural high concentrations 1366
    neonatal toxicity 1217, 1218
    plant root uptake 1369
    renal injury 680–1
    reproductive effects 1146, 1350
    screening methods 1497, 1554
    in soils 1329
    toxicology 257
helanine 1519
helenaline 1519
heleurine 1519

heliotrine 1519
HEMASTIX 496
hemlock 1489, 1490
heparin 357, 1511
hepatitis B vaccine 1966
heptachlor 392, 1145, 1244, 1329, 1343, 1523, 1995
heptane 2022, 2034
herbal products 757, 1550, 1552
heroin 223, 814–15, 942, 944, 946
heterocyclic amines 271–4, 276, 1039, 1981, 1982
2,2´,4,4´,5,5´-hexabromobiphenyl 142
hexacarbon 1430
hexachlorobenzene 142, 557, 870, 1226, 1864–5, 1901, 1907
hexachlorobiphenyls 131, 1870
hexachlorobutadiene 121, 133, 569, 690, 690–1
γ-hexachlorocyclohexane
  see lindane
hexachloroethane 2036
hexachlorophene 638–9, 639, 1147, 1430
hexaconazole 2001, 2003
hexadimethrine bromide 985
hexafluoroisopropanol 614
hexahydrophthalic anhydride 1845
hexamethylene diisocyanate 707
hexamethylenetetramine (HMT) 2014, 2016, 2099–100
hexamethylmelamine 992
hexamethylphosphoramide 232
hexamine see hexamethylene tetramine
hexandiones 637
hexane 2034
  biomonitoring 1901
  biotransformation 2031
  characteristics 2035
  CNS effects 1455
  eye toxicity 756
  metabolism 2032
  metabolites, toxicity 637
  with methyl n-butylketone 149
  neuropathy 131, 1475
  neurotoxicity 637
  PBPK modelling 142
  toluene interaction 2033
  toxicity 2030, 2031
  uses 2034
hexane-2,5-dione 131, 149, 654, 1907, 2031, 2033, 2035
2-hexanol 199, 637, 2034–5

2-hexanone 131, 149, 637, 1902, 1907, 2031, 2035
hexobarbital 255
hexobarbitone 110, 111, 226
hexylhydrophthallic anhdyire 2020
HI see hippuric acid
HI-6 430
hippuric acid (HI) 1130, 1904, 1907, 1989, 2038, 2039
hisidine 974
histamine
  cardiac toxicity 823
  circadian toxicology 262–3
  cutaneous toxicity 834
  elevated levels 1554
  eye toxicity 764
  fish poisoning 2193
  H_1/H_2 antagonists 1124, 1131, 2184
  haematotoxity 384
  pathological studies 344
  peroral toxicity 546
Hjorton's powders 1428
HMT see hexamethylenetetramine
HN1 see nitrogen mustard
Hoechst 33258 185
homocysteate 634
homocysteine 234, 430
hormone substitutes 1964
HS see sulphur mustard
human follicle stimulating hormone 1965
human growth hormone 1964, 1965, 1966, 1970, 1973
  see also growth hormone
human insulin 1965
  see also insulin
Hun Stoff see sulphur mustard
hyaluronic acid 829
hycanthone methanesulphonate 1046
hydantoin 226, 2001, 2002
hydralazine 101, 103, 108, 112, 2188
hydrazides 105
hydrazine hydrate 1863
hydrazines 101, 1144, 1455, 1901, 1907, 1981
hydrocarbons 161, 257–8, 731–2, 1464
  see also aliphatic hydrocarbons; chlorinated hydrocarbons
hydrochloric acid
  in chemical warfare 2097

as combustion product 1821, 1822, 1917, 1927
  from volcanoes 1815
  peripheral sensory irritation 616
  peroral toxicity 545
  PVC 1915, 1918, 1925
  in rubber 2018
hydrochlorothiazide 253, 795, 807
hydrocodone 220
hydrocortisone 758
hydrocyanic acid see hydrogen cyanide
hydrofluoric acid see hydrogen fluoride
hydrogen 563, 1815, 1917
hydrogen chloride see hydrochloric acid
hydrogen cyanide
  see also cyanide
  absorption 17
  biomonitoring 1908
  and chemical warfare 2100–2
  with CO 1924
  as combustion product 1922–4, 1927
  endocrine toxicology 990
  eye toxicity 760
  in fires 1821, 1822
  food poisoning 1983–4
  forensic toxicology 1489
  management of poisoning 2101
  as natural poison 34
  nitrogen-containing polymers 1919
  pancreatic toxicity 900, 918
  physicochemical properties 2100
  polyacrylonitrile 1918, 1923
  polymer 1917
  prophylaxis 2102
  PU 1918, 1919
  and smoking 28
  symptoms and signs of poisoning 2101
  terrorist use 1724
  toxicity 2100–1
hydrogen fluoride 1455, 1815, 1821, 1822, 1831, 1918
hydrogen peroxide 158, 185, 190, 199, 1275, 1455, 1511, 2021–2
hydrogen sulphide 28, 34, 1516–17, 1815, 1817
hydromorphone 1491, 1504
hydroprene 1999–2000
hydroquinone 100, 240, 395, 1986, 2190

hydroxocobalamin 428
hydroxquinone 990
3α-hydroxy bile acids 360
N-hydroxy-2-acetylaminofluorene
metabolism 102
hydroxyalkenals 158, 1868
hydroxyamines 393, 556
1-hydroxyaminonaphthalene 876
4-hydroxyamphetamine 220
p-hydroxybenzoic acid 1989
3-hydroxybutyrate 365
hydroxychloroquine 764, 945
hydroxycobalamin *see* vitamin B12
hydroxycoumarins 231, 231
4-hydroxycyclophosphamide 729
4-hydroxydebrisoquine 112, 222
8-hydroxydeoxyguanosine 1845,
1867, 1868, 2015
6-hydroxydopamine 641
β-hydroxyethoxyacetic acid 84
2-hydroxyethyl mercaptoethanol
1865
N_3-(2-hydroxyethyl)adenine 1885
hydroxyethyl amines 2115
N-(2-hydroxyethyl)valine 1845,
1884
2-hydroxy-5-hexanone 2035
hydroxyhippuric acid 1989
5-hydroxyindol-3-ylanic acid 236
hydroxylamines 104, 109, 161, 413,
426, 429, 1883, 2094, 2119
11β-hydroxylase 370
4-hydroxymethamphetamine 220
N-(3′-hydroxy-4i-methoxyphenyl)-
2-chloroamides 612
R-4′-hydroxy-*N*-methylphenytoin
226
5-hydroxymethyluracil 235, 1845
N-hydroxy-2-naphthylamine 134
4-hydroxynonenal 184, 764, 896
hydroxyochratoxin 2156
4-hydroxyphenoxy)benzoic acid
466
2-hydroxyphenylacetaldehyde 231,
231
2-hydroxyphenylacetic acid 231
2-hydroxyphenylethanol 231
hydroxyproline 722
4-hydroxypropranolol metabolism
100
2-(hydroxypropyl)amine 2115
3-hydroxypropylmercaptouric acid
1865
1-hydroxypyrene 1905, 1927

4-hydroxy-1-(3-pyridyl)butan-1-one
1883
8-hydroxyqunilines 1565–6
3β-hydroxy-5β-steroids 236
hydroxytamoxifen 284–5
5-hydroxytryptamine antagonists
763
hydroxyurea 258
1′-hydroxyversicolorone 2151
hymenoxon 1519
hyoscyamine 1521
hyoscyamus 1489
hypericin 1523
hypochlorite 737, 905
hypoxanthine 103

I

ibotenate 634, 641, 1513
ibufenac 132
ibuprofen 263, 1550
ICI 162 1124
ICI 164,384 1395
ICI 182,780 764, 1403
ifosfamide 262, 727, 1862
imazalil 2001, 2003
imidazoles 1147, 1429
3,3′-iminodipropionitrile 637, 638
imipenem 686
imipramine
acute toxicity 325
cardiac toxicity 805
eye toxicity 756
forensic screening tests 1497
pharmacogenetics 222, 232, 233
post-mortem changes 1495
site-dependent blood
concentrations 1495
systemic pulmonary toxicity 730
indigo dyes 1987
indinavir (Crixivan) 1427
indium 2063
indium arsenide 2063
indocyanine green 361
indolcarbazoles 163
indol-3-carboxylic acid scopine
ester 763
indoles 132, 222–3, 2131
indol-3-ylmethanal 238
indomethacin 184, 253, 254, 807,
1427, 1428, 1917
indoprofen (Flosint) 1427
indoramin 220
inosinic acid 1988

inositol triphosphate (PIP3) 808,
896
insulin-like growth factor 1972
interferons 1964, 1965, 1966,
1971–2
intermidine 1519
inulin 362, 1462
iodide 2102
iodine 1328, 1329, 1365, 1551,
1552, 1969
iodoacetamide 167
iodochlorohydroxy quinoline 413
iodoquinol (Yodoxin, Moebiquin),
adverse effects 1566
iodothalamate 362
2-iodo-3,7,8-trichlorodibenzo-*p*-
dioxin 90, 142
ioxynil 2003, 2005
ipecacuanha 2, 546
4-ipomeanol 132, 726–8, 727
iprindole 730
iprodione 2000, 2002
iproniazid 114
irinotecan 262
iron 2064–5, 2066
in ancient Indian writings 1489
bioavailablity in drinking water
1381
biomonitoring 1905
cardiac toxicity 822
cartilage and bone toxicity 973
chelation 634, 2068
deficiency 1551, 2053
ferric *see* iron(III)
fortification 1223, 1552
haematotoxicity 384
hepatotoxicity 870
ligand exchange 1369
metabolism 1863
neonatal toxicity 1217
stains for 867
transport, as biomarker 1864
iron(II) sulphide 2050
iron(III) 2065
iron(III) mitoxantrone 184
iron(III) oxide 2017
isobutanol 1298
isocyanates 701, 1004, 1475, 1927,
2014, 2021
isoeugenol 708, 711
isofenphos 142
isoflavonoids 570, 1398, 1984
isofluorophate 760
isoflurane 2030
isoleucine 229

isolinoleic esters 1428
isomyl alcohol 142
isoniazid 28, 105, 108, 112, 113, 119–20, 325, 390, 756, 1430
isonicotinic acid 119
isopentane 1867
isophorone 692
isophthalic anhydride 2020
isoprenaline (isoproterenol) 58, 430, 808, 810, 814, 1430
isoprene rubber 2013, 2015
isopropanol 237, 2041
isopropyl alcohol see isopropanol
isoprpyly ethylphosphonofluoridate (GE) 2089
isoprostanes 1867, 1868
isoproterenol see isoprenaline
isoquinolones 191
isoretinoin 1430
isosasafrole 1866
isosorbide dinitrate 460
isosorbide mononitrate 460
isothiocyanates 234, 1430
isotretinoin see 13-*cis*-retinoic acid
itraconazole 1429
ivermectin 1648, 1994, 1999

J

jacobine 1519
jacodine 1519
jervin 1521

K

kainate 634, 634, 641
kallikreinogen 897
kanamycin 128, 129–30, 685, 787, 789, 792, 795, 1430
kaolin 1475, 2022
Kepone see chlordecone
kerosene 315, 920, 922, 2087
ketoconazole 38, 50, 1147, 1403, 1427, 1429
ketones 103, 104, 362, 911, 1383, 1418, 2023, 2032
  see also individual chemicals
ketoprofen 263
kinesin 631
King's yellow 2050
kohl 759

L

β-lactam antibiotics 686–8, 1049
lactate 563, 806, 939, 969

LAL see limulus amoebocyte lysate
laminin 342–3
landrin 1347
lanolin 605
lantadine 1519
lanthanides 870
lanthanum 805, 822
lasiocarpine 883, 1519
latex 510–11, 828, 1667, 1674
lathyrogens 1983
α-latrotoxin 640
lauric acid 101
lazaroid U-78517F 954
lead 2054–7, 2066
  age effects 1417
  animal toxicoses 1343, 1513, 1515, 1518, 1523–4
  anthropogenic emissions 1370
  antidotal studies 426, 433
  behavioural toxicity 650, 654, 658, 661, 665–6
  binding values (EU) 1595
  biomarker 1844, 1848, 1864
  biomonitoring 1485, 1780, 1899, 1901, 1904, 1905, 1907, 1909, 1910, 1911
  cardiac toxicity 821, 822
  cartilage and bone toxicity 973, 974, 2068
  central neurotoxicity 1378, 1523
  chelation therapy 2068
  CNS symptoms 1523
  in contaminated cattle feed 1554
  and DALAD 1343, 1345
  developmental toxicity 1487
  in drinking water 1377, 1378, 1382
  exposure routes 606
  eye toxicity 759
  forensic analysis 1491
  in gull feathers 654
  haematology 390–2
  haematotoxicity 1513
  hepatotoxicity 880
  historical aspects 1482, 1489
  in home environment 1417
  human studies data 463
  and idiopathic environmental illness 1711, 1712
  industrial exposure 683
  ingestion 1340
  interaction with smoking 1417
  and lung disease 1474
  mitochondria sensitivity 683
  neonatal toxicity 1227, 1248

nephrotoxicity 683
  nestling studies 1349
  neurotoxicity 633, 638–9, 639, 1518
  not taken up by plant roots 1369
  ototoxicity 784
  PBPK modelling 142
  in precipitation 1370, 1377
  reproductive toxicity 1145, 1146, 1156, 1464, 1465, 1466, 1467
  risk assessment 1777
  in river Rhine 1370
  in sewage sludge 1372
  in soil 1329, 1371, 1373, 1375
  storage sites 17
  susceptibility 29
  systemic effects 1475
  teratogenicity 1205
  threshold levels 1378
  and Wilms' tumour 1464
lead arsenate 2050, 2055
lead compounds
  binding values (EU) 1595
  in leaded petrol 1266, 1267
  marketing controls 1595
  in plastics industry 2022, 2023
  rubber additive 2014, 2017
  therapeutic use 1451
lead nitrate 184
lead oxide 1446, 2055
lead shot, waterfowl poisoning 1523
lead sulphide (galena) 252, 1366, 2054, 2056
leather 564
lecithin 619
lecithin/sphingomyelin ratio 1216
lectin 338, 343
leptophos 1345, 1997
levamisole 692
lewisite 427, 1724, 2068, 2081, 2082, 2088–9
licorice 945
lidocaine see lignocaine
light hydrocarbons 691
lignans 570, 1984
lignocaine (lidocaine) 254, 265, 366, 522, 529, 555, 640, 817, 947, 956
  toxicity 265
lime salts 972
d-limonene 136, 692, 1757
linamarin 918, 1984
lincomycin 1438

lindane 1994, 1995
  biomonitoring 1901, 1907
  haematotoxicity 389, 392
  hepatotoxicity 879
  hexachlorocyclohexane (HCH)
    879, 1127, 1244, 1995
  human studies 460
  neonatal toxicity 1226
  neurotoxicology 641
  PBPK modelling 142
  persistence in environment 1510
  placental toxicity 1244
  toxicity to poultry 1523
  varied uses 1548
  in waste disposal site 1372
linoleic acid 534, 1979–80, 1981
linolenic acid 1979–80
linseed oil 911
linuron 2003, 2005
lipopolysaccharides 184, 536
lipoproteins 253, 367
lithium 989, 1205–6, 1218, 1382
lithium heparinate 357
lithocholic acid 360, 567
lithostatin 897
lobelidine 1521
lobeline 1521
lomustine 727
loop diuretics 784, 785, 795–6
loperamide 220
lorazepam 252
lotaustralin 918, 1984
lovastatin 946
loxidine 1124, 1125
LSD see lysergic acid diethylamide
lubricating oils 920–2
luminal acid 525
lupanine 1521
lupinine 1521
lycopene 1982
lycopsamine 1519
lymphokines 1972
lysergic acid diethylamide (LSD)
  763, 1146, 1491, 1495, 1545,
  1550, 2081, 2082
lysine 637, 764
lysine–diazepam 2095
lysophosphatidylcholine 191, 2191

M

machining fluids 1456
macrolide antibiotics 1429
magenta 463

magnesium 200, 364, 366, 823,
  940, 973, 974, 1328, 1381, 1382
magnesium carbonate 1985
magnesium compounds 2014, 2017,
  2068
magnesium ions, and apoptosis
  187, 192
magnesium oxide 1985
magnesium sulphate 1216
magnetite 2064
maitotoxin (MTX) 819–20, 2191
malachite green 1648
malaoxon 1996
malathion 1994, 1995
  aquatic toxicity 1316
  behavioural effects 1348
  cardiac toxicity 824
  circadian toxicology 259
  differential toxicity 110, 1335,
    1342, 1523
  human studies 460
  mixtures 21
  poultry toxicity 1342, 1523
  varied uses 1548
maleic anhydride 2020
malondialdehyde 1042, 1867, 1868
manadione 159
mancozeb 2000, 2001
mandelic acid 1485, 1907, 1910,
  2020, 2040
mandelonitrile 566
maneb 2001, 2002
manganese
  behavioural toxicity 668
  bioavailablity in drinking water
    1381
  biomonitoring 1909
  cardiac toxicity 822
  cartilage and bone toxicity 965,
    968, 974, 2068
  ligand exchange 1369
  risk assessment 1777
  sperm evaluation studies 1467
mannitol 792, 795, 2192
MAOIs see monoamine oxidase
  inhibitors
maprotoline 220, 1495
marcain see bupivacaine
marijuana see cannabis
margarines 922, 1552
3-MC see 3-methylcholanthrene
MCPA see 2-methyl-4-
  chlorophenoxyacetic acid
MDA see 4,4′-diaminodiphenyl-
  methane

MDI see diphenylethane-4,4′-
  diisocyanante
MDMA see 3,4-methylene-
  dioxymethamphetamime
MDP see methoxydihydropyran
mechlorethamine 527
mecoprop 1907, 2003, 2005
melamine 1922, 2018
melanin 830
melatonin 222, 257
melittin 820
melphalan 185, 191, 727, 1537
menadione 156, 184, 199
menocil 815
menotrophin 538
meperidine 1495
mephenytoin 226, 227
S-mephenytoin 226
mephobarbitone 226, 227
mepivacaine 1216
meprobamate 1496, 1503
mercaptobenzothiazole 2014, 2016
mercaptoethanol 109
N-(2-mercaptoethyl)propane-1,3-
  diamine 200
2,3-mercaptopropanol antidote
  2068
3-mercaptopropionate 641
6-mercaptopurine 261, 390, 727,
  1153
mercapturic acid see N-acetylcysteine (NAC)
mercurials 816, 1341, 1346, 1557
mercury 2057–60, 2066
  see also mercury chloride;
    mercury sulphide;
    methylmercury
  and acid precipitation 1377
  acute overdose 1496
  antidotal studies 427
  aquatic toxicity 1310
  biomarker 1861, 1864, 1869
  biomonitoring 1485, 1901–2,
    1904, 1905, 1907, 1908, 1910
  cardiac toxicity 821
  chelation therapy 2068
  circadian toxicity 257
  early research 1482
  entry to renal tubular cells 681
  as environmental pollutant
    1378–9
  food poisoning 1724, 1824–6,
    1828
  forensic analysis 1491
  fulmonate 2057

mercury (*Contd.*)
  gastro-intestinal microflora 570
  hepatotoxicity 870
  history 2
  in home environment 1418
  human data studies 460
  immunotoxicity 1003, 1004
  inorganic 681, 1355, 2058, 2066
  interactions with selenium 1351
  ion binding 128
  kidney response 681, 683
  marketing controls 1595
  metallothionein and 2067
  in mine tailings 1355
  neonate toxicity 1226
  neurotoxicity 633, 643, 1564–5
  not taken up by plant roots 1369
  organic 1343, 1355, 1994
  ototoxicity 784
  peripheral neuropathy 1475
  reproductive toxicity 1156
  in sewage sludge 1372
  in soils 1329, 1373
  speciation 1365–6, 1378
  sperm evaluation studies 1467
  and spontaneous abortion 1465
  subchronic testing 1344
  toxicity 1344–5
  transplacental transport 1464
mercury(I) chloride 2000, 2001, 2057
mercury(II) chloride (corrosive sublimate) 257, 267, 681, 682, 822, 1490, 1528, 1861, 2001, 2057, 2059
mercury(II) sulphide 2057
merphos 1512, 2006
mesna 809
mestranol 568
metala 2049–78
metal chelates 1867
metaldehyde 2006
metal ions, binding 128
metalloids 2049
metallothioneins 367, 533, 682, 684, 1317, 1461
metals 104, 1952, 2000, 2001, 2014, 2016, 2023, 2049–78
  see also heavy metals and individual elements
metam 2000, 2001
metamizol (novaminosulfon) 1427, 1428
metamphetamine 1491
metapramine 805

metaprolol 760
metaraminol 220
methacarbamol 2186
methacholine 512
2-methacryloxypropyltrimethoxy-silane 27
methadone 114–15, 220, 1145, 1154, 1497, 1503, 1504
methaemoglobin-generating substances 28, 426
methaemoglobin inhibitors 1902
methamidophos 1997
methamphetamine 184, 220, 814, 1495
methanamine hexamethylene tetramine
methandrostenolone 815
methane 1516–17, 1917, 1927, 2034
methanediol 2040
methanol 2040
  antidotes 425–6, 429
  biomonitoring 1902, 1907
  with carbon tetrachloride 149
  as combustion product 1927
  eye toxicity 755, 765
  forensic analysis 1491
  from wood burning 1918
  GLC 1503
  inhalation 1419
  LD_{50} 15
  metabolism 103, 119, 2032
  microdiffusion 1497
  PBPK modelling 142
  pharmacogenetics 237
  steam distillation 1497
  toxic reactions 1430
methapyriline 878, 1127, 1128
β-methasone 758
methenyl trichloride 2036
methimazole 232
3-methindole 731–2
methiocarb 1336, 1347, 1998, 2006
methionine 426, 430, 644, 793, 972, 1970, 1973
methoprene 1999–2000
methotrexate
  and apoptosis 185
  carcinogenicity 1455
  circadian toxicology 261
  cytotoxicity 1454–5
  eye toxicity 755
  haematotoxicity 390, 391
  metabolism 16
  mutagenicity 1053, 1054

neonatal toxicity 1219
  systemic pulmonary toxicity 727, 728, 729
methoxsalen 1537
methoxyacetic acid 142, 2041
methoxyamphetamines 220
methoxychlor 1145, 1153–4, 1243–4, 1329, 1396
methoxydihydropyran (MDP) 26
5-methoxy-*N,N*-dimethyltryptamine 222–3
2-methoxyethanol 142, 583–4, 2030, 2033, 2041
  and radiofrequency radiation 1419
methoxyethylmercury 2058
methoxyfluorane 357, 387, 498, 818, 1430
methoxyphenamine 100, 220
8-methoxypsoralen 415, 762, 1430
2-methylacrolein 1919
methylacrylamidoglycolate methyl ether 554
N-methylamino-L-alanine 634
methylarsenic compounds 267, 1907
methylating agents 1881
methylazooxymethane 876
methylazoxymethanol 184, 566, 569, 635–6, 876, 877
methylbenzene *see* toluene
methylbenzoic acid 793, 2039
methylbromide 615, 755
methyl-1-(butylcarbamoyl) benzimidazol-2-ylcarbamate 758
methyl *iso*-butyl ketone 1907, 2018
methyl butyl ketone *see* 2-hexanone
methyl *tert*-butyl ether, PBPK modelling 142
N-methylcarbamoylmercaptouric acid 1865
methylchloroform *see* 1,1,1-trichloroethane
methyl chlorosulphonate 2102
3-methylcholanthracene 258, 279, 280, 283, 395, 525, 549, 763
3-methylcholanthrene (3-MC) 113, 114, 118, 866, 910
methylcobalamin 2064
S-methylcysteine sulphoxide 1522
methylcysteine sulfoxide 234
7-methyl-2′-deoxyguanosine-3′-monophosphate 225
2-methyl-4-chlorophenoxyacetic acid (MCPA) 1907

morphine 114, 184, 198, 556, 568, 569, 1430, 1491
   see also opiates
morpholines 2001, 2004
morsodren 1336, 1337
motilin 547
moulds *see* mycotoxins
moxidectin 1642
4-MP *see* 4-methylpyrazole
6-MP *see* 6-mercaptopurine
MPDP⁺ 132, 133

MPDP$^+$ 132, 133
MPP$^+$ 132, 133, 224
MPTP *see* methylphenyltetra-hydropyridine
muconic acid 607
mumps vaccines (Pluserix-MMR, Immravax) 1427
β-muricholate 360
muromonab 1965
muscimol 1513
musk ambrette 1430
Mus m 1 allergen 511
Mus m 2 allergen 511
mustard gases 1035, 1444
   see also nitrogen *or* sulphur mustard
MX mutagen 1383
MXT *see* maitotoxin
mycophenolate 1130
mycotoxins 2145–76
   biological activity 2146
   in biological warfare 2082
   characterization 2148
   as chemical warfare agent 2104
   in diet 58, 1982
   in mouldy food 1554
   placental toxicity 1251–4
   produced by non-storage fungi 2148–9
   structures 2145, 2146
   toxicity 1339, 1340, 1515–16, 1520, 1524
mydriatics 1548
myelin 636–7
myricetin 571

N

nabam 990
NABQI *see* N-acetyl-p-benzoquinoneimine
NAC *see* N-acetylcysteine
nafenopin 1127
nafoxidine 762
naloxone 426, 430, 433

2-naphthalene sulphonate 2018
naphthalene 108, 731, 763, 1455
naphthalene dihydrodiol 763
naphthalene diisocyanate 2021
naphthaquinones 358
naphthazoline 738
naphthoflavones 113, 763, 918, 925, 990
naphthotriazoles 2023
naphthoxylacetic acid 100, 228
α-naphthyl isothiocyanate (ANIT) 882, 1860, 1861
naphthylamines
   biochemistry 134
   carcinogenicity 1537, 2015, 2017
   extrapolation studies 1952
   in humans 463
   metabolism 120
   rubber additive 2014
   toxic reactions 1430
α-naphthylthiourea (ANTU) 724, 1511
NAPQI *see* N-acetyl-p-benzoquinoneimine
naringenin 22
natamycin 1642
neamine 792
neocarzinostatin 527
neomycin 129–30, 685, 787, 788, 791–2, 795, 819, 1455
neoprontosil 565
neostigmine bromide 2181
neostygmine 951
neriine 821
netilmicin 685
netropsin 163
neurotrophic factors 1972
Neutral Red 753, 753
ngaione 872, 877
niacin 972
nicarbazine 1521
nickel 2062–3, 2066
   anthropogenic emissions 1370
   and apoptosis 188–9
   biomarker 1849
   biomonitoring 1902, 1904, 1907, 1909, 1910
   carcinogenicity 1537, 1539
   cardiac toxicity 808
   cutaneous toxicity 835
   genotoxicity 200
   PBPK modelling 142
   placental toxicity 1249–50
   in sewage sludge 1372

   in soils 1329, 1373
   teratogenicity 127–9, 1206–9
nickel carbonyl 758
nickel chloride 664
nickel sulphate 413
nicotinamide 190, 200
nicotine
   biomonitoring 1905
   circadian toxicity 265
   extraction from tissues 1490
   favourable effects 1452
   metabolism 238, 239
   PBPK modelling 142
   peroral toxicity 548
   as pesticide 1994, 1999
   pharmacogenetics 220–1, 231, 233, 238–9
   risk acceptance 1960
   steam distillation 1497
   toxicity 265
nicotinic alkaloids 1520, 1521
nifedipine 188, 817
nimodipine 22
nitrates 2111–43
   air pollution 1266
   animal toxicoses 1509, 1514, 1519, 2135
   carcinogenic 1382
   conversion to nitrite 1383
   dose levels expression 2111
   endogenous synthesis 2118–21, 2133
   epidemiological studies 2129–31
   fertilizer, in soil 1960
   human body burdens 2133–4
   human dietary intakes 2115–18
   interspecies differences 1509, 1519
   leaching 1371
   levels in food and beverages 2112–14
   reduction 566–7
   RfD 1760
   toxicokinetics and metabolism 2121–3
nitrenium ions 161
nitric acid 1275, 1376, 1477
nitric oxide 104, 158, 199, 634, 808, 1266, 1274–5, 2119, 2121
nitric oxide radical 896, 903
nitrile rubber 2013
nitriles 2003, 2005
nitrites 2111–43
   carcinogenic 1383
   dose levels expression 2111

nitrites (*Contd.*)
    endogenous synthesis 2120, 2134
    epidemiological studies 2131–2
    haematotoxicity 390
    human body burdens 2134
    human dietary intakes 2115–18
    levels in food and beverages 2112–14
    susceptibility 28
    toxicokinetics and metabolism 2121–2, 2123, 2125–8
    toxicological data in animals 2135
4-nitroacetophenone 243
nitroalkanes 2023
nitroamines 1883
nitroarenes 1883
nitroaromatics 238, 1867
nitroarsenilic acid 1515
nitrobenzaldehyde 243
nitrobenzenes 104, 565, 572, 585, 1902
6-nitrochrysene 565
nitro compounds 565
nitrofen 990, 1557
nitrofurans 1642
nitrofurantoin 726, 1430
nitrogen 563, 1372
    see also urea
nitrogen/argon inhalation 498
nitrogen-based fertilizers, toxicity 1514
nitrogen dioxide
    acute toxicity 50, 51
    air pollution 1266
    ambient concentration effects on humans 1279
    biochemical and histopatho-logical effects 1278–6
    in fires 1821
    mixtures 314
    in plastics industry 2021
    respiratory effects 1279
    and response to allergens 1279–80
    silo filler's disease 1517
    toxicokinetics 1278
    transport 158
nitrogen mustard 199, 258, 2083, 2085
nitrogen oxides 1266, 1267, 1297, 1376, 1927
nitrogen poisoning, rumen microflora 1514

nitrogen trichloride 626
nitroglutethimide 1122
nitroglycerine 460, 527, 545, 1475, 1722–3, 1902, 2187
nitroimidazoles 1090
3-nitromalonate 635
1-nitronaphthalene 731, 876
nitrophenazide 1521
p-nitrophenol, biomonitoring 1907
3-nitropropionate 634, 635, 636
nitropyrene 130, 565, 569, 1038
nitroquinoline oxide 104, 240, 1047
nitrosamides 1982, 1989
nitrosamines
    biomarkers 1880, 1882
    carcinogenicity 2128–9
    cytogenicity 1079
    in diet 1981, 1982, 1989
    DNA adducts 1885, 1886
    genotoxicity 7
    in German food and drink 2118
    hepatotoxicity 876, 877
    mixtures 305, 314
    mutagenicity 1039
    pancreatic toxicity 902, 911, 920, 924, 925, 926
    rubber additives 2014, 2016–17
    in tobacco smoke 2115
nitroschloramphenicol 390
N^1-nitrosoanabasin 2115
N^1-nitrosoanatabine 2115
nitrosobenzene 565
N-nitrosobis(2-hydroxypropyl) amine (BOP) 922, 923–4, 927
nitroso compounds
    carcinogenic 1383
    in chemical warfare 2111
    endogenous synthesis 2120–1, 2134
    epidemiological studies 2132–3
    and gastro-intestinal microflora 562, 566
    human studies 2115–18, 2134–5, 2137
    rubber additives 2014
    toxicokinetics and metabolism 2121–2, 2123, 2128–9
    toxicological data in animals 2135–6
nitrosodiethanolamine 274, 2115, 2121, 2123
nitrosodimethylamine 232, 234, 2115, 2118, 2121, 2123, 2132
nitrosodiphenylamine 2016, 2017
nitrosohydroethylglycine 2121

nitrosomethylurea (NMU) 1030, 1100
nitrosomorpholine 2121
N′-nitrosonornicotine *see* 4-(*N*-methylnitrosoamino)-1-(3-pyridyl)butan-1-one (NNK)
nitrosopiperidine 2120, 2123
nitrosoproline (NPRO) 2120, 2123
nitrosopyrrolidine 2115, 2120, 2123
nitrosothiioproline 2123
nitrosoureas 7, 1885
β-nitrostyrene 612
nitrous oxide 390, 1151
nivalenol 2104, 2149
NMU *see* nitrosomethylurea
NNK *see* 4-(*N*-methylnitrosoamino)-1-(3-pyridyl)butan-1-one
nocodazole 199
nomifensine (Merital) 1427, 1438
nonane 2034
non-steroidal anti-inflammatory drugs (NSAIDs) 51, 132, 136, 167, 229–30, 458, 940, 1427, 1428, 1550
nonylphenol 1396, 1397
nordoxepin 1495
norephedrine *see* phenylprop-anolamine
norepinephrine (noradrenaline) 730, 1348
norethisterone 879, 1127
norethynodrel 879
norfluoxetine 1495
norgestimate 1428
normeperidine 1495
norpropoxyphene 1495, 1504
norsolorinic acid 2151
nortriptyline 220, 819, 1495
noscapine 220
NO_x *see* nitrogen oxides
NSAIDs *see* non-steroidal anti-inflammatory drugs
nucleic acid
    extractants 1454, 1455
    identification chemicals 1454
    sequencing reagents 1454, 1455
nux vomica *see* strychnine
nylon 1922, 2022

O

obidoxime 426, 429, 2094
OCDD *see* 2,3,7,8-tetrachloro-*p*-dibenzodioxin octochloroanalog

ochratoxins 2145
analogues 2155–7
analysis 2157–8
animal toxicoses 1515–16, 1524
A (OTA) 197, 1253, 2156, 2157
B 2155, 2156
biological activity 2146,
2154–62
C 2156
chemical characteristics and
biosynthesis 2154–5
chemical structures 2146, 2156
genotoxicity 2160
immunotoxicity 2160
isolation and purification 2157
mechanisms of action 2161–2
pharmacokinetics 2160–1
production, isolation and
purification 2157
toxicity 1516, 2157
OC *see* organochlorines
octadecysilane 1455
octane 2034
octanoic acid 1298
octanol 199
octylphenol 1404–5
17β-oestradiol
assay 1402
clearance rates 1408
developmental effects 1406
and gastro-intestinal microflora
568, 569, 570
grapefruit interaction 22
natural oestrogen 1392
normal levels 1398
as reference substance 1397
structure 1396
testosterone metabolite 1395,
1406
toxicity and reproduction studies
1404, 1405
use in assay 1403
oestrogens *see Subject Index*
oestrogens, synthetic
see dithethystilboestrol
oestrogen sulphate 568
oil, detection by histology 534
oil of Bergamot 413
oil spill control agents 1313
OK-432 184
okadaic acid 186, 199, 817, 2193
olanzapine 220
olaquindox 1648
oleandrin 821
oleates 534, 731–2, 2022

olefins 2034
oligomycin 816
olive oil 58
oltipraz 278, 1887
omeprazole 227–8, 1124
ondansetron 220
OP *see* organophosphates
opiates
acute overdose 1496
controlled drug 1545
forensic analysis 1491, 1495,
1503, 1504
heroin injection 814–15, 942,
944, 946
maternal addiction 1224, 1256–7
pancreatic toxicity 901
reproductive toxicity 1145
skeletal muscle toxicity 942
opium 1489, 1490
OPP *see* 2-phenylphenol
Orange II 565
orcinol 990
organic acids *see* acids
organic solvents 2029-47
aliphatic 2034-7
aromatic hydrocarbons 2037-40
biological monitoring 1906
chlorinated aliphatic 2035-7
combustion toxicology 1919,
1928
enzyme induction 2032-3
metabolism 2032, 2033-4
mixtures 2033, 2042
toxicity 2030-3
behavioural 651
narcosis 8
occupational 1418, 1487
ototoxicity 794-5
organoarsenicals 3, 56, 1426, 1427
organochlorines (OC)
biomarker 1848
biomonitoring 1902
and breast cancer 1400
chronic intake 82
environmental 1370, 1553–4
human studies 460
as mixtures 2007
molecular interactions 163
oestrogenic effects 1398
persistence 1392, 1548, 1553–4,
1599
as pesticides 2, 1994, 1995,
1996–8
placental toxicity 1243–4
prohibited 1557

organohalides 1366, 1457
organomercurials 681–2, 1824–5,
2000
see also mercurials;
methylmercury
organometallic compounds,
fungicide 2001
organophosphates (OP)
see also nerve agents *in Subject
Index*
acute poisoning 34
additive effects 50
age/maturation effects 1337
antidotes 431
behavioural effects 662, 1348
biochemical disturbances 63
biological effect monitoring
1485
biomarker 1848
biomonitoring 1900, 1906
and brain cholinesterase levels
1343, 1523
cardiac toxicity 807, 823–4
cholinesterase inhibition 114,
951–5, 1345, 1475, 1554, 1866,
1900
differential toxicity 1328, 1335
domestic animal toxicity 1510,
1512
effect of formulation 1339
equine toxicity 1518
extrapolation of acute effects 51
fungicides 2001, 2003
herbicides 1512, 2003, 2006
history 2, 3
immunotoxicity 1004, 1006,
1010
insecticides 466, 1996–8
lability 1329
long-term exposure 1487
metabolism by HMOs 1334
as mixtures 2007
neurotoxicology 23, 43, 55,
637–8, 1333
pancreatic toxicity 917
pesticides 578
phytometabolism 1341
placental toxicity 1242–3
in plastics industry 2023
poultry toxicity 1523
repeated exposure 1418
reproduction testing 1351
rubber additive 2014
species sensitivity differences
110

organophosphates (OP) (*Contd.*)
  sulphoxide and sulphone
    metabolites 1341
  toxicity 426, 429, 432
  varied uses 1548
  wildlife toxicity 1337, 1338,
    1341
organophosphonate 635
organosilicones 751
organotins 523, 1004, 1006, 2000,
  2001, 2022
orpiment 2050
osmosin 1427, 1428
OTA *see* ochratoxin A
ouabain 265, 807, 821
oxalates 97, 973, 1518, 1522, 2032
oxaliplatin 260–1
oxamniquine 882
β-*N*-oxatylamino-L-alanine 634
oxazepam 114
oxazolone 707, 711
oxides of nitrogen *see* nitrogen
  oxides (NO_x)
oximes 3, 426, 429–30, 516, 1998,
  2093, 2094–5
oxiranes 130
oxmetidine 1124
8-oxo-dG adducts 1890
2-oxothiazolidine-4-carboxylic acid
  689
oxprenolol 220
oxybisbenzenesulphonyl hydrazides
  2023
oxybuprocaine 741
oxychlordane 1343
oxycodone 1491, 1504
oxygen 238, 429, 430, 516, 590,
  1417, 2099
oxygen free radical(s) 792, 793,
  807, 809
  biology 903–4
  oxidation products (FROPS) 896
  pathology *see* oxidative stress
oxyphenbutazone 807, 1427
oxytetracycline 534, 537
oxytocin 537
oxytotic drugs 220
ozone
  air pollution 1267, 1268, 1273–4
  behavioural toxicity 653, 665
  biochemical and histopatho-
    logical effects 1276
  causing apoptosis 184
  effects on human health 1276–8,
    1283

ethics 1960
mixtures 314, 315, 316
and nitric oxide 1274–5
occurrence and production 1275
pancreatic toxicity 922
and sulphuric acid, comparison of
  factors 1280
toxicokinetics 1275
transport 158

P

PAF *see* lysophospholipid
PAHs *see* polycyclic aromatic
  hydrocarbons
paint(s) 918, 1295
paint thinners 918, 922
palladian catalysts 563
palmitic acid 813
palytoxin 820, 2104
2-PAM *see* pyridine-2-aldoxime
  methyl chloride
PAN *see* peroxyacetyl nitrate
pancuronium 947
papaverine 817
paper products 1298
PAPP *see* 4-aminopropiophenone
paraffins 2034
paraoxon 50, 102, 656, 1996
paraquat 2003, 2004
  action 127
  acute toxicity 34
  antidotes 428
  behavioural effects 1346
  biomarker 1867
  cardiac toxicity 821
  cationic 1369
  developing countries 1512
  inducing enzymes 1866
  LD_{50} 51
  mechanism of toxicity 125
  pancreatic toxicity 904
  systemic pulmonary toxicity
    723–4
  tissue take-up 128
  toxic reactions 1430
parathion 1994
  biomonitoring 1902
  birds, toxicity 1336, 1337, 1342,
    1523
  cardiac toxicity 824
  effect on invertebrate food source
    1355
  metabolism 101, 102
  oxidative desulphuration 1329

PBPK modelling 142
percutaneous absorption 578
and predation behaviour 1348
reduced sensitivity 1342
regional differences in
  percutaneous absorption 578
reproductive effects 1351
secondary poisoning 1342
parathion-methyl
  behavioural effects 1348–9, 1352
  birds, toxicity 1336, 1337
  effect on invertebrate food source
    1355
  human studies 466
  placental toxicity 1243
paroxetine 220
PAS *see* p-aminosalicylic acid
patulin 2146
PBBs *see* polybrominated biphenyls
PCBs *see* polychlorinated biphenyls
PCP *see* phencyclidine
peanut oil 911
peanuts, roasted 1005
pectin 572
pegaspargase 1965
pemoline (Volital) 1427
penchloromethane 2035–6
penciclovir 239
penconazole 2001, 2003
penethamate 1642
D-penicillamine 427, 552, 755,
  942, 1430, 1513, 1514–15, 2068
penicillins
  biomarker 1849
  cardiac toxicity 807
  in chemical warfare 2099
  eye toxicity 756
  haematotoxicity 390
  immunotoxicity 1004
  irritation 413
  nephrotoxicity 686
  neurotoxicology 641
  parenteral toxicity 532
  peroral toxicity 547
penitrem A 2146, 2147
pennyroyal oil 731
S-(1,2,3,4,4-pentachloro-1,3-
  butadienyl) glutathione 690
pentachloroethane 142
pentachlorophenol 6, 917, 1902,
  1907, 2001, 2002
pentaerythritol 460
pentagastrin 1548
pentamidine 915, 992
pentane 2022, 2034

2,4-pentanedione 15, 26
pentanol 199
pentazocine 942
pentobarbital *see* phenobarbitone
pepleomycin 727
peptides 265, 1964, 2082
peptidoglycans 571
perbenzoates 2022
perchloric acid 1455
perchloroethylene
 see tetrachloroethylene
perfluorodecanoic acid 869
perfluorophenyl isothiocyanate
 1883, 1884
perfluorophenylthiohydantoin 1884
perfluoropropene 1915
perfumes 230
perhexiline 220, 221
periciazine 220
perlolidine 1521
perloline 1521
Perls' Prussian Blue 867
permethrin 460, 651, 1244, 1245,
 1994, 1998, 1999
peroxides 160, 2014, 2023, 2106
peroxisomes 344, 680
peroxyacetyl nitrate (PAN) 1278
peroxyacyl nitrates 1275
peroxynitrite 160, 199, 633, 634
perphenazine 220
perthane 1243–4
pertussis toxin 819
PE *see* polyethylene
pethidine 366, 1491, 1497, 1504
petroleum ether 920
petroleum hydrocarbons 691–2,
 1310, 1313
petroleum jelly, for mustard gas eye
 damage 2087
petroleum pollutants, avian embryo
 bioassay 1334
petroleum products
 car exhaust 606
 contamination 1373
 fractionation 920–2
 gasoline 607, 658, 2034
 groundwater contamination 1772
 interactions 2034
 lead additive 2054–5
 methanol in 2040
 paternal workplace exposure
 1464
 petrol/diesel fumes 917, 918,
 919, 1215
 in plastics industry 2023

underground storage tanks 1372
 unleaded petrol 692
phalloidin 782, 870, 1513
phasin 1518
phenacetin 103, 105, 390, 569, 569,
 1427, 1428, 1438
phenanthridine 239
o-phenanthroline 200
phencyclidine (PCP, angel dust)
 89, 942, 1491, 1495, 1503, 1545,
 1550
phenelzine 112
phenformin 112, 125, 220, 1430,
 1438
phenindione 241, 807
p-phenitidine 103
phenitrothion 259
phenobarbital *see* phenobarbitone
phenobarbitone
 bromobenzene toxicity and 118
 carcinogenicity 1127
 cardiac toxicity 818
 circadian toxicology 267
 DNA damage and 126
 endocrine toxicology 990
 and gastro-intestinal microflora
 566, 569
 hepatotoxicity 866, 867, 872,
 880
 increased 117
 inducing GSTs 1866
 LD$_{50}$ 51
 metabolism 106, 113, 114, 119
 pancreatic toxicity 910, 918, 925
 peroral toxicity 548
 use in assay 1403
phenol–formaldehyde composite
 1709, 2018
phenolphthalein 1427, 1429
phenols
 biomonitoring 1902, 1903, 1907
 fungicides 2001, 2002
 and gastro-intestinal microflora
 568–9
 haematotoxicity 395
 human studies 463
 metabolism 98, 100, 107, 111
 microdiffusion 1497
 parenteral toxicity 535
 percutaneous toxicity 585
 rubber additive 2014, 2016
 steam distillation 1497
 toxic hazard 1455
phenolsulphonphthalein 546

phenothiazines
 cardiac toxicity 819
 forensic analysis 1491, 1497
 haematotoxicity 395
 hepatotoxicity 884
 mutagenicity 1042
 parenteral toxicity 536
 reproductive toxicity 1146
 tissue specificity 129
 toxic reactions 1430, 1438
phenoxyacetates 2104
phenoxybenzamine 684
3-phenoxybenzoic acid 466, 569
phenoxy herbicides 2004–5
phentermine 730, 815, 1427, 1501
phenylacetone 102
phenylacetone oxime 102
phenylalanine 1518, 1989
phenylalanine mustard 527
phenylarsonic aresenicals 1515
phenylbutazone 253, 390, 756, 807,
 1438
S-phenylcysteine 607
phenyldiamines 413, 1861
phenylenediamines 1849, 2014,
 2020
phenylephrine 738
R-5-phenyl-5-ethylhadantoin 226
phenylglyoxylic acid 1907, 1910,
 2040
phenylhydroxylamine 393, 565
phenylimidazopyridine 1881, 1886
phenylisopropylamine 1501
phenyl isothiocyanate (PITC) 1883,
 1884
phenylmercapturic acid 2037
phenylmercury 2058
phenylnaphthylamine 2014, 2017
2-phenylphenol 2001
 sodium salts (OPP/SOPP)
 1129–30
3-phenylpropan-1-ol 101
phenylpropanolamine (PPA) 814,
 1501
phenyl sulphate 98
phenylthiohydantoin 1883, 1884
phenylthiourea 724
phenylureas 990
phenytoin
 cardiac toxicity 807, 817
 circadian toxicity 252, 254, 265
 disaster 1427
 endocrine toxicology 989, 991,
 992
 eye toxicity 760

phenytoin (*Contd.*)
   metabolism, genetic factors 112
   neonatal toxicity 1215, 1218, 1228
   peroral toxicity 555
   pharmacogenetics 220, 228
   skeletal muscle toxicity 948
phlorizin 816
phloroglucinol 990
phomopsins 870, 877, 2145, 2146, 2147, 2148–9
phorate 1335, 1341
phorbol esters 126
phorone 1863
phosacetim 523
phosgene
   absorption 2096
   in chemical warfare 2082, 2097–100
   as combustion product 1917, 1927
   exposure mode 2096
   gas 1724
   histopathology of lung damage 2098
   long-term effects 2100
   management of poisoning 2099–100
   mechanism of action 2097–8
   metabolism 2036
   nephrotoxicity 689–90
   physicochemical properties 2096
   symptoms and signs of exposure 2098–9
   toxicity 2096–7
phosmet 1335
phosphate esters 2022
phosphates 355, 357, 972, 973, 1369, 1371, 1985
phosphatidylinositol 808
phosphatidylinositol 4′,5′-bisphosphate (PhIP2) 791–2
phosphide 2006
phosphine 2006
phosphoinositol metabolites 982
phosphonates 973, 1996
phosphonofluoridates 1996
N-phosphonomethylglycine
   see glyphosate
phosphoramide mustard 729
phosphoric acid 1996
phosphorothioates 21, 1995, 1996
phosphorus 807, 1371, 1372
   see also white phosphorus;
      yellow phosphorus

phosphorus-based fire retardants 1917
Photomirex 879
phthalates 7, 125, 523, 1866, 2014, 2022
phthalazine 103, 239
phthalazinone 103
phthalic anhydride 1915, 2016, 2020
phthalimides 2022
phthalocyanines 2023
phylloerythrin, excretion 2148
physostigmine 142, 951, 2093
phytates 530, 973, 974
phyto-estrogens 570–1
phytolaccin 1518
phytolaccotoxin 1518
phytomenadione *see* vitamin K$_1$
picrotoxin 641
pigments
   bismuth 2061
   chromium 2062
   in plastics industry 2023
   in rubber industry 2014, 2017
pimozide 663
pinacolyl methylphosphono-fluoridate (GD, soman, VX)
   ageing 2092
   antidotes 426, 428
   cardiac toxicity 823
   LD$_{50}$ 50
   management 2093, 2094–5
   military use 2089, 2090
   PBPK modelling 142, 150
   as pesticide 1996–7
   physicochemical properties 2090
   temperature effects 1724, 1726
   terrorist use 1724, 1726, 2090
   toxicity 2091
pindolol 220
PIP$_2$ *see* 4,5-bisophosphate
PIP$_3$ *see* inositol 1,4,5-triphosphate
piperazine 2121
piperidine 1455
piperonyl butoxide 114
piretanide 785, 795
pirimicarb 1998
piroxicam 2161
pitch 463
PITC *see* phenyl isothiocyanate
pitressin tannate 534
plant dyes 965, 973
plant flavonoids 571
plant glycosides 565–6
plant toxins 215, 820–1, 1444, 1513

plastic film 466, 1130
plasticizers 523, 1565
plastics 564, 1456, 1654, 1655, 1657, 1662, 1669
   see also specific plastics
platelet-derived growth factor 1972
platinum 257, 701
Plexiglas *see* poly(methyl methacrylate)
plutonium 974
podophyllotoxin 186
polamides 2018
polpylene glycol alginate 1985
polyacrylamides 637, 2021
polyacrylate rubbers 2013
polyacrylonitrile 1918, 1921, 1922
polyamide fibre 2022
polyaromatic hydrocarbons
   see polycyclic aromatic hydrocarbons
poly-L-aspartic acid 685
polybrominated biphenyls (PBBs) 879, 1595
polybutadiene rubber 2013
polycarbonates 2018
polychlorinated aromatic compounds 163
polychlorinated biphenyls (PCBs)
   see also Arochlor
   and apoptosis 197
   aquatic toxicity 1316, 1317
   behavioural effects 665, 1348
   biomonitoring 1780
   bioremediation 1373
   cardiac toxicity 810–11
   as combustion product 1929
   diagnostic brain residues 1343
   endocrine toxicology 990
   environmental oestrogen effects 1565
   excretion 97
   genotoxicity 24
   hepatotoxicity 1554
   immunotoxicity 1005–6
   inducing enzymes 1866
   industrial use 1554
   in lake sediments 1371
   litigation 1949
   marketing controls 1595
   metabolism 131
   molecular interactions 163
   natural 1366
   nestling studies 1349
   neurotoxicology 642–3
   pancreatic toxicity 924

polychlorinated biphenyls (PCBs)
(*Contd.*)
  PBPK modelling 142
  peroral toxicity 549
  persistence 1370, 1392, 1553–4
  placental toxicology 1251
  risk assessment 1756, 1770,
    1777, 1778
  risk management 1588
  in sewage sludge 1372
  sorbed to humus 1369
  toxicity 1554
  transplacental transport 1464
polychloroprenes 2013
polycyclic aromatic hydrocarbons
(PAHs)
  adducts 162, 1880, 1887
  air pollutants 1267, 1300
  analysis 1883
  and apoptosis 197, 198
  aquatic toxicity 1316, 1317
  atmospheric deposition 1376
  biomarkers 1848, 1870, 1880,
    1882, 1886
  biomonitoring 1904–5
  bioremediation 1373
  circadian toxicology 271
  as combustion product 1927,
    1929
  cutaneous toxicity 27
  in diet 1982
  genotoxicity 7
  hepatic monoesterase (HMO)
    induction 1345
  hepatotoxicity 876, 879
  induction 113
  interspecies variation in toxicity
    278
  metabolism 1883
  mixtures 315
  mutagenicity 1026–7
  neonatal toxicity 1226
  oil spillages 1826–7
  pancreatic toxicity 917, 920
  persistence 1370, 1376
  reaction with DNA 161
  reproductive toxicity 1142, 1144,
    1145, 1146, 1150, 1153
  risk assessment 1756, 1791
  in rubber 2017
  in sewage sludge 1372
  and smoking 28
  in soils 1369, 1370, 1376
polycyclic aromatic hydrocarbon-
type inducer 113

polydimethylsiloxane 1985
polyesters 1922, 2018, 2020
polyether 1922
polyethylene (PE) 1130, 1918,
  1919, 2018, 2019
polyethylene glycols 533–4, 740,
  744, 748, 750, 908, 2023
polyfluorocarbons 2018
polyglycols 2022
polyhalogenated biphenyls 1956,
  1982
  see also polybrominated
    biphenyls; polychlorinated
    biphenyls
polyhydric alcohols 1989
polyhydroxyphenols 990
polymers, combustion products
  1922–3
poly(methyl methacrylate) 2018,
  2019
polymyxin B 537, 538
polyols 1989
  brominated 2022
polyphenolics 1984
polypropylene 1918–19, 2018,
  2019
polypropylene glycol 552
polypropylene homopolymer 626
polypropylene-polyethylene
  copolymer 626
polysaccharides 571, 1981
polystyrene 2018
polytetrafluoroethylene (PTFE)
  1282, 1915, 1918
polythene *see* polyethylene
polyunsaturated fats 807
polyunsaturated fatty acids (PUFA)
  634, 904–5
polyurethanes (PU) 1918, 1919,
  1922, 1923, 1925, 2013, 2018,
  2021
poly(vinyl chloride) (PVC) 2018,
  2019
  see also vinyl chloride
  combustion products 1918, 1925,
    1928
  film, allergy 1915
  hot wire cutting 1915
  human studies 466
  PBPK modelling 1770–1
  peripheral sensory irritation 626
  waste from chimneys 1960
poly(vinylidine chloride) 2018
Ponceau MX 879, 1127
Pondimin *see* fenfluramine

potassium 355, 357, 364, 366, 370,
  463, 1430, 1979
potassium arsenite 460
potassium ascorbate 2087
potassium cyanide 635, 1724
potassium (KS+s) 808, 940, 941
  see also sodium/potassium
PPA *see* phenylpropanolamine
practolol 1427, 1428, 1438, 1439,
  1549
pralidoxime *see* pyridine-2-
  aldoxime methyl chloride
praseodymium 870
pravastatin 946
praziquantel 1642
prazocin 2188
prednisolone 758, 969
prednisone 22, 552, 758, 1455
5-pregnenolone 370
pregnenolone-16α-carbonitrile 113,
  285
prenalterol 426, 430
prenylamine 809
primaquine 391, 393
primidone 390, 391
printing inks 564
probenecid 691
procainamide 103, 105, 108, 112,
  218, 220, 221, 265, 817
procaine 105
procarbazine 727, 1145
procarcinogens 231
prochlorperazine 220
proflavine sulphate 415
proglycem *see* diazoxide
proguanil 227
promazine 730
promethazine 188, 220
prontosil 104, 325, 565
propachlor 569, 2003, 2005
propafenone 220
propandiol 237, 1438
propane 1867
propane thiosulphonate 428
propanil 390, 393, 1845, 2003,
  2005
propanol 553, 612, 626, 1298,
  1417, 1491, 1503, 1706, 1902
propanolol 1495
proparacaine 762
propellants 460, 1985
propionaldehyde 237, 613
propionic acid 554, 1989
propionitrile 1922

propofol (Diprivan) 234, 1427
propoxyphene 1495–6, 1500, 1503, 1504
propranolol 100, 228, 252, 254, 265, 555, 760
N-propylamine 220, 222
propylbenzene 101
propylene 2019
propylene glycol 460, 533, 740, 1426, 1427, 1428, 2020
propyleneimine 680
propylene oxide 21, 1880, 1884
propyl gallate 1985
propyl methanesulphonate 1145
n-propyl disulphide 1522
2-n-propylpent-4-enoic acid 121
propylthiouracil (PTU) 941, 989, 1121, 1403
prostaglandins 241, 243, 361, 525, 657, 741, 786, 845, 1981, 2161
prostigmine 951
proteins
    see also mycotoxins
    allergens 702
    in animal poisons 2184, 2186
    binding 253–4
    catalytic activities 217
    in food toxicology 1983
    hepatic metabolism tests 359
    metabolites 568
    nephropathy marker 678
    neuronal synthesis 631
    phosphorylation 982
    tests 355, 362, 370
    toxicities 265
proteoglycans 364
protoanemonin 1518
proton-pump inhibitor 227
Prussian blue 391
pseudoephedrine 1501
psoralens 22, 1043, 1523
PTFE see polytetrafluoroethylene
PTU see propylthiouracil
pulegone 1655
puromycin 184, 869
PU see polyurethane
putrescine 103, 128, 2193
PVC resin manufacturing company 457
pyrazole 429
pyrazophos 2001, 2003
pyrene 1886, 1907
pyrenol (1-hydroxypyrene) 1905, 1907

pyrethrins 34, 524, 534, 1510, 1994, 1998–9
pyrethroids
    behavioural toxicity 651
    domestic animal poisoning 1510
    human studies 460
    hydrolysis 524
    insecticides 465
    neurotoxicology 639
    parenteral toxicity 524, 534
    placental 1244–5
    sodium channel action 639
    synthetic 465, 1994, 1998–9
pyrethrum 259, 1642, 1994
pyridazinones 990
pyridine 109, 221, 1455, 1919, 1922
pyridine-2-aldoxime methyl chloride (2-PAM) 429, 955, 1510, 1998, 2094
pyridinium oximes 429
pyridostigmine 1995, 2081, 2093
pyridoxine see vitamin B$_6$
pyromellitic dianhydride 2020
pyrrole, oxidation 637
pyrrolidine dithocarbamate 926
pyrrolizidine alkaloids 133, 730, 872, 873, 881, 882, 1981
pyruvate 806
pyruvate decarboxylase 427

Q

quartz see silica
quaternary amines 69
quaternary ammonium salts 2023
quercetin 241, 566, 571
quercetin-O-rutinoside see rutin
quinacridones 2023
quinalphos 1243
quinidine 22, 395, 817–18
quinine 395, 784, 785, 787
quinolinate 641
quinolines 2014, 2017
quinols 100
quinoneimine 71
quinone methides 725
quinones 240, 835, 1043
    and apoptosis 199
    biomarker 1867
    and calcium homeostasis 156
    cell prolferation stimulation 165
    metabolism 104
    and oxidative stress 160
    redox cycling 127, 691

Quintox see cholecalciferol
quintozene 2001
3-quinuclidinyl benzoate 1082

R

radium 974
radon 28, 252, 259, 260, 1293, 1538, 1827, 1959
raloxifene 1392
ranitidine 572
Rat n 1A allergen 511
Rat n 1B allergen 511
realgar 2050
recombinant-methionyl human brain-derived neurotrophic factor 1972
red squill 1511
Redux see dexfenfluramine
refrigerants 460
reserpine 1403
resins, absorbent 2161
resmethrin 1244, 1998
resorcinol 100, 990, 2014
respiridone 220
retarders, rubber industry 2014, 2016–17
13-cis-retinoic acid 236, 867, 946, 1188, 1189, 1218
retinoids 197, 755, 972, 1549
retinol 236, 642
retrorsine 872
RG12195 763
rhodanese 426, 428–9
riboflavins 972, 1987
ribonucleic acid (RNA) 1988
ribostamycin 789
rice oil 1005–6, 1226
ricin 184, 1518, 1726, 1727, 2082, 2104
rickettsia 2082
rifampicin 273, 1455
ristocetin 395
ritodrine 1216
ritonavir (Norvir) 1427
road oil 922
robin 1518
robitin 1518
ronidazole 1642
rotenone 807, 1994, 1999
rubber see Subject Index
rubidium 805
rubratoxins 1253
rubril 565

rutin 566
ryanodine 806, 808

S

S100 protein 347
SA *see* sodium ascorbate (SA)
SAC *see* acid saccharin
D-saccharic acid-1,4-lactone 568
saccharin 81, 1537, 1553, 1653,
 1658, 1989
safrole 526, 569, 879, 1981
salazopyrin 390
salicylates 524, 553, 756, 969, 989,
 991, 992
 see also aspirin
 acute overdose 1496
 ATP synthesis and 127
 cartilage and bone toxicity 969
 endocrine toxicology 989, 991,
  992
 eye toxicity 756
 forensic screening tests 1497
 metabolism 115
 ototoxic effects 784, 785–7
 parenteral toxicity 524
 peroral toxicity 553
 in plastics industry 2022
 rubber additive 2014, 2016
 teratological effects 971, 1223
salicylazosulphapyridine 565
salt *see* sodium chloride
salvarsan 1426
saponins 759, 1519, 1521
saquinavir (Invirase) 22, 1427
sarafotoxin 812
sargramostim 1965
sarin (GB)
 ageing 2092
 cardiac toxicity 824
 L(Ct)$_{50}$ 2091
 management 2094
 military use 2089, 2090
 mixed routes of exposure 605
 physicochemical properties 2090
 regulations 1555
 safety 1444
 skeletal muscle toxicity 955
 terrorist use 1721, 1723, 1725–6,
  1728, 1729, 1730, 1827, 2092
 toxicity 2091
satumomab 1965
saxitoxins 639, 816, 818, 1554,
 2082, 2104, 2192
SBP *see* sulphobromophthalein

scaritoxin 2191
scombrotoxins 1554, 2193
scopolamine 527, 1430, 1521
scorpion toxins 818, 820, 898
SDZICT 322 763
sea anemone toxins 816, 818, 820
sebacates 549, 2017, 2022
secalonic acid D 1253–4
secoisolariciresinol 570
secretin 547
Seldane *see* terfenadine
selenites 870
selenium 2065, 2066
 accumulation in plants 1515
 in agricultural drainwater 1351
 as antioxidant 158, 1983
 biomarker 1868
 biomonitoring 1902, 1907
 cardiac toxicity 823
 in drinking water 1382
 hepatotoxicity 877
 pancreatic toxicity 908, 911
 poisoning in food-producing
  animals 1515
 rubber additive 2014, 2016
 in soils 1328, 1329, 1371, 1380
 toxicity to horses 1518–19
selenomethionine 1351, 1354
semustine 727
sequestrene *see* ethylene diamine
 tetra-acetic acid
sertraline 220
sesbanine 1518
sevoflurane 2030
shale 605
shale oils 1537
shellfish toxin 816
SHI *see* sodium hippurate
sialomucin 897
sialoproteins 974
silica
 causing apoptosis 184
 early research 1482
 from volcanoes 1815, 1817
 irritant effects 1455
 and lung cancer 1457
 in mines 1827
 in plastics industry 2022
 in rubber 2017
 silicosis 1475
silicates 1985
silicon 1382, 1905
silicones 1662, 1674, 2013, 2014
siloxanes 1585
silver 1489, 1765, 2087, 2089

silybin 870
simazine 2003, 2006
simvastatin 946
sincamidine 1519
sinigrin 234
sirolimus 1130
SKF93479 1124
smoke 919–20, 1266, 1446
 see also tobacco smoke
smoke flavourings 1654, 1655,
 1657
snake venoms 428, 812, 820, 956,
 957–8
sodium
 cardiac action potential 805, 816
 food toxicology 1979, 1990
 forensic toxicology 1504
 mineralocorticoid action 370
 in soils 1367
 in tests 355, 358, 364, 366
sodium aluminosilicate 2153
sodium ascorbate (SA) 1130
sodium azide 1046, 1047
sodium bentonite 2153
sodium bicarbonate 546
sodium birate 618
sodium chlorate 51, 390, 393, 2003,
 2004
sodium chloride 528, 537, 685,
 1517, 1522–3
sodium chromate 463
sodium chromoglycate 513
sodium citrate 2087
sodium cyanide 50, 760, 1331,
 1725, 1726
sodium 2,3-dimercaptopropane-
 sulphonate *see* dimercaprol
sodium edetate 427, 1513
sodium ethane thiosulphonate 428
sodium fluoride 357, 1994
sodium fluoroacetate (compound
 1080) 6, 34, 325, 643, 1510–11
sodium hippurate (SHI) 1130
sodium iodoacetate 821
sodium lactate 1709
sodium lauryl sulphate 842, 844
sodium β-mecaptopyruvate 428
sodium metabisulphite 535
sodium monofluorate 1524
sodium nitrate 428
sodium nitrite 393, 426, 429, 433,
 1519
 for hydrogen cyanide poisoning
  2102
sodium nitroprusside 185, 2188

sodium phosphate 821
sodium saccharine (SSAC) 1130
sodium salicylate 263, 525, 528
sodium thiosulphate 426, 428, 433, 1519
   for hydrogen cyanide poisoning 2102
sodium valproate 917
solanine 1521, 1554, 1984
solochrome cyanine 342
solvents
   see also organic solvents
   animal studies 1222
   and blood–testis barrier 1463
   eye toxicity 737
   and female reproductive disorders 1465
   as food additives 1552
   indoor source 1295
   neonatal toxicity 1215
   neurotoxicity 127
   occupational exposures 1463
   pancreatic toxicity 918, 920, 922
   and *ras* oncogene activation 1457
   reproductive toxicity 1146
   in sewage sludge 1372
soman *see* pinacolyl methylphosphonofluoridate
somatomedins 950
somatostatin 346
somatotropin 1965, 1970
somatrem 1965
sophorine 1520
SOPP *see* 2-phenylphenol
sorbic acid 1989
sorbinol 763
sorbitol 764, 1653
sorivudine 1565
soya 184, 925, 1392, 1398, 1553
soya bean oil 2022
sparsomycin 765
sparteine 112, 218, 220, 222
spider toxins 820–1
spiramycin 1645, 1648
spironolactone 807, 985, 988, 1151
sporidesmins 877, 881, 882, 883, 2145, 2146, 2147, 2148
SSAC *see* sodium saccharine
stainless steel 1674
Stalinon 1427, 1428
stannous chloride 2023
staphylococcal enterotoxin B 2104
staurosporine 191, 197, 199
stearates 1980, 2014, 2022

stearic acid 813
sterigmatocystin 533, 1043, 2151
sterilants, chemical 1455, 1667
steroids 105, 113, 346, 372, 1645
   see also corticosteroids
stilbamidine 882, 883
stilboestrol *see* diethylstilboestrol
straight-run gas oils 315
streptomycin 21, 522, 532, 537, 572, 685, 787, 807, 1025, 1042, 1455
streptozotocin 128, 132–3, 924, 991, 992
strontium 17, 973, 974
strychnine (nux vomica) 498, 641, 1490, 1510–11, 1524
styrene–butadiene rubber 2013
styrene–O^6-guanine, biomarker 1845
styrene oxide 2020, 2040
styrene (vinylbenzene) 2039–40
   biomarker 1845
   biomonitoring 1902, 1907, 1910
   characteristics 2035
   eye toxicity 756
   Hb adduct levels 1880, 1884
   metabolism 2032
   ototoxicity 784, 795
   PBPK modelling 142
   percutaneous absorption 19–20
   in plastics industry 2019
   in rubber industry 2015
succimer (DMSA) 1513
succinylcholine 97
sucrose 1989
sugar alcohols 1989
sugars 548
sulfanilamide elixir 1426, 1427, 1444, 1544, 1562, 1634
sulindac 132
sulphacetamide 621, 761
sulphadiazine 807
sulphaemoglobin 392–3
sulphamethazine 274
sulphamethoxazole 393
sulphamethoxypyridazine 1438
sulphanilamide 2, 104, 108, 460–1, 1637
   see also sulfanilamide elixir
sulphapyridine 565
sulphasalazine 565, 1146, 1147
sulphate esters 7
sulphides 1497
sulphinamide 1883
sulphisoxazole 807

sulphites 1653, 1987
sulphmethaemoglobin 392
sulphobromophthalein (SBP) 910, 913
sulphonamides
   adverse drug reactions 1439
   endocrine toxicology 993
   eye toxicity 756, 761
   and gastro-intestinal microflora 565
   hepatotoxicity 390–1, 395
   mixtures 49
   mutagenicity 1025
   parenteral toxicity 532, 534
   poultry toxicity 1520–1
   regulations 1426
   renal toxicity 131
   rubber additive 2014
   solubility 98
   tissue take-up 128, 129
sulphones 102, 131, 428, 1341
N-sulphonyloxymethyl-4-aminoazobenzene 130
sulphonylureas 390, 391, 807, 992
sulphorhodamine B 746, 750
5-sulphosalicylic acid 546
sulphotidine 1124
sulphoxides 102, 104, 1341
sulphur compounds 1917, 2014, 2016
sulphur dioxide
   air pollution 1265, 1266
   in animal husbandry 1517
   as combustion product 1927, 1928
   dangerous dose 1831
   effects on humans 1280
   in fires 1821
   inhalational toxicity 589
   mixtures 314
   in particulate complex 1268–73, 1281
   peripheral sensory irritation 616
   as preservative 1653
   toxicokinetics 1280
   volcanic 1815
   wood burning 1917
sulphuric acid 1266, 1280–1, 1376, 1475, 2006
sulphur mustard
   absorption 2084
   bone marrow 2086
   clinical investigations 2086
   eye 2085
   haematotoxicity 395

sulphur mustard (*Contd.*)
  histopathology of skin effects 2085
  history 2079, 2080, 2081
  management of casualites 2087
  mechanism of action 2084–5
  physicochemical properties 2083
  prognosis for casualties 2087–8
  respiratory tract 2086
  symptoms and signs of exposure 2086
  terrorist use 1724
  toxicity 2084
sulphur oxides, precursors of acid rain 1376
superoxide radicals 633, 726, 807, 866, 872
suprofen (Suprol) 1427
surfactants 39
suxamethonium 1547
sweeteners 1985, 1989–90

T

T-2 mycotoxin 184, 394, 1254, 1515–16, 1520, 2104, 2147, 2149
2,4,5-T *see* 2,4,5-trichlorophenoxy-acetic acid
tabun (GA) 429, 1724, 1726, 2080, 2089, 2090, 2091, 2092, 2094
tacrolimus 764
talc 2014, 2017, 2022
tallysomycin 727
tamoxifen 135, 220, 271, 284–5, 755, 756, 764, 1129, 1392, 1395
tannic acid 882, 883, 1518, 1522
tannins 1984
tar products 2017
tartaric acid 1985
tartrazine 1653, 1986
taurine 361
taxine 1522
taxol 637, 638, 727
TBTO *see* tributyltin oxide
TCDD *see* 2,3,7,8-tetrachloro-dibenzo-*p*-dioxin
TCE 200
TCP *see* tricresyl phosphate
p,p-TDE *see* 1,1-dichloro-2,2-bis(p-chlorophenyl)ethane
TDI *see* toluene diisocyanate
TDMAS *see* tris(dimethylamino)silane
TEAS+s *see* tetraethylammonium
tebuconazole 2001, 2003

tebufenozide 1994, 2000
teflubenzuron 1642
tellurium 638, 2014, 2016
temephos 1335
teniposide 727
terfenadine (Triludan, Seldane) 22, 38, 50, 125, 1427, 1429
terolidine (Micturin) 1427
terpenes 1298
testosterone 371–2, 569, 653, 1395, 1403, 1406, 1407
tetanus toxin 633, 640
TETD *see* disulfiram
tetrabromobisphenol A 2022
2,3,7,8-tetrabromodibenzo-*p*-dioxin 142
tetracaine 529
1,1,2,2-tetrachlorethane 877
tetrachlorobenzene 1818
2,3,7,8-tetrachlorodibenzo-*p*-dioxin (Agent Orange TCDD)
  see also dioxins
  behavioural toxicity 653
  bioaccumulation 284
  cardiac toxicity 821
  in chemical warfare 2105
  cutaneous toxicity 838
  developmental toxicity 1188–9
  endocrine toxicology 990
  environmental endocrine toxicity 1395
  hepatotoxicity 879
  immunosuppressive effects 283
  interspecies differences in toxicity 281–5
  intoxication signs 283
  mixtures 21
  neurotoxicology 642
  placental toxicity 1250–1
  reproductive toxicity 1145
  responsiveness as autosomal dominant trait 282
  as tumour promoter 281
2,3,7,8-tetrachlorodibenzofuran 142
tetrachloroethane 810
tetrachloroethylene 2035, 2037, 2041
  biomonitoring 1903, 1907
  hepatotoxicity 877
  Monte Carlo analysis 1784, 1785, 1786
  neonatal toxicity 1216, 1226
  nephrotoxicity 678, 691
  occupational hazard 1417
  PBPK modelling 142, 150

tetrachloromethane 2035–6
tetrachlorophenol 1907
tetracyclines 366, 531, 537, 549, 552, 807, 869, 973, 992, 1025
12-*O*-tetradecanoylphorbol 13-acetate (TPA) 184, 191
tetraethylammonium (TEAS+s) 679, 816, 817, 822
tetraethyl lead 1866
tetraethylthiuram disulphide (TETD) *see* disulfiram
tetrafluoroethylene 691
tetrafluoroethylenecysteine (TFEC) 167
L-Δ⁹-tetrahydrocannabinol *see* cannabis
α-tetrahydrocannibol *see* cannabis
tetrahydrofolates 119, 391
tetrahydrofuran 1903, 2014, 2018
1,2,3,4-tetrahydroisoquinoline 232
tetrahydrotriamcinolone 758
tetrahydroxybutyl imidazole 1987
tetrahydrozoline 738
tetraiodotyrosine *see* thyroxine
N,N,N′,N′-tetrakis(2-pyridylmethyl)ethylenediamine 200
tetramethrin 1244
tetramethylbutanediamine 738
tetramethylenediamine 1455
tetramethylethylenediamine 738
tetramethylthiuram disulphide *see* thiram
tetramethylthiuram monosulphide 2016
2,3,5,6-tetra-*p*-phenylenediamine 1860, 1861
tetrodotoxin 34, 639, 816, 818, 2104, 2193
TFEC *see* tetrafluoroethylene-cysteine
6-TG *see* 6-thioguanine
thalidomide
  developmental 1167, 1170
  disaster 2, 125, 1426
  ethics and 1956
  exposure 1444
  metabolism, diet and 115
  neonatal toxicity 1218
  regulations 1427, 1429
  reproductive toxicity 1137
  toxic reactions 1430
  tragedy 1561, 1634
thallium 1467, 1491, 1496, 1511
thallium sulphate 1994
thapsigargin 197

THC *see* cannabis

Δ⁹-THC *see* cannabis

theobromine 823

theophylline 200, 252, 256, 433, 552, 816, 823, 911, 917

thermoplastic resins 626

thiabendazole 2000, 2001, 2002

thiazoles 2016

thiazopyr 990

thioacetamide 184, 233, 257, 881, 882, 883, 1860, 1861, 1862

thioacetic acid 134

thioamides 990

thiobarbituric acid 757

thiobenzamide 184

thiocyanate 566, 1822, 1905, 1907, 1927, 2100

thioglycollic acid 134

6-thioguanine (6-TG) 24, 261, 985, 1052

thiols 2014, 2052, 2054

thiomersal 1642

thiopentone sodium 522

thiophanate 2000, 2002

thiophanate-methyl 2000, 2002

thiophosphorus insecticides, oxidative desulphuration 1329

thioredoxin 199, 200

thioridazine 129–30, 220, 819, 1146, 1495

thiotepa 231

2-thiothaizolidine-4-carboxylic acid 1907

thiouracil 1121

thioureas 233, 724–5, 1121, 2003, 2005

thiram 1415, 2001, 2002, 2014, 2016

thorium 974

thorium dioxide 881

thorotrast *see* thorium dioxide

thromboxanes, carcinogenesis and 1981

thymidine glycol 1867, 1868

thyrocalcitonin 968

ticrynafen *see* tienillic acid

tienillic acid 229, 1439

tilidine fumarate 882

tilmicosin 1645

timolol 220, 760–1, 760–1, 761

tin 1489

tiotidine 1124

TIQ *see* 1,2,3,4-tetrahydroiso-quinoline

tissue plasminogen activator 1970

titanium dioxide 1280, 1282, 2014, 2017, 2023

TMA *see* trimethylamine

TMT *see* trimethyltin

tobacco smoke
  carcinogenicity 1538
  chemical constituents 224, 1278, 1296, 1297, 1298
  epidemiology 1537
  and gastro-intestinal microflora 565
  indoor source 1293
  in vitro tests 417
  mixtures 305, 314
  neonatal toxicity 1215, 1218, 1224
  pancreatic toxicity 911, 917, 919, 920, 926
  particulate matter 1299
  passive smoking 1267, 1293
  placental function and amino acid transport 1255–6
  reproducitve toxicity 1151, 1153
  source of cadmium 1377

tobramycin 685

toclofos-methyl 2001, 2003

tocopherols *see* vitamin E

tolbutamide 228–9

o-tolidine 463, 565, 1587

tolrestat 763

toluene 2038–9
  abuse 2029
  behavioural toxicity 651, 657, 660
  with benzene 149, 1445–6
  biomonitoring 1903, 1904, 1907
  characteristics 2035
  CNS effects 1455, 2030, 2031
  as combustion product 1927
  and *o*-cresol excretion 1417
  enzyme induction 2033
  ethanol interaction 2033, 2034
  exposure routes 607, 613
  from PU 1918
  genotoxicity 1456
  hepatotoxicity 1456
  neurotoxicity 634
  and noise 1419
  occupational hazards 510, 515
  ototoxicity 784, 794, 795, 1418
  PBPK modelling 142, 149
  reproductive toxicity 1156
  rubber additive 2014, 2018
  with *m*-xylene 149

toluene diisocyanate (TDI) 413, 616, 705, 707, 709, 711, 1456, 1712, 2021

toluidine blue 344, 393

o-toluidine 1484

o-tolyl diguanidine 2016

torsemide 229

toxaphene 879, 1244, 1316, 1336, 1346, 1995

TPA *see* 12-*O*-tetradecanoylphorbol 13-acetate

trace elements 1370, 2049, 2062, 2063–6

traclimus 1130

tramadol 220

transferrin 254, 363, 367, 634, 678

trematoxin 877

tremetol 1520

triacetyloleandomycin 114

trialkyl phosphorothioate 21

trialkyltin salts 882

triamcinolone 758, 969

triaryl phosphates 986

triazines 990, 1042, 1369, 1511–12, 2003, 2006

triazolam (Halcion) 22, 252, 1427, 1428, 1438

triazoles 1123, 2003, 2006

tributylin 186, 188–9, 197

S,S,S-tributyl phosphorotrithoate (DEF) 2006

tributyltin oxide (TBTO) 1007–8, 2000, 2001

tributyltins 200, 1407

tricaine/benzocaine injection 498

tricarboxylic acid 632

trichlorethylene 917

trichlorfon 635, 636, 824, 1341, 1352

trichloroacetic acid 566, 1383, 1485, 1908, 2037

1,1,1-trichloroethane 206, 2035, 2037
  biomonitoring 1903, 1908
  cardiac toxicity 810
  eye toxicity 750
  genotoxicity 24
  mixed routes of exposure 607
  PBPK modelling 142
  in rubber 2017

trichloroethanol 1908, 2036, 2042

trichloroethanol glucuronide 2037

trichloroethylene 2036–7
  anaesthesia 2030
  biomonitoring 1903

trichloroethylene (*Contd.*)
  cardiac toxicity 810
  CNS effects 1475
  and degreasers' flush 1415
  with dichloroethylene 148
  enzyme induction 2033
  with ethanol 149, 2033
  and gastro-intestinal microflora
    566
  human studies 463
  impurities 1445
  nephrotoxicity 691
  ototoxicity 784, 794, 795
  PBPK modelling 142, 1770–1
  peroral toxicity 551
  protein adducts 1887
  rubber additive 2014, 2018
  systemic pulmonary irritation
    731
  with vinyl chloride 149
trichlorofluoroethane 1908
trichlorofluoromethane 461, 2023
trichloromethane 2036
trichloromethyl, free radical 2036
trichloronat 1997
2,4,5-trichlorophenol 281, 1818
2,4,5-trichlorophenoxyacetic acid
  (2,4,5-T) 879, 1222, 2003, 2005,
  2104
1,1,1-trichloropropene-2,3-oxide
  279
1,1,2-trichloro-1,2,2-trifluoroethane
  142
trichothecenes 390, 391, 394, 525,
  1254, 2104, 2145, 2146, 2149
  see also T-2 mycotoxins
tri-*o*-cresyl phosphate (TOCP)
  637–8, 1554, 1824, 1997
tricresyl phosphate (TCP) 986,
  2014, 2017
tricyclic antidepressants 1495, 1504
tridemorph 2001, 2004
triethanolamine 2014
triethylamine 738, 1903, 1908,
  2020
triethylenemelamine 1145
tri(2-ethylhexyl)phosphate 750
triethyltin 638–9, 639, 2001
triethyltin bromide 274
trifluoperazine 819
3-trifluormethylpyridine 590
trifluoroacetic acid 101, 102, 1908
trifluoroacetyl chloride 102, 104
triglycerides 361, 367, 548, 939
1,2,3-trihydroxybenzene 100

3,4,5-trihydroxybenzoic acid 109
Triludan *see* terfenadine
trimellitic anhydride (TMA) 706,
  709, 1004, 2022
trimethoprim 390, 391, 532
trimethoxysilane 15, 16
trimethylamine 102, 103, 220,
  233–4
trimethylamine oxide 679, 2127
1,2,4-trimethylbenzene, interactions
  2033
2,2,4-trimethyl-2-dihydroquinolone
  2017
trimethylolpropane 1925
2,2,4-trimethylpentane 692
3-[2(2,4,6-trimethylphenyl)thiothyl]-
  4-methylsydnone 870
trimethyltin 642, 784, 794, 2001
trimipramine 221, 1495, 1497
triparanol 730, 1430, 1634
triphenylmethane 531, 1987
triphenylmethane triisocyanate
  2021
triphenyltin chloride 274
tris(chloroalkyl) phosphate esters
  2022
tris(2,3-dibromopropyl) phosphate
  2022
tris(dimethylamino)silane (TDMAS)
  26–7
trolitazone 992
tropicamide 759
tropisetron 221
troponins 366, 812
tryptamine 222, 223, 225
Tryptan Blue 565
tryptophan 22, 283, 395, 942, 946,
  1552, 1553, 1568
tryptophol 222, 236
tubocurarine 34, 954, 955
Tween 80 1086
Tween 20 551
Tylenol *see* acetaminophen
tylosin 1648
tyramine 21, 103, 114, 823, 1518

U

unsaturated fats 823
uracil 235, 990
uranium 1475, 1866
uranium oxide 1820
urates 363
urea 355–6, 362, 1455, 1514, 2003,
  2005

urea–formaldehyde 1922
urethane 881, 1035, 1922
uric acid 1983

V

valeric acid 1125
valinomycin 819
valium *see* diazepam
valproic acid 121, 254, 258, 869,
  993, 1189, 1216
vanadate 822
vanadium 823, 1370, 1382, 1908
vanadium pentoxide 1903
vedaprofen 1642
vegetable oils 534, 551, 823, 2014
vehicle emissions 1265–6, 1267,
  1268, 1273, 1274
  see also petrol/diesel fumes
verapamil 22, 188, 198, 809, 817,
  1495, 2190
veratridine 639, 816, 818
veratrosin 1521
veratrum 821
vermillion *see* mercury(II) sulphide
versicolorins 2151
versiconal 2151
villin 894
vinblastine 186, 199, 262, 942,
  1146
vinca alkaloids 638, 942, 943, 992,
  1152, 1153
vinclozolin 2001, 2002
vincristine 199, 262, 522, 637, 638,
  942, 943, 1455
vinegar, for jellyfish stings 2190
vinorelbine 262
vinyl acetate 550, 2019
vinylbenzene *see* styrene
vinyl chloride 2019
  see also poly(vinyl chloride)
    (PVC)
  age effects 1417
  binding values (EU) 1595
  biomonitoring 1903
  carcinogenicity 1417, 1456,
    1475, 1536, 1537, 1538, 1551
  as combustion product 1928
  DNA adducts from 1881
  extrapolation studies 1952
  from polymers 1917
  hepatotoxicity 881
  human studies 457, 463
  metabolism 100–1
  mixtures 21

vinyl chloride (*Contd.*)
    monomer 2019
    Monte Carlo analysis 1784
    pancreatic toxicity 922
    rat toxicity 1417
    reproductive toxicity 1145
    sperm evaluation studies 1467
    and spontaneous abortion 1464
    threshold limit value 1475
    toxic reactions 1430
    with trichloroethylene and 1,2-
      dichloroethylene 149
4-vinylcyclohexene diepoxide 184
vinylidene fluoride 142
vinylidine chloride 2019
L-5-vinyl-2-thiooxazolidone 1121
Vioform 1565
virginiamycin 1648
vitamin(s)
    see also food supplements *in
      Subject Index*
    deficiency, effect on metabolism
      115
vitamin(s) 548, 938, 972, 1217,
    1223, 1552, 1690, 1985, 2161
vitamin(s)
    A 127, 316, 864, 946, 969, 972,
      1430, 1551, 1552, 1982
    B_6 1430, 1552, 1987
    B_{12} 391, 428, 1548, 2064
    C 127, 158, 191, 200, 491,
      1982–3, 1985, 2131, 2132,
      2161
    D_2 2068
    D_3 (cholecalciferol) 1511, 2068
    D 316, 949–50, 968, 972, 973,
      983, 1430, 2068
    E
      as antioxidant 158
      and apoptosis 191, 200
      cardiac toxicity 809
      food toxicology 1978, 1982,
        1983, 1985, 1986
      human studies 2132, 2137
      nephrotoxicity 681
      parenteral toxicity 532
      toxicokinetics 2121
      toxic response moderation
        127

    K 229, 1524
    K_1 1511, 2006
vitellogenin 1407, 1408
V nerve agents 2090
volatile organic compounds (VOCs)
    1266–7, 1292, 1295, 1297–8,
    1299, 1300, 1302
volvatoxin A 820
vomitoxin *see* deoxynivalenol
VP-16 186, 195
VX *see* pinacolyl methylphosphono-
    fluoridate

W

Warbex 1342
warfarin 114, 229, 243, 569,
    1510–11, 2006
white oils 920
white phosphorus 1340–1, 1475,
    1511
white spirit 2018
wood dusts 701
WR 2721 792

X

xylenes 2033, 2039
    biomarker 1844
    biomonitoring 1903, 1908
    characteristics 2035
    CNS effects 1475
    enzyme induction 2033
    interactions 2033–4
    irritation 1475
    laboratory occupational hazard
      510, 515
    mixed routes of exposure 607
    ototoxicity 784, 795
    PBPK modelling 142
    rubber additive 2014, 2018
    skin effects 1475
    with toluene 149
xylitol 1653
xylose 107, 365
xylyl bromide 2102

Y

yellow phosphorus 1523–4
Yellow Rain 2080

Z

zearalenone 1515–16, 2145, 2146,
    2147
zenarestat 764
zeranol 284
zidovudine (AZT) 942, 946
zimeldine (Zelmid) 1427, 1438
zinc 2066
    anthropogenic emissions 1370
    and apoptosis 188
    apoptosis and 200
    associated cadmium 1374
    biomarker 1864, 1869
    cartilage and bone toxicity 965,
      968, 972, 973, 974, 2068
    circadian toxicology 257
    depletion 757
    in diet, cadmium toxicity and
      2054
    domestic animal toxicoses 1513
    fortification 1552
    from mining sites 1373
    fungicide 2001
    in Greenland snow cover 1370
    hepatotoxicity 870
    as impurity in fertilizer 1371
    metallothionein and 2067
    plant root uptake 1369
    in plastics 2022
    in sewage sludge 1372
    soil reference values 1373
    in soils 1329
    in water distribution systems
      1377
zinc carbonate 2052
zinc chloride 1475
zinc dimethyl dithiocarbamate
    see ziram
zinc naphthenate 917
zinc nitrate 2018
zinc oxide 2014
zinc phosphide 1346–7, 1510–11,
    2006
zineb 990, 2000, 2001
zinostatin 727
ziram 990, 2001, 2002, 2016, 2017
zoalene (3,5-dinitro-*o*-toluamide)
    1521
zomepirac (Zomax) 1427, 1428
zuclopentixol 221
zygacine 1522